THE PHARMACEUTICAL CODEX

Principles and Practice of Pharmaceutics

THE
PHARMACEUTICAL
CODEX

Twelfth Edition

Principles and Practice of Pharmaceutics

Editor: Walter Lund

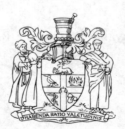

*Published by direction of the Council of the Royal Pharmaceutical Society of
Great Britain and prepared in the Pharmaceutics Division of the Society's
Department of Pharmaceutical Sciences*

London
THE PHARMACEUTICAL PRESS
1994

The Pharmaceutical Press
(publications division of the Royal Pharmaceutical Society
of Great Britain)
1 Lambeth High Street, London SE1 7JN

Australia
The Australian Pharmaceutical Publishing Co. Ltd.
40 Burwood Road, Hawthorn, Victoria 3122
and
The Pharmaceutical Society of Australia
Pharmacy House, PO Box 21, Curtin, ACT 2605

Germany, Austria, Switzerland
Deutscher Apotheker Verlag
Postfach 10 10 61, Birkenwaldstrasse 44, D-7000 Stuttgart

Japan
Maruzen Co. Ltd.
3-10 Nihonbashi 2-chome, Chuo-ku, Tokyo 103
or
PO Box 5050, Tokyo International, 100-31

New Zealand
The Pharmaceutical Society of New Zealand, Pharmacy House,
124 Dixon Street, PO Box 11640, Wellington

USA.
Rittenhouse Book Distributors, Inc.
511 Feheley Drive, King of Prussia, Pennsylvania 19406

A catalogue record for this book is available from the British Library.

Typeset in Great Britain by Alden Multimedia, Northampton
Printed and bound by The Bath Press, Bath, Avon

CONTENTS

Part I Preparation and Presentation of Drugs as Medicines

Section 1 Dosage Forms 1

Section 2 Product Design, Development, and Presentation 177

CONTRIBUTORS

NA Armstrong, PhD, FRPharmS
Senior Lecturer, Division of Pharmaceutics, Welsh School of Pharmacy, University of Wales College of Cardiff.
Oral Solids

ND Barber, BPharm, PhD, MRPharmS
Professor of the Practice of Pharmacy, The Centre for Pharmacy Practice, The School of Pharmacy, University of London.
Statistics

MI Barnett, PhD, MRPharmS
Senior Lecturer, Division of Pharmaceutics, Welsh School of Pharmacy, University of Wales College of Cardiff.
Particulate Contamination

NDS Bell, BSc, PhD, FRPharmS
Microbiology Services Manager, Organon Laboratories Ltd.
Aseptic Processing (principal author); Cleanrooms for Pharmaceutical Production

G Buckton, PhD, MRPharmS
Senior Lecturer in Pharmaceutics, Centre for Materials Science, The School of Pharmacy, University of London.
Preformulation

C Clark, MRPharmS
Director of Pharmacy, Hope Hospital, University of Manchester School of Medicine.
Parenteral and Enteral Nutrition Fluids

JA Clements, PhD, MRPharmS
Head of Scientific and Technical Services Division, Department of Pharmaceutical Sciences, Royal Pharmaceutical Society of Great Britain.
Biopharmaceutics and Pharmacokinetic Principles

JH Collett, BSc, PhD, DSc, FRPharmS
Reader in Pharmacy, Department of Pharmacy, University of Manchester.
Modified-release Drug Delivery Systems

RS Cook, MSc, PhD
Quality Assurance Manager (GMP), Rhône-Poulenc Rorer, Dagenham Research Centre.
Validation

I Couper, MSc, MRPharmS
Principal Pharmacist, Area Quality Control Laboratory, Knightswood Hospital, Glasgow.
Medical Gases; Pyrogens

T Deeks, BSc, MSc, PhD, MRPharmS
Head of Formulation, Marion Merrell Dow, Winnersh Research Centre.
Parenterals

C Glover, BSc, MRPharmS, MIPharmM
Community Pharmacist.
Homoeopathic Pharmacy

LB Hakes, BPharm, PhD, MRPharmS
Manager, Clinical Trial Supply Operations, Lilly Research Centre, Windlesham.
Process Development

G Halbert, BSc, PhD, CChem, MRSC, MRPharmS
Director, Cancer Research Formulation Unit, Department of Pharmaceutical Sciences, University of Strathclyde.
Control of Microbial Contamination and the Preservation of Medicines

N Harvey, BPharm, MRPharmS
Production Manager, Roussel Laboratories Ltd, Swindon.
Design Criteria for Production Facilities

M Heward, BPharm, MRPharmS
Strategic Studies Manager, Roussel Laboratories Ltd, Swindon.
Design Criteria for Production Facilities

EG John, MPhil, MRPharmS, MInst Pkg (Dip)
Senior Manager, Clinical Supplies, Merck Sharp & Dohme Research Laboratories.
Pharmaceutical Packaging

SC Kendall-Smith, BPharm, MPharm, MRPharmS
Principal Pharmacist, Aseptic Services, St James's University Hospital, Leeds.
Infusion Fluids: Admixtures and Administration

M Lynch, MRPharmS
Senior Department Head, Pharmaceutical Operations, Syntex Research Centre.
Electrolyte Powders and Oral Rehydration Fluids; Pharmaceutical Aspects of Clinical Trials

TM MacLeod, PhD, CChem, FRSC, FRPharmS
Formerly Principal Pharmacist, Quality Assurance, Tayside Pharmaceuticals, Ninewells Hospital and Medical School, Dundee.
Peritoneal Dialysis and Haemodialysis Preparations

IA Marshall, BSc, MIHSM, FRPharmS
Director of Pharmacy and Supplies, St James's University Hospital, Leeds.
Infusion Fluids: Admixtures and Administration

A Millar, MRPharmS
Principal Pharmacist, Radiopharmacy, Royal Infirmary of Edinburgh.
Radiopharmaceuticals

T Murray, MSc, PhD, MRPharmS
Principal Pharmacist, Radionuclide Dispensary, Western Infirmary, Glasgow.
Radiopharmaceuticals

AS Pinkus, BPharm, MRPharmS
Homoeopathic Pharmacist.
Homoeopathic Pharmacy

JA Rees, BPharm, MSc, PhD, MRPharmS
Senior Lecturer, Department of Pharmacy, University of Manchester.
Storage

AB Selkirk, PhD, MRPharmS
Vice-President, Director of Pharmaceutical Sciences and Site Operations, Syntex Research Centre, Heriot-Watt University, Edinburgh.
Formulation

CJ Soper, BPharm, MSc, PhD, MRPharmS
Senior Lecturer in Pharmaceutical Microbiology, School of Pharmacy and Pharmacology, University of Bath.
Sterilisation

G Smith, PhD, MRPharmS
Formerly Senior Lecturer in Pharmaceutics, Heriot-Watt University.
Stability of Medicinal Products; Incompatibility

W Whyte, BSc
Lecturer, Building Services Research Unit, Department of Mechanical Engineering, University of Glasgow.
Cleanrooms for Pharmaceutical Production (principal author); Aseptic Processing

AJ Winfield, BPharm, PhD, MRPharmS
Head of Pharmacy Practice, Faculty of Health and Food, School of Pharmacy, The Robert Gordon University, Aberdeen.
Rheology

D Wiseman, PhD, MRPharmS
Senior Lecturer in Pharmaceutics, The School of Pharmacy, University of Bradford.
Ophthalmic Products

PREFACE

In 1903 the Council of the Pharmaceutical Society decided to produce a book of reference that supplied authoritative guidance to those engaged in the prescribing and dispensing of medicines throughout the British Empire. The first edition of this book was published in 1907 under the title *The British Pharmaceutical Codex (BPC)* and subsequent editions were published at regular intervals. The early editions of the *British Pharmaceutical Codex* were designed to supplement the information in the *British Pharmacopoeia* by providing information on the actions and uses of drugs; they also provided formulae and standards for a range of materials that were not included in the Pharmacopoeia. However, in 1972, the Medicines Commission (formed as a result of the Medicines Act 1968) recommended that there should be only one compendium of standards for all medicines in the United Kingdom, and that this should be the *British Pharmacopoeia*; the provision of standards in the *BPC* was therefore discontinued. A major reconstruction of the *BPC* was undertaken, resulting in the publication of the 11th Edition, known as *The Pharmaceutical Codex*. The prime function of the 1979 edition was as a compendium of drug information arranged in encyclopaedic style.

In the mid-1980s the Council considered the content of all of the Society's publications. In view of the coverage of actions and uses of drugs and medicines in *Martindale: The Extra Pharmacopoeia* and the *British National Formulary* it was decided to discontinue those aspects of the *Codex*. Consequently, the content of the *Codex* was changed to reflect some of the core areas of pharmacy identified by the Nuffield Report on Pharmacy. These include the materials of pharmacy, the preparation and presentation of drugs as medicines, and the biological fate of drugs as medicines. The more patient orientated aspects of pharmacy that appeared in *The Pharmaceutical Codex* and the former *Pharmaceutical Handbook* were developed in the *Handbook of Pharmacy Health-care: Diseases and Patient Advice* (1990) and *Handbook of Pharmacy Health Education* (1991).

This 12th Edition, now retitled *The Pharmaceutical Codex: Principles and Practice of Pharmaceutics* is produced by direction of the Council of the Royal Pharmaceutical Society of Great Britain.

The practice of pharmacy has changed considerably since the publication of the previous *Codex*. The extent of extemporaneous dispensing undertaken in pharmacies has been greatly reduced in favour of the presentation of medicaments as unit dosage forms. Nevertheless, it is well recognised that the pharmacist has a unique and central role in the provision of effective modern dosage forms.

The objective of the augmented and redesigned *Codex* is to provide a reference source on those aspects of pharmaceutical science and technology that are applied in the development and provision of therapeutically active dosage forms.

The underlying themes of the chapters are the multidisciplinary nature of pharmaceutics, which draws on physical, biological, engineering, and material sciences in the development of drug delivery systems, and how quality is built into medicines from conception and development to production and use. The chapters are supplemented by an extensive collection of data on the pharmaceutical aspects of 154 drugs, drawn from the files of the Pharmaceutics Division of the Royal Pharmaceutical Society in Edinburgh, and arranged in monograph form.

The Pharmaceutical Codex: Principles and Practice of Pharmaceutics, like its predecessors, represents a valuable reference source to any person with an interest in the preparation and presentation of medicines including pharmaceutical scientists engaged in formulation, development, or production; preregistration pharmacy graduates; students of pharmacy and related subjects; and all pharmacists—both in the United Kingdom and overseas.

ARRANGEMENT

Part I of *The Pharmaceutical Codex: Principles and Practice of Pharmaceutics* comprises six sections, which consider the essential aspects of the **Preparation and Presentation of Drugs as Medicines**. The chapters in each section broadly encompass the pharmaceutics content of the syllabus for pharmacy undergraduates and also provide direction and support for the continuing education of graduates, with special emphasis on the requirements of those associated with product development and innovation.

The majority of chapters in Part I were contributed by authors with specialist knowledge and experience, ensuring the provision of information that is accurate, topical, and relevant, and which also provides an insight into developments and future directions.

Section 1 describes the characteristics, formulation, and preparation of different types of **Dosage Forms** including oral solids, oral liquids, parenterals, inhalation products, topical semi-solids, topical liquids and powders, ophthalmic products, and rectal and vaginal products. The physicochemical aspects of these types of preparation are described in the chapters on solution properties, suspensions, emulsions, and aerosols.

Section 2 addresses the subjects associated with **Product Design, Development, and Presentation**. The section includes reviews of the biopharmaceutics, pharmacokinetics, and stability of medicinal products, and also encompasses such topics as preformulation, formulation, rheology, incompatibility, packaging, storage, and modified-release drug delivery systems. The section also considers the pharmaceutical aspects of clinical trials and the application of statistics.

Section 3 provides information on the **Preparation and Supply of Medicines**, including the design criteria necessary for production facilities, process development, and validation. Good manufacturing practice and licensing are covered in many of the chapters of the *Codex*; the principal aspects of these topics are summarised. An account of dispensing procedures and practice-related guidelines is provided, which includes information on homoeopathy. In addition, the section encompasses radiopharmaceuticals, medical gases, paediatric preparations, immunological products, information on the admixture and administration of infusion fluids, and precautions to be taken when handling cytotoxic drugs.

Pharmaceutical Microbiology, Sterile Processing, and Contamination Control constitute the main subject matter covered in Section 4. The section includes a comprehensive account of sterilisation as well as chapters on particulate contamination, control of microbial contamination and the preservation of medicines, and pyrogens. The important aspects of aseptic processing, cleanrooms, and the application of disinfectants and antiseptics are discussed. An overview of pharmaceutical microbiology is also provided. The chapters in Section 5 detail **Electrolyte Replacement, Nutrient Fluids, and Dialysis Solutions**.

Section 6 comprises **Nomenclature and Miscellaneous Data**. It includes a revised and updated account of the nomenclature of organic compounds and provides a valuable explanation of the principles and conventions associated with the approved names of pharmaceutical substances.

A Miscellaneous Data section comprising tables of useful reference data concludes Part I of the book.

Part II contains **Monographs on Drug Substances**. The monographs describe the pharmaceutics-related aspects of 154 active substances (most of which are included in the World Health Organization *Model List of Essential Drugs*). In addition to relevant physicochemical data, the monographs include abstracts from key papers on topics that range across stability, storage, incompatibility, formulation, dosage form development, excipients, bioavailability, and processing. The monographs were compiled from a detailed evaluation of material obtained by an extensive search of the relevant literature and standard sources.

ACKNOWLEDGEMENTS

The publication of *The Pharmaceutical Codex: Principles and Practice of Pharmaceutics* is overshadowed by the fact that the Editor, Mr Walter Lund, did not live to see its completion. After gaining wide experience in pharmacy, he joined the Society's pharmaceutics laboratory in Edinburgh in 1967. As Head of Pharmaceutics Division, the breadth and depth of his knowledge and experience of pharmaceutics and pharmaceutical technology were put to good use in the planning and development of the *Codex* from 1986 onwards. From July 1992 until the completion of the book, Dr John Martin, Editor, Handbook of Pharmacy Practice series, was seconded to the *Codex* project. His contribution throughout the later stages of production has been invaluable. The contributions, in both an advisory and editorial capacity, of Dr Geoffrey Smith, Sara B Williamson, and Professor Malcolm S Parker are gratefully acknowledged. The content of each monograph in Part II was reviewed by Dr Geoffrey Smith who made many useful suggestions.

The *Codex* staff are indebted to Dr Colin Cable, Acting Head of the Pharmaceutics Division, for responding to our queries and for providing helpful advice on many aspects during the preparation of the book. The support and guidance offered by Ainley Wade, General Editor of Scientific Publications, and Dr W Gwynne Thomas (deceased), former Director of the Department of Pharmaceutical Sciences, and other members of the Society's staff are also appreciated.

Thanks are due to David Wilson for his advice and assistance during the preparation of the Pharmaceutical Microbiology chapter and to Peter Mulholland for allowing the reproduction of the table entitled 'Reconstitution and Dosage Guidelines for Powder Injections' in the Miscellaneous Data Section. We are grateful to Allen & Hanbury Ltd and to 3M Health Care Ltd for providing illustrations for the Aerosols and Inhalation products chapters.

The preparation of this 12th Edition of the *Codex* has involved a team of dedicated editorial and clerical staff and it is a pleasure to acknowledge the commitment and enthusiasm of Wendy M Grant, Mary Stewart, Jane E Virden, Margaret L Sutherland, and Janice M Robertson. The contributions of Dr Heather J Barcroft, M Regina C Brophy, Anne Gilchrist, Vivien Moffat, Bernadette Stamper, Scott Wilson (deceased), Dr Stuart Young, and Sandra Hannen (deceased) in the earlier stages of production are also acknowledged.

Thanks are also due to Bernard Yates, the Society's publisher, the staff of the Society's Law Department, Dorothy Barker, of the Library at the Scottish Department, and Rena Adamson.

In order to assist in the preparation of future editions of the *Codex*, the reader is invited to send any constructive comments and relevant data to the Pharmaceutics Division, The Royal Pharmaceutical Society of Great Britain, 36 York Place, Edinburgh EH1 3HU.

Millicent M Bichan
September 1993

GENERAL NOTICES

Legal Aspects

Substances and their preparations described in the *Codex* may be subject to legal control in the United Kingdom or in other parts of the world in which the *Codex* is used. This control may be concerned with preparation, labelling, and standards.

In the United Kingdom, regulations under the Medicines Act 1968 require the licensing of the manufacture of medicinal products and the approval of new products by the Committee on Safety of Medicines before they are marketed. It should not be assumed that medicinal products prepared in accordance with the recommendations of the *Codex* will necessarily have been approved by the Committee on Safety of Medicines.

Licence to manufacture substances or products protected by Letters Patent is neither conveyed nor implied by the inclusion of information on such substances in the *Codex*.

Monograph Titles

In selecting the titles of monographs preference has been given to British Approved Names, United States Adopted Names, and International Nonproprietary Names. The titles of salts or esters of the monograph substance are also included with the relevant authorities, which are abbreviated as BAN, rINN, pINN, or their modified forms, and USAN.

Atomic and Molecular Weights

Molecular weights are given corrected to one place of decimals or to four significant figures for relative weights of less than 100. Atomic weights are based on the table of Atomic Weights as revised in 1983 by the Commission on Atomic Weights and Isotopic Abundance, International Union of Pure and Applied Chemistry based on the ^{12}C scale.

Preparations listed in Part II

Relevant preparations of the BP and USP are listed. Proprietary preparations available in the UK are listed with details of manufacturer, dosage forms, and available strengths. Supplementary information from manufacturers' data sheets is included. Although the dilution convention for oral liquids was abolished in 1992, information about diluents provided in the data sheet is included.

Substance combinations with BAN status are described; products commercially available in the UK are listed.

Compendial formulae from the *British Pharmacopoeia* and from the *British Pharmaceutical Codex 1973* (if relevant) are presented under the heading Formulation. Excipients that have been used in presentations of the drug are listed under the appropriate dosage form and drug substance. The excipients have been collected from UK and international sources and not all the excipients are necessarily present in any one product.

CAS Registry Numbers

Chemical abstracts service (CAS) registry numbers are provided, where available, in the monographs to assist readers to refer to other information systems. Numbers for various forms of the monograph substance are listed with the variation in form given in parentheses.

Solubility

Where solubility is given in words, the following terms describe the solubility ranges:

very soluble	less than 1
freely soluble	1–10
soluble	10–30
sparingly soluble	30–100
slightly soluble	100–1000
very slightly soluble	1000–10 000
practically insoluble or insoluble	10 000 and over

The figures given for solubility in each monograph have generally been obtained from the pharmacopoeias in which the substance is described. The values are subject to the methods and conditions of determination.

Dissociation constant(s)

Numerous methods can be used for the determination of dissociation constants, and there are often differences in the various values reported in the scientific literature. The pK_a values given in the monographs have been taken from published data. The temperature at which the determination was made is given where known.

Temperatures

Unless otherwise indicated, temperatures are expressed in degrees Celsius (centigrade).

Trade marks

In Part I, names followed by the symbol ™ are or have been used as proprietary names. These names may in general be applied only to products supplied by the owners of the trade marks.

ABBREVIATIONS

A number of units, terms, and symbols are not included in this list as they are defined in the text. Common abbreviations have been omitted. The titles of journals are abbreviated according to the general style of *Index Medicus*.

$\approx$ – approximately equals.

° – degrees (angular) *or* degrees Celsius (centigrade). Unless otherwise indicated in the text, temperatures are expressed in this thermometric scale.

ABPI – Association of the British Pharmaceutical Industry.

ADI – acceptable daily intake.

AIDS – acquired immune deficiency syndrome.

Ala – alanine.

a.m. – *ante meridiem*, 'before noon'.

AMA – American Medical Association.

APF – Australian Pharmaceutical Formulary and Handbook.

Arg – arginine.

Asn – asparagine.

Asp – aspartic acid.

ATCC – American Type Culture Collection.

ATP – adenosine 5′-triphosphate.

AUC – area under the curve.

β^+ – beta particles: positrons.

β^- – beta particles: electrons.

B. – *Bacillus, Bacteroides,* or *Bordetella.*

BAN – British Approved Name.

BANM – British Approved Name Modified.

BMA – British Medical Association.

BNF – British National Formulary.

b.p. – boiling point.

BP – British Pharmacopoeia 1993.

BP (Vet) – British Pharmacopoeia (Veterinary) 1993.

BPC – British Pharmaceutical Codex.

Bq – becquerel(s).

Br. – British or *Brucella.*

BS – British Standard (specification).

BSI – British Standards Institution.

C. – *Campylobacter, Candida, Chlamydia,* or *Corynebacterium.*

CAS – Chemical Abstracts Service.

cfu – colony forming unit(s).

Ci – curie(s).

Cl. – *Clostridium.*

cm – centimetre(s).

cm^2 – square centimetre(s).

cm^3 – cubic centimetre(s).

cmc – critical micelle concentration.

CNS – central nervous system.

COSHH – Control of Substances Hazardous to Health.

cP – centipoise(s).

CRM – the former Committee on the Review of Medicines (UK).

CSF – cerebrospinal fluid.

CSM – Committee on Safety of Medicines (UK).

cSt – centistoke(s).

Cys – cysteine.

D&C – designation applied in USA to dyes permitted for use in drugs and cosmetics.

Da – dalton(s).

dB – decibel(s).

DHSS – the former Department of Health and Social Security (UK).

DIN – Deutsche Industrie-Norm (German Industrial Standards).

DNA – deoxyribonucleic acid.

DOE – Department of the Environment (UK).

DoH – Department of Health (UK).

DPF – Dental Practitioners' Formulary (UK).

DSC – differential scanning calorimetry.

DTA – differential thermal analysis.

E. – *Enterococcus* or *Escherichia.*

EC – European Community.

ECG – electrocardiogram.

ECT – electroconvulsive therapy.

ed. – edition.

EDTA – edetic acid.

EEC – European Economic Community.

EEG – electro-encephalogram.

e.g. – *exempli gratia*, 'for example'.

et al – *et alii*, 'and others'.

eV – electronvolt(s).

EVA – ethyl vinyl acetate.

FAC – Food Additives and Contaminants Committee of the Ministry of Agriculture, Fisheries and Food (UK).

FAO – Food and Agriculture Organization of the United Nations.

FAO/WHO – Food and Agriculture Organization of the United Nations *and the* World Health Organization.

FDA – Food and Drug Administration of USA.

FdAC – Food Advisory Committe of the Ministry of Agriculture, Fisheries and Food (UK).

FD&C – designation applied in USA to dyes permitted for use in foods, drugs, and cosmetics.

FEV_1 – forced expiratory volume in one second.

FIP – Fédération Internationale Pharmaceutique.

fl.oz – fluid ounce(s).

f.p. – freezing point.

FPA – Family Planning Association (UK).

ft – foot (feet).

ft^2 – square foot (feet).

g – gram(s).

gal – gallon(s).

GC – gas chromatography.

GC-MS – gas chromatography-mass spectrometry.

GFR – glomerular filtration rate.

GLC – gas-liquid chromatography.

Gln – glutamine.

Gly – glycine.

GMP – Good Manufacturing Practice.

Gy – gray(s).

h – hour(s).

H. – *Haemophilus* or *Helicobacter*.

Hb – haemoglobin.

HDL – high-density lipoproteins.

HDPE – high-density polyethylene.

HEPA – high efficiency particulate air.

Hib – *Haemophilus influenzae* type b.

His – histidine.

HIV – human immunodeficiency virus.

HLA – human lymphocyte antigen.

HLB – hydrophile-lipophile balance.

HSE – Health and Safety Executive (UK).

IARC – International Agency for Research on Cancer.

ibid. – *ibidem*, 'in the same place (journal or book)'.

i.e. – *id est*, 'that is'.

Ig – immunoglobulin.

Ile – isoleucine.

in – inch(es).

in^2 – square inch(es).

INN – International Nonproprietary Name.

INNM – International Nonproprietary Name Modified.

IR – infrared.

ISO – International Organization for Standardization.

IUPAC – International Union of Pure and Applied Chemistry.

J – joule(s).

K – kelvin.

kBq – kilobecquerel(s).

kcal – kilocalorie(s).

keV – kiloelectronvolt(s).

kg – kilogram(s).

kJ – kilojoule(s).

Kleb. – *Klebsiella*.

kPa – kilopascal(s).

kW – kilowatt(s).

L – litre(s).

L. – *Legionella* or *Listeria*.

LAL – *Limulus* amoebocyte lysate.

lb – pound(s) avoirdupois.

LD50 – a dose lethal to 50% of the specified animals or micro-organisms.

LDL – low-density lipoproteins.

LDPE – low-density polyethylene.

Leu – leucine.

lx – lux.

Lys – lysine.

m – metre(s).

m^2 – square metre(s).

m^3 – cubic metre(s).

M – molar.

MAFF – Ministry of Agriculture, Fisheries and Food (UK).

MAG3 – mercaptoacetyltriglycine.

MAOI – monoamine oxidase inhibitor.

max. – maximum.

MBq – megabecquerel(s).

MCA – Medicines Control Agency (UK).

mCi – millicurie(s).

mEq – milliequivalent(s).

Met – methionine.

MeV – megaelectronvolt(s).

mg – milligram(s).

MIBG – metaiodobenzylguanidine.
MIC – minimum inhibitory concentration.
min – minute(s).
min. – minimum.
MJ – megajoule(s).
mL – millilitre(s).
mM – millimolar.
mm – millimetre(s).
mm^2 – square millimetre(s).
mm^3 – cubic millimetre(s).
mmHg – millimetre(s) of mercury.
mmol – millimole(s).
mN – millinewton(s).
mol – mole(s).
mol. wt. – molecular weight.
mosmol – milliosmole.
m.p. – melting point.
mPa – millipascal(s).
Mrad – megarad.
MRC – Medical Research Council (UK).
μCi – microcurie(s).
μg – microgram(s).
μL – microlitre(s).
μm – micrometre(s).
N – newton(s) *or* normal (concentration).
N. – Neisseria.
nCi – nanocurie(s).
NCTC – National Collection of Type Cultures (Central Public Health Laboratory, London, England).
ng – nanogram(s).
nm – nanometre(s).
NMR – nuclear magnetic resonance.
NRPB – National Radiological Protection Board, Harwell, Oxfordshire, England.
NSAID – non-steroidal anti-inflammatory drug.
ORS – oral rehydration salts.
ORT – oral rehydration therapy.
o/w – oil-in-water.
o/w/o – oil-in-water-in-oil.
oz – ounce(s).
P – probability.
Pa – pascal(s).
pCO_2 – plasma partial pressure (concentration) of carbon dioxide.
p_aCO_2 – arterial plasma partial pressure (concentration) of carbon dioxide.
PE – polyethylene.

PET – poly(ethylene terephthalate) *or* positron emission tomography.
pg – picogram(s).
pH – the negative logarithm of the hydrogen ion concentration.
Phe – phenylalanine.
pINN – Proposed International Nonproprietary Name.
pINNM – Proposed International Nonproprietary Name Modified.
pK_a – the negative logarithm of the dissociation constant.
p.m. – *post meridiem*, 'afternoon'.
pO_2 – plasma partial pressure (concentration) of oxygen.
p_aO_2 – arterial plasma partial pressure (concentration) of oxygen.
PP – polypropylene.
ppm – parts per million.
Pr. – Proteus.
Pro – proline.
PS – polystyrene.
Ps. – Pseudomonas.
PSGB – The Pharmaceutical Society of Great Britain. Now the Royal Pharmaceutical Society of Great Britain.
PVC – polyvinyl chloride.
q.s. – *quantum sufficit*, 'as much as suffices'.
R – röntgen.
rad – radiation absorbed dose.
RDA – recommended dietary allowance (USA).
RH – relative humidity.
rINN – Recommended International Nonproprietary Name.
rINNM – Recommended International Nonproprietary Name Modified.
RNA – ribonucleic acid.
rpm – revolutions per minute.
RPSGB – The Royal Pharmaceutical Society of Great Britain.
s – second(s).
S. – Salmonella or *Serratia.*
SEM – scanning electron microscopy *or* standard error of the mean.
Ser – serine.
Sh. – Shigella.
SI – Statutory Instrument *or* Système International d'Unités (International System of Units).

SLE – systemic lupus erythematosus.

sp. – species (plural spp.).

SPECT – single photo emission computed tomography.

Staph. – Staphylococcus.

Str. – Streptococcus.

Suppl – supplement(s).

Sv – sievert.

$t_{10\%}$ – time for 10% decomposition.

$t_{50\%}$ – time for 50% decomposition.

TGA – thermogravimetric analysis.

Thr – threonine.

TLC – thin layer chromatography.

TPN – total parenteral nutrition.

Trp – tryptophan.

TWA – time weighted average.

Tyr – tyrosine.

UK – United Kingdom.

UNICEF – United Nations International Children's Emergency Fund.

US *and* USA – United States of America.

USAN – United States Adopted Name.

USP – The United States Pharmacopeia XXII, 1990, and Supplements 1 to 7.

UV – ultraviolet.

V – volt(s).

V. – Vibrio.

Val – valine.

var. – variety.

VLDL – very low-density lipoproteins.

vol(s) – volume(s).

v/v – volume in volume.

v/w – volume in weight.

WHO – World Health Organization.

w/o – water-in-oil.

w/o/w – water-in-oil-in-water.

wt – weight.

w/v – weight in volume.

w/w – weight in weight.

Y. – Yersinia.

Part I Preparation and Presentation of Drugs as Medicines
Section 1 Dosage Forms

Oral Solids

The term 'oral solids' refers to three major groups of dosage forms, the compressed tablet, the hard shell capsule, and the soft shell capsule, together with other less frequently used dosage forms such as the powder. When considered together, they are easily the most popular group of dosage forms. They account for in excess of 70% of all dispensed National Health Service prescriptions dispensed in the United Kingdom, as well as a significant proportion of 'over-the-counter' sales, and a similar degree of usage is encountered world-wide. Of the three dosage forms to be discussed in this chapter, the tablet is the most commonly used, followed by the hard shell capsule and then the soft shell capsule, the ratio being about 65:30:5.

There are several reasons for the popularity of this group of dosage forms:

- they all employ the oral route of administration, which is generally the most acceptable route
- they permit a high accuracy of dosage
- the dose of the active drug is contained in a relatively small volume. Thus a concentrated dosage form is produced, leading to ease of packaging, transport, storage, and eventual administration.
- all three dosage forms are essentially water-free and hence loss of potency due to hydrolysis should be minimised. Packaging of the products into strip or blister packs should also enhance stability.

Although the manufacture of all three dosage forms requires the use of specialised equipment, all can be manufactured in large quantities over relatively short time periods. For example, it is possible to manufacture tablets at the rate of one million per hour and to fill hard shell capsules at a rate of 150 000 per hour.

Appropriate formulation results in the production of a dosage form that rapidly releases the drug contained within it. In addition, alternative formulations are available that promote controlled drug release.

This chapter will survey the formulation, manufacture, and usage of the tablet, the hard shell capsule, and the soft shell capsule, as well as some other related dosage forms.

Tablets

The *British Pharmacopoeia* states that tablets are solid preparations each containing a single dose of one or more active ingredients and are obtained by compressing uniform volumes of particles. The tablet is undoubtedly the most popular mode of presentation for solid dosage forms intended for oral administration.

Although references to products that appear to have resembled tablets can be found in tenth century Arab medical literature, the tablet as it is currently recognised was introduced in the middle of the 19th century. As a dosage form, it rapidly became popular as it lent itself to mass manufacture by mechanical means, a more favourable approach than the labour-intensive production of solid dosage forms such as the pill. As it is impractical for individual pharmacists to prepare small numbers of tablets, the tablet contributed greatly to the move to concentrate pharmaceutical manufacture at relatively few industrial sites.

A further reason for its popularity is that when properly formulated and prepared, the tablet offers a stable, highly concentrated and convenient dosage form, which contributes towards accurate dosage and rapid dispensing, and encourages good patient compliance.

The preparation of virtually all tablets involves a compression stage during which uniform volumes of particulate solid are poured into a die and then compressed between two punches. The applied force brings the particles into close proximity to each other so that interparticulate forces of attraction can cause cohesion; this results in the formation of compacted masses which have low porosity.

TABLET PRESSES

Tablet presses are categorised as either eccentric or rotary. The former are also known as single punch presses.

Eccentric Presses

An eccentric press has only one set of tooling, that is, one die and one pair of punches. A diagram of an eccentric press is shown in Fig. 1.

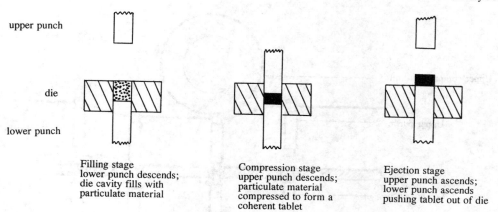

Fig. 1
Cycle of operation of an eccentric tablet press.

The cycle of operations of an eccentric press is as follows:

The Filling Stage. The lower punch moves downwards in the die leaving a cavity into which particles flow by gravity from a hopper or shoe. Although tablets are conventionally described in terms of weight, the die is filled by a volumetric process; the volume is determined by the depth to which the lower punch descends, which in turn is controlled by the 'weight'-adjusting screw.

The Compression Stage. The feed shoe moves away from the die and the upper punch descends producing gradual consolidation of the powder bed. As the particles come into ever closer contact, interparticulate bonds develop and a coherent structure is obtained. In an eccentric press, the lower punch remains stationary during the compression stage. The further the upper punch penetrates into the die, the greater the force to which particles are subjected and hence the greater the degree of consolidation.

The Ejection Stage. Both the upper punch and the lower punch move upwards, forcing the tablet from the die. After ejection, the tablet is swept aside, usually by the feed shoe as it moves towards the die ready to begin the next cycle.

Eccentric presses are usually only used for small scale production, research, and development as their rate of output is limited (rarely greater than 100 tablets per minute). There is only restricted scope for increasing the rate of ouput by means of an increase in the speed of operation of the press.

Rotary Presses

The rotary press has more than one set of tooling. The dies and their corresponding pairs of punches are arranged around a circular rotating turret (Fig. 2). Each individual die, with the lower punch in its lowest position, passes under the powder bed which is contained within a feed frame, which in turn is fed from a hopper. The die is completely filled under gravity, flow sometimes being assisted by rotating fingers in the feed frame. The quantity of solid in the die is corrected as the lower punch passes over a weight-controlling cam; any excess powder is swept off. The punches then pass compression rollers which cause the upper punch to descend and the lower punch to rise. Thus the powder is actively compressed from both top and bottom faces. The top punch then withdraws and the lower punch ascends as it passes over an ejection cam. In some rotary presses, precompression rolls are fitted, which are positioned before the main compression rolls so that the powder is in effect compressed twice.

The rate of output of a rotary press is governed by the number of tooling sets and the speed of rotation of the die table. Punches with multiple tips are available, and on some presses, the circumference of the turret is sufficiently large to accommodate two or more feed frames and sets of compression rollers. An example of a rotary press is the Manesty Rotapress Mark IV, which has 75 sets of tooling; the turret rotates 67 times per minute, and in each rotation, two tablets are produced from each die; thus output can reach 10 000 tablets per minute. Details of a number of commercial presses are given in Table 1.

Many modern presses are designed to operate automatically. For any given formulation and punch face separation, the force applied is governed by the mass of particles in the die, that is,

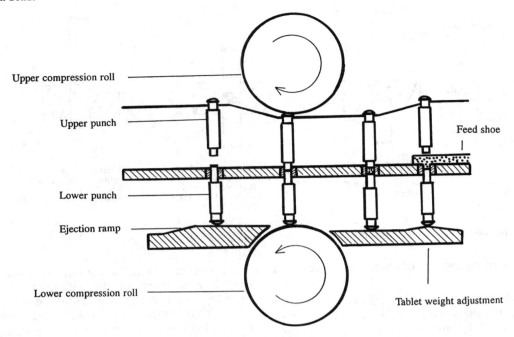

Fig. 2
Cycle of operations of a rotary tablet press.

the weight of the tablet. The force is measured by transducers attached to the press, often in the axles or bearings of the compression rollers; these in turn emit an electrical signal which can be used to alter the weight control cam so that the force is maintained within specified limits. Thus the weight of the tablets is controlled. In addition automatic sampling devices can measure tablet weight, thickness, and crushing strength, and such data are automatically stored to form part of the batch records. The shape and diameter of the tablet is governed by the design of the die and the punch faces. Tablet dies and punches are almost invariably made of stainless steel. The majority of tablets are circular in cross section but other shapes (for example, oval or angular) are available. Punch faces can be flat, bevelled, or concave and may be embossed to produce engraving on the tablet surface such as breaklines or the name of the manufacturer. Tablet shape and decoration together with diameter and weight form valuable means of identification.

METHODS OF TABLET PRODUCTION

Before it can be tableted, particulate matter must possess the ability to:

- flow uniformly and quickly into the die of the tablet press
- cohere when subjected to a compressing force
- ensure that the finished tablet will be ejected from the die of the press quickly and easily.

Few substances possess all three of these properties and hence few powders can be made directly into tablets without some preliminary treatment and the addition of one or more excipients. There are three principal methods of converting powders

Table 1
Details of a number of commercial tablet presses (Manesty Machines Ltd., Liverpool)

Model	Single/ Double sided	Number of sets of tooling	Maximum tablet diameter (mm)	Rotations per minute	Output per minute
Rotary presses	Single	16	15.8	44	700
B3B		23	11.1	44	1000
Novapress	Single	37	25.4	100	3700
		45	15.8	100	4500
		61	11.1	100	6100
Rotapress	Double	45	25.4	67	6000
Mk IV		55	15.8	67	7330
		75	11.1	67	10 000
Eccentric presses F3	–	1	22.2	85	85

into a form suitable for tableting; these are wet granulation, direct compression, and precompression.

Wet Granulation

The wet granulation method of tablet production is essentially a process of size-enlargement, sticking particles of drug and excipient together using an adhesive to produce a granular product with improved flow properties and an increased ability to cohere under pressure. A flow chart of the process is shown in Fig. 3.

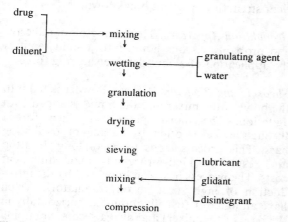

Fig. 3
The wet granulation process of tablet manufacture.

Mixing

The purpose of the mixing stage is to ensure homogeneity of drug content. A blend of solid particles is produced such that when a sample is removed, the relative proportions of ingredients in that sample are the same as in the whole of the mixture. Unlike molecules in a liquid, solid particles do not undergo spontaneous diffusion but remain in their relative positions; thus to bring about mixing of solid particles, work must be put into the system.

The first step in the mixing process is to dilate the powder bed which in turn allows relative particle motion. As the mixing process proceeds, the mixture becomes progressively more random. In a **random mixture** there is an equal chance of any given particle being at a given point at any one time. The deviation of a given mixture from randomness is expressed as the **index of mixing**; this is the ratio between the calculated variation among samples taken from a random mixture of a given composition and the actual variation seen among samples from the same mixture.[1] The degree of mixing normally increases with time, but under certain conditions, segregation may occur where the mixture shows a tendency to separate back into its components. Segregation is most common in mixtures which have marked variation in particle size between the components; differences in particle shape and density are further contributing factors. Segregation is particularly likely to occur if the motion of the mixing device is regular as patterns of particle movement may be established. It is therefore desirable that an irregular mixing motion is adopted.[2]

Ordered mixing occurs when small particles of one component become lodged in surface irregularities of much larger particles of another component. Such mixtures cannot be considered random as the particles do not behave independently of each other. The concept of ordered mixing is particularly useful in the manufacture of tablets which contain highly potent materials with direct compression diluents.[3]

Mixing Equipment. The underlying function of mixing equipment is to cause particles to move relative to one another. Free flowing materials are usually mixed in some form of rotating container, for example cube or Y-cone blenders (Fig. 4), the function of which is to raise the powder bed until

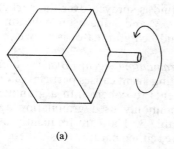

(a)

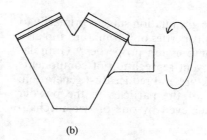

(b)

Fig. 4
(a) Cube blender, (b) y-cone blender.

its angle of repose is exceeded and flow occurs. The asymmetry of their design imparts a lateral movement to the solid as well as a tumbling action. These mixers are often fitted with baffles that break up regular patterns of particle flow.

Diluent. A tablet that weighs less than 50 mg is difficult to handle, but many drugs are administered at doses much less than this; in such cases a diluent (or filler) must be used to bulk the tablet up to a convenient size. The ideal diluent would be chemically and physiologically inert, cheap, and would not complicate the tableting process. Details of some tablet diluents are shown in Table 2.

Table 2
Tablet diluents

Diluent	Comments
Calcium carbonate	insoluble in water
Glucose	hygroscopic, reducing sugar
Calcium hydrogen phosphate	insoluble in water, good flow properties
α-Lactose	inexpensive, relatively inert, the most common diluent
Mannitol	freely water soluble, cool taste, popular for chewable tablets
Microcrystalline cellulose	excellent compression properties, may not need lubricant, some disintegrant action, highly stable
Sodium chloride	freely soluble, used in solution tablets, taste problems
Sucrose	hygroscopic, sweet taste, used in lozenges in conjunction with lactose

By far the most common diluent used in tableting is lactose.[4] A disaccharide produced from whey, a by-product of the cheese industry, lactose can be used in a variety of forms, but is most commonly used as α-lactose monohydrate. It is not a reducing sugar, hence it is reasonably stable, although it can take part in the Maillard reaction[5] to give highly coloured products, especially under alkaline conditions. Other diluents are used in specific situations; these will be addressed where appropriate.

Granulation

The purpose of the granulation stage is primarily to improve the flow properties of the mixture and also to improve its compression properties.[6] Granulation may also prevent segregation of components of the powder mixture and reduce dust generation. Size enlargement of the particles in the powder mixture can be achieved by one of two mechanisms:

- use of an adhesive substance which sticks adjacent particles together or,

- particle dissolution in the granulating fluid, followed by bridge formation between adjacent particles on evaporation of the granulating fluid; this mechanism obviously depends on the solubility of the solid in the granulating fluid.

The rate of granule formation is a function of the amount of granulating fluid present, maximum granulation being achieved when all the pores in the powder bed are filled with liquid.

To form granules, bonds must be formed between powder particles so that they adhere with sufficient strength to prevent breakdown.[7,8]

Granulation Apparatus. The mixing of an adhesive and probably viscous liquid into a solid requires the application of a considerable shearing force.

Shearing and Planetary Mixers. Powder is fed into the bowl of the mixer and the liquid is added with agitation. The moist material is then forced through a sieve, often by means of oscillating bars. This process tends to be of long duration and results in high processing and equipment costs. The process has been improved by the introduction of high speed mixer/granulators, which have an agitator (usually mounted horizontally in the base of the mixer) and also a second chopping blade which rotates in the vertical plane (Fig. 5). Thus mixing, massing, and granulation all take place in the same piece of apparatus; massing takes place rapidly and as there is a danger that the solid can be overmassed, the granulation process is often monitored (for example, by measuring the electrical power consumption of the impeller).[9]

Fluid Bed Granulation. A fluid, usually air, is passed into the powder bed from below. If the air velocity is sufficient, the particles become suspended in the air and move relative to one another; this is termed fluidisation and gives effective mixing. Granulating liquid is sprayed over the particles, which become sticky and adhere on collision. A diagram of a fluid-bed granulator is shown in Fig. 6.

Granulating Agent (Binder, Adhesive). The granulating agent causes particles of drug and other excipients to cohere into a granular form. Details of commonly used granulating agents are given in Table 3. They are frequently of a polymeric nature, either natural or synthetic, and are normally used as aqueous solutions or dispersions. Alternatively, they can be mixed with the other dry ingre-

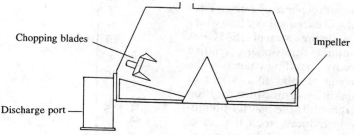

Fig. 5
High speed mixer-granulator.

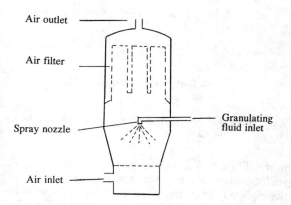

Fig. 6
Fluidised bed granulation.

Table 3
Granulating agents used in the wet granulation process

Adhesive	Concentration in granulating fluid (% w/v)	Comments
Acacia mucilage	up to 20	gives very hard granules
Glucose	up to 50	strong adhesive, hygroscopic
Gelatin	5–20	used as warm solution as it forms gel when cold; strong adhesive
Povidone (PVP)	2–10	soluble in water and some organic solvents, can be used in non-aqueous granulation
Starch mucilage	5–10	a common adhesive
Sucrose	up to 70	hygroscopic, tablets harden on storage
Tragacanth mucilage	up to 20	gives very hard granules
Water		suitable for easily wetted and soluble materials

dients and water added to the mixture. Water itself can be used as a granulating agent with hydrophilic and water-soluble materials.

Substances which react in the presence of water may require the use of an anhydrous granulating fluid; povidone dissolved in isopropanol is the usual choice. However, the additional expense, and the environmental problems associated with the use and subsequent evaporation of an inflammable liquid cannot be ignored.

Drying

After granulation, the product exists as a damp mass. It is sieved through a relatively coarse screen to produce wet granules, which must be dried. The drying process involves removal of liquid by the application of energy, usually heat energy, but occasionally microwave radiation is used.

The relationship between a solid and water is important in a variety of situations. Many drug substances and excipients are susceptible to hydrolysis and hence the water content of pharmaceutical preparations is often a matter of importance. A drying stage is essential to the wet granulation process of tablet manufacture. Unless moisture is removed, the required flow properties will be lost. Furthermore many tablet formulations appear to have an optimal water content which is believed to be related to the porosity of the tablet when under its maximum compressive force.[10]

The relative humidity of the atmosphere is expressed by the following ratio:

$$\frac{\text{Vapour pressure of water vapour in the air} \times 100\%}{\text{Saturated vapour pressure in air at the same temperature}}$$

It follows that the relative humidity is related to temperature; as the latter rises, the amount of water required to saturate the atmosphere also rises and so the relative humidity falls, even though the quantity of water vapour actually present in the atmosphere remains unchanged. Conversely a reduction in temperature may cause the relative humidity to exceed 100%, leading to precipitation of water.

If a solid is placed in an atmosphere of a given relative humidity, the solid will either gain or lose water until an **equilibrium moisture content** (**EMC**) is achieved. A change in the atmospheric relative humidity will cause a corresponding change in the EMC. Thus by exposing a solid to a series of increasing relative humidities, a moisture sorption isotherm can be constructed. If the relative humidity is then progressively reduced, then the corresponding desorption isotherm will be obtained. Sorption and desorption isotherms do not necessarily coincide. The relative humidities in such studies are most readily achieved by storing the solids over saturated electrolyte solutions. The relative humidities obtained from a number of electrolyte solutions are listed in Table 4.[11]

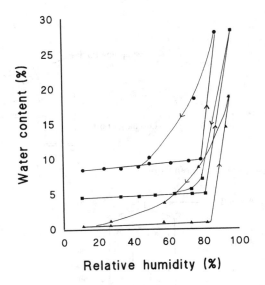

Fig. 7
Water adsorption-desorption isotherms of glucose (●), lactose (■), and sucrose (▲)

Table 4
*Relative humidities of some saturated electrolyte solutions at 25°
(abstracted from Reference 11)*

Electrolyte	Relative humidity (%)
Chromium trioxide	40.0
Cupric chloride	68.0
Lithium chloride	11.3
Lithium sulphate	87.8
Magnesium bromide	30.7
Potassium acetate	21.6
Sodium chloride	75.3
Sodium dichromate	59.4

Note. For further values at various temperatures, see the Miscellaneous Data section.

The adsorption-desorption moisture isotherms for a number of sugars are shown in Fig. 7. It is apparent that until the relative humidity exceeds a certain value (for example, 85% for sucrose or 95% for lactose) the water content of the solid remains relatively low.

The mechanism of drying should now be apparent. If the atmosphere above a wet solid is heated, the relative humidity falls and the solid will lose water until it comes into equilibrium with the lower relative humidity. If this lost water is removed, it follows that the solid cannot return to its former water content, even when the temperature of the atmosphere has decreased again.

Attainment of the EMC can sometimes be a protracted process which depends largely on the surface area exposed to the atmosphere. Water loss takes place primarily from the water-atmosphere interface. As water is lost from the solid surface, more water diffuses from the interior of the solid to replace it. Therefore, as the water content of the solid decreases, it will become progressively more difficult for the water concentration at the surface to be maintained; the degree of difficulty depends on the depth of the powder bed and hence the distance over which the water must diffuse. The smaller this distance, the more rapid the drying process.

Drying Equipment. The requirements for rapid drying can be summarised as a heat supply to increase the temperature, a system that allows the removal of evaporated liquid from the atmosphere, and minimisation of the distance over which the water must diffuse before evaporation.

For drying tablet granules, two types of drying equipment are commonly used: tray driers and fluid bed driers. In the tray drier, air (which is repeatedly heated) flows over a series of shelves on which the wet material is spread. The rate of evaporation is governed by the area available for heat transfer, the temperature difference between the wet solid and the drying air, and the thickness of the layers of wet material.

In fluid bed driers, the solid is fluidised from below as described earlier under Granulation (see Fig. 6), but hot air is used. In effect, each particle is surrounded by a current of hot air and so rapid drying ensues. Further advantages are that the temperature of the bed can be precisely controlled and a free flowing product is obtained. The same apparatus can be used for mixing, granulating, and drying and so handling costs are reduced. A disadvantage associated with the use of fluid bed driers is that movement of particles in hot dry air can lead to the generation of static electricity with attendant risk of explosion, especially if inflammable liquids have been used in the granulation process. A recent development in drying has been the use of microwaves. Microwaves are electromagnetic radiation in the wavelength range 10 mm to 1 m, although the wavelengths used for drying are limited to 122 mm and 312 mm (equivalent to frequencies of 2450 MHz and 960 MHz) to avoid interference with radio and television transmissions. As microwaves fall on materials such as water, electrons resonate rapidly in sympathy with the radiation and this results in the generation of heat and the evaporation of water. Microwave driers usually operate under vacuum and this removes the water vapour. The advantages of microwave drying are rapid drying at low temperatures, and the particle bed is stationary so interparticle attrition may be avoided. Microwave driers can be combined with high speed granulators. Transport of water to the drying surface will also involve the movement of any substance dissolved in the water. This poses few problems when each granule is dried individually as in fluid-bed drying, but with tray driers migration of solutes can occur between neighbouring granules. This can lead to non-uniform drug content and, if coloured substances such as dyes are involved, uneven coloration of the tablet surface.[12]

Second Mixing Stage

After granulation and a second sieving stage, a final mix is usually needed. At this stage, several other ingredients can be added:

Lubricant. The inclusion of a lubricant is essential in virtually every tablet formula. Friction occurs between the formed tablet and the wall of the die, and this resists expulsion of the tablet from the die. A layer of lubricant between the tablet and the die wall deforms preferentially when the tablet is moved, and thus ejection is facilitated. Some tablet lubricants are listed in Table 5; in practice magnesium stearate is by far the most commonly used lubricant. Many of these substances depend on hydrophobic groups for their lubricant effect; however, these can cause the tablets to become water repellent, and hence delay breakdown after ingestion. The physical strength of the tablet can also be impaired. All these effects may be governed by the mixing process; the longer the mixing time, and/or the more vigorous the mixing process, the

Table 5
Tablet lubricants

Substance	Concentration in tablet (%w/w)	Comments, commercial name
Fumaric acid	5	water soluble
Hydrogenated vegetable oil	0.5–2.0	Lubritab™
Liquid paraffin	up to 5	dispersion problems
Magnesium lauryl sulphate	1–2	water soluble
Macrogol 4000 and 6000	2–5	water soluble
Sodium benzoate	5	water soluble, taste problems
Sodium lauryl sulphate	0.5–5.0	wetting agent, often used in conjunction with stearates
Sodium stearyl fumarate	1–2	soluble in hot water, Pruv™
Stearates calcium magnesium stearic acid	0.25–1.0	very effective lubricants, prolong disintegration time, reduce tablet crushing strength

more thoroughly each granule will become coated with lubricant.[13]

Disintegrant. It is a paradox of tablet manufacture that considerable ingenuity is used to make individual particles form a coherent structure and yet further ingenuity is then often required to ensure the breakdown of that structure into its individual components after ingestion. This is achieved by the incorporation of a disintegrant, examples of which are given in Table 6.

Although all disintegrants may not act by the same mechanism, their general role is to provide a hydrophilic network within the structure of the tablet through which water may diffuse.[14] This can be assisted by the use of wetting agents, especially if the tablet has been partly waterproofed by a hydrophobic lubricant.

Glidant. A further ingredient added if necessary at this stage is a glidant, the function of which is to facilitate flow of the granular material into the die cavity. Though a number of substances have been suggested as being suitable (Table 7), almost invariably the glidant of choice is finely divided silica (Aerosil™). Colours and flavours can also be added at this stage if required.

Direct Compression

Direct compression is the process by which tablets are compressed directly from mixtures of the drug and excipients without any preliminary treatment; the process is outlined in Fig. 8. The mixture to be compressed must have adequate flow properties

Table 6
Tablet disintegrants

Substance	Concentration in tablet (%)	Comments, commercial name
Alginic acid, sodium alginate	2–10	
Aluminium magnesium silicate	up to 10	Veegum[TM]
Carbon dioxide		created *in situ* in effervescent tablets
Carmellose sodium	1–2	Nymcel[TM]
Cationic exchange resins	up to 10	Amberlite[TM] IRP-88
Croscarmellose sodium	2	Ac-Di-Sol[TM]
Crospovidone		cross-linked povidone, Polyplasdone XL[TM]
Microcrystalline cellulose	up to 10	lubricant properties, directly compressible, Avicel[TM]
Modified starch		starch 1500, Sta-Rx[TM] 1500
Sodium lauryl sulphate	0.5–5.0	wetting agent
Sodium glycine carbonate		source of carbon dioxide
Sodium starch glycollate	1–10	Primojel[TM]; Explotab[TM]
Starch	2–10	potato and maize starches most commonly used

Table 7
Tablet glidants

Glidant	Concentration in tablet (%)	Comments, commercial name
Colloidal silica	0.1–0.5	excellent glidant, Aerosil[TM]; Cab-O-Sil[TM]
Talc	1–2	insoluble but not hydrophobic

Table 8
Tablet diluents used in the direct compression process

Diluent	Proprietary Name	Comments
Calcium hydrogen phosphate	Emcompress[TM]	good flow properties, insoluble in water
Dextrates	Emdex[TM]	
Lactose anhydrous spray-dried	DCL 30[TM] Fast-Flo[TM] Zeparox[TM]	good flow properties, high bulk density
Microcrystalline cellulose	Avicel[TM] Emcocel[TM]	highly compressible, forms strong tablets, low bulk density
Microfine cellulose	Elcema[TM]	
Modified starch	Sta-Rx[TM] 1500	good disintegrant
Sucrose-dextrin co-precipitate	Di-Pac[TM]	good flow properties, moisture sensitive

and cohere under pressure, thus making pretreatment such as wet granulation unnecessary. Few drugs can be directly compressed into tablets of acceptable quality, but a number of materials are available which are directly compressible and which can serve as tablet diluents. Details of some are given in Table 8, and their use has been discussed by Shangraw *et al.*[15]

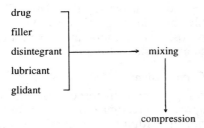

Fig. 8
The direct compression process of tablet manufacture.

Since the direct compression properties usually derive from the diluent, it follows that only relatively potent drugs whose tablets require a diluent can be tableted by this method. The apparent simplicity of the direct compression process is obvious and it is, therefore, not surprising that it has been extensively studied. In practice, although the direct compression approach offers considerable savings in energy, equipment, and materials handling, the wet granulation process still predominates. One reason for this is that in wet granulation, the properties of the individual particles are, at least in part, lost due to the effects of the granulating agent. With direct compression, the original individual particles are still present, and so there is a premium on obtaining diluents with minimal batch-to-batch variation. Further disadvantages of direct compression are that segregation of the components of the mixture is possible and also dust formation is more likely to occur.

Many direct compression diluents are considerably more expensive than their counterparts used for wet granulation or precompression and so increased expenditure on ingredients must be balanced against reduced equipment and handling cost. The additives used in direct compression (for example, lubricant or disintegrant) are the same as those used in the wet granulation process.

The most frequently used direct compression diluent is microcrystalline cellulose (for example, Avicel[TM]). This is a powder of low bulk density and is highly compressible to form strong compacts which disintegrate readily in water.

An important feature of direct compression diluents is their **capacity** or **dilution potential**. This is the amount by which they can incorporate substances which are not directly compressible and yet still produce acceptable tablets. The capacity will depend on the properties of the solid that is to be mixed with the diluent, but objective methods have been developed using ascorbic acid or paracetamol.[16]

Precompression

An alternative to the wet process for making a granular product is precompression, sometimes referred to as double compression or 'slugging' (Fig. 9). In this, the lubricated components of the tablet are compressed and the resultant aggregate is broken down to a granular mass which is then recompressed. Precompression takes place in either a tablet press, or via a roller compactor. In the former case, the tablets will be poorly formed and of variable weight due to poor flow properties of the powder mixture. Though not widely used, this process is a useful alternative when neither direct compression nor wet granulation are feasible.

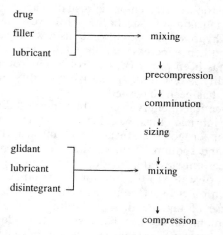

Fig. 9
Tablet production by precompression.

Reworking

A single batch of tablets may total several million, and the cost of active ingredients can be extremely high. Therefore, if a batch of tablets fails to meet predetermined specifications, a considerable financial loss can accrue. It may be possible to recover the active principle by an extraction process, but this itself is costly and produces active material by another route, leading to the possibility that solvent residues may be present; in addition the products of the extraction process may have different impurity profiles to those of the original ingredients. A potentially simpler method is to mill the tablets into a powder, perhaps modify the formula in some minor way, and then compress again. This is termed **reworking**.

The process of reworking involves exposing the constituents of the tablet to a second compression. Recompression generally reduces the physical strength of the tablet obtained at any given compression pressure. This is attributed to work hardening of the particles at the first compression producing, after comminution, granules that have increased resistance to consolidation when compressed again. It follows that materials in which the major mechanism of consolidation is plastic deformation, for example cellulose derivatives, are more likely to be affected by a second compression stage than those solids that tend to fragment on compression.[17]

Changes in physical strength of the tablets after reworking can be quantified by calculating the reworking potential, which is derived from the tablet strength-compression pressure profiles of the original and recompressed tablets.[18]

Because of the lower physical strength of the recompressed tablets, it might be expected that reworking would decrease disintegration time. This is not the case, and it has been shown that reworked tablets often require the addition of extra disintegrant to reattain their former disintegration times.[19]

A loss of physical strength does not occur when wet granulation has been used to prepare the original tablets, provided the comminuted material is wetted before recompression. This is because wetting reactivates the binder in the formulation, thereby providing increased adhesional properties.[20]

An alternative to the recompression of a whole batch of faulty tablets is to comminute the batch and then redistribute the product among several subsequent batches.

Although reworking is a useful means of relieving a potentially costly situation, it is not without its drawbacks. Any form of reworking involves a departure from the standard manufacturing procedure, and documentation must accurately record the reworking processes that have been carried out. Any reworked material that might affect product quality, safety, or efficacy must not be used, and the reprocessing of rejected products should therefore be exceptional.[21]

THE EFFECT OF FORMULATION ON TABLET PROPERTIES

Since all tablets are made by compression, the demands of the tableting process have a major influence on the choice of excipients, for example the necessity for granulation and lubrication. Most tablets are expected to be swallowed intact and then disintegrate in the gastro-intestinal tract thus necessitating the incorporation of a disintegrant. However, there are a number of other methods of presenting tablets, and these also influence the formulation and method of manufacture.

Lozenges

Lozenges are large tablets that are intended to stay in the mouth for relatively long periods (perhaps 10 to 15 minutes) while they dissolve or erode, often releasing an antibacterial agent or anaesthetic which produce a local effect on the mouth or throat. Lozenges contain no disintegrant, but the choice of diluent must be considered carefully to ensure the preparation of a product with a smooth texture and pleasant taste. Many sugars (for example, sucrose and glucose) especially in their directly compressible forms, can be used as diluents for lozenges. If a sugar-free diluent is required, mannitol or sorbitol may be suitable. A comprehensive list of diluents suitable for lozenges is given by Peters.[22]

Chewable Tablets

In contrast to lozenges, chewable tablets are designed to be broken down rapidly in the buccal cavity by the action of the teeth. Here too, taste is an important consideration. Mannitol is the diluent of choice, due to its negative heat of solution which produces a cooling sensation in the mouth and acts as an effective mask for unpleasant tastes. A flavouring agent is also frequently included in the formulation. A disintegrant is not necessary and there is no need for all ingredients to be water soluble. Common examples of chewable tablets are those containing antacids such as aluminium hydroxide.[23]

Solution Tablets

These are formulated to dissolve completely in cold water; all ingredients must therefore be freely soluble in water.

Dispersible Tablets

Dispersible tablets disintegrate rapidly in cold water to produce a suspension suitable for ingestion. Although there is no need for all the ingredients to be totally water soluble the need for a disintegrant which is effective in cold water is paramount.

Effervescent Tablets

These tablets effervesce when added to cold water to produce a clear, sparkling solution. The effervescence is almost invariably carbon dioxide, generated by the reaction between an acid (usually citric or tartaric acids) and a bicarbonate (usually sodium or potassium). The effervescence gives rapid disintegration and increases palatability. As the formulation is unstable in the presence of water, conventional wet granulation cannot be used for manufacture. However, granulation can be achieved by a fusion method as follows: the acid component is citric acid monohydrate; on heating, part of the water of crystallisation is released and this acts as the granulating fluid; in addition the reaction between acid and alkali generates further water which also aids granulation. Alternatively, anhydrous citric acid can be used, in which case a little water is added to the powder mixture. A further possibility is to use anhydrous granulation. Sweetening is usually achieved by the inclusion of saccharin. However, sucrose, being hygroscopic, can also act as a water scavenger and hence increase stability. Once the granulation has been prepared, control of environmental humidity is essential. A relative humidity of 25% at 25° has been suggested.[24]

Lubrication of effervescent tablets poses difficulties as the lubricant must be completely soluble. Micronised macrogol, fumaric acid, sodium stearyl fumarate, and sodium lauryl sulphate have been used. Magnesium stearate, in addition to slowing down access of water to the interior of the tablet, leaves a scum on the surface of the water. Alternatively, the use of tapered dies and punches faced with chromium alloys has been suggested. Common examples of effervescent tablets are those containing aspirin or ascorbic acid.[24, 25]

Sublingual and Buccal Tablets

These are designed to be held either under the tongue or in the buccal pouch for short periods. During this time, the drug is directly absorbed through the mucosa and passed via the jugular vein to the superior vena cava. Thus the gastro-intestinal tract and the liver are by-passed. Such tablets should not disintegrate, as it is likely that fragments of the tablet would then be swallowed. Rapid dissolution is required, although it is not essential that every component is freely soluble in water. However, unpleasant tastes should be avoided. An example of such a formulation is glyceryl trinitrate tablets.[26]

COATED TABLETS

For a variety of reasons, many tablets are coated after compression. Coating can protect the tablet from environmental factors such as light and mechanical damage, mask an unpleasant flavour, aid product identification, and enhance the appearance of the tablet. Coating can also provide a means of controlled drug release.

Three methods of coating are available: sugar coating, film coating, and compression coating.

Sugar Coating

This is the traditional coating method. Essentially a coating of sucrose is applied to the tablet core. The apparatus is almost invariably a circular coating pan the diameter of which may range from 15 to 200 cm (Fig. 10a). The tablets cascade in the pan as it rotates; the interior is often fitted with baffles to ensure adequate mixing. The coating material is added as an aqueous solution or dispersion. The excess liquid phase must then be removed, usually by hot air. However, as air enters and leaves the pan via the same aperture, drying is inefficient; in addition only a low drying rate is achieved because evaporation occurs only from the surface of the tablet bed.

Within the sugar coating process there are several stages.

Sealing Stage. For efficient coating, tablet cores should have deeply convex faces and minimal edge thickness. As the tablet cores are to be coated with an aqueous solution, it is essential that they do not begin to disintegrate during the coating process; therefore, to prevent water penetration, they are first protected by the addition of a water-insoluble polymer dissolved in a non-aqueous solvent. Examples are cellacephate, polyvinyl acetate phthalate, and shellac. All these materials can form coatings which are resistant to gastric juice, and so as little as possible is applied at this stage.

Subcoating. This stage produces a completely rounded shape free from sharp edges. A gum solution (for example, acacia or gelatin) is applied, followed by dusting with a dry powder (such as calcium carbonate, starch, sucrose, or talc). This is repeated ten to twenty times until the required shape is obtained. Alternatively, all these ingredients can be added together as an aqueous suspension.

Sugar Coat. Syrup is now applied and the water evaporated to give a coating of sucrose over the tablet. Again this step is repeated many times. By

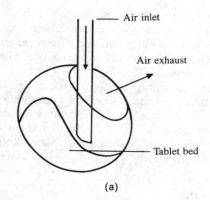

(a)

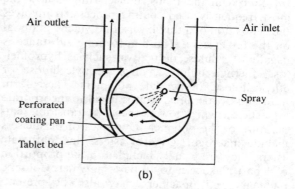

(b)

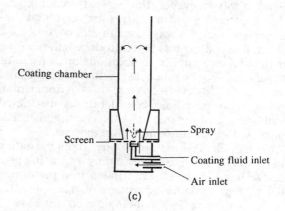

(c)

Fig. 10
Tablet coating apparatus: (a) coating pan, (b) spray coater, (c) air suspension coater.

using dyes (usually in the form of insoluble lakes or pigments) dispersed in the syrup, the colour of the tablet can be changed at this stage, and titanium dioxide can be used as an opacifier. If dyes are used, water must be evaporated slowly, otherwise the dye can migrate with the solvent to give uneven coloration on the surface of the tablet.

Polishing. Up to this point, the tablets have a matt finish. They are transferred to a separate pan, often lined with canvas impregnated with wax, and more wax such as beeswax or carnauba wax applied in an organic solvent.

The sugar coating process is protracted, a single batch taking several days to complete, and it requires a high level of skill. The mass of the tablet is greatly increased (often doubled) and surface features of the tablet cores, such as breaklines, are totally obscured.

Film Coating

Introduced in the 1950s, film coating is now the most frequently used coating process. It involves the deposition of a thin layer of polymeric material on the tablet core. The film-forming substance is usually a cellulose derivative, such as hypromellose, methylcellulose, hydroxypropylcellulose or ethylcellulose, or acrylate polymers. These form hard and brittle films, so it is usual to incorporate a plasticiser which lowers the glass transition temperature of the polymer. Examples of plasticisers include macrogol, glycerol esters, and phthalate esters; they are usually included in the proportion of 1 part plasticiser to 10 parts polymer. Colours, pigments and opacifiers may also be present. Because solvent evaporation is rapid, colour migration is often a problem if dyes are used, and pigments are almost always used in film coating.

When film coating was first introduced, the coating materials were applied as solutions or dispersions in organic liquids such as methyl chloride and methanol. However, because of environmental, safety, and economic considerations associated with the use of organic solvents, coating materials dispersed in water are now more popular.[27,28]

Although film coating can be carried out in coating pans, the film is usually applied by a spraying process, while the tablets are rotated in a perforated drum (Fig. 10b). An advantage of this apparatus is that incoming and outgoing air do not have to use the same aperture in the drum; drying air is fed through the perforations directly on to the tablet surface and extraction takes place underneath the tablet bed, thus ensuring efficient drying. Process variables relate to the apparatus (design, speed, load), the air (temperature, flow rate), and the spray (spray rate, pattern, distance from nozzle to powder bed); all need to be controlled for a reproducible product.

Alternatively fluidised bed coating equipment can be used. This must have provision for atomising the spray liquid and agitating the tablet so that all pass through the spray (Fig. 10c).

Advantages of film coating are that the process is rapid, lends itself to automation and can readily be made to comply with Good Manufacturing Practice regulations. The increase in tablet mass is small (2% to 3%) and surface features of the tablet remain visible through the coating.

Film coating provides a useful means of achieving controlled drug release from the tablet. This has been most successful in the area of gastric resistant coating (enteric coating), which allows the tablet to pass intact through the stomach and to disintegrate in the small intestine. It follows that the coating material should be resistant to gastric fluids, but readily permeable to those of the intestine. This may be desirable to protect acid-labile drugs, prevent nausea, and to delay release. Traditional materials such as shellac can be used, but the most widely used substance is cellacephate (cellulose acetate phthalate, CAP) which dissolves at a pH of about 6. Other enteric coating materials include acrylate polymers (Eudragit™) and hypromellose phthalate.[29]

Compression Coating

In this process, tablet cores are compressed and then surrounded by granular coating material and compressed again. The obvious advantage is that the process is dry and therefore does not require heat to evaporate the coating fluid; hence it may be useful for thermolabile and water-sensitive materials. Specialised presses are needed and, with the increased popularity of film coating, compression coating is now of diminishing importance.

QUALITY CONTROL AND MEASUREMENT OF TABLET PROPERTIES

Tablets are subject to a number of test procedures, some of which are pharmacopoeial.

Pharmacopoeial Tests

The *British Pharmacopoeia 1993* contains standards and test methods for the following tablet properties:

- uniformity of weight
- content of active ingredient
- uniformity of content
- disintegration
- dissolution.

The first three standards are designed to control the amount of active material in the tablet and the last two control the ability of that drug to be released from the tablet.

In the **uniformity of weight** test, 20 tablets taken from a batch are individually weighed and the mean calculated. Not more than two tablets are permitted to deviate from the mean by more than the percentage given in Table 9 and none by more than double that percentage.

Table 9
Uniformity of weight test; permitted variations

Average weight of tablet	Percentage deviation
80 mg or less	10
More than 80 mg but less than 250 mg	7.5
250 mg or more	5

The **content of active ingredient** is determined, again from a sample of 20 tablets, by crushing the tablets and subjecting an aliquot of the resultant powder to the stipulated assay procedure. The result of the assay gives the average drug content of the 20 tablets but gives no indication of the variation of drug content among the individual tablets. Gross variation would be excluded by the uniformity of weight test only if the drug comprises the bulk of the tablet; this would be true of relatively non-potent drugs which do not require dilution before tableting. Content variation among tablets of high potency drugs, in which most of the tablet will be diluent, cannot be picked up by a combination of these two tests. In such cases, the uniformity of content must be established by individual tablet assays. Ten tablets are assayed by the specified method. The preparation being examined fails to comply if more than one tablet is outside the range of 85% to 115% of the average value or if any tablet is outside the range of 75% to 125% of the average. If one tablet is outside the 85% to 115% range, then a further 20 tablets are assayed and no more tablets outside this range should be found. To comply with the standards of the *British Pharmacopoeia* the uniformity of content test must be applied to all tablets which have a drug content of less than 2 mg or when the active ingredient comprises less than 2% of the total tablet weight.

The *United States Pharmacopeia XXII* adopts a somewhat different approach. It permits uniformity to be demonstrated by either weight variation or content uniformity, but accepts that weight variation is not an adequate test when the active substance is a minor component of the tablet formulation. Hence weight variation can only be used when there is 50 mg or more of active ingredient present which comprises at least 50% of the weight of the dosage form. A sample of 30 tablets is randomly selected. Ten are weighed and the average calculated. From the results of the assay, the content of active ingredient is calculated, assuming homogeneous distribution of the drug among the tablets.

Content uniformity is also established using a random sample of 30 tablets. Ten are assayed and the mean content and relative standard deviation (RSD) calculated. If one tablet is outside the range 85% to 115% of the claimed content but within the range 75% to 125%, or the RSD is greater than 6% or both, the remaining 20 tablets are assayed. No further tablets outside the 85% to 115% range may be present, but an RSD of not greater than 7.8% is now permitted.

Until comparatively recently, the only pharmacopoeial standard relating to the release of drug from a tablet was a simple tablet **disintegration test**. One tablet is placed in each of six tubes of specified dimensions, each tube being closed at the lower end by a screen of 2 mm nominal aperture. The tubes are raised and lowered in a bath of fluid maintained at 37°. The fluid is water unless otherwise specified and for most tablets the permitted disintegration time is 15 minutes. Tablets are said to have disintegrated if no fragment (other than fragments of coating) remains on the screen or, if particles remain, they are soft without an unwetted core. Full details are given in the *British Pharmacopoeia*.

The above test is applied to tablets which are designed to disintegrate in the gastro-intestinal tract. If this is not the case, the test may be modified. For example, dispersible tablets must disintegrate in water at 19° to 21° within three minutes, and effervescent tablets must disintegrate in 200 mL of non-agitated cold water at 15° to 25° within five minutes.

Although tablet disintegration is monitored by this test, a drug must be in solution before it can be absorbed from the gastro-intestinal tract. It therefore follows that a tablet may meet disintegration standards yet be therapeutically inactive. Hence where there may be problems in dissolving the active ingredient, the tablet is subjected to a **dissolution test**. The *British Pharmacopoeia 1993* permits three types of apparatus, the 'rotating basket', the 'paddle', and the 'flow-through cell' methods; the precise form of the test, including the medium to be used, is specified in the relevant monograph. In general, acidic media are used with basic drugs (for example, 0.1M hydrochloric acid with quinine sulphate), more alkaline media with acidic drugs (for example, pH 6.8 buffer with phenoxymethylpenicillin) and water for non-ionising molecules such as digoxin. Unless otherwise specified, a sample is removed from the dissolution fluid after 45 minutes and analysed. The most common standard is that 70% of the stated amount of drug must be in solution after this time has elapsed. The approach of the *United States Pharmacopeia* to disintegration and dissolution is slightly different, although the apparatus used is virtually identical. In the disintegration test, six tablets are used, and if after the specified time one or two have not disintegrated, another 12 are tested. Not less than 16 of the 18 should disintegrate fully. In the dissolution test, the relevant monograph specifies details of the apparatus and test fluid. The test can take place in up to three stages, using the acceptance criteria shown in Table 10.

Table 10
The USP test for tablet dissolution; acceptance criteria

Stage	Number of tablets	Acceptance criteria
S1	6	Q ± 5%
S2	6	mean of (S1 + S2) greater than or equal to Q; no unit less than Q − 15%
S3	12	mean of (S1 + S2 + S3) greater than or equal to Q; not more than two units less than Q − 15%; no unit less than Q − 25%

Q is the amount of dissolved active ingredient specified in the individual monograph, expressed as a percentage of the labelled content.

Non-pharmacopoeial Tests

A wide variety of non-pharmacopoeial tests are applied to tablets, both as in-process controls and as part of quality assurance programmes. Thus individual tablet weights, thicknesses, and diameters are routinely and often automatically measured.

Mechanical strength measurements are also important. The most common is that of **crushing strength**; this is the compressional force which, when applied diametrically to the tablet, just causes it to fracture. A number of commercial instruments are available (CT40, Erweka, Monsanto, Pfizer, Strong Cobb, Schleuniger) which work on similar principles. A moving plunger presses on the edge of the tablet, which is held either vertically or horizontally, and the applied force is measured by a transducer. It has been shown that the rate at which force is

applied can affect the measured value of the crushing strength, and so more accurate results are obtained if the force is applied at a uniform rate by mechanical or electromechanical means rather than manually.

The size of the tablet affects the force needed to break it. To correct for this, the tablet tensile strength (T_s) can be calculated[30] using the formula:

$$T_s = \frac{2P}{\pi d t}$$

where P is the breaking force, d is tablet diameter, and t is tablet thickness.

An alternative method of expressing tablet tensile strength corrects for the porosity (E) of the tablet:[31]

$$T_s = \frac{2P}{\pi d t (1 - E)}$$

The tablet must fail in tension for tensile strength calculations to be valid.

Another variant is to calculate **tablet toughness** or **work of tablet failure**, in which the movement of the plunger as well as the applied force is measured. The toughness is the area under the curve of a plot of force against plunger movement.[32]

Although the crushing strength is a useful measurement which can be obtained easily, it could be argued that a tablet is more likely to be subjected to a large number of small impacts, perhaps during coating or packaging, than to one catastrophic blow. Therefore, tablets may be subjected to **friability tests** which measure the resistance of the tablet to abrasion. Tablets are subjected to a standardised level of agitation for a given time, and friability is expressed as percentage weight loss.

STUDIES ON POWDER COMPACTION AND TABLET FORMATION

A considerable number of parameters have been devised which attempt to describe the process of powder compaction, both to elucidate underlying principles and also to enable predictions to be made regarding compaction properties of solids. Some of these parameters are summarised in Table 11, and the field has been comprehensively reviewed.[43,44]

Tablet Press Instrumentation

All the parameters listed in Table 11 require knowledge of the force which is being applied to the powder bed and some also require the position of the punches applying that force to be known. Therefore, significant progress in tableting research did

Table 11
Techniques used to characterise the compaction process

Technique	Reference
Brittle fracture propensity	33
Compression pressure cycles	34
Elastic recovery	35
Force-displacement curves	36
Multiple compression	37
Power of compaction	38
Pressure-density relationships	39, 40
Strength-compression pressure profiles	41
Surface hardness	42
Tensile strength-compression pressure profiles	31
Work of tablet failure	32

not develop until force and punch position could be measured accurately. The topic was transformed by the introduction of the 'instrumented tablet machine'.[45] In this device, strain gauges are attached to parts of the press, such as the upper punches. At its simplest, the strain gauge is a network of wires through which an electric current is passed. Application of force to the punch causes it to deform, the magnitude of the deformation (the strain) being governed by a combination of the applied force (the stress) and the Young's modulus for the material from which the punch is made. The wire of the strain gauge is also deformed and hence its electrical resistance changes. If the strain gauge forms part of a Wheatstone bridge circuit, a small voltage change occurs which can be ampli-

fied and recorded. The size of the signal from the strain gauge is thus proportional to the amount of deformation, which in turn is a function of the applied force. Hence after appropriate calibration, force can be expressed in terms of voltage. Punch position can be determined by displacement transducers. There are several varieties of these, but all emit an electrical signal whose magnitude is governed by the position of a sensing device in relation to a fixed reference point. Signals from the transducers may be fed into an oscilloscope, or a chart recorder or, alternatively, stored electronically and subsequently manipulated by computer.
Instrumentation of a rotary press is more difficult than for an eccentric press if transducers are to be fitted directly to the punches. Due to the rotation of the turret, a fixed connection between the transducers and the recording apparatus is impracticable. Alternatives to fixed connections are radiotelemetry and slip rings, a further option is to fit the force transducers to more remote parts of the press which do not rotate. Tablet press instrumentation has been fully reviewed by Ridgway-Watt.[46]

Data From Instrumented Tablet Presses

A set of results from an eccentric press fitted with force and displacement transducers on both punches is shown in Fig. 11.

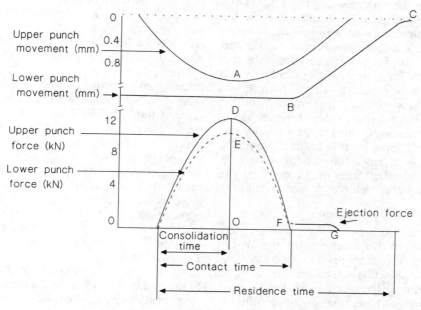

Fig. 11
Data from instrumented tablet press.

Displacement Data

Upper punch displacement describes a path which is symmetrical about the point of maximum penetration (Point A). The lower punch remains at the same level until the compression stage is over. Then it begins to rise (Point B) and as it does, it ejects the tablet from the die. The maximum height reached by the lower punch is where its tip is level with the top of the die (Point C), after which it begins to descend again ready for the next filling stage. It follows that at any given point in time, the distance between the punch faces can be measured. Up to Point A, this corresponds to the height of the powder bed, and hence the porosity of the latter can be calculated.

Force Data

As the upper punch descends into the die, the applied force increases to a maximum (Point D), although it is noticeable that the punch penetrates a considerable distance into the die before a measurable force is detected. The time at which Point D is reached usually coincides with maximum upper punch penetration, though slight deviations from this may occur, depending on the nature of the solid.

Force is transmitted through the powder bed to the lower punch. The changes in lower punch force with time follow a similar pattern to those of the upper punch, but the force is always slightly lower (Point E) during the compression stage; this is due to some of the force being transmitted to the die wall, where it appears as die wall friction.

After the maximum force has been achieved and the upper punch begins to withdraw from the die, the upper punch force does not immediately fall to zero as might be expected. This is because the tablet expands and remains in contact with the ascending punch for a short time. However as the upper punch accelerates, contact is eventually lost and upper punch force returns to zero (Point F). At this point, lower punch force is not zero as die wall friction holds the tablet in the die, and the lower punch must apply a force to eject it (Point G).

Mechanisms of Tablet Formation

Attractive forces exist between two particles; these may be non-specific (for example, van der Waal's forces) or specific forces brought about by features of the particles' molecular structures (for example, hydrogen bonding). Irrespective of their nature, these forces enable the formation of a coherent tablet. However, with particles of the mass of a powder particle, the force will be so weak that a significant degree of interparticulate attraction is only obtained when the particles are actually touching each other or are in very close contact. Thus anything that increases the area of interparticulate contact will favour tablet formation.

Consider a large number of particles in a die to which a compressing force is applied. A series of events will occur, perhaps sequentially but more likely with overlap.

The particles undergo rearrangement to form a less porous structure. As particles slide past each other, some rough points will be abraded. The force needed to achieve rearrangement is hardly detectable. The particles have now reached a stage where further rearrangement is impossible, even though the porosity may still be considerable. A further increase in force will cause particle fragmentation and/or deformation although, for any given solid, one of these two mechanisms will predominate. This will result in a further decrease in porosity and will increase the amount of interparticulate contact.

After the maximum force has been applied, the effect of removing the force must be considered. If particles have fragmented, then they cannot recombine. However, if particles have deformed elastically rather than plastically, they will attempt to return to their former shape. This will reduce interparticulate contact and hence reduce tablet strength. Most solids exhibit both plastic and elastic behaviour, but it is desirable that plastic behaviour should predominate.

As stated earlier, the force detected from the lower punch of an eccentric press is less than that applied by the upper punch. However, this reduction in force is not uniform on descent through the bed[47] (Fig. 12). Significant features are zones of high force at the periphery near the moving punch and much lower on the central axis of the tablet. Conversely, a zone of lower force occurs on the axis just below the top surface. Since tablet strength depends on porosity, which in turn depends on the applied force, it follows that some parts of the tablet will be weaker than others. If a tablet is to be disrupted, this will occur first at its weakest point which is near the top surface; this gives rise to a well-known phenomenon of tablet manufacture called **capping**.

For many years, capping was considered to be due to the entrapment of air in the tablet. However it is now recognised that the fundamental cause of capping is variation in porosity within the tablet,

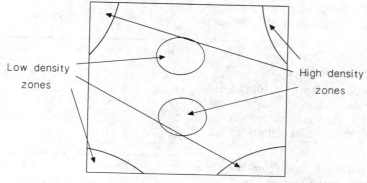

Fig. 12
Density distribution within a powder bed under compression.

although if pores contain entrapped air at elevated pressure, this will assist disruption of the tablet structure.[48]

Assessment of Lubricant Action

The reduction in force between upper and lower punches is due to loss of force to the die wall, this is reduced by lubrication. Thus the ratio between lower and upper punch forces affords a measure of lubricant action. This method of assessment, first suggested by Higuchi and co-workers,[45] defines the force ratio (usually denoted as R) as the ratio between lower and upper punch maximum forces (OE/OD from Fig. 11). The maximum value is unity, and evaluation of the action of the tablet lubricant involves measurement of the ejection force, that is, the force needed to remove the tablet from the die after the compressing force has been removed (see Fig. 11).

Mathematical Treatment of Compression Data

Data obtained from curves such as those illustrated in Fig. 11 have been used in a variety of ways in attempts to represent the compression process in mathematical form.

A number of equations have been derived to link the applied forces to the density of the resultant tablet. The most commonly used of these is the Heckel equation:[40]

$$\ln 1/(1 - D) = kP + A$$

where D is the apparent density of the tablet, hence $(1 - D)$ is the porosity, P is the applied pressure, k and A are constants.

If this relationship is valid, then a graph of $\ln 1/(1 - D)$ against P should be rectilinear with slope of k and intercept A. The reciprocal of the slope is related to the yield pressure of the substance, and this equation has been used to distinguish materials which fragment from those which deform on compression.

It must be emphasised that all compression equations are simply attempts to mathematically describe the experimentally derived relationship between porosity and applied pressure. They do not have an underlying physical basis.

Data from Fig. 11 can also be used to obtain the so-called **force-displacement curve**, a plot of the force applied on the ordinate against the corresponding punch displacement on the abscissa (Fig. 13). The area bounded by the curve has units of force multiplied by distance, which dimensionally is equal to work. Therefore, the force-displacement curve has

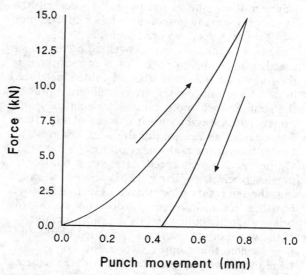

Fig. 13
Force-displacement curve using data derived from Fig. 11.

been used to calculate work of compression and also to quantitatively distinguish plastic from elastic deformation.[36]

Time-dependent Compression Effects

References to compression time in the literature are often confused, both in relation to the duration of force application and to the precise definition of the time involved. A number of useful definitions are as follows:

- *consolidation time*: the time from the force ceasing to be zero to maximum force
- *dwell time*: time at maximum force. This is zero for eccentric presses, but has a finite value for rotary presses due to the geometry of the punch head
- *contact time*: time during which a force is detected at the upper punch
- *ejection time*: time during which ejection occurs.

All these are shown in Fig. 11. Changing the operating speed of the press has a proportional effect on the duration of these events.

The rate at which the powder is compressed has, in many cases, an important effect on tablet strength. In general, the more important that deformation is in the consolidation mechanism of a solid, the more likely are the tablets of that solid to be affected by rate of compression. Thus microcrystalline cellulose is rate dependent whereas dicalcium phosphate, which consolidates chiefly by fragmentation, shows hardly any speed sensitivity. Speed sensitivities of a number of common tablet ingredients have been reported.[49]

The rate of consolidation is governed by the punch speed. For any given press this is proportional to the output of the press (that is, tablets produced in unit time) but to compare two different presses, the actual punch speed must be calculated. Equations which describe punch movement as a function of time, and hence punch speed, are available for both eccentric and rotary presses.[50]

Output and punch speed data for a number of presses is given in Table 12. It should be noted that though rotary presses have a much higher output than eccentric presses, it does not necessarily follow that the punch speeds are much greater.

If the work of compression is divided by the time over which the compressive event takes place, then the power of compression with dimensions of Joules/time or Watts is obtained.[50] This permits compression events on different tablet presses

Table 12

Output and punch speed data for a number of Manesty tablet presses

Press	Maximum production rate per die (tablets/min)	Time for punch to descend final 5 mm (msec)	Punch speed at first contact (mm/sec)	Dwell time (msec)
F3	85	68.6	139	0
B3B	44	61.4	163	10.84
Express	100	26.7	416	3.94
Unipress	121	19.1	485	3.16
Novapress	100	10.0	720	2.14

to be compared quantitatively. A dimensionally equivalent way of calculating power of compression is to multiply the force by the speed of the punch when that particular force was applied. Again this can be obtained from data obtained from Fig. 11.

Tablet Press Simulators

Since tablet quality may be dependent on the type of press on which the tablets are made, it is desirable to carry out compression studies on the press which will be used for large scale production of the tablets. This will almost invariably be a rotary press. However, such presses require large quantities of raw materials which may not be available, especially during development of new drug substances. It is for this reason that tablet press simulators have been introduced; these are sophisticated hydraulic presses, the platens of which are equipped with punches. The platens can be made to follow any predetermined path, and so the pattern of punch movement for any press can be simulated, forces being recorded as they do so. Simulators make single tablets, and so are economical with raw material, while imitating conditions which apply during large scale manufacture. The construction and uses of tablet press simulators have been reviewed.[51]

Capsules

Capsules are defined as solid preparations with hard or soft shells, of various shapes and capacities, containing a single dose of active ingredient. They are intended for oral administration. Among the advantages associated with the capsule as a dosage form are elegance, ease of swallowing, and the ability to mask an unpleasant taste. Hard shell capsules are also used for powders such as pancreatin to be sprinkled on food and for powders to be inhaled from devices such as sodium cromoglycate.

HARD SHELL CAPSULES

The hard shell capsule as a dosage form consists of two distinct parts, the shell and the contents. The shell is almost invariably composed of gelatin, and comprises two sections, the body and the cap. Both are cylindrical, sealed at one end. The body is filled with a particulate solid and the capsule then closed by bringing cap and body together. Hard shell capsules are produced by dipping steel pins into a hot aqueous gelatin solution, a film of which adheres to the surface of the pin. The film is dried and then stripped from the pins. The resultant cap and body sections are trimmed and united. The capsule shell will often bear projections or some similar feature to ensure that the body and cap do not inadvertently become separated.

The shell is rigid and has a water content of 12% to 16%, although this is affected by environmental humidity since the gel is hygroscopic. If required, dyes and opacifiers can be incorporated and an identification mark can be printed on the shell.

Capsule Contents and Filling Apparatus

The contents of the hard shell capsule are usually powders, although granules, pellets, and semi-solids can be used. A variety of methods are available to transfer the powder to the shell. On a small scale, capsule bodies are held in a plate, and the powder poured in. To achieve a satisfactory uniformity of fill, good flow properties are essential. This can be achieved by using a glidant such as finely divided silica. As the shells are filled by gravity, particle packing is loose and as the process is manual, production rates are limited. Examples of this type of apparatus are the Feton and Tevopharm capsule fillers.

On a larger scale, powder is transferred to the body of the shell by a dosator or tamping device. In the former, a dosating tube is plunged into the powder bed and a small plug of powder is formed inside the tube. The dosating tube is positioned over the body of the capsule, and a piston located within it ejects the plug. The upper part of the capsule is then applied. A very free-flowing powder is not required as a cohesive plug would not then form inside the dosator tube. However, the powder cannot be too cohesive since the powder bed must be maintained at a reasonably uniform depth. A lubricant such as magnesium stearate may be required. Examples of machines using this technique are the MG2 and Zanasi (Fig. 14). A variety of models are available with a maximum output of about 150 000 capsules per hour.

In the tamping type of machine, exemplified by the Hofliger and Karg, powder is fed from a supply hopper into the filling chamber, then pressed into the holes of a perforated disc by a tamping finger. The plugs of powder are then pushed into the capsule bodies (Fig. 15). Maximum output is also of the order of 150 000 capsules per hour.

Capsule filling machinery can be fitted with force transducers. For example the dosator of a Zanasi machine has been fitted with strain gauges[52] and a capsule machine simulator constructed.[53] A high sensitivity transducer is required, since the maximum force exerted at the dosator is usually less than 100 N, compared to the 10 to 40 kN in a tablet press. See also below.

Capsule Filling

Hard shell capsules are available in eight sizes, although the smallest and two largest are rarely used (Fig. 16). Hence the contents must be formulated so that one dose is contained in the volume represented by a given capsule size. The degree of dilution is determined by the bulk density of the

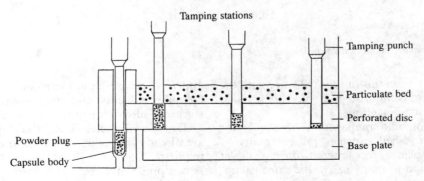

Fig. 14
Capsule filling by dosator tube method.

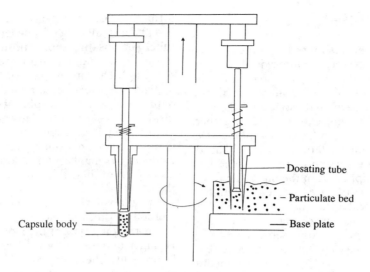

Fig. 15
Capsule filling by tamping method.

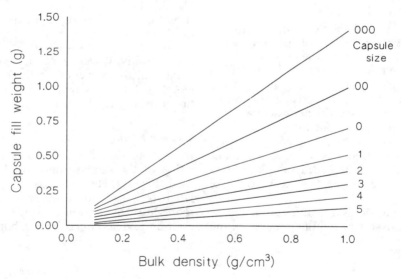

Fig. 16
Weights of solid required to fill capsule shells.

ingredients, although this in turn will vary with the degree of compression brought about by the particular type of filling machine.

The formulation and preparation of blends for filling into hard shell capsules present many of the same problems encountered during tablet manufacture, and in many cases, the same excipients and equipment are used. Thus the same considerations of mixing and particle segregation apply. Lactose and calcium phosphate are common diluents and magnesium stearate and silica are also frequently used as a lubricant and glidant respectively. Since the capsule contents are already in powder form, disintegrants are not required.

A comprehensive review of hard shell capsules is available[54] and formulation aspects have been described by Newton and Razzo[55] and Shek et al.[56]

The Fitting of Transducers to Capsule Filling Machinery

In contrast to the amount of work carried out on the instrumentation of tablet presses, relatively few developments have taken place in the field of capsule machine instrumentation. This is because the compressive forces utilised in capsule filling are much lower (a few hundred Newtons) than those used in tablet compression, and so an extremely sensitive system of force transducers is required. Furthermore capsule filling machinery affords few positions for the siting of transducers from which reliable measurements can be made.

A dosator type machine (Zanasi LZ64) was fitted with force transducers by Small and Augsburger[57] and later with displacement transducers by Mehta and Augsburger.[58] A typical force-time record is shown in Fig. 17. Point A represents a precompression force developed on the dosator piston as the dosator tube plunges into the powder bed. The larger peak (point B) is caused by a tamp being applied to the powder by the piston. This force decays rapidly but a residual force remains (point C) until after the plug is ejected (point D) by further movement of the piston. As the piston retracts to its original position, a drag force (point E) is detected.

A simulator based on a dosating piston type of machine, the Macofar, has been described by Britten and Barnett.[59] This apparatus, operated pneumatically, is fitted with force transducers on the dosator piston and dosator funnel, and the relative movements of powder bed and dosator are monitored by displacement transducers.

Because of its mode of construction, instrumentation of an mG2 type of machine is extremely difficult, and consequently simulators have been devised. The work by Jolliffe and Newton[60] and Tan and Newton[61] is particularly noteworthy.

Liquid and Semi-solid Hard Shell Capsule Fills

Filling of liquids into hard shell capsules causes problems because of the tendency of the contents to leak where the body and the cap join. However, if the formulation is liquid during filling but then forms a semi-solid, then a satisfactory product can be achieved. The fill may be liquefied by melting, and then congeal after filling. Alternatively, a thixotropic formulation may be used; this liquefies by the application of a shearing force as it is pumped into the capsule shell, and the viscosity of the mixture increases again later. A thixotropic system can be achieved by incorporating finely divided silica into the formulation.[62]

Pharmacopoeial Standards for Hard Shell Capsules

Hard shell capsules are subject to standards similar to those for tablets. **Uniformity of weight** and **content of active ingredient** tests are carried out, and a standard for **uniformity of content** is applied if the content of active ingredient is less than 2 mg or less than 2% by weight of the total weight of the capsule fill. The disintegration test is also similar to that for tablets, the capsules being expected to disintegrate within 30 minutes unless otherwise specified, the disintegration fluid being either water or hydrochloric acid. In a few cases, capsules are subjected to a dissolution test; again the basis of the test is the same as that for tablets.

SOFT SHELL CAPSULES

Soft capsules are used primarily as oral dosage forms, but they may also be used rectally or vaginally. In addition they are widely used in the food and cosmetic industries. The soft capsule consists of a solid flexible shell surrounding a liquid or semi-solid fill. They offer a number of interesting advantages: they permit liquid drugs to be presented as solid dosage forms; inter-capsule variation of dose is low since accuracy is a function of pumping a liquid rather than depending on powder flow; problems encountered when mixing solids and during compression are avoided; and as the drug is protected from water and oxygen

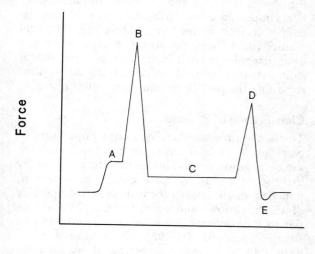

Fig. 17
Force-time relationship from an instrumented Zanasi LZ64 capsule filling machine.

by a hydrophobic liquid, stability is enhanced.
The shell is composed of gelatin, a plasticiser (usually glycerol), and water, plus preservatives, dyes, and opacifiers as required. A typical composition before filling and drying would be gelatin 43%, glycerol 37%, and water 20%.

Capsule Contents

As the contents of the soft capsule are usually liquid, they are in intimate contact with the shell. Consequently, materials which interact with shell components cannot form part of the fill. Water will diffuse into the shell, as will any water-soluble material, and volatile solvents such as ethanol will pass through the shell and be lost. For these reasons, most soft shell capsules are filled with hydrophobic liquids such as fractionated coconut oil. In some cases, the active ingredient itself is oily (for example, fish liver oils) and can act as the fill.

If a more hydrophilic fill is required, low molecular weight macrogols can be used although these, being hygroscopic, may scavenge water from the capsule shell.

As the capsule fill is usually hydrophobic, it follows that the number of active ingredients which will actually dissolve in such oils is limited. Nonetheless, if a solution can be made, significant advantages ensue in terms of content homogeneity. Alternatively, a suspension of the drug in the liquid is used. In such cases, the viscosity of the fill may be increased by adding a solid hydrophobic substance such as paraffin wax.

Capsule Filling

Although a number of methods have been described for making soft shell capsules, the majority are made by the rotary die process. The gelatin shell materials are melted and held in tanks at a temperature of about 60°. They then flow across the surface of cooled drums, there forming two ribbons. These are drawn together and flow over heated die rollers which have impressions of the shape of the capsule cut into their surfaces. As the ribbons flow over these dies, they are drawn down to fill the cavities and fill material is injected between them. The heated rollers cause the two halves of the capsule shell to adhere, trapping pockets of the fill material. The sealed capsules are then cut out of the ribbons, washed, and dried to a water content of between 5% and 10%.

The field of soft capsules has been extensively reviewed.[63]

Powders

A powder may be defined as solid material in a finely divided state.

Most dosage forms contain ingredients which, in their pure state, are solids, and these are almost invariably present as particles or powders. These particles may then be dissolved in a liquid, or remain in the solid state as constituents, for example, of tablets and capsules.

In solid dosage forms, the size of the powder particle is often of vital importance. In tablet manufacture, particle size governs the volume occupied by a given mass of solid. Since in a tablet press the quantity per tablet is measured volumetrically, it follows that the particle size controls the mass of the tablet. A similar situation applies to the filling of hard shell capsules. Furthermore, following oral administration, the dissolution rate of a drug is governed by its surface area, which in turn is linked to the particle size.

It follows that a knowledge of particle size and how it may be controlled is essential in the manufacture of efficacious medicines.

Particle Dimensions

The size of a large regular object, for example a block of wood, can be completely determined by measuring it in three dimensions perpendicular to each other. These dimensions are usually described as the length, breadth, and height of the object. However, most particles of pharmaceutical importance are irregular, and cannot be defined in such simple terms. Therefore, statistical methods have been developed to express the size of an irregular particle in terms of a single dimension, usually referred to as its diameter, thus regarding the particle as equivalent to a sphere.

Classification of Particles

This is the process whereby a large population of particles is divided into groups possessing the same range of sizes. This is usually achieved by the use of sieves. A sieve comprises a woven, punched, or electrically formed mesh, the aperture of which is known and which forms a physical barrier to the particles. All sieves should conform to British Standard 410:1986 (International Standard ISO 565), and are designated by numbers indicating the nominal mesh aperture in micrometres. The diameter of the wire forming the sieve is also specified. An alternative, though outdated, method of designation is to use a sieve number which represents the number of openings per linear inch of mesh. It follows that in the latter convention, the larger the number, the finer the sieve. Sieves listed in the *British Pharmacopoeia 1993* are shown in Table 13, together with their equivalent sieve number.

Table 13
Mesh sizes of sieves in the British Pharmacopoeia 1993 and their equivalent sieve numbers

Nominal dimension of aperture (micrometres)	Sieve number (meshes per inch)
11 200	—
8000	—
5600	—
4000	4
2800	6
2000	8
1700	10
1400	14
1000	18
710	22
500	30
355	44
250	60
180	85
125	120
90	170
63	230
45	325
38	400

The *British Pharmacopoeia* contains a series of definitions of powders, most of which are derived from sieve sizes or, where the use of sieves is inappropriate, they are defined in terms of particle size as determined by microscopy. The following terms are used:

Coarse Powder. A powder all the particles of which pass through a sieve with a nominal mesh aperture of 1700 micrometres and not more than 40% by weight pass through a sieve with a nominal aperture of 355 micrometres.

Moderately Coarse Powder. A powder all the particles of which pass through a sieve with a nominal mesh aperture of 710 micrometres and not more than 40% by weight pass through a sieve with a nominal aperture of 250 micrometres.

Moderately Fine Powder. A powder all the particles of which pass through a sieve with a nominal mesh aperture of 355 micrometres and not more than 40% by weight pass through a sieve with a nominal aperture of 180 micrometres.

Fine Powder. A powder all the particles of which pass through a sieve with a nominal mesh aperture of 180 micrometres and not more than 40% by weight pass through a sieve with a nominal aperture of 125 micrometres.

Very Fine Powder. A powder all the particles of which pass through a sieve with a nominal mesh aperture of 125 micrometres and not more than 40% by weight pass through a sieve with a nominal aperture of 45 micrometres.

Microfine Powder. A powder of which not less than 90% by weight of the particles pass through a sieve with a nominal mesh diameter of 45 micrometres.

Superfine Powder. A powder of which not less than 90% by number of the particles are less than 10 micrometres in size.

It should be appreciated that each of these definitions embraces a wide range of particle sizes. The first five have a maximum size but no minimum, and the last two have neither a maximum nor a minimum size included in the definition.

Comminution

Few solids exist naturally in the optimal size and shape for processing into pharmaceutical dosage forms, and hence some form of size reduction or comminution process is usually necessary. If enough energy is applied to a particle, then it will break, breakage occurring at flaws or points of weakness. Large particles will have more flaws in their structure than small particles, and so it requires less energy to fracture a large particle than a small one, and as the size reduction process proceeds, a progressively larger amount of energy is required. However, only a small fraction of the energy consumed during the milling process can be accounted for by the energy of the new surfaces produced.

The properties of a solid dictate its ability to resist size reduction and they also govern the choice of equipment used. Relevant properties include the hardness of the material, its physical nature (whether it is fibrous or friable), and its water content. Milling equipment suitable for pharmaceutical use has been described by Parrott.[64,65]

Particle Size Distribution and its Measurement

The quoted value of the size of a given particle is very much dependent on the method of measurement. For a particle to pass through the aperture of a sieve, at least two of its three dimensions must be less than the sieve aperture. It therefore follows that the third dimension can be considerably greater than the sieve aperture. However, if the same particles are sized using a method that involves the particles moving in a fluid, then a different result is obtained. Thus with an electrical resistivity method, conductivity falls because a volume of electrolyte equal in volume to that of the particle has been displaced. The diameter recorded is that of a sphere, the volume of which is equal to that of the particle. With light scattering methods, in which the particles rotate in a fluid (either liquid or gaseous), the size is that of a circle described by the rotation of the largest dimension, whereas with sedimentation methods, the reported size is that of a sphere that would move through the fluid at the same speed as the particle.

The most direct method of size measurement is microscopy, using a microscope fitted with a scaled eyepiece or graticule. The method is laborious (British Standard 3406 recommends counting at least 625 particles), and is subject to operator bias in the selection of the particles to be measured. However, the use of photomicrographs and automatic scanning devices can reduce operator fatigue.

Members of a group of particles are unlikely to have identical sizes and shapes. Thus a statement that a population of particles has a diameter of 100 micrometres almost certainly does not mean that all the particles are identically sized spheres, 100 micrometres in diameter. There will be a range of particle sizes. For this reason, it can be misleading to quote a single number to represent the mean diameter of a population of particles without further definition.

Comprehensive surveys of methods used to determine particle size and treatment of particle size data are available.[66, 67]

POWDERS AND GRANULES AS DOSAGE FORMS

Powders are mixtures of finely divided solids intended for oral administration, and comprise the active ingredients plus excipients (such as diluents, sweeteners, and dispersing agents) where necessary. They are usually mixed with water or other suitable liquid before administration.

Powders containing non-potent materials are often supplied in bulk, with directions to administer a specific volume as a dose. An alternative use for bulk powders is as the basis for the preparation of liquid mixtures (see Oral Liquids chapter), the solid ingredients in the powder being in the same proportions as they occur in the liquid preparation. Thus the packaging and transport costs of

the liquid ingredients are avoided. Powders for mixtures may be presented in bulk, from which the appropriate quantity of powder is weighed, or in packs, each pack containing sufficient powder to prepare a given volume of mixture. Because of the possibility of segregation occurring within bulk powders during storage or when subjected to vibration, care must be taken to ensure homogeneity before use. The label must state that the powder is for use in preparing a mixture, the name of the mixture, and the names and quantities of the remaining ingredients to be added to the powder in order to prepare the mixture. Examples include powders for Kaolin Mixture BP and Magnesium Trisilicate Mixture BP.

For more potent drugs, or where accuracy of dosage is more important, individually packaged powders (either in sheets of paper or in sachets) are used. The minimum weight of such powders is 120 mg, and so dilution of the drug, usually with lactose, is often necessary. Though not a frequently encountered dosage form, the individually wrapped powder offers the opportunity for administration of potent drugs in doses that are not commercially available in tablet or capsule form. Because of their method of manufacture, tablets and capsules are only produced in large quantities, and hence only in those doses which are most frequently used. Hence, extemporaneously prepared powders are often prepared from crushed tablets or the contents of hard shell capsules, together with an appropriate amount of a suitable diluent.

Unless otherwise justified, individually wrapped powders are subject to a uniformity of weight test, or a uniformity of content test if each dose contains less than 2 mg of active ingredient or the content of active ingredient represents less than 2% of the total weight.

By choosing appropriate ingredients, powders may be soluble, dispersible, or effervescent.

Granular materials may also be used as dosage forms for oral administration, being either swallowed as such, chewed, or dispersed in water or a suitable liquid before consumption. They too can be presented as bulk packs or as individually packaged doses. The granules are made by the methods described earlier (see Methods of Tablet Production), and may be uncoated, effervescent, or coated to give products that are gastric resistant or that have modified-release properties.

A particular use of powders and granules as dosage forms is in the preparation of liquid medicines containing drugs that hydrolyse or are otherwise unstable in the presence of water. By presenting the drug as a dry product which is readily dispersed in water, a liquid preparation of short but adequate shelf-life is obtained. Such products may be presented as single-dose medicines, when the solid ingredients are packed in sachets, or as multidose preparations. In the latter case, the solid ingredients are presented in a bottle, to which a specified volume of water is added, and the solids dispersed in it. Such a preparation would normally have a shelf-life of about one to two weeks, depending on storage conditions; this is long enough for antibiotic preparations, where the course of treatment is usually only a few days. A prerequisite of this type of formulation is that the final product is physically stable for the duration of its intended life. Thus if the final product is a suspension, then easy redispersion is necessary. Such considerations do not apply to single-dose products that are to be consumed immediately.

Oral liquids may contain a variety of other ingredients, such as: preservatives; buffering, suspending, and dispersing agents; and flavours, colours, and sweeteners. It follows that such ingredients must be included in the powder or granule formulation. Furthermore, all these ingredients must be readily soluble or dispersible in cold water. This requirement in particular rules out some common suspending agents such as methylcellulose and sodium alginate, which need heat and/or vigorous agitation before they can be dispersed in water.

The ingredients may be mixed as a dry powder or may be pregranulated. Dry product mixes demand less equipment, and no heat or liquid is involved. However, unless all solids possess the same particle size distribution, segregation may occur during filling. Granulated products are usually prepared by wet granulation. This is more expensive, and can result in chemical degradation of ingredients. On the other hand, there are fewer segregation problems, less dust is generated, and improved flow properties usually result. The formulation and preparation of dry syrup preparations has been reviewed by Ryder[68] and a formula giving the required amount of water for a specified formulation has been devised by Gibbins and James.[69]

Spheronisation

In certain circumstances, there may be a need for the production of regular spherical granules. These have been claimed to produce stronger tablets, and their regular shape is obviously desirable if the granules are to be used as the basis of a coated modified-release system, since the coating material will be expected to adhere more closely to a relatively smooth surface.

The traditional method for building up cores into spherical granules is by use of a coating pan. This process is slow and usually requires skilled personnel. An alternative method is fluidisation; the bowl of a conventional fluid-bed granulator is replaced by a bowl that has a rapidly revolving base. The rotational movement rounds the granules as they are produced to give a spherical product.

A third alternative is to use an extrusion process followed by spheronisation. The solids are wetted with water or a binder solution to give a mass of similar consistency to that used for the wet granulation method of tablet production. The mass is then forced through a perforated plate, to produce cylindrical segments. These are chopped into short lengths, which are then rolled into solid spheres on a rapidly rotating roughened plate. The pieces must, therefore, be plastic enough to withstand rolling. Equipment available for the production of spherical pellets or granules has been surveyed.[70]

Water content and spheroniser speed were found to be the two process variables that had the most significant effects on the properties of the product (flow rate, bulk density, size, friability) and also on properties of tablets made from the product.[71, 72]

Drug release from granules prepared in pans has been shown to be much faster than from those made by extrusion.[73]

MICROENCAPSULATION

Microcapsules consist of a solid or liquid core containing one or more drugs enclosed in a coating, usually in the size range 1 to 2000 micrometres. Products smaller than this are referred to as **nanocapsules**.

There are a number of reasons for employing the process of microencapsulation. The major use of microcapsules in pharmacy is as a means of achieving modified release of a medicament. In addition, because the dose of drug is contained in a large number of individual units, failure of a few of these units to release the drug will not have a major effect on the total amount released. Other possible advantages of microencapsulation include the conversion of liquid drugs to a solid form, taste masking, and enhanced stability.

The process involves the application of thin coatings to small particles of solid or droplets of liquid. Methods available include air suspension, coacervation phase separation, pan coating, spray drying, and congealing and pan coating. A number of substances have been suggested as suitable coating materials; these include water-soluble materials (gelatin and povidone), water-insoluble materials (ethylcellulose, polyamides, and copolymers of lactic and glycollic acids), waxes (paraffin wax and fatty acids), and gastric-resistant materials (such as cellacephate).

The materials and techniques used to prepare microcapsules and the pharmaceutical applications of the process have been fully described by Deasy.[74]

BIOAVAILABILITY AND USAGE CONSIDERATIONS

Most solid dosage forms are designed to be swallowed intact and following ingestion the drug should be released in the gastro-intestinal tract. Ulceration with occasionally fatal results has been associated with dosage forms becoming lodged in the oesophagus[75] and so it is recommended that all solid dosage forms be swallowed with a draught of liquid.

Tablets

When a drug is made into a tablet, a large reduction in effective surface area occurs and hence disintegration or deaggregation is a necessary preliminary. This procedure is more prolonged if the tablet has been coated, since the coating must be disrupted before disintegration of the core can begin.

In the gastro-intestinal tract, drug release is preceded by tablet disintegration and drug dissolution, both of which can be influenced by formulation. Disintegration is controlled by the use of disintegrants (Table 6). A number of methods of studying in-vivo disintegration have been described[76], but the most useful is probably gamma scintigraphy. The dosage form is labelled with a gamma-emitting isotope such as technetium-99m or indium-111 and the progress of the dosage form along the gastro-intestinal tract is followed by a gamma camera.[77] The intact dosage form is seen as a bright spot which becomes more diffuse as disintegration occurs.

Most drugs are absorbed by a process of passive diffusion across biological membranes, but before absorption can occur, the drug substance must dissolve. The rate of dissolution of a solid can be expressed by means of the Nernst-Brunner form of the Noyes-Whitney equation:

$$\frac{\mathrm{d}W}{\mathrm{d}t} = \frac{DS(C_s - C)}{h}$$

where W is the mass of solid dissolved at time t, D is a diffusion coefficient, S is the surface area, C is the concentration at time t, C_s is the concentration of a saturated solution, and h is the thickness of a stationary liquid diffusion layer around the particle.

The surface area of a solid is governed by the size of the particles and hence small particles dissolve more quickly than large particles of the same solubility. It follows that the bioavailability of materials of low water solubility may be improved by a reduction in particle size.[78]

The different regions of the gastro-intestinal tract have varying pH values. The solubility of neutral compounds is not affected by pH, but for substances capable of ionisation, their solubility will vary with progression down the gastro-intestinal tract.

The crystalline state of the drug may also affect bioavailability. Many drugs exhibit polymorphism, and in general, the least stable polymorph is the most soluble. The bioavailability of chloramphenicol palmitate has been shown to depend on the polymorphic state of the drug.[79]

Formulation and manufacturing variables can affect drug availability from tablets; the choice of diluent, disintegrant, lubricant, wetting agent, and compression pressure can all have an effect, interaction between factors often giving a complex overall picture.[80]

Hard Shell Capsules

These might intuitively be expected to show more rapid dissolution and hence perhaps higher bioavailability than tablets, as once the shell is broken or dissolved, the contents are already in particulate form. Factors which relate to the drug itself (such as particle size or solubility) will still apply. However, it has been shown that formulation and processing variables (for example, diluent or lubricant) also play a role in determining bioavailability.[81]

Soft Shell Capsules

The shell of a soft capsule can be expected to dissolve readily after ingestion, releasing its contents into the gastro-intestinal tract.

The vehicle within a soft shell capsule can be either hydrophilic (for example, macrogol) or hydrophobic (for example, vegetable oil). If the vehicle is hydrophilic, this will disperse in the gastro-intestinal fluid, liberating the drug either as a solution or a fine suspension, depending on its solubility in the gastro-intestinal environment.

If the drug is dissolved in oil, then partitioning must occur between the oil and the aqueous luminal contents before the drug can be absorbed. If the drug is dispersed in the oil as a suspension, then the particles must cross the interfacial barrier to form an aqueous solution. The rate of this process is governed by the aqueous solubility of the drug, the interfacial tension, and the size of the drug particles.[82] As in any partitioning process, the area of the interface between oil and water plays an important role, and drug release will be facilitated if the oil can be subdivided by the action of emulsifiers.

For drugs dissolved in digestible and hence absorbable oils, absorption directly into the lymphatic system may occur without the need for partitioning into an aqueous medium. The bioavailabilities of several drugs such as griseofulvin and flufenamic acid have been enhanced by their administration as an oily solution. The whole field of drug absorption from oily media has been surveyed.[83]

REFERENCES

1. Staniforth JN. Int J Pharm Tech Prod Mfr 1982;3(Suppl):1–12.
2. Campbell H, Bauer WC. Chem Eng 1966;Sept 12th:179–84.
3. Crooks MJ, Ho R. Powder Technol 1976;14:161–7.
4. Vromans H, deBoer AH, Bolhuis GK, Lerk CF. Acta Pharm Suec 1985;22:163–72.
5. Eskin NAM, Henderson HM, Townsend RJ. The Biochemistry of Foods. New York: Academic Press, 1971.
6. Seager H, Burt I, Ryder J et al. Int J Pharm Tech Prod Mfr 1979;1(1):36–44.
7. Newitt DM, Conway-Jones JM. Trans Inst Chem Engrs 1958;36:422–9.
8. Capes CE, Danckwerts GC. Trans Inst Chem Engrs 1965;43:T116-24, T125–30.
9. Leuenberger H. Pharm Acta Helv 1982;57:72–82.
10. Armstrong NA, Jones TM, Patel AN. Int J Pharmaceutics 1988;48:173–7.
11. Nyquist H. Int J Pharm Tech Prod Mfr 1983;4(2):47–8.
12. Armstrong NA, March GA. J Pharm Sci 1976;65:198–200, 200–4.
13. Miller TA, York P. Int J Pharmaceutics 1988;41:1–19.
14. Lowenthal W. J Pharm Sci 1972;61:1695–1711.
15. Shangraw RF, Wallace JW, Bowers FM. Pharmaceut Technol 1981;September:69–78.
16. Minchom CM, Armstrong NA. J Pharm Pharmacol 1987;39:69P.
17. Armstrong NA, Lowndes DHL. Int J Pharm Tech Prod Mfr 1984;5(5):11–14.
18. Malkowska S, Khan KA. Drug Dev Ind Pharm 1983;9(3):331–47.
19. Gould PL, Tan SB. Drug Dev Ind Pharm 1985;11(2&3):441–60.
20. Malkowska S, Khan KA, Lentle R, Marchant J, Elger G. Drug Dev Ind Pharm 1983;9(3):349–61.
21. Commission of the European Communities. The rules governing medicinal products in the European Community, Vol IV. Good manufacturing practice for medicinal products. Luxembourg: The Commission, 1992.
22. Peters D. Medicated lozenges. In: Lieberman HA, Lachman L, Schwartz JB, editors. Pharmaceutical dosage forms: tablets; vol 1. New York: Marcel Dekker, 1989:419–582.
23. Mendes RW, Anaebonam AO, Daruwala JB. Chewable tablets. In: Lieberman HA, Lachman L, Schwartz JB, editors. Pharmaceutical dosage forms: tablets; vol 1. New York: Marcel Dekker, 1989:367–417.
24. Mohrle R. Effervescent tablets. In: Lieberman HA, Lachman L, Schwartz JB, editors. Pharmaceutical dosage forms: tablets; vol 1. New York: Marcel Dekker, 1989:285–328.
25. Sendall FEJ, Staniforth JN, Rees JE, Leatham MJ. Pharm J 1983;230:289–94.
26. Conine JW, Pikal MJ. Special tablets. In: Lieberman HA, Lachman L, Schwartz JB, editors. Pharmaceutical dosage forms: tablets; vol 1. New York: Marcel Dekker, 1989:329–66.
27. Banker G, Peck G, Jan S, Pirakitikulr P, Taylor D. Drug Dev Ind Pharm 1981;7:693–716.
28. Hogan JE. Int J Pharm Tech Prod Mfr 1982;3(1):17–20.
29. Healey JNC. Enteric coatings and delayed release. In: Hardy JG, Davis SS, Wilson CG, editors. Drug delivery to the gastro-intestinal tract. Chichester: Ellis Horwood 1989:83–96.
30. Rudnick A, Hunter AR, Holden FC. Materials research and standards 1963;3:284–99.
31. Newton JM, Rowley G, Fell JT, Peacock DG, Ridgway K. J Pharm Pharmacol 1971;23:195S–201S.
32. Rees JE, Rue PJ. Drug Dev Ind Pharm 1978;4:131–56.
33. Hiestand EN, Wells JE, Peot CB, Ochs JF. J Pharm Sci 1977;66:510–19.
34. Huckle PD, Summers MP. J Pharm Pharmacol 1985;37:722–5.
35. Huffine CL, Bonilla CF. AIChE Journal 1962;8:490–3.
36. de Blaey CJ, Polderman J. Pharm Weekbl 1971;105:241–50.
37. Armstrong NA, Abourida NMAH, Krijgsman L. J Pharm Pharmacol 1982;34:9–13.
38. Armstrong NA, Abourida NMAH, Gough AM. J Pharm Pharmacol 1983;35:320–1.
39. Kawakita K, Ludde K-H. Powder Technol 1970/71;4:61–8.
40. Heckel RW. Trans Metall Soc AIME 1961;221:671–5.
41. Higuchi T, Rao AN, Busse LW, Swintosky JV. J Am Pharm Assoc (Sci) 1953;42:194–200.
42. Aulton ME. Pharm Acta Helv 1981;56:332–6.
43. Krycer I, Pope DG, Hersey JA. Drug Dev Ind Pharm 1982;8:307–42.
44. Hiestand EN, Smith JF. Powder Technol 1984;38:145–59.
45. Higuchi T, Nelson E, Busse LW. J Am Pharm Assoc (Sci) 1954;43:344–8.
46. Ridgway-Watt P. Tablet machine instrumentation in pharmaceutics. Chichester: Ellis Horwood, 1988.
47. Train D. Trans Inst Chem Engrs 1957;35:258–66.
48. Mann SC, Roberts RJ, Rowe RC, Hunter BM, Rees JE. J Pharm Pharmacol 1983;35:44P.
49. Roberts RJ, Rowe RC. J Pharm Pharmacol 1985;37:377–84.
50. Armstrong NA. Int J Pharmaceutics 1989;49:1–13.
51. Bateman SD. Pharm J 1988;240:632–3.
52. Cole GC, May G. J Pharm Pharmacol 1975;27:353–8.
53. Britten JR, Barnett MI. Int J Pharmaceutics 1991;71:R5–R8.

54. Ridgway K, editor. Hard capsules; development and technology. London: Pharmaceutical Press, 1987.
55. Newton JM, Razzo FN. J Pharm Pharmacol 1977;29:294–7.
56. Shek E, Ghani M, Jones RE. J Pharm Sci 1980;69:1135–41.
57. Small LE, Augsburger LL. J Pharm Sci 1977;66:504–9.
58. Mehta AM, Augsburger LL. Int J Pharmaceutics 1980;4:347–51.
59. Britten JR, Barnett MI. Int J Pharmaceutics 1991;71:R5–R8.
60. Jolliffe IG, Newton JM. J Pharm Pharmacol 1982;34:293–8.
61. Tan SB, Newton JM. Int J Pharmaceutics 1990;61:145–55.
62. Walker SE, Ganley JA, Bedford K, Eaves T. J Pharm Pharmacol 1980;32:389–93.
63. Jimerson RF. Drug Dev Ind Pharm 1986;12:1133–44.
64. Parrott EL. Milling. In: Lachman L, Lieberman HA, Kanig JL. Theory and practice of industrial pharmacy. 3rd ed. Philadelphia: Lea and Febiger, 1986:21–67.
65. Parrott EL. In: Swarbrick J, Boylan JC. Encyclopaedia of pharmaceutical technology; vol 3. New York: Marcel Dekker, 1990:101–21.
66. Washington C. Particle size analysis in pharmaceutics and other industries: Theory and practice. Chichester: Ellis Horwood, 1992.
67. Allen T. Particle size measurement. 3rd ed. London: Chapman Hall, 1981.
68. Ryder J. Int J Pharm Tech Prod Mfr 1979;1(1):14–25.
69. Gibbins LB, James KC. Int J Pharmaceutics 1980;4:353–5.
70. Gamlen MJ. Mfg Chem 1985;56(6):55–9.
71. Malinowski HJ, Smith WE. J Pharm Sci 1974;63:285–8.
72. Malinowski HJ, Smith WE. J Pharm Sci 1975;64:1688–92.
73. Zhaug G, Schwartz JB, Schnaare RL. Drug Dev Ind Pharm 1990;16:1171–84.
74. Deasy PB. Microencapsulation and related drug processes. New York: Marcel Dekker, 1984.
75. Howard PJ, Heading RC. The role of oesophageal transit in relation to drug delivery. In: Hardy JG, Davis SS, Wilson CG, editors. Drug delivery to the gastro-intestinal tract. Chichester: Ellis Horwood,1989:27–36.
76. Steinberg WH, Frey GH, Masci JN, Hutchins HH. J Pharm Sci 1965;54:747–52.
77. Christensen FN, Davis SS, Hardy JG, Taylor MJ, Whalley DR, Wilson CG. J Pharm Pharmacol 1985;37:91–5.
78. Fincher JH. J Pharm Sci 1968;57:1825–35.
79. Aguiar AJ, Krc J, Kinkel AW, Samyn JC. J Pharm Sci 1967;56:847–53.
80. Marlowe E, Shangraw RF. J Pharm Sci 1967;56:498–504.
81. Tyrer JH, Eadie MJ, Sutherland JM, Hooper WD. Br Med J 1970;4:271–3.
82. de Blaey CJ, Polderman J. Rationales in the design of rectal and vaginal delivery forms of drugs. In: Ariens EJ, editor. Drug design; vol 9. London: Academic Press, 1980:237–66.
83. Armstrong NA, James KC. Int J Pharmaceutics 1980;6:185–93, 195–204.

Oral Liquids

Oral liquids are homogeneous preparations containing one or more active ingredients in a suitable vehicle and are intended to be swallowed either undiluted or after dilution. There are three main types of oral liquids: solutions, suspensions, and emulsions. In addition, a few oral liquids may comprise a liquid active constituent (for example, liquid paraffin) without additives. The physicochemical aspects of these dosage forms are dealt with in the chapters on Solution Properties, Suspensions, and Emulsions. Some solutions and suspensions may be prepared from granules or powder by reconstitution immediately before issue for use.

The presentation of drugs as liquid formulations has some advantages over those of solid dosage forms:

- the drug is more readily available for absorption
- liquids are more easily swallowed than tablets or capsules and are therefore especially suitable for children and the elderly
- gastric irritation, caused by certain drugs when they are administered as a solid dosage form, may be reduced or avoided by formulating the drug as a liquid preparation.

There are also some disadvantages associated with the use of liquid preparations:

- the drug may be less stable in a liquid formulation than in tablets or capsules, especially in solutions; this disadvantage may be partly overcome by the formulation of a suspension or, for drugs susceptible to hydrolysis, by the use of appropriate surfactants or non-aqueous solvents
- liquids, especially aqueous preparations, are susceptible to microbial contamination that may be unavoidably present from the time of manufacture; however, the proliferation of micro-organisms can be controlled by adding a preservative
- masking the unpleasant taste of a drug in solution is more difficult than when the drug is in a solid dosage form
- liquid preparations tend to be bulky and therefore inconvenient to store and transport

- administration of the correct dose is less precise since it involves the use of a 5 mL spoon, an oral syringe, or sometimes a volumetric dropper
- suspensions and emulsions have the added drawback that they must be thoroughly shaken to allow accurate dosing.

ORAL SOLUTIONS

Oral solutions contain one or more active ingredients dissolved in a suitable vehicle. The aqueous solubility of insoluble or sparingly soluble drugs can be enhanced by the addition of water-soluble cosolvents such as ethanol, glycerol, or propylene glycol, which are suitable for oral administration. The solubility of poorly soluble drugs may also be improved by the addition of solubilising agents such as the nonionic surfactants, by the addition of acid or alkali to form salts, or by complexation.

Draughts

The term 'draught' has been applied to oral solutions (and suspensions) intended to be administered as a single large dose such as 50 mL.

Elixirs

Elixirs are clear, flavoured liquids for oral administration. They contain one or more active ingredients dissolved in a vehicle that usually contains a high proportion of sucrose or a suitable polyhydric alcohol or alcohols. Elixirs may also contain ethanol. Traditionally, the term 'elixir' was often applied to sweetened liquid preparations of potent or unpalatable drugs.

Linctuses

Linctuses are viscous liquids for oral administration intended for use in the treatment of cough; they should be sipped and swallowed slowly without the addition of water. They contain one or more active ingredients in a vehicle that usually contains a high proportion of sucrose, other sugars, or a suitable polyhydric alcohol or alcohols.

Mixtures

The term 'mixture' is often applied to traditional oral solutions (and suspensions).

Oral Drops

The term 'oral drops' is sometimes applied to oral solutions (and suspensions) that are intended to be administered in small volumes with the aid of a suitable measuring device.

OFFICIAL EXAMPLES OF ORAL SOLUTIONS:
Alkaline Gentian Oral Solution BP
Ammonium and Ipecacuanha Oral Solution BP
Ammonium Chloride Oral Solution BP
Ammonium Chloride and Morphine Oral
  Solution BP
Chloral Mixture BP
Chloral Elixir, Paediatric BP
Ephedrine Elixir BP
Ipecacuanha Emetic Mixture, Paediatric BP
Opiate Squill Linctus BP
Phenobarbitone Elixir BP
Piperazine Citrate Elixir BP
Potassium Citrate Mixture BP
Sodium Salicylate Mixture BP
Simple Linctus BP
Simple Linctus, Paediatric BP

ORAL SUSPENSIONS

Oral suspensions contain one or more active ingredients suspended in a suitable vehicle. A suspension formulation may be used to mask the unpleasant taste of certain drugs such as paracetamol.
Sedimentation of suspended solids in suspensions may occur gradually on standing but redispersion should occur easily on shaking. The suspended particles should be small, uniformly sized, and evenly distributed in order to obtain accurate and reproducible doses; it may be necessary to add flocculating, suspending, and viscosity-enhancing agents.

Draughts

The term 'draught' has been applied to oral suspensions (and solutions) intended to be administered as a single large dose such as 50 mL.

Mixtures

The term 'mixture' is often applied to traditional oral suspensions (and solutions).

Oral Drops

The term 'oral drops' is sometimes applied to oral suspensions (and solutions) that are intended to be administered in small volumes with the aid of a suitable measuring device.

OFFICIAL EXAMPLES OF ORAL SUSPENSIONS:
Aromatic Magnesium Carbonate Mixture BP

Kaolin and Morphine Mixture BP
Magnesium Trisilicate Mixture BP

The term 'gel' is sometimes applied in pharmacy to semi-solid, aqueous, colloidal suspensions of insoluble inorganic compounds such as aluminium hydroxide. However, most pharmaceutical gels are semi-solid preparations intended for application to the skin or mucous membranes (see Topical Semi-solids chapter).

ORAL EMULSIONS

Oral emulsions are stabilised oil-in-water dispersions, either or both phases of which may contain dissolved solids. They contain one or more active ingredients. Solids may also be suspended in oral emulsions. Emulsions are a convenient means for the presentation, in a diluted and possibly flavoured form, of oils and fats or oily solutions of water-insoluble or unpalatable drugs. As oral emulsions are potentially viscous preparations they should be supplied in wide-mouthed bottles.

OFFICIAL EXAMPLES:
Liquid Paraffin and Magnesium Hydroxide Oral
  Emulsion BP
Liquid Paraffin Oral Emulsion BP

The term 'emulsion' is sometimes applied in pharmacy to emulsified preparations of liquids used as ingredients in oral liquids, especially for flavouring purposes (for example, concentrated peppermint emulsion).

FORMULATION

Oral liquids may contain antimicrobial preservatives and antioxidants as well as excipients such as dispersing, suspending, emulsifying, stabilising, flavouring, colouring, and sweetening agents.

Vehicles

Vehicles commonly used in the preparation of oral liquids include water, aromatic waters, and syrups. The choice of vehicle depends on the intended use of the preparation and on the nature and physicochemical properties of the active ingredients.

Water

Potable water is mainly derived from surface sources such as lakes, rivers, and streams or from underground sources such as springs or wells. Its chemical composition depends upon the source from which it is drawn. Potable water that is palatable and of satisfactory microbiological and chemical quality for drinking is available in many areas and may be used in preparations that are not intended to be sterile, provided that the mineral impurities that it contains do not react with the medicaments or other ingredients; the use of this potable water is described under Water for Preparations (below). Where potable water containing mineral substances is not acceptable, purified water is used but, as it is likely to be contaminated with micro-organisms, it is boiled and cooled before use.

Distilled Water. Purified water that has been prepared by distillation. Purified water (see below) is supplied when distilled water is ordered.

Purified Water (Syn. Aqua Purificata). Water prepared from suitable potable water by distillation, by treatment with ion-exchange materials, or by any other suitable method. A standard for purified water is given in the *European Pharmacopoeia*. It is used as a solvent and vehicle.

The ion-exchange materials used in the preparation of purified water are known as 'de-ionising resins' and consist of hard organic polymer particles, each containing ionised functional groups of a single type distributed throughout the mass of the material. The potable water is passed through two columns containing a cation-exchange resin and an anion-exchange resin, respectively, or through a single column containing a mixture of the two resins.

Resins that may be used include a strong cation exchanger containing sulphonic acid functional groups ($R.SO_3^-H^+$, where R represents the resin structure) and a strong anion exchanger containing quaternary ammonium groups ($R.NZ_3^+OH^-$, where Z represents an aliphatic group).

Micro-organisms may multiply in ion-exchange columns, but their growth can be minimised by using the column continuously and regenerating regularly after a thorough backwashing. It is inadvisable to use the ion-exchange method for preparing purified water unless facilities are available for controlling the quality of the water.

Purified water should be stored in well-closed containers that do not alter the properties of the water.

Water for Preparations. Water for preparations is potable or freshly boiled and cooled purified water. It is used in preparing oral liquid preparations that are not intended to be sterile but for which water of good bacteriological quality is required.

Potable water is drawn freshly from a public supply and must be safe and palatable for drinking; water obtained from the supply via a local storage tank is unsuitable for this purpose. If such stored water is the only source of mains water, freshly boiled and cooled purified water should be used instead. Freshly boiled and cooled purified water should also be used when the potable water in the pharmacy is unsuitable for a particular preparation because of the presence of impurities that might interact with active or other ingredients of the preparation. For example, the colour of mixtures containing compound cardamom tincture, which is prepared with cochineal (an indicator), depends upon the pH of the water. An unsightly fine precipitate is formed if compound sodium chloride mixture (which contains sodium bicarbonate) is made with a hard water; similarly in other mixtures containing sodium bicarbonate, the use of a hard water may result in precipitation. The sol viscosities and gel strengths of alginate and pectin dispersions may be affected by the concentration of calcium in the water.

Aromatic Waters. Aromatic waters are saturated aqueous solutions of volatile oils or other aromatic or volatile substances that are often used as solvents and vehicles in oral liquids especially in extemporaneously prepared mixtures. Some aromatic waters have a mild carminative action but they are used mainly for their flavouring properties. Chloroform water is used mainly as an antimicrobial preservative. The preparation of aromatic waters may involve the dilution of a concentrated ethanolic solution of the aromatic substance with water.

OFFICIAL EXAMPLES:
    Anise Water, Concentrated BP
    Camphor Water, Concentrated BP
    Chloroform Water BP
    Chloroform Water, Double-strength BP
    Chloroform Water, Concentrated (BPC 1959)
    Cinnamon Water, Concentrated BP

Juices

Juices are aqueous liquids expressed from fruits and other plant parts and are used in the preparation of some syrups. Pectinase is added to the juice to destroy the pectin and the juice is then clarified by filtration. Sucrose and a preservative may be added. Concentrated fruit juices are often used in the preparation of syrups. Juices have now been largely replaced by artificial flavours because of problems of microbial growth.

Syrups

Syrups are concentrated aqueous solutions of sucrose, other sugars, or sweetening agents that are used as vehicles for their flavouring and sweetening properties. Glycerol, sorbitol, or other polyhydric alcohols may be added to retard crystallisation of sucrose or to increase the solubility of the other ingredients. Syrups usually contain aromatic or other flavouring materials and may also contain suitable antimicrobial preservatives such as benzoic acid, hydroxybenzoate esters, or sorbic acid.

OFFICIAL EXAMPLES:
    Black Currant Syrup BP
    Syrup BP
    Tolu Syrup BP

Syrups are now defined as flavouring vehicles and are not intended to be used directly as oral liquids. Nevertheless the term 'syrup' has been applied to certain sweetened oral preparations; the term 'syrup' may be included in the subsidiary title of an individual compendial monograph for an Oral Liquid where that preparation was formerly known by an official title that included that term.

OFFICIAL EXAMPLE:
    Compound Fig Elixir BP
    (Aromatic Fig Syrup)

Spirits

Spirits are solutions of one or more substances, usually of a volatile nature, in ethanol 96% or a dilute ethanol; they may contain a proportion of water. Aromatic Ammonia Spirit BP is prepared by a distillation process, but other spirits in current use are prepared by simple solution in ethanol. Care should be taken when spirits are added to aqueous media as their high ethanolic content may result in either the precipitation of salts from the aqueous media or separation of material dissolved in the spirit itself.

OFFICIAL EXAMPLES:
    Benzaldehyde Spirit BP
    Lemon Spirit BP

Oils

Suitable vegetable oils such as fractionated coconut oil or arachis oil have been employed as vehicles for fat-soluble substances, particularly in vitamin preparations such as Calciferol Oral Solution BP.
Oils have also been used as vehicles for the suspension of drug substances, including penicillins that are unstable in aqueous media. However, this use has been largely superseded by the formulation of granules for reconstitution.

Suspending Agents

Individual agents are described in detail in the chapter on Suspensions. Suspending agents that can be used in oral liquid preparations include carbomer, carmellose sodium, microcrystalline cellulose, methylcellulose, povidone, sodium alginate, tragacanth, and xanthan gum.

Emulsifying Agents

Acacia and methylcellulose (or other cellulose ethers) are commonly used as emulsifying agents, especially for small-scale preparation. Other emulsifying agents used in the preparation of oral emulsions include glycerol esters, polysorbates, and the sorbitan esters. The properties and uses of emulsifying agents are discussed in detail in the chapter on Emulsions.

Antimicrobial Preservatives

Microbial contamination is inevitable during the period of use of an oral liquid preparation when the container is opened for the removal of doses, often several times in one day. As most oral liquids, especially aqueous preparations, provide suitable conditions for the growth of microorganisms an effective antimicrobial preservative should be included in formulations. Only a limited number of antimicrobial preservatives are appropriate to oral administration and few of these are active at alkaline pH. Antimicrobial preservatives that have been used in oral liquid preparations include chloroform, ethanol, benzoic acid, sorbic acid, the hydroxybenzoate esters, and syrup. Benzoic acid and sorbic acid are only active at low pH. Microbial growth in syrups with a sucrose concentration greater than 65% w/w is usually retarded due to osmotic effects; at this strength however, crystallisation of the sucrose may occur. Crystallisation can be minimised by the use of invert syrup mixed in suitable proportions with syrup.
Chloroform has several disadvantages:

- high volatility leads to loss of chloroform when the container is opened
- permeation through some plastics, for example polyvinyl chloride, can cause distortion of containers
- reported carcinogenicity in animals has led to concern about the safety of chloroform and to the withdrawal of chloroform in sev-

eral countries including the USA; in the UK medicinal products are limited to a chloroform content of not more than 0.5% (w/w or w/v).

The continued use of chloroform as a preservative, despite these problems, reflects the lack of a suitable alternative, particularly for alkaline preparations. More detailed information on individual antimicrobial preservatives is given in the Control of Microbial Contamination and Preservation of Medicines chapter.

Antoxidants

It may be necessary to include an antioxidant in oral liquid preparations that contain ingredients such as oils liable to degradation by oxidation. The ideal antioxidant is non-toxic, non-irritant, effective at low concentration under the expected conditions of storage and use, soluble in the vehicle, and stable (to reactions other than oxidation). In emulsions the antioxidant should usually be preferentially soluble in the oily phase. Inclusion in a liquid preparation for oral administration requires an antioxidant that is both odourless and tasteless. Antioxidants that have been used in oral liquid preparations include ascorbic acid, citric acid, sodium metabisulphite, and sodium sulphite. Details of the mechanisms of action of antioxidants and chelating agents, are given in the Stability of Medicinal Products chapter.

Viscosity-enhancing Agents

Viscosity-enhancing agents may be added to oral liquids to improve palatability and ease of pouring. The addition of sugars in relatively high concentration leads to an increase in viscosity and they also serve as sweetening agents.

Sweetening Agents

Traditionally, oral liquid medications have been sweetened with various forms of sugar including glucose, sucrose, syrups, and honey. Sucrose forms colourless solutions that are stable over the pH range 4 to 8. In the high concentrations required to produce a sweet taste that masks the bitterness or saltiness of some drugs, sucrose not only enhances the viscosity of oral liquids but imparts a pleasant texture to them in the mouth; for this reason syrups are widely used in cough medicines in spite of their cariogenic properties. The prolonged use of oral liquid medications containing sugars increases the incidence of dental caries; this is a particular problem when children receive long-term therapy. Sugar-free formulations of many medications are now available and, because of increasing concern about dental caries, it is likely that the demand for such preparations will grow.

The sugar content of oral liquid formulations is also of concern to diabetic patients who should either use alternative preparations or be made aware of the precise sugar content of a medicine in order to modify their diet, or insulin dose, if necessary. Preparations sweetened with fructose or hydrogenated glucose syrup must be used with care in diabetic patients as fructose is metabolised to form glucose, and hydrogenated glucose syrup is broken down to glucose and sorbitol; similarly isomalt is partly metabolised in the small intestine to glucose, mannitol, and sorbitol.

Sorbitol, mannitol, and xylitol have been used as sweetening agents. In large doses, these substances have been shown to cause diarrhoea. Artificial sweeteners are sometimes known as 'intense sweeteners' because, unlike sugars, they effectively sweeten preparations at a low concentration; those that have been used in oral liquid preparations include the sodium and calcium salts of saccharin, aspartame, acesulfame potassium, and thaumatin. The saccharin salts have been widely used for many years; they are very soluble in water to form stable solutions over a wide pH range. Aspartame has become increasingly used as a sweetening agent in recent years especially for sweetening foods and drinks. It hydrolyses in solution especially when heated at high temperatures with a resulting loss in sweetness; excessive use should be avoided by patients with phenylketonuria. Less commonly used are acesulfame potassium, which does not appear to be affected by heating at high temperatures, and thaumatin, which is probably the sweetest of these compounds. Artificial sweeteners tend to impart a bitter or metallic after-taste and, for this reason, they are sometimes used in conjunction with sugars. In the UK, lists are published in the pharmaceutical press giving details of the sugar content of commercially available preparations. If the sugar content of a particular preparation cannot be found from such a source then the information should be readily obtainable from the manufacturer.

Flavouring Agents

Flavouring agents are used to mask unpleasant tastes and make medicines more acceptable to patients, especially children. The type of flavour is usually chosen according to the taste to be disguised or masked but the selection of a flavour for a particular liquid medicine is difficult because of the highly subjective nature of taste preferences; panels of volunteers are often used to evaluate the effectiveness of a flavour in masking the unpleasant taste of a drug. The age of patients for whom the medicine is intended should be taken into account. Children may prefer sweet or fruit-flavoured medicines whereas some adults choose acidic flavours.

Fruit flavours help to disguise acid or sour tastes; butterscotch, liquorice, and cinnamon are said to be effective with salty tastes whereas chocolate, anise, and various fruit syrups may disguise bitter tastes. A flavour that is usually associated with the type of taste to be disguised may be preferred by some patients; for example orange or gentian is useful for solutions of bitter drugs. Emulsions that may have a sweet taste are often flavoured with benzaldehyde or vanillin. Chloroform or menthol may exert a mild local anaesthetic action on the sensory taste receptors on different areas of the tongue. Flavour-enhancing agents such as citric acid, salt, and monosodium glutamate are sometimes useful. Some improvement in acceptability may be achieved by adjusting the sweetness and viscosity of preparations and by incorporating a colour associated with the flavour used. In addition, certain flavours may be associated with particular medicinal uses; for example, peppermint flavour is traditionally associated with antacid medicines administered for the treatment of dyspepsia.

Flavours for oral liquid medicines are presented in several different forms including juices (raspberry or other fruits), extracts (liquorice), spirits (orange, lemon, and benzaldehyde), syrups (blackcurrant), tinctures (ginger), and aromatic waters (anise, dill, and cinnamon).

Flavours that have traditionally been obtained from natural sources are increasingly being replaced by synthetic materials. Natural flavours may vary widely in composition and taste and some batches may be contaminated with microorganisms; in particular, mould spores may abound in fruit juices and syrups. Some synthetic flavours are more chemically stable than the corresponding natural materials.

Flavouring agents may be chemically unstable because of oxidation, reduction, or hydrolysis and the stability may be affected by pH.

Colouring Agents

Colouring agents may be added to oral liquid preparations to mask an unpleasant appearance or to increase the acceptability of the preparation to the patient. Acceptability may be enhanced by inclusion of a colour that is closely associated with the flavour of the preparation. Colours are also added in order to produce a consistent appearance from raw materials of variable colour. Occasionally, oral liquid preparations are coloured distinctively as an aid to identification; for example, a green colour (green S and tartrazine) is used in methadone mixture (previously DTF).

Dyes should be non-toxic, non-irritant, and compatible with the active and other ingredients of the preparation. The selection of a colouring agent requires an in-depth knowledge of the physicochemical properties of both the dye and all other excipients. The solubility, stability, compatibility, and required concentration of the dye in the particular preparation must be considered. The colour stability of dyes is often pH-dependent; for example, sunset yellow FCF is stable at acidic pH but may be precipitated or change colour at alkaline pH.

The dyes selected must be permitted for use in orally administered medicines in the country or countries concerned. In the European Community (EC) colours used in human and animal medicinal products must be selected from those permitted in foodstuffs, designated by E numbers 100 to 180. Colours certified by the United States Food and Drug Administration are described by FD&C numbers. Most of the colours commonly used in pharmaceutical preparations have both an E number and an FD&C number; for example, tartrazine is E102 and FD&C yellow number 5. Some colouring agents, including tartrazine, amaranth, and lissamine green are subject to further restrictions or bans in some countries of the EC.

Colouring agents can be classified into three categories: mineral pigments, natural colourants, and synthetic organic dyes. Mineral pigments such as iron oxides are used mainly in solid pharmaceutical dosage forms and in preparations for external use; their use in oral liquids is restricted by the very low solubility of these minerals in water. Natural colourants comprise a wide variety of materials isolated, extracted, or derived from plants or animals; they include anthocyanins, carotenoids, chlorophylls, xanthophylls, riboflavine, saffron, red beetroot extract, cochineal, and caramel (from sucrose and other edible sugars). Disadvantages of natural colourants may include variation in composition and colour between batches. Some solutions of natural colourants have limited stability to light and pH and to oxidising and reducing agents; certain natural colourants are used mainly for colouring oily or fatty products.

Synthetic organic dyes are commonly known as 'coal-tar' dyes and are often preferred to natural colourants for oral liquids because they provide a wider range of bright and stable colours of more uniform intensity; however they are seldom pure compounds. There are two main types of synthetic dyes: acid dyes and basic dyes. Acid dyes form salts with bases, the coloured ion being negatively charged; basic dyes form salts with acids, the coloured ion being positively charged. Most synthetic colouring agents used in oral liquids are acid dyes; nearly all are sodium salts of sulphonic acids and many are azo compounds. Because of their chemical structure, such acid dyes may interact in solution with large cations to form insoluble compounds; thus they may be incompatible with many alkaloids, phenothiazine derivatives, and antihistamines.

Recent concern about adverse reactions to colouring agents, particularly tartrazine and other azo dyes, in preparations intended for paediatric use has led to a demand for formulations free from colours. For example, tartrazine is a permitted colour in the UK but reports of rare allergic reactions have caused its removal from many commercial preparations. Official formulations that in the past contained tartrazine have been amended to open formulae. A further problem is that the presence of dyes in liquid medicines has confused the diagnosis of disease; for example, green or red dyes in vomit have been wrongly assumed to be bile or blood.

Galenical Preparations of Crude Drugs

Traditionally, many liquid medicines for oral administration contained tinctures or other preparations derived by the extraction of crude drugs of plant origin with a suitable solvent. Such preparations of active constituents are often known as 'galenical preparations' or 'galenicals'; sometimes however, the term 'galenical' is applied to any pharmaceutical preparation including dosage forms.

Extracts

Extracts are concentrated products containing the active principles of crude drugs of natural origin. The choice of extraction method depends on the chemical and physical properties of the material being extracted. Maceration and percolation are the two main methods, but extracts may also be prepared by decoction, digestion, or infusion processes.

Liquid extracts are prepared by maceration or percolation with suitable solvents followed by concentration; they are usually of such a strength that one part by volume of the product is equivalent to one part by weight of the crude drug. If, however, the active principle is potent and can be assayed, the liquid extract is adjusted to a definite strength.

Dry extracts and **soft extracts** are prepared by evaporating the extractive from the crude drug either to dryness, usually under reduced pressure, or until a soft mass is obtained.

OFFICIAL EXAMPLES:
   Belladonna Dry Extract BP
   Ipecacuanha Liquid Extract BP
   Liquorice Liquid Extract BP

Tinctures

Tinctures are alcoholic liquids usually containing, in comparatively low concentration, the active principles of crude drugs. They are generally prepared by maceration or percolation or obtained by dilution of the corresponding liquid or soft extract. The term 'tincture' is also applied to some preparations made from volatile oils (or other volatile substance) or the active constituent of a crude drug.

OFFICIAL EXAMPLES:
   Aromatic Cardamom Tincture BP
   Belladonna Tincture BP
   Chloroform and Morphine Tincture BP
   Ginger Tincture, Strong BP
   Ipecacuanha Tincture BP

Infusions

Infusions are dilute solutions that contain the readily soluble constituents of crude drugs. Traditionally, fresh infusions were made by pouring boiling water on the drug, in a suitable state of comminution, and macerating for a short time. Now infusions are usually prepared by diluting 1 volume of a concentrated infusion to 10 volumes with water. Concentrated infusions are usually made by maceration of the drug with ethanol (25%). For dispensing purposes, infusions should be used within 12 hours of preparation from concentrated infusions.

OFFICIAL EXAMPLES:
   Compound Gentian Infusion BP
   Orange Peel Infusion BP

Oxymels

Preparations of acetic acid and honey are known as oxymels and have been used as vehicles or solvents for crude drugs. In Squill Oxymel, squill is extracted with diluted acetic acid by maceration and honey is added to the extract; it is used in expectorant medicines.

OFFICIAL EXAMPLE:
  Squill Oxymel BP

Dry Powders and Granules for Reconstitution

Medicines may be formulated as powders or granules for subsequent reconstitution if a liquid preparation has a limited shelf-life because of physical or chemical instability. In addition, oral liquid preparations formulated in oily vehicles can be unpalatable; the use of powders or granules for reconstitution with water permits the presentation of the final product in an aqueous vehicle and makes taste masking easier. Such powders and granules are sometimes known as 'dry syrups' and may be formulated as powder mixtures or as granules.

Powder Mixtures

Among the types of formulation intended for reconstitution, powder mixtures are the simplest and most economical preparations to manufacture. They present few stability problems as no heat or solvents are involved in their production. A practical problem is that it is difficult to ensure an even distribution of the drug within the mixture. Ideally, the excipients should have uniform particle size, otherwise surface interaction between the drug and the excipients will lead to uneven drug distribution.

Granules

Granules for the preparation of oral liquids are of two types, wholly granulated products and partly granulated products.

In wholly granulated preparations the active ingredient is either blended with the other dry ingredients before incorporation or it may be dissolved in the granulating fluid before granulation. The granules are screened to break down or remove oversize lumps. A detailed discussion of granulation techniques can be found in the Oral Solids chapter. A disadvantage associated with the preparation of granules is that it involves more processing, exposure to heat, and contact with solvents than the production of powder mixtures and there is, therefore, an increased risk of chemical instability. When a formulation includes ingredients that are incompatible, because of interactions when stored for long periods, the preparation of multi-layered granules may be necessary. Granulated products have a more elegant appearance than powder mixtures; they also have improved flow properties and generate less dust on handling. A disadvantage is that granulated products are less dense than simple mixtures and therefore require larger containers.

Partly granulated products may be prepared if some ingredients of a formulation will not stand up to the physical or chemical stresses of granulation. Suitable excipients are included at the granulation stage and the remaining ingredients are mixed with the granules before packaging of the product.

Excipients

Oral liquids prepared by the reconstitution of powders or granules contain the same categories of excipients as ready-prepared oral liquids. However, additional substances may be required to produce a satisfactory reconstituted product; for example the addition of a solid diluent, granule binder, moisture scavenger, glidant, granule disintegrant, or release-retarding agent may be necessary. Liquid excipients are either dissolved in the granulating fluid or adsorbed onto a carrier. The choice of excipients is restricted by the need for reconstitution and possibly granulation. Substances that cannot be adequately dispersed without soaking, heating, or high shear mixing will not produce an acceptable oral liquid preparation on the addition of cold water at the dispensing stage. Several preservatives (for example, benzoic acid and hydroxybenzoates) that are often used in oral liquid preparations dissolve too slowly in cold water and therefore cannot be used in products for reconstitution. In addition, compounds that are active only at high concentrations (for example, alcohols and glycerol) are not suitable for inclusion in these mixtures or granules. Preservatives that may be suitable for powders or granules for reconstitution include sucrose, potassium sorbate, sodium benzoate, and sodium methyl hydroxybenzoate.

The number of excipients that may be required in a dry preparation is potentially large. It is, therefore, desirable to use excipients that can fulfil more than one role. Sucrose is often included as a diluent; however, it can also act as a sweetening agent, a viscosity-increasing agent, and an antimicrobial agent (at high concentrations).

Presentation

Powders or granules for reconstitution may be presented as multidose, single-dose, or bulk powder products.

Multidose products are reconstituted by the pharmacist at the dispensing stage, by the addition of a specified volume of cold water to produce a stated volume of liquid, which is then taken in 5-mL or other specified doses by the patient. These products are then assigned an expiry date; for reconstituted antibiotic syrups this date is usually seven days from the date of reconstitution.

Single-dose products are packed in individual sachets and reconstituted by the patient immediately before administration.

Bulk solids are also reconstituted by the patient immediately before administration; individual doses are measured by volume from a bulk container of granules or powder. In this instance thorough mixing of the bulk powder is particularly important to ensure accuracy of dosage.

Diluent Volume

The volume of water that must be added to a powder or granules to produce a specific volume of final product (often 100 mL) varies between formulations. The amount of water displaced by the active ingredient and excipients must be calculated. The major components of powders and granules are usually sugars and the active ingredients; other excipients are present in relatively low concentrations. Gibbins and James described a method (see Further Information below) for the calculation of the amount of water displaced by 1 gram of solid, similar to the calculation of displacement values for medicaments in suppository bases. A slight alteration by the manufacturer of the sugar content of the formulation enables the required diluent volume to be a multiple of 10 mL, a convenient volume for the dispensing pharmacist.

Reconstitution of Multidose Products

The reconstitution of portions of granules or powders intended for multidose use, in order to produce smaller volumes or different concentrations, is not recommended. Subdivision does not give a uniform concentration because of possible segregation of the active ingredient within the granules. Dilution to volumes other than those recommended by the manufacturer may compromise the stability of the final product.

Compendial Requirements

Certain compendial requirements are applied to the formulation and manufacture of oral liquids including those mixtures that may be prepared extemporaneously in the pharmacy. However, the *British Pharmacopoeia* does not specify a precise shelf-life for extemporaneously prepared oral liquids. Pharmacists have to make their own decisions on an appropriate shelf-life for a particular product. Guidance is given under Stability of Extemporaneously Prepared Mixtures in the chapter on Stability of Medicinal Products.

Manufacture and Extemporaneous Preparation of Oral Liquids

Certain oral liquids are defined in the *British Pharmacopoeia* only in terms of the principal ingredients; whatever method of manufacture is used, the product must comply with the pharmacopoeial requirements.

Other oral liquids are defined by means of a full formula and, for some, directions for their preparation. No deviation from the stated formula is permitted except for the use of alternative antimicrobial preservatives. Where directions are given these are intended for the extemporaneous preparation of relatively small quantities for short-term supply and use and, when so prepared, no deviations from those directions are permitted. Deviations from the stated directions are permitted for such a preparation, however, if manufactured on the large scale with the intention that it be stored, provided that it retains the essential characteristics of the preparation made in accordance with the directions and that it complies with the pharmacopoeial requirements.

A third category comprises monographs for oral liquids that include a definition in terms of the principal ingredients and also a full formula, sometimes with directions for preparation. The full formula and the directions are intended for the extemporaneous preparation of relatively small quantities for short-term supply and use, and no deviations from the formula and directions are permitted. However, if manufactured on the large scale, deviations in the formula and directions are permitted provided that the product complies with the pharmacopoeial requirements and that it retains the essential characteristics of the preparation made in accordance with the formula and directions.

Practical Problems in Dispensing Oral Liquids

Although most oral liquids are now manufactured on the large scale, community and hospital pharmacists may occasionally be called upon to prepare extemporaneously mixtures (or other products) for individual patients; preparation may involve solving problems of chemical, physical, or microbiological stability. In addition, it is good pharmaceutical practice when dispensing medicines to counsel patients about all aspects of their medicinal treatment including expiry dates and storage of medicines in the home. Guidance on the application of knowledge of pharmaceutics to the stability of medicines is given under Stability of Medicines in Pharmaceutical Practice in the chapter on Stability of Medicinal Products.

Incompatibilities are not often encountered in dispensing oral liquids but failure to detect interactions between potent drugs and other drugs or excipients may have serious clinical consequences. Examples of incompatibilities arising from the admixture of oral liquids or the addition of a drug to an oral liquid are given under Incompatibilities in Pharmaceutical Practice in the chapter on Incompatibility.

Problems in the selection and use of containers and closures for oral liquids are considered in the chapter on Pharmaceutical Packaging.

FURTHER INFORMATION

Preservatives. Lynch M, Lund W, Wilson D. Chloroform as a preservative in aqueous systems. Losses under 'in-use' conditions and antimicrobial effectiveness. Pharm J 1977;219: 507–10.

Flavouring Agents. Love DW, Foster TS, Bradley DL. Comparison of the taste and acceptance of three potassium chloride preparations. Am J Hosp Pharm 1978;35:586–8.

Schumacher GE. Palatability of bulk compounded products. Am J Hosp Pharm 1967;24:588-9, 713–14.

Short GRA. Flavours and colours in medicines. Pharm J 1960;2:565–9.

Swinyard EA, Lowenthal W. Pharmaceutical necessities: coloring, flavoring and diluting agents. In: Gennaro AR, editor. Remington's pharmaceutical sciences. 18th ed. Easton: Mack, 1990:1288–1300.

Sweetening Agents. Greenwood J. Sugar content of liquid medicines. Pharm J 1989;243:553–7.

Hobson P. Sugar based medicines and dental disease. Community Dental Health 1985;2:57–62.

Jones R. Sugar free medicines. Drug Information Letter. Mersey Regional Drug Information Service 1992;90:1–7.

Sheiham A. Sugars and dental decay. Lancet 1983;1:282–4.

Colouring Agents. American Pharmaceutical Association and The Pharmaceutical Society of Great Britain. Pharmaceutical coloring agents. In: Handbook of pharmaceutical excipients. 1st ed. London: Pharmaceutical Press, 1986:81–90.

D'Arcy PF. Adverse reactions to excipients [tartrazine] in pharmaceutical formulations. In: Florence AT, Salole EG, editors. Topics in pharmacy. Formulation factors in adverse reactions; vol 1. London: Wright,1990:4–6.

Pollock I, Young E, Slater N, Wilkinson JD, Warner OJ. Survey of colourings and preservatives in drugs. Br Med J 1989;299:649–51.

Reconstitution from Dry Powders or Granules. Gibbins LG, James KC. Calculating quantities in dispersible powders containing antibiotics. Int J Pharmaceutics 1980;4:353–5.

Hempenstall JM, Irwin WJ, Li Wan Po A, Andrews AH. Antibiotic granules for reconstitution as syrups: product uniformity and stability dependent upon reconstitution procedure. Int J Pharmaceutics 1985;23:131–46.

Ryder J. The formulation of dry syrup preparations. Int J Pharm Tech Prod Mfr 1979;1:14–25.

Solution Properties

Solutions are thermodynamically stable homogeneous mixtures of two or more components; they comprise one or more solutes molecularly dispersed (dissolved) in one or more solvents. The solutes and solvents may be gases, liquids, or solids. In pharmaceutical practice, gas in liquid, liquid in liquid, and solid in liquid systems are the most widely used.

Gases in Liquids

The quantity of gas dissolved in a liquid is, in general, governed by Henry's Law. This states that at a given temperature the weight of gas dissolved is proportional to its pressure. However, Henry's Law only holds for sparingly soluble gases and breaks down completely when used to describe very soluble gases. Nearly all gases are soluble in liquid media to some extent; their solubility, however, decreases with increasing temperature.

Liquids in Liquids

A liquid may be totally miscible, miscible only in certain proportions, or totally immiscible with another liquid medium. For liquids with limited mutual solubilities, a phase diagram may be constructed to illustrate the solubility of one liquid in another at various temperatures (Fig. 1).

The critical solution temperature is the temperature above which a homogeneous solution results regardless of the relative concentrations of the two media. Nicotine/water systems have two critical solution temperatures, one above which and one below which miscibility occurs, irrespective of the relative proportions of the media.

Systems that comprise three liquids are more complex and may be depicted by an equilateral triangle. The corners of the triangle represent the pure components, the sides binary mixtures, and the interior ternary mixtures (Fig. 2).

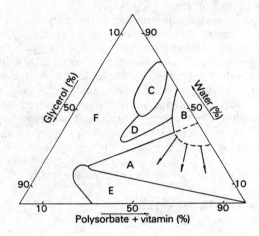

Fig. 2
Phase solubility profile of a ternary system. Vitamin A, polysorbate 80, glycerol, water system (Boon *et al.* 1961). A, transparent single phase; B, semi-solid; C, faintly opalescent; D, markedly opalescent; E, two transparent phases; F, emulsions.

Solids in Liquids

The majority of pharmaceutical solutions comprise a solid material dissolved in a liquid vehicle. The principles involved in the dissolution of a solid are discussed under Solubility, below. Many of these aspects are equally applicable to gas in liquid and liquid in liquid systems.

SOLUBILITY

When a solid is placed in contact with a solvent, molecules or ions detach themselves from the surface of the solid and diffuse throughout the solvent; these ions or molecules therefore become

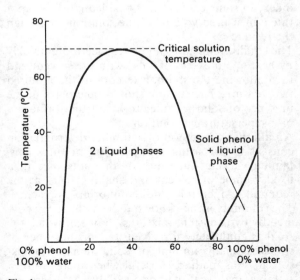

Fig. 1
Phase solubility profile of two liquids with limited mutual solubility.

molecularly dispersed. However, some of the solute may return to the surface of the solid and therefore pass back out of solution. The process will continue until the solubility limit of the material is exceeded, at which point an equilibrium is reached between the dissolved and undissolved material. The resulting solution is a **saturated solution** and the concentration of the solute, at the temperature used, is the solubility of the substance in the solvent. Saturated solutions are normally prepared by adding an excess of solute to a solvent and applying heat. The prepared solution is then cooled to room temperature in the presence of the undissolved material. Alternatively, the solubility of the compound may be obtained from the literature and the saturated solution prepared by dissolving the requisite quantity of the compound in the solvent, usually with the aid of heat, and making up to volume.

Supersaturated solutions are formed by dissolving the solute to a level in excess of its solubility in a particular solvent with the aid of heat. By cooling the solution in the absence of any undissolved material or extraneous particulate matter, the system may remain stable even at temperatures below its saturation temperature. Supersaturated solutions may, however, be broken down readily by excessive shaking, by scratching the container sides that are in contact with the solution, or by adding dust particles or crystals of the dissolved material to act as nuclei for crystal growth.

Solubility Thermodynamics

Dissolution can be described by:

$$\Delta G = \Delta H - T\Delta S$$

where ΔG is the free energy change, ΔH and ΔS are the enthalpy and entropy changes respectively, and T is the temperature (K). For any process to be thermodynamically favourable, ΔG must be negative.

The enthalpy of dissolution is governed by three factors. The first factor relates to the cohesive forces operating between solute molecules, the second to the forces operating between solvent molecules, and the third to the resultant interactions between the dissolved solute and solvent molecules after dissolution. During dissolution, solute cohesive forces must be overcome in order to provide individual molecules suitable for dispersion; the interactions between solvent molecules must also be overcome to provide spaces in which the dispersed solute molecules can fit. These two processes require

energy. This energy requirement can be fully or partly offset by the third factor that arises from the resultant interactions between the dissolved solute and the solvent. For dissolution to be thermodynamically feasible, any large positive enthalpy change must be offset by a more positive $T\Delta S$ term. This can often be achieved by an increase in temperature.

As well as enthalpy and temperature, the entropy of the system is an important determinant of the thermodynamics of dissolution. During dissolution, the solute molecules become randomly spread throughout the medium. This results in greater disorder and in an increase in the entropy associated with the system. A special case occurs when non-polar molecules are dissolved in water; hydrophobic associations may lead to a structuring of the aqueous environment and to a decrease in entropy. By combining the overall ΔS and ΔH terms, ΔG can be calculated. The thermodynamic feasibility of dissolution is governed by the result of this calculation.

Determination of Solubility

The simplest method of determining solubility for most compounds is to shake an excess of the finely powdered substance with the solvent at the required temperature until equilibrium is reached. The solution is then filtered and the concentration of the dissolved material determined by a suitable method such as a quantitative chemical or physical method, or by use of a physical characteristic of the solution such as specific gravity or refractive index. In some cases it may be adequate to evaporate a measured volume of the solution and weigh the residue.

The equilibrium state can be reached more quickly by heating an excess of solid with the solvent and then allowing the solution to cool to the required temperature. The cooling should take place in the presence of solid in order to avoid the formation of a supersaturated solution.

An alternative method of solubility determination consists of preparing a number of mixtures containing varying quantities of the substance in a fixed volume of solvent and shaking them at the required temperature until equilibrium is reached. The solubility is then known to be in the range covered by two adjacent mixtures, in one of which the solid is completely dissolved and in the other of which a small amount of solid remains undissolved. This method is useful when there is not a suitable analytical method available or where the solvent is volatile.

Factors Affecting Solubility

The balance between the hydrophilic and lipophilic groups within a molecule determines its overall polarity. In general, compounds with similar polarities are mutually soluble. For example, compounds that are predominantly non-polar tend to be more soluble in non-polar solvents, such as chloroform. Polar compounds tend to be more soluble in polar solvents, such as water and ethanol. Within this general rule, however, other factors may also influence solubility.

Nature of the Solute

Solid particles must first disintegrate for dissolution to occur. Solubility is, therefore, largely determined by the size of the intermolecular forces that hold solid lattices together. In a series of chemically related compounds, it is generally observed that as the **molecular weight** of a material increases, intermolecular forces also increase, and solubility subsequently falls. **Melting points** reflect the size of intermolecular interactions; therefore, compounds with high melting points tend to have low solubilities. Yalkowsky and Valvani[1] developed a method to estimate the aqueous solubility of organic non-electrolytes from their structures and melting points only. Intermolecular forces are also influenced by **crystal structure** and by **solvation**. Compounds that demonstrate polymorphism or that can exist with different numbers of solvated solvent molecules in their crystal lattice may display markedly different solubilities for each chemical form. The solubility of a solid is also influenced by possible interactions with the solvent. A reduction in the **particle size** to molecular dimensions markedly increases the surface free energy of a solid. This increase in free energy may lead to an increase in solubility when a critical diameter is reached. To increase solubility, the size and shape of the solute molecule should be appropriate for maximal interaction with the solvent. Of geometric isomers, the more compact *cis* form is usually the more water soluble.

Nature of the Solvent

The term **dipole moment** is used to quantify polarity. Polar solvents possess a large dipole moment because the electrical charge distributed in their bonds is not equally shared between the constituent atoms. The bond is therefore polarised, with one atom being partially positively charged and the other partially negatively charged. On addition of an ionic material to a polar solvent, ion pairs form between the additive and the solvent. This process is termed solvation, or hydration if the solvent happens to be water, and results in the rapid dispersion of the ionic material. Polar solvents may also break covalent bonds in polar solutes to allow solvation of the liberated anions and cations. Polar solvents possess large dielectric constants. The **dielectric constant** is a measure of the ease with which a medium can separate ions of opposite charge. Non-polar solvents have small dielectric constants; they facilitate dissolution by interactions between induced dipoles (van der Waals interactions). The dielectric constants of the commonly used pharmaceutical solvents are listed in Table 1. The dielectric constant, however, is only one determinant of the solubility profile of a solvent; dissolution also depends upon other factors such as hydrogen bonding and the degree of ionisation. The solubility behaviour of water, for example, can be explained by both dipole and hydrogen-bonding effects.

Table 1
Dielectric constants of some pharmaceutical solvents

Solvent	Dielectric constant	Temperature (°C)
Acetone	20.7	25
Arachis oil	3.0	20
Butanol	17.8	20
Carbon tetrachloride	2.2	20
Chloroform	4.8	20
Cottonseed oil	3.1	20
Dichloromethane	9.1	20
Ethanol	24.3	25
Ethyl acetate	6.0	25
Glycerol	46.0	20
Isopropanol	18.3	25
Liquid paraffin	2.1	20
Methanol	33.6	20
Olive oil	3.1	20
Propylene glycol	32.0	20
Sesame oil	3.0	20
Water	80.4	20

pH

Many of the organic drugs and adjuvants now used in pharmacy are weak acids or bases. As a result their ionisation is determined by the pK_a value of the compound and the pH of the medium, the ionised form being more water soluble than the unionised derivative. Tables 2 and 3 provide a rapid check on the likely solubility of a drug at a given pH.

Temperature

Most compounds demonstrate increased solubility at higher temperatures, but this is not always the

Table 2
The relationship between pH and solubility for a weakly acidic drug

$pH - pK_a$	Approximate mole fraction of ionised drug	Aqueous solubility
< −2	< 0.01	insoluble
−1	0.09	insoluble
0	0.50	soluble at low concentrations
1	0.91	soluble except at very high concentrations
> 2	> 0.99	soluble

Table 3
The relationship between pH and solubility for a weakly basic drug

$pH - pK_a$	Approximate mole fraction of ionised drug	Aqueous solubility
< −2	> 0.99	soluble
−1	0.91	soluble except at very high concentrations
0	0.50	soluble at low concentrations
1	0.09	insoluble
> 2	< 0.01	insoluble

case; calcium hydroxide, for example, is more soluble in cold than in hot water. This behaviour is controlled by the heat of solution (ΔH). If ΔH is positive, heat is absorbed during the dissolution process and solubility increases with increasing temperature. However, if ΔH is negative, as is the case with calcium hydroxide, heat is evolved during dissolution and solubility decreases with increasing temperature. When negligible heat is absorbed or given off, as is the case with sodium chloride, temperature has little influence on solubility.

Solution Additives

Additives can either increase or decrease the solubility of a solute in a given solvent.

Salting Out. This phenomenon occurs when an electrolyte is added to an aqueous solution. The salt competes with the solute for water molecules to allow hydration; this effectively reduces the solubility of the dissolved material.

Salting In. Several salts that are very soluble in water and that possess large anions or cations have the ability to increase the solubility of non-electrolytes. This process is also known as *hydrotropism* (see below).

Common Ion Effect. Dissolution is an equilibrium process operating between the dissolved and non-dissolved material. By adding a common ion, for example, magnesium sulphate to a solution of polymyxin B sulphate, the equilibrium becomes disturbed as the concentration of sulphate increases. To regain equilibrium, the concentration of dissolved polymyxin B sulphate must therefore fall.

Methods of Increasing Solubility

Chemical Modification

Solubility can be improved by chemical modification; for example, aqueous solubility can be improved by increasing the number of polar groups in a molecule. This is often achieved by salt formation; for instance, the aqueous solubility of chlorpromazine hydrochloride is about 20 000 times greater than that of the free base. Alternatively, a molecule may be modified to produce a new chemical entity or **prodrug**. The aqueous solubility of chloramphenicol sodium succinate, for example, is about 400 times greater than that of chloramphenicol. Prodrugs, however, must revert to the parent molecule after administration.

Complexation

The addition of a third substance that is capable of forming intermolecular complexes with a solute may increase the apparent solubility of the solute. After complexation, solubility is determined by the new chemical environment in which the solute finds itself. A number of compounds, such as nicotinamide and β-cyclodextrin, have been investigated as possible agents to increase the solubility of poorly water-soluble drugs.

Cosolvency

The solubility of weak electrolytes and non-polar molecules in water may be considerably enhanced by the addition of cosolvents such as ethanol, glycerol, propylene glycol, or sorbitol. These agents may work by decreasing the interfacial tension between the hydrophobic solute and the aqueous environment or by altering the dielectric constant of the medium.

Hydrotropism

Hydrotropism is the term used to describe the increase in aqueous solubility achieved by large concentrations (20% to 50%) of certain additives. The additives tend to be extremely water soluble and have large anions or cations; examples include sodium acetate, sodium benzoate, sodium tosylate, and sodium salicylate. The solubility of caffeine, for example, can be increased by the addition of sodium benzoate. Hydrotropism is rarely applied to pharmaceutical formulations, as the increase in aqueous solubility is generally inadequate.

The mechanism by which hydrotropic agents increase aqueous solubility is unclear; solute molecules may become dispersed in aggregates of the hydrotrope, the increase in solubility may arise through complexation, or the hydrotropic agent may alter the physicochemical properties of the solvent.

Solubilisation

Surfactants are used as solubilising agents in many pharmaceutical applications. They effect dissolution by a process known as micellar solubilisation. Micelles form because surfactant molecules possess distinct and separate hydrophilic and lipophilic areas, and they have a reasonably balanced hydrophile-lipophile character; complete dissolution would occur in an aqueous medium if the molecule were predominantly hydrophilic and, conversely, precipitation would occur if the molecule were predominantly lipophilic.

On addition to a liquid, surfactant molecules first accumulate at the air/solvent interface; further addition then leads to their dispersion as monodisperse units throughout the liquid bulk. At a certain concentration, the **critical micelle concentration** (cmc), the dispersed surfactant molecules aggregate to form micelles of colloidal dimensions. A dynamic equilibrium operates between the molecules resident in the micelle and those singly dispersed in the bulk phase.

In aqueous media, the hydrophilic areas of the surfactant molecule orient themselves towards the solvent for maximum hydration while the lipophilic groups reside in the micelle interior. In non-polar solvents, micelles form with the lipophilic regions protruding into the solvent phase and the hydrophilic areas forming the micelle interior. Micelle interiors therefore provide relatively hydrophobic environments in aqueous media and relatively hydrophilic environments in non-polar media. They may therefore be used to dissolve otherwise insoluble materials. The dissolved compound may reside in the micelle interior, be adsorbed onto the micelle surface, or sit at some intermediate point depending on the polarity of the compound. The dimensions of a micelle enlarge when material is incorporated.

Surfactants that are used as solubilising agents generally have **hydrophile-lipophile balance** (HLB) values in excess of 13; nonionic polyoxyethylated surfactants such as polysorbate 20, polysorbate 80, polyoxyl 40 stearate, and nonoxinol 9 are widely used. In a homologous series their solubilising power increases with decreasing oxyethylene chain length. Ionic surfactants such as soaps have also been used; their solubilising power increases with increasing hydrocarbon chain length.

Solubilising agents should be non-toxic and stable, possess good solubilising power, and be compatible with other formulation ingredients; if they are intended for oral use, they should also have an agreeable taste and odour. An added complication of micellar systems is that a preservative may preferentially partition into the aggregates. This may reduce the effective concentration of the preservative in the liquid bulk.

Factors Affecting Solubilisation. There is a marked increase in solubility of the solute when the surfactant concentration reaches the critical micelle concentration. Solubility continues to increase at higher concentrations of surfactant because of the increasing size of the micelles.

The solubilising potential of a homologous series of surfactants for hydrocarbons in aqueous media is generally increased by an increase in alkyl chain length and decreased by chain branching. The degree of solubilisation is influenced by the polarity and molecular geometry of the molecule. For a range of simple compounds, the extent of solubilisation is generally greater for unsaturated molecules and for those molecules that possess short alkyl chain lengths and a high degree of cyclisation. Electrolytes increase the solubilising power of surfactants by reducing their critical micelle concentration and by increasing the size of the resultant micelles.

Applications of Solubilising Agents in Pharmacy. Solubilising agents allow water-soluble and oil-soluble materials to be formulated in a single phase. They have been used to dissolve a number of therapeutic agents including analgesics, anticoagulants, antimicrobials, barbiturates, corticosteroids, non-steroidal anti-inflammatory agents, oil-soluble vitamins, and phenolic disinfectants.

Dissolution Rate

The process of dissolution involves molecules migrating from the solid to the liquid phase. On leaving the solid, molecules first form a concentrated layer around the particle; this layer is called the stagnant layer. The stagnant layer moves with the particle in the solvent. Any dissolved molecules must traverse this layer to reach the liquid bulk; diffusion across the stagnant layer is often the rate determining step in the dissolution process.

Factors Affecting the Dissolution Rate

Concentration Gradient. Fick's first law of diffusion states that the dissolution rate is directly proportional to the concentration gradient across the stagnant layer. It can be represented by:

$$\frac{dm}{dt} = -DA\frac{dc}{dx}$$

where the mass of the substance, dm, diffusing across a cross section of area A in time dt is proportional to the concentration gradient dc/dx and D is a proportionality constant, the diffusion coefficient. The negative sign arises because the concentration decreases as the distance x increases. The value of D is not completely independent of the concentration.

Stirring Rate. Increased stirring causes a reduction in the thickness of the stagnant layer and therefore, a subsequent rise in the dissolution rate. The stagnant layer can never be removed completely.

Particle Size. A reduction in particle size increases the surface area and surface free energy of a solute and so increases its dissolution rate.

Solubility. Highly soluble compounds dissolve faster than poorly soluble compounds.

Viscosity. Dissolution rates decrease as viscosity increases. Diffusion from a solid to a liquid phase is more difficult in viscous media.

UNITS OF CONCENTRATION, MILLIMOLES, AND MILLIEQUIVALENTS

In the International System of Units, concentrations may be expressed either as mass concentration or amount of substance concentration. The SI recommends that, wherever possible, concentrations should be expressed as 'amount of substance concentration' and that ratios and units such as %, mg%, microgram %, per thousand, parts per million (ppm), and parts per billion (ppb) should be avoided. It is claimed that they may be ambiguous. In pharmacy it is still common and practical to express concentrations in terms of % w/v for solids in liquids, % v/v for liquids in liquids, % v/w for volatile oils in crude drugs, and % w/w for gases in liquids and solids in solids.

It has been the practice in pharmacy and medicine for over a century that, unless otherwise specified, liquids be measured by volume and solids by weight. Care is needed in expressing concentrations of liquids such as liquid paraffin and glycerol which are often more conveniently weighed than measured when included in semi-solid preparations such as creams.

Mass concentration is used by SI for substances with an indefinite or unknown molecular weight (relative molecular mass), and is usually expressed as kg per m³ or kg per litre or as thousand-fold multiples or submultiples of these units. Prescribing, manufacturing, and dispensing of most drugs and medicines continue to be carried out in terms of mass concentration and this is unlikely to change since materials have to be weighed in mass units and volumes measured.

Amount of substance concentration should be used in SI for substances with a defined molecular weight (relative molecular mass) and may be expressed as mol per m³, mol per kg, mol per litre, or as thousand-fold multiples or submultiples of these units. In clinical chemistry, laboratory results are usually reported in terms of mol per litre (mmol per litre, µmol per litre). Two exceptions are haemoglobin and plasma protein, which are usually stated in terms of g per 100 mL or g per litre respectively. The composition of parenteral electrolyte infusions and dialysis solutions is usually stated in terms of mmol per litre, although in some countries milliequivalents are still used. Apart from electrolytes, drugs are prescribed and administered by mass, by volume, or by units, for example, enzymes. In general, concentrations of endogenous substances, such as creatinine or cholesterol, are measured and reported in mmol per litre and drug concentrations in body fluids in mg or g per litre.

Moles and Millimoles

The **mole** (mol) is the SI base unit for amount of substance. A mole is defined as the amount of substance of a system which contains as many elementary entities as there are atoms in 12 g of carbon-12. When the mole is used the elementary entities must be specified and may be atoms, molecules, ions, electrons, other particles, or specified groups of such particles. A **millimole** (mmol) is one thousandth of this amount. For practical purposes, one mole is equal to the mass in grams of Avogadro's number of particles, that is, the atomic, ionic, or molecular weight in grams.

EXAMPLE

The atomic weight of Ca^{2+} is 40.08

$$1 \text{ mol } Ca^{2+} \equiv 40.08 \text{ g of calcium}$$
$$1 \text{ mmol } Ca^{2+} \equiv 40.08 \text{ mg of calcium}$$

The **molality** of a solution is the number of moles of solute per kilogram of solvent, whereas the **molarity** is the number of moles of solute per litre of solution. Although it has been recommended that the term molarity should be avoided because of possible confusion with molality, it is commonly used in analysis and in the pharmaceutical sciences and will continue to be used because of the convenient practice of making solutions up to a fixed volume. Molarity should preferably be expressed in terms of mol per litre. The use of the term 'molar' and the symbol M to describe solutions is not recommended by SI (for example, a 0.1M hydrochloric acid solution contains 0.1 mol per litre) but they remain in extensive use, particularly in the analytical literature.

The amount of substance concentration is sometimes called the molar concentration, but this term should not be used, as in SI the meaning of molar is restricted to 'divided by amount of substance'.

Methods of Calculation

To calculate the number of millimoles contained in 1 gram of substance the following formula may be applied:

$$\text{mmol} = \frac{1000 \times \text{no. of specified units in one atom/molecule/ion}}{\text{atomic, molecular, or ionic weight}}$$

EXAMPLES

(i) For Ca^{2+} (atomic weight 40.08):

$$\text{mmol in 1 g of calcium} = \frac{1000 \times 1}{40.08}$$
$$= 24.95 \text{ mmol}$$

that is, each g of calcium represents 24.95 mmol.

(ii) For $CaCl_2$, $2H_2O$ (molecular weight 147):

$$\text{mmol of } Ca^{2+} \text{ in 1 g of } CaCl_2, 2H_2O = \frac{1000 \times 1}{147}$$
$$= 6.8 \text{ mmol}$$

$$\text{mmol of } Cl^- \text{ in 1 g of } CaCl_2, 2H_2O = \frac{1000 \times 2}{147}$$
$$= 13.6 \text{ mmol}$$

$$\text{mmol of } H_2O \text{ in 1 g of } CaCl_2, 2H_2O = \frac{1000 \times 2}{147}$$
$$= 13.6 \text{ mmol}$$

that is, each g of $CaCl_2$, $2H_2O$ represents 6.8 mmol of calcium, 13.6 mmol of chloride, and 13.6 mmol of water of crystallisation.

(iii) For $CaCl_2$, $6H_2O$ (molecular weight 219.1):

$$\text{mmol of } Ca^{2+} \text{ in 1 g of } CaCl_2, 6H_2O = \frac{1000 \times 1}{219.1}$$
$$= 4.56 \text{ mmol}$$

$$\text{mmol of } Cl^- \text{ in 1 g of } CaCl_2, 6H_2O = \frac{1000 \times 2}{219.1}$$
$$= 9.13 \text{ mmol}$$

$$\text{mmol of } H_2O \text{ in 1 g of } CaCl_2, 6H_2O = \frac{1000 \times 6}{219.1}$$
$$= 27.4 \text{ mmol}$$

that is, each g of $CaCl_2$, $6H_2O$ represents 4.56 mmol of calcium, 9.13 mmol of chloride, and 27.4 mmol of water of crystallisation.

(iv) For anhydrous glucose (molecular weight 180.2):

$$\text{mmol per g of anhydrous glucose} = \frac{1000}{180.2}$$
$$= 5.55 \text{ mmol}$$

that is, each g of anhydrous glucose represents 5.55 mmol.

To calculate the number of milligrams of substance containing 1 millimole of a specified particle the following formula may be applied:

mg of substance containing 1 mmol of molecular weight

$$= \frac{\text{molecular weight}}{\text{no. of specified particles in 1 molecule of substance}}$$

EXAMPLES

(i) For $CaCl_2$, $2H_2O$ (molecular weight 147):

mg of $CaCl_2$, $2H_2O$ containing 1 mmol Ca^{2+}

$$= \frac{147}{1} \text{ mg}$$
$$= 147 \text{ mg}$$

that is, 147 mg of $CaCl_2$, $2H_2O$ contains 1 mmol of calcium.

(ii) For atropine sulphate, $(C_{17}H_{23}NO_3)_2$, H_2SO_4, H_2O (molecular weight 694.8):

mg of atropine sulphate containing 1 mmol of atropine

$$= \frac{694.8}{2} \text{ mg}$$

$$= 347.4 \text{ mg}$$

that is, 347.4 mg of atropine sulphate contains 1 mmol of atropine.

Conversion Equations

Conversion of mEq to mmol:

$$\text{mmol} = \frac{\text{mEq}}{\text{valency}}$$

Conversion of percentage strength w/v to mmol per litre:

mmol per litre

$$= \frac{\text{percentage strength w/v} \times 10\,000}{\text{mg of substance containing 1 mmol}}$$

Conversion of mmol per litre to percentage strength w/v:

percentage strength w/v

$$= \frac{\text{mg of substance containing } 1 \text{ mmol} \times \text{mmol per litre}}{10\,000}$$

Conversion of mg per litre to mmol per litre:

mmol per litre

$$= \frac{\text{mg per litre}}{\text{mg of substance containing 1 mmol}}$$

Conversion of mmol per litre to mg per litre:

mg per litre = mmol per litre × mg of substance containing 1 mmol

Milliequivalents

The concentration of electrolytes in biological fluids and solutions for parenteral use was formerly expressed in terms of milliequivalents. Since the adoption of the mole as the SI base unit for amount of substance, such solutions are now described in terms of millimoles (see Tables 4 and 5). The use of the equivalent is, however, still valid when discussing chemical equivalence. For example, body fluids are electrically neutral and when all ionic constituents are expressed as milliequivalents the sum of the concentrations of anions should equal the sum of the concentrations of cations. Equivalents are applicable only to ionic substances; nonionic compounds such as glucose cannot be expressed in terms of milliequivalents.

The **gram equivalent** of an ion is that mass, expressed in grams, which combines with or displaces 1.0079 g of hydrogen, that is, the ionic weight, expressed in grams, divided by the valency of the ion. The **milliequivalent** (mEq) of an ion is one thousandth of the gram equivalent of that ion.

$$\text{One mEq} = \frac{\text{ionic weight in mg}}{\text{valency}}$$

EXAMPLES

The atomic weight of Ca^{2+} is 40.08

$$1 \text{ mEq } Ca^{2+} = \frac{40.08}{2} \text{ mg of calcium}$$

$$= 20.04 \text{ mg of calcium}$$

The atomic weight of Cl^- is 35.453

$$1 \text{ mEq } Cl^- = \frac{35.453}{1} \text{ mg of chloride}$$

$$= 35.453 \text{ mg of chloride}$$

Normality expresses the concentration of a solute in a solution. A **normal** (1.0 N) solution contains 1 gram equivalent per litre. The terms normal and normality should no longer be used. However, the use of 'normal' in the synonym 'Normal Saline' has caused confusion between doctors, nurses, and pharmacists on numerous occasions and any prescriptions or orders bearing the word 'normal' should be carefully checked to establish which meaning is intended.

Methods of Calculation

To calculate the number of milliequivalents contained in 1 gram of substances the following formula may be applied:

$$\text{mEq} = \frac{\text{valency} \times 1000 \times \text{no. of specified units in one atom/molecule/ion}}{\text{atomic, molecular, or ionic weight}}$$

EXAMPLE

(i) For $CaCl_2, 2H_2O$ (molecular weight 147.0):

$$\text{mEq } Ca^{2+} \text{ in } 1 \text{ g of } CaCl_2, 2H_2O = \frac{2 \times 1000 \times 1}{147}$$

$$= 13.6 \text{ mEq}$$

$$\text{mEq } Cl^- \text{ in } 1 \text{ g of } CaCl_2, 2H_2O = \frac{1 \times 1000 \times 2}{147}$$

$$= 13.6 \text{ mEq}$$

that is, each g of $CaCl_2, 2H_2O$ represents 13.6 mEq of calcium and 13.6 mEq of chloride.

Table 4
Millimoles and milliequivalents–Electrolytes

Ion	Weight of a millimole (mg)	Weight of a milliequivalent (mg)	Salt	Milligrams of salt containing 1 mmol | 1 mEq of specified ion	
Ca^{2+}	40.08	20.04	Calcium acetate, $C_4H_6CaO_4$	158.2	79.1
			Calcium chloride, $CaCl_2,2H_2O$	147.0	73.51
			Calcium gluconate, $C_{12}H_{22}CaO_{14},H_2O$	448.4	224.2
			Calcium lactate, $C_6H_{10}CaO_6,5H_2O$	308.3	154.1
			Calcium laevulinate, $C_{10}H_{14}CaO_6,2H_2O$	306.3	153.2
K^+	39.1	39.1	Potassium acetate, $C_2H_3KO_2$	98.14	98.14
			Potassium bicarbonate, $KHCO_3$	100.1	100.1
			Potassium chloride, KCl	74.55	74.55
			Potassium citrate, $C_6H_5K_3O_7,H_2O$	108.1	108.1
			Potassium gluconate $C_6H_{11}KO_7$	234.2	234.2
Mg^{2+}	24.31	12.15	Magnesium acetate, $C_4H_6MgO_4,4H_2O$	214.5	107.2
			Magnesium chloride, $MgCl_2,6H_2O$	203.3	101.7
			Magnesium sulphate, $MgSO_4,7H_2O$	246.5	123.2
Na^+	22.99	22.99	Sodium acetate, $C_2H_3NaO_2,3H_2O$	136.1	136.1
			Sodium acid citrate, $C_6H_6Na_2O_7,1\frac{1}{2}H_2O$	131.6	131.6
			Sodium acid phosphate, $NaH_2PO_4,2H_2O$	156.0	156.0
			Sodium bicarbonate, $NaHCO_3$	84.01	84.01
			Sodium chloride, $NaCl$	58.44	58.44
			Sodium citrate, $C_6H_5Na_3O_7,2H_2O$	98.03	98.03
			Sodium hydroxide, $NaOH$	40.0	40.0
			Sodium lactate*	112.1	112.1
			Sodium phosphate, $Na_2HPO_4,12H_2O$	179.1	179.1
			Sodium salicylate, $C_7H_5NaO_3$	160.1	160.1
			Sodium sulphate, $Na_2SO_4,10H_2O$	161.1	161.1
NH_4^+	18.04	18.04	Ammonium chloride, NH_4Cl	53.49	53.49
Cl^-	35.45	35.45	Ammonium chloride, NH_4Cl	53.49	53.49
			Calcium chloride, $CaCl_2,2H_2O$	73.51	73.51
			Magnesium chloride, $MgCl_2,6H_2O$	101.7	101.7
			Potassium chloride, KCl	74.55	74.55
			Sodium chloride, $NaCl$	58.44	58.44
			Hydrochloric acid, HCl	36.46	36.46

Table 4—*Continued*

Ion	Weight of a millimole (mg)	Weight of a milliequivalent (mg)	Salt	Milligrams of salt containing 1 mmol | 1 mEq of specified ion	
$C_2H_3O_2^-$ (Acetate)	59.04	59.04	Calcium acetate, $C_4H_6CaO_4$	79.1	79.1
			Magnesium acetate, $C_4H_6MgO_4,4H_2O$	107.2	107.2
			Potassium acetate, $C_2H_3KO_2$	98.14	98.14
			Sodium acetate, $C_2H_3NaO_2,3H_2O$	136.1	136.1
$C_6H_5O_7^{3-}$ (Citrate)	189.1	63.0	Sodium citrate, $C_6H_5Na_3O_7,2H_2O$	294.1	98.03
$C_6H_6O_7^{2-}$ (Acid citrate)	190.1	95.1	Sodium citrate, acid, $C_6H_6Na_2O_7,1\frac{1}{2}H_2O$	263.1	131.6
$C_3H_5O_3^-$ (Lactate)	89.07	89.07	Calcium lactate, $C_6H_{10}CaO_6,5H_2O$	154.1	154.1
			Sodium lactate*	112.1	112.1
HCO_3^-	61.02	61.02	Potassium bicarbonate, $KHCO_3$	100.1	100.1
			Sodium bicarbonate, $NaHCO_3$	84.01	84.01
HPO_4^{2-}	95.98	47.99	Sodium phosphate, $Na_2HPO_4,12H_2O$	358.1	179.1
$H_2PO_4^-$	96.99	96.99	Sodium acid phosphate, $NaH_2PO_4,2H_2O$	156.0	156.0

*Prepared in solution by neutralising lactic acid with sodium hydroxide; 1 mL of a solution containing sodium lactate 1 mol per litre contains 112.1 g.

Table 5
Millimoles–Non-electrolytes

Substances	Molecular weight	Weight of a millimole (mg)	Amount of substance per g (mmol)
Glucose, anhydrous, $C_6H_{12}O_6$	180.2	180.2	5.55
Glucose, monohydrate, $C_6H_{12}O_6,H_2O$	198.2	198.2	5.05
Ethanol, C_2H_5OH	46.07	46.07	21.7
Lactose, $C_{12}H_{22}O_{11},H_2O$	360.3	360.3	2.78
Fructose, $C_6H_{12}O_6$	180.2	180.2	5.55
Sorbitol, $C_6H_{14}O_6$	182.2	182.2	5.49
Sucrose, $C_{12}H_{22}O_{11}$	342.3	342.3	2.92

Conversion Equation

Conversion of mmol to mEq:

$$mEq = mmol \times valency$$

Use of Tables of Millimoles and Milliequivalents

EXAMPLE
To prepare a solution containing 67 mmol sodium, 6 mmol potassium, 2 mmol calcium, and 77 mmol chloride.

Millimoles required				Salts and quantities used
Ca^{2+}	K^+	Na^+	Cl^-	
2			4	Calcium chloride 2×147 mg $= 0.294$ g
	6		6	Potassium chloride 6×74.55 mg $= 0.4473$ g
		67	67	Sodium chloride 67×58.44 mg $= 3.916$ g

ISOTONIC AND ISO-OSMOTIC SOLUTIONS

When a solute is dissolved in a solvent certain properties of the solution differ from those of the pure solvent. The presence of solute particles results in lowering of the vapour pressure, elevation of boiling point, depression of freezing point, and osmotic pressure. These phenomena are called **colligative properties** and they are dependent on the total number of particles in the solution irrespective of whether they are ions, molecules, or both. These colligative properties are directly and quantitatively inter-related. The most important of these in the pharmaceutical sciences is osmotic pressure, which relates particularly to fluid transfer across physiological membranes.

Osmotic Pressure

If two solutions of different concentrations are separated by a membrane permeable to the solvent but not to the solute, that is, a **semipermeable membrane**, the solvent will move from the solution of lower concentration to the solution of higher concentration. This process is called **osmosis**, and the force that causes this movement is called the **osmotic pressure**. If two solutions of the same osmotic pressure are separated by a perfect semipermeable membrane they will be in osmotic equilibrium and there will be no net movement of solvent across the membrane. Such solutions are said to be **iso-osmotic**.

Isotonic Solutions

In biological systems, semipermeable membranes are never impermeable to all solutes and invariably permit the passage of the solute particles of some substances. When two solutions, separated by such a membrane, are in osmotic equilibrium they are said to be **isotonic** with respect to that membrane. Solutions that are iso-osmotic, therefore, can only be considered isotonic when they are separated by a biological membrane that is impermeable to and is not otherwise affected by all their solute particles.

In the case of blood, the membrane of the erythrocyte acts as a semipermeable membrane. Solutions isotonic with blood have the same osmotic pressure as blood serum and the solutes present do not penetrate or adversely affect the erythrocyte membrane. Some solutions, however, that are iso-osmotic with blood serum (for example, ammonium chloride 0.8% w/v, glucose 0.505% w/v, or urea 1.63% w/v) are not isotonic because they can pass through the membrane of the erythrocyte and cause haemolysis.

Hypo-osmotic solutions (hypotonic solutions) have a lower osmotic pressure than blood serum, due to a lower concentration of ions and undissociated molecules. On administration, liquid passes from the solution into the erythrocytes to achieve osmotic equilibrium and they eventually burst, this process of haemolysis being irreversible. **Hyperosmotic solutions** (hypertonic solutions) have a higher osmotic pressure than blood serum, due to a higher concentration of ions and undissociated molecules. On administration, they cause passage of liquid out of the erythrocytes which shrink and become crenated, the process being reversible.

Pharmaceutically, the need for isotonicity of injections is governed by the route of administration. Solutions for **subcutaneous injection** are of small volume and need not necessarily be made isotonic, although isotonicity reduces pain on injection. Solutions for **hypodermoclysis**, the administration of large volumes of fluid by subcutaneous injection, should be isotonic. Solutions for **intramuscular injection** should be isotonic, or slightly hypertonic to promote exosmosis and penetration of the surrounding tissue. Aqueous depot formulations should be isotonic. Solutions for **intravenous injection** are usually of large volume and should generally be isotonic. Hypo-

tonic solutions may cause haemolysis of erythrocytes and hypertonic solutions may damage the walls of the veins. When therapeutically necessary, small volumes of hypertonic solutions may be administered slowly into a vein, or a large volume may be administered through a cannula into one of the large vessels, such as the vena cava, where it will be rapidly diluted. Solutions for **intrathecal injection** require strict isotonicity as the osmotic pressure of the small volume of cerebrospinal fluid is considerably altered by the injection of a hypotonic or hypertonic solution. (See also the Parenterals chapter.) **Eye drops** are rapidly diluted by tears and so isotonicity is not essential. **Eye lotions** are preferably made isotonic with the lachrymal secretion because of the large volumes involved. **Nasal drops** are usually made isotonic with nasal secretion although this is not essential.

Osmolality and Osmolarity

Solute concentration is sometimes expressed in terms of osmoles (osmol or Osm) or milliosmoles (mosmol or mOsm). An osmole represents one mole of osmotically active particles; a milliosmole is one thousandth of this amount. These osmotically active particles may be either molecules or ions. For an ideally behaving non-electrolyte, one mole of solute would produce one osmole of osmotically active particles; a monovalent electrolyte that dissociated completely would produce two osmoles of particles (one osmole of anions and one osmole of cations) from one mole of solute. However, under non-ideal conditions, factors such as solvation and particle interactions reduce the number of osmotically active particles in solution. It is, therefore, difficult to predict the osmotic strength of concentrated solutions; experimental methods are usually needed to measure the osmolality or osmolarity of complex mixtures such as protein hydrolysate injection.

Osmolality is the concentration of a solution expressed as moles of solute particles *per kilogram of water*. The osmolality of a solution can be determined using an osmometer, which measures either freezing point depression or vapour pressure. The instruments are calibrated so that osmolality is read directly.

Osmolarity is the concentration expressed as moles of solute particles *per litre of solution*. The osmolarity may be calculated from measured osmolality or by summing the particle concentration of each constituent. Some osmometers are calibrated to read osmolarity directly. In dilute solutions osmolality is approximately equal to osmolarity but in concentrated solutions the mass of solute particles becomes significant.

Particle interaction also becomes significant in concentrated solutions. The calculated osmolarity of Sodium Chloride Injection (9 g per litre; 154 mmol each of Na^+ and Cl^- per litre) is 308 mmol per litre, representing 308 mosmol per litre, but the measured osmolarity is about 286 mosmol per litre. The theoretical osmolality of plasma calculated from its constituents is about 325 mmol per kg, representing 325 mosmol per kg, while the measured osmolality is about 291 mosmol per kg. The difference probably results from incomplete dissociation of electrolytes and protein binding of constituents.

There are a number of equations that may be used to estimate the osmolarity of simple solutions.

Non-electrolytes

$$\frac{\text{grams/litre}}{\text{molecular weight}} \times 1000 = \text{mmol/litre}$$

Strong Electrolytes

Osmolarity depends on the number of individual particles present in solution. Sodium chloride, for example, dissociates into sodium ions and chloride ions. The relevant equation is:

$$\frac{\text{grams/litre}}{\text{molecular weight}} \times n \times 1000 = \text{mmol/litre}$$

where n is number of ions into which an electrolyte dissociates. The osmolarity of each individual ion can be estimated using the following equation:

$$\frac{\text{grams of ion/litre}}{\text{ionic weight}} \times 1000 = \text{mmol (of ion)/litre}$$

Osmolality and osmolarity are also discussed in the Parenterals chapter.

Preparation of Iso-osmotic Solutions

Aqueous solutions are usually made iso-osmotic with body fluids by adding some therapeutically inactive solute if the solution is hypo-osmotic or by dilution if it is hyperosmotic. Glucose or sodium chloride is usually added to hypo-osmotic solutions for intravenous use. Sodium chloride or boric acid is usually added to hypo-osmotic ophthalmic solutions. Solutions are adjusted so that they are iso-osmotic with a solution of sodium

chloride 0.9%, and thus in most cases isotonic with body fluids. The adjusting substance must be compatible and non-toxic. Since the amount of solute or the dilution required to render a solution isotonic cannot be calculated, estimates may be made by four methods: from the freezing point depression, the sodium chloride equivalent, the amount of substance concentration (molar concentration), or the osmolarity. (See also the Parenterals chapter.)

Calculations based on Freezing Point Depression

The freezing point of both blood serum and tears is −0.52°. Therefore any other aqueous solution that freezes at −0.52° will have the same osmotic pressure as these body fluids. Hypo-osmotic solutions have a higher freezing point and require an additional solute to depress the freezing point to −0.52°.

It should be noted that the freezing point depression of an electrolyte solution is not strictly proportional to the concentration. For instance, atropine sulphate 1% has a freezing point depression of 0.073° while a solution containing 5% has a freezing point depression of 0.311°, not $5 \times 0.073° = 0.365°$. This fact may have to be taken into account when precise adjustments of isotonicity are necessary for solutions at concentrations greater than 1%.

From the depression of freezing point values in Table 6, the concentrations of solutions iso-osmotic with blood serum and tears can be calculated, as can the depression of freezing point caused by a given concentration of a substance in a solution, and the amount of adjusting substance required to make a hypo-osmotic solution iso-osmotic.

The second and third columns of Table 6 give the concentration of the substance that is iso-osmotic with blood serum in g per litre and %w/v, respectively; in the succeeding columns, the sodium chloride equivalents are the values first listed; the freezing point depression values are in *italic* numerals, for example, 0.135° (see Preparation of Iso-osmotic Solutions above).

The amount of adjusting substance required may be calculated from the equation:

$$W = \frac{0.52 - a}{b}$$

where W is the concentration in grams per 100 mL (or % w/v) of the adjusting substance in the final solution; a is the freezing point depression of the unadjusted hypo-osmotic solution, calculated by

Table 6
Sodium chloride equivalents and freezing point depressions

Substance	Concentration iso-osmotic with blood		NaCl equivalents and freezing point depressions				
	g per litre	% w/v	0.5%	1%	2%	3%	5%
Acetazolamide sodium	38.5	3.85	0.24 *0.068°*	0.23 *0.135°*	0.23 *0.271°*	0.23 *0.406°*	
Acetylcysteine	45.8	4.58	0.20 *0.055°*	0.20 *0.113°*	0.20 *0.227°*	0.20 *0.341°*	
Adenosine phosphate			0.50 *0.140°*	0.41 *0.234°*			
Adiphenine hydrochloride			0.28 *0.083°*	0.22 *0.126°*	0.17 *0.194°*	0.15 *0.250°*	0.12 *0.346°*
Adrenaline acid tartrate	57	5.7	0.18 *0.050°*	0.18 *0.098°*	0.17 *0.190°*	0.16 *0.281°*	0.16 *0.458°*
Adrenaline hydrochloride	34.7	3.47	0.30 *0.088°*	0.29 *0.165°*	0.27 *0.311°*	0.26 *0.451°*	
Adrenalone hydrochloride	42.4	4.24	0.30 *0.086°*	0.27 *0.154°*	0.24 *0.275°*	0.22 *0.387°*	
Alphaprodine hydrochloride	49.8	4.98	0.19 *0.053°*	0.19 *0.105°*	0.18 *0.212°*	0.18 *0.315°*	
Amantadine hydrochloride	29.5	2.95	0.31 *0.090°*	0.31 *0.180°*	0.31 *0.354°*		
Ametazole hydrochloride	19.1	1.91	0.54 *0.158°*	0.51 *0.294°*			
Amethocaine hydrochloride			0.20 *0.062°*	0.18 *0.109°*	0.17 *0.189°*	0.15 *0.261°*	0.12 *0.358°*
Amikacin base			0.06 *0.016°*	0.05 *0.031°*	0.05 *0.062°*	0.05 *0.091°*	0.05 *0.153°*
Aminacrine hydrochloride			0.20 *0.052°*	0.17 *0.097°*			
Aminoacetic acid	22	2.2	0.42 *0.119°*	0.41 *0.235°*	0.41 *0.470°*		
Aminocaproic acid	35.2	3.52	0.26 *0.075°*	0.26 *0.148°*	0.26 *0.297°*	0.26 *0.444°*	
p-Aminohippuric acid			0.13 *0.035°*	0.13 *0.075°*			
Aminophylline			0.18 *0.056°*	0.17 *0.100°*			
Amitriptyline hydrochloride			0.24 *0.070°*	0.18 *0.100°*	0.11 *0.125°*	0.08 *0.147°*	0.06 *0.177°*
Ammonium chloride	8	0.8	1.16 *0.331°*				
Amphetamine phosphate	34.7	3.47	0.38 *0.114°*	0.34 *0.196°*	0.30 *0.338°*	0.27 *0.466°*	
Amphetamine sulphate	42.3	4.23	0.22 *0.066°*	0.22 *0.128°*	0.22 *0.251°*	0.21 *0.371°*	
Ampicillin sodium	57.8	5.78	0.16 *0.045°*	0.16 *0.090°*	0.16 *0.181°*	0.16 *0.272°*	0.16 *0.451°*
Amydricaine hydrochloride	57.4	5.74	0.28 *0.080°*	0.24 *0.136°*	0.20 *0.231°*	0.18 *0.316°*	0.16 *0.467°*
Amylobarbitone sodium	36	3.6	0.26 *0.074°*	0.25 *0.144°*	0.25 *0.293°*	0.25 *0.440°*	
Amylocaine hydrochloride	49.8	4.98	0.24 *0.067°*	0.22 *0.126°*	0.20 *0.233°*	0.19 *0.338°*	
Antazoline hydrochloride			0.25 *0.073°*	0.23 *0.131°*	0.21 *0.245°*		
Antazoline phosphate			0.20 *0.062°*	0.20 *0.112°*	0.18 *0.204°*	0.17 *0.291°*	0.15 *0.445°*
Antimony potassium tartrate			0.22 *0.065°*	0.18 *0.106°*	0.15 *0.174°*	0.13 *0.232°*	0.10 *0.331°*
Antimony sodium tartrate	79	7.9	0.14 *0.039°*	0.13 *0.074°*	0.13 *0.142°*	0.12 *0.208°*	0.12 *0.338°*
Apomorphine hydrochloride			0.14 *0.041°*	0.14 *0.080°*	0.14 *0.155°*		
Arecoline hydrobromide	38.8	3.88	0.30 *0.084°*	0.27 *0.155°*	0.25 *0.286°*	0.24 *0.413°*	
Arginine glutamate	53.7	5.37	0.17 *0.048°*	0.17 *0.097°*	0.17 *0.195°*	0.17 *0.292°*	0.17 *0.487°*

Table 6—*Continued*

Substance	Concentration iso-osmotic with blood g per litre	% w/v	NaCl equivalents and freezing point depressions 0.5%	1%	2%	3%	5%
Ascorbic acid	50.4	5.04	0.20 *0.053°*	0.18 *0.105°*	0.18 *0.209°*	0.18 *0.311°*	0.18 *0.516°*
Atropine methobromide	70.3	7.03	0.15 *0.045°*	0.15 *0.086°*	0.14 *0.162°*	0.14 *0.236°*	0.13 *0.380°*
Atropine methonitrate	65.2	6.52	0.20 *0.055°*	0.18 *0.101°*	0.16 *0.185°*	0.15 *0.264°*	0.14 *0.412°*
Atropine sulphate	88.5	8.85	0.14 *0.039°*	0.13 *0.073°*	0.12 *0.136°*	0.11 *0.196°*	0.11 *0.311°*
Aurothioglucose			0.03 *0.007°*	0.03 *0.014°*	0.03 *0.028°*	0.03 *0.044°*	0.03 *0.073°*
Azovan blue			0.06 *0.017°*	0.06 *0.033°*	0.06 *0.061°*	0.05 *0.091°*	0.05 *0.148°*
Bacitracin			0.06 *0.016°*	0.05 *0.028°*	0.05 *0.052°*	0.04 *0.075°*	0.04 *0.120°*
Barbitone sodium	31.2	3.12	0.32 *0.087°*	0.30 *0.171°*	0.29 *0.336°*	0.29 *0.500°*	
Benzalkonium chloride			0.18 *0.048°*	0.16 *0.091°*	0.15 *0.170°*	0.14 *0.245°*	0.13 *0.388°*
Benzethonium chloride			0.08 *0.022°*	0.05 *0.028°*	0.03 *0.037°*	0.02 *0.043°*	0.02 *0.051°*
Benzpyrinium bromide			0.20 *0.061°*	0.20 *0.114°*	0.19 *0.213°*	0.18 *0.309°*	0.17 *0.483°*
Benztropine mesylate			0.26 *0.073°*	0.21 *0.115°*	0.15 *0.170°*	0.12 *0.203°*	0.09 *0.242°*
Benzyl alcohol			0.18 *0.049°*	0.17 *0.095°*	0.16 *0.182°*	0.15 *0.266°*	
Benzylpenicillin potassium	54.8	5.48	0.18 *0.052°*	0.18 *0.101°*	0.17 *0.197°*	0.17 *0.290°*	0.16 *0.474°*
Benzylpenicillin sodium			0.18 *0.052°*	0.18 *0.100°*	0.17 *0.190°*	0.16 *0.280°*	0.16 *0.451°*
Bethanechol chloride	30.5	3.05	0.50 *0.140°*	0.39 *0.225°*	0.32 *0.368°*	0.30 *0.512°*	
Bismuth sodium tartrate	89.1	8.91	0.14 *0.041°*	0.13 *0.075°*	0.13 *0.139°*	0.12 *0.199°*	0.11 *0.312°*
Borax	26	2.6		0.42 *0.241°*			
Boric acid	19	1.9	0.52 *0.146°*	0.50 *0.283°*			
Bretylium tosylate			0.16 *0.043°*	0.14 *0.081°*	0.13 *0.148°*	0.12 *0.208°*	0.11 *0.327°*
Brompheniramine maleate			0.10 *0.026°*	0.09 *0.050°*	0.08 *0.084°*		
Bupivacaine hydrochloride	53.8	5.38	0.17 *0.048°*	0.17 *0.096°*	0.17 *0.193°*	0.17 *0.290°*	0.17 *0.484°*
Butacaine sulphate			0.26 *0.073°*	0.20 *0.114°*	0.16 *0.175°*	0.13 *0.223°*	0.10 *0.304°*
Butethamine hydrochloride			0.28 *0.079°*	0.25 *0.141°*	0.22 *0.251°*		
Caffeine			0.08 *0.025°*	0.08 *0.048°*			
Caffeine and sodium benzoate	39.2	3.92	0.28 *0.077°*	0.26 *0.146°*	0.25 *0.278°*	0.23 *0.405°*	
Caffeine and sodium salicylate	57.7	5.77	0.24 *0.065°*	0.21 *0.118°*	0.18 *0.213°*	0.17 *0.300°*	0.16 *0.460°*
Calcium chloride (2H$_2$O)	17	1.7	0.50 *0.145°*	0.51 *0.298°*			
Calcium chloride (6H$_2$O)	25	2.5	0.34 *0.097°*	0.35 *0.200°*	0.36 *0.414°*		
Calcium folinate			0.06 *0.013°*	0.05 *0.026°*	0.05 *0.052°*	0.04 *0.077°*	0.04 *0.126°*
Calcium gluconate			0.18 *0.050°*	0.16 *0.091°*	0.15 *0.167°*	0.14 *0.237°*	
Calcium lactate	45	4.5		0.23 *0.13°*		0.12 *0.36°*	

Table 6—*Continued*

Substance	Concentration iso-osmotic with blood		NaCl equivalents and freezing point depressions				
	g per litre	% w/v	0.5%	1%	2%	3%	5%
Calcium laevulinate			0.30	0.27	0.26	0.25	
			0.080°	*0.155°*	*0.304°*	*0.442°*	
Calcium pantothenate	56	5.6	0.20	0.19	0.18	0.17	0.16
			0.055°	*0.105°*	*0.201°*	*0.293°*	*0.470°*
Camphor				0.21			
				0.12°			
Capreomycin sulphate			0.04	0.04	0.04	0.04	0.04
			0.011°	*0.020°*	*0.042°*	*0.063°*	*0.106°*
Carbachol	28.2	2.82	0.40	0.36	0.34		
			0.108°	*0.203°*	*0.383°*		
Carbenicillin sodium	44	4.4	0.20	0.20	0.20	0.20	
			0.059°	*0.118°*	*0.236°*	*0.355°*	
Carmellose sodium			0.03	0.03			
			0.007°	*0.017°*			
Cefoxitin sodium			0.18	0.16	0.15	0.14	0.13
			0.050°	*0.092°*	*0.166°*	*0.238°*	*0.384°*
Cephaloridine			0.09	0.07	0.06	0.06	0.05
			0.023°	*0.041°*	*0.074°*	*0.106°*	*0.145°*
Cephalothin sodium	68	6.8	0.18	0.17	0.16	0.15	0.14
			0.050°	*0.095°*	*0.179°*	*0.259°*	*0.400°*
Cephamandole nafate			0.16	0.14	0.12	0.11	0.10
			0.045°	*0.079°*	*0.137°*	*0.187°*	*0.290°*
Cephazolin sodium			0.14	0.13	0.12	0.11	0.11
			0.042°	*0.074°*	*0.132°*	*0.190°*	*0.303°*
Cetrimide			0.10	0.09	0.09	0.09	0.08
			0.030°	*0.051°*	*0.105°*	*0.148°*	*0.233*
Chloramine	41	4.1	0.24	0.23	0.22	0.22	
			0.064°	*0.129°*	*0.255°*	*0.383°*	
Chloramphenicol				0.10			
				0.06°			
Chloramphenicol sodium succinate	68.3	6.83	0.14	0.14	0.14	0.13	0.13
			0.038°	*0.078°*	*0.154°*	*0.230°*	*0.382°*
Chlorbutol			0.24				
			0.071°				
Chlordiazepoxide hydrochloride	55	5.5	0.24	0.22	0.19	0.18	0.17
			0.068°	*0.125°*	*0.220°*	*0.315°*	*0.487°*
Chloroprocaine hydrochloride			0.20	0.20	0.18		
			0.054°	*0.108°*	*0.210°*		
Chloroquine phosphate	71.5	7.15	0.14	0.14	0.14	0.14	0.13
			0.039°	*0.082°*	*0.162°*	*0.242°*	*0.379°*
Chloroquine sulphate			0.10	0.09	0.08	0.07	0.07
			0.028°	*0.050°*	*0.090°*	*0.127°*	*0.195°*
Chlorpheniramine maleate			0.17	0.15	0.14	0.13	0.09
			0.048°	*0.085°*	*0.165°*	*0.220°*	*0.265°*
Chlorpromazine hydrochloride			0.18	0.10	0.06	0.05	0.03
			0.052°	*0.058°*	*0.069°*	*0.078°*	*0.100°*
Chlortetracycline hydrochloride				0.10	0.10	0.10	
			0.030°	*0.061°*	*0.121°*		
Cinchocaine hydrochloride			0.14	0.13	0.12	0.11	0.08
			0.040°	*0.076°*	*0.139°*	*0.188°*	*0.223°*
Citric acid	55.2	5.52	0.18	0.18	0.17	0.17	0.16
			0.050°	*0.098°*	*0.193°*	*0.287°*	*0.472°*
Clindamycin phosphate	107.3	10.73	0.08	0.08	0.08	0.08	0.08
			0.022°	*0.046°*	*0.095°*	*0.144°*	*0.242°*
Cocaine hydrochloride	63.3	6.33	0.16	0.16	0.16	0.15	0.14
			0.047°	*0.091°*	*0.175°*	*0.256°*	*0.416°*
Codeine phosphate	72.9	7.29	0.14	0.14	0.13	0.13	0.13
			0.040°	*0.078°*	*0.151°*	*0.223°*	*0.362°*
Colistin sulphomethate sodium	68.5	6.85	0.16	0.15	0.14	0.14	0.13
			0.045°	*0.087°*	*0.161°*	*0.235°*	*0.383°*
Congo red			0.05	0.05	0.05	0.05	0.05
			0.015°	*0.030°*	*0.059°*	*0.092°*	*0.151°*
Copper sulphate	68.5	6.85	0.20	0.18	0.16	0.15	0.14
			0.054°	*0.098°*	*0.179°*	*0.254°*	*0.396°*

Table 6—*Continued*

Substance	Concentration iso-osmotic with blood		NaCl equivalents and freezing point depressions				
	g per litre	% w/v	0.5%	1%	2%	3%	5%
Cyclopentamine hydrochloride	26.8	2.68	0.36 0.104°	0.36 0.204°	0.35 0.392°		
Cyclopentolate hydrochloride	53	5.3	0.22 0.061°	0.20 0.117°	0.19 0.218°	0.18 0.319°	0.17 0.499°
Cyclophosphamide			0.10 0.031°	0.10 0.061°	0.10 0.125°		
Cytarabine	89.2	8.92	0.11 0.034°	0.11 0.066°	0.11 0.134°	0.11 0.198°	0.11 0.317°
Decamethonium bromide	50	5.0	0.29 0.084°	0.25 0.144°	0.22 0.256°	0.20 0.350°	0.18 0.52°
Demecarium bromide			0.14 0.038°	0.12 0.069°	0.10 0.108°	0.08 0.139°	0.07 0.192°
Desferrioxamine mesylate			0.09 0.023°	0.09 0.047°	0.09 0.093°	0.09 0.142°	0.09 0.241°
Dexamethasone sodium phosphate	67.5	6.75	0.18 0.050°	0.17 0.095°	0.16 0.180°	0.15 0.260°	0.14 0.410°
Dexamphetamine sulphate			—	0.134°			
Dexpanthenol	56	5.6	0.20 0.53°	0.18 0.100°	0.17 0.193°	0.17 0.283°	0.16 0.468°
Diatrizoate sodium	105.5	10.55	0.10 0.025°	0.09 0.049°	0.09 0.098°	0.09 0.149°	0.09 0.248°
Dibutoline sulphate			0.18 0.049°	0.16 0.093°	0.15 0.175°	0.15 0.259°	0.14 0.416°
Dichlorophenarsine hydrochloride	16.4	1.64	0.55 0.150°	0.55 0.310°			
Dicloxacillin sodium (1H$_2$O)			0.10 0.030°	0.10 0.061°	0.10 0.122°	0.10 0.182°	
Diethanolamine	29	2.9	0.31 0.089°	0.31 0.177°	0.31 0.358°		
Diethylcarbamazine citrate	62.9	6.29	0.14 0.042°	0.14 0.083°	0.14 0.166°	0.14 0.248°	0.14 0.415°
Dimethindene maleate			0.13 0.039°	0.12 0.070°	0.11 0.120°		
Dimethyl sulphoxide	21.6	2.16	0.42 0.122°	0.42 0.245°	0.42 0.480°		
Diodone	92.1	9.21	0.12 0.036°	0.11 0.067°	0.11 0.127°	0.11 0.185°	0.10 0.298°
Diphenhydramine hydrochloride			0.34 0.099°	0.27 0.158°	0.22 0.256°	0.20 0.338°	0.17 0.477°
Diphenidol hydrochloride			0.16 0.045°	0.16 0.090°	0.16 0.180°		
Diprophylline	108.7	10.87	0.14 0.038°	0.12 0.069°	0.11 0.124°	0.10 0.176°	0.09 0.270°
Disodium edetate	44.4	4.44	0.24 0.070°	0.23 0.132°	0.22 0.248°	0.21 0.360°	
Dopamine hydrochloride	31.1	3.11	0.30 0.085°	0.30 0.170°	0.29 0.335°	0.29 0.502°	
Doxapram hydrochloride			0.12 0.035°	0.12 0.070°	0.12 0.140°	0.12 0.210°	
Dyclonine hydrochloride			0.26 0.073°	0.24 0.135°	0.17 0.190°		
Ecothiopate iodide			0.16 0.045°	0.16 0.090°	0.16 0.179°		
Edrophonium chloride	33.6	3.36	0.32 0.093°	0.31 0.175°	0.29 0.326°	0.27 0.473°	
Emetine hydrochloride			0.12 0.033°	0.10 0.062°	0.10 0.118°	0.10 0.171°	0.10 0.274°
Ephedrine hydrochloride	32	3.2	0.32 0.087°	0.30 0.169°	0.29 0.331°	0.28 0.489°	
Ephedrine sulphate	45.4	4.54	0.24 0.070°	0.23 0.132°	0.22 0.247°	0.20 0.355°	
Ergometrine maleate			0.20 0.055°	0.16 0.089°	0.13 0.143°		

Table 6—*Continued*

Substance	Concentration iso-osmotic with blood g per litre	% w/v	NaCl equivalents and freezing point depressions 0.5%	1%	2%	3%	5%
Erythromycin gluceptate			0.08	0.07	0.07	0.07	0.07
			0.021°	*0.042°*	*0.081°*	*0.120°*	*0.194°*
Erythromycin lactobionate			0.08	0.07	0.07	0.07	0.06
			0.020°	*0.040°*	*0.078°*	*0.115°*	*0.187°*
Ethanolamine	17	1.7	0.53	0.53			
			0.154°	*0.306°*			
Ethylenediamine			0.46	0.44	0.43		
			0.130°	*0.255°*	*0.501°*		
Ethylmorphine hydrochloride	61.8	6.18	0.16	0.16	0.15	0.15	0.15
			0.045°	*0.088°*	*0.173°*	*0.257°*	*0.423°*
Ethylnoradrenaline hydrochloride	33.2	3.32	0.36	0.32	0.29	0.28	
			0.104°	*0.188°*	*0.334°*	*0.477°*	
Floxuridine	84.7	8.47	0.14	0.13	0.13	0.12	0.12
			0.040°	*0.076°*	*0.147°*	*0.213°*	*0.335°*
Fluopromazine hydrochloride			0.10	0.09	0.05	0.04	0.03
			0.031°	*0.051°*	*0.061°*	*0.073°*	*0.092°*
Fluorescein sodium	33.4	3.34	0.36	0.31	0.29	0.27	
			0.099°	*0.182°*	*0.332°*	*0.472°*	
Fluphenazine hydrochloride			0.14	0.14	0.12	0.09	
			0.041°	*0.082°*	*0.145°*	*0.155°*	
Fructose	50.5	5.05	0.18	0.18	0.18	0.18	0.18
			0.050°	*0.100°*	*0.205°*	*0.310°*	*0.516°*
Furtrethonium iodide	44.4	4.44	0.24	0.24	0.22	0.21	
			0.070°	*0.133°*	*0.250°*	*0.360°*	
Galactose, anhydrous	49.2	4.92	0.18	0.18	0.18	0.18	
			0.053°	*0.105°*	*0.210°*	*0.316°*	
Gallamine triethiodide			0.08	0.08	0.08	0.08	0.08
			0.022°	*0.046°*	*0.091°*	*0.136°*	*0.227°*
Gentamicin sulphate			0.05	0.05	0.05	0.05	0.05
			0.015°	*0.030°*	*0.060°*	*0.093°*	*0.153°*
D-Glucuronic acid	50.2	5.02	0.20	0.20	0.19	0.19	0.18
			0.061°	*0.115°*	*0.220°*	*0.323°*	*0.517°*
Glucose, anhydrous	50.5	5.05	0.18	0.18	0.18	0.18	0.18
			0.050°	*0.100°*	*0.205°*	*0.310°*	*0.516°*
Glucose monohydrate	55.1	5.51	0.16	0.16	0.16	0.16	0.16
			0.045°	*0.091°*	*0.184°*	*0.279°*	*0.470°*
Glycerol	26	2.6	0.36	0.35	0.35		
			0.104°	*0.202°*	*0.403°*		
Glycine	21.9	2.19	0.41	0.41	0.41		
			0.118°	*0.235°*	*0.470°*		
Heparin sodium	122	12.2	0.07	0.07	0.07	0.07	0.07
			0.021°	*0.042°*	*0.084°*	*0.128°*	*0.213°*
Hetacillin potassium	55	5.5	0.17	0.17	0.17	0.17	0.17
			0.048°	*0.095°*	*0.190°*	*0.284°*	*0.474°*
Hexafluorenium bromide			0.12	0.11			
			0.033°	*0.065°*			
Hexamethonium bromide	49.9	4.99	0.24	0.22	0.20	0.19	
			0.069°	*0.126°*	*0.233°*	*0.330°*	
Hexobarbitone sodium	38.8	3.88	0.28	0.26	0.25	0.24	
			0.078°	*0.148°*	*0.282°*	*0.409°*	
Hexylcaine hydrochloride			0.28	0.26	0.24	0.22	
			0.084°	*0.151°*	*0.270°*	*0.380°*	
Histamine acid phosphate	41	4.1	0.28	0.25	0.24	0.23	
			0.080°	*0.148°*	*0.274°*	*0.394°*	
Histamine hydrochloride	22.4	2.24	0.40	0.40	0.40		
			0.115°	*0.233°*	*0.466°*		
Homatropine hydrobromide	56.7	5.67	0.18	0.17	0.17	0.16	0.16
			0.049°	*0.096°*	*0.189°*	*0.280°*	*0.461°*
Hyaluronidase			0.01	0.01	0.01	0.01	0.01
			0.004°	*0.007°*	*0.013°*	*0.020°*	*0.033°*
Hydralazine hydrochloride			0.44	0.37			
			0.126°	*0.213°*			
Hydromorphone hydrochloride	63.9	6.39	0.26	0.22	0.19	0.17	0.15
			0.073°	*0.124°*	*0.211°*	*0.288°*	*0.429°*

Table 6—*Continued*

Substance	Concentration iso-osmotic with blood g per litre	% w/v	NaCl equivalents and freezing point depressions				
			0.5%	1%	2%	3%	5%
Hydroxyamphetamine hydrobromide	37.1	3.71	0.28 *0.083°*	0.26 *0.156°*	0.26 *0.298°*	0.25 *0.435°*	
Hydroxystilbamidine isethionate			0.20 *0.060°*	0.16 *0.090°*	0.12 *0.137°*	0.10 *0.170°*	0.07 *0.216°*
Hydroxyzine hydrochloride	63.2	6.32	0.26 *0.075°*	0.25 *0.138°*	0.22 *0.251°*	0.20 *0.345°*	0.16 *0.458°*
Hyoscine hydrobromide	78.5	7.85	0.12 *0.034°*	0.12 *0.068°*	0.12 *0.135°*	0.12 *0.201°*	0.12 *0.333°*
Hyoscine methonitrate	69.5	6.95	0.18 *0.049°*	0.16 *0.091°*	0.15 *0.171°*	0.14 *0.244°*	0.13 *0.387°*
Imipramine hydrochloride			0.20 *0.058°*	0.20 *0.110°*			
Indigo carmine			0.30 *0.085°*	0.30 *0.172°*			
Isometheptene mucate	49.5	4.95	0.18 *0.048°*	0.18 *0.095°*	0.18 *0.196°*	0.18 *0.302°*	
Isoniazid	43.5	4.35	0.28 *0.079°*	0.25 *0.144°*	0.23 *0.266°*	0.22 *0.378°*	
Isoprenaline sulphate	66.5	6.65	0.14 *0.039°*	0.14 *0.078°*	0.14 *0.156°*	0.14 *0.234°*	0.14 *0.389°*
Kanamycin sulphate			0.08 *0.021°*	0.07 *0.041°*	0.07 *0.083°*	0.07 *0.125°*	0.07 *0.210°*
Lactic acid	23	2.3	0.44 *0.124°*	0.41 *0.237°*	0.39 *0.457°*		
Lactose	97.5	9.75	0.06 *0.019°*	0.07 *0.040°*	0.08 *0.088°*	0.08 *0.139°*	0.09 *0.246°*
Leptazol	49.1	4.91	0.24 *0.069°*	0.22 *0.127°*	0.21 *0.236°*	0.19 *0.337°*	
Levallorphan tartrate	94	9.4	0.13 *0.036°*	0.13 *0.073°*	0.13 *0.143°*	0.12 *0.210°*	0.12 *0.329°*
Levorphanol tartrate			0.12 *0.033°*	0.12 *0.067°*	0.12 *0.136°*	0.12 *0.203°*	
Lignocaine hydrochloride	44.2	4.42	0.22 *0.065°*	0.22 *0.125°*	0.21 *0.243°*	0.21 *0.358°*	
Lincomycin hydrochloride	66	6.6	0.16 *0.045°*	0.16 *0.090°*	0.15 *0.170°*	0.14 *0.247°*	0.14 *0.400°*
Lobeline hydrochloride			0.16 *0.047°*	0.16 *0.091°*	0.16 *0.174°*		
Magnesium chloride	20.2	2.02	0.48 *0.136°*	0.45 *0.260°*	0.45 *0.515°*		
Magnesium sulphate	63	6.3	0.18 *0.049°*	0.17 *0.094°*	0.16 *0.178°*	0.15 *0.261°*	0.15 *0.419°*
Mannitol	50.7	5.07	0.16 *0.047°*	0.17 *0.099°*	0.17 *0.200°*	0.17 *0.304°*	0.18 *0.514°*
Meglumine	50.2	5.02	0.20 *0.057°*	0.20 *0.111°*	0.18 *0.214°*	0.18 *0.315°*	0.18 *0.517°*
Meglumine diatrizoate	121	12.1	0.09 *0.024°*	0.08 *0.047°*	0.08 *0.093°*	0.08 *0.137°*	0.08 *0.222°*
Menadiol sodium diphosphate			0.27 *0.078°*	0.25 *0.142°*	0.23 *0.262°*	0.21 *0.372°*	
Menaphthone sodium bisulphite	50.7	5.07	0.20 *0.057°*	0.20 *0.110°*	0.19 *0.213°*	0.18 *0.315°*	0.18 *0.511°*
Menthol				0.21 *0.12°*			
Mephenesin			0.19 *0.055°*	0.19 *0.108°*			
Mephentermine sulphate	47.4	4.74	0.24 *0.069°*	0.22 *0.131°*	0.21 *0.245°*	0.20 *0.346°*	
Mepivacaine hydrochloride	46	4.6	0.21 *0.060°*	0.21 *0.116°*	0.20 *0.230°*	0.20 *0.342°*	
Mepyramine maleate			0.24 *0.072°*	0.18 *0.106°*	0.14 *0.156°*	0.11 *0.195°*	0.09 *0.258°*
Mercaptomerin sodium			0.19 *0.056°*	0.18 *0.107°*	0.18 *0.206°*	0.18 *0.308°*	0.17 *0.494°*

Table 6—*Continued*

Substance	Concentration iso-osmotic with blood g per litre	% w/v	NaCl equivalents and freezing point depressions 0.5%	1%	2%	3%	5%
Mersalyl acid	90.6	9.06	0.14 / *0.041°*	0.12 / *0.063°*	0.11 / *0.122°*	0.11 / *0.181°*	0.10 / *0.294°*
Metaraminol tartrate	51.7	5.17	0.20 / *0.060°*	0.20 / *0.112°*	0.19 / *0.210°*	0.18 / *0.308°*	0.17 / *0.505°*
Methacholine chloride	32.1	3.21	0.34 / *0.099°*	0.32 / *0.181°*	0.30 / *0.338°*	0.28 / *0.494°*	
Methadone hydrochloride	85.9	8.59	0.22 / *0.060°*	0.18 / *0.101°*	0.15 / *0.171°*	0.14 / *0.232°*	0.12 / *0.344°*
Methicillin sodium	60	6.0	0.18 / *0.050°*	0.18 / *0.099°*	0.17 / *0.192°*	0.16 / *0.281°*	0.15 / *0.445°*
Methiodal sodium	38.1	3.81	0.24 / *0.068°*	0.24 / *0.136°*	0.24 / *0.274°*	0.24 / *0.410°*	
Methocarbamol			0.10 / *0.030°*	0.10 / *0.060°*			
Methotrimeprazine hydrochloride			0.12 / *0.034°*	0.10 / *0.060°*	0.07 / *0.077°*	0.06 / *0.094°*	0.04 / *0.125°*
Methoxamine hydrochloride	38.2	3.82	0.28 / *0.078°*	0.26 / *0.148°*	0.25 / *0.281°*	0.24 / *0.416°*	
Methylamphetamine hydrochloride	27.5	2.75	0.38 / *0.112°*	0.37 / *0.208°*	0.34 / *0.388°*		
Methyldopate hydrochloride	42.8	4.28	0.21 / *0.063°*	0.21 / *0.122°*	0.21 / *0.244°*	0.21 / *0.365°*	
Methylergometrine maleate			0.10 / *0.028°*	0.10 / *0.056°*			
Methylphenidate hydrochloride	40.7	4.07	0.22 / *0.065°*	0.22 / *0.127°*	0.22 / *0.258°*	0.22 / *0.388°*	
Methylprednisolone sodium succinate			0.10 / *0.025°*	0.09 / *0.051°*	0.09 / *0.102°*	0.08 / *0.143°*	0.07 / *0.200°*
Metoclopramide hydrochloride			0.16 / *0.045°*	0.15 / *0.084°*	0.13 / *0.155°*	0.12 / *0.216°*	0.11 / *0.315°*
Minocycline hydrochloride			0.10 / *0.030°*	0.10 / *0.058°*	0.09 / *0.107°*	0.08 / *0.146°*	
Morphine hydrochloride			0.16 / *0.044°*	0.15 / *0.086°*	0.15 / *0.168°*	0.14 / *0.248°*	
Morphine sulphate			0.16 / *0.046°*	0.14 / *0.078°*	0.12 / *0.131°*	0.11 / *0.178°*	0.09 / *0.258°*
Nafcillin sodium			0.14 / *0.039°*	0.14 / *0.078°*	0.14 / *0.158°*	0.13 / *0.219°*	0.10 / *0.285°*
Nalorphine hydrochloride	63.6	6.36	0.24 / *0.070°*	0.21 / *0.121°*	0.18 / *0.210°*	0.17 / *0.288°*	0.15 / *0.434°*
Naloxone hydrochloride	80.7	8.07	0.14 / *0.042°*	0.14 / *0.083°*	0.14 / *0.158°*	0.13 / *0.230°*	0.13 / *0.367°*
Naphazoline hydrochloride	39.9	3.99	0.30 / *0.084°*	0.27 / *0.155°*	0.25 / *0.286°*	0.24 / *0.413°*	
Neomycin sulphate			0.14 / *0.041°*	0.12 / *0.067°*	0.10 / *0.112°*	0.09 / *0.154°*	0.08 / *0.223°*
Neostigmine bromide			0.23 / *0.065°*	0.22 / *0.123°*	0.20 / *0.230°*	0.19 / *0.333°*	
Neostigmine methylsulphate	52.2	5.22	0.22 / *0.056°*	0.20 / *0.108°*	0.18 / *0.208°*	0.18 / *0.306°*	0.17 / *0.500°*
Nicotinamide	44.9	4.49	0.30 / *0.083°*	0.26 / *0.148°*	0.23 / *0.264°*	0.21 / *0.371°*	
Nicotinic acid			0.26 / *0.074°*	0.25 / *0.145°*			
Nikethamide	59.4	5.94	0.20 / *0.053°*	0.18 / *0.100°*	0.17 / *0.190°*	0.16 / *0.276°*	0.15 / *0.443°*
Noscapine hydrochloride			— / *0.058°*				
Novobiocin sodium			0.10 / *0.025°*	0.08 / *0.046°*	0.08 / *0.086°*	0.07 / *0.122°*	0.07 / *0.190°*
Oleandomycin phosphate	108.2	10.82	0.08 / *0.017°*	0.08 / *0.038°*	0.08 / *0.084°*	0.08 / *0.129°*	0.08 / *0.255°*
Orphenadrine citrate			0.13 / *0.037°*	0.13 / *0.074°*	0.13 / *0.144°*	0.12 / *0.204°*	0.10 / *0.285°*

Table 6—*Continued*

Substance	Concentration iso-osmotic with blood g per litre	% w/v	NaCl equivalents and freezing point depressions				
			0.5%	1%	2%	3%	5%
Oxacillin sodium	66.4	6.64	0.18 0.050°	0.17 0.095°	0.16 0.177°	0.15 0.257°	0.14 0.408°
Oxybuprocaine hydrochloride			0.20 0.061°	0.18 0.104°	0.15 0.175°	0.14 0.239°	
Oxymetazoline hydrochloride	49.2	4.92	0.22 0.063°	0.22 0.124°	0.20 0.232°	0.19 0.335°	
Oxytetracycline hydrochloride			0.17 0.052°	0.14 0.081°	0.11 0.113°	0.08 0.141°	
Papaverine hydrochloride			0.10 0.028°	0.10 0.060°	0.10 0.121°		
Paraldehyde	36.5	3.65	0.25 0.071°	0.25 0.142°	0.25 0.288°	0.25 0.430°	
Pentazocine lactate			0.15 0.042°	0.15 0.085°	0.15 0.169°	0.15 0.253°	0.15 0.420°
Pentobarbitone sodium			0.26 0.076°	0.25 0.143°	0.24 0.270°	0.23 0.393°	
Pentolinium tartrate			0.18 0.050°	0.17 0.097°	0.16 0.186°	0.15 0.268°	0.15 0.440°
Pethidine hydrochloride	48	4.8	0.24 0.066°	0.22 0.124°	0.21 0.235°	0.20 0.340°	
Phenacaine hydrochloride			0.22 0.061°	0.20 0.108°			
Phenazone	68.1	6.81	0.18 0.050°	0.17 0.094°	0.16 0.174°	0.14 0.250°	0.14 0.394°
Phenethyl alcohol			0.25 0.070°	0.25 0.141°	0.25 0.283°		
Pheniramine maleate			0.18 0.052°	0.16 0.095°	0.15 0.173°	0.14 0.247°	0.13 0.383°
Phenobarbitone sodium	39.5	3.95	0.24 0.069°	0.24 0.135°	0.23 0.267°	0.23 0.396°	
Phenol	28	2.8	0.38 0.104°	0.35 0.199°	0.33 0.381°		
Phentolamine mesylate	82.3	8.23	0.18 0.052°	0.17 0.096°	0.16 0.173°	0.14 0.244°	0.13 0.364°
Phenylbutazone sodium	53.4	5.34	0.19 0.054°	0.18 0.104°	0.17 0.202°	0.17 0.298°	0.17 0.488°
Phenylephrine hydrochloride	30	3.0	0.34 0.096°	0.32 0.184°	0.31 0.354°	0.30 0.520°	
Phenylpropanolamine hydrochloride	26	2.6	0.40 0.117°	0.38 0.218°	0.35 0.406°		
Physostigmine salicylate			0.16 0.045°	0.16 0.090°			
Physostigmine sulphate	77.4	7.74	0.14 0.040°	0.13 0.076°	0.13 0.146°	0.12 0.214°	0.12 0.344°
Pilocarpine hydrochloride	40.8	4.08	0.24 0.069°	0.24 0.134°	0.23 0.262°	0.22 0.387°	
Pilocarpine nitrate			0.24 0.070°	0.23 0.131°	0.21 0.247°	0.20 0.355°	
Piperacillin sodium			0.11 0.032°	0.11 0.063°	0.11 0.123°	0.10 0.175°	
Polymyxin B sulphate			0.10 0.033°	0.09 0.049°	0.07 0.075°	0.06 0.098°	0.04 0.131°
Polysorbate 80			0.02 0.005°	0.02 0.010°	0.02 0.020°	0.02 0.032°	0.02 0.055°
Potassium acid phosphate	21.8	2.18	0.48 0.133°	0.44 0.252°	0.42 0.480°		
Potassium chloride	11.9	1.19	0.76 0.219°	0.76 0.439°			
Potassium iodide	25.9	2.59	0.34 0.104°	0.34 0.205°	0.34 0.402°		
Potassium nitrate	16.2	1.62	0.58 0.163°	0.56 0.323°			
Potassium permanganate			0.39 0.112°	0.39 0.224°	0.39 0.449°		

Table 6—*Continued*

Substance	Concentration iso-osmotic with blood		NaCl equivalents and freezing point depressions				
	g per litre	% w/v	0.5%	1%	2%	3%	5%
Potassium phosphate	20.8	2.08	0.48	0.46	0.44		
			0.139°	*0.265°*	*0.501°*		
Povidone			0.01	0.01	0.01	0.01	0.01
			0.004°	*0.008°*	*0.010°*	*0.017°*	*0.035°*
Pralidoxime chloride	28.7	2.87	0.32	0.32	0.32		
			0.092°	*0.183°*	*0.364°*		
Pramoxine hydrochloride			0.18	0.18	0.17	0.15	0.10
			0.056°	*0.104°*	*0.196°*	*0.253°*	*0.281°*
Prilocaine hydrochloride	41.8	4.18	0.22	0.22	0.22	0.22	
			0.062°	*0.125°*	*0.250°*	*0.375°*	
Procainamide hydrochloride			0.24	0.22	0.20	0.19	0.17
			0.071°	*0.128°*	*0.231°*	*0.330°*	*0.505°*
Procaine hydrochloride	50.5	5.05	0.24	0.21	0.20	0.19	0.18
			0.065°	*0.122°*	*0.227°*	*0.327°*	*0.515°*
Procaine penicillin				0.10			
				0.06°			
Prochlorperazine edisylate			0.08	0.06	0.05	0.03	0.02
			0.020°	*0.033°*	*0.048°*	*0.056°*	*0.065°*
Promazine hydrochloride			0.18	0.13	0.09	0.07	0.05
			0.050°	*0.077°*	*0.102°*	*0.112°*	*0.137°*
Promethazine hydrochloride			0.28	0.18	0.12	0.10	0.07
			0.084°	*0.112°*	*0.151°*	*0.180°*	*0.224°*
Propantheline bromide			0.11	0.11			
			0.032°	*0.064°*			
Propiomazine hydrochloride			0.18	0.15	0.12	0.10	0.08
			0.050°	*0.084°*	*0.133°*	*0.165°*	*0.215°*
Propoxycaine hydrochloride			0.22	0.19	0.17	0.16	0.15
			0.063°	*0.112°*	*0.199°*	*0.281°*	*0.425°*
Propranolol hydrochloride			0.20	0.20	0.20		
			0.060°	*0.122°*	*0.230°*		
Propylene glycol	20	2.0	0.45	0.45	0.45		
			0.131°	*0.262°*	*0.520°*		
Pyridostigmine bromide	41.3	4.13	0.22	0.22	0.22	0.22	
			0.062°	*0.125°*	*0.250°*	*0.377°*	
Pyridoxine hydrochloride			0.41	0.36	0.32	0.29	
			0.118°	*0.208°*	*0.367°*	*0.512°*	
Quinidine gluconate			0.14	0.12	0.11	0.10	
			0.037°	*0.069°*	*0.124°*	*0.178°*	
Quinine dihydrochloride	50.7	5.07	0.26	0.23	0.20	0.19	0.18
			0.072°	*0.129°*	*0.232°*	*0.330°*	*0.513°*
Quinine hydrochloride			0.16	0.14	0.13	0.11	
			0.043°	*0.077°*	*0.140°*	*0.197°*	
Resorcinol	33	3.3	0.28	0.28	0.28	0.27	
			0.082°	*0.161°*	*0.319°*	*0.473°*	
Riboflavine phosphate (sodium salt)			0.08	0.08	0.08	0.08	
			0.022°	*0.047°*	*0.098°*	*0.510°*	
Rolitetracycline			0.11	0.11	0.10	0.09	0.07
			0.032°	*0.064°*	*0.113°*	*0.158°*	*0.204°*
Rose bengal	149	14.9	0.08	0.07	0.07	0.07	0.07
			0.020°	*0.040°*	*0.083°*	*0.124°*	*0.198°*
Silver nitrate	27.4	2.74	0.33	0.33	0.33		
			0.095°	*0.190°*	*0.380°*		
Silver protein			0.12	0.08	0.06	0.05	0.04
			0.033°	*0.047°*	*0.066°*	*0.081°*	*0.107°*
Silver protein, mild	55.1	5.51	0.17	0.17	0.17	0.17	0.16
			0.047°	*0.095°*	*0.189°*	*0.283°*	*0.472°*
Sodium acetate	20.3	2.03	0.47	0.46	0.45		
			0.136°	*0.267°*	*0.513°*		
Sodium acetrizoate	96.4	9.64	0.10	0.10	0.10	0.10	0.10
			0.027°	*0.055°*	*0.109°*	*0.163°*	*0.273°*
Sodium acid phosphate (1H$_2$O)	24.5	2.45	0.44	0.40	0.38		
			0.123°	*0.228°*	*0.434°*		
Sodium acid phosphate (2H$_2$O)	27.7	2.77	0.40	0.36	0.34		
			0.109°	*0.202°*	*0.384°*		

Table 6—*Continued*

Substance	Concentration iso-osmotic with blood g per litre	% w/v	NaCl equivalents and freezing point depressions 0.5%	1%	2%	3%	5%
Sodium acid phosphate, anhydrous	21	2.1	0.50 *0.142°*	0.46 *0.263°*	0.43 *0.499°*		
Sodium aminosalicylate	32.7	3.27	0.30 *0.086°*	0.29 *0.169°*	0.29 *0.326°*	0.28 *0.479°*	
Sodium ascorbate	29.9	2.99	0.34 *0.097°*	0.32 *0.186°*	0.30 *0.350°*		
Sodium aurothiomalate			0.10 *0.032°*	0.10 *0.061°*	0.10 *0.111°*	0.09 *0.159°*	0.09 *0.250°*
Sodium benzoate	22.5	2.25	0.40 *0.116°*	0.40 *0.232°*	0.40 *0.464°*		
Sodium bicarbonate	13.9	1.39	0.68 *0.197°*	0.65 *0.381°*			
Sodium borate	26	2.6	0.48 *0.137°*	0.42 *0.241°*	0.37 *0.421°*		
Sodium calciumedetate	45	4.5	0.21 *0.061°*	0.21 *0.120°*	0.21 *0.240°*	0.20 *0.357°*	
Sodium chloride	9	0.9	1.00 *0.289°*	1.00 *0.576°*			
Sodium citrate	30.2	3.02	0.32 *0.091°*	0.31 *0.178°*	0.30 *0.349°*	0.30 *0.518°*	
Sodium diatrizoate	105.5	10.55	0.10 *0.025°*	0.09 *0.049°*	0.09 *0.098°*	0.09 *0.149°*	0.09 *0.248°*
Sodium folate			0.14 *0.040°*	0.12 *0.069°*	0.11 *0.120°*	0.10 *0.166°*	
Sodium glucosulphone			0.18 *0.049°*	0.16 *0.089°*	0.14 *0.162°*	0.13 *0.233°*	0.13 *0.366°*
Sodium iodide	23.7	2.37	0.41 *0.113°*	0.39 *0.223°*	0.39 *0.441°*		
Sodium iodohippurate	59.2	5.92	0.16 *0.047°*	0.16 *0.091°*	0.16 *0.180°*	0.15 *0.267°*	0.15 *0.442°*
Sodium lactate	17.2	1.72	0.58 *0.164°*	0.55 *0.315°*			
Sodium metabisulphite	13.8	1.38	0.70 *0.206°*	0.67 *0.389°*			
Sodium nitrite	10.8	1.08	0.86 *0.248°*	0.84 *0.481°*			
Sodium nitroprusside	33.0	3.30	0.30 *0.086°*	0.29 *0.167°*	0.28 *0.322°*	0.28 *0.475°*	
Sodium phosphate, dibasic (2H$_2$O)	22.3	2.23	0.44 *0.127°*	0.42 *0.244°*	0.41 *0.470°*		
Sodium phosphate, dibasic (12H$_2$O)	44.5	4.45	0.24 *0.064°*	0.22 *0.126°*	0.21 *0.242°*	0.21 *0.358°*	
Sodium propionate	14.7	1.47	0.62 *0.177°*	0.61 *0.353°*			
Sodium salicylate	25.3	2.53	0.38 *0.106°*	0.36 *0.209°*	0.36 *0.412°*		
Sodium succinate	29	2.9	0.32 *0.092°*	0.32 *0.184°*	0.31 *0.361°*		
Sodium sulphate	39.5	3.95	0.28 *0.079°*	0.26 *0.148°*	0.25 *0.280°*	0.23 *0.405°*	
Sodium sulphate, anhydrous	16.1	1.61	0.62 *0.179°*	0.58 *0.336°*			
Sodium thiosulphate	29.8	2.98	0.32 *0.092°*	0.31 *0.180°*	0.31 *0.354°*		
Sorbitol (½H$_2$O)	54.8	5.48	0.16 *0.045°*	0.16 *0.094°*	0.16 *0.191°*	0.16 *0.288°*	0.16 *0.488°*
Sparteine sulphate	94.6	9.46	0.10 *0.030°*	0.10 *0.056°*	0.10 *0.111°*	0.10 *0.167°*	0.10 *0.277°*
Spectinomycin hydrochloride	56.6	5.66	0.16 *0.045°*	0.16 *0.092°*	0.16 *0.185°*	0.16 *0.280°*	0.16 *0.460°*
Stibophen			0.20 *0.059°*	0.18 *0.107°*	0.17 *0.196°*	0.16 *0.281°*	0.15 *0.435°*
Streptomycin sulphate			0.08 *0.020°*	0.07 *0.038°*	0.07 *0.072°*	0.06 *0.108°*	0.06 *0.177°*

Table 6—*Continued*

Substance	Concentration iso-osmotic with blood		NaCl equivalents and freezing point depressions				
	g per litre	% w/v	0.5%	1%	2%	3%	5%
Strychnine hydrochloride			0.20	0.18	0.14		
			0.060°	*0.099°*	*0.160°*		
Sucrose	92.5	9.25	0.08	0.08	0.09	0.09	0.09
			0.023°	*0.047°*	*0.099°*	*0.154°*	*0.268°*
Sulphacetamide sodium	38.5	3.85	0.24	0.23	0.23	0.23	
			0.066°	*0.133°*	*0.268°*	*0.406°*	
Sulphadiazine sodium	42.4	4.24	0.26	0.24	0.23	0.22	
			0.073°	*0.137°*	*0.262°*	*0.381°*	
Sulphadimidine sodium			0.22	0.21	0.20	0.19	0.18
			0.066°	*0.122°*	*0.225°*	*0.324°*	*0.511°*
Sulphafurazole diethanolamine			0.20	0.18	0.16	0.15	
			0.059°	*0.104°*	*0.186°*	*0.262°*	
Sulphamerazine sodium	45.3	4.53	0.24	0.23	0.22	0.21	
			0.069°	*0.132°*	*0.248°*	*0.361°*	
Sulphathiazole sodium	48.2	4.82	0.23	0.22	0.21	0.20	
			0.067°	*0.124°*	*0.236°*	*0.340°*	
Sulphobromophthalein sodium			0.07	0.06	0.05	0.05	0.04
			0.019°	*0.034°*	*0.060°*	*0.084°*	*0.123°*
Suramin			—	*0.058°*			
Suxamethonium chloride	44.8	4.48	0.20	0.20	0.20	0.20	
			0.059°	*0.117°*	*0.233°*	*0.353°*	
Tartaric acid	39	3.9	0.26	0.25	0.24	0.23	
			0.075°	*0.144°*	*0.278°*	*0.406°*	
Terbutaline sulphate	67.5	6.75	0.14	0.14	0.14	0.14	0.13
			0.042°	*0.082°*	*0.161°*	*0.238°*	*0.390°*
Tetracycline hydrochloride			0.16	0.14	0.12	0.10	
			0.046°	*0.078°*	*0.128°*	*0.172°*	
Tetrahydrozoline hydrochloride			0.30	0.28	0.25	0.23	
			0.090°	*0.162°*	*0.285°*	*0.406°*	
Theophylline			0.10				
			0.028°				
Theophylline sodium glycinate	29.4	2.94	0.32	0.31	0.31		
			0.090°	*0.180°*	*0.355°*		
Thiamine hydrochloride	42.4	4.24	0.26	0.25	0.23	0.22	
			0.074°	*0.139°*	*0.262°*	*0.378°*	
Thiethylperazine maleate			0.10	0.09	0.08	0.07	0.05
			0.030°	*0.050°*	*0.089°*	*0.119°*	*0.153°*
Thiopentone sodium	35	3.5	0.28	0.27	0.27	0.26	
			0.079°	*0.155°*	*0.302°*	*0.447°*	
Thiotepa	56.7	5.67	0.16	0.16	0.16	0.16	0.16
			0.045°	*0.090°*	*0.182°*	*0.278°*	*0.460°*
Ticarcillin sodium	46.2	4.62	0.20	0.20	0.20	0.19	
			0.056°	*0.113°*	*0.226°*	*0.339°*	
Timolol maleate			0.14	0.13	0.12		
			0.038°	*0.077°*	*0.146°*		
Tobramycin			0.08	0.07	0.07	0.07	0.06
			0.019°	*0.038°*	*0.075°*	*0.112°*	*0.187°*
Tolazoline hydrochloride	30.5	3.05	0.36	0.34	0.31	0.30	
			0.107°	*0.194°*	*0.358°*	*0.512°*	
Triethanolamine	40.5	4.05	0.20	0.21	0.22	0.22	
			0.050°	*0.121°*	*0.252°*	*0.383°*	
Trifluoperazine hydrochloride			0.18	0.18	0.13		
			0.052°	*0.100°*	*0.144°*		
Trimeprazine tartrate			0.10	0.06	0.04	0.03	0.02
			0.023°	*0.035°*	*0.045°*	*0.052°*	*0.061°*
Trimetaphan camsylate			0.12	0.10	0.10	0.09	0.09
			0.033°	*0.060°*	*0.111°*	*0.158°*	*0.248°*
Trimethobenzamide hydrochloride			0.12	0.10	0.10	0.09	0.08
			0.033°	*0.062°*	*0.108°*	*0.153°*	*0.232°*
Tripelennamine hydrochloride			0.38	0.30	0.24	0.20	
			0.110°	*0.173°*	*0.268°*	*0.353°*	
Trometamol	34.1	3.41	0.26	0.26	0.26	0.26	
			0.075°	*0.152°*	*0.305°*	*0.458°*	

Table 6—*Continued*

Substance	Concentration iso-osmotic with blood		NaCl equivalents and freezing point depressions				
	g per litre	% w/v	0.5%	1%	2%	3%	5%
Tropicamide			0.10	0.09	0.030°	0.050°	
Tryparsamide	46.2	4.62	0.20	0.20	0.20	0.20	
			0.057°	0.113°	0.225°	0.339°	
Tuaminoheptane sulphate	34	3.4	0.28	0.27	0.27	0.27	
			0.078°	0.154°	0.304°	0.466°	
Tubocurarine chloride			0.14	0.13	0.11	0.10	0.09
			0.042°	0.077°	0.124°	0.175°	0.269°
Urea	16.3	1.63	0.64	0.59			
			0.188°	0.341°			
Vancomycin hydrochloride			0.06	0.05	0.04	0.04	0.04
			0.015°	0.028°	0.049°	0.066°	0.098°
Vinbarbitone sodium	35.5	3.55	0.26	0.26	0.26	0.25	
			0.074°	0.148°	0.294°	0.440°	
Viomycin sulphate			0.08	0.08	0.08	0.07	0.07
			0.025°	0.047°	0.087°	0.126°	0.199°
Warfarin sodium	61	6.1	0.18	0.17	0.16	0.15	0.15
			0.049°	0.095°	0.181°	0.264°	0.430°
Xylometazoline hydrochloride	46.8	4.68	0.22	0.21	0.20	0.20	
			0.065°	0.121°	0.232°	0.342°	
Zinc chloride			0.66	0.61			
			0.190°	0.354°			
Zinc sulphate	76.5	7.65	0.16	0.15	0.14	0.13	0.12
			0.045°	0.085°	0.157°	0.226°	0.355°

multiplying the freezing point depression of a 1% w/v solution by the concentration of the unadjusted solution expressed as % w/v; b is the freezing point depression produced by 1% w/v of the adjusting substance.

EXAMPLES

A. The strength of a solution of sodium chloride iso-osmotic with blood serum and tears may be calculated by simple proportion.

A 1% w/v solution of sodium chloride depresses the freezing point of water by 0.576°. Thus, the strength of sodium chloride that will depress the freezing point by 0.52°

$$= \frac{1 \times 0.52}{0.576} = 0.9\% \text{ w/v} = 9 \text{ g per litre}$$

B. Suppose a solution for intravenous injection containing 0.18% w/v of sodium chloride is required to be made iso-osmotic with blood serum by the addition of anhydrous glucose.

From Table 6:

A 1% w/v solution of sodium chloride depresses the freezing point of water by 0.576°.

The depression of the freezing point of the unadjusted solution of sodium chloride will therefore be $0.18 \times 0.576 = 0.1037°$ *(a)*.

A 1% w/v solution of anhydrous glucose depresses the freezing point of water by 0.10° *(b)*.

Substituting these values for a and b in the formula:

$$W = \frac{0.52 - 0.1037}{0.1} = \frac{0.4163}{0.1} = 4.2$$

The intravenous solution thus requires the addition of 4.2% w/v of anhydrous glucose to make it iso-osmotic with blood serum.

Calculations Based on Sodium Chloride Equivalents

The sodium chloride equivalent of a substance is the mass (in grams) of sodium chloride that has an effect on the freezing point depression equivalent to that produced by 1 g of substance. The sodium chloride equivalent is obtained by dividing the value for the freezing point depression produced by a solution of the substance by the value for the freezing point depression produced by a solution of sodium chloride of the same concentration.

The concentration of sodium chloride (g per litre) required to make a solution iso-osmotic with blood serum is the difference between the concentration of a solution of sodium chloride iso-osmotic with body fluids (9 g per litre) and the concentration of substance multiplied by its sodium chloride equivalent:

concentration of NaCl required (in g per litre) = 9 − (concentration of substance × NaCl equivalent)

The sodium chloride equivalents provide a simple method of determining the amount of sodium chloride required to render a hypo-osmotic solution iso-osmotic with body fluids. In calculations, the equivalent should be employed that represents the concentration nearest to the desired concentration of medicinal substance used.

EXAMPLES—as examples A and B under Calculations based on Freezing Point Depression

A. With this method the strength of a solution of sodium chloride iso-osmotic with blood serum and tears is 0.9% w/v, as sodium chloride equivalents are calculated directly from the freezing point depression values on the basis of a 1% w/v solution of sodium chloride depressing the freezing point of water by 0.576°—see example A under Calculations based on Freezing Point Depression

B. Quantity of sodium chloride present = 1.8 g per litre
Concentration of sodium chloride required to render the solution iso-osmotic = 9 − 1.8 = 7.2 g per litre
From Table 6:
1 g of anhydrous glucose is equivalent to 0.18 g of sodium chloride
Therefore, 7.2 g of sodium chloride

$$= \frac{1}{0.18} \times 7.2$$

$$= 40 \text{ g per litre}$$

Calculations Based on Amount of Substance Concentration (Molar Concentration)

In ideal solutions the freezing point is lowered by 1.858° for each mole of solute particles per kilogram of water. Blood serum and tears have a freezing point of −0.52°.
Thus, by proportion, the amount of nonionising substance required to make 1 litre of solution iso-osmotic with blood serum and tears is:

$$\frac{1 \times 0.52}{1.858} \text{ mol} = 0.280 \text{ mol}$$

$$= 280 \text{ mmol}$$

Therefore a solution containing 280 mmol per litre of an undissociated solute is iso-osmotic with blood serum and tears.
When a substance ionises, the amount of substance required to make 1 litre of solution iso-osmotic with blood serum and tears is:

$$\frac{280}{n} \text{ mmol}$$

where n is the number of ions that one molecule of the substance forms in aqueous solution, assuming complete ionisation.
In terms of mass concentration, the concentration of a solution iso-osmotic with blood serum and tears is:

$$W = \frac{280 \times M}{n \times 1000}$$

where W is the concentration (g per litre) of a solution iso-osmotic with blood serum and tears; M is the molecular weight of the substance; n is the number of ions that one molecule of the substance forms in aqueous solution, assuming complete ionisation.

EXAMPLES—as examples A and B under Calculations based on Freezing Point Depression
A. The concentration of a solution of sodium chloride iso-osmotic with blood serum and tears may be calculated thus:
Molecular weight of sodium chloride (M) = 58.44
In solution, 1 molecule of sodium chloride dissociates into 2 ions (n). Therefore:

$$W = \frac{280 \times 58.44}{2 \times 1000} = 8.2 \text{ g per litre}$$

B. The unadjusted solution contains 1.8 g per litre of sodium chloride.
An iso-osmotic solution of sodium chloride contains 8.2 g per litre (see example A, above).
The unadjusted substance thus requires the addition of 8.2 − 1.8 = 6.4 g per litre of sodium chloride or its equivalent.
The adjusting substance is anhydrous glucose, the molecular weight (M) of which is 180.2.
In solution, the glucose molecule is undissociated, thus $n = 1$.
Therefore, by proportion, the equivalent quantity of glucose required for adjustment is:

$$\frac{6.4}{\left(\frac{58.44}{2}\right)} \times 180.2 = 39.5 \text{ g per litre}$$

Calculations Based on Serum Osmolarity

The theoretical osmolarity of serum, calculated from its known constituents, is approximately 305 mmol per litre. Therefore a solution iso-osmotic with blood serum and tears has an osmolarity of approximately 305 mmol per litre. The concentration of adjusting substance can be calculated by means of the equation:

$$a = 305 - b$$

where a is mmol per litre of adjusting substance (molecules and ions) and b is mmol per litre of dissolved substance (molecules and ions).

EXAMPLES—as examples A and B under Calculations based on Freezing Point Depression

A. A solution of sodium chloride which has an osmolarity of 305 mmol per litre will contain:

$$\frac{305 \times 58.44}{2 \times 1000} = 8.9\,\text{g of sodium chloride per litre}$$

B. The unadjusted solution contains 1.8 g per litre (0.18% w/v) of sodium chloride

$$\frac{1800}{58.44} = 30.8\,\text{mmol of sodium chloride per litre}$$

$$= 30.8\,\text{mmol of Na}^+ \text{ and } 30.8\,\text{mmol of Cl}^-$$

$$= 61.6\,\text{mmol of solute particles per litre}$$

and $a = 305 - 61.6 = 243.4$

Thus, 243.4 mmol of glucose will be required to make the solution iso-osmotic (glucose does not ionise). Molecular weight of anhydrous glucose $= 180.2$

$$243.4\,\text{mmol per litre} = \frac{243.4 \times 180.2}{1000}\,\text{g per litre}$$

$$= 43.9\,\text{g per litre}$$

The 1.8 g per litre solution of sodium chloride thus requires the addition of 43.9 g per litre of anhydrous glucose to make it iso-osmotic with blood serum.

Comparison of Results

Calculations based on	Example A	Example B
1. depression of freezing point	9 g per litre	42 g per litre
2. sodium chloride equivalent	9 g per litre	40 g per litre
3. amount of substance concentration (molar concentration)	8.2 g per litre	39.5 g per litre
4. serum osmolarity	8.9 g per litre	43.9 g per litre

Calculations based on the depression of freezing point are accurate enough for most clinical purposes as long as the concentration of the substance is reasonably close to that for which the freezing point depression has been determined. Sodium chloride equivalents are based on freezing point determinations and may be conveniently used when the concentration of drug approximates to one of the concentrations for which equivalents are given in Table 6. Calculations based on the amount of substance concentration (molar concentration) and serum osmolarity are reasonably accurate for dilute solutions of molecules that dissociate completely or for those that do not dissociate at all. Calculations based on serum osmolarity have the added advantage of being simple and rapid.

It should be realised that iso-osmotic concentrations that are calculated from data derived from determination of freezing point depressions or by similar methods are not necessarily isotonic, and that for some substances iso-osmotic solutions may cause haemolysis of erythrocytes.

BUFFERED SOLUTIONS

Buffers are compounds or mixtures of compounds which, when in solution, resist changes in the pH of the solution upon addition of acid or alkali, upon dilution with the solvent, or when there is a temperature change. In buffer (or buffered) solutions the hydrogen ions are in dynamic equilibrium with one or more substances capable of combining with or releasing hydrogen ions. Water and solutions of neutral salts (such as sodium chloride) have no ability to resist changes in pH on addition of weak acid or base. For example, uptake of carbon dioxide by water to form carbonic acid can produce a twenty-fold increase in hydrogen ion concentration.

A solution containing a strong acid or a strong base does have buffering capacity, but only at the extremes of pH. Most buffers consist of a mixture of a weak acid and one of its salts or a weak base and one of its salts. Buffer solutions should be prepared using freshly boiled and cooled water. They should be stored in containers of alkali-free glass and discarded no later than three months from the date of manufacture.

The buffer equation, that is, the Henderson-Hasselbalch equation, allows the pH of a buffer solution containing a weak acid and its salt to be calculated:

$$pH = pK_a + \log_{10}\frac{[\text{salt}]}{[\text{acid}]}$$

where pK_a is the common logarithm of the reciprocal of the dissociation constant of the acid, [salt] is the concentration of the salt, and [acid] is the concentration of the acid, both in mol per litre.

EXAMPLE
The pK_a value for acetic acid is 4.8. A buffer solution containing acetic acid 0.1 mol per litre and sodium acetate 0.2 mol per litre has a pH given by:

$$pH = 4.8 + \log_{10}\left(\frac{0.2}{0.1}\right)$$

$$= 5.1$$

The pH of this buffer solution is over two pH units greater than that of acetic acid 0.1 mol per litre alone and arises because of the suppression of ionisation of the acetic acid by the common acetate ion introduced as the sodium salt. The addition of an acid to this buffer causes a momentary drop in pH, but the hydrogen ions combine with acetate ions to form unionised acetic acid and the pH rises. The addition of an alkali causes a momentary rise in pH, but the hydroxyl ions combine with hydrogen ions and acetic acid ionises to form hydrogen ions and acetate ions so that the pH falls.

In a buffer solution containing a weak base and salt, the pH is given by:

$$pH = pK_a + \log_{10} \frac{[base]}{[salt]}$$

where pK_a is the common logarithm of the reciprocal of the dissociation constant of the conjugate acid produced by the base, [base] is the concentration of the base, and [salt] is the concentration of the salt, both in mol per litre.

Buffer solutions often contain polybasic acids or polyacidic bases, and in calculating the expected pH of solutions containing these substances the appropriate value for pK_a must be selected. Thus, in a buffer solution containing equimolar quantities of phosphoric acid and sodium hydroxide,

$$H_3PO_4 + NaOH \rightleftharpoons NaH_2PO_4 + H_2O$$

addition of a small quantity of acid would involve the first replaceable hydrogen atom ($pK_a = 2.1$),

$$NaH_2PO_4 + H^+ \rightleftharpoons Na^+ + H_3PO_4$$

whereas addition of a small quantity of alkali would involve the second replaceable hydrogen atom ($pK_a = 7.2$).

$$NaH_2PO_4 + NaOH \rightleftharpoons Na_2HPO_4 + H_2O$$

If two equivalents of alkali were added to one equivalent of phosphoric acid, disodium hydrogen phosphate would be formed.

$$H_3PO_4 + 2NaOH \rightleftharpoons Na_2HPO_4 + 2H_2O$$

Addition of any further alkali would involve the third replaceable hydrogen atom ($pK_a = 12.7$).

$$Na_2HPO_4 + NaOH \rightleftharpoons Na_3PO_4 + H_2O$$

Buffer Capacity

The buffer capacity (buffer index; buffer efficiency) of a solution is a measure of its resistance to change

in pH. The buffer capacity (β) is equal to the amount of strong acid or strong base, expressed as moles of hydrogen or hydroxyl ion per litre, required to change the pH of the buffer system by one unit. A solution has a buffer capacity of 1 when 1 litre requires 1 mol of hydrogen or hydroxyl ions to change the pH by 1 unit. Therefore the smaller the pH change in a solution after the addition of a specified amount of acid or base, the greater the buffer capacity of the solution. A buffer solution containing a weak acid and its salt has a maximum buffer capacity (β_{max}) when the pH is equal to the pK_a value for the weak acid. At this pH, the value of β_{max} may be approximated by:

$$\beta_{max} \approx \frac{2.303}{4} c$$

where c is the total buffer concentration in mol per litre. For most buffer systems, a total buffer concentration of between 0.5 and 0.05 mol per litre gives an adequate buffer capacity over a pH range of about 2 units. In practice, inter-ionic effects impose an upper limit of about 0.2 on the buffer capacity.

Selection of a Buffer System

The choice of a suitable buffer system is governed by the pH range and buffer capacity desired and the purpose for which it is required. Compatibility and low toxicity are important requirements for buffers used in medicines.

Toxicity

Boric acid and borates are non-irritant and stable and have a good buffer capacity; they are used in preparations applied externally such as eye drops. The composition of boric acid buffer solutions iso-osmotic with tears is shown in Table 7. These

Table 7
Borate buffer

pH (25°)	Boric acid H_3BO_3 g per litre	Borax $Na_2B_4O_7.10H_2O$ g per litre	Sodium chloride to make iso-osmotic g per litre
6.8	12.03	0.57	2.7
7.2	11.66	1.15	2.7
7.4	11.16	1.91	2.7
7.7	10.54	2.87	2.6
7.8	9.92	3.82	2.6
8.0	9.30	4.78	2.5
8.1	8.68	5.73	2.4
8.2	8.06	6.69	2.3
8.4	6.82	8.60	2.1
8.6	5.58	10.51	1.9
8.7	4.96	11.46	1.8
8.8	3.72	13.37	1.4
9.0	2.48	15.28	1.1
9.1	1.24	17.20	0.7

compounds are toxic and cannot be used in injections or where absorption into the systemic circulation may occur, such as areas of abraded skin.

Incompatibility

Borate and phosphate buffers are incompatible with many inorganic compounds including the salts of silver, iron, magnesium, and zinc. Borate buffers form chelates with many polyols including glycerol, catecholamines, phenols, and carbohydrates.

Range of Buffering Action

General buffers usually contain only a single salt and have an effective buffer range of about two pH units. The buffer system giving the best buffer action will be that containing an acid with a pK_a closest to the desired pH of the solution. The composition of Sørensen's modified buffer solution is shown in Table 8; it has a maximum buffer capacity of 0.04 at a pH of 7.2. At this pH it is equally resistant to the addition of acid and alkali.

Table 8
Phosphate buffer (Sørensen, modified)

pH	Sodium acid phosphate $NaH_2PO_4,2H_2O$ g per litre	Sodium phosphate $Na_2HPO_4,12H_2O$ g per litre	Sodium chloride to make iso-osmotic g per litre
5.9	9.4	2.4	5.2
6.2	8.3	4.8	5.1
6.5	7.3	7.2	5.0
6.6	6.2	9.5	4.9
6.8	5.2	11.9	4.8
7.0	4.2	14.3	4.6
7.2	3.1	16.7	4.5
7.4	2.1	19.1	4.4
7.7	1.0	21.5	4.3
8.0	0.5	22.7	4.2

If the solution is liable, through manufacture or storage, to become more acidic it may be preferable to increase the ratio of dibasic salt to monobasic salt. Conversely, if alkalinity is liable to increase on storage, this ratio should be decreased. In general, higher resistance to acidity is achieved by the use of a high ratio of base to salt, or salt to acid, whereas higher resistance to alkalinity is achieved by the use of a high ratio of salt to base, or acid to salt.

Solutions of 'universal' buffers contain two or more buffer systems and give a buffering action over a relatively wide range of pH values. Their buffer capacity is lower than that of the general buffers at the same concentration. The citrate-phosphate

Table 9
Citrate-phosphate buffer (McIlvaine)

pH	Sodium phosphate $Na_2HPO_4,12H_2O$ g per litre	Citric acid $C_6H_8O_7,H_2O$ g per litre
2.2	1.4	20.6
2.4	4.4	19.7
2.6	7.8	18.7
2.8	11.4	17.7
3.0	14.7	16.7
3.2	17.7	15.8
3.4	20.4	15.0
3.6	23.1	14.2
3.8	25.4	13.6
4.0	27.6	12.9
4.2	29.7	12.3
4.4	31.6	11.7
4.6	33.5	11.2
4.8	35.3	10.7
5.0	36.9	10.2
5.2	38.4	9.7
5.4	39.9	9.3
5.6	41.5	8.8
5.8	43.3	8.3
6.0	45.2	7.7
6.2	47.3	7.1
6.4	49.6	6.5
6.6	52.1	5.7
6.8	55.3	4.8
7.0	59.0	3.7
7.2	62.3	2.7
7.4	65.1	1.9
7.6	67.1	1.3
7.8	68.6	0.9
8.0	69.7	0.58

buffer system (McIlvaine) covers the range from pH 2.2 to pH 8.0 (see Table 9).

Biological Buffers

Phosphate, carbonate, and borate buffers are not suitable for biological pH control as they precipitate calcium or enter into reactions with other components of the media or with the biological system. Buffer solutions suitable for pH control in biological media are either of the fixed-pH type, where the solution is buffered to a pH of 7.3 to 7.4, or variable-pH type where the pH of the buffer solution can be altered by addition of acid or alkali. Krebs solution and Ringer-Locke solution are examples of fixed-pH solutions (see Table 10). Variable pH buffer solutions in common use are those containing imidazole (see Table 11), tris(hydroxymethyl)aminomethane (trometamol) (see Table 12), or N-2-hydroxyethylpiperazine-N'-2-ethanesulphonic acid (HEPES) (see Table 13).

Miscellaneous Factors Influencing Buffer pH

The pH of a buffer solution may be altered by dilution with the solvent, by addition of a solution of a neutral salt, or by a change in temperature.

Table 10
Physiological salt solutions

	Krebs		Ringer-Locke	
	mmol per litre	g per litre	mmol per litre	g per litre
Sodium chloride (NaCl)	118.07	6.90	154.00	9.00
Potassium chloride (KCl)	4.69	0.35	5.63	0.42
Magnesium sulphate (MgSO$_4$,7H$_2$O)	1.18	0.29	—	—
Potassium acid phosphate (KH$_2$PO$_4$)	1.18	0.16	—	—
Glucose (C$_6$H$_{12}$O$_6$)	10.09	2.00	5.04	1.00
Sodium bicarbonate (NaHCO$_3$)	24.97	2.10	5.95	0.50
Calcium chloride (CaCl$_2$,2H$_2$O)	2.52	0.37	1.09	0.16

Table 11
Imidazole buffer. Contains imidazole 3.40 g per litre (50.0mmol per litre) and specified amount of hydrochloric acid

pH (25°)	Hydrochloric acid	
	mmol per litre	g per litre
6.2	42.9	1.56
6.4	39.8	1.45
6.6	35.5	1.29
6.8	30.4	1.11
7.0	24.3	0.89
7.2	18.6	0.68
7.4	13.6	0.50
7.6	9.3	0.34
7.8	6.0	0.22

Table 12
Tris buffer. Contains Tris (trometamol) 6.06 g per litre (50.0 mmol per litre) and the specified amount of hydrochloric acid

pH	Hydrochloric acid	
	mmol per litre	g per litre
7.2	44.7	1.63
7.4	42.0	1.53
7.6	39.3	1.43
7.8	33.7	1.23
8.0	27.9	1.02
8.2	22.9	0.83
8.4	17.3	0.63
8.6	13.0	0.47
8.8	8.8	0.32
9.0	5.3	0.19

Table 13
HEPES buffer. Contains HEPES 11.92 g per litre (50.0 mmol per litre) and the specified amounts of sodium hydroxide and sodium chloride

pH	Sodium hydroxide		Sodium chloride	
	mmol per litre	g per litre	mmol per litre	g per litre
6.6	5.0	0.200	95.0	5.552
6.7	6.2	0.248	93.8	5.482
6.8	7.5	0.300	92.5	5.406
6.9	9.1	0.364	90.9	5.312
7.0	11.0	0.440	89.0	5.201
7.1	13.1	0.524	86.9	5.078
7.2	15.4	0.616	84.6	4.944
7.3	18.0	0.720	82.0	4.792
7.4	20.7	0.828	79.3	4.634
7.5	23.6	0.944	76.4	4.465
7.6	26.4	1.056	73.6	4.301
7.7	29.3	1.172	70.7	4.132
7.8	32.0	1.280	68.0	3.974
7.9	34.6	1.384	66.4	3.822
8.0	36.9	1.476	63.1	3.688
8.1	39.0	1.560	61.0	3.565
8.2	40.9	1.636	59.1	3.454
8.3	42.5	1.700	57.5	3.360
8.4	43.8	1.752	56.2	3.284
8.5	45.0	1.800	55.0	3.214

Dilution of an aqueous buffer solution with water in moderate quantities has only a small effect on the pH, and in most cases the pH moves towards neutrality. The **dilution value** is the change in pH when the buffer solution is diluted with an equal volume of water. The dilution values for most common buffer systems are usually less than 0.1 pH unit. Addition of neutral salts changes the pH by altering the ionic strength. Provided the final concentration of neutral salt is no greater than that of the buffer system, the change in pH will be less than about 0.1 unit.

The temperature of the buffer solution has some influence on the pH. A temperature increase will lower the pH of buffer solutions containing boric acid and sodium borate and will raise the pH of those containing acetic acid and sodium acetate. The **temperature coefficient of pH** is the change in pH per degree rise in temperature. Its value is greater for cationic buffers such as the aliphatic amines than for those containing inorganic salts; the pH of tris(hydroxymethyl)aminomethane buffer decreases by about 0.04 pH unit per degree, whereas the decrease for Sørensen's phosphate buffer is less than 0.003 pH unit per degree. Extremes of temperature may produce large changes in pH; in solutions at or near 0° the change may be caused by crystallisation of a buffer component.

After preparation of a buffer solution the pH should be measured after the addition of all other components of the solution and at the appropriate temperature. Changes in pH upon storage may occur if moulds grow in the buffer solution or if crystals of a component of the buffer system are deposited.

PARTITION COEFFICIENTS

A partition coefficient is a solubility ratio that is a measure of the distribution of a solute between two immiscible phases. For most purposes these phases are an organic solvent and water.

Partition coefficients are most frequently determined in attempts to correlate the relative lipophilic character of a drug substance with biological properties. A drug substance can exert its influence only if it can reach the active site by a transfer process that involves passage through both hydrophilic and lipophilic barriers in the biological system. The **partition coefficient** (P) of a solute is defined as the ratio of the concentrations in the two phases at equilibrium, and it is usual to present the ratio as that in favour of the organic phase:

$$P = \frac{C_o}{C_w}$$

where C_o is the concentration of the solute in the organic phase, and C_w is the concentration of the solute in the aqueous phase. Owing to the widespread use of partition coefficients in structure-activity studies, it is often convenient to use log P, the logarithm of the partition coefficient, instead of the partition coefficient itself.

The above equation assumes that the compound, if it is an ionisable molecule such as an acid or a base, is fully unionised under the conditions of the measurement. This usually requires the use of an acidic aqueous phase for an acidic compound, or of an alkaline phase for a base. However, it may be desirable to measure a partition coefficient under conditions where the compound is partially ionised, for example by using a pH 7.4 buffer. In this case, the ratio is termed the **apparent partition coefficient** to distinguish it from the real partition coefficient for the totally unionised compound. The term **distribution coefficient** (D) is also used for this quantity. The apparent partition coefficient (P_{app}) is related to the proportion of drug present in solution as the unionised species, which in turn depends upon the pH of the aqueous phase used.

$$P_{app} = Pf_u$$

where f_u is the fraction of molecules present in the unionised form.

For a monobasic acid,

$$f_u = \frac{1}{(1 + 10^{pH - pK_a})}$$

For a monoacidic base,

$$f_u = \frac{1}{(1 + 10^{pK_a - pH})}$$

Hence, for an acid,

$$P_{app} = \frac{P}{(1 + 10^{pH - pK_a})}$$

and for a base,

$$P_{app} = \frac{P}{(1 + 10^{pK_a - pH})}$$

Thus knowledge of the pK_a and true partition coefficient of a molecule allows calculation of the apparent partition coefficient at any pH. For example, the basic drug amphetamine has a pK_a of 9.7 and an n-heptane/water partition coefficient of 3.4. Using the final equation, its apparent partition coefficient at pH 7.4 is 0.017.

It is assumed here that ions are not extracted into the organic layer. This can occur under some circumstances and precautions have to be taken to prevent it occurring during the determination of the apparent partition coefficients.

Determination of Partition Coefficients

The Shake-flask Method

Partition coefficients are usually determined by the traditional shake-flask method. In this method the compound is dissolved in one phase, the other phase added, the mixture is shaken, allowed to stand, and the phases separated; the concentration of solute in each phase is then determined by a suitable analytical method.

Effect of Temperature. Partition coefficients are usually measured at room temperature. Although the values will vary with temperature, the effect is usually of the order of 0.01 log unit per degree (either positively or negatively) and, in general, is not large enough for normal fluctuations in room temperature to be significant.

Determination of Concentration of Solute. A prerequisite for the determination of partition coefficients is the availablity of a suitable sensitive method of assaying the compound in one (or preferably both) phases.

Adjustment of Concentration. In an ideal determination the following conditions are met: the two phases are transparent to ultraviolet radiation, the solute is a neutral molecule with a strong ultraviolet absorption spectrum, and the ratio of concentration of equilibrium lies within the ratio of 5 to 1 either way. In this situation, absorbances can be measured directly in both phases, the concentrations calculated, and the partition coefficient obtained.

However, partition coefficients well outside this range often occur and, with compounds with very high or very low partition coefficients, the equilibrium concentration in the less favoured phase may be below or close to the limits of detection. Modifications to the ideal situation are therefore required.

Choice of Solvent. A large number of different solvent-water systems have been used for the determination of partition coefficients in connection with drug design and structure-activity studies. In this context the solvent is intended as a model for the lipophilic phase of biological systems, and the water as a model for the hydrophilic phase.

The Significance and Use of Partition Coefficients

Body membranes are mainly lipoid in nature and consequently are more easily penetrated by lipophilic molecules than by hydrophilic molecules. As the partition coefficient between organic solvent and water is an index of the lipid solubility of a compound, there is often a relationship between this and the rate of transfer of a molecule across a biological membrane; this may be evident particularly within a series of structurally related compounds. The **pH-partition hypothesis** of drug absorption is described in the Biopharmaceutics and Pharmacokinetic Principles chapter.

REFERENCES

1. Yalkowsky SH, Valvani SC. J Pharm Sci 1980;69:912–22.
2. Boon PFG, Coles CLJ, Tate M. J Pharm Pharmacol 1961;13:200T.

FURTHER INFORMATION

Atkinson HC, Duffull SB. Prediction of drug loss from PVC infusion bags. J Pharm Pharmacol 1991;43:374–6

Badwan AA, El-Khordagui LK, Saleh AM, Khalil SA. The solubility of benzodiazepines in sodium salicylate solution and a proposed mechanism for hydrotropic solubilization. Int J Pharmaceutics 1983;13:67–74.

Bodor N, Huang MJ. Partition coefficients–of over 300 drugs. J Pharm Sci 1992;81(3):272–81.

Cassidy SL, Lympany PA, Henry JA. Lipid solubility of a series of drugs and its relevance to fatal poisoning. J Pharm Pharmacol 1988;40:130–2.

Duchene D, Vaution C, Glomot F. Cyclodextrins, their value in pharmaceutical technology. Drug Dev Ind Pharm 1986;12:2193–2215.

Grant DJW, Abougela IKA. A synthetic method for determining the solubility of solids in viscous liquids. Int J Pharmaceutics 1983;16:11–21.

Grass GM, Cooper ER, Robinson JR. Mechanisms of corneal drug penetration III: modeling of molecular transport. J Pharm Sci 1988;77(1):24–6.

Grouls R, Ackerman E, Machielson E, Casparie R, Korsten H. Partition coefficients of local anaesthetics measured by HPLC. Pharm Weekbl (Sci) 1992;14(5):F27.

Higuchi T, Shih F-M L, Kimura T, Rytting JH. Solubility determination of barely aqueous-soluble organic solids. J Pharm Sci 1979;68:1267–72.

Láznicek ML, Kvetina J, Mazák J, Krch V. Plasma protein binding-lipophilicity relationships: interspecies comparison of some organic acids. J Pharm Pharmacol 1987;39:79–83

Leahy DE, De Meere ALJ, Wait AR, Taylor PJ, Tomenson JA, Tomlinson E. A general description of water-oil partitioning rates using the rotating diffusion cell. Int J Pharmaceutics 1989;50:117–32.

Lovgren T, Lundberg B, Blomqvist C, Sjoblom L. Solubilisation of spironolactone and flumedroxone acetate. Acta Pharm Suec 1978;15:233–6.

Muller BW, Brauns U. Solubilization of drugs by modified β-cyclodextrins. Int J Pharmaceutics 1985;26:77–88.

Patel MS, Elworthy PH, Dewsnup AK. Solubilisation of drugs in nonionic surfactants. J Pharm Pharmacol 1981;33:64P.

Pitha J, Pitha J. Amorphous water soluble derivatives of cyclodextrins: nontoxic dissolution enhancing excipients. J Pharm Sci 1985;74:987–90.

Pitha J, Szente L, Greenberg J. Poly-l-methionine sulphoxide: a biologically inert analogue of dimethyl sulfoxide with solubilizing potency. J Pharm Sci 1983;72:665–8.

Saleh AM, El-Khordagui LK. Hydrotropic agents: a new definition. Int J Pharmaceutics 1985;24:231–8.

Stanaszek WF, Ecanow B. Anaesthetic gas absorption properties of surfactant systems. J Pharm Sci 1972;61:860–2.

Sung C, Raeder JE, Merrill EW. Drug partitioning and release characteristics of tricyclic antidepressant drugs using a series of related hydrophilic-hydrophobic copolymers. J Pharm Sci 1990;79(9):829–36.

Takács-Novák K, Jozan M, Hermecz I, Szasz G. Lipophilicity of antibacterial fluoroquinolones. Int J Pharmaceutics 1992;79:89–96.

Tayar NE, Tsai NE, Testa B, Carrupt P-E, Leo A. Partitioning of solutes in different solvent systems: the contribution of hydrogen-bonding capacity and polarity. J Pharm Sci 1991;80(6):590–7.

Truelove J, Bawarshi-Nassar R, Chen NR, Hussain A. Solubility enhancement of some developmental anti-cancer nucleoside analogs by complexation with nicotinamide. Int J Pharmaceutics 1984;19:17–25.

Walkling WD, Chrzanowski FA, Mamajek RC, Fegely BJ, Mobley NG, Ulilli LA. Solubilisation of zomepirac. J Parenter Sci Technol 1982;36:190–3.

Wan LSC, Lee PFS. CMC of polysorbates. J Pharm Sci 1974;63:136–7.

Suspensions

A suspension is a two-phase system comprising solid particles (the disperse phase) dispersed in a liquid (the continuous phase or dispersion medium). Suspensions may be divided into **colloidal suspensions**, which are similar in appearance to solutions, and **coarse suspensions**, which contain visible solid particles.

Colloidal suspensions contain particles that are not visible to the naked eye, the particles being 1 nanometre to 1 micrometre in diameter. They can be subdivided into **lyophilic colloidal suspensions**, which form spontaneously when agents with a high affinity for the continuous phase are dispersed, and **lyophobic colloidal suspensions** which are thermodynamically unstable. Lyophobic colloids are formed either by the comminution of large particles or by the aggregation of small particles. The physicochemical properties of colloidal suspensions are primarily determined by the extensive interfacial area provided by the two phases.

The vast majority of pharmaceutical suspensions are coarse suspensions containing particles that are greater than 1 micrometre in diameter. As a dosage form, a suspension possesses many attributes. Suspensions allow the formulation of drugs that have a very low solubility in pharmaceutically acceptable liquids. In addition, suspensions in non-aqueous solvents provide a useful form of administration for drugs that degrade rapidly in aqueous solution. Suspensions can provide palatable mixtures of an insoluble derivative of a drug that in its soluble form has a highly unpleasant taste. An insoluble derivative may also be administered in suspension form to prolong the action of the drug. A wide range of pharmaceutical preparations are formulated as suspensions.

OFFICIAL EXAMPLES:
   Amitriptyline Oral Suspension BP
   Benorylate Oral Suspension BP
   Biphasic Insulin Injection BP
   Calamine Lotion BP
   Dithranol Ointment BP
   Hydrocortisone Acetate and Neomycin Ear
     Drops BP
   Insulin Zinc Suspension BP
   Magnesium Hydroxide Mixture BP
   Paracetamol Oral Suspension BP

Procaine Penicillin Injection BP
Selenium Sulphide Scalp Application BP

The desirable properties of a pharmaceutical suspension include:

- pourability and the easy removal of a dose
- ready redispersion of a settled preparation
- constant particle size distribution
- elegant smooth appearance
- resistance to microbial contamination.

Ideally, suspensions should display **thixotropic** properties; that is, they should be highly viscous at rest but thin readily on shaking. This behaviour prevents sedimentation during storage and allows the easy withdrawal of accurate dose volumes after agitation. For more information on thixotropic behaviour, see the Rheology chapter.

Suspensions are normally prepared using dispersion techniques. Shear must be applied during the dispersion process; this is often achieved, on a large scale, by using a colloid mill or ultrasound equipment, and on a small scale, with a mortar and pestle. Suspensions may also be prepared by chemical reaction or by altering the solvent, temperature, or pH conditions experienced by a previously dissolved material.

SUSPENSION THEORY

Small suspended particles confer a relatively large surface area to suspension systems. Suspensions are, therefore, associated with high interfacial tension and large surface free energy. Surface free energy may be decreased if the interfacial area afforded by the suspended particles is reduced, for example, by simple aggregation. Concentrated suspensions are particularly prone to aggregation because the suspended solid particles have an increased chance of collision. Although interparticulate interactions should ideally be avoided, most suspension formulations are a compromise. Particles with like charge avoid interaction by simply repelling each other. A charge can arise from ionisable groups on the solid surface or by the adsorption of ionic surfactants or electrolytes from the liquid medium. The anionic surfactant sodium oleate, for example, can coat solid particles to give a net negative charge, the hydrophobic portion of the surfactant binding to the solid and the hydrophilic portion oriented in close proximity to the continuous aqueous phase. The surface charge attracts ions of opposite polarity and repels ions of like polarity. The surface potential is reduced, but not completely balanced, by a layer of counter ions, known as the **Stern layer**. A **diffuse double layer** (which comprises positively-charged and negatively-charged ions, with an excess of counter ions) exists to completely balance the surface potential. The Stern layer and diffuse double layer comprise the **electrical double layer** (see Fig. 1).

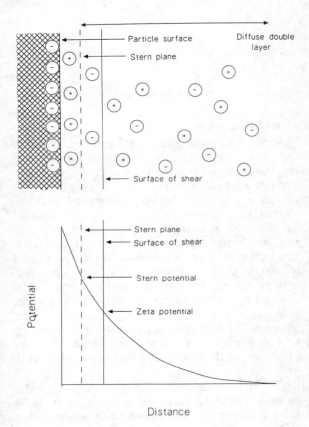

Fig. 1
Schematic representation of the electrical double layer around a negatively charged particle and the changes in potential with distance from the surface of the particle.

The ions in the Stern layer plus bound solvent molecules move with the particle and are usually considered to be part of the disperse phase. The **plane of shear** is the boundary between the Stern layer with its bound solvent molecules and the liquid bulk. The net charge at this boundary is termed the **zeta potential**, the magnitude of which determines the stability of the disperse system. Electrophoresis is used to measure the electrophoretic mobility of particles, from which the zeta potential can be calculated.

As two particles approach, several interactive forces act to determine whether the particles will collide and remain in contact, or whether they will rebound. The main forces of interaction are van der Waals (or electromagnetic) attractive forces and electrostatic repulsive forces. The repulsive forces arise from interactions of the electrical double layers; the magnitude of this repulsive force is determined by the zeta potential. These forces of attraction and repulsion are additive; the total potential energy of interaction is shown in Fig. 2.

In addition to electrostatic and van der Waals forces other types of forces can influence the interaction between particles. Such forces include: repulsive hydration or solvation forces; Born repulsive forces, which are short range and due to the overlap of atomic orbitals; and steric repulsive forces, which depend on the size, geometry, and conformation of molecules (for example, adsorbed surfactants) at the interface of particles.

Flocculation

The properties of a suspension depend to a large extent on the degree and nature of aggregation of the dispersed particles. In general, if the zeta potential lies within the range $\pm 25\,\text{mV}$, the electrical repulsive forces become insufficient to overcome the attractive van der Waals forces; the suspended system therefore becomes unstable, particles clump together, and flocculation occurs. Flocculated systems contain particles that are bound together, at the secondary minimum (see Fig. 2), in a lattice arrangement of loose aggregates or **floccules**.

The forces holding the particles together are weak and the floccules can be easily broken up and particles resuspended by simple shaking. Floccules cannot pack easily and therefore processes such as **coagulation** and **caking** are inhibited.

Flocculation can occur by a number of processes. Addition of an electrolyte may reduce the magnitude of the zeta potential of the dispersed particles and so result in flocculation. The ability of an electrolyte to reduce the value of the zeta potential is governed by the **Schulze-Hardy rule**. This states that the greater the valence of the electrolyte, the lower the concentration required to reduce the zeta potential. The Schulze-Hardy

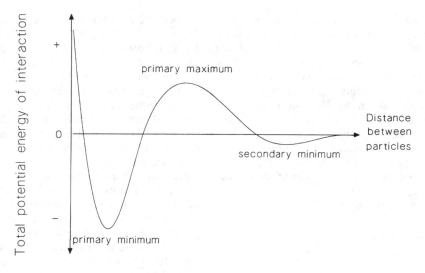

Fig. 2
Schematic representation of the total potential energy of interaction against distance between the surfaces of two particles.

rule only holds if there is no chemical interaction between the added electrolyte and the ions of the double layer.

Deflocculation

A flocculated system may become deflocculated by the continued addition of an electrolyte. At high concentration, the added electrolyte inverts the sign of the zeta potential; deflocculation occurs when the electrical repulsive force associated with the charge is of sufficient magnitude to overcome the van der Waals attractive forces.

Suspensions in which the particles remain discrete are known as deflocculated suspensions. Oily suspensions of drugs are usually deflocculated.

Deflocculated suspensions settle slowly but can cause serious redispersion problems on storage. The concentrated solid, settled at the bottom of the container, may become dilatant and extremely difficult to redisperse, a phenomenon known as **claying** or **caking**. Caking occurs at the primary minimum (see Fig. 2). Caking may be aggravated by crystal growth at the junction points between particles; this may result in a completely indispersible solid mass. Crystal growth will also lead to the formation of larger particles and perhaps bring about modifications in the bioavailability of the product. Growth is accentuated by temperature fluctuation and may, therefore, be retarded by storing the product at an even temperature. The addition of traces of nonionic surfactants may also retard crystal growth.

Flocculating Agents

Flocculating agents, such as electrolytes, are often used in pharmaceutical suspensions to prevent caking. Polymers, such as starch, sodium alginate, and carbomer, which are capable of anchoring onto the surface and bridging between suspended particles, also make good flocculating agents. Flocculated suspensions, however, sediment at an increased rate, which may cause the rapid formation of separate inelegant layers. **Controlled flocculation** is used to maximise the sedimentation volume while preventing caking. The rate of sedimentation can be reduced by increasing the viscosity of the suspension.

Microbial contamination can also cause flocculation, either by reducing the zeta potential or by interfering with a controlled flocculation process.

Sedimentation

In most pharmaceutical suspensions the particles are too large to remain permanently suspended in water as a consequence of Brownian movement. These suspensions will therefore sediment and the rate of sedimentation is related to the particle radius, the density of both the particle and the liquid, and the viscosity of the medium. These relationships are described by **Stokes' law**:

$$v = \frac{2r^2(\rho_1 - \rho_2)g}{9\eta}$$

where v is the sedimentation rate (cm/s), r is the particle radius (cm), $(\rho_1 - \rho_2)$ is the density difference between the solid and the liquid (g/cm^3), g is the acceleration due to gravity (cm/s^2), and η is the viscosity of the dispersion medium (1 poise = 10^{-1} Pa s).

The equation only holds for particles that are spherical, of uniform size, that settle at a velocity that produces no turbulence, and that exert no effect upon each other or upon the walls of the container. Particles should also exceed a critical radius, which is typically 2 to 3 micrometres for most drugs. The critical radius is the size at which gravitational forces dominate thermal forces in their influence on particle movement. Particles that are smaller than the critical radius are influenced more by thermal effects than by gravitational forces and so Brownian movement maintains the particles in suspension.

Diffusible solids, such as light kaolin and magnesium trisilicate, sediment sufficiently slowly to enable a dose to be satisfactorily removed after redispersion. Indiffusible solids, such as chalk and sulphadimidine, sediment too rapidly and require the addition of other materials to reduce the sedimentation rate to an acceptable level.

As with emulsions, the settling rate may be lowered by reducing the particle size of the solids. Although size reduction may reduce the irritancy of a solid, care must be taken to select the size for optimum bioavailability where this is important. Settling rates may also be reduced by increasing the viscosity of the vehicle. This may be achieved by the addition of viscosity-increasing agents, such as tragacanth and cellulose derivatives, or by the use of 'structured vehicles' such as bentonite, alginates, and carbomers (in higher concentration than used for flocculation). In these instances, the materials can form thixotropic gels, which may become semi-solid on standing but flow readily after agitation of the suspension. The gel network reforms quickly and prevents excessive sedimentation of the solid.

Wetting

The production of a suspension may be a problem when the solid is hydrophobic and cannot be readily wetted; air becomes entrapped in the solid particles, which float on the surface of the preparation and cling to the upper parts of the container walls. To facilitate wetting, the interfacial tension between the solid and the dispersion medium must be reduced. This can be achieved by using surfactants with HLB values (see Emulsions chapter) between about 7 and 9, such as the polysorbates or sorbitan esters, or by the addition of hydrophilic colloids such as acacia or tragacanth. Care is required when using these agents as they may promote deflocculation; in addition, surfactants may cause foaming. Solvents, such as ethanol, glycerol, and the glycols, also facilitate wetting. Only the lowest possible concentration of wetting agent should be used.

SUSPENSION STABILITY

The stability of suspensions is complex; the balance between flocculation and deflocculation is readily disturbed by small changes in pH, temperature, electrolyte and polymer concentration, and the concentration of other additives such as flavouring and colouring agents. Suspensions are adversely affected by both high and low temperatures. Refrigerators and freezers, for example, are unsuitable locations in which to store suspension systems as their cold environments can promote aggregation. Fluctuation in temperature should be avoided as this may accelerate crystal growth and lead to the formation of increasingly large particles. Very small particles may dissolve more readily than larger particles in solution; in such instances the smaller particles will go into solution and recrystallise on the larger particles. This causes coarsening of the suspension and is known as **Ostwald ripening**.

Each suspension must be considered individually and the mixing of a preformulated suspension with other materials of any kind should be avoided unless detailed information on its formula and characteristics is available.

Evaluation of Suspension Stability

To allow the rapid accumulation of data on suspension stability, a number of techniques have been used to cause the premature ageing of samples, including storage at a range of temperatures, freeze-thaw cycling techniques, and centrifugation. The following methods have been used to assess suspension stability.

Measurement of Sedimentation Volume. This involves placing a thoroughly mixed suspension in a cylinder and measuring the sedimentation volume, V, at appropriate intervals; the initial sedimentation volume (V_o) is taken to equal the total volume of the suspension. The ratio V/V_o is plotted against time and the slope of the graph used to assess stability. A zero slope, for example, indicates zero sedimentation; such a system will remain suspended over a long period and require the minimum of shaking to resuspend it. However, a suspension with a large negative slope may pose problems in that its sedimentation may be so rapid that the withdrawal of an accurate dose may be impossible.

A second test, often linked to sedimentation volume measurement, is the number of standard shakes it takes to completely resuspend a system after storage.

Rheological Techniques. Rheological measurements should be carried out on undisturbed samples at low shear rates. The instrument most commonly employed is the Brookfield viscometer. The test involves lowering a T-bar spindle through the suspension and measuring the resistance it encounters at various depths. By repeating the test at different levels, changes in aggregation can be followed.

Electrophoretic Methods. Electrophoretic methods involve the measurement of migration velocity of suspended particles under the influence of an electric field. They have been used to estimate the zeta potential.

Particle Size Analysis. Samples are subjected to particle sizing at suitable intervals using microscopic or photographic techniques. Particle sizing can only be performed on diluted suspensions, although dilution may affect the aggregation behaviour of the samples.

Miscellaneous Techniques. A number of other methods have been developed to study sedimentation, caking, and flocculation phenomena. These include measurement of filtration rates,[1] quantification of particle charges using streaming current techniques,[2] and conductance studies.[3]

SUSPENDING AND VISCOSITY-INCREASING AGENTS

Suspending and viscosity-increasing agents are used to maintain a uniform dispersion of particles that would otherwise settle rapidly to form a closely packed sediment and prevent the removal of an accurate dose. Some are also flocculating agents. The agents prevent caking either by increasing the apparent viscosity of the vehicle, thereby interfering with the sedimentation process, or by forming a physical barrier to aggregation. Suspending and viscosity-increasing agents can be categorised under five broad headings: natural polysaccharides, semi-synthetic polysaccharides, clays, synthetic agents, and miscellaneous compounds.

Natural Polysaccharides

Acacia. Acacia in aqueous solution is used as a suspending agent, usually with tragacanth, in mixtures containing resinous tinctures or powders that do not readily disperse. A mucilage may be prepared by dissolving 40 g of acacia tears, previously rinsed, in 60 mL of chloroform water. The mucilage deteriorates rapidly on storage. Solutions of acacia have remarkably low viscosity, a 30% w/v aqueous solution having a typical viscosity of only 200 centipoises (0.2 Pas), but they have a marked activity as a protective colloid, hence their use to stabilise particulate dispersions by affording protection against coagulation. The viscosity of solutions may be increased by incorporation of tragacanth as indicated above. The viscosity of acacia dispersions is greatest between pH 5 and 9; maximum stability is achieved at pH values between 3 and 9.

Acacia, being a natural product, is frequently contaminated with micro-organisms such as *Escherichia coli* and *Salmonella* species. Preservatives, such as chloroform water, benzoic acid, or hydroxybenzoates, should therefore be included in formulations.

Agar. Agar is insoluble in cold water but soluble in boiling water. Solutions demonstrate maximum stability at pH values between 4 and 10.

Carrageenan. Carrageenan is soluble in 30 parts of water at 80° forming a viscous clear or slightly opalescent solution. Dispersion is more readily achieved when an initial mixture is prepared using ethanol, glycerol, or syrup. Maximum stability is achieved at pH values between 4 and 10.

Guar Gum. Guar gum disperses in hot and cold water to form a colloidal solution. A 1% aqueous dispersion has a similar viscosity to acacia mucilage; a 3% dispersion has a similar viscosity to tragacanth mucilage. Guar gum is a poor suspending agent for insoluble powders. It is employed as a thickener in lotions in concentrations of up to 2.5%. Maximum stability is achieved at pH values between 3 and 9. Dispersions can be preserved with benzoic acid 0.2%.

Sodium Alginate. Various grades are available which yield aqueous solutions having viscosities covering the range 20 to 400 centipoises (0.02 to 0.4 Pa s) in 1% solution at 20°. Sodium alginate is slowly soluble in water. It is normally used in concentrations of between 1% and 5%. Sodium alginate has the advantage of being less variable in composition than other natural suspending agents. A 1% solution has suspending properties similar to those of tragacanth mucilage. Maximum stability is achieved at pH values between 4 and 10.

Preparation of a dispersion may be aided by first mixing the sodium alginate with a suitable dispersing agent such as sucrose, ethanol, glycerol, or propylene glycol. The solution should be prepared with a high-speed stirrer. Warming the solution to temperatures above 70° causes depolymerisation and a subsequent loss of viscosity.

Starch. Starch is usually used in combination with other suspending agents. It is an ingredient of Compound Tragacanth Powder BP 1980, see below.

Tragacanth. Tragacanth is widely used as a suspending agent in the form of tragacanth mucilage or as compound tragacanth powder. Dispersion of tragacanth alone in water is facilitated by first wetting the gum with a little ethanol, in which it is completely insoluble. The compound powder gives an easily dispersible suspending agent suitable for extemporaneous use.

COMPOUND TRAGACANTH POWDER BP 1980

Tragacanth, finely powdered	150 g
Acacia, finely powdered	200 g
Starch, finely powdered	200 g
Sucrose, finely powdered	450 g

TRAGACANTH MUCILAGE BPC 1973

Tragacanth, finely powdered	1.25 g
Ethanol (90%)	2.5 mL
Chloroform water to	100 mL

Mix the tragacanth with the ethanol in a dry bottle, add as quickly as possible, sufficient of the chloroform water to produce 100 mL, and shake vigorously.

Commercial samples of tragacanth vary considerably in their suspending properties, but some indication of these properties may be obtained from the apparent viscosity of the mucilage. Tragacanth forms highly viscous solutions and gels even at relatively low concentrations; the viscosity of a 1% solution of a high grade sample may be over 3500 centipoises (3.5 Pa s). Tragacanth gels are non-thixotropic; although stable at pH values as low as 2.5, they are most stable at pH values between 3 and 9. Tragacanth is non-toxic and almost tasteless, and is widely used to modify the continuous phase of suspensions for oral use in order to prevent settling. Its colloidal nature also modifies the flocculation characteristics, increasing the sedimentation volume and assisting resuspension.

Like all natural gums, tragacanth is likely to be heavily contaminated with bacteria. Energetic methods to reduce contamination, such as irradiation and dry heat, may seriously impair the suspending properties of the gum. A suitable quality may, however, be achieved by gassing with ethylene oxide or slurrying with ethanol/water mixtures under appropriate conditions. Preservatives must be included in the formulation of mucilages to allow long-term storage.

Xanthan Gum. Xanthan gum is soluble in hot and cold water; a 1% solution has a viscosity of about 1000 centipoises (1 Pa s). Solutions of xanthan gum demonstrate maximum stability at pH values between 4 and 10. Xanthan gum has been used as an alternative to tragacanth in the preparation of suspensions from crushed tablets.[4] Compared with tragacanth, xanthan gum was found to be easier to use and capable of preparing suspensions of better quality and of improved consistency.

Semi-synthetic Polysaccharides

The semi-synthetic polysaccharides are derivatives of the natural polysaccharide, cellulose.

Carmellose Sodium. Carmellose sodium is the sodium salt of carboxymethylcellulose. Different grades are available which yield 1% aqueous solutions with viscosities in the range 6 to 4000 centipoises (0.006 to 4 Pas). It is used at concentrations ranging from 0.25% to 1% in suspension dosage forms designed for oral, topical, and parenteral use; mucilages are most stable within the pH range 3 to 10. Carmellose is anionic and is therefore incompatible with cationic compounds. Aqueous preparations that are likely to be stored for long periods should contain an antimicrobial preservative.

Carmellose sodium can be sterilised in the dry state by maintaining at 160° for 1 hour, but this leads to a substantial decrease in viscosity and some deterioration in the other properties of solutions prepared from the sterilised material.

Sterilisation of solutions by heating also causes some lowering of viscosity, but this is much less marked. When a solution is autoclaved at 125° for 15 minutes and allowed to cool, the viscosity may be expected to decrease by about 25%; allowance should therefore be made for this when calculating the amount of carmellose sodium to be included in a preparation that is to be sterilised. See also Dispersible Cellulose below.

Hydroxyethylcellulose. Hydroxyethylcellulose is used as a viscosity-increasing agent. Various grades are available that differ in their aqueous solution viscosities. Solutions display maximum stability in the pH range 2 to 10.

Hydroxypropylcellulose. Hydroxypropylcellulose is used as a viscosity-increasing agent for oral and topical use. A wide range of grades are available that differ in their aqueous solution viscosities. Maximum stability is demonstrated at pH values between 2 and 10.

Hypromellose. Hypromellose is the hydroxypropyl derivative of methylcellulose; it has properties similar to those of methylcellulose but produces aqueous solutions with higher gel-points (for example, a 2% solution of methylcellulose 4500 gels at about 50° and a 2% solution of hypromellose 4500 gels at about 65°). Various grades are available that differ in their aqueous solution viscosities.

Methylcellulose. Methylcellulose is used as a suspending and viscosity-increasing agent. Various grades are available and are classified according to the viscosity of a 2% solution at 20°. The use of the lower viscosity grades is preferred at concentrations up to 5%. Methylcellulose disperses slowly in cold water to form a viscous colloidal solution. A mucilage may be prepared by adding the methylcellulose to about one-third the required amount of boiling water and when the powder is thoroughly hydrated, adding the remainder of the water preferably in the form of ice and stirring until homogeneous.

Methylcellulose is nonionic and is stable over a wide range of pH values. Although methylcellulose mucilages keep well, stored solutions should be adequately preserved. Suitable preservatives include phenylmercuric acetate, phenylmercuric nitrate, and chloroform water.

Microcrystalline Cellulose. Microcrystalline cellulose is widely used as a suspending agent, either alone, or in conjunction with other cellulose derivatives such as carmellose sodium or hypromellose or with clays such as bentonite.

There are two pharmaceutical grades of microcrystalline cellulose commercially available: one is a colloidal water-dispersible powder with a small average particle size and the other is a non-dispersible powder of larger average particle size. Although the particle size of the colloidal type is small, disaggregation in water by high shear produces particles of sub-micron size that interact as a network to form thixotropic gels when the concentration exceeds 1%. The degree of shear-mix-

ing required to produce a gel varies with the grade used, and the rheology of a particular grade depends on the intensity of mixing. Gel rheology does not vary greatly with temperature, permitting sterilisation by autoclaving.

The colloidal type of powder may contain a small percentage of carmellose sodium. The function of this, and other agents used to aid dispersion, is to act as a protective colloid. Unlike some naturally occurring suspending agents, microcrystalline cellulose is free from heavy microbial contamination. **Dispersible cellulose** is used as a suspending agent; it is a colloid-forming, attrited mixture of microcrystalline cellulose and carmellose sodium. Dispersions demonstrate maximum stability at pH values between 3 and 10.

Propylene Glycol Alginate. Propylene glycol alginate is used as a suspending agent. Solutions demonstrate maximum stability in the pH range 3 to 7.

Clays

Clays are inorganic materials derived from natural sources; they are predominantly hydrated silicates. Clays form highly thixotropic gels. The gels must be preserved with suitable antimicrobial agents as clays are liable to heavy contamination with microbial spores.

Aluminium Magnesium Silicate. Aluminium magnesium silicate is used as a suspending and viscosity-increasing agent, usually at a concentration of between 0.5% and 2.5%. A number of different grades are available, which are distinguished by the degree of alkalinity and the viscosity of an aqueous dispersion. For example, a dispersion prepared using an average pharmaceutical grade of aluminium magnesium silicate in water has a pH of about 9 and the viscosity of a 5% dispersion is about 250 centipoises (0.25 Pa s). Dispersions in water are thixotropic, and at a concentration of 10% a firm gel is formed. The viscosity of dispersions is increased by heating, by the addition of electrolytes, and at higher concentrations by ageing.

When aluminium magnesium silicate is used in conjunction with other suspending agents, such as methylcellulose or carmellose sodium, the dispersions produced have an enhanced viscosity; it can also be used in conjunction with natural gums such as acacia.

Bentonite. Bentonite absorbs water readily to form either sols or gels depending on its concentration; a preparation containing about 7% of bentonite is just pourable. Sols, containing between 0.5% and 5.0% bentonite, are suitable for suspending powders in aqueous preparations such as calamine lotion. Dispersions display maximum stability at pH values between 3 and 10.

In aqueous sols and gels, bentonite particles have negative charge and flocculation results if electrolytes or suspensions with positive charge are added. Sols or gels may conveniently be prepared by sprinkling portions of bentonite on the surface of hot water; when all the bentonite has become thoroughly wetted, it is left to stand for about 24 hours (with occasional stirring). Water should not be added to bentonite alone, but a satisfactory dispersion in water may be effected if the bentonite is first triturated with glycerol or powders such as calamine or zinc oxide. Bentonite is sterilised by dry heat, after previously drying at 100°; aqueous suspensions are sterilised by heating in an autoclave.

Synthetic Agents

The quality of synthetic agents tends to be less variable than that of suspending agents derived from natural sources.

Carbomer. Carbomer is an acrylic acid polymer; it disperses in water to form an acidic colloidal solution of low viscosity, which produces a highly viscous gel on neutralisation. The powder should be dispersed in water with the aid of a high-speed stirrer, and care taken to avoid the formation of indispersible lumps. The solution is then neutralised, usually with a solution of sodium hydroxide, but other bases such as triethanolamine, ammonia, and di-isopropylamine are sometimes used; each gram of carbomer requires 400 mg of sodium hydroxide for neutralisation. During preparation of the gel, the solution should be agitated slowly with a broad paddle-like stirrer and care taken to avoid the introduction of air bubbles.

Carbomer gels are most viscous between pH 6 and 11. The viscosity is reduced if the pH is less than 3 or greater than 12; electrolytes also reduce the viscosity. Carbomer is readily oxidised and formulations should be stabilised with appropriate antoxidants and chelating agents (for example, edetic acid). Suitable antimicrobial preservatives for carbomer gels include chlorocresol 0.1% and thiomersal 0.01%; higher concentrations of these substances may reduce the viscosity of the gels. Benzoic acid is not a suitable preservative since it reduces the viscosity.

Carbomer is used in the form of a neutralised gel as a suspending agent in preparations for internal and external use. The proportion depends upon the required flow properties of the preparation, the other ingredients, and the pH; carbomer 0.1% to 0.4% is usually sufficient. Gels containing 0.5% to 5% are used as aqueous ointment bases. Aqueous gels are sterilised by heating in an autoclave.

Colloidal Anhydrous Silica. Colloidal anhydrous silica acts as a suspending agent by forming a network of hydrogen-bonded particles on dispersion; this network inhibits sedimentation. It forms thixotropic gels at concentrations between 2% and 10%. However, suspensions prepared using colloidal anhydrous silica tend to cake on sedimentation.

Polyvinyl Alcohol. A range of polyvinyl alcohols of varying viscosity and saponification value are available. They are used as viscosity-increasing agents in ophthalmic preparations.

Povidone. Povidone is the pharmaceutical grade of polyvinylpyrrolidone. It is used in concentrations up to 10% as a suspending and dispersing agent. The viscosities of solutions increase with increasing molecular weight of the polymer, although the viscosities of aqueous solutions containing up to 10% of many grades do not differ significantly from water. The viscosity of solutions is not influenced by pH except in extreme cases; concentrated hydrochloric acid increases the viscosity but strong alkali will precipitate the polymer, which redissolves on the addition of water. An increase in temperature causes a significant reduction in viscosity. Aqueous solutions of povidone are stable and can be stored for long periods in suitable containers. Such solutions should contain a suitable antimicrobial preservative, such as benzoic acid or the hydroxybenzoate esters.

Miscellaneous Agents

Gelatin. Gelatin is used as a suspending and viscosity-increasing agent. Solutions demonstrate marked variations in viscosity between batches; maximum stability is achieved at pH values between 5 and 8. Gelatin is stable in air when dry, but putrefies rapidly when moist or in solution. It can be sterilised by dry heat.

Suspending Agents Suitable for Extemporaneous Dispensing

Suspensions may have to be prepared from crushed tablets or the contents of capsules for patients who are unable to swallow solid dosage forms. Such suspensions usually require a suitable suspending agent to produce a product that is not only elegant and stable but also capable of delivering the drug to the systemic circulation at an appropriate rate.

The criteria for the ideal suspending agent for extemporaneous dispensing were listed by Farley and Lund.[5] An ideal suspending agent should be:

- capable of being easily incorporated into the material to be suspended
- readily dispersed on mixing with an appropriate vehicle without recourse to special techniques
- capable of providing a uniform and stable suspension which is readily redispersed and which does not cake
- inert with regard to the absorption rates and profiles of suspended active materials
- non-toxic and compatible with other formulation ingredients
- of an acceptable odour, colour, and taste
- free of microbial contamination
- readily available and inexpensive.

Tragacanth is the most widely used suspending agent in extemporaneous dispensing. It is, however, variable in composition, unstable to heat sterilisation, and prone to microbial contamination. Pregelatinised starch, sodium starch glycollate, carmellose sodium, microcrystalline cellulose, alginate salts, and aluminium magnesium silicate were studied by Farley and Lund[5] as possible alternatives to tragacanth for use in extemporaneous dispensing. The prepared suspensions were assessed with respect to their ease of manufacture, sedimentation characteristics, and ease of redispersion. Of the materials studied, sodium starch glycollate was most suitable as a general-purpose suspending agent.

Trevean[6] studied a number of suspending agents (carmellose sodium, tragacanth, carbomer 934, carbomer 940, aluminium magnesium silicate, sodium alginate, methylcellulose, and guar gum) and assessed their properties with respect to rheology, sedimentation, caking, and drug delivery. Of the suspending agents studied, tragacanth, carmellose sodium, and guar gum were found to be the most suitable for extemporaneous use.

SMALL-SCALE PREPARATION OF SUSPENSIONS

Crystalline and granular solids should be finely powdered and intimately mixed with any solid suspending agent. A small portion of the liquid vehicle or suspending mucilage should be added and the mixture thoroughly triturated until a smooth creamy paste free from lumps is formed. Where viscous liquids such as glycerol or syrups are included in the formulation it is advantageous to use them to form the paste. Any wetting agents should also be added at this time. Soluble solids should be dissolved in the remainder of the vehicle, which should then be added gradually; the mixture should be triturated to a smooth consistency between each addition.

REFERENCES

1. Dakkuri A, Ecanow B. J Pharm Sci 1976;65:420–3.
2. Shah DG, Sheth BB. Drug Dev Ind Pharm 1978;4:209–23.
3. Ecanow B, Webster JM, Blake MI. J Pharm Sci 1982;71:456–7.
4. Pharm J 1986;237:665.
5. Farley CA, Lund W. Pharm J 1976;216:562–6.
6. Trevean MA. NZ Pharm 1981;1:42–9.

FURTHER INFORMATION

Suspension theory. Kayes JB. Pharmaceutical suspensions: micro-electrophoretic properties. J Pharm Pharmacol 1977;29:163–8.

Rawlins DA, Kayes JB. Steric stabilisation of suspensions. Drug Dev Ind Pharm 1980;6:427–40.

Flocculation. Heyd A, Dhabhar D. Particle shape effect on caking of coarse granulated antacid suspensions. Drug Cosmet Ind 1979;125:42–5, 146–7.

Hiestand EN. Physical properties of coarse suspensions. J Pharm Sci 1972;61:268–72.

Kayes JB. Pharmaceutical suspensions: relation between zeta potential, sedimentation volume and suspension stability. J Pharm Pharmacol 1977;29:199–204.

Schott H. Controlled flocculation of coarse suspensions by colloidally dispersed solids. I. Interaction of bismuth subnitrate with bentonite. J Pharm Sci 1976;65:855–61.

Van Mil PJJM. Flocculation of coarse suspensions in non-polar media. Pharm Weekbl (Sci) 1984;6:121–2.

Zatz JL, Lue R-Y. Flocculation of suspensions containing nonionic surfactants by sorbitol. J Pharm Sci 1987;76:157–60.

Suspension stability. Law SL, Kayes JB. Stability of suspensions in the presence of nonionic water-soluble cellulose polymers. Drug Dev Ind Pharm 1984;10:1049–69.

Plaizier-Vercammen JA, Janssens E. A universal method to obtain stable and easily redispersible suspensions. Labo Pharma Probl Tech 1984;32:583–7.

Rohdewald P. Quality of suspensions. Cosmet Perfum 1975;90:35–45.

Zatz JL. Physical stability of suspensions. J Soc Cosmet Chem 1985;36:393–411.

Zatz JL, Lue R-Y. Effect of polyols on physical stability of suspensions containing nonionic surfactant. J Soc Cosmet Chem 1982;33:149–55.

Suspending and viscosity-increasing agents. Altagracia M, Ford I, Garzon ML, Kravzov J. A comparative mineralogical and physicochemical study of some crude Mexican and pharmaceutical grade montmorillonites. Drug Dev Ind Pharm 1987;13:2249–62.

Barry BW, Meyer MC. The rheological properties of carbopol gels. I. Continuous shear and creep properties of carbopol gels. Int J Pharmaceutics 1979;2:1–25.

Campbell M. Some incompatibilities of methyl cellulose and sodium carboxymethylcellulose [carmellose sodium]. Australas J Pharm 1957;38:1029.

Hartman AW, Nesbitt RU, Smith FM, Nuessle NO. Viscosities of acacia and sodium alginate after sterilisation by cobalt-60. J Pharm Sci 1975;64:802–5.

Haugen P, Tung MA, Runikis JO. Steady shear flow properties, rheological reproducibility and stability of aqueous hydroxyethylcellulose dispersions. Can J Pharm Sci 1978;13:4–7.

Huikari A. Effect of heat sterilisation on the viscosity of methylcellulose solutions. Acta Pharm Fenn 1986;95:9–17.

Huikari A, Hinkkanen R, Michelsson H, Uotila J, Kristoffersson E. Effect of heat sterilisation on the molecular weight of methylcellulose, determined using high pressure gel filtration chromatography and viscometry. Acta Pharm Fenn 1986;95:105–11.

Huikari A, Kristoffersson E. Rheological properties of methylcellulose solutions: general flow properties and effects of added substances. Acta Pharm Fenn 1985;94:143–54.

Jacobs GP, Simes R. The gamma irradiation of tragacanth: effect on the microbial contamination and rheology. J Pharm Pharmacol 1979;31:333–4.

Levy G, Schwarz TW. The role of residual calcium in the viscosity changes of sodium alginate solutions. J Am Pharm Assoc Sci Ed 1958;47:455–7.

Levy G, Schwarz TW. Tragacanth solutions. I. The relation of method of preparation to the viscosity and stability. J Am Pharm Assoc (Sci) 1958;47:451–4.

McCarthy TJ, Myburgh JA. The effect of tragacanth gel on preservative activity. Pharm Weekbl 1974;109:265–8.

Marshall K, Sixsmith D. Some physical characteristics of microcrystalline cellulose. Drug Dev Commun 1974-5;1:51–71.

Myburgh JA, McCarthy TJ. The influence of suspending agents on preservative activity in aqueous solid/liquid dispersions. Pharm Weekbl (Sci) 1980;2:143–8.

Schwarz TW, Levy G. A report on the oxidative degradation of neutralised carbopol. J Am Pharm Assoc (Sci) 1958;47:442–3.

Schwarz TW, Levy G. Viscosity changes of sodium alginate solutions after freezing and thawing. J Am Pharm Assoc (Sci) 1957;46:562–3.

Schwarz TW, Levy G, Kawagoe HH. Tragacanth solutions. III. The effect of pH on the stability. J Am Pharm Assoc (Sci) 1958;47:695–6.

Tempio JS, Zatz JL. Flocculation effect of xanthan gum in pharmaceutical suspensions. J Pharm Sci 1980;69:1209–14.

Tillman WJ, Kuramoto R. A study of the interaction between methylcellulose and preservatives. J Am Pharm Assoc (Sci) 1957;46:211–14.

Zatz JL, Knapp S. Viscosity of xanthan gum solutions at low shear rates. J Pharm Sci 1984;73:468–71.

Zatz JL, Sarpotdar P, Gergich G, Wong A. Effect of surfactants on the flocculation of magnesium carbonate suspensions by xanthan gum. Int J Pharmaceutics 1981;9:315–19.

Emulsions

An emulsion consists of two immiscible liquid phases, one of which is finely subdivided and uniformly dispersed as droplets in the other. This thermodynamically unstable system is stabilised by the presence of emulsifying agents.

In pharmaceutical emulsions, one phase is usually water and the other an oil, fat, or waxy substance. Systems in which oil is the disperse, discontinuous, or internal phase and water is the continuous phase, dispersion medium, or external phase are termed **oil-in-water** emulsions. Conversely, **water-in-oil** emulsions are those in which the aqueous phase is dispersed in the oil. The ratio of the disperse phase volume to the total volume is known as the **phase volume** or **phase volume ratio**. Emulsions can vary in viscosity from liquid to semi-solid. In pharmaceutical practice, it has been generally accepted that the title 'emulsions' is applied to liquid preparations intended for oral administration. Emulsions for external application are usually referred to as creams (semi-solids), lotions, or liniments (liquids). Several of the emulsifying agents described in this chapter are only suitable for inclusion in products intended for external use.

Emulsions for oral ingestion are almost invariably of the oil-in-water type. For oils with a disagreeable taste or unpleasant consistency, the external aqueous phase of an oil-in-water emulsion may provide a degree of taste masking. Intestinal absorption may be enhanced when globules are homogenised to below one micrometre in diameter. Sterile oil-in-water emulsions, particularly of soya bean oil, may be used with other nutrients to feed patients intravenously (see Parenteral and Enteral Nutrition Fluids chapter). The oil globules in such emulsions must be about one micrometre and not greater than five micrometres in diameter, and the emulsifying agent must be carefully selected.

Emulsified systems have also been used successfully in X-ray diagnostic work, in the formulation of depot preparations for intramuscular administration, and in the formulation of perfluorohydrocarbons for use as oxygen carriers in blood replacement therapy.

Emulsions typically contain globules ranging from 0.1 to 100 micrometres in diameter. **Micro-emulsions**, however, contain globules that have diameters of less than 0.1 micrometre. Droplets of such dimensions cannot refract light and, as a result, are invisible to the naked eye. Micro-emulsions are, therefore, transparent systems. They may also be unstable as Brownian movement of the colloidal particles and subsequent collision may lead to coalescence and the formation of larger globules of reduced mobility.

EMULSION THEORY

Two distinct layers form when two immiscible liquids are placed together in a container. Molecules at the interface experience a larger attractive force from molecules of their own kind than from molecules of the other liquid. Interfacial molecules, therefore, experience a force pulling them away from the other liquid phase. This creates an **interfacial tension**, the strength of which depends on the immiscibility of the two media.

Agitation of the interface leads to the dispersion of one liquid as droplets in the other. This leads to an increase in the interfacial area of the system and to a rise in free energy. The system is, therefore, thermodynamically unstable and the two phases will reform when the agitation stops.

Stabilisation of the emulsion system may be achieved at the interface by the addition of an emulsifying agent. The question of which immiscible liquid will form the disperse phase and which the continuous phase depends on a number of factors including the properties of the liquids and of the emulsifying agent employed. Simplistically, the liquid present in the greater quantity will tend to form the continuous phase.

STABILITY OF EMULSIONS

There are two principal requirements to ensure the stability of emulsions. First, there should be no appreciable change in either the mean particle size or the size distribution of the droplets of the disperse phase throughout the shelf-life of the product. Secondly, there should be a homogeneous distribution of the emulsified droplets throughout the system.

Flocculation

Flocculation is the clumping together of globules into loose aggregates. The aggregates can often be redispersed by shaking as the interfacial films do not necessarily break. However, it is usual for flocculation to precede **coalescence**. Whereas flocculation is influenced by the electrical potential on the surface of the droplets, coalescence depends upon the structure of the interfacial film.

Creaming

Creaming occurs in oil-in-water emulsions when the dispersed oil globules move upwards and accumulate at the top. In water-in-oil emulsions, sedimentation occurs owing to the accumulation of water droplets at the bottom. A creamed emulsion can usually be redispersed by agitation; however, creaming is undesirable because the closeness of the droplets in the cream favours breakdown of the oil/water interface and coalescence of the droplets. Since large droplets cream rapidly and coalesce more readily in the cream layer, the emulsion may eventually crack (see below).

Reducing the particle size of the dispersed globules, equalising of the densities of the oil and water phases, and increasing the viscosity of the system are methods by which the rate of creaming can be reduced. The viscosity of an emulsion may be increased by homogenisation, by increasing the concentration of the disperse phase, by increasing the concentration of the emulsifying agent, by adding solid or semi-solid materials to the disperse phase, or by adding viscosity-increasing agents to oil-in-water emulsions.

Cracking

Rupture of the interfacial film can lead to coalescence of the globules in the disperse phase. Coalescence may lead eventually to the complete and irreversible separation of the two phases; the term cracking is applied to such phase separation.

Film breakdown can often arise from chemical incompatibility of the emulsifying agent with other constituents of the system; it may also be induced by exposure to increased or reduced temperatures or by the action of contaminant micro-organisms. Systems with a large phase volume and a closely packed disperse phase are prone to cracking.

Phase Inversion

Phase inversion is the process by which the disperse phase of an emulsion becomes the continuous phase, and the continuous phase becomes the disperse phase. Following phase inversion, an oil-in-water emulsion, for example, becomes a water-in-oil emulsion.

Phase inversion may occur in a number of ways. If the amount of the disperse phase is increased until it approaches or exceeds the theoretical maximum of 74% of the total volume, the emulsion may invert; alternatively, the emulsion may break down completely. Temperature changes, or the addition of a material that changes the solubility of the emulsifying agent, may also cause phase inversion. Phase inversion occurs at the phase inversion temperature. Inversion may also occur in systems manufactured using dirty equipment or prepared using incorrect mixing procedures.

Evaluation of Emulsion Stability

Emulsion stability may be assessed after storage of the product for the proposed shelf-life; this, however, is time-consuming and most workers rely on accelerated tests to provide information on long-term stability. Accelerated tests involve placing the emulsion under stress; this is normally applied using agitation, centrifugation, or temperature manipulation techniques.

Agitation increases the rate at which droplets meet and therefore decreases the time-scale over which collisions occur. **Centrifugation** rapidly induces creaming or coalescence in potentially unstable systems. Conditions should be carefully chosen to prevent distortion of the droplets or disruption of the interfacial film. **Temperature** manipulations, such as alternating between high and low temperatures, are the most commonly employed type of accelerated stability tests. Extremes of temperature, however, should be avoided.

Various physical parameters including phase separation, viscosity, electrophoretic properties, particle size, and particle counts are used to monitor the stability of emulsions during these tests.

FORMULATION

Antoxidants

In an emulsion where air may be incorporated during preparation and there is a large oil/water interface, conditions can be suitable for oxidation of the unsaturated organic compounds present in the vegetable oils, mineral oils, vitamin oils, and steroidal materials that are common constituents of emulsions. Inhibition of the rancidity and spoilage that can result from oxidation can be achieved by the inclusion of antoxidants such as the alkyl gallates, butylated hydroxyanisole, butylated hydroxytoluene, and tocopherols. Antoxidants and chelating agents are discussed in the chapter on Stability of Medicinal Products.

Preservation

Adequate preservation of emulsions is necessary as micro-organisms can proliferate in emulsified systems with a high water content, particularly if carbohydrates, proteins, or steroidal materials are also present. Contamination may occur during preparation from raw materials or equipment, or during the use of the product. Emulsions must therefore be adequately preserved.

The polymorphic nature of emulsions presents special problems in preservation due to partitioning of the preservative between the oily and the aqueous phases. To protect the product it is necessary to have an effective bactericidal and fungicidal concentration of preservative in the aqueous phase; however, in order to achieve this the total concentration of preservative required may be clinically unacceptable if the preservative has a high partition coefficient between the particular oil and water.

Examples of antimicrobial agents used to preserve emulsion systems include chlorocresol, chloroform, hydroxybenzoate esters, organic acids such as sorbic acid and benzoic acid, organic mercurials such as phenylmercuric acetate and phenylmercuric nitrate, phenoxyethanol, quaternary ammonium compounds such as cetrimide, and sodium benzoate.

Other problems in emulsion systems can arise from interactions between preservatives and constituents of the emulsion. The presence of nonionic emulsifying agents such as polysorbates or compounds with polyoxyethylene groups can inhibit or inactivate phenolic preservatives, while hydroxybenzoate esters can be partially inactivated by binding with polysorbates, povidone, certain macrogols, methylcellulose, and gelatin. Complexation of methylcellulose with hydroxybenzoates has also been reported.

Emulsifying Agents

Emulsifying agents prevent coalescence of the dispersed globules in emulsified systems by forming barriers at the interface; they may also facilitate the initial dispersion of globules by reducing interfacial tension. The stability of a prepared emulsion is primarily determined by the strength and nature of the interfacial film formed. It is important to use only the minimum concentration of the chosen emulsifying agent as any excess may result in the formation of a foam.

The ideal emulsifying agent for pharmaceutical purposes should be stable, inert, and free from toxic and irritant properties; it should be odourless, tasteless, colourless, and low concentrations should produce stable emulsions of the desired type. Although emulsifying agents of natural origin are widely used in pharmaceutical emulsions, the number of synthetic emulsifying agents that can be used in emulsions for oral ingestion is relatively small.

Emulsifying agents can be broadly classified into three groups: surfactants, those derived from natural products, and finely divided solids.

Surfactants

Surfactants contain both hydrophilic and lipophilic regions in their molecular structure. An efficient emulsifying agent should have both lipophilic and hydrophilic properties in reasonable balance, such that at the interfaces of the system, the lipophilic non-polar groups of the surfactant, which are attracted to the oil phase, and the hydrophilic polar groups, which are oriented towards the water, should form a stable film. The interfacial film is believed to comprise a lamellar liquid crystal structure in which the water, the emulsifying agent, and the oil alternate in consecutive layers. This film acts as a mechanical barrier to coalescence by physical or chemical effects due to the adsorbed emulsifying agent, by the repulsive effect of electrically charged groups, or by a combination of the two.

Cationic, anionic, and ampholytic surfactants provide a surface charge to dispersed globules; the concept of dispersed charged particles is treated in the Suspensions chapter. The location of the surface activity on dissociation can be used to divide the surfactants into four groups:

- anionic,
- cationic,
- nonionic, and
- ampholytic.

Anionic Surfactants. Soaps formed from long-chain (C_{12} to C_{18}) fatty acids, sulphated alcohols, and sulphonates comprise many of the anionic emulsifying agents in common use. On dissociation, the long-chain anion imparts surface activity, while the cation is inactive. Soaps and similar anionic agents are unsuitable for emulsions intended for internal use because of their unpleasant taste and irritant action on the intestinal mucosa.

Fatty acids, such as stearic acid, are useful emulsifying agents. They are normally used after partial neutralisation with inorganic or organic bases.

Alkali metal and ammonium soaps comprise the ammonium, potassium, and sodium salts of long-chain fatty acids. Good oil-in-water emulsions can be prepared from the alkali soaps, but they become unstable below pH 10 and are incompatible with acids and polyvalent inorganic and long-chain organic cations. An example of this group of emulsifying agents is sodium stearate.

Soaps of divalent and trivalent metals, such as calcium, magnesium, zinc, and aluminium are water-insoluble and form water-in-oil emulsions; an example is calcium stearate.

Amine soaps yield oil-in-water emulsions and are made *in situ* by reaction between amines such as ethanolamine, diethanolamine, triethanolamine, or isopropanolamine and fatty acids such as oleic acid; they are less alkaline than alkali soaps (about pH 8) and more resistant to the presence of calcium ions or changes in pH.

Alkyl sulphates are the esters formed when fatty alcohols react with sulphuric acid. Examples include sodium lauryl sulphate, sodium ceto-stearyl sulphate, and triethanolamine lauryl sulphate. The alkyl sulphates form oil-in-water emulsions, but the dispersions usually require a secondary emulsifying agent to achieve adequate stability. Such emulsions have a pH of approximately 7 and are fairly resistant to pH change. Alkyl sulphates are liable to hydrolysis so pH control is important. They are widely used as wetting agents.

Alkyl phosphates are the esters formed when fatty alcohols react with phosphoric acid; they have similar properties to the alkyl sulphates.

Alkyl sulphonates are less liable to hydrolysis than the alkyl sulphates. Docusate sodium, for example, is an effective wetting agent and forms oil-in-water emulsions preferentially when supplemented with a secondary emulsifying agent.

Carbomer, a synthetic carboxyvinyl anionic polymer, can be used to prepare oil-in-water emulsions for both internal and external use. It is usually used in combination with other emulsifying agents.

Cationic Surfactants. Cationic surfactants dissociate to yield a surface-active cation and an inactive anion (see also the Disinfectants and Antiseptics chapter). Like the anionic surfactants, they require to be ionised to be effective. Quaternary ammonium compounds, such as **cetrimide**, **benzalkonium chloride**, and **domiphen bromide**, are the most important cationic surfactants. They are used in combination with secondary emulsifying agents to prepare oil-in-water emulsions for external application; such emulsions are stable over the pH range 3 to 7. Cationic agents are compatible with divalent inorganic anions, but incompatible with inorganic anions of higher valency and with long-chain organic anions.

Nonionic Surfactants. The nonionic surfactants constitute the largest group of surface active compounds and are used to produce oil-in-water and water-in-oil emulsions for both external and internal administration.

The advantages of nonionic derivatives include their resistance to the effects of electrolytes, their compatibility with other surfactants, and their stability, in general, between pH 4 and 9. Surfactants containing ester groups, however, may hydrolyse rapidly at pH values above 9. Emulsions made with nonionic surfactants are usually less irritant than those made with ionic derivatives. Some agents, such as polysorbates and sorbitan esters, are therefore suitable for inclusion in emulsions intended for oral administration.

A disadvantage of nonionic surfactants is their tendency, when present in excess, to bind or to inactivate preservatives having phenolic or carboxylic acid groups. Nonionic surfactants can be made, often by the use of long-chain ethylene oxide polymers, in different physical forms with varying hydrophilic and lipophilic characteristics. The type of emulsion produced can depend on the hydrophilic-lipophilic balance of the surfactant and this may be defined by the HLB number (see below).

Esters of polyhydric alcohols include the glycol and glycerol esters. Glyceryl monostearate is a typical glyceryl ester, being predominantly lipophilic and insoluble in water; it is a poor emulsifying agent, but an effective stabiliser. Examples of glycol esters include propylene glycol alginate, propylene glycol diacetate, and propylene glycol monostearate.

Macrogol esters form oil-in-water and water-in-oil emulsions that are less resistant to pH changes than those prepared with macrogol ethers. Examples include polyoxyl 8 stearate, polyoxyl 40 stearate, and polyoxyl 50 stearate; the numbers refer to the approximate number of oxyethylene subunits that make up the polymer. Cetostearyl alcohol is often used as a stabiliser in systems emulsified by macrogol esters. Polyoxyl 35 castor oil and polyoxyl 40 hydrogenated castor oil are prepared by reacting ethylene oxide with either glycerol ricinoleate or glycerol trihydroxystearate, respectively.

Sorbitan esters such as sorbitan monolaurate, sorbitan mono-oleate, sorbitan monopalmitate, and sorbitan monostearate, which have predominant lipophilic elements, produce water-in-oil emulsions. They are often used in combination with polysorbates to stabilise both water-in-oil and oil-in-water systems.

The **polysorbates** are polyoxyethylene sorbitan fatty acid esters; they are formed by copolymerising 20 moles of ethylene oxide with one mole of a mixture comprising the partial fatty acid esters of sorbitol and its mono- and di-anhydrates. By altering the type of fatty acid and the number of oxyethylene groups contained within the molecule a wide range of products can be formed. Examples include polysorbate 20 (polyoxyethylene 20 sorbitan monolaurate), polysorbate 60 (polyoxyethylene 20 sorbitan monostearate), polysorbate 80 (polyoxyethylene 20 sorbitan mono-oleate). The polysorbates yield oil-in-water emulsions of good stability that are resistant to pH changes and electrolytes.

Macrogol ethers (polyoxyethylene alkyl ethers) produce stable emulsions that are capable of withstanding contact with acids and alkalis; they are often used in combination with a long-chain alcohol. Examples include cetomacrogol 1000, polyoxyl 10 oleyl ether, and polyoxyl 20 cetostearyl ether.

Long-chain alcohols act as weak water-in-oil emulsifying agents. Their main function, however, is to act as stabilisers of oil-in-water systems. Examples include cetostearyl alcohol, cetyl alcohol, oleyl alcohol, and stearyl alcohol.

Poloxamers are macrogol-polyoxypropylene-macrogol copolymers; they are available in a number of grades, each represented by a three-digit number, for example, poloxamer 188. The first two digits represent the approximate average molecular weight of the polyoxypropylene portion of the molecule divided by 10, and the last digit represents the percentage by weight of the polyoxyethylene portions divided by 10. Water solubility increases as the polyoxyethylene content of the molecule increases.

Polyvinyl alcohols are prepared by the hydrolysis of polyvinyl acetate. A range of polyvinyl alcohols are available commercially with different viscosity and saponification values. They are used as emulsion stabilisers.

Ampholytic Surfactants. Ampholytic surfactants are not widely used as emulsifying agents; their chief applications are as bactericidal detergents (see the Disinfectants and Antiseptics chapter) or in shampoos that are not irritant to the eyes. The ionic characteristics of ampholytic emulsifying agents depend on the pH of the system; below a specific acid pH for each agent they are cationic and above a defined alkaline pH they are anionic, while at intermediate pH they behave as zwitterions.

Ampholytic surfactants may be incompatible with long-chain organic ions because of their ionic nature. The main types of ampholytic substances are available as fatty acid derivatives, amino acids, and long-chain betaines.

Surfactant Selection. Generally, a surfactant with a large hydrophilic group compared with the nonpolar lipophilic portion of the molecule favours formation of an oil-in-water emulsion. A surfactant with a relatively larger lipophilic group tends to produce a water-in-oil emulsion. The degree to which the surfactant is soluble in each phase may give an indication of the type of emulsion that will be formed, although other factors such as viscosity and phase volume ratio will also have an influence.

The HLB System. The balance between the hydrophilic and lipophilic moieties of a surface-active molecule has been used as the basis for a more rational means of selecting and classifying emulsifying agents than the empirical methods traditionally used. In the HLB (hydrophile-lipophile balance) system, which was originally developed for nonionic surfactants, each emulsifying agent is assigned a number between 1 and 20. In the case of nonionic substances the number is calculated from the hydrocarbon chain length and the number of polar groupings; for other surfactants HLB values have been derived from other characteristics such as water solubility, dielectric constant, interfacial tension, and cloud points, as a rough guide. Surfactants with HLB values of between 3 and 6 are lipophilic and form water-in-oil emulsions, while values of 8 to 18 indicate predominantly hydrophilic characteristics and the formation of oil-in-water emulsions. See Table 1.

Table 1
The relationship between HLB numbers and surfactant properties

HLB range	Property
4–6	emulsifying agents (water-in-oil)
7–9	wetting agents
8–18	emulsifying agents (oil-in-water)
13–15	detergents
10–18	solubilising agents

Extensive lists of HLB values for emulsifying agents have appeared in the literature. In addition, many oils and waxy materials used in emulsions have been given a 'required HLB' value, determined by experiment, to facilitate the selection of the appropriate emulsifying agent. See Table 2.

Table 2
Required HLB values for oils and waxes

| | Emulsion type | |
	oil-in-water	water-in-oil
Beeswax	12	5
Castor oil	14	—
Cetyl alcohol	15	—
Cottonseed oil	9	—
Paraffin, hard	10	4
Paraffin, liquid	12	4
Paraffin, soft	12	4
Stearic acid	16	—
Wool fat	10	8

Since HLB values can be added it is possible to calculate the amounts required for a mixture of two surfactants, one of low HLB and the other of high HLB value in order to obtain a blend of appropriate HLB for the oil to be emulsified. Greater efficiency is often obtained by using a blend of surfactants in this manner instead of a single substance. The following example illustrates the method used to determine the proportions of two surfactants.

Polysorbate 80 (HLB = 15) and sorbitan mono-oleate (HLB = 4.3) are to be used as the emulsifying agents in the following oil-in-water system:

Liquid paraffin (required HLB = 12)	30 g
Wool fat (required HLB = 10)	5 g
Emulsifying agents (polysorbate 80)	
(sorbitan mono-oleate)	5 g
Water	to 100 g

1. Required HLB for the oily phase

$$= \frac{30}{35} \times 12 + \frac{5}{35} \times 10 = 11.7$$

2. Proportion of emulsifying agents required can then be calculated. If X is the percentage of polysorbate 80 in the blend $100 - X$ is the percentage of sorbitan mono-oleate.

Required HLB

$$= 11.7 = \frac{X}{100} \times 15 + \frac{(100 - X)}{100} \times 4.3$$

$$X = 69\%$$

Therefore, in the final formulation the content of polysorbate 80 is 3.45 g and of sorbitan mono-oleate is 1.55 g.

The HLB system was originally devised for non-ionic surfactants, but it has since been extended to include anionic and cationic substances. Some modification has been necessary and in the case of sodium lauryl sulphate, which has marked hydrophilic activity, an HLB number of 40 has been allocated.

HLB values may not be precise and several pairs of different surfactants with the same HLB numbers may not produce similar emulsions. It is often necessary to prepare a series of emulsions in order to determine the optimum combination. Moreover, the HLB calculations do not take into account the total concentration of surfactants to be used. As a guide, 2% is considered optimum, and 5% maximum, but again a series of samples may have to be prepared to determine the optimum concentration.

Emulsifying Agents Derived from Natural Products

Many traditional emulsifying agents are derived from plant or animal sources. Such substances are often complex and of undefined or variable chemical composition; they are thus subject to considerable variation in emulsifying power. In most cases, the mode of action of natural emulsifying agents is more dependent on increasing the viscosity of the aqueous phase than on surface activity at the interface and they are frequently used as stabilisers in conjunction with a primary emulsifying agent.

The presence of microbial contamination is a major limitation of many natural emulsifying agents and this can lead to rapid spoilage unless adequate preservatives are included. Some vegetable materials may hydrolyse on storage with consequent reduction in emulsifying power.

Polysaccharides. Polysaccharides, derived from vegetable sources, are prone to hydrolysis and depolymerisation. Degradation results in loss of emulsifying power, especially at high pH or when grossly contaminated with micro-organisms (for which they provide good culture media).

In this group, **tragacanth** and **acacia** have been the most widely used, particularly in emulsions for internal use. Acacia yields stable emulsions of low viscosity which are often thickened with other gums such as tragacanth or agar. Emulsions of tragacanth alone are less stable and of coarser texture than those of acacia. **Agar** is a poor emulsifying agent but produces viscous mucilages or gels; it is included in concentrations of about 1% as a stabiliser in acacia emulsions. **Starch** is also a poor emulsifying agent but acts as a stabiliser by forming a continuous phase of high viscosity. **Pectin** has also been used as an emulsion stabiliser.

Carrageenan is a more effective viscosity-increasing agent than primary emulsifying agents. Other emulsifying agents derived from seaweed include the salts of alginic acid, such as **sodium alginate**, which are available in a range of viscosity grades of reasonable consistency. They are used at a concentration of about 1% as thickeners and stabilisers, but tend to precipitate at pH values below 5 or in the presence of heavy metal ions.

Carmellose sodium (sodium carboxymethylcellulose), **hydroxypropylcellulose**, and **methylcellulose** are commonly used as emulsifying and viscosity-increasing agents; they are available in various viscosity grades. Methylcellulose and hydroxypropylcellulose are nonionic while carmellose sodium is anionic.

Steroidal Materials. Steroidal emulsifying agents derived from animals include **wool fat**, **wool alcohols**, **beeswax**, **cholesterol**, and the bile salts **sodium glycocholate** and **sodium taurocholate**. Wool fat and wool alcohols are used in topical preparations; they absorb water and form water-in-oil emulsions with other oils and fats. Wool alcohol is a more effective emulsifying agent than wool fat but both substances can be chemically modified to liquid or solid forms with different solvent and surface-active characteristics.

Mineral oil and lanolin alcohols, a mixture also used as an emulsifying agent, is obtained by dissolving, in liquid paraffin, the surface active alcohols derived from the fractionation of saponified wool alcohols. It forms water-in-oil emulsions but can be used as a stabiliser of oil-in-water systems.

Cholesterol and related sterols are the principal emulsifying agents in lanolin products and beeswax; cholesterol also emulsifies the fatty substances in the human diet in conjunction with the bile salts and pancreatic fluids.

Glycerides. **Monoglycerides** and **diglycerides** have been used as emulsifying agents.

Phospholipids. The chief phospholipid is **lecithin**, present in egg-yolk and soya bean oil. Lecithin shows surface activity and yields oil-in-water emulsions; it also has antoxidant activity but degrades rapidly in unpreserved systems. In oil-in-water emulsions made with egg-yolk the hydrophilic effect of lecithin exceeds the lipophilic affinity of the cholesterol and a high degree of stability is obtained. One egg-yolk will emulsify approximately 60 mL of volatile oil or 120 mL of fixed oils; such emulsions must contain a preservative.

Proteins. **Gelatin** and **casein** are only of limited value as emulsifying agents, particularly in small-scale production; however, oil-in-water emulsions can be produced and improved by homogenisation. If type A (cationic) gelatin is used, acidic emulsions of pH 3 can be prepared, while for emulsions of pH 8 and above, type B gelatin is used.

Saponins. **Saponins** are effective primary emulsifying agents with marked surface activity, which have only limited use in pharmacy in the form of quillaia liquid extract. The use of saponins in medicines for internal administration has aroused controversy because of their irritant and haemolytic effects.

Finely Divided Solids

Colloidal particles are not easily wetted; they accumulate at oil/water interfaces to yield solid interfacial films. A number of colloidal clays and several inorganic substances are effective emulsifying agents when in the finely divided state and although the emulsions that result are often of coarse texture they show good stability and are less prone to microbial spoilage than many of those made with natural emulsifying agents. The texture of the emulsions may be improved by the addition of surfactants.

Of the colloidal clays, one of the most widely used in pharmacy is **bentonite**; others are **aluminium magnesium silicate**, **attapulgite**, **colloidal anhydrous silica**, and **hectorite**. The clays absorb considerable amounts of water to form gels, and in concentrations of 2% to 5% usually form oil-in-water emulsions, although bentonite will stabilise emulsion systems of either type.

Insoluble hydroxides and oxides of aluminium and magnesium can be absorbed at oil/water interfaces and are, therefore, of value as emulsifying agents though relatively high concentrations are required. **Hydrated aluminium oxide** will emulsify oils in a disperse phase containing ethanol and will also stabilise water-in-oil emulsions. **Magnesium hydroxide** and **magnesium oxide** will form oil-in-water emulsions that usually require homogenisation.

Mixed Emulsifying Agents

More rigid interfacial films can often be achieved by the use of two emulsifying agents. Ionic surfactants, for example, form expanded films when used alone and produce relatively poor emulsions. They may, however, form complexes with nonionic compounds and produce charged condensed complex films which act as electrical energy barriers to coalescence. These nonionic secondary emulsifying agents or stabilisers are usually long-chain alcohols, steroidal materials, or nonionic surfactants of low HLB number, all of which are themselves water-in-oil emulsifying agents. Examples are cetostearyl alcohol, beeswax, and glyceryl monostearate.

Complexes may also be formed between nonionic surfactants of high and low HLB numbers; the emulsions produced are superior to those formed from a single surfactant. It is often found that the best results are obtained from pairs of compounds that have the same hydrocarbon chain length. If the secondary emulsifying agent is added in quantities exceeding those needed to form a complex, the viscosity of the emulsion may be increased with a consequent improvement in stability.

Examples of mixed emulsifying agent systems are the emulsifying waxes.

EMULSIFYING WAX BP (ANIONIC EMULSIFYING WAX)

Emulsifying Wax BP contains cetostearyl alcohol and either sodium lauryl sulphate or sodium salts of similar alkyl sulphates. An example of a suitable formulation is:

Cetostearyl alcohol	90 g
Sodium lauryl sulphate	10 g
Purified water	4 mL

CETOMACROGOL EMULSIFYING WAX BP (NONIONIC EMULSIFYING WAX)

Cetostearyl alcohol	800 g
Cetomacrogol 1000	200 g

IDENTIFICATION OF EMULSION TYPE

The results from one test should not be taken to be conclusive and the identity of an emulsion type should always be confirmed by at least one of the other test procedures.

Cobalt Chloride Test. Filter paper soaked in a cobalt chloride solution and allowed to dry turns from blue to pink on exposure to oil-in-water emulsions. The test may not work for unstable emulsions.

Conductivity Test. An emulsion with an aqueous continuous phase will transmit an electrical current whereas one with an oily continuous phase will not. Conductivity tests, however, may give false results with nonionic oil-in-water emulsions.

Dilution Test. The type of emulsion may be determined by examining the miscibility of the continuous phase when shaken or stirred with oil or water. An oil-in-water emulsion, for example, will readily disperse in an aqueous solvent whereas a water-in-oil emulsion will not. Care must be taken during dilution as phase inversion may occur.

Direction of Creaming Test. The direction of creaming precisely identifies the emulsion type if the densities of the aqueous and oil phases are known. Water-in-oil emulsions normally cream downwards as oil is usually less dense than water. Oil-in-water emulsions normally cream upwards.

Dye Test. When an oil-in-water emulsion is mixed with a water-soluble dye such as amaranth and examined under a microscope, the continuous phase should be coloured. Similarly, the continuous phase of a water-in-oil emulsion would be coloured by an oil-soluble dye such as Sudan III.

Filter Paper Test. This test is based on the fact that an oil-in-water emulsion will spread out rapidly when dropped onto filter paper. In contrast, a water-in-oil emulsion will migrate only slowly. This method should not be used for highly viscous creams.

Fluorescence Test. A drop of the emulsion is exposed to ultraviolet radiation and observed under a microscope. Because many oils fluoresce under ultraviolet light, a water-in-oil emulsion should show continuous fluorescence, while in an oil-in-water type only the globules fluoresce.

PREPARATION OF EMULSIONS

Before an emulsion is prepared, the oil-soluble and water-soluble constituents are separately dissolved if necessary in the appropriate phase; a suitable emulsifying agent is selected for the type of emulsion required, and this is also dissolved in either the aqueous or the oil phase. Ideally, the disperse phase volume should be between 40% and 60% of the total volume; lower phase volumes increase the tendency to cream or sediment, while higher volumes tend to cause inversion in emulsions of high viscosity. If it is necessary to melt or to heat constituents to maintain a fluid state in either phase, the other phase should be brought to a similar temperature before mixing and emulsification.

Generally, the dispersed phase is gradually added to the continuous phase; often a more viscous primary concentrated emulsion is formed before the main bulk of the continuous phase is incorporated. Alternatively, the continuous phase may be added gradually to the disperse phase; while the disperse phase is in excess it will constitute the continuous phase of the first emulsion formed but as addition continues the first emulsion should invert to form the required type.

In a less frequently used method, all the emulsifying agent is mixed with a portion of one phase and then a portion of the other phase is incorporated. Successive additions of each phase are made until all have been included.

Emulsions for external application (creams, applications, liniments, and lotions) often include waxy solids that require melting before mixing; the order of mixing is less important. When soaps are included as emulsifying agents these can be prepared at the interface by bringing together the fatty acid in the oil phase and the alkali in the aqueous phase.

Equipment

The mortar and pestle is a simple and inexpensive piece of equipment for the extemporaneous preparation of small quantities of emulsions, although its efficiency is limited. Electric mixers can also be used on the small scale although care must be taken to avoid excessive entrapment of air. On the larger scale, more controlled agitation and greater shearing forces can be obtained by using mechanical stirrers, although their value may be limited for viscous emulsions.

Emulsions prepared by hand or by means of mechanical mixers usually consist of droplets in the 1 to 50 micrometre range; the particle size range may be reduced to between 1 and 3 micrometres by further homogenisation. Colloid mills are suitable for continuous processing and produce high rates of shear and globules of very low particle size; the equipment may need cooling during operation.

Homogenisers are made for small-scale and large-scale production and may be used both to mix and to emulsify a product, or to improve the quality of a coarse emulsion pre-mixed in other equipment. The shearing forces produced can often be adjusted if the emulsion is to be recirculated through the equipment; small ranges of particle size are produced.

By using oscillating devices, ultrasonic vibrations can be set up within coarse emulsions to induce cavitation and thus reduce the particle size of globules; equipment of this type is available for large-scale and small-scale production.

MULTIPLE EMULSIONS

Simple multiple emulsions consist of oil-in-water or water-in-oil emulsions dispersed in another liquid medium. An oil-in-water-in-oil emulsion, for example, consists of very small droplets of oil dispersed in the water globules of a water-in-oil emulsion. More complex systems, such as water-in-oil-in-water-in-oil-in-water emulsions, have also been developed.

Preparation

The preparation of multiple emulsions involves two stages. For example, a water-in-oil-in-water emulsion is prepared by first forming a water-in-oil system. The second stage involves dispersion of this primary emulsion in a second aqueous phase. A high stress method of emulsification should not be used at the second stage as this may result in the complete breakdown of the internal aqueous phase.

Stability

Multiple emulsions contain many sites capable of demonstrating instability. The addition of drugs or excipients may further upset the delicate stability balance; electrolytes for example may alter the osmotic forces operating between the water and oil phases of a water-in-oil-in-water system. Multiple emulsions are unstable to heat and should therefore not be sterilised by autoclaving.

Potential Uses

Multiple emulsions have been proposed as possible sustained-release dosage forms. A drug trapped in the internal phase of an oil-in-water-in-oil emulsion, for example, must pass through two other phases before being released and ultimately absorbed.

FURTHER INFORMATION

Emulsion Stability. Akers MJ, Lach JL. Evaluation of emulsion stability by diffuse reflectance spectroscopy. J Pharm Sci 1976;65:216–22.

Garrett ER. Prediction and evaluation of emulsion stability with ultracentrifugal stress. J Soc Cosmet Chem 1970;21:393–415.

Garti N, Magdassi S, Rubinstein A. A novel method for rapid non destructive determination of o/w creams stability. Drug Dev Ind Pharm 1982;8:475–85.

Horie K, Tanaka S, Akabori T. Determination of emulsion stability by spectral absorption. 1. Relation between surfactant type, concentration, and stability index. Cosmet Toilet 1978;93:53-4,56-8,60,62.

Holtan R, Pickard JF. Laser diffraction as a method for the particle size analysis of pharmaceutical emulsions. J Pharm Pharmacol 1985;37:120P.

Merry J, Eberth K. Ultrasonic preparation of pharmaceutical emulsions. Droplet size measurements by quasi-electric light scattering. Int J Pharmaceutics 1984;19:43–52.

Rambhau D, Phadke DS, Dorle AK. Evaluation of o/w emulsion stability through zeta potential — 1. J Soc Cosmet Chem 1977;28:183–96.

Reiger MM. The predictive determination of emulsion stability. Cosmet Toilet 1982;97:27–31.

Schott H, Royce AE. Improved microscopic techniques for droplet size determination of emulsions. J Pharm Sci 1983;72:313–15.

Yalabik-Kas HS. Stability assessment of emulsion systems. STP Pharma 1985;1:978–84.

Preservation. Kazmi SJA, Mitchell AG. Correlation of mathematically predicted preservative activity with antimicrobial activity. J Pharm Sci 1978;67:1260–6.

Mitchell AG, Kazmi SJA. Chemical preservation of emulsified and solubilized disperse systems. Cosmet Toilet 1977;92:33–4,36,38,40,43.

Patel NK, Romanowski JM. Influence of partitioning and molecular interactions on *in vitro* biologic activity of preservatives in emulsions. J Pharm Sci 1970;59:372–6.

Wan LSC, Kurup TRR, Chan LW. Partition of preservatives in oil/water systems. Pharm Acta Helv 1986;61:308–13.

Emulsifying Agents. Donbrow M, Azaz E, Pillersdorf A. Autoxidation of polysorbates. J Pharm Sci 1978;67:1676–81.

Fost DL. Cationic emulsification in creams and lotions. Drug Cosmet Ind 1985;137:58,60,94–8.

Zatz JL. Effect of formulation additives on flocculation of dispersions stabilised by a non-ionic surfactant. Int J Pharmaceutics 1979;4:83–6.

HLB System. Bonadeo I, Lodi V. Formulation of stable emulsions according to recent achievements in emulsology. Riv Ital Essenze Profumi, Piante Off, Aromi, Saponi, Cosmet, Aerosol 1980;62:179–88.

Marszall L. Determination of the required HLB of oil-in-water emulsions by a simple phase-inversion titration. Cosmet Perfum 1975;90:37–9.

Emulsion Type. Bhargava HN. The present status of formulation of cosmetic emulsions. Drug Dev Ind Pharm 1987;13:2363–87.

Bonadeo I, Lodi V. Formulation of stable emulsions according to recent achievements in emulsology. Riv Ital Essenze, Profumi, Piante Off, Aromi, Saponi, Cosmet, Aerosol 1980;62:179–88.

Lin TJ. Low energy emulsification. II. Evaluation of emulsion quality. J Soc Cosmet Chem 1978;29:745–56.

Lin TJ. Low-energy emulsification principles and applications. J Soc Cosmet Chem 1978;29:117–25.

Shapiro WB. Thickening oil in water emulsions. Cosmet Toilet 1982;97:27–30,32–3.

Multiple Emulsions. Abd-Elbary A, Nour SA, Mansour FF. Efficacy of different emulsifying agents in preparing o/w/o or w/o/w multiple emulsions. Pharm Ind 1984;46:964–9.

Adeyeye CM, Price JC. Effect of non-ionic surfactant concentrations and type on the formation and stability of w/o/w multiple emulsions: Microscopic and conductimetric evaluations. Drug Dev Ind Pharm 1991;17:725–36.

Florence AT, Whitehill D. The formulation and stability of multiple emulsions. Int J Pharmaceutics 1982;11:277–308.

Florence AT, Whitehill D. Stabilisation of water/oil/water multiple emulsions by polymerisation of the aqueous phases. J Pharm Pharmacol 1982;34:687–91.

Law TK, Florence AT, Whateley TL. Release from multiple w/o/w emulsions sterilised by interfacial complexation. J Pharm Pharmacol 1984;36(Suppl):50P.

Omotosho JA, Whateley TL, Florence AT, Bell G. Release of cytotoxic agents from multiple w/o/w emulsions. J Pharm Pharmacol 1987;39(Suppl):38P.

Omotosho JA, Whateley TL, Law TK, Florence AT. The nature of the oil phase and the release of solutes from multiple w/o/w emulsions. J Pharm Pharmacol 1986;38:865–70.

Rosoff M. Specialized Pharmaceutical Emulsions. In: Lieberman HA, Rieger MM, Banker GS, editors. Pharmaceutical dosage forms: disperse systems; vol. 1. New York: Marcel Dekker, 1988.

Whitehill D. Multiple emulsions and their future uses. Chemist Drugg 1980;213:130,132,135.

Whitehill D, Florence AT. Mechanism of instability in w/o/w multiple emulsions. J Pharm Pharmacol 1979;31(Suppl):3P.

Parenterals

Parenteral products are intended for administration by injection or implantation through the skin, or other external layers such as the stratum corneum, and directly into body fluids, tissues, or organs. From the site of administration the medicament is then readily transported to its site of action. The term **parenteral** is derived from the Greek words 'para' and 'enteron' meaning outside of the intestine, that is, by-passing the enteral route of administration. However, it is commonly used to imply administration by injection or infusion.

Parenteral products can be solutions, suspensions, or emulsions in a suitable aqueous or non-aqueous vehicle. They may contain one or more medicaments and they are always presented as sterile products. Parenterals may produce a localised response such as local anaesthetics, a sustained response as with depot injections of corticosteroids, or an extremely rapid general response by direct systemic administration, for example general anaesthetics. Parenteral products may also be administered in a slow controlled manner in order to titrate the medicament against a physiological response, as in the case of many antiarrhythmic drugs, in order to maintain electrolyte balance, as with sodium chloride infusion, or to provide nutrition for patients who are unable to absorb nutrients via the enteral route, as is the case with parenteral nutrition solutions (see Parenteral and Enteral Nutrition Fluids chapter).

The parenteral route of administration is generally adopted for medicaments that cannot be given orally, either because of patient intolerance (for example, nausea in patients undergoing chemotherapy) or because of instability, therapeutic inactivity, or poor absorption via the enteral route. Injections are often preferred for use in emergency therapy because they can produce an extremely rapid and effective response. In the unconscious patient parenteral administration is the only safe, effective means of administering medicaments. Parenteral therapy also gives the physician control of the drug regimen, since the patient must return for continued treatment in most cases, thus aiding compliance in patients who cannot be relied upon to take oral medication.

ROUTES OF ADMINISTRATION

Injections are often classified according to their route of administration. These are as follows:

Intravenous injections are administered directly into a prominent vein, normally in the forearm. They are usually aqueous solutions, but may also be oil-in-water emulsions in which the droplet size is carefully controlled. Water-in-oil emulsions and suspensions must not be given by this route. The volume of the injection may vary widely from 0.5 mL to 1 litre. Volumes of up to 10 mL are normally given via a syringe as a bolus dose. Larger volumes are given either by slow intravenous injection (10 to 50 mL), via a syringe in a syringe-driver (which pushes the plunger of the syringe at a slow, controlled rate), or by intravenous infusion from an infusion bag (50 mL to 1 litre).

The intravenous route is the most commonly used route for parenterals. It has significant advantages in certain clinical situations. A rapid response can be elicited, bioavailability of the medicament in the blood is always 100%, and doses can be readily titrated against a physiological response.

Intramuscular injections are administered into a muscle mass. A common site is the deltoid muscle of the upper arm, into which as much as 2 mL may be injected.[1] Larger volumes, up to 5 mL, may be administered into the gluteal medial muscle of each buttock.[1] Absorption is relatively rapid following administration via the intramuscular route in comparison to the subcutaneous route (see below), but intramuscular administration will not mediate the rapid response that is possible via the intravenous route. Absorption of a drug from the intramuscular route can be delayed or prolonged by administration of the drug as a suspension in an aqueous or oily vehicle. If administered too rapidly, intramuscular injections can cause considerable pain around the site of the injection.

Subcutaneous injections are administered into the loose tissue immediately below the dermis layer of the skin. The most popular sites for subcutaneous injections are the arm and thigh. Absorption after subcutaneous administration is slower than that following intramuscular administration. Injections are normally aqueous solutions or suspensions. This route is frequently used for the administration of local anaesthetics and it has the advantage that a relatively low dose of drug can be used to elicit a significant local response without large quantities of drug reaching the blood stream, thus avoiding the adverse cardiac effects of some local anaesthetics.

Injection volumes do not normally exceed 1 mL. However, tissue permeability is enhanced by the enzyme hyaluronidase and concomitant administration will allow much larger volumes to be injected subcutaneously in cases where intravenous administration is contra-indicated. This technique is known as hypodermoclysis, but it is used only in rare circumstances.

Intradermal injections are injected into the skin between the epidermis and the dermis. This route is also referred to as the intracutaneous route. Injection volumes should not exceed 0.2 mL and 0.1 mL is the most common volume. This route is used for diagnostic test injections for allergy or immunity. A limited number of vaccines are also administered by this route. Absorption from intradermal injections is prolonged with slow onset of drug action. Consequently, allergens used in diagnostic tests are taken into the blood very slowly in very small quantities which are less likely to elicit a major allergenic response in the body. Thus the allergenic response is contained around the site of administration.

Intra-arterial injections are similar to intravenous injections except that the drug is administered directly into an artery rather than a vein. They are sometimes used to target a particular organ which the artery serves, for example, the heart. Because of the large flow of blood through the arteries, the drug is rapidly diluted throughout the blood system. This is an advantage in the administration of radio-opaque materials for diagnostic purposes, such as arteriograms. Some cytotoxic drugs such as methotrexate can also be administered by this route. However, administration via the intra-arterial route can be hazardous and arterial spasm and subsequent gangrene can result.[1] Intra-arterial injections must not contain a bactericide.

Intracardiac injections are aqueous solutions injected directly into either the cardiac muscle or a ventricle. They are used in emergency treatment only. However, due to the growing success of intensive care for patients with coronary heart disease or cardiac arrest, the use of this route of administration is increasing. Again these injections must not contain a bactericide.

Intraspinal injections are also aqueous solutions injected into particular areas of the spinal column. Volumes should not exceed 20 mL and solutions should not contain bactericides or antoxidants. They should be presented in single-dose containers; in many instances there is a preference for ampoules that are sterilised in a transparent outer wrap that maintains the sterility of the external ampoule surfaces. This maintains the sterility of the outside of the ampoule, while allowing particulate inspection before use. This preference stems from the need to exercise extreme care to avoid contamination of the solution during administration, since the spinal fluid contains no natural body defence mechanism.

Intraspinal injections are further sub-divided according to the area of the spinal cord into which the injection is given. These are intrathecal or subarachnoid, intracisternal, and epidural or peridural injections. In some cases the specific gravity of the solution is adjusted in order to localise the action of the medicament. Local anaesthetics may have a very high specific gravity to prevent the anaesthetic from spreading up the spinal column. The epidural route is commonly used for the administration of such preparations.

Intra-articular injections are aqueous solutions or suspensions that are injected into the synovial fluid in a joint cavity.

There are a number of injections designed for ophthalmic use. These must be aqueous solutions or suspensions and the volume injected is generally small (not exceeding 1 mL). The most common ophthalmic injections are **subconjunctival** injections, which are administered beneath Tenon's capsule, close to the eye but not into it. This route is commonly used for the administration of local anaesthetics used in eye surgery. **Intracameral** injections are administered into the anterior chamber, **intravitreous** injections into the vitreous humour, and **retrobulbar** injections into the posterior segment of the globe.

The use of antimicrobial preservatives is permissible in subconjunctival injections but not in intracameral or intravitreous injections. The inclusion of antoxidants should be avoided because of their irritant effects on the eye. In all cases, extreme care should be taken to avoid contamination during the administration of ophthalmic injections because of the high risk of infection of the eye.

There are several other sites available for the administration of injectable products. These include the peritoneum (intraperitoneal), the amniotic fluid (intra-amniotic), the lymph (intra-lymphatic), the ureter (ureteral), and the pleural cavity (intrapleural). This list is not exhaustive.

In veterinary medicine, drugs are sometimes administered as **intramammary** injections, in the form of solutions or suspensions, by introduction into the mammary gland through the teat canal. Such products fall into two types, those administered to lactating animals and those administered to non-lactating animals. The former type are formulated for rapid dispersion of the medicament into the mammary tissue and they are not excreted in the milk. The latter type are formulated to release the medicament over a longer period of time and are referred to as slow release products. The *British Pharmacopoeia (Veterinary) 1993* gives examples of these products. Cloxacillin Sodium Intramammary Infusion BP (Vet) is a sterile suspension of cloxacillin sodium in an oily base intended for rapid dispersion. Cloxacillin Benzathine Intramammary Infusion BP (Vet) is a sterile suspension of cloxacillin benzathine in oil for slow release.

TYPES OF PARENTERALS

Parenteral products can also be classified according to their presentation. It has already been mentioned that some presentations are specifically required for certain routes of administration.

Aqueous Solutions

The simplest and most convenient form of presentation of an injectable product is as an isotonic aqueous solution, which has a pH close to that of blood and body tissues (pH 7.4). The inclusion of buffers in the formulation may be necessary to stabilise the injection at a suitable pH. Such a presentation is suitable for all routes of administration provided that the active ingredients are sufficiently soluble to ensure that the required dose is dissolved in an injection volume appropriate to the desired route. This consideration is of particular importance for medicaments intended for administration by the intradermal, subcutaneous, or subconjunctival routes where the injection volume must be small. However, medicaments administered by these routes are generally intended to mediate a local effect and therefore doses are usually small.

If the medicament is susceptible to oxidation, antioxidants must be added to stabilise the product. The use of antioxidants is dealt with in greater detail in the section of this chapter dealing with preformulation. The use of antioxidants in injection formulations is not permissible for a number of parenteral routes of administration because of their toxic or irritant properties. If injected into the spinal column they interact with the nerve endings causing traumatic effects, which can include paralysis. Many antioxidants are also irritant to mucous membranes and to the eye.

Injectable solutions can be presented in either single-dose or multidose containers. Multidose containers are normally glass vials with rubber stoppers suitable for multiple withdrawal. The major pharmacopoeias require multidose injections to contain an antimicrobial preservative. However, because of the toxicity of most antimicrobial preservatives and the potential for contamination of multidose containers, multidose injection formulations are normally only developed for products for which the normal indication of the product requires such presentations. Such products might be required for multiple self-administration by the patient, for example, insulin preparations, or for multiple administration in a specific clinical situation, such as the injection of vaccines. In the UK and in a number of other EC countries, the use of multidose injections is increasingly regarded as poor pharmaceutical practice. Consequently, the majority of newly developed parenteral products are single-dose preparations, which should not contain an antimicrobial preservative. The use of preservatives is also dealt with in greater detail in the section of this chapter dealing with preformulation.

Infusion fluids are aqueous solutions that are presented in larger volumes than those normally administered by intravenous injection. Injection volumes range from 50 mL to 1 litre and they are normally presented in polyvinyl chloride infusion bags. Products presented as infusions include preparations used for:

- basic nutrition, for example, glucose injection
- restoration of electrolyte balance, for example, compound sodium chloride injection, which contains sodium, potassium, and calcium ions
- fluid replacement, for example, a combination such as glucose and sodium chloride injection
- a number of special uses, such as parenteral hyperalimentation.[1]

Local anaesthetics for spinal injection are formulated at different specific gravities in order to target the portion of the spinal column where nerve block is required. The position at which the anaesthetic acts will depend on both the specific gravity of the solution and the positioning of the patient. **Hypobaric** solutions have a specific gravity lower than that of the cerebrospinal fluid and thus move upwards after administration. **Isobaric** solutions have approximately the same specific gravity as the cerebrospinal fluid and exert their effect at about the same level as the injection site. **Hyperbaric** solutions have a greater specific gravity than the cerebrospinal fluid and exert their effects at sites lower than the injection site. Amethocaine, bupivacaine, lignocaine, mepivacaine, and prilocaine have all been formulated in this way for spinal anaesthesia usually by the addition of glucose.

Suspensions

Aqueous Suspensions

Parenterals can be presented as aqueous suspensions of insoluble medicaments or with the medicament adsorbed onto an insoluble matrix to promote modified release of the medicament. Isophane Insulin Injection BP, Insulin Zinc Suspension BP, Procaine Penicillin Injection BP, and Tetracosactrin Zinc Injection BP are all examples of pharmacopoeial injectable products that are formulated in this way. Zinc salts have found wide application in this respect. The aqueous vehicle can be complex, containing a number of additives, which must be non-toxic and capable of sterilisation.

The particle size of solids in suspension is normally small and the particle size distribution must be carefully controlled to ensure that the particles pass readily through a hypodermic needle during administration. Particle size must not increase and caking must not occur during storage.

Surfactants such as lecithin, polysorbate 80, and sorbitan esters may be included in the formulation. Gel-forming agents such as carmellose sodium, methylcellulose, and gelatin may also be included to increase viscosity and hence aid the stability of the suspension. Ideally, the vehicle should provide a stable dispersion during storage and be sufficiently fluid to allow administration via a syringe. A thixotropic (see Rheology chapter) vehicle may, therefore, be desirable.

Further examples of injectable aqueous suspensions are Hydrocortisone Acetate Injection BP, Methylprednisolone Acetate Injection BP, Sterile Medroxyprogesterone Acetate Suspension USP, Propyliodone Suspension BP, and Spectinomycin Injection BP. These products are all formulated in an aqueous vehicle; the vehicle for Spectinomycin Injection also contains 3% v/v benzyl alcohol. Chloramphenicol Injection BP (Vet) or USP is also a sterile suspension in an aqueous vehicle, but it can also be presented simply as a sterile (micronised) powder, which can be reconstituted to an injectable suspension, for example, Sterile Chloramphenicol USP.

All of the above examples are intended for intramuscular administration only. Suspensions should never be administered by the intravenous or intra-arterial routes, nor as intraspinal, intracardiac, or ophthalmic injections.

Oily Suspensions

Injectable suspensions can also be presented in an oily vehicle, although such preparations are far less common than aqueous suspensions. They can provide an effective slow release or depot mechanism by the deep intramuscular route. Aluminium monostearate is sometimes included in oily vehicles to produce thixotropic gels, for example in Sterile Penicillin G Procaine with Aluminum Stearate Suspension USP.

Oily Injections

There are a number of lipophilic products that are formulated as oily solutions. Oily solutions are also intended primarily for intramuscular administration and, under normal circumstances, they should not be administered by other routes. The vehicle used varies widely from vegetable oils such as arachis oil (used with benzyl benzoate in Dimercaprol Injection BP) and sesame oil (used in the depot injections Fluphenazine Decanoate Injection BP and Fluphenazine Enanthate Injection BP) to simple esters such as ethyl oleate, which is relatively non-toxic and therefore very popular. Ethyl oleate may be used as the vehicle in a range of pharmacopoeial products such as Nandrolone Decanoate Injection BP, Oestradiol Injection BP, and Testosterone Propionate Injection BP. However, not all steroidal products are formulated in ethyl oleate and the *British Pharmacopoeia* recommends 'a suitable fixed oil' for use in Hydroxyprogesterone Injection.

Emulsions

Medicaments that are lipophilic can also be presented as oil-in-water emulsions. The medicament may be dissolved in an oily solution and then emulsified or it may be an oil itself. Some nutrient intravenous infusions are formulated in this way, for example, Intralipid™. As with particle size in suspensions, the oil droplet size must be carefully controlled and the emulsion must be formulated so that it will not crack on storage. The ideal droplet size is 3 micrometres in diameter.

Intravenous infusions formulated as emulsions normally contain up to 15% of emulsified vegetable oil and glucose. They are used for parenteral nutrition in patients who may rely entirely on intravenous feeding (as a means of delivering essential fatty acids and fat soluble vitamins) for long periods of time. In these instances the fat soluble vitamins are added to the parenteral nutrition bag on the prescription of the physician. Additives may be small volume intravenous injections in an oily base or they also may be formulated as emulsions, for example, Vitlipid N™ and Diazemuls™. In these instances it is important to have a knowledge of any interactions between the additive and the nutrient emulsion in order to avoid cracking the emulsion. This can easily happen with surfactants that are incompatible. More information on the formulation of intravenous nutrition fluids is given in the Parenteral and Enteral Nutrition Fluids chapter.

Emulsifiers and stabilisers for intravenous emulsions must be non-toxic. Such materials include lecithin, polysorbate 80, gelatin, methylcellulose, and serum albumin.

Colloidal Solutions

There are instances where medicaments have been formulated as sterile colloidal solutions for injection. These preparations are sterilised by heating in an autoclave since they may be retained on bacterial filters. Iron Dextran Injection BP and Iron Sorbitol Injection BP are two such preparations. Iron Dextran Injection BP contains dextrans complexed with ferric ions, and Iron Sorbitol Injection BP contains sorbitol, dextrins, and citric acid complexed with ferric ions. Both are given by deep intramuscular injection.

Mixed Solvent Systems

In many clinical situations it is necessary to formulate a true solution, which is readily and completely miscible with serum for intravenous administration. If the medicament is poorly water soluble, formulation can be difficult. For weak acids and bases selection of the most appropriate salt or formulation at a high or low pH value can be very successful. However, for some medicaments it is necessary to formulate the product in a mixed solvent system. In these instances a cosolvent is added in order to reduce the polarity of the vehicle and render the medicament more soluble. Ethanol, propylene glycol, and glycerol have all been used as cosolvents. The choice of cosolvent is restricted due to the danger of toxicity and the concentrations of such cosolvents must be restricted to ensure that there is a safe quantity of cosolvent being administered in the maximum recommended injection volume. In many cases the formulator must strike a fine balance between the concentration of cosolvent and the injection volume required. Some formulations contain a number of cosolvents thus avoiding the use of a toxic quantity of a single cosolvent.

Injections that are formulated as mixed solvent systems are often incompatible with intravenous fluids, bags, giving sets, or plastic syringes. They should be used with care in patients with impaired liver function since clearance of the cosolvent may be impaired. The use of mixed solvent systems is therefore normally restricted to a small number of products that are required to be administered intravenously in critical clinical circumstances.

The most common examples of injections formulated in mixed solvent systems are Digoxin Injection BP, which has a mixture of ethanol, propylene glycol, and water as vehicle, and Ergotamine Injection BP, which has a vehicle that comprises ethanol and glycerol.

Although it is not strictly a mixed solvent vehicle, Phenol and Glycerol Injection BP can be included in this group of products since it is miscible with serum and is intended for intravenous administration.

Concentrated Solutions

Some medicaments, for example potassium chloride, are required to be administered at a low concentration over a long period of time, because rapid administration of a concentrated solution can elicit a toxic effect. In the case of potassium chloride, concentrated solutions are cardiotoxic. However, it is a considerable disadvantage to present the medicament as a large volume of dilute solution, particularly where the medicament is highly soluble and can be presented in a small volume. In these cases the medicament is presented as a concentrate, which can be diluted or added to an intravenous infusion before administration. The advantages of such a presentation are economies in manufacture and transport, and ease of handling in the clinic.

Powders for Injection

Some medicaments are not sufficiently stable in solution to be presented as parenteral solutions. Such compounds are presented as powders for injection. These can be dry-filled powders in vials or lyophilised (freeze-dried) products. Dry-filled powders must be sterilised as powders, before filling, either by dry heat or by gamma irradiation. Dry-filled powders are not common since many medicaments that are unstable in solution are also unstable on exposure to heat or irradiation. In these circumstances the product must be sterilised in solution by filtration and subsequently lyophilised.

Lyophilised parenterals form a large percentage of all injectable dosage forms. There are many groups of medicaments that are formulated in this way ranging from relatively simple molecules such as penicillins and cephalosporins, to corticosteroids, aminoglycoside and glycopeptide antibiotics, and large molecular weight peptides. Many diagnostic agents, blood products, immunological products, and vaccines are presented as lyophilised products. Lyophilisation is an ideal way of preserving a large percentage of the activity of vaccines, particularly live cells and large peptides whose tertiary structure is critical for their activity.

Lyophilisation renders the product very hydrophilic and it is normally more readily reconstituted, using an aqueous diluent, than a dry-filled powder. Storage and transport become easier as a result of the removal of water and the product can be presented as a very elegant, sterile, and particle-free preparation.

The major disadvantages associated with lyophilisation are the high cost of the process and the need to maintain sterility following sterile filtration. Lyophilisation is addressed in greater detail later in the chapter.

Implants

Implants have been developed as a means of slow, delayed, or controlled delivery of medicaments that cannot be given via the oral route. Products for hormone replacement therapy are commonly administered in this way, for example, Testosterone Implant BP and Hexoestrol Implant and Progesterone Implant BP (Vet). However, implants have found other applications and their use in bone infections has recently been reported.[2-5]

The *British Pharmacopoeia* states that 'Implants are sterile solid preparations of size and shape suitable for implantation into body tissues'. They frequently contain the medicament and no other substance and are produced either by fusion or heavy compression. However, medicaments may also be incorporated into a matrix in order to achieve slow release. Materials suitable for use in such matrices are cross-linked polydimethylsiloxane (PDMS),[2] polymethylmethacrylate (PMMA),[4] and other polymers.[3,6] The release rate of lipophilic drugs, such as progesterone and testosterone, from silicone polymers has been reported to be several orders of magnitude higher than that from organic polymers.[7] However, the release rate of hydrophilic drugs from silicone matrices is low. The addition of hydrophilic compounds, such as glycerol, to the polymer matrix greatly enhances the release rate of several hydrophilic drugs.[8-11]

RELEASE OF MEDICAMENT FROM PARENTERALS

Measurement and optimisation of release of medicaments form an integral part of the formulation development of all pharmaceutical products. Medicaments administered by the intravenous or intraspinal routes usually produce a rapid therapeutic effect since no absorption mechanism is involved before the medicament is transported to the body fluids. For other routes of administration there may be a delay in absorption of the medicament into the blood or in transport to the site of action. Subcutaneous, intradermal, and intramuscular injections may act fairly rapidly, but absorption of the medicament and transport to the site of action must occur in these instances. The rates at which such absorption occurs follow similar kinetics to those for orally administered medicaments.

Absorption from subcutaneous and intramuscular injections is normally by simple diffusion into blood capillaries and the lymphatic system. There is also some evidence that, following injection, drug molecules may be transported by phagocytes. However, there are a number of widely used drugs that are incompletely absorbed after intramuscular injection, including ampicillin, cephradine, chlordiazepoxide, diazepam, digoxin, insulin, and phenytoin.[12] In the last three cases, clinically important problems have resulted from incomplete absorption.

A number of physicochemical parameters influence absorption from subcutaneous and intramuscular injections. Molecular weight is one of the more significant parameters. Small molecules will diffuse more rapidly and will pass more readily through capillary walls. Larger molecules and colloids appear to be primarily absorbed and transported via the lymphatic vessels. Other factors that influence the rate and extent of absorption include capillary blood flow, hydrostatic and osmotic pressure differences, body movement, the extent of dissociation of the medicament, and the nature of the vehicle. The water solubility and lipophilicity of the molecule are also very important factors.

Where sustained release is required from a parenteral formulation it can be achieved by modifying the absorption of the medicament from the site of injection. Alternatively, for intravenous formulations it can be achieved by slow infusion. Slow absorption can be produced by chemical modification of the medicament, for example, aminophylline which hydrolyses to produce theophylline, or by modifications to the formulation. Intramuscular drugs which are formulated in water-miscible solvents such as propylene glycol may precipitate on dilution by tissue fluids, thus retarding absorption. Drugs formulated in oily solution will normally be absorbed very slowly from intramuscular injections. This is the basis of depot injections. In many cases the medicament for the depot injection must be chemically modified to find the most suitable ester, for example, testosterone propionate.

Adsorption of the medicament onto an insoluble material, for example, adsorption of insulin onto zinc salts, formation of colloids with dextran, and the use of implants have all been used as means of modifying the release of medicaments from intramuscular and subcutaneous injections.

Absorption of any medicament, presented as a suspension or dispersion and injected into the tissues, will be affected by the physicochemical characteristics of both the medicament and the vehicle. Polymorphic form, crystal size and habit, size distribution, surface area and concentration of the solid component, volume, pH, tonicity, viscosity, and the presence of adsorbents in the vehicle can all affect the rate of release of the medicament. Additives can also retard absorption. Adrenaline is often administered in conjunction with lignocaine as it causes a reduction in capillary blood flow, thus prolonging the local anaesthetic activity.

PREFORMULATION AND FORMULATION

Preformulation

During the development of a suitable formulation for the parenteral administration of a medicament, the physical, chemical, and biological properties of the medicament need to be assessed in order to make rational decisions on the following: selection of a suitable vehicle (aqueous or non-aqueous); selection of added substances or excipients (preservatives, antioxidants, buffers, solubilising agents, chelating agents, and tonicity adjusters); and the selection of containers and closures. Preformulation tests will normally include solubility measurements, analysis of the effects of common excipients on solubility and stability, measurement of the oxidation potential of the medicament, determination of the pH-stability profile, measurement of the osmolarity of the medicament in water over a range of concentrations, and assessment of the stability of the medicament to heat sterilisation.

pH

The solubility and stability of the medicament in water can be greatly affected by the pH of the solution. Many drugs that are administered parenterally are the salts of organic acids or bases. These salts are selected because of their water solubility. However, in these cases it is essential that extensive pH-solubility and pH-stability profiles are undertaken in order to determine the optimum pH for the formulation. Many organic salts (for example, acetate, mesylate, or sodium salts) have a considerable buffering capacity at higher concentrations. Nevertheless, many compounds are particularly susceptible to pH changes, which can be brought about by heat sterilisation, contact with containers and closures, degradation of the medicament, or dissolution of carbon dioxide from the headspace of the container. In these cases it is necessary to introduce a buffer.

The ideal pH of a parenteral product is 7.4, the pH of blood. Extreme deviation from this pH can cause complications.[13] Above pH 9, tissue necrosis often occurs, whereas below pH 3 extreme pain is experienced at the site of injection. The acceptable pH range (3 to 10.5) for intravenous preparations is wider than the acceptable range for other routes (pH 4 to 9). This is because blood itself is an excellent buffer and it can dilute and distribute the solution throughout the circulatory system very rapidly. However, when administering intravenous parenterals at the extremes of the pH range care must be taken to avoid extravasation—accidental injection of the solution into the tissue surrounding the injection site—since this will also give rise to necrosis or pain.

Determination of the desired pH for a particular product will normally determine the choice of buffer. For optimum solubility the pH of the buffer will be at least 2 pH units away from the pK_a of the salt being considered. However, this may not be the optimum pH for stability or for biological activity. When considering biological activity it must be remembered that once the product has been diluted and distributed to its site of action it will be exposed to physiological pH 7.4. In fact it is quite common for the active species to be the free base or even a metabolite of the species that has been administered. The pH for optimum biological activity is, therefore, very rarely a primary consideration in parenteral formulations. The desired pH is normally a compromise between the optimum for solubility, the optimum for stability, and the ideal of pH 7.4.

The most common buffers used in parenterals are acetate buffers (pH range 4 to 6), phosphate buffers (pH range 6 to 8), glutamate buffers (pH range 2 to 5 and 8.5 to 10.5), and citrate buffers (pH range 2 to 6). Buffers exert their greatest buffering capacity when the pH is equal to the pK_a of the buffer. Buffers are normally selected with a pK_a within 1 pH unit of the desired pH. Glutamate and citrate buffers have more than one pK_a, hence the wide pH range over which they may be used. The *British Pharmacopoeia* gives guidance on the selection of buffers for parenteral products and the subject is generally well covered in the literature.[13]

The Henderson–Hasselbalch equation is used to calculate the quantities of buffer species required to provide the desired pH:

$$pH = pK_a + \log \frac{C_{salt}}{C_{acid}}$$

where C_{salt} and C_{acid} are the molar concentrations of the salt form and acid form, respectively.

Oxidation and Antioxidants

Many drugs in aqueous solution are subject to oxidative degradation. Therefore, parenteral products that contain such drugs will frequently require the addition of an antioxidant. An antioxidant is an agent that has a lower oxidation potential than the drug and can be preferentially oxidised, until all of the oxygen present has been taken up, thus providing protection from oxidation for the drug molecule. A loss of antioxidant, during processing and during the first few weeks of storage of the product, is normally seen. The extent and the rate of this loss will be dependent upon the amount of oxygen present in the container and the redox potential of the antioxidant. For a description of the types,

choice, and effectiveness of antioxidants, see the Stability of Medicinal Products chapter.

For some medicaments that are susceptible to oxidation it may not be necessary to add an antioxidant and for some routes of administration (for example, intraspinal injections) the inclusion of antioxidants in the formulation is not permissible. The use of antioxidants can sometimes be avoided by reducing the amount of oxygen dissolved in solution and the amount present in the container headspace. This is achieved by sparging solutions with an inert gas, such as nitrogen, to displace the oxygen in solution before filling and by purging the container with inert gas both before and after filling. The amount of oxygen present will depend upon the efficiency of sparging and purging and on the speed with which the container is sealed after purging. The manufacturing process can be closely monitored by specialised equipment for monitoring dissolved and headspace oxygen.

Additionally, if the concentration of medicament is high in relation to the dissolved oxygen concentration and the injection volume is low, that is, less dissolved oxygen for a given concentration, then the amount of oxidation that might be expected will be small as a percentage of the total quantity of medicament. In these instances the loss of activity will be acceptably small and if the degradates do not have significant toxic effects the use of an antioxidant can be avoided.

Where the inclusion of an antioxidant in the formulation is necessary, it must have a lower oxidation potential than the medicament itself, otherwise oxygen will preferentially attack the medicament. The oxidation process involves the transfer of electrons and protons. A chemical oxidation-reduction reaction can be expressed as an equation:

Reduced form $\rightleftharpoons$ oxidised form + n electrons

Oxidation-reduction reactions are usually reversible and can be made to proceed in either direction. During an oxidation process there must be an electron donor and an electron acceptor. In any mixture of oxidation-reduction reagents the substance that has the greatest tendency to lose electrons is itself oxidised and, in addition, reduces all other substances. The tendency to lose electrons is determined by measuring the electromotive force. The Nernst equation defines the standard potential (E°) for an oxidation-reduction system:[14]

$$E = E^\circ - \frac{2.303RT}{nF} \log \frac{(B)^\beta}{(A)^\alpha}$$

where (A) and (B) are the activities of reactants A and B in the oxidation-reduction system, R is the gas constant, T is the absolute temperature, n is the number of equivalents of the reacting substance, F is the Faraday constant, α is the number of moles of reduced form A which are converted to B, β is the number of moles of the oxidised form B, and E is the measured electromotive force. When the activities and concentrations of the reactants and products are equal then $E = E^{\circ}$.

When comparing two substances and their potential for oxidation, the substance with the higher E° value will be the substance that will be oxidised, whereas the substance with the lower E° will accept those electrons and be reduced.[14] Table 1 lists the standard oxidation potentials for some common drugs, antioxidants, and other reagents. It is clear from the data presented in Table 1 that it is important to screen antioxidants during preformulation studies on parenteral solutions. Such screening is described elsewhere.[15]

Table 1
*Standard oxidation potentials for various substances**

Substance	E° (V)	pH	Temperature (°C)
Acetylcysteine	−0.293	7.0	25
Adrenaline	−0.380	7.0	30
Ascorbic acid	+0.003	7.0	25
	−0.115	5.2	30
	−0.136	4.58	30
Dithiothreitol	+0.053	7.0	30
Hydroquinone	−0.673	—	—
Methylene blue	−0.011	7.0	30
Phenol	−1.089	—	—
Propyl gallate	−0.199	7.0	25
Resorcinol	−1.043	—	—
Riboflavine	+0.208	7.0	30
Sodium bisulphite	−0.117	7.0	25
Sodium metabisulphite	−0.114	7.0	25
Sodium thiosulphate	+0.050	7.0	30
Thiourea	+0.029	7.0	30
Vitamin K	−0.363	—	20

*E° values correspond to the reaction (reduced) $\rightleftharpoons$ (oxidised) $+ \text{e}^{-}$

The other factor that influences the choice of antioxidant is toxicity. Regulatory authorities publish guidelines on the compounds that are regarded as acceptable for use as excipients in medicines; the number of antioxidants that are universally acceptable is limited.

The process of oxidation in parenterals involves a reaction between oxygen and the medicament. The process is spontaneous and is often referred to as **autoxidation**. Autoxidation is a chain reaction involving free radicals formed by the loss of

a hydrogen atom. It may be catalysed by variations in temperature or hydrogen ion concentration, the presence of trace metals or peroxides, or exposure to light.[14] While the solubility of oxygen is less at higher temperatures[16] the rate of oxidation will increase as temperature is increased. Conversely, the storage of oxygen-sensitive drugs in solution at low temperatures will result in increased oxygen concentrations in the solution.

Hydrogen ion concentration has a direct effect on the Nernst equation, as shown below:

$$E = E^{\circ} - \frac{RT}{nF}\left(\ln\frac{(ox)}{(red)} - pH \right)$$

As pH increases, the oxidation potential of the system increases. For example, at pH 4.58 ascorbic acid has an E° of −0.136 V and at pH 5.20 this increases to −0.115 V.[14] Therefore, many oxygen-sensitive compounds, provided they are still soluble, are formulated at lower pH values to increase their resistance to oxidation. However, the salts of sulphur dioxide are most effective at varying pH values. Metabisulphite is used as antioxidant at low pH, bisulphite at intermediate pH, and sulphite at higher pH values.

Metals can react directly with oxygen and with hydroperoxides to form free radicals which could initiate the chain reaction of autoxidation. Copper and iron are the most active catalysts.[14] Accordingly, antioxidants are often used in combination with chelating agents such as edetic acid and its sodium and calcium salts.

Exposure to light will also catalyse autoxidation reactions. Low wavelength (high energy) light has the greatest effect and oxygen-sensitive products are least stable in ultraviolet light.

In addition to chelating agents, there are other additives that are used in parenteral solutions as antioxidant synergists.[14] Citric, phosphoric, and tartaric acids are used to reduce the pH of the solution and povidone, lecithin, glycerol, and propylene glycol are used to increase viscosity and thus reduce the rate of diffusion of oxygen. Surfactants, such as polysorbates, and certain amino acids such as glycine, cysteine, and tryptophan have also been used as antioxidant synergists.

Osmolality and Osmolarity

Osmolarity is a measure of the osmotic potential of a solution, that is, its potential to move water through a semi-permeable membrane from a solution of lower osmotic potential (see also the Solution Properties chapter). Solutions that have the same osmolarity as erythrocytes are **isotonic** ('in tone with erythrocytes'). Solutions with higher osmolarity than the blood are hypertonic and solutions with lower osmolarity are hypotonic. The normal units of osmolarity are osmols and milliosmols (mosmol). An osmol is the weight of a chemical substance, dissolved in one litre of water that exerts an osmotic pressure equal to that exerted by a gram-molecular weight of an unionised substance dissolved in one litre of water. One osmol contains the same number of particles as a one molar solution of an unionised substance. For example, 1M of glucose is the same as 1 osmol of glucose since it does not ionise.[1]

Where osmolarity is the concentration expressed as moles of solute particles per litre of water, **osmolality** is the concentration expressed as moles of solute particles per kilogram of water. At standard temperature and pressure (STP) one litre of water weighs approximately one kilogram and this approximation is accepted for practical calculations and measurements of tonicity of solutions. Therefore, in dilute solutions osmolality is approximately equal to osmolarity, but in concentrated solutions the mass of solute particles becomes significant. In most cases parenteral solutions are dilute solutions. However, in complex mixtures, such as protein hydrolysate injection, the theoretical osmolarity cannot be readily calculated.[17]

For electrolytes the particles formed by ionisation must be considered in osmotic relationships. One mole of sodium chloride is fully ionised in aqueous solutions to give 1M of sodium and 1M of chloride. Thus one mole of sodium chloride in one litre has an osmolarity of 2 osmol. Electrolyte concentrations in parenteral solutions are normally expressed in milliequivalents, where the equivalent weight takes into account the valency of the ionised species.

The osmolarity of plasma is reported as 306 mosmol/litre.[1] Parenteral solutions that have osmolarities which deviate significantly from this value can cause haemolysis of blood cells, tissue irritation, pain on injection, and electrolytic shifts. Intravenous administration of hypotonic solutions causes swelling of erythrocytes and haemolysis, whereas hypertonic solutions cause crenation of the erythrocytes. Ideally, parenteral solutions should be formulated to be approximately isotonic. Large volume intravenous parenterals are normally formulated in this way. Glucose 5% infusion has an osmolarity of 280 mosmol/litre and sodium chloride infusion has an osmolality of 308 mosmol/litre. Other large volume intravenous solutions have values within the range of 260 to 340 mosmol/litre.

If a parenteral solution is hypotonic an osmolarity adjustment is made, using, in most cases, either sodium chloride, glucose, or mannitol to make the solution isotonic. Drug solutions that are already hypertonic cannot be adjusted and there are some hypotonic drug solutions that cannot be adjusted, either for clinical reasons or because of the likelihood of incompatibility. In these circumstances the product must be administered slowly in small volumes or into a large vein, such as the subclavian, where distribution and dilution occur rapidly.[1] Alternatively, these products may be diluted immediately before administration. Intramuscular and subcutaneous administration of solutions that are not isotonic should be avoided. The amount of sodium chloride required to make a product isotonic is calculated simply by referring to the sodium chloride equivalent of the excipient. See the Solution Properties chapter for examples of the calculation.

Where an alternative excipient is used for adjusting tonicity, for example, mannitol, the sodium chloride equivalent of the excipient is calculated thus:

$$C_e = (9 - C_m X_m) X_e$$

where C_e is the concentration of the excipient (g per litre), X_e is the sodium chloride equivalent of the excipient, C_m is the concentration of medicament (g per litre), and X_m is the sodium chloride equivalent of the medicament.

The sodium chloride equivalent of the medicament is determined experimentally by measuring the osmolarity of the medicament over the concentration range used in formulations.

Where a number of excipients are incorporated into a formulation, or a number of medicaments are formulated together, the contributions of the individual components are additive as shown below:

$$C_e = [9 - (C_1 X_1 + C_2 X_2 + C_3 X_3 \ldots)] X_e$$

where C_1, C_2, C_3 ... are the concentrations of components 1, 2, 3 ..., and X_1, X_2, X_3 ... are the sodium chloride equivalents of components 1, 2, 3 ...

For some components of a parenteral formulation, such as preservatives, the contribution to the tonicity of the solution is insignificant and can, for all practical purposes, be ignored. However, the contribution of additives such as buffer salts and antoxidants can be large and these must be considered during the development of the formulation. A comprehensive list of sodium chloride equivalents is given in the Solution Properties chapter.

Calculations for the adjustment of tonicity can also be made by three other methods. These are based on:

- freezing point depression
- molar concentrations, and
- serum osmolarity.

All of these calculations are illustrated in the Solution Properties chapter.

During preformulation studies, it is necessary to determine the osmotic contribution of the medicament, usually as the sodium chloride equivalent. It is also necessary to measure the osmolarity of the formulation following tonicity adjustment, to ensure that the theoretical calculation has held true in practice. There are two instrumental methods by which osmolarity can be measured and these are both dependent upon the colligative properties of solutes, (the lowering of vapour pressure, elevation of boiling point, depression of freezing point, and osmotic pressure).

The colligative properties are all interrelated and the two that are commonly employed to measure osmolarity are lowering of vapour pressure and depression of freezing point. Measurement of vapour pressure can be difficult and costly; however, only microlitre quantities of solution are required and results are often more reliable. The measurement of freezing point depression is relatively simple, less costly, and can be carried out on the laboratory bench using about 100 microlitres of solution. It is important to note that the two methods may give slightly different results for a given solution because of instrumentation and temperature differences during measurement. Measurement of osmolarity is briefly described in the *United States Pharmacopeia XXII*.

Sodium chloride is the excipient that is most frequently used to adjust osmolarity. However, other excipients may be preferred for inclusion in products used for clinical indications in which the electrolyte balance is important, for example, cardiac therapy. The solubility of the medicament can be greatly affected by the addition of sodium chloride, possibly causing a 'salting out' of the medicament as a precipitate. This can occur as a result of the common ion effect or simply as a result of displacement of an ionised species by sodium or chloride ions.

In such cases it can be extremely difficult to redissolve the medicament. The reduction in solubility can lead to larger injection volumes being required for a given dose and it is often advisable to select another excipient for adjustment of osmolarity. If 'salting out' occurs, an assessment of the physical compatibility of the medicament with sodium chloride infusion must be made since the addition of parenterals to sodium chloride infusions is common practice in parenteral therapy. Glucose and mannitol are excipients that have far less potential for reducing the solubility of the medicament; if 'salting out' is a problem these excipients are preferred. However, both glucose and mannitol are chemically incompatible with some medicaments. Chemical incompatibility is less likely with sodium chloride.

Other excipients that have been used for adjusting osmolality include glycerol, propylene glycol, and sodium sulphate. Buffer salts will also contribute to the osmolarity of the solution and these must be considered when adding osmolarity adjusters.

Antimicrobial Preservatives

Antimicrobial preservatives must be included in parenteral products that are presented in multidose containers unless their inclusion is prohibited by the monograph of the product, or unless the formulation itself can be shown to be bacteriostatic by meeting the requirements of the pharmacopoeial preservatives efficacy tests. However, good pharmaceutical practice dictates that multidose containers should only be used where the clinical use of the product warrants such a presentation. An example of such circumstances would be in insulin therapy where the patients themselves administer repeated doses, normally at home.

It is not considered professionally acceptable to present a product in a multidose container with the intention of withdrawing doses for a number of different patients over a prolonged time period, since, despite the presence of a preservative, this practice involves a significantly higher risk to the patient due to the danger of microbial contamination of the product. Cross-contamination between patients could also be a major concern in these circumstances. Regulatory authorities require applicants to provide adequate justification for presenting parenterals in multidose containers.

Where the inclusion of an antimicrobial preservative is deemed to be necessary in a formulation, consideration must be given to the stability and effectiveness of the preservative in combination with the active ingredient and other added substances. Many papers have been published describing the incompatibilities or binding of preservatives with surfactants, medicaments, and rubber closures. Selection of an appropriate rubber formulation will minimise the absorption of preservative from solution and will thus prevent a loss of preservative efficacy during the shelf-life of the product. The effectiveness of antibacterial agents can be tested by challenging the product with selected organisms to evaluate the bacteriostatic or bactericidal activity in a formulation. Such tests are described in the *British Pharmacopoeia* and the *United States Pharmacopeia*.

Preservative challenge tests should be performed throughout the projected shelf-life of the product and near the expiry date of the product to ensure that adequate levels of preservative are still available. Consequently, preservative efficacy tests are routinely included in stability testing protocols for formulations containing preservatives. However, with the availability of accurate and selective analytical methods for measuring low preservative concentrations in the presence of high concentrations of medicaments, it is more convenient and more economical to perform chemical assays for preservatives provided that such assays can be related to preservative efficacy. The United States Food and Drug Administration (FDA) stability testing guidelines require that preservative efficacy testing is carried out yearly during stability testing protocols, but preservative assays are normally performed at more frequent intervals.

Consideration must also be given to the relative tonicity of the preservative used. This consideration is increasingly restricting the choice of preservatives available in formulations. Table 2 shows a list of commonly used preservatives and the concentrations in which they are normally used to provide effective bacteriostasis. However, the Food and Drug Administration and European regulatory authorities produce their own lists of preservatives and other excipients suitable for use in parenterals.

Table 2
Commonly used preservatives in parenteral products

Preservative	Usual concentration (% w/v)
Benzalkonium chloride	0.01
Benzethonium chloride	0.01
Benzyl alcohol	2.0
Chlorbutol	0.5
Chlorocresol	0.1–0.3
Cresol	0.3–0.5
Methyl hydroxybenzoate	0.18
Phenol	0.5
Phenethyl alcohol	0.5
Phenylmercuric nitrate and acetate	0.002
Propyl hydroxybenzoate	0.5
Thiomersal	0.01

The pH of the formulation can sometimes affect the efficacy of the preservative and the chemical stability of the preservative itself. Some preservatives are active in the unionised form, for example, phenolics and benzoic acid, which are inactivated at high pH. Others are preferentially active as the anion or cation. Cationic antibacterials such as quaternary ammonium compounds are more active at alkaline pH. Chlorbutol is less active above pH 5.0 and unstable above pH 6.0. The best preservative is one which is active at the pH of the formulation and is not affected by small changes in pH. More information on preservatives is given in the chapter on Control of Microbial Contamination and the Preservation of Medicines.

Solubilising Agents

To enhance the solubility of drugs, in addition to the use of organic solvents which are miscible with water, other substances may be used as **solubilisers**. Surfactants, especially the nonionic types, are used to solubilise drugs such as vitamins. Ethylenediamine is required in aminophylline injections to maintain the theophylline in solution. Creatinine, nicotinamide, and lecithin have all been used for solubilising steroids in the free-alcohol form. The use of the salt or ester of these steroids or vitamins eliminates the need to use solubilisers but requires other additives to ensure stability.

Suspending Agents

It has already been stated that parenteral suspensions must be of a regular small particle size and must not cake during storage. Parenteral suspensions should also be easy to resuspend and inject through an 18- to 20-gauge hypodermic needle. In order to achieve these parameters it is necessary to control the degree of crystallisation, the particle size range, and the method of sterilisation of the drug substance. Micronisation may be necessary. The processes involved in wetting the drug, aseptic dispersion and milling, and filling into final containers must all be carefully controlled. Uniform distribution of the drug is required to ensure that a controlled and adequate dose is administered to the patient. Suspending agents play a vital role in controlling these processes. Carmellose sodium, povidone, and gelatin are all commonly used as suspending agents in parenterals. Gelatin and carmellose sodium are derived from natural sources and consequently must be carefully monitored for microbial contamination during routine production.

Process Development

Before transferring a parenteral formulation to routine manufacture, the ability of the formulation to withstand manufacture and storage must be evaluated. This involves an evaluation of the stability of the formulation to heat sterilisation, the suitability of (and compatibility with) various types of filters, microbiological challenge to the sterilisation process presented by the formulation, the selection of the most suitable containers and closures for the product, and the stability of the formulation in its chosen packaging during transport and storage. Additionally, information is required on suitable procedures for sterility and pyrogen or endotoxin testing and on rate of drug release for slow-release formulations. The optimisation and development of parenteral formulations can therefore be very time consuming and expensive and involves careful planning. The key elements of the developmental process are described in this section.

Sterilisation and Sterilisation Validation

Sterilisation is the process of killing or removing micro-organisms. It may be effected by killing the micro-organisms by physical or chemical methods or removal by filtration. Parenteral products can either be sterilised in their final container, or as bulk solution, or by sterilisation of the components which are then mixed aseptically (aseptic processing). Sterilisation in the final container is often referred to as 'terminal sterilisation'. Products that are not terminally sterilised must be transferred aseptically to their final container, which must also be sterile (aseptic filling). Terminal sterilisation methods are the preferred methods of sterilising parenteral products, since they are more easily controlled, monitored, and quantified than aseptic processes. Processes involving heat are the most reliable and should be used whenever possible. Aseptic processes involve a risk of contamination which varies depending upon the environment, the processing operations, the processing time and, most importantly, the operators.

The choice of sterilisation method is also governed by the type of product and the stability of the product to the process under consideration. In order to make this choice and carry out the necessary validation procedures, it is necessary to understand more fully what is involved in the various methods of sterilisation. These are dealt with, in detail, in the Sterilisation chapter. To recap, the methods that are principally employed in the manufacture of parenterals are dry heat sterilisation, heating in an autoclave, filtration, and ethylene oxide sterilisation. Heating with a bactericide is rarely used. It is no longer specified as an acceptable method in the *British Pharmacopoeia* or the *United States Pharmacopeia*, and consequently its use would require extensive justification and validation.

Dry heat sterilisation also has limited applications in parenteral manufacture. Various combinations of temperature and time are recommended depending upon the material to be sterilised. The *British Pharmacopoeia* recommends cycles of a minimum of 180° for not less than 30 minutes, a minimum of 170° for not less than 1 hour, or a minimum of 160° for not less than 2 hours. However, it also states that other combinations of time and temperature may be necessary for certain preparations. Whatever combination is selected, the process must be fully validated both for efficacy of sterilisation and for product stability. The *United States Pharmacopeia* requires manufacturers to challenge dry heat sterilisation cycles with heat-resistant spores such as *Bacillus subtilis*. A 12 log reduction in the number of spores is desirable.[18] Where non-pharmacopoeial cycles are employed they should, in any case, be validated by spore challenge tests. Such validation is normally required by the Food and Drug Administration and can be performed during formulation development.

Dry heat sterilisation can be used for sterilisation of oily injections and implants, for sterilisation of oily vehicles for injections, which are subsequently processed aseptically, and for sterilisation of glassware, for parenterals manufacture, and containers. Fixed oils such as ethyl oleate, liquid paraffin, and glycerol require lower temperatures, whereas glassware and containers will withstand much higher temperatures. Glassware and containers are often sterilised at temperatures of up to 250° for 2 hours in order to effect simultaneous depyrogenation. Depyrogenation of glassware and containers also requires full validation. This can be done independently of the product and is undertaken by inoculating the glassware or containers with 1000 or more *USP* units of bacterial endotoxin. After heating, an endotoxin test is carried out with Limulus Amoebocyte Lysate (the LAL test, described later in this chapter) to demonstrate that the endotoxin has been inactivated. A minimum 3 log reduction in endotoxin levels is required. The procedure for this validation technique is well documented.[18]

Dry heat sterilisation is not suitable for injections formulated in an aqueous base or a cosolvent system. The method of choice for these products is

heating in an autoclave. (This is the most commonly employed method in the sterilisation of parenterals.) It has the great advantage that it is relatively easy to control and the efficiency of sterilisation can be readily measured.

The recommended temperatures and minimum holding times to effect sterilisation can be found in the Sterilisation chapter. The most frequently used sterilising temperatures are 115° to 118° and 121° to 124°. At 121° the *British Pharmacopoeia* requires a minimum holding time of 15 minutes, whereas the *United States Pharmacopeia* requires 30 minutes. In order to satisfy all regulatory authorities the latter holding time is normally adopted. However, a longer holding time also needs to be justified with respect to the stability of the product and it is normal to conduct stability studies on products following sterilisation at 121° for up to one hour. Such studies are normally done during formulation development in order to ensure that an optimally stable formulation has been selected.

The holding times specified do not include the time required for the product to attain sterilisation temperature. The heating-up and cooling-down periods are dependent upon the thermal properties of the product, the volume of the product in the container, and the heat transfer properties of the container. The heating-up time must therefore be determined for each product individually and must be performed in the autoclave or autoclaves that will be used in routine batch production. These heat penetration studies are normally done during scale-up to the production batch size and are carried out using thermocouples or other calibrated temperature probes as described in the Sterilisation chapter. Three production-scale batches are normally required to be validated in this way and subsequent revalidation is normally carried out on at least one batch every six months.

It must be established that new formulations do not protect micro-organisms from steam sterilisation; such protection can occur in some parenteral vehicles. This is done by measuring the **D-value** for a given organism in the parenteral solution. The D-value is a measure of the amount of heat required to kill a certain micro-organism. For a given organism, it is defined as the time (in minutes) required to reduce the population by 90%, or 1 log cycle, at a specific temperature. The organism normally chosen is *Bacillus stearothermophilus* spores, with a minimum D-value of 1.5. The D-value is normally measured at 121°, thus at 121° it takes 1.5 minutes for a 1 log reduction of *Bacillus stearothermophilus*

spores under a given set of experimental conditions. This procedure is well documented.[19]

If the D-value is significantly increased when measured in the parenteral formulation under development, it can be concluded that the formulation is providing some protection against autoclaving and the autoclave cycle must be modified accordingly. This is done by measuring the F_0 **value** for the autoclave cycle (see the Sterilisation chapter). For an organism with a D-value of 1.5, a sterilisation cycle with an F_0 value of 1.5 is required to give a 1 log reduction of the organism. The F_0 value for a given autoclave cycle must be sufficient to give a level of sterility assurance of less than one contaminated container in one million, that is, a **Sterility Assurance Level** (SAL; see Sterilisation chapter) of 10^{-6}. Thus, if each container in the autoclave load contains 100 micro-organisms (10^2), it would require an 8 log reduction of organisms to give an SAL of 10^{-6}. For an organism with a D-value of 1.5 this equates to a minimum sterilisation cycle of 12 minutes at 121°.

The measurement of D-values is susceptible to the conditions under which an organism is cultured and stored and this must be borne in mind when such work is undertaken.

Organisms used for measuring the effectiveness of the sterilisation cycle are commonly referred to as **biological indicators**. It is essential that the resistance of the biological indicator used is greater than that of the natural microbial flora found in the parenteral product before sterilisation. The type and number of organisms found in a product before sterilisation is known as the **bioburden**. Measurement of bioburdens is dealt with elsewhere in this chapter.

Often medicaments are unstable to pharmacopoeial sterilisation cycles and in some instances the containers selected will not withstand the high temperatures required. Many medicaments are unstable at 121°, but are relatively stable at lower temperatures, as are some polymers used in parenteral containers. In other cases it is the duration of the holding time, rather than the high temperature, which causes instability. In these instances the manufacturer is faced with a choice between a reduced temperature/time combination or an alternative method of sterilisation. A reduced heat sterilisation cycle is still the method of choice provided that it can be demonstrated, by suitable validation methods, to render the product sterile. It is in these instances that application of the F_0 concept is most useful. However, reduced heat cycles are commonly used in order to reduce energy consumption in large-scale production.

Where non-pharmacopoeial cycles are used, the parameter that will determine the acceptability of the cycle is the measured F_o value. Measurement of the F_o value normally starts at about 80°, thus there is a contribution to the F_o value during the heating-up and cooling-down phases of the cycle. This contribution can be quite significant for large volume parenterals.

Many parenteral products cannot be sterilised by heat sterilisation even at reduced temperature/time combinations. Many steroids, antibiotics, and peptides fall into this category. There are also many parenteral suspensions and emulsions that cannot be heat sterilised since heat will affect the physical properties of the formulation. In these instances an alternative method of sterilisation must be chosen. **Ethylene oxide sterilisation** and irradiation are sometimes used for medicaments, excipients, or containers, but neither method has found wide application in the sterilisation of parenteral products. These methods are hazardous, difficult to control, and less effective than heat sterilisation methods, yet they are often just as destructive to the product. Additional restraints on the use of ethylene oxide are the limited ability of the ethylene oxide gas to diffuse to the innermost areas of the product that require sterilisation, and the toxicity of the gas.

can our produce withstand?

Validation of Aseptic Processes

Parenteral products that will not withstand heat sterilisation normally require some form of aseptic processing. Products that are clear solutions can be sterilised by filtration and then filled aseptically into sterile containers. Suspensions and emulsions may have to be compounded aseptically, following sterilisation of the components, and then aseptically filled. Aseptic compounding demands additional controls and great care to ensure that sterility is not compromised. See also the Aseptic Processing chapter.

Sterilisation by filtration must be fully validated, just as methods of heat sterilisation are validated, on a product by product basis. Selection of filter type is governed by the physical and chemical properties of the product. The filter selected must be tested for sterilisation efficiency and for physical and chemical compatibility with the product being filtered.

Sterilising filters are normally made of cellulose derivatives, such as cellulose nitrates and acetates, or suitable polymeric materials. Nylon, polyvinyl chloride, and polypropylene are also commonly used. A pore size of 0.2 micrometre is normally used. Filters with larger pore sizes may be used for clarification before heat sterilisation, but they will not normally provide the sterilising efficiency provided by 0.2 micrometre filters. If the solution to be filtered contains large numbers of particulates, pre-filtration, using filters of up to 5 micrometres pore size, may be necessary.

Pore size can be affected by the pH, viscosity, or ionic strength of the solution being filtered. This in turn will affect the sterilising efficiency of the filter. The effect that these varying physical properties will have is also dependent upon filtration pressure and flow rate of solution. Some of the modern polymeric materials are less affected by variations in physical properties of solutions than the more traditional cellulose derivatives.

Filter manufacturers can often provide good advice on the selection of filter materials for a particular product. However, the choice may also be influenced by the physical and chemical compatibility of the product with the filter during filtration. Components of the solution being filtered may be adsorbed onto the surface of the filter. Adsorption is more significant in dilute solutions and solutions containing minor components such as preservatives. It is also more significant when depth filters are used. Depth filters are sometimes used for pre-filtration. For a high concentration of a relatively particle-free solution passing through a membrane filter, adsorption may occur at levels that are undetectable and, therefore, insignificant. However, at a lower concentration the degree of adsorption may become significant.

Another factor affecting the choice of filter is the chemical compatibility of the product with the filter, for example, certain amines are known to interact with cellulose derivatives causing degradation. Degradation mechanisms may also be catalysed by trace chemicals present on the filter. Chemical stability studies should therefore be carried out on the product that has been filtered. Modern polymeric materials are normally superior with respect to chemical compatibility but are expensive compared to the cellulosic filters, which are perfectly suitable for many solutions.

Validation of filter efficiency can be done using a bacterial challenge test. Various test organisms have been used for this type of test;[20] an example is *Pseudomonas diminuta*, which is ellipsoidal in shape, 0.75 to 1.0 micrometre long and 0.25 micrometre in diameter. However, the actual size changes with the nutritional state of the organism and is influenced by the growth medium and incubation conditions. Therefore, the test conditions must be carefully controlled. The *United States Pharmacopeia* recommends this organism for challenge testing (ATCC No. 19146) and most manufacturers claim that a 0.2 micrometre filter will sterilise solutions containing 10^{12} organisms.

In addition to filter efficiency the integrity of the filter must be checked during aseptic processing. This can be done before filtration, to ensure that the filter is acceptable before use, and again after filtration, to ensure that no damage has occurred during filtration. One method used is the **bubble point test**. This consists of applying gas pressure to the upstream side of a wetted filter to determine the minimum pressure required to force bubbles of gas through the wetted filter (minimum displacing pressure). This test measures the size of the largest effective pores in the filter but also provides a useful safeguard against leaks in the filtration system as a whole. If the gas pressure is allowed to build up slowly until there is a slow steady stream of bubbles, the maximum effective pore diameter (d) is given by:

$$d = 4\sigma \frac{\cos \theta}{P}$$

where P is the minimum displacing pressure, σ is the surface tension of the liquid used in the test, and θ is the angle of wetting of the solid surface by the liquid.

For a given liquid, for example water, the pressure P is constant for a particular filter. Filter manufacturers will supply the value for P when measured using water. If the bubble point is measured using a solution with a significantly different surface tension than water (that is, $\cos \theta$ is significantly different) then a different result is given. The bubble point for a given solution must therefore be established on a product by product basis or the bubble point test must be conducted using water as the wetting liquid and the product must be thoroughly washed from the filter, with water, after filtration. The bubble point test is gradually being superseded by instrumental methods, which measure the pressure differential across the filter. Again this can be performed either on water or on the product and the same considerations apply. This method is more precise and reproducible and it gives a quantitative measurement, which can be related to filter pore size. It has the added advantage that the same equipment can be used to test the integrity of hydrophobic filters used for vacuum release in lyophilisers and air inlets in porous load autoclaves. In these cases the filter is wetted using isopropanol. The equipment used for this method is expensive and is normally supplied by filter manufacturers, who can also provide technical support for the evaluation of integrity testing of new products.

Sterility Testing

Methods employed for sterility testing are well documented in the pharmacopoeias. However, for any new product the detailed test conditions must be validated to ensure recovery of a range of contaminating organisms, to ensure that any antimicrobial preservatives in the product have been neutralised and to ensure that the product itself is not affecting the ability of the sterility test filter to entrap the organisms and transfer them to the incubation medium. This validation will also provide information on the most suitable incubation medium and temperature for the organisms that are the most likely contaminants. The validation procedure involves challenging the test method with small inocula (10^2) of the selected organisms. A positive validation is given by the growth and identification of each organism.

Pyrogens and Pyrogen Testing

Pyrogens are substances which, when injected, produce a pyrogenic response, that is, a rise in body temperature. The most common pyrogens in parenterals are endotoxins formed from the outer membrane of Gram-negative bacteria. Endotoxins also elicit other undesirable responses when injected, such as erythema at the injection site, pain in the legs and back, and general discomfort. (See also the Pyrogens chapter.)

The presence of pyrogens in parenteral products must be controlled to ensure that a pyrogenic response is not induced during administration. This is achieved by a combination of controls on the components of the product and on the manufacturing process. These are detailed in the section on parenterals manufacture.

The traditional method of testing for pyrogens is detailed in the *British Pharmacopoeia*. It involves the administration of the product to laboratory *rabbits* and measurement of the resulting rise in body temperature. The dose administered is dictated on a mg/kg basis by the maximum recommended dose of the product. This method does not quantify the amount of bacterial endotoxin present in the product and, as is common with biological tests, it suffers from wide experimental variability. It is also expensive, time consuming, and may cause discomfort to laboratory animals.

In recent years an alternative method of measuring bacterial endotoxin has been developed. This method utilises the activity of an enzyme extracted from the horseshoe crab, *Limulus polyphemus* and is known as the Limulus Amoebocyte Lysate (LAL) test, after the enzyme concerned. In the presence of bacterial endotoxin this enzyme gels. The degree of gelling can be quantified and related to the amount of endotoxin present. There are a number of instrumental methods now available for measuring the gelling reaction, including colorimetric and turbidimetric methods. This test can be used to accurately quantify the amount of bacterial endotoxin present in a product and consequently provides better information on the quality of the product than the *rabbit* pyrogen test. It is also quicker, more economical, and does not use laboratory animals.

The LAL test is preferred for new products and can be readily validated on pilot batches. Data on three batches of product are normally sufficient. For products whose registered specification involves the *rabbit* test, it is normally necessary to validate the LAL test against the *rabbit* test for a number of batches, to demonstrate equivalent, or better, sensitivity.

Validation of Bioburden Testing

Most sterilisation processes are designed to give a reduction in organisms far in excess of that required by the pharmacopoeias and regulatory authorities. However, it is desirable to keep the number of viable organisms in the product, before sterilisation, as low as possible. In this way the challenge to the sterilisation process and, more importantly, the potential for production of endotoxins, which are not removed by sterilisation, are minimised. Bioburden testing is carried out on parenteral solutions before sterilisation and the methodology must be validated in a similar manner to that for sterility testing. The bioburden is the total number and type of viable organisms present in the product, per unit volume or mass of product, before the final sterilisation process. It is the challenge that is presented to the sterilisation process. Bioburdens can be measured either by membrane filtration followed by incubation of the filter on an agar plate (a modification of the *British Pharmacopoeia* sterility test), or by direct inoculation into agar and then transferring the agar to a 'pour plate'. In either case the medicament or one of the excipients may be bactericidal or bacteriostatic

and the validation process must demonstrate that this activity has been neutralised or eliminated. The number of viable organisms (the viable count) is the bioburden and is usually measured in colony forming units (cfu) per millilitre or per gram.

The bioburden of the product will be dictated by the contamination levels of the components. Therefore, in order to control the bioburden, it is necessary to measure and control the viable counts in the medicament, in all of the excipients, in the injection vehicle, and in the containers and closures. Water is the main contributor to the bioburden of the product but medicaments and excipients from natural sources, for example, insulin, gelatin, or mannitol, may contain large numbers of viable organisms. It is therefore necessary to develop methods for measuring viable counts on all new medicaments and excipients.

CONTAINERS AND CLOSURES

Ampoules and Vials

The overwhelming majority of small volume parenterals are currently presented in glass ampoules or vials. Ampoules have a number of advantages over vials and some disadvantages. One of the advantages is that they can be filled at higher speeds than vials. Ampoules can also be bought as sealed units that are practically particle-free and sterilised; this reduces the amount of washing, rinsing, and sterilisation required at the manufacturing site. Such ampoules are blown from tubular glass and sterilised in purpose-built premises. Ampoules can be filled, purged with nitrogen if necessary, and sealed in one quick operation, thus reducing the risk of contamination during the process. Ampoules provide a more reliable seal, which can be readily leak tested and which will not deteriorate during the lifetime of the product. Ampoules are also lighter for transport and occupy less storage space than corresponding sizes of vials.

The disadvantages of ampoules relate to their handling. Of greatest concern are the hazards associated with opening them. This can result in spicules of glass being drawn into the ampoule and consequently being injected into patients. It can also result in lacerations to the fingers of those trying to open ampoules. Ampoules are now designed with a 'snap-off' ring around the neck of the ampoule where the glass is at its weakest and this should break more easily. Various types of openers are also available. These can be inserted over the top of the ampoule and will retain the broken top once the ampoule has been opened. However, these improvements do not prevent the ingress of spicules. The significance of this problem is the subject of wide debate.

Despite the disadvantages of ampoules they are still the most common container type used for small volume parenterals in Europe. The advantages they offer in terms of filling speed, cost, and simplicity, far outweigh other considerations. In the USA, however, there is currently a market preference for vials, probably based on the perception of greater safety.

Many of the disadvantages of ampoules are eliminated by the use of vials. Vials are not generally hazardous to open and they are not prone to contamination by glass spicules. However, when a hypodermic needle is inserted through the stopper into the product, there is a risk of particulate contamination from the stopper. Closure integrity relies on the fit between the neck of the vial and the stopper, held in place by a metal crimp. The seal is less reliable than that of an ampoule.

Leak Testing of Ampoules and Vials

Leak testing of vials and ampoules can be carried out by a variety of methods.[21] Previously, leak testing of vials was carried out as a quality control test on a statistical sample of containers and closures before manufacturing. But it is now increasingly being carried out on 100% of containers, after batch processing is complete. The methods used include the 'dye bath test', liquid loss tests, and high voltage detection methods. The **'dye bath test'** involves subjecting the containers to vacuum and/or pressure while immersed in a dye bath. The force applied will cause dye solution to enter through any hole or break in the container, or any defective seal. **Liquid loss tests** also involve pulling a vacuum, but without the dye, resulting in a loss of liquid. This method has the advantage of avoiding the risk of contamination from the dye. **High voltage detection** involves very costly electronic equipment, which applies a high voltage across the length of the ampoule and measures the resistance of each container. Ampoules with cracks or holes give a significantly lower resistance because the fluid in the ampoule, which has a much greater conductivity than glass, will flow into the crack or hole. This method is extremely sensitive in comparison to other methods. It is also faster, does not rely on visual observation, can be used on coloured containers and coloured

solutions, and there is no risk of undetected contaminated containers. However, the initial capital cost is high. The method has been applied successfully to vials.[21]

The integrity of the closure is a critical factor in the quality and safety of small volume parenterals. Because of the difficulties of demonstrating closure integrity during storage, the Food and Drug Administration now recognises that stability testing protocols on parenterals in vials include sterility tests at least annually. However, it can be argued that this is unnecessary for ampoules.

Types of Glass Used in Parenteral Containers

Regardless of the type of container used, containers for parenteral preparations must be made from materials that are sufficiently transparent to permit visual inspection of the contents, that do not adversely affect the quality of the contents and that do not permit diffusion of foreign substances into the product. The last two criteria also apply to stoppers.

The type of glass used in ampoules and vials is normally borosilicate glass, such as that specified as Type I by the *United States Pharmacopeia*. The *United States Pharmacopeia* also specifies Type II and Type III glass. Type II glass is sulphur dioxide-treated soda-lime glass and is less expensive than Type I. It is also suitable for products that remain below pH 7.0 for their shelf-life. However, its use is declining, its main application being bottles for large volume parenterals. Type III glass has been found to be acceptable for some dry powders that are subsequently dissolved to make a buffered solution and for liquid formulations that prove to be insensitive to alkali. It is not normally used for terminally-sterilised products. (See also the Pharmaceutical Packaging chapter.)

Design of Parenteral Containers

Glass containers may be moulded or made from tubular glass. Tube-blown containers are of a more regular wall thickness and are consequently preferred for lyophilised products. All major suppliers manufacture their products to meet international standards; however, the design and physical dimensions are generally tailored to the requirements of the modern, high-speed filling equipment that is available. Containers must be of a sufficient capacity to allow for a slight excess in the fill volume, such that the nominal injection volume can be drawn up into a syringe. The *United States Pharmacopeia* gives recommendations for excess volumes. The *British Pharmacopoeia* simply specifies that the excess should be sufficient to permit withdrawal of the nominal volume.

Closures for Vials

Stoppers for vials must also be chosen with great care, to avoid interactions with the vial contents. Absorption of medicaments and excipients, such as preservatives and antoxidants, into the stopper can occur. Chemical degradation of the product arising from interactions with, or catalysed by the extractives from, the stopper can occur.

In addition to preventing the access of microorganisms and other contaminants, the closure must permit the withdrawal of a part of, or the whole of, the contents of the container, without removal of the closure. The plastic materials or elastomers of which the closure is composed must be sufficiently firm and elastic to allow the passage of a needle with minimal shredding of particles and, for multidose containers, to ensure that the puncture is resealed when the needle is withdrawn. Closures are also frequently siliconised before use to aid insertion. This treatment is known to give rise to many subvisible particles and modern elastomeric materials do not require siliconisation.

A number of butyl, chlorobutyl, and bromobutyl rubber formulations have been developed in recent years for use in closures. They contain fewer extractives, give rise to less particulate contamination, and cause fewer interactions with products than traditional materials. The selection of the most suitable closure formulation depends upon the chemical and physical properties of the formulation. One important consideration is pH. Some formulations are preferred for lyophilised products since they retain less moisture after preparation. The selection of closures for vials was reviewed in a publication by the US Parenteral Drug Association.[22]

Containers for Lyophilised Products

Vials are generally preferred for lyophilised products, although ampoules are sometimes used. The advantage of vials is that they can be filled and loaded into the lyophilisation chamber with the stoppers half inserted. The stoppers are designed such that sublimation can occur through gaps between the stopper and the neck of the vial, created by grooves in the stopper. When lyophilisation is complete the vacuum can be released or partially released using an inert gas such as nitrogen or helium. The stoppers can then be fully inserted, via

a ram in the chamber, in an inert and sterile atmosphere and if necessary under a partial vacuum.

When ampoules are used for lyophilisation, they must be filled and loaded into the lyophilisation chamber unsealed. When lyophilisation is complete they must be removed from the chamber and transported back to the filling line for sealing. This means that the unsealed ampoules are at risk of contamination during three separate operations and may have to stand unsealed for long periods of time before being sealed. Ampoules have been designed that will accommodate rubber stoppers of a similar type to those used in vials undergoing lyophilisation. These stoppers can be fully inserted via the ram. The ampoules are then removed and sealed as normal, by drawing off the top part of the ampoule neck with the stopper inserted. These ampoules have had limited success. Because of the small aperture through which sublimation can occur, lyophilisation is slow and the depth of fill of the pre-lyophilisation solution limits the fill volume possible for a given ampoule size.

Plastics used in Parenteral Containers

Glass ampoules and vials are regarded as the most commonly used types of container for small volume parenterals. However, the recent innovation of plastic ampoules has found applications in a number of products such as water for injections, sodium chloride injection, and lignocaine injection.

Plastic ampoules are produced by a technology known as **Blow, Fill, Seal** (BFS) technology. Beads of polypropylene or polyethylene are melted and blown into a mould. The moulded ampoule is then filled with the product and sealed. The entire process is complete in a few seconds and takes place within a confined area in the filling machine. The polymers used are free from plasticisers and will withstand heat sterilisation at about 100°.

Plastic ampoules offer significant advantages to the user of the product and to the manufacturer. They are unbreakable, and cause neither glass spicules in the product nor lacerations of the fingers. They are lighter for transport purposes and are inert to many products. Adsorption of medicaments from parenteral solutions onto polyethylene is far less common than with polyvinyl chloride. Plastic ampoules are also more economical than glass; however, BFS technology requires large initial investment in filling equipment and specialised ballasted autoclaves.

Novel Developments in Parenteral Containers

From the clinical viewpoint, the ideal presentation of a small volume parenteral is one that is ready to use and does not require the product to be drawn up into a hypodermic syringe. A number of novel presentations exist to overcome this problem. Pre-filled syringes are the most common and have found wide application, particularly in products used for cardiac arrest and intensive care therapy, where the product may be needed quickly. A very recent development in prefilled syringes is a syringe that has two chambers. One chamber contains a lyophilised product and the other contains the diluent. The critical design factor for such products is to ensure that the diluent only comes into contact with the product when required, otherwise the product is rendered unstable. The two chambers are separated by a rubber septum which is pushed forward to a point where the barrel of the syringe is widened. This allows the diluent to bypass the septum and reconstitute the lyophilised product. However, the rubber septum must prevent passage of diluent or water vapour during storage. The rubber type, design, and dimension tolerances for this septum are therefore critical.

There are also patented systems available, which contain a lyophilised product in a specially designed vial. The vial is connected to an infusion bag in such a way that the infusion solution can be reconstituted and the product transferred back to the infusion bag without coming into contact with the atmosphere or a non-sterile surface. The vial may be presented already connected to the bag. Such presentations have found wide application in North America, where intravenous solutions are commonly administered by slow intravenous infusion rather than bolus injection via a syringe. However, the relatively high cost of these presentations, coupled with some initial reservations when first introduced, has limited their use in Europe. The initial problems have now been resolved, but there is a reluctance to use, and a limited need for, such products in the UK.

Large Volume Parenterals

The use of polyvinyl chloride bags for large volume parenterals is well established and the overwhelming majority of infusion fluids are presented in this way. The normal presentation volumes are 50 mL and 100 mL 'minibags' and 500 mL and 1 litre bags. Total parenteral nutrition (TPN) solutions are presented in bags of up to 3 litres. Infusion bags are designed with a port for the attachment of the delivery set and an additives port for addition of small volume parenterals, which are required to be given by slow infusion. Nutritional supplements such as intravenous vitamins and minerals may also be added to TPN bags via this port.

STABILITY TESTING OF PARENTERALS

Accelerated stability testing of parenteral solutions, in order to select those which are optimally stable, can produce good shelf-life predictions for the formulation under study. This is because the physical and chemical properties of the medicament and excipients in solution tend to follow more predictable patterns at elevated temperatures in solution than in the solid state.

This is not necessarily true of suspensions, emulsions, or lyophilised products, where parameters such as particle or droplet size and reconstitution time are important and may vary widely at elevated temperatures.

Long-term stability data are nevertheless required for all parenteral products and most regulatory authorities will only accept 'real time data' for shelf-life predictions, that is, data generated from the storage of the product at a controlled temperature, which reflects the recommended storage conditions, over the entire shelf-life of the product. Primary stability data submitted to regulatory authorities must be provided on the product in the same container and closure type as that which will be used for the commercial product. Stability batches can normally be a mixture of pilot-scale and production-scale batches. The proposed EC guideline recommends two pilot batches and one production batch. The Food and Drug Administration guideline, on the other hand, currently requires data on three production-scale batches of each strength or container size.

There are a number of discrepancies in the requirements for stability testing between the three major regulatory authorities (the FDA, the EC, and the Japanese Ministry of Health). These differences, together with many other differences in the quality, safety, and efficacy requirements for product registration are currently being considered by the International Conference on Harmonisation (ICH). The ICH is sponsored by regulatory bodies and pharmaceutical manufacturers organisations from the USA, the EC, and Japan.

When designing stability-testing protocols the requirements of the various regulatory bodies must be considered. The type of parenteral and the container and closure must also be considered. It is important to demonstrate that the container/closure combination will not only provide adequate stability for the product, but that it will also maintain sterility throughout the shelf-life of the product. Batches used for stability tests must therefore be manufactured under the conditions that will apply in commercial production and must be sterilised in the same way. For heat-sealed ampoules, it is probably sufficient for stability batches to be fully leak tested and sterility tested following sterilisation. It is not normally necessary to carry out sterility testing throughout the stability testing protocol. However, it may be desirable to perform a sterility test on each batch on completion of a stability study, to give added assurance that the ampoules have maintained their seal during storage.

For vials and other presentations where the container is sealed by a rubber stopper or septum, it will be necessary to perform sterility tests on stability batches during storage. This is normally done annually, rather than at every time station. The tests are normally only carried out on samples stored under the conditions of long-term storage. The integrity of the seal on vials is dependent upon the aluminium crimp which holds the stopper in place. Stoppers and crimps may deteriorate during storage, leading to a loss of seal integrity. This deterioration is the main justification for performing sterility tests during stability studies. Selection of the most appropriate stopper and seal combination is very important in this respect. Antimicrobial preservative efficacy tests and tests for the presence of particulate matter are other parameters that are routinely measured during the stability testing of parenterals. Tests for the assessment of antimicrobial preservative efficacy may be carried out annually, whereas antimicrobial preservative assays may be required at every time station and under all storage conditions. It is possible to reduce antimicrobial preservative efficacy testing to initial testing and testing at the end of the shelf-life, if a clear correlation can be demonstrated between preservative efficacy and preservative concentration. (See also the chapter on Control of Microbial Contamination and the Preservation of Medicines.)

Tests for particulate contamination may be necessary for a number of reasons. Where the liquid product is in contact with rubber or plastic components, it may be necessary to demonstrate that particulates are not being generated during storage due to an interaction between the product and component. For parenteral solutions where the medicament concentration is near to its maximum solubility, particulate tests may be required to show that no precipitation has occurred during storage, especially at lower temperatures. It may also be necessary to show that there are no insoluble degradates being precipitated from the solution. This can be avoided by determining the solubility of the degradates as they are identified. (See also the chapter on Particulate Contamination.)

Sterility testing and particulate matter tests are applied specifically to parenteral product stability testing. In addition, stability testing protocols must include the normal physical parameters and chemical analysis necessary to show that the product is not deteriorating during storage. These include pH, chemical assays, and degradate assays. There are a wide range of tests, which form part of the product specification, that are not affected by storage conditions. These tests do not need to be performed as part of stability protocols and include fill volume, specific gravity, excipient concentrations other than antimicrobial preservatives, and antioxidants. Antioxidant concentrations need to be monitored during storage; however, it must be remembered that they are present in the formulation to protect the medicament from oxidation by preferentially reacting with and removing oxygen from solution. In performing their function there will be an initial loss in concentration, which should reduce and cease altogether once all the dissolved oxygen has been utilised. If the loss of antioxidant continues to the point where there is no longer an effective concentration, it will be necessary either to modify the manufacturing process in order to further reduce the initial level of dissolved oxygen, or to increase the concentration of antioxidant in the formulation. All compounds, medicaments, excipients, and degradates are 100% bioavailable in the blood when given by the intravenous route. Thus, where there are unknown degradates or degradates of unknown toxicity, it is important to keep the acceptance limits for these degradates as low as can be practically achieved during the formulation development of the product. Where little is known about the degradates the normal limits set are 0.5% (by weight or by peak area on an HPLC trace) for individual degradates and 2.0% for total degradates. However, peak area percentage on an HPLC trace can be very misleading where the degradate is chemically very different from the parent compound. This is because the HPLC detector response may change significantly, for example, due to a significant change in ultraviolet chromophore. Limits on most physical parameters are determined either by pharmacopoeial test limits, for example, particulates, or by the clinical requirements of the product, for example, pH.

Stability testing of parenterals must also determine the ability of the formulation to withstand heat sterilisation, possibly at a range of temperatures and holding times. For medicaments that are generally regarded as heat stable, it is quite normal to subject the formulation to sterilisation holding times two or three times longer than those normally applied. This will determine whether re-autoclaving of production batches is feasible in the event of a faulty cycle. For less stable products, studies should be conducted to determine whether reduced temperatures and holding times could be applied. 'Minimum kill' sterilisation cycles will give better sterility assurance levels than aseptic processing can and must therefore be preferred.

MANUFACTURE OF PARENTERALS

The scale of parenteral manufacture ranges from small-scale manufacture of a wide variety of products in small, non-dedicated cleanrooms, in hospitals or small private companies, to large-scale batch production in specially designed facilities. These facilities may be dedicated to a single product or a related group of products, such as the penicillins. The manufacture of parenterals cannot be undertaken as a continuous process and must be regarded as a batch process. During large-scale production some products are manufactured in campaigns, thus reducing the amount of preparation and cleaning of facilities and equipment between batches. Antibiotics are often manufactured on a campaign basis. The need for extensive cleaning between batches is forcing many manufacturers to reassess their manufacturing strategies.

Whatever the scale of operation, however automated the process is, and no matter how dedicated or otherwise the facilities are, the manufacturing conditions for all parenterals must comply with certain basic rules relating to quality. These are given in the European Community Guide to Good Manufacturing Practice and the *Guide to Good Pharmaceutical Manufacturing Practice* (the 'Orange Guide'). The Food and Drug Administration also publish their own rules which relate to pharmaceutical good manufacturing practices.

The Food and Drug Administration guidelines are mandatory for companies wishing to export products to the USA. The EC guidelines and the 'Orange Guide' are intended as guidance. However, any departure from these guidelines must be justified by scientifically generated validation data, which show that the alternative procedures or processes used 'achieve the same objective' as the guidelines.

The GMP guidelines give detailed recommendations regarding facilities, procedures, documentation systems, quality control and quarantine arrangements, recall procedures, training requirements and responsibilities of key people within the manufacturing operation. It is not the intention to discuss these topics in detail in this section, but rather to draw attention to key factors currently relating to the manufacture of parenterals.

The first of these factors is the **environmental requirements for cleanrooms**; these are detailed in the Cleanrooms for Pharmaceutical Production chapter. Manufacturers who wish to manufacture parenterals for the European and the US markets are required to meet both the standard of the EC guidelines and the Food and Drug Administration requirements. The more exacting standard is Federal Standard 209E, owing to the extensive and detailed particulate monitoring required by this standard.

Cleanroom standards also give requirements for air pressure differentials between different classes of room. These pressure differentials are primarily intended to ensure that the appropriate level of environmental cleanliness is maintained during the use of cleanrooms. Thus any contamination that occurs is literally blown from a higher grade room to a lower grade room and eventually out of the manufacturing suite altogether. The engineering and design of cleanrooms is a very specialised area of knowledge, and is addressed in the Cleanrooms for Pharmaceutical Production chapter.

The operating and entry procedures for personnel and the control of contamination in cleanrooms are discussed in the Aseptic Processing chapter.

Cleanroom procedures demand a knowledge and practical application of aseptic technique. During training of cleanroom operators, aseptic technique can be demonstrated by performing aseptic transfer operations using sterile nutrient broth. However, this is not the same as aseptic process validation. Cleanroom operators should also understand the ways by which contamination is created and transferred in a cleanroom environment. This essentially involves minimising movement and air turbulence; contact with non-sterile surfaces should be discouraged. It is impossible to sterilise all surfaces within a cleanroom. The best compromise is strict adherence to hygiene and cleaning procedures, coupled with regular spraying or swabbing of contaminated surfaces using appropriate hard surface disinfectants or alcohol sprays.

Wherever possible, equipment should be sterilised by dry heat or by autoclaving; it should never be stored wet.

The **water** used in parenteral manufacture is of vital importance to the quality of the product. It must be of a quality which meets the chemical specifications for Water for Injections BP, EP, or USP. This effectively means that it must be distilled from potable or Purified Water BP. The *United States Pharmacopeia* also permits purification by reverse osmosis. This is not currently the case in the *British Pharmacopoeia*. Water for parenteral manufacture must meet stringent requirements for microbial contamination and bacterial endotoxins. The microbial contamination limits applied vary between regulatory authorities but it is not difficult to achieve a bioburden of less than 10 colony forming units (cfu) per millilitre; 100 cfu per mL would give cause for concern and probably an investigation.

In small-scale manufacturing water is often freshly distilled and collected on the day of manufacture. However, large-scale processes require large volumes of water, which would take a long time to collect and would be heavily contaminated by the time it was required. In these circumstances water is normally stored at elevated temperatures (65° to 80°) to prevent microbial growth. The water is normally fed to the processing areas via a ring main, which must contain no 'dead legs' where water could be allowed to cool and stagnate. This is particularly a problem at draw-off points on the main, where heat-exchangers are required to reduce the temperature of the water collected.

Water for parenterals manufacture must meet the same requirements for bacterial endotoxins as those required for the product itself. This is because bacterial endotoxins cannot be removed from solutions during processing. The pharmacopoeial pyrogen tests can be applied, but it is more common and more economical to perform LAL testing for routine monitoring purposes.

Water, active components, and other excipients must all be carefully monitored to minimise the microbial contamination level of the product before sterilisation, that is, the bioburden challenge to the sterilisation process itself. Solutions must not be stored for prolonged periods before sterilisation because of the risk of a high bioburden and high endotoxin levels. Active components and other excipients can be monitored by measuring the number of viable organisms per gram or per millilitre of the material. The method used for viable counts must be capable of eliminating bacteriostatic properties of the material and must be validated for recovery of organisms, as has been referred to previously.

Some excipients, such as antimicrobial preservatives, sodium hydroxide, alcohols, and even sodium chloride are incapable of supporting the growth of vegetative cells. If these materials come from a chemical source it may not be necessary to monitor them. However, if they come from a natural (animal, vegetable, or mineral) source, they may require monitoring because of the possible presence of pathogenic organisms that they may have acquired from their natural source. The acceptable limit for actives and excipients might be less than 100 organisms per millilitre or per gram. In addition, all components of injectable products must be free of pathogens.

Process Validation

In addition to the normal process validation, which is required for all pharmaceutical products, the sterilisation process must be fully and thoroughly validated. All parts of the manufacturing process contribute to the overall quality of the product, but validation of the sterilisation method and subsequent maintenance of sterility in the product are the areas that require the greatest validation effort. See also the Validation and Sterilisation chapters. For terminally sterilised products, the validation process entails demonstrating that the product reaches sterilisation temperature for the specified time. This has been described previously in the section on Process Development. Temperature mapping and heat penetration studies, as they are often called, are carried out every three to six months during normal production. A minimum of twelve thermocouple probes are normally distributed throughout the steriliser load. More probes may be used in larger sterilisers to give a better heat distribution pattern. The procedures recommended for this work are well documented.[19]

Filtration processes are monitored on a batch to batch basis by performing integrity testing on the filter, both before and after filtration of the product. This can be done using either the 'Bubble Point Test' or by the forward flow test. Additionally, sterile filtration and aseptic filling must be validated by process simulations with nutrient broth (media fills). Media fills are normally used to simulate the compounding, filtration, collection, storage, and filling processes. Currently the only published guidelines for media fill validation are those published by the Parenteral Drug Association.[23]

Once a product has been filled into its final container, it is necessary to demonstrate that the container will provide an airtight seal which will maintain the sterility of the product. This can be achieved by carrying out leak testing on the entire batch of product. A recent publication by the Parenteral Society gives authoritative guidance on procedures, which can be used for leak testing.[21]

Other parts of the manufacturing process that must be validated include compounding and mixing, fill volumes, and lyophilisation processes. These processes are normally monitored by in-process testing. However, lyophilisation processes require extensive validation to ensure reproducibility of heat transfer and vapour loss (see Lyophilised Products, below).

Labelling of Parenterals

Parenteral containers vary greatly in size from 1-mL ampoules to 3-litre bags. It is difficult to put much information on a label intended for a 1-mL ampoule and it is important not to completely obliterate the product from view. The user must be able to see the product before administration in case a faulty container has escaped detection by normal inspection and testing procedures. The *United States Pharmacopeia* states that the label must leave a sufficient area of the container uncovered for its full length or circumference to permit inspection of the contents. The information on the container label is often limited to that which is essential and more information is contained on the label for the outer pack or on the package insert.

The *British Pharmacopoeia* requires that where appropriate the label must state the strength of the preparation in terms of the amount of active ingredient in a suitable dose-volume. The label must also state the name of any added substance, the expiry date, and the storage conditions. Statements of storage conditions are becoming increasingly important, based on the temperature at which long-term stability data have been generated. In order to claim an unspecified room temperature storage, European regulatory authorities require stability data generated at 25° and 60% relative humidity. The Food and Drug Administration currently require data at 30° and 60% relative humidity. The requirement varies for different markets depending upon the climatic conditions that prevail in each region (or 'climatic zone').

The label for a single-dose parenteral product states that any portion of the contents remaining should be discarded.

The *United States Pharmacopeia* currently accepts the strength of the preparation either as the percentage content of drug or the amount of drug in a specified volume. The requirement of the *British Pharmacopoeia* for the amount of drug in a suitable dose-volume therefore covers the requirements for both the European and the US markets. On the other hand, the *United States Pharmacopeia* requires more information regarding added substances. It requires the percentage content of each ingredient or the amount of each ingredient in a specified volume, with the exception that ingredients added to adjust the pH or to make the solution isotonic may be declared by name and a statement as to their effect. Quantities in these cases need not be given. The *United States Pharmacopeia* also requires the route of administration to be stated.

For intravenous infusions the *British Pharmacopoeia* requires the label to state the nominal volume of the contents. The *British Pharmacopoeia* also requires that the label on powders for injection states:

- that when dissolved or suspended, the contents of the sealed container are intended for parenteral use
- the amount of active ingredient contained in a sealed container
- the directions for the preparation of the injection or intravenous infusion.

If a container of the liquid for reconstitution is supplied, the label of the container should state the composition of the liquid. The requirements of the *United States Pharmacopeia* for powders for injection are more detailed and, in this instance, if a product meets the labelling requirements of the *United States Pharmacopeia* it is probably suitable for both European and US markets.

The *British Pharmacopoeia* also has specific requirements for concentrated solutions for injections. In these instances the label must state the name of the concentrated solution, that the solution must be diluted, and the directions for preparation of the injection or infusion. The *United States Pharmacopeia* also has some specific requirements which relate to dialysis, haemofiltration, or irrigation solutions. Veterinary injections must be clearly labelled as to their intended use in all markets.

PARENTERALS IN USE

Great care is taken to ensure that the quality of parenteral products is suitable for their intended purpose. However, the quality of the product upon leaving the factory is not necessarily the quality of the product that is ultimately administered. This also depends upon the care taken during handling, storage, and administration of the product. These considerations are probably more important for parenterals than for any other dosage forms.

Because many parenteral products are presented in glass containers and an airtight seal is vital for maintenance of sterility, great care must be applied to packaging for shipment and during handling to prevent damage. Damage may not be immediately obvious since hairline cracks may develop in ampoules and damaged crimps may lead to the seals on vial closures being broken. Careless handling may also generate particles from contact between parenteral solutions and rubber stoppers and it may also cause physical changes such as cracking of emulsions and sedimentation of suspensions. Careful inspection of containers is therefore advisable before dispensing and administration.

Storage of products under the recommended storage conditions is also vitally important. Parenteral solutions and suspensions are particularly vulnerable to extremes of temperature. High temperatures may lead to degradation and low temperatures may result in precipitation of dissolved medicaments and excipients.

Immediately after the seal is broken on a parenteral container the contents are exposed to microbial and particulate contamination. Great care must be taken during withdrawal of the product and its administration to the patient, in order to minimise the degree of contamination. This is particularly important for parenterals that are to be administered into a body cavity where there is no natural defence against invading organisms, such as the spinal cord. For this reason intrathecal and epidural injections are often overwrapped and re-sterilised, such that the outer surface of the ampoule is also sterile. The overwrap is removed by the anaesthetist or nurse wearing sterile disposable gloves. An alternative to this is to swab or spray the outer surface of the ampoule with an alcoholic disinfectant (for example, chlorhexidine in ethanol 70%).

Also because of the risk of microbial contamination and growth, it is normally recommended that parenteral solutions should not be stored for more than 24 hours after opening, either in their original container or in a syringe. European regulatory authorities will not permit companies to recommend a longer shelf-life after opening even when supported by chemical stability data. Parenteral solutions that are stored after opening should be kept in a refrigerator to restrict microbial growth, provided that this does not cause precipitation or other physical changes in the product. Additionally, parenteral solutions that are readily oxidised will rapidly degrade once opened. It is therefore not recommended practice to store parenteral products after they have been opened. However, this is a practice that is often undertaken for practical reasons. It occurs in hospitals that offer centralised intravenous additive (see chapter on Infusion Fluids: Admixture and Administration) and cytotoxic reconstitution services. These services are provided in order to eliminate the handling risks to nurses and medical staff associated with antibiotics and cytotoxics. However, centralised services such as these do not operate on a 24 hour, 7 days per week basis. Antibiotics and cytotoxics are therefore reconstituted or prepared and drawn up into syringes ready for use in small batches, under aseptic conditions similar to those used for parenterals manufacture. It may be necessary to store parenteral products, ready for use in syringes, for up to 48 hours and if there is a high demand for the service it may be desirable to make batches large enough for usage over a period of 7 to 14 days. Where such practices are in operation the aseptic procedures must be fully validated using monitoring procedures similar to those used in aseptic processing (see the Aseptic Processing chapter). The shelf-life of the product in the syringe must also be supported by chemical stability data. These data are often generated in hospital pharmaceutical quality assurance laboratories and the Regional Pharmaceutical Officers' Quality

Control Sub-Committee maintains a database of this information.

The pharmaceutical industry and regulatory authorities are alert to the potential risks associated with the handling, storage, and administration of parenteral products. Many developments have taken place to reduce such risks. Among these are in-use and freeze-thaw test protocols, which have been introduced to simulate some of the stresses a product will experience during handling, shipping, and storage. Plastic is being substituted for glass in many presentations. The use of polyvinyl chloride infusion bags is now standard practice and the use of plastic ampoules is well established in the UK. Perhaps the most important innovations in reducing both handling and administration risks are the ready-to-use presentations, which have been discussed previously, such as prefilled syringes and specialised vials.

One innovation, which has found wide application, is the use of in-line filters. These are small 0.2 micrometre membrane filters that are placed in infusion lines or in lines from syringe drivers to filter the parenteral solution immediately before it goes into the blood. These filters will remove both particulate and adventitious microbial contamination. The use of in-line filters is now standard practice in intravenous therapy involving paediatric and immuno-compromised patients.

As with other registration requirements regulatory authorities are currently looking at the guidelines relating to labelling.[24]

LYOPHILISED PRODUCTS

Lyophilisation or freeze-drying is a process by which water is removed from a frozen solution, by sublimation, under a vacuum. The water removed is condensed into ice and subsequently thawed and drained away. This normally results in a 'cake' or 'plug' of very porous and hydrophilic material, in the ampoule or vial, which has a low moisture content. This renders the product more stable than it is in solution and it can be rapidly reconstituted by adding water, sodium chloride solution, or some other suitable aqueous diluent.

The process is applicable to a wide range of pharmaceuticals, biologicals, sera, and hormones which are thermolabile or otherwise unstable in aqueous solution for prolonged storage periods. The product in solution is frozen to below its eutectic point, a vacuum is pulled, and the water is removed by sublimation. Because of the loss of latent heat during sublimation, heat must be applied to the product. The drying step consists of two distinct phases; primary drying, which constitutes the bulk of the sublimation process to form the 'cake', and secondary drying which removes the remaining solvent. The two phases can be followed by monitoring the temperature of the product. At the end of the primary drying phase there is a noticeable increase in product temperature because of the reduced latent heat loss.

The success of the process depends upon keeping the product below its eutectic temperature. Temperature control is governed by the rate of heat input to the product and the rate of vapour loss. Heat input can be greatly affected by the thermal contact between the ampoules or vials and the shelves of the lyophilisation chamber, the thickness and type of glass, the thermal contact with the surrounding ampoules or vials, and depth of fill of the product. If the depth of fill is large there is a greater distance between the surface of the product, where water vapour escapes, and the base of the container, where most of the heat is input. This can set up a large temperature gradient across the product and in order to produce a reasonable rate of vapour loss the temperature at the base of the container must be relatively high. This can lead to a phenomenon known as 'melt-back', whereby the product melts and the 'cake' structure is lost. This occurs when the product temperature exceeds the eutectic point.

Vapour loss is also dependent upon a number of factors. The structure of the frozen product and the porosity of the dried 'cake' above the frozen interface are the main factors and these will be determined by the formulation itself.[25] Another factor is the depth of the fill. If the depth of fill is too large, the vapour must escape through a greater depth of 'cake' when the frozen interface moves towards the bottom of the vial.

When vials are used they are normally stoppered within the lyophilisation chamber by closing the shelves together with a mechanical ram. The stoppers are therefore placed on top of the vials after filling, but are not pressed home. The stoppers are designed with special grooves to allow vapour to escape. The design of the stoppers can have a profound effect on the rate of vapour loss and a change of stoppers can affect the process parameters dramatically.

One further pitfall associated with lyophilisation is the phenomenon of 'collapse'.[26] This is similar to 'melt-back', but occurs in the partially dried 'cake' rather than in the frozen mass. It occurs due to the product temperature exceeding the collapse temperature. The collapse temperature is normally different from, and often lower than, the eutectic point. However, not all products experience collapse.

For any product that is to be manufactured by a lyophilisation process, the eutectic point and the collapse temperature for the formulation must be known. Containers and closures must be carefully selected and the process must be carefully controlled. Process control will also depend upon the capacity, capability, and loading pattern of the lyophilisation chamber. Modern lyophilisers are normally automatically controlled, often by microprocessors. They are generally sterilised by steam sterilisation. The chambers are, therefore, pressure vessels similar to autoclaves. Steam sterilisation cycles must be validated using similar methods to those applied to autoclaves and filling of containers must be evaluated using media fills. The most critical parts of the process are loading and vacuum release, which must also be evaluated using media fills. The vacuum is normally released by letting air or inert gas into the chamber through a 0.2 micrometre hydrophobic filter. The integrity of this filter must be tested *in situ*.

In addition to validating processes for maintenance of sterility, it is also necessary to carry out temperature distribution studies on products, sublimation rate studies, and other measurements of equipment performance.[27]

Because of the complexity of the process, the level of development and validation work required, the cost of equipment, and the energy input required by the process, lyophilisation is an extremely expensive technique. It is normally reserved for products that are unstable in aqueous solution and cannot be formulated in any other way. However, lyophilised products are relatively easy to handle, are sometimes very stable, are light for shipping purposes, and are often very elegant preparations.

BIOTECHNOLOGY PRODUCTS

Modern developments in recombinant-DNA technology have produced a wide range of pharmaceutical products. These are collectively referred to as **biotechnology products** and include vaccines, pharmacologically active peptides, genetically engineered hormone molecules, diagnostic products, and antibiotics. They can be large molecules, cell fragments, or even live cells, and are normally administered parenterally. They represent a major challenge to traditional methods of parenteral

manufacture and formulation. They can be difficult to purify and to filter and are generally unstable to heat sterilisation. In addition, the processes by which the new medicaments are produced are difficult to control and involve cultures of microbial organisms. The challenge which these products present have been well reviewed by Chen.[28] Biotechnology products are viewed differently by regulatory authorities because of the difficulties involved in manufacturing operations and because of their specialised nature. However, the essential regulatory requirements for validation and GMP apply.

The greatest challenge of all is sterility assurance. Biotechnology products currently marketed are, almost without exception, lyophilised products. The normal method of sterilisation is therefore filtration. However, products with active constituents that are cells, or cell fragments, cannot be filtered through a sterilising filter, since this process would also remove the active constituent. Proteins and large peptides are also difficult to filter as they often adhere to the filter material.

Where filtration is impossible the product must be produced via a process involving aseptic techniques at every step from initiation of the cell culture through to filling of the final product. Monitoring of such processes involves sampling at every step and testing for purity of the culture. The methods developed to monitor such processes are often highly specific to the particular process being monitored.

REFERENCES

1. Turco S, King RE. Sterile dosage forms, their preparation and clinical application. Philadelphia: Lea and Febiger, 1974.
2. Dash AK, Suryanarayanan R. Pharm Res 1992;9(8):993–1002.
3. Sampath S, Robinson DH. Pharm Res 1991;8:5–194.
4. Robinson DH, Sampath S. Drug Dev Ind Pharm 1989;15:2339–57.
5. Goodell JA, Flick AB, Herbert JC, Howe JG. Am J Hosp Pharm 1986;43:1454–61.
6. Sampath SS, Garvin K, Robinson DH. Int J Pharmaceutics 1992;78:165–74.
7. Kincl FA, Benagiano G, Angee I. Steroids 1968;11:673–80.
8. McGinity JW, Hurke LA, Combs AB. J Pharm Sci 1979;68:662–4.
9. DiColo G, Carelli V, Nannipieri E, Sarafini MF, Vitale D, Bottari F. Il Farmaco 1982;37:377–89.
10. Carelli V, DiColo G. J Pharm Sci 1983;72:316–17.
11. Hsich DST, Mann K, Chien YW. Drug Dev Ind Pharm 1985;11:1391–410.
12. Florence AT, Attwood D. Physicochemical principles of pharmacy. London: Macmillan, 1981:345–54.
13. DeLuca PP, Rapp RP. Parenteral-drug delivery systems. In: Banker GS, Chalmers RK, editors. Pharmaceutics and pharmacy practice. Philadelphia: Lippincott, 1982:238–78.

14. Akers MJ. J Parenter Sci Technol 1982;36(5):222–7.
15. Akers MJ. J Parenter Drug Assoc 1979;33:346.
16. Lachman L, Liebermann HA, Kanig JL. The theory and practice of industrial pharmacy. 1st ed. Philadelphia: Lea and Febiger, 1970:687.
17. Wade A, editor. Pharmaceutical handbook. London: Pharmaceutical Press, 1980:244–63.
18. Parenteral Drug Association. Technical Monograph No.3. Validation of dry heat processes used for sterilisation and depyrogenation. Philadelphia: The Association, 1981.
19. Parenteral Drug Association. Technical Monograph No.1. Validation of steam sterilisation cycles. Philadelphia: The Association, 1978.
20. Kartinos NJ, Groves MJ. Manufacturing of large volume parenterals. In: Avis KE, Lachman L, Liebermann HA, editors. Pharmaceutical dosage forms: parenteral medications; vol 1. New York: Marcel Dekker, 1984:298.
21. Parenteral Society. Technical Monograph No.3. The prevention and detection of leaks in ampoules, vials and other parenteral containers. Swindon: The Society, 1992.
22. Parenteral Drug Association. Technical Methods Bulletin No.2. Elastomeric closures: evaluation of significant performance and identity characteristics. Philadelphia: The Association, 1981.
23. Parenteral Drug Association. Technical Monograph No.2. Validation of aseptic filling for solution drug products. Philadelphia: The Association, 1980.
24. Kelly S, Greenberg E. Mfg Chem 1992;63(10):55–7.
25. Franks F. Cryo-Letters 1990;11:93–110.
26. MacKenzie AP. Collapse during freeze drying–qualitative and quantitative aspects. In: Goldblith SA, Rey L, Rothmayer WW, editors. Freeze drying and advanced food technology. London: Academic Press Inc, 1975:277–307.
27. Trappler EH. Pharmaceut Technol 1989;13(1):56–7.
28. Chen T. Drug Dev Ind Pharm 1992;18:1311–54.

Aerosols

The true definition of an aerosol is a dispersion of solid or liquid particles in a gas. However, pharmaceutical 'aerosol' presentations generally consist of solutions, emulsions, or suspensions of medicaments in a mixture of inert propellants which are held under pressure until required. For the purpose of this discussion the term aerosol will be used to describe these pharmaceutical presentations. There are three types of aerosol:

- **Space sprays** produce a dispersion of particles, which remain in the air for prolonged periods. The particles of the spray are usually less than 50 micrometres in size.
- **Surface coating sprays** produce a film on the surface treated. This type of aerosol is relatively coarse: the particles range in size from 50 to 200 micrometres.
- **Foams** are formed when expansion of propellant within an emulsion results in the production of small bubbles.

Aerosols have many pharmaceutical applications. Topical preparations have included antiseptics, antifungals, local anaesthetics, anti-inflammatory agents, and antibiotics as well as novel products such as spray-on protective films. However perhaps the greatest use of aerosols is in inhalation therapy (see Inhalation Products chapter), where they are utilised for the delivery of bronchodilators and corticosteroids.

An aerosol package provides protection against environmental factors such as oxygen and moisture and can thus enhance the stability of the preparation. In addition, protection is provided against contamination and aerosols provide a convenient method of presenting sterile products.

COMPONENTS

There are four component parts of an aerosol product: the propellant, the container, the valve and actuator, and the active ingredient concentrate.

Propellants

The function of the propellant in an aerosol system is to produce a pressure such that the medicament is expelled when the valve is opened. The propellant, depending on the type, can also function as a solvent for the active substance, and can affect the characteristics of the expelled product. There are two classes of aerosol propellant: liquefied gases and compressed gases. The liquefied gases are further subdivided into chlorofluorohydrocarbons (such as trichloromonofluoromethane, dichlorodifluoromethane, and dichlorotetrafluoroethane) and hydrocarbons (such as butane, propane, and isobutane). Gases that can be used for compressed gas systems include nitrous oxide, carbon dioxide, and nitrogen.

Vapour Pressure

When a liquefied propellant is used, the force that is responsible for expelling the preparation from the aerosol package is the vapour pressure. In a sealed aerosol container the propellant will evaporate into the head space, producing a vapour pressure. This increases until an equilibrium is established between the liquid and the vapour, at which point the vapour pressure becomes constant.

In general, an aerosol preparation consists of propellants, solvents, and solutes. Under ideal conditions the vapour pressure of a mixture is the sum of the vapour pressures of the individual components (Dalton's Law).

For a mixture of two propellants, x and y:

$$p_x = \frac{m_x}{m_x + m_y} p_x^0 = M_x p_x^0 \quad \text{(Raoult's Law)}$$

where p_x is the partial vapour pressure of the propellant x, p_x^0 is the vapour pressure of pure propellant x, m_x is the number of moles of propellant x, and M_x is the mole fraction of propellant x.

The vapour pressure of propellant y is calculated similarly.

$$p_y = \frac{m_y}{m_y + m_x} p_y^0 = M_y p_y^0$$

Thus the vapour pressure of the whole system (P) can be calculated according to Dalton's Law from:

$$P = p_x + p_y$$

Ideal behaviour is only approached at relatively low concentrations. Aerosol systems are never ideal, but calculations based on the above equations are usually adequate for most purposes. Mixing propellants in varying proportions results in a range of vapour pressures, and mixtures of propellants are generally used in pharmaceutical aerosols. The pressure within an aerosol container filled with liquefied gases remains constant, because as propellant is lost through actuation, more vapour is formed within the container, and equilibrium is re-established. The vapour pressure is therefore independent of the quantity of liquefied gas used, but it does vary with temperature. Compressed gases, as their name suggests, are used in the gaseous state and as such there is a drop in pressure during use. This occurs because as the concentrate is expelled from the container, the head space increases and the gases expand causing a decrease in pressure.

Chlorofluorohydrocarbon (CFC) Propellants

Although there are several chlorofluorohydrocarbon propellants, trichloromonofluoromethane (propellant 11), dichlorodifluoromethane (propellant 12), and dichlorotetrafluoroethane (propellant 114) have been the most widely used in pharmaceutical aerosols. Increased use of chlorofluorohydrocarbons has been implicated in the depletion of the ozone layer of the earth's atmosphere; attempts are, therefore, being made to reduce the use of chlorofluorohydrocarbon propellants (see below).

The numerical designation of the propellants is explained by the following:

- Saturated propellant compounds are designated by three digits except when the first digit would be zero, when only two digits are used.
- The first digit represents the number of carbon atoms in the molecule, less one. If there are only two digits then the molecule is a methane derivative, that is the first digit would be zero $(1 - 1)$. If the first digit is one then the propellant is an ethane derivative $(2 - 1)$.
- The second digit is one more than the number of hydrogen atoms in the molecule.
- The third digit represents the number of fluorine atoms in the molecule.
- The difference between the sum of the fluorine and hydrogen atoms and the number of atoms required to saturate the carbon chain is the number of chlorine atoms.
- Isomers of a compound have the same number, the most symmetric being indicated by number alone and degrees of asymmetry are designated by the letters a, b, c, and so on, following the number.

- For cyclic derivatives, the letter C is used before the identifying number.
- In the case of unsaturated propellant compounds, the number one is used as the fourth digit from the right to indicate an unsaturated double bond.

FOR EXAMPLE:

Propellant 152 (1,2-difluoroethane)

first digit = 1,   number of C atoms = 2

second digit = 5,   number of H atoms = 4

third digit = 2,   number of F atoms = 2

number of Cl atoms = $6 - (4 + 2) = 0$

The Montreal Protocol, modified in June 1992, recommended that CFC production be phased out by the year 2000 and that hydrochlorofluorocarbon (HCFC) production be phased out by 2020. Furthermore, EC environment ministers recommended a ban on CFC production by the end of 1995, although pharmaceutical aerosols are to be exempt.

At present, CFCs are used extensively in pressurised metered-dose inhalers used for the treatment of asthma. Alternative non-CFC propellants will require extensive toxicological testing and clinical trials before receiving regulatory approval.

Hydrocarbon Propellants

The most commonly used hydrocarbon propellants are n-butane, isobutane, and propane. As with the chlorofluorohydrocarbon propellants, they are usually blended to obtain the desired properties. The advantages of hydrocarbon propellants are their ability to dissolve a wide range of medicaments, their chemical and physical stability, lack of odour, low cost, and low toxicity. Hydrocarbon propellants are immiscible with water and so they can be used for three-phase aerosols. Hydrocarbons are less dense than water and thus they stay above the aqueous layer and push the aerosol contents out of the container.

Compressed Gas Propellants

Nitrous oxide, carbon dioxide, and nitrogen have been used as aerosol propellants.

Containers

Five different materials have been used for the construction of aerosol containers: tin-plated steel, aluminium, stainless steel, glass, and plastic.

Tin-plated steel is used for most aerosols, as it is light, inexpensive and durable. It is steel that has been plated on both sides with tin. An additional coating of an organic material is usually also present as this protects the container from the corrosive activity of water and other substances. Tin-plated steel containers are of two types, two-piece or three-piece. The two-piece container body is seamless, consisting of a drawn cylinder; the base of the container is held in place with a double seam. The three-piece container has a side-seam, the base being attached as for the two-piece container; the top has a 2.54 cm (1 inch) opening and is joined to the body by double seaming. **Aluminium** containers are more resistant to corrosion than tin-plated steel. Aluminium is, however, subject to corrosion by water and ethanol and therefore may be coated with organic substances to provide protection. Aluminium containers are produced by an extrusion process and hence have no seams. **Stainless steel** is very resistant to corrosion and generally no coating is required. Stainless steel containers can also withstand high pressures. However, they are expensive. **Glass** containers are often coated with plastic, the coating giving protection from impact and serving to contain any broken fragments. The coating can be bonded to the glass or provided as a cover which fits over the container. Glass has the advantage over the other container materials of being transparent, so the contents can be viewed. Glass is also virtually inert. **Plastic** materials have not been extensively used for aerosol containers. However, polyethyleneterephthalate (PET) has been used commercially for a non-pharmaceutical presentation.

Choice of Container Material

Container choice is dependent on the pressure of the system, whether the product is aqueous or not, the pH of the product, and other physicochemical characteristics of the preparation. Metal containers can generally be used at higher pressures than glass containers.

If the product is non-aqueous, an unlined tin-plated steel container is suitable. However, metal containers for aqueous preparations must be coated internally (unless stainless steel). Epoxy or vinyl linings are suitable for low pH preparations. These coating materials can also be used together, with a vinyl coat next to the container, and an epoxy coat on top of that. Epoxy resin is more stable to heat.

When a preparation contains a soap, lead must not be included in the container, as insoluble lead salts form and can cause clogging of the valve. Lead is most frequently found in the soldering material for the side-seam, therefore welded side-seams are more suitable. Polar solvents, especially anhydrous ethanol, attack aluminium containers, but this reaction can be inhibited by the addition of 2% to 3% water. Attack by ethanol can also be prevented by anodising the container.

Valves

There are two classes of valve commonly used in pharmaceutical aerosols, the conventional or continuous spray valve, and the metered-dose valve.

Continuous Spray Valve

The continuous spray valve, as its name suggests, allows the product to be released for as long as the valve is opened. Valves are available that can disperse the product as a spray, foam, powder, or semi-solid stream. Six basic components make up the continuous spray valve.

The **ferrule (mounting cup)** is used to attach the valve to the container. The ferrule is made of tin-plated steel or very occasionally of aluminium. A coating is applied to protect against corrosion. The ferrule is attached to the container by curling under the lip of the container.

The **valve housing** has an opening of 0.033 to 0.20 cm at the point of attachment to the dip tube. A second opening known as the vapour tap may also be present. This allows vaporised propellant and liquid product to escape. It also produces a fine particle size, prevents valve clogging in the presence of insoluble substances, and reduces the flame extension produced by hydrocarbon propellants. The chilling effect of propellants on the skin is also reduced and expulsion from inverted containers aided.

The **gasket** is made of synthetic rubber and provides a seal between the valve and container.

The **spring** is usually made of stainless steel, and holds the gasket in place. It also serves to return the valve to the closed position after actuation.

The inside diameter of the **dip tube** is normally between 3.0 and 3.2 mm, but may range from 1.3 to 5.0 mm. The dip tube diameter is chosen with regard to the viscosity of the product and the desired delivery rate. It is usually made of polyethylene or polypropylene.

When the **stem** is pressed, the product is emitted from the container. The stem may have one orifice of 0.33 to 0.76 mm or up to three orifices of 1 mm each.

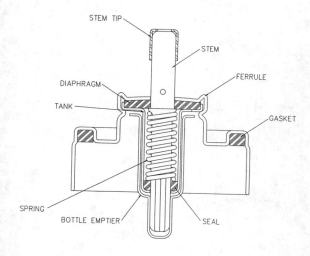

Fig. 1
Metered-dose valve.

Metered-dose Valves

Metering valves (see Fig. 1) are essentially the same as continuous spray valves except that they contain a separate chamber constructed of stainless steel or plastic. The dimensions of this chamber determine the quantity of medicament delivered. Metered-dose valves have been developed which are capable of dispensing some of the more potent topical medications, such as corticosteroids, for inhalation (see Inhalation Products chapter).

Actuators

Actuators allow for easy opening and closing of the valve. The design of the actuator determines whether a spray, foam, or solid stream is produced. Actuators are available which facilitate delivery of medication to a specific site (for example, the throat or the vagina).

In order to produce a spray that consists of small particles, the product can be passed through up to three orifices ranging in diameter from 0.4 to 1.0 mm. The orifice must not be too small though, as clogging may occur. Factors such as quantity and nature of the propellant can also contribute to the spray characteristics.

When the aerosol is intended for oral administration adaptors can be used which allow the propellant to evaporate and thus produce a dispersion of small particles. Another device which can be used when a spray aerosol is desired but there is insufficient propellant to achieve this, is a mechan-

ical break-up actuator. Channels in the actuator cause the stream to break-up into a spray.

Foam actuators have large chambers where the product expands before release. The orifice size, typically 1.8 to 3.2 mm, is larger than that for spray actuators.

Semi-solids are delivered using solid-stream actuators which have a larger orifice.

AEROSOL SYSTEMS AND FORMULATION

Liquefied Gas Systems: Two Phase

The simplest aerosol system is the two-phase or solution system (see Fig. 2). It consists only of a vapour phase and a liquid phase and is a solution of the active ingredient in liquid propellant, or liquid propellant plus solvent if the active ingredient is not soluble in the propellant alone.

Two-phase systems normally utilise propellants 11, 12, and 114, n-butane, isobutane, or propane. A formulation containing a large proportion of propellant 12 will produce a rapidly evaporating dry spray, and consequently fine particles of sizes as low as 1 micrometre. The particle size is influenced by the concentration of non-volatile components, initial droplet size, and rate of droplet evaporation. Increasing the proportion of propellant 11 (which has a relatively high boiling point), reducing the quantity of low boiling point propellants, introducing solvents such as ethanol, propylene glycol, glycerol, acetone, or ethyl acetate (which decrease the vapour pressure), or increasing the proportion of active ingredients, will result in a spray that is much wetter and coarser. The particle sizes in such a system can range from 50 to 200 micrometres.

Liquefied Gas Systems: Three Phase

When some of the components of an aerosol are immiscible with, or insoluble in, the liquefied propellant, a three-phase system results (see Fig. 2). This occurs particularly where water is included in the formulation. The non-vapour phases can be two liquid layers, a dispersion or suspension, or an emulsion.

The three phases of a two-layer system typically comprise an aqueous solution of the active ingredients, the liquid propellant, and vaporised propellant. If a chlorofluorohydrocarbon propellant is used, the propellant layer lies beneath the aqueous layer as the propellants are denser than water. Hydrocarbon propellants, in contrast, are less

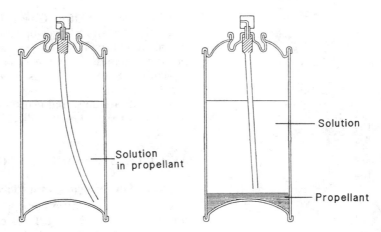

Fig. 2
Two-phase and three-phase systems.

dense than water. The dip-tube of the container must reach down into the aqueous region. When the valve is opened, the pressure of the vapour forces the aqueous liquid up the tube, but no liquefied propellant escapes. As no liquefied propellant is emitted to break up the droplets, and because of the low vapour pressure and low volatility of the solution of the active ingredient, a mechanical break-up actuator is required to reduce the size of the droplets.

Modifications to this type of formulation can produce a more efficient spray. The use of water with another solvent (for example, ethanol) gives a system which, when shaken, forms a dispersion of the active ingredient plus solvents in the propellant. When the valve is depressed some of the propellant is emitted together with the active ingredient; the rapid evaporation of the propellant results in a small particle size. Surfactants may also be included in the formulation, at a concentration of 0.5% to 2.0%.

Suspensions and emulsions also constitute three-phase systems. In a suspension system, the finely-divided active ingredient is suspended in the liquefied propellant. In an emulsion system, the propellant is incorporated into the emulsion, and the product is a foam which can be quick-breaking or stable.

Suspension systems are largely employed to avoid the use of a cosolvent, but they do have their own inherent problems. The physical stability of the suspension is the main concern and aggregation must be controlled. Aggregation can give rise to valve blockage and hence inaccuracy of dosage. To prevent aggregation it is desirable that the moisture content of the aerosol system be below 300 ppm (0.03%), and that a derivative of the active substance that is poorly soluble in the propellant be chosen. A high moisture content leads to aggregation, and substances that are soluble in the propellant can be subject to particle growth. If the density of the suspended substance and that of the vehicle are similar, the rate of settling of the suspended particles will be decreased and hence the propensity for aggregation reduced. The physical stability of suspension systems can also be increased by ensuring that the particle size of the active ingredient is in the 1 to 5 micrometre range. The inclusion of a surfactant in a suspension formulation, particularly for metered-dose aerosols, can also be useful as it exerts a valve lubricating effect.

Emulsion aerosols are of three types: aqueous foams, non-aqueous foams, and quick-breaking foams. Aqueous foams, as the name suggests, contain water in the formulation. The emulsion is formed in much the same way as a non-aerosol emulsion, with the liquefied propellant constituting part of the internal phase (typically 3% to 5% by weight of the formulation). Increasing the proportion of propellant results in the production of a stiffer dryer foam. Non-aqueous aerosols are produced by replacing the water of aqueous emulsions with various glycols, and by using emulsifying agents such as glycol esters.

Quick-breaking foams have the propellant in the external phase. Surfactants of any charge can be used in quick-breaking foam formulations, but as ethanol is sometimes included in such systems, a surfactant that is soluble in both ethanol and water is preferred.

Compressed Gas Systems

Compressed gases can be used to dispense a product as a semi-solid, a wet spray, or a foam. The gases used are nitrogen, carbon dioxide, or nitrous oxide. Nitrogen is insoluble in, and immiscible with, the active ingredient concentrate, whereas carbon dioxide and nitrous oxide are slightly soluble in the concentrate. Nitrogen has application where the product is to be dispensed in an unchanged form, for example a semi-solid. Also nitrogen can be used where the liquefied gases may be irritant to the condition being treated or where they interact with the active substance.

The gases that are slightly soluble in the concentrate can cause some change in the product on emission from the container. For this reason the soluble gases are used in dispensing foams. The gas dissolved in the product is released on exposure to the air, causing foam to form. The product must be shaken before release in order to disperse the gas through the concentrate. If a spray is to be dispensed, the container must be fitted with a mechanical break-up actuator as the compressed gases have very little dispersing power.

Compressed gas propellants are relatively inert. As they replace the air in the head space above the product, the stability of drugs liable to oxidation can be improved.

Other Systems

A polyethylene piston fitted into an aluminium container can be used to ensure that semi-solids are completely removed from the container. The propellant lies below the piston, and the product above. When the valve is actuated the propellant pushes up the piston, scraping the sides of the container and forcing out the product.

MANUFACTURE AND PACKAGING

Preparation of the product concentrate is similar to the preparation of any equivalent pharmaceutical product. However, the overall process is unique, in that part of the manufacturing procedure for pressurised products takes place during packaging. There are two modes of filling: the cold-filling process and the pressure-filling process.

Cold Filling

Low temperatures, in the range $-34°$ to $-40°$, are required for the cold-filling process, so this method is not suitable for aqueous products or for preparations that are adversely affected by low temperatures.

The product concentrate is chilled and added to the open container followed by the chilled propellant. Alternatively, the concentrate and propellant can be chilled together and the mixture added to the container. The temperature of the components must be carefully controlled to prevent loss due to evaporation. A valve is then crimped into place and the container passed through a heated test bath ($54.4°$) as a check for leakage and container strength.

Pressure Filling

The pressure-filling process can be used for all types of aerosols, although it can only be applied to metered-dose products if a specially designed container is used. The product concentrate is added to the container at room temperature and the valve crimped into place. The propellant is then added, under pressure, through the valve stem or through the actuator and around the sealing gaskets.

A second technique, the 'under-the-cap' method, is also used. The product concentrate is added to the container and the valve placed in position. A seal is formed around the shoulder of the container and, using a vacuum, the valve cup is raised slightly from the can and the propellant added. The valve is then crimped into place.

For all pressure-filling techniques, air can be purged from the headspace before adding the propellant. This serves to protect oxygen-sensitive products. The completed container is passed to the test tank as in the cold-filling process.

EVALUATION AND QUALITY CONTROL

Physicochemical Properties

Standards are specified for the physicochemical properties of an aerosol, including the vapour pressure, density, and moisture content.

Vapour pressure must be constant from container to container, and several methods of measurement are available. A gauge that has been calibrated to the pressure of the system, a water-bath test, and a container-puncturing device can all be used. The container and its contents should be brought to a constant temperature in a water-bath before measurement.

Specially adapted procedures using hydrometers and pycnometers are utilised to measure the **density** of aerosol systems.

As with the determination of water in other preparations, the Karl Fischer method of determining **moisture content** has been used for aerosol systems. It is also possible to employ gas chromatography for this purpose.

Aerosol Performance

In order to determine if an aerosol is functioning to accepted standards various tests are carried out. These include measuring the contents of the container (usually by weighing before and after filling). Filled containers are passed through a water bath to test for leaks. The rate of discharge through the valve may also be tested, and the pattern of the spray examined.

Specific Tests for Metered-dose Aerosols

The **quantity of active ingredient** delivered by a metered-dose valve is determined by discharging the aerosol into a solvent and assaying the resulting solution. A method for such a procedure is given in the *British Pharmacopoeia*.

The **number of deliveries** is measured simply by actuating the valve at intervals of not less than five seconds until the container is spent. The number of deliveries should be not less than that stated on the label. Further details of this test are given in the *British Pharmacopoeia*.

Particle Size Determination

Particle sizing may not be necessary for most aerosol products, but it is essential for inhalation aerosols, and for some topical preparations. A variety have been employed for the determination of particle size.

Microscopy

Microscopic examination is the method given in the *United States Pharmacopeia* and in the *British Pharmaceutical Codex 1973* for the determination of particle size of aerosol products. The aerosol is actuated onto a glass slide after priming of the valve, and the slide rinsed with carbon tetrachloride, avoiding loss of particulate matter. The slide is allowed to dry, and then examined under a microscope. Limits on the size of the particles are given. Limitations of this method are that larger droplets tend to spread, and small particles are difficult to see.

Cascade Impaction

The most common method of determining particle size is by use of a cascade impactor, although light-scattering methods also enjoy some popularity.

A cascade impactor is capable of measuring particles in the size range 0.2 to 20.0 micrometres. The aerosol passes through a series of nozzles of decreasing diameter, under the influence of a vacuum. After each stage there is a glass slide coated with a viscous fluid. Those particles with the largest aerodynamic diameter have the largest momentum and hence become trapped on the first glass slide. Smaller particles flow around the glass slide and pass through the second nozzle. The narrower bore of the second nozzle causes the particles to increase in velocity and a further fraction is collected on the second plate. The remaining particles pass through yet narrower nozzles and any remaining after the final plate are captured by a filter. The size distribution of the aerosol can then be determined; if required, the quantity of active ingredient present in each size range can be measured.

For aerosol inhalations, cascade impaction is either carried out at relatively high humidity, or the size distribution is corrected to account for the growth of particles that would occur under the humid conditions of the respiratory tract. A problem with the use of the cascade impactor is that material can be lost to the walls of the apparatus. A modification of the cascade impactor is the multi-stage liquid impinger. The design of this instrument is very similar to the cascade impactor, but the sintered-glass collection plates are wet and the final nozzle is at a tangent to the foot of the apparatus. A terminal filter is included.

Light-scattering Methods

Light-scattering methods can measure particles in the size range 0.1 to 20 micrometres. They can utilise either white light or laser light and work on the principle that particles suspended in air will cause a scattering of light which can be monitored by a photodetector. Concentration is a critical factor when using light scattering methods: too concentrated a sample will cause saturation of the electronic counters, while dilution of the sample may result in loss of large particles and may also alter initial droplet size. Another limitation of light-scattering methods is that it is not possible to determine if the particles counted contain active ingredient.

A detailed discussion of the stability testing of pharmaceuticals is given the chapter Stability of Medicinal Products.

The stability of an aerosol product can be affected by interactions between the component parts of the container and the concentrate/propellant mixture. Aerosols under test are stored on their sides so that there is maximum contact between the product and the container/valve.

Controls are prepared using glass containers. The following characteristics may be assessed during the test period: colour, odour, pH, vapour pressure, density, refractive index, and viscosity of the concentrate; assay of active principles, total weight; integrity of the container and the valve; and valve performance.

FURTHER INFORMATION

Developments in Aerosol Technology. Aerosol beats CFC problem. Chemist Drugg 1988;230:493.
Alternative propellants [editorial]. Mfg Chem 1988;58:61.
Bagging the can [an alternative aerosol pack from which only product is released]. Mfg Chem 1988;59:79.
Dalby RN, Byron PR, Shepherd HR, Papadopoulos E. CFC propellant substitution: P134a as a potential replacement for P-12 in MDIs. Med Dev Technol 1990;1(2):37–41.
First edible whip product in USA [editorial]. Mfg Chem 1987;57:19.
Containers. Shattock G. Petasol–the fibrenyle PET aerosol. Mfg Chem 1987;57(11):33–4.
Milnes J. PET aerosols for saline solutions. Mfg Chem 1988;59(11):77.
Formulation. Byron PR. Some future perspectives for unit dose inhalation aerosols. Drug Dev Ind Pharm 1986;12:993–1015.
Dalby RN, Byron PR. Comparison of output particle size distributions from pressurised aerosols formulated as solutions and suspensions. J Pharm Pharmacol 1987;39(Suppl):72P.
Hickey AJ, Gonda I, Irwin WJ, Fildes FJT. Effect of hydrophobic coating on the behaviour of a hygroscopic aerosol powder in an environment of controlled temperature and relative humidity. J Pharm Sci 1990;79:1009–14.
Hickey AJ, Jackson GV, Fildes FJT. Preparation and characterization of disodium fluorescein powders in association with lauric and capric acids. J Pharm Sci 1988;77:804–9.
Luongo M, Sciarra JJ, Ward CO, De Paul Lynch V, Feinstein W. A comparative study of the *in vitro* and *in vivo* release of dexamethasone from a spray-on bandage and timed release aerosol [including formulation details]. Drug Dev Ind Pharm 1981;7:497–523.
Luongo M, Sciarra JJ, Ward CO. *In vivo* method for determining effectiveness of spray-on bandages containing anti-infectives [including formulation details]. J Pharm Sci 1974;63:1376–9.
Sanders PA. Aqueous alcohol aerosol foams. Drug Cosmet Ind 1966;99:56–58,60–61,142–143,146–154,170–75.
Sanders PA. Molecular interactions in aerosol emulsion systems. III. Pearlescent structures. J Soc Cosmet Chem 1969;20:577–93.
Sciarra JJ, Iamacone A, Mores L. An evaluation of dispersing agents in aerosol formulations. I. Synthetic esters. J Soc Cosmet Chem 1976;27:209–20.
Woodford R, Barry BW. Bioavailability and activity of topical corticosteroids from a novel drug delivery system, the aerosol quick break foam. J Pharm Sci 1977;66:99–103.
Manufacture and packaging. Fults K, Cyr TD, Hickey AJ. The influence of sampling chamber dimensions on aerosol particle size measurement by cascade impactor and twin impinger. J Pharm Pharmacol 1991;43:726–8.
Page D. The electrostatic hazard of powder-based aerosols. Mfg Chem 1990: 61(4):30–3.

Sciarra JJ. Quality control for pharmaceutical and cosmetic aerosol products. In: Cooper MS, editor. Quality control in the pharmaceutical industry; vol 2. New York: Academic Press, 1973:1–54.
Specific tests for metered-dose aerosols. Bell JH, Brown K, Glasby J. Variation in delivery of isoprenaline from various pressurised inhalers. J Pharm Pharmacol 1973;25(Suppl):32P–36P.
Benjamin EJ, Kroeten JJ, Sherk E. Characterisation of spray patterns of inhalation aerosols using thin-layer chromatography. J Pharm Sci 1983;72:380–5.
Cutie A, Burger J, Clawans C, Dolinsky D, Feinstein W, Gupta B. Test for reproducibility of metered-dose aerosol valves for pharmaceutical solutions. J Pharm Sci 1981;70:1085–7.
Davies PJ, Amin KK, Mott GA. Particle size of inhalation aerosol systems. I. Production of homogeneous dispersions. Drug Dev Ind Pharm 1980;6:645–51.
Davies PJ. Size analysis of suspension inhalation aerosols. Pharm Int 1981;2:110–3.
Dhand R, Malik SK, Balakrishnan N, Verma SR. High-speed photographic analysis of aerosols produced by metered dose inhalers. J Pharm Pharmacol 1988;40:429–30.
Fiese EF, Gorman WG, Dolinsky D, Harwood RJ, Hunke WA, Miller NC. Test method for evaluation of loss of prime in metered-dose aerosols. J Pharm Sci 1988;77:90–3.
Groom CV, Gonda I. Cascade impaction: the performance of different collection surfaces. J Pharm Pharmacol 1980;32(Suppl):93P.
Hallworth GW, Andrews UG. Size analysis of suspension inhalation aerosols by inertial separation methods. J Pharm Pharmacol 1976;28:898–907.
Hallworth GW, Clough D, Newnham T, Andrews UG. A simple impinger device for rapid quality control of the particle size of inhalation aerosols delivered by pressurised aerosols and powder inhalers. J Pharm Pharmacol 1978;30(Suppl):39P.
Hickey AJ. Practical aspects of aerosol characterization in an environment of controlled temperature and relative humidity. Drug Dev Ind Pharm 1988;14:337–52.
Miszuk S, Gupta BM, Chen FC, Clawans C, Knapp JZ. Video characterisation of flume patterns of inhalation aerosols. J Pharm Sci 1980;69:713–17.
Moren F, Jacobsson S-E. *In vitro* dose sampling from pressurised inhalation aerosols. Investigation of procedures in BPC and NF. Int J Pharmaceutics 1979;3:335–40.
Sciarra JJ. Pharmaceutical and cosmetic aerosols. J Pharm Sci 1974;63:1828–31.
Swift DL. Aerosol characterisation and generation. In: Moren F, Newhouse MT, Dolovich MB, editors. Aerosols in medicine. Principles, diagnosis and therapy. Amsterdam: Elsevier, 1985:62–3.
Stability. Halliday JA, Johnson JR, Smith IJ, Wyatt DA. The physical stability of betamethasone 17-valerate suspension in metered dose inhaler formulations. J Pharm Pharmacol 1987;39(Suppl):76P.
Richman MD, Shangraw RF. A study of pressurized foams with emphasis on rheological evaluation. II. Foam stability and effect of shear. Aerosol Age 1966;11:45-6,109–10.

Inhalation Products

Inhalation products are designed to deliver therapeutic agents to the respiratory tract for either local or systemic effect. Drugs delivered in this way include sodium cromoglycate, beta-adrenoceptor agonists, corticosteroids, and volatile materials such as menthol. Steam vaporisers and humidifiers are used to deliver moisture.

The Respiratory Tract

The respiratory system in man is responsible for the processes of gaseous exchange between the atmosphere, the circulation, and the cells of the body; the homoeostatic maintenance of blood pH; and the provision of vocal expression.

When air is inhaled through the nose, it passes through the nasal cavity and the **pharynx** and then past the epiglottis to the **trachea**. The nasal cavity acts as a filter to prevent the entry of large particles, as well as warming and humidifying the airstream.

On passing through the trachea, air enters the lungs via the bronchi, bronchioles, and alveoli. The **bronchi** walls contain rings of cartilage interspersed throughout smooth muscle and their inner surface is lined by cilia whose roots are in the mucous membrane. The rings of cartilage prevent the collapse of the bronchi when the internal pressure changes, and the beating cilia assist in the upward and outward movement of unwanted fine particles.

The **bronchioles** are narrower versions of the bronchi, usually of less than 1mm diameter. However, unlike the bronchi, their walls are not reinforced with cartilage, and they may open and narrow to modify the resistance to the passage of air. Deeper within the lung, the bronchioles repeatedly branch, giving rise to terminal bronchioles. The terminal bronchioles divide further into the respiratory bronchioles, which possess end outgrowths, the **alveoli**. The walls of the respiratory bronchioles and the alveoli are thin, covered in a network of fine capillaries, and are the sites of gaseous exchange.

The upper regions of the respiratory tract, from the lower epiglottis to the terminal bronchioles, are lined with ciliated epithelium, which secretes mucus and is involved in the removal of particulate matter. Any particles that become trapped in the mucus are transported by the action of the beating cilia to the pharynx where they are swallowed. For most drugs administered by inhalation, the desired site of action lies deep in the respiratory tract, in the bronchioles and alveoli.

Deposition of Inhaled Particles

Inhalation products usually deliver the active ingredient in the form of aerosol droplets or solid particles. The particular site at which deposition of these droplets or particles occurs depends largely on their **aerodynamic diameter**. The aerodynamic diameter is defined as the diameter of the perfect sphere that would fall through air at the same speed as the particle in question. Large particles with an aerodynamic diameter greater than 10 micrometres tend to be deposited in the upper regions of the respiratory tract, where they are removed by the ciliated epithelium. Only the smallest particles (approximately 2 micrometres) are capable of reaching the alveoli. The proportion of the delivered dose that reaches its site of action may only be 5% to 20%.

The relative humidity of the respiratory tract is approximately 99.5%. Inhaled particles of water-soluble materials may therefore absorb some of this moisture, dissolve, and grow in size. Growth may continue until the vapour pressures on the surface of the particle and in the respiratory tract are the same, a process that may take only milliseconds to complete.

Deposition Mechanisms

Particles may be deposited on the mucosa of the respiratory tract in one of three ways:

Inertial Impaction. The airstream with associated particles must manoeuvre around the various branches of the respiratory tract in order to reach the deeper areas of the lungs. Particles that possess high momentum, however, cannot change direction easily and tend to collide with the walls of the tract immediately ahead of them. This process is known as inertial impaction. Inertial impaction provides an efficient mechanism for the removal of large, fast-moving particles in the upper parts of the respiratory tract.

Sedimentation. A suspended particle is influenced by gravity and settles at a rate dependent on its aerodynamic diameter. In the upper airways, however, settling may be retarded by the force of the airflow. In the lower respiratory tract the velocity of the airflow may be insufficient to maintain a particle in suspension. Particles may therefore be deposited by gravitational forces. Sedimentation is an important method for the deposition of particles in the 0.5 to 3.0 micrometre range.

Diffusion. Particles below 0.5 micrometre in diameter display Brownian motion and move from areas of high to low particle concentration. They leave the airstream and deposit on the walls of the respiratory tract; the rate of this diffusion increases with decreasing particle size.

Deposition Studies

In-vitro Studies. Deposition studies *in vitro* utilise simulated respiratory systems. These systems vary considerably in their complexity, ranging from simple tubes to pieces of apparatus consisting of several chambers linked by angled tubes.

The *British Pharmacopoeia* specifies two pieces of apparatus to assess the deposition of the emitted dose from a pressurised inhalation. The dose is drawn through a series of angled tubes and an impingement chamber, and the drug remaining in the airstream at the end is collected and measured.

In-vivo Studies. Radionuclide tracer studies have been used to assess the deposition of particles in healthy subjects. Short-life radionuclides that emit gamma-radiation, such as ^{99m}Tc, are particularly useful for this purpose.

Inhalations

Inhalations are solutions or suspensions of one or more active ingredients which, when vaporised in a suitable manner, are intended to be brought into contact with the lining of the respiratory tract. The ingredients may be volatile at room temperature, in which case they may be inhaled from an absorbent pad on which they have been placed, or they may require to be added to hot water (about 65°) and the vapour inhaled. Inhalations intended to be added to hot water may consist of alcoholic solutions or of mixtures with water to which a diffusing agent such as light magnesium carbonate has been added.

OFFICIAL EXAMPLES:
    Benzoin Inhalation BP
    Menthol and Benzoin Inhalation BP
    Menthol and Eucalyptus Inhalation BP 1980

Vitrellae

Vitrellae consist of thin-walled glass capsules containing a volatile medicament such as amyl nitrite; they are protected by a wrapping of fabric or other suitable material. They are intended for use by crushing the glass and inhaling the vapour.

Pressurised Inhalations (Metered-dose Aerosols)

Pressurised inhalations consist of solutions, suspensions, or emulsions of one or more active ingredients with suitable propellants or suitable mixtures of propellants held under pressure in an aerosol dispenser. They are fitted with a metering valve and are intended to be inhaled in controlled amounts. Pressurised metered-dose inhalers are used for the administration of bronchodilators, corticosteroids, and sodium cromoglycate.

The formulation and design of the delivery device should be such that an adequate proportion of the active ingredient is made available for inhalation when the product is used in accordance with the manufacturer's instructions; the quantity available is less than that released by actuation as some of the active ingredient is deposited on the inner surface of the actuator.

The propellants may be either liquefied gases such as chlorofluorohydrocarbons or compressed gases such as carbon dioxide. Suitable combinations may be used to give the required pressure, delivery, or spray characteristics. Pressurised inhalations may also contain excipients such as solvents, solubilising agents, suspending agents, emulsifying agents, and lubricating agents. They should be prepared in conditions designed to prevent microbial and particulate contamination. Further information on the formulation and packaging of aerosols can be found in the Aerosols chapter. An example of a metered-dose pressurised inhaler device is illustrated in Fig. 1.

A problem with the use of conventional metered-dose pressurised inhalers is the need to coordinate actuation of the device and inspiration of air. Many patients, through lack of skill, tuition, or understanding, do not employ the most efficient technique for using metered-dose inhalers. Poor inhaler technique results in reduced efficacy of the administered medication. The difficulty experienced by these patients is that of manually actuating the metering valve to release medication in synchrony with inhalation. The development of a breath-actuated delivery system (such as the Aerolin™ Autohaler) has reduced the difficulty of hand-breath coordination.

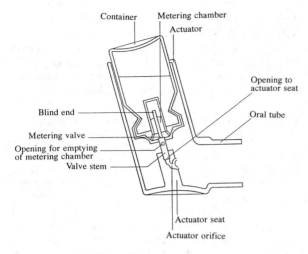

Fig. 1
A metered-dose pressurised inhaler.

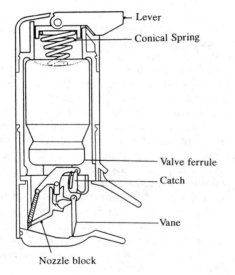

Fig. 2
A breath-actuated metered-dose inhaler.

The breath-actuated pressurised inhaler (see Fig. 2) ensures that the drug is delivered synchronously with inhalation. The inhaler is primed by raising a latching lever on the top of the adaptor. This applies pressure to the base of the aerosol can via a spring. Before inhalation, downward movement of the can to actuate the metering valve in response to the spring force is prevented by the blocking action of a precision-moulded triggering mechanism. As soon as the patient starts to inhale, a small vane positioned within the mouth-piece rotates in the air stream to release the mechanism. This allows the spring to move the can sufficiently to actuate the valve and deliver drug as the patient inhales.

Extension devices (spacers) that also obviate the need for coordination have been developed. These act as reservoirs for the actuated dose and allow inspiration after actuation. The devices range from the Bricanyl Spacer™, a collapsible extended mouthpiece, to larger spacing models with a one-way valve (Nebuhaler™, Rondo™, Volumatic™). Some devices allow the dose to be inhaled over several breaths. Extension devices also improve drug delivery to the deeper regions of the lungs. This extra distance allows the eva-poration of more of the propellant, which causes a reduction in particle size. In addition, the parti-cles decelerate during transit and lose momentum. Fewer particles are therefore lost through inertial impaction in the oropharynx.

Powder Inhalations

A powder inhalation consists of a means to contain or meter the powder, and a device from which the dose is inhaled. The dose consists of powdered medicinal substances often diluted with a suitable inert powder such as lactose. Powder inhalations are breath-actuated and contain no propellants. The flow of powder is controlled by the patient's own inspiratory effort. The term **insufflation** is used to describe certain simple powder inhala-tions. Examples of drugs administered as powder inhalations include bronchodilators, corticoster-oids, and sodium cromoglycate. Many products are available as both pressurised aerosol and pow-der formulations.

The particle size of powder inhalations should be sufficiently small to maximise administration to the deeper regions of the lungs. The small particle size, however, is associated with a large surface area; to minimise the resulting large surface free energy, particles tend to aggregate and adhere to surfaces with which they come in contact. Hygro-scopic particles will increase in size when water is absorbed. For this reason, powder inhalations are less efficient than pressurised inhalations. How-ever, as powder inhalers are simpler to use and do not require coordination of inhalation with manual operation they may deliver more drug than a pressurised aerosol used incorrectly. Pow-der inhalers usually incorporate a means of break-ing up any aggregates that form; either a mesh or a propeller driven by airflow.

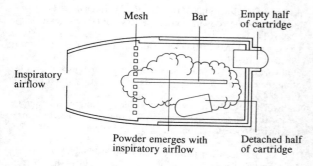

Fig. 3
A unit-dose powder inhaler.

Powder inhalations may be supplied as single doses in hard capsules (cartridges) or as multidose devices. An example of a single dose powder inhaler is shown in Fig. 3.

The Diskhaler™ (Fig. 4) is a multidose powder inhalation device. Each metered dose of the drug is contained within one of either four or eight foil blisters on a circular aluminium foil disk, which is inserted in the device. Each blister is pierced in turn to free the contents for inspiration. After inhalation of the dose, the Diskhaler™ is prepared for the next inhalation by sliding the tray out and in once. The disk incorporates an indicator, which shows the number of remaining doses. After the last dose the disk is removed from the device and replaced with a new one.

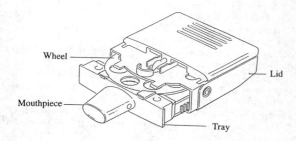

Fig. 4
A diskhaler™ device.

The Bricanyl Turbohaler™ is a disposable inhaler preloaded with sufficient drug powder to produce 200 doses. It contains no diluent or lubricant. A dose is measured by volume just before use. The dosing unit consists of a disc with a group of conical holes. Powder is pushed into the holes by specially designed scrapers on rotation of the dosing

unit. A red-indicator warns the patient when only 20 doses remain in the device.

Nebulisers

Nebulisers are devices that are used to generate a mist of fine particles from a drug solution or suspension. This method of drug administration may be used to deliver higher doses of a drug than is usual with standard inhaler therapy. Nebulisers are useful for the treatment of patients who are in respiratory distress or cannot inhale effectively.

It has been estimated that only 10% of a nebulised solution reaches the respiratory system; the remainder being deposited on the tubing and mouthpiece.

The nebulised particles should be of uniform shape, size, and density, and in the respirable size range. These factors are characterised by the mass median diameter (MMD). Most nebulisers produce particles with an MMD of up to 5 micrometres, which penetrate deep within the bronchi. In addition, there are nebulisers designed to produce an aerosol mist with particles of up to 2 micrometres for delivering nebulised drugs to the alveolar region.

The time required to administer a dose by nebuliser may be considerable. Becotide™ suspension, for example, is only suitable for children and infants because the large volumes required by adults would take too long to nebulise.

Nebuliser Solutions

Nebulisers are used for the administration of antimicrobial drugs, as well as bronchodilators, corticosteroids, and sodium cromoglycate. Nebuliser solutions should be isotonic in order to prevent irritation and to prevent the growth or diminution of aerosol particles in the humid environment of the respiratory tract. Multidose nebuliser solutions require adequate preservation and stabilisation. However, preservatives such as benzalkonium chloride and stabilising agents such as edetic acid, sulphites, and metabisulphite have been reported to cause bronchoconstriction. Benzalkonium chloride may also cause partial paralysis of ciliary movement. The efficient use of almost all inhalation products involves considerable care and expertise. The patient requires clear instructions from the pharmacist.

Jet Nebulisers

Jet nebulisers operate by forcing a compressed gas, such as air or oxygen, through a narrow-bore inlet and across the top of a capillary tube, the lower end of which is immersed in the liquid to be nebulised. As the gas expands on leaving the inlet, the resulting negative pressure draws the liquid up the capillary and into the gas stream. This, in turn, breaks the liquid into droplets, the largest of which are removed by baffles and returned to the liquid bulk. Small droplets are carried by the gas stream and delivered to the patient via a face mask or mouthpiece.

Nebulisers can use a variety of power sources. Electrically driven air compressors vary in power rating and may generate flow rates of between 6 and 15 litres per minute. Domiciliary compressors usually provide a continuous airflow. It is important that air compressors are used according to the manufacturers' instructions and are serviced regularly. All accessories, including air filters, should be replaced at regular intervals.

Compressed gas stored in a cylinder may also be suitable as the power source for nebuliser therapy. The use of oxygen rather than air may have a beneficial effect.

A foot-operated pump may be suitable when a power supply is not available.

Ultrasonic Nebulisers

Ultrasonic nebulisers produce an aerosol using the high frequency vibrations generated by a piezoelectric crystal; they do not require the use of a carrier gas. The particle size range produced is dependent on the conditions of operation and the properties of the liquid to be nebulised. However, aerosols can be produced containing particles in the respirable size range. Heat generation may be a problem with such devices.

FURTHER INFORMATION

Byron PR, Davis SS, Bubb MD, Cooper P. Pharmaceutical implications of particle growth at high relative humidities. Pestic Sci 1977;8:521–6.

Clarke JG, Farr SJ, Wicks SR. Technetium-99m labelling of suspension type pressurised metered dose inhalers comprising various drug/surfactant combinations. Int J Pharmaceutics 1992;80:R1–R5.

Clay MM, Pavia D, Newman SP, Clarke SW. Factors influencing the size distribution of aerosols from jet nebulisers. Thorax 1983;38:755–9.

Crompton GK. Use of nebulisers in asthma. Pharm J 1985;235:237–8.

Davies PJ, Hanlon GW, Molyneux AJ. An investigation into the deposition of inhalation aerosol particles as a function of air flow rate in a modified 'Kirk Lung'. J Pharm Pharmacol 1976;28:908–11.

Davis SS, Bubb MD. Physico-chemical studies on aerosol solutions for drug delivery. III. The effect of relative humidity on the particle size of inhalation aerosols. Int J Pharmaceutics 1978;1:303–14.

de Boer AH, Buitendijk HH, Lerk CF, Vermeulen J. Development of dry powder inhalation systems. Pharm Weekbl (Sci) 1989;II:D6.

Dry powder inhalers–the shape of things to come? Pharm J 1992;248:816–17.

Hallworth GW, Malton CA. Recent in-vivo methods for evaluating the deposition of aerosols in the respiratory tract. Pharm Int 1984;5:61–5.

Hallworth GW, Westmoreland DG. The twin impinger: a simple device for assessing the delivery of drugs from metered dose pressurized aerosol inhalers. J Pharm Pharmacol 1987;39:966–72.

Horsley M. Nebuliser therapy. Pharm J 1988;240:22–4.

Johnson CE. Principles of nebulizer-delivered drug therapy for asthma. Am J Hosp Pharm 1989;46:1845–55.

Karig AW, Peck GE, Sperandio GJ. Evaluation of inhalation aerosols using a simulated lung apparatus. J Pharm Sci 1973;62:811–15.

Kirk WF. Aerosols for inhalation therapy. Pharm Int 1986;7:150–4.

Kirk WF. In-vitro method of comparing clouds produced from inhalation aerosols for efficiency in penetration of airways. J Pharm Sci 1972;61:262–5.

Lippmann M, Yeates DB, Albert RE. Deposition, retention, and clearance of inhaled particles. Br J Ind Med 1980;37:337-62.

Livingstone C, Livingstone D. Inhalation therapy. Pharm J 1988;241:476–8.

Meakin BJ, Stroud N. An evaluation of some metered dose aerosols using a twin stage impinger sampling device. J Pharm Pharmacol 1983;35(Suppl):7P.

Moren F, Draco AB. Dosage forms and formulations for drug administration to the respiratory tract. Drug Dev Ind Pharm 1987;13:695–728.

Moren F. Drug deposition of pressurized inhalation aerosols. 1. Influence of actuator tube design. Int J Pharmaceutics 1978;1:205–12.

Moren F. Pressurised aerosols for inhalation. Int J Pharmaceutics 1981;8:1–10.

Najafabadi AR, Ganderton D. The effect of suspension concentration of aerosols produced by metered dose inhalers. J Pharm Pharmacol 1991;43 (Suppl):66P.

Nebuliser solutions and paradoxical bronchoconstriction. CSM Current Problems, No. 22, May 1988.

Newman SP, Clark AR, Talaee N, Clarke SW. Lung deposition of 5mg Intal from a pressurised metered dose inhaler assessed by radiotracer technique. Int J Pharmaceutics 1991;74:203–8.

Newman SP, Pavia D, Moren F, Sheahan NF, Clarke SW. Deposition of pressurised aerosols in the human respiratory tract. Thorax 1981;36:52–5.

Phipps PR, Gonda I, Bailey DL, Borham P, Bautovich G, Anderson SD. Comparison of methods for the measurement of regional aerosol deposition. J Pharm Pharmacol 1987;39(Suppl):73P.

Sciarra JJ, Cutie A. Simulated respiratory system for in vitro evaluation of two inhalation delivery systems using selected steroids. J Pharm Sci 1978;67:1428–31.

Smith D, Erskine D, Steele J, Hills D. Gazzard B. Comparison of nebuliser efficiency for aerosolizing pentamidine. J Pharm Pharmacol 1992;44:7–9.

Vidgren M, Kärkkäinen A, Karjalainen P, Paronen P, Nuutinen J. Effect of powder inhaler design on drug deposition in the respiratory tract. Int J Pharmaceutics 1988;42:211–16.

Vidgren M, Paronen P, Vidgren P, Vainio P, Nuutinen J. Radiotracer evaluation of the deposition of drug particles inhaled from a new powder inhaler. Int J Pharmaceutics 1990;64:1–6.

Vidgren MT, Paronen TP, Kärkkäinen A, Karjalainen P. Effect of extension devices on the drug deposition from inhalation aerosols. Int J Pharmaceutics 1987;39:107–12.

Zainudin BMZ, Tolfree SEJ, Biddiscombe M, Whitaker M, Short MD, Spiro SG. An alternative to direct labelling of pressurised bronchodilator aerosol. Int J Pharmaceutics 1989;51:67–71.

Zanen P, van Spiegel PI, van der Kolk H, Tushuizen E, Enthoven R. The effect of the inhalation flow on the performance of a dry powder inhalation system. Int J Pharmaceutics 1992;81:199–203.

Topical Semi-solids

Topical semi-solids are preparations designed to exert local activity when applied to the skin or mucous membranes. The main medicinal applications of semi-solids are as protective, emollient, and therapeutic agents; they include such dosage forms as **creams**, **gels**, **ointments**, **pastes**, and **poultices**. **Ophthalmic ointments** are dealt with in the chapter on Ophthalmic Products.

Through the centuries topical semi-solid dosage forms have evolved with little understanding of skin physiology or of absorption mechanisms. These factors may be largely unimportant when action at the skin surface is desired but the skin is not an impenetrable barrier and the diffusive penetration of a potent therapeutic agent may result in serious systemic side-effects.

CLASSIFICATION OF TOPICAL SEMI-SOLIDS

The development of topical semi-solids owes more to cosmetic considerations than to scientific thought; as a result the factors that traditionally distinguished an ointment from a cream were ill-defined and the two terms are almost interchangeable. For example, Hydrous Ointment BP is often referred to as Oily Cream. Flow, adhesion, and stiffness are important characteristics of topical semi-solids and rheological properties have therefore provided a useful aid to classification.

Creams

The term 'cream' should be restricted to preparations intended for external use.

Creams are viscous semi-solids and are usually oil-in-water emulsions (aqueous creams) or water-in-oil emulsions (oily creams). Certain other water-miscible bases that have a complex matrix-like structure are also known as 'creams', although these bases are usually anhydrous or contain only a small proportion of water. They are similar in appearance and consistency to traditional emulsion-type cream bases. Creams are used to apply solutions or dispersions of medicaments to the skin for therapeutic or prophylactic purposes where a highly occlusive effect is not necessary. Bland creams may also be applied for their emollient, cooling, or moistening effects upon the skin.

As emulsified creams are usually non-Newtonian systems, their rheological properties vary with the shear forces applied (see Rheology chapter). Creams are usually pseudoplastic and exhibit low yield values. Viscosity and flow characteristics may change in accordance with the degree to which the systems are homogenised or with the amount of shear applied during processing either in mechanical devices or by a spatula. Flow may also increase during application to the skin by hand. The microstructure of oil-in-water creams may comprise several phases, such as a viscoelastic gel with fixed water, dispersed oil, free water, and crystalline material from the fatty alcohol. Rigidity can be increased by the inclusion of higher concentrations of emulsifying agents, which are usually admixtures of cetyl and stearyl alcohol and a surfactant. In most emulsified systems, the overall viscosity of the microstructure may be increased by increasing the viscosity of the continuous phase, by increasing the content of a single emulsifying agent, or by reducing the globule size, for example by homogenisation.

Gels

Gels are transparent or translucent semi-solid or solid preparations, consisting of solutions or dispersions of one or more active ingredients in suitable hydrophilic or hydrophobic bases. They are made with the aid of a suitable gelling agent. Usually gels exhibit pseudoplastic flow properties and those made with synthetic or semi-synthetic polymers with a high degree of cross-linking have relatively high yield values and low viscosity. Gels are often non-greasy and are generally applied externally. The term 'gel' has also been applied in pharmacy to some viscous suspensions for oral use, for example, aluminium hydroxide gel. As well as being used as delivery vehicles for local anaesthetics, spermicides, and dermatological agents, gels are used for lubrication of gloves and instruments, as film-formers in patch testing, and for conductivity enhancement on the terminals of electrocardiograph leads. Gels used as lubricants for catheters or devices inserted into internal organs are required to be sterile.

As vehicles for the presentation of water-soluble medicaments, gels are ideal because of their high water content. Products tend to be smooth, elegant, and produce cooling effects because of evaporation of water; they may also dry out to form films. Films adhere well to the skin and are usually easily removed by washing; gelatin-containing films may be less readily removed. For the presentation of insoluble materials hydrophilic gels have the limitation that the resultant products may lack clarity and smoothness.

Non-aqueous liquids may also be formed into gels. For example, liquid paraffin gelled with low-density polyethylene is the base for a commercial ointment basis; softer gels of liquid paraffin can be obtained using colloidal silica. Vegetable oils form gels with aluminium stearate, and cellulose derivatives are used as gelling agents for mixtures of ethanol and propylene glycol.

A solid gel produced by cooling a hot solution of gelatin into which the medicament has been incorporated is Zinc Gelatin BPC 1968 (Unna's Paste); for application, it is melted and applied with a brush.

Ointments

Ointments are semi-solid preparations intended to adhere to the skin or certain mucous membranes; they are usually solutions or dispersions of one or more medicaments in non-aqueous bases.

Ointment bases are often anhydrous and include fats, oils, and waxes of animal, vegetable, or mineral origin; non-oleaginous and synthetic substances are also incorporated in bases.

Ideally, an ointment basis should not produce irritation or sensitisation of the skin, nor should it retard wound healing; it should be smooth, inert, odourless, physically and chemically stable, and compatible with the skin and with dermatological medicaments.

Ointments are used as vehicles for medicaments intended to produce a pharmacological effect at, or near, the application site; they are also applied as emollients and skin protectives.

The rheological behaviour of ointments is closely related to their structure; for example, at microscopic level soft paraffins consist of solid and liquid fractions in the form of a fibrous crystal matrix of the waxy components to which the liquid components are held by sorption.

A gel-like matrix can also form in the continuous phase of emulsified bases and in absorption bases, especially those that contain emulsifiers based on surfactants and long-chain alcohols. The flow properties of ointments are controlled mainly by the rigidity of the matrix and the concentration of the waxy constituents. When shear stress is applied, ointments usually exhibit a relatively high yield value and then behave as viscoelastic materials.

Pastes

Pastes are much stiffer than ointments and are used principally as absorbents, antiseptics, protectives, or to soothe broken skin surfaces; they are often applied thickly on dressings rather than spread on the skin. Pastes usually consist of finely ground insoluble powders (at concentrations of 20% to 60%) dispersed in hydrocarbon or water-miscible bases. Basis materials that have been used in the preparation of pastes include soft and liquid paraffins, glycerol, mucilages, and emulsifying waxes and ointments. High yield values and dilatant flow properties are typical rheological characteristics of pastes.

Poultices

Poultices have a long history of use in medicine. Traditionally, poultices consisted of moistened masses of vegetable materials or clay that were sometimes heated before application. Only one poultice is now officially recognised, Kaolin Poultice BP, which is a dense, nearly solid mass with hygroscopic properties and good heat retention. It is spread thickly on a dressing and applied hot, with the objective of reducing inflammation and allaying pain.

PERCUTANEOUS ABSORPTION

In products applied topically for therapeutic effect it is necessary that the medicament is released from the base and penetrates the skin at a suitable rate and in sufficient quantity to maintain an effective concentration at the site of action. **Percutaneous absorption** is the term used to describe the penetration of a substance through the skin and subsequent movement into the systemic circulation. It should be recognised that skin penetration is not always a necessary requirement for a topically applied medicament. A surface film of the active substance is often intended for skin protection, for example, against sunlight or loss of moisture, for emollient effect, or for antimicrobial activity in skin disinfection.

When skin penetration for local activity is the aim, it is desirable that the active substance should be retained for as long as possible in the viable epidermis and dermis with only slow or minimal elimination by the systemic circulation. Achievement of these conditions cannot be assured, but may be optimised by appropriate formulation.

In contrast, the more recently developed techniques of transdermal drug delivery rely on the optimal transport of the active substance through the skin into the systemic vasculature.

An understanding of the nature, properties and functions of human skin is an essential preliminary to a study of the routes and mechanisms by which medicaments penetrate the skin barrier.

Skin Anatomy and Physiology

The skin serves a number of invaluable functions. It is involved in the regulation of body temperature and blood pressure and acts to some degree as a barrier against damage by radiation, physical action, chemical agents, and micro-organisms. Anatomically, the skin may be considered as three tissue layers: the epidermis, the dermis, and the subcutaneous fat layer or hypodermis. Fig. 1 shows a simplified section through the skin with the associated blood vessels, hair follicles, nerves, and glands.

Epidermis

The epidermis is about 110 micrometres in thickness and is pierced by hair follicles and sebaceous glands; it is non-vascular. The outermost layer of the epidermis is called the **stratum corneum** or horny layer. Kligman[1] described it as a transparent, tough, coherent membrane with viscoelastic properties. It is composed of dense overlapping laminates of dead cells, each packed with keratin filaments in an amorphous matrix of proteins with lipids and water-soluble substances. The cells are polygonal when viewed perpendicularly and are arranged in layers about 15 cells deep. Lipid materials are mainly found in the intercellular region. Resistance to the diffusion of chemicals is greater in the stratum corneum than in the underlying living skin tissues. The stratum corneum is therefore recognised as the rate-limiting barrier to the ingress of materials and is the tissue predominantly responsible for the remarkable impenetrability of the skin. However, the layer is not an absolute barrier and trace amounts of penetrants can be detected. Contact sensitisers such as nickel or chromium ions are known to penetrate, as are toxic insecticides such as parathion, and certain toxic gases.

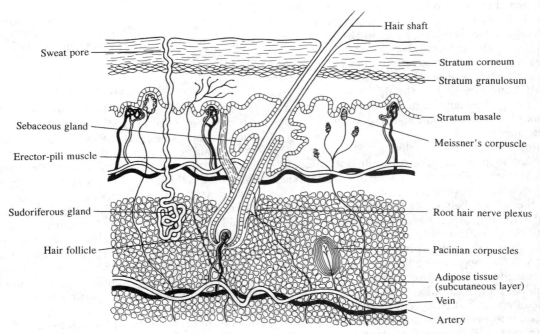

Fig. 1
Skin section.

The thickness of the stratum corneum varies: it is thick on the plantar and palmar areas and thin behind the ear and on the eyelid. Although the stratum corneum is normally about 10 micrometres thick when dry, it can swell four- or five-fold when fully hydrated. The stratum corneum takes up water by a reversible process; a balance is normally maintained at about 20% by weight of water. At a water content of 10% or less, skin loses its suppleness and the cells of the stratum corneum become shrunken and distorted; the barrier may become damaged. Dry stratum corneum contains 15% to 20% lipid material. An emulsion of lipids, with a pH of about 5, permeates the outer layers of the stratum corneum; it arises from the secretions of the sebaceous glands and is thought to modify water transport and aid absorption of anionic substances.

The living cells of the epidermis are located immediately below the stratum corneum. Lying directly above the dermis is a single layer of cells called the **stratum basale** which constantly divides to produce keratinocytes. Mitosing cells from the stratum basale migrate slowly upwards towards the **stratum granulosum** where they flatten, their content becomes granular and keratin forms. Ultimately, through oxygen and nutrient deprivation, the cells shrink and die to become the cells of the stratum corneum. Within the stratum corneum, the cells become more compacted as they proceed towards the surface, until they are eventually lost by abrasion. To maintain mechanical protection the stratum corneum is therefore much thicker in those regions of the body that are either constantly abraded or bear weight.

Dermis

Below the epidermis is the dermis or corium. Convolutions in the boundary between the two layers increase the area of contact between the epidermis and the dermis with its numerous blood vessels, nerves, and lymphatics, and bring the blood supply closer to the skin surface. The dermis is about 3.2 mm thick and is the largest of the three skin layers. It is predominantly connective tissue and the few cells it contains are principally involved in the secretion of elastin and collagen.

Subcutaneous Fat Layer

The final layer of skin, the subcutaneous fat layer or hypodermis, contains adipose cells which serve principally as an energy source. Additionally, the tissue cushions the outer skin layers from impact and its insulation properties contribute to the temperature regulation function of the skin.

Skin Appendages

The blood supply, nerves, and lymphatics that maintain the functions of the dermis also support skin appendages located in the dermis and hypodermis, some of which penetrate the epidermis as ducts or follicles.

Hair Follicles. Hair follicles are sebum-filled openings from which keratinous hair filaments protrude; follicles occupy about 0.1% of the skin surface area but are absent from plantar and palmar surfaces, the red areas of the lips, and parts of the genitalia. Follicles are well served with nerve fibres to maintain the sensory function of the hair. Ducts into each hair follicle transport sebum secreted by one or more sebaceous glands; collectively, the follicle and gland make up a **pilosebaceous unit**. About 100 sebaceous glands per square centimetre is the usual level of distribution but on the more hairy regions of the body they number between 400 and 900 per square centimetre. Breakdown of cells from the sebaceous glands yields sebum which consists of 95% lipids, principally triglycerides, wax esters, squalene, cholesterol esters, and cholesterol.

Sweat Glands

The sweat glands are coiled tubules in the dermis which open onto the skin surface; they can be sub-divided into two classes, **eccrine glands** and the larger **apocrine glands**.

Eccrine sweat glands are involved in the regulation of body temperature by water elimination. There are about two million eccrine sweat glands on the average human body; they predominate on the hairless surfaces of the hands and feet. Sweat secreted by eccrine glands varies in composition with the stimulus, the rate of sweating, and the site; it is a clear watery liquid of acid pH containing electrolytes, trace elements, and organic substances.

Apocrine sweat glands are larger than eccrine but fewer in number; they are mainly located in the hairier regions of the axillae and around the nipples. Apocrine sweat differs in composition from eccrine and may be cloudy and coloured.

Absorption Mechanisms

Early empirical studies, in which the skin was stripped, indicated that the stratum corneum was the predominant barrier to penetration of the skin by topically applied chemicals. However, the effects of absorbed toxic chemicals and contact sensitisers, together with histological observations and measurements with radiolabelled or skin-blanching compounds have amply affirmed the permeability of human skin to some substances. Attempts to make generalised predictions of the penetration potential of drug molecules on the basis of physico-chemical characteristics such as lipid-solubilising, diffusion, or partition coefficients have not been entirely successful. The mechanisms by which percutaneous absorption takes place are not yet fully understood and the processes involved are still the subject of argument and debate. Of the many theories for drug penetration that have been advanced, the two that are most widely accepted are the **transappendageal theory** and the **trans-epidermal theory**.

Transappendageal Penetration

The transappendageal theory proposes that the barrier afforded by the stratum corneum is circumvented and that there is relatively rapid ingress via eccrine sweat glands and hair follicles. Of the two routes, the eccrine sweat glands are probably the least important because increased permeability has not been demonstrated in areas where they predominate and they represent only a tiny proportion of the skin surface. Furthermore, drug diffusion would be against the outflow of sweat which appears to be controlled within the gland.

Penetration via hair follicles has been taken seriously by some workers. The absence of keratinised cells and the direct ingress of the follicles to the dermis and hypodermis certainly suggest an easy pathway for the diffusion of topically applied medicaments. It is postulated that lipophilic drugs diffuse into the sebum of the pilosebaceous unit before being absorbed directly into the dermis. As with the sweat glands the negligible surface area taken up by hair follicles tends to limit their significance as a major route of penetration. However, the follicles have high permeability in comparison with the stratum corneum and absorption of a substance may initially be predominantly through the hair follicles with a lag time before absorption through the stratum corneum. For large molecules with low diffusion constants or poor solubility, transfollicular penetration may be the sole absorption mechanism.

Transepidermal Penetration

The unbroken epidermis constitutes the larger surface for absorption and is widely regarded as the major, but not the exclusive, pathway for the percutaneous absorption of many compounds. It appears that initial transient diffusion through appendages may be supplemented or followed by a steadier phase of diffusion through the epidermis. The factors that govern the route and rate of penetration are complex and variable. Identification of a particular route by experiment is difficult to achieve.

Passive diffusion is recognised as the transport mechanism through the epidermis and there is little evidence of active transport within the inviable cells of the stratum corneum.

There are two possible routes for the transepidermal absorption of drugs. The first involves a tortuous course between the cells of the stratum corneum and the second is the direct diffusion of the drug through the cells. These two pathways are respectively called the intercellular and intracellular routes. Because of the difficulty in designing experiments to demonstrate which of the two routes is predominant, there is still much argument as to their relative merits.

Intercellular Diffusion. The intercellular spaces account for only a small proportion, up to 1%, of the stratum corneum; however, absorption by this route should be assisted by the lower resistance to diffusion in the intercellular spaces. The width of intercellular spaces has been disputed and there is some evidence to suggest that they may be an important route for the diffusion of small molecules.

Intracellular Diffusion. Many workers now believe that the intracellular route is the dominant pathway. Their evidence supports an inverse relationship between the thickness of the stratum corneum and its permeability. Penetration rates have progressively increased as layers of stratum corneum are removed by stripping. The theory has also been supported by measurements of drug distribution in skin removed by adhesive tape stripping.

The difficulty in predicting penetration behaviour of lipophilic and hydrophilic substances, and between those of high and low molecular weight, is compounded by regional variation in thickness and permeability of the stratum corneum and the altered permeability of damaged skin surfaces. Among the mechanisms offered to explain the molecular penetration of intact stratum corneum is the possibility that lipid-rich lamellae associated with the keratin fibrils permit the diffusion of lipophilic compounds and that the degree of hydration of the protein-containing keratinised cells influences the flux of hydrophilic compounds.

There is little doubt that the dense keratinised cells of the stratum corneum present high diffusional resistance to any penetrating drug. Against this limitation it must be remembered that the epidermis constitutes a surface area 100 to 1000 times greater than the appendageal routes.

Most substances that penetrate the stratum corneum meet negligible resistance on entering the viable epidermis and the upper layers of the dermis. The profuse capillary network ensures rapid entry into the circulation and residence times in the dermis may be of only a few minutes. For a few substances, such as certain electrolytes, testosterone, and highly lipophilic drugs, there is evidence of retention in the dermis or a rate-limiting barrier to absorption at the epidermal-dermal junction.

It is believed that any drug arriving in the dermis is rapidly cleared by the blood vessels thus maintaining classical 'sink' conditions. In this way, topically applied substances reach the general circulation but, because of slow penetration rates and extensive dilution, blood concentrations are usually insufficient to cause serious or evident side-effects. This is not always the case, as Cushing's syndrome is a recognised side-effect of long-term topical steroid therapy. Guy and Maibach[2] present evidence that certain drugs applied topically may be retained in the subcutaneous tissue and deeper muscle below the dermis.

Reservoir Effects

Evidence that reservoirs or depots of drug substance can exist within the stratum corneum was presented by Vickers,[3] although the phenomenon had been observed earlier.[4,5]

By occluding the skin surface after the application of a corticosteroid, vasoconstriction was achieved after 16 hours. At intervals of up to 14 days after a single application, vasoconstriction could be reinduced at the original site solely by the application of an impermeable film. Vickers confirmed by experiment that the reservoir was in the stratum corneum and demonstrated the importance of occlusion in providing the flux necessary to achieve a reservoir of the corticosteroid. Examples of other drugs that have been associated with depot effects are griseofulvin, benzocaine, oestradiol, hexachlorophane, and hyoscine. Reservoir-forming drugs tend to be of low aqueous solubility and/or poor penetration capacity; depots have

been formed by the use of penetrating solvents such as dimethyl sulphoxide. The therapeutic potential of reservoirs is restricted to highly potent compounds because of the relatively small amounts that can be retained in the stratum corneum.

Factors that affect Percutaneous Absorption

Transdermal kinetics appear to follow Fick's law of diffusion:

$$J_s = \frac{K_m D C_s}{E}$$

where J_s is the steady state flux of solute, K_m is the distribution coefficient of the drug between the solvent or vehicle and the stratum corneum, C_s is the concentration difference of solute across the membrane, E is the thickness of the stratum corneum, and D is the average membrane diffusion coefficient for the solute in the stratum corneum.

Therefore, the quantity of drug absorbed over unit area in unit time depends on:

- the drug's solubility and distribution characteristics
- the concentration difference of the drug across the membrane
- the nature of the solvent or vehicle in which the drug is presented
- the thickness of the stratum corneum.

The factors that control percutaneous absorption and gastro-intestinal absorption are essentially the same. Skin penetration can be considered under three main headings: condition of the skin; physicochemical characteristics of the active substances; and the effects due to the vehicle.

Condition of the Skin

Damage and Disease. Intact skin presents a barrier to absorption that can be reduced considerably when the skin is damaged or is in a diseased state. Skin can be damaged by dryness, irritation, allergic reactions, or by abrasion. Bronaugh and Stewart[6] demonstrated the enhanced percutaneous absorption of nicotinic acid and cortisone afforded by skin injury. The skin was damaged by stratum corneum removal, hypodermic needle abrasion, or ultraviolet irradiation. The greatest increase in penetration was observed after removal of the stratum corneum by adhesive tape stripping.

Age. Although the ultrastructure of infant skin is indistinguishable from that of an adult, blood concentrations of topically applied drugs can be much higher. This difference is because the skin is a much larger organ, relatively, in infants than in adults and because the epidermal enzymes capable of metabolising applied medicaments may not be fully developed. The skin of pre-term infants may be even more permeable as the stratum corneum is not completely formed until the end of gestation. Old age can also affect permeability of the skin through changes in the elasticity, ultrastructure, chemical composition, and barrier properties.

Temperature and Humidity. Absorption is influenced by environmental factors such as skin temperature and surface humidity. Diffusion can be accelerated by raising surface temperature, for example, by occlusion.

Skin Site. Fick's law of diffusion states that the diffusion of a solute will be inversely proportional to the thickness of the stratum corneum. In the plantar and palmar areas keratinised layers are thick and absorption rates are consequently slow; on the face, and particularly behind the ear, absorption is more rapid. However, factors other than thickness also play a role in deciding the extent of percutaneous absorption at a particular body site: these include the size and lipid composition of the cells in the stratum corneum, their number of layers and associated stacking pattern, and the depth and distribution of the appendages.

Hydration. The keratinised cells of the stratum corneum have the ability to hold water; their degree of hydration, which is also related to the environmental humidity and the extent of perspiration, affects the pliancy of the skin. Absorption of active substances is enhanced as the skin becomes more hydrated; this is the principle involved in the use of occlusive dressings, where loss of moisture from the skin is retarded by the application of a film of low permeability.

Sex and Race. There is no evidence to suggest that the permeability characteristics of male and female skin differ. However, Behl *et al*[7] demonstrated that skin penetration may be influenced by race; propranolol was found to be absorbed by Negroid skin at a rate that was forty times slower than that demonstrated by Caucasian skin *in vitro*.

Miscellaneous Aspects. The application of vasoconstrictors such as steroids to the skin surface may slow penetration because of the reduced blood supply. However, Bucks *et al*[8] suggested that the long-term application of hydrocortisone may have the opposite effect and that percutaneous absorption may be enhanced as the barrier properties of the stratum corneum could be damaged by the long-term use of the steroid.

Physicochemical Characteristics of the Active Substance

A number of mathematical terms are used to describe the percutaneous absorption of active substances; the most commonly employed are the permeability constant and the thermodynamic activity (chemical potential). The permeability constant is the product of the stratum corneum/vehicle partition coefficient and the degree of diffusion of the compound in the skin. A substance that is very soluble in a particular vehicle will tend to have a low permeability constant and will, therefore, be poorly absorbed. The thermodynamic activity describes the potential of a substance to be absorbed; compounds diffuse from regions of high activity to areas of low activity.

Both the permeability constant and the thermodynamic activity of an active substance are influenced by its ionisation constant and by the pH of the skin and of aqueous vehicles. The lipid-soluble unionised species of many substances are more rapidly absorbed than their water-soluble salts.

Molecular Modification. Molecular modification of active substances can have marked effects on their activity. Changes in functional groups that alter the solubility and the partition coefficient of the substance between the vehicle and the skin barrier may retard or enhance skin penetration. For example, when applied topically, most of the esters of the fluorinated corticosteroids have considerably greater activity than hydrocortisone.

A novel variation in the use of molecular modification to enhance percutaneous absorption is the formation of prodrugs that undergo **cutaneous biotransformation**. In this case, the modification is designed to be reversed by the enzyme activity of the epidermis or dermis after the derivatised drug has crossed the stratum corneum. This technique is potentially useful for poorly absorbed compounds that can be prepared as inactive prodrugs. A greater understanding of the enzyme systems involved is required before the full potential of this technique can be realised. Bodor *et al*[9] used the technique to increase the dermal delivery of cromoglycic acid.

Partition Coefficient. A partition coefficient that approaches unity aids penetration of the skin barrier, which has both hydrophilic and hydrophobic properties.

Concentration. An increase in the concentration of an active substance in a vehicle usually produces an increase in the thermodynamic activity of the system and a subsequent increase in the quantity of the material absorbed. The thermodynamic activity is the product of the concentration of the active substance in the vehicle and an activity coefficient. However, as concentration increases and the particles become more closely packed, there is an increased chance of interactions. Particle-particle interactions may reduce the activity coefficient of the preparation and limit the amount of active substance absorbed. In dilute solutions, the activity coefficient approximates to unity but at high concentrations the value may fall.

Molecular Size and Shape. Molecules of small size in high concentration tend to penetrate more readily than large molecules. However, for a range of chemically equivalent molecules with similar molecular weights, there is little correlation between their size and absorption potential.

Particle Size. The rates of dissolution and subsequent penetration of a substance may be influenced by its particle size. It is important to ensure that different batches of a preparation contain particles of equivalent size to prevent problems of bioinequivalence. Particle size reduction has been used to enhance the percutaneous absorption of poorly soluble drugs such as hydrocortisone or hydrocortisone acetate.

Polymorphism. Physical properties such as solubility may vary greatly between different polymorphs. Ideally, where polymorphic forms of a substance occur, the form with physical characteristics most suitable for penetration should be selected.

Effects due to the Vehicle

Although the nature of the vehicle can affect the release of an active substance, the thermodynamic activity of the substance and its potential for absorption by the skin are more important factors in percutaneous absorption than the ability of the vehicle to penetrate the skin. For most substances, the rate-determining step in skin penetration is the diffusion of the substance through the stratum corneum. For certain steroids that have a very low solubility in the vehicle, the release of the drug from the vehicle is the rate-determining step. The nature of the vehicle can influence not only the amount of active substance that is dissolved or suspended in it but also the diffusion coefficient of the substance and its partition coefficient between the vehicle and the skin. Substances that have a high affinity for the vehicle have a low thermodynamic activity and are released slowly; their lipid/water partition coefficients are often low. By reducing the solubility of the substance in the vehicle, conditions more favourable for release can usually be obtained. In some instances, the high affinity of the active substance for the vehicle may be due to complexation or 'binding' to constituents of the vehicle.

The state of hydration of the skin can also be affected by the vehicle. Increased hydration is achieved, clinically, by reducing evaporation with an occlusive layer. Emulsified creams are less occlusive than oleaginous ointment bases, but the water-in-oil creams have some occlusive properties.

Traditionally, when a medicament was formulated as a topical dosage form the vehicle was chosen on empirical grounds based on compatibility, stability, and cosmetic aspects rather than its potential influence on percutaneous absorption. However, vehicles are now being studied in greater depth with particular attention to their influence on penetration rates.

Lippold and Schneemann[10] have studied the influence of different vehicles on the bioavailability of betamethasone-17-benzoate. Two types of bases were studied: solution and suspension bases. In solution bases, where the drug is molecularly dispersed, the bioavailability was found to be poor in those vehicles with a high affinity for the steroid. The high affinity results in a low stratum corneum/vehicle partition coefficient and the drug consequently remains in the vehicle and does not penetrate the skin. Dugard and Scott[11] developed a method that predicts the percutaneous absorption rates from different vehicles using solubility data and knowledge of the rate in a single vehicle system.

Effect of Viscosity. DiColo *et al*[12] reported that the release of benzocaine from suspension hydrogels was dramatically reduced in vehicles of high viscosity. The diffusion coefficient of a drug was inversely proportional to viscosity; thus a reduction in viscosity enhanced diffusion.

Effect of pH. In systems where a weakly ionised active substance is present in the aqueous phase of an oil-in-water emulsion, adjustment of the pH to values above or below the pK_a value will influence the degree of ionisation with consequent effect on both activity and release. Swarbrick *et al*[13] found that the permeability coefficients of the unionised chromone-2-carboxylic acids were approximately 10 000 larger than those of the corresponding ionised species.

Effect of Volatility. Volatile components have been used to increase penetration. Their evaporation on application to the skin surface increases the local concentration of the active ingredient and so helps maximise the thermodynamic activity of the system.

Effect of Excipients. Excipients can affect penetration by either altering the hydration state of the stratum corneum or by modifying the stratum corneum/vehicle partition coefficient. For example, humectants may decrease hydration by extracting moisture from the skin itself. Insoluble powders also decrease hydration by disrupting the continuity of oily films at the skin surfaces and by providing an increased surface area for evaporation. Propylene glycol and ethanol have been included in vehicles as solvents for steroids; if their concentration in such systems is carefully controlled they can favourably influence lipid/water partition coefficients to aid penetration.

Umer[14] found that the addition of macrogol 400 and dimethyl sulphoxide to hydrocarbon ointment bases increased the absorption of hydrocortisone acetate. Such compounds are called penetration enhancers and are discussed in greater detail later in this chapter. Okamoto *et al*[15] studied the effects of β-cyclodextrin and di-0-methyl-β-cyclodextrin on the percutaneous absorption of butyl hydroxybenzoate, indomethacin, and sulphanilic acid. Although the absorption of the latter compound was increased by di-0-methyl-β-cyclodextrin, both butyl hydroxybenzoate and indomethacin demonstrated decreased skin permeation *in vitro* under the influence of the two agents.

Surfactants can influence percutaneous absorption in two opposing ways: disruption of the barrier properties of the stratum corneum causing an increase in penetration; or by increasing the solubility of drugs in the vehicle, thereby reducing the stratum corneum/vehicle partition coefficient, and indirectly decreasing penetration. Surfactants have been principally used to stabilise topical systems in order to maintain homogeneous, elegant, and rheologically stable products. However, in the formulation of new semi-solid preparations, the possible influence they may have on percutaneous absorption should be fully realised.[16]

In conclusion, the main function of a vehicle is to carry and release the active substance. In view of the complexity of the absorption mechanisms, the extent to which the vehicle can penetrate the skin is an unreliable basis on which to attempt to predict the effectiveness of the vehicle in enhancing the penetration of the active substance.

Methods of Estimating or Measuring Percutaneous Absorption

A number of elegant methods have been devised to measure the degree of systemic absorption after topical application. These methods have helped elucidate routes of penetration and identify specific barriers to absorption. Both *in-vitro* and *in-vivo* methods have been used.

In-vitro Methods

Model Systems. The earliest experiments used unrepresentative model systems such as agar gel. The effectiveness of antibiotic ointment formulations, for example, was assessed by cutting cups in an agar plate, filling these with the ointment under investigation, and measuring the zones of inhibition caused by the antibacterial agent on the growth of a sensitive micro-organism.

A mixture of solvents such as ethanol and water, in which the drug is fairly soluble, has also been utilised to model skin penetration. The skin is represented by the interface between these two solvents and another immiscible solvent, such as chloroform or isopropyl myristate. The latter solvents serve as the sink and the partitioning behaviour of a compound is used to furnish information on percutaneous absorption.

Membrane Systems. Although model membranes such as cellulose films have been developed to simulate skin,[17] much work on percutaneous absorption *in vitro* has been carried out on excised animal or human integument. Tape-stripping techniques, for example, have been employed to remove sheets of stratum corneum for use in such experiments, and both post-mortem and post-surgical human skin can be obtained with relative ease. In addition, excised skin can be frozen and stored indefinitely without significantly disturbing the barrier properties of the stratum corneum.

A simple design for studying percutaneous absorption involves stretching human skin over a funnel and measuring the passage of materials from the epidermal surface through the membrane to a receptor phase. Most experiments use a more complex system such as a Franz-type diffusion cell but the principle is much the same.

A number of workers have criticised such experiments saying that the experimental design does not take into account vasoconstriction effects, surface desquamation, and the sink conditions afforded by living skin. In addition, *in-vitro* techniques do not allow for depot effects or the metabolism of the compound in the viable epidermis.

There are a number of advantages of *in-vitro* experimentation: the greater control over environmental conditions; the increased precision of the test design; and the lowered chance of experimental error. Kligman[1] has argued that *in-vitro* studies should accurately represent the situation *in vivo* provided that circumstances are equivalent. Sink conditions should operate and only the epidermis should be used; the dermis is the site of the sink and its inclusion in the experimental design may introduce variables that are not relevant to the situation *in vivo*.

In-vivo Methods

In-vivo methods can involve the use of either animals or human volunteers. There has been a great debate on the relevance of animal experiment results, as absorption has been found to vary markedly with different species. Efforts have been made to identify an animal species whose skin closely resembles that of humans but such endeavours have met with little success. Penetration through the skin of small animals, for example, is consistently greater than that of humans. The closest model would appear to be the skin of either the *pig* or the *rhesus monkey*.

Analysis of Body Fluids and Histological Methods. A more accurate method involves the analysis of body fluids or tissues after topical application. The concentration of absorbed penetrants are most often assayed in urine samples but alternatively small specimens of skin can be obtained by biopsy. Samples may be analysed by any of the normal chemical procedures although gas chromatographic methods, radioactive and fluorescence techniques, and specific colour reactions are the most popular. Radioactive techniques are the most sensitive.

Radioisotope work involves applying a radiolabelled medicament to the skin surface. Measurements can be made either in the body fluids or on the surface where the radioactivity will fall as absorption proceeds. In the former case the technique should be combined with a chemical identification test to ensure that the compound has not been metabolised and that the radioactivity actually represents the material under investigation. The disadvantage of using concentrations in urine to assess percutaneous absorption is that the applied agent may be concentrated in a body compartment other than the urinary system. A steady state between absorption and excretion needs to be reached before measurement of urinary-drug concentrations can be accepted.

A novel method to quantify penetration rates can be applied to animals. The animal is first 'calibrated' by administering a penetrant at a known rate by slow intravenous injection. The blood-penetrant concentrations are then plotted against time for various administration rates. By comparing these blood-penetrant concentrations with those produced after topical application, the particular penetration rate should be calculable. Other histological and body fluid studies make use of dyes, fluorescent tracers, and autoradiography. The application of dyes has been extensively used because their routes of penetration can be easily followed. However dyes do not necessarily follow the same route or indeed penetrate at the same rate as the compounds that they are meant to be labelling. Fluorescent labels possess the same problems but if the compound under investigation is itself fluorescent, techniques such as fluorescence microscopy or the measurement of the diminution of fluorescence at the skin surface may be used with confidence. Some drugs cause alterations in epidermal sulphydryl groups and these changes can be used to follow the permeation process. Radioactive tracers have also been used. The selection of a radionuclide of the compound under investigation produces the most accurate representation of the rate and route of penetration.

Autoradiography is used to derive information on specific routes of penetration. However, the routes are often difficult to identify because of shadowing and scattering, which are often associated with this technique. In addition, penetration cannot be quantified by this technique because of the difficulty of handling the preparations.

Physiological Responses. Many agents are able to elicit a response in the skin when they are applied topically. This response can be used to determine the extent of penetration. Examples of possible responses include sweat secretion, vasoconstriction (blanching), vasodilatation, keratolysis, pigmentation, and changes in vascular permeability.

Blanching, for example, caused by the topical application of steroids, is the basis of a vasoconstrictor assay. The assay involves using the extent of blanching elicited by the application of different corticosteroids, or different formulations of the same corticosteroid, to assess relative potencies.

Other physiological responses to topical application include the reversal of sweat secretion blockade by antimuscarinic agents, the keratolysis induced by salicylic acid, and the vasodilatation promoted by the administration of histamine, methyl nicotinate,[18] and nicotinic acid. Each of these responses can be used to assess the influence of vehicle composition.

Release Rates from Vehicles

Dissolution testing has become an indispensable technique for the evaluation of tablets and has been applied to the study of topical semi-solid preparations. Behme, Kensler, and Brooke,[19] for example, described a dissolution technique for evaluating the release of oestradiol from cream formulations. The cream was spread on an 80-mesh stainless steel screen and immersed in water. This technique could be applied to a wide range of drugs and cream formulations.

The release of salicylic acid from ointment bases has been studied using a mathematical model by Bialik.[20] Similar studies have been performed *in vivo* and *in vitro* using infrared measurements by Lehky *et al*.[21] Tanaka *et al*[22] studied the release of hydrocortisone butyrate propionate into silicone rubber (as a skin model) from cream and gel formulations containing volatile constituents. Release rates were compared after storage under open and closed conditions to assess the effects of evaporation. Open conditions were found to increase the release rates as both the concentration of the steroid and the thermodynamic activity of the system were increased by evaporation.

Pharmacokinetic Models

The physicochemical characteristics of the drug and vehicle and the physiological condition of the skin are major influences on the extent of percutaneous absorption (as discussed earlier). Any model that purports to describe penetration *in vivo* must therefore make allowance for parameters such as the age of the skin and its state of hydration, the temperature and humidity conditions, the concentration, partition coefficient and particle size of the drug substance to be absorbed, and formulation aspects of the vehicle such as the pH and viscosity.

Guy, Hadgraft, and Maibach[23] developed a pharmacokinetic model to describe percutaneous absorption. This model involves four first-order rate constants: k_1 represents the rate of diffusion of the drug across the stratum corneum, and k_2 the equivalent term for further penetration into the deeper regions of the skin. The term k_3 is used to take into account any reservoir effects and k_4 is simply the elimination rate constant. This model was further refined to allow for such factors as metabolism within the epidermis[24] and drug loss at the skin surface.[25] Most importantly the model was enlarged to take into account the release characteristics of a topical formulation.[26]

Penetration Enhancers

Penetration enhancers (sorption promoters or accelerants) improve absorption by penetrating the skin and interfering with the barrier properties of the stratum corneum. A mixture of two parts chloroform and one part methanol, for example, if used to pre-treat the skin will increase the penetration of any medicament subsequently applied. It is presumed that the solvents disrupt the structure of the stratum corneum through the removal of lipids.

Little is known about the mode of action of most of the penetration enhancers used, but increased permeability can be achieved by increasing the water content of the stratum corneum or by simply damaging its barrier properties. Water is the simplest and most commonly employed penetration enhancer, as evidenced by the widespread use of occlusive dressings and vehicles. Examples of other penetration enhancers include sulphoxides, amides, pyrrolidones, organic solvents, laurocapram (Azone™), and calcium thioglycollate. Propylene glycol can also be thought of as a penetration enhancer where it increases the thermodynamic potential and therefore the penetration of steroids when used at a concentration just sufficient to dissolve the drug.

A penetration enhancer should be non-toxic, non-irritant, non-allergenic, and devoid of any pharmacological activity. Its action should be rapid, predictable, and reversible, and it should not facilitate the loss of any material from the skin or underlying layers. In addition, the penetration enhancer should be compatible with a wide variety of drugs and excipients. Whitworth and Stephenson[27] studied water, dimethyl sulphoxide, and ethanol as possible penetration enhancers for the diffusion of atropine sulphate from various ointment bases. In each of the bases studied, diffusion was increased by the inclusion of a penetration enhancer; the increase was greatest for polar bases with a high aqueous content. It was much less for water-in-oil emulsions and for non-polar bases such as hydrogenated cottonseed oil.

Sulphoxides and Amides

Dimethyl sulphoxide (DMSO) passes readily through the stratum corneum and has consequently been used in commercial preparations as a penetration enhancer. The antiviral agent, idoxuridine, for example, is presented as a 5% solution in DMSO (Herpid™, Boehringer Ingelheim). High concentrations of DMSO (at least 60%) are required to enhance absorption perceptibly. Increased penetration has been demonstrated both *in vivo* and *in vitro* for a wide variety of compounds including water, dyes, barbiturates, steroids, griseofulvin, phenylbutazone, salicylic acid, local anaesthetics, amphetamine sulphate, antibiotics, and quaternary ammonium compounds.

Dimethylacetamide (DMA) and dimethylformamide (DMF) have similar actions to DMSO but their effectiveness as penetration enhancers is not as great. All three agents are hygroscopic and they may, therefore, accelerate penetration simply by increasing the water content of the stratum corneum. In addition, dimethyl sulphoxide may alter the protein structure of the stratum corneum either by substituting itself for integral water molecules or by extracting soluble materials from the skin matrix. Alternatively, DMSO may cause swelling in the stratum corneum and a subsequent opening of pores. DMSO has an added advantage as a penetration enhancer in that it can establish a reservoir of usually poorly absorbed non-polar compounds in the stratum corneum. Unfortunately, DMSO can be both irritant and toxic in excess, and on application it confers a garlic-like odour to the breath.

Other examples of sulphoxides or amides that have been studied as penetration enhancers include the non-polar surfactant, n-decyl-methylsulphoxide and the amide, N,N-diethyl-m-toluamide.

Urea

In the stratum corneum a dynamic equilibrium exists between bound water and free water. Urea, by favouring the conversion of bound water to free water, may cause the skin to hydrate. This, in turn, may enhance the penetration potential of simultaneously applied materials; urea may also act as a mild keratolytic.

Pyrrolidones

Both 2-pyrrolidone and N-methyl-2-pyrrolidone have been studied as penetration enhancers. Southwell and Barry[28] found that 2-pyrrolidone increased the topical absorption of aspirin and caffeine.

Azone

Azone (1-dodecylazacycloheptan-2-one; laurocapram) has been used to enhance the percutaneous absorption of a number of drugs including 5-fluorouracil, clindamycin, erythromycin, griseofulvin, and metronidazole.[29] Its safety in human volunteers has been studied by Wiechers *et al*;[30] the conclusion drawn was that at the relatively low concentration used (2% to 10%), laurocapram should be safe for human use.

Surfactants

Surfactants are used in pharmaceutical formulations as solubilisers, emulsion and suspension stabilisers, and wetting agents. In dilute aqueous solutions they can also act as penetration enhancers. Two theories have been proposed to explain their activity: surfactants may either facilitate transappendageal absorption by lowering interfacial tension or they may alter the protein structure of the skin. Anionic surfactants, for example, bind strongly to skin protein and may cause a reversible denaturation. This may lead to a gross expansion of the tissue and to an increased capacity of the integument to absorb hydrophilic materials. The penetration enhancement achieved by anionic surfactants is greater than that by cationic surfactants, probably because of their irritancy potential. Nonionic surfactants appear to be relatively inert.

Sarpotdar and Zatz[31] studied the influence of polysorbates on the percutaneous absorption of hydrocotrisone *in vitro* through hairless *mouse* skin. These nonionic surfactants were observed to have a synergistic effect with large concentrations of propylene glycol and increased penetration dramatically.

Novel Delivery Systems

Barker and Hadgraft[32] have proposed a facilitated transport process for the absorption of those anionic drugs that are poorly absorbed. The process involves utilising the acidic pH of the sebum to protonate a carrier molecule (for example, an N-substituted di-isopropanolamine) at the skin surface. The carrier then forms a dimer with the anionic drug and the uncharged lipophilic complex diffuses relatively easily through the stratum corneum. On reaching the deeper layers of the epidermis (at pH 7.4), the carrier is deprotonated and the drug released. It is proposed that the carrier then diffuses back to the skin surface where the process can be repeated. The process was demonstrated using methyl orange as the model drug substance.

BASIS CLASSIFICATION

Bases for topical semi-solids can be classified in terms of their physicochemical properties into four main types: fatty or oleaginous, absorption, emulsion, and water-soluble.

Fatty Bases

Fatty bases are usually anhydrous and may contain water-insoluble vegetable oils, animal fats and waxes, hydrocarbons, silicones, or certain synthetic esters. They are not absorbed, but exert an occlusive effect by limiting the evaporation of moisture. Fatty bases have a low capacity to absorb water and are usually used as emollients or as inert vehicles. Because of their greasiness, they tend to be cosmetically unattractive and they are difficult to remove after treatment because of their immiscibility with water. Their stickiness, however, helps maximise contact times. Fatty bases are suitable for sterile products as they are stable to dry heat sterilisation and do not provide a good medium for the growth of micro-organisms.

Absorption Bases

A vehicle that absorbs water is described as an absorption basis; the name does not describe the mode of action of the basis. Absorption bases are often anhydrous and, typically, consist of a hydrophobic fatty basis in which a water-in-oil emulsifier has been incorporated to render it hydrophilic. Examples of emulsifying agents used include wool fat (anhydrous lanolin), wool alcohols (the emulsifying fraction of wool fat), beeswax, and cholesterol. Additional water can be incorporated into the basis to form the internal phase of an emulsion with a consequent increase in the viscosity of the system. Bases of this type are used as vehicles for aqueous liquids or solutions of medicaments; they are not always easily removed from the skin. Absorption bases are easily spread and less occlusive than fatty bases.

Emulsion Bases

Absorption bases to which water has been added to give water-in-oil emulsions are termed emulsion bases. Examples of such systems include Hydrous Ointment BP and hydrous wool fat (lanolin). Hydrous wool fat contains wool fat (70%) and water (30%) and Hydrous Ointment BP includes Wool Alcohols Ointment BP and water in approximately equal parts. Water-in-oil bases have occlusive properties and because of their oily external phase are less readily removed by water than oil-in-water bases. They are generally easier to spread on the skin and are cosmetically more acceptable than either fatty or absorption bases.

Emulsion bases need not necessarily be water-in-oil emulsions as there are many examples of oil-in-water systems. The oil-in-water (o/w) variety are generally regarded to be the most cosmetically elegant; they are easily spread on the skin and readily form vanishing-type creams on admixture with water. There are three official emulsifying ointments that are used to form oil-in-water emulsion bases: Emulsifying Ointment BP (anionic); Cetrimide Emulsifying Ointment BP (cationic); and Cetomacrogol Emulsifying Ointment BP (nonionic). They all contain an oil-in-water emulsifying agent.

Aqueous Cream BP and Buffered Cream BP are prepared with Emulsifying Ointment BP. Cetomacrogol Emulsifying Ointment BP is used in the preparation of Chlorhexidine Cream BP 1988, and Aqueous Calamine Cream BP.

Water-soluble Bases

Most water-soluble ointment bases are made by blending macrogols (polyethylene glycols) of high and low molecular weights. Macrogols conform to the general formula:

$$H(OCH_2CH_2)_nOH$$

Water is not usually included in the formulation of water-soluble bases, as it dissolves the macrogol base and promotes softening. Consistency is varied by adjusting the proportion of the liquid and solid macrogols. Water-soluble medicaments can usually be dissolved in macrogol bases but because these bases are less occlusive than absorption or fatty bases, rates of drug release from them may differ and this may require evaluation.

Water-soluble bases have no protective or emollient properties and their hydrophilicity means they are easily washed from the skin surface by perspiration. They can be sterilised by heat: dry heat for solids and heating in an autoclave for liquids.

An example of a water-soluble basis is Macrogol Ointment BP:

Macrogol 4000	350 g
Macrogol 300	650 g

Macrogol 300 is added to molten macrogol 4000 and the mixture stirred until cold.

Water-soluble macrogol bases have a number of advantages and disadvantages. Advantages include their high water-solubility and consequent ease of removal after use, and their good absorption characteristics; in addition, they are stable, compatible with most drugs and excipients, and non-greasy. Unfortunately, macrogol bases cause a reduction in the potency of certain antimicrobial agents (for example, phenols, hydroxybenzoates, quaternary ammonium compounds, penicillin, and bacitracin) and dissolve certain plastics such as polyethylene and Bakelite. The latter points make the choice of container and closure critical. In addition macrogols produce bland preparations that cannot accommodate large quantities of water.

MICROSTRUCTURE OF TOPICAL SEMI-SOLIDS

A greater understanding of the microstructure of topical semi-solid preparations should improve manufacturing techniques and lead to the development of products with improved cosmetic and therapeutic properties. A number of techniques have been employed to study microstructure and these have been reviewed by Eccleston.[33]

Oil-in-water creams have been studied by Junginger[34] using techniques such as differential scanning calorimetry, X-ray diffraction, and electron microscopy. The creams were observed to be composed of two gel phases: a hydrophilic gel and a lipophilic gel. The water was observed to be either bound in the hydrophilic phase or part of the bulk environment, the two situations being in dynamic equilibrium.

Rowe and Bray[35] used techniques such as thermogravimetric analysis, differential scanning calorimetry, ultracentrifugation, and scanning electron microscopy to study the water distribution of cream formulations containing cetostearyl alcohol and cetrimide. The water was found to be associated with crystalline networks located either around oil droplets or in the bulk. Further studies on cream formulations involving cetrimide and cetostearyl alcohol have employed cryogenic scanning electron microscopy[36] and light-scattering techniques.[37]

Radebaugh and Simonelli[38] used a non-destructive technique to characterise the viscoelastic properties of powder-filled semi-solids. A mathematical model was constructed to describe the behaviour of such systems under the influence of shear and temperature.

FORMULATION

There is an enormous range of potential ingredients available to the formulator of a dermatological dosage form. These include not only the numerous bases required to dilute the chosen medicament but also a vast array of emulsifiers, humectants, antioxidants, stabilisers, preservatives, and penetration enhancers, which are often used to facilitate a particular topical effect. The excipients may be derived from natural, synthetic, or semi-synthetic sources.

Constituents of Topical Semi-solids

Hydrocarbons (Hard, Soft, and Liquid Paraffins)

Paraffins are the most widely used constituents of ointment bases. They are relatively inert and show few incompatibilities with dermatological medicaments.

Soft paraffin is easily spread at normal temperature but its rheological properties can change after heating and cooling, or after mechanical treatment; the consistency can be modified by the addition of liquid paraffin or hard paraffin. A form of soft paraffin is commercially available which exhibits a 'fibrous' internal appearance. The 'long fibre' type is considered to enhance stability in emulsified systems and to produce better occlusion than the 'short fibre' type.

Liquid paraffin can be mixed with hard paraffin to form semi-solid bases, some of which tend to become crystalline on storage; it has also been formed into an ointment-like gel (Plastibase™) by heating with polyethylene and cooling under special conditions.

Vegetable Oils

These include almond oil, arachis oil, castor oil, coconut oil, cottonseed oil, maize oil, olive oil, persic oil (peach or apricot kernel oil), and soya oil. Except for coconut oil, these are all liquids. They are used to modify the consistency of ointments and for their emollient properties. Vegetable oils tend to vary in composition and they are readily oxidised, especially if contaminated with trace metals. Butylated hydroxyanisole, butylated hydroxytoluene, or alkyl gallates are often incorporated to retard oxidation, sometimes in conjunction with organic acids (citric, phosphoric, and tartaric) to chelate metal ions; these are usually added by the suppliers of vegetable oils.

Wool Fat

Wool fat has both emollient properties and the ability to absorb about 30% of water. Thus, wool fat and its derivatives, for example, lanolin oil, are widely used in absorption bases. Limitations on the use of wool fat are its tendency to oxidise, its sticky texture, its odour, and its capacity to induce skin sensitivity in some patients.

Fatty Acids and Alcohols

These include the fatty acids, such as stearic acid and oleic acid; and the fatty alcohols, including cetostearyl, stearyl, and cetyl alcohols. The fatty acids are of natural origin and, because of this, their composition tends to vary. They are mainly used with alkalis as soap emulsifiers; in excess, fatty acids can increase the stiffness and change the appearance of emulsified systems.

Fatty alcohols act as secondary emulsifiers and also as bodying agents; stearyl alcohol tends to form harder bases than cetyl alcohol. They are non-greasy, have excellent emollient characteristics, and readily penetrate the skin. In addition, fatty alcohols readily allow the incorporation of water and hydrophilic materials, and are resistant to oxidation.

Synthetic Esters

Synthetic esters such as glyceryl monostearate, isopropyl myristate, isopropyl palmitate, isopropyl lanolate, butyl stearate, and butyl palmitate have been employed as fatty bases. They are all resistant to oxidation and hydrolysis and, being synthetic, can be prepared to stringent standards.

Isopropyl myristate is a colourless liquid that can be mixed with hydrocarbons, fixed oils, or up to 50% wool fat to form semi-solid bases; it is insoluble in water. Although isopropyl myristate is compatible with soft paraffin, mixtures with liquid paraffin are unstable. On application, it is readily absorbed by the skin and is relatively non-toxic.

Silicones

Oily silicones, for example, dimethicone and cyclomethicone, have been used as hydrophobic oils and as constituents of barrier creams because of their water-repellent properties.

Emulsifiers

The emulsifier system is an important aspect of cream formulation. More information on emulsion theory and individual emulsifying agents can be found in the chapter on Emulsions. Aqueous (oil-in-water) creams are commonly stabilised with surfactants; these can be anionic, cationic, or nonionic. By a judicious selection of surfactant, it is possible to formulate creams that are compatible with most active substances. The water-in-oil emulsions that form oily creams are commonly stabilised using metallic soaps, beeswax, wool fat and its derivatives, and some synthetic nonionic substances; wool fat and beeswax owe their emulsifying properties to their sterol content.

Semi-solid emulsions usually require to be stabilised with more than one emulsifier: for example, a surfactant such as triethanolamine stearate is often used in combination with an oil-soluble auxiliary emulsifier like cetyl alcohol. Chester and Dixon[39] described how the formulation of water-in-oil creams can be simplified by reducing the number of added ingredients.

Anionic Emulsifiers. Anionic emulsifiers are incompatible with cations and may be irritating on application to the skin. The most widely used anionic surfactants are the alkyl sulphates, which include sodium lauryl sulphate and sodium cetostearyl sulphate. Other anionic emulsifiers are the amine soaps such as triethanolamine stearate, and the metallic soaps such as calcium oleate. The alkyl sulphates are more acid-stable than the soaps and they conveniently allow the pH of emulsion systems to be adjusted to that of human skin (pH 4.5 to 6.5).

Cationic Emulsifiers. Cationic emulsifiers such as the quaternary ammonium compound, cetrimide, are incompatible with anionic species. They are often used in combination with fatty alcohols such as cetostearyl alcohol. Cationic emulsifiers have an intrinsic antimicrobial activity and therefore often abrogate the need for the inclusion of additional antimicrobial preservatives in an emulsion formulation. They are also most stable within the pH range 3 to 7 and are therefore suitable for topical products. However, cationic emulsifiers may prove irritating when applied to the skin or eyes.

Nonionic Emulsifiers. Nonionic emulsifiers are used for both oil-in-water and water-in-oil emulsion systems. They are compatible with many drug substances and electrolytes and tend to be stable and non-irritant.

Condensation products of ethylene oxide groups and long-chain hydrophobes are often used as nonionic emulsifiers. The hydrophilic characteristics, and therefore the hydrophile-lipophile balance (HLB; see Emulsions chapter), are determined by the number of oxyethylene groups.

Examples of nonionic emulsifiers are the glycol and glycerol esters, higher fatty alcohols, the macrogol esters (for example, the polyoxyl stearates), the macrogol ethers (for example, cetomacrogol 1000), the sorbitan esters (for example, sorbitan monostearate), the polysorbates, the poloxalkols, and the polyvinyl alcohols.

Gelling Agents

Most topical gels are prepared from organic gelling agents, whether of natural or synthetic origin; some inorganic clays will also form suitable gels with water.

Aluminium Magnesium Silicate. In dispersions of up to 5%, aluminium magnesium silicate (Veegum^{TM}) is used as an emulsion stabiliser or suspending agent but at 10% it will form firm thixotropic gels. The viscosity of dispersions is affected by heat, electrolytes, and ageing. It is compatible with ethanol, glycerol, propylene glycol, and macrogols of high molecular weight.

Bentonite. Bentonite, a montmorillonite clay, swells in water to form thixotropic gels that tend to be coloured and opalescent. Concentrations of bentonite between 7% and 20% in water readily allow the incorporation and suspension of solids; higher concentrations may be used to gel ethanol, glycerol, or glycols. Bentonite gels have a pH of about 9; magnesium oxide is often added to improve gelling properties. Bentonite may be contaminated with pathogenic spores and should be sterilised before use in preparations applied to open wounds; aqueous dispersions may be autoclaved. Chemically modified bentonites (bentones) are used to form thixotropic gels in organic liquids.

Carbomers. Carbomers are carboxyvinyl polymers of high molecular weight, extensively cross-linked with polyalkylsucrose; an aqueous dispersion (1%) is acidic (approximately pH 3) and forms a gel on neutralisation with a suitable base. Viscosity is reduced at pH values below 3 or above 12. Relatively low concentrations of carbomers are normally sufficient to produce a gel. For lubricant gels, typical concentrations are 0.3% to 1%; for medicated gels, 0.5% to 2%. Aqueous carbomer gels are usually clear and translucent; similar gels can be formed with ethanol, glycols, and other organic solvents provided that an appropriate base is used for neutralisation. During preparation, precautions are necessary to prevent the entrapment of air bubbles which can aid oxidation in the presence of light. An antoxidant, a chelating agent (for example, disodium edetate), and an antimicrobial agent may be incorporated in carbomer gels. The rheological properties of carbomer gels are retained at elevated temperatures and under steam sterilisation conditions; such gels are therefore widely used for sterile products. The adverse effect on viscosity of sterilisation by irradiation can be reduced by the inclusion of 5% to 10% ethanol.

Cellulose Derivatives. Cellulose derivatives used as gelling agents are synthetic or semi-synthetic ethers of varying molecular weight in which the cellulose chain has been subjected to different degrees of substitution. Solubility characteristics in water vary between compounds. Viscosity increases with concentration but the higher molecular weight grades tend to be the most viscous. The viscous mucilages formed in water are usually nonionic, clear, translucent, and relatively free from fibres. Some grades change from mucilages to gels on heating to temperatures between 50° and 90° whereas others can be autoclaved with only small viscosity changes.

Examples of cellulose derivatives include methylcellulose, carmellose sodium (sodium carboxymethylcellulose), hypromellose (hydroxypropylmethylcellulose), hydroxyethylcellulose, and microcrystalline cellulose. Both carmellose sodium and hydroxyethylcellulose are more readily dissolved in water than either methylcellulose or hypromellose. Hydroxyethylcellulose loses viscosity on heating but carmellose sodium solution can be autoclaved with only a small viscosity change. Hypromellose is more commonly used in admixture with other cellulose derivatives. Microcrystalline cellulose is insoluble in water but in aqueous dispersions of high concentration or in commercially available mixtures with carmellose sodium (Avicel^{TM} RC and CL) it forms thixotropic gels. Carmellose sodium is used in concentrations of 1.5% to 5% to form lubricant gels. Medicated gels are prepared using 5% carmellose sodium.

Gelatin. Gelatin dissolves in hot water to form heat-reversible elastic gels at temperatures below 40°. Concentrations of 2% to 15% produce gels suitable for dermatological use. Gelatin gels have adhesive properties but are easily removed from the skin. Aqueous preparations should be sterilised before application to skin surfaces, but gel strength can be considerably reduced by prolonged heating above 80°. A traditional use for gelatin has been to prepare very stiff medicated gels such as Zinc Gelatin BPC 1968.

Pectin. Pectin is a purified carbohydrate with high gelling power, but only in acidic media; it is degraded by alkalis. Pectin gel formulations require the addition of preservatives and possibly a hygroscopic material such as glycerol as they are subject to microbial spoilage and water loss.

Polyvinyl Alcohols. The nonionic polyhydric alcohols, to which the generic term polyvinyl alcohol is applied, are formed from polymerised vinyl acetate. By hydrolysing the polymer under controlled conditions grades are obtained that differ in their properties according to the degree of hydrolysis and the molecular weight. Viscosity is greatest in those grades that display high molecular weight and extensive hydrolysis; from such grades gels are formed at concentrations of 8% to 15% in water. Gel formation is enhanced by the inclusion of low concentrations of borax.

Alginates. Gels can be formed from sodium alginate in cold water by the inclusion of a calcium salt (for example, calcium hydrogen phosphate) together with sodium citrate and adipic acid. In this instance sodium alginate is partly converted to the corresponding calcium salt. A gel can also be produced by the addition of a soluble borate. Calcium content affects the gel structure, which can be either thixotropic or irreversible after shear-thinning. Concentrations of sodium alginate used in gels vary from 1.5% to 2% for lubricants and 5% to 10% for medicated gels depending upon the grade. Propylene glycol alginate is not gelled or precipitated by calcium or other polyvalent metal ions; it is used in concentrations up to 5%.

Starch. A translucent gel can be formed by incorporating starch as an aqueous suspension in heated glycerol, but the product has a relatively short shelf-life.

Carrageenans. The solubility of carrageenans in water varies between grades but in hot water they form transparent elastic gels of low yield value. Viscosity is generally increased in the presence of calcium, potassium, sodium, and ammonium ions. Gels are of pH 7 to 9.5 and are degraded in acidic conditions; preservation is essential. The usual concentration for gels is 1.5% to 2%.

Tragacanth. Tragacanth is a complex polysaccharide of natural origin; it is therefore variable in its rheological properties and its microbiological quality. It must be pre-wetted with ethanol or glycerol before dispersion in water. Yield values and rheological properties of gels are affected by the shear forces applied during processing, and by the presence of citrates or edetates. Tragacanth is used in concentrations from 2% to 3% in lubricants and approximately 5% in medicated gels. An antimicrobial preservative should be included.

Xanthan Gum. Xanthan gum is a mixed salt (sodium, potassium, or calcium) of a partially acetylated polysaccharide of very high molecular weight. Aqueous solutions have enhanced pseudoplastic characteristics and are unaffected by pH changes, heating to 100°, or exposure to enzymes. Gelation occurs in the presence of low concentrations of borate ions but only in the presence of other soluble salts. Commercial products combine xanthan gum with galactomannans such as locust bean gum or guar gum to form heat-reversible gels at concentrations of only 1% total gum. Cationic dyes and preservatives are incompatible with xanthan gum.

Poloxamers. Grades of poloxamers (polyoxyethylene-polyoxypropylene block polymers) such as Pluronic™ F-127 form clear colourless and thermally reversible gels when dissolved in water at concentrations between 20% and 30%. Other grades of poloxamers have been mixed and co-polymerised to form three-dimensional cross-linked hydrogels. Both types of gels have been evaluated for their potential as drug delivery systems.

Other Gelling Agents. Among other gelling agents that have been used commercially are polyoxyethylene oleyl ethers, which form clear gels with liquid paraffin, water, and non-polar solvents.

Agar forms opaque gels and viscous mucilages in water but its main application in pharmaceutical products is as an emulsion stabiliser.

Humectants

Humectants are used to minimise water loss from semi-solid preparations; they prevent drying-out and add to the overall acceptability of products by improving their rubbing qualities and general consistency.

The choice of humectant is based not only on its properties regarding water disposition but also on the effects it may have on the viscosity and consistency of the final product. Compounds that have been utilised as humectants in cream and gel formulations include glycerol, propylene glycol, sorbitol, and the lower molecular weight macrogols.

Insoluble Powders

Insoluble powders may be included in topical formulations: such products are often referred to as pastes. The powders should be uniformly dispersed and should not confer any feeling of grittiness to the preparation. This impalpability is usually achieved by milling the solid dispersant until particles less than 74 micrometres are produced. Some powders, however, tend to aggregate owing to surface electrical charges and are, therefore, difficult to disperse. This is especially true for particles smaller than 5 micrometres.

Many drug substances, for example prednisolone, exist in several polymorphic forms; with regard to percutaneous absorption, each form has a different thermodynamic activity. The choice of crystalline form and the maintenance of that form once incorporated in a topical dosage form are, therefore, of the utmost importance.

Antoxidants

Natural fats and oils and certain emulsifying agents are susceptible to oxidation by atmospheric oxygen; these materials therefore require the addition of one or more antoxidants to prevent decomposition. A full account of antoxidants is given in the Stability of Medicinal Products chapter. The particular antoxidant system should be chosen with regard to such factors as colour, odour, potency, irritancy, toxicity, stability, and compatibility. Edetic acid and certain other organic and inorganic acids (for example, citric, maleic, tartaric, or phosphoric) may also be added to the formulation in order to chelate trace metals that could act as catalysts for the oxidation process.

Microbial Contamination

Semi-solid preparations may become contaminated with micro-organisms from raw materials, particularly natural ingredients like wool fat or water, from carelessly cleaned equipment, or via closures. Microbial contamination can reduce the potency of a preparation, and adversely affect the stability of the formulated product. The presence of pathogenic organisms may also pose a risk of infection, particularly when the product is used on damaged skin. The presence of *Pseudomonas aeruginosa*, for instance, in corticosteroid creams can present a risk to patients because of the reduced resistance to local infection caused by the steroid.

Microbial contamination can be overcome by sterilisation, where appropriate. Bacterial filtration or sterilisation by exposure to dry heat for one hour at a temperature not lower than 150°, for example, can be applied to some anhydrous ointments or their constituents, but these procedures are not usually practicable for polybasic ointments or for those that contain water. For the latter, an aseptic technique is usually required. Although sterilisation may avoid the problems of microbial contamination, pyrogens, which have allergenic potential, may remain in the preparation.

Antimicrobial Preservatives

It is not usual to include antimicrobial preservatives in anhydrous ointments because micro-organisms, while they may survive, rarely proliferate in such systems. However, in polyphasic ointments that contain water, in aqueous gels, and in creams (particularly emulsions of the oil-in-water type) antimicrobial systems should be included to prevent both spoilage and the growth of pathogenic organisms.

It must be remembered that preservatives themselves may provoke a physiological response when applied to the skin; an effective concentration of preservative may, therefore, produce undesirable clinical side-effects and the concentration selected will then be, of necessity, a compromise. This limitation means that less reliance than usual can be placed on preservatives for the prevention of microbial growth in topical semi-solids and consequently there is an even greater need for high standards of cleanliness during the preparation and handling of these products.

A preservative should ideally be non-toxic and non-allergenic, have a bactericidal rather than a bacteriostatic action, and be active against a wide range of micro-organisms. As well as being inexpensive and potent it should also possess a high resistance to attack by micro-organisms, be stable under a wide range of storage conditions, be free from unpleasant odour or strong colour, and be unaffected by other formulation ingredients and packaging materials.

Preservation requires the efficient operation of the antimicrobial agent in the often complex milieu of pharmaceutical ingredients. Plastic containers may sorb preservatives and thereby reduce their effective concentration. Conversely, perfumes and high concentrations of glycerol or electrolytes can reduce the preservative requirements of a preparation by themselves making the semi-solid environment less favourable for microbial growth.

Important factors that can reduce antimicrobial action in polybasic systems are the partitioning of the antimicrobial agent between the oil and water phases, and the inactivation of the antimicrobial agent in the presence of surfactants, especially non-ionic surfactants. In the investigation of formulae it is usual to assess the effectiveness of a system by submitting the preserved product to challenge tests with appropriate pathogenic and spoilage organisms.

The following are the most widely used preservatives in commercial creams, gels, and ointments containing water: chloroform; organic acids, for example, benzoic acid and sorbic acid; chlorocresol; phenethyl alcohol; phenoxyethanol; quaternary ammonium compounds, for example, cetrimide; and organic mercurials such as phenylmercuric nitrate and phenylmercuric acetate.

The hydroxybenzoate esters (methyl, ethyl, propyl, and butyl) are stable, odourless, and virtually non-toxic. However, they have a low aqueous solubility and show weak activity against Gram-negative bacteria; they have also been associated with allergic reactions. Propylene glycol, in sufficient concentration, can also function as a preservative. Benzalkonium chloride and chlorhexidine salts have been used to preserve aqueous gels. Further information can be found in the chapter on Control of Microbial Contamination and the Preservation of Medicines, and also in reviews by Wedderburn[40] and by Parker.[41]

Stability Factors

Major factors that affect the stability of topical semi-solids are temperature, cohesive and gravitational forces, the physical and surface properties of any oily constituents and, if relevant, the relative densities, viscosities, and concentrations of the two phases of an emulsion system. In formulating topical semi-solids, the chemical and physical properties of the active substance must also be considered carefully: for instance, anionic substances are incompatible with cationic emulsifying agents; hydrolysis of an active substance may be enhanced if an aqueous base is used instead of an anhydrous base; and electrolytes can react with emulsifying agents or may induce gel formation.

Garti, Magdassi, and Rubinstein[42] have developed a non-destructive method to determine the stability of oil-in-water creams. This involves measuring conductivity differences in cream formulations after short heating-cooling-heating cycles. The differences in the conductivity measurements after repeated cycles are assumed to reflect the likely stability of the emulsion system during storage.

Formulation Problems

Preparations for Use in Tropical Climates

The high temperatures associated with many areas of the world may necessitate alterations in the formulation of those topical semi-solid preparations designed for use in more temperate climates. For example, the official ointment bases are intended for use at the temperatures usually encountered in the UK and it may be necessary to increase the proportions of higher melting point ingredients such as hard paraffin or beeswax in order to produce a preparation of suitable consistency for use in tropical climates. General permission for such adjustment is given in the *British Pharmacopoeia* provided that the amount of active ingredient is unchanged.

Skin Sensitisers

Possible skin sensitisers present in topical corticosteroid formulations include butylated hydroxyanisole, chlorocresol, ethylenediamine, the hydroxybenzoates, hydrous wool fat (lanolin) and its derivatives, propylene glycol, sorbic acid, and various fragrances.

Formulation of Steroid Preparations

Corticosteroids such as fluocinolone acetonide pose interesting formulation problems in that, although they are absorbed more readily through hydrated skin, they are insoluble in emollient bases such as soft paraffin. However, steroids can be presented to the skin in hydrocarbon bases, either as well-dispersed microfine powders or as more complex systems in which the drug is dissolved using a suitable solvent. The latter method is usually chosen, as greater penetration levels are achieved if the steroid is molecularly dispersed, and dissolution eliminates the problems involved in using microfine powders.

Usually in steroid preparations, the drug is dissolved in an organic solvent that is itself immiscible with soft paraffin; this solvent should ideally be non-volatile and required only in small volumes to dissolve the drug. Propylene glycol is the most widely used solvent for this purpose. It is dispersed in the hydrophobic phase, usually with the aid of wool fat or hydrogenated lanolin. Maximum release of the steroid is obtained when the quantity of propylene glycol used is the minimum needed to dissolve the steroid: release rates from the vehicle are dramatically reduced when greater amounts of the solvent are used.

The increased penetration of corticosteroid observed with these systems may be caused by the propylene glycol acting as an efficient reservoir for the release of the dissolved drug. An alternative mechanism, whereby the propylene glycol penetrates the skin and carries the steroid with it, has also been proposed. Similar improvements in the absorption of topically applied corticosteroids were noted for an anhydrous fatty alcohol-propylene glycol (FAPG) cream base. This vehicle was developed by Syntex, and although it bears a physical resemblance to a gel, it is more like a cream in overall appearance and consistency: it does not dry out, or oxidise at room temperature, and is resistant to spoilage. FAPG base contains stearyl alcohol, a macrogol, and glycerol; propylene glycol again dissolves the drug and ensures an even dispersion. A further advantage of propylene glycol systems is that the drug solution can be sterilised by filtration.

PREPARATION

Preparation of Ointments

The method selected for the preparation of ointments usually depends on the properties of the medicament, the type of basis, and the quantity of ointment required. For small quantities of a relatively soft ointment, trituration on a slab with a spatula of flexible metal or plastic is one of the easiest methods for the mixing and incorporation of liquids or solids. Steel spatulas are suitable for most substances but should not be used for preparing ointments that contain mercuric salts, tannic acid, salicylic acid, or iodine.

Before incorporation, insoluble powders must be finely powdered and levigated, either with some of the melted basis or with a suitable liquid. Wool fat, glycerol, and polyoxyl 8 stearate are good levigating agents and are sometimes included in the basis in order to obtain a smoother product. Water-soluble salts should be dissolved in the minimum amount of water and incorporated with the aid of a small amount of lanolin. A mortar and pestle is more convenient when liquids are to be incorporated or for the preparation of larger amounts of ointment.

Fusion is the method usually adopted for large-scale manufacture or for ointments in which waxes or solids of high melting point are to be mixed with semi-solids or oils; it is also used when large volumes of water are to be incorporated. Constituents are melted successively in decreasing order of melting point and the fluid mixture stirred until cooled, avoiding aeration. If not stirred effectively, fatty alcohols and acids may crystallise

from systems that contain paraffins. Volatile medicaments are usually added when the ointment has cooled to below 40°. Insoluble powders in the form of a levigated dispersion are often incorporated when the ointment begins to thicken. Soluble solids that are heat-stable can be dissolved in the melted basis before it congeals. For quantities of less than 500 g, further treatment of the ointment to improve homogeneity may not be feasible, but for larger amounts, roller mills or colloid mills aid the uniform distribution of insoluble solids and the elimination of particles larger than about 50 micrometres.

Preparation of Semi-solid Emulsions

Emulsified creams that contain waxes or fatty solids are prepared by heating to 70° to 75° the oil-soluble or oil-miscible constituents, together with the emulsifying agent, if it is oil soluble. Water-soluble or water-miscible constituents, dissolved in or incorporated with the aqueous phase, are heated to a similar temperature and the two phases are mixed. If the dispersed phase occupies only a small volume, it is usual to add this to the continuous phase, otherwise the order of mixing is of little importance. The important factors are that the two phases should be at similar temperatures and addition should be steady, without splashing or vortexing, in order to avoid the entrapment of air. Subsequent cooling should be slow, with stirring that is adequate to ensure homogeneity yet minimise aeration. Sudden cooling or excessive aeration can lead to a granular product. After cooling to 30° to 40°, the cream can usually be homogenised.

All apparatus used in preparation and the final containers should be thoroughly cleaned before use and rinsed with freshly boiled and cooled purified water before drying.

Hygiene during Preparation

For small-scale dispensing, a number of procedures should be adopted: freshly boiled and cooled purified water should be used where applicable; work surfaces should be scrupulously cleaned; clean overgarments should be worn; operators' hands should be scrubbed; and at all stages during the manufacturing process the highest standards of hygiene should be adopted.

Preparation from Another Dosage Form

When topical administration is required and the pure drug substance cannot be obtained, a pharmacist may have to resort to another dosage form to obtain a source of the active material: injectable solutions, powders for injection, suspensions, and tablets have been used for this purpose. Vehicles have to be chosen that allow incorporation of not only the drug substance but also any excipients. Aqueous solutions, for example, have to be compounded with vehicles that allow the incorporation of water. If tablets are to be used, they should be crushed and powdered before being incorporated in the chosen vehicle. In some cases, the tablet coating materials may need to be dissolved or broken down before the tablet can be incorporated into the vehicle. The biopharmaceutics of such preparations, and the levels of percutaneous absorption achieved, will be largely unknown.

Dilution of Preparations

If a topical semi-solid preparation is prescribed with a content of active substance that is less than that available from a manufacturer, the manufacturer's product may be diluted with a suitable diluent. Suitable diluents are specified in official monographs. Particular care should be taken in the dilution of steroid preparations, which are normally manufactured under sterile or 'near sterile' conditions. Further information on their dilution can be found in articles by Tanner and Woodford,[43] Smith,[44] Wilcock,[45] and Deeks.[46] The dilution of anhydrous ointments may present a lesser problem than the dilution of creams since the former do not promote the growth of micro-organisms.

Dilution of Creams

Any creams used as diluents and the dilutions themselves should be prepared under hygienic conditions, and the stability and the bactericidal properties of the original cream should not be reduced on dilution.

The use of an unsuitable diluent may yield a product of limited bactericidal efficiency because the diluent either does not contain a preservative or contains one that is inactive or incompatible on admixture. A diluent that differs in pH from the original cream may promote chemical breakdown or inactivation of the active substance. Physical breakdown may occur when a system formed by an anionic emulsifier is mixed with a cationic-based emulsion or with a system that contains cationic active substances. The extent of release or the release rate of an active substance from a cream could be altered by admixture with a diluent of a different emulsion type or with a diluent that

changed the physical form or the complexation behaviour of the active substance. It is inadvisable, therefore, to make dilutions in the absence of information on the suitability of the diluent.

Diluted creams must be freshly prepared without the application of heat; they are usually given an expiry period of two weeks from the date of issue.

Dilution of Ointments

For certain specific ointments, when the strength prescribed is not available from a manufacturer, a stronger ointment should be diluted to the required strength with the recommended diluent. When the specified diluent is soft paraffin, a portion of it may be replaced by hard paraffin or liquid paraffin to obtain an ointment of suitable consistency.

Industrial Processing

The manufacture of topical semi-solid preparations on an industrial scale involves the same procedures as those described for small-scale dispensing. However, unseen problems can arise when batch sizes are increased. The subject has been reviewed by Idson and Lazarus.[47]

Some indication of the parameters governing large-scale production can be gained from small-scale trials using equipment similar to full size plant. However, after scaling-up it will be necessary to adjust the timing, temperature, and degree of agitation of the different processes. The speed of mixing may need to be altered to avoid problems caused by air entrapment as a result of too rapid mixing or poor emulsion formation resulting from inadequate mixing.

Analytical Methods

Van der Vaart et al[48,49] developed a thin layer chromatographic technique to separate and identify excipients commonly used in creams. Lake et al[50] used high performance liquid chromatography, without prior sample clean-up, to quantify the active components of oil-in-water emulsions.

CONTAINERS AND STORAGE

Topical semi-solid preparations should be supplied in well-closed containers that prevent evaporation and contamination of the contents. The materials of construction should be resistant to sorption or diffusion of the contents. Plastic containers may be unsuitable for preparations that contain methyl salicylate, phthalate esters, or similar substances. Collapsible tubes of metal, conforming to British Standard 4230:1967(1986), or flexible plastic tubes may be used. The internal surface of metal tubes may be coated with a lacquer of a heat-cured epoxy resin. Collapsible tubes may also be lined near the base with a suitable pressure-sensitive sealing coat.

Uncoated aluminium tubes may be treated with a phosphate buffer such as that provided by a mixture of 0.1% of disodium hydrogen phosphate (anhydrous) and 0.2% of sodium dihydrogen phosphate (dihydrate), if this is specified in the compendial entry describing the cream. The buffer is intended to inhibit corrosion of the aluminium and to reduce the possibility of hydrogen formation. Aluminium tubes are not suitable for creams preserved with organic mercury compounds unless adequately protected by a suitable internal lacquer. Topical semi-solids may also be supplied in wide-mouthed glass or plastic jars fitted with plastic screw caps with impermeable liners or with close-fitting slip-on lids. Collapsible tubes reduce the risk of bacterial contamination during use and should be used in preference to wide-mouthed jars. Creams should preferably be stored in a cool place.

LABELLING

The container should be labelled 'for external use only' with the strength of the active ingredient given as a percentage, by weight or by volume. The label on the container of a diluted product should also state that the contents should not be used later than two weeks after issue, unless otherwise stated. If a preservative is included, the name and concentration should appear on the label.

REFERENCES

1. Kligman AM. Drug Dev Ind Pharm 1983;9:521–60.
2. Guy RH, Maibach HI. J Pharm Sci 1983;72:1375–80.
3. Vickers CFH. Arch Dermatol 1963;88:20.
4. Malkinson FD, Ferguson EH. J Invest Dermatol 1955;25:281.
5. Guillot M. J Physiol 1954;46:31.
6. Bronaugh RL, Stewart RF. J Pharm Sci 1985;74:1062–6.
7. Behl CR, Mann KV, Bellantone NH. APhA Abstracts 1984;14(1):58(Abstract No.32).
8. Bucks DAW, Maibach HI, Guy RH. J Pharm Sci 1985;74:1337–9.
9. Bodor N, Zupan J, Selk S. Int J Pharmaceutics 1980;7:63–75.
10. Lippold BC, Schneemann H. Int J Pharmaceutics 1984;22:31–43.
11. Dugard PH, Scott RC. Int J Pharmaceutics 1986;28:219–27.
12. DiColo G, Carelli V, Giannaccini B, Serafini MF, Bottari F. J Pharm Sci 1980;69:387–91.
13. Swarbrick J, Lee G, Brom J, Gensmantel NP. J Pharm Sci 1984;73:1352–4.
14. Umer S. Acta Pol Pharm 1985;42:172.
15. Okamoto H, Komatsu H, Hashida M, Sezaki H. Int J Pharmaceutics 1986;30:35–45.
16. Ashton P, Hadgraft J, Walters KA. Pharm Acta Helv 1986;61:228.
17. Hadgraft J. Int J Pharmaceutics 1983;16:255–70.
18. Guy RH, Wester RC, Tur E, Maibach HI. J Pharm Sci 1983;72:1077–9.
19. Behme RJ, Kensler TT, Brooke D. J Pharm Sci 1982;71:1303–5.
20. Bialik W. Acta Pol Pharm 1985;42:74.
21. Lehky M, Stravratjev M, Szucsova S, Stubna J. Farm Obz 1982;51:13.
22. Tanaka S, Takashima Y, Murayama H, Tsuchiya S. Int J Pharmaceutics 1985;27:29–38.
23. Guy RH, Hadgraft J. Maibach HI. Int J Pharmaceutics 1982;11:119–29.
24. Guy RH, Hadgraft J. Int J Pharmaceutics 1984;20:43–51.
25. Guy RH, Hadgraft J. J Soc Cosmet Chem 1984;35:103.
26. Guy RH, Hadgraft J. Int J Pharmaceutics 1986;32:159–63.
27. Whitworth CW, Stephenson RE. Can J Pharm Sci 1975;10:89.
28. Southwell D, Barry BW. Int J Pharmaceutics 1984;22:291–8.
29. Wotton PK, Møllgaard B, Hadgraft J, Hoelgaard A. Int J Pharmaceutics 1985;24:19–26.
30. Wiechers JW, de Zeeuw RA, Drenth BFH, Jonkman JHG. Pharm Weekbl (Sci) 1986;8:329.
31. Sarpotdar PP, Zatz JL. Drug Dev Ind Pharm 1986;12:1625–47.
32. Barker N, Hadgraft J. Int J Pharmaceutics 1981;8:193-202.
33. Eccleston GM. Pharm Int 1986;7:63–70.
34. Junginger HE. Pharm Weekbl (Sci) 1984;6:141–9.
35. Rowe RC, Bray D. J Pharm Pharmacol 1987;39:642–3.
36. Rowe RC, McMahon J. Int Pharm J 1987;1:91–3.
37. Rowe RC, Patel HK. J Pharm Pharmacol 1985;37:222–5.
38. Radebaugh GW, Simonelli AP. J Pharm Sci 1984;73:590–4.
39. Chester J, Dixon M. Mfg Chem 1986;57:59.
40. Wedderburn DL. Preservation of emulsions against microbial attack. In: Bean HS, Beckett AH, Carless JE, editors. Advances in pharmaceutical sciences; vol 1. London: Academic Press, 1964:195.
41. Parker MS. J Appl Bact 1978;44:SXXIX.
42. Garti N, Magdassi S, Rubinstein A. Drug Dev Ind Pharm 1982;8:475–85.
43. Tanner AC, Woodford R. Br J Pharm Pract 1981;3(3):29–34.
44. Smith JF. J Clin Hosp Pharm 1982;7:137–40.
45. Wilcock M. Pharm J 1985;234:170–1.
46. Deeks T. Br J Pharm Pract 1985;7(6):134–40.
47. Idson B, Lazarus J. Semi-solids. In: Lachman L, Lieberman HA, Kanig JL, editors. The theory and practice of industrial pharmacy. 3rd ed. Philadelphia: Lea and Febiger, 1986:554.
48. Van der Vaart FJ, Hulshoff A, Indemans AWM. Pharm Weekbl (Sci) 1983;5:109–13.
49. Van der Vaart FJ, Hulshoff A, Indemans AWM. Pharm Weekbl (Sci) 1983;5:113–19.
50. Lake OA, Hulshoff A, Van der Vaart JF, Indemans AWM. Pharm Weekbl (Sci) 1983;5:15–21.

Topical Liquids and Powders

This chapter includes discussions on various dosage forms intended for application to the skin and for use in the ears, nose, and oral cavity. A detailed treatment of skin physiology and the mechanisms of percutaneous absorption can be found in the Topical Semi-solids chapter.

Topical liquid formulations may be formulated as solutions, suspensions, or emulsions in either aqueous or non-aqueous vehicles. The physicochemical properties of these dosage forms and the general principles of formulation and preparation are discussed in the chapters entitled Solution Properties, Suspensions, and Emulsions, respectively. Topical liquid preparations may contain various excipients including emulsifying and suspending agents, tonicity and viscosity adjusting agents, stabilisers, buffers, and solubilising agents. The choice of excipient will be influenced by the integrity of the skin surface.

Precautions must be taken to avoid the proliferation of micro-organisms in topical liquid preparations. Preservatives have two functions: to reduce the bioburden in the dispensed product and to prevent growth of micro-organisms introduced during the period of product use. Solutions of some antiseptics have been shown to support the growth of certain organisms including *Pseudomonas* species. Further information on microbial contamination is given in the Control of Microbial Contamination and the Preservation of Medicines chapter. The particular problems of preservation of topical preparations are examined in more detail in the Topical Semi-solids chapter.

The traditional classification of the various types of preparation has been retained, although it is appreciated that in several instances the distinctions are not clear. In particular, applications, liniments, and lotions have similar characteristics and a particular preparation may be known by more than one title.

LIQUID PREPARATIONS

Lotions and Applications

Lotions are liquid or semi-liquid solutions, suspensions, or emulsions intended for application, without friction, to unbroken skin. They contain one or more active ingredients in suitable vehicles and are used for the treatment of skin diseases, or as antiseptics, antipruritics, astringents, or protectives.

Applications have similar physicochemical properties, but have traditionally been used to administer antiparasitic medications.

Many lotions are simple solutions, but others (for example, shake lotions) contain insoluble powders such as calamine, sulphur, or zinc oxide. The advantage of a lotion formulation is that it leaves a thin coating of medicament on the skin surface after solvent evaporation. Evaporation can also lead to cooling of the skin, which may ease inflammation. The inclusion of ethanol in a lotion accentuates this cooling effect; conversely, the inclusion of glycerol keeps the skin moist for a considerable time. The contact time between an applied medicament and the skin surface can be prolonged by the inclusion of a semi-synthetic polysaccharide, such as carmellose sodium or methylcellulose. Bentonite and carmellose sodium are commonly used to suspend insoluble substances like calamine; the addition of a surfactant such as sodium lauryl sulphate promotes the dispersion of substances such as sulphur, which are not readily wetted. More detailed information on the formulation of suspensions can be found in the Suspensions chapter.

OFFICIAL EXAMPLES:
Aminobenzoic Acid Lotion BP
Benzyl Benzoate Application BP
Calamine Lotion BP
Lindane Application BP
Salicylic Acid Lotion BP
Sulphur Lotion, Compound, BPC
Zinc Sulphate Lotion BP

Liniments

Liniments are liquid or semi-liquid preparations intended to be applied, with friction, to unbroken skin. They may contain one or more active ingredients with local analgesic, rubefacient, soothing, or stimulant properties. The vehicle may be alcohol, oil, or soap based.

OFFICIAL EXAMPLES:
Turpentine Liniment BP
White Liniment BP

Topical Solutions

Topical solutions are liquid preparations containing one or more soluble ingredients usually dissolved in water. They are intended for external use or for instillation into body cavities. Some solutions are simply applied to the skin, but many are used in large volumes as irrigations. The solute is usually non-volatile although **aromatic waters**, such as hamamelis water, have been used externally.

Topical solutions may be issued either sterile or unsterilised, depending on the purpose for which they are intended. Solutions for application to broken skin, eyes, or body cavities should be sterilised.

OFFICIAL EXAMPLES:
  Chloroxylenol Solution BP
  Alcoholic Iodine Solution BP
  Coal Tar Solution BP

Solution-tablets are compact products containing one or more active ingredients in compressed form and are intended, after being dissolved in water, to be used externally or on mucous surfaces. Solution-tablets may be prepared by the methods described in the Oral Solids chapter, but any lubricant or diluent used should be readily soluble in water. Sodium chloride is normally used as a diluent, but such preparations become less readily soluble on storage. Solution-tablets should be completely soluble in water.

Collodions

Collodions are liquid preparations usually consisting of a solution of pyroxylin (a nitrocellulose) in a mixture of organic solvents, usually ether and ethanol. They are intended for local external application and are applied by painting onto the skin and allowing to dry; a flexible film forms when the solvent evaporates. Flexibility is conferred by the inclusion of castor oil in the formulation. Suitable drugs, such as salicylic acid, can be dissolved in the base to form medicated collodions. Collodions may be used to seal off minor cuts and wounds or as a means of holding a dissolved medicament in contact with the skin for long periods. Care must be used in handling and applying collodions as they are inflammable.

OFFICIAL EXAMPLES:
  Flexible Collodion BP
  Salicylic Acid Collodion BP

Paints

Paints are solutions or dispersions of one or more active ingredients intended for application with a brush to the skin or mucous membranes. They are usually medicated with substances possessing antiseptic, astringent, caustic, or local analgesic properties. Paints containing crystal violet are no longer recommended for application to broken skin or mucous membranes because of concern at possible *animal* toxicity.

Often the vehicle is volatile, for example, ethanol, so that evaporation is rapid and a film of drug is left on the skin surface. **Throat paints** and other paints for application to mucous surfaces are usually formulated in a liquid of high viscosity such as glycerol to hold the drug at the site of application.

OFFICIAL EXAMPLE:
  Compound Podophyllin Paint BP

Glycerins, Spirits, and Tinctures

Glycerins, spirits, and tinctures may be used directly, or as ingredients in other preparations. Glycerins are liquid preparations containing medicinal substances in glycerol, with or without the addition of water.

Spirits are solutions of one or more substances in ethanol. They may contain a proportion of water.

OFFICIAL EXAMPLES:
  Soap Spirit BP
  Surgical Spirit BP

Tinctures are alcoholic liquids that usually contain, in low concentration, the active principles of crude drugs. They are generally prepared by maceration or percolation or obtained by dilution of the corresponding liquid or soft extract.

OFFICIAL EXAMPLE:
  Compound Benzoin Tincture BP

Gargles and Mouthwashes

Gargles are aqueous solutions, usually in concentrated form, intended for use, after dilution with warm water, in the prophylaxis or treatment of throat infections. Antiseptics are often included in formulations but the concentrations normally employed are insufficient to give a useful antibacterial effect. A quantity of the gargle is taken and suspended in the throat by slowly exhaling through it. The liquid is then rejected, unless the patient has been directed to swallow it after gargling. The process of gargling is intended to bring the liquid into intimate contact with the membranous lining of the throat. A gargle is not intended to act as a protective covering to the membrane, and therefore oily substances that require a suspending agent and drugs of a mucilaginous nature should not be used.

Mouthwashes are aqueous solutions, in concentrated form, of one or more active ingredients with deodorant, antiseptic, local analgesic, or astringent properties. They are similar preparations to gargles but are used on the mucous membranes of the oral cavity rather than in the throat. Mouthwashes are usually diluted with warm water before use. Many mouthwashes are also used as gargles. However, gargles tend to contain higher concentrations of active ingredients. **Throat sprays** are intended for local effect.

OFFICIAL EXAMPLES:
   Phenol Gargle BPC
   Compound Sodium Chloride Mouthwash BP

Ear Drops

Ear drops are solutions, suspensions, or emulsions of one or more active ingredients in water, diluted ethanol, glycerol, propylene glycol, or other suitable vehicle. They are intended for instillation into the ear. Ear drops presented in multidose containers must also contain appropriate concentrations of suitable antimicrobial preservatives, unless the product itself possesses sufficient antimicrobial activity.

OFFICIAL EXAMPLES:
   Aluminium Acetate Ear Drops BP
   Sodium Bicarbonate Ear Drops BP

Nasal Preparations

Nasal drops are liquid preparations for instillation into the nostrils by means of a dropper. They are usually aqueous solutions containing substances with antiseptic, local analgesic, or vasoconstrictor properties. Liquid medications are also applied to the nasal mucosa in the form of sprays and aerosols.

Nasal drops should be non-irritating and should not interfere with ciliary transport. Oily vehicles and several preservatives have been found to stop cilial movement. Chlorhexidine gluconate and thiomersal appear to have little effect on ciliary activity. In order to prevent deleterious effects on cilial action, the viscosity, tonicity, and pH of nasal drops should be as near as possible to those of natural secretions; adjustment may be made by the addition of hypromellose, sodium chloride, and buffers.

OFFICIAL EXAMPLE:
   Ephedrine Nasal Drops BP

Intranasal solutions are solutions of active ingredients intended for systemic effect. They may contain suitable buffering agents and preservatives. The nasal mucosa may be suitable for the administration of drugs that, after oral administration, either undergo hydrolysis in the gastro-intestinal tract or are susceptible to first-pass metabolism in the liver.

DUSTING POWDERS

Dusting powders contain one or more substances in fine powder. They are intended to be applied externally in the prophylaxis or treatment of skin disorders or for lubricant purposes. They should be free from grittiness. Dusting powders may be presented as single-dose or multidose preparations. When presented in pressurised containers, dusting powders may contain suitable excipients such as propellants; lubricating agents may also be used to prevent valve clogging. Propellants used are either liquefied gases under pressure or compressed gases. Suitable liquefied gases are, for example, halogenated hydrocarbons (especially chlorofluoromethanes and chlorofluoroethanes). A suitable compressed gas is, for example, carbon dioxide. Mixtures of these propellants may be used to obtain optimal solution properties and desirable pressure, delivery, and spray characteristics.

Dusting powders should be sterile when intended for application to large open wounds or to severely injured skin. They should not be used on areas that exude large volumes of fluid as hard crusts may form. Materials such as zinc oxide and starch are included in dusting-powder formulations to absorb moisture; talc is used for its lubricant properties. Talc, kaolin, and other natural mineral ingredients are liable to be heavily contaminated with bacteria, including *Clostridium tetani*, *Cl. perfringens (Cl. welchii)*, and *Bacillus anthracis*. Such ingredients should be sterilised by dry heat. This procedure is not necessary when the final product is subjected to a sterilisation process.

OFFICIAL EXAMPLES:
   Chlorhexidine Dusting Powder BP 1988
   Talc Dusting Powder BP

FURTHER INFORMATION

Batts AH, Marriott C, Martin GP, Bond SW. Influence of preservatives on ciliary movement. J Pharm Pharmacol 1987;39(Suppl):92P.

Duchateau GSMJE, Zuidema J, Albers WM, Merkus FWHM. Nasal absorption of alprenolol and metoprolol. Int J Pharmaceutics 1986;34:131–6.

Duchateau GSMJE, Zuidema J, Basseleur SWJ. Influence of some surface active agents on nasal absorption in *rabbits*. Int J Pharmaceutics 1987;39:87–92.

Duchateau GSMJE, Zuidema J, Merkus FWHM. Bile salts and intranasal drug absorption. Int J Pharmaceutics 1986;31:193–9.

Fisher AN, Brown K, Davis SS, Parr GD, Smith DA. The effect of molecular size on the nasal absorption of water-soluble compounds in the albino *rat*. J Pharm Pharmacol 1987;39:357–62.

Hardy JG, Lee SW, Wilson CG. Intranasal drug delivery by sprays and drops. J Pharm Pharmacol 1985;37:294–7.

Harris AS, Hedner P, Vilhardt H. Nasal desmopressin by sprays and drops. J Pharm Pharmacol 1987;39:932–4.

Harris AS, Nilsson IM, Wagner ZG, Alkner U. Intranasal administration of peptides: nasal deposition, biological response and absorption of desmopressin. J Pharm Sci 1986;75:1085–8.

Harris AS, Ohlin M, Svensson E, Lethagen S, Nilsson IM. Effect of viscosity on the pharmacokinetics and biological response to intranasal desmopressin. J Pharm Sci 1989;78:470–1.

Parr GD. Nasal delivery of drugs. Pharm Int 1983;4:202–5.

Su KSE. Intranasal delivery of peptides and proteins. Pharm Int 1986;7:8–11.

Van de Donk. Nasal medication and ciliary movement. Pharm Weekbl (Sci) 1983;5:32–3.

Visor GC, Schuessler B, Thompson J, Ling T. Nasal absorption of the calcium antagonist nicardipine in rats and rhesus monkeys. Drug Dev Ind Pharm 1987;13:1329–43.

Ophthalmic Products

Medicinal ophthalmic products are preparations designed for application to the eye either for the treatment of disease, for the relief of symptoms, for diagnostic purposes, or as adjuncts to surgical procedures.

Ophthalmic preparations may be categorised into a number of groups:

- liquid preparations for application to the surface of the eye (for example, eye drops and eye lotions)
- semi-solid dosage forms (for example, ointments, creams, and gels) for application to the margin of the eyelid or for introduction into the conjunctival sac
- solid dosage forms intended to be placed in contact with the surface of the eye to produce modified release of medication
- devices for surgical implantation within the eye to give modified release of medicament over a prolonged period
- parenteral products for subconjunctival or intraocular (intracorneal, intravitreous, or retrobulbar) injection
- liquid products for irrigation of the eye during surgical procedures.

Most liquid ophthalmic products are prepared using aqueous vehicles, whereas semi-solid dosage forms may be based on paraffins, water, or water-in-oil emulsions. Solid modified-release products either have the drug enclosed within a diffusion membrane, or are hydrophilic gels or matrices from which the active ingredient is slowly released. All ophthalmic products are required to be sterile and free from extraneous particulate matter. They should not contain non-essential ancillary ingredients.

Liquid and semi-solid preparations may be presented as either single-use or multi-use products and, in common with parenteral dosage forms, the multidose preparations are required to contain appropriate antimicrobial agents to combat in-use contamination.

DRUGS USED IN OPHTHALMIC PRODUCTS

Drugs used in the eye may be categorised as follows: miotics, mydriatics, cycloplegics, anti-inflammatory agents, anti-infective agents, antiglaucoma drugs, diagnostic agents, and surgical adjuvants such as local anaesthetics.

The medicaments contained in products intended for administration to the surface of the eye may be required either to act at that surface or to penetrate through the surface structures to act within the interior of the eyeball.

Some ophthalmic products contain no pharmacologically active ingredients; examples are lotions used for washing contaminated eyes or artificial tears for the treatment of dry eye conditions.

ANATOMY OF THE EYE

The outermost layer of the globe of the eye or eyeball is a tough pliable but non-stretchable structure that is maintained in its shape by the internal pressure exerted by the **aqueous** and **vitreous humours**. The front facing part of the boundary layer is clear and colourless and is called the **cornea**. The cornea contains no blood vessels but is richly supplied with nerve endings. The other part of the boundary layer of the eye is the **sclera** which is opaque and white in colour and contains most of the blood vessels that nourish the anterior tissues of the eyeball. The outer surface of the sclera is loosely covered by the **conjunctival membrane** which is continuous with the lining of the inner surface of the eyelids. The conjunctival and corneal surfaces are continually lubricated by a film of fluid secreted by the conjunctival and lachrymal glands. The lachrymal glands secrete tears, a clear watery fluid containing mineral salts, glucose, other low molecular weight organic compounds, and protein.

Sebaceous glands on the margins of the eyelids secrete an oily fluid which spreads over the tear film, reducing the rate of evaporation from the exposed surfaces of the eye.

The tear film in the eye is constantly being replenished; this process is assisted by blinking which spreads the film evenly over the surface of the eye and sweeps any excess fluid into the triangular lachrymal lake which lies at the angle of the inner junction of the eyelids. Excess tears are drained from the lachrymal lake into the lachrymal sac which is activated as a pump, by blinking, to drain the tears via the nasolachrymal duct into the nose and ultimately down the back of the throat into the gastro-intestinal tract.

The film of fluid covering the eye maintains the optical efficiency of the cornea which must remain moist in order to function correctly. The composition of this precorneal film is complex and comprises a three-layered structure: a lipid outer layer, a watery middle layer, and a mucoid inner layer that is in contact with the corneal epithelium.

DRUG PENETRATION INTO THE EYE

One of the main problems associated with the treatment of ocular disease is the difficulty in achieving a sufficient concentration of the drug at the required site of action. When medicated ophthalmic preparations are administered systemically, the lack of vascularity in the cornea and the chambers of the eye, together with the relatively non-permeable nature of the capillaries in the retina and iris, limits diffusion of drug from the blood into the aqueous and vitreous humours. It is therefore necessary to consider alternative, non-systemic means of delivering drugs to ocular targets.

For the treatment of superficial eye diseases, such as conjunctivitis, topical application is clearly the appropriate route of administration, but when the intended site of action is within the globe of the eye, the ocular barrier presents penetration problems for topically applied preparations. When topically applied products come into contact with the surface of the eye they first encounter the cornea and the conjunctiva; these surfaces represent the primary barriers to drug penetration.

For the purposes of drug penetration the cornea can be considered to consist of three layers: the **external epithelium**, the **stroma**, and the **internal endothelium**. Both the epithelium and the endothelium are lipid-rich layers and represent significant barriers to water-soluble compounds whilst allowing the relatively easy passage of lipid-soluble compounds. The stroma, however, is an aqueous barrier which is permeable to water-soluble compounds but not to lipid-soluble compounds. This combination of lipid and aqueous barriers dictates that ionisable drugs are most suited to penetration across the cornea; solutions of these drugs contain water-soluble ions in equilibrium with lipid-soluble free bases or acids. Ideally, such drugs should have pK_a values close to physiological pH so that solutions at the pH of tears will contain equal fractions of the ionised and unionised species. In practice, compounds with a wide range of pK_a values are usually acceptable.

The sclera is a relatively porous structure but the overlying conjunctiva presents a significant permeability barrier to most drugs. In addition, the vascular systems of the conjunctiva and sclera tend to transport the penetrating drug away from the eye into the general circulation. It is generally considered, therefore, that the cornea is a more favourable route than the conjunctiva for the penetration of topically applied drugs into the interior of the eye. However, this is a somewhat simplistic view and conjunctival penetration followed by vascular transport may be a significant route for the administration of drugs reaching the iris.[1]

FORMULATION OF OPHTHALMIC PRODUCTS

Eye Drops

The *British Pharmacopoeia* defines eye drops as 'sterile aqueous or oily solutions or suspensions of one or more active ingredients intended for instillation into the eye'. Most therapeutic agents used in eye products are water-soluble compounds or can be formulated as water-soluble salts and most eye drops consist essentially of aqueous solutions, although some are suspensions of poorly soluble drugs or oily solutions. In comparison with multi-phase systems, solutions produce potentially more favourable uniformity of dosage, better bioavailability, and greater ease of handling of the product during the final stages of commercial production.

The main physicochemical considerations associated with the selection of salts for formulation as ophthalmic solutions are: solubility, stability, the required pH and buffering capacity of solutions, and compatibility with other ingredients in the formulation.

Most drugs used for ophthalmic preparations are weak bases and the salts most commonly employed are hydrochlorides, sulphates, and nitrates, although acetates, phosphates, hydrobromides, and others are also used. In the case of acidic drugs, the use of the sodium salt is most common. The solubility of a few drugs administered as eye drops is too low to allow their formulation as solutions; in these cases aqueous or oily suspensions can be used. The solid particles must be very finely divided to prevent irritation of the cornea; there are pharmacopoeial limits for the number of particles greater than the stated size permitted in ophthalmic products.

Drop Size and Dosage

Eye drops are unlike most liquid dosage forms in that there is a considerable degree of imprecision associated with the dose administered. The volume delivered as a single drop by most commercial eye droppers is of the order of 50 microlitres but patients often instil more than one drop, either inadvertently or because of uncertainty as to whether the first drop entered the eye. Occasionally, drops may only partially enter the eye or they may even miss it completely.

The mean volume of tears in the human eye under normal conditions is about 7 microlitres, whereas the maximum volume that can be held in the cul-de-sac without spillage is about 30 microlitres. The potential drainage rate from the eye is normally far greater than the lachrymation rate and it can therefore usually cope with the increase in tear volume above 30 microlitres that normally follows instillation of a single eye drop dose. Blinking rapidly reduces the tear volume to the normal value of about 7 microlitres. Because of this drainage effect a drop size greater than 25 microlitres or multiple-drop application has little effect on the amount of drug left in the tear film within seconds of administration. Although the drainage of excessively large doses of eye drops into the nasal cavity and ultimately into the gastro-intestinal tract prevents local overdosage in the eye, it can result in significant systemic absorption of drugs, which may be undesirable. For example, the use of eye drops containing beta-blocking agents for the treatment of glaucoma can cause problems in patients with heart disease or with bronchial asthma.

Studies of the effect of drop size on the ocular bioavailability of drugs have indicated that a decrease in drop size to below 20 microlitres decreases the drainage rate and thus increases residence time and bioavailability.[2]

Mitra[3] applied an interesting mathematical treatment to the analysis of the effect of drop size on ocular bioavailability.

In theory, a high concentration of a therapeutic agent in a small drop volume would appear to be the ideal objective in eye drop formulation; however, in practice, patients have difficulty in detecting the entry of very small drops into the eye, and the design of serviceable and safe droppers that will deliver volumes as small as 5 or 10 microlitres presents problems.

Following instillation of even a small drop into the eye, normal lachrymation will immediately begin to dilute and wash away the therapeutic agent and the normal tear production rate can easily result in a 20% decrease in drug concentration per minute. In practice, even the most favourably formulated

eye drops are likely to cause an increase in lachrymation rate with a resultant increase in the rate of removal. It has been suggested that as little as 1% of a dose of drug applied as eye drops typically penetrates into the aqueous humour.[4]

As increasing the volume of eye drops administered has minimal effect on the actual amount of drug penetrating the cornea, consideration must be given to alternative methods of increasing the dose of drug reaching the target site. The simplest technique is to increase the concentration of drug in each drop; this may be successful to some extent because corneal penetration increases, within limits, with increasing concentration. However, increasing the concentration of a drug in eye drops is not always an available option: the drug may have limited solubility, and even if it is sufficiently soluble the higher concentrations used may result in unacceptable systemic activity following drainage of any excess drop volume.

An alternative approach is to attempt to improve the ocular bioavailability from eye drops by increasing the residence time of the product in the eye. Several methods have been used to achieve this whilst retaining the traditional drop as the dosage form. The most common method used has been to increase the viscosity of the drops. Other methods include the formulation of suspensions of relatively insoluble drugs or of drug/carrier particles.

Viscosity-increasing Agents

Studies of the effects of adding viscosity-increasing substances to eye drops have produced some conflicting results, although it is generally agreed that an increase in viscosity increases residence time in the eye. The main areas of controversy are whether there is an upper limit to this effect and whether increased residence time is associated with increased penetration.

Early reports suggested that there would be little advantage, in terms of drug bioavailability, in increasing viscosity beyond 15 to 20 cP and many eye drops are formulated at this level.[5] Examples of viscosity-enhancing agents used include methylcellulose derivatives, polyvinyl alcohol, povidone, dextran, and macrogol. The results of more recent studies of drug penetration rather than residence time have suggested that ocular bioavailability increases with an increase in the viscosity of the preparation, even up to viscosities as high as 1000 cP.[1,4]

It has been reported that, in addition to the level of viscosity of the preparation, the nature of the viscosity-increasing agent is also important. In particular, mucoadhesive polymers (for example, hyaluronic acid and its derivatives, or carbomer) appear to be significantly more effective than non-mucoadhesive polymers at equiviscous concentrations.[6, 7]

The viscosity of eye drops is a complex subject to study; a factorial analysis approach to eye drop formulation has suggested that a change in pH can also affect the activity of viscosity-increasing agents.[8]

Some of the problems associated with the use of products with high viscosity are that they are not always well tolerated in the eye; they can leave a deposit or crust on the eyelid; they do not mix readily with tears; and they may interfere with drug diffusion.

Most commercial eye drops have their viscosities adjusted to be within the range 15 to 25 cP by the addition of hypromellose or polyvinyl alcohol. Some higher viscosity products are also being produced using both well established and newer viscosity-increasing agents such as the acrylate polymers.

Suspensions

Suspensions of drugs are sometimes used as eye drops either due to the lack of availability of soluble forms of the drug or because of toxicity or stability problems associated with soluble formulations. Achromycin has, in the past, been presented as an aqueous suspension, and some eye drops containing corticosteroids are still formulated as suspensions.[9]

The cornea of the normal eye is an extremely sensitive surface and the application of particles in suspension usually produces irritation and increases the rate of lachrymation and blinking. This irritancy problem can largely be overcome by the use of suspensions with very small particles formulated from micronised drug powders.

One possible advantage of suspension formulations is that the presence of particles of drug may result in a prolonged residence time in the eye, allowing time for dissolution in the tears with a resulting increase in bioavailability and therapeutic effect. This effect does seem to occur but only with particles larger than those presently accepted for ophthalmic suspensions. Drugs in the form of particles smaller than 10 micrometres are just as rapidly removed from the eye as are drugs in solution.

A potential problem associated with ophthalmic suspensions is the possibility of a change in particle size during storage of the product, which could result in the presence of unacceptable numbers of large particles.[9]

If residence time in the eye is not increased significantly by the presence of particles it may be argued that the use of suspensions has no advantage over the use of saturated or near-saturated solutions of low solubility drugs.

Investigations into the use of nanoparticle drug carriers in eye drops have produced encouraging results.

pH and Buffering Capacity

Human tears normally have a pH of about 7.2 with a good buffering capacity and, despite the sensitivity of the cornea, unbuffered solutions with pH values of between 3.5 and 10.5 can usually be tolerated with little discomfort. Outside this pH range irritation of the eye usually occurs and increased lachrymation will be induced, particularly with alkaline solutions.

Ideally, eye drops should be formulated to be at physiological pH but in practice drug solubility or stability considerations often necessitate deviation from this ideal. Eye drops formulated at particular pH values for solubility or stability reasons require the addition of buffering agents to minimise pH changes during storage. The concentrations at which buffering agents are used should be controlled to ensure that sufficient buffer is present to stabilise the pH of the product during storage but buffer concentration must not be high enough to significantly change the pH of the tear film within the eye.

The buffering agents most frequently used in eye drops are borate, phosphate, and citrate buffers.

Tonicity

To minimise irritation of the sensitive tissues of the eye, ophthalmic solutions should ideally be isotonic with lachrymal secretions; to achieve this eye drops should theoretically have tonicities equivalent to a 0.9% solution of sodium chloride.

In practice, the eye is usually tolerant of solutions with a fairly wide range of tonicities and eye drops are normally acceptable if their tonicities lie within a range equivalent to between 0.7% and 1.5% sodium chloride. Sodium chloride is the most commonly used agent for the adjustment of tonicity although potassium chloride, glucose, glycerol, and buffers can also be used. Formulation of hypotonic eye drops can therefore be avoided by the use of these agents, although preparation of hypertonic solutions is sometimes unavoidable due to the high concentrations of active drug required in some products.

Stabilisers

A number of drugs used in the eye are susceptible to oxidative decomposition in the presence of air and ophthalmic solutions containing such drugs may require the inclusion of antoxidants to improve their stability. The most common antoxidants used in eye drop formulations are sodium metabisulphite and sodium sulphite; however, ascorbic acid and acetylcysteine are also used, particularly in phenylephrine formulations.

Oxidative degradation is often catalysed by the presence of heavy metal impurities and chelating agents such as disodium edetate, which are often included in preservative systems, can act as stabilising agents by complexing with such impurities. Antoxidants are discussed in greater detail in the Stability of Medicinal Products chapter.

The use of plastic dropper bottles, which in some instances are permeable to gases, has increased the significance of oxidative deterioration during storage of eye drops. Formulators must be aware of this potential hazard during formulation and also during the selection of a suitable container for the product.

Wetting and Spreading Agents

Surface active compounds can disturb the integrity of the tear film and are not often included in eye drop formulations except in the form of antimicrobial preservatives. However, some suspension formulations require the inclusion of surface active additives to facilitate the dispersion of the finely divided powdered drug. Nonionic surfactants are less toxic to the eye than are the anionic and cationic compounds; the agent most frequently used is the nonionic surfactant polysorbate 80. Macrogol is used in some artificial tear formulations to facilitate spreading over the surface of the eye; dextran and polyvinyl alcohol can serve the same purpose.

Preservatives

The surface of the eye normally presents an efficient barrier to the entry of bacteria and other micro-organisms; however, if this barrier is penetrated by, for example, physical trauma, the eye will be susceptible to microbial attack because of the relative lack of vascularity of the interior of the eyeball. The limited vascularity of the eye also makes systemic antibiotic treatment of ocular infections difficult and it is therefore important that products applied to diseased, irritated, or traumatised eyes should be free from micro-organisms. The bioburden (see Sterilisation chapter) in unopened products is minimised by the sterilisation methods used during manufacture; however, maintenance of sterility during the use of multidose preparations depends upon the inclusion of appropriate antimicrobial compounds.

The in-use contamination of eye drops with a variety of micro-organisms is a well recognised problem; therefore, eye drops in multi-use containers should contain suitable antimicrobial agents. However, there are strict constraints on the use of antimicrobials in eye drop preparations as the cornea can be easily damaged by the application of chemical agents. Eye drops may have to be used at the same site several times per day over a period of many years.

Compounds suitable for use as antimicrobial preservatives in eye drops include quaternary ammonium compounds and chlorhexidine (often in combination with edetic acid), organic mercurial compounds, aromatic or chlorinated alcohols, benzoates, boric acid, or borax.

The most widely used antimicrobial is benzalkonium chloride, which is present in over 70% of all commercially produced eye drops. Edetic acid is also included in about a third of the products preserved with benzalkonium chloride. Organic mercurial compounds are the next most commonly used antimicrobial agents but these have been losing favour over recent years and are being phased out, where possible, by some manufacturers.

Antimicrobial preservatives are discussed in detail in the Control of Microbial Contamination and Preservation of Medicines chapter.

Benzalkonium Chloride. Benzalkonium chloride is a mixture of alkylbenzyldimethylammonium compounds. The mixture contains compounds of different alkyl chain lengths containing even numbers of carbon atoms between 8 and 18, with the C12 and C14 compounds predominating. Benzalkonium chloride is a surface active compound but it is well tolerated in the eye at concentrations up to 0.02% and is normally used in eye drops at a concentration of 0.01%. It is non-volatile and is stable to autoclaving.

The compound is bactericidal against a wide range of Gram-positive and Gram-negative bacteria at the pH values of ophthalmic solutions. Its activity is reduced in the presence of a range of materials, for example, methylcellulose derivatives, multivalent metal ions such as magnesium and calcium, anionic and nonionic surfactants, and large anionic molecules. It is incompatible with fluorescein and with nitrates. The activity of benzalkonium chloride is increased in the presence of some chelating agents and it can be used at a concentration as low as 0.004% in the presence of 0.02% disodium edetate.

The surface activity of benzalkonium chloride can be exploited to increase the corneal penetration of some non-lipid drugs but the same property can disturb the outer oily layer of the tears. This latter effect is of little significance in most instances but if blinking is suppressed it can lead to breakdown of the precorneal film, drying of the eye, and irritation of the cornea. Inclusion of benzalkonium chloride should therefore be avoided in eye drops that contain local anaesthetics (which suppress blinking) unless they are short-acting compounds. As with most preservatives, some people can show hypersensitivity to benzalkonium chloride.

Chlorhexidine. Chlorhexidine is a bisbiguanide bactericide that is effective (at a concentration of 0.01%) against most bacteria. Chlorhexidine is used in only a few commercially produced eye drops but it is extensively used in contact lens solutions, often in combination with benzalkonium chloride and with disodium edetate.

Chlorhexidine is a cationic agent and although it does not have the surface active properties of benzalkonium chloride its antibacterial activity is reduced by the same range of metal ions and anionic compounds. It forms insoluble salts with some inorganic anions and is incompatible with sulphates. Its activity is increased in the presence of disodium edetate. Some organic salts of chlorhexidine have good solubility properties and the acetate and gluconate are the salts of choice in the formulation of eye products. Chlorhexidine is not as stable to autoclaving as benzalkonium chloride.

Organic Mercurial Compounds. Phenylmercuric acetate, phenylmercuric nitrate, and thiomersal are all organic mercurial compounds that are used as preservatives in eye drops. The phenylmercuric salts are most commonly used at a concentration of 0.002% and thiomersal at 0.005%.

These agents exert an inhibitory effect against a wide range of bacteria and fungi over a wide range of pH values; at the concentrations used they are non-irritant and do not disrupt the tear film. Use of these compounds over a prolonged period can result in the intraocular deposition of mercury; allergic reactions can also occur, particularly with thiomersal. The use of mercurial compounds as preservatives has declined over recent years.

Chlorbutol. Chlorbutol is a substituted alcohol that is effective (at a concentration of 0.5%) against most bacteria and against fungi. It is well tolerated in the eye and is compatible with most drugs used in ophthalmic products. In common with most preservatives it is incompatible with fluorescein.

Chlorbutol can be a useful preservative for eye drops but it is volatile and can be lost from solutions stored in plastic containers. It is only stable in acidic solution and even then it will not withstand autoclaving without significant loss in activity.

Eye Lotions

Eye lotions are intended for application to the eye in relatively large volumes to mechanically remove foreign materials and to relieve irritation. The control of pH and tonicity in eye lotions is of more importance than it is in eye drops because of the large volumes administered. Eye lotions can also be used to impregnate eye dressings. Where possible, eye lotions should be formulated to have a neutral pH and to have a tonicity equivalent to a 0.9% solution of sodium chloride.

Most eye lotion preparations are intended for use on one occasion only and may not require the addition of antimicrobial preservatives. Any product intended for multi-occasion use should contain suitable antimicrobial preservatives.

Eye Ointments

The *British Pharmacopoeia* defines eye ointments as 'sterile semi-solid preparations of homogeneous appearance intended for application to the conjunctiva'.

Many of the drugs that are used in eye drops can also be formulated as eye ointments. Such ointments are normally paraffin based and are usually designed to have a melting point close to body temperature. These products can in some ways be considered as extreme cases of increased viscosity eye drops and are particularly useful where a prolonged duration of activity is required. As for eye drops, eye ointments are required to be sterile and free from extraneous particulate matter. Single-dose and multidose products are available and preservatives capable of dealing with in-use microbial contamination may need to be included in multidose products.

The paraffin basis used for eye ointments is non-irritant and chemically inert and it can be used as an anhydrous medium for the delivery of moisture-sensitive drugs. Drugs may be added to anhydrous eye ointments either by direct solution in the oily basis or by the incorporation of very finely powdered drug into the basis. An example of a basis for dissolution or dispersion of the active ingredient is Simple Eye Ointment BP (Eye Ointment Basis).

The incorporation of aqueous solutions of drugs into eye ointments may require the addition of hydrous wool fat or aliphatic alcohols to the basis to increase its emulsifying capacity. Incorporation of aqueous phases into eye ointments may necessitate the addition of buffering agents and antoxidants and the inclusion of antimicrobial preservatives is essential in multidose products.

Preservation of multiphase systems is particularly difficult and this, together with the need to avoid irritant materials, limits the choice of preservative systems. Preservatives commonly used in eye ointments are chlorbutol, phenethyl alcohol, p-hydroxybenzoates, and organic mercurials.

Gels

Studies of the effects of increased viscosity on the residence time of eye drops led to investigations into the use of water-based gels as alternatives to traditional ointment bases and several gel-based products are now available.

The distinction between eye drops and semi-solid dosage forms is no longer clear. Some gel formulations are designed to liquefy and some liquid formulations are designed to gel on contact with the eye.[10]

Some gel-based products are claimed to extend the time of drug action to such an extent that they are described as prolonged-release products.

Several types of gelling agent have been investigated for use in eye products, examples include polyacrylic acid compounds, hypromellose, carbomer, and gellan gums. Anhydrous but water-miscible ocular bases have also been made using macrogol-based formulations (for example, Albucid Eye Ointment).

Ocular Inserts

Research into means of achieving prolonged release of drugs into the eye, particularly for the treatment of conditions such as glaucoma, has been ongoing for many years and a variety of solid dosage forms have been designed for use in contact with the surface of the eye to produce slow release of drug over a prolonged period of time.

Gelatin-based lamellae have been used but two main approaches are now used: products such as Ocuserts™ in which a reservoir of drug is contained within a diffusion membrane which allows

a constant controlled release of drug for up to seven days; and products in which the drug is bound within an erodible matrix composed of materials such as hyaluronic acid, carbomer, polyacrylic acids,[11] or polyvinyl alcohol.[12] For example, a Novel Ophthalmic Delivery System (NODS™)[12, 13] has been developed for the delivery of tropicamide.

Injections

Drugs can be administered to the eye by intraocular (intracorneal, intravitreous, or retrobulbar) or subconjunctival injection. Preparations may be formulated as injection solutions or as sterile powders for reconstitution before use.

CONTAINERS

In the past liquid eye products were packed in glass containers, with glass droppers fitted with rubber teats for eye drops. Semi-solid products were packed in collapsible tin tubes. Glass containers for liquid products have largely been replaced by flexible plastic containers made of polyethylene or polypropylene, with built-in droppers for eye drops. For semi-solid ophthalmic products, however, plastic tubes have proved unsuitable owing to their non-collapsible nature which causes air to enter the tube after withdrawal of each dose. Because of this, tin tubes are still used for packing eye ointments although they are being replaced by collapsible tubes made from laminates of plastic, metal foil, and paper.

Plastic eye drop bottles have several advantages over glass ones but also have some disadvantages. Plastic bottles are cheap, light in weight, relatively non-fragile, and, because of the built-in dropper, are easier to use and less likely to be contaminated during use than are glass dropper bottles. However, polyethylene containers cannot withstand autoclaving and are usually sterilised by irradiation or by ethylene oxide before being filled aseptically with pre-sterilised product. Polypropylene bottles are much less flexible than polyethylene ones but are less permeable and, if desired, they can be sterilised by autoclaving after filling with the product.

Plastic bottles can sorb some preservatives and may be permeable to volatile compounds, water vapour, and oxygen; on prolonged storage, loss of preservative, drying of the product (especially in single-dose containers), and oxidative degradation of unstable drugs can occur.

Where benzalkonium chloride is included in the eye drops, it is preferable when using glass dropper bottles to use teats made of silicone rubber or other types of rubber that are known to be compatible with this preservative. Silicone rubber has the disadvantage that it is relatively permeable to water vapour so that gradual loss of water may occur from solutions. Where a silicone rubber teat is fitted to a dropper bottle, storage of the eye drops should be limited to three months. Bottles for eye drops should preferably be regarded as disposable containers and treated soda-glass bottles should not be reused. Metal caps should not be used with eye drops containing phenylmercuric salts.

Compendial Requirements

The *European Pharmacopoeia* and *British Pharmacopoeia* require that containers for eye drops are made from materials that do not cause deterioration of the preparation as a result of diffusion into or across the material of the container or by yielding foreign substances to the preparation. They may be of glass or other suitable material. The package and container of a single-dose preparation are such as to maintain sterility of the contents and the applicator up to the time of use. Eye ointments should be supplied in small, sterilised collapsible tubes fitted or provided with a nozzle. The content of such containers should not be more than 5 g of the preparation. Eye ointments may also be supplied in suitable single-dose containers. Eye lotions should be supplied in suitable containers. Unless otherwise justified and authorised, containers for multidose eye lotions should not contain more than 200 mL of the preparation.

In addition, the following requirements are specified for preparations that are the subjects of monographs in the *British Pharmacopoeia*. Eye drops should be supplied in tamper-evident containers. The compatibility of plastics or rubber components should be confirmed before use. Containers for multidose eye drops should be fitted with an integral dropper or with a sterile screw cap of suitable materials incorporating a dropper and rubber or plastic teat. Alternatively, such a cap assembly is supplied, sterilised, separately. Single-dose containers for eye ointments, or the nozzles of tubes, should be of such a shape as to facilitate administration without contamination. The former type of container is individually wrapped. Tubes should be tamper-evident.

LABELLING

The *European Pharmacopoeia* and *British Pharmacopoeia* specify the following requirements for the labelling of ophthalmic preparations.

Eye Drops. The label should state the name and concentration of any antimicrobial preservative or other substance added to the preparation. For multidose containers the label should state the period after opening the container after which the contents should not be used. This period does not exceed four weeks unless otherwise justified and authorised. Single-dose containers that, because of their size, cannot bear a label are marked with an indication of the nature and concentration of the active ingredient in the preparation.

Eye Ointments. The label should state the name and concentration of any antimicrobial preservative or other auxiliary substance added to the preparation.

Eye Lotions. The label should state the name and concentration of any antimicrobial preservatives added to the preparation. For single-use containers the label should state that the contents are to be used on one occasion only. For multidose containers the label should state the period after opening the container after which the contents should not be used. This period should not exceed four weeks unless otherwise justified and authorised.

In addition, the following requirements are specified for preparations that are the subjects of monographs in the *British Pharmacopoeia*.

Eye Drops. The label should state: the names and percentages of the active ingredients; the date after which the eye drops are not intended to be used; and the conditions under which the eye drops should be stored. Single-dose containers that, because of their size, bear only an indication of the active ingredient and the strength of the preparation do so by use of an approved code (see below), together with an expression of the percentage present. When a code is used on the container, the code is also stated on the package. For multidose containers the label should state that care should be taken to avoid contamination of the contents during use.

Eye Ointments. The label should state: the names and percentages of the active ingredients; the date after which the eye ointment is not intended to be used; and the conditions under which the eye ointment should be stored.

Codes for Eye Drops in Single-dose Containers

The following codes are approved for use on single unit doses of eye drops where the individual container may be too small to bear all of the appropriate labelling information. If such codes are used, the outer package should be labelled in accordance with the requirements for eye drops.

Eye Drops	Code
Adrenaline, neutral	ADN
Amethocaine	AME
Atropine sulphate	ATR
Benoxinate	BNX
Betamethasone	BET
Carbachol	CAR
Castor oil	CASOIL
Chloramphenicol	CPL
Cocaine	CCN
Cyclopentolate	CYC
Fluorescein	FLN
Gentamicin	GNT
Homatropine	HOM
Hydrocortisone	HCOR
Hydroxyethylcellulose and sodium chloride	HECL
Hyoscine	HYO
Hypromellose	HPRM
Lachesine	LAC
Lignocaine and fluorescein	LIGFLN
Metipranolol	MPR
Neomycin	NEO
Phenylephrine	PHNL
Phenylephrine and cyclopentolate	PHNCYC
Physostigmine	ESR
Pilocarpine	PIL
Prednisolone	PRED
Proxymetacaine	PROX
Rose bengal	ROS
Sulphacetamide	SULF
Thymoxamine	THY
Tropicamide	TRO
Zinc sulphate	ZSU

The term 'saline' may also be used as a code on the inner container of single unit doses of eye drops and as such indicates that the contents are a sterile 0.9% w/v solution of sodium chloride.

ADMINISTRATION AND USE OF OPHTHALMIC PREPARATIONS

During the use of eye drops it is inevitable that some microbiological contamination will occur and the preservative systems included in multi-use products are designed to deal with such in-use contamination. During long-term use, however, the preservative systems in even the best formulations will ultimately break down because of repeated contamination.

For normal domiciliary use the recommended expiry date is four weeks after opening and the user should be warned of the need to avoid contamination during application. When the eye drops are dispensed for use in hospital wards, individual supplies of previously unopened containers should be provided for each patient. When both eyes are being treated, a separate container should be used for each eye. Single-dose forms are required in all circumstances in which the dangers of infection are high. When single-dose forms are specified but are not available, multiple-application containers may be used, provided that the same principle is adhered to, that is, use of a previously unopened container for one patient on one occasion only.

Eye drops used in hospital wards should be discarded not later than 7 days after first opening the container. When used for treating a patient before an operation on the eye, they should be discarded at the time of the operation and, if treatment with eye drops is continued after the operation, fresh supplies should be provided. Similarly, at the time of discharge of the patient from the hospital, eye drops in use should be discarded and, if treatment is to be continued, fresh supplies should be given to the patient.

Eye drops for use in outpatient departments, except fluorescein eye drops, may be supplied and used in multiple-application containers. The contents of opened containers should be discarded at the end of each day. A patient who undergoes outpatient surgery which requires the use of eye drops should be treated with a separate supply of eye drops from a previously unopened container and given a further fresh supply, if prescribed, after the operation.

Eye drops for use in clinics for external eye diseases and ophthalmic accident and emergency departments should be supplied in single-dose form or, if this is not possible, in multiple-application containers used for one application only.

Eye drops for use in operating theatres should be supplied in single-dose form or, if this is not possible, in multiple-application containers used for one application only. When possible, the outer surface of containers should be sterile and supplied with a sterile overwrap, or else the outer surface of the packs should, as far as possible, be rendered free from contamination by a suitable method such as washing with sterile purified water or by spraying with an antiseptic solution just before the packs are taken into the operating theatre for use.

Some medicaments can be sorbed to soft hydrophilic contact lenses with consequent modification of the intensity and duration of the therapeutic action; also, sorption of a preservative to the contact lens may lead to eye irritation. Wherever possible, wearers of such lenses should remove them before administration of therapeutic ophthalmic preparations but if this is not practicable the use of a single-dose form may be preferable. In addition, systemic administration of some drugs, for example rifampicin and sulphasalazine, cause discoloration of soft contact lenses.

When using eye ointments, precautions should be taken to avoid contamination. For domiciliary use, the ointment is best applied directly from the tube or with the aid of a clean glass rod. When used in hospital wards, a single-application pack should be opened, if necessary, with a sterile instrument and the eye ointment applied directly to the eye. When a multiple-application container is used, the eye ointment should be applied to the eye with a sterile applicator. Sterile applicators should preferably be supplied singly in sealed packs and should each be used for one application only. Unless otherwise specified, eye drops should be stored in a cool place but preferably not in a refrigerator and eye ointments should be stored at a temperature not exceeding 25°.

REFERENCES

1. Li VHK, Robinson JR. Int J Pharmaceutics 1989;53:219–25.
2. Ludwig A, Van Ooteghem. Drug Dev Ind Pharm 1986;12:2231–42.
3. Grove J, Durr M, Quint MP, Plazonnet B. Int J Pharmaceutics 1990;66:23–8.
4. Chrai SS, Robinson JR. J Pharm Sci 1974;63:1218–23.
5. Saettone MF, Giannaccini P, Chetoni P, Toracca MT, Monti D. Int J Pharmaceutics 1991;72:131–9.
6. Davies NM, Farr SJ, Hadgraft J, Kellaway IW. J Pharm Pharmacol 1988;40:15P.
7. Vulovic N, Primorac M, Stupar M, Ford JL. Int J Pharmaceutics 1989;55:123–8.
8. Keister JC, Cooper ER, Missel PJ, Lang JC, Hager DF. J Pharm Sci 1991;80:50–3.
9. Patel JP, Marsh K, Carr L, Nequist G. Int J Pharmaceutics 1990;65:195–200.
10. Rozier A, Mazuel C, Grove J, Plazonnet B. Int J Pharmaceutics 1989;57:163–8.
11. Saettone MF, Chetoni P, Toracca MT, Burgalassi S, Giannaccini B. Int J Pharmaceutics 1989;51:203–12.
12. Fitzgerald P, Wilson CG, Greaves JL, Frier M, Hollingsbee D, Gilbert D et al. Int J Pharmaceutics 1992;83:177–85.
13. Pharm J 1993;250:174.

FURTHER INFORMATION

Edman P, editor. Biopharmaceutics of ocular drug delivery. Boca Raton: CRC Press, 1993.

Hecht G, Roehrs RE, Cooper ER, Hiddemen JW, Van Duzee BF. Design and evaluation of ophthalmic pharmaceutical products. In: Banker GS, Rhodes CT, editors. Modern pharmaceutics. 2nd ed. New York: Marcel Dekker, 1990.

Mitra AK, editor. Ophthalmic drug delivery systems. New York: Marcel Dekker, 1993.

Rectal and Vaginal Products

Products may be administered via the rectum or vagina for local or systemic effect. Rectal and vaginal products may be solid or liquid unit dosage preparations, or creams, ointments, gels, or foams.

RECTAL PRODUCTS

Systemic administration via the rectum is particularly useful for medicaments that may not be tolerated orally; on occasion it may also be regarded as a comparatively easy alternative to the parenteral route.

Anatomy and Physiology of the Rectum

The rectum is about 150 to 200 mm in length and forms the lower part of the gastro-intestinal tract. It is lined with a single epithelial layer, composed of cylindrical cells and mucus-producing goblet cells. The rectum normally contains about 2 to 3 mL of mucus, which has a pH of about 7.4 and little buffering capacity. The rectal tissues are drained by the inferior, middle, and superior haemorrhoidal veins, but only the superior vein connects with the hepatic-portal system. The terminal 20 to 30 mm of the rectum is called the anal canal; the opening of the anal canal to the exterior is called the anus. The anus is controlled by an internal sphincter of smooth muscle and an external sphincter of skeletal muscle. Medicaments absorbed in the lower part of the rectum are delivered directly into the systemic circulation, thus avoiding any first-pass metabolism of the drug in the liver. However, it has been found that suppositories can settle high enough in the rectum to allow at least some drug absorption into the superior vein.

Suppositories

Suppositories are solid unit dosage forms containing one or more active ingredients for local or systemic effect. Locally acting drugs that are often given rectally include astringents, local anaesthetics, laxatives, and corticosteroids. Medicaments that are administered rectally for systemic effect include anti-emetics, antipsychotics, drugs used in the treatment of migraine, and non-steroidal anti-inflammatory agents.

The active ingredients are dissolved or dispersed in a suitable basis that should either melt at body temperature, or dissolve or disperse in the mucous secretions of the rectum. Suppositories may also contain suitable excipients such as absorbents, absorption enhancers, diluents, lubricants, preservatives, and surfactants. They are usually made in moulds and weigh between 1 and 3 g. The shape, volume, and consistency of suppositories should be such that the preparation is suitable for rectal administration.

The ideal suppository basis should melt or otherwise deform or dissolve to release its drug content at 37°; it should be non-irritant, non-toxic, and non-sensitising. It should be compatible with a wide range of drugs and should be readily moulded or formed into stable rigid shapes that maintain uniform drug release characteristics on storage. In addition, although the basis should remain molten for a sufficient period of time to allow pouring into moulds, it should solidify sufficiently rapidly to minimise sedimentation of any dispersed solid material. Ideally, the basis should also contract on cooling to allow easy withdrawal of the suppositories from the mould.

When the liquid content is sufficiently high to reduce the rigidity of the suppository, an inert powder such as starch or magnesium oxide may be introduced. If the plasticity of the suppository mass is reduced because of the inclusion of a high concentration of powders, it may be restored by the addition of a small amount of vegetable oil. The use of water for this purpose in fatty bases can lead to drug incompatibility or crystallisation, microbial spoilage, or rancidity of the bases.

Fatty Suppository Bases

Theobroma Oil. Theobroma oil (cocoa butter) is a bland material that softens and melts between 30° and 35°. It is a mixture of solid and liquid triglycerides, chiefly 2-oleopalmitostearin and 2-oleodistearin. Theobroma oil has the disadvantage that it shrinks only slightly on solidification; a mould lubricant is therefore required. It exists in four polymorphic forms with different melting points (18.9°, 23.0°, 28.0°, and 34.5°). In order to minimise the formation of the unstable low melting point forms, theobroma oil should only be heated for short periods and at temperatures below 36°. When the melting point of theobroma oil has been reduced by the addition of drugs such as volatile oils or chloral hydrate, it may be raised by the addition of 3% to 5% of beeswax.

Theobroma oil has a low absorptive capacity for water, but this can be increased by adding surfactants such as cholesterol 2%, emulsifying wax up to 10%, polysorbates 5% to 10%, or wool fat 5% to 10%. However, the addition of a surfactant may lead to a drug-base interaction or affect the release of drug from the suppository.

Theobroma oil is prone to air oxidation; this can be partly overcome by storage in a cool, dark place. In common with other natural products, theobroma oil may vary in consistency, odour, and colour depending on its source. The low melting point of theobroma oil suppositories may pose storage problems in hot climates.

Hard-fat Alternatives to Theobroma Oil. These include hard fat and the esterified, hydrogenated, or fractionated vegetable oils. Hard fat is a mixture of the mono-, di-, and tri-glycerides of saturated fatty acids (C_{10} to C_{18}). The hydroxyl value of a basis is determined by the proportions of mono- and di-glycerides contained within it. A higher hydroxyl value indicates that the basis can absorb water more readily and is therefore less suitable for formulations containing drugs that are easily hydrolysed. Bases with higher hydroxyl values (for example, Witepsol^{TM} S51) have longer solidification times. This renders products less friable and these bases are more suited to formulations that require rapid cooling. Most of the bases have the advantages of freedom from polymorphism and a low risk of rancidity. The solidification temperatures of these bases are unaffected by overheating and there is only a small temperature difference between melting and solidification; thus the sedimentation of suspended insoluble drugs is minimised. Mould lubrication is unnecessary since these bases show marked contraction on cooling. The water-absorbing capacity of hard fats can be improved (to about 25% or 30% w/w) by the inclusion of glyceryl monostearate. A tendency to fracture when poured into chilled moulds can be overcome by including very small quantities of polysorbate 80.

On prolonged storage, semi-synthetic suppository bases have been shown to be subject to crystallisation, which causes hardening of the suppository and lengthens the melting time. The degree of crystallisation can be reduced by storage in a cold place. The hard-fat alternatives to theobroma oil are available in various grades with different melting ranges, hydroxyl values, and other physicochemical characteristics; examples include the fractionated palm kernel oils, *Extracoa*^{TM} (Loders and Nucoline, UK) and *Supercoa*^{TM} (Loders and Nucoline, UK) and the hard fats, *Massa Estarinum*^{TM} (Hüls, UK), *Massuppol*^{TM} (Loders and Nucoline, UK), *Suppocire*^{TM} (Alfa, UK), and *Witepsol*^{TM} (Hüls, UK).

Water-soluble Suppository Bases

Glycerol. Glycerol suppository basis is prepared using the formula for Glycerol Suppositories BP:

Gelatin	14 g
Glycerol	70 g
Purified water,	a sufficient quantity

The final product should weigh 100 g.

In tropical and subtropical countries the proportion of gelatin may be increased to 18% w/w. Glycerol suppository basis has a physiological laxative effect. The water-soluble basis dissolves slowly in the mucous secretions of the rectum. Factors that influence the dissolution rate include the relative proportions of the constituents, the type of gelatin used and its reaction with the active drug. Gelatin is a purified protein obtained either by partial acid hydrolysis (type A) or by partial alkaline hydrolysis (type B) of animal collagen. Type A is cationic and is compatible with substances such as boric acid, lactic acid, and bismuth subnitrate. Type B is anionic and can be used with ichthammol and zinc oxide. Gelatin BP may be a mixture of types A and B. Gelatin should be appropriately labelled to indicate whether the material is suitable for the preparation of suppositories or pessaries and, if so, state the Jelly strength, often expressed as 'Bloom strength' or 'Bloom rating'.

Glycerol suppository basis requires protection from heat and moisture. In use, its hygroscopic nature may cause dehydration of the rectal mucosa and subsequent irritation. Glycerol suppository basis may support microbial growth and the inclusion of preservatives may be necessary; methyl and propyl hydroxybenzoates have been recommended.

Macrogols. Water-soluble macrogols (polyethylene glycols) of various molecular weights have been blended to produce suppository bases that differ in their melting point ranges, physical characteristics, and dissolution rates. Macrogols have the advantages of stability, inertness, high water capacity, and freedom from rancidity; they are useful as vehicles for drugs such as chloral hydrate and ichthammol, which tend to lower the melting points of other bases. Usually no mould lubricant is required, but macrogol suppositories may be brittle unless the molten basis is poured into the mould at as low a temperature as possible. Brittleness can be reduced by the addition of surfactants or plasticisers such as castor oil or propylene glycol. Macrogol bases that melt above body temperature are available; they offer less risk of leakage from body cavities and present fewer storage problems than lower melting point bases. Because macrogol bases usually dissolve readily in body fluids their drug release rates tend to differ from those obtained from fatty or glycerol bases. Substances that are incompatible with macrogols include some bacitracins, benzocaine, penicillin, phenols, plastics, quinine salts, salicylic acid, silver salts, sorbitol, sulphonamides, and tannic acid. Suspended solid materials may display crystal growth in macrogol bases; such crystals may show delayed dissolution and cause irritation of the rectum.

Dehydration of the rectal mucosa with consequent irritant effects can arise from the administration of macrogol bases formulated without water. Such irritant effects can be reduced by immersing the suppository in water before insertion or by the application of coatings of cetyl or stearyl alcohol, although these may retard dissolution.

The following combinations of macrogols have been used as suppository bases:

(1) Macrogol 1000   96%
    Macrogol 4000   4%

A low melting point basis that is useful if relatively rapid dissolution is desired. It may require refrigeration during the summer months.

(2) Macrogol 1000   75%
    Macrogol 4000   25%

A more stable formulation than basis 1 above; it can be used if the suppository is to be subjected to extreme storage conditions.

(3) Macrogol 6000   50%
    Macrogol 1540   30%
    Macrogol 400   20%

A good general purpose basis.

(4) Macrogol 6000   50%
    Macrogol 1540   30%
    Water and medicament 20%

This formulation contains water to facilitate the incorporation of medicaments soluble in water but not in macrogols.

Hydrophilic or Water-dispersible Suppository Bases

Hydrophilic or water-dispersible bases contain mainly nonionic surfactants, either alone or mixed with vegetable oils or waxy solids. The most frequently used surfactants are the polysorbates, polyoxyl stearates, and sorbitan fatty acid esters. These bases can be handled at higher temperatures; they are non-toxic and do not support microbial growth. Hydrophilic bases are compatible with a wide range of drugs but they have a potential for interaction because of their surfactant content. Such interactions may increase or decrease the rate or extent of drug absorption.

Methods of Suppository Preparation

Although cold compression has been used on a small scale, the most common method of small-scale or large-scale preparation is by pouring the melted mass into suitable moulds (pour moulding).

Cold Compression

Cold compression involves incorporating the active material into the grated basis using a mortar and pestle; the active ingredient is usually finely powdered, dissolved in a little water, or mixed with a small amount of wool fat. The mass is then shaped into suppositories by hand or forced into moulds by machine.

Pour Moulding

The finely divided suppository basis is heated to just above its melting point; for small batches, an evaporating dish is a suitable vessel. Insoluble drugs are finely powdered and levigated with a little of the melted basis; immiscible liquids are treated similarly. The mixture is then added to the bulk of the melted basis. Soluble solids in powder form, and miscible liquids are added directly to the basis. Special care is required in the case of suppositories containing chloral hydrate (or other medicaments that lower the melting point of the basis) in both theobroma oil and synthetic bases.

After incorporation or dissolution of the medicament, the melted basis should be stirred as little as possible to avoid the formation of air bubbles. When the medicated mass has been adequately mixed and is of a suitable consistency, it is poured into the moulds, which have been lubricated, if appropriate. Suppositories based on theobroma oil or hard fat may be slightly overfilled to allow for subsequent contraction, and the excess mass trimmed off after cooling. When pouring glycerol-based suppositories, the mould cavities should not be overfilled since the cooled mass does not contract.

Large-scale manufacture of suppositories involves automated pour moulding and forced cooling techniques. The basis selected must be suitable for rapid cooling, with no tendency to become brittle.

Moulds. Traditionally, metal moulds made from stainless steel, nickel, brass, or plated metal have been used. These allow suppositories to set quickly due to their efficient heat transfer and thus reduce the risk of sedimentation of suspended solids. Although metal moulds are usually marked with a nominal weight, it is advisable to calibrate the mould before use by preparing suppositories using only the basis and taking their mean weight as the capacity of the mould. For large-scale manufacture, metal moulds have been replaced, to a considerable extent, by cheaper disposable moulds of plastic materials in which the suppositories are cast and remain enclosed until removal by the patient.

Disposable plastic moulds are also available for the production of small batches.

Moulds can be pre-formed from semi-rigid films of polyvinyl chloride, polyethylene, or aluminium; more rigid plastic moulds are also available. After sealing within such moulds, suppositories will withstand tropical conditions or high storage temperatures without distortion. When selecting packaging of this type, care must be taken to ensure that the material is compatible with, and impermeable to, both the active constituents and the other ingredients in the suppository. Metal foils may not be suitable for suppositories containing acidic substances.

Lubricants. The adhesion of theobroma oil to metal moulds can be minimised by the application of lubricants or 'release agents' such as alcoholic solutions of soft soap and glycerol, silicones, or sodium lauryl sulphate in aqueous solution or in propylene glycol. The silicones can be applied, on the large scale, by a spraying technique. For macrogol-based suppositories a mineral oil may be used, whereas for glycerol bases a mineral or vegetable oil is suitable.

Displacement Values. Because the density of the medicament affects the amount of basis required for the suppository it is necessary to make an allowance for each medicament in terms of the particular basis. This allowance, termed the displacement value, is the quantity of medicament that displaces one part of the basis. Displacement

values for a range of medicaments in theobroma oil are shown in Table 1. The same figure may be used for other fatty bases. For glycerol suppository basis, about 1.2 g occupies the same volume as 1 g of theobroma oil. A displacement value of 1.0 is generally adopted for liquids. Each mould should be calibrated with the particular basis before the displacement due to the medicament is calculated. If the displacement value is not available for a particular drug, it may be calculated using the following method:

Prepare six suppositories using the basis alone; the weight of these six suppositories = a mg.
Prepare six suppositories using the basis and a known percentage (b) of the active substance; the weight of these six suppositories = c mg. These six suppositories will contain d mg (where $d = \frac{b}{100} \times c$) of the active substance and e mg of the basis (where $e = c - d$).
The displacement value of the active substance =

$$\frac{d}{a - e}$$

The following example demonstrates the practical application of displacement values:

EXAMPLE
Prepare 12 suppositories each containing zinc oxide 0.3 g with theobroma oil as the basis. Capacity of mould, 1 g of theobroma oil; displacement value for zinc oxide, 4.7; calculate quantities for 14 suppositories.

Weight of basis required =

$$\text{weight of 14 suppositories} - \frac{\text{weight of active ingredient}}{\text{displacement value}}$$

$$= (14 \times 1) - \left(\frac{14 \times 0.3}{4.7}\right) = 13.11 \text{ g}$$

If glycerol suppository basis were to be used, an allowance has to be made for the higher density of the basis (1.2 relative to theobroma oil). The quantity of glycerol suppository basis required in relation to the last example would therefore be:

$$1.2\left[(14 \times 1) - \left(\frac{14 \times 0.3}{4.7}\right)\right] = 15.73 \text{ g}$$

Testing of Suppository Formulations

Suppositories may be subjected to tests with regard to their appearance, disintegration and softening times, uniformity of weight, mechanical strength,

Table 1
Displacement values of medicaments in theobroma oil

Medicament	Displacement value
Alum	1.8
Aminophylline	1.3
Aspirin	1.1
Barbitone	1.2
Barbitone sodium	1.2
Beeswax, white	1.0
Bismuth subgallate	2.7
Bismuth subnitrate	5.0
Boric acid	1.5
Camphor	0.7
Castor oil	1.0
Chloral hydrate	1.4
Cinchocaine	1.5
Cinchocaine hydrochloride	1.0
Cocaine hydrochloride	1.4
Codeine phosphate	1.1
Dimenhydrinate	1.3
Diphenhydramine hydrochloride	1.3
Glycerol	1.6
Hamamelis dry extract	1.5
Hydrocortisone	1.5
Hydrocortisone acetate	1.5
Ichthammol	1.0
Iodoform	4.0
Menthol	0.7
Metronidazole	1.7
Morphine hydrochloride	1.6
Morphine sulphate	1.6
Paracetamol	1.5
Paraffin	1.0
Pentobarbitone sodium	1.2
Peru balsam	1.2
Pethidine hydrochloride	1.6
Phenobarbitone	1.1
Phenobarbitone sodium	1.2
Phenol	1.1
Podophyllum resin	1.3
Potassium iodide	4.5
Procaine hydrochloride	1.2
Quinalbarbitone sodium	1.2
Quinine hydrochloride	1.1
Resorcinol	1.5
Salicylic acid	1.3
Sulphanilamide	1.7
Sulphathiazole	1.6
Sulphur	1.6
Tannic acid	1.3
Theophylline sodium acetate	1.7
Zinc oxide	4.7
Zinc sulphate	2.4

and content of active substance. Further tests may be carried out on the drug-release characteristics of the suppository formulation. These often take the form of dissolution tests and may be divided into non-membrane methods and membrane methods. Non-membrane methods are based on the dissolution test apparatus developed for tablets. Membrane methods employ a synthetic dialysis or natural dialysis membrane, inside which the suppository is placed. The concentration of the drug outside the bag is measured as a function of time.

Factors Influencing Absorption

Physicochemical Drug Properties. The first stage in the release of a drug from a fatty basis is the partitioning of the active ingredient between the melting basis and the mucosal secretions of the rectum. As the drug must subsequently partition into the lipid membrane of the mucosal wall, an intermediate value for the oil/water partition coefficient will favour absorption.

After the base has melted, the factor that limits absorption of a drug from a water-soluble basis is its transport through the rectal mucosa. A drug with a high oil/water partition coefficient is likely to be absorbed more rapidly from a water-soluble basis. Absorption through the rectal mucosa proceeds in accordance with the pH-partition hypothesis. At the slightly alkaline pH of the rectal mucosa weakly basic drugs will exist in their lipid-soluble unionised form and be readily absorbed.

Particles suspended in a suppository are released on melting with dissolution occurring in the rectal fluid; reducing the particle size of the suspended powder increases the surface area for dissolution and so improves absorption.

Absorption Enhancers. Agents such as medium-chain glycerides,[2,3] salicylate derivatives,[4] and sodium decanoate[5] have been observed to increase the absorption of rectally administered drugs. Surfactants may improve absorption by aiding the dissolution of the drug. However, complexes may form between the surfactant and the active material which may delay absorption.

Modified Release. Modified-release suppositories have been formulated using water absorbable polymers or microencapsulation techniques.

Double Layer Suppositories. In such formulations, the active ingredient is contained in an outer layer surrounding a core that consists of the basis alone. More rapid release of medicament has been demonstrated from double layer suppositories.[1]

Rectal Conditions. Rectal absorption gives more variable plasma-drug concentrations than oral administration. The rate and extent of absorption is influenced by the pH of the rectal fluid, anorectal physiology, and the quantity of faecal material in the rectum at the time of administration.

Rectal Capsules

Rectal capsules (shell suppositories) are soft gelatin capsules shaped like suppositories. The contents should be solid at room temperature, as with conventional suppositories. Vegetable oils, solid fats, and their derivatives together with surfactants such as glyceryl monostearate and polysorbates may be used in formulations. Rectal (soft) gelatin capsules are suitable for use in tropical climates, provided that containers are hermetically sealed. Special machinery is used for the production of these capsules.

Enemas

Enemas are aqueous or oily solutions or suspensions for rectal administration. Enemas normally display good absorption characteristics as no melting or dissolution is required before drug release. They are usually given for their anti-inflammatory, purgative, or sedative effects, or for X-ray examination of the lower bowel.

Retention enemas rarely exceed 100 mL in volume; they should preferably be used after defaecation. Retention enemas should be administered slowly with the patient lying on one side. The patient should then lie prone and retain the enema for at least 30 minutes to allow distribution and absorption of the medicament. **Micro-enemas** are single-dose small-volume solutions or dispersions; they are presented in plastic containers with a nozzle to aid insertion into the rectum. **Large-volume enemas** should be warmed to body temperature before administration.

VAGINAL PRODUCTS

Vaginal products are normally administered for their local effect. Creams, ointments, or foams designed for rectal or vaginal administration are available with an appropriate applicator to ensure effective distribution.

Anatomy and Physiology of the Vagina

The vagina is a muscular, tubular organ lined with mucous membrane and measures about 100 mm in length, extending from the cervix to the vestibule. The mucosa of the vagina contains large amounts of glycogen, which decomposes to produce organic acids. These acids create a low pH environment that retards microbial growth. The vagina possesses a good blood supply and may be utilised for systemic delivery; drugs pass directly into the systemic circulation following absorption and thus by-pass the liver.

Pessaries

Pessaries are solid preparations suitably shaped for vaginal administration and contain one or more medicaments that are usually intended to act locally. Pessaries may be prepared by moulding or by compression and by methods designed to minimise microbial contamination; they usually weigh between 1 and 15 g.

Moulded pessaries may be of various shapes but are usually smooth ovoids. Fatty bases, such as theobroma oil or hard fat, or water-soluble bases, such as glycerol suppository basis or macrogol mixtures, may be used. Bases containing gelatin should be maintained at 100° for one hour, replacing any water lost by evaporation, before incorporating the other ingredients. Bases should be formulated so that the pessaries melt at, or slightly below, 37°.

Vaginal Capsules

Vaginal capsules (shell pessaries or ovules) are modified forms of soft gelatin capsules differing only in their size and shape; they are usually ovoid with a smooth appearance.

Vaginal Tablets

Vaginal tablets (compressed pessaries) are usually prepared in the form of a diamond, almond, wedge, disk, or other suitable shape that provides a large surface area. They are similar to uncoated tablets although they are generally larger and heavier. Vaginal tablets may be manufactured by the moist-granulation or direct-compression techniques using diluents, disintegrating agents, moistening agents, and lubricants.

Other Vaginal Preparations

Vaginal contraceptives or spermicides contain a surfactant to immobilise sperm. Spermicides are contained in a variety of dosage forms: foams, creams, gels, pessaries, and films. These preparations are usually deposited high in the vagina, near the cervix. A disposable polyurethane contraceptive sponge, which is permeated with a spermicide is also available. The sponge is moistened with water and is inserted into the vagina so that the concave side covers the vagina.

Creams, pessaries, and vaginal tablets containing an oestrogen are used for the topical administration of the hormone. Creams, water-miscible or water-soluble gels, and medicated tampons are also used in antifungal treatment. Vaginal douches are used as cleansing and antiseptic solutions.

The characteristics of creams, ointments, and foams are discussed in the chapter entitled Topical Semi-solids.

The mineral or vegetable oil content of some rectal and vaginal products may damage latex rubber condoms or contraceptive diaphragms and reduce their efficiency.

REFERENCES

1. Deshmukh AA, Thwaites PM. Drug Dev Ind Pharm 1989;15:1289–1307.
2. Van Hoogdalem EJ, Stijnen AM, de Boer AG, Breimer DD. J Pharm Pharmacol 1988;40:329–32.
3. Watanabe Y, van Hoogdalem EJ, de Boer AG, Breimer DD. J Pharm Sci 1988;77:847–9.
4. Hauss DJ, Ando HY. J Pharm Pharmacol 1988;40:659–61.
5. Van Hoogdalem EJ, de Boer AG, Breimer DD. Pharm Weekbl(Sci) 1988;10:76–9

FURTHER INFORMATION

Formulation of Suppository Bases. American Pharmaceutical Association and The Pharmaceutical Society of Great Britain. Suppository bases. In: Handbook of pharmaceutical excipients. London: Pharmaceutical Press, 1986.
Banakav U, Speake W. Fats and waxes in pharmaceuticals. Mfg Chem 1990 Sept;61(9):43–6.
Coben LJ, Lordi NG. Physical stability of semi-synthetic suppository bases. J Pharm Sci 1980;69:955–60.
Fulper LD, Cleary RW, Harland EC, Hikal AH, Jones AB. Liquefaction times of fatty-type suppositories with and without progesterone. Am J Hosp Pharm 1990;47:602–3.
Muller BW, Hassan I, Heers W. Studies on the thermal conditions of glycerides. Pharm Ind 1989;51:681–5.
Schumacher GE. Chloral hydrate suppositories. Am J Hosp Pharm 1966;23:110.
Testing of Suppository Formulations. Ackermann P, Fischer FX. Device for the automatic determination of the melting time of suppositories. Pharm Ind 1988;50:1295–7.
McElnay JC, Nicol AC. The comparison of a novel continuous-flow dissolution apparatus for suppositories with the rotating basket technique. Int J Pharmaceutics 1984;19:89–96.
Palmieri A. Suppository dissolution testing: apparatus design and release of aspirin. Drug Dev Ind Pharm 1981;7:247–59.
Roseman TJ, Derr GR, Nelson KG, Lieberman BL, Butler SS. Continuous flow bead-bed dissolution apparatus for suppositories. J Pharm Sci 1981;70:646–51.
Tukker JJ, de Blaey CJ. Membranes in dissolution testing: a good choice? Drug Dev Ind Pharm 1983;9:383–98.
Factors which Influence Absorption. Armstrong NA, James KC. Drug release from lipid-based dosage forms. Int J Pharmaceutics 1980;6:185–93.
Grant DJW, Liversidge GG. Influence of physicochemical interactions on the properties of suppositories. III. Rheological behaviour of fatty suppository bases and its effect on spreading in rats. Drug Dev Ind Pharm 1983;9:247–66.

Hauss DJ, Ando HY. The influence of concentration of two salicylate derivatives on rectal insulin absorption enhancement. J Pharm Pharmacol 1988;40:659–61.
Nishihata T, Rytting JH, Higuchi T. [letter]. Enhancement of rectal absorption of drugs by adjuvants [lignocaine and theophylline by salicylate]. J Pharm Sci 1980;69:744–5.
Rutten-Kingma JJ, de Blaey CJ, Polderman J. Biopharmaceutical studies of fatty suspension suppositories. II. Influence of particle size and concentration on in vitro release of readily water-soluble compounds. Int J Pharmaceutics 1979;3:179–86.
Schoonen AJM, Moolenaar F, Huizinga T. Release of drugs from fatty suppository bases. I. The release mechanism. Int J Pharmaceutics 1979;4:141–52.
Stuurman-Bieze AGG, Moolenaar F, Schoonen AJM, Visser J, Huizinga T. Biopharmaceutics of rectal administration of drugs in man. II. Effect of particle size on absorption rate and bioavailability. Int J Pharmaceutics 1978;1:337–47.
Stuurman-Bieze AGG, Schoonen AJM, Heuy AF-VD, Peeters-Udding LM, Huizinga T. Effect of suppository bases on rectal absorption rate of drugs. Pharm Weekbl (Sci) 1980;2:172–8.
Van Hoogdalem EJ, de Boer AG, Breimer DD. Rectal absorption enhancement of rate-controlled delivered ampicillin sodium by sodium decanoate in conscious rats. Pharm Weekbl (Sci) 1988;10:76–9.
Van Hoogdalem EJ, Wackwitz ATE, de Boer AG, Cohen AF, Breimer DD. Rate-controlled rectal absorption enhancement of cefoxitin by co-administration of sodium salicylate or sodium octanoate in healthy volunteers. Br J Clin Pharmacol 1989;27:75–81.
Drug Absorption. Arima H, Irie T, Uekama K. Differences in the enhancing effects of water soluble β-cyclodextrins on the release of ethyl 4-biphenyl acetate, an anti-inflammatory agent from an oleagenous suppository base. Int J Pharmaceutics 1989;57:107–15.
Moes AJ. Suppositories formulation and drug release. Boll Chim Farm 1989;128:5–12.
Modified Release. Böttger WM, Schoonen BJM, Moolenaar F, Visser J, Meijer DKF. A study on the buffering activity of the human rectum. Pharm Weekbl (Sci) 1989;11:9–12.
De Boer AG, de Leede LGJ, Breimer DD. Rectal drug administration partial examination of hepatic first-pass elimination. Pharm Int 1982;3:267–9.
Nishihata T, Tsutsumi A, Ikawa C, Sakai K. Sustained release suppository of sodium diclofenac: use of water absorbable polymer. Drug Dev Ind Pharm 1990;16:1675–86.
Safwat SM, El-Shanawany S. Evaluation of sustained release theophylline and oxyphenbutazone. J Controlled Release 1989;9:65–73.
Rectal Capsules. Hardy JG, Feely LC, Wood E, Davis SS. The application of gamma-scintigraphy for the evaluation of the relative spreading of suppository bases in rectal hard gelatin capsules. Int J Pharmaceutics 1987;38:103–8.
Senior N. Review of rectal suppositories. Pharm J 1969;203:703–6.
Enemas. Hardy JG, Lee SW, Clark AG, Reynolds JR. Enema volume and spreading. Int J Pharmaceutics 1986;31:151–5.
Wood E, Wilson CG, Hardy JG. Spreading of foam and solution enemas. Int J Pharmaceutics 1985;25:191–7.

Section 2 Product Design, Development, and Presentation

Preformulation

Following the identification of a new chemical entity that is suitable for development, the formulator will be called upon to produce dosage forms. Initially, this may involve the production of an injectable form suitable for early efficacy and toxicity testing and subsequently there will be a need to develop the final dosage form, which generally will not be an injection. The challenge for the formulator is to develop the initial and final dosage forms to the highest quality in the shortest time. This process is best achieved when certain physicochemical properties of the drug substance are investigated, understood, and effectively utilised: this is preformulation.

Preformulation studies include investigations of chemical form (for example, salts), crystal form (for example, polymorphism and habit), solubility, dissociation (pK_a), partitioning, mechanical properties, stability, and excipient compatibility. The number of experiments that could be performed is extremely large and it is necessary to balance the value of the results against the time taken to obtain them. There is also a need to obtain as much information as possible at the earliest stage. However, the quantities of drug available will be extremely limited until the synthesis has been scaled up, and also the changes in the chemical production process may result in changes in the physicochemical properties of the drug, for example, different crystal forms (which is discussed below). Thus, there must be careful thought about the experiments that will be performed and the stage at which they should be considered. The development scientist should, if possible, be involved at an early stage in the discussion on choice of synthetic route for the bulk production of drug substance, especially the final crystallisation step. Furthermore, the range of tests to be performed will vary depending upon the desired route of administration and dosage form selected. Thus, only for tableted products would one consider material compression properties. Such compression tests would usually be left to the later stages, simply on the basis of balancing material supply with the requirements of the test.

As preformulation covers such a large range of subject areas, the scope of this chapter has been restricted to an introduction to the concepts of preformulation, with the aim being to highlight the tests that are available and to draw attention to relevant texts for further reading.

The order of the sections below does not represent any chronological order in which the experiments are performed. For example, solubility experiments have a higher priority than investigations of some aspects of crystal form; however, it is easier to describe the solubility of polymorphs after introducing the concepts of polymorphism and that is the basis on which the chapter is arranged.

ORGANOLEPTIC PROPERTIES

With the Control of Substances Hazardous to Health (COSHH) safety regulations it would be unusual for preformulation scientists to routinely taste new chemical entities. In the following section, the need for accurate analysis is discussed; however, there are occasions when organoleptic aspects provide useful information. When an oxidation reaction produces a coloured degradation product it will often be detected by the human eye before the breakdown product has reached a sufficiently high concentration to be detected by chemical analysis. Equally, problematic crystal transitions can often be detected by simple light microscopy, where even qualitative observations on particle shape and approximate size distribution can also be a valuable guide to potential problems (for example, a wide size distribution would alert the worker to the possibility of Ostwald ripening in suspensions; acicular shaped crystals to potential problems with flow). Smell can be an efficient method by which chemical and microbiological instabilities can be detected. With the wide range of erudite techniques available to the scientist it is easy to forget that careful organoleptic observations and thorough note taking can be valuable tools by which to monitor changes in a drug and to make decisions about subsequent preformulation tests, as well as formulation and processing factors.

ANALYSIS

An essential part of preformulation is to be able to assay the drug. Analysis is a subject that is too large to be adequately addressed here; however, assays are commonly undertaken by high performance liquid chromatography (HPLC), thin layer chromatography (TLC), or gas chromatography (GC), which can allow the drug and degradation products or related substances to be monitored (a stability-indicating assay). It is also useful to have a simple assay (based on an ultraviolet (UV)-absorbing chromaphore that obeys a Beer-Lambert plot) to allow easy and rapid quantification of the preformulation experiments. Users should be aware of the limitations of an assay, for example, whether it is stability-indicating or whether the breakdown product absorbs at the same wavelength, or if other ingredients in the formulation (for example, excipients) interfere with the assay by absorbing at the same wavelength.

CRYSTAL PROPERTIES

The majority of drug substances are regarded as crystalline materials; the molecules are packed in an ordered and reproducible manner. Excipients vary from crystalline materials to amorphous polymers. However, few samples will be entirely homogeneous, polymers will be partially crystalline and drugs at least partially amorphous. The extent of crystallinity of compounds will greatly affect their physical properties.

Polymorphism

Changes in the crystallisation process can affect not only the degree of crystallinity, but also the way in which the molecules are packed. When a particular solid has been shown to exist in more than one packing arrangement, it is said to exhibit polymorphism. There are two types of polymorphism. Monotropic polymorphs are those for which only one form is stable (irrespective of temperature and pressure) and the metastable form will revert to the stable form with time. Enantiotropic polymorphs are those for which different forms are stable under different experimental conditions, such that a change in pressure or temperature may alter the form that is stable.

Different monotropic polymorphs often have different melting points, with the most stable form generally having the highest melting point (see Thermal Methods below). They also exhibit different X-ray diffraction patterns and infrared (IR) spectra. At any one particular temperature and pressure, there will be only one stable polymorph, all other forms that exist for any detectable period of time (and there may be several) are termed metastable. Metastable polymorphs will have a faster dissolution rate than the stable form, and apparently have a greater equilibrium solubility, thus the bioavailability from a metastable form can be considerably greater than from the stable form of that drug. This type of behaviour is due to the fact that the melting point is an indication of the lattice energy of the crystal, so the most stable crystals will have the largest lattice energy, the highest melting point, and the lowest rate of solution, and *vice versa*. However, by definition, the metastable form is not stable and will tend to revert to the stable polymorph. Transitions in polymorphic form can occur gradually as a function of time, and can be accelerated by changes in storage conditions (such as increases in temperature and humidity) or energetic treatment (processing) of the powder. Thus, unit processing such as mixing, milling, and tableting can cause changes in crystal type and consequently change the physical, and potentially the biopharmaceutical, properties of a drug. It follows that great care must be taken to determine which polymorph is present, and under what conditions and for how long it will be stable. A useful stress test for a drug substance is to ball mill it for a defined time and then to check for any change in polymorphic form, perhaps by use of differential scanning calorimetry (see Thermal Methods below).

Pseudopolymorphism

Changes in crystallisation processes can also result in inclusion of molecules of the solvent in the crystal, producing solvates (or in the unique case where water is included, hydrates). These crystals have different properties from the non-solvated sample, in a similar manner to different polymorphic forms, and are thus often termed 'pseudopolymorphs'. It has been shown that different solvates of the same drug can produce different blood concentrations following administration of a solid oral dosage form. However, whereas with polymorphs it is the form with the lowest melting point that will produce the highest blood concentrations, for solvates it can sometimes be the hydrate and for other drugs the anhydrous form that produces the highest concentrations.[1]

Crystal Habit

Habit is the term given to the outward appearance of a crystal. It is possible to change polymorphic form without altering habit and equally to change habit while maintaining the same polymorphic form; the two parameters are independent. Habit can be described by variations on the theme of seven systems (cubic, tetragonal, orthorhombic, monoclinic, triclinic, trigonal, and hexagonal, see Table 1). The pharmaceutical significance of changes in habit can be an alteration in dissolution rate, powder flow, and compressibility; thus it can influence processing (for example, flow and compression during tableting[2]) and use of dosage forms. Dissolution rates are affected by the surface to volume ratio, while terms such as 'needle' (to describe the shape of acicular crystals) will indicate those that will have poor flow properties.

Table 1
Angles and lengths of axes that describe crystal habits

Crystal (synonym)	Angles of axes	Length of axes	Example
Cubic (regular)	$\alpha = \beta = \gamma = 90°$	$x = y = z$	sodium chloride
Tetragonal	$\alpha = \beta = \gamma = 90°$	$x = y \neq z$	nickel sulphate
Orthorhombic	$\alpha = \beta = \gamma = 90°$	$x \neq y \neq z$	potassium permanganate
Monoclinic	$\alpha = \beta = 90° \neq \gamma$	$x \neq y \neq z$	sucrose
Triclinic (asymmetric)	$\alpha \neq \beta \neq \gamma \neq 90°$	$x \neq y \neq z$	copper sulphate
Trigonal (rhombohedral)	$\alpha = \beta = \gamma \neq 90°$	$x = y = z$	sodium nitrate
Hexagonal	z at 90° to base	—	silver nitrate

Habit can be altered by changes in the crystallisation process. The habit is determined by the rate of growth of the different faces of the crystal. The fastest growing faces will tend to grow out of existence, and will, therefore, be the smallest faces on the final crystal, whereas the slow growing faces will dominate the final structure. As different faces can exhibit different proportions of the functional groups that make up the drug molecule, changes in the crystallising solvent may preferentially favour the interaction with different faces and consequently alter habit. The presence of impurities can result in adsorption at certain faces, which in turn can prevent (or slow) drug deposition to these faces, thus altering the growth rates of the exposed areas. Such adaptations can be accidental, due to impurities, breakdown products, or synthetic precursors in the crystallisation mixture, or deliberate due to the specific addition of impurities (such as surfactants). A well cited example of this is the modification of adipic acid crystals by Fairbrother and Grant.[3,4] The preformulation scientist should consider the optimum form of habit and, if possible, influence crystallisation procedures to ensure optimum properties are not due to serendipity, but rather a consequence of crystal engineering. Crystal habit and morphology are best investigated by microscopy. Standard light microscopes fitted with polarising filters and phase contrast facilities can allow crystals to be visualised with ease, and habit and size to be quantified (for further detail on size, see Physicomechanical Properties below).

Crystal Defects

Bulk crystallisation of drug substances will be prone to produce imperfect crystals. The imperfections will be due to point defects and dislocations during the packing of the lattice. The addition (or accidental presence) of low concentrations of impurities will increase the disruption in the lattice. Disruptions in the crystal lattice can result in major changes in the ease of processing, chemical reactivity, and dissolution rate, and hence bioavailability.[5] York and Grant[5,6] have described a method by which it is possible to define a disruption index to quantify the disorder induced by additives and/or impurities in crystals. The disruption index can be calculated from differential scanning calorimetry measurements or from calorimetric measurements of the enthalpy of solution (see Thermal Methods for further details of these instruments).

Optical Isomers

Historically, attempts were not generally made to separate optical isomers for most compounds. However, drugs with one or more chiral centres are now given special consideration, as the preferred isomer must be identified and any other isomers regarded as impurities. It is important to identify the correct isomer and to eliminate all others. Considerable effort is being invested in the development of column-based systems for the separation of isomers.

Summary of Tests Relating to Crystal Properties

Standard tests should include melting point (to provide an indication of purity and crystal form) and thermal analysis (see separate section). It is usual to obtain a photomicrograph or for very small particles a scanning electron micrograph, from which comment about habit can be made. For the photomicrograph, image enhancement may be utilised (for example, polarised light). The tests described under Physicomechanical Properties are also relevant to crystal form. The aims are to identify the polymorph, solvate, habit, and optical isomer and to monitor the changes in properties against subsequent batches of drug.

Conclusions

The crystallisation process will influence the behaviour of the drug, in terms of its physical and chemical stability, its processability, and its bio-pharmaceutical performance. Inappropriate crystallisation procedures can make a successful formulation unnecessarily difficult to achieve. There are precedents for the selection of appropriate crystallisation procedures to yield optimum properties for the drug.[7] Subsequent to crystallisation, the processing of the drug substance will also potentially alter its physical properties (see Physicomechanical Properties below). The influence of physical changes in materials upon processing and bioavailability cannot be overemphasised.

PHYSICOMECHANICAL PROPERTIES

The important physicomechanical properties of a drug are its particle size distribution, density, surface area, wettability, hygroscopicity, flow, and compression properties. Many of these properties are influenced or controlled by crystallisation procedures, however, it is equally true that processing (such as milling) can affect many or all of these critical parameters.

Particle Size Analysis

The size of particles can affect processability and dissolution rate. For high potency drugs, it can be advantageous to have small particle sizes to maximise the number of particles in order to allow adequate mixing and dose uniformity. However, static charges can be of greater significance with small particles and this can result in aggregation and, ironically, poor mixing; thus it is important to balance the desired properties. Obtaining a particle size distribution for a powder is easy, a range of instruments being available for the task. However, the result that is given may require careful interpretation and may not be a true reflection of the particle size of the powder. For many systems, sizing is not as straightforward as it may seem. The first approach to sizing is to use a microscope with a calibrated graticule in order to estimate the size with which to compare the result of the automated system. Care should be taken with the presentation of particle size data, which may, for example, be 'by number' or 'by mass'. Microscopy will give a 'by number' result in which each particle is measured and the numbers in each predefined size band are counted. On a 'by number' distribution, if a sample of 500 particles contained 495 small particles and 5 large particles, the large particles would be 1% of the distribution by number. Other techniques often have data presentation 'by weight', whereby a sample with many small particles and only a few large particles may, in fact, have a high percentage of large particles by weight (for example, 40%), as one large particle contains the equivalent weight of material of many small particles. The 'by weight' distributions are more useful in describing the particle size distribution of pharmaceutical systems.

The automated sizing techniques, which have the advantage of giving distributions by weight, can present problems as they assume spherical particles and make no allowance for aggregation. Many pharmaceutical crystals are acicular and few are spherical, thus the error can be significant, depending upon the aspect ratio of the particle. Drugs tend to aggregate in suspension, especially small particles (with a high electrostatic charge density). Aggregation can be worse if the particles are not adequately dispersed in the suspending solvent (for example, partially hydrophobic solids in water). Surfactants are often used to aid dispersion, in which case care must be taken to ensure that the smaller (more rapidly soluble) particles are not dissolved in preference to the large particles in a solubilising medium. The relationship between particle size and the apparent solubility of a drug (S_r) is obtained from the Gibbs Kelvin relation, which for submicron particles demonstrates that the true equilibrium solubility (that of an infinitely large particle, S_∞) of the drug can be exceeded due to the high interfacial energy that exists between the solid and the liquid (γ_{SL}) for very small particles, of radius r:

$$\log\left(\frac{S_r}{S_\infty}\right) = \frac{2\gamma_{SL}M}{2.303\,RT\rho r}$$

where M is the molecular weight, R is the gas constant, T is the absolute temperature, and ρ is the density of the solid.

There are two popular types of automated sizing instruments, the Coulter counter and those that use laser light diffraction (for example, Malvern). The Coulter counter method involves the dispersion of particles in an electrolyte (it can be difficult to find a suitable electrolyte for samples that cannot be dispersed in aqueous liquids). The instrument draws the electrolyte through a small orifice, and detects the conductance through the liquid. As particles pass through the orifice the conductance is changed and the response is proportional to the size of the particle that passes through. The approximate powder size must be known in order to select an appropriate size of tube orifice. The Malvern type of instrument detects diffraction of a laser light, the dispersion of which is inversely proportional to the size of the particle that passes through the beam.

A value for a median size is not an adequate description of a sample; some indication of the distribution around the median is needed. This is often obtained by quoting an interquartile range. Having obtained the size of the material, the data is presented as a distribution. This is conventionally done by plotting a cumulative percentage oversize (or undersize) as a function of log of size, which will yield a sigmoidal graph that can be linearised (to aid the calculation of interquartile range) by plotting it on log probability paper.

Surface Area

One of the reasons for controlling particle size is that changes will alter the available surface area and consequently affect dissolution and potentially bioavailability. In this respect, size is a crude indication of surface area. Most automated sizing instruments will give a value for the surface area of the sample. This is calculated assuming that the particles are spheres and as this is almost always untrue the result will be a crude estimation of the true surface area. A more appropriate test for surface area is by a BET (Brunauer, Emmett, and Teller) gas adsorption experiment.[8] It is usual to adsorb nitrogen gas onto a packed column of powder. This is done by passing nitrogen over the sample and detecting the output, and then quenching the sample in liquid nitrogen, such that the nitrogen gas inside the column will adsorb onto the available surface; from the reduced output of nitrogen gas the amount adsorbed is assessed and from the cross-sectional area of a nitrogen molecule the surface area of the solid is estimated using the BET isotherm equation. Similar experiments can be undertaken using krypton (giving improved accuracy) and some workers utilise water sorption to provide an indication of the effective surface area available to water molecules.

Wetting

The degree of wetting of a solid by a liquid can control its effective surface area. A finely divided powder (high surface area) that is poorly wetted will have a limited interface with the liquid, because the powder will tend to aggregate[9] and air will be trapped at the powder surface preventing contact with the liquid. Wells[10] states that wetting is an important factor in controlling solubility and can be influenced by changes in salt form and by recrystallising to change habit. Wetting is indeed influenced by chemical variation of the molecule and

as different faces of a crystal can express different proportions of the functional groups that make up the molecule, wetting will also be influenced (to some extent) by crystallisation. However, a significant factor that affects wetting is that of physical processing. Buckton et al[11] have demonstrated that significantly different wettabilities can be observed by changes in the processes used to mill a drug. These changes are undoubtedly a function of disordering the outer molecules of the crystal, possibly causing changes in the degree of crystallinity of the surface. Thus, the duration of changes in wettability will be linked to the tendency for the surface to recrystallise (for example, humidity and storage temperature) and the crystal form that is produced upon surface recrystallisation. There is no doubt that changes in the physical processing of materials can cause sufficiently large changes in properties to completely alter the subsequent processing or the functional performance of the product.

The use of wettability data to predict product performance has been a central issue of a number of publications.[9, 12–15] The concept is that during preformulation studies, the wettability of the drug is assessed and this is utilised to estimate the surface energy and polarity. These values are then compared with a library of data for commonly used excipients and the most logical choice of adjuvants is then made, rather than resorting to a trial and error approach. This concept forms the starting point for 'expert systems', whereby computer-aided formulation should allow the development of an initial formulation on the basis of physicochemical characteristics of the drug (preformulation).

Determining Values for Contact Angle and Surface Energies

While it is possible to assess wettability by use of calorimetric methods,[16] the most utilised method is to determine the value of a contact angle. For powdered systems this is not straightforward and the available techniques are all flawed.[16] Most workers use an approach whereby a drop of liquid is placed upon the surface of a presaturated powder compact and the angle is either measured directly (difficult due to dynamic effects), photographed and measured, or the maximum height of liquid drop measured from which the contact angle can be calculated.[17] A contact angle (θ) is formed due to a balance of the interfacial forces between the solid/liquid (γ_{SL}), the liquid/vapour (γ_{LV}), which is the surface tension of the liquid, and the solid/vapour (γ_{SV}), and is expressed by Young's equation:

$$\gamma_{LV} \cos \theta = \gamma_{SV} - \gamma_{SL}$$

While it is impossible to measure directly the terms for solid interfacial energy, it is possible to estimate values for them by measuring contact angles for two liquids of known surface tension on the unknown solid. If the surface tension is divided into two components (polar and dispersion), it is also possible to calculate the polarity of the solid (see Zografi and Tam[18] for detail of calculation method). Having determined the polar (p) and dispersion (d) components for the surface energy of the solid, it is possible to compare these with similar values for any other potential component of the formulation by calculation of a spreading coefficient (λ), which is shown here for the general case of phase 1 spreading over phase 2:

$$\lambda_{1,2} = 4 \left[\frac{\gamma_1^p \cdot \gamma_2^p}{\gamma_1^p + \gamma_2^p} + \frac{\gamma_1^d \cdot \gamma_2^d}{\gamma_1^d + \gamma_2^d} - \frac{\gamma_1}{2} \right]$$

A positive value for the spreading coefficient of phase 1 over phase 2 will indicate that phase 1 will indeed spread over phase 2; such a situation may be desirable in the example of a binder for use in wet granulation. Thus, having determined the surface energy and polarity of the drug, the correct binder can be selected before attempting to make the formulation. The value of spreading coefficients of binders over drugs has been shown to correlate with the properties of the subsequent tablet.[14] Equally, this approach can be used to predict the tendency for a drug to aggregate in suspension[9, 15] and to alert the formulator to any potential difficulties regarding drug loss due to adhesion to the container wall.[9] This form of physicochemical profiling of drug substances offers great advantages if correctly utilised during preformulation. Although the use of surface energies and their constituent polar and dispersion components has been shown to have advantage in pharmaceutical material characterisation, the theory has now been developed and it is deemed more appropriate to consider surface energies in three distinct terms: dispersion, Lewis acid, and Lewis base. The acid/base components are an alternative way of describing interactions that were previously deemed to be polar; they allow more adequate differentiation between materials.[19, 20]

Hygroscopicity and Water Sorption

The vast majority of pharmaceutical materials sorb water from the atmosphere in different amounts, as a function of atmospheric conditions (temperature and relative humidity (RH)). This is true for even the most 'hydrophobic' of pharmaceutical materials. For example, magnesium stearate, which is acknowledged as a hydrophobic lubricant, contains in excess of 3% equilibrium moisture content at ambient conditions. It follows that there is a paradox regarding wettability. It is often desirable to have good wetting by water, to allow for rapid drug dissolution, but equally this could lead to significant hygroscopicity and thus instability. With a high content of sorbed water, stability problems can be both chemical and microbiological. Even tableted products will show mould growth if the relative humidity and water sorption are high enough. As described above, the wettability of a drug, and hence hygroscopicity, can be influenced by changes in salt form, crystallisation process, and physical manipulation (such as milling). It is, of course, possible to change the wettability to promote dissolution and then to package the product to limit water vapour sorption.

Water sorption can be due to either adsorption to the solid surface or absorption within the solid. It has been shown that even multilayer adsorption equates to no more than 3 to 5 layers of water molecules around the solid and that is likely to be too low a water content to affect stability. Amorphous solids take up water by absorption, and it is likely that recently milled surfaces will be partially amorphous, and thus will absorb water. The water content of amorphous regions can be far more significant than that of adsorbed water. Simple considerations for water content per unit weight of material can give totally misleading impressions of the effects of water sorption, as the water will not be evenly distributed. Ahlneck and Zografi[21] describe this amplification of water content by considering a solid which contains 0.5% w/w of water. For such a solid it can reasonably be assumed that the majority of that water is in amorphous regions. Thus it is possible that if the amorphous component is 5%, then the water content in the amorphous region will be 10% and if the amorphous material is only 0.5% of the total weight then the water content in this region will be 100% (that is, 100 mg water for each 100 mg of amorphous material in the solid). It is this process of amplification that is responsible for the drastic effects of water in solids. For example, this water may then allow some local dissolution and subsequently result in surface recrystallisation and by extension result in the surface only adsorbing rather than absorbing water. Thus, the storage conditions after processing can influence the properties of the solid surface; even if the conditions are not optimised to ensure the surface behaves in its most suitable manner, storage conditions should at least be rigidly controlled (to prevent batch to batch variation).

If a solid is crystalline and still takes up substantial quantities of water, it is likely that the water is in the form of a non-stoichiometric hydrate. Modelling of crystal structures has revealed that certain solids contain channels into which water can position itself without significantly affecting the X-ray pattern of the crystal. Such water is loosely associated, readily removed, and consequently may present problems in formulations. It is likely that the water associated with magnesium stearate is in this form.

Powder Flow

Good flow properties of powders are essential for uniform filling into dies of tableting machines and for easy movement of materials around a production facility. Flow properties are affected by particle size and shape, with larger more rounded particles giving improved flow. Flow is difficult to measure with the small amount of material that is present at the start of preformulation studies, but if measured it will be a good indicator of changes that are occurring as chemical manufacture of the drug is scaled up.

The angle of repose is one method by which flow is measured. Here the powder is allowed to fall under gravity and the angle of incline of the formed cone that is produced is assessed (by measuring the height and having a fixed size base). The better the flow properties, the lower the angle (less than 30° would constitute good flow).

An alternative test is to determine the Carr's index, which relates the poured (often termed 'fluff') density of the material (the volume occupied by a certain mass when gently poured into a measure) to the tapped density (the volume occupied by that same mass of powder after a standard tapping of the measure):

Carr's index =

$$\frac{\text{tapped density} - \text{poured density}}{\text{tapped density}} \times 100$$

Values below 15 would indicate excellent flow, whereas powders with values over 20 to 30 would have poor flow. The Hausner ratio is a similar index, which is calculated simply by dividing the tapped density by the poured density.

Compression Characteristics

The acquisition of information on the compression properties of a drug involves the use of considerable quantities of powder. As drug supply is likely to be limited, the value of compressibility tests must be weighed against the fact that many other tests may not be possible if so much of the drug has been devoted to this investigation. The benefit to be derived from compression testing is an indication of whether the drug is elastic, plastic, or brittle. In order to make a good tablet, there is a need for brittle fracture and plastic flow; elasticity is also often present, but is not a desirable property. It is advisable to determine the properties of the drug, and attempt to match these with the complimentary diluent. For example, if the drug is a plastic material the diluent should compact by brittle fracture (for example, lactose). If the drug is a brittle material it is best to mix it with a plastic excipient, such as microcrystalline cellulose. This is only necessary for fairly high dose products which are to be made by direct compression, for high potency drugs compression aids can effectively mask the drug's compression properties. For granulated products, the properties of the binder can become critical.

A simple method has been reported[10] by which it is possible to assess the plastic or brittle compaction properties of a drug; arguing that three 500 mg aliquots of drug should be weighed, two of these (1) and (2) should be blended with magnesium stearate 1% for 5 minutes, and the other (3) for 30 minutes, in a tumbler mixer. Formulations (1) and (3) should be compressed for one second, and (2) for 30 seconds. Each compact should be stored overnight in a sealed container. The force (F) required to break each tablet should be measured. If F is greater for (2) than (1); greater for (1) than (3); and if F for (2) is greater than (1), which is greater than (3), then the drug is likely to be plastic. If all the values of F are essentially the same, then it is likely to be brittle. Elastic materials will tend to laminate, especially (1) and (3). The reasons for the changes in behaviour are that plastic materials, unlike fracturing solids, do not form new surfaces on compaction, so they will tend to be more susceptible to the degree of lubricant mixing. Equally, plastic materials tend to show a greater influence of dwell time.

The use of instrumented tableting machines and compaction simulators allows a considerable body of data to be collected regarding compaction mechanisms, and thus allows a plan for formulation development. Instrumented machines afford a method of determining compaction mechanisms,[22] which provide a predictive capability of tablet strength (and maybe even dissolution), and create a database from which it is possible to detect changes in drug properties due to bulk manufacture processes. Instrumented machines (or compaction simulators) seem to be the most appropriate method by which to monitor compaction and by which to develop and then monitor a formulation after it is in production. Tableting machine instrumentation has been reviewed extensively.[23]

Summary of Tests Relating to Physicomechanical Properties

The following information should be recorded: particle size (median and distribution), there may be more than one set of data depending upon the methods used (for example, Malvern and microscopy); surface area (perhaps before and after milling); presence or absence of static charge; angle of repose; bulk density and tapped bulk density, and derived indices; compressibility; hygroscopicity (as weight gain/loss at defined time intervals, in days, at defined temperatures); contact angle (and possible derived parameters).

SOLUBILITY

An understanding of the solubility of a drug can be regarded as the most important aspect of preformulation testing. Drugs are generally less stable when in solution and, consequently, it is often desirable to limit aqueous solubility in a liquid dosage form.

Factors Affecting Solubility

When a solute (solid or liquid) dissolves in a solvent (liquid), the liquid volume does not increase by as much as would be expected by additivity. It follows that the solute must be fitting into 'cavities' within the liquid structure. The simplest model of solubility is that the process can be divided into three parts: firstly, it is necessary to remove a molecule from the solute; secondly, it is necessary to prepare a cavity in the solvent in which to house the dislodged solute molecule; and thirdly, the solute molecule is positioned in the cavity. On the basis of this simple model, solubility is related to the strength of solute-solute bonds (that is, lattice energy for crystals, which is often mirrored by melting point), the solvent-solvent bond strength (ease of making a cavity, which may be linked to the boiling point), the size of the solute molecule

(larger molecules require larger cavities), and finally, the interaction between the solute and solvent. If this model is expressed in terms of work involved, then the work required to dissolve each molecule of solid solute (W) will be:

$$W = W_{SS} + W_{LL} - 2W_{SL}$$

where W_{SS}, W_{LL}, and W_{SL} are the bond strengths between two solid (solute) molecules, two liquid molecules, and a detached solute molecule and a liquid molecule respectively. On the basis of this model, solubility will depend upon the lattice energy of the solid (for example, polymorphism, crystal defects), the nature of the liquid (which can be adjusted with additives, such as cosolvents), and the interaction between the two. The interaction between a solute and a solvent will depend upon chemical and physical properties of the solute and solvent. The chemical aspects determine the polarity of the molecule, which can be considered on the generalisation that 'like dissolves like'. The physical properties of the molecule relate to ionisation, the extent of which will greatly influence the interaction with a solvent. Ionised species are much more soluble in water than unionised, whereas the opposite is true for non-polar solvents.

pK_a

Most drug molecules contain ionisable groups, existing either as weak acids or weak bases.

Solubility of Weak Acids

Weak acids, such as the non-steroidal anti-inflammatory drugs, will dissociate in water:

$$HA \rightleftharpoons H^+ + A^-$$

The solubility (S) of the weak acid will relate to the solubility of the unionised (S_{HA}) and the ionised (S_A) form:

$$S \rightleftharpoons S_{HA} + S_{A^-}$$

From this equation, the dissociation constant K_a is given by

$$K_a = \frac{[H^+][A^-]}{[HA]}$$

Substituting $[A^-] = S_A = S - S_{HA}$; and $[HA] = S_{HA}$ into the above equation and rearranging

$$\frac{K_a}{[H^+]} = \frac{S - S_{HA}}{S_{HA}}$$

Taking logarithms, and remembering that pH $= -\log_{10}[H^+]$, and p$K_a = -\log_{10} K_a$

$$pH - pK_a = \log\frac{S - S_{HA}}{S_{HA}}$$

Thus, if solubility is measured at a point where only the unionised form of the drug is present, then $S = S_{HA}$, the pK_a of the drug can be calculated. Having determined the pK_a, it is possible to calculate the solubility at any other pH using the same equation. This allows a prediction of the range of pH over which it is possible to achieve a desired concentration of drug in solution, and conversely, pH values at which a drug will precipitate. S_{HA} is often termed the 'intrinsic solubility' of the drug and is often given the symbol C_0.

Solubility of Weak Bases

Basic drugs (which can be represented as $R-NH_2$) are ionised, and thus more soluble in acidic solutions. The expression for the solubility (S) of a base is the sum of the intrinsic solubility (C_0) (solubility of the undissociated form $R-NH_2$), and the solubility of the ionised form. The expression of solubility and intrinsic solubility as a function of pH can be determined exactly as above and is found to be:

$$pH - pK_a = \log\left(\frac{C_0}{S - C_0}\right)$$

Solubility of Amphoteric Drugs

Amphoteric drugs, such as oxytetracycline, exhibit both acidic and basic groups and the dissociation can be represented as follows:

$$R-X-COOH \rightleftharpoons R-X-COO^- \rightleftharpoons R-X-COO^-$$
$$\underset{\text{at low pH}}{\overset{|}{NH_3^+}} \qquad \overset{|}{NH_3^+} \qquad \underset{\text{at high pH}}{\overset{|}{NH_2}}$$

In this case, two dissociation constants can be defined, one from the cation (which will be present at low pH) to the zwitterion, and the other from the zwitterion to the anion (which will be present at high pH). The zwitterion will exist at the isoelectric point, which will be the point of minimum solubility (C_0). The solubility can be predicted for solutions at pH values above and below the isoelectric point by use of the equations above. For amphoteric drugs, there will not be a single value for pK_a, for example, oxytetracycline has three different values, reflecting the three different ionisable regions on the molecule.

Salts

The value obtained for the intrinsic solubility will identify potential bioavailability problems for a drug molecule. Kaplan[24] stated that an aqueous solubility of less than 10 mg/mL over a pH range of 1 to 7 at 37° is indicative of potential difficulties and that a value of less than 1 mg/mL would indicate that consideration should be given to salt formation. The particular salt form that is selected will alter the chemical and physical properties of the drug, for example, the pK_a of the drug and its interaction with the solvent will change. Wells[10] has shown that changes in salt form can result in increases in solubility by nearly two orders of magnitude (for example, chlordiazepoxide from 2 to 165 mg/mL).

Other Factors Affecting Solubility
Temperature

The variation of solubility (expressed as mole fraction dissolved—x) with temperature (T) for an ideal system (one in which there is no solute-solvent interaction) is given by:

$$\log x = \frac{-\Delta H_f}{2.303\,R}\left(\frac{T_m - T}{T_m T}\right)$$

where ΔH_f is the enthalpy of fusion of the crystal, T_m is the melting point and R is the gas constant. Very few systems follow ideality, most deviate significantly due to solute-solvent interaction. Most crystalline solids do have a higher solubility at higher temperatures, although the extent to which solubility increases for any given temperature rise is dependent upon the solid and the solvent. Rarely, some solids are more soluble at low temperatures (for example, some polymers such as hypromellose).

Common Ion Effect

As the solubility of electrolytes has been shown to depend upon their degree of ionisation, factors that reduce ionisation will reduce the solubility. Thus, weak electrolytes in the presence of a common ion, such as a hydrochloride salt of a weak acid in the stomach, will show significantly lower solubility than at an equivalent pH with the common ion absent.[25]

Solubilisation

On occasions it may be desirable to measure the solubility of a drug after first having overcome an adverse wettability by adding a surfactant to the solvent. In aqueous solutions, above a certain concentration (the critical micelle concentration, cmc) surfactant molecules self associate to internalise the hydrophobic portion of their molecules. In such circumstances drug solubility can be elevated by incorporation within this hydrophobic core. If the desired effect is to increase wetting, and not to alter solubility, surfactants should only be used at concentrations below the cmc.

Crystal Purity

During the earliest stages of development, the drug substance will be in its most pure state; almost without exception the process of scale-up of bulk drug manufacture will result in lower purity. Furthermore, the impurity profile may change upon scale-up. The presence of impurities can alter the solubility of the drug by, for example, solubilisation or the common ion effect. It may be advisable to deliberately add possible impurities (for example, breakdown products) into the early batches before preformulation, otherwise limits set on the high purity material (regarding solubility and stability) will be impossible to achieve in full scale production.

Measurement of Solubility

Equilibrium solubility is measured by shaking an excess of the solid solute in the presence of the solvent, in a sealed container at a defined temperature. After equilibration, a sample is withdrawn, the solid is filtered off, and the liquid assayed. This process is repeated until the concentration measured does not rise on successive measurements. The problems that occur include difficulties in filtering out colloidal particles of solid (which interfere with analysis) and instability of the solute in the solvent. Solids are normally much less stable when wet and often a compromise must be reached, whereby solubility is measured before it has truly come to equilibrium, in order to prevent excessive degradation. If the solvent is highly volatile or if the solution has been equilibrated at elevated temperatures, precipitation can occur during filtration and assay; this must be avoided.

Flow-through methods of solubility determination can speed the time taken to reach equilibrium. In such methods the solvent is circulated and allowed to percolate through a bed of the solid supported on a filter. The effluent can be collected and then passed directly through a flow-through ultraviolet (UV) spectrophotometer.

Rate of Drug Dissolution

When considering the drug release from a solid oral dosage form, it is the rate at which it goes into solution that is often of greater interest than the equilibrium solubility. In the majority of cases, however, dissolution rate (expressed as the rate of change of mass with time, dm/dt) is directly proportional to equilibrium solubility under sink conditions (where sink conditions refer to the concentration in solution (C) being very much lower than the equilibrium solubility (C_s), which is often defined as C being no more than 10% to 20% of C_s) as indicated by the Noyes-Whitney relationship:

$$\frac{dm}{dt} = \frac{DA(C_s - C)}{h}$$

where D is the diffusion coefficient of the dissolving solute moving away from the solid, A is the surface area of the solid, and h is the thickness of the thin stationary film of solution around the surface of the solid (the diffusion layer). In order to obtain a value for dissolution rate that is related to a property of the material, it is necessary to force A to be constant. This is achieved by preparing a cylindrical compact of the drug and coating all but one circular face with wax. The compact is then secured (to a flat metal stirrer) and rotated at 100 rpm, 20 mm from the bottom of a one-litre compendial dissolution flask, with fluid at 37°. The standard vessel geometry and stirring rate will yield constant hydrodynamic regimens for constant geometry discs. As long as the disc does not swell or disintegrate, dm/dt will give an intrinsic dissolution rate (mg/mm^2).

Solvent

As described above, the solvent plays a major role in controlling solubility. It may be desirable to use solvents to either increase (for example, to form an intravenous solution) or decrease (to form a more stable suspension) solubility of a drug. It is also possible to attempt to alter physiological solvents, such as adding components to formulations that buffer the local environment around a dosage form. Another reason for considering other solvents may be to facilitate extraction of a drug for analysis. Solvents that are used can conveniently be divided into three groups: those that are mixed with water in formulation, those that are mixed with water for extraction and analysis, and those that do not mix with water. The first group are termed 'cosolvents' and their function is to mix with the water in order to alter its physical properties. The aim of cosolvency will either be to make poorly soluble drugs of low polarity more soluble or polar unstable drugs less soluble (although this a comparatively rare approach). Examples of cosolvents are ethanol, glycerol, macrogols, and propylene glycol. The second class of solvents include organic compounds that are miscible with water, but are not suitable for use in a formulation on toxicity grounds (for example, methanol). Methanol is a good solvent in which to dissolve poorly water-soluble drugs and is used widely for extraction and analysis. Preformulation studies should involve investigations into solubility in these non-aqueous systems.

The final group of solvents are the oils (for example, liquid paraffin, arachis oil, fractionated coconut oil, isopropyl myristate). These would be used in two-phase systems such as emulsions and creams. Multiple phase formulations are useful to remove unstable non-polar drugs from an aqueous environment. However, interest in solvents that are immiscible with water is also central to calculation of partition coefficients.

Partition Coefficient

When a drug is dissolved in an aqueous liquid and then brought into contact with a non-aqueous liquid, there will be a partitioning of the solute between the two liquid phases until the activities of the drug in both phases are equal. The concentration that partitions to the non-aqueous phase will depend upon the relative interactions between the drug and water, and the drug and the 'oil'. In effect, the partition coefficient will provide an indication of the hydrophilic/lipophilic balance of the molecule. This may well be different from the wettability of the drug crystal as the crystal exhibits functional groups in its surface in a manner related to the crystallising solvent and the subsequent physical processing of the solid, which may not be in proportion to the sum of the functional groups of the molecule itself.[26] The following uses are extracted and adapted from a list of applications of partition coefficients that was presented by Wells:[10]

- assessment of the solubility in aqueous and mixed solvents
- indication of biological response
- extraction of drug from aqueous fluids (especially blood and urine)
- aid the choice of column or mobile phase for chromatographic analysis
- establish levels of drug and/or preservative in the aqueous phase of emulsions
- predict the release of drug from semi-solids, such as ointment bases.

Choice of Partitioning Solvent

As listed above, one of the major advantages of partition coefficients is that they offer a prediction of the tendency for a drug to move from an aqueous compartment into a membrane, and consequently have been found to correlate well with biological response.[27–29] It is conventional to use octanol as the non-aqueous solvent for such experiments, however, the question must be addressed as to whether this solvent is the best model of a biological membrane. Octanol contains a moderately long lipophilic chain and a polar (hydrophilic) head group, thus molecules will align in a manner similar to that of a membrane structure. The Collander equation relates the water/solvent partitioning behaviour of a solute in one system (P_1) to the value obtained for the same solute partitioning from water to a different solvent (P_2):

$$\ln P_1 = a + b \ln P_2$$

The Collander equation is a simple and indeed simplistic method of relating partition in different solvents; it is by no means universally applicable. However, the values obtained for the constants a and b are usable for homologous series of solutes and often for similar solvents (that is, those of similar polarity, hydrogen bonding capacity, etc.). It has been suggested that the value of the constant a reflects the solvent lipophilicity and the water content of the solvent at saturation.[30] The values of b are reported to reflect the similarity of the solvent environment with respect to the solute.[31, 32] For non-polar solvents, values of b are higher than for polar solvents. Beezer et al[33] reported values of the gradient b for a number of solvents and some liposomes (as model biological membranes) (see Table 2). In this example, all solvent systems were scaled with reference to octanol/water partitioning. Assuming that liposomes are a reasonable model of biological membranes, then it is probable that a log P between water and octanol will not be a perfect indication of partition into a membrane.

Table 2

Values of b calculated for partitioning between water and various solvents and liposomes, using water/octanol as partitioning system 2 in the Collander equation

Solvent system 1 Water	Solute	b
Propylene carbonate	m-Alkoxy phenols	0.36
Liposome ($T < T_c$)	21-Alkyl esters of hydrocortisone	0.546
Isopropyl myristate	21-Alkyl esters of cortisone	0.582
Liposome ($T > T_c$)	21-Alkyl esters of hydrocortisone	0.616
Isopropyl myristate	21-Alkyl esters of hydrocortisone	0.625
Liposome ($T < T_c$)	21-Alkyl esters of cortisone	0.672
Octanol	All solutes, by definition	1.0
Heptane	m-Alkoxy phenols	1.04
Diethyl ether	21-Alkyl esters of cortisone	1.30
Diethyl ether	21-Alkyl esters of hydrocortisone	1.53

(T_c—lipid phase transition temperature of the liposome)

The success of a partition coefficient in predicting biological response is likely to depend upon the solubility of water in the non-aqueous solvent used. The solvents (including the liposomes) with lower b values (see Table 2) have a higher water content than octanol, as do, for example, the lower chain length alcohols. Such solvents (relatively polar, compared to octanol) are likely to provide a better, and more discriminating, indication of biological response. Conversely, less polar solvents such as hydrocarbons will be less discriminating and consequently provide a poor indication of biological response. However, despite the non-ideality of octanol as a solvent to predict biological response, in terms of preformulation testing, on the basis of consistency and due to the enormous body of data that already exists, it undoubtedly remains as the partitioning solvent of choice.

Solubility Parameter

The intermolecular forces that act within a non-polar solvent are often described in terms of a solubility parameter (δ_1), which is defined as:

$$\delta_1 = \left[\frac{\Delta_{\text{VAP}} H - RT}{V} \right]^{\frac{1}{2}}$$

where $\Delta_{\text{VAP}} H$ is the enthalpy of vaporisation and V is the molar volume of the solvent. The solvent capacity is related to the energy required to remove a molecule of the liquid from the liquid, thus the solubility parameter is essentially the cohesive energy density to the power $\frac{1}{2}$. It is possible to calculate the value of a solubility parameter for a solid (δ_2) by substituting a lattice energy term in the above equation, for example the enthalpy of fusion. Florence and Attwood[34] report on data that demonstrate that the square of the difference between the solubility parameters for the solute and the solvent forms a linear relationship with the log of the solubility:

$$\log S = c + m(\delta_2 - \delta_1)^2$$

where c and m are constants. Surprisingly, solubility parameters have been found to correlate well with membrane absorption and biological processes.[35]

Rowe[36] has used partial solubility parameters (dividing the solubility parameter into contribution for polar and dispersion interactions) to calculate the interactions between different phases of formulations as a preformulation screen (similar to that described for surface energies under Wetting).

Summary of Tests Relating to Solubility

The following should be recorded: solubility of different observed polymorphs/crystal forms; intrinsic solubility; pH-solubility profile, pK_a and other solubility data; selection of salt form (if required); solubility profiles of preferred crystal form in selected solvents at different temperatures; effect of, for example, surfactants on solubility; determination of partition coefficient; and particulate dissolution profile (as a function of pH if necessary).

STABILITY

A detailed account of drug stability is addressed in the chapter Stability of Medicinal Products.

As with many aspects of preformulation, stability studies should be considered in two ways: firstly, it is necessary to develop a profile for the drug substance and secondly, at an early stage, it is necessary to consider possible interactions between the drug and the excipients that are candidates for inclusion in the desired formulation. This will include, or develop into, studies between the drug/excipients and the package. Many of the tests undertaken on the drug alone will be repeated following the inclusion of excipients; this repetition is essential. In this respect, the aims of preformulation testing are to identify routes of degradation of the active substance, indicate the types of excipients that would improve stability (for example, antoxidants), and to screen other excipients that will be necessary for product manufacture to ensure that they will not adversely affect the product stability. In general, the aim of the formulator will be to produce a product with a shelf-life in the order of five years, during which time the original stated drug content should not have fallen to below a predetermined level (often 90 to 95%).

Kinetics and Order of Reaction

Any understanding of stability and the ability to define a shelf-life will depend upon an understanding of the order of reaction and the kinetics of that reaction. Kinetic theory allows the calculation of a rate constant for a reaction, which in turn allows the prediction of the future rate of change of concentration with time, provided that the order of reaction is known.

Many pharmaceutical processes, including certain degradation reactions, do not fit into any simple model of reaction kinetics. However, most degradation processes do fit to either first-order or zero-order equations. First-order reactions are described by an exponential fall in concentration of the reactant (drug) with time, the first-order rate constant (k_1) being obtained from the gradient of a semi-logarithmic plot:

$$\ln\left(\frac{C_t}{C_i}\right) = -K_1 t$$

where C_i and C_t are the molar concentration at the onset of the experiment and after time t, respectively. It follows that in absolute terms the amount of drug that is degraded will depend upon the initial drug concentration (C_i). The time taken for half of the remaining concentration to be degraded ($t_{50\%}$) will be constant and will be equal to ($0.693/k_1$). The majority of all definable rate processes resulting in degradation are first-order. However, while the hydrolysis of, for example, aspirin solution fits a first-order mechanism, the degradation of aspirin suspension is a better fit to a zero-order process.

Zero-order reactions are those in which the amount of drug degraded in any fixed time period will remain the same until the reaction stops (due to exhaustion of a reactant). This can be represented as:

$$C_i - C_t = k_0 t$$

The zero-order rate constant (k_0) can then be obtained as the gradient of the plot of amount remaining (often expressed as a percentage) as a function of time.

Chemical Stability

The primary causes of chemical instability of drug substances are hydrolysis and oxidation. These processes, especially oxidation, are often catalysed by light (photolysis), trace metal impurities, or both.

Solutions

Hydrolysis. Water is the major cause of drug instability. The process of hydrolysis can be affected by changes in temperature and pH.

Temperature. In general, a 10° increase in temperature will result in an approximately three-fold increase in rate constant. Changes in rate of reaction with temperature are often found to fit the Arrhenius relationship, which can be expressed in the form:

$$\ln k = \ln A - \frac{E_a}{RT}$$

in which A is the pre-exponential factor or the collision number, and E_a is the activation energy and is the energy that must be exceeded if the reaction is to take place. Thus a plot of the natural logarithm of the rate constant (k) as a function of $1/T$ will have a gradient of E_a/R. The higher the value of E_a the greater will be the influence of temperature upon the reaction. The Arrhenius equation can be used to obtain a prediction of shelf-life at lower temperatures (for example, room or below room temperature) from more rapid experiments involving degradation at higher temperatures. For this purpose, degradation rates are measured at elevated temperature (where the reaction will be significantly faster), and a plot of $\ln k$ as a function of $1/T$ is constructed. This line is then extrapolated to give a rate constant at room temperature, which in turn can be used to estimate a shelf-life for the product. Apart from experimental inaccuracies, the problem with such an approach is that the assumption is made that the reaction that is being monitored at an elevated temperature is the same reaction that will occur at room temperature; this is not necessarily so, as it is possible to pass activation barriers by increasing to a temperature below which there would be no reaction. Although it would be very unusual for any worker to rely on such accelerated storage tests for anything other than a rough estimation of product stability, surprisingly, many workers seem happy to do just that when differential scanning calorimetry is used instead of chemical analysis (see Thermal Methods below). Furthermore, although Arrhenius plots appear linear over the narrow temperature ranges that are used in pharmaceutical stability studies, they are in reality curvi-linear, as E_a is a temperature-dependent constant.[37] While accelerated tests have their value, the real time tests at ambient conditions are the only true indication of shelf-life.

Ionic Strength. The ionic strength (I) of a solution of any one salt is a dimensionless number that depends upon the valence of the ions present, as shown in Table 3. Thus the ionic strength of a salt M_2X_4 (which is $M^{4+}_2X^{2-}_4$) of molality m, would have an ionic strength of $12\,m/m^\ominus$ (where $m^\ominus$ is the standard state). Further details may be found in standard physical chemistry textbooks.[38] The Bronsted-Bjerrum equation, provides a linear relationship between the logarithm of the rate constant and the square root of I. The larger the value of I the faster the reaction rate. Ionic strength is often changed as a consequence of adjusting pH (with buffers) or by adding sodium chloride to adjust the tonicity of injections.

Table 3
Demonstration of ionic strengths of multivalent ions of molal concentrations

I	X^-	X^{2-}	X^{3-}	X^{4-}
M^+	1	3	6	10
M^{2+}	3	4	15	12
M^{3+}	6	15	9	42
M^{4+}	10	12	42	16

pH. The effect of pH on drug degradation is via a catalysis of reactions involving H^+ or OH^- ions. Ionic materials are more susceptible to hydrolysis than the undissociated form. Hydrogen and hydroxyl ions will act as catalysts for any type of hydrolysis and it is not necessary for the drug to bear the same, or indeed a different, charge to the solvent. This creates one of a number of dilemmas for the formulator; the drug will be most soluble when ionised, thus one would change pH to facilitate ionisation, however, this may result in conditions for poor stability. In such situations, it may be necessary to consider alternative methods of increasing solubility than pH changes; such a method may involve the addition of a cosolvent.

Solvent Effects on Stability

As mentioned in the section on solubility, solvents such as ethanol, glycerol, and propylene glycol can be added to a formulation to improve solubility. It is possible that making drugs soluble by changes in solvent, rather than pH, may assist in producing more stable solutions; this effect is related to the dielectric constant of the solvent (which in turn is related to solvent polarity). If both the drug and the solvent ion have the same charge (that is, hydrogen ions as a catalyst for cationic drugs or hydroxyl ions for anionic drugs) then adding solvents of low dielectric constant will lower the decomposition rate. Water and ethanol, for example, have dielectric constants of 80.4 and 25.7, respectively, at 20°. Conversely, if the charges are opposite, adding a solvent of a low dielectric constant will not aid stability. An alternative way of considering this situation is that if the reaction products are more polar than the drug, then the solvent should be made non-polar, and *vice versa*, thus minimising the existence of the breakdown product.

Alternative approaches to improving stability by changing the solvent include the addition of non-aqueous phases, for example, the production of oil-in-water emulsions that allow a drug to partition into the oil phase, but which retain the essential properties of an aqueous dosage form. Surfactants can be used at concentrations above their cmc in order to remove drug from solution (by solubilisation into the micelle). Solvents can be added to suppress solubility, thus allowing the formulation of a suspension that is often much more chemically stable than a solution.

Solid State

Drugs are generally more stable in the solid state than when dissolved. However, both hydrolysis and oxidation can still be a problem. In ordinary environmental conditions, hydrolysis of solid material occurs, as solids will sorb water vapour from the atmosphere. It is often observed that, while hydrolysis in solution will tend to follow first-order kinetics, hydrolysis in the solid state (due to moisture sorption) will tend to be analogous to degradation from a concentrated (or saturated) solution and follow zero-order kinetics. The change in kinetic mechanism demonstrates that it is unwise to extrapolate from observations in dilute solution in order to predict the stability in the solid state, as dilute and saturated solutions are completely different in their behaviour. Although all solid oral dosage forms contain some moisture, which may often be a desirable property (for example, compaction is aided by the presence of small percentages of moisture), excessive water sorption can be prevented by either adjustments to the formulation (to alter hygroscopicity) or by changes in packaging (for example, impervious blister packing).

The crystal form of the drug will affect stability,[1] due to a change in lattice energy. In this respect, changes in salt form, polymorphic form, and solvates will all alter the tendency for drugs to degrade. Weaker lattice energies (assessed by enthalpies of fusion and, approximately, by melting point) will tend to lead to greater instability.

Oxidation

Certain chemical entities are prone to oxidation. A characteristic of oxidative reactions is that they often result in coloured products, thus even in situations where the degradation product is non-toxic the product may be spoiled by a colour change. Such reactions will obviously be influenced by the amount of oxygen that gains access to the drug, and can be limited by packaging and by the addition of antoxidants. Antoxidants work by being readily oxidised themselves and thus removing free radicals before the drug can be degraded. Sodium metabisulphite is an example of an antoxidant. The presence of trace metal impurities and light can often act as a catalyst for the oxidation. The concentrations of trace metals can be ascertained by simple analysis and consequent limits can be set and maintained; the effect of light is harder to investigate.

Photolysis

Temperature is a uniform variable that is easy to control; however, light is not so straightforward. The damaging effects of light are related to intensity and inversely related to wavelength. Thus 'natural light' is not a single variable, as it is made up of light of many wavelengths and differing intensities. Consequently 'natural light' conditions vary widely depending upon geographical location. Electric lighting will have different wavelengths and intensities and it is important to know, and to control, these factors if storage tests are to be carried out. Any testing cabinets that are used should mimic daylight in terms of wavelength, but intensities can be varied in order to accelerate reactions. Unlike any other form of stability testing, the effect of light has no defined regulatory requirements at the present time.

Stability Testing Regimens

Accelerated isothermal storage regimens (suitable for progression to, but not sufficient to comply with all international requirements for, registration) may typically be 40°/75% relative humidity for up to six months, with other samples stored at 30° and 25° for longer durations. Samples would be sealed in the presence and absence of air, and also in a suitable light box.

It is important to realise that elevated storage testing can produce misleading results as activation steps may be passed by elevating temperature and allow reactions to proceed that would not occur at room temperature. Certain materials can change their physical state under stressed conditions,[21] for example, povidone is plasticised by water vapour, such that the glass transition temperature is changed from close to 100° at 40% relative humidity to below 40° at 75% relative humidity. Thus for povidone, storage at 40°/75% relative humidity will result in stability testing of the rubber form of the polymer, while at more usual humidities the polymer will be in its glassy state. It may be appropriate to investigate the properties of both the glass and rubber states, but not appropriate to assume that tests in the rubber state relate to ambient conditions.

ACTIVE COMPOUND AND EXCIPIENTS

Preformulation essentially relates to the characterisation of the physicochemical properties of the drug substance, but almost invariably this will be continued to consider some aspects of excipient compatibility and allow the formulator to proceed with a reasonable knowledge base. In this respect the dividing line between preformulation and formulation is inexact, probably because there is no need for such a dividing line in the practical situation. It is appropriate, therefore, to consider the influence of excipients on solubility, stability, and physicomechanical properties under the heading of preformulation. The true role of excipients will be to produce a stable, uniform product of high quality, and in some cases to influence the delivery of a drug to the desired location at the desired rate; thus excipients have a major impact on the field of biopharmaceutics.

Excipients and Solubility

Excipients may be used to alter solubility, by changing pH, cosolvency, solubilisation, and common ion effects, as described above. Equally, excipients can be used to alter the rate of solution, for example, by adding a surfactant to improve wetting or by adding a disintegrant to increase rapidly the available surface area for dissolution. Conversely, magnesium stearate (a commonly used tableting lubricant) is an example of a hydrophobic excipient that can potentially slow dissolution, causing a dilemma regarding factors that are important for ease of production of a high quality product and those which relate to product biopharmaceutics. An understanding of the physicochemical properties of the drug and careful consideration of the consequences of adding different excipients will allow the areas of potential difficulties, with respect to dissolution, to be highlighted at an early stage. The biopharmaceutical implications of excipient effects on drug solubility (in aqueous and non-aqueous media) may be considerable.

Excipients and Stability

Under the heading of preformulation, perhaps the most important aspect relating to excipients is their effect on drug stability. Excipients can accelerate the existing instabilities of drug substances or entirely new problems can arise due to a chemical incompatibility between the excipient and the drug. On occasion, instabilities occur as a consequence of a mixture of more than one excipient and the drug, whereby the three component system is unstable, but any binary mixture of the three is stable. It follows that screening, and in particular rapid screening, of excipients for potential interactions is a difficult study in which it is possible to obtain both false-positive and false-negative results. While the types of experiments described below are valuable, in order to highlight potential problems at an early stage, it must be stressed that they do not replace the need for storage of the full formulation under ambient conditions.

Possible Screening Methods

Many workers use thermal analysis techniques to screen for excipient/drug interactions. Such applications of thermal analysis are considered, along with their wider use, in the following section. It is apparent that certain thermal analysis investigations can give misleading results (see below), so it is unwise to rule out excipients for which there is no good alternative at an early stage simply on the basis of thermal analysis. Magnesium stearate is an example of an excipient that is used in very low concentrations in the final product and for which there are no good alternatives. These combined effects would make it worth confirming whether the observed threat of an interaction is going to become a serious problem in the final formulation at ambient conditions. However, if a diluent is implicated as having a potential interaction, it may be easy to select an alternative and this would be a wise precaution even if the original excipient may not present real difficulties.

One of the problems with screening excipients for incompatibilities is that, in order to be able to detect the interaction, it is usual to mix 50:50 proportions of drug and excipient. These concentrations are often totally unrealistic and can be the cause of problems in terms of false-positive results. Conversely, mixtures of realistic concentrations (for example, magnesium stearate at 0.5%) may result in little detectable change over the time scale of the experiment and yield false-negative results. In a powder mixture, the number of contact points and thus potentially particle size can influence the result. This can be overcome by preparing compacts of the 50:50 mixture in an infrared press. In order to speed any reactions that occur, it is usual to store the mixtures (or compacts) at an elevated temperature (for example, 50°) for a number of weeks before analysis by a chromatographic method. Stresses of humidity (75% relative humidity) can also be investigated, as can the presence and absence of oxygen and light.

Other Aspects Relating to Stability

Microbiological

The potential for microbial spoilage of pharmaceuticals is something that must be considered from an early stage. The process used to prepare sterile products will be selected on the basis of the stability of the product. Reaction rates are increased with heat and drugs that are liable to degradation will not survive a heat sterilisation process. The control of microbial contamination of non-sterile products is dependent upon the bioburden of raw materials and the extent to which contamination is introduced during processing. For naturally occurring materials, it is advisable to be aware of bioburden from an early stage. Many non-sterile products are protected from spoilage by the use of antimicrobial preservative agents. The preformulation scientist should be aware of how the physicochemical properties of the drug/excipients, and hence the type of dosage form, are likely to affect the efficacy of antimicrobial agents. Particular care should be given to multiphase systems where partitioning may prove to be a problem, perhaps leaving the aqueous phase unpreserved; this can also occur with adsorption/partitioning onto, or into, plastic containers. The microbial control of non-sterile products has been reviewed.[39]

Thermal Methods

Methods of thermal analysis find application in a number of areas of preformulation testing and include:

- the characterisation of the material (for example, polymorphic form)
- the interaction between the drug and excipients
- purity determination.

Most workers seem to rely heavily on differential scanning calorimetry (DSC), although other techniques are available for some of these functions and indeed may be more appropriate for certain applications.

Thermal Analysis Instrumentation

A wide variety of thermal analysis instruments exist, but discussion will be restricted to DSC, thermogravimetric analysis (TGA), isothermal microcalorimetry, and hot stage microscopy. The principles of these techniques are outlined briefly below, but for further reading, see Ford and Timmins[40] (for DSC and TGA) and Buckton and Beezer[41] (for isothermal microcalorimetry).

Differential scanning calorimeters work by raising (or lowering) a sample and reference pan from one temperature to another at a constant rate of change of temperature. If the contents of the sample pan behave in a different manner to the reference (usually an empty pan), perhaps due to an endothermic response for melting of a solid, then at some stage the signal will be out of balance. This differential of response is monitored and presented as the result. Routinely the sample would be in the order of 10 mg of powder. The result obtained is sensitive to the sample preparation (for example, weight, particle size, type of pan). With TGA, the sample is again heated at a constant rate, and in this case the weight change is recorded as, for example, water is driven off the solid. Isothermal microcalorimetry offers significantly greater sensitivity than DSC. The sample (up to 1 g) is housed in a cell and held at a constant temperature. Any changes that spontaneously occur in the sample (such as a degradation) will be detected as a thermal event (as all chemical and physical processes result in a change of heat content). The output is detected as the rate of change of heat with time (power) as a function of time.

Material Characterisation

Purity Determination

DSC is often used to estimate the purity of a material, by utilising the colligative property that an impurity will depress the melting point of a substance. A van't Hoff relationship is used to assess the mole fraction of impurity (x_2) from a plot of T (the sample temperature at that time) as a function of $1/F_m$ (where F_m is the fraction molten at temperature T):

$$T = T_0 - \left(\frac{RT_0^2 x_2}{\Delta_{FUS} H_0 F_m} \right)$$

where T_0 is the melting point of the pure substance and $\Delta_{FUS} H_0$ is enthalpy of fusion of the pure substance. A schematic DSC trace for a substance with different levels of impurity is shown in Fig. 1.

Polymorphism

Polymorphic forms usually have different melting points, thus DSC offers a convenient method by which it is possible to identify which polymorphic form, or potentially, what proportions of mixed polymorphs are present. A schematic DSC trace showing polymorphic transitions is shown in Fig. 2. Investigations of polymorphic transitions by DSC should always be confirmed by use of hot

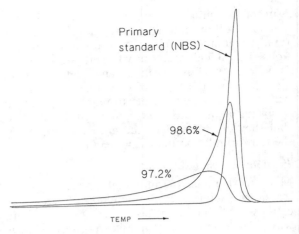

Fig. 1
Effect of purity on DSC melting peak shapes and melting temperature of benzoic acid.

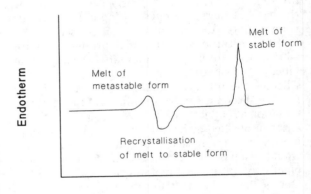

Fig. 2
Schematic DSC trace of polymorphic transitions.

stage microscopy. If the sample is mounted in oil on the stage of a microscope and heated at the same rate as in the DSC then the melt of the metastable polymorph will be seen, followed by the recrystallisation and melt of the stable form. If, however, the DSC transition is due to loss of a solvate then bubbles will be distinctly visible as the vaporised solvent is driven off.

Thermal Analysis and Solvates

Solvates will show a response on a DSC trace that is similar to a polymorphic transition; the solvate can be studied by hot stage microscopy to confirm the observation. A more appropriate assessment of solvates is to use TGA, as the loss of the solvate will result in weight reduction. The first derivative of a TGA trace will provide peaks to indicate whether a sample is, for example, a monohydrate or a dihydrate, and also whether it contains free (loosely bound) water. Such an investigation will prove a valuable quality assurance specification for subsequent production and will alert the preformulation scientist to changes in properties during the scale up of bulk drug manufacture, as well as a valuable indicator of product stability (for example, free water would tend to lead to instability). The use of thermal methods for the characterisation of pharmaceuticals has been discussed.[42]

Thermal Methods for Excipient Compatibility Screening

A number of approaches have been described by which kinetic information about drug instability can be derived from DSC studies.[40] While it is straightforward to calculate such information, its reliability is often open to question. Very few quantitative reports on the use of thermal analysis to assess drug stability have appeared in the pharmaceutical literature. Considerably more work has been published on the use of DSC to screen for drug/excipient interactions. The use of conventional HPLC or TLC assays to monitor for drug/excipient incompatibilities would normally involve storage of the mixtures at elevated temperatures and humidities, and assaying for drug content at different time intervals. This process will often take months and will certainly take some weeks to complete. It is, therefore, not surprising that the use of DSC to screen for possible incompatibilities has gained favour, as a result is available in minutes or hours.

For a DSC screen, the drug and the excipient is prepared in a 50:50 mix, often with size reduction to ensure good particle/particle contact. However, it should be noted that size reduction techniques can change crystal properties in terms of degree of crystallinity and polymorphic form, and consequently may alter the potential for interaction. The mixtures are then filled into a pan (about a 10 mg sample size) and heated at a rate of, for example, 5 or 10 degrees/min. An interaction is suspected if a significant difference is observed between the response for the mixture and the responses for the two powders when run separately; for example, the loss of a peak, the presence of a new peak, changes in peak shape, significant changes in peak onset temperature or peak maxima, and changes in the relative heights of peaks. For a rapid screen it is often unnecessary to consider why changes are seen, but simply worthwhile eliminating those excipients that can readily be substituted if problems are indicated. It is perfectly possible that vast changes may be seen in the thermogram of the mixture, suggesting an incompatibility, but that the actual mixture at ambient (or near ambient) conditions may prove to be adequately stable. Equally, it is possible that DSC responses may show no indication of interaction, but the final product may prove unstable. The reasons for this are that DSC transitions are seen at temperatures significantly above ambient, in the regions where drugs and excipients are seen to melt. Interactions at these temperatures may not relate to any chemical or physical processes that occur under normal storage conditions. False-negative results may be due to factors such as inadequate particle/particle contact, or too fast a scan rate. It follows that DSC experiments for excipient screening are a rapid, but rough guide. In all cases analytical data, from mixtures stored at more realistic temperatures, will be required. The single advantage of a DSC screen is that analytical time can be reduced by eliminating excipients that can readily be substituted.

An alternative to DSC for excipient screening is the use of isothermal microcalorimetry. The microcalorimeter is more sensitive than conventional DSC instruments and can be expected to show evidence of interactions at a defined temperature that is rather closer to room temperature. It has been demonstrated that the isothermal microcalorimeter has an effective sensitivity four orders of magnitude greater than DSC.[41] Thus for a reaction with an activation energy of 50 kJ/mol it would be necessary to raise the temperature by almost 240° (to 265°) to observe an interaction in a DSC that could be observed at 25° in the isothermal microcalorimeter. It is obviously more reliable to use the isothermal instrument at near ambient temperatures than to use DSC and it is probable that isothermal calorimetry will prove suitable for screening drug/excipient mixtures at temperatures only marginally above ambient (perhaps 30° to 60°). The advantage being that a result (that is, an indication of presence or absence of reaction) will be available within a few hours, rather than weeks or months. However, the output of an isothermal microcalorimeter is a function of the concentration of reactants, the enthalpy of reaction, and the rate of reaction. Thus from one experiment it is possible to confuse slow reactions of high enthalpy (which may not be a serious problem for stability) with fast reactions of low enthalpy (which may be a serious problem). Thus, isothermal microcalorimetry seems to be a more reliable screening method than DSC, but will not replace the ultimate need for chemical analysis. The methods have been extensively reviewed.[43-48]

Thermal Methods in Product Development

The measurement of an enthalpy of solution in an isothermal (or isoperabol) calorimeter has been shown to be of value in material characterisation.[42] The interaction between solids, which may be excipients or drugs, and a liquid (water) provides a valuable way of characterising a material. For example, microcrystalline cellulose from different suppliers often has an identical specification, but different performance in the product;[42] the performance of the excipient is related to the enthalpy of immersion for the material in water. There is considerable scope for characterising materials in this manner. Isothermal calorimetry in physical pharmacy has been reviewed.[41] The use of thermal methods in the physical characterisation of materials may well be the most valuable application of such techniques.[41-48]

PRODUCT SPECIFIC ASPECTS

At a certain point, preformulation tests will no longer be a physicochemical screen of the drug, but will develop into tests that relate specifically to a desired dosage form. For example, compression properties of a drug are not a high priority test for a topical product. Thus, the boundary between preformulation and formulation is an indistinct one.

Ideally, the development of a formulation should be as a consequence of decisions that are based on the results obtained from the preformulation testing procedures. In order to use the preformulation data to best effect, it is necessary to consider the important properties that are required of the dosage form that is to be made. Such properties will relate to ease of manufacture, optimisation of stability, and bioavailability. For many dosage forms there will be conflicting needs between the ideal properties for manufacture, stability, and bioavailability. For example, with solid dosage forms it may be necessary to optimise flow by having a large particle size (for example, granulation), but also to have a very small size to speed dissolution. With liquid dosage forms, it is often found that a pH that optimises solubility results in the least stable product as the increased ionisation will increase both solubility and the tendency to hydrolyse. Many such dilemmas will face the for-

mulator. However, if a sound understanding of the physicochemical properties of the drug substance exists, it will be possible to consider logical compromises or alternatives.

There are few preformulation tests that are truly product specific. In the section that follows, the tests that are directly related to certain classes of products are noted. Many of these tests have already been discussed above.

Solid Dosage Forms

As described above, it is necessary to consider solubility, partitioning, and if necessary, changes in particle size and even crystal form, in order to promote absorption. However, it is also necessary to consider the method of manufacture. Stability during granulation should be predictable and flow optimisation should be considered, as should mixing. On occasions, the method of production will impose conflicting demands to those of absorption enhancement, for example, micronisation for improved dissolution and particle size increase (through granulation) for improved flow. A further area that has not been addressed is that of mixing. To comment on concepts of mixing (see Oral Solids chapter) would be outside the scope of this chapter, however, it is clear that small particles (with high static charge) will present special problems. Preformulation testing will at least indicate the tendency for good or poor mixing.

Oral Liquids

For oral liquids, organoleptic properties are of great importance and taste masking becomes essential. For solutions, the stability and solubility will be critical. For suspensions, the viscosity of the continuous phase is important, and the interfacial interactions between the disperse phase and the continuous phase will be vital.

Semi-solids

Surface and interfacial science relating to creams (and emulsions) cannot be covered with a passing comment, but it is obvious that such complex systems are dependent upon consistency of the manufacturing process and material source.

Parenterals

Specific problems exist with parenteral manufacture; the most obvious being the need to ensure sterility. It is necessary to assess the effect that a heat sterilisation process will have on a drug and also whether excipients will affect the stability. Many products are aseptically prepared and others are subjected to lyophilisation, to remove water and consequently improve stability. The implications of the addition of tonicity adjusters must also be considered, particularly with respect to ionic strength. When considering the addition of preservatives, products may also be screened for their intrinsic antimicrobial activity.

Inhalations

A unique test for inhalations is the need to assess aerodynamic particle size rather than simply to rely on the traditional methods of sizing. Aerodynamic size is usually determined by impactors or impingers (impactors have dry surfaces and impingers have liquid covered surfaces), which are calibrated to determine the respirable fraction of the inhaled dose.

The need to prepare products with small particle sizes makes inhalation development a formulation challenge. Suspension aerosols (as metered dose inhalers) must allow delivery of non-aggregated particles and must not allow adhesion to the container wall. Parsons et al[9] have modelled the tendency to aggregate and adhere to containers in terms of surface energies. Dry powder inhalations consist either of a powder that is loosely adhered to a large carrier particle (lactose), and which is dislodged during inhalation, or of fine particles that have been stabilised (in terms of surface energy optimisation) to allow delivery of a non-aggregated particle cloud. The ideal properties of particles can be produced by manipulation and determined by preformulation testing.

Summary

Preformulation testing can, at best, provide the necessary physicochemical/physicomechanical profile of drug and excipient substances to allow a logical, scientific approach to formulation optimisation. The best products can be regarded as being those that are simple, elegant, and robust. There is a greater chance of achieving such a product if the correct foundations are laid and an understanding of the potential problems has been obtained by rigorous preformulation testing.

REFERENCES

1. Shefter E, Higuchi T. J Pharm Sci 1963;52:781–91.
2. York P. Int J Pharmaceutics 1983;14:1–28.
3. Fairbrother JE, Grant DJW. J Pharm Pharmacol 1978;30:19P.
4. Fairbrother JE, Grant DJW. J Pharm Pharmacol 1979;31:27P.
5. York P, Grant DJW. Int J Pharmaceutics 1985;25:57–72.
6. Grant DJW, York P. Int J Pharmaceutics 1986;28:103–12.
7. Nyqvist H, Gaffner C. Acta Pharm Suec 1986;23:257–70.
8. Brunauer S, Emmett PH, Teller E. J Am Chem Soc 1938;60:309–19.
9. Parsons G, Buckton G, Chatham SM. Int J Pharmaceutics 1992;83:163–70.
10. Wells JI. Pharmaceutical preformulation: the physicochemical properties of drug substances. Chichester: Ellis Horwood, 1988.
11. Buckton G, Choularton A, Beezer AE, Chatham SM. Int J Pharmaceutics 1988;47:121–8.
12. Rowe RC. Int J Pharmaceutics 1989;53:75–8.
13. Rowe RC. Int J Pharmaceutics 1989;56:117–24.
14. Rowe RC. Int J Pharmaceutics 1990;58:209–14.
15. Young SA, Buckton G. Int J Pharmaceutics 1990;60:235–41.
16. Buckton G. Powder Technol 1990;61:237–49.
17. Heertjes PM, Kossen NWK. Powder Technol 1967;1:33–42.
18. Zografi G, Tam SS. J Pharm Sci 1976;65:1145–9.
19. van Oss CJ, Good RJ, Chaudhury MK. Langmuir 1988;4:884–91.
20. Fowkes FM. Ind Eng Chem 1964 Dec:40–52.
21. Ahlneck C, Zografi G. Int J Pharmaceutics 1990;62:87–95.
22. Marshall K. Drug Dev Ind Pharm 1989;15:2153–76.
23. Ridgeway Watt K. Tablet machine instrumentation in pharmaceutics: principles and practice. Chichester: Ellis Horwood, 1978.
24. Kaplan SA. Drug Metab Rev 1972;1:15.
25. Serajuddin AM, Sheen P-C, Augustine MA. J Pharm Pharmacol 1987;39:587–91.
26. Buckton G, Bulpett R, Verma N. Int J Pharmaceutics 1991;72:157–62.
27. Leo A, Hansch C, Elkins D. Chem Rev 1971;71:525–73.
28. Kubinyi H. Prog Drug Res 1979;23:97–136.
29. Tomlinson E. Int J Pharmaceutics 1983;13:115–44.
30. Leo A, Hansch C. J Org Chem 1971;36:1539–44.
31. Katz Y, Diamond JM. J Membrane Biol 1974;17:87–98.
32. Katz Y, Diamond JM. J Membrane Biol 1974;17:101–12.
33. Beezer AE, Gooch CA, Hunter WH, Volpe PLO. J Pharm Pharmacol 1987;39:774–9.
34. Florence AT, Attwood D. Physicochemical principles of pharmacy. London: Macmillan, 1981.
35. Khalil SA, Abdullah DY, Moustafa MA. Can J Pharm Sci 1976;11:26–30.
36. Rowe RC. Int J Pharmaceutics 1988;41:223–6.
37. Krug RR, Hunter WG, Greiger RA. J Phys Chem 1976;80:2335–42.
38. Atkins PW. Physical chemistry. 3rd ed. Oxford: University Press, 1986.
39. Bloomfield SF, Baird R, Leak RE, Leech R. Microbial quality assurance in pharmaceuticals, cosmetics and toiletries. Chichester: Ellis Horwood, 1988.
40. Ford JL, Timmins P. Pharmaceutical thermal analysis. Chichester: Ellis Horwood, 1989.
41. Buckton G, Beezer AE. Int J Pharmaceutics 1991;72:181–91.
42. Pharm J 1990;245:183–4.
43. Angberg M, Nystrom C, Castensson S. Acta Pharm Suec 1988;25:307–20.
44. Angberg M, Nystrom C, Castensson S. Int J Pharmaceutics 1990;61:67–77.
45. Angberg M, Nystrom C, Castensson S. Int J Pharmaceutics 1991;73:209–20.
46. Angberg M, Nystrom C, Castensson S. Int J Pharmaceutics 1991;77:269–77.
47. Pikal MJ, Dellerman KM. Int J Pharmaceutics 1989;50:233–52.
48. Hansen LD, Lewis EA, Eathough DJ, Bergstrom RG, DeGraft-Johnson D. Pharm Res 1989;6:20–7.

Formulation

The medicines that patients take are usually formulations of drugs in suitable materials, which are processed in a suitable manner to produce the required dosage form or medicine. Any drug may exist in a number of dosage forms, for example, tablets, capsules, injections, ointments, and creams. This chapter provides an overview of the formulation development process of the medicine. Many of the specific areas are covered in greater depth in other chapters.

When a pharmaceutical product is being developed it is usual for more than one formulation to be devised. Thus formulations may be developed for toxicological studies, early clinical studies, and metabolism studies, as well as that which will become the marketed product. However, it is only this last formulation which will be considered here.

FORMULATION OBJECTIVES

There are several reasons why drugs are formulated. The prime objective is to ensure that the correct amount of the active ingredient reaches the correct site in the body for the desired length of time. This will differ depending on whether the drug is required to exert a local effect (for example, a topical preparation) or a systemic effect. The formulation may be used to modify drug activity in a temporal or a spatial manner; in the former case, the release rate of the drug is controlled to provide the required release characteristics (for example, a sustained-release dosage form). In the latter case, the drug may be formulated in a manner that facilitates transport to a specific site in the body before release. Cytotoxic drugs have been the focus of much attention, in this respect, in an attempt to reduce their toxicity.[1]

In many cases the intensity and duration of the pharmacological response can be correlated with the plasma concentration of the circulating drug. A typical plasma-drug concentration versus time curve is represented in Fig. 1.

The plasma-drug concentration initially increases with time due to the rate of absorption of the drug exceeding its rate of elimination. The faster the absorption rate the steeper the slope of the initial part of the curve and generally the faster the onset of action. When the plasma-drug concen-

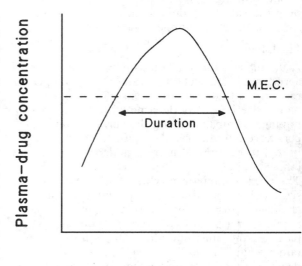

Fig. 1
Typical plasma-drug concentration versus time curve.

tration reaches its peak the absorption rate and elimination rate are equal and usually absorption is largely complete. Subsequently, the plasma-drug concentration decreases as the drug is eliminated from the body. For the drug to exert a therapeutic effect there is often a minimum plasma-drug concentration or minimum effective concentration (MEC) that must be exceeded. The duration of response is determined by the length of time the MEC is exceeded. Too high a plasma-drug concentration may result in unwanted side-effects. Finally, the area under the plasma-drug concentration versus time curve gives a measure of the extent of systemic absorption of the drug. The formulation of a drug significantly affects all these parameters.[2]

Drug formulation is designed to offer a medicine that is acceptable to patients and convenient for prescribing by doctors. In this respect, the most common types of dosage form that have stood the test of time (for example, tablets, capsules, ointments, creams, suppositories, injections) are still the primary forms of choice. However, with the newer drugs such as polypeptides and other biotechnology products, newer delivery systems have been devised. These will be considered later in this chapter.

Similarly, for convenience and compliance, it is preferable that medicines should not be administered more than once or twice daily. Although there are still many exceptions, this is a clearly discernible trend in formulation and has led to a proliferation of modified-release preparations.

In addition to convenience of administration, it is essential that the medicine is stable throughout its shelf-life. Compatibility studies are carried out using the drug and a range of excipients[3] with a view to choosing those that, in addition to conferring suitable bioavailability properties to the dosage form, render it sufficiently stable. Indeed, excipients may be added to the formulation to improve the stability of an otherwise unstable drug. This is discussed in greater detail in the Stability of Medicinal Products chapter.

From a pharmaceutical production viewpoint, it is essential that the dosage form can be made easily, economically, and reproducibly. The yield must be good, few if any batches should fail to meet specifications, standard equipment is preferable, and where possible, well characterised excipients should be used. However, there is little justification for designing bioavailable, stable, and elegant formulations if they cannot be made on a routine basis in production. In this respect, it is important to select and validate the final formulation and manufacturing process as early as possible in the development programme. Subsequent clinical supplies should then preferably be manufactured at the identified production site. This will facilitate both the launch of the product and the Food and Drug Administration pre-approval inspections in which European sites are increasingly involved.

PREFORMULATION

A full account of the stages that constitute the preformulation of a product is described in the Preformulation chapter.

Before formulation development can begin, the formulator must ascertain background information on the pharmacological nature of the drug, its intended use, the preferred routes of administration, and any other relevant information. The formulator should then interact with the medicinal chemists who synthesised the compound to obtain basic information regarding the properties of the molecule. Such information should include whether the compound has one or more chiral centres, and if so, whether a specific isomer or a race-

mate is to be developed. In the present regulatory and scientific climate the former case is the more likely. For ionisable compounds the pK_a should be determined and salt selection should be discussed (see below). In some instances, it is better to develop a prodrug than the drug itself. Such prodrugs may be developed for stability, taste, or other purposes or indeed it may transpire that what was thought to be the active compound is actually a prodrug which undergoes metabolic activation. The use of prodrugs have been widely reviewed.[4, 5]

Salt Selection

Hydrochloride salts may give a metallic taste and di- or trihydrochloride salts are generally hygroscopic and pose corrosion problems with manufacturing equipment. Berge *et al*[6] have reviewed various pharmaceutical salts, covering most of the aspects necessary for the formulator to consider. Salt selection is a crucial aspect for the development programme. In addition to imparting desirable physicochemical characteristics to the drug, it is important to ensure the salt selected will not lead to other real or potential problems. Mesylate salts, for example, must be checked to ensure minimal levels or preferably the absence of methyl and ethyl esters of methane sulphonic acid as these impurities are carcinogenic. A further example is that the quinine bisulphate salt is hydrated to a greater extent than the sulphate salt. Once a potential salt of the drug has been identified, other data required for formulation development include an assessment of solubility as a function of pH, determination of the hygroscopic properties of the salt, its melting point, an evaluation of its potential to show polymorphism, its chemical stability under a range of stressed conditions and as a function of pH, measurement of its bulk density, and particle size distribution. In addition, determination of its flow properties and intrinsic dissolution are useful.

The desirable characteristics of a good salt are as follows:

- acceptable organoleptic properties
- easily synthesised
- good flow and compaction properties
- minimal hydration
- non-irritant to veins
- non-hygroscopic
- non-polymorphic
- non-toxic
- reproducible particle size
- stable

- suitable aqueous solubility and intrinsic dissolution
- suitable bulk density
- suitable and sharp melting point.

Excipient Selection

Initially, the formulator should carry out a series of experiments to determine the compatibility of the drug with an appropriate range of excipients. The choice of excipients depends on the intended dosage form. For example, compatibility studies with lubricants, binders, disintegrants, and commonly used diluents would be appropriate for tablets or capsules, while tonicity agents, antoxidants, buffers, and potential preservatives would be more appropriate for parenteral dosage forms. Considerable care should go into the design of these compatibility studies to ensure meaningful results. Stability studies at stress conditions that are too severe may give results that cannot be extrapolated to the dosage forms when exposed to normal storage conditions.

SOLID ORAL DOSAGE FORMS

The formulation development of solid oral dosage forms is primarily concerned with the formulation of tablets and capsules. Capsules can consist of hard gelatin capsules or soft gelatin capsules. In the former case the capsule usually contains solid material although viscous liquids or semi-solids have been successfully used. In the latter case, liquids are filled into the capsules.

Tablet Formulation

For a chemically stable drug the main determinant in the formulation of a tablet is the dose. For low dose drugs a direct compression formulation would probably be preferred since this reduces the number of operations involved. It is important to ensure adequate powder mixing and no subsequent segregation to give acceptable dose uniformity. The materials used in direct compression and details of their processing are described in greater detail in the Oral Solids chapter. However, they should preferably be described in the monographs of the appropriate pharmacopoeias to ensure worldwide acceptance.

Tablet lubrication is still largely restricted to the use of magnesium stearate and stearic acid. The former has been found to vary considerably from one supplier to another[7] and many regulatory authorities are now strict about limiting the number of suppliers that can be used. It is important

not to prolong the mixing of the lubricant as this may lead to bioavailability problems.[8] The consequences of prolonged mixing may be lessened by using a colloidal silica (Aerosil™) mix[9] and are generally not apparent when talc and stearic acid mixes are used.

The traditional starch disintegrants have now been largely superseded by the newer so-called super disintegrants such as sodium starch glycollate (Explotab™ or Primojel™) or croscarmellose sodium (Ac-Di-Sol™); these are efficient disintegrants. Finally with 'sticky' drugs it may be necessary to incorporate a glidant such as colloidal silica to ensure sufficient flow properties during tablet compression.

At higher doses (for example, above 100 mg) it is probably necessary to granulate the formulation; at doses of 250 mg and above it is likely that the great majority of the granulate will compose of drug, thereby necessitating good salt selection. Under the latter conditions, dose uniformity is rarely a problem but tablet compaction may present a difficulty. Similar excipients can be used for the granulated materials with the addition of binders such as povidone. The lubricant should be added as an extragranular excipient while the super disintegrants are often added both as intra- and extra-granular excipients.

The shape and extent of embossing of tablets is usually decided by marketing groups. A case can be made from a production and a packaging viewpoint for some standardisation in size and shape of the tablets.

The choice of excipient and its concentration is fundamental. Numerous papers[10] have discussed statistical techniques for optimisation of formulations and determination of key excipients. Used properly these can be of significant value, but used improperly they can result in complex and largely redundant formulation exercises.[11] The choice of excipient is also often significantly influenced by previous formulations within a company. Apart from the experience gained with these excipients it is of advantage to production to have common excipients thus reducing the inventory. Thus many formulation exercises will start with a standard set of excipients and will not change unless problems are encountered.

In recent years some tablets have been made by lyophilisation techniques.[12] These are the Zydis™ formulations and although they may be more friable than other tablets they offer the advantage of instant dissolution.

Tablets may be coated or uncoated. Coating may be carried out to improve stability, especially if hygroscopicity or light instability is a problem; to mask unpleasant tastes; to change the release characteristics (for example, enteric coating); and to reduce dustiness during packaging. Film coating has now replaced sugar coating for virtually all new products although several older products on the market are still sugar coated. Several reviews have described in detail the process of film coating[13] especially in the areas of modified-release technology.

Capsule Formulation

Hard gelatin capsules are essentially prepared in an identical manner to that of tablets with the exception of the final stage where capsule filling replaces compaction. In general, these formulations are simpler than tablets because compression forces are much lower. If a powder blend has a reasonable cohesiveness and forms a bed of even bulk density then it should fill if adequately lubricated. In addition, fewer complications with respect to scale-up are generally found with capsule formulations. Low doses of drug can again often be accommodated by simple powder fills; high doses may need to be granulated.

The use of high doses in capsules is more limited as capsules larger in size than size 1 are unpopular with marketing personnel, and capsule sizes larger than size 0 are not acceptable to the patient, leading to reduced compliance. Thus doses over 250 to 400 mg may not be able to be encapsulated in a single capsule and as such may be limited to tablet formulations. However, where capsules do offer an advantage over tablets is in the variety of materials that can be filled into them and the relative ease of changing the dose by changing the fill weight.

Hard gelatin capsules can be filled with powders, granules, pellets, tablets if necessary, or semi-solid solutions of materials like Labrafils™ or Gelucires™ (which are mixtures of glyceride and macrogol esters). Many capsule filling machines can fill more than one of these components and some can fill three components. Thus both powder and pellets can be filled separately into one capsule shell as could a liquid, a powder, and a small tablet. This permits considerable flexibility in formulating medicines in hard gelatin capsules.

There is a bridge from hard gelatin capsules to soft gelatin capsules with the use of liquid or semi-solid filled materials. This may offer an advantage for poorly soluble compounds, some otherwise unstable compounds, or where modified-release of the drug is required.[14,15] In many cases where liquids or semi-solids are formulated in hard gelatin capsules it may be necessary to band the capsules. This consists of the application of a thin gelatin band around the junction of the cap and body of the capsule, which ensures there is no leakage of the contents. High speed machines are now available for such banding. Banding also has the advantage of making the capsule tamper resistant.

Soft gelatin capsules are manufactured and filled in a single operation. They are primarily of use for liquids and suspensions.[16] The equipment and processing techniques used for such dosage forms is specialised and soft gelatin capsules are normally manufactured by a limited number of manufacturers. They are of particular use with drugs that have poor aqueous solubility, but which are soluble in solvents such as arachis oil, or Neobees™ (medium chain triglycerides).

Coloration of Solid Dosage Forms

The colouring of tablets or capsules allows ease of recognition. It also gives marketing groups the opportunity to develop distinctive trade marks. Research[17] has indicated some colours may be more psychologically beneficial for certain conditions than others, for example, red for cardiovascular compounds. The downside to this is that the worldwide acceptability of colours is confused. Many dyes are acceptable in some countries but not others, with only titanium dioxide, indigo carmine, and some iron oxides being widely accepted. Thus the same coloured tablets or capsules may contain different dyes in different countries.

PARENTERAL DOSAGE FORMS

If a drug is sufficiently soluble in water, then in theory, the formulation of injections for intravenous, intramuscular, or subcutaneous administration is simple; in practice this is rarely so. This section will concentrate on intravenous injections but the principles equally apply to the other routes.

The basic ingredients for an injection are the drug, an aqueous solvent, a tonicity agent, and a suitable container. On occasions a buffer may also be used but as a general rule the simpler the formulation the better.

Again the initial stage in the formulation exercise is to decide on the dose or dose range and also the route of injection as this will significantly affect the concentration and volume of the injection.

Resistance to autoclaving should then be tested in a series of formulations because a formulation that can be terminally sterilised is desirable both from a safety and ease of registration viewpoint. Resistance to autoclaving and stability on storage must be assessed both from physical and chemical criteria. In the former case, the presence of particulate matter can give rise to unacceptable formulations that give acceptable potency assays. The majority of formulation failures caused by particulate matter occur during the manufacturing stage but it is possible that contamination by such matter may occur during storage. As a result, injections that pass the test for particulate matter immediately after manufacture may fail a similar test 3 to 6 months later. In this respect, it should be appreciated that the composition of Type I glass varies significantly from one manufacturer to another especially between Europe and the USA. It is predictable that weak acids may precipitate with di- or trivalent metals leachable from the glass. Edetic acid or citrates may complex metals, for example, calcium and magnesium.

Tonicity agents should be chosen with care as it may be necessary for some medical conditions to have sugar-free formulations thus precluding the use of agents such as glucose or sorbitol. Similarly, agents like sodium chloride may reduce the solubility of hydrochloride salts of active ingredients due to a common ion effect.

Once a potential formulation has been established it is essential to determine if it is to be given by intravenous infusion or as a bolus injection. In the former case, compatibility testing with appropriate infusion fluids and with giving sets is necessary. While the former is obvious, the latter is also important as adsorption onto giving sets has been found with some drugs and may be significant even at very low drug concentrations; an event likely to be more common with the general increase in potency of new drugs.

If the drug is to be given as a single dose, decisions have to be made on suitable containers (see Pharmaceutical Packaging chapter). Glass ampoules are generally favoured in Europe, whereas single- or multiple-dose vials are favoured in the USA. In the latter case, compatibility studies are necessary with the stopper of the vial. In addition, the USA favours the inclusion of preservatives in the formulation while the UK does not. It is an obvious advantage if the injection has its own bacteriostatic properties, for example, as a result of the pH of the formulation. Formulations in the pH range of 3 to 4 are generally acceptable to the patient and often have bacteriostatic properties. These can be tested by the use of the pharmacopoeial preservative efficacy tests. There is a discrepancy between the *British Pharmacopoeia* and *United States Pharmacopeia*, with the *British Pharmacopoeia* test being far more stringent, so that it is not unusual for a formulation to pass the *United States Pharmacopeia* test but fail the *British Pharmacopoeia* test. A new *European Pharmacopoeia* test is in preparation and the topic is high on the list of international harmonisation initiatives.

In some circumstances an injection may be needed in an emergency. Therefore, it may be desirable to formulate it in a prefilled syringe. Many such systems are available; however, most of them are not capable of terminal sterilisation within the syringe. One exception to this is the Dupharject™ system,[18] which can be terminally sterilised in a properly ballasted autoclave.

A final issue that must be evaluated early in the programme is the potential of the injection to cause vein irritation. Some evidence of this may be obtained in the early intravenous toxicity studies, but a number of other models may also be used. In many cases vein irritation may be minimised by reformulation, but some compounds may possess intrinsic irritant properties making such formulations difficult. One possible approach in these circumstances is the use of materials such as cyclodextrins, which will minimise the contact of the drug with the biological constituents at the site of injection.

SCALE-UP AND PROCESS VALIDATION

Early formulation development is frequently carried out at a laboratory scale using batches often of one kilogram or less. Initial formulations can thus be developed with minimal use of the drug, which is usually in short supply at that time. Once an initial formulation has been selected, both the formulation and the subsequent production process that will be used to make it must be validated. It is, therefore, essential to receive early input from production personnel as to the likely processes to be employed (for example, fluid bed granulation or wet massing and screening) and also the equipment to be used.

Planetary mixers such as Hobart mixers usually give significantly different results from high shear mixers, necessitating the use of different binder volumes. Similarly, a high shear mixer of the Diosna/TK Fielder™ type can give a different product to other high shear mixers like the Littleford Lodige™. It is, therefore, essential that pilot-scale equipment used for any process validation is comparable with that to be subsequently used in production. The validation of the formulation and processing conditions is an area where sensible use of multivariate statistical design can be used.[19] This will permit determination of critical ingredients and processing parameters, which can then be suitably controlled. Stability studies at the extremes of the formulation and possibly at extremes of processing conditions will permit further confidence in the overall product.

This work should be completed before the start of large international Phase III clinical trials. These trials can then be supplied from an identified production site to the final product specifications. This approach familiarises the production site with the formulation and process before preparation of launch batches and should significantly facilitate any Food and Drug Administration pre-approval inspections by the authorities. It also allows registration stability studies to be carried out early, on what are essentially production batches.

STABILITY

The intention of this section is to briefly review the place of stability in the overall development process. The theory and applications of stability testing are covered in the Stability of Medicinal Products chapter. Stability studies are either carried out on the active raw material or on formulations of that material.

Raw material stability methodology should be developed and stability studies carried out as early as possible in the development programme. It is desirable to have stability data on compounds before development has started in order to assist drug discovery research and to provide an input into whether the compound should be developed. Assuming that the drug is sufficiently stable to be developed, long-term stability studies at both ambient and stressed conditions should be initiated. The stressed conditions should include thermal and light stress together with studies at elevated humidities.

Stability of drug solutions should be determined as a function of pH. Extreme stressing of the drug will allow evaluation of potential degradation products. Further stability testing would normally be carried out for each new batch of drug received. The extent of this testing is dependent on the results of previous batches and would obviously be considerably more extensive for less stable compounds.

Finally, registration stability studies must be carried out on raw material made at the chemical production site by the proposed final route of synthesis. Guidelines for such regulatory studies are usually supplied by the authorities. These guidelines will also cover the formulations for registration.

Stability testing is carried out on all formulations developed during the programme. This includes formulations for toxicological and clinical testing as well as prototype and final marketing formulations. The conditions of testing and the tests carried out depend on the dosage forms. In all cases potency and purity assays are included, but dissolution testing is likely to be included for solid dosage forms while particulate matter and pH determinations would be included for parenteral solutions. Similarly, elevated humidity storage conditions would be included in solid dosage form evaluations whereas freeze-thaw cycling may be included for parenterals, and possibly semi-solids such as gels and creams. In all these cases, it is essential to evaluate the effect of the container on the stability of the product. The container should preferably add protection to the stability of the product, but at the least, it should not contribute to its degradation.

Coloured glass bottles, high-density polyethylene (HDPE) containers, and polypropylene containers (for example, Securitainers™) will protect an oral solid dosage form against light and humidity conditions. Such protection is significantly reduced by the use of polyvinyl chloride blister packaging although the use of secondary packaging may alleviate light degradation problems as may the use of opaque or amber materials in the blister composition. If humidity conditions are problematic other blister materials such as polyvinylidene chloride (PVDC) and Aclar™ may offer some additional protection[20] but this is still likely to be less than with the bottles listed above. If unit packing is required a foil-foil pouch type of packaging may be necessary to give the required protection. Humidity apart, product packaging interactions are rare for solid dosage forms, but they are more common for liquid and semi-solid dosage forms.

Glass, even Type I borosilicate glass, may release alkaline ions into solution, changing the pH and, therefore, the stability of the product.[21] Thus, acid washing may be employed to minimise this interaction. In addition, different lots of Type I glass contain significantly different ratios of mono-, di-, and tri-valent metal ions such as Ca^{2+} and Cr^{3+}. These can leach from the glass and may also interact with the product to its detriment, for example, by forming an insoluble precipitate causing particulate matter to appear in injections on storage.

The position is potentially worse with plastics and many regulatory authorities require details of the resins and other components in the plastic containers proposed for use. One other problem with some plastic containers is the potential for migration of liquid through the container. This can give rise to high assay results for solutions stored at elevated temperatures due to the evaporation of the solvent. There have even been examples of solutions stored in plastic bottles interacting with printing inks and label adhesives on the outside of the bottle.[22] Differences in the composition of laminated tubes for ointments and creams can give rise to instability problems. There are a number of reviews of the stability of pharmaceuticals.[23]

In addition to chemical stability, physical stability should be evaluated where appropriate. Thus the performance of pulmonary delivery systems and some newer systems like nasal pumps should be subject to stability investigations.

A final concern about stability of medicines is the potential for toxicity of the degradation products. As a general rule degradation products greater than 0.1% of the parent compound as determined by area normalisation on high pressure liquid chromatographs should be identified and quantified, while those over 0.5% should have their potential for toxicity evaluated. This will vary from compound to compound but is a potential problem that must be evaluated in the development programme. This topic is the subject of a future harmonisation initiative by the regulatory authorities of Europe, the USA, and Japan; more definitive guidelines are likely to emerge.

FUTURE DEVELOPMENTS IN FORMULATION TECHNOLOGY

Although all the previous dosage forms, optimisation processes, and stability testing protocols are continually being updated the most significant advances to come in the area of formulation technology are likely to be in the areas of modified release and novel dosage forms. The latter term simply means dosage forms different from those already described in this chapter and in many cases are modified-release dosage forms. See also the Modified-release Drug Delivery Systems chapter.

MODIFIED-RELEASE DOSAGE FORMS

Spatial Modified-release Dosage Forms

Spatial release forms are designed to release the drug at a specific site in the body. Spatial dosage forms are also often referred to as targeted dosage forms. They have been the subject of much research,[24] often with respect to cytotoxic drugs that often have associated toxicity problems. The two main lines of approach have essentially focussed on using immunological principles to target the drug via antibody-antigen interactions or the use of carriers such as liposomes. The successes that have been reported to date are largely restricted to laboratory experiments and *in-vitro* situations and have often not been repeated in the clinical setting. There are a number of reasons for this. It is extremely difficult to qualitatively differentiate tumour cells from normal cells. None of the carriers to date can be administered successfully by the oral route, thus the predominant route of choice is by intravenous injection. Drug carriers that have a small enough particle size to be administered by this route are quickly sequestered by the reticulo-endothelial system, primarily in the spleen and liver. Thus such targeting is only likely to be effective if these are the target organs. Tumour cells generally have lower blood flow further restricting ingress of these targeted formulations.

Temporal Modified-release Dosage Forms

Temporal dosage forms are those where release is a controlled function of time. The temporal release of drugs from dosage forms can be principally achieved by the oral, transdermal, and parenteral routes although some control by inhalation, ocular, and buccal administration may be possible.

There is a bewildering array of modified-release dosage forms especially for oral administration. With a few notable exceptions like the Alza GITS™ system and Pennwalt's Penkinetic™ ion exchange resin system, they can all be explained by their effect on dissolution as described by the Noyes-Whitney equation.[25]

$$\frac{dW}{dt} = \frac{D}{h} S (C_s - C)$$

where dW/dt is the rate of dissolution, D is the diffusion coefficient, h is the thickness of the diffusion layer, S is the surface area available for dissolution, and $C_s - C$ is the concentration gradient (Fig.2). In *in-vivo* conditions where absorption is rapid (sink conditions) the value for C is much less than that of C_s and the equation reduces to:

$$\frac{dW}{dt} = \frac{D}{h} S C_s$$

Diffusion can be affected by the use of viscosity inducing agents such as hypromellose and other

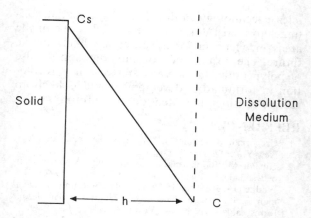

Fig. 2
Dissolution rate model as described by the Noyes-Whitney equation.

similar materials. The surface area for dissolution can be controlled by either formulating non-disintegrating tablets or non-porous beads of a fixed size range. In the former case dissolution can occur by surface erosion or by leaching of the drug from an insoluble matrix when dissolution is described by the Higuchi equation:[26]

$$Q = \left[\left(\frac{D \epsilon C_s}{\tau} \right) (2A - \epsilon C_s) \, t \right]^{\frac{1}{2}}$$

where Q is the amount of drug released per unit surface area after time t, D is the diffusion coefficient, τ is the tortuosity of the matrix, ϵ is the porosity of the matrix, C_s is the solubility of the drug in the elution medium, and A is the initial drug loading dose in the matrix.
Spherical, non-porous particles of fixed diameter can be prepared by coating inert materials such as non-pareil seeds,[27] an extrusion-spheronisation process,[28] or spherical agglomeration using roto-granulators like the Freund.[29] The concentration gradient can be affected by many different resources, such as using salts of different solubility, excipients whose solubility is affected by pH, or complexation techniques. The formulation of modified-release dosage forms will often utilise two or more of these techniques, for example, preparation of spherical granules of a less soluble salt. The multiparticulate conglomerates can also be made sufficiently small to permit formulation of a liquid dosage form; a significant advantage to many people at either end of the age spectrum who may have difficulty swallowing solid oral dosage forms.

In general, oral modified-release dosage forms are either multiparticulate or single nondisintegrating entities. For either of these to act they must be formulated to release the drug throughout the gastro-intestinal tract and the drug must then be absorbed. This is especially so with respect to colonic absorption which in the past has been reported to be poor. More recent studies have shown that some drugs, for example, nicardipine hydrochloride[30] have excellent colonic absorption.
It is therefore obvious that stomach emptying and gastro-intestinal transit rates are critical in evaluating the potential for oral modified-release dosage forms. Transit rates have been extensively studied by a number of techniques of which gamma ray scintigraphy is the most important.[32] Using this non-invasive technique the movement of radiolabelled material through the gastro-intestinal tract can be monitored after the administration of the dosage form under investigation. It is also possible to relate this transit time to plasma-drug concentrations, giving a far better picture of the in-vivo situation.
Food is the major factor affecting the rate of gastric emptying of dosage forms. Gastric emptying is probably the major factor controlling the absorption of drugs and is especially important for modified-release drugs. This extends even to liquid dosage forms, although it is most marked with large single-unit dosage forms.[33] Indeed some dosage forms are designed to resist emptying from the stomach.[34] Once in the small intestine, most dosage forms have a fairly uniform transit time of 3.5 ± 1 hour regardless of their nature; on reaching the colon wide differences are observed.
Some dosage forms are designed not to release their drug until after they have left the stomach. This is usually achieved by coating with an enteric material, that is, one soluble in alkali but not in acid. Such a procedure may be used to protect the drug against an acid environment, to protect the stomach against the drug, or to slow the release of the drug if it is poorly soluble at alkaline pH but readily soluble in acidic pH conditions.
There are other techniques being adopted to delay drug release that are being used in colonic delivery systems. One such system relies on the swelling of a polymer plug in an insoluble capsule shell. As the polymer swells it becomes detached from the shell thus releasing the contents at a predetermined time after administration.[35] The concept of triggered dosage forms has been evaluated by Theeuwes.[36]

The parenteral route has been used for modified release, especially from implants or intramuscular injections.[37] One of the more interesting advances is in the area of microencapsulated products using biocompatible polymers. These systems have been commercially applied to the administration of polypeptide drugs.[38]

FORMULATION OF PREPARATIONS FOR OTHER ROUTES OF ADMINISTRATION

Ocular Administration

Advances have been made in the formulation of ocular dosage forms. Significant research has gone into ocular absorption and methods of retaining drugs in the eye.[39,40] The Alza Ocusert[TM 41] although not a commercial success probably had much to do with a renaissance in ocular formulation.

Nasal Administration

Nasal administration used to be essentially restricted to nasal decongestant preparations and the treatment of allergic rhinitis. However, with the advent of potent polypeptides that cannot be administered orally, the nasal route has received increased attention.[42] It is now one of the main routes of choice for these materials.[43]

Pulmonary Administration

The pulmonary route has been, and continues to be, one of the two major routes of administration for drugs used in the treatment of asthma. The balance between the inhalation route and the oral route varies between countries, with the UK preferring the inhalation route. The major problems with inhalation therapy relate to forming and maintaining a fixed particle size following atomisation and ensuring the administration of the dose coincides with inspiration of breath by the patient. Significant work[44] is continuing in these areas to maximise the fraction inhaled.

Following the Montreal protocol, the use of chlorinated fluorocarbons (CFCs) has been significantly reduced resulting in reappraisal of the propellant systems used for these inhalation dosage forms.[45]

FUTURE DEVELOPMENTS IN FORMULATION

The 'conventional' dosage forms such as tablets, capsules, and creams will continue to be major forms for the foreseeable future. Advances in formulation will continue to be made to ensure that products are stable, bioavailable, and readily amenable to high speed production. Modified-release technology, both temporal and spatial, continues to increase in importance and is one of the areas in which major advances are likely in the future. The upsurge of biotechnology and the use of polypeptides has already started a new revolution in formulation development and is likely to receive considerable attention in the future.

REFERENCES

1. Gregoriadis G, Senior J, Tronet A. Targeting of drugs. New York: Plenum Press, 1982.
2. Gibaldi M. Biopharmaceutics and clinical pharmacokinetics. 2nd ed. Philadelphia: Lea and Febiger, 1977.
3. Wadke DA, Jacobson H. Preformulation testing. In: Lachman L, Lieberman HA, editors. Pharmaceutical dosage forms: tablets; vol 1. New York: Marcel Dekker, 1989.
4. Higuchi T. Prodrugs: principles and practice. In: Prescott LF, Nimmo W, editors. Drug absorption—Proceedings of Edinburgh International Conference. Balgowlah: Adis Press, 1979.
5. Svennson LA, Tunek A. Drug Metab Rev 1988;19:165–95.
6. Berge SM, Bighley LD, Monkhouse DC. J Pharm Sci 1977;66:1–19.
7. Frattini C, Simioni L. Drug Dev Ind Pharm 1984;10(7):1117–30.
8. Chowhan ZT, Li-Hua Chi. J Pharm Sci 1986;75:542–5.
9. Lerk CF, Bolhuis GK, Smedama SS. Pharm Acta Helv 1977;52:33–44.
10. Stetsko G. Drug Dev Ind Pharm 1986;12:1109–23.
11. Shek E, Ghani M, Jones RE. J Pharm Sci 1980;69:1135–41.
12. Virley P, Yarwood R. Mfg Chem 1990;61(2):36–7.
13. Kawashima Y, Takeuchi H, Handa T, Thiele WJ, Deen DP, McGinty JW. Aqueous-based coatings in matrix tablet formulations. In: McGinty JW, editor. Aqueous polymeric coatings for pharmaceutical dosage forms. New York: Marcel Dekker, 1989.
14. Walker SE, Bedford K, Eaves T. UK patent 7745755. 1977.
15. Cuine A, Francois D. UK patent 1590864. 1978.
16. Stanley JP. Soft gelatin capsules. In: Lachman L, Lieberman H, Kanig J, editors. Theory and practice of industrial pharmacy. 3rd ed. Philadelphia: Lea and Febiger, 1986:398–412.
17. Buckalew LW, Coffield KE. J Clin Psychopharmacol 1982;22:245–8.
18. DupharJect. Solvay Duphar BV, Medical Devices. PO Box 900, 1380 DA Weesp, The Netherlands.
19. McGurk JG, Lendrem DW, Potter CJ. Drug Dev Ind Pharm 1991;17:2341–58.
20. Guise W. Mfg Chem 1984 Nov;55:28.
21. Bacon FR. Glass containers for parenterals. In: Avis E, Lieberman HA, Lachman L, editors. Pharmaceutical dosage forms: parenteral medications; vol 2. New York: Marcel Dekker, 1986.
22. Chrai S, Gupta S, Brychta K. Bull Parenter Drug Assoc 1977;31:195–200.
23. Connors KA, Amidon SL, Kennon L, editors. Chemical stability of pharmaceuticals. New York: John Wiley & Sons, 1979.
24. Tomlinson E, Davis SS, editors. Site specific drug delivery. Chichester: John Wiley & Sons, 1986.
25. Noyes A, Whitney J. J Am Chem Soc 1897;19:930.
26. Higuchi T. J Pharm Sci 1963;52:1145.
27. Rekhi GS, Mendes RW, Porter SC, Jambhekar SS. Pharmaceut Technol 1989;13:112–25.

28. Conine JW, Hadley HR. Drug Cosm Ind 1970;106:38–41.
29. Runakoshi Y, Funakoshi Y, Yamamoto M, Matsumura Y, Komeda H. Powder Technol 1980;27:13–21.
30. Selkirk A. Personal Communication.
31. Bieck PR. Drug absorption from the human colon. In: Hardy JG, Davis SS, Wilson CG, editors. Drug delivery to the gastro-intestinal tract. Chichester: Ellis Horwood, 1989.
32. Davis SS. Evaluation of the gastro-intestinal transit and release characteristics of drugs. In: Johnson P, Lloyd-Jones JG, editors. Drug delivery systems, fundamentals and techniques. Chichester: Ellis Horwood, 1987.
33. Wilson CG, Washington N. The stomach: its role in oral drug delivery. In: Physiological pharmaceutics. Chichester: Ellis Horwood, 1989.
34. Hoffman La Roche. UK patent 1546448. 1976.
35. Davis SS. Physiological factors in drug absorption. In: Hrushesky WJM, Langer R, Theeuwes F, editors. Temporal control of drug delivery; vol 618. Annals of New York Academy of Sciences, 1991.
36. Theeuwes F. Triggered, pulsed and programmed drug delivery. In: Prescott LF, Nimmo WS, editors. Novel drug delivery and its therapeutic application. Chichester: John Wiley & Sons, 1989.
37. Chien YW. Novel drug delivery systems. New York: Marcel Dekker, 1982.
38. Langer R. Pharmaceut Technol 1989;13(8):18–32.
39. Lee VHL. Practical ocular drug delivery: approaches to minimise the systemic side-effects of ocularly applied drugs. In: Prescott LF, Nimmo WS, editors. Novel drug delivery and its therapeutic application. Chichester: John Wiley & Sons, 1989.
40. Greaves JL. Ocular drug delivery. In: Wilson CG, Washington N, editors. Physiological pharmaceutics. Chichester: Ellis Horwood, 1989.
41. Michaels AS, Mader WJ, Manning CR. New concepts and standards of quality control as applied to controlled drug delivery systems. In: Deasy PB, Timoney RF, editors. The quality control of medicines. Amsterdam: Elsevier, 1976.
42. Prescott LF, Nimmo WS, editors. Novel drug delivery and its therapeutic application. Chichester: John Wiley & Sons, 1989.
43. Medical Economics Company. Physicians' desk reference. 46th ed. Oradell: Edward R. Barnhart, 1992:2300.
44. Byron PR. Pharmaceut Technol 1987;11(Part 5):42–54.
45. Fisher FX, Hess H, Sucher H, Byron P. Pharmaceut Technol 1989;13(9):44–52.

Modified-release Drug Delivery Systems

Modified-release dosage forms are prepared using substances or procedures which, separately or together, are designed to modify the rate or the place at which active ingredient or ingredients are released in the body.

The plasma-drug concentration range over which there is a therapeutic effect without unwanted toxic effects is represented by a therapeutic window. If a drug has a wide therapeutic index, that is, the difference between effective and toxic plasma-drug concentrations is large, then the control of plasma-drug concentrations is not critical. However, if the drug has a narrow therapeutic index then it is necessary to exercise close control on plasma-drug concentrations.

After the oral administration of a conventional dosage unit that exhibits first-order kinetics there is a transient increase in plasma-drug concentration to a peak followed by an exponential decay. The magnitude of the plasma-drug concentration is influenced by the dose administered, the dosage interval, and the rates of drug absorption, distribution, metabolism, and elimination (see Biopharmaceutics and Pharmacokinetic Principles chapter). In order to achieve a predetermined kinetic profile of plasma-drug concentration, it may be necessary to modify conventional dosage forms or dose regimens.

There has been considerable effort directed towards the design of drug delivery systems capable of eliminating the cyclical plasma-drug concentrations obtained following the administration of conventional dosage forms. An ideal dosage form should be capable of delivering a known amount of drug to a specific site in the body at a predetermined rate or combination of rates in order to produce an optimum therapeutic effect.[1] Many terms have been used to describe modified-release drug delivery systems:

- delayed release—the drug is released at a time other than immediately after administration
- repeat action—the drug is released in small amounts at intermittent intervals after administration
- sustained release—the drug is released slowly at a rate governed by the delivery system
- controlled release—the drug is released at a constant rate and the drug concentrations obtained after administration of the system are invariant with time.

The first three classes of delivery system will be designated 'extended release' in this chapter.

The most commonly cited advantage of modified-release products is the reduction of the characteristic 'peak and valley' fluctuations in plasma-drug concentration observed after repeated dosing with conventional formulations; these fluctuations can result in the patient being exposed to toxic or non-therapeutic drug concentrations. Further advantages of modified-release systems include reduced dosing frequencies, possible improvement in the selectivity of pharmacological activity, and the achievement of a more constant or prolonged therapeutic effect. The advantages of extended-release and controlled-release dosage systems over conventional dosage forms have been well documented.[2-5]

The formulation of a drug with a short *in-vivo* half-life as an extended-release system may result in a reduction in the frequency of administration of the drug. From a therapeutic standpoint, less frequent dosing should improve patient compliance.

There are several potential problems or disadvantages associated with the use of extended-release drug delivery systems. These delivery systems are, in essence, multidose preparations and there is the possibility of 'dose-dumping' occurring, in which the total drug load of the system is suddenly released. Furthermore, the virtue of a longer therapeutic action can become a drawback in cases of unusual drug response or side-effects, when rapid elimination of drug from the body may be desired. The more uniform plasma-drug concentration seen after administration of extended-release systems is not always an advantage. Physiological tolerance caused by continuous therapeutic plasma-drug concentrations[6] can result in a loss of clinical efficacy of the administered drug. Furthermore, non-uniform plasma-drug concentrations can be a desirable therapeutic feature in disease states influenced by factors such as circadian rhythms. Nonetheless, it should be possible to adjust the rate of drug release from a truly controlled-release delivery system. The rate of release may be modified as a response to a physiological stimulus, such as blood-glucose concentrations or an externally applied stimulus, such as ultrasonic waves.[7] However, the cost and technical requirements of developing these controlled-release formulations and satisfying regulatory authorities pose further challenges to the formulator.

Not all drugs are suitable for presentation in extended-release delivery systems; the physiological and biological properties of some drugs restrict their applicability. For example, prolonged duration of action is seen with drugs that have long half-lives due to extensive binding to plasma protein[6, 8–10] and in such cases the drug delivered from an extended-release system would accumulate in the body tissues resulting in toxicity. While extended-release delivery systems are ideal for use with drugs with short half-lives, the half-life of each particular drug must not be so short that prohibitively large amounts of active ingredients are required in the dosage form. Potent low-dose drugs may present formulation problems due to their restricted flexibility in dosage adjustment. In addition, since potent drugs have a low margin of safety, the risk of dose-dumping must be considered.

PRELIMINARY CONSIDERATIONS

Extended-release drug delivery systems are administered mainly by the oral and percutaneous routes for systemic effects; however, the potential of the buccal, nasal, ophthalmic, and intrauterine routes of administration is yet to be fully realised and may be significant. A variety of factors influence the design of delivery systems. These include pharmaceutical considerations, the physicochemical and biological properties of the drug, patient/ disease factors, and the required pharmacokinetic profile.

Pharmaceutical Considerations

In general, the route of administration and total dose administered determine the type of delivery system required. For example, if the duration of action for one dose is more than one day, it is unlikely that oral delivery will be used. In addition, for oral dosage forms, the compatibility (within the formulation) and acceptability (to the patient) of excipients must be considered.

Physicochemical Properties

These are closely linked to the pharmaceutical considerations. These properties include the drug's aqueous solubility, pK_a, partition coefficient, molecular size and diffusivity, and protein binding capacity.[3] It may be necessary to modify the physicochemical properties of the drug to prevent interactions with excipients (for example, by the formation of stable insoluble salts). After selecting the appropriate form of the drug with the desired physicochemical properties and acceptable excipients, it is not unusual to find that the technical manipulations involved in processing may present insurmountable problems.

Biological Properties

The choice of route of administration may be constrained by physiological factors including hepatic first-pass metabolism, the biological half-life of the drug, and possible side-effects of the drug. Consideration of biological factors is particularly important during the formulation of drugs that are susceptible to acidic environments such as that of the stomach (for example, proteins and peptides). Therefore, there has been extensive research into exploiting other routes including nasal, pulmonary, and percutaneous administration.[11, 12]

Patient/Disease Factors

Patient/disease factors have a significant role in the design of suitable drug delivery systems. The age and physiological state of the patient must be considered along with a knowledge of whether acute or chronic therapy is required. Further, the degree of mobility of the patient must also be considered. During the development of novel delivery systems it may be possible to make use of changes in the pathological state of cells during the course of disease. For example, the differences between normal and malignant cells could be used to attain preferential specific drug delivery.[13] Similarly, higher concentrations of plasminogen activators[14] and tyrosinase[15] in melanoma cells may be exploited for their role in the bioconversion of prodrugs.

ENTERAL SYSTEMS

Mechanisms of Drug Release

Following oral administration of a dosage form, the principal mechanisms involved in controlling drug release are diffusion and dissolution. If a drug dissolves under 'sink' conditions, that is, the concentration in the bulk solution does not exceed 10% of its saturation solubility, then a plot of concentration of dissolved drug in the bulk solution as a function of time should produce a straight line with the gradient equal to the zero-order rate constant. Such a dissolution profile would be ideal for an extended-release product. In general, drug release is not zero order due to the difficulty of ensuring that release occurs from a constant surface area of drug. A drug with low aqueous solubility is likely to have an in-built potential for extended release in that the dissolution rate will be slower than the rates of absorption through a biological membrane. It is possible to modify, by chemical means, highly water-soluble drugs to less water-soluble forms, thereby reducing dissolution rate and extending the period of release. However, a more usual approach to retarding release is to incorporate the drug into a biodegradable or non-biodegradable system. Systems designed to give zero-order release can be prepared by embedding the drug in a polymer or material matrix with specialised dissolution properties.

Diffusion is the spontaneous flow of particles from a region of high concentration to one of low concentration resulting in a reduction in the concentration difference between the two regions. The driving force in diffusion is the gradient of chemical potential, although it is more usual to regard the diffusion process as a concentration gradient. The expression relating the flow of a component to the concentration gradient is known as Fick's first law and can be written for steady-state conditions as:

$$J = -D\frac{[dc]}{[dx]}$$

In terms of a drug crossing a membrane, J is the flux of particles across a plane membrane, dc/dx is the concentration gradient across a membrane and D is the diffusion coefficient of the drug across the membrane. The negative sign is indicative of diffusion occurring in the direction of decreasing concentration.

Diffusion in pharmaceutical systems is usually concerned with changes of concentration with time and distance. For such systems, the above equation is converted to a second-order partial differential equation known as Fick's second law:

$$\frac{\delta c}{\delta t} = D\frac{\delta^2 c}{\delta x^2}$$

According to Fick's second law, the change of concentration with time in a volume element in a diffusional field is related by a constant D, the diffusion coefficient, to the change of concentration with time at a point in the field.

The form of Fick's law describing diffusion from a particular system depends on the boundary conditions. For example, the steady-state diffusion and release from a reservoir-type extended-release system is described generally by Fick's second law.

The oral route is usually the preferred route of administration. The clinical performance of drugs administered by the oral route is influenced by the inherent physiological variables in the gastro-intestinal tract. These variables include gastro-intestinal motility and transit time. In addition, the presence of mucus and intestinal flora along with changes in luminal content and pH all contribute to considerable inter- and intra-individual variation in the *in-vivo* properties of dosage forms.

Gastro-intestinal Transit

If an extended-release delivery system is not in the body for the required period of time, it can only be of limited success as a means of controlling the amount of drug available for absorption. The transit time of solid oral dosage forms through the gastro-intestinal tract is usually approximately 24 hours although transit can take only 6 hours[16] or up to 60 hours.[17] Unless the residence time of the dosage form is modified, it may be expelled having delivered only a fraction of its drug content.

Gastro-intestinal transit is one of the most important physiological factors to be considered when designing extended-release dosage forms for oral administration. The gastro-intestinal transit time, like motility, is dependent on whether the gastro-intestinal tract is in the fed or fasted state.[18] Variations in gastro-intestinal transit time have implications for absorption of drugs that are only absorbed at specific areas of the tract, known as 'absorption windows'. The bioavailability of drugs presented as extended-release systems may be reduced if the drug cannot be held in the specific region of the gastro-intestinal tract where maximum absorption occurs. As a general indication, tablets, capsules, and particles have similar transit patterns to those of food material. The rate of gastric emptying exerts control on gastro-intestinal transit time and food intake appears to be the main contributing factor.[16, 19]

Non-disintegrating tablets have a residence time of between two and six hours in a full stomach, and less than 90 minutes when the stomach is in the fasted state. Multiparticulates have longer and more reproducible gastro-intestinal transit patterns than single-unit delivery systems. However, disintegrating dosage forms have been found to empty from the stomach along with food particles. Single and multidose units have been shown to empty rapidly from the stomach except in the presence of a heavy meal.[20]

The transit time of dosage forms through the small intestine is approximately three hours irrespective of food intake or gastro-intestinal transit time.[21, 22] The overall transit time of dosage forms in humans from the stomach to the ileocaecal junction is approximately six hours in the fasted state and about ten hours in the fed state. The implication of these transit times is that the maximum exposure time, during which the drug can be absorbed from the small intestine, is ten hours. There have been numerous attempts at mitigating the influence of gastro-intestinal transit on the efficiency of dosage forms in delivering drugs to the gastro-intestinal tract. One such system is the elementary osmotic pump (OROS) (see Fig. 7 in the Biopharmaceutics and Pharmacokinetic Principles chapter).[23] In its simplest form the pump is a tablet core consisting of drug and an osmotically active agent surrounded by a non-swelling semi-permeable membrane polymer. The aqueous content of the gastro-intestinal tract permeates the membrane and dissolves the osmotically active agent thus increasing the pressure inside the system and forcing drug out of the laser hole at a constant rate. There are several modifications of the design, which include coating the membrane with biodegradable polymer[24] or the inclusion of moveable partitions.[25] However, the main principle is that the drug is dissolved at a constant rate as the delivery system absorbs moisture while passing along the gastro-intestinal tract. The system can deliver drugs of any molecular weight and generally at a faster rate than diffusion-controlled reservoir systems. There are osmotic pumps with no orifice and these burst when the osmotic pressure reaches a certain level, thus releasing the drug.[26]

Other approaches aimed at overcoming the limiting effect of gastro-intestinal transit on the efficiency of dosage forms in delivering a drug for gastro-intestinal absorption have relied mainly on altering gastric residence time via modification of the density or buoyancy of the delivery system. High-density systems may be single or multiple units and include high-density excipients in the formulation. However, the results of one study[27] indicated that although the density of the systems was markedly increased, the transit time of the single-unit capsules and tablets was influenced more by the intake of food.

Low-density single-unit systems are designed to float on the stomach contents. They are formulated as 'hydrodynamically balanced systems' containing one or more hydrocolloids, the rationale being that the hydrocolloids swell on contact with water to form a gel layer. This layer presents a low-density system that floats on the gastro-intestinal contents. Bi-layer tablet formulations have been prepared in which one layer has carbon dioxide-generating ingredients to help flotation.[28] However, there are reports that capsules and tablets formulated as low-density systems do not show prolonged gastric residence.[29, 30]

A further approach has been to design delivery systems that are capable of adhering to the gastro-intestinal tract at specified sites, the principle being that there would be a subsequent improvement in the bioavailability of drugs with a narrow absorption window.[31] However, there are problems associated with the location of delivery systems at specific sites by the use of mucoadhesive additives. The mucoadhesives may adhere directly to surfaces either by binding to specific tissues or, alternatively, by complexing with the mucous coat of the tissue surface. Polycarbophil and carbomer have been used as agents capable of producing mucoadhesion. Multiple unit pellet formulations containing polycarbophil have shown prolonged gastric residence compared to a similar formulation with no bioadhesive.[31] Pellets containing carbomer have been reported to exhibit prolonged residence times and this effect was attributed to mucoadhesion.[32]

Another method used to modify the release characteristics of solid dosage forms is the Zydis™ system, which produces tablets that disperse rapidly when placed in the mouth—so-called melt-in-the-mouth tablets. The manufacturing process involves dissolving or suspending the drug in an aqueous matrix that is then filled into preformed cavities in a blister pack. The solution or suspension is then frozen and the water removed by lyophilisation. An extensive network of pores in the tablet allows buccal fluids to enter rapidly and disperse the Zydis™ unit.

pH Effects

In addition to problems associated with gastro-intestinal transit, the gastro-intestinal contents and environment influence drug absorption. The gastro-intestinal tract has extremes of pH and this can influence the stability and dissolution rate of many drugs. Particular problems arise when the drug shows maximum solubility in a region of the tract where absorption does not occur.

The effect of food on products that have pH-dependent dissolution properties must be determined during the development of modified-release preparations. The increase in hepatic blood flow and gastro-intestinal motility that follows food intake can also affect the bioavailability of dosage forms that release the drug in a pH-independent manner.

Design of Modified-release Systems

Several approaches have been applied to the design of modified-release drug delivery systems and each method has been based on the principle of modifying or controlling the availability of drug in solution to the body. The classification used here is based on chemical and physicochemical approaches.

Chemical Approach

The aims of the chemical approach are: firstly, to modify the structure of the drug molecule without influencing its therapeutic action in order to ensure that it is neither susceptible to unwanted metabolism nor poorly absorbed at unpredictable rates;[33] and secondly, to modify the solubility and selectively change the pharmacodynamics of the molecule to enhance its therapeutic action.

Two principal approaches have been used in the chemical modification of drug molecules.[9] The first approach involves preparing synthetic analogues of the parent compound, the philosophy being to develop an analogue that either enhances the required properties or decreases the undesirable properties of the parent compound. The second approach is to complex the active molecule to an inert carrier by covalent bonds that are susceptible to biodegradation. These complexed molecules are intended to have different lipophilicity from the original parent drug molecules enabling them to cross membranes. Alternatively, the complexed molecule may take part in an active transport system.[34, 35]

Physicochemical Approach

There were reports as long ago as 1860 of attempts to disperse drug into insoluble waxes and to partially coat tablet surfaces to delay release. In general, the release rate was unpredictable and the materials used were toxic.

It is possible to categorise delivery systems based on the physicochemical approach into two groups depending on the mechanism of drug release. There are diffusion-controlled delivery systems, where the principal mechanism of release is diffusion, and chemically controlled systems, where cleavage of drug-excipient bonds results in bioerosion of excipient molecules and subsequent drug release.

The majority of extended-release products are solid dosage forms for oral drug delivery. Liquid suspension preparations are not common since the controlling mechanism for release is dissolution or diffusion and when the drug comes into contact with an aqueous environment it is possible that a liquid formulation containing an aqueous vehicle would release drug during storage. However, a controlled-release morphine suspension is available (MST Continus suspension^{TM}) in which morphine is incorporated into beads of ion exchange resin. Following administration, sodium and potassium ions in the gastro-intestinal tract displace morphine from ionic sites in the resin; morphine at the surface of the resin is released quickly whereas morphine bound to sites inside the resin is released more slowly as it takes longer for the sodium and potassium ions to reach these sites. Each dose of the suspension is prepared immediately before administration.

Solid oral dosage forms may be presented as either single units or multiple units. Single units can include soluble and insoluble matrix tablets, coated tablets, or capsules. Multiple units are generally presented as drug particles or drug-loaded beads contained within an outer unit such as a capsule.

As noted earlier, it is desirable to have zero-order release from single- or multiple-unit dosage forms. However, it is more common for the delivery system to exhibit first-order or pseudo-first-order release kinetics. These systems do provide amounts of drug for absorption over extended periods of time but the concentration decreases with time. It is possible to consider the way in which extended release is achieved by controlling dissolution or diffusion of the active drug in the delivery system. Such a consideration is an over-simplification in that the performance of a system may be governed by a combination of mechanisms.

Dissolution-controlled Systems. Two groups of oral delivery system, encapsulated and matrix systems, rely on dissolution of the drug or components as the rate-controlling process in release. If dissolution is dependent on the surrounding environment, the amount of drug available for absorption may change as the delivery system passes through the gastro-intestinal tract.

Encapsulated systems are drug particles or drug coated non-pareil seeds surrounded by a slowly dissolving film layer.[36, 37] The time for dissolution of the layer depends on its thickness and composition, that is, whether soluble coatings such as carbohydrates, cellulose coatings, or less soluble wax-based coatings are used.[10] Theoretically, pareils may be prepared with a series of several different coat thicknesses in the same dosage unit. In this way it should be possible to have a combination of several dissolution rates. In practice, usually two or three pareils are used.[10]

Matrix systems are of two types, those in which drug particles are embedded in a soluble matrix and those where solid drug is dispersed uniformly in an insoluble matrix. The system in which drug is dispersed in a soluble matrix depends on the slow dissolution of the matrix for extended release. The most commonly used components of such matrices are fats and waxes,[38] but synthetic polymers are used for more sophisticated systems.[39] A major problem associated with the use of soluble matrices is that the surface area of the matrix decreases as dissolution takes place with a concomitant decrease in dissolution rate.

When the drug is dispersed in an insoluble matrix the solvent must reach the drug particle by penetrating the matrix before dissolution ensues. The dissolved drug must then diffuse through the pores of the matrix before release. Such a system has limitations for drugs with low aqueous solubility.[38] A series of hydrophobic polymers has been used in insoluble matrices. The delivery systems can take the form of tablets,[40] or beads or pellets.[41-48] However, zero-order drug release is only achieved if dissolution is the rate-limiting step and the undissolved area of drug is constant.

Diffusion-controlled Systems. Membrane reservoir systems and certain drug-dispersed matrix systems are two types of extended-release delivery systems from which drug diffusion is the rate-limiting step. The controlling mechanism is clearly diffusion in the reservoir systems but is less well differentiated in the matrices. Membrane reservoir systems are usually single dosage units and comprise a reservoir of drug surrounded by a water-insoluble polymer membrane that is applied by an air suspension technique.[10] There are reports of multiple unit systems but these are prepared by a microencapsulation process.[49, 50] The water-insoluble polymer is the rate-controlling membrane surrounding the drug which may be in solution or in the form of a particle. Release occurs after the drug partitions into the membrane, diffuses to the exterior, and exchanges with the environment surrounding the membrane. The drug release is diffusion-controlled and the rate-limiting step is the diffusivity of the drug through the polymer membrane, which is related to the area of the membrane and its thickness. The delivery systems may take the form of capsules,[51] microcapsules,[52] seeds,[51] or hollow fibres.[53]

Zero-order release can be maintained if: firstly, the area of the membrane does not change, that is, it does not swell or disintegrate; secondly, saturated drug concentrations are maintained in the interior of the membrane structure; and thirdly, sink conditions exist at the exterior of the system. However, there may be a 'lag time' or reduced rate of drug release for a period of time after administration until steady-state conditions are established in the membrane. In some formulations the membrane may have been saturated with drug during storage and release of drug from the membrane results in a 'burst effect'.

Polymers suitable for preparing non-porous homogeneous membranes for use in reservoir systems include ethylene vinyl acetate copolymers, ethylcellulose, and silicone networks.[54] These polymers are suitable as membranes for controlling the release of drugs of molecular weight less than 600.[55] Specific 'microporous' polymers may be used as a reservoir membrane that permits diffusion of dissolved drug through fluid-filled pores.[56] The micropores are innate or may be created by incorporating a soluble component into the membrane. In such cases drug release is controlled by the dissolution of the soluble component then diffusion of dissolved drug through the pores.

Diffusion-controlled matrix systems comprise drug dispersed uniformly in an insoluble polymer matrix. They may be of several forms: drug dissolved in matrix, drug dispersed in a non-porous matrix, or drug dispersed in a porous matrix. The release characteristics of the systems are based on the assumption that the matrix is a slab and that the drug is released under sink conditions.

The release of drug from a system in which the drug is dissolved in a matrix is related to the square root of time after the initial release. This time dependency applies for approximately 60% of the drug loading, but after this the amount of drug released is constant with time.[57]

When a drug is dispersed in a non-porous matrix, the mechanism of release involves dissolution of the drug followed by diffusion through the polymer. It is possible to devise equations relating the amount of drug released to the drug diffusion coefficient.[58] For example:

$$M_t = A_s[D_x t C_x (2C_o - C_x)]^{\frac{1}{2}}$$

where M_t is the amount of drug released at time t, A_s is the surface area of the slab, D_x is the drug diffusion coefficient in the matrix, C_x is the drug solubility in the matrix, C_o is the total drug concentration in the matrix.

The equation can be modified to take account of assumptions made about the conditions of release such as the constant drug diffusion coefficient,[59] non-steady-state conditions,[60] and absence of boundary layers.[57, 60, 61]

If the polymer is porous, matrix porosity and the tortuosity of the diffusion path within the pore structure of the matrix must be considered. The release of drug from matrices other than those in which the drug is dissolved decreases with time as a result of the increased diffusional path of the drug. Several attempts have been made to maintain constant release rates. One concept involved increasing the area of the diffusional front, thereby compensating for the increase in diffusional distance.[62] The design of the delivery device was based on the application of an impermeable coating on hemispheres or cylinders excluding a small area on the surface of the hemisphere or a small cavity in the cylinder. The impermeable coating or rate-limiting barrier on the surface of a diffusion-controlled matrix changes the release mechanism control from diffusion to dissolution.

Other techniques aimed at compensating for the decrease in release rate with time include the preparation of systems with non-uniform drug concentrations in the matrix[63, 64] or preparing systems with concentric layers of differing drug concentration.[65]

NON-ENTERAL SYSTEMS

Two major developments gave added impetus to the design of extended-release, and particularly controlled-release, products for administration by routes other than the oral route. Firstly, biological and informational molecules became commercially available. The second development was the availability of specialised polymers with known and reproducible physicochemical characteristics, which enabled polymers to be selected for a specific system.

The potential for delivering drugs by way of mucosal cells other than those of the gastro-intestinal tract has received considerable attention in recent years. Administration of drugs to the ocular, nasal, buccal, rectal, and vaginal cavities presents the opportunity to deliver drugs directly to the site of action or, alternatively, to avoid hepatic first-pass metabolism.

Ocular Delivery

The ocular route is not suitable for the systemic delivery of drugs. In fact absorption of drugs from eye drops can lead to unwanted side-effects. Eye drops and ointments are intended for local action. However, unless eye drops are formulated correctly they are not even an efficient method for local delivery since lachrymal secretions and blinking cause only a fraction of a single dose to reach the target site seconds after a large and variable initial dose (see Ophthalmic Products chapter). The appropriate formulation of drugs suspended in pharmaceutical vehicles prolongs the contact with the corneal surface. The vehicles used are generally solutions of viscosity-enhancing agents such as methylcellulose.

The use of drug pre-soaked hydrogels increases drug contact time over that seen with eye drops. These hydrogels could be looked upon as the forerunners of the ocular inserts known as the Alza Ocusert[TM] system.[66, 67] The Ocusert[TM] system consists of a core reservoir of drug complexed with alginic acid retained by two sheets of a transparent ethylene vinyl acetate copolymer membrane. The system is placed in the conjunctival sac of the eye and lachrymal secretions pass through the lipophilic membrane. Drug molecules dissolve and the drug in solution is released from the device at a zero-order rate. This delivery system avoids frequent dosing and has been found to promote good patient compliance.

Another method of ocular drug delivery is the Novel Ophthalmic Delivery System (NODS[TM]). The device contains the drug in a water-soluble polyvinyl alcohol (PVA) flag, which is attached to a stiffened paper handle by a soluble membrane. The unit is applied to the surface of the lower conjunctival sac. Contact with the moist eye causes the membrane to hydrate and the flag to detach and dissolve, thus releasing the drug. Reduced rate of clearance with NODS[TM] allows for greater ocular penetration.

Nasal Delivery

Nasal delivery has the potential for development as a route of administration for extended-release products. The anatomical and physiological characteristics of the nasal cavity make it an ideal candidate for investigation. Administration is easy and convenient, the region is well vascularised and hepatic first-pass metabolism is avoided. Drugs with presystemic metabolism such as progesterone, hydralazine, and propranolol have shown higher bioavailability in *animals* when administered nasally rather than orally. A more interesting development is that of delivering peptides and proteins by this route. The delivery of peptides is governed by molecular size and partition coefficient. In addition, nasal residence time and formulation factors have considerable influence. The most likely peptide candidates for nasal delivery are those with a broad therapeutic index and a relatively low cost such as desmopressin, lypressin, oxytocin, and nafarelin acetate.

Vaginal Delivery

Intravaginal modified-release drug delivery systems have the potential to deliver drugs for local action or systemic action without the drawback of hepatic first-pass metabolism. The drugs administered most commonly by this route are contraceptive steroids, which are delivered from biocompatible silicone vaginal rings. Drug release occurs over a period of three months.

Intra-uterine devices (IUDs) were developed for contraceptive use in the early 1920s and were made from silkworm gut and metal wire. These devices were unreliable and produced physiological complications. Later IUDs were prepared using inert biocompatible polymers and the intra-uterine plastic spiral and loop were developed. These devices worked principally on a mechanical basis and produced biological damage. Later, T-shaped polyethylene devices were developed containing contraceptive agents such as copper or progestogens. Progesterone-releasing IUDs such as Progestasert™ are plastic T-shaped devices containing progesterone. The main advantage of these devices over conventional oral products is that progesterone is delivered locally to the uterus rather than through systemic delivery.

Transdermal Delivery

Several transdermal drug delivery systems have been marketed. Their development was to some extent prompted by the discovery that continuous administration of some drugs through intact skin could produce many of the benefits of intravenous infusion associated with the control of plasma-drug concentrations while avoiding some of the hazards.[68] Furthermore, the skin is the most accessible and probably the most extensive organ of the body. It is well vascularised, elastic, and self-regenerating. The anatomy and physiology of the skin is discussed in the Topical Semi-solids chapter.

Not all drugs are suitable or desirable for use in transdermal delivery systems; for example, the phy-sicochemical properties of the drug may be unsuitable, or there may not be a justifiable clinical need. Some drugs have inadequate transdermal permeability, others cause irritation, sensitisation, or are metabolised in transit. In certain cases the required therapeutic effect can be achieved more adequately by conventional drug delivery.

The most common extended-release delivery system is the transdermal patch, which offers continuous therapy, good patient compliance, and convenience in use. Transdermal patches are usually polymeric multi-layered devices. A drug reservoir or a drug polymer matrix is fixed between two laminated layers of polymer. One layer is the backing, which is impermeable in order to prevent loss of drug and protect the matrix or reservoir. The other polymer laminate is the adhesive or the rate controlling membrane for the drug. For convenience of description transdermal delivery systems can be categorised as reservoir or matrix systems.

Release from **reservoir systems** (Fig. 1) is controlled by diffusional resistance across a polymeric membrane. The drug in the reservoir is either dissolved in an appropriate solvent or distributed uniformly in a solid polymer matrix such as polyisobutylene, which is suspended in a viscous liquid such as silicone fluid. The polymer membranes used are non-porous or microporous and the patch is attached to the skin by a hypoallergenic adhesive. The drug release rate can be modified by selection of appropriate reservoir formulations or changes in the characteristics of the rate-controlling membrane. Transiderm Nitro™, Transiderm Scop™, and Catapres TTS™ are based on reservoir systems.

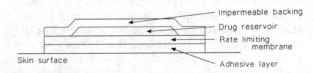

Fig. 1
The reservoir system.

In **matrix systems** the drug is either dispersed or dissolved in a polymer. Matrix patches can be regarded as belonging to one of three types depending on the type of matrix used. The drug may be homogeneously dispersed in a hydrophilic or hydrophobic matrix reservoir, which is mounted on an impermeable backing membrane. Adhesive polymer is only required as a strip around the system. The Nitro-Dur™ system used for angina pectoris is based on this approach. A more elegant system can be prepared by directly dispersing the drug in an adhesive polymer such as polyacrylate, which can be used as a pressure sensitive polymer. Nitro-Dur II™ systems are based on this technology. The Deponit™ system for glyceryl trinitrate is a reservoir gradient-controlled matrix system (Fig. 2) designed to compensate for non-zero-order drug delivery from matrix systems. The delivery system is prepared from layers of matrix. The amounts of drug in each layer decrease with distance from the impermeable backing at time zero. The philosophy behind this system is that as the drug is lost from the layer with the lowest amount of drug then drug diffuses down the diffusional path from the layer with the largest amount.

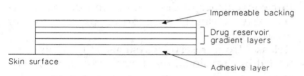

Fig. 2
The reservoir gradient-controlled matrix system.

Delivery systems have been marketed based on a combination of reservoir and matrix dispersions. The Nitrodisc™ system depends on this technology. A drug reservoir containing drug solids dispersed in an aqueous solution of drug solubiliser is dispersed in a hydrophobic polymer using high shear rate. The dispersion is then stabilised by cross-linking the polymer *in situ* before mounting on the impermeable base layer.

The choice of reservoir or matrix formulation is influenced by the required rate of drug transport. If the rate of transport across the skin is greater than the rate required to produce a therapeutic steady state, then control of the delivery rate is required and a reservoir delivery system would be used. Alternatively, if permeation through the stratum corneum controls the rate of delivery to the body then a matrix delivery system can be used. It would not be advisable to present a drug with a narrow therapeutic index in a matrix delivery system because variability in permeation characteristics of the stratum corneum may lead to the production of toxic drug concentrations in the body.

The transdermal patch is not the only novel device for controlling the release of drugs for transfer across the skin. For example, electrical current has been used to activate and control the movement of ionised drug molecules across various biological membranes. The technique of iontophoresis has been used to enhance the transfer of drugs such as polypeptides across the skin.[69]

Parenteral Drug Delivery

Parenteral drug delivery, particularly by the intravenous route, is the least appealing route of drug delivery to patients. However, in circumstances where a carefully specified route of administration is required to provide a therapeutic effect for designated periods of time there may be few alternatives available. The route is particularly useful for delivering biological molecules that are susceptible to hepatic first-pass metabolism or where administration via the gastro-intestinal route provides poor bioavailability. The formulation, preparation, and administration of parenteral products are discussed in detail in the Parenterals chapter.

Parenteral depot delivery systems have many of the benefits associated with intravenous drug infusion. The depot may be formulated in an aqueous or an oily basis or as a thixotropic suspension. The drug may be used in its original form or derivatised as a salt or complex. The form of the drug and the vehicle used are particularly important in controlling release rates. Many depot formulations have been developed, for example procaine penicillin suspensions, insulin zinc suspensions, and medroxyprogesterone acetate (Depo-Provera™).

More recently, the dispersion of drugs in polymeric biodegradable, biocompatible polymers has become a commercial reality. A luteinising hormone releasing hormone (LHRH) analogue, goserelin, has been marketed (Zoladex™) for use as an implant in the treatment of prostatic carcinoma. The successful action of this injectable implant product depends largely on the biodegradation of a novel lactide-glycolide polymer.[70]

It is likely that many more biological molecules will be administered by this route. An added advantage of this route is that it offers the possibility of judicious implantation near the site of action. However, a drawback is that once the implant is sited, removal generally requires surgical procedures.

Liposomes are small vesicles with phospholipid bilayers surrounding an aqueous core. As a result of their structure they may be used as carriers of both lipid-soluble and water-soluble drugs. In the intravenous infusion AmBisome™, amphotericin is incorporated into liposomes prepared from phospholipids and cholesterol. A reduction in toxicity with the liposomal formulation is achieved as amphotericin is already bound to liposomal steroid and is less likely to interact with host cell membranes while maintaining its affinity for fungal sterols when released at the site of action.

In cytotoxic therapy, liposomal encapsulation of anthracyclines and the sequestration of vincristine in low density lipoprotein (LDL) particles has been attempted. Complexation of vincristine into LDL particles may be considered a means of drug targeting, by taking advantage of the high concentration of LDL receptors and LDL receptor internalisation found in some tumour cells relative to normal tissue.

Acknowledgements—Thanks to Dr S. Nicholson and Mr H. Huatan for assistance with literature work and Mrs B. Thorne for preparation of the manuscript.

REFERENCES

1. Bagnall RD. Biomat Med Dev Art Org 1977;5:355.
2. Hsieh DST. Controlled release systems: Fabrication technology; vol I. New York: CRC Press, 1986.
3. Chien YW. In: Chien YW, editor. Novel drug delivery systems; vol 14. New York: Marcel Dekker, 1982.
4. Li VH, Lee VH, Robinson JR. Influence of drug properties and routes of drug administration on the design of sustained and controlled release systems. In: Robinson JR, Lee VH, editors. Controlled drug delivery: Fundamentals and applications; vol 29. 2nd ed. New York: Marcel Dekker, 1987.
5. de Duve C. Foreword. In: Gregoriadis G, editor. Drug carriers in modern medicine. New York: Academic Press, 1979.
6. Ritschel WA. Drug Dev Ind Pharm 1989;15:1073–103.
7. Theeuwes F. Triggered, pulsed and programmed drug delivery. In: Prescott LF, Nimmo WS, editors. Novel drug delivery. Chichester: John Wiley & Sons, 1989.
8. Li VH, Lee VH, Robinson JR. Influence of drug properties and routes of drug administration on the design of sustained and controlled release systems. In: Robinson JR, Lee VH, editors. Controlled drug delivery: Fundamentals and applications; vol 29. 2nd ed. New York: Marcel Dekker, 1987.
9. Rubenstein A, Robinson JR. Prog Clin Med 1987;4:71-107.
10. Conrad JM, Robinson JR. Sustained drug release from tablets and particles through coating. In: Lieberman HA, Lachman L, editors. Pharmaceutical dosage forms: Tablets; vol 3. New York: Marcel Dekker, 1982.
11. O'Hagan DT, Illum L. Drug carrier systems; vol 7. New York: CRC Press, 1990:35–97.
12. Fisher AN, Farray NF, O'Hagan DT, Jabbal-Gill I, Johansen BR, Davis SS et al. Int J Pharmaceutics 1981;74:147–99.
13. Gregoriadis G, Senior J, Poste G. Targeting with synthetic drug carrier systems; vol 113. New York: Plenum Press, 1986.
14. Chakravarty PK, Carl PL, Weber MJ, Katzenellerge JA. J Med Chem 1983;26:633.
15. Chakravarty PK, Carl PL, Weber MJ, Katzenellerge JA. J Med Chem 1983;26:864.
16. Davis SS. [Chapter 10]. In: Johnson P, Lloyd-Jones JG. Drug delivery systems. Chichester: Ellis Horwood, 1987.
17. Hinton JM, Lennard-Jones JE, Young AC. Gut 1969;10:842.
18. Quigly S, Phillips SF, Dent J. Gastroenterology 1984;87:836.
19. Wilson CG, Washington N. Drug Dev Ind Pharm 1988;14,211–81.
20. Christensen FN, Davis SS, Hardy JG, Taylor MJ, Whalley DR, Wilson CG. J Pharm Pharmacol 1985;37:91–5.
21. Davis SS, Hardy JG, Taylor MJ, Whalley DR, Wilson CG. Int J Pharmaceutics 1984;21:167–77.
22. Davis SS, Hardy JG, Taylor MJ, Whalley DR, Wilson CG. Int J Pharmaceutics 1984;21:331–40.
23. Theeuwes F. J Pharm Sci 1975;64:1987–91.
24. Methods for administering drug to the gastrointestinal tract. US patent 4096238. 1978.
25. Osmotic system for the control and delivery of agent over time. US patent 4111202. 1978.
26. Bechgaard H, Christensen FN, Davis SS, Hardy JG, Taylor MJ, Whalley DR et al. J Pharm Pharmacol 1985;37:718–21.
27. Bechgaard H, Ladefoged K. J Pharm Pharmacol 1978;30:690–2.
28. Ingani HM, Timmermans J, Moes AJ. Int J Pharmaceutics 1987;35:157-64.
29. Muller-Lissner SA, Blum AL. New Engl J Med 1981;304:1365–6.
30. Sangekar S, Vadino WA, Chaudry I, Parr A, Beihn R, Digenis G. Int J Pharmaceutics 1987;35:187–91.
31. Langer MA, Ch'ng HS, Robinson JR. J Pharm Sci 1985;74:406–11.
32. Fell JT, Harris D, Sharma HL, Taylor DC. Polym Prepr (Am Chem Soc Div Polym Chem) 1987;28:145–6.
33. Langer R. Science 1990;249:1527–33.
34. Bodor N, Simpkins JW. Science 1983;222:221–5.
35. Kumagan AK, Pardridge WM. J Biol Chem 1987;262:1524.
36. Chandrasekaran SK, Paul DR. J Pharm Sci 1982;71:1399–402.
37. Peppas NA. J Biomed Mater Res 1983;17:1079–87.
38. Ritschel WA. [Chapter 2]. In: Ariens EJ, editor. Drug design; vol 4. New York: Academic Press, 1973.
39. Heller J. Use of polymers in controlled release of active agents. In: Robinson JR, Lee VH, editors. Controlled drug delivery: Fundamentals and applications; vol 29. 2nd ed. New York: Marcel Dekker, 1987.
40. Gould PL, Holland SJ, Tighe BJ. Int J Pharmaceutics 1987;38:231–7.
41. Bodmeier R, Chen H. J Pharm Sci 1989;78(10):819–25.
42. Benita S, Benoit JP, Puisseux F, Thies C. J Pharm Sci 1984;73(12):1721–4.
43. Brophy MRC, Deasy PB. Int J Pharmaceutics 1986;29:223–31.
44. Kishida A, Dressman JB, Yoshioka S, Aso Y, Takeda Y. J Controlled Release 1990;13:83–9.
45. Izumikawa S, Yoshioka S, Aso Y, Takeda Y. J Controlled Release 1990;15:133–40.
46. Bodmeier R, Oh KH, Chen H. Int J Pharmaceutics 1989;51:1–8.
47. Holland SJ, Yasin M, Tighe BJ. Biomaterials 1990;11:206–15.
48. Gangrade N, Price JC. J Microencapsulation 1991;8(2):185-202.
49. Luzzi LA. J Pharm Sci 1970;59:1367–76.
50. Li SP, Kowarski CR, Feld KM, Grim WM. Drug Dev Ind Pharm 1988;14:353–76.
51. Pitt CG, Gratzi MM, Jeffcoat RA, Zweidainger R, Schnider A. J Pharm Sci 1979;68:1534–8.
52. Ogawa Y, Yamamoto M, Takada S, Okada H, Shimamoto T. Chem Pharm Bull 1988;36:1095–103.
53. Eeink MJD, Feijen J, Olijslager J, Abers JH, Reike JC, Greidamus PJ. J Controlled Release 1987;6:225–47.
54. Passi WJ. Prog Polym Sci 1989;14:629–77.

55. Langer R. Chem Eng Commun 1980;6:1–48.
56. Langer RS, Peppas NA. J Macromol Sci 1983;C23:61–126.
57. Baker RW, Lonsdale HK. In: Tanquary AC, Lacey RE, editors. Controlled release of biologically active agents. New York: Plenum Press, 1974:15–71.
58. Higuchi T. J Pharm Sci 1963;52:1145–9.
59. Cardinal JR. In: Anderson JM, Kim SW, editors. Recent advances in drug delivery systems. New York: Plenum Press, 1984:229–48.
60. Paul DR, McSpadden SK. J Memb Sci 1976;1:33–48.
61. Roseman TJ, Cardarelli NF. [Chapter 2]. In: Kydonieus AF, editor. Controlled release technologies: Methods, theory and applications; vol 1. Boca Raton: CRC Press, 1980.
62. Hsieh DST, Rhine WD, Langer R. J Pharm Sci 1983;72:17–22.
63. Lee PI. Polymer 1984;25:973–8.
64. Lee PI. J Controlled Release 1986;4:1–7.
65. Ganderton D. [Chapter 9]. In: Johnson P, Lloyd-Jones JG, editors. Drug delivery systems. Chichester: Ellis Horwood, 1987.
66. Shell J, Baker R. Ann Ophthalmol 1974;6:1037.
67. Shell J. Ophthalmic Surg 1974;5:73.
68. Kydonieus AF. In: Kydonieus AF, Berner B, editors. Fundamentals of transdermal drug delivery in transdermal delivery of drugs; vol 1. Boca Raton: CRC Press, 1987.
69. Burnette RR, Marreo D. J Pharm Sci 1986;75:738.
70. Hutchinson FG, Furr BJA. J Controlled Release 1990;13:279.

FURTHER INFORMATION

Junginger HE, editor. Drug targeting and delivery: Concepts in dosage form design. Chichester: Ellis Horwood, 1992.
Tomlinson E, Davis SS, editors. Site-specific drug delivery: Cell biology, medical and pharmaceutical aspects. Chichester: John Wiley & Sons, 1986.
Tyle P, editor. Specialized drug delivery systems: Manufacturing and production technology. New York: Marcel Dekker, 1990.

Biopharmaceutics and Pharmacokinetic Principles

Medicinal compounds exert their pharmacological activity in a variety of ways. Many act by occupying a receptor site, that is, a specific group of macromolecules in tissue cells, and the result is an interaction that elicits a pharmacological response. Other drugs act by altering or interfering with homoeostatic mechanisms in the body; for example, by a stimulation or a reduction in the production of endogenous compounds. For a drug to act in any of these ways, it must be distributed within the body. In contrast, some treatments require only a local application of the drug; for example, skin conditions and infestations are usually treated topically. Nevertheless, most treatments require the transfer of drug from the site of administration to the site of action. The transfer of drug utilises the systemic blood circulation or the lymphatic system, or both, for transport of the compound to the vicinity of the drug receptor or site of action.

Medicines are conventionally applied to the body at various sites. The most common sites are the gastro-intestinal tract, following oral administration; muscle and subcutaneous tissues, following injection; and the lungs, following delivery from an aerosol.

Transport of drug from the administration site to the blood or lymphatic system is the process of **absorption** and requires the transfer of drug molecules across a membrane. Drugs given by direct injection into a vein do not require absorption.

Immediately following absorption, the drug is transported away from the region of the administration site. The process of **distribution** occurs via the systemic circulation and by the subsequent diffusion into tissues and fluids of the body. The drug may bind to proteins present in blood plasma and this initially aids distribution; however, the subsequent transfer into tissues can only occur if the drug uncouples from the plasma proteins; the drug-protein complex itself is too large to diffuse through the blood capillary membrane and remains within the systemic circulation.

The processes of **excretion** and **metabolism** act to reduce the amount of drug in the body. These **elimination** processes lead to termination of drug action as the drug concentration falls, although the metabolites of the drug may themselves exert a pharmacological effect.

The events that follow absorption, namely, distribution and elimination, are known collectively as drug **disposition**. Each process is, inevitably, quite complex and may involve many individual mechanisms. The relationships are shown in a simplified form in Fig. 1. An equilibrium exists between the unbound (free) drug in plasma and the drug at the sites of action, drug stored in body tissues, and that bound to proteins in the plasma.

There are several mechanisms by which drug transfer can occur. However, with few exceptions the

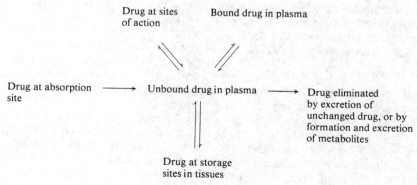

Fig. 1
Schematic representation of drug disposition.

driving force for drug movement is passive diffusion (see below) from the region of high drug concentration around the site of application to regions of negligible concentration elsewhere in the body. Diffusion takes place through tissue, such as the epidermis and dermis of the skin, but often a body membrane must be crossed. For example, transfer of drug between cell tissue and blood plasma occurs through the layer of endothelial cells forming the wall of a blood capillary. The rate at which transmembrane movement of drug takes place is largely dependent on the physicochemical properties of the drug itself, the rate at which the tissue is perfused by blood, and the inherent permeability of the membrane.

ABSORPTION

Mechanisms of Drug Transport

The processes of absorption, distribution, and excretion all involve the transfer of the drug across biological membranes. Biological membranes are complex lipoprotein structures which vary from a single membrane, such as a cell membrane, to several layers of cells, such as the skin. Membranes also vary in their intrinsic ability to allow molecules to transfer, some being more 'open' structures than others; the gastro-intestinal membrane is an example of a relatively 'closed' structure.

Five mechanisms of membrane transfer have been identified. Fig. 2 illustrates some of these. **Passive diffusion**, the most important mechanism, requires the compound to be of low molecular weight and to be lipophilic; also, there must be a concentration gradient. The concentration gradient across the membrane (dc/dx) is approximately equal to the difference in concentrations across the membrane (Δc) divided by membrane thickness.

The rate of transport across a membrane by passive diffusion is derived from the classical equation for the First Law of Diffusion of Fick. The rate is dependent upon the membrane surface area (A) and the permeability constant (P).

$$\text{Rate of transport} = P \times A \times \Delta c$$

For drugs that do not meet the requirements for passive diffusion, other transfer mechanisms may be operative. There are a few drugs with structural similarities to naturally occurring compounds, which are transported by special biological systems. These systems transport amino acids, sugars, and weak organic acids through a carrier mechanism. The drug binds temporarily to the carrier and the complex crosses the membrane. In

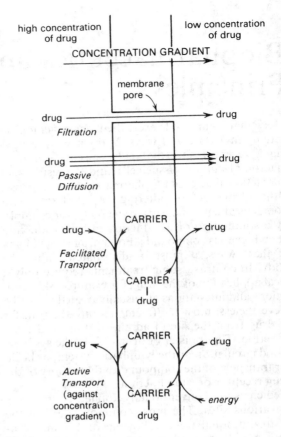

Fig. 2
Main mechanisms of membrane transfer.

facilitated transport, the transfer is always in the direction of the concentration gradient. In **active transport**, transfer can be against the concentration gradient and the compound can accumulate in high concentrations. There is an energy requirement for active transport. The main features of these three mechanisms are given in Table 1.

Water-soluble compounds of low molecular weight, for example, urea, and small ions, such as sodium and potassium, can pass through membrane pores. This process, **filtration**, requires a concentration gradient and a relatively 'open' membrane structure, such as is found in the kidney tubule.

In the process of **pinocytosis**, extracellular material is enveloped by the cell membrane and absorbed into the cell. After the encapsulated material has been transported, it is expelled from the cell. This mechanism allows relatively large molecules, such as proteins, to cross membranes although transfer is likely to be slow.

Table 1
Comparison of mechanisms of drug transport

	Facilitated transport	Active transport	Passive diffusion
Carrier substance required	yes	yes	no
Concentration gradient required	yes	no	yes
Specific	yes	yes	no
Saturable	yes	yes	no
Sensitive to metabolic inhibitors	yes	yes	no
Energy requirements	only to maintain cell integrity	to effect transport against concentration gradient	only to maintain cell integrity
Examples of transfer across gastro-intestinal mucosa	quaternary ammonium compounds	many L-amino acids (L-dopa); some mono-saccharides (glucose and galactose); some pyrimidines and 5-fluorouracil; some water-soluble vitamins	most compounds

Absorption of Drugs by Passive Diffusion

From the results of many studies of the transfer of drugs through mammalian cell membranes, several features of passive diffusion can be stated. These form the basis of the theory that has become known as the **pH-partition hypothesis**.

Cell membranes, including the lining of the gastro-intestinal mucosa, behave as though they were a 'lipoidal sieve', allowing the transfer of lipid-soluble materials and preventing the transfer of water-soluble, ionised materials. Consequently the transfer of small unionised organic molecules is favoured.

Where a drug molecule is capable of dissociating into ions an equilibrium exists between the ionised and unionised species. However, it is only the unionised form that is appreciably absorbed. Because the proportion of ionised and unionised forms of weak acids and bases varies with the hydrogen ion concentration, pH changes can alter markedly their rates of absorption. A strong acid or strong base will exist in the ionised form at all pH values and will be poorly absorbed through membranes. For weak acids and bases the proportions of unionised absorbable species and ionised non-absorbable species can be calculated at any pH if the dissociation constant (or ionisation constant, K_a) for the acid or base is known. The dissociation constant of a weak acid (HA) ionising to give hydrogen ions (H^+) and ions of the conjugate base (A^-) is defined by:

$$K_a = \frac{[H^+][A^-]}{[HA]}$$

where $[H^+]$, $[A^-]$, and $[HA]$ are the concentrations of the hydrogen ions, conjugate base, and unionised acid, respectively. The pK_a value for an acid is the common logarithm of the reciprocal of the dissociation constant K_a, and is a measure of acid strength. A pK_a value below 2.5 indicates a strong acid. Weak acids have a pK_a value in the range 2.5 to 8 and very weak acids a pK_a greater than 8. The relative proportions of ionised (A^-) and unionised (HA) species can be calculated from the Henderson-Hasselbalch equation:

$$\log_{10} \frac{[A^-]}{[HA]} = pH - pK_a$$

For a moderately weak acid such as salicylic acid (pK_a 3.0) the proportions of ionised and unionised forms are shown in Table 2. There are equal concentrations of ionised and unionised acid when the pH is equal to the pK_a of the weak acid. Below this pH the unionised form predominates and above it the acid is mainly in the ionised form. Because the pH scale is a logarithmic one, a small pH change produces a large change in the composition of the mixtures of species; a change of one pH unit leads to a ten-fold change in the proportion of ionised to unionised form.

Table 2
Effect of pH on the degree of ionisation of salicylic acid

pH of medium	Ratio ionised:unionised	Percentage of unionised form
1	0.01	99.0
3	1	50.0
5	100	1.0
7	10 000	≈0.0

The general conclusion is that for weak acids the unionised form predominates at a pH below the pK_a value. Consequently the absorption of a weak acid proceeds more rapidly at low pH than at high pH, and this has been demonstrated in practice for many medicinal compounds.

The ionisation of a weak base (B) may be represented as producing hydroxyl ions (OH^-) and ions of the conjugate acid (BH^+):

$$B + H_2O \rightleftharpoons BH^+ + OH^-$$

The dissociation constant (K_b) for the weak base may be defined as:

$$K_b = \frac{[BH^+][OH^-]}{[B]}$$

However, it is usual to express the strength of a weak base in terms of strength of the conjugate acid it produces, that is in terms of the equilibrium:

$$BH^+ \rightleftharpoons B + H^+$$

so that

$$K_a = \frac{[B][H^+]}{[BH^+]}$$

Since a strong base gives rise to a weak conjugate acid and *vice versa*, a high pK_a value indicates a strong base and a lower value indicates a weak base. If the pK_a for the conjugate acid is below about 11.5 the base that gives rise to the conjugate acid is considered to be a weak base. For example, atropine (pK_a 9.65) is stronger than codeine (pK_a 8.2), although both are weak bases. The relative proportions of the ionised (BH^+) and unionised (B) forms can be calculated from the Henderson-Hasselbalch equation:

$$\log_{10} \frac{[BH^+]}{[B]} = pK_a - pH$$

This equation predicts that the proportion of ionised species is increased by a decrease in pH. This is the reverse of the behaviour shown by weak acids.

In summary it is seen that the formation of a high proportion of the unionised species of a weak acid is favoured by a low pH whereas the formation of a high proportion of the unionised species of a weak base is favoured by a high pH. Consequently the absorption of weak acids occurs more readily from acidic solutions than from alkaline solutions and the converse is true for weak bases.

It should not be supposed that all compounds existing predominantly in the unionised form are absorbed through cell membranes at equal rates. An important factor controlling the rate of transmembrane movement is the lipid solubility of the unionised species. This in turn is governed primarily by the chemical structure of the compound and can be illustrated by reference to homologous series of compounds. The lipid solubility is usually expressed as the oil-in-water partition coefficient (P) which for most compounds can be written as:

$$P = \frac{\text{concentration of compound in organic phase}}{\text{concentration of compound in aqueous phase}}$$

where the concentrations are measured after the solute (in monomeric form) has reached a distribution equilibrium between the two immiscible liquids and do not approach the solubility in either phase. A high lipid solubility is indicated by a high value for the partition coefficient and is favoured by an increase in the number of alkyl or aryl groups, the absence of strongly ionising groups, the presence of sulphur atoms in preference to oxygen, and the presence of halogen atoms in the molecule. Table 3 shows how changes in the substituents of the barbiturate molecule markedly alter the partition coefficient.

Table 3
The effect of different substituents of the barbiturate molecule on the partition coefficient

Compound	Substituents	Partition coefficient	pK_a	Comments
Barbitone	$R_1 = CH_3CH_2-$ $R_2 = O=$	0.07	8.0	predominantly water-soluble
Phenobarbitone	$R_1 = C_6H_5-$ $R_2 = O=$	0.4	7.4	increased lipid solubility due to phenyl group
Thiophenobarbitone	$R_1 = C_6H_5-$ $R_2 = S=$	14	—	marked effect of replacing oxygen atom by sulphur atom
Thiopentone	$R_1 = CH_3CH_2CH_2- C(CH_3)H-$ $R_2 = S=$	90	7.6	predominantly lipid-soluble

The pK_a values for these compounds are similar. The large differences in their rates of penetration of membranes are due almost entirely to differences in lipid solubility; the effects of lipid solubility, and the dissociation of weak acids and bases into ions cannot be considered separately. Thus, rapid transmembrane movement by passive diffusion is favoured by a high proportion of drug molecules being in the unionised form at the pH conditions prevailing and a high oil-in-water partition coefficient. Slow penetration of a membrane may be the result of a low proportion of unionised molecules or a small value for the oil-water partition coefficient, or a combination of the two.

Main Routes of Drug Absorption

Absorption from the Gastro-intestinal Tract

The oral route of administration is the most popular and convenient, and is effective for many drugs. Physiological properties of the gastro-intestinal tract that favour absorption are the relatively large volume of fluid available for dissolution of the drug, the peristaltic movement of the stomach and small intestine which promotes some mixing of the luminal contents, the large mucosal area over which absorption can occur, and the extensive blood flow through the mesenteric circulation. Less desirable are the extremes of pH and the variety of enzymes to which the drug is exposed.

Gastric and intestinal fluids are produced in normal healthy adult individuals in copious quantity, with about 5 litres being formed in 24 hours. In healthy subjects, typical pH values of fluids in various segments of the gastro-intestinal tract are: stomach, pH 2; duodenum, jejunum and ileum, pH progressively increasing from 6.5 to 7.5; caecum, pH falling to 5.5 but thereafter progressively rising to 6.0 (transverse colon), 7.2 (descending colon), and 7.5 (rectum).

The pH influences the extent to which weak acids and weak bases exist in the unionised, lipid-soluble state. Under the acid conditions in the stomach, weak acids will exist largely in the unionised form, and weak bases in the ionised form. In the less acid fluid of the small intestine, weak acids will be predominantly ionised and weak bases mainly unionised. This is illustrated for a few compounds in Table 4. Saccharin and dexamphetamine being a strong acid and a strong base, respectively,

will be extensively ionised at pH 2 and pH 7. The oral absorption of ionised compounds, such as hexamethonium and pentolinium has been shown to be poor and irregular. However, some compounds, such as dexamphetamine, imipramine, and bethanidine are well absorbed even though they are strong bases showing that the pH-partition hypothesis is not fully predictive of drug absorbability. Furthermore, the pH-partition hypothesis predicts that the stomach will be the main site for absorption of weak acids, but that weak bases will not be absorbed until they encounter the higher pH conditions of the small intestine. Other factors, such as drug dissolution and the limited surface area of the stomach, are important in influencing the absorption site.

Although weak acids are absorbed more rapidly from an acidic medium, drug dissolution is favoured by a high pH. In contrast, weak bases dissolve readily in the acid gastric juice, and are favourably absorbed in the less acid environment of the small intestine. Since dissolution must precede absorption from solid dosage forms, in theory the absorption from a powdered acidic drug will not occur until after it has dissolved in the fluids of the small intestine, and absorption may therefore be incomplete. In practice, there are several other factors that make this simple model inappropriate. First, dissolution of an acidic drug will occur to a limited extent in stomach acid, and the upper small intestine, being slightly acidic, provides a site for absorption. Second, weak acids may be administered as a sodium or calcium salt, which has a higher water solubility than the acid form. The salt dissolves readily in the gastric juice, although the free acid may then be precipitated. However, gastric mucin inhibits or delays precipitation and any crystals formed are probably small and dissolve readily on dilution with more fluid. Finally, the rate of absorption is dependent upon the available mucosal area. The stomach with its limited surface area is a poor site for absorption. In contrast, the unique morphological structure of the duodenum gives it a surface area many times greater than that of a simple cylinder of the same dimensions. There is considerable evidence that the small intestine is the main site of absorption for many drugs, including weak acids. For this reason the gastric residence time of the drug (or the medicine containing it) has a large influence upon the time of onset of absorption.

Gastro-intestinal Motility.
The upper small intestine is the main site of dissolution and absorption

Table 4

The effect of pH on the ionisation of weak acids and bases

| Compound | pK_a | Percentage unionised | |
		Stomach (pH 2)	Small intestine (pH 7)
Weak acid			
Acetylsalicylic acid	3.5	97	0.03
Benzylpenicillin	2.8	86	0.004
Phenylbutazone	4.4	99.6	0.25
Saccharin	1.6	29	0.001
Weak base			
Colchicine	1.9	56	99.99
Dexamphetamine	9.9	0	0.13
Lignocaine	7.9	0	11.1
Mecamylamine	11.3	0	0.005
Reserpine	6.6	0.002	71

of oral dosage forms. The retention of drug in the stomach will delay the onset of activity, because of poor absorption from the stomach, and may lead to hydrolytic degradation of acid-labile compounds. The residence time of an oral formulation in the stomach will depend on the rate of emptying of the gastric contents. Measurements of gastric emptying of the liquid and solid components of ingested materials can be made by labelling them with suitable gamma- emitting isotopes (for example, ^{131}In and ^{99m}Tc, respectively) and external scintigraphic monitoring of the subject using a gamma camera or scintiscanner.

Gastric emptying patterns are substantially different in the fed and fasted (or interdigestive) states. The difference arises from the physiological control of transfer of gastric contents through the pyloric sphincter into the duodenum in the two conditions. After food, the pyloric sphincter relaxes intermittently to allow the passage of chyme and food particles. Recent studies have shown in healthy volunteers that food particles up to 7 mm in diameter are emptied. Consequently, the components of multi-particulate delivery systems, as well as small and intermediate-sized intact tablets, can pass into the duodenum together with digested food. Larger tablets will undergo disintegration or erosion until of a small enough size to empty from the stomach. Non-disintegrating tablets of about 10 mm or larger (such as enteric-coated tablets) will not empty from the stomach in the fed state.

The rate of emptying of drug particles mixed with food has been shown to depend on the size of the meal; times for emptying of half of the contents were from 1.5 hours after a light breakfast to 3.5 hours after a heavy breakfast. Because absorption occurs mainly after the drug has passed out of the stomach, rates of absorption will be lower in the presence of food, as has been observed for many drugs. Large non-disintegrating tablets remain in the stomach while food is present, being unable to pass through the pyloric sphincter. In the fasted condition, however, the motility pattern in the gastro-intestinal tract changes such that a powerful contraction sweeps the length of the tract every two hours. This occurs during Phase 3 of the 'migrating myoelectric complex'. The effect is to sweep large objects out of the stomach. These factors explain why the onset of absorption from single-unit, enteric-coated tablets is highly variable under conditions of food ingestion.

The subsequent transit of drug through the small intestine is independent of physiological factors (such as the presence of food) or the dosage form (solution, pellets, or intact tablets). Transit varies between individuals, and transfer from the pylorus to the ileo-caecal sphincter occurs in 1 to 5 hours. Total transit times (mouth to anus) for non-disintegrating, modified-release products are highly variable between individuals. After dosing at breakfast time, the mean total transit time is 25 hours in healthy subjects but varies from 6 to 72 hours. In most subjects, therefore, these products reside for longer in the large intestine than in the remainder of the gastro-intestinal tract. There is, however, evidence that absorption of drug from the dosage form does occur from the colonic regions of the gastro-intestinal tract for most drugs studied to date. Indeed, a major part of the total dose may be absorbed from the colon.

Transit of single non-disintegrating dose units through the large intestine may be quite rapid. If the total transit time for a modified-release formulation is short then there is concern that drug release may be incomplete. Total transit times as short as six hours have been observed. Low bioavailability has been observed for a product containing oxprenolol in subjects in whom total transit time was short.

Much of the information on the transit of dosage forms and drug absorption from the gastro-intestinal tract is obtained from studies in healthy subjects. The influence of gastro-intestinal disorders, such as Crohn's disease, coeliac disease, and physiological changes, such as constipation and diarrhoea, have not been investigated to any great extent.

Food and Concomitant Drug Therapy. The administration of oral dosage forms at some fixed time in relation to food has been shown to improve compliance to the dosage regimen by acting as a reminder to the patient. However, concurrent food intake can alter drug absorption (see above). In addition, a number of drugs are known to affect gastro-intestinal motility and can therefore alter absorption of a second drug taken concomitantly. The effect of food is commonly to slow drug absorption. The extent of absorption may also be reduced or, for some drugs, increased. The mechanisms involved include the following:

- *Reduced gastric emptying*. Consequently, the transfer of drug to the absorbing surfaces of the small intestine is slowed and absorption is slower. When a rapid onset of action is desirable, as for analgesics, sedatives, and hypnotics, administration under fasting conditions is preferable.

Prolonged residence in the acid environment of the stomach is undesirable for acid-labile drugs, such as penicillins, erythromycin (base and stearate), and cephalosporins because of loss of part of the dose by hydrolysis.

In contrast, for a few drugs, prolonged gastric residence of the formulation may increase the extent of absorption. This effect is seen for drugs that are poorly or slowly soluble, where the longer residence period and increased volume of gastric secretion aid dissolution. Also, fat components of the diet may dissolve drugs (such as griseofulvin), which are almost insoluble in water, and facilitate absorption through the normal mechanisms for lipid absorption.

- *Drug binding and complexation.* A few drugs undergo binding or complexation with dietary components to form products of low aqueous solubility with a reduction in the extent of absorption. The first-generation tetracyclines were found to complex with calcium ions, and concurrent administration of tetracycline and dairy products was found to reduce absorption of the antibiotic.
- *Splanchnic blood flow.* The flow of blood through the splanchnic bed is increased in response to food intake. This effect, together with concurrent changes in absorption rate, plasma protein binding, and the activity of drug-metabolising enzymes, may reduce the extent of first-pass loss, thus increasing the extent of absorption. This effect has been observed for several β-adrenergic blocking drugs (such as propranolol) and hydralazine.

The effect of food on the bioavailability of some drugs is shown in Table 5.

Some drugs should be administered under fasting conditions. For several other drugs, absorption may be improved by concurrent food intake. However, for all drugs, the patient should be encouraged to take the medicine at a fixed time in relation to food intake to minimise any food-related effects.

One drug may alter the absorption of a second drug given at the same time. There are two main mechanisms:

- the interfering drug adsorbs or complexes with the drug in the gastro-intestinal lumen
- the interfering drug exerts a pharmacological effect upon gastro-intestinal tract motility

and muscle tone; thus, parenterally administered drugs may also interfere with absorption.

Adsorption may be unintentional, as when antacid or antidiarrhoeal mixtures are co-administered with other drugs, or intentional, as in the treatment of poisoning or a drug overdose. Charcoal has been recommended for the latter purpose, but is only effective when treatment is prompt. Aluminium hydroxide, activated attapulgite, kaolin, and magnesium trisilicate are components of antacid and antidiarrhoeal mixtures. Interference with absorption *in vivo* has been shown for a number of drugs including chloroquine, isoniazid, phenytoin, and rifampicin. Adsorption of steroid hormones and other potent drugs may be anticipated although little information is available. For some drugs, diminished rate of absorption may be partially due to slow gastric emptying caused by the antacid. However, absorption may sometimes be enhanced by the antacid as for dicoumarol given with magnesium hydroxide.

The complexation of tetracyclines with polyvalent cations is well known (see above) and concurrent administration of antacids containing calcium, magnesium, or aluminium, or preparations containing ferrous salts should be avoided. The usual advice is to separate administration by two hours.

Most drugs that affect gastro-intestinal motility decrease the rate of gastric emptying either by reducing gastric motility or by interfering with normal peristalsis and increasing the tone of smooth muscle, including the pyloric sphincter. Effects on gastric emptying are often quite marked; for example, the opioid analgesics produce a 5-fold to 10-fold decrease in emptying rate, and the onset of action of an orally administered drug is often correspondingly delayed. Other drug groups that delay gastric emptying are antimuscarinic drugs, phenothiazines, and sympathomimetic drugs.

Prokinetic drugs increase the gastric emptying rate; examples include metoclopramide and domperidone. Sumatriptan, a drug used for the treatment of migraine, has been shown to hasten gastric emptying. Drugs such as cimetidine, ranitidine, and omeprazole that reduce gastric acid secretion do not appear to alter the absorption of co-administered drugs to any important extent. Table 6 lists examples of drugs that affect gastric emptying in man. Autonomic dysfunction may cause motor abnormalities in the gastro-intestinal tract, including

Table 5
The effect of food on absorption of some drugs

Drug or drug group	Reported effect	Comments
Reduced absorption		
Atenolol	food decreases the extent of absorption	a reduction of about 20% has been reported
Captopril	food decreases the extent of absorption	reduction is 35.5% to 40% and may alter the therapeutic effect
Cephalosporins	the rate of absorption and amount absorbed are reduced	
Digoxin	absorption delayed but total amount not reduced	the lower rate of absorption is not important for this chronically administered drug; concurrent food intake does not alter the plasma concentration in patients on maintenance therapy
Erythromycin (base and stearate)	the rate of absorption and amount absorbed are reduced	the extent of absorption of the base and stearate is reduced in the fed state because of acid hydrolysis. For the more stable estolate derivative, the extent of absorption is higher in the fed state
Isoniazid	extent of absorption reduced by food	
Ketoconazole	extent of absorption reduced by food	effect seen with high carbohydrate, low fat meal
Penicillins	the rate of absorption and amount absorbed are reduced	the penicillins vary widely in their susceptibility to acid hydrolysis. Loss of drug by extended gastric residence is greater for readily hydrolysed penicillins (including benzyl-penicillin, methicillin, and oxacillin) than for more stable ones (such as amoxycillin and ampicillin)
Rifampicin	the rate of absorption and amount absorbed are reduced	this expensive drug is used in developing world countries and ideally should be given in the fasted state
Sulphonamides	absorption delayed but total amount not reduced	most sulphonamides are readily absorbed from the gastro-intestinal tract and are stable in gastric juice. Food extends the period over which absorption takes place
Tetracyclines	the rate of absorption and amount absorbed are reduced	first-generation tetracyclines are irregularly absorbed and food reduces the total amount absorbed. Milk and milk products taken concurrently substantially reduce the amount absorbed. Doxycycline hydrochloride is better absorbed than most tetracyclines and least affected by food
Increased absorption		
Dicoumarol	extent of absorption is increased by food	
Griseofulvin	absorption enhanced by concurrent ingestion of a fatty meal	may be due to dissolution in fat components and absorption through fat uptake mechanisms
Mebendazole, flubendazole, and halofantrine	extent of absorption increased when taken with fatty foods	
Nitrofurantoin	absorption enhanced by concurrent ingestion of a fatty meal	
Phenytoin	food appears to increase the rate and extent of absorption	changes in the extent of absorption can be dangerous because of the saturable hepatic metabolism
Propranolol, metoprolol, labetalol, and hydralazine	absorption greater in fed than fasted state	the low systemic availability, due to extensive first-pass metabolism, is increased by 50% or more
Propafenone	food increases the extent of absorption	effect is large (six-fold difference) in 'fast metabolisers' but activity resides also in an active metabolite. Clinical significance not clear
Riboflavine	absorption may be delayed but amount is increased	food extends the period over which this vitamin is at the site of active transport in the small intestine. The carrier mechanism does not approach saturation and absorption is more complete
Warfarin and phenindione	no important changes in absorption with food	

Table 6
Drugs affecting gastric emptying rate

Decrease gastric emptying rate	Increase gastric emptying rate
Antihistamines	Anticholinesterases
	Neostigmine
Antimuscarinic drugs	Physostigmine
Atropine	
Propantheline	Cisapride
Chloroquine	Dopamine antagonists
Ganglion-blocking drugs	Domperidone
Hexamethonium	Metoclopramide
Opioid analgesics	Iproniazid
Diamorphine	
Buprenorphine	Reserpine
Meptazinol	
Morphine	Sodium bicarbonate
Nalbuphine	
Nefopam	Sumatriptan
Pentazocine	
Pethidine	
Phenothiazines	
Sympathomimetics	
Isoprenaline	
Dopamine	

gastroparesis, which may be asymptomatic. Gastric stasis, when this occurs, is usually evident from a feeling of fullness and distension of the stomach.

Absorption from the Buccal Cavity

The lining of the buccal cavity and the tongue are highly vascular and provide sites for the absorption of some drugs. Saliva secreted by the sublingual, submandibular, and parotid glands is available to dissolve the drug although the volume of fluid is quite small. Drugs administered to the buccal cavity may be used either for a local action in the mouth or throat or for a systemic effect.
The two areas used for drug therapy are the buccal and the sublingual sites. For buccal absorption a tablet is allowed to dissolve in the buccal sulcus, between the cheek and the gum of the lower jaw. Alternatively, the tablet is formulated to adhere to the sulcus and to release drug slowly from the matrix. For sublingual absorption a tablet is placed beneath the tongue; this route is preferable for patients who wear dentures. The patient should retain the tablet in position until it has completely dissolved, and should try to avoid swallowing saliva although the salivation induced by the drug or the tablet can make this difficult. If local activity is required, such as in treating mouth ulcers, the tablet or lozenge is allowed to dissolve in the affected area.

In adults, mixed saliva is only slightly acid, with a pH of about 6.4. Drugs that are prone to hydrolysis in the gastro-intestinal tract may be stable under the comparatively mild pH conditions found in the buccal cavity. Furthermore, the venous blood leaving the buccal mucosa does not pass to the liver and this site of metabolism is avoided. Most drugs cannot be given by this route because they are poorly absorbed or have a bitter taste. For a few drugs, however, rapid absorption occurs and when rapid onset of action is desired this may be the preferred route. Some examples of such systemically acting drugs that are absorbed from the buccal cavity are given in Table 7.
Absorption occurs by passive diffusion from the saliva, through the buccal mucosa into blood capillaries and lymph channels. The drug should be in

Table 7
Systemically acting drugs absorbed from the buccal cavity

Drug	Comments
Alkaloids	Absorption rates are variable since many alkaloids have unfavourable oil-water partition coefficients or are largely ionised in saliva; alkaloids of ergot (such as ergotamine tartrate) and the dihydrogenated ergot alkaloids (such as dihydroergotoxine mesylate) are well absorbed and give more rapid onset of action and more predictable response than when swallowed.
Barbiturates	Although well absorbed in most cases, their bitter taste makes this route inappropriate.
Enzymes	A few enzymes such as chymotrypsin and streptokinase with streptodornase are absorbed well from the buccal cavity.
Glyceryl trinitrate; Erythrityl tetranitrate	These two vasodilators are better absorbed from the buccal cavity than from the gastro-intestinal tract; they are rapidly absorbed after sublingual administration and this is the preferred route for prophylaxis and treatment of angina of effort.
Isoprenaline	A tablet allowed to dissolve under the tongue without sucking produces bronchodilatation within about 4 minutes. Inhalation produces a more rapid effect than sublingual administration.
Nifedipine	This calcium channel blocking agent is absorbed buccally. Biting open the capsule formulation gives earlier relief than does swallowing the intact capsule; the contribution of gastro-intestinal absorption of swallowed solution to this process is uncertain.
Steroid hormones	Several steroid hormones that are well absorbed from the buccal cavity have been commercially available (ethinyloestradiol, methyltestosterone, progesterone, stanolone and testosterone); ethisterone is better absorbed sublingually than when swallowed; deoxycortone acetate is destroyed in the gastro-intestinal tract and has been given sublingually.

the lipid-soluble, unionised form for rapid absorption. For example, sodium pentobarbitone is not as effectively absorbed as the free acid. It has been suggested that for satisfactory absorption the oil-water partition coefficient of a drug should be not less than 40. However, a very high oil-water coefficient (greater than 2000) renders the drug almost insoluble in saliva so that absorption is limited by the low concentration. Oil-water partition coefficients are most commonly measured *in vitro* using *n*-heptane or *n*-octanol.

Absorption from the Rectum

Drugs are administered rectally as enemas and suppositories usually for local medication, as in the treatment of haemorrhoids. They may also be administered to obtain a systemic effect, and the rectal route is a useful method of administering drugs to patients who are vomiting or unable to take drugs by mouth.

Absorption through the rectal mucosa is in accordance with the pH-partition hypothesis. At the slightly alkaline pH of the rectal mucosa, weakly basic drugs will exist in their lipid-soluble, unionised form and be readily absorbed. However, complete rectal absorption of weak acids under favourable conditions has been observed; rectal fluids have a low buffer capacity and the pH in the lumen is governed by the pH of the enema or suppository contents.

Rectal administration avoids the destruction of acid-labile drugs that occurs in the stomach, and there may be less degradation by liver enzymes than when drugs are absorbed from higher regions of the gastro-intestinal tract. The unpleasant effects of drugs causing nausea when given orally may be avoided by rectal administration. However, drugs that are irritant to the gastric mucosa will usually cause irritation of the rectum. The degree of irritation depends upon the rate of release from the suppository; a moderately low rate causes less irritation but can result in incomplete release of the administered dose. When given in suppository form, a drug may be released slowly over a period of time.

Rectal absorption gives more variable plasma-drug concentrations than oral administration of an aqueous solution, and absorption from a suppository is more variable than from a rectal solution. The rate and extent of absorption is influenced by the quantity of faecal material in the rectum at the time of administration. Patients should be encouraged to defaecate before insertion of the suppository.

Suppositories are prepared either from fatty bases, such as theobroma oil or proprietary semi-synthetic glycerides, which melt at body temperature, or from water-miscible bases such as macrogols and their esters and ethers, and glycerol-gelatin mixtures. The water-miscible bases slowly dissolve in the mucosal secretions of the rectum. The drug may be incorporated in the basis as a solution or as a suspension.

Drug release from a solution in a fatty basis proceeds by partitioning between the melting basis and the mucosal secretion. As the drug must subsequently partition between mucosal secretion and the lipid membrane of the mucosal wall, an intermediate value for the oil-water partition coefficient will favour transfer.

Suppositories containing suspended drug particles release them on melting, and dissolution of the drug occurs at the mucosal surfaces. The extent to which the drug dissolves in the basis and partitions between basis and mucosal fluid will be governed by the properties of the basis. The scarcity of controlled trials in human subjects and the difficulty in designing realistic tests *in vitro* make the selection of a satisfactory formula a difficult task. Suppository bases that are irritant should clearly be avoided; the macrogol bases are known to be irritant in some subjects and may promote defaecation and loss of the drug. Diazepam is available as a rectal solution, which is useful in situations where absorption from a suppository would be too slow (for example, febrile convulsions, status epilepticus). Drugs that have been administered rectally for their systemic effect include aminophylline, chlorpromazine, morphine, and paracetamol.

Absorption from the Lungs

The intake of drugs by inhalation into the trachea, bronchi, and alveoli has long been practised. For a long time, relief from attacks of asthma was sought by inhaling the smoke from smouldering mixtures of powdered lobelia and stramonium, and relief from the common cold by inhalation of aromatic vapours and sprays. Hand-operated atomisers or nebulisers and spray solutions have been replaced by aerosols dispersed from pressurised containers. Antibiotics, such as colistin sulphomethate sodium, have been used for their local pulmonary action in the treatment of bacterial infections of the respiratory tract. Salbutamol and ipratropium bromide produce bronchodilatation by their local action when applied as a spray. However, the concentration of the solution used is critical if unwanted systemic effects are to be avoided.

Inhalation of sprays containing surfactants, proteolytic enzymes, or acetylcysteine have been used in the treatment of respiratory infections and bronchospasm by lowering the viscosity of tenacious mucus. Aerosol therapy with corticosteroids in chronic bronchial asthma is preferred to oral administration because a smaller dose can be used and many side-effects are avoided.

The pulmonary route of drug administration for systemic effect has been used relatively little. As with the sublingual route, the drug reaches the systemic circulation without being exposed to the acidic environment of the stomach or to the enzyme activity of the gastro-intestinal tract and the liver.

The lungs are constructed for the rapid exchange of gases and vapours, particularly oxygen and carbon dioxide, between the blood and the air in the alveoli. The total area of the alveolar membrane through which the exchanges occur is very large indeed, about one square metre per kilogram body-weight. Further, the membrane is only about one micrometre in thickness. Anaesthetic gases (such as halothane, enflurane, isoflurane, and nitrous oxide) diffuse rapidly across this membrane and through the blood capillary walls, favoured by their relatively high oil-water partition coefficient.

Some drugs are absorbed well by the pulmonary route. From the small amount of data available, it appears that (like other mucosal surfaces) the alveolar membrane behaves as a lipoidal sieve, and the pH-partition hypothesis applies. Transfer of drug molecules may be facilitated by endogenously produced 'surfactant' (containing phospholipids, mucopolysaccharide, and possibly protein), which lowers the surface tension of mucosal secretions. Absorption of some relatively large unionised molecules (such as the polysaccharide inulin) has been observed and suggests that pores exist in the membrane.

Drugs given as aerosol sprays or from nebulisers can be absorbed extremely rapidly and the speed of action may be comparable with that of intravenous injection. Consequently the pulmonary route is particularly useful when self-medication is necessary for acute crises in a chronic illness. Table 8 lists drugs that have been given by this route.

Particles of solid or liquid droplets inhaled from an aerosol spray are deposited in the lungs by impaction. The depth of penetration into the bronchopulmonary tree and the extent of retention both depend on the particle size. Particles greater than about 50 micrometres are mostly deposited in the

Table 8
Drugs administered by inhalation into the lungs

Drug	Comments
Corticosteroids	Beclomethasone dipropionate, betamethasone valerate, and triamcinolone acetonide used for relief in bronchial asthma.
Ergotamine tartrate	Ergotamine tartrate is available as a pressurised aerosol preparation. Relief from migraine is achieved much faster than from oral preparations.
Sympathomimetics	Fenoterol, rimiterol, salbutamol, salmeterol, and terbutaline are well absorbed from the lungs giving early relief from asthmatic attacks.
Oxytocin	Irregular absorption from the lungs makes the intravenous route preferable.
Sodium cromoglycate	Well absorbed from the lungs when administered as a fine powder or spray but poorly absorbed from the gastro-intestinal tract. Inhalation of the powder may cause bronchospasm; isoprenaline may be given concurrently to minimise this effect.

mouth and trachea, and may be absorbed from these sites. Oral absorption from swallowed saliva has also been noted.

Particles of 20 micrometres diameter are deposited throughout the regions of the mouth, pharynx, trachea, and primary and secondary bronchi, but not in the lower respiratory tract. Most of the particles in the range of 2 to 5 micrometres are retained in the bronchioles and alveoli, and rapid absorption of systemically acting drugs occurs here. Particles of about 0.5 micrometre are largely lost in exhaled air, but very fine particles (0.01 micrometre) are retained in the alveoli.

Both conventional aerosol packs and hand-operated nebuliser sprays produce particles in the range 0.5 micrometre to 50 micrometres. 'Micro-aerosol' preparations producing particles between 0.005 micrometre and 0.5 micrometre have been manufactured. In theory, the desired type of action, systemic or local, can be achieved by control of particle size, but droplet size changes due to solvent evaporation make this difficult in practice.

The quantity of drug retained from a spray can be increased by synchronising the operation of the spray with inhalation and by training the patient to hold the breath after administration. Young children may find it difficult to achieve a sufficient degree of synchronisation. Medicinal aerosols for inhalation must be equipped with a metering valve to provide accurate and reproducible dosage, to within ±5% to 10%. Experience over the past 25 years has shown that inhalation therapy is of great benefit to many patients, notably asthmatics. The unique advantages of this route for administering systemically acting drugs have yet to be fully explored.

Absorption from Injection Sites

From the definition of drug absorption it is clear that absorption is not involved when a drug is injected intravenously or intrathecally, since drug is delivered directly into a fluid of distribution.

Drugs given by subcutaneous, intradermal, and intramuscular injection reach the systemic circulation by diffusion through body tissue and penetration of the walls of blood capillaries and lymphatic vessels. It is these processes that are referred to as **parenteral absorption**.

The subcutaneous region and muscle tissue are both richly supplied with blood capillaries. Lymph vessels occur extensively in the subcutaneous region, in connective tissue sheaths, and where fascial planes enter the muscle, but only in small numbers in muscle tissue itself. Ions and small molecules can readily pass through the capillary wall; transfer into the lymphatic system is not an important route for their absorption. Large molecules, such as proteins, and colloidal particles are absorbed into the lymph vessels. There is some evidence that small particles and fluid can cross the endothelial tissue of blood capillaries and lymph vessels by transport in small vesicles that cross the membrane, a process called **cytopemphis**. The contribution of this mechanism of transfer to the absorption of injected drugs is not known.

Subcutaneous and intramuscular injections may be either solutions or suspensions; intradermal injections, being mainly for diagnostic purposes, are usually solutions.

Drugs that are destroyed by the acidic gastric secretion, or hydrolysed by enzymes of the gastro-intestinal tract or the liver may be given by intramuscular or subcutaneous injection. Injection into deep muscle tissue can provide a depot from which drug is released over an extended period.

Factors Affecting Absorption from Injections. Drug absorption from intramuscular and subcutaneous injections of aqueous solutions is usually quite rapid and similar to absorption from an oral preparation. The rate of absorption from an injected solution depends mainly upon the surface area of the walls of blood capillaries and lymphatic vessels and the rate of flow of fluid through them.

Aqueous solutions given intramuscularly spread along the muscle fascias (the thin sheets of connective tissue enclosing bundles of muscle fibres) and provide contact with a large area of capillary and lymphatic wall. Absorption is usually complete within about 30 minutes, although factors such as degree of ionisation and lipid solubility, volume of solution, and osmolality are known to influence the drug absorption rate. The rate of absorption from subcutaneous injection is, for most drugs, about the same as from intramuscular injection but the volume of solution tolerated is smaller.

Blood flow through skeletal muscle may be increased more than ten-fold during exercise. Muscular movement also encourages the flow of lymph through lymphatic vessels and increases the rate of absorption of high molecular weight compounds such as snake venom. It has been shown that immobilisation of the limb after injection of snake venom prolongs the life of test animals. Muscular activity has been shown also to increase the absorption rate from subcutaneous implants.

Speed and duration of local anaesthesia has been increased by the inclusion of a vasoconstrictor, such as adrenaline, in the formulation, particularly in dental practice. The adrenaline constricts arteries, arterioles, capillaries, and venules. Blood flow is diminished and the rate of removal of local anaesthetic from the region surrounding the injection site is greatly reduced. In some cases the injected drug itself may alter the capillary blood flow. The cholinergic action of methacholine chloride given by subcutaneous injection causes vasodilatation and the systemic effects are seen within 1 to 2 minutes.

Subcutaneous indurations caused by repeated injection of insulin lead to diminished vascularity and blood flow and therefore to lower absorption rates. Subcutaneous injections have been found to be more rapidly absorbed from the arm than from the thigh, presumably due to differences in blood flow and vascularity.

Conditions leading to diminished circulation, for example low temperatures, shock, cardiac disease, and myxoedema, can result in decreased absorption rates. Thus emergency drugs cannot be given by intramuscular or subcutaneous injection to patients in shock. Conversely, massage or application of heat increases blood flow and absorption rate. In the UK, an exception to this is adrenaline injection, which is administered by intramuscular injection for allergic emergencies; the intravenous route is used for cardiac resuscitation only.

The enzyme hyaluronidase, sometimes added to subcutaneous and intramuscular formulations, increases spreading rate by hydrolysing the hyaluronic acid present in the interstices of the protein chains of connective tissue. In this way, large volumes of fluid can be given subcutaneously by hypodermoclysis.

Absorption from the Skin

Drugs applied to the skin are used almost exclusively for their local effect on the outer layers of the epidermis. The skin offers greater resistance to penetration by drugs than do other mucosal surfaces used as absorption sites. To be absorbed, drug molecules must pass through the several layers that form the epidermis. The main barrier is the stratum corneum, the outermost horny layer composed of dead keratinised flattened cells. The sebum that coats some areas of the stratum corneum does not hinder absorption of drugs. The epidermal layer is an effective barrier, and topical doses of various drugs need to be much greater than intradermal doses.

Transfer across the stratum corneum is by passive diffusion and for most drugs occurs only very slowly. The tissue consists of aggregates of closely-packed cells, and contains both lipid and aqueous regions. Lipid-soluble drugs can pass readily through lipid regions of the cell membranes whereas water-soluble drugs pass through because of hydrated protein particles within the cell wall. There is some evidence that compounds with both lipophilic and hydrophilic properties, that is, with an oil-water partition coefficient close to unity, are best able to pass through the stratum corneum. Water-soluble ions and molecules, unless very small, do not pass through. Gases readily pass through the stratum corneum and this may account for the good penetration found for volatile drugs.

Some drugs are retained in small quantities within the stratum corneum for periods of several days after topical application. The therapeutic implications of the reservoir or depot formed in this manner are not yet fully understood. Substances that pass through the stratum corneum move freely through the lower epidermal strata, and into the dermis. From here the compound reaches the systemic circulation by diffusion through the walls of blood vessels or lymphatic vessels.

Alternative routes to the dermis are via the skin appendages, namely the hair follicles and the sweat ducts. These communicate directly with the dermis and subcutaneous fatty tissue, so that drugs penetrating in this way by-pass the stratum corneum. The space between the hair shaft and the follicular wall communicates with the sebaceous gland and it is filled with sebum. Drugs which are sufficiently lipid-soluble can pass through the sebum by diffusion to the sebaceous glands and also through the follicular walls. However, the area available for absorption by these routes is small when compared to that of the total epidermal surface, and percutaneous absorption via the appendages is important only for compounds that penetrate the stratum corneum very slowly. There is some evidence for appendageal penetration of certain corticosteroids. When the epidermis has been broken or destroyed by wounds, burns, or abrasion, drugs are able to pass freely into the dermis.

The absorption of drug from a topical preparation is highly variable and depends on physiological factors associated with the subject, the physicochemical properties of the drug, and the properties of the basis or vehicle.

Physiological Factors Influencing Percutaneous Absorption. The percutaneous absorption from a topically applied preparation is governed by several factors. These include the area of body selected, the age and temperature of the skin, the degree of skin hydration, and the rate of blood flow through the dermis. The thickness of the stratum corneum varies considerably, being greatest in the palmar and plantar regions and least in the facial and post-auricular regions. Thus penetration rates from a site behind the ear are greater than from the palm of the hand in any one subject, but large differences can exist between subjects.

Vasoconstriction caused by topically applied corticosteroids slows penetration by decreasing the rate of drug loss from dermal tissue. An increased rate of drug penetration following vasodilatation does not appear to have been demonstrated.

Percutaneous absorption of most drugs is enhanced by hydration of the epidermis. Moisture loss is greatly reduced by occlusive dressings applied to the skin. The highly impermeable film retains water diffusing from lower epidermal layers and from perspiration. The water content of the stratum corneum rises and it becomes more permeable to drugs. Upon hydration the stratum corneum becomes less compact and the size of the pores increases. The penetration of some corticosteroids may be increased 100-fold by using occlusive plastic films in place of conventional dressings; the dosage must be adjusted accordingly to avoid systemic toxicity.

Physicochemical Properties of the Drug. Although the penetration of the stratum corneum is often enhanced by increased lipid solubility, some water solubility is desirable. The activities of highly water-soluble and highly oil-soluble molecules are less than those of drugs with a more evenly balanced solubility behaviour.

Weak acids and bases are absorbed more readily in their lipid-soluble, unionised form, in accordance with the pH-partition hypothesis. Percutaneous absorption of water-soluble salts is poor compared to that of the free acid or base. Modification of molecular structure to change the partitioning and solubility characteristics of the compound and alter the rate of penetration through the epidermis has been used extensively for corticosteroids. As a general rule, for good absorption the drug should have an oil-water partition coefficient close to unity and a moderately high water solubility. Among many esters of betamethasone tested the highest topical activity was found for the 17-valerate ester, which exhibited these properties.

An increase in concentration of the drug in the vehicle increases the amount absorbed percutaneously during a given interval of time. Where the drug has a low solubility in the vehicle (and is suspended in the vehicle) the release rate is proportional to the square root of the concentration; for example, to achieve a doubling of the rate a four-fold increase in concentration is required. However, penetration can often be enhanced by particle size reduction before dispersion in the ointment basis. Among compounds such as steroids that show polymorphism, selection of a metastable high-activity form may provide increased penetration rates from topical suspensions.

Properties of the Vehicle. The vehicle or basis provides a convenient means of maintaining the drug at, or close to, the topical absorption site. It is doubtful if vehicles used for dermatological preparations can promote the absorption of drugs that are not themselves absorbable, but the composition of the vehicle can markedly affect the absorption of absorbable drugs.

The nature of the vehicle controls the drug activity, the rate of diffusion in the vehicle, and the partition coefficient between the vehicle and skin. A high affinity of the basis for the drug is not desirable. Drugs that complex or 'bind' to components of the vehicle are released into the skin very slowly. Release of drug is favoured by using a vehicle that is a poor solvent for the drug. A high stratum corneum-vehicle partition coefficient encourages the process of transfer of drug into the epidermis. The partition coefficient may be altered by including various solvents (such as ethanol and propylene glycol) in the vehicle. Other solvents such as dimethyl sulphoxide, dimethylformamide, and dimethylacetamide rapidly penetrate the epidermis and in doing so aid the absorption of drugs dissolved in them; however, their use has been limited by fear of toxic effects when used at the relatively high concentrations that effectively promote absorption.

Hydrocarbon ointment vehicles have an occlusive action on the skin but emulsion bases are less occlusive. Insoluble powders, such as zinc oxide, reduce the occlusive properties by their uptake of water and by providing a large surface area for evaporation.

Although the various factors that influence percutaneous absorption of drugs are becoming better understood, it is not yet possible to select the best vehicle for a new drug solely from a knowledge of their respective physicochemical properties. The vehicle is chosen on the basis of practical experience with selected formulations using a quantitative or semi-quantitative measurement of drug penetration.

Percutaneous Absorption of Drugs. Application to the skin is rarely used to elicit a systemic effect. Percutaneous absorption is generally slower and less reliable than absorption from the gastro-intestinal tract, although the extent of metabolism is less. Topical application is generally reserved for treatment of superficial layers of the skin; some diseases of the lower epidermis and the dermis are better treated systemically. Sometimes percutaneous absorption is an undesirable consequence of topical application for a local effect, as observed on occasions for lindane and neomycin. Many drugs have been shown to be absorbed from the skin. These include the oil-soluble vitamins (A,D,E, and K) and some water-soluble vitamins (ascorbic acid and the components of the B complex). Interest in transdermal drug delivery has led to the development of systems comprising a drug-loaded patch for systemic delivery. Examples include a glyceryl trinitrate patch that is applied to the chest for control of anginal attacks, a hyoscine-releasing patch used for motion sickness, oestradiol-releasing patches for the management of menopausal symptoms, and nicotine patches for cessation of smoking.

In **iontophoresis**, an ionised drug in solution is placed on the skin and an electrical potential difference established, so driving the ions into the skin; hydrocortisone and methacholine have been administered in this way. Although absorption is quite efficient, the technique is clearly not of wide application.

Absorption from the Eye

Drugs applied to the eye for local effects are administered either as an aqueous solution or suspension, an oily solution, or in an ointment basis. Absorption occurs mainly into the cornea, conjunctiva, sclera, and aqueous humour of the eye. Upon instillation eye drops are continuously diluted by lachrymal secretion, and unabsorbed drug is lost by drainage into the nasolachrymal duct. The pH of eye drops can affect absorption because absorption is faster when a weak acid or weak base is in the unionised form. However, the diminished absorption of weak bases from acidic solutions may be partly due to increased lachrymation caused by the low pH of the solution. The rate of lachrymation is lower at slightly alkaline pH values but poor stability may preclude the presentation of eye drops in solutions of pH 8.

Polymeric materials, such as hypromellose and polyvinyl alcohol, may be included in eye drops to increase their viscosity. This reduces the rate of loss of instilled solution from the precorneal region and extends the period of absorption. A similar but more pronounced effect is achieved with ophthalmic ointments from which release usually occurs over several hours. Release from ophthalmic ointments of poorly lipid-soluble drugs (such as pilocarpine) is, however, about the same as from aqueous solutions.

The eye is not used as a route of systemic administration. However, absorption from eye drops into the systemic circulation may sometimes occur, probably at the mucosal surfaces of the nose after drainage from the eye through the nasolachrymal duct.

A device has been developed to provide treatment over an extended period. The Ocusert™ device consists of a reservoir of drug solution surrounded by a polymeric membrane that limits the rate of drug release. When placed into the conjunctival cul-de-sac, the drug is released at a near-constant rate for seven days. The use of a device containing pilocarpine is reported to increase compliance in many patients because the episodes of blurred vision resulting from frequent instillation of eye drops are avoided; overnight therapy of glaucoma is also improved.

Intranasal Absorption

The observation that application of drugs to the nasal mucosa led to systemic side-effects stimulated an interest in the use of this route for drug delivery. The nasal route may provide an alternative route for those drugs which currently are administered by injection because of poor absorption following oral administration.

Peptides up to ten amino acids appear to be able to penetrate the nasal mucosa. Examples include vasopressin, desmopressin, gonadorelin, buserelin, leuprorelin, nafarelin, and oxytocin. Calcitonin is available as a nasal spray in some countries. Other drugs that have been investigated for administration by the nasal route include: insulin, progesterone, glucagon, somatorelin, and propranolol. Bioavailability is usually low but may be increased by the incorporation of surfactant materials as absorption promoters. It appears that use of a spray is preferable to nasal drops.

DRUG DISTRIBUTION

After a drug has been absorbed into the blood circulation it will, inevitably, be distributed into a variety of body tissues and fluids to varying extents. Indeed, in order to exert its effect, the drug will usually have to leave the systemic circulation to reach its site of action. The main factors affecting the extent of distribution of a drug are: plasma protein binding, blood flow rate to individual tissues, ability to cross membranes, and tissue binding.

Plasma Protein Binding

In the circulatory system, drugs distribute between erythrocytes, leucocytes, plasma proteins, and plasma itself. The binding of a drug to plasma proteins can influence the distribution of the drug, the rate at which it passes through membranes, the pharmacological effect, and the rate of elimination from the body. Many different types of drugs bind to plasma proteins, mainly to albumin, but sometimes to globulins. There is considerable variation in the type of bond formed between the drug and the plasma protein; bond formation is dependent upon the molecular structure of the drug. The extent of protein binding is also variable; antibiotics (such as penicillins and tetracyclines), non-steroidal anti-inflammatory drugs, barbiturates and sulphonamides all exist to varying extents as reversibly bound albumin complexes. Basic drugs, in contrast, generally bind to globulin components (such as α_1-acid glycoprotein) of the plasma. The fraction of bound drug may be concentration dependent.

An equilibrium is set up in the circulatory system between bound and unbound drug. It is generally the unbound drug that is pharmacologically active. Bound drug molecules are retained in plasma because the high molecular weight of the plasma protein complex prevents their passage across the capillary walls. Thus only the unbound portion of the dose is able to reach the sites of action in the tissues. Bound drug molecules are not filtered in the kidney glomeruli, but renal tubular secretion and metabolic processes can often decouple the drug from the plasma protein.

Drug interactions may occur if two drugs that compete for binding sites on the same plasma protein are administered concurrently. For example, the activity of coumarin anticoagulants is enhanced following the administration of aspirin; the coumarin anticoagulant is displaced by aspirin from its binding site on plasma albumin leading to increased plasma concentrations of unbound, active anticoagulant. Other drugs with the same ability to displace the coumarin anticoagulants include phenylbutazone, mefenamic acid, and nalidixic acid.

Membrane Transfer

Almost all drugs, when not bound to plasma proteins, can readily leave the capillaries and become rapidly diluted in the interstitial fluid. Lipid-soluble drugs readily cross the capillary membrane, while water-soluble drugs and some proteins are filtered through the intercellular pores in the capillary membrane at a rate inversely proportional to their molecular weight. Similarly, transfer of most drugs from interstitial fluid to tissue cells occurs by passive diffusion. Thus lipid-soluble drugs diffuse freely into cells across cell membranes, while small water-soluble molecules (molecular weight less than 50) or ions can pass through aqueous channels or pores in the membrane. Larger water-soluble drugs cannot enter cells except by special transport mechanisms.

Tissue Binding

The pharmacological effects of some drugs are exerted by binding to specific macromolecules, known as **receptors**, in the cells and tissues. Receptors may be enzymes, genetic material, or membrane structures. The bonds formed when a drug interacts with its receptor are similar to those formed when the drug binds to other macromolecules in cells and to plasma proteins. The amount of drug at a receptor is very small compared to the amount bound to pharmacologically inactive sites.

Some drugs bind specifically to tissue in which there are no receptors, and this binding may be irreversible, thus resulting in storage of drugs in the body in an inactive form. Some drugs such as tetracyclines are deposited in bones and teeth; this process appears irreversible as the blood supply to these tissues is so poor that loss of drug from the tissue binding site back into the blood is very slow.

Occasionally, active transport processes may result in the concentration of a drug in a particular type of tissue; for example, the active transport of the antihypertensive agent guanethidine into cardiac muscle.

Binding to tissue components may be useful therapeutically; for example, chloroquine interacts with nucleic acids in cell nuclei, and may achieve a concentration in the liver which is much greater than the plasma concentration. When chloroquine is used in antimalarial therapy, adequate plasma concentrations are only attained when the process of binding in the liver is saturated. However, in hepatic amoebiasis, the accumulation of chloroquine in the liver is therapeutically useful.

Blood Flow Rate

Transfer of drug to tissues occurs through the tissue blood supply and therefore the transfer rate depends on the blood perfusion rate of the tissues. There is wide variation in the blood perfusion rates of various tissues (Table 9) and in the time blood remains in the tissue.

Table 9
Blood flow rates in body tissues of man

	Tissue	Percent of body-weight	Percent of cardiac output	Blood flow (mL/100 g tissue per minute)
Highly perfused	Adrenals	0.02	1	550
	Kidney	0.4	24	450
	Thyroid	0.04	2	400
Moderately perfused	Liver-hepatic	2	5	20
	-portal	0	20	75
	Portal-drained	2	20	75
	Heart (basal)	0.4	4	70
	Brain	2	15	55
Poorly perfused	Skin	7	5	5
	Muscle (basal)	40	15	3
	Connective tissue	7	1	1
	Fat	15	2	1

After Butler TC. In: Brodie BB and Erdos EG, editors. Proceedings of the First International Pharmacological Meeting; vol 4. London: Pergamon Press, 1962: 197.

Fat Content of Tissues

Lipid-soluble drugs will be taken up into tissues with a high fat content by simple partitioning. The anaesthetic agents thiopentone and halothane are highly lipid soluble and will partition favourably into adipose tissue, such that concentrations much higher than in plasma water are achieved.

Time-course of Drug Uptake into Tissue

Because of the wide differences in perfusion rates, tissues take up the drug at different rates. Moderate and highly perfused tissues are exposed to the drug in high concentrations soon after administration. Transfer of drug to poorly perfused muscle tissue and to fat (which is very poorly perfused) occurs subsequently. Uptake into fat will only occur if the drug is lipid soluble.

The changes in concentration of thiopentone with time in various tissues shown in Fig. 3 illustrate the successive uptake and redistribution which is a result of the tissue perfusion rates.

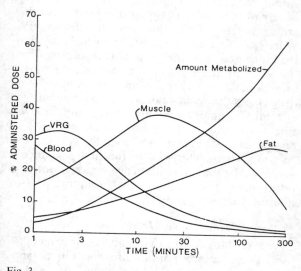

Fig. 3
Changes in concentration of thiopentone with time in various tissues (VRG = vessel rich group; includes brain, heart, kidney, splanchnic bed (including liver), and endocrine glands) (after Eger EI. editor. Anaesthetic Uptake and Action. Baltimore: Williams & Wilkins, 1974).

Drug held in muscle and fat exerts no pharmacological effect but is part of a 'pool' or 'reservoir' from which drug may redistribute into the blood circulation. The 'reservoir' effect is of clinical importance when repeated doses of a stored drug are administered. Drugs that are less lipid soluble than thiopentone do not distribute into fat to any extent. The distribution of drugs which are rapidly eliminated is much less extensive because they reach the poorly perfused tissues in low concentrations.

Blood-brain Barrier

The blood-brain barrier is a term which has been introduced to explain the lack of uptake from blood of some substances by the brain. The capillaries in the brain differ from those found in other parts of the body. They are composed of continuous sheets of endothelial cells with no pores between them. Lipid-soluble unionised drugs are transferred rapidly from blood to brain by passive diffusion but water-soluble ionised drugs, which usually pass through the intercellular pores in the peripheral capillaries, are excluded. Water-soluble substances required for cell metabolism, for example, glucose, are transported into the brain by active transport processes; it is possible that foreign compounds of similar molecular structure to these substances are taken up by the same active transport processes.

The rate at which a drug is taken into brain tissue depends on its lipid solubility and its degree of ionisation in plasma. Highly lipid-soluble, unionised drugs enter the brain rapidly and the onset of pharmacological action is correspondingly fast. For example, the onset of action of thiopentone occurs within minutes as equilibrium is rapidly attained between the plasma and brain fluids. Less lipid-soluble barbiturates such as phenobarbitone have a much slower onset of action. However, thiopentone is rapidly redistributed from the brain to poorly perfused tissues, such as adipose tissue, which have a greater affinity for the lipid-soluble drug. Thus concentrations in the central nervous system decrease and the hypnotic effect is of short duration, although the drug is not metabolised or excreted from the body very rapidly. The duration of action of phenobarbitone is considerably longer, as it is not concentrated to the same extent by adipose tissue, and termination of effect only occurs when a sufficient amount of the dose has been metabolised or excreted.

Benzylpenicillin exists in an ionised, water-soluble form that is also extensively protein bound at plasma pH. It does not readily penetrate into the central nervous system, despite increased permeability of the blood-brain barrier in meningeal infections. However, benzylpenicillin remains one of the drugs of choice for bacterial meningitis.

Placental Transfer of Drugs

The membranes separating foetal capillary blood from maternal blood have permeability characteristics similar to those of cell membranes in other parts of the body. Many drugs of moderate to high lipid solubility can be detected in foetal blood or tissues after administration to the mother.

DRUG ELIMINATION

Elimination of drugs from the body occurs by metabolism and by excretion of the parent drug and its metabolites. The major routes of elimination are hepatic metabolism and renal excretion. The rates of metabolism and excretion determine the duration and intensity of drug action and may be altered in disease states and by the concurrent administration of drugs which affect the elimination processes.

Drug elimination occurs as the drug traverses an 'organ of elimination', for example, the liver or kidney, in the blood flow. A proportion of the drug arriving at the organ is removed by the elimination process. If the drug is one which is extensively eliminated (greater than 70%) during its passage through the organ then it has a high extraction ratio; if only a small amount is eliminated (less than 30%) the drug has a low extraction ratio (see Drug Clearance below).

The rate of drug elimination is clearly dependent on the extraction ratio. However, it also depends upon the extent of distribution. For example, if the drug binds extensively to tissue proteins then the fraction of the total body load that is circulating in blood and available for elimination is low. Thus, elimination is slower than if only limited distribution into tissues occurs. Drugs with high lipid solubility distribute extensively into adipose tissue and may be eliminated only very slowly.

The binding of drug to plasma proteins will protect the drug from elimination processes only if it is a low extraction ratio drug. High extraction drugs are effectively decoupled from the binding proteins in the elimination processes.

Drug Metabolism

Some drugs are not metabolised by the body; they are excreted unchanged or retained in the body for a long period. For example, digoxin is excreted in the urine mainly as unchanged drug. However, the majority of drugs are metabolised to some extent before being excreted as metabolites. Several metabolites may be formed from a single drug. Drug metabolism occurs predominantly in the liver, although other tissues such as the kidneys

and the lungs have some ability to metabolise drugs. Metabolism may also occur in the gastro-intestinal fluid or in the gastro-intestinal wall during the absorption process. The metabolising enzymes are localised in the hepatic microsomes, a cellular fraction derived from the endoplasmic reticulum of the parenchymal cells of the liver. These microsomal enzymes include oxidases, reductases, esterases, and several enzymes which take part in conjugation (Phase II) reactions. Enzyme systems are also found in mitochondria and in the soluble fraction of hepatic cells.

Metabolism usually decreases or destroys the pharmacological activity of a drug. However, a significant number of drugs are converted to pharmacologically active compounds. For example, codeine is converted to morphine and phenacetin is converted to paracetamol. Metabolism also renders drugs more suitable for excretion by the liver and the kidneys, as their metabolites are generally more water soluble. In the absence of metabolism, the rate of excretion of lipid-soluble drugs would be very low. Highly lipid-soluble drugs are widely distributed throughout the body; also they are reabsorbed from the urine by the kidneys. Water-soluble metabolites are less widely distributed in the body and their rate of reabsorption from the urine by the kidneys is also lower, favouring excretion. After absorption an orally administered drug enters the hepatic portal vein, passing into the systemic circulation only after traversing the liver. For some drugs a large proportion of the dose may be metabolised and not reach the systemic circulation. This is referred to as the 'first-pass' loss; it accounts for the large difference between oral and intravenous doses, as is seen for morphine (see Pharmacokinetics below).

Factors Affecting Drug Metabolism

There are many factors that influence drug metabolism. These factors result in differences in metabolism between individuals, but some also lead to differences in metabolism in an individual, depending on the physiological or pathological state. Factors known to affect drug metabolism include genetic differences, age, sex, nutritional status, physiological factors (such as stress, pregnancy and hormonal activity), and disease states. Furthermore, the concurrent administration of a second drug that alters the level of activity of hepatic enzymes, will change the rate of metabolism.

Genetics. Genetic differences can account for variation in metabolic rates between individuals. For some drugs there is a discontinuity in the distribution of metabolic rates, referred to as **polymorphism**, such that recognisable phenotypes exist. The best known examples are the polymorphism of acetylation and hydroxylation reactions, each under the control of a single gene.

Isoniazid is metabolised by acetylation and two groups exist in the population. One group (about 50% of Caucasians) acetylate the drug rapidly, the other group acetylate it slowly. Polymorphism has also been demonstrated in the acetylation of dapsone, caffeine, phenelzine, sulphadimidine, and sulphamethoxypyridazine. About 5% to 10% of the Caucasian population have a restricted ability to hydroxylate phenytoin. Other drugs that exhibit polymorphism in the hydroxylation reaction include debrisoquine, metoprolol, dextromethorphan, and propafenone. A further example of genetic polymorphism is the activity of plasma cholinesterases on suxamethonium. For phenacetin, a single family was shown to have a deficiency of the enzymes which de-ethylate the compound to form paracetamol. Instead, the toxic metabolite hydroxyphenetidine was formed.

The evidence for continuous variations associated with genetic composition has come from studies on identical and non-identical twins with dicoumarol, nortriptyline, phenazone, and phenylbutazone.

Species. The metabolic fate of a compound is highly dependent on the animal species, reflecting differences in the presence and activity of enzyme systems. Elimination routes that are particularly species dependent are aromatic hydroxylations, conjugate formation, and biliary excretion. Consequently, data obtained in laboratory animals are of limited predictive value in man and early evaluations of new compounds require careful investigations of metabolic routes in humans.

Age. Metabolic enzyme systems are not fully developed at birth and metabolism in neonates is usually slower than in the adult. In advanced age, hepatic enzyme activity can be diminished.

Differences in renal excretion patterns may be found with age because of the immaturity of renal function in the first few weeks of life and the deterioration that occurs in later life. For both groups, particular care must be taken in repeat dosing with drugs that have a low therapeutic margin of safety.

Sex-linked Differences. Sex-linked variations in the metabolism of methadone, nicotine, and pentazocine have been reported in man. However, it appears that no differences have been identified that are significant enough to require a dose adjustment.

Nutritional Status. Diets low in protein adversely affect microsomal enzyme activity and also reduce amino acid conjugation. High protein diets lead to production of relatively acidic urine and in this manner diet can alter the pH-dependent excretion of drugs.

Physiological Factors. Factors such as stress, pregnancy, and hormonal activity may influence drug metabolism. However, these factors have not been studied systematically in humans; the finding that stress can enhance metabolic activity in laboratory animals for a few drugs may have no important implications for man.

In pregnancy, the placenta forms an extra membrane barrier through which a drug may pass. Placental transfer is controlled mostly by passive diffusion but there is evidence of an active transport system for certain drugs, for example ampicillin. Many drugs cross the placenta; those that readily cross the placenta include alcohol, aminoglycosides, barbiturates, chlorpromazine, etretinate, tetracyclines, morphine, and certain antibiotics. The *British National Formulary* provides guidance on the use of drugs during pregnancy. Drug metabolism may also be affected by pregnancy; the conjugation of drugs with glucuronic acid is reduced and the metabolism of pethidine is decreased.

In the obese patient, metabolic enzyme differences appear to be less important than the increase in distribution of lipophilic drugs into adipose tissue, leading to a longer elimination half-life.

Disease. It might be supposed that metabolism would be diminished in patients with liver disease. Whereas this may be generally true, there are few data to substantiate the existence of a difference. Also, a distinction should be made between chronic liver disease, such as cirrhosis and chronic active hepatitis, and acute disease, such as acute viral hepatitis. The enzyme systems affected may depend on the underlying disease state.

In addition, in chronic liver disease, patients often have a reduced rate of protein synthesis. The plasma-albumin concentration in these patients is lower so that the distribution volume (see Pharmacokinetics below) for a drug that binds to albumin will be higher than in healthy subjects. For amylobarbitone, the half-life in patients with cirrhosis has been found to be about double that in healthy subjects. The difference is largely due to the reduction in metabolic activity. In contrast, the half-life of tolbutamide is shorter in acute viral hepatitis. This difference is not due to any change in metabolic activity, but to an elevated fraction of unbound drug, caused by hyperbilirubinaemia, which occurs in this condition; the bilirubin competes with tolbutamide for plasma-protein binding sites. In kidney disease, the half-life of some drugs that are eliminated in the urine may be substantially prolonged and accumulation may occur if dosage schedules are not changed. A useful measure of renal function is the clearance of creatinine (which is formed by the catabolism of muscle tissue). Based on this parameter, adjustment of dose schedules is necessary for drugs such as the aminoglycosides and cephalosporins. Nomograms have been published for the adjustment of dosage regimens in patients with diminished renal function. The *British National Formulary* provides guidance on the use of drugs in patients with renal impairment.

Concurrent Drug Administration. The activity of liver enzymes can be altered by administered drugs, either through changes in the amount of enzyme formed or in the intrinsic enzyme activity. There are examples both of an increase and a decrease in enzyme activity, through changes in enzyme synthesis or in enzyme catabolism. Enzyme activity may be affected by:

- the concentration of the substrate or product of the reaction
- isosteric inhibition, where the catalytic site of the enzyme is blocked
- allosteric inhibition, where the catalytic site is free, but where the activity of the enzyme is moderated by binding to another site on the enzyme molecule.

There are several important examples of the increased enzyme activity or **enzyme induction** produced by administered drugs. The effect of enzyme induction on some drugs is to increase its metabolic clearance. Some drugs, such as glutethimide, carbamazepine, and meprobamate can induce their own metabolism. Examples are given in Table 10. A reduction in enzyme activity, **enzyme inhibition**, has been found in both microsomal and non-microsomal enzymes. An example of non-microsomal inhibition occurs with the monoamine oxidase inhibitors (such as phenelzine), which increase sensitivity to some sympathomimetic amines. An example of microsomal inhibition is the action of cimetidine, which inhibits the metabolism of com-

Table 10
Examples of enzyme induction in man

Drug affected	Enzyme inducer
Carbamazepine	Carbamazepine
Coumarin anticoagulants	Phenobarbitone and some other barbiturates
Digitoxin	Phenobarbitone and some other barbiturates
Glutethimide	Glutethimide
Hydrocortisone	Phenobarbitone and some other barbiturates, phenylbutazone, phenytoin, dicophane
Meprobamate	Meprobamate
Oral contraceptives	Rifampicin
Phenytoin	Phenobarbitone and some other barbiturates
Testosterone	Phenobarbitone and some other barbiturates
Tolbutamide	Alcohol
Warfarin	Glutethimide

pounds and increases their activity, including theophylline, warfarin, lignocaine, nifedipine, procainamide, propranolol, quinidine, and some benzodiazepines.

There are two groups of reactions by which drugs are metabolised. **Phase I reactions** involve the oxidation, reduction, or hydrolysis of drugs and usually either add functional groups to the molecule or expose functional groups through cleavage. **Phase II reactions** involve the conjugation of the drug molecule, often via the functional group introduced by Phase I reactions, with substances such as glucuronic acid, the amino acids glycine and glutamine, and sulphate moieties.

Phase I (Pre-conjugation) Reactions

Oxidation. Oxidative changes to drugs are a common pathway of metabolism. In the endoplasmic reticuli of the liver 'mixed function oxidases' (of which there are several) are found, each able to catalyse the oxidation of a number of drugs. To be active, the enzymes require a supply of oxygen and reduced nicotinamide-adenine dinucleotide phosphate (NADPH). The enzymes take part in an electron transport chain in which cytochrome P450 is an important terminal oxygen-transferring enzyme system to which the drug binds.

Non-microsomal oxidations are catalysed by enzymes in mitochondria (for example, amine oxidases) and plasma (for example, amidases, esterases, hydrolases and amine oxidases). Sites on the molecule at which oxidation can occur include carbon, nitrogen, sulphur, and oxygen atoms. Some illustrative examples are provided in Fig. 4.

Reduction. Reduction reactions are less common than oxidation reactions and may lead to the formation of more lipid soluble, relatively toxic products (such as the amine products of azoreduction). Reductions are carried out by both microsomal and non-microsomal enzymes. Microsomal reductases are flavoproteins, with flavine-adenine dinucleotide (FAD) as their

At carbon atoms,
  Aliphatic oxidation (for example, glutethimide, tolbutamide, meprobamate, chloral hydrate, and amylobarbitone)

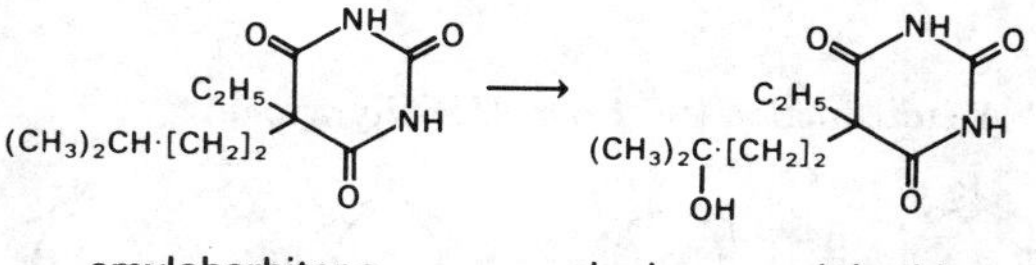

amylobarbitone   hydroxyamylobarbitone

Aromatic oxidation (for example, phenobarbitone and phenylbutazone)

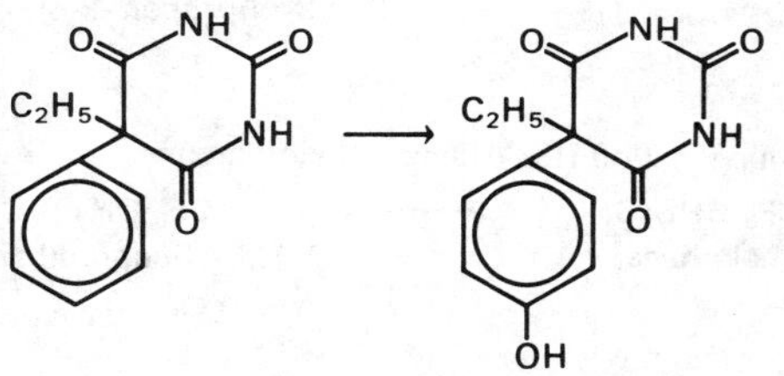

phenobarbitone   *p*-hydroxyphenobarbitone

Alicyclic oxidation (for example, cyclobarbitone and hexobarbitone)

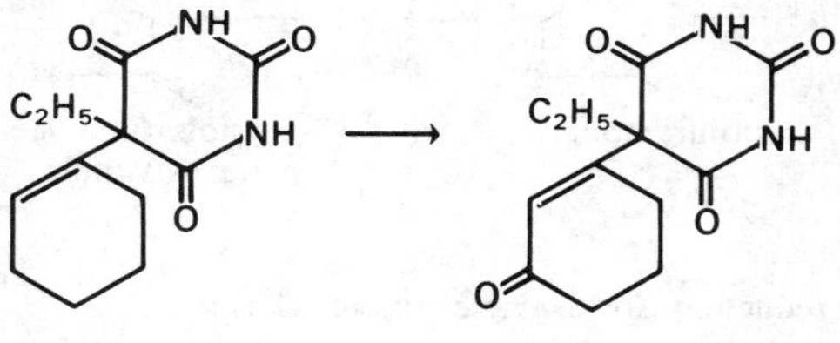

cyclobarbitone   ketocyclobarbitone

Epoxidation (for example, cyproheptadine, in rats)

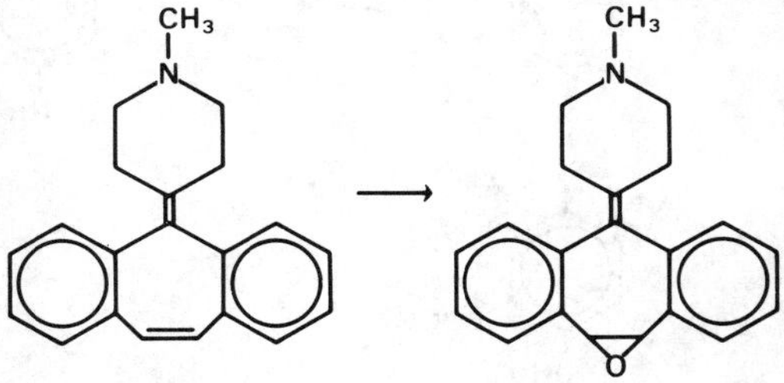

cyproheptadine   cyproheptadine epoxide

At nitrogen atoms,
  Primary *N*-oxidation (for example, amphetamine)

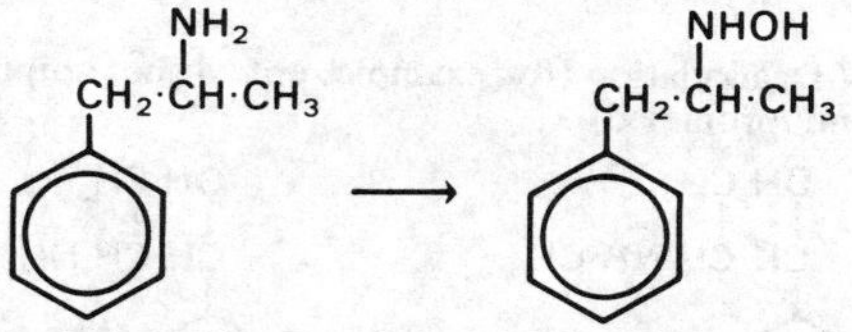

amphetamine   *N*-(1-phenylprop-2-yl)hydroxylamine

At oxygen atoms,
  O-Dealkylation (for example, diamorphine and phenacetin)

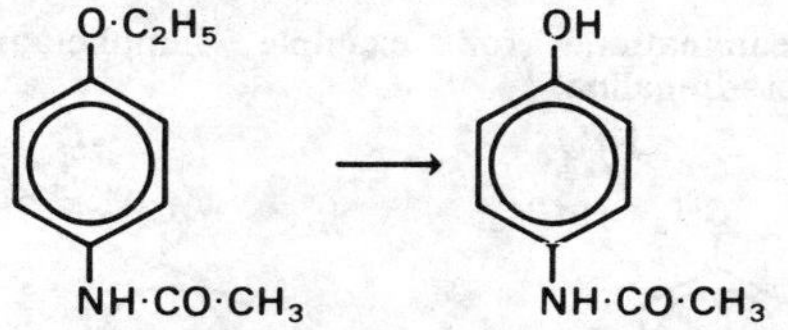

phenacetin   paracetamol

Other oxidation reactions,
  Ring fission (for example, catechol)

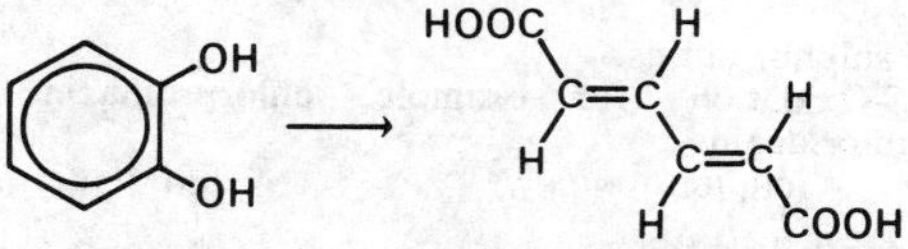

catechol   *trans-trans*-muconic acid

Ring formation (for example, proguanil)

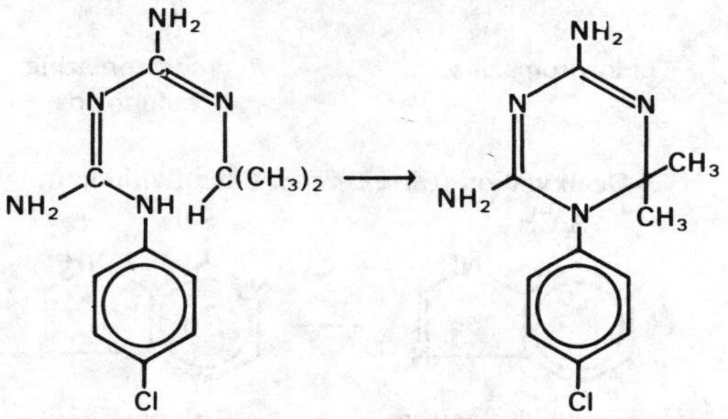

proguanil   cycloguanil

Tertiary *N*-oxidation (for example, chlorpromazine)

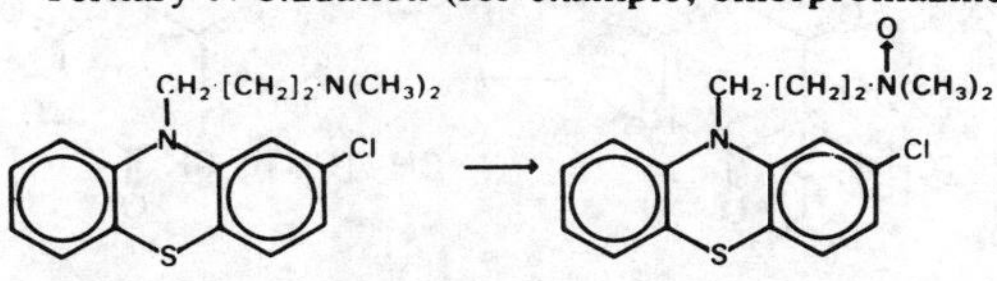

chlorpromazine   chlorpromazine *N*-oxide

Fig. 4
Oxidation reactions.

Fig. 4—*Continued*

prosthetic group; these too require NADPH to be active. It is possible that the reaction mechanism involves the reduction of FAD by the enzyme, using NADPH or NADH (reduced nicotinamide-adenine dinucleotide) as a cofactor, and then the

reduction of the drug occurs non-enzymatically by a reaction with reduced FAD. Non-microsomal enzymes include those which occur in the gastro-intestinal flora. Reduction reactions may occur at carbon, nitrogen, and sulphur atoms. Illustrative examples are given in Fig. 5.

N-Dealkylation (for example, ephedrine, imipramine, and iproniazid)

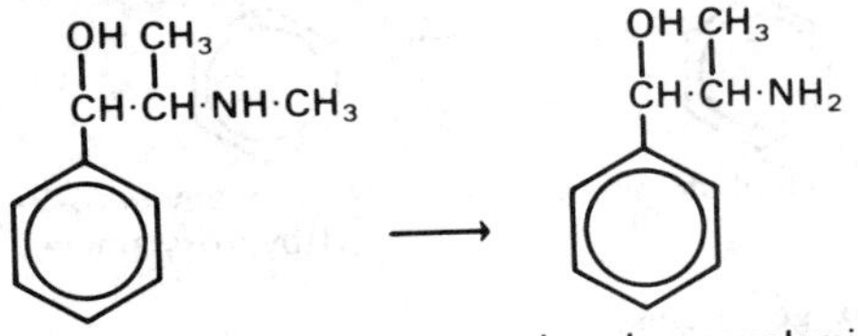

ephedrine → phenylpropanolamine

Deamination (for example, amphetamine and noradrenaline)

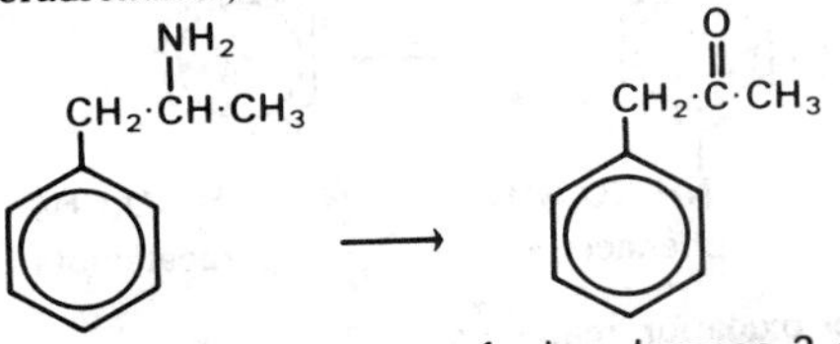

amphetamine → 1-phenylpropan-2-one

At sulphur atoms,
S-Oxidation (for example, chlorpromazine and thioridazine)

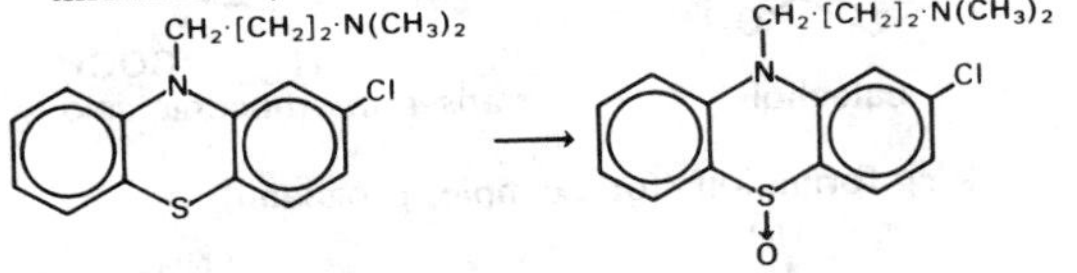

chlorpromazine → chlorpromazine sulphoxide

S-Dealkylation (for example, 6-methylthiopurine)

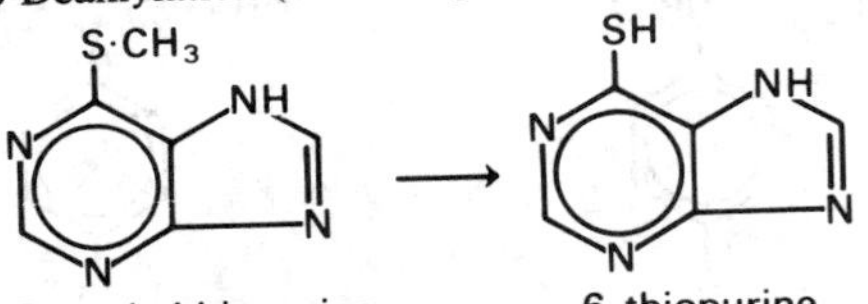

6-methylthiopurine → 6-thiopurine

Desulphuration (for example, thiopentone)

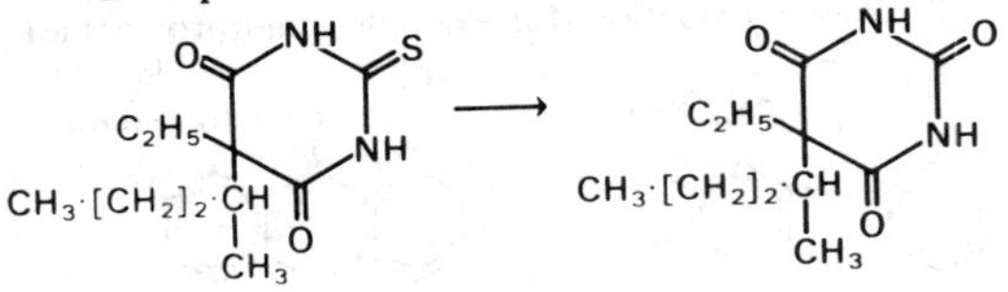

thiopentone → pentobarbitone

Fig. 4—Continued

At carbon atoms,
Aldehyde reduction (for example, chloral)

$$CCl_3 \cdot CHO \longrightarrow CCl_3 \cdot CH_2OH$$

chloral   trichloroethanol

Ketoreduction (for example, metyrapone)

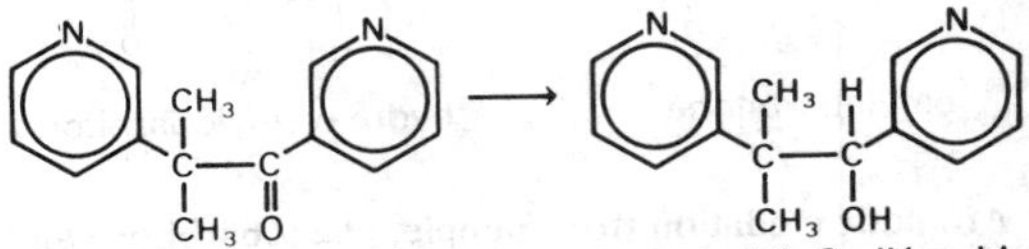

metyrapone → 2-methyl-1,2-di(pyrid-3-yl)propan-1-ol

Dehalogenation (for example, halothane)

$$CF_3 \cdot CHBrCl \longrightarrow CF_3 \cdot CH_3$$

halothane   1,1,1-trifluoroethane

At nitrogen atoms,
Nitroreduction (for example, nitrofurantoin)

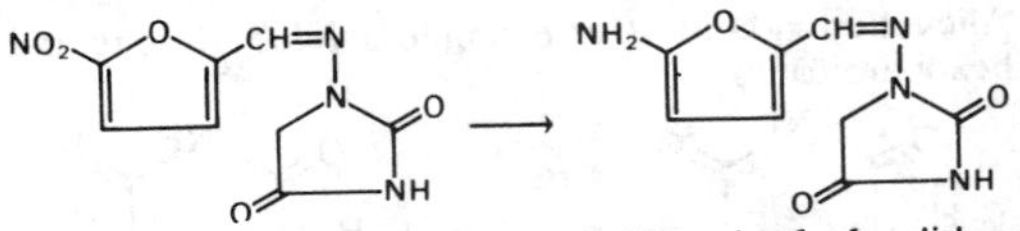

nitrofurantoin → 1-(5-aminofurfurylidene-amino)hydantoin

Azoreduction (for example, sulphasalazine)

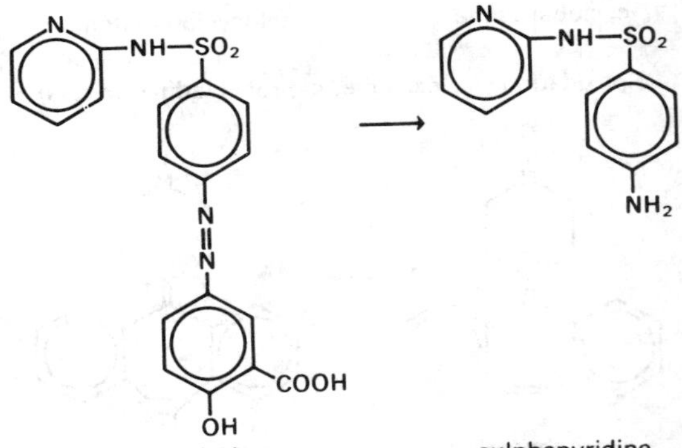

sulphasalazine → sulphapyridine

Fig. 5
Reduction reactions.

Hydroxamic acid reduction (for example, salicyl hydroxamic acid)

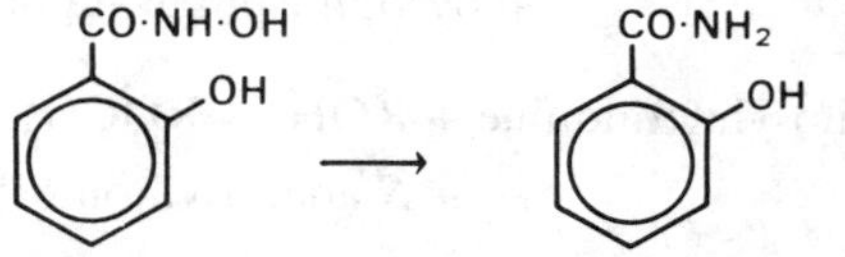

salicylhydroxamic acid → salicylamide

At sulphur atoms,
  sulphoxide reduction (for example, dimethyl sulphoxide)

$$(CH_3)_2SO \longrightarrow (CH_3)_2S$$

dimethyl sulphoxide   dimethyl sulphide

Disulphide reduction (for example, disulfiram)

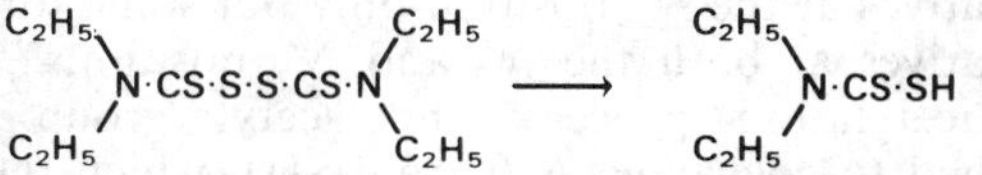

disulfiram → diethyldithiocarbamic acid

Fig. 5—*Continued*

Hydrolysis. Hydrolysis is a common metabolic reaction of esters and amides. The responsible enzymes are found in the microsomes of the liver, gastro-intestinal wall and other tissues, and in blood plasma. Illustrative examples are given in Fig. 6.

Phase II (Conjugation) Reactions

In conjugation reactions, an endogenous chemical group combines with the drug (or its metabolite). Generally, the products have increased polarity and higher water solubility, which renders them more readily excreted by the kidneys.

In many conjugation reactions the conjugating group is transferred to the drug or metabolite from an activated coenzyme through the mediation of a transferase enzyme; this mechanism operates for the formation of glucuronides, sulphates, and methyl and acetyl conjugates. Amino acid conjugates, however, are formed through the initial production of a coenzyme-drug complex before the conjugating group is added. In contrast, glutathione and thiocyanate conjugates do not require coenzymes.

Glucuronide Formation. Glucuronide formation is an important conjugation reaction because of the wide range of compounds that are metabolised in

Ester hydrolysis (for example, pethidine, procaine, and suxamethonium)

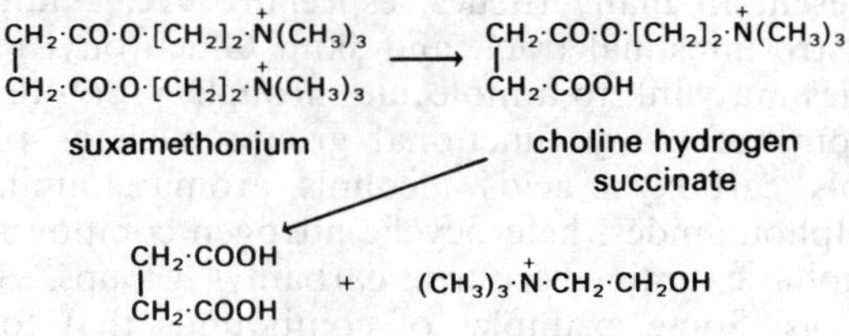

suxamethonium → choline hydrogen succinate → succinic acid + choline

Amide hydrolysis (for example, salicylamide)

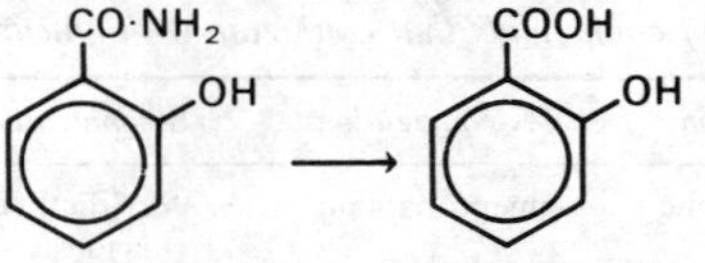

salicylamide → salicylic acid

Hydrazide hydrolysis (for example, isoniazid and phenelzine)

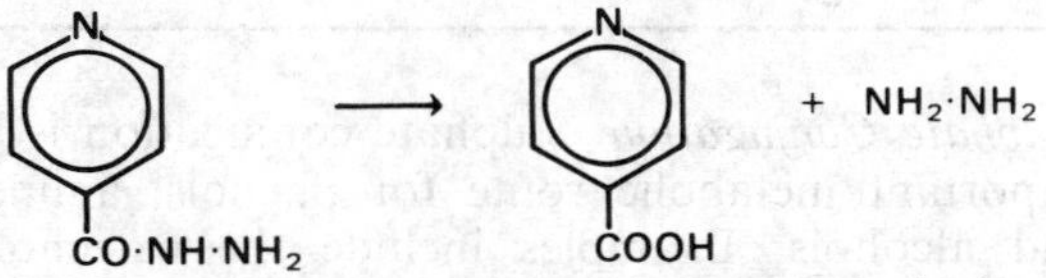

isoniazid → isonicotinic acid + hydrazine

Carbamate hydrolysis (for example, meprobamate)

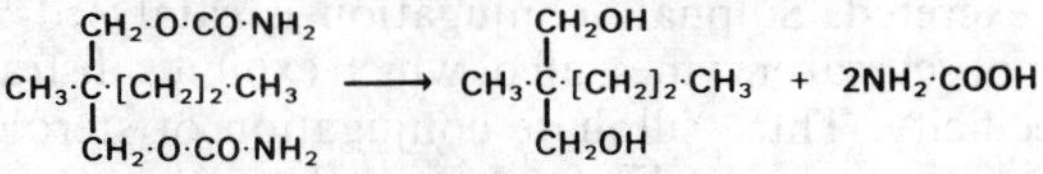

meprobamate → 2-hydroxymethyl-2-methylpentan-1-ol + carbamic acid

Deacetylation (for example, phenacetin)

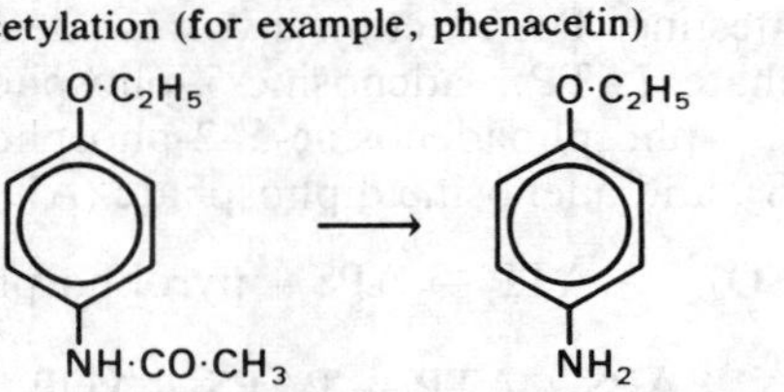

phenacetin → *p*-ethoxyaniline

Hydrolytic ring fission (for example, hexobarbitone and phenytoin)

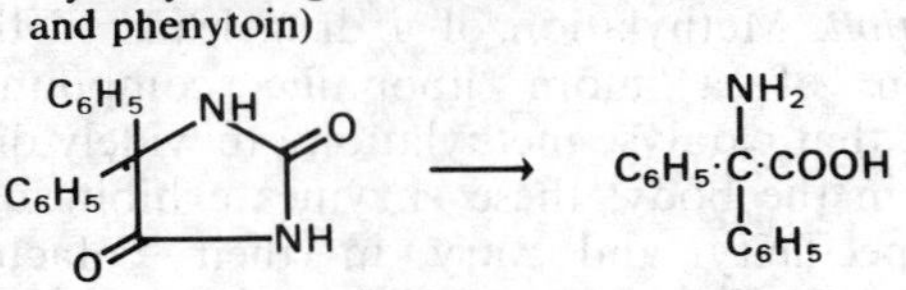

phenytoin → α-aminodiphenylacetic acid

Fig. 6
Hydrolysis reactions.

this manner. The enzyme glucuronyl transferase is present in many tissues, especially liver, kidney, gastro-intestinal tract, and skin. Glucuronyl residues may link to a molecule through N-, O- or S-atoms of many functional groups such as phenols, carboxylic acids, alcohols, aromatic amines, sulphonamides, heterocyclic nitrogen compounds, aliphatic amino groups, carbamyl groups, and thiols. Some examples of compounds that form glucuronides are given in Table 11.

Table 11
Examples of compounds that conjugate with glucuronic acid

O-*conjugation*	N-*conjugation*	S-*conjugation*
hydrocortisone	meprobamate	*N,N*-diethyldithiocarbamic acid
4-hydroxycoumarin	sulphadimethoxine	2-mercaptobenzothiazole
indomethacin	sulphafurazole	
morphine	sulphathiazole	
nicotinic acid		
salicylic acid		

Sulphate Conjugation. Sulphate conjugation is an important metabolic route for phenols, amines, and alcohols. Examples include the catecholamines, steroids (such as oestrone), paracetamol, 3-hydroxycoumarin, and chloramphenicol. The conjugates are relatively strong acids and are readily excreted. Sulphate conjugation is catalysed by one of several enzymes, all of which exhibit substrate specificity. Thus, sulphate conjugation of steroids occurs only in the liver whereas there is evidence (from studies *in vitro*) that phenols are sulphated in the soluble fraction of the liver and in the kidney and intestine. The reaction involves adenosine triphosphate (ATP), adenosine-5'-phosphosulphate (APS), phosphoadenosine-5'-2-phosphosulphate (PAPS), and adenosine diphosphate (ADP):

$$SO_4^{2-} + ATP \rightarrow APS + \text{pyrophosphate}$$

$$APS + ATP \rightarrow PAPS + ADP$$

$$PAPS + ROH \rightarrow ROSO_2H + ADP$$

Methylation. Methylation of a drug leads to the formation of a more lipophilic compound. Enzymes that catalyse methylation are widely distributed in the body; these enzymes exhibit substrate specificity and vary in their cofactor requirements. Examples of drugs that undergo methylation include some phenols and thiols such as noradrenaline, isoprenaline, dihydroxybenzoic acid, and thiouracil. The reaction is:

$$\text{Methionine} + ATP \rightarrow S\text{-adenosylmethionine}$$
$$+ \text{pyrophosphate} + \text{phosphate}$$

$$S\text{-adenosylmethionine} + ROH \rightarrow ROCH_3$$
$$+ S\text{-adenosylhomocysteine}$$

The methylated products may undergo a Phase I hydrolysis reaction to yield the original compound and consequently this metabolic pathway may not always be evident.

Acetylation. Acetylation has been found to occur mainly in the liver but also in spleen, lungs, and other tissues. Classes of compounds which are acetylated are primary aromatic and primary aliphatic amines, hydrazines, hydrazides, and sulphonamides. Thus, isoniazid is extensively metabolised. Most sulphonamides form acetyl derivatives at the N^4 position only but some form derivatives at both the N^1 and N^4 positions. In the acetylation process, the acetyl group is attached to coenzyme A (CoA—SH), which then reacts with the drug:

$$CH_3CO—S—CoA + RSO_2NH_2$$
$$\rightarrow RSO_2NHCOCH_3 + CoA—SH$$

Conjugation with Amino Acids. Aromatic and heterocyclic carboxylic acids and some aliphatic acids with aromatic substituents conjugate with glycine, or in some instances with taurine or glutamine. Aliphatic acids that lack aromatic substituents are readily oxidised and so conjugation does not occur. The amino acid conjugates are strongly acid, with pK_a values of about 3; they are susceptible to hydrolysis under alkaline conditions. Unlike most other reactions, amino acid conjugation occurs in the mitochondria. The acid substrate is converted to an active form, attached to coenzyme A and then converted to the amide:

$$RCO_2H + ATP \rightarrow RCO—AMP + \text{pyrophosphate}$$
$$RCO—AMP + CoA—SH \rightarrow RCO—S—CoA$$
$$+AMP$$

$$RCO—S—CoA + NH_2CH_2CO_2H \rightarrow$$
$$RCONHCH_2CO_2H + CoA—SH$$

Glutathione Conjugation and Mercapturic Acid Formation. Compounds containing electrophilic centres (such as ethacrynic acid) and some unsaturated hydrocarbons and their halides and nitro-compounds may be conjugated with glutathione. The glutathione conjugate may be excreted in bile, together with catabolites formed by the stepwise removal of glutamate and glycine, followed by acetylation of the free amino group formed. The resulting mercapturic acid metabolite (*N*-acetylcysteine derivative) is excreted in urine and bile. Aromatic hydrocarbons are first converted to an epoxide before conjugation with glutathione. The enzymes responsible for both the conjugation and the removal of the amino acid are located mainly in the liver and kidneys.

Thiocyanate Formation. Cyanide ions are conjugated by endogenous thiosulphate, a sulphur-donating compound, to form thiocyanates. This reaction is important as a detoxification mechanism because the products have much reduced toxicity.

$$CN^- + S_2O_3^{2-} \rightarrow SCN^- + SO_3^{2-}$$

Drug Excretion

The most important organs involved in the excretion of drugs are the kidneys and the liver, although other routes of excretion may be important for some drugs.

Renal Excretion

The urine is the major vehicle for the excretion of drugs and their metabolites from the body. Some drugs, such as digoxin, are excreted in urine mainly as unchanged drug, whereas other drugs, such as propranolol, are almost completely metabolised before being excreted in the urine. Many drugs are excreted by the kidney as a mixture of unchanged and metabolised forms. Renal excretion of drugs occurs through three processes: glomerular filtration, passive tubular diffusion, and active transport into the renal tubules.

Glomerular filtration is the simple ultrafiltration of the blood plasma. Substances with a molecular weight below about 66 000 pass through the glomerular filter and appear in the tubular fluid. Molecules bound to plasma proteins are thus excluded from renal tubular fluid and only the unbound fraction is available for filtration.

Lipid-soluble compounds may be excreted into the distal portion of the renal tubule by passive diffusion providing that there is a concentration gradient and a urinary pH which favours the unionised form. Lipid-soluble compounds already in the glomerular filtrate may be reabsorbed by the same process. Highly lipid-soluble compounds are therefore excreted slowly.

Because the reabsorption of weak electrolytes from the glomerular filtrate is pH-dependent, with only the unionised lipid-soluble form able to cross the renal tubular wall, the rates of urinary excretion of weak electrolytes will be dependent upon the urinary pH, which varies over the range 5 to 8. Weak acids having pK_a values in the range 3.0 to 7.5, such as the salicylates and phenobarbitone, will be more readily excreted in alkaline urine, while weak bases having pK_a values in the range 7.5 to 10.5, such as amphetamines, will be more readily excreted in acid urine. The effect of pH on overall drug excretion, however, is only significant if the drug is excreted mostly in the unmetabolised form since most drug metabolites are polar and therefore not readily reabsorbed by passive diffusion.

Active transport is associated with the proximal tubule of the kidney and is involved in the secretion of some acids and bases. These compounds are highly ionised and are readily excreted with little or no tubular reabsorption. Active transport mechanisms exist for the excretion of endogenous substances. Separate mechanisms exist for acidic drugs such as probenecid, penicillins, thiazides, and glucuronic acid conjugates, and basic drugs including quaternary ammonium compounds. Competitive inhibition of secretion of one drug by another can occur, and may be useful therapeutically. For example, probenecid competitively inhibits active transport of some penicillins into urine and therapeutic plasma concentrations of penicillins are thus maintained for a longer period.

Biliary and Faecal Excretion

Bile is formed from blood plasma by secretion of bile salts, water, and solutes at a rate of 0.5 to 0.8 mL/minute. Whereas all drugs will pass into bile, this route of excretion only becomes important where the biliary-drug concentration greatly exceeds the plasma-drug concentration. Some drugs, and their metabolites, achieve biliary concentrations of up to 1000 times the plasma concentration through active secretion processes.

There appear to be separate mechanisms for the active secretion of acids, bases, and unionised compounds. Drugs excreted in bile are polar, water-soluble compounds of relatively high molecular weight, generally exceeding 250 daltons (although the value in man appears not to have been defined). Drugs excreted in bile, include carbenoxolone, cromoglycate, digitoxin, norethynodrel, pancuronium, and sulphobromophthalein. However, biliary excretion is more important for the excretion of metabolites, particularly the water-soluble conjugates such as glucuronide and glutathione conjugates.

Drugs and metabolites excreted into bile pass into the intestine and may be excreted with faecal material. Strongly polar compounds such as cromoglycate and propantheline are excreted in faeces after biliary excretion. However, the compounds may be reabsorbed from the intestine and some may be excreted again in the bile. This cycle of excretion and reabsorption, the enterohepatic circulation, prolongs the period during which the drug is in the body.

Glucuronide conjugates excreted in the bile may not be absorbed *per se*. However, biliary enzymes or gastro-intestinal flora may hydrolyse the conjugates, leaving the parent compound to be reabsorbed; the enterohepatic circulation of chlorpromazine involves the formation of the glucuronide, hydrolysis of the conjugate in the gastro-intestinal tract, and the reabsorption of chlorpromazine.

Excretion in Sweat and Tears

Sulphonamides, some amines, and urea are excreted in sweat by passive diffusion. Some drugs (for example, rifampicin and sulphasalazine) are excreted in lachrymal secretions and may cause discoloration of soft contact lenses.

Excretion in Milk

Excretion in milk occurs primarily by passive diffusion, the extent being dependent upon the pK_a and lipid solubility of the drug, the pH value of the milk or colostrum, and the concentration gradient between the blood and milk. Milk is more acid than blood (pH value about 6.8) and accumulates weak bases.

Most drugs administered to a nursing mother will be excreted in milk, either as the drug or as a metabolite. The degree of harm to which the infant is exposed will depend on the dose and frequency of administration and the potency of the drug. Although concentrations in milk will be low, drug accumulation may occur in the nursing infant because of a low rate of elimination.

Drugs known to be excreted in relatively high concentrations in milk include sulphafurazole (which may cause kernicterus), chloramphenicol (which has toxic effects on accumulation), and metronidazole. Examples of other drugs excreted in milk in significant amounts are: anticoagulants, aspirin, barbiturates, benzodiazepines, caffeine, erythromycin, morphine, nicotine, penicillins, quinine, steroidal hormones, sulphonamides, and tetracyclines. If a drug is known to be excreted in quantities that may place the infant at risk, a clinical judgement as to whether to discontinue breast-feeding or drug therapy will be required. The *British National Formulary* provides guidance on the use of drugs during breast-feeding.

Excretion in Expired Air

Gases and volatile liquid anaesthetics are absorbed and excreted through the lungs. Some other drugs (such as paraldehyde, alcohol, and dimethyl sulphoxide metabolites) are excreted in expired air but this represents only a minor elimination route.

Excretion into the Gastro-intestinal Tract

Drugs in the blood circulation can be excreted into the gastro-intestinal tract in saliva, into the stomach, and into the intestine.

Excretion into saliva occurs by passive diffusion. Examples are the sulphonamides, phenobarbitone, clonidine, and many amines. There is some evidence that the excretion of penicillin into saliva occurs through an active transport process. If a drug is excreted in saliva in measurable quantities this fluid may be used to monitor drug concentration in the body. The drug excreted in saliva is swallowed and may be reabsorbed from the gastro-intestinal tract.

Some basic drugs, such as morphine, quinine, and nicotine, are excreted into the stomach in relatively large amounts by pH-dependent passive processes. The compounds are 'ion-trapped' in the acid of the stomach contents although reabsorption will occur in the intestine. Excretion into the intestine may occur directly or by biliary excretion.

BIOAVAILABILITY

The bioavailability of a medicine is defined as the rate at which the drug becomes available to the body and the extent to which the dose is ultimately absorbed after administration. The bioavailability of a drug is dependent upon the formulation of the medicine containing the drug. Poor or inappropriate formulation can result in a product which releases the drug at too slow a rate, or fails to release a proportion of the contents, or leads to unacceptable variations in the performance of the individual dose units.

Fast absorption is generally desirable to provide a rapid onset of action or to achieve high drug concentrations, for example, of an analgesic or antianginal drug. Slow absorption may sometimes be necessary to extend the period of action or to minimise undesirable systemic or local effects such as the emesis produced by nitrofurantoin or the gastro-intestinal ulceration caused by potassium chloride.

Many medicines contain a drug in particulate form. It is necessary, therefore, to examine the factors that influence the process of dissolution of drug, in order to understand how formulation factors can influence bioavailability.

Dissolution of Solid Drug Particles

Absorption of a drug at an absorption site occurs invariably from a simple solution of the drug. However, medicines very often contain the drug suspended in a dispersion medium (as in oral suspensions, some ointments, and some intramuscular injections) or in powder mixtures with a variety of adjuvants (as in tablets, capsules, and lozenges); dissolution of the solid drug particles must precede absorption and the dissolution rate will usually control the overall absorption process. For the drug particles to dissolve there must be available at the absorption site a quantity of liquid in which the drug particles are soluble. The volume of liquid available may sometimes be quite small, as in the case of a sublingual tablet or a subcutaneous implant.

The main factors influencing the rate of dissolution are contained in the equation of Noyes and Whitney:

$$\text{Rate of dissolution} = k \times A \times (C_s - C)$$

where A is the area of solid wetted by the dissolution medium, C_s is the solubility of the drug in the dissolution medium, C is the drug concentration in the bulk solution, and k is the dissolution constant. The value of k is governed by the size of the diffusion coefficient of the drug molecules in the dissolution medium and the extent of agitation. After a medicine is administered, transport of dissolved drug away from the absorption site is usually quite rapid so that the concentration (C) does not rise much above zero. The concentration of drug in the surrounding fluid remains close to zero and dissolution occurs under what are referred to as 'sink' conditions.

The total wetted surface area (A) may be increased by reducing the size of the drug particles. The specific surface or surface area per gram (S_{sp}) for spherical particles of diameter d and density ρ is found from:

$$S_{sp} = \frac{6}{\rho d}$$

Some values for the specific surface of spherical particles of density equal to 2.0 g per cm³ with various particle diameters are shown below.

Particle diameter μm	Specific surface cm² per g
100	300
10	3000
1	30 000

For non-spherical particles in a polydisperse system d is a mean particle diameter and the value of the numerator of the equation will differ from six. Nevertheless the specific surface will still be inversely related to mean particle diameter. The total wetted surface area will usually be smaller than the value calculated from the specific surface and the weight of powder because of particle aggregation. Incomplete dispersal of drug particles in the dissolution medium is often found to occur with powders of small particle size; wetting agents in solution aid in de-aggregation of the particles and are found in gastric juice and biliary secretion.

Under 'sink' conditions the rate of dissolution is directly proportional to the solubility of the drug in the medium. Solubility is not an invariant property of a compound but is dependent on such factors as the temperature, pH, and physicochemical nature of the solvent, the presence of surfactants, and the polymorphic or crystalline form of the drug.

The pH of the dissolution medium can alter drug solubility markedly when the drug is either a weak acid or a weak base. For a weak acid (HA), the total solubility (C_T) is equal to the sum of the concentrations of the unionised acid (HA) and of the conjugate base (A⁻) in a saturated solution.

$$C_T = [\text{HA}] + [\text{A}^-]$$

$$\text{Since } K_a = \frac{[\text{H}^+][\text{A}^-]}{[\text{HA}]}$$

$$\text{then } [\text{A}^-] = K_a \frac{[\text{HA}]}{[\text{H}^+]}$$

$$\text{or } \quad C_T = [\text{HA}] + \frac{K_a[\text{HA}]}{[\text{H}^+]}$$

For a weak acid, therefore, a decrease in hydrogen ion concentration [H⁺] (increase in pH) will increase the solubility. It should be noted that a pH increase of one unit can lead to a large increase in total solubility.

The corresponding equation for a weak base is:

$$C_T = [\text{B}] + \frac{[\text{H}^+][\text{B}]}{K_a}$$

Thus weak acids are more soluble at high pH values but weak bases are more soluble at low pH values. The solubility of a neutral compound is little affected by pH change. Amphoteric compounds can behave as an acid and a base and so have a minimum solubility at intermediate pH values. In addition to the characteristic properties of the drug itself the release, dispersal, and dissolution of the drug also depend on the properties of adjuvants, excipients, and other components present in the formulation and on the manufacturing processes used in its preparation.

Formulation Factors Affecting Absorption from the Gastro-intestinal Tract

The rate and extent of absorption can both be influenced by the pharmaceutical dosage form in which the drug is administered. The orally administered dosage forms can be listed in order of decreasing ability to make the drug available: solutions; suspensions; oil-in-water emulsions; capsules and tablets; sustained-action and delayed-action capsules and tablets.

An aqueous solution taken on an empty stomach will rapidly reach the duodenum, and absorption starts almost immediately. The particles in a suspension start to dissolve upon dilution with gastro-intestinal fluids. Increasing the viscosity of the suspension reduces the rate of absorption either by prolonging gastric emptying time or by slowing the dissolution of particles.

Emulsions, being little used oral dosage forms, have received scant attention. However, it is apparent that absorption from oil-in-water emulsions is quite rapid, and is favoured by the use of digestible oils. Absorption is by pinocytosis through the mucosa into the lymphatic vessels, so by-passing the liver.

Release of drug from conventional tablets and hard gelatin capsules follows their disintegration in the stomach and small intestine. The site of disintegration will depend upon the characteristics of the dosage form, the amount of fluid available, and the gastric emptying time. Disintegration probably starts in the stomach and the individual drug particles pass through the pylorus. The increased surface area of drug in contact with the luminal fluids allows rapid dissolution to occur. Dissolution may start in the stomach and continue in the small intestine, depending upon the nature of the drug.

The disintegration and dissolution properties of tablets and hard gelatin capsules can be altered greatly by changes in their formulation and manufacture. For a tablet these variables include the nature and quantity of the diluent, the disintegrant, the lubricant, any wetting agent, the size of granules and their method of manufacture, the compressional pressure and speed of compression used in tableting, and the conditions of storage and age of the finished product. After release of the drug particles the dissolution rate depends on their wettability by the fluids, their particle-size distribution, the salt form, and the polymorph used (where more than one crystalline form exists).

The incomplete release from solid dosage forms observed for several potent drugs may lead to under-dosage and failure of the treatment. When drug therapy involves adjustment of the dose to the requirements of a particular patient, a change in the dosage form or brand of medicine can lead to either under- or over-dosage. Similarly, changes in the formulation of a brand of tablet or capsule by a manufacturer may cause considerable problems and danger to patients, as has happened with phenytoin capsules and digoxin tablets.

Incidents of variable release have predictably been observed most often for drugs with a well recognised or quantifiable pharmacological effect. The problem is greatest for potent drugs of low aqueous solubility and those known to be absorbed in an irregular fashion from the gastro-intestinal tract. A few selected examples of drugs which have on specific occasions shown variable absorption behaviour are shown in Table 12.

Table 12
Some drugs for which variable absorption has been observed

Drug	Observation	Cause
Chloramphenicol palmitate	inactive suspension	use of inactive polymorph (Form A) rather than active one (Form B)
Cortisone acetate	change in brand of tablets precipitated an Addisonian crisis	drug particles in ineffective tablets were aggregated and dissolved only very slowly
Digoxin	enhanced activity of tablets	change in method of production
Griseofulvin	tablets inactive in some patients	particle size of this sparingly soluble drug was too large
Phenytoin sodium	drug intoxication 'epidemic'	manufacturer changed adjuvant in capsule from calcium sulphate to lactose
Tolbutamide	loss of diabetic control due to change in brand of tablet	poor dissolution of drug from one brand

The Disintegration Test for Solid Oral Dosage Forms (*European Pharmacopoeia*) and the Dissolution Test for Tablets and Capsules (*British Pharmacopoeia*) are examples of tests that set minimum standards for drug release *in vitro*. Failure of a product to comply with the test requirement is an indication that slow or incomplete release is likely to occur after ingestion.

Alteration of Release of Drug in the Gastro-intestinal Tract

It may be desirable to modify the rate of release of a drug from the oral dosage form compared with that achieved from a conventional product. If the drug has a low aqueous solubility, **enhanced release** may be achieved by one or more of the following methods:

- formulation as a solution in a water-miscible solvent mixture
- reduction of particle size of the powdered drug
- use of a salt in preference to the weak acid or base
- use of a water-soluble prodrug derivative
- selection of a metastable crystalline form, if the compound exhibits polymorphism
- selection of a solvated form, if the compound exists in non-solvated and solvated forms
- formulation as a molecular dispersion in a water-soluble inert carrier. Large-scale production difficulties limit the use of this approach.

Delayed onset of release may be achieved by various means including enteric-coating of capsules and tablets. This method has been used for substances producing nausea or irritation of the gastric mucosa. The various coating materials that have been used include keratin, salol, shellac, fatty acids, fats, waxes, synthetic resins, and cellulose derivatives (especially cellacephate). The dissolution of these coating materials in a medium of pH 1 to 3 is slow, but proceeds rapidly at the less acid pH of the small intestine. The decline in use of enteric-coated products is due in part to the introduction of sustained-release preparations that avoid the local irritation of the duodenal mucosa that occurs after the enteric coating has dissolved away. Also, the time of onset of absorption from enteric-coated tablets and capsules is highly variable, being dependent upon the rate of gastric emptying. Some enteric coating materials become less soluble with age and fail to release the drug.

A reduced rate of release may be desirable for several reasons. Where a prolonged action is required it is desirable that the dosage form provides a slow and constant supply of the drug. The active component is given in a larger dose and released at a rate which is safe and which maintains therapeutic blood concentrations for a prolonged period. Where a high local concentration of an irritant drug causes tissue necrosis and ulceration of the mucosal wall, damage can largely be prevented by reducing the rate of drug release.

Many dosage forms have been developed to achieve these aims. They are variously described as 'sustained-release', 'prolonged-action', 'timed-release', 'controlled-release' or other similar terms. The *European Pharmacopoeia* and *British Pharmacopoeia* definition of modified-release capsules or tablets covers preparations that have been designed in such a way that the rate or the place at which the active ingredients are released has been modified. All these terms are qualitative and give no indication of intended quantitative release patterns. In most preparations, the rate of diffusion of drug molecules is limited by applying a suitable coating to drug particles or by embedding the particles in a wax or plastic matrix. Drug particles (or sugar granules coated with the drug) can be coated with one of a variety of materials including natural and synthetic oils, fats, waxes, resins, and cellulose derivatives. Various thicknesses of coat are applied to batches of material, blended with uncoated material, and then filled into capsules. Some coating materials such as ethylcellulose allow the granules to be compressed into tablets without rupture of the coat. Drugs embedded in a slowly eroding wax matrix or a non-disintegrating plastic matrix are presented in tablet form; some contain an outer compression-coat or separate layer of immediately available drug.

Polystyrene cationic exchange resins have been used to prepare drug-resin complexes (resinates) of basic drugs such as amphetamines and alkaloids. The drug-resin complex is then formulated in a tablet, capsule, or suspension. The drug is exchanged in the presence of cations in the gastric and intestinal fluids but release is usually incomplete.

Chemical modification of the drug molecule to yield a compound of lower solubility has been used to give a sustained-release effect. Benzathine penicillin is a less soluble salt of benzylpenicillin. Compared with benzylpenicillin the peak blood concentration is produced less rapidly but effective levels are maintained for much longer. The effect of the palmitate ester of chloramphenicol is more sustained than that of the free alcohol. The free alcohol is absorbed, but not the sparingly water-soluble ester, which undergoes slow hydrolysis in the gastro-intestinal tract.

Other attempts to produce a sustained-release effect have been based on the low aqueous solubility of the polygalacturonate salt of a basic drug, such as quinidine; embonate and tannate salts have also been used. The success of this approach has been marginal, presumably because the salts tend to dissociate at the low gastric pH and dissolve more rapidly than indicated by the equilibrium solubility measurement.

One disadvantage of systems that rely on diffusional transfer of drug from a matrix is that release is often too slow.

In the 'osmotic pump' system for drug delivery, shown in Fig. 7, there is a mixture of drug and an osmotically active constituent surrounded by a selectively permeable coating. Water is taken up by osmotic action and the dissolved drug is discharged through a small orifice in the coating. With this system, relatively high release rates are possible; in addition, the rate of release is largely independent of the degree of agitation in the vicinity of the device. As a result, it is usual to find that release rates *in vivo* are close to those *in vitro*. Examples of drugs that have been included in osmotic pump systems are indomethacin and salbutamol.

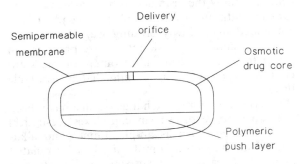

Fig. 7
'Osmotic pump' drug delivery system.

Experience with the system containing indomethacin showed that the solution discharged from the orifice was capable of causing local tissue necrosis in the gastro-intestinal tract and the product was withdrawn from use. Osmotic pump systems containing less irritant substances are not expected to cause local gastro-intestinal irritation.

Formulation Factors Affecting Absorption from Injections

The pH of injected aqueous solutions can greatly affect drug absorption. Unlike intravenous injections, subcutaneous and intramuscular injections are only diluted quite slowly by tissue fluids. The pH of the solution changes gradually from its initial value to that of interstitial fluid (pH 7.2 to 7.4).

In accordance with the pH-partition hypothesis of drug absorption, basic drugs are more rapidly absorbed by these routes when a significant proportion of the drug exists as the free base, that is, when the environmental pH is greater than the pK_a value of the drug. It is known that some amines, including procaine and other local anaesthetics, are better absorbed from slightly alkaline solution. However, they are not sufficiently stable at these pH values for storage purposes, and so acidic solutions are still used.

The rate of absorption of some weakly acidic drugs from intramuscular injections may be substantially lower than from an oral preparation. Solutions of sodium salts of weak acids have a pH value greater than about 8.5 and this slowly decreases to pH 7.2 to 7.4 after injection, due to dilution with interstitial fluid. Particles of the free acid may precipitate and their subsequent slow dissolution limits the rate of absorption of the drug. The concentration of drug in blood plasma may, therefore, be lower than expected. Intramuscular injections of phenytoin sodium have failed to control seizures because the rate of dissolution of precipitated phenytoin in muscle tissue is low.

The slow absorption from aqueous suspensions of drug particles may be desirable when rapid elimination from the body would otherwise make frequent injections necessary. Salts of penicillin with low aqueous solubility (benzathine penicillin and procaine penicillin) injected intramuscularly as a suspension form a depot from which the penicillin is slowly leached. The rate of release is governed by their solubility in tissue fluids and the surface area of the drug particles.

Several corticosteroids are injected intramuscularly as aqueous suspensions and are released over several days; intra-articular injection into rheumatoid or osteoarthritic joints is used to produce a local anti-inflammatory action.

The effects of particle size and crystallinity upon the absorption rate from subcutaneous injections of insulin are utilised to provide the flexibility of treatment required by diabetics. The duration of activity is governed by the size and the amorphous or crystalline nature of the suspended particles. The *British Pharmacopoeia* specifies the size and shape of particles in Biphasic Insulin Injection, Isophane Insulin Injection, and three injections of Insulin Zinc Suspensions.

Some drugs exist in several polymorphic or crystalline forms. A metastable, high-energy form has a greater solubility than the stable polymorph and so should be absorbed more rapidly. In practice, a metastable form in a suspension is liable to undergo solvent-mediated reversion to the stable form during manufacture or storage, usually accompanied by crystal growth. This undesirable phenomenon is avoided by using the stable polymorph. Drugs may crystallise from a variety of solvents as solvates. Several steroids form solvates with ethanol, acetone, and chloroform. The tertiary butylacetate esters of prednisolone and hydrocortisone form solvates with ethanol that are absorbed several times more rapidly than the non-solvated forms.

Oily intramuscular injections are sterile solutions or suspensions in a suitable oil such as arachis oil. Being more viscous than aqueous solutions, these do not spread along muscle fascias but form a depot in the muscle tissue. The drug must partition into, or dissolve in, the aqueous tissue fluid, and so release occurs very slowly.

The need for long-term therapy with steroid hormones has generated much research into intramuscular and subcutaneous preparations of these drugs. Chemical modification of the molecule to produce an oil-soluble compound is often necessary; for example, testosterone propionate ester. These derivatives are poorly water soluble and dissolve in tissue fluid over an extended period of time; in some cases a single dose lasts up to one month. Some antipsychotic agents have been prepared as long-acting intramuscular injections. An intramuscular injection of the decanoate ester of fluphenazine in sesame oil provides an antipsychotic effect for two to five weeks, and patient compliance is much better than with daily doses of fluphenazine hydrochloride.

Procaine penicillin has been formulated as an oily suspension containing aluminium stearate as a gelling agent. The sustained action of preparations containing aluminium stearate depends on their high viscosity. Also, there is some evidence that a chemical interaction occurs between the stearate and the surface of the procaine penicillin particles so that, contrary to expectation, the use of finer drug particles enhances the prolongation of action.

Formulation Factors affecting Absorption from Implants

Subcutaneous pellets or implants provide drug depots that may maintain satisfactory blood concentrations over several months. Slow release is due to the use of a drug or prodrug with low aqueous solubility and to the small surface area of the implant. As absorption proceeds the surface area decreases and the absorption rate falls. To minimise this effect, cylindrical implants are used, typically 8 mm long and 3 mm in diameter. They are inserted subcutaneously during a minor surgical operation.

The presence of diluents in implants could affect the release rate. If the diluent is more readily soluble than the drug in tissue fluids, it disappears more rapidly, leaving particles of drug exposed to tissue fluids; drug surface area and release rate would both increase. The main use of implants is in long-term therapy with steroid hormones.

Assessment of Bioavailability

The rate and extent of absorption can be determined from measurements of drug concentration in various body fluids including whole blood, plasma or serum, urine, or saliva. The analytical method of measuring drug concentration should be appropriate for the intended purpose; some analytical methods do not distinguish between inactive metabolites and the parent compound and are therefore unsatisfactory. If a metabolite is pharmacologically active, an analytical method which also measures it is desirable.

Drug Concentration in Blood

As shown in Fig. 8, the changes of drug concentration in blood plasma with time may be used to construct a plasma concentration-time profile. There are methods for calculating the apparent absorption rate constant from the data. However, the time to peak concentration and the peak concentration itself are useful indices of the absorption rate.

The fraction of dose absorbed (F) can be found by measurement of the total area under the curve (AUC) of the concentration-time profile from time zero to time infinity. The area is related to the administered dose D_{admin} by:

$$\text{Total area under the curve} = \frac{F \times D_{admin}}{\text{Total body clearance}}$$

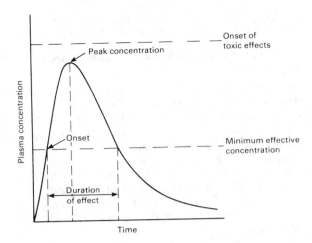

Fig. 8
Plasma-drug concentration–time profile.

so that if on successive occasions an individual receives a drug in the same dose by intravenous bolus injection (where $F = 1$) and via an absorption site, measurement of the areas under the curves allows F to be calculated as:

$$F = \frac{\text{AUC after administration via absorption site}}{\text{AUC after administration as intravenous bolus injection}}$$

The areas are corrected for the doses used if these are different. The value of F, usually expressed as a percentage, is the **'absolute' bioavailability** of the drug from the dosage form. If the drug cannot be given intravenously the area term in the denominator of the equation relates to the drug given as an aqueous solution, or as an established commercial preparation of known clinical effectiveness that serves as a standard; from this the **'relative' bioavailability** is calculated.

Absorption may often be incomplete, and the size of the administered dose is established through clinical experience. Changes in the fraction absorbed are undesirable especially when the drug has a low therapeutic index, as a small increase in the fraction of the dose absorbed may lead to toxic effects.

Because the area under the curve also depends upon the total body clearance value, studies on bioavailability should be based on a crossover design, where the test animal or subject receives, on separate occasions, each preparation being evaluated. The bioavailability from different commercial preparations can be compared in randomised complete crossover studies conducted in healthy volunteers. In this study design, all subjects receive both (or all) the formulations on separate occasions, in random order, with a 'wash-out' period between administrations.

Therapeutic activity may be expected to rise with increasing concentration of the drug in blood. For various reasons this may not be the case in practice; for example the plasma concentration-time profile may not reflect the changing amounts of drug at the site of drug action. The purpose of tests *in vivo* is to establish whether there is satisfactory drug release and absorption from a dosage form.

Drug Concentration in Urine

Measurements of drug or metabolite concentration in urine can be used in bioavailability studies. Collection of urine samples is safer and is easier and less traumatic for the subject than is collection of blood samples. Urine has lower concentrations of protein and some endogenous materials and usually has higher drug concentrations so that analytical procedures are often simpler. The method is only applicable when a drug or rapidly formed metabolite is extensively excreted in urine. The concentrations of drug (or metabolite) in discrete urine samples may be used to calculate the rate of urinary excretion and the cumulative amount excreted. If the rate of drug excretion is proportional to the concentration in blood plasma the curve obtained by plotting urinary excretion rate against time is of the same shape as the plasma concentration-time curve. This proportionality does not hold if:

- the compound is actively secreted into the distal kidney tubule
- the compound is a weak acid or base and urine pH is fluctuating
- or the excretion rate is urine flow-dependent.

Urinary excretion rate measurements may be unsatisfactory for estimating the apparent absorption rate constant because of the difficulty in collecting frequent discrete urine samples in man. The cumulative urinary excretion over a sufficient period (usually from 0 to 48 or 72 hours) may be used to calculate the absolute bioavailability (F):

$$F = \frac{U_{abs}}{U_{iv}} \times 100$$

where U_{abs} and U_{iv} are the cumulative amounts excreted after administration via an absorption site and by intravenous injection respectively, corrected for the dose administered if necessary. The relative bioavailability of two oral formulations can be determined in a similar manner from the cumulative amounts excreted. A practical difficulty encountered is that of incomplete collection of urine samples from individuals during the test period.

Drug Concentration in Saliva

Some drugs are excreted into saliva in moderate quantities and for most of these it has been shown that the concentration in mixed saliva is proportional to that in blood plasma. These drugs include: digoxin, isoniazid, lignocaine, lithium, mexiletine, paracetamol, phenazone, phenytoin, salicylates, and some sulphonamides. The measurement of salivary excretion rate provides an alternative method for the assessment of bioavailability. Sample collection is simple and non-invasive. The rate of salivary excretion may be expected to be dependent upon saliva pH and this has been confirmed for procainamide. The bioavailabilities of some orally administered preparations have been measured by this method; care must be taken with liquid or uncoated solid preparations to minimise contamination of early saliva samples with drug retained in the mouth after administration.

Bioequivalence and Bioinequivalence

In the development of a new medicinal product, bioavailability of the active constituent must normally be demonstrated to be satisfactory. In general, products which release substantially less than the total content are considered unacceptable. A programme of development of a new compound should include an assessment of bioavailability in man.

Before a new product, or a new formulation of an existing product, can be introduced into clinical use, regulatory authorities will require evidence of satisfactory bioavailabilty. In general, the data required will be from a bioequivalence study in man in which the bioavailability of the new product is compared with that of an existing product containing the same active ingredient. Detailed requirements of regulatory authorities differ from one country to another. However, it is generally accepted that a requirement for a bioequivalence study must be considered in the following circumstances:

- a new product is introduced by one manufacturer and a similar product is already licensed to another manufacturer
- the manufacturer of a licensed product wishes to vary the excipients used or the process of manufacture

- a new product is introduced that is not identical to an existing licensed product although it contains the same chemical entity or a closely-related compound, such as a salt (of an acid or base), an isomer, a hydrate, or a solvate
- when a new product is introduced for which specific claims are made for the rate of drug release. All sustained-release products must be evaluated in bioequivalence studies.

Evidence of bioequivalence of products is required when inequivalence would be hazardous to the patient because of efficacy or safety considerations. A hazard may exist in the following circumstances:

- the active ingredient has a narrow therapeutic margin such that a change of product may lead to an increased bioavailability and to the development of an increased incidence of recognised adverse events or new adverse events or other signs of toxicity in patients
- there are serious consequences for the patient in the event of inefficacy of the product. Therapeutic agents used for the treatment or prevention of serious disease, condition, or symptoms must be scrutinised closely and the degree of inequivalence tolerated will depend upon the seriousness of the hazards involved
- the patient group for which the product is primarily intended is particularly at risk. Groups will include children and the elderly
- there is evidence from the scientific literature that some products containing the active ingredient have shown bioinequivalence and that this has led to an important clinical problem in the treatment of patients
- a drug is formulated in a modified-release form such that it contains more drug than constitutes a normal single dose. The rapid release of a large proportion of the content through failure of the modified-release mechanism may lead to the absorption of an overdose. This 'dose-dumping' effect has been observed with some oral modified-release products when taken with food and appears to occur because of changes in gastric pH.

Tests of the bioequivalence of products are typically carried out in a group of 12 to 24 healthy young volunteers who are within ±10% of their ideal body weight. Each product is administered in random order as a single dose under fasting conditions on separate occasions in a crossover design. The requirements are that the study must have sufficient power (usually 80% or greater) to detect a difference in AUC values of $\pm 20\%$ with a probability level of 95%. Other differences may be appropriate, however, as for warfarin products ($\pm 10\%$), anti-arrhythmic agents ($\pm 25\%$), and antipsychotic agents ($\pm 30\%$).

There are some circumstances under which bioequivalence studies may not be considered necessary. For example, if accumulated evidence has shown that a dissolution test is an accurate predictor of performance in vivo then the test in vitro will suffice. Also, there are no requirements for the bioequivalence testing of intravenous or topical preparations.

In summary, in considering the need to conduct a bioequivalence study on a new product, consideration must be given to the accumulated information on the therapeutic agent, the dosage form and its formulation, and the disease entity being treated. This approach is preferable to one in which the test is applied to all new products.

Clinical Equivalence of Medicines

The bioequivalence of two (or more) products may be established through tests in vivo of the type described under Assessment of Bioavailability, above. However, to ensure that products from different sources or manufacturers can be used interchangeably requires that the products be shown to be equivalent in clinical practice, that is, to produce the same therapeutic effect, as measured by control of the disease or its symptomatic relief.

Assessment of clinical equivalence is inevitably more difficult to assess than bioequivalence because of confounding factors such as uncertain diagnosis, partial remission of the disease, or the presence of other disease states. It is possible for products that are not bioequivalent to be clinically equivalent. If the effect is observed over a wide plasma-drug concentration range, and any toxic effects are seen only at high concentrations, many concentration-time profiles may be satisfactory. In contrast, for drugs with a low therapeutic index where careful control of plasma-drug concentration is required, clinical equivalence can only be achieved with products that are bioequivalent.

These considerations show that it is not possible to predict what plasma-drug concentration-time profile is desirable. However, when clinical experience with a product has established that a particular product, given in accordance with a stated dose regimen, provides satisfactory drug therapy then it is reasonable to demand bioequivalence of any products subsequently introduced into clinical practice.

Attention has been drawn to the question as to whether bioequivalent products are necessarily clinically equivalent. Inevitably two products will differ to a small degree in rate or extent (or both) of drug release. The consequences of these small differences have not been fully assessed.

If a metabolite of the administered drug is active, then the rate of formation of the metabolite after administration of the product should be assessed as part of the bioequivalence study.

In vivo-In vitro Correlation

Although the dissolution test in vitro provides valuable information on the release characteristics of solid dosage forms, the test conditions do not allow an extrapolation to the release of drug under conditions in vivo. Whereas it is possible to mimic in vitro some of the parameters (such as temperature and the pH, viscosity, and surface tension of gastro-intestinal fluids) the type and intensity of mixing and interaction of drug with food or food residues cannot be reproduced.

It is common, therefore, to find that the dissolution rate in vitro differs from that in vivo. Laboratory-based tests are therefore not predictive of the release rate in absolute terms from a formulation in vivo. However, experience over 25 years with testing the same formulations in dissolution tests and bioavailability studies has shown that formulations that have poor release characteristics in vitro often have low bioavailability in a clinical study, and the converse is also true.

In dissolution tests a profile of the percentage of the nominal (or label) content released against time can be used to characterise the release rate (Fig. 9).

Single-point indices of the profile include, for example, the percentage dissolved in 30 minutes or the time taken for 75% to dissolve. When a series of formulations of a compound is tested, indices of the dissolution rate will vary considerably between products. Where the same products have also been tested in bioavailability studies it is useful to seek a correlation between the results from the two types of tests. The results for an evaluation of 11 oral formulations of prednisone are shown in Fig. 10.

If a good correlation is obtained between the indices of performance in vitro and in vivo in a representative number of products available, then

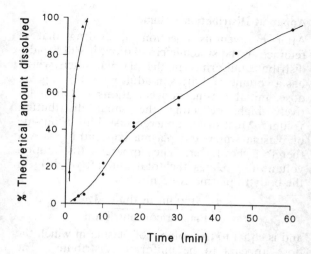

Fig. 9 Dissolution of drug from capsules: drug/calcium phosphate/magnesium stearate 2% in simulated gastric fluid (▲) and water (●) (after Samyn JC, Jung WY. J Pharm Sci 1970;59(2):169–75).

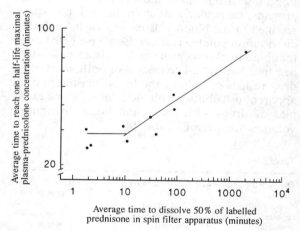

Fig. 10
Correlation of average time to reach half-maximal plasma concentration of prednisolone with average time to dissolve 50% of labelled amount of prednisone in spin filter apparartus (after Sullivan *et al.* J Biopharm Pharmacokinetics 1976;4:173–81).

it may be acceptable to use the relation in a prospective manner. From Fig. 10 it is apparent that a product that takes more than 50 minutes for 50% of the labelled content of prednisone to dissolve will take longer than 35 minutes for plasma concentrations of prednisolone (the active metabolite) to reach half the maximum concentration. This approach to the evaluation of oral formulations has only been confirmed for a few therapeutic agents and is not generally applicable. For most

compounds the close correlation of results *in vitro* and *in vivo* has not been established.

PHARMACOKINETICS

The subject of pharmacokinetics is the study of the quantitative changes of absorption, distribution, metabolism, and excretion of a drug with time, following its administration to man or animals. The measurement of the pharmacokinetics of a drug or its dosage forms may provide information on the onset of action and the intensity, and duration of a pharmacological effect. Where a drug or dosage form fails to elicit an effect, investigation of the pharmacokinetics of the drug may identify the cause of failure as being due to poor absorption or to rapid elimination. If the drug is present in high concentrations but fails to produce a response, this may be attributable to insensitivity of the receptors, that is, to **pharmacodynamic factors**.

In **clinical pharmacokinetics**, pharmacokinetic data are applied to the design of safe and effective therapeutic regimens for an individual patient. This implies a knowledge of the effect of various disease states upon the pharmacokinetics of the drug. The four component processes of absorption, distribution, metabolism, and excretion have been discussed previously. In quantitative terms, the decline in amount of drug at an absorption site is accompanied by increasing amounts distributed in the body and undergoing elimination. After direct intravenous injection the pharmacokinetic properties of a drug are dependent upon two variables, the **clearance** and the **apparent distribution volume** of the drug.

Drug Clearance

Clearance of a drug occurs when it is removed irreversibly from the systemic circulation or body tissue by metabolism or excretion. With the exception of drugs that undergo elimination through breakdown within the blood, clearance occurs during the transit of drug in blood through an 'organ of elimination', such as the liver or kidneys. During transit, a proportion of the drug presented to the organ of elimination is removed. For convenience, **low extraction drugs** are arbitrarily defined as those where less than 30% of the drug is extracted, and **high extraction drugs** are those where more than 70% is lost; the extraction ratios are 0.3 and 0.7, respectively.

Clearance may be defined as the volume of blood from which drug is totally removed per unit of time and has units of measurement of millilitres per minute. Clearance is related to blood flow (Q) through the organ and the extraction ratio (E) by:

$$Clearance = Q \times E$$

Table 13 shows examples of low and high extraction drugs cleared by the liver and kidney and their clearance values; clearances are described as **hepatic clearance** or **renal clearance**, depending on the organ of elimination. When these two sites are the only sites of drug removal, the **total clearance** is calculated as:

Total clearance = Hepatic clearance
+ Renal clearance

Table 13
Clearance and extraction

Organ	Drug	E	Clearance (mL/min)
Kidney	cephazolin	0.05	55
	inulin	0.1	120
	penicillin	0.42	500
Liver	theophylline	0.04	60
	amitriptyline	0.3	450
	lignocaine	0.74	1100

Renal blood flow = 1200 mL/minute
Hepatic blood flow = 1500 mL/minute

Direct measurement of clearance from the organ blood flow and the extraction ratio is impracticable in man. However, mathematically, total clearance can be calculated from the relationship:

$$Total\ clearance = \frac{Dose\ absorbed}{AUC}$$

where AUC is the total area beneath the curve of plasma-drug concentration plotted against time after administration of the drug dose. The AUC is estimated by adding the areas of individual trapezia, which approximate to the shape of the concentration-time profile. The above relationship between clearance, dose, and AUC is only valid when the drug is eliminated in accordance with first-order kinetics. The clearance may be used to calculate the rate of drug elimination because:

Rate of drug elimination

= Clearance × Plasma-drug concentration

During the elimination phase the rate of drug elimination declines as the drug concentration falls.

Apparent Distribution Volume

After intravenous injection of a drug that is retained in the systemic circulation, it will rapidly distribute uniformly in the plasma water, which has a volume of 3 litres in adult man. For a given dose, initial plasma concentrations will be relatively high, reflecting the small distribution volume. Most drugs undergo distribution outside of plasma water and plasma concentrations will therefore be lower. The apparent distribution volume (V) relates the total amount of drug in the body to plasma concentration:

$$V = \frac{Amount\ in\ the\ body}{Plasma\ concentration}$$

and is equal to the volume of plasma in which the dose appears to be uniformly distributed. The volume of distribution does not correspond to an actual volume of body fluid, but depends upon the extent to which the drug distributes into and binds to various tissues.

For those drugs that bind extensively to plasma proteins, particularly albumin, most of the drug is retained in the blood plasma and so the apparent distribution volume is small. Conversely, for drugs that bind to plasma proteins to only a small extent, or which bind avidly to tissues, or both, most of the drug resides outside of the blood plasma and the apparent distribution volume is large. Some examples of drugs with small and large distribution volumes are given in Table 14.

Table 14

Drugs with volumes of distribution less than 200 mL/kg

aspirin	diflunisal	probenecid
carbenicillin	flurbiprofen	salicylic acid
cephamandole	frusemide	tolbutamide
cephazolin	ibuprofen	tolmetin
chlorothiazide	ketoprofen	valproic acid
chlorpropamide	naproxen	warfarin
clofibric acid	oxyphenbutazone	
dicloxacillin	piperacillin	

Drugs with volumes of distribution greater than 2 litres/kg

amphetamine	mepacrine	procainamide
desipramine	nortriptyline	propranolol
digoxin	pentamidine	
ethchlorvynol	pethidine	

The extent of distribution of drugs can vary widely. This has implications in the use of haemodialysis for the treatment of drug overdosage. The effectiveness of haemodialysis treatment of patients who have taken a drug in overdose depends to a large extent on the apparent distribution volume. Those drugs with a low apparent distribution, present in blood plasma in relatively high concentrations, are generally more effectively cleared by haemodialysis.

Pharmacokinetic Models of Drug Absorption and Disposition

A model of the processes of drug absorption, distribution, and elimination may serve to understand the changes in the quantities of drug within the body. The human body is a highly complex system of physiological and biochemical processes that act upon, and in turn may be altered by, xenobiotic substances. Models of varying degrees of complexity may be used in an attempt to describe various processes. However, pharmacokinetic models may be quite simple while retaining an ability to describe the kinetics of the individual processes.

A pharmacokinetic model that has been found to be useful is depicted in Fig.11. In this model of drug absorption and disposition, the drug is seen to transfer from the site of absorption to a central compartment. A proportion of the drug is eliminated whereas some drug undergoes distribution into a peripheral compartment, from which it returns by redistribution into the central compartment. In this model, ultimately, all the drug returns from the peripheral compartment and is eliminated from the central compartment.

another. For drugs with limited tissue distribution, such as gentamicin, it may be disregarded. In contrast, for drugs that distribute widely, the peripheral compartment may assume a larger role and, in some instances, it may be necessary to extend the model to include separate 'shallow' and 'deep' peripheral compartments, a total of three body compartments.

The model that applies for a particular drug can be deduced from the plasma-drug profile after intravenous injection. The distribution and redistribution processes profoundly affect the profile. Pharmacokinetic profiles also depend upon route of drug administration, and profiles following direct intravenous injection, extravascular administration, and constant-rate intravenous infusion will be considered.

Direct intravenous injection produces relatively high concentrations within a few minutes. Thereafter, concentrations decline as a result of the combined effects of distribution and elimination. For drugs that undergo extensive distribution, the curve is biphasic. In the first phase, the decline in concentration is a result of the combined effects of distribution and elimination (Fig. 12). In the second phase, the decline is much slower because of redistribution from the peripheral tissue. In this 'terminal' phase, elimination often occurs

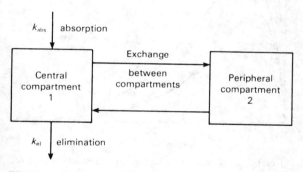

Fig. 11
A two-compartment model.

The compartments are not identifiable as specific tissues or organs. However, it is apparent that the central compartment usually includes those tissues that are rapidly accessed by the drug and are well-perfused by blood. The peripheral compartment includes tissues that are slowly accessed, as occurs with poorly perfused tissues. Examples of well-perfused and poorly perfused tissues are given in Table 9. The influence of the peripheral compartment on the pharmacokinetic profile varies from one drug to

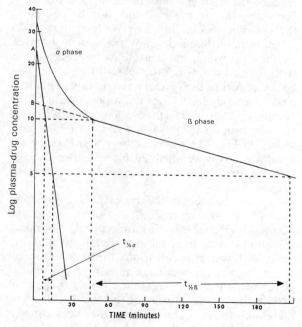

Fig. 12
Semilogarithmic plot of plasma-drug concentration versus time for a drug distributed within 2 compartments.

exponentially and is characterised by the **half-life**. The half-life, variously referred to as apparent, terminal, or biological, is defined as the time taken for the concentration to fall from any value to half that value. The half-life of a drug is an important parameter. It is related to the clearance and apparent distribution volume by:

$$\text{Half-life} = \frac{0.693 \times \text{Apparent distribution volume}}{\text{Clearance}}$$

For individual drugs, half-life values can vary widely, from a few minutes (for drugs with high clearance and small volume) to many days (for drugs with low clearance and large volume). From the equation, it is seen that half-life is governed by the two parameters, clearance and apparent distribution volume. Half-life values for drugs in healthy individuals and in a variety of disease states are reported in standard texts. The half-life of a drug in individuals with diseases of the liver or kidney failure is almost always longer than in healthy subjects. This has important consequences when drugs are used in repeated doses (see below). Systemically acting drugs administered by an extravascular route need to undergo absorption before entering the circulation. The pharmacokinetic profile differs from that found after intravenous injection in two important respects. Firstly, drug reaches the systemic circulation at a lower rate. Secondly, the absorption may not be complete; the systemic availability may be less than 100% of the administered dose. When a drug is given by the oral route, the anatomical arrangement is such that all the drug must pass through the liver before reaching the systemic circulation. The first-pass effect may lead to loss of a proportion of the administered dose. The profile achieved after extravascular administration has a characteristic shape shown in Fig. 13. Where activity and toxicity are associated with well-defined plasma-drug concentrations, the period of onset and duration may be defined.

Effects of changes in absorption and elimination kinetics are shown in Fig.14. Compared to the plasma-drug concentration-time profile (a), curve (b) shows that a reduced systemic availability leads to lower concentrations throughout; in (c) faster absorption produces an earlier and higher peak concentration with earlier termination of activity; in (d) a shortening of the half-life (by increased clearance) produces a lower peak concentration and faster fall in concentrations.

The corresponding changes in AUC can be predicted from the equation:

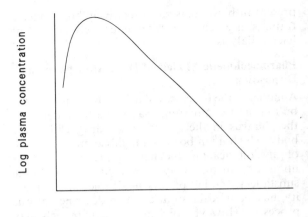

Fig. 13

Semilogarithmic plot of plasma-drug concentration as a function of time after oral administration.

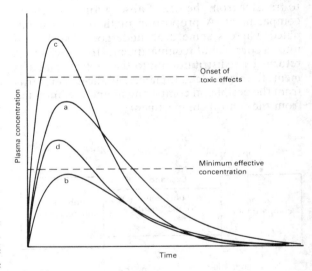

Fig. 14

The plasma-drug concentration–time profile (a) may be altered by decreasing the fraction of dose absorbed (b), by increasing the apparent absorption rate constant (c), or by increasing the apparent elimination rate constant (d).

$$\text{AUC} = \frac{F \times \text{Dose administered}}{\text{Total clearance}}$$

which demonstrates: (b) a reduced AUC due to a lower absorbed dose; (c) no change in AUC; (d) a decrease in AUC because of the higher clearance. Under most circumstances, absorption proceeds relatively rapidly. Occasionally, absorption is slow and may exert a controlling effect on the elimination rate. This effect is observed, for example, for drugs given by deep intramuscular injection to achieve a prolonged, slow release. The pharmacokinetic profile will show a terminal half-life that reflects the absorption process and the calculated half-life is not the true half-life for drug elimination. It is recognised that, in these circumstances, elimination is rate-limited by the absorption process.

First-pass Effect

After oral administration, a drug is absorbed from the intestinal lumen into the hepatic portal vein. Before the drug reaches the systemic circulation, however, it must pass through the liver. If the drug is readily metabolised in the liver a large fraction of the absorbed drug may be inactivated, substantially reducing the quantity of drug reaching the systemic circulation. The 'first-pass loss' of drugs can account for the large difference between an oral and an intravenous dose required for activity. In addition, the extent of formation of a metabolite may be greater after oral than intravenous administration. Thus concentrations of 4-hydroxypropranolol are much less after intravenous administration of propranolol than after oral ingestion. Examples of other drugs that undergo substantial first-pass loss include imipramine, lignocaine, and nortriptyline.

Intravenous infusion at a constant rate produces increasing concentrations with time, as shown in Fig. 15. If infusion is continued for a sufficient period, concentrations reach a constant level (steady state) or plateau concentration. At this point rates of infusion and elimination exactly balance, such that:

Rate of infusion
$$= \text{Clearance} \times \text{Steady state concentration}$$

Rearrangement of the equation gives:

$$\text{Clearance} = \frac{\text{Rate of infusion}}{\text{Steady state concentration}}$$

which provides another practical method for the measurement of clearance. Alternatively, the relationship can be used to estimate the steady-state concentration achieved with a particular rate of infusion when the clearance is known for an individual. The duration of infusion required to virtually achieve steady-state is approximately equal to five elimination half-lives. After termination of the infusion, the half-life of the drug can be estimated from the elimination phase as for direct intravenous injection. If the infusion is terminated before the plateau is reached, such that clearance cannot be estimated from the previous equation, then a value for clearance can be estimated as:

$$\text{Clearance} = \frac{\text{Infused dose}}{\text{AUC}}$$

where the AUC is as previously defined.

There are other circumstances in which a drug enters the systemic circulation at a constant (zero-order) rate. For example, the oral osmotic pump system and the transdermal patch system are both designed to provide drug at a constant rate. Although the rate of drug release may be well-characterised, it cannot be assumed that the systemic availability is 100% of the total content of the system and the drug clearance cannot be calculated from the penultimate equation.

Multiple-dose Regimens

Some therapeutic regimens require the administration of a single dose or only a small number of doses. For other regimens, administration of the dose is repeated on a regular basis over several weeks, months, or years. It is useful to consider the pharmacokinetic profile that results from the repeated administration of a fixed dose of drug at regular intervals. In a multiple-dose regimen, the amount of drug present in the systemic circulation will depend on the following:

- the number and frequency of previous doses
- the elimination half-life of the drug
- the interval since the last dose.

In simple terms, the amount of drug in the body at any time is equal to the sum of the amounts of drug remaining from all the administered doses. For a

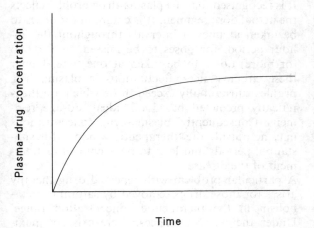

Fig. 15
Plot of plasma-drug concentration as a function of time during an intravenous infusion at constant rate.

drug with a short half-life given at infrequent intervals, the amount present depends almost entirely on the quantity remaining from the most recent dose. Conversely, for a drug with a long half-life given at short intervals the amount present is the sum total of residual amounts from several or many preceding doses.

In the latter example, the amount present after several doses may be many times that provided by a single dose and this effect is referred to as **drug accumulation**. In a multiple-dose regimen, concentrations do not rise indefinitely but reach a plateau (or steady state). There is an analogy with the constant rate infusion because the multiple-dose regimen provides the drug at a constant rate. Just as for an intravenous infusion at constant rate, the terms of interest are:

- the average plasma-drug concentration at the plateau
- the time taken from the start of the regimen to reach the plateau.

The average plasma-drug concentration can be calculated in the same way as for an infusion at constant rate, with the infusion rate being replaced by the **dosing rate**, which is given by:

$$\text{Dosing rate} = \frac{\text{Absorbed dose}}{\text{Interval between doses}} = \frac{F \times \text{dose}}{T}$$

Therefore:
Average plasma-drug concentration

$$= \frac{\text{Absorbed dose}}{\text{Clearance} \times \text{Interval between doses}}$$

Naturally, the plasma-drug profile in a multiple-dose regimen has a characteristic 'saw-tooth' appearance because of the discrete dose administrations (Fig.16).

The period of treatment before the plateau is reached is approximately equal to five times the half-life of drug elimination. This implies that for a drug with a long half-life, several days or weeks of treatment may elapse before the plateau is reached and this is clearly undesirable. Under these circumstances, one (or more) loading doses may be given at the start of the treatment period to elevate plasma-drug concentrations and shorten the interval before the plateau is reached. Delays in the onset of drug action may thus be avoided.

Drugs given in multiple-dose regimens are usually administered orally. The effects of changes in the rate and extent of absorption therefore merit consideration.

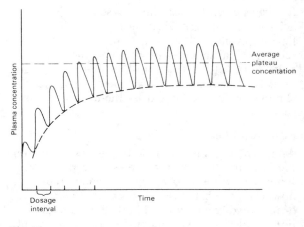

Fig. 16
Plasma-drug concentration–time profile following administration of multiple doses.

In regimens where drug accumulation occurs, plasma-drug concentrations at the plateau considerably exceed the concentration from a single dose. Changes in the rate of absorption from an orally administered product produce only minor changes in the profile and are therefore of little or no clinical importance. In contrast, unanticipated changes, whether an increase or decrease, in the extent of absorption directly affect the average plasma-drug concentration in the plateau. There are examples of therapeutic failures from unexpectedly high plasma-drug concentrations (such as with phenytoin and digoxin) and from unexpectedly low concentrations (such as with theophylline).

It is recognised that the plasma-drug profile reflects the actual dose regimen. It is common for doses to be taken at uneven intervals throughout the 24-hour period, for doses to be missed, or for two (or more) doses to be taken at one time. Under these circumstances, fluctuations in plasma-drug profiles substantially exceed those which are theoretically predicted based on 'ideal' dosage regimens. Consequently, plasma-drug concentrations may lie outside the 'therapeutic window' for substantial periods and lead to poor control or treatment of the disease.

A particular problem with repeated drug therapy arises for those drugs removed by saturable metabolism in the therapeutic concentration range. Under these circumstances, there exists a maximum rate of drug metabolism. If the rate of administration closely approaches or exceeds the maximum rate, then plasma-drug concentrations do not reach a plateau but continue to rise throughout the period of drug administration. Concentrations may rise to levels associated with severe toxicity and side-effects, unless these are recognised and there is a therapeutic intervention. Phenytoin, salicylates (in high doses), and ethanol are examples of drugs which exhibit saturable metabolism.

FURTHER INFORMATION

Adou HM. Dissolution, bioavailability and bioequivalence. Easton: Mack, 1989.

Davis SS. Assessment of gastrointestinal transit and drug absorption. In: Prescott LF, Nimmo WS, editors. Novel drug delivery and its therapeutic application. Chichester: John Wiley & Sons, 1989.

Rowland M, Tozer TN. Clinical pharmacokinetics: Concepts and applications. 2nd ed. Philadelphia: Lea and Febiger, 1989.

Rheology

Rheology is the study of the deformation of materials including flow. As a science it may be traced back to Newton who, in Principia Mathematica (1687), attempted to quantify flow by stating that 'The resistance which arises from the lack of slipperiness originating in a fluid, other things being equal, is proportional to the velocity by which the parts of the fluid are being separated from each other'. It is now recognised that rheology involves more than flow. Its applications in pharmacy are wide ranging including liquids, semi-solids, gels, solid deformation, coatings, and packaging materials.

CONCEPTS AND DEFINITIONS

All matter deforms when a stress is applied, the resulting deformation being the strain. Stress is measured as a force per unit area, usually Pascals (Pa) and is designated F. Various other symbols are used in the literature (for example τ, S). The extent of deformation is called strain, γ, and has no units, but in flow it is called the shear rate, with units of time, usually per second. Stress may be applied as an elongation, compression, bending, twisting, or shearing. Only the latter produces flow in liquids.

If the material regains its original shape and position when the stress is removed it is said to be elastic. Solids can deform elastically under all five ways of applying stress, but liquids are only elastic under compression. If the material does not recover, it has flowed. Thus, as a simplification, solids are elastic and liquids flow.

The elastic modulus is a measure of the difficulty in obtaining a deformation. For each method of applying the stress, the modulus has the same form:

$$\text{Modulus of elasticity } (G) = \frac{\text{stress}}{\text{strain}}$$

The reciprocal, called the compliance, J, is the ease of deformation. Liquids do not have a modulus of elasticity under normal circumstances. To measure the ease or difficulty of flow, compliance is considered by measuring the rate of shear strain $(d\gamma/dt)$ under an applied stress (F). Thus for an ideal (that is, viscous) liquid:

$$\frac{d\gamma}{dt} = \frac{1}{\eta} F$$

where η is the viscosity (units usually Pa s).

Some materials will show both elasticity and flow and are referred to as being viscoelastic.

The different types of behaviour may be demonstrated by considering the strain produced by an applied stress with the passage of time. Fig. 1 shows the ideal behaviour for flow. There is a linear increase in strain with time for the whole time during which the stress is applied. When the stress is removed the system remains in its new location. A mechanical model of this behaviour is the dashpot (Fig. 2). A force applied to the piston causes it to move through a viscous medium, the speed being a function of force and viscosity. Removing the force leaves the piston where it is. The material has flowed. Fig. 3 shows the behaviour of an elastic material. On application of the force, there is an immediate and complete deformation which remains constant throughout the application of the force. On removal, there is an immediate and

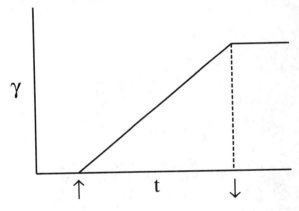

Fig. 1
Ideal flow behaviour. During application of the stress, indicated by the arrows, strain develops linearly with time.

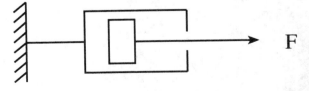

Fig. 2
The dashpot—a mechanical model for ideal flow. During the application of a force F, the piston will move out linearly with time.

260

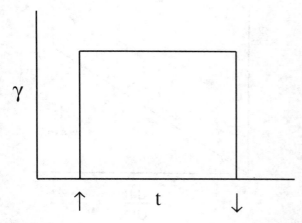

Fig. 3
Ideal elastic behaviour. During the application of the stress, indicated by the arrows, there is a complete unchanging strain, followed by a complete recovery on removal of the stress.

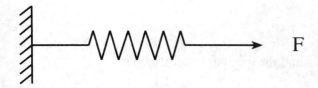

Fig. 4
The spring—a mechanical model for ideal elastic behaviour. During the application of a force F, the spring extends and returns to its rest position when the stress is removed.

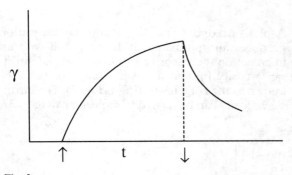

Fig. 5
Simple viscoelastic behaviour. During application of the stress, indicated by the arrows, strain develops non-linearly with time and recovery is also non-linear.

complete recovery to original shape. Elastic behaviour may be modelled by a spring (Fig. 4). A force causes immediate and complete response, the extent of lengthening depending on the force and the 'elasticity' of the spring. Removal of the force allows an immediate return to the starting position. Fig. 5 represents a simple viscoelastic

behaviour pattern, although real systems may be more complex. When the force is applied there is a non-linear change in strain which may become linear over longer times of observation. Removal of the force results in a gradual recovery, which may or may not be complete. Models can be built using springs and dashpots to describe viscoelastic behaviour as discussed later.

RHEOLOGY OF SOLIDS

All materials can show some form of elasticity although it is generally regarded as a property of a solid. Thus a solid particle may be expected to be an ideal elastic body. Allowing for inertia, it deforms reversibly with a strain proportional to stress and recovers to its original shape immediately on release of the stress. The ratio of stress to strain is called the elastic modulus. For a totally anisotropic solid, no less than 21 moduli are required to define its elastic behaviour. In practice many are ignored, and four constants are commonly used, corresponding to the common types of deformation. These are:

- Youngs modulus (Y)—elongation stress
- shear or rigidity modulus (G)—tangential stress
- bulk modulus (K)—compression stress
- Poisson's ratio (μ)—ratio of lateral contraction to extension in tension

From a theoretical standpoint, only small deformations are accommodated. However, it is usual to allow larger strains, although this may lead to some non-linearity, when each is referred to as an apparent modulus. Because for an ideally elastic, isotropic body only two elastic moduli are required, the relationship between the moduli can be established:

$$Y = 3K(1 - 2\mu) = 2G(1 + \mu)$$

Thus the ratio of moduli varies with Poisson's ratio. The ratio Y/G is approximately 2.5 for rigid solids and 3 for rubber-like materials, while for rubbery solids which thin on elongation ($\mu = 0.5$), Y and G must be several orders of magnitude less than K. When very large deformations are allowed, the elastic limit of the solid may be exceeded and flow will result. The elastic limit is referred to as the **yield point**; the flow being referred to as plastic deformation. This is an important process in tablet compression. When the powder is perfectly elastic, the application of an axial force (δ) will result in the transmission of a radial force (τ) of the same magnitude, which will be completely reversible and the tablet will be free to move out of the die, so long as the yield point is not exceeded. However, if the yield point is exceeded in axial force, the material will flow. Removal of the axial force will allow some elastic recovery, but the radial force will remain higher than the axial force, so a residual force of $2S$ will remain against the die wall, where S is the yield stress in shear. An alternative type of behaviour occurs if the powder behaves as a Mohr body. In this case the yield stress is a function of the normal stress on the plane of shear, and involves a friction-like factor. Rather than flowing under pressure the particle may fracture, the difference in behaviour being shown by using Heckel plots. The Heckel equation assumes a first-order-like reaction in which filling in of the pores present in the powder bed represents progression of the process. The equation is:

$$\log \frac{1}{\epsilon} = K_y P + K_r$$

where ϵ is porosity, K_y is $1/3S$, K_r is related to the initial packing (that is, ϵ_0), and P is the applied pressure. Thus, log porosity plotted against the compressional force should produce a straight line showing that, after initial packing, soft plastic materials will compact by plastic deformation producing a fairly steep line, while harder, more brittle, materials will compact by fracture producing a fairly shallow slope.

FLOW CHARACTERISTICS OF FLUIDS

Newtonian Flow

Newton recognised that the rate of flow of a liquid is proportional to the stress (F) applied (Fig. 6), the constant of proportionality being called the (dynamic) viscosity (η). It is now recognised that adherence to Newton's Law is relatively uncommon, materials that deviate from it being referred to as non-Newtonian. The units of viscosity are dynes/cm^2, Poise (P) (cgs units), or Pa s (SI units). It is more usual to use reduced forms of the units, so that 1 mPa s is the same numerically as 1 cP. The kinematic viscosity (ν) is the dynamic viscosity divided by the density of the liquid, with units of m^2/s (SI), cm^2/s (cgs units), or centistoke (cSt $= 10^{-6}$ m^2/s). The dynamic viscosity of water at 20° is about 1 mPa s (1 cP) and the kinematic viscosity of water is 10^{-6} m^2/s (1 cSt).

Solution Viscosity

The viscosity of a dilute solution (η) is always greater than that of the solvent (η_0) so that the relative viscosity (η_r) is:

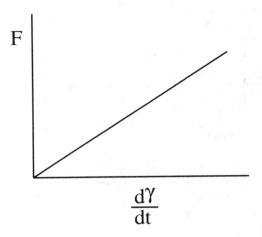

Fig. 6
Newtonian flow. The graph of shear stress against shear rate is a straight line passing through the origin with a slope equal to the Newtonian viscosity.

$$\eta_r = \frac{\eta}{\eta_0}$$

and the specific viscosity (η_{sp}) is:

$$\eta_{sp} = \eta_r - 1$$

The specific viscosity increases with concentration, c, the effect being compensated for in calculating the reduced viscosity (η_{red}):

$$\eta_{red} = \frac{\eta_{sp}}{c}$$

A plot of reduced viscosity against concentration produces an approximately linear graph with an intercept on the viscosity axis known as the intrinsic viscosity $[\eta]$ and a positive slope of value k_2 known as the Huggins constant (Fig. 7). The intrinsic viscosity can be related to molecular weight, M,

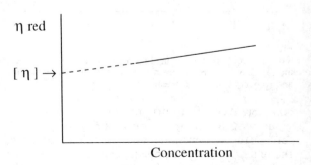

Fig. 7
A plot of reduced viscosity against concentration gives a straight line, intercepting the axis at the intrinsic viscosity.

in dilute colloidal systems using the Mark-Houwink equation:

$$[\eta] = K M^{a}$$

and can be used in quality control, as for example with dextran injections. The constants K and a may be related to molecular shape. The Huggins constant gives an indication of polymer-solvent interactions and may be used in their investigation.

Non-Newtonian Flow

Deviations from Newton's Law are frequently demonstrated using rheograms (graphs of shear rate against shear stress). Several different types of deviation are found.

Plastic Flow

This is sometimes called **Bingham flow** and a material showing it, a **Bingham body**. The characteristic of plastic flow shown in Fig. 8, is a straight line with an intercept on the shear stress axis. Thus, below this stress, no flow will occur, while above it, flow increases linearly with applied stress. The intercept is called the yield value (f). The behaviour may be expressed by the equation:

$$U = \frac{(F - f)}{d\gamma/dt}$$

where U is the plastic viscosity.
The yield value arises from the breaking of interactions of similar strength within the system. This type of behaviour is often found with high concentration or flocculated suspensions and with some suspending agents.

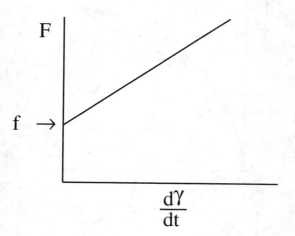

Fig. 8
Plastic flow. The graph of shear stress against shear rate is a straight line intercepting the shear stress axis at the yield value (f).

Pseudoplastic Flow

The rheogram is usually a smooth curve (Fig. 9). Since the slope of the line represents the viscosity, it can be seen that the material becomes thinner the faster it is stirred. For this reason pseudoplastic flow is sometimes called **shear rate thinning**. The viscosity calculated from the slope is not the Newtonian viscosity but the apparent viscosity (η') and requires a shear rate (or shear stress) to be quoted for it to have significance. It is, therefore, difficult to adequately quantify pseudoplastic flow. The usual equation is:

$$F = \eta' \left(\frac{d\gamma}{dt}\right)^{N}$$

where N is the index of pseudoplasticity.

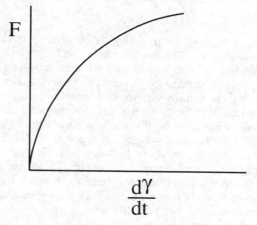

Fig. 9
Pseudoplastic flow. The graph of shear stress against shear rate is a curve passing through the origin.

Frequently, at higher shear rates, the graph becomes linear, so that the equation is often no more than an approximation. This type of flow is very common pharmaceutically, occurring in aqueous dispersions of many suspending agents and with emulsions and creams. It may be regarded as arising from the wide spectrum of interaction strengths within the system.

Dilatant Flow

The rheogram of a dilatant system is the reverse of that for pseudoplastic flow (Fig. 10), indicating that the system becomes thicker as stirring is increased, hence the alternative name of **shear rate thickening**. The behaviour may be quantified using the same equation as for pseudoplastic

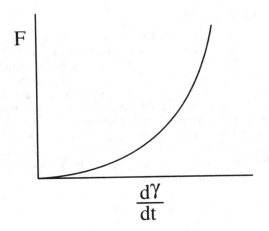

Fig. 10
Dilatant flow. The graph of shear stress against shear rate is a curve passing through the origin and becoming steeper as shear rate increases.

flow, although in this case N is greater than 1, increasing as dilatancy increases. While relatively uncommon, the appearance of dilatancy can be important, especially during pharmaceutical processing. It usually occurs in highly concentrated, deflocculated suspensions and so can arise when small volumes of liquids are being used to disperse powders. It occurs because there is inadequate liquid to fill the voids between particles as they separate to move past each other. This gives rise to frictional and surface tension forces, which impair flow. It is most acute with high speed blenders and mills, but can also occur with a pestle and mortar or spatula.

Other Behaviour

Other intermediate types of behaviour can also occur. The most common is a yield value that leads to pseudoplastic-type flow before becoming linear. Various alternative equations have been devised for these systems, one of the most useful pharmaceutically being the Herschel-Bulkley equation:

$$F = f + \eta' \left(\frac{d\gamma}{dt} \right)^N$$

Time-dependent Flow

Non-Newtonian flow arises because of interactions within the systems. At any given point, an equilibrium is established between breakdown and build-up of these interactions. However, if these interactions take longer to form or break, then a non-equilibrium observation may be made. On a rheogram, this will show as a difference between the curves obtained when increasing and decreasing the speed (or stress).

Thixotropy

Thixotropy is a time-dependent flow that indicates a relatively slow recovery of the viscosity lost on shearing a plastic (Fig. 11) or pseudoplastic (Fig. 12) system. The down curve is always at a lower shear stress for a given shear rate than the up curve (Fig. 12). The area enclosed between the up curve

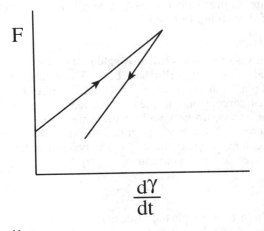

Fig. 11
Thixotropy superimposed on plastic flow. The down-curve occurs at a lower value of stress for any shear rate than the up-curve and may either intercept the stress axis at a yield value or pass through the origin.

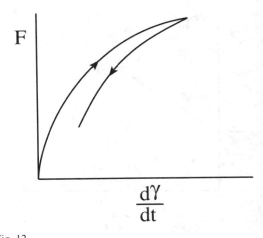

Fig. 12
Thixotropy superimposed on pseudoplastic flow. The down-curve occurs at a lower value of stress for any shear rate than on the up-curve and will return to the origin.

and down curve is the hysteresis loop and gives an indication of the extent of thixotropy. Because the down curve is showing a delay in the reformation of a structure, the time-scale of the experiment will affect the actual position of the line. If the determination is carried out sufficiently slowly, the down curve will become superimposed on the up curve, as seen with non-time-dependent flow. Thus, in any comparative work, it is necessary to specify the time-scale of measurement.

Quantitative measurement of thixotropy is difficult. The most commonly used figure is the hysteresis loop area (the index of thixotropy). It has been shown that, in many instances, the breakdown and build-up of structure is an exponential function of time, so that the slope of a plot of log shear stress (at fixed shear rate) against log time is linear. A variation on this approach is the coefficient of thixotropic breakdown (B) in which differences in shear stress (S_1 and S_2) after times t_1 and t_2 at an arbitrary fixed shear rate are compared:

$$B = \frac{S_1 - S_2}{\ln(t_2/t_1)}$$

Thixotropy is a fairly common phenomenon pharmaceutically, occurring with many suspending agent dispersions, pastes, emulsions, and creams. In some systems (for example, ointment bases and clay-type suspending agents), complex rheograms may be produced with one or more bulges or spurs on the up-curve (Fig. 13). The ones at the lower shear rates are associated with structural interaction breakdown, while those at higher shear rates are associated with molecular reorientation (for example, slippage of planar hydrated clay molecules).

Some materials (for example, gels), when stirred will thin with time, but on standing will not regain their original structure. This is called 'false thixotropy' and will frequently arise with molecules in which hydrogen-bond cross-linking produces a three-dimensional structure. Shearing will move the groups into new positions which prevents the re-establishment of the original bonds.

Rheopexy

There is some confusion in the literature about the precise definition of rheopexy. Just as thixotropy is a time-dependent loss and recovery of structure, so rheopexy is a time-dependent gain and loss of structure in a dilatant system. Therefore, it only occurs in concentrated suspensions such as Milk of Magnesia (USP) and is a rare occurrence. Techniques used with thixotropy are used to quantify rheopexy.

Temperature Effects

The viscosity of most liquids is closely related to temperature by an inverse relationship that is usually quantified using an Arrhenius-type equation:

$$\eta = A\mathrm{e}^{E/RT}$$

where A is related to molecular size and E is akin to the activation energy. Because of this relationship, close temperature control is required during rheological measurement, the more accurate the instrument, the closer the control required. Where a temperature-dependent chemical or physical reaction is possible, a more complex viscosity-temperature relationship may arise. Examples include the setting of resins or suspending agent dispersions, which demonstrate a lower critical solution temperature.

VISCOELASTICITY

Viscoelasticity may be measured by imposing a deformation and measuring the stress required to maintain it with time (stress relaxation), or by applying a small stress and measuring the resulting deformation with time (creep). Both methods give information about the viscous and elastic elements of the rheological behaviour.

Stress Relaxation

Imposing a deformation on a viscoelastic material will require a force. As the deformation is maintained, the required force will decline with time.

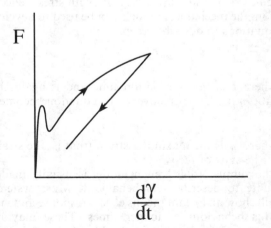

Fig. 13
Abnormal flow. The up-curve shows a single spur; others may have a series of spurs or bulges on the up-curve.

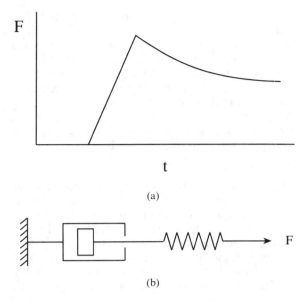

(a)

(b)

Fig. 14
(a) A typical stress relaxation graph showing that a finite time is required to apply the force (and extend the system) following which, the stress required to maintain the extension decays with time; (b) The Maxwell model of stress relaxation.

Fig. 14(a) shows a typical behaviour assuming a short, finite time to apply the force. This type of behaviour can be represented by a mechanical model of spring and dashpot arranged in series, this being known as the Maxwell model (Fig. 14(b)). A pull of force F will cause an immediate elastic deformation of the spring. The force is transmitted through to the dashpot and the piston moves outwards, allowing the spring to contract again thereby reducing the force required to maintain the extension. An example of this behaviour is an elastic bandage which 'relaxes' when it is left on for a few hours. Similar effects are found with catgut.

Using the equations for the spring and dashpot, it is possible to develop mathematical expressions to describe the behaviour observed. For stress relaxation the equation is:

$$F = F_0 e^{(-Gt/\eta)}$$

where F is the force required to maintain the extension at time t, and F_0 is the force at the initial extension. G and η are the elastic and viscous moduli respectively. The ratio η/G is indicative of the balance of viscous and elastic properties and is called the relaxation time (τ), representing the time taken for the force to decay to $1/e$ of its original value (approximately 37%). Thus the equation is usually written in the form:

$$F = F_0 e^{(-t/\tau)}$$

As with non-Newtonian flow, the time-scale of observation is important. When the whole experiment is carried out quickly, the dashpot may not have time to respond to any measurable extent so only elastic behaviour is observed. If, however, the extension is applied very slowly the dashpot may produce the total response, so that the spring will not extend and hence only fluid behaviour will be observed. The Deborah Number (D) which is defined as:

$$D = \frac{\text{retardation time}}{\text{experimental time}}$$

may be used to estimate suitable experimental times because for viscoelastic materials D should be approximately 1.

Creep
A constant force is applied to a sample and the resulting strain is measured. It is necessary to distinguish creep, where the values of strain are very small, from flow, where the strain is very large.

At its most simple, the strain increases with time in a non-linear manner, becoming linear with longer times (Fig. 15(a)). When the stress is removed there is a time-dependent recovery of strain. The mechanical models can be used in parallel to mimic this behaviour – the **Voigt-Kelvin model** (Fig. 15(b)). In the rigid frame, the extension of the spring is retarded by the drag of the dashpot, hence the term retardation is applied to this type of behaviour. Thus, during application of the force there will be a gradual extension and on its removal, a gradual recovery. As with stress relaxation, the mechanical models can be used to develop equations to describe creep:

$$\gamma = \frac{F}{G} [1 - e^{(-t/\tau)}]$$

where τ is the retardation time and is again the ratio η/G. Under recovery, the equation becomes:

$$\gamma = \gamma_0 e^{(-t/\tau)}$$

where γ_0 is the maximum strain (that is, the strain at the start of recovery).

The simple Voigt-Kelvin model is usually inadequate to describe real behaviour. Most systems will show an instantaneous elastic response and viscous behaviour at longer times. These may be accounted for by putting the Maxwell and Voigt-Kelvin models together as shown in Fig. 16 – the **Burgur model**. The overall compliance (J) of such

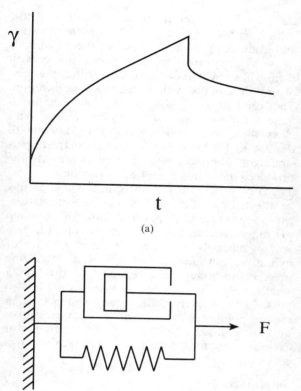

(a)

(b)

Fig. 15
(a) A typical creep graph showing an instantaneous compliance, the non-linear and linear changes in strain with time and the early stages of recovery; (b) The Voigt-Kelvin model of creep.

a system will be made up of the compliance of each part of the model:

$$J = J_1 + J_2 + J_3$$

so that:

$$J = \frac{F}{\gamma} + J_2[1 - e^{(-t/\tau)}] + \frac{t}{\eta_3}$$

In more complex systems a range of values of J_2 and τ occur, so that a number of different Voigt-Kelvin units are required. This produces the **generalised Voigt model** (Fig. 17) in which as many Voigt-Kelvin units as necessary may be added, although it is usually shown as having three i = 2, 3, or 4. The generalised equation is:

$$J = J_1 + \sum_{i=2}^{4} J_i[1 - e^{(-t/\tau_i)}] + \frac{t}{\eta_5}$$

Modern computer-controlled instruments perform the necessary curve stripping in order to elucidate the different constants. Viscoelastic behaviour is common in pharmaceutical systems although its significance is, in the main, not appreciated. The balance between elastic (solid-like) and viscous (liquid-like) behaviour must be important in any situation where flow or deformation is involved. Thus, for example, pourability, ease of packaging, the spreadability of an external semi-solid, and squeezing from a tube are all situations where detailed studies would be beneficial. Equally, many biological systems (for example, mucus and sputum) display viscoelastic phenomena, which can

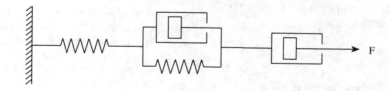

Fig. 16
The Burgur model of creep, which allows for instantaneous elastic compliance, flow, and one retardation time.

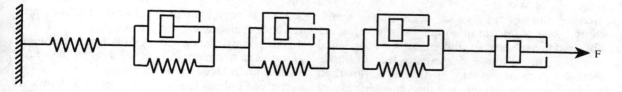

Fig. 17
The Generalised Voigt model of creep, which allows for instantaneous elastic response, flow, and three different retardation times. Voigt-Kelvin units may be added or removed in order to fit the experimental data.

be modified by the presence of other materials such as drugs. In the field of polymer science, results from creep studies may be related to molecular models describing molecular interactions. Such interpretations have not been developed for pharmaceutical systems to any marked extent.

SOME PHARMACEUTICAL APPLICATIONS OF RHEOLOGY

Potentially, rheological properties play an important role in many pharmaceutical situations, but to a large extent they are either little studied or ignored. The main exceptions to this generalisation concern the flow of liquid-type formulations and, to a lesser extent, the consistency of topical semi-solids, and the compression of tablet ingredients.

It is important to have some appreciation of the relationship between conditions experienced in practice and those appertaining to instrumental analysis. In the early 1960s approximations were produced for the shear rates of some common pharmaceutical operations. Thus, the shear rate for pouring from a bottle is below 100 per second, squeezing from a plastic squeezy bottle will be at about 1000 per second, putting an ointment on the skin about 120 per second, whilst rubbing it in can vary from 100 to 10 000 per second depending on the technique. During processing higher shear rates are likely to be encountered; 1000 to 100 000 per second during pumping, 1000 to 12 000 per second in roller milling rising to more than 100 000 per second in a colloid mill. High speed filling in a packing line can also reach 100 000 per second and is dependent on the rate of packing and the orifice size.

Liquid Dosage Forms

Thickening Agents

A wide range of materials can be used to increase the viscosity of water-based formulations. These are often classified, according to their origin, into natural, semisynthetic, synthetic, and mineral materials. A wide range of natural gums may be used as thickening agents (for example, tragacanth, guar gum, xanthan gum). Alginates are obtained from seaweed and gelatins from animal sources. The cellulose derivatives (for example, methyl, carboxymethyl, hydroxypropylmethyl) are among the most common thickeners in current use. Synthetic thickeners include carbomer, povidone, polyvinyl alcohol and, like the semisynthetic materials, are available in different grades. Various

clays swell in water to increase viscosity. These include bentonite, Veegum^{TM}, montmorillonite, and attapulgite. Although each of these materials has unique properties, dispersions made with them will show pseudoplastic flow with some thixotropy developing with increasing concentration. The pseudoplastic viscosity increases approximately exponentially with concentration. With clays there is a tendency for a yield value to develop and for viscosity to increase as the dispersion ages. Abnormal flow rheograms may also be produced indicating complex interactions.

The viscosities of thickening agent dispersions may be affected by other additives to the formulation. Most are sensitive to pH and have an optimum pH range. Salts and high concentrations of hygroscopic materials will compete for the water of hydration, causing a reduction in viscosity. Some preservatives have been reported to produce a small increase or decrease in viscosity. It is also possible to thicken non-aqueous systems. High melting point waxes (for example, cetostearyl alcohol), or multivalent alkali salts of fatty acids (for example, aluminium stearate), can achieve this effect.

Suspensions

Einstein indicated in 1906 that the viscosity of a dispersion of rigid spheres will increase with concentration, ϕ:

$$\eta = \eta_0 \left(1 + 2.5\,\phi\right)$$

Various other mathematical expressions have been postulated, some of which accommodate different shapes of particle. While these equations may be of interest, they do not apply to highly concentrated dispersions because hindered settling will occur. It has also been demonstrated that the larger the particle, the higher the viscosity, probably due to electrical interactions. This latter observation has implications in flocculated suspensions, which have a higher viscosity, but in highly flocculated systems interactions between flocs may also occur causing a further increase in viscosity. Such interactions will produce yield values and thixotropy. At very high solid content, dilatancy may develop as discussed previously.

In designing a suspension formulation, the aim is to obtain a uniform quantity of solid each time a dose is measured. Due to sedimentation this may not be achieved unless the viscosity of the liquid is increased. By increasing the Newtonian viscosity, sedimentation will be reduced, but there is a limit beyond which pouring and measuring the dose are impaired. The use of a pseudoplastic suspending agent will impart a high viscosity at rest which can be decreased by shaking or pouring. Thixotropy will enhance this effect. The use of a plastic suspending agent system offers the prospect of a non-sedimenting suspension. This occurs if the force exerted by a particle is less than the yield value of the dispersion. Similar results, though not as effective, may be produced using suspending agents with abnormal flow patterns.

Apart from these effects it appears that suspending agents may have a direct bearing on the clinical efficacy of a drug. Non-steroidal anti-inflammatory drugs suspended in different systems have been shown to produce both different physical characteristics and different extents of gastric erosion in *rats*.

Emulsions

Like suspensions, emulsions are dispersed systems and so show many similar properties. However, they do not readily flocculate and remain stable. The presence of emusifying agents produces an approximately linear increase in viscosity with concentration. However, the surfactant may alter the viscosity in other ways. Of particular importance is the formation of liquid crystalline phases, usually on the addition of a long-chain molecule such as cetostearyl alcohol or glyceryl monostearate. This is referred to as self-bodying. Liquid crystalline phases have viscoelastic properties and are discussed under Ointments and Creams. Similar effects can arise with smaller molecules in micellar systems.

Other Liquid Formulations

Injections are subjected to high shear rates as they pass through the needle, (up to 10 000 per second). Plastic, pseudoplastic, or thixotropic systems are subjected to structure breakdown under these conditions. Early work in the 1950s showed that thixotropic behaviour of procaine penicillin injection suspensions was advantageous in producing a depot effect, thus the greater the shear stress required to establish early flow, so the greater was the prolongation of action. Clearly there is a practical limit to this yielding stress; if it is too large, flow can not be initiated in the syringe, as has been demonstrated with similar suspensions which have aged on storage.

Some vaccines can be prepared as water-in-oil (w/o) emulsions, the oil acting as a diffusion barrier. Viscosity of the emulsion is important in these vaccines because if it is too large it cannot be injected, but if too low, instability will lead to rapid antigen release. Rheological properties are important with many other liquids. Dosing efficiency of eye drops is related to solution viscosity, clearance rates of nasal sprays are inversely related to viscosity, and the spreadability of contraceptive foams is increased by materials that reduce viscosity.

Solid Dosage Forms

Discussion of the flow characteristics of bulk powders is outside the scope of this chapter, but is important in the context of mixing, granulation, and in the flow of granules into the tablet machine die. When wet granulation techniques have to be used, the power consumption, as the granulating fluid is blended into the powder mass, is an important factor in optimising the process. Results indicate that the liquid content dictates the properties of the mass during granulation and spheronisation and that end-points, which can be indicated by the rheological properties of the mass, may also be related to process performance.

Some aspects of the rheological behaviour of solids under compression were discussed earlier (see Rheology of Solids above). Unless the tablet is fully elastic there will be a residual pressure on the die wall, which will produce friction and possible adhesion. Instrumented tablet machines enable the transmission of forces during and after compression to be quantified; the ejection force being indicative of the residual forces. However, ejection force itself varies, being at a peak when the initial tablet/die wall adhesions are broken. Lubrication of the tablet is required in order to minimise this effect. An ideal lubricant will bind strongly to both tablet and die-wall, but will have very low shear strength in the direction of shear. In this way shear failure occurs in the lubricant layer, not in the tablet structure. In addition, because of the time-dependent nature of the plastic and viscoelastic processes occurring within tablets during compression and release, the profile of stress with time will be significant.

Coatings may be used on tablets for a variety of reasons: improving palatability, increasing stability, producing a controlled availability of drug, or producing an elegant product. These coats may be based on sugar, which markedly increases tablet weight, or be a surface film. With the latter, a polymer is applied together with a plasticiser, such as diethyl phthalate, to prevent brittleness on ageing. Enteric coatings tend to be based on cellacephate with a plasticiser such as castor oil or butyl stearate. It is essential that the coating solution adheres to the tablet surface. For relatively dilute coating solutions, tackiness is a function of viscosity, although this is not a linear relationship. For more concentrated solutions, such as occur during the drying process, tackiness is more dependent on viscoelastic properties of the coating and may render the separation of tablets which stick together at this stage more difficult.

A recent development has been the interest in using mucoadhesion to attach a dosage form to a surface mucous layer in the body. Mucin, the main component of mucus, has many sialic and sulphonic acid residues on its surface producing an anionic charge. Neutral or charged polymers can form non-covalent bonding to the surface when the polymer chains entangle and produce a level of interaction between polymer and mucin that is greater than between mucin molecules themselves. The rheology of these interactions has not been fully elucidated.

Semi-solid Systems

Ointments and Creams

Ointments and creams show complex rheological behaviour including irreversible shear breakdown, thixotropy, viscoelasticity, and various anomalous behaviours that are reliant on the previous history of the sample. High shear measurements (such as viscometry) cause significant levels of structural breakdown and are useful for predicting behaviour under processing conditions. However, low shear, creep, or oscillatory measurements give information on their behaviour under clinical use conditions or in their 'ground state'.

Early work, using flow measurement, established that ointment bases such as white soft paraffin produce anomalous up-curves probably arising from chain entanglements, are thixotropic and, because of a slow recovery, produce variable rheograms dependent on previous handling. In emulsified systems, the concentration of emulsifier produced marked changes in thixotropic loop area which could be related to sensory assessment. These rheological properties appear to change as internal interactions occur. Thus, cetostearyl alcohol/polyoxyethylene (POE) alkyl ether nonionic surfactant systems age and have high consistencies with large POE chains. This type of study has established the importance of the development of liquid crystalline gel-like phases between dispersed phase globules as a result of surfactant-water interactions. This is called the gel network theory and explains many of the consistency changes seen in oil-in-water (o/w) creams, in particular the slow development of the gel-structure as the penetration of the surfactant, fatty acid, and water occurs.

More extensive work has been undertaken to evaluate semi-solids as viscoelastic systems using creep tests or oscillatory measurements. These have enabled an investigation of the structural aspects of some formulations, which cannot be obtained from flow studies. Thus, for example, it has been shown that there is a non-linear relationship between the elastic modulus and the amount of polyethylene used to thicken a paraffin basis, indicating changes in the gel structure within the base. As with flow studies, viscoelastic analysis shows marked variations between batches and on processing. Significant changes have also been noted with changing temperature, which may be important in clinical use.

While these findings are of intrinsic interest, their influence on the 'feel' of the product in use is of great importance. It has been suggested that spreadability is related to the shear stress, and stickiness to the time required to separate finger and skin with the product between. Also of significance to the patient will be the ease of removing the ointment or cream from a tube. This is influenced by the force required and the elastic recoil back into the tube, the latter being of great importance when small quantities are required, as with eye ointments.

Gels

Gels are two-component systems of a semi-solid nature that have a high liquid content. The gelling agent, which may be an organic polymer or a clay, forms a solid-phase structure which is responsible for the high consistency. At low concentrations, gels are pseudoplastic, becoming plastic at higher concentrations, and some have high thixotropy when studied by flow. These studies have demonstrated relationships between formulation and rheological parameters such as thixotropic area. However, the viscoelastic nature of gels suggests that creep studies, which have minimal effects on structure, would be better for elucidating changes in gel structure, although relatively little work appears in the literature.

More recently, pharmaceutical interest has grown in the use of hydrogels as drug delivery systems. The term is open to varying interpretation, but is usually taken to refer to systems based on synthetic cross-linked polymers of various types.

Viscoelastic and flow studies have been used to examine the process of cross-linking in hydrogels and the elastic properties of polyhydroxyethyl-methacrylate confirmed the presence of high level ordering in the polymer network.

Drug Availability

The diffusion rate of a drug is an inverse function of the viscosity of the medium and this is significant in a number of situations connected with the bioavailability of a drug. Thus, diffusion is assumed to be rapid in liquids, such as in the gastro-intestinal tract, in dissolution apparatus, and in topical liquid preparations. While the basic relationship is shown to be correct, closer examination suggests the situation is more complex. In the gastro-intestinal tract, the mucous lining has non-Newtonian behaviour which has been shown to significantly delay diffusion with methylcellulose suspensions. This is also true of the dissolution process, where it is the effective viscosity in the stationary layer, not the bulk liquid, which will influence the Noyes-Whitney equation (see Preformulation chapter). In a gel-like system, diffusion will be through the continuous phase, and it is the micro-viscosity of this liquid that will affect diffusivity. Similarly in creams, diffusion through liquid crystalline regions will be important. The systems are complex and little published work exists relating drug availability to specific rheological parameters.

Biorheology

Most biological materials either flow or deform and some abnormalities in their normal behaviour may cause, or be indicative of, disease.

The greatest volume of published material is concerned with blood. Whole blood behaves as an approximately Newtonian liquid, although with some anomalies. Thus, at low shear rates (below about 70 per second), the erythrocytes stack to form 'rouleaux', which cause an increase in viscosity to the range of 50 to 150 mPa s (at 0.1 per second). The rouleaux tend to be in the centre of the blood vessels where shear rate is lowest, giving rise to plug flow and a yield value. Higher shear rates cause the rouleaux to separate and the viscosity falls to about 5 mPa s. Single erythrocytes can deform to allow passage through capillaries at higher shear rates. There is also evidence that towards the edges of blood vessels there is a lower concentration of erythrocytes, thus producing easier flow, perhaps also aided by a coating of a fibrin-like protein on the inside of the vessels—the so called endo-endothelial layer.

Blood clots behave as viscoelastic gels. With time there is a re-orientation of fibrin within the gel to produce clot retraction and syneresis.

The erythrocyte sedimentation rate (ESR) is used as a routine test in medical laboratories because abnormal values, although not diagnostic, are indicative of pathologies (for example, infection, inflammation, malignancy, and ankylosing spondylitis).

Mucus is a viscoelastic material that occurs at many sites around the body including the nose, ear, mouth, respiratory tract, gastro-intestinal tract, and cervix. It varies in its constituents and detailed chemical nature, as well as in its quantity and properties. In the gastro-intestinal tract it is thought to have a mainly protective role, acting as a physical and chemical barrier to prevent injury, but will also have an effect on drug absorption. For small molecules it will reduce the diffusion rate, as discussed earlier, but it has been suggested that it prevents macromolecule absorption because of the exclusion volume effect of precipitation when two macromolecules are placed in the same system.

In the respiratory tract, the layer of mucus is about 5 micrometres thick, trapping airborne particles and bacteria. Cilia then move the mucus towards the throat for swallowing. It has been estimated that a turnover of about one litre per day is involved in this defence mechanism. The mucus is viscoelastic with a yield value; both can change with disease. In bronchitis, the mucus is much thicker and can overload the cilia and make a cough non-productive. In cystic fibrosis, physiotherapy is required to aid the patient in removing the excessive quantities of very thick mucus. Various materials may alter the consistency of mucus, making it easier to remove. Some surfactants appear to work *in vivo* by altering surface tension, while other materials break disulphide bridges within the mucin molecules.

Cervical mucus changes during the menstrual cycle, reaching a minimum consistency at 15 days (ovulation) and just before menstruation. Consistency is elevated in pregnancy. The changes at ovulation aid the passage of sperm. At other times, the high consistency mucus has a protective function. Complex enzymatic activity in semen is responsible for initial gelling, then liquefaction following ejaculation. Abnormalities in these processes are associated with low fertility.

Synovial fluid has been studied as a rheological material and as a 'mechanical lubricant'. At low frequencies, corresponding to gentle movement, it behaves as a viscous liquid, while at high frequencies, corresponding to high stress situations, the elastic properties predominate. Steroid injections have been shown to increase both viscous and elastic moduli of synovial fluid.

Miscellaneous

The consistency of a liquid being swallowed is important. Not only is this true from an acceptability point of view, where it has been shown that the sensory response is proportional to a rheological property, but also from that of the ability of the patient to manage the medicine. Some dysphagic patients have difficulty in swallowing due to a delay in triggering the swallow reflex. The time taken for the liquid to drain from the vallecular space can make the difference between a successful swallow and aspiration of the liquid into the lungs. Dysphagia appears to be increasing and requires careful control of the viscosity of fluids to assist the patient.

The integrity and efficiency of closures on bottles and vials is a function of the viscoelastic properties of the materials used to make up the seal. These are usually high molecular weight polymers with a glass transition temperature well below ambient temperature. Their viscous properties allow them to 'flow' and conform to any irregularities on the surfaces to be sealed, while the elastic component maintains a force against the surface, ensuring a tight seal with time.

VISCOMETRY AND RHEOMETRY

From the foregoing sections it is clear that experimental methods are available for measuring flow and viscoelasticity. For the former, relatively large forces are applied and the resulting flow rates are determined or conversely, a system is made to flow at a known speed and the force required to achieve this measured. For viscoelasticity, the forces or strains are usually very much smaller. For stress relaxation, a known strain is imposed and the stress required to maintain it with time is measured, while for creep, a stress is applied and the strain produced with time is determined.

In addition to these fundamental methods, which produce quantitative data identifiable in terms of the equations discussed earlier, there are a range of empirical methods designed to measure a specific property, often in a particular context.

Viscometry

Not all instruments are equally able to quantify their total flow behaviour. Where a liquid is known to be Newtonian, it is adequate to measure the flow rate at a single stress because direct proportionality exists, irrespective of the flow rate or stress used. However, with non-Newtonian systems this is not the case and a single determination is inadequate to describe the behaviour. It may be argued that only two points are required for plastic flow, but ideal behaviour is rare, invalidating this suggestion. Multiple point determination is far more reliable and employed in most sophisticated instruments. For time-dependent flow there is an additional requirement—the ability to control the duration of the experimental determinations.

Single-point Instruments

Capillary Viscometers. The *British Pharmacopoeia 1993* makes use of a number of single-point instruments for measuring the viscosity of some fluids or dilute colloidal solutions, all of which are taken to be Newtonian. All of these instruments apply a stress and measure the resulting movement. Two of them use the flow of a liquid through a capillary tube under the influence of gravity, although artificially applied pressures can be used to allow multi-point measurement. Abnormalities in the flow within the capillary make it unsuitable for non-Newtonian systems.

The Ostwald capillary viscometer (Fig. 18) is the simplest, where the time (t) taken for a known volume of liquid (V) to flow through a capillary tube is measured. The narrower the radius (r), or the longer the length (l) of the tube, the longer the flow takes. A suitable instrument should be selected to give a time of at least 200 seconds. The volume is identified as the volume between two graduation marks. The force applied (P) is taken to be $\rho g h$ (ρ is the density of the liquid, g is gravity and h is the difference in the height of meniscus in the two arms of the instrument), but the height of the liquid reduces during the experiment and the back pressure increases as the liquid collects in the receiving arm. The flow through the capillary tube is described by Poiseuille's equation:

$$\eta = \frac{\pi r^4 t P}{8lV}$$

The values of r, l, and V are not normally known, but may be incorporated into a constant by using

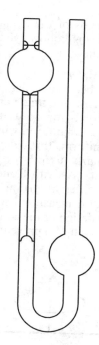

Fig. 18
The Ostwald capillary viscometer. Liquid in the upper bulb flows through the capillary tube, the meniscus being timed between the two graduations.

a calibrating fluid. While P varies, it is taken to be a constant variation which can also be taken into the instrumental constant (K'). Thus the equation simplifies to:

$$\eta = K't\rho$$

While instruments may be purchased ready calibrated, their use is usually to compare two liquids in the same viscometer. In this situation it is not necessary to know K', and the relative viscosity (η/η_0) may be measured directly:

$$\frac{\eta}{\eta_0} = \frac{t\rho}{t_0\rho_0}$$

as may the kinematic viscosity (ν)

$$\frac{\nu_1}{\nu_0} = \frac{t_1}{t_0}$$

The suspended level viscometer has a third arm, to allow liquid to be removed after it has flowed through the capillary tube, thus reducing the effect of back pressure. The equations are the same. Other capillary viscometers exist, some of which angle the capillary to reduce the effect of gravity (for example, the Cannon-Fenske viscometer). As all capillary viscometers are precision instruments, good temperature control, preferably to ±0.01°, is essential.

Falling Sphere Viscometer. A sphere of diameter d and density ρ_s will fall through a liquid of density ρ_l at a speed (v) described by the Stokes equation, from which the viscosity may be calculated:

$$\eta = d^2 g \frac{(\rho_s - \rho_l)}{18v}$$

The method involves timing the movement of the steel sphere between two graduation marks as it falls through the test liquid. A variation on this principle uses a sphere of a similar size to the tube, which rolls down the inclined tube. This method enables the viscosity of gases to be measured.

Extrusion Rheometers. Instead of gravity, external mechanisms can be used to force a liquid to flow through a capillary. This can be achieved either by imposing a linear velocity onto a piston or by applying a known pressure. Examples of the two methods are the Instrom and the Cannon-Manning, respectively. The equations discussed above are used.

Rather than use a capillary tube, a short tube or orifice may be used. In these situations a shear rate cannot be calculated and empirical results only are obtained. Instruments such as the FIRA-NIRD Extruder, devised for testing butter and other dairy products, can be applied to pharmaceutical semi-solids and tablet granulations.

Penetrometers. These instruments were developed to measure the consistency of more rigid semi-solids such as greases and waxes. A cone or needle of known weight is allowed to fall through the test material. The depth of penetration in a fixed time is inversely related to the consistency, a cone giving a smaller penetration than a needle. Again the results are not fundamental, but are consistent, and provide useful comparisons between similar materials.

Multipoint Instruments

A rotational viscometer measures the viscous drag exerted by a fluid on a body that is rotated in it. A known stirring rate can be applied and the force required to maintain this rate determined, or a known force can be applied and the resulting speed of rotation measured. There are also two basic geometries used for holding the sample. In one, concentric cylinders are used (Couette systems) and in the other, a cone-plate arrangement is employed.

Concentric Cylinder Viscometers. The first rotational instrument was described by Couette in 1890, using a rotating cup and an inner cylinder mounted on a torsion wire. The principle of using two concentric cylinders of different diameters was thus established and is the basis of all 'cup and bob' rotational viscometers (Fig. 19). Many variations in size, shape, area of contact, gap width, method of drive, and detection of viscous drag have been devised over the years. By using a range of pre-set speeds or stresses, or by using programmed sweeps of speed or stress, the instrument can be made multipoint and time controlled.

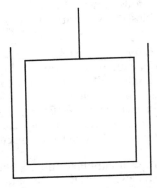

Fig. 19
The arrangement of a concentric cylinder viscometer. Different instruments employ different shapes of cylinder and different methods of driving and measuring the response.

In order to obtain values of viscosity it is necessary to calculate the shear rate and the shear stress. For a cylinder of height h, rotating at a constant speed Ω, under torque (M) with a difference in radius between the two cylinders $(R_2 - R_1)$, it can be shown that the viscosity (η) is given by the equation:

$$\eta = \frac{M(R_2^2 - R_1^2)}{4\pi \Omega h\, R_1^2\, R_2^2}$$

For a given measuring system an instrumental constant (K) allows the equation to be simplified to:

$$\eta = K\frac{M}{\Omega}$$

A closer examination of the behaviour of the liquid in the gap indicates that these equations are an over simplification, because the shear rate varies across the gap. This can give rise to anomalous flow behaviour, such as plug flow with plastic materials. There are also problems with end effects, due to the drag on the ends of the cylinders. These can be controlled by using hollow cylinders. Turbulent flow can also occur.

Cone-Plate Viscometers. In these viscometers, the sample is placed between a flat plate and a low angle cone (Fig. 20). The angle and radius of the cone may be varied; for accurate readings, the angle should be less than 3° in which situation the shear rate is uniform throughout the sample, which is particularly useful for non-Newtonian flow measurements. As with Couette viscometers, there are many different arrangements of drive and torque/rotation measurement in commercial instruments. The design of the cone may be refined by truncation of the tip, to prevent any tendency to 'drill' the plate.

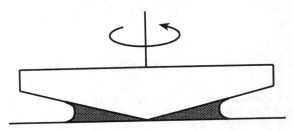

Fig. 20
The arrangement of a cone-plate viscometer.

The equation for calculating viscosity is:

$$\eta = \frac{3M\theta}{2\pi r^3 \Omega}$$

where θ is the cone angle and r the cone radius.

Rheometry

The distinction between viscometry and rheometry lies in the ability of the latter to quantify viscoelastic behaviour in addition to flow. While these are discussed separately, several modern instruments are capable of multimode operation using computer control, data capture, and processing.

Controlled Stress Rheometers

As the name implies, stress is applied to the sample, the resulting strain being measured. A very wide range of stress values is usually available (for example from $5\,mN/m^2$ to $2 \times 10^3\,N/m^2$) with sensitive strain detection (usually down to 10^{-4} radians) allowing either creep studies (low stress) or flow determination (higher stress). Measurement system geometry can be of the Couette, cone-plate, or parallel plate type. The latter uses one fixed

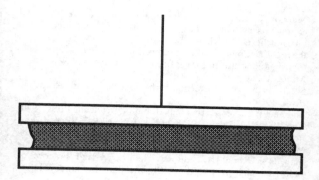

Fig. 21
The arrangement of a plate-plate (parallel plate) viscometer.

and one moving plate with the sample held in the gap between (Fig. 21), the gap always being small compared to the plate diameter. The viscosity of a sample at the edge of the gap is given by the equation:

$$\eta = \frac{2ML}{\pi r^4 \omega}$$

where M is the torque, L is the gap width, r is the radius of the plate, and ω is the angular velocity (speed = ωr).

Oscillatory Rheometers

Instead of imposing the stress in a constant direction, these instruments use an oscillation of one part of the measuring system. Couette, cone-plate, or plate-plate configurations may be used, although the latter predominates. The particular advantages of oscillatory measurement are that very small displacements (amplitudes) are used, so that structural elements are not destroyed and measurement can be made relatively quickly, allowing the monitoring of time-dependent changes such as gelling of starch dispersions.

Elastic and viscous materials behave in different ways under oscillation. The oscillation is imposed by alternating application and removal of stress to produce a sine wave. Since, in an elastic body the modulus is stress/strain, the maximum strain occurs at the maximum stress (the peak and trough of the sine waves). An elastic body produces a strain curve exactly in phase with the stress curve. In a viscous liquid the transmitted stress is a function of the rate of shear. This is at a maximum when the applied stress is at zero and the sine curves are exactly 90° out of phase. The number of degrees out of phase is called the phase angle δ. Viscoelastic materials have a phase angle

between 0° and 90°. Thus, with viscoelastic materials, during the course of a complete oscillation, part of the energy is stored elastically to be released on the counter swing, while part of the energy is lost and is not recovered. The elastic modulus is derived from the former and the viscosity from the latter. It is difficult to separate the observed complex modulus into its two constituent moduli mathematically, not least because they have different dimensions. This process is achieved by multiplying the viscous modulus (G''—also called loss modulus) by the imaginary number, i ($i = -1^{1/2}$), so that the complex moulus G^* is:

$$G^* = G' + i\,G''$$

where G' is the elastic modulus (storage modulus). From this G''/G' is ∞ if $\delta = 90°$ and 0 if $\delta = 0°$. This is a property of a tangent so:

$$\tan \delta = \frac{G''}{G'}$$

Using this relationship, a vector diagram can be used to determine individual values of G' and G''. From these moduli, values for dynamic viscosity (η') and dynamic elasticity (η'') can be obtained by dividing by the angular velocity (ω). The term 'dynamic' is rather confusing, especially for viscosity because the movement in these determinations is much less than in conventional measurement of viscosity by flow.

Other Instrumentation

Many of the instruments discussed above will yield rheological parameters, but many of them have not been correlated to the properties of the material in use. For this reason many empirical instruments have been devised for specific applications.

The rigidity of gels can be monitored by a variety of tests. Some use a mercury manometer in contact with a stressed gel contained in a tube. Others monitor the gel under extension and by rotating a disc on the surface. Various tests are available to measure the stickiness of semi-solids by measuring the force required to separate a moveable plate in contact with the test material. These instruments are known as 'tackometers'. Attempts have been made to quantify spreadability of semi-solids by moving devices through or over them, or by observing their spread under controlled compression. The hardness of a material can be measured by a variety of techniques that tend to rely on measuring an indentation left on a flat surface by a cone, sphere, or other shape. The food industry, in particular, has a wide range of tests for monitoring consistency of, for example, doughs, biscuits, fruit, and toughness of meat. These may have applications in specific pharmaceutical situations.

FURTHER INFORMATION

Barry BW. Dermatological formulations: percutaneous absorption. New York: Marcel Dekker, 1983.

Barry BW. Rheology of pharmaceutical and cosmetic semisolids. In: Bean HS, Beckett AH, Carless JE, editors. Advances in pharmaceutical sciences; vol IV. London: Academic Press, 1974:1–72.

Florence AT, Attwood D. Physicochemical principles of pharmacy. 2nd ed. London: Macmillan, 1988.

Marriott C. Rheology and the flow of fluids. In: Aulton ME, editor. Pharmaceutics: the science of dosage form design. Edinburgh: Churchill Livingstone, 1988:17–37.

Parrott EL. Compression. In: Lieberman HA, Lachman L, editors. Pharmaceutical dosage forms: tablets; vol II. New York: Marcel Dekker, 1981:153–84.

Scott Blair GW. Elementary rheology. London: Academic Press, 1969.

Sherman P. Industrial rheology. London: Academic Press, 1970.

Van Wazer JR, Lyons JW, Kim KY, Colwell RE. Viscosity and flow measurement. New York: Interscience Publishers, 1963.

Wood JH. Pharmaceutical rheology. In: Lachman L, Lieberman HA, Kanig JL, editors. The theory and practice of industrial pharmacy. 3rd ed. Philadelphia: Lea and Febiger, 1986:123–45.

Stability of Medicinal Products

A medicinal product is designed to possess certain desirable properties of which the following are of major importance. When the product is administered by the specified route, the active constituent should achieve the required rate and extent of bioavailability. The product itself should be efficacious, safe, and acceptable to the patient; it should be convenient in use and stable. The **stability** of a product relates to its resistance to the various chemical, physical, and microbiological reactions that may change the original properties of the preparation during transport, storage, and use. Other criteria of stability are the effects of such changes on the fitness of the product for use as a medicine.

Stability is often expressed in quantitative terms as the **shelf-life**, that is the time during which the medicinal product is predicted to remain fit for its intended use under specified conditions of storage. The shelf-life of a medicinal product kept in its closed container under specified conditions is commonly defined as the time from manufacture or preparation until the original potency or content of active constituent has been reduced by 10%. This time is known as the $t_{10\%}$; in some books and papers, the term $t_{90\%}$ (or t_{90}) is used in place of $t_{10\%}$. For most products, this 10% limit of chemical degradation is usually considered to be acceptable in practice but more stringent limits may need to be imposed if the degradation products are more toxic or irritant than is the drug.

Although it is often convenient to express shelf-life solely in terms of the chemical stability of the active constituent, it is essential that the other desirable properties of the product are retained during storage. For example, a lotion that contains a corticosteroid in an oil-in-water emulsion basis may be highly stable in terms of chemical stability of the corticosteroid but the basis may thicken so much on storage that the patient cannot pour the lotion from the bottle. Similarly, an elixir containing dextromethorphan may be chemically stable in respect of the drug yet unacceptable for use because of changes in odour and flavour as a result of oxidation of the volatile oils used as flavouring agents. Another example is that of physical changes in chemically stable tablets and other solid dosage forms on storage that may occasionally lead to a decrease in dissolution rate and bioavailability and thus possibly in efficacy.

The first section in this chapter comprises an outline of the general principles of chemical kinetics. Although the theory of kinetics was originally derived to express quantitatively the order and rate of chemical reactions, the principles of kinetics are sometimes applied also to certain physical and microbiological reactions that may occur in medicines. The chemical, physical, and microbiological aspects of the stability of medicinal products are considered in separate sections together with an account of the principles, methods, and limitations of stability tests. In addition, this chapter includes a section on problems associated with the shelf-life of medicines prepared and dispensed in community and hospital pharmacies.

CHEMICAL KINETICS

Chemical kinetics is concerned with the rate and mechanism of chemical reactions. Application of the theory of chemical kinetics enables the rate of degradation of a drug substance or excipient to be calculated from the results of stability experiments conducted under specified conditions. Useful information can be obtained on the nature and number of intermediate steps in a degradation reaction and on the effects of factors such as concentration of reactants, temperature, pH, and surfactants. Chemical kinetics can be applied not only to the chemical stability of substances in solution but also to that of substances in suspensions, emulsions, solid dosage forms, and semi-solid preparations. The rate of kill of micro-organisms by antimicrobial preservatives and the rate of some physical reactions (for example, viscosity changes) can also be assessed by chemical kinetics. A knowledge of chemical kinetics is also of value to the pharmacist in community and hospital practice who may be called upon to solve practical stability problems or to make decisions on the shelf-life of medicines.

Rate Expression

The theory of chemical kinetics is based upon the law of mass action. In accordance with this law, the rate of chemical change in a reaction varies directly as the active molar concentrations of the reacting substances. For the homogeneous reaction:

$$mA + nB \rightarrow \text{products}$$

in which the active concentrations of A and B are equal to their actual concentrations in the system, the **rate of reaction** is expressed as:

$$-\frac{d[A]}{dt} = k[A]^m [B]^n$$

This mathematical equation is known as the **rate expression** or **general rate equation**. The proportionality constant k is the **rate constant** for the reaction. Since the concentrations of the reactants [A] and [B] decrease as the reaction progresses, the rate of reaction must decrease with time. Thus the rate constant is more convenient and useful than is the rate of reaction at a particular time as a measure of the progress of the reaction with time. It is sometimes more convenient to express the rate of reaction as the increase in concentration per unit time of one of the degradation products rather than the decrease in concentration per unit time of one of the reacting substances. If the initial concentration of a reactant (for example, a drug) in solution is a (mol/L) and after time t (s) assay of the solution shows that x (mol/L) has reacted, then the concentration remaining is $a - x$ (mol/L). Since the initial concentration a is constant:

$$-\frac{d[A]}{dt} = -\frac{d(a - x)}{dt}$$

$$-\frac{d[A]}{dt} = \frac{dx}{dt}$$

Order of Reaction

The sum of the exponents of the concentration terms in the rate expression is known as the **order of reaction**. In the example given above the exponent of [A] is m and that of [B] is n. The overall order of reaction is the sum of the exponents of [A] and [B], that is $m + n$; thus the overall reaction is said to follow $(m + n)$-order kinetics. The order of reaction can also be described as m-order in respect of [A] and n-order in respect of [B].
The rate of reaction may depend on a smaller number of concentration terms than that predicted by the overall stoichiometric equation or the molecularity of the reaction; that is the number of molecules or atoms that must collide simultaneously to form the reaction products. The rate may be determined by the slowest or rate-determining step. The order of a particular reaction should therefore be determined by experiment. For some reactions the experimentally determined order of reaction may be fractional or zero. Methods for

the determination of the order of a reaction are described in textbooks on pharmaceutics (see Further Information).

$t_{10\%}$

The $t_{10\%}$ of a medicinal product is defined in the introduction to this chapter. The method of calculating the $t_{10\%}$ under specified conditions of storage depends on the order of reaction; calculations are given in the sections on zero-order and first-order reactions.

$t_{50\%}$

The rate of a chemical reaction can also be expressed as the $t_{50\%}$ ($t_{\frac{1}{2}}$ or half-life); that is the time taken for one-half of the reactant to degrade. Values for the $t_{50\%}$ calculated from the results of experiments at elevated temperatures can be used in the determination of the order of reaction. The term 'half-life' is widely used to express the rate of decay of a radioactive isotope and to express the rate of irreversible loss of a drug from the blood (biological half-life). Methods for the calculation of $t_{50\%}$ values follow the general principles of the methods used to calculate $t_{10\%}$ values.

Zero-order Reactions

In a zero-order reaction the rate is constant and is independent of the concentrations of any of the reactants.
The rate expression is:

$$-\frac{d[A]}{dt} = k$$

Since

$$-\frac{d[A]}{dt} = \frac{dx}{dt}$$

$$\frac{dx}{dt} = k$$

or

$$dx = k\,dt$$

At $t = 0$, $x = 0$

$$\int_0^x dx = k \int_0^t dt$$

$$x = kt$$

$$(a - x) = a - kt$$

Thus a graph of the reactant concentration against time is rectilinear with a slope of $-k$ and an intercept at $t = 0$ of a (see Fig.1). The zero-order rate

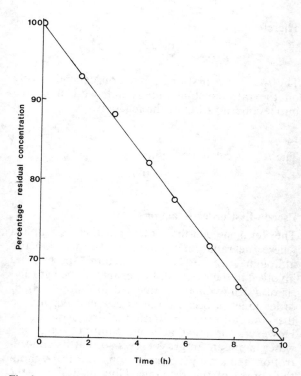

Fig. 1
Zero-order plot of percentage residual concentration against time for a model drug in aqueous suspension at constant pH and temperature.

constant k can be calculated from the regression equation of the straight line. For a zero-order reaction, k has the dimensions of concentration per time and is often expressed as $mol\,L^{-1}\,s^{-1}$.

$t_{10\%}$

The $t_{10\%}$ of a zero-order reaction is derived by rearrangement of the preceding equation.
Since

$$t = \frac{a - (a - x)}{k}$$

$$t_{10\%} = \frac{a - 0.9a}{k} = \frac{0.1a}{k}$$

Note that the $t_{10\%}$ for a zero-order reaction depends on both the initial reactant concentration and the rate constant.

$t_{50\%}$

The $t_{50\%}$ is calculated similarly:

$$t_{50\%} = \frac{0.5a}{k}$$

EXAMPLES

Some photochemical reactions follow zero-order kinetics; an example is the photochemical degradation of chlorpromazine in aqueous solution. Reactions that are catalysed by enzymes may follow zero-order kinetics in the presence of an excess of substrate. Zero-order reactions are also commonly encountered in aqueous suspensions of sparingly soluble drugs such as aspirin. Part of the drug exists as a saturated solution in water and is subject to hydrolysis by a first-order reaction. As hydrolysis proceeds, however, some of the suspended particles of drug will dissolve so that the solution remains saturated. Since the concentration of drug in solution remains constant, if instant dissolution is assumed, the rate of degradation is independent of drug concentration; thus hydrolysis of such suspensions follows zero-order kinetics.

First-order Reactions

In a first-order reaction the rate is proportional to the concentration of one of the reactants.
The rate expression is:

$$-\frac{d[A]}{dt} = k[A]$$

Since

$$[A] = (a - x) \text{ and } -\frac{d[A]}{dt} = \frac{dx}{dt}$$

$$\frac{dx}{dt} = k(a - x)$$

or

$$\frac{dx}{(a - x)} = k.dt$$

At $t = 0$, $x = 0$, hence

$$\int_0^x \frac{dx}{(a - x)} = k \int_0^t dt$$

Therefore

$$\ln \frac{a}{(a - x)} = kt$$

or

$$k = \frac{1}{t} \cdot \ln \frac{a}{(a - x)}$$

If common logarithms are used in place of natural logarithms,

$$k = \frac{2.303}{t} \cdot \log \frac{a}{(a - x)}$$

By rearrangement

$$\log (a - x) = \log a - \frac{kt}{2.303}$$

Thus a graph of the logarithm of the reactant concentration against time is rectilinear with a slope of $-k/2.303$ and an intercept at $t = 0$ of $\log a$ (Fig.2). The first-order rate constant k can be calculated from the regression equation of the straight line. For a first-order reaction, k is often expressed as reciprocal seconds.

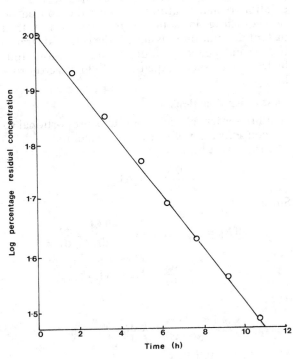

Fig. 2
First-order plot of log percentage residual concentration against time for a model drug in aqueous solution at constant pH and temperature.

$t_{10\%}$

The $t_{10\%}$ of a first-order reaction is derived by rearrangement of the above equation.
Since

$$t = \frac{2.303}{k} \cdot \log \frac{a}{(a - x)}$$

$$t_{10\%} = \frac{2.303}{k} \cdot \log \frac{1}{0.9}$$

Therefore

$$t_{10\%} = \frac{0.105}{k}$$

The $t_{10\%}$ for a first-order reaction depends solely on the rate constant and is independent of the initial concentration of the reactant.

$t_{50\%}$

The $t_{50\%}$ is calculated similarly:

$$t_{50\%} = \frac{0.693}{k}$$

Pseudo-first-order Reactions

The term **pseudo-first-order reaction** is applied where degradation follows first-order kinetics although two or more reactant species are involved in the reaction. For example, the hydrolysis of a drug would be expected to follow second-order kinetics because the rate would depend on the concentrations of both the drug and water. However, for most aqueous solutions of drugs, water is present in gross excess so that its concentration remains practically constant throughout the course of the reaction. Thus in practice, the rate of degradation depends solely on the concentration of the drug and pseudo-first-order kinetics are followed.

EXAMPLES
Many drugs (for example, aspirin, procaine hydrochloride) and excipients (for example, methyl hydroxybenzoate) in aqueous solution degrade by first-order or pseudo-first-order kinetics. Degradation in solid or semi-solid dosage forms is often complex but sometimes follows first-order or pseudo-first-order kinetics.

Second-order Reactions

In a second-order reaction the rate is proportional to the concentrations of the two reactants.
The rate expression is:

$$-\frac{d[A]}{dt} = k[A][B]$$

If the initial concentrations [A] and [B] are a and b respectively,

$$\frac{dx}{dt} = k(a - x)(b - x)$$

where x is the decrease in the concentrations [A] and [B] after time t.
Acid-catalysed and base-catalysed hydrolysis reactions of drugs and excipients may follow second-

order kinetics. An example is the hydrolysis of chlorbutol in aqueous solution containing sodium hydroxide; the rate depends on the concentrations of both chlorbutol and hydroxide ions. In practice, however, conditions are usually such that second-order reactions appear to follow first-order kinetics (see Pseudo-first-order Reactions above). For this reason, second-order kinetics are not considered in detail.

Complex Kinetics

Reactions of an order higher than second-order are rarely encountered since they involve the simultaneous collision of more than two reactants. However, degradation may comprise a number of intermediate steps (for example, hydrolysis of idoxuridine) or may proceed simultaneously by parallel reactions that involve more than one pathway (for example, simultaneous oxidation and isomerisation of vitamin A); some reactions may be reversible (for example, epimerisation of tetracycline) or may comprise parallel reactions, some of which are reversible (for example, degradation of chlorothiazide). In such instances, the kinetic equations used to express the rates of degradation are often complex. Fractional orders of reaction may be observed occasionally; for example, in the heat-catalysed oxidation of promethazine in aqueous solution at certain drug concentrations where some molecules of the drug may be present in the form of micelles. The kinetics of degradation in a semi-solid basis (for example, a cream or gel) or in a solid dosage form may be especially complex because of the physical nature of the preparation.

Effect of Temperature on the Rate Constant

For most reactions other than photochemical or radiation-induced processes, a rise in temperature increases the rate. In many hydrolysis reactions, for example, the rate may increase 2 or 3 times for a 10° rise in temperature.

The effect of temperature on the rate constant of a reaction can be described by the Arrhenius equation:

$$k_T = A \exp \left(-\frac{E_a}{RT} \right)$$

where, k_T is the rate constant at a particular thermodynamic (absolute) temperature T for the particular order of reaction (determined by experiment); A is the Arrhenius frequency factor (or pre-exponential factor) associated with the frequency of collisions between the reacting molecules and with the entropy of reaction; E_a is the energy of activation that molecules must possess in order that collision can lead to reaction; and R is the universal gas constant. Units for both k and A are those for the particular order of reaction, for example, reciprocal seconds for a first-order reaction; units for E_a, R, and T are J/mol, J mol^{-1} K^{-1}, and K, respectively. For application to the stability of drug substances or medicinal products, the Arrhenius equation is more usefully expressed in logarithmic form:

$$\ln k_T = \ln A - \frac{E_a}{RT}$$

$$\log k_T = \log A - \frac{E_a}{2.303RT}$$

A graph of the logarithm of the rate constant against the reciprocal of temperature is rectilinear with a slope of $-E_a/2.303R$ and an intercept at $1/T = 0$ of log A (Fig. 3).

The Arrhenius equation is widely applied to the results of accelerated stability tests on drug substances and medicinal products in order to predict the stability at room temperature from that at elevated temperatures (see Accelerated Stability Tests below).

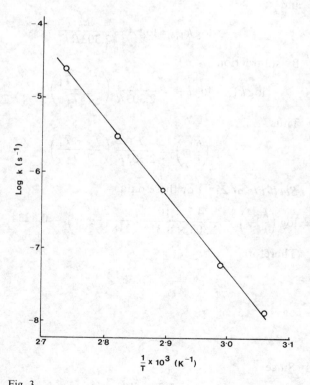

Fig. 3
Arrhenius plot of log first-order rate constant against the reciprocal of temperature (1/T) for a model drug in aqueous solution at constant pH.

Prediction of Shelf-life from Kinetic Data

Knowledge of the activation energy of the degradation reactions and of the rate constant at a particular temperature enables the shelf-life ($t_{10\%}$) of a product at another temperature to be predicted by application of the Arrhenius equation.

Consider an oral liquid containing an antibiotic in aqueous solution buffered at pH 6.5. The activation energy is 74.7×10^3 J/mol and the first-order rate constant for hydrolysis of the antibiotic at 45° is 7.27×10^{-7} s^{-1}. The universal gas constant R is 8.314 J mol^{-1} K^{-1}. It is assumed that the pH is independent of temperature and that there are no deviations from the Arrhenius equation. What is the shelf-life at 25° and at 5°?

For the calculation of a rate constant k_{T_1} at absolute temperature K_1 from the rate constant k_{T_2} at T_2, the logarithmic form of the Arrhenius equation is used.

From the preceding equation:

$$\log k_{T_2} = \log A - \frac{E_a}{2.303 R T_2}$$

and

$$\log k_{T_1} = \log A - \frac{E_a}{2.303 R T_1}$$

By subtraction

$$\log k_{T_2} - \log k_{T_1} = \frac{E_a}{2.303 R} \left(\frac{T_2 - T_1}{T_2 T_1} \right)$$

Thus

$$\log \left(\frac{k_{T_2}}{k_{T_1}} \right) = \frac{E_a}{2.303 R} \left(\frac{T_2 - T_1}{T_2 T_1} \right)$$

Shelf-life at 25°. For these data,

$$\log \left(\frac{k_{45°}}{k_{25°}} \right) = \frac{74.7 \times 10^3}{2.303 \times 8.314} \left(\frac{20}{318 \times 298} \right) = 0.8234$$

Therefore

$$\frac{k_{45°}}{k_{25°}} = 6.66$$

or

$$k_{25°} = \frac{k_{45°}}{6.66}$$

Since

$$k_{45°} = 7.27 \times 10^{-7} \, \text{s}^{-1}$$

$$k_{25°} = 1.09 \times 10^{-7} \, \text{s}^{-1}$$

The equation for a first-order reaction is:

$$t_{10\%} = \frac{0.105}{k}$$

Hence at 25°

$$t_{10\%} = \frac{0.105}{1.09 \times 10^{-7}} \, \text{s}$$
$$= 9.63 \times 10^5 \, \text{s}$$
$$= 268 \, \text{h}$$
$$\approx 11 \, \text{days}$$

Thus the shelf-life of the product at 25° is about 11 days.

Shelf-life at 5°. By a similar calculation:

$$\frac{k_{45°}}{k_{5°}} = 58.2$$

Therefore

$$k_{5°} = 1.25 \times 10^{-8} \, \text{s}^{-1}$$
$$t_{10\%} = 8.40 \times 10^6 \, \text{s}$$
$$= 2330 \, \text{h}$$
$$\approx 97 \, \text{days}$$

Thus the shelf-life of the product at 5° is about three months.

CHEMICAL STABILITY

Chemical degradation of the active constituent in a medicinal product often results in a loss in potency; for example, hydrolysis of the β-lactam ring of benzylpenicillin results in a lower antimicrobial activity. In a few instances the degradation products of a drug may be toxic (for example, epianhydrotetracycline formed from tetracycline or free amines produced by degradation of iodipamide) so that clinical use of preparations may be unacceptable if the extent of decomposition is relatively great. Degradation of an excipient can pose problems of physical or microbiological stability. For example, hydrolysis of a sorbitan ester may result in sufficient loss in its ability to produce an interfacial film that a formulated emulsion may crack; hydrolysis of an antimicrobial preservative such as methyl hydroxybenzoate can so reduce the concentration that it no longer inhibits the growth of micro-organisms. Marked discoloration of solutions that contain adrenaline may represent only a very slight change in drug content but is unacceptable to the patient, pharmacist, physician, and nurse. In general, chemical reactions proceed more readily in the liquid state than in the solid state so that serious stability problems are more commonly encountered in liquid medicines; the stability of suspensions of solid drugs in water or other liquid is usually greater than that of solutions. In this section, the various types of reaction that cause chemical degradation of medicines are considered together with the principal factors that affect the rate; general methods by which degradation can be minimised are suggested. Interactions between the drug, excipient, and packaging may also occur; such interactions are described in the chapter on Incompatibility.

Chemical Reactions that Cause Degradation

A variety of chemical reactions can result in the degradation of drug substances and excipients; the most common reactions are oxidation and hydrolysis. Sometimes more than one reaction may occur at the same time; for example, pilocarpine in aqueous solution degrades simultaneously by base-catalysed hydrolysis and epimerisation. Degradation may also involve consecutive reactions as with the anticholinesterase ester, physostigmine; in aqueous solution, this alkaloid first hydrolyses relatively slowly to form a colourless phenolic compound, eseroline, which is devoid of anticholinesterase activity. In the presence of oxygen, eseroline is then rapidly oxidised to rubreserine and other highly coloured, inactive products. In this instance, the initial hydrolysis represents the slower or rate-determining step in the degradation of the alkaloid; it also represents the step at which pharmacological activity is lost.

Hydrolysis

Hydrolysis involves the reaction of a molecule with water that results in cleavage. Pharmaceutical examples of substances that degrade by hydrolysis include: esters such as amethocaine, aspirin, and chlorbutol; amides such as chloramphenicol and ergometrine; lactams such as the penicillins and nitrazepam; and oximes such as pralidoxime. Hydrolysis may occur not only in aqueous solutions of drugs but also in aqueous suspensions of sparingly soluble drugs. In tablets and other solid dosage forms there may be sufficient water to allow hydrolysis of the drug to proceed. In addition, enzyme-catalysed hydrolysis may take place in drugs of natural origin; for example, enzymes catalyse the hydrolysis of cardiac glycosides in digitalis leaf.

Dehydration

Dehydration reactions occur occasionally in drugs. An example is atropine, which not only hydrolyses in aqueous solution to tropine and tropic acid but also dehydrates to form apoatropine.

Oxidation

The term oxidation is applied to reactions in which either one or more electropositive atoms, radicals, or electrons are lost or one or more electronegative atoms or radicals are gained. Many drugs (for example, morphine, dopamine) and other substances used in pharmaceutical formulation (for example, fixed oils and fats) are prone to degrade by oxidation.

Redox Reactions. Some oxidation reactions are redox reactions that involve the reversible loss of electrons without the addition of oxygen. Examples in pharmacy include the oxidation of ferrous sulphate (and other ferrous salts), ascorbic acid, adrenaline, and riboflavine. In certain instances, the susceptibility of a substance to such reversible oxidation can be predicted from a knowledge of its standard oxidation-reduction potential E_0. For a substance in solution at constant temperature, the oxidation-reduction potential E_h depends on the standard oxidation-reduction potential, the number of electrons n transferred per ion, and the logarithm of the ratio of concentrations of the oxidised and reduced forms:

$$E_h = E_0 + \frac{0.06}{n} \log \frac{[\text{oxidised form}]}{[\text{reduced form}]}$$

Substances with a high value for E_0 are more resistant to oxidation than are those with a low E_0 value. Thus in an aqueous solution of ascorbic acid and adrenaline, at pH 4.7, the oxidation of ascorbic acid ($E_0 = +0.14$ V) will occur preferentially to that of adrenaline ($E_0 = +0.52$ V); for this reason, ascorbic acid can be used to protect solutions of adrenaline from oxidation.

Autoxidations. In the manufacture and storage of medicinal products autoxidations are more common than redox reactions. An autoxidation is an irreversible chain reaction in which a substance becomes slowly oxidised in the presence of atmospheric oxygen. Such chain reactions which involve the formation of free radicals occur in fixed oils and fats that contain unsaturated linkages. Autoxidations are also common in essential oils in which darkening and changes in odour and flavour may occur together with the deposition of solid resins. In anaesthetic ether, autoxidation leads to the formation of peroxides that have caused explosions in operating theatres. Phenols, alcohols and aldehydes are also susceptible to auto-oxidation. Particularly hazardous is the slow oxidation in atmospheric oxygen of paraldehyde; the acetic acid that forms can cause severe corrosion of mucous membranes. Thus the use of old stocks of paraldehyde kept in partly-filled containers can be dangerous.

Chain reactions, for example, in a fixed oil or fat, comprise three steps: initiation, propagation, and termination.

Initiation involves conversion of an organic compound RH to a free radical R$^\bullet$; this step may be activated by light, heat or traces of heavy metals.

$$RH \rightarrow R^\bullet + H^\bullet$$

In the **propagation** step, the free radical R$^\bullet$ reacts with oxygen to form a peroxy radical ROO$^\bullet$; this free radical then removes H from another molecule of RH to form a hydroperoxide ROOH and a new free radical R$^\bullet$ which enables the chain reaction to proceed.

$$R^\bullet + O_2 \rightarrow ROO^\bullet$$
$$ROO^\bullet + RH \rightarrow ROOH + R^\bullet$$

Hydroperoxides are odourless and tasteless but degrade to form aldehydes, ketones and short-chain fatty acids that result in an oil or fat developing a rancid odour and taste.

Propagation may continue until all the organic compound or the oxygen has been consumed but usually **termination** of the chain reaction occurs because some of the free radicals combine with each other to form inactive products.

$$R^\bullet + R^\bullet \rightarrow$$
$$ROO^\bullet + ROO^\bullet \rightarrow \quad \text{Inactive Products}$$
$$R^\bullet + ROO^\bullet \rightarrow$$

During initiation of the chain reaction, oxidation is very slow so that there is a period of induction or 'lag phase'.

Propagation leads to a logarithmic increase in the rate of oxidation. Finally termination slows down the reaction until it practically stops.

Isomerisation

Isomerisation is the conversion of a substance into its geometric or optical isomers; these have the same structural formula but differ in stereochemical configuration.

Geometric Isomerisation. This conversion involves changes in the relative spatial configuration of atoms or groups around ethylenic double bonds or cyclic compounds. Different geometric isomers may possess different potencies. For example, the most active form of vitamin A is the all-*trans* configuration; when solubilised in aqueous solution, vitamin A palmitate not only oxidises but also isomerises to form the less active 6-mono-*cis* and 2,6-di-*cis* isomers.

Optical Isomerisation. Changes in the optical rotation of a substance as a result of the presence of one or more chiral centres are described as optical isomerism; chiral centres usually comprise asymmetric carbon atoms. Chirality may also be due to restricted rotation about bonds (atropisomerism) but this is uncommon in drugs; an example is methaqualone. Two types of optical isomerisation can be distinguished: racemisation and epimerisation.

Racemisation in solution involves the conversion of an optically active drug with one chiral centre into an isomer whose structure is a mirror image of the original molecule; such optically active pairs of optical isomers are known as enantiomers. The reaction continues until the concentrations of the two enantiomers are equal; at this stage the solution of the racemic mixture no longer rotates the plane of polarised light. An example is the laevo-form of adrenaline which racemises in aqueous solution to form a mixture of equal parts of the laevo- and dextro-forms. The pharmacological activity of the laevo-form is about fifteen times that of the dextro-form; thus the activity of a solution of the racemic mixture is just over half that of the original solution. Recent work has shown that racemisation of some drugs may lead to more complex pharmacological or toxicological effects. It is possible, for example, that enantiomers may differ in their affinity for receptors or they may have opposite effects; one isomer may be principally responsible for the desired therapeutic action and the other isomer for the toxicity or side-effects of the drug. There is enhanced interest in the clinical action of different enantiomers of drug substances which is concomitant with developments in stereospecific asymmetric synthesis and in the separation of racemates.

Where there is more than one chiral centre in a molecule **epimerisation** can occur in which there is selective racemisation at one centre. Equilibrium between the two epimers may not represent equal concentrations of each since the presence of other chiral centres may favour the formation of one epimer rather than the other. For this reason and since the optical rotations of the two isomers are not equal and opposite, the optical activity of the mixture of epimers at equilibrium will not be zero. Pharmaceutical examples of epimerisation include tetracycline which epimerises in acidic solution to form 4-epi-tetracycline which has much lower antimicrobial activity than the original antibiotic. Similarly ergometrine in aqueous solution undergoes epimerisation at carbon atom 8 to ergometrinine which possesses very little pharmacological activity.

Polymerisation

The combination of two or more identical molecules of a substance to form a more complex molecule is known as polymerisation. For example, storage in the cold of an aqueous solution of the hydrate of formaldehyde may result in the appearance of a white deposit that consists of paraformaldehyde, formed by polymerisation. Often, polymerisation follows a primary degradation process. Sterilisation of glucose intravenous infusion by autoclaving leads first to the formation of 5-hydroxyfurfural, which then polymerises to various straw-coloured products. Ampicillin and other amino-penicillins degrade not only by hydroxide-ion catalysed hydrolysis but also by self-aminolysis to form dimers; higher polymers may also form. It is thought that certain skin rashes sometimes produced after administration of amino-penicillins are hypersensitivity reactions associated with the presence of such polymers.

Photochemical Reactions

When exposed to light many drugs and excipients are susceptible to degradation by a variety of photochemical reactions; the photo-oxidation of chlorpromazine is a typical example. Ultraviolet light may initiate the chain reaction in autoxidation. Among the photoreduction reactions that occasionally occur in pharmaceutical preparations are those reported for aqueous solutions of ferrous gluconate. In sunlight, the content of ferrous iron is actually increased beyond that originally present as a result of the small amount of ferric iron present being reduced to ferrous iron. Storage of colchicine injection in the light may result in the crystallisation of isomers of the drug, known as lumicolchicines. In general, photochemical reactions are highly complex and few mechanisms have been fully elucidated. Other substances that are unstable to light under certain conditions include chloroform, erythrosine (and other colouring agents), frusemide, methotrexate, phenols, and sodium nitroprusside.

Radiation-induced Reactions

Degradation by complex mechanisms may result from exposure of products (for example, insulin injection) to ionising radiation during sterilisation procedures.

Decarboxylation

Decarboxylation is a reaction where carbon dioxide is removed from a substance. Thus aminosalicylic acid (and its salts) in aqueous solution degrade to form 3-aminophenol which is then oxidised to various coloured products. Sodium bicarbonate decarboxylates to sodium carbonate when aqueous solutions are sterilised by autoclaving. Decarboxylation may also occur as a secondary degradation reaction; for example, in acidic solution, procaine hydrochloride hydrolyses to 4-aminobenzoic acid; this acid decarboxylates to form aniline which then darkens if exposed to light. Carbon dioxide may be lost from effervescent tablets and granules due to condensation of water on the product during storage.

Absorption of Carbon Dioxide

Solutions of the sodium salts of hexobarbitone and other barbiturates are alkaline and readily take up carbon dioxide so that the pH is lowered and the free acid form is precipitated. Absorption of carbon dioxide also occurs, for example, in solutions of calcium hydroxide; formation of calcium carbonate results in the solution becoming turbid on storage.

Factors that may affect Chemical Stability

The rate of chemical reaction of a drug or excipient in a medicine may be affected by physicochemical factors such as pH, ionic strength, or the physical state of the product. The nature and concentration of other drugs and excipients may also influence the rate of degradation. Temperature, intensity of light, relative humidity, and other environmental conditions often affect the chemical stability of medicinal products during manufacture, storage, and use.

pH

In reversible oxidations the standard oxidation-reduction potential may depend on pH; thus pH may affect the tendency of a drug to be oxidised. The rate of oxidation of drugs that contain phenol groups (for example, adrenaline and dopamine) or sulphydryl groups (for example, captopril) is highly sensitive to pH since it is mainly the ionised form of these drugs that is oxidised. Hydrolysis reactions

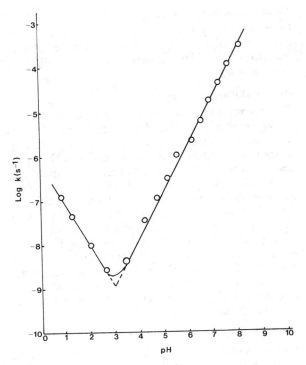

Fig. 4
Plot of log first-order rate constant (log k) against pH for a model drug in aqueous solution at constant temperature.

are often catalysed by both hydrogen ions and hydroxide ions. Since hydroxide ions usually exert a greater catalytic effect than hydrogen ions, the minimum degradation rate (that is maximum stability) of many drugs is in the range pH 2 to 5. In addition temperature may modify the effects of pH. For example, the minimum rate of hydrolysis of physostigmine sulphate in aqueous solution is at pH 3.7 at 25° and at pH 3.1 at 75°. The rate of other reactions such as isomerisation may be influenced by pH. An example is the hydroxide-ion catalysis of the epimerisation of pilocarpine. The dehydration of atropine to apoatropine occurs mainly at pH 2 to 4.

Typical effects of pH on the chemical stability of a model drug are shown in Fig. 4. The effects of pH may be more complex because of the presence of several ionic forms of the drug. Pipkin[1] described in detail the influence of pH on the stability of aztreonam for which three ionisation constants have been determined.

General Acids and Bases

In addition to catalysis by hydrogen ions and hydroxide ions (specific acid-base catalysis), cer-

tain hydrolysis reactions are catalysed by other acidic and basic species (general acid-base catalysis) such as those in salts used to buffer solutions of drugs. For example, the rate of hydrolysis of chloramphenicol is practically independent of pH in the range pH 2 to 7 but is catalysed by some general acids and bases, which include monohydrogen phosphate ions, monohydrogen and dihydrogen citrate ions, and unionised acetic acid; however, the rate is not affected by the presence of dihydrogen phosphate ions.

Ionic Strength

Addition of an inert electrolyte to an aqueous solution of a drug may exert a direct effect on stability even though there is no chemical interaction between the drug and the electrolyte. Such **primary salt effects**, which depend on the concentration of the added salt and on the charges borne by the reacting ions, have been reported for a number of drugs (for example, ampicillin and thiamine) and excipients (for example, methyl hydroxybenzoate). If the ions bear the same charge, the addition of a salt increases the rate of degradation. In contrast, when ions are of opposite charge, the rate is decreased. When one of the reactants is not charged, addition of a salt should not affect stability of the drug (for example, chloramphenicol) provided that the drug concentration is below 0.01M; a primary salt effect may be observed in more concentrated solutions.

Electrolytes may also indirectly influence the rate of reaction by modifying the ionisation constant of weak acids or bases present in buffer solutions and thus enhancing or reducing catalysis by general acids and bases. Such effects are known as **secondary salt effects**.

Nature of the Solvent

The influence of the solvent on the rate of degradation of a drug depends largely on the dielectric constant of the solvent and on the electrical charge on the drug. Where the charges on the drug and the attacking ion are the same, part or complete replacement of the water (high dielectric constant) by alcohol, propylene glycol, or glycerol (lower dielectric constants) usually lowers the rate of degradation; an example is the hydroxide-ion catalysis of the hydrolysis of aspirin anions. Where the charges are opposite (for example, hydrogen ions and aspirin anions), reduction in dielectric constant of the solvent would be expected to increase the rate of degradation. However, in the hydrogen-ion catalysed degradation of protonated chloramphenicol in various propylene glycol-water mixtures, a decrease in dielectric constant results in an increase in the rate of degradation although the charges on the drug and the attacking ion are the same. The reason is that the rate-determining step is an ion-dipolar molecule reaction between hydrogen ions and the hydrated amide.

Drug Concentration

The effects of drug concentration on degradation depend on the order of reaction. For example, if the reaction follows first-order kinetics, the **rate** is directly proportional to drug concentration but the **time** for a certain proportion (for example, 10%) to decompose is independent of concentration. For rate equations in respect of zero-order, first-order, and second-order reactions see the section on Chemical Kinetics above.

Where the mechanism of degradation and order of reaction depend on drug concentration, the kinetics are complex. In dilute solution, ampicillin degrades by pseudo-first-order kinetics but in more concentrated solutions the reaction becomes third-order; concentrated solutions of this drug degrade much more rapidly than dilute solutions.

For the degradation of those drugs where the molecules associate with each other at a critical concentration to form micelles, the order of reaction may depend on drug concentration. Meakin, Stevens, and Davies[2] showed that the thermal degradation in the dark of promethazine hydrochloride in aqueous solution appeared to follow first-order kinetics at concentrations below 0.5% but zero-order kinetics at concentrations above 3.0%; at intermediate concentrations the data could not be fitted to a simple kinetic equation. The change in apparent order was attributed to the formation of micelles and the results were interpreted in terms of the kinetics of two simultaneous processes; first-order for degradation of the monomer and half-order for the solubilised drug in the micelles.

Surfactants

Surfactants are commonly used as excipients in the formulation of medicines, especially as dispersing, emulsifying or solubilising agents. The effects of surfactants on the stability of drugs may depend on factors such as concentration, solubility, chemical nature, and chain-length of the surfactant, the mechanism of degradation of the drug, its site of solubilisation, and the charge on the attacking ion. In oxidation reactions the physical state of the product is important. Carless and Nixon[3] showed that in a simple dispersion in water, the autoxidation of

the oil methyl linoleate was very slow because very little oil was soluble. Addition of potassium laurate resulted in the formation of an emulsion in which part of the methyl linoleate was solubilised in micelles of the surfactant and part was present as oil droplets. Autoxidation of the emulsion was rapid since the micelles provided especially favourable conditions for initiation of the reaction; the free radicals formed then migrated from the micelles into the water and diffused into the oil droplets where propagation proceeded rapidly. Further addition of the surfactant resulted in more oil molecules becoming solubilised until the solubilisation process was complete; at this stage, the rate of autoxidation was much lower because there were no oil droplets present to enable rapid propagation to occur. At high concentrations of the surfactant, the autoxidation rate was further reduced; this effect was attributed to a smaller number of methyl linoleate molecules in each micelle.

The effects of various surfactants on the rate of hydroxide-ion catalysed hydrolysis of benzocaine were reported by Riegelman.[4] As the concentration of an anionic or cationic surfactant was increased a higher proportion of benzocaine was solubilised in the micelles under the polar head group; the hydrolysis rate was decreased because of protection in the micelles from the attacking hydroxide ions. Less protection was given by nonionic than by ionic surfactants since benzocaine was solubilised in the hydrated polyoxyethylene palisade layer of the nonionic micelles, where it was easier for hydroxide ions to attack the drug.

Peroxides

The presence of highly labile peroxides may catalyse the initiation and propagation stages of autoxidations since these substances easily form free radicals. Peroxides are commonly formed in fixed oils and fats and in diethyl ether.

Heavy Metal Ions

Traces of heavy metal ions often catalyse autoxidation reactions; for example, as little as 0.05 ppm of cupric ions may be sufficient to initiate the oxidation of fatty acids and to enhance the rate of propagation of the chain reaction. In stability experiments the effect of heavy metals is demonstrated by shortening of the lag phase. The mechanism of action of heavy metal ions appears to be associated with the rapid formation of free radicals and is thought to be due to the ability of such cations to change readily from one valency state to another, for example, cupric to cuprous.

Sources of heavy metal ions include metal manufacturing equipment, water, drugs of natural origin, excipients, and chromic acid solution used to clean glassware. Although heavy metals present in coloured glass ampoules or other containers are strongly bound in the matrix of the glass, traces of such cations may be released to aqueous solutions of drugs; the rate of oxidation of amitriptyline in buffered aqueous solution has been reported to be greater in amber glass than in colourless glass ampoules. If water that contains heavy metal ions is stored in plastic or glass vessels, some heavy metal ions may be lightly adsorbed on the surface and subsequently released into a product.

Oxygen

Many oxidation reactions that occur in the ingredients of medicines are autoxidations where oxygen is necessary for propagation of the chain reaction. Often a low concentration of oxygen in the product is sufficient to permit considerable oxidation to take place. The partial pressure of oxygen in the air in a container may be important; for example, the rate of oxidation of sulpyrine in the solid state has been shown to depend on the partial pressure of oxygen as well as the presence of water. Entrapped air in viscous emulsions and creams can enhance the oxidation rate of the oily phase.

Carbon Dioxide

The partial pressure of gaseous carbon dioxide in the container or its concentration in the product may affect the rate and extent of reactions that involve the uptake of this gas.

Water

Drug substances, excipients (especially starches), and solid dosage forms such as tablets and capsules may contain small amounts of water. Since substances and solid dosage forms are sometimes kept at a relatively high relative humidity they may sorb water on the surface which may lead to dissolution of the drug and to degradation. In a study of the hydrolysis of aspirin in the solid state, Leeson and Maddocks[5] showed that degradation depended on water vapour pressure. The probable mechanism is that water is rapidly sorbed as a monolayer or multilayer on the surface of the drug particles; the amount being a function of water vapour pressure. Some of the aspirin then dissolves in the sorbed water to form a saturated solution. As the aspirin in solution hydrolyses to acetic and salicylic acids, more of the solid aspirin dissolves so that the solution remains saturated. Thus hydrolysis under these conditions follows zero-order kinetics. When only about 20% to 30% of the drug remains, however, the particles tend to stick together so that the physical state changes and the simple mechanism no longer operates. This example is typical of the hydrolysis of many drugs in the solid state when kept at a high relative humidity. Storage under damp conditions may cause loss of carbon dioxide from effervescent products. The rate of oxidation (or other reaction) may be enhanced similarly by high relative humidity; examples are the oxidation of ferrous sulphate and captopril.

Crystal form, size, and habit (external shape) can also affect the rate of degradation. The effects of moisture on the stability of drugs in formulated solid dosage forms are often difficult to predict because of the complex physical structure of solid products. Monkhouse[6] has presented a comprehensive review of stability aspects of preformulation and formulation of solid pharmaceuticals and discusses in detail the effect of moisture. The application of chemical kinetics to the stability of solids and solid dosage forms is discussed by Carstensen.[7] The uptake of water on solids is discussed further in the section on Physical Stability.

Temperature

For many reactions an increase in temperature enhances the rate constant and the effects can often be described by the Arrhenius equation (see Chemical Kinetics above). Detailed knowledge of these effects is especially critical in the formulation and manufacture of injections, ophthalmic solutions, and other products that are sterilised by moist or dry heat. Information on the effects of temperature is also important in the prediction of shelf-life of products marketed in the tropics. The effects of temperature on some oxidation reactions in aqueous products may operate in opposing directions. Although a rise in temperature results in a higher degradation rate it also decreases the solubility of oxygen in water; thus where oxygen concentration affects the rate of oxidation, the effects of temperature do not follow the Arrhenius equation. Storage at low temperatures may adversely affect the stability of some medicines, for example, the polymerisation of formaldehyde in aqueous solution proceeds more rapidly below $15°$. The effects of freezing solutions are considered in the section on Stability of Medicines in Pharmaceutical Practice.

Light

Photochemical reactions involve the absorption of light of a particular wavelength in the ultraviolet or visible regions of the spectrum. Each molecule that undergoes chemical change absorbs one quantum of radiant energy; the unit of radiant energy that is equivalent to one quantum is the photon. The radiant energy must exceed a threshold before the reaction will occur. However, not all absorbed light leads to a reaction, since some may be converted to heat or transferred to molecules of another substance (photosensitisation), or emitted at the same or different wavelength.

Radiation in the ultraviolet region has the highest energy; as the wavelength increases there is a decrease in radiant energy. Hence sunlight and light from fluorescent tubes have a greater effect on photochemical reactions than light from tungsten-filament bulbs. In practice, the radiation that strikes a light-sensitive substance in a medicinal product depends not only on the source of radiation but also on the light-filtering activity of other constituents and the packaging.

For solid dosage forms photochemical degradation is usually most rapid during the early stages of exposure to light because the reaction occurs mainly at the surface of the product.

Ionising Radiation

The use of ionising radiation to sterilise medicinal products may result in decomposition. At the radiation dose (25 kGy) commonly recommended for sterilisation, the nature or extent of degradation of many substances in aqueous solution (for example, heparin injection, insulin injection, and cyanocobalamin injection) is unacceptable. A particular problem is that irradiation of water produces hydrogen peroxide and various free radicals that can initiate and propagate chain reactions. Drug substances (for example, atropine sulphate) if free from moisture are often more stable to radiation than are their solutions (for example, atropine sulphate injection) although some substances (for example, choramphenicol and polymyxin sulphate) may become discoloured.

Mechanical Processes

Grinding can cause drug solvates or hydrates to become more chemically unstable since it weakens the bonding force between a drug molecule and its water of crystallisation; thus liberated water molecules can take part in hydrolysis reactions.

Methods of Stabilisation

Enhancement of the chemical stability of a medicinal product demands a sound knowledge of the nature of the degradation reactions that are likely to occur during manufacture and storage and of the factors that may influence the rate of degradation. The many stages at which such knowledge has to be applied include preformulation; excipient selection; processing development; packaging evaluation; the application of quality controls; and in the recommendation of appropriate storage conditions. Since most medicines are complex in physicochemical terms, much experimental work is necessary to achieve acceptable chemical stability and to predict the shelf-life of the product. This section includes brief descriptions of the principal methods used to enhance chemical stability.

Antoxidants

Many pharmaceutical preparations deteriorate on storage because of oxidation of one or more of the ingredients on exposure to atmospheric oxygen (see below). Such autoxidation reactions are often catalysed by light, temperature, hydrogen ion concentration, the presence of trace metals (for example, copper, iron, heavy metals) or peroxides.[9]

Pharmaceutical substances that are especially susceptible to oxidation include unsaturated oils and fats, and compounds with aldehyde groups or phenolic groups (see Table 1). Excipients such as colourings, flavourings, and sweeteners are prone to oxidation,[10] and plastics and rubber used in containers and closures also tend to oxidise on sto-

Table 1
Examples of substances that degrade by oxidation

adrenaline	heparin	paraldehyde
amikacin sulphate	hyaluronidase	pentazocine
amitriptyline	hydrocortisone	phenylephrine
amphotericin	hydrogen peroxide	phenylbutazone
apomorphine	isoamyl nitrite	physostigmine
ascorbic acid	isoprenaline	prednisolone
benzyl alcohol	kanamycin	prednisone
betamethasone	local anaesthetics	promethazine
captopril	6-mercaptopurine	reserpine
chlorpromazine	metaraminol	resorcinol
cysteine	methyldopa	riboflavine
dexamethasone	metoclopramide	rifampicin
dobutamine	morphine	streptomycin
edrophonium	neomycin	sulphacetamide sodium
ergometrine	netilmicin	thiothixene
ergotamine	noradrenaline	tobramycin
ferrous sulphate	novobiocin	tubocurarine
folic acid	nystatin	unsaturated fats and oils
gentamicin	oleyl alcohol	vitamin A
glucose	para-aminobenzoic acid	volatile oils

rage. Autoxidation reactions can be inhibited by the addition of small amounts of substances known as antoxidants.

An account of oxidative degradation and the use of antoxidants in injectable preparations is described in the Parenterals chapter.

Antoxidants are usually classified in accordance with their reputed mode of action into three groups: true antoxidants, reducing agents, and antoxidant synergists. Knowledge of their mode of action is, however, incomplete. Table 2 lists some of the antoxidants used in pharmaceutical products and the food industry, and their properties.

The Antoxidants in Food (Amendment) Regulations 1991 (SI No 2540) was introduced to amend The Antoxidants in Food Regulations 1978 and The Antoxidants in Food (Scotland) Regulations 1978.

True antoxidants are thought to block chain reactions by reacting with free radicals; thus the period of induction of the autoxidation reaction is prolonged. These substances are effective in the inhibition of autoxidations but are not effective in reversible oxidation (redox) reactions. True antoxidants, singly or in admixture are widely used to retard the autoxidation of oils and fats. Often an antoxidant synergist is added (see below).

Reducing agents are substances that have a lower redox potential than the drug or adjuvant that they are intended to protect against oxidation. Thus reducing agents are more readily oxidised than the drug or adjuvant and are effective in the presence of oxidising agents. Reducing agents may also be effective in blocking chain reactions that take place in the autoxidation of drugs and adjuvants.

Antoxidant synergists are substances that enhance appreciably the effects of antoxidants although if used alone most synergists have little antoxidant activity. Edetic acid (EDTA) and its calcium disodium salt or disodium salt[11] form chelates with ions of heavy metals, which often catalyse autoxidation, and are sometimes used as synergists in aqueous solutions of drugs, such as neomycin, that oxidise to form coloured solutions. The mode of action of other synergists, such as citric acid and phosphoric acid, is a subject of controversy. It is thought that these synergists, which are often used in conjunction with true antoxidants in oils and fats, may form chelates with ions of heavy metals or may provide hydrogen for the regeneration of inactivated radicals of the antoxidant.

An ideal antoxidant for a pharmaceutical product would possess the following properties:

- effective in low concentration in retarding the oxidation of a variety of substances used in pharmacy over a wide range of temperature and pH
- readily soluble at the concentration used
- stable (chemically and physically) over a wide range of temperature and pH values
- compatible with other components of the preparation
- compatible with plastics, rubber, and other materials used in containers and closures
- free from objectionable odour, taste, or colour
- free from toxic, carcinogenic, irritant, or sensitising effects at the concentration used.

Similar criteria are applied to antoxidants in foods and cosmetics. The use of antoxidants in these products may pose serious problems of safety since they are sometimes eaten or applied to the skin in large amounts for many years.

All antoxidants have limitations. The choice of antoxidant for a particular medicine depends upon the route, dose, and frequency of administration, the chemical and physical properties of the preservative, the various constituents of the medicine, and the properties of the container and closure. Since it is often not possible to predict the effectiveness of an antoxidant in a particular preparation, the choice of concentration should be determined by experiment.

If an antoxidant is added to a material or preparation after oxidation has progressed beyond the period of induction, many free radicals will be present and the antoxidant will be quickly destroyed. Under these conditions, autoxidation may be retarded only for a very short time. It is important therefore to add the antoxidant as early as possible in the preparation of the product. Care should also be taken to ensure that the antoxidant is effectively incorporated into the product.

An increase in concentration of the antoxidant usually leads to an enhanced antoxidant effect until an optimum concentration is attained. At higher concentrations, however, the antoxidant may be less effective; this 'pro-oxidative' effect has been attributed to the reaction of hydroperoxides with the antoxidant to form free radicals. The optimum concentration for a particular material or preparation must be determined by experiment.

The effectiveness of antoxidants may be reduced in formulated products especially in polyphasic

Table 2

True antoxidants, reducing agents, and antoxidant synergists

Antoxidant	Serial number	Solubility				Typical concentration (%)	Additional information
		water	alcohols	oils	others		
True antoxidants							
Acetylcysteine		sol	sol	insol		0.1–0.5	
Alpha tocopherol acetate		insol	sol	sol		up to 0.001	Up to 10 ppm may be added to liquid paraffin
d-Alpha tocopherol (natural)	E306	insol	sol	sol	sol in acetone, chloroform, ether	0.05–0.075	ADI up to 2 mg/kg body-weight. Stable to heat and alkali
dl-Alpha tocopherol (synthetic)	E307	insol	sol	sol			
Ascorbyl palmitate	E304	sl sol	sol	sl sol		0.01–0.2	ADI up to 1.25 mg/kg body-weight
Butylated hydroxyanisole (BHA)	E320	insol	sol	sol	sol in arachis oil, chloroform, ether, propylene glycol	0.005–0.02	ADI up to 0.5 mg/kg body-weight. See below*
Butylated hydroxytoluene (BHT)	E321	insol	sol	sol	sol in chloroform, ether, liquid paraffin	0.005–0.02	Temporary ADI up to 125 micrograms/kg body-weight. See below†
Cysteine		sol	sol	insol		0.1–0.5	
Cysteine hydrochloride	920	sol	sol	insol	sol in acetone	0.1–0.5	
Delta tocopherol (synthetic)	E309	insol	sol	sol			Also used as a synergist
Dithiothreitol		sol	sol	insol			
Dodecyl gallate	E312	insol	sol	sol	sol in acetone, ether	0.01–0.1	
Ethyl gallate		sl sol	sol	insol	sol in ether		
Gamma tocopherol (synthetic)	E308	insol	sol	sol			
Glutathione		sol					
4-Hydroxymethyl-2,6-di-tert-butylphenol							Present in pharmaceutical formulations and food products
Nordihydroguaiaretic acid (NDGA)		insol	sol	sol		0.001–0.01	Used in fats and oils
Octyl gallate	E311	insol	sol	sol	sol in acetone, propylene glycol, ether		
Propyl gallate	E310	sl sol	sol	sl sol	sol in ether, propylene glycol	0.001–0.15	ADI up to 2.5 mg/kg body-weight. Prevention of deterioration and rancidity of fats and oils
tert-Butyl-hydroquinone (TBHQ)							Present in pharmaceutical formulations and food products
Thiolactic acid		sol					
Thiosorbitol		sol					
2,4,5-Trihydroxy-butyrophenone (THBP)							Present in pharmaceutical formulations and food products
Reducing agents							
Acetone sodium bisulphite						0.2–0.4	
Ascorbic acid	E300	sol	sol	insol	sol in glycerol, propylene glycol	0.01–0.5	Also used as a synergist. Unstable in solution; solutions exhibit maximum stability at about pH 5.4. Oxidation is accelerated by light and heat and catalysed by traces of copper and iron.
Calcium ascorbate	E302	sol					
Calcium bisulphite	E227	sol					
Calcium sulphite	E226	sol					
Isoascorbic acid (erythorbic acid)		sol	sol	insol			
Potassium metabisulphite	E224	sol	insol			0.1–1.0	
Sodium ascorbate	E301	sol	sl sol	insol			
Sodium bisulphite	E222	sol	sl sol	insol		0.05–0.15	See below‡
Sodium formaldehyde sulphoxylate		sol	sl sol			0.005–0.15	
Sodium metabisulphite	E223	sol	sl sol	insol	sol in glycerol	0.01–1.0	See below‡. Incompatible with sympathomimetics and related compounds and chloramphenicol. Glucose decreases stability. Has anti-microbial properties. Decomposes in air
Sodium sulphite	E221	sol	insol	insol		0.01–0.2	See below‡

Table 2—*Continued*

Antoxidant	Serial number	Solubility				Typical concentration (%)	Additional information
		water	alcohols	oils	others		
Sodium thiosulphate		sol	insol				See below[‡]. Unstable in solution
Sulphur dioxide	E220	sol	sol	sol	sol in chloroform, ether		ADI up to 700 micrograms/kg body-weight. Has antimicrobial properties
Thioglycerol		sol	sl sol			0.1–1.0	
Antoxidant synergists							
Citric acid	E330	sol	sol			0.005–0.01	Incompatible with potassium tartrate, alkali, acetates, and sulphites
Edetic acid (EDTA) and salts		sl sol				0.002–0.1	Incompatible with polyvalent metal ions. Chelates traces of metal ions, particularly copper, iron, and manganese[§]
Hydroxyquinoline sulphate		sol	sl sol				
Phosphoric acid	E338	sl sol	sl sol			0.005–0.01	
Sodium citrate	E331	sol	insol				
Tartaric acid	E334	sol	sol			0.01–0.02	

sol = soluble
sl sol = slightly soluble
insol = insoluble
ADI = Acceptable Daily Intake
*has antimicrobial activity, mainly against moulds and Gram-positive bacteria. Light and trace quantities of metals cause discoloration and loss of activity. Used to delay or prevent oxidative rancidity of fats and oils and to prevent loss of activity of oil-soluble vitamins.
[†]has antimicrobial activity. Refer to butylated hydroxyanisole for effect of light and trace quantities of metals, and uses.
[‡]ADI as for sulphur dioxide.
[§]may also exert a bacteriostatic effect by chelating trace metals necessary for growth.

preparations such as emulsions and suspensions. For example, the concentration of antoxidant in the oily phase of an emulsion depends upon the partition coefficient of the substance and upon the extent of solubilisation by the surfactant. In suspensions, the antoxidant may be adsorbed onto particles of the drug or may interact with the suspending agent.

Reduction in antoxidant effectiveness may also occur by sorption on to containers or closures, especially those made with components of plastics or rubber, or by interaction with substances leached from those materials.

Control of pH

Knowledge of the effects of pH on degradation rate enables the formulator to adjust or buffer the pH near that corresponding to maximum stability. Thus oxidation of adrenaline injection is minimised by use of the acid tartrate so that the pH (2.8 to 3.6) is close to the pH of maximum stability (3.2 to 3.4). Cyanocobalamin injection is adjusted to pH 4 with acetic acid or hydrochloric acid and is sufficiently stable to be sterilised by autoclaving. Buffers are sometimes employed; sodium phosphate (0.45%) and citric acid monohydrate (0.075%) are used in digoxin injection to buffer the solution to pH 7. However, formulation of a solution near the pH of maximum stability is not always possible because solubility, absorption by the tissues, efficacy, and irritant effects must also be considered. For example, weak alkaloidal bases such as homatropine used as eye drops are most stable in acidic solution (pH 3 to 4) but possess maximum therapeutic activity in the eye when applied in slightly alkaline solution because the free base has enhanced lipid solubility; irritant effects are minimised at pH 7.4. In such solutions it is often possible to select an intermediate pH (for example, pH 5) as a compromise to achieve adequate stability, efficacy and comfort to the patient. For those drugs that are sensitive to ionic strength (for example, ampicillin) or general acid-base catalysis (for example, chloramphenicol), special care should be taken in the adjustment of tonicity or pH to minimise the effects of added salts. When an increase in pH during storage is undesirable, aqueous solutions should be packed in bottles made of neutral glass (Type I) or surface-treated soda glass (Type II) rather than soda glass (Type III) from which alkali is leached.

Change of Solvent

The use of organic solvents in place of part or all of the water in an aqueous vehicle can enhance the stability of solutions of certain drugs. An injection of phenobarbitone sodium in a mixture of propylene glycol and water (9:1 v/v) can be sterilised by autoclaving, whereas an aqueous solution of the drug degrades appreciably. The polymerisation of formaldehyde in aqueous solution can be retarded by the addition of 10% to 15% (v/v) of methanol.

Control of Drug Concentration

Drug concentration in a medicine is usually determined by therapeutic considerations but it is sometimes possible to enhance stability by modifying the concentration. Where zero-order kinetics are followed, as in suspensions of sparingly soluble drugs such as aspirin, the $t_{10\%}$ can be prolonged by increasing the drug concentration although the concomitant increase in viscosity restricts the application of this approach. For ampicillin, dilute solutions are more stable than are concentrated solutions because of the complex kinetics of degradation.

Conversion to Sparingly Soluble Salts

It is sometimes possible to convert a relatively unstable, soluble drug to a sparingly soluble drug that can be formulated as a stable suspension; an example is procaine benzylpenicillin injection.

Formation of a Complex

Protection from degradation can sometimes be achieved by the formation of a complex; for example, the hydrolysis of procaine can be retarded by the addition of caffeine to form a water-soluble complex. In recent years, cyclodextrins have been used to enhance the stability of drugs by forming inclusion complexes (clathrates). Cyclodextrins (α-, β-, and γ-) are cyclic oligosaccharides whose structure is doughnut-shaped with a hydrophobic cavity in which drug molecules can be trapped; externally the ring formed by cyclodextrins is hydrophilic. The rate of oxidation of vitamin D_3 is reported to be reduced by complexing with β-cyclodextrin and the sensitivity to light of clofibrate is lowered by β- or γ-cyclodextrin. For hydrolysis and other reactions, the effects depend on the type of cyclodextrin, the chemistry of the drug and pH. The hydrolysis of aspirin at pH 1 is not affected by α-cyclodextrin since the cavity of the α-form is too small to accommodate the drug but β-cyclodextrin retards degradation appreciably since the aspirin molecule fits snugly in the cavity; γ-cyclodextrin retards degradation only moderately because aspirin fits loosely into the cavity so that there is a void into which a proton or molecule of water can easily penetrate. Inclusion complexation may result in greater degradation. In alkaline solution, the degradation of hydrocortisone is accelerated by β-cyclodextrin yet α- and γ-cyclodextrins do not influence the rate. Cyclodextrins can also affect physical stability, solubility, and bioavailability. Duchêne, Vaution and Glomot[8] have reviewed comprehensively the uses and value of cyclodextrins in pharmaceutical technology.

Control of Surfactant Concentration

In medicines such as emulsions it may be necessary to control surfactant concentrations to enhance the chemical stability of the active constituents.

Control of Peroxides

To minimise autoxidation especially of oils and fats care should be taken to use ingredients with concentrations of peroxides that are as low as possible.

Control of Heavy Metals

Where the drug or other ingredients are prone to degrade by oxidation the content of heavy metal ions should be kept as low as possible. Manufacturing equipment should be made of stainless steel, glass, or other materials from which heavy metal ions are not leached. Equipment made of cast iron or copper should be lined with suitable materials.

Control of Oxygen Content

To minimise oxidation, it may be sufficient to recommend storage of the substance or product in well-filled, airtight containers (for example, peppermint oil) or well-filled, well-closed containers (for example, calciferol oral solution). Some products (for example, promethazine injection) are required to be prepared with water for injections free from dissolved air; the water is boiled for at least 10 minutes with as little exposure to air as possible and cooled with precautions to exclude air. For ampoules and other sealed, single-dose containers the air can be displaced by oxygen-free nitrogen or other inert gas although complete removal of air is difficult. Carbon dioxide has been used since it is a heavy gas and does not escape from the container as easily as nitrogen; however, in some neutral or alkaline products, the use of carbon dioxide may result in an undesirable reduction in pH. The process of manufacture of viscous emulsions and creams should be devised to minimise entrapment of air.
The use of antioxidants in pharmaceutical preparations is covered above.

Control of Carbon Dioxide Content

Where instability of a product involves uptake of carbon dioxide, precautions should be taken to remove the gas as far as possible. Aminophylline injection is prepared in water for injections free from carbon dioxide; the water is boiled for at least 10 minutes as described above for the control of oxygen.

In contrast, carbon dioxide is passed through solutions of sodium bicarbonate before sterilisation to reduce decarboxylation to sodium carbonate.

Control of Water Content

Drugs for oral use (for example, many antibiotics) that are highly unstable in solution or suspension are often formulated as powder or granules for extemporaneous reconstitution with water. Similarly, unstable drugs for injection (for example, diamorphine hydrochloride) are presented as sterile powders so that solutions can be made immediately before administration. Protection against moisture during manufacture can be achieved by many approaches that include: lyophilisation of powders; dry compression processes; formulation of hard tablets; coating of tablets; microencapsulation with hydrophobic materials; and the use of excipients that do not readily take up water.

Stringent quality control of the water content of ingredients must be exercised where the dosage form is sensitive to moisture. Control of manufacturing and packaging is important; for example, lyophilised powders should be distributed into containers at a low relative humidity. The design and materials of packaging should be chosen to minimise the ingress of water vapour through the container and closure; sometimes a desiccant such as silica gel is enclosed in the package. Storage under dry conditions is an added safeguard for those products such as effervescent tablets that are highly sensitive to moisture.

Control of Temperature

Precise control of temperature and time of heat-sterilisation processes is especially important for thermolabile products (see Sterilisation chapter). Knowledge of the activation energies of both drug degradation and bacterial death can aid the choice of sterilisation temperature and time. For certain drugs (for example, procaine) where the activation energy of degradation is significantly lower than that of killing most thermally resistant bacteria, it may be preferable to sterilise solutions by autoclaving for a very short time at a very high temperature rather than by prolonged heat-ing at a lower temperature; by this means sterilisation can be achieved with minimal product degradation. The temperature of drying of heat-sensitive drug substances may have to be controlled carefully. Some medicines are required to be stored at a low temperature to prolong the shelf-life; for example, insulin injections that are stored at 2° to 8° may be expected to retain their potency for at least two years. Aqueous solutions such as intravenous infusions or eye drops that contain thermolabile drugs are sometimes frozen to enhance their stability. The physicochemical effects of freezing solutions are often complex and may not be predictable by simple application of the Arrhenius equation; such effects are considered in the section on Stability of Medicines in Pharmaceutical Practice.

Protection from Light

Medicinal products that are sensitive to light are usually protected from light by suitable packaging. Coloured glass or opaque plastic containers are commonly used. The proportion of light transmitted depends on the nature and thickness of the material used to make the container; amber containers are commonly employed since little light is transmitted at wavelengths below 400 nm. Coloured containers may be unsuitable for clear solutions for injection because of the difficulty in detecting discoloration or precipitation. An alternative method is to wrap clear containers in a suitable light-resistant material such as a coloured plastic film which contains a substance that absorbs ultraviolet light; packaging clear containers in light-resistant cartons is another approach. Protection from light can also be conferred by skilful formulation, for example, by coating tablets with an opaque material or using opaque shells for capsules.

Control of Ionising Radiation

A minimum absorbed dose of 25 kGy is used for the sterilisation of some materials. Where this dose causes unacceptable degradation it may be possible to use a lower dose of radiation provided that appropriate microbiological tests are done to validate the sterilisation process.

Control of Mechanical Processes

Where grinding promotes chemical degradation the process can be avoided by using wet granulation provided that the solvent does not induce polymorphic changes in the drug. Encapsulating the drug rather than making tablets is sometimes preferable.

PHYSICAL STABILITY

Many medicinal products are complex physico-chemical systems that may be subject to a diverse variety of physical changes during the period from preparation to administration. Like reactions that cause chemical degradation, physical reactions may result in diminished bioavailability and efficacy or may adversely affect other properties such as dispersibility, acceptability to the patient and convenience for use. This section includes examples of physical reactions that are commonly encountered in medicines; factors that affect stability; and methods of avoiding or minimising physical reactions.

Physical interactions between drugs or excipients and packaging materials are discussed in the chapter on Incompatibility.

Volatility of Constituents

Drugs, solvents, and excipients with high vapour pressure can be lost from medicinal products during manufacture and storage. Some drugs are used largely because of their volatility; for example, menthol, benzoin, and eucalyptus oil are ingredients of inhalations. Such drugs and products should be kept in well-closed or airtight containers to avoid loss of active constituent.

The volatility of glyceryl trinitrate is clinically important since tablets of this drug lose potency rapidly at elevated temperatures especially if packed in loosely closed containers or in contact with plastics or cotton wool. The ways in which pharmacists can minimise the loss of glyceryl trinitrate are discussed in the section on the Stability of Medicines in Pharmaceutical Practice.

Occasionally, a degradation product in tablets (for example, salicylic acid in aspirin tablets) may sublime and appear as a deposit on the tablet surface or on the walls of the container. In recent years, cyclodextrins have been used to reduce the volatility of drugs by the formation of inclusion complexes.[8] An example is the preparation of a complex of isosorbide mononitrate with β-cyclodextrin to prevent the formation of needles of the volatile drug on the surface of tablets during storage as well as to reduce chemical degradation. Volatility of ethanol used as a solvent in a solution of morphine and opium alkaloids has led to a potentially hazardous concentration of the preparation especially in poorly closed, partly-filled containers kept in a dry warm place. Loss of water by evaporation from aqueous solutions in warm dry conditions may result in crystallisation of the drug or excipients. Similarly creams may lose water and form a skin on the surface; the emulsion may crack. Chloroform, a volatile antimicrobial preservative, is widely used as a 0.25% aqueous solution in oral liquids. Although little chloroform is lost from mixtures in well-filled, unopened bottles, greater losses may occur from opened stock solutions; this problem is discussed further in the section on Stability of Medicines in Pharmaceutical Practice.

Changes in the Water Content of Solids

Water can be sorbed on many solid drugs, excipients, and medicinal products. In many substances water is bound rather than unbound. Bound water interacts physically with the solid and its equilibrium vapour pressure is less than that of unbound water; bound water may be entrapped in pores or may be molecularly bound to form a crystalline hydrate. Isotherms for the sorption of water on solids are discussed by Stewart and Tucker.[12] Many materials (for example, glycerol, sodium cromoglycate, dry extracts) are hygroscopic, that is they gain (or lose) water in accordance with the relative humidity; some (for example, potassium hydroxide) are deliquescent, that is they take up water and dissolve. In contrast, some salts (for example, sodium sulphate) are efflorescent; their tendency to lose water to form a lower hydrate or the anhydrous salt depends on relative humidity and temperature. Information on the effects of relative humidity on the equilibrium moisture content of excipients is given in the *Handbook of Pharmaceutical Excipients*;[13] moisture sorption-desorption isotherms are included for some materials.

Storage of hard gelatin capsules at a high relative humidity may result in the capsules becoming sticky and distorted due to a loss in mechanical strength. In very dry conditions water is desorbed from the capsule shells, which shrink and become brittle.

In filled capsules, moisture may be transferred from the shell to its contents if the drug or excipients are hygroscopic. Such moisture transfer could result in chemical degradation, formation of hydrates, or the production of a hard cement-like mass from which the drug would be only slowly released after administration; thus bioavailability could be reduced. Soft capsules are especially sensitive to conditions of relative humidity greater than 60% since irreversible softening may occur; the capsules may also become tacky and bloated. The uptake or loss of water from some solid dosage forms can result in undesirable changes in properties such as tablet hardness, disintegration time, dissolution rate, bioavailability, and efficacy. Dry powders and granules may become aggregated to form a cake. Special care should be taken in the formulation and development of these products to minimise such changes.

Sorption

Sorption of drugs or excipients such as antimicrobial preservatives from solution on to solid drug particles, containers, or closures is discussed in the chapter on Incompatibility.

Changes in Crystal Properties

Changes in crystal form, habit, and size of a solid can affect not only the physical properties of a medicine but also its bioavailability.

Crystal Form

Some drugs (for example, cortisone acetate, chloramphenicol palmitate, and riboflavine) can exist in several crystal forms or polymorphs, which represent different arrangements of molecules within the crystal lattice; although chemically identical, polymorphs differ in physical properties because of differences in free energy. At a given temperature and pressure in a particular solvent, only one form is thermodynamically stable; other metastable forms tend to be converted to the stable form. Metastable forms have higher free energies, higher solubilities and dissolution rates and lower melting points than have the thermodynamically stable form. Amorphous forms exist for some substances (for example, digoxin and novobiocin) in which there is no ordered arrangement of molecules. Other drugs (for example, tertiary butyl esters of prednisolone) can be crystallised as a solvate from ethanol or other organic solvent. Many substances (for example, ampicillin and theophylline) can form hydrates.

Conversion of a metastable form to the stable form of a drug usually occurs more rapidly in suspensions than in solid dosage forms and is often associated with crystal growth (for example, cortisone acetate), which may lead to caking of the suspended particles.

Effects of crystal growth and polymorphic changes in suspensions during storage may be appreciable. Identification of the different forms of a drug is therefore crucial in the formulation of a product. Conversion of amorphous novobiocin to the less soluble and poorly absorbed crystalline form results in a considerable reduction in bioavailability. For these suspensions, judicious choice of solvent and manufacturing process is desirable to ensure that the intended bioavailability is achieved. Stringent quality control is required. For chloramphenicol palmitate oral suspension, for example, the method of manufacture must ensure that the content of polymorph A, which is biologically inactive, is within the pharmacopoeial limit. Large fluctuations in storage temperature should be avoided to minimise changes in crystal form of a drug.

Polymorphic changes can also occur during mechanical treatment of solid drugs. For example, grinding phenylbutazone at high amplitude in a vibratory ball mill or compressing it into tablets at high pressure can cause polymorphic changes. Grinding crystalline digoxin may result in conversion to the amorphous form which has a higher dissolution rate and biological activity. Care should be taken in the development of a manufacturing process for a solid dosage form to avoid adverse changes in crystal form of the active constituent.

Crystal Habit

The same crystal form of a substance may exist in different habits or external shapes; examples are the prismatic, tabular, and isometric habits of an orthorhombic crystal form. Changes in habit in a suspension can affect physical properties such as dissolution rate and the ability to flow through a syringe needle. Sound knowledge of possible changes in crystal habit of the drug is important in the formulation of a suspension. Large fluctuations in storage temperature should be avoided where habit changes are likely to occur.

Crystal Growth

Crystals of a drug, for example nitrofurantoin, may grow in suspension because of temperature fluctuations; dissolution of small crystals occurs when the temperature is raised followed by deposition on to large crystals during cooling. Even at constant temperature crystal growth may occur in suspensions of drugs such as corticosteroids that contain very small particles (<1 micrometre). Because such tiny crystals have a higher solubility they dissolve in water but deposit on the larger crystals. Growth may be associated with polymorphic changes (for example, cortisone acetate).

Crystal growth can be minimised by addition of surfactants or polymers in low concentration, by use of a narrow size range of particles, by increasing viscosity of the vehicle and by avoiding large fluctuations in the temperature of storage.

Crystallisation from Solution

Crystals of a drug may be deposited from solutions because of a fall in temperature or a change in pH. Supersaturated solutions are especially likely to deposit crystals. Calcium gluconate injection contains 20% w/v of the drug; it is a supersaturated solution but is relatively stable at 20° unless particles (for example, dust) are present to act as nuclei for crystallisation. A stabiliser such as calcium D-saccharate is used to reduce the risk of crystallisation of calcium gluconate.

Precipitation in Galenicals

Inert matter derived from the contents of plant cells may coagulate in galenicals such as liquid extracts and tinctures; this precipitation is often known as 'pitching'. In manufacturing practice such preparations may be stored for several months before filtration to remove the precipitate. Traditional mixtures that contain galenicals may form precipitates if kept for more than a few weeks; these mixtures are intended to be recently prepared.

Physical Changes in Emulsions

The physical instability of emulsions occurs in four main forms: flocculation where the dispersed globules aggregate to form clumps but where the interfacial film is not broken; 'cracking' where the globules coalesce because of rupture of the interfacial film; 'creaming' where the globules move towards the surface of the product; and sedimentation where the movement of globules is downwards. These changes are often accompanied by changes in viscosity of the emulsion. A reduction in viscosity is sometimes caused by degradation of polymers such as cellulose derivatives used as emulsifying agents. Adverse physical changes in emulsions can be avoided only by careful formulation especially in the choice of emulsifying agent to reduce the interfacial tension between the oily and aqueous phases and to form a strong mechanical film at the interface. For further information see the Emulsions chapter.

Physical Changes in Suspensions

The physical state of particles of a solid drug in suspension in a liquid depends largely on the magnitude of the opposing forces of attraction and repulsion; attraction between particles occurs because of relatively weak London-van der Waals forces whereas repulsion is caused by the electrical double layer that surrounds each particle. If the forces of repulsion are greater than those of attraction, the suspension is deflocculated, that is, each particle settles slowly and individually to form a sediment; sometimes in a compact sediment the particles may aggregate to form an indispersible cake. In contrast, if attractive forces predominate, the particles come together to form loose flocculate that settle rapidly to produce a readily dispersed sediment; the suspension is said to be flocculated. In the formulation of pharmaceutical suspensions, the degree of flocculation should be controlled to avoid the extremes of caking and too rapid sedimentation by the addition of low concentrations of electrolytes, surfactants, polymers, or a combination of these agents; polymers in higher concentration can be used to enhance viscosity of the preparation. Other stability problems that are associated with crystal form, habit, and growth in suspensions are discussed under Changes in Crystal Properties above.

Other Physical Changes

Signs of other physical changes in dosage forms may be observed. In some instances, the changes may be affected by more than one factor (for example, mechanical treatment, water, and temperature) and the cause is not always precisely known. Examples are given of physical signs that are commonly encountered in dispensed medicinal products. Such physical changes can be avoided by special care in formulation.

Semi-solids

Ointments, creams, and pastes may soften, harden, or become granular or gritty during storage. Syneresis (separation of liquid) may occur in both aqueous and non-aqueous gels because of elastic contraction of the polymeric molecules of the gelling agent. Suppositories and pessaries may soften, harden, or shrivel; oil stains may appear on packaging material.

Uncoated Tablets

Tablets may crumble or break especially during packaging or transport to produce powder or pieces at the bottom of the container; cracks or chips may be evident in tablet surfaces. Changes in hardness, disintegration rate, or dissolution rate may occur. A mottled appearance in coloured tablets may be caused during manufacture by intragranular migration of the dye during wet granulation. After drying, the granules have a colourless core surrounded by an intensely coloured outer zone; compression of the granules results in granule fracture so that coloured fragments can be seen against a colourless background to give a mottled appearance.

Coated Tablets

Signs of physical changes during manufacture include clumping of film-coated tablets where inadequate drying of the coat results in a tacky tablet that sticks to neighbouring tablets. Similarly inadequate drying of sugar-coated tablets can lead to blotchiness. The coating on tablets may crack under tropical conditions or by abrasion during transport.

MICROBIOLOGICAL STABILITY

Many liquid medicines can support the growth of micro-organisms. Aqueous preparations such as solutions, suspensions and oil-in-water emulsions are especially susceptible to microbial growth; in water-in-oil emulsions proliferation is more difficult because the oily continuous phase impedes the spread of micro-organisms. Growth may also occur in those tablets and other solid dosage forms that contain some water.

Contamination of products with bacteria, moulds or yeasts may occur during manufacture, dispensing, storage or use and may be derived from water and from drug substances or excipients, particularly those of natural origin; other sources include packaging materials, premises, equipment, clothing, workers, and the atmosphere.

Proliferation of micro-organisms in medicinal products is unacceptable for two reasons. First, the presence of pathogenic bacteria, moulds, yeasts or endotoxins can be hazardous to the patient particularly in solutions or emulsions administered by intravenous infusion or in solutions introduced into the anterior chamber of the eye during surgical procedures. Second, contamination with non-pathogenic micro-organisms can result in spoilage of the product.

This section includes: a short account of the effects of growth of pathogenic micro-organisms; a brief description of the spoilage of products by micro-organisms; a summary of the use of antimicrobial preservatives and other means by which microbial growth can be controlled.

More detailed information on factors that affect the growth of micro-organisms and on the properties and uses of antimicrobial preservatives is included in the chapters on Control of Microbial Contamination and the Preservation of Medicines.

Effects of Growth of Pathogenic Micro-organisms

Pathogenic bacteria include *Pseudomonas aeruginosa, Staphylococcus aureus, Escherichia coli*, and various species of *Salmonella*. Other pathogens that may contaminate medicinal products are *Candida albicans* (a yeast) and various species of *Aspergillus* (moulds).

Acute systemic infections and deaths have resulted from the use of intravenous infusions contaminated with micro-organisms. Fortunately, such serious cases are rare but local infections near the site of infusion have occurred. Causes of infection include inadequate control of autoclaves and contamination during infusion of the solution. The addition of drugs to intravenous infusions is associated with a higher risk of contamination especially where drugs are added in the hospital ward rather than under strict aseptic conditions. The presence in intravenous infusions of pyrogenic substances (usually lipopolysaccharides) released from Gram-negative bacteria can cause not only an appreciable rise in body temperature but also acute discomfort, pain, and erythema at the site of infusion.

The use of ophthalmic solutions contaminated with *Pseudomonas aeruginosa* has resulted in severe infections in abraded or damaged eyes; rapid spread of infection after surgery has led to loss of sight. Particularly hazardous is the introduction of contaminated solutions into the anterior chamber of the eye. Fluorescein sodium eye drops, used as a diagnostic agent in ophthalmology, readily support the growth of pathogenic pseudomonads so that the use of multidose containers for this preparation is unacceptable.

In dermatological wards, the application of creams or ointments contaminated with *Pseudomonas aeruginosa* is reported to have caused serious skin infections in a number of patients receiving treatment for psoriasis and other diseases; poor preservation, the use of contaminated ointment jars, and the application of the product to more than one patient have been suggested as possible causes.

Infections of the urinary tract have resulted from irrigation using contaminated solutions. The presence of *Aspergillus* species in solutions instilled in the ear constitutes a risk to patients with perforated ear drums.

The contamination of aqueous mixtures and other oral preparations with opportunist pathogens such as *Pseudomonas aeruginosa* is unlikely to cause severe infections except in patients who are seriously debilitated. With acute pathogens such as *Salmonella* species, however, oral administration of contaminated products may give rise to severe infection. *Salmonella* infections have been reported following oral ingestion of contaminated carmine capsules used as a 'marker' in metabolism tests. The use of defatted thyroid powder in tablets has led to salmonellosis in Sweden.

Spoilage due to Growth of Micro-organisms

The presence of low levels of microbial contamination may not be detectable but proliferation often results in spoilage of medicinal products. An early sign of spoilage may be microbial growth on the surface of a liquid or cream or on the condensed film of moisture on the surface of a solid product or on a lid. Evidence of growth may be manifested as turbidity, discoloration, development of unpleasant odours, gas formation, loss in viscosity, or formation of a slime ('ropiness'). In oil-in-water creams and emulsions, micro-organisms would proliferate rapidly unless an effective antimicrobial preservative is present; the surfactant, especially if nonionic, may be subject to microbial attack and the emulsified preparation may separate into its oil and water phases or become gritty or lumpy.

Degradation of drugs may occur because of microbial growth; for example, a batch of atropine sulphate eye drops lost much of its antimuscarinic activity. Similarly aspirin, paracetamol, benzylpenicillin and chloramphenicol can be metabolised by certain micro-organisms. Fungi growing on the surface of tablets or creams containing hydrocortisone and other corticosteroids may cause decomposition of the drug.

Excipients often act as growth media. Polymers such as starches, carmellose sodium, tragacanth, pectin, and dextran are subject to depolymerisation by extracellular enzymes in micro-organisms. Oils and fats may be attacked by lipolytic fungi. Although concentrated sugar solutions are unlikely to support the growth of most micro-organisms because of the low water activity of syrups, osmophilic yeasts (for example, *Zygosaccharomyces rouxii*) may proliferate; growth of other micro-organisms may occur later to cause gross spoilage. Peppermint water is a good growth medium for some bacteria (including pseudomonads) and yeasts. The methyl and propyl esters of 4-hydroxybenzoic acid are commonly employed as antimicrobial preservatives but at relatively low concentrations (such as formerly used in eye drops) may be metabolised by bacteria such as pseudomonads.

Crude drugs and excipients of natural origin (for example, digitalis, tragacanth, and kaolin) may be contaminated with micro-organisms and thus may contaminate preparations. During storage, Gram-negative bacteria (for example, pseudomonads) can multiply rapidly in distilled water in which there is sufficient nutrient for growth; water purified by passage through ion-exchange resins is even more prone to bacterial multiplication.

Factors that affect spoilage include the physicochemical nature of the medicine, the inoculum size and species of micro-organisms present, the moisture content, and the redox potential. In general, bacteria grow best in solutions at pH 6 to 8 whereas most moulds and yeasts proliferate in more acidic preparations (pH 4 to 6).

Nevertheless, some species of bacteria, moulds, and yeasts proliferate at pH values outside these ranges; for example, species of *Aspergillus* can grow at pH 1.5 to 2.0. Many but not all bacteria grow best at 35° to 40° but can survive over a wide range of temperature; in contrast, moulds and yeasts generally show optimum growth at 20° to 30°.

Control of Microbial Contamination and Growth

Several approaches are usually necessary to stop or restrict the contamination and growth of micro-organisms in medicinal products; methods must be based on knowledge of the likely sources of contamination and the factors that affect growth. For a particular medicine, the clinical need for sterility or for limitation of the level of micro-organisms must be carefully assessed particularly in relation to the route of administration. Approaches may involve: care in formulation especially in choice of ingredients and packaging; selection of processes of manufacture including sterilisation where appropriate; good manufacturing practice; and recommendations for storage.

Formulation and Packaging

Where possible, excipients that are likely to be contaminated with micro-organisms should be avoided. For example, attempts should be made to formulate suspensions with a cellulose derivative rather than tragacanth as suspending agent; synthetic flavours are preferable to fruit syrups in this respect. However, other physicochemical properties of the formulated preparation must be taken into consideration in deciding whether to include an excipient that may be contaminated. Choice of packaging may also be important; in particular, multidose containers and closures (for example, for eye drops) should be designed to minimise contamination of the product in use.

Addition of Antimicrobial Preservatives

Antimicrobial preservatives are substances that are added to kill or inhibit the growth of micro-organisms in medicines. Preservatives must never be used to mask contamination that arises from unsatisfactory manufacturing procedures or inadequate packaging.

Medicines that require an antimicrobial preservative can be placed into two categories. The first category includes those injections, eye drops, eye ointments, irrigation solutions, preparations for application to wounds (including some creams), and any other medicines that are required to be supplied or dispensed as sterile products in multi-dose containers. The function of an antimicrobial preservative in these sterile products is to maintain sterility to ensure safety in use. The second category comprises preparations that are not supplied or dispensed as sterile products and includes many liquid and semi-solid preparations that are administered by mouth, applied to the skin or instilled into the ear. Traditionally, preservatives have been added to these non-sterile preparations primarily to minimise proliferation of micro-organisms that may cause spoilage. However, it is also important that preservatives should kill pathogenic micro-organisms, which may contaminate such preparations during storage and use.

An ideal antimicrobial preservative for a particular medicine should be rapidly effective in low concentration against a variety of bacteria, moulds, and yeasts over a wide range of pH and temperature. It should be readily soluble in the vehicle, chemically and physically stable, devoid of toxic and irritant effects, colourless, and free from an objectionable odour and taste; it should also be compatible with the drug and other constituents and with the materials used to fabricate the container and closure. No preservative fully meets these criteria.

The choice of preservative for a particular medicine depends on: the route, dose and frequency of administration; the physicochemical properties of the preservative, drug and other constituents; and the nature of the packaging materials. Incompatibility problems associated with antimicrobial preservatives especially in polyphasic preparations are discussed in the chapter on Incompatibility. Information on the properties of different preservatives is given in the chapter on Control of Microbial Contamination and the Preservation of Medicines; suitable tests and specifications for the efficacy of antimicrobial preservatives are also discussed.

Good Manufacturing Practice

It is essential that adequate precautions be taken in the manufacture and packaging of medicines to minimise the access of micro-organisms. Raw materials, especially those of natural origin, may need to be treated to remove or reduce the microbial load without adversely affecting their properties. Good manufacturing practice also embraces control of the atmosphere and careful design of premises and equipment. Strict control of contamination during manufacture is essential; measures include the provision of suitable protective clothing and appropriate education for all staff engaged in the manufacture of medicines. Inspection of materials, processes, packaging, and the final product must be rigorously enforced. In dispensing practice, pharmacists should inspect medicines thoroughly for evidence of microbial growth; for sterile products special care should be taken to confirm the integrity of seal of the container.

Storage Conditions

In general, microbial growth in medicines can be minimised by avoiding storage in warm places although the bactericidal activity of preservatives usually increases with a rise in temperature.

STABILITY TESTS

Tests on the chemical, physical, or microbiological stability of a drug substance, excipient, or formulated medicine involve the application of a suitable stress or challenge over a period of time and the assessment of the effects of that stress on a particular chemical, physical, or microbiological property at appropriate intervals. Examples of commonly used stresses are temperature, light, relative humidity, gravity and micro-organisms. The choice of stress is based on the physicochemical nature of the substance or medicinal product and the conditions that are likely to be encountered during transport, storage, and use. For some medicinal products it may be necessary to determine the effects of a number of stresses. Some effects can be assessed by observation of changes in properties such as colour, odour, taste, clarity, degree of flocculation, dispersibility, or microbial growth. Wherever possible, however, changes in properties are determined quantitatively. Examples of determinations are: content of drug; content of a degradation product; sediment volume of a suspension; reflectance of a tablet surface; dissolution rate of a tablet; yield value of a gel; globule-size distribution in an emulsion; and rate of kill of suitable micro-organisms by an antimicrobial preservative. Special care should be taken in the choice of methods for measuring chemical, physical and microbiological changes since quantitative stability tests and the prediction of shelf-life depend on the use of accurate, precise, and sensitive techniques. In chemical stability tests, it is particularly important to devise a 'stability-indicating' assay; that is, the assay must be specific for the drug in the presence of degradation products, impurities, and any other substances present.

High performance liquid chromatography is now widely used in stability-indicating assays where the extent of degradation is low (for example, less than 10%), and it is often preferable to determine the increase in concentration of a degradation product since the increase in concentration is very large compared with the small decrease in concentration of the drug. Determination of degradation products is desirable where highly toxic substances are formed on storage.

Three principal types of stability tests are described in this section: long-term storage tests; 'field' tests; and accelerated tests. The principles, methods, and limitations of accelerated stability tests are considered in detail. In addition, a short account is given of the application of stability tests at different stages in the development and marketing of a medicine.

Long-term Stability Tests

These are stability tests that are conducted in the laboratory under controlled stresses similar to those likely to be encountered during storage. Typical stresses are 25° at 75% relative humidity to represent temperate conditions and 38° at 90% relative humidity to represent tropical conditions. In practice, of course, fluctuations occur in the conditions of storage; for this reason, stability tests are sometimes carried out where the temperature or the relative humidity or both are programmed to rise and fall in a regular sinusoidal cycle. Carstensen and Rhodes[14] suggest that if the mean loss of drug after the expiry date (for example, three years) at a constant temperature (25°) is m%, then cyclic storage at $25° \pm 5°$ will result in a loss of 1.1 m%; it is assumed that the Arrhenius plot is linear over the range 20° to 30° and that the activation energy of the degradation reaction is within the range (60 to 120 kJ/mol) usually encountered in liquid medicines.

Field Tests

In 'field' tests, the packaged medicinal product is sent by various means of transport (for example, aircraft, ship, and lorry) to the countries in which it is to be sold; it is stored in a warehouse, trans-

ferred to a typical pharmacy, and then returned to the manufacturer's laboratory for examination and analysis. Such realistic tests provide information of value since the conditions are those encountered when the product is marketed.

Accelerated Stability Tests

In accelerated stability tests, the substance or medicinal product is challenged by a controlled, exaggerated stress over a short time so that the rate of reaction is enhanced. Since results are obtained relatively rapidly, accelerated tests are of particular value in providing information on stability to the formulator in the early stages of product development.

Accelerated Chemical Stability Tests

Examples of exaggerated stresses used in accelerated chemical tests are elevated temperature, high intensity of light, high partial pressure of oxygen, and high relative humidity.

Tests at Elevated Temperature. Two types of test are used. In the traditional application of this accelerated test by the **isothermal** approach, a series of experiments is carried out at a number of elevated temperatures. The rate constant is determined at each temperature and the linear form of the Arrhenius equation applied to the results. In the section on Chemical Kinetics, the following equation is quoted:

$$\log k_T = \log A - \frac{E_a}{2.303RT}$$

Thus from a graph (see Fig.3) of the logarithm of the rate constant against the reciprocal of absolute temperature, the pre-exponential factor (A) and the energy of activation (E_a) can be calculated and the rate constant (k_T) at a particular storage temperature (for example, 25°) can be predicted.

Careful design of experiments is important especially in the selection of elevated temperatures and the sampling intervals. In practice, at least four elevated temperatures (for example, 40°, 50°, 60°, and 70°) are chosen and several replicate experiments are conducted at each temperature.

The line of best fit (the regression line) of the data when plotted in accordance with the linear form of the Arrhenius equation can be calculated by the method of least squares. In practice, however, it is highly unlikely that the estimates of log k at different temperatures will be known with equal precision; sometimes the reproducibility gets worse as degradation proceeds. To overcome this problem the values of log k can be weighted in inverse proportion to their variance. Limits of confidence of the predicted rate constant at a particular temperature can then be calculated from the weighted Arrhenius plot. The mathematical interpretation of stability data using kinetic models of degradation has been well documented in a review of the evaluation of drug stability by Ferguson.[15] The effects of errors in the assay and in the measurement of temperature have been examined statistically by Davies and Budgett.[16]

The **non-isothermal** approach is also based on the Arrhenius equation; in place of a series of experiments at different temperatures there is a single experiment in which the temperature is made to rise in accordance with a pre-determined programme. An example is the method of Rogers[17] in which the reciprocal of temperature varies logarithmically with time. The increasing availability of computer-controlled equipment to enable precise programming of temperature to be achieved together with the ready availability of computers for calculations of stability parameters may result in enhanced use of these less time-consuming non-isothermal methods. In a comprehensive review of non-isothermal stability testing, Tucker[18] commented that such methods have been applied mainly to solutions and suggests that their application to heterogeneous liquids and to solid dosage forms should be further explored.

The uses and limitations of **tests at elevated temperatures** require consideration. The Arrhenius equation represents a simplification of a complex relationship and is not strictly correct; the Arrhenius frequency factor (A) is certainly not independent of temperature and the activation energy (E_a) may not necessarily be independent of temperature. Nevertheless, within the relatively small range of temperatures used in the stability testing of drugs and medicines, errors in the application of the Arrhenius equation are usually negligible provided that there is no change in the reaction mechanism. Such changes are observed with peptides in biological products; hydrolysis and oxidation tend to take place at lower temperatures whereas at higher temperature denaturation occurs.

Application of the Arrhenius equation is most suitable for substances in aqueous solution at constant pH and where the activation energy of the reaction is about 60 to 120 kJ/mol. Accelerated temperature tests are of little value for photolytic reactions in which the activation energy is low (typically 8 to 12 kJ/mol) since temperature has very little effect on reaction rate, or pyrolytic reactions (activation energy 200 to 300 kJ/mol) where the degradation rate is high at elevated temperatures but negligible at room temperature.

Examples of causes of deviations from the Arrhenius equation are: pH changes during degradation; changes in the solubility of a drug with temperature; and loss of oxygen at elevated temperatures. The stability of a drug in frozen solutions is often difficult to predict from the results of tests at elevated temperatures (see section on Stability of Medicines in Pharmaceutical Practice). Although the kinetics of degradation of drugs in solid dosage forms are usually complex it is often possible to apply the Arrhenius equation to the results of stability experiments at elevated temperatures. In some instances, however, the limits of confidence of a predicted rate constant may be much wider than those for the rate constant of a drug in aqueous solution at constant pH; for example, moisture loss from tablets or capsules at higher temperatures may lead to deviations from the Arrhenius equation.

In some solid dosage forms degradation may approach an equilibrium rather than proceed to completion. In such instances, stability prediction may be better accomplished by application of the Van't Hoff equation rather than the Arrhenius equation; this was shown by Carstensen, Johnson, Spera, and Frank[19] for vitamin A acetate or vitamin E succinate in lactose-base tablets. In the Van't Hoff approach, the logarithm of the equilibrium constant is plotted against the reciprocal of absolute temperature; the logarithm of the equilibrium constant at a particular storage temperature is calculated from the slope of the graph.

Tests at High Intensity of Light. Artificial light of high intensity can be used to accelerate photochemical reactions in drugs and medicinal products. The energy distribution of the light source should resemble that of sunlight; Lachman, Swartz, and Cooper[20] reported that daylight fluorescent tubes are suitable for this purpose. Very high intensities of light from a xenon lamp are used sometimes in photochemical studies.

In practice, the photochemical efficiency or quantum yield (the ratio of number of molecules that react per unit volume in unit time to the number of photons absorbed) is usually less than unity. Light may be absorbed by excipients or packaging and may not penetrate to drug molecules below the surface of solid preparations. The relationship between light intensity and rate of reaction depends on the composition of the particular formulated product and its packaging. Another problem is defining the flux of light that would be expected to reach the preparation during storage. For these reasons, precise prediction of the stability of a product to light is very difficult to achieve from accelerated tests. The value of light testing is questionable where the product in its container is to be packed in a light-resistant carton. Such tests are of particular value, however, in preformulation studies and in the early stages of product development especially in comparative tests on the light stability of different formulations.

Tests at a High Partial Pressure of Oxygen. Accelerated tests using high partial pressures of oxygen can provide useful information to the formulator in the early stages of product development. Where the rate of oxidation is directly proportional to the partial pressure of the gas, accelerated tests can be used to predict stability under the expected conditions of storage. However, precise prediction is usually difficult because of uncertainty about the access of oxygen to the drug or medicine under the usual storage conditions. The presence of an antoxidant that simply acts by removing oxygen until the antoxidant is used up can make valid prediction of the shelf-life unrealistic.

Tests at High Relative Humidity. The principal use of accelerated tests at high relative humidities is to aid the selection of suitable packaging for moisture-sensitive, solid dosage forms. Such accelerated tests can only be of value in the prediction of shelf-life if the relationship between relative humidity and degradation rate for the preparation is known in detail; the relationship is usually complex. An example of quantitative prediction is a study of the stability of a dispersion of nitrazepam in microcrystalline cellulose by Genton and Kesselring[21] who used an empirical regression equation to establish a relationship between relative humidity, temperature, and the rate constant.

Accelerated Physical Tests

It is not usually possible to apply general methods to accelerated physical tests because of the diversity of physical reactions in different preparations. Experiments have to be designed for particular products by consideration of their physical properties, the stresses likely to be encountered during transport, storage and use, and the physical effects of those stresses. In most instances, the relationship between the magnitude of the stress and the effect will not be known although an empirical relationship can sometimes be derived for a particular product. It is usually assumed that if negligible physical effects occur after the application of an exaggerated stress then the product will be physically stable. Examples are given to illustrate how accelerated physical tests can be applied to medicines.

Accelerated Tests on Emulsions. The physical stability of emulsions can be assessed by various means including measurements of globule size, viscosity, dielectric properties, and the volumes of the disperse and continuous phases. Elevated temperatures (for example, 45° to 70°) can be used as an exaggerated stress to accelerate creaming or cracking of the emulsion and, for most emulsions, to decrease viscosity; however, emulsions made with methylcellulose become thicker as the temperature is raised. Misleading results may be obtained from accelerated tests; the emulsion may crack rapidly at elevated temperatures but be stable for prolonged periods at room temperature. Another accelerated test is to cycle the temperature between extremes that represent greater fluctuations than normal; the number of freeze-thaw cycles a product can withstand under specified conditions has been used as an index of emulsion stability.

The effects of gravity can be greatly exaggerated by centrifuging emulsions to accelerate the rate of creaming, but the results of such tests should be interpreted with caution. For example, an emulsion made from oil and aqueous phases that differ appreciably in density might be highly stable under normal conditions yet would cream rapidly when centrifuged at high speed. Groves[22] has presented a useful review of the accelerated stability testing of emulsions.

Accelerated Tests on Suspensions. Methods for assessing the physical stability of suspensions include measurements of sedimentation rate; the ratio of final sediment volume (or height) to the original volume (or height) of the suspension; ease of redispersion of the sediment; rheological properties; and size distribution of the dispersed particles. Centrifuging at a force several hundred times that of gravity (*g*) has been used as an exaggerated stress to enhance the sedimentation rate but such treatment may break down the structure of flocculated suspensions to yield an indispersible sediment; this effect would not occur under gravity even on prolonged storage. However, low-speed centrifuging at 4*g* can be a useful stress in comparing the stability of some suspensions.

Experiments at elevated temperatures have limited value; in contrast, tests in which fluctuations in temperature are applied to suspensions at a greatly increased frequency are useful in accelerating crystal growth. The lines of approach and limitations of accelerated tests on the physical stability of suspensions and other products are discussed in a review by Carless.[23]

Accelerated Tests on Tablets. The physical stability of tablets can be assessed by a variety of measurements which include: reflectance, colour, moisture uptake, friability, disintegration time, dissolution rate, hardness, tensile strength, and crushing strength. High relative humidities (for example, 75%) or elevated temperatures (for example, 45°) are commonly used as exaggerated stresses. Such accelerated tests are useful in comparisons of the physical stability of tablets made to different formulations or kept in different packaging.

Various experiments have been designed to enable the physical stability of tablets during storage to be predicted. For example, Amidon and Middleton[24] have used a physical model to predict the moisture uptake and crushing strength of tablets in various blister packs kept at constant or fluctuating relative humidities.

Accelerated Microbiological Tests

In general, challenge tests to determine the efficacy of an antimicrobial preservative in a product are conducted under conditions that are intended to simulate those encountered during storage and use. However, tests in which a cream packed in a jar is kept at rapidly fluctuating temperatures can be considered to be accelerated; under such conditions, a film of water containing little or no preservative may be formed on the surface so that microbial growth may occur readily. Similarly challenge by a very high inoculum of a highly resistant micro-organism could represent an exaggerated stress.

Stability Tests During Product Development and Marketing

Stability tests must be conducted at different stages in the development and marketing of a medicinal product. The primary aim of a programme of tests must be assurance of the quality of the product in respect of efficacy and safety. It is important to define precisely the objectives of the tests at each stage and to design each test with great care to meet those objectives. For each stage Cartwright[25] has indicated minimum requirements for stability

data presented for licensing in the United Kingdom; in addition, he has considered the design of stability studies and has drawn attention to the need for data on the stability of products that are required to be diluted by the pharmacist before issue to the patient or hospital ward. Guidance on the objectives and design of protocols for the evaluation of stability is given by Hill and Khan;[26] particular attention is drawn to tests on relatively unstable drugs. Stewart and Tucker[27] have also reviewed procedures used in stability tests. A review by Ferguson[15] on the evaluation of drug stability considers requirements in the USA and includes useful guidelines for stability testing together with sound advice on mathematical methods for interpretation of data. Factorial design experiments are often of value in stability testing where different factors may interact; for example, the effects of temperature and relative humidity on the chemical stability of a drug in tablets can be evaluated from the results of experiments in which both factors are varied.

It is essential that manufacturers obtain guidance on the stability data required by the appropriate licensing authority in the countries in which the product is to be marketed.

Stages at which Stability Tests are Conducted

Preformulation studies include chemical and physical stability tests on the drug substance and on solutions in suitable solvents; accelerated tests are of particular value in providing data on the mechanism and kinetics of degradation. Several batches of substance should be tested; each batch should be synthesised by the route likely to be used in large-scale manufacture. See also the chapter on Preformulation.

In **early formulation studies**, accelerated tests are useful in comparisons of the stability of different formulations. Data must be obtained to confirm that simple formulations used in trials on healthy volunteers and in early clinical trials are sufficiently stable for the duration of the trials. Stability experiments in the **main formulation studies** are conducted to aid the development of the final product. At this stage, a programme of chemical, physical, and microbiological stability tests is needed to enable the shelf-life of the product to be predicted (see under Expiry Dating of Medicines below). Toxicological experiments may be required where toxic degradation products may be formed or where additives to plastics may be leached into solutions; special precautions have to be taken with intravenous infusions. After a product licence has been granted for a product, it may be necessary to modify the formulation; **post-marketing studies** that involve stability tests may be required. Accelerated stability tests are sometimes applied to batches of medicines made by routine processes to confirm that the stability is the same as that of the original batch.

Expiry Dating of Medicines

The expiry date of a product is the date after which the product is not intended to be used. Before a medicinal product in its packaging can be labelled with an expiry date, a shelf-life under specified conditions of storage must be assigned to the product. Chemical, physical, and microbiological data from a programme of accelerated, long-term, and field tests have to be interpreted in relation to the conditions likely to be encountered in the countries in which the product is to be marketed. Guidance on the labelling requirements for expiry date should be obtained for each country.

As stated in the introduction to this chapter all the desirable properties of a medicine should be retained within acceptable limits during transport, storage, and use; it is not sufficient to assign a shelf-life solely in terms of the time for 10% (or other limit) of the active constituent to degrade. Assignment of the shelf-life should allow for uncertainties in knowledge of the storage conditions actually encountered by the product. A slight, specified excess or 'overage' of the active constituent may be included in the product especially where it is not possible to achieve a long shelf-life, as in some liquid multivitamin preparations. Special care has to be taken in the quality assurance of such products to ensure that the amount of drug is within specified analytical limits; overage is undesirable where a slight excess of drug could be harmful to the patient. Where the product may be required to be diluted when dispensed, the manufacturer should devise appropriate stability tests so that data are available on the stability of dilutions in suitable vehicles. Examples of products that may require dilution are some creams, oral liquids, and injections (for intravenous infusion). Similarly, stability tests are required to establish the shelf-life of those relatively unstable products (for example, ampicillin oral suspension) that are prepared freshly by dispersing dry ingredients in the vehicle.

Expiry Dating of Special Hospital Formulations

Hospital pharmacists are sometimes asked to formulate and prepare extemporaneously special medicines for particular patients; a short shelf-life (for example, seven days) is usually assigned in the absence of rigorous testing. A limited programme of stability tests is desirable where demand grows for a special formulation. Tight limits should be specified for potentially toxic degradation products formed during storage. For such products a shelf-life of not more than three months is reasonable as a goal but the possible benefits and risks to the patient of using stored products must be assessed carefully. For an example, see the protocol devised by Stewart, Doherty, Bostock, and Petrie[28] to test the stability of six paediatric formulations of indomethacin in aqueous suspension.

STABILITY OF MEDICINES IN PHARMACEUTICAL PRACTICE

The ways in which pharmacists in community and hospital practice can apply their knowledge of pharmaceutics to the stability of medicines are discussed in this section and examples of practical problems are presented. Possible future developments arising from extensions of the pharmacist's role are indicated.

Applications in Pharmaceutical Practice

Community and hospital pharmacists may be called upon to advise, solve problems, or make decisions on the stability of medicines. Evidence of incorrect storage conditions (for example, a faulty refrigerator) or of changes in the appearance or characteristics of a product (or packaging) can alert the vigilant pharmacist to the possibility of instability. By careful observation, and recording of changes that occur during the storage of medicines under particular conditions, pharmacists can provide valuable information to manufacturers especially on recently introduced products. In store rooms, dispensaries, and wards, special vigilance is required to keep products under the recommended storage conditions, to check expiry dates, and to ensure that old stock is used first.

Although original pack dispensing is becoming more common, some products are still required to be repackaged before issue to the patient or ward. Stability problems can arise especially with aqueous liquids where repackaging may result in an increased susceptibility to oxidation or other chemical reaction as well as to microbial contamination and growth; inadequate repackaging of tablets and capsules can lead to physical or chemical changes due to a greater uptake of moisture.

Where appropriate, such repackaged products should be labelled with storage recommendations and an expiry date. In assigning an expiry date, the pharmacist should consider: any recommendation made by the manufacturer; the expiry date of the product in its original packaging; the nature of the product; the nature of the original container (and closure) and that used for dispensing; the expected storage conditions in the home or ward; and the expected duration of the course of treatment. Because of uncertainty about the actual storage conditions of a dispensed product in the home, a short shelf-life (for example, a few weeks) may be assigned to products that are particularly susceptible to chemical, physical, or microbiological changes.

It is good pharmaceutical practice to counsel patients about their medicinal treatment and this affords an opportunity to give advice on expiry dates and on the best ways of keeping medicines stable and safe in the home. At the same time, encouragement and help can be given to the patient for the safe disposal of old medicines.

Hospital pharmacists may be required to devise stability tests for special formulations; see under Expiry Dating of Medicines above.

Examples of Stability Problems in Pharmaceutical Practice

Stability of Glyceryl Trinitrate Tablets

Because of an unusual form of physical instability that may result in a serious loss in potency, difficult problems are posed in the formulation, packaging, dispensing, storage, and use of glyceryl trinitrate tablets. The drug is not only volatile but is also soluble in some plastics and other organic materials used in packaging. These physicochemical problems may be compounded by the manner of use of the tablets. Some patients transfer tablets to their own containers and carry these about the person for ready access if an anginal attack occurs; therefore, for much of the time that the tablets are in use, their temperature may be close to that of the body.

At room temperature glyceryl trinitrate has a low but significant vapour pressure. Thus the pores in the tablet structure and the air surrounding the tablets become saturated with glyceryl trinitrate vapour. At 25°, the concentration of drug in the air is less than 7 micrograms per litre so that losses in potency are small provided that the containers are tightly closed. In contrast, if the closures are loose (possibly because of lack of resilience in the liner) or if the containers are opened frequently, glyceryl trinitrate vapour will be lost from the air-space in the container; then more drug from the tablets will be vaporised so that equilibrium is maintained. However, losses at room temperature are usually slight.

Lagas and Duchateau[29] postulate that the rate of evaporation of glyceryl trinitrate from tablets is controlled not only by the vapour pressure and diffusion coefficient of the drug but also by a 'matrix effect' that is associated with the porous structure of the tablet matrix. At first, the drug escapes by vaporisation from the outer layers; tablets with the lowest vapour pressure are the most stable. After the drug has escaped from the outer layers, however, the rate of evaporation decreases with time because of collisions of drug molecules in the vapour phase with the tablet matrix. At this stage the rate depends largely on the nature of the porous matrix; the retarding effect of the matrix is greater for compressed tablets than for moulded tablets.

Vaporisation can also cause migration of the drug between tablets by capillary condensation shortly after the tablets have been packed in the container; this process may result in poor uniformity of content of the tablets in a container. Inter-tablet migration may be retarded but not eliminated by the inclusion of stabilisers (for example, povidone) in the formulation.

Glyceryl trinitrate may be lost when the vapour dissolves in plastic containers or is sorbed by cork or paperboard liners of screw-caps or by stuffing materials (fillers) such as cotton wool, lambswool, or rayon. Russell, Lund, and Lynch[30] demonstrated that drug losses could be reduced markedly from tablets in screw-capped bottles by insertion of a liner made of aluminium foil over the ceresin-faced cork liner supplied with the screw-cap.

The greatest losses of glyceryl trinitrate from tablets (including stabilised formulations) are caused by elevated temperatures such as those encountered when tablets are carried about the person. Although the inclusion of a stabiliser in the formulation reduces inter-tablet migration and sorption on materials, serious losses in potency may still occur at elevated temperatures. An additional problem was noted by Pikal, Lukes, and Conine[31] who showed that some stabilisers at high concentrations decreased the chemical stability of glyceryl trinitrate, particularly at high temperatures. It is usually assumed that hydrolysis of the drug does not contribute significantly to losses in potency of tablets.

Guidelines for the packaging, storage and shelf-life of glyceryl trinitrate tablets are given below so that pharmacists can avoid or minimise problems of physical instability.

Packaging and Storage. Repackaging of glyceryl trinitrate tablets from bulk containers into dispensing containers is undesirable. For some years, the *British Pharmacopoeia* and *United States Pharmacopeia* have required that these tablets be issued to patients in containers of not more than 100 tablets. A glass container fitted with a screw-cap lined with aluminium or tin foil should be used without cotton wool or other additional packing materials that sorb the drug. The tablets should be stored protected from light at a temperature not higher than 25°.

Shelf-life on Dispensing. The Council of the Royal Pharmaceutical Society recommends that glyceryl trinitrate tablets be labelled with an indication that they should be discarded after 8 weeks in use. The recommendation applies to dispensed tablets and to tablets sold over-the-counter. It is assumed that the packaging is as described above. The recommendation of an arbitrary shelf-life of 8 weeks is based on an assumption that the tablets will be kept by the patient under the worst possible conditions, that is at body temperature and opened regularly.

Stability of Diluted Topical Preparations

Pharmacists may be asked to dispense extemporaneously dilutions of topical preparations; especially those that contain corticosteroids. Busse[32] indicated how an unsuitable diluent can adversely affect bioavailability as well as stability. In particular, an unsuitable diluent can markedly reduce the microbiological stability of creams especially if the diluent does not contain a preservative or contains one that is incompatible with the product. It is especially important that in diluted creams, the preservative should be partitioned sufficiently in favour of the water phase so that the antimicrobial activity is adequate.

Chemical stability may also be decreased by inappropriate dilution. For example, Yip and Li Wan Po[33] showed that dilution of betamethasone valerate ointment with a neutral or alkaline basis results in rapid isomerisation of the 17-ester to the less active 21-ester. Physical instability may occur where the composition of the diluent differs markedly from that of the original preparation; an extreme example is the cracking of a cream when diluted with a basis made with an emulsifier of different ionic type (see Incompatibility chapter).

Only diluents known to be appropriate for a particular product should be used. Guidance on suitable diluents should be obtained from the manufacturer of the product; the *British National Formulary* recommends that dilution be avoided.

Shelf-life of Diluted Corticosteroid Products. Dilutions should be freshly prepared using precautions to minimise microbial contamination. Extemporaneously diluted products should be discarded not more than two weeks after issue. However, now that ready-made dilutions of a few corticosteroid products are commercially available the problems of dilution in the pharmacy may be avoided.

Stability of Extemporaneously Prepared Mixtures

Although some traditional mixtures are now manufactured on a large scale with a modified formula and an extended shelf-life, pharmacists may still be called upon to prepare mixtures extemporaneously. The *British Pharmacopoeia* does not specify a shelf-life for mixtures that are made extemporaneously in accordance with the specified formula and directions but states that these mixtures are to be 'recently prepared'; this term indicates that deterioration is likely where the mixture is kept for more than about four weeks at 15° to 25°. Thus pharmacists are required to make decisions on an appropriate expiry date for a particular mixture. Such decisions can only be made by careful consideration of the likely stability problems of the particular formulation, the nature of the container and closure and the expected storage conditions.

A few mixtures (for example, chloral mixture and paediatric ferrous sulphate mixture) are known to degrade chemically. In some batches of certain suspensions, the drug particles may settle to form a hard, compact sediment that is difficult to redisperse; an example is magnesium trisilicate mixture. Precipitation may occur in mixtures (for example, ammonia and ipecacuanha mixture) that contain tinctures and other galenicals.

Mixtures are aqueous and will generally support the growth of micro-organisms; thus an antimicrobial preservative is usually included in the formulation. The adequacy of preservation of many mixtures is, however, uncertain. Despite the presence of chloroform (0.25% v/v) in most extemporaneously prepared mixtures in the UK, microbial growth is sometimes observed especially after the container has been opened a number of times;

growth is usually attributed to the loss of chloroform by volatilisation.

Lynch, Lund, and Wilson[34] reported that losses of chloroform from mixtures in unopened, well-closed containers kept for 8 weeks under ambient conditions were negligible. In contrast, stock mixtures in 2.5-litre bottles, opened twice daily for the removal of 50-mL portions to simulate use in the pharmacy, showed losses of 30 to 40% of the original content of chloroform in four weeks. Losses from 150-mL dispensing bottles, opened once, twice, or thrice daily for removal of 5-mL doses to simulate use by the patient, depended on the frequency of removal of doses and the period of storage; after two weeks, losses in all mixtures tested were roughly 20%. It was also observed that in mixtures containing suspended drugs, some of the chloroform appeared to be sorbed or otherwise bound to the solid particles. From the results of microbiological tests, these workers suggested that for mixtures prepared with precautions to minimise microbial contamination, a reasonable level of preservation against vegetative bacteria could be achieved provided that the chloroform concentration did not fall below 0.2%.

Guidelines on the shelf-life of extemporaneously prepared mixtures containing chloroform have been suggested by Lynch, Lund, and Wilson[34] and with minor modification are outlined below. The main criterion is microbiological quality; it is assumed that the chemical and physical stability is adequate and that mixtures are stored at ambient temperatures.

Shelf-life in the Pharmacy

Non-sedimented Mixtures or Aqueous Solutions of Chloroform. Stock preparations in well-filled, well-closed containers may be kept for not more than two months. Once the container has been opened and portions removed for dispensing, the stock preparation should be discarded after two weeks.

Sedimented Mixtures. Ideally, sedimented mixtures should be prepared freshly, possibly using pre-mixed powders; alternatively such mixtures should be pre-packed in the final dispensing containers and kept for not more than two months before issue.

Shelf-life in the Home or Ward

Dispensed mixtures should be discarded two weeks from the date of issue. This arbitrary period is in line with the generally accepted shelf-life of diluted mixtures.

Extension of Shelf-life by Freezing

The shelf-life of unstable solutions such as intravenous infusions that contain antibiotics can often be enhanced by freezing at temperatures such as $-10°$ to $-25°$. In some instances, the stabilising effect of very low temperatures may be greater than that predicted by the Arrhenius equation because of changes in pH. For example, Larsen[35] reported that a special formulation of homatropine eye drops (adjusted to pH 7.4 with disodium monohydrogen phosphate and monosodium dihydrogen phosphate) was unstable at room temperature (41% loss in 6 weeks) but was stable for 21 weeks at $-10°$ without detectable degradation. The remarkably enhanced stability was attributed to a fall in pH from 7.4 to 3.6, close to the pH of maximum stability of the alkaloid; the fall in pH resulted from crystallisation of disodium monohydrogen phosphate as the temperature was reduced. Such pH changes on freezing may, however, result in lower stability; for example, frozen solutions of benzylpenicillin buffered with phosphates at pH 6.5 are less stable at $-5°$ than at 20° because at the final pH (3.6), this antibiotic degrades more rapidly. Freezing may also increase the degradation rate of ampicillin sodium in dilute solutions containing glucose or sodium chloride. The ampicillin and other substances are concentrated in pockets of liquid water which are entrapped in an ice lattice; in such concentrated solutions the degradation rate of ampicillin is enhanced. Thawing of frozen solutions must be complete before use but should be performed carefully to ensure that localised overheating does not result in rapid degradation of the drug. Thomas, Tredree, and Barnett[36] have discussed the problems associated with the use of microwave ovens to thaw solutions.

Freezing of emulsions, suspensions, or gels may result in undesirable physical changes. In oil-in-water emulsions, formation of ice crystals can disrupt the interfacial film of emulsifier surrounding the oil globules and cause the emulsion to crack. Electrolytes present in the aqueous phase may be concentrated in pockets of unfrozen water and so affect the charge density on the globules; in addition at very low temperatures some emulsifiers may be precipitated. Drug particles in frozen suspensions (for example, insulin suspensions) may clump when the product is thawed; for injections, this can lead to blockage of hypodermic needles. Freezing of suspensions may also reduce the solubility of the drug in the vehicle; this can result in crystal growth and difficulty in redispersion. Gels should not be frozen since irreversible structural changes may occur.

Stability at Room Temperature of Products Recommended for Cold Storage

Some medicinal products (for example, insulin injections) are recommended to be kept at a particular range of temperature (for example, 2° to 8°). Pharmacists may be asked about their suitability for use if such products are kept at room temperature; for example, a refrigerator may break down, delivery of the product may be delayed, or the product may be placed in a handbag during the working day. Before making a decision on the suitability for use of a product, the pharmacist should seek guidance from the manufacturer or data sheet and should check the shelf-life that remains before the expiry date and the storage history.

Longland and Rowbotham[37] have tabulated information from manufacturers on 280 products marketed in UK in 1989; shelf-lives are given at the recommended storage temperature and, where known, at room temperature (18° to 25°).

Longland and Rowbotham have suggested that an old concept based on Q_{10} values could be useful for estimating the shelf-life at room temperature of such products. The Q_{10} value is the factor by which a rate constant increases for a 10° rise in temperature; for rough estimates, a Q_{10} value is often assumed to be 2 (for an optimistic estimate) or 4 (for a pessimistic estimate). Calculations are based on the following equation:

$$t_{s(T_2)} = \frac{t_{s(T_1)}}{Q_{10}^{\left(\frac{T_2 - T_1}{10}\right)}}$$

where $t_{s(T_1)}$ and $t_{s(T_2)}$ are the shelf-lives at temperatures T_1 and T_2.

Consider a product that has a remaining shelf-life of 1 year at 2° to 8° (mean 5°) before the expiry date. Assume that $Q_{10} = 4$. From the above equation:

$$t_{s(25°)} = \frac{365}{4^2} = 23 \text{ days}$$

Thus the remaining shelf-life at 25° is estimated to be 23 days. If Q_{10} is assumed to be 2, the remaining shelf-life would be 91 days. In practice, it is safer to take a pessimistic view and use a Q_{10} value of 4. The Q_{10} approach should be used with caution. Values of Q_{10} may not be 2 to 4 and may vary with the particular 10° range of temperature chosen: their use may give misleading results, for example, where the mechanism of reaction changes with temperature or where the manufacturer bases the shelf-life on physical or microbiological stability. Such information is not usually available to the practising pharmacist. The Q_{10} approach is not suitable for the more precise predictions of shelf-life required in the development of a new product (see under Stability Tests above).

Future Applications in Pharmaceutical Practice

As more medicines are dispensed in original packs, fewer stability problems will arise from the repackaging of products. However, with an extended clinical role, pharmacists should have more opportunities of giving advice to patients or to the staff of nursing and residential homes on the storage and expiry dates of medicines. Those community pharmacists who collaborate with general medical practitioners in the development of formularies for individual practices will be able to provide guidance on all pharmaceutical aspects of prescribing including the stability and storage of medicines. Increasing direct clinical involvement of some community pharmacists in the chemotherapy of cancer patients in the community, in enteral nutrition, and in the supply of medicines for the terminally ill should result in a more detailed application of knowledge on stability. Similarly, hospital pharmacists should be able to expand their present role in providing pharmaceutical information to doctors, nurses, and other professionals. It is likely that more complex problems of stability (and compatibility) will need to be tackled particularly in the formulation and administration of parenteral and enteral solutions (see chapter on Parenteral and Enteral Nutrition Fluids). Investigations on the stability of cytotoxic drugs in intravenous infusions may increase in extent and complexity so that efficacy can be enhanced and side-effects reduced; in some instances such work may be associated with detailed studies on pharmacokinetics in individual patients. It is to be hoped that more hospital pharmacists will be able to join or advise the ethics committees that review either experiments with new substances on healthy volunteers or clinical trials on patients. Such work provides an ample opportunity to apply knowledge of formulation and stability at a critical stage in the development of a new medicine.

REFERENCES

1. Pipkin JD. Monograph on Aztreonam. In: Connors K, Amidon GL, Stella VJ. Chemical stability of pharmaceuticals: A handbook for pharmacists. 2nd ed. New York: John Wiley & Sons, 1986:250–6.

2. Meakin BJ, Stevens J, Davies DJG. J Pharm Pharmacol 1978;30:75–80.
3. Carless JE, Nixon JR. J Pharm Pharmacol 1960;12:348–59.
4. Riegelman S. J Am Pharm Assoc (Sci) 1960;49:339–43.
5. Leeson LJ, Maddocks AM. J Am Pharm Assoc (Sci) 1958;47:329–33.
6. Monkhouse DC. Drug Dev Ind Pharm 1984;10:1373–1412.
7. Carstensen JT. J Pharm Sci 1974;63:1–14.
8. Duchêne D. Vaution C, Glomot F. Cyclodextrins, their value in pharmaceutical technology. In: Rubinstein MH. editor. Pharmaceutical technology. Drug stability. Chichester: Ellis Horwood, 1989:9–23.
9. Akers MJ. J Parenter Sci Technol 1982;36(5):222–8.
10. Lachman L. Drug Cosmet Ind 1968;102:36–40,146–7.
11. Johnson DM. In: Swarbrick J, Boylan JC, editors. Encyclopaedia of pharmaceutical technology; vol 1. New York: Marcel Dekker, 1988: 433.
12. Stewart PJ, Tucker IG. Aust J Hosp Pharm 1985;15:236–46.
13. American Pharmaceutical Association and the Pharmaceutical Society of Great Britain. Handbook of pharmaceutical excipients. London: Pharmaceutical Press, 1986.
14. Carstensen JT, Rhodes CT. Drug Dev Ind Pharm 1986;12:1219–25.
15. Ferguson LD. FDA By-Lines 1976;6:281–320.
16. Davies OL, Budgett DA. J Pharm Pharmacol 1980;32:155–9.
17. Rogers AR. J Pharm Pharmacol 1963;15:101T–5T.
18. Tucker IG. Pharmaceut Technol 1985;9:68–78.
19. Carstensen JT, Johnson JB, Spera DC, Frank MJ. J Pharm Sci 1968;57:23–7.
20. Lachman L, Swartz CJ, Cooper J. J Am Pharm Assoc (Sci) 1960;49:213–8.
21. Genton D, Kesselring UW. J Pharm Sci 1977;66:676–80.
22. Groves MJ. Pestic Sci 1970;1:274–8.
23. Carless JE. Pestic Sci 1970;1:270–3.
24. Amidon GE, Middleton KR. Int J Pharmaceutics 1988;45:79–89.
25. Cartwright AC. Int J Pharm Tech Prod Mfr 1982;3:43–6.
26. Hill SA, Khan KA. Int J Pharmaceutics 1981;8:73–80.
27. Stewart PJ, Tucker IG. Aust J Hosp Pharm 1986;16:35–43.
28. Stewart PJ, Doherty PG, Bostock JM, Petrie AF. Aust J Hosp Pharm 1985;15:55–60.
29. Lagas M, Duchateau AMJA. Pharm Weekbl(Sci) 1988;10:246–53.
30. Russell VA, Lund W, Lynch M. Pharm J 1973;211:466–8.
31. Pikal MJ, Lukes AL, Conine JW. J Pharm Sci 1984;73:1608–12.
32. Busse MJ. Pharm J 1978;220:25–6.
33. Yip YW, Li Wan Po A. J Pharm Pharmacol 1979;31:400–2.
34. Lynch M, Lund W, Wilson DA. Pharm J 1977;219:501–10.
35. Larsen SS. Arch Pharm Chemi (Sci) 1973;1:61–8.
36. Thomas PH, Tredree RL, Barnett MI. Br J Intraven Ther 1983;4:14-21.
37. Longland PW, Rowbotham PC. Pharm J 1989;243:589-95.

FURTHER INFORMATION

Carless JE. Drug Stability. In: Rawlins EA, editor. Bentley's textbook of pharmaceutics. 8th ed. London: Bailliere Tindall, 1977:140–70.

Connors K, Amidon GL, Stella VJ. Chemical stability of pharmaceuticals: a handbook for pharmacists. 2nd ed. New York: John Wiley & Sons, 1986.

Ferguson LD. Evaluation of drug stability. FDA By-Lines 1978;6:281–320.

Florence AT, Attwood D. Physicochemical principles of pharmacy. 2nd ed. London: Macmillan, 1987:445–93.

Rácz I. Drug formulation. Chichester: John Wiley & Sons, 1989:28–175.

Richards JH, Aulton ME. Kinetics and stability testing. In: Aulton ME, editor. Pharmaceutics: The science of dosage form design. London: Churchill Livingstone 1988:119–28.

Special issue on expiration dating for pharmaceuticals. Drug Dev Ind Pharm 1984;10(No. 8 & 9).

Stella VJ. Chemical and physical bases determining the stability and incompatibility of formulated injectable drugs. J Parenter Sci Technol 1986;40:142–63.

Young WR. Accelerated temperature pharmaceutical product stability determinations. Drug Dev Ind Pharm 1990;16(4):551–69.

Incompatibility

Incompatibilities can be classified as physicochemical or therapeutic.

Physicochemical incompatibilities are unintentional interactions that occur *in vitro* between drugs and other components of medicinal products during their preparation, storage, or administration. Drug-drug, drug-excipient, excipient-excipient, drug-packaging, and excipient-packaging are all interactions that may cause adverse effects on bioavailability, efficacy or toxicity. Additionally, interactions may induce changes in physicochemical properties and stability, which may diminish the acceptability of the product to the patient or its convenience in use. Among the interactions readily detected by the senses are those which result in turbidity, coagulation, precipitation, crystallisation, crystal growth, aggregation, solidification, liquefaction, phase separation, discoloration, thickening, or changes in odour and taste. Other interactions are known as 'hidden' or 'masked' since they can only be detected by physical or chemical analysis; an example is the sorption of diazepam on to plastic components of certain administration equipment.

Intentional or deliberate interactions can be exploited by pharmaceutical formulators to retard or enhance the release and absorption of drugs. For example, complexes of drugs with ion-exchange resins are used in the formulation of slow-release products. Caffeine may be added to ergotamine tartrate to enhance its dissolution rate, its absorption, and its efficacy in products used for the treatment of migraine. Intentional interactions are not considered to represent incompatibilities and are not discussed further in this chapter.

Therapeutic incompatibilities are unintentional pharmacodynamic or pharmacokinetic interactions that take place *in vivo* after the administration of medicinal products; these incompatibilities are usually known as **drug interactions**. Pharmacodynamic interactions occur between drugs that possess similar or antagonistic pharmacological effects or side-effects. In pharmacokinetic interactions, one drug alters the absorption, distribution, metabolism or excretion of another drug; such interactions may be associated with physicochemical reactions *in vivo* such as protein binding, chelation, complex formation, and adsorption. For information on the principles and mechanisms of drug interactions, see Stockley[1] and Hansten and Horn.[2] An updated list of drugs and their interactions is included in the *British National Formulary*. The first section of this chapter comprises an account of the types of physicochemical incompatibility that may be encountered in the formulation, manufacturing, packaging, storage, and dispensing of medicinal products. Prediction and the detection of incompatibilities are considered in the second section with special reference to compatibility tests on solid dosage forms. The chapter also includes a section on incompatibility problems which may be encountered in community and hospital practice.

TYPES OF PHYSICOCHEMICAL INCOMPATIBILITY

Precipitation of Unionised Acids and Bases

Many drugs and excipients are weak organic acids (for example, frusemide, phenobarbitone, benzoic acid) or bases (for example, neomycin, diphenhydramine, lignocaine) or their salts. The ionised salt is usually very soluble in water whereas the unionised acid or base is often sparingly soluble. For solutions of weak acids or their salts, a reduction in pH results in an increase in the proportion of the unionised drug; precipitation will occur if the concentration of unionised acid exceeds its solubility. In contrast, in solutions of weak bases or their salts, the proportion of unionised drug is increased if the pH is raised; precipitation will occur if the concentration of unionised base exceeds its solubility.

For a **weak acid**, the relationship between pH, pK_a, S_0 (solubility of the unionised drug in water), and S (total solubility of the drug) is described by the following equation:

$$pH = pK_a + \log\left[\frac{S - S_0}{S_0}\right]$$

For a **weak base**, the corresponding equation is:

$$pH = pK_a + \log\left[\frac{S_0}{S - S_0}\right]$$

Thus for a weak acid, the pH below which precipitation is likely to occur can be predicted from the first equation. Similarly application of the second equation allows prediction of the pH above which precipitation of a weak base is likely to occur. If the solubility of the unionised form of a drug is not known it may be assumed that it is insoluble in water. As an approximate guide to the likely solubility of the drug at a given pH, reference can be made to Table 1 (weak acids) or Table 2 (weak bases).

Table 1
Effects of pH and pK_a on the solubility in water of a weakly acidic drug

$pH - pK_a$	Approximate mole fraction of ionised drug	Solubility in water
< −2	< 0.01	insoluble
−1	0.09	insoluble
0	0.50	soluble at low concentrations
1	0.91	soluble except at very high concentrations
> 2	> 0.99	soluble

Table 2
Effects of pH and pK_a on the solubility in water of a weakly basic drug

$pH - pK_a$	Approximate mole fraction of ionised drug	Solubility in water
< −2	> 0.99	soluble
−1	0.91	soluble except at very high concentrations
0	0.50	soluble at low concentrations
1	0.09	insoluble
> 2	< 0.01	insoluble

To illustrate the method of calculation, an example of the effects of pH on the solubility of a weak acid (for example, frusemide) is presented below in the section on Incompatibilities in Intravenous Infusions. Other examples of calculations, including those for basic and amphoteric drugs, are given by Florence and Attwood.[3] Although application of the above equations may predict precipitation, a supersaturated solution of a substance may occasionally be produced; in such supersaturated solutions crystallisation can begin any time during storage.

Precipitation on Dilution of Solutions which contain Cosolvents

The formulation of solutions for oral or parenteral use which contain drugs such as diazepam or digoxin that are only sparingly soluble in water can sometimes be achieved by the use of water-miscible cosolvents such as ethanol, glycerol, or propylene glycol. A particular problem in oral liquids is that cosolvents may reduce the solubility of other constituents, for example, gums, polymers, inorganic salts, or sugars.

Dilution of cosolvent-containing solutions with water (or infusion fluids) may result in precipitation of the active substance unless the extent of dilution is such that the final concentration is below its solubility in water (or the infusion fluid). Prediction of drug precipitation may be difficult because the relationship between solubility and the proportion of cosolvent is often complex.

Precipitation by 'Salting-out'

The solubility of an organic compound or excipient may be reduced by addition of a salt. For example, sodium chloride or potassium chloride decrease the solubility of benzoic acid; in concentrated solutions some benzoic acid may be precipitated. The reconstitution of lyophilised erythromycin lactobionate with sodium chloride injection instead of water for injections may result in precipitation or gel formation. Such 'salting-out' phenomena may be attributed to the effects of the ionic size and valency of salts on the structure of water or to competition between salts and organic solutes for water molecules. Addition of salts initially increases the viscosity of methylcellulose mucilages because of 'salting-out' of the cellulose ether. In very high concentrations of a salt, methylcellulose may be precipitated.

Ionic Interactions

In active substances which ionise in solution interactions between cations and anions represent a common type of incompatibility that may lead to precipitation. Examples of cationic-anionic interactions are promethazine hydrochloride-thiopentone sodium, kanamycin sulphate-sulphadiazine sodium, and erythromycin lactobionate-heparin sodium. Partial inactivation of the drugs may occur even in the absence of precipitation.

Drug-excipient ionic interactions also abound. Carmellose sodium, an anionic polymer, reacts with large cations such as neomycin and chlorpromazine in solution; formation of a precipitate depends upon the conditions and especially on the concentrations of each substance. Emulsions made with anionic polymers may 'crack' in the presence of a large cation. Benzalkonium chloride and other cationic antimicrobial preservatives are inactivated to varying degrees in the presence of carbomer and other anionic polymers. Gelatin, which is amphoteric, may interact with either cationic substances (for example, veratrum alkaloids) or anionic substances (for example, sodium lauryl sulphate); the extent of interaction depends upon pH and the concentrations of the reactants.

Precipitation of sparingly soluble inorganic salts can occur by ionic reactions. An example is the interaction between calcium ions and phosphate ions in preparations for total parenteral nutrition.

Formation of Complexes

Molecules of an active compound may interact reversibly with excipients to form complexes whose physicochemical properties differ from those of the parent compound; the solubility and bioavailability of a complex may depend upon its stability constant and molecular size.

Although complexation interactions have been used to enhance solubility and stability in medicinal products when solubility is reduced they can produce less desirable effects. Tetracycline derivatives form stable chelates with metal ions of calcium, magnesium, and ferric iron; the absorption of tetracycline from these chelates is reduced markedly. Excipient-excipient interactions are also common. Phenolic preservatives may be partly inactivated in complexes formed with derivatives of macrogols. The nonionic excipient povidone may form complexes with other excipients (for example, anionic or cationic dyes) or with drugs (for example, chlorpromazine hydrochloride, chloramphenicol). Gels made with povidone may increase in viscosity as a result of complexation with 8-hydroxyquinoline sulphate or thiomersal sodium. Starches form complexes with acidic drugs and excipients such as salicylic acid, benzoic acid, and p-aminobenzoic acid.

Effects of Excipients on Drug Stability

The chemical stability of a drug can be reduced by the presence of an excipient (or another drug). For example, sodium metabisulphite rapidly inactivates cisplatin. Even when the excipient itself is inert, its impurities can affect drug stability; traces of ferric iron in clays catalyse the oxidation of hydrocortisone adsorbed on the clay particles. Propylene glycol and macrogols catalyse the degradation of benzoyl peroxide to benzoic acid and carbon dioxide. Carbohydrates in intravenous infusions catalyse the degradation of penicillins including ampicillin.

Changes in pH caused by the addition of another substance commonly cause adverse effects on chemical stability. Addition of coal tar, which is alkaline, to betamethasone valerate cream catalyses conversion of the 17-valerate to the less active 21-valerate. Tar (pine tar) is acidic and produces a more stable product when added to betamethasone valerate cream.

Other Chemical Interactions

Carbon dioxide liberated from mixtures by reaction of bicarbonates or carbonates with any acid or acidic substance which are stronger acids than the weak and unstable carbonic acid can cause bottles to explode; fortunately such reactions are now rare. Interaction may occur between sodium bicarbonate intravenous infusions and acidic additives such as ascorbic acid injection, insulin injection, or methadone injection.

In tablets that contain both aspirin and phenylephrine, acetic acid formed by hydrolysis of aspirin can then interact with phenylephrine to form an acetylated compound; transacetylation may also occur between aspirin and paracetamol.

A common incompatibility which may be enhanced after heat sterilisation of solutions or high temperature storage of solid dosage forms is the Maillard reaction between the aldehyde groups of glucose (or other reducing sugars) and primary amines (for example, amino acids, pheniramine, or dexamphetamine) to form brown products.

Eutectic Mixtures of Powders

The melting points of certain solid substances are lowered when the substances are mixed; the eutectic mixture may become moist or even liquefy if the melting point of the mixture is below room temperature. Ibuprofen forms such eutectic mixtures with stearic acid, stearyl alcohol, calcium stearate, and magnesium stearate. A mixture of phenol with chloral hydrate, menthol, or thymol tends to form a liquefied mass. Where liquefaction is undesirable for the clinical use of the preparation, the individual constituents can be sorbed on inert solids such as magnesium carbonate, magnesium oxide, lactose, or starch.

Partitioning of Substances Between Aqueous and Oily Phases

In emulsified preparations active constituents and excipients are distributed between the aqueous and oily phases. Such partitioning may seriously affect the preservation of emulsions if the concentration of an antimicrobial preservative in the aqueous phase which is available to kill or inhibit the growth of micro-organisms is much lower than the total concentration in the emulsion as a whole. The partition coefficients of phenolic preservatives so favour distribution into vegetable oils that they have little antimicrobial activity in emulsions made with these oils. The preservative may also be inactivated by solubilisation or by complexation with the surfactant. The preservation of emulsified products is discussed in the chapter on Preservation of Medicines and the Control of Microbial Contamination.

Adsorption on Solid Particles

Molecules of a drug or excipient may be adsorbed from solution in water or other solvent on to the surface of solid particles. In **physical adsorption** the adsorbate molecules are bound to the surface of the adsorbent by relatively weak van der Waals forces. Physical adsorption may sometimes involve formation of more than one molecular layer of adsorbate on the surface; binding is usually rapid and reversible. In **chemisorption** the adsorbate is bound to the surface in a monolayer by stronger, specific valence forces; an ion-exchange mechanism often operates especially in the adsorption from solution of ionised substances on clays. Chemisorption is often slow and not readily reversible since the heat of adsorption is much higher than that for physical adsorption. Adsorption from solution can often be described by the Langmuir equation; the physicochemical principles of adsorption and the factors which affect the process are described by Florence and Attwood.[4]

Mixtures which contain clays such as kaolin, aluminium magnesium silicate, attapulgite, or suspended antacids may pose incompatibility problems due to adsorption. El-Masry and Khalil[5] showed that about 93% of the original content of hyoscyamine in magnesium trisilicate and belladonna mixture (BPC 1973) was adsorbed on the solid particles; it was suggested that desorption *in vivo* after administration of the mixture was unlikely. A variety of other drugs including antidepressants, antihistamines, beta-blockers, and benzodiazepines may be adsorbed *in vitro* on clays and antacids. Adsorption of cyanocobalamin by talc, a tablet lubricant, may diminish absorption of this vitamin from the gastro-intestinal tract.

Adsorption *in vivo* is responsible for a number of therapeutic incompatibilities in the body after the co-administration of different medicines. Examples are: digoxin (tablets), oxyphenonium bromide (tablets), or rifampicin (capsules or oral suspension) adsorbed on magnesium trisilicate (oral suspensions, powders, or tablets); and lincomycin (capsules or syrup) adsorbed on kaolin (oral suspensions or powders).

Adsorption of antimicrobial preservatives on to drug or excipient particles may lead to loss of antimicrobial activity. Adsorbents that may result in the loss of activity of antimicrobial preservatives include clays, antacids, talc, aluminium magnesium silicate, corticosteroids, and procaine benzylpenicillin.

Sorption on Filters

The possibility of loss by sorption of active substances or excipients from solutions passed through filters has long been recognised; anions are often sorbed on positively charged surfaces of filters made of porcelain or diatomaceous earth whereas cations may be sorbed on negatively charged filter surfaces such as cellulose. In recent years there has been concern about sorption of substances on membrane filters particularly where these are employed for the in-line filtration of intravenous infusions.

Membrane filters for in-line filters are commonly made of a mixture of acetate and nitrate esters of cellulose or of nylon. In general, only drugs administered in very low concentrations (less than 5 micrograms per mL) or in small total amounts (less than 5 mg) over a 24-hour period are likely to pose incompatibility problems with the filter. Butler et al[6] used simulated conditions of infusing intravenous fluids to test commonly used drugs in these categories for potential binding to filters that contained a mixture of acetate and nitrate esters of cellulose; glucose 5% and sodium chloride 0.9% solutions were used as intravenous fluids. Substantial sorption was observed with digitoxin, insulin, mithramycin, and vincristine sulphate; there were no measurable losses of bleomycin sulphate, cyanocobalamin, ergometrine maleate, folic acid, heparin, noradrenaline acid tartrate, oxytocin, and vinblastine sulphate. In a similar investigation using cellulose ester and nylon filters, De Muynck et al[7] showed that there was a marked reduction in the amount of digoxin or diazepam delivered to the patient in the first 20 to 60 minutes of infusion; a slight loss of dopamine was observed but no fentanyl was sorbed on the filters. Another incompatibility was noted by Richards et al[8] who attributed impaired treatment of a baby with gentamicin to sorption of the antibiotic on an in-line filter.

For direct sterilisation by filtration of medicinal products, a wide variety of membranes is used which includes polycarbonate, acrylic polypropylene, polysulphone, hydrophilic polyvinylidene fluoride, and polytetrafluoroethylene (Teflon) in addition to nylon and cellulose esters. A particular problem is the sterilisation of solutions of protein or peptides which tend to be readily sorbed on filters. Pitt[9] showed that binding of porcine insulin, human chorionic gonadotrophin, bovine serum albumin, and sheep immunoglobulin G was least on hydrophilic polyvinylidene fluoride, slightly greater on polysulphone, and much greater on nylon and on mixed cellulose esters. Sorption of luteinising hormone releasing hormone, bovine serum albumin, and gammaglobulin was shown by van den Oetelaar et al[10] to be very slight on polyvinylidene fluoride, slight on nylon but appreciable on cellulose nitrate. Since adsorption followed time-dependent saturation kinetics, the largest amounts of protein were lost from the first few millilitres of solution.

Antimicrobial preservatives present in low concentration in medicinal products may be lost by sorption, especially on nylon filters. Significant losses of phenol, benzalkonium chloride, methyl hydroxybenzoate, and propyl hydroxybenzoate on five types of nylon filter were noted by Guilfoyle et al.[11]

Interactions with Packaging

Incompatibilities between drugs or excipients and glass, rubber (elastomers) or plastics components of packaging are discussed briefly in four categories, sorption, leaching, permeation and interactions with metals in packaging. A detailed account of these interactions with particular reference to those encountered in the formulation and packaging of sterile pharmaceutical products has been presented in a comprehensive review by Wang and Chien.[12] See also the Pharmaceutical Packaging chapter.

Sorption on Packaging

Some drugs may be adsorbed on the surface of glass containers, for example macromolecular drugs such as proteins, globulins, insulin; smaller molecules such as chloroquine (soda glass only); and surfactants such as benzalkonium chloride. The addition of another macromolecule such as human serum albumin reduces the loss of insulin from solution by competitive adsorption.

With elastomers and plastics, adsorption of substances on the surface is often followed by absorption into the matrix of the material. In published work, a clear distinction between adsorption and absorption is not always made and it is preferable to use the term 'sorption'.

Losses of antimicrobial preservatives from multi-dose injections or eye drops or rubber elastomeric closures can have serious consequences. According to Royce and Sykes,[13] the primary mechanism is interfacial partitioning of the preservative between the rubber and the solution followed by diffusion into the matrix of the rubber and finally volatilisation into the atmosphere. The equilibrium is disturbed and more preservative absorbs and permeates. The former practice of presoaking and autoclaving rubber closures in double-strength solutions of the preservative has limited value in preventing sorption during storage.

The clinical importance of unwanted sorption of drugs on plastic bags and tubing for intravenous infusions is well recognised. A useful summary of the results of sorption experiments by numerous workers has been tabulated by Wang and Chien.[12] Losses of drug from aqueous solution by sorption occur commonly on polyvinyl chloride. Examples of drugs sorbed by polyvinyl chloride are glyceryl trinitrate, warfarin sodium, isosorbide, chlorpromazine, vitamin A, thiopentone sodium, and various benzodiazepines. In general, fewer sorption problems occur with administration sets made of polyethylene, polypropylene or polybutadiene but polyvinyl chloride is still widely used because of its physical and mechanical properties. De Muynck et al[14] showed that the sorption on polyvinyl chloride tubing of isosorbide dinitrate from infusions of sodium chloride (0.9%) or glucose (10%) depended largely on the hardness of the tubing, which is inversely related to the proportion of plasticiser; the greater the hardness the lower the sorption. The nature of the plasticiser (di-2-ethylhexylphthalate or triethylhexyltrimelitate) did not affect sorption of the drug provided that the hardness of the tubing was the same. Sorption was much less for tubing made of polyethylene or polybutadiene. With laminates of polybutadiene with polyvinyl chloride, however, sorption of isosorbide dinitrate was appreciable and varied inversely with the molecular weight of the polybutadiene; for glucose infusion only, sorption depended also on the hardness of the laminate.

Leaching from Packaging

The term 'leaching' is applied to the migration of a substance from packaging material into a medicine. Examples are the leaching of alkali from Type III soda-glass bottles and the leaching of zinc salts, used as activators, from rubber closures. Barium ions leached from borosilicate glass may react with sulphates of drugs (for example, kanamycin, atropine, or magnesium) to form barium sulphate crystals; the presence of sulphurous acid salts as antoxidants in solutions may result in the formation of crystals. Similar incompatibilities may occur with calcium ions leached from glass. Di-2-ethylhexylphthalate (DEHP), a plasticiser used in relatively high concentration in flexible bags of polyvinyl chloride is readily leached into lipophilic products such as blood or fat emulsions. Migration into blood or fat emulsions can be avoided by the use of bags made of ethyl vinyl acetate (EVA) which contain practically no plasticiser. Although much less DEHP is leached from polyvinyl chloride into aqueous solutions, colloidal globules of the plasticiser may be detected in solutions stored in polyvinyl chloride bags especially when the bags are shaken vigorously.

Permeation Through Packaging

A common problem in pharmaceutical packaging is permeation of gases, vapours, or liquids. For example, water vapour permeates through rubber, especially silicone rubber, and to varying degrees through plastics, particularly polyvinyl chloride and polystyrene. Benzyl alcohol and chloroxylenol are lost to the environment following permeation through polyethylene containers. Certain organic liquids, such as methyl salicylate and dibutyl phthalate, act as plasticisers and attack polystyrene while chloroform will soften and permeate rigid polyvinyl chloride. Factors that affect permeation are discussed in detail by Wang and Chien.[12]

Interaction with Metals in Packaging

The presence of metals or metallic salts in packaging components can cause incompatibility problems with medicinal products. Bacitracin is precipitated from solution by heavy metal salts. Benzoates may react with ferric, lead, barium, manganese, silver, and mercury salts to form precipitates. Mercury salts produce a white precipitate with benzalkonium chloride. Aluminium displaces platinum from cisplatin in solution with the formation of a black precipitate and evolution of a gas. Traces of heavy metals may catalyse the degradation of adrenaline, phenylephrine, nitrafurantoin, and other drugs.

PREDICTION AND DETECTION OF INCOMPATIBILITIES

Judicious application of the principles of pharmaceutical chemistry may enable incompatibilities to be predicted. In particular, knowledge of the chemical structure and ionisation properties of sub-

stances is important. Thus precipitation of weak organic acids or bases from aqueous solution because of pH shifts in admixtures can be readily predicted from theory. Double decomposition is expected to occur between an alkaloidal base and the sodium salt of a carboxylic acid of high molecular weight. Similarly the effects of pH on the chemical stability of many drugs are well known. Adsorption of a large cation on particles of a negatively charged clay is known to be likely. Many other interactions that may be predictable are considered in the section on Types of Physicochemical Incompatibility.

Care should be taken in predicting interactions between two substances since in many instances the conditions in a medicinal product are unsuitable for a reaction to proceed. For example, interaction between an organic acid and an alcohol to form an ester is unlikely in dilute aqueous preparations at room temperature. In addition, because of the complexity of composition and physical structure of many medicinal products, it may not be possible to predict precisely the extent or even the nature of interactions. Useful guidance on the prediction of incompatibilities is given by King.[15]

Unfortunately some incompatibilities reported in the literature are based on single observations or on scanty evidence; the physicochemical nature of the reaction may not be known. Data on incompatibility should be interpreted carefully in relation to conditions such as concentration of the reactants, pH, ionic strength, temperature, physical state of the product, and the nature of materials used in containers and closures; the route of administration, frequency of dosage, and clinical uses of the product should also be considered.

Experiments to detect incompatibilities and to determine the nature, rate and extent of interactions between drugs and excipients are usually conducted at the preformulation stage in the development of a medicine; compatibility tests of drugs and excipients with packaging materials are often carried out at a later stage. To illustrate the uses and value of different experimental approaches in the selection of excipients in pharmaceutical formulation, compatibility tests for solid dosage forms are considered.

Compatibility Tests for Solid Dosage Forms

A variety of excipients is usually required in the formulation of solid dosage forms. For example, tablets may contain diluents, moistening agents, binding agents, glidants, lubricants, disintegrating agents, colours, and flavours; additionally materials to retard or delay release of the drug or to coat the tablets may be included. Thus the possibility exists of multiple interactions between excipients as well as between the drug and the excipients. Some excipients, notably the lubricant magnesium stearate, may affect not only the solid-state stability of the active compound, especially after compaction, but also its dissolution rate from the product.

A typical programme of compatibility tests involves the preparation of binary mixtures of the drug with each excipient in powder form; for each excipient, mixtures (in a fixed weight ratio) are prepared with and without moisture. Pairs of excipients can be mixed under the same protocol. The admixtures are stored at an elevated temperature (for example, 50°) and examined at appropriate times for signs of visual deterioration. Thin-layer chromatography may detect chemical changes but where possible, specific chemical methods are used to determine the extent of degradation or interaction.

Interactions in simple admixtures can be detected rapidly by changes in the phase diagrams produced by differential thermal analysis (DTA) or by differential scanning calorimetry (DSC). In DTA the difference in temperature is measured between the sample in a closed pan and a reference pan when both are heated at a constant rate. In DSC measurements are made of the energy required to keep the sample in a pan and the reference pan at the same temperature. The applications of thermal analysis in detecting incompatibilities are discussed by Ford and Timmins.[16] Diffuse reflectance spectroscopy has been used in studies of solid-solid compatibility to measure changes in reflectance at a particular wavelength; this technique is simple and rapid but lacks specificity.

Problems in the Design of Compatibility Tests for Solid Dosage Forms

Compatibility tests are widely used but the results should be interpreted with caution. Problems in the design of tests and the main limitations of tests have been pointed out by Monkhouse and Maderich.[17] For example, DTA and DSC may indicate incompatibilities that do not take place in the final formulation or may fail to detect interactions that occur during the process of manufacture. Whether or not an interaction is detected may depend upon the ratio of the two substances under test but the final ratio in the dosage form is not usually known at this stage of product development. It is impractical to test numerous ratios for each pair of substances although the number of experiments can

be reduced by a factorial design such as that proposed by Leuenberger and Becher.[18]

In a report concerned with accelerated tests of the compatibility of lubricants (magnesium stearate and glyceryl behenate) with an ester, Davies *et al*[19] conclude that for such excipients test sample ratios should be based upon surface area rather than weight since interactions would be likely to occur at points of contact between the surfaces of drug and lubricant. These workers also recommend that in addition to tests at elevated temperatures, tests should always be made at 25° since the effect of temperature on the reaction may not necessarily follow the Arrhenius equation. Relative compatibilities predicted from studies on binary mixtures can be different in the final formulation because of the presence of other excipients; multiple interactions may occur.

Another problem is that mechanical processes such as grinding, mixing, granulation, and compaction during dosage form manufacture can affect interactions, especially those which involve crystalline substances. Such interactions may not be predicted by conventional compatibility tests. Monkhouse and Maderich[17] recommend an alternative programme of tests in which a series of pre-mixed combinations of excipients are used as bases for prototype formulations of the drug; among the properties of the pre-mixed bases evaluated in detail are their interactions with acidic, alkaline and low-melting materials. The compression characteristics of the excipient bases and the drug should be recorded. Monkhouse and Maderich[17] acknowledge that conventional tests on drug-excipient interactions are of value in investigating problems where the prototype formulations are unstable.

INCOMPATIBILITIES IN PHARMACEUTICAL PRACTICE

Incompatibilities in Oral Liquids

Since few prescriptions require extemporaneous preparation for individual patients, incompatibilities are infrequently encountered in dispensing oral liquids. Nevertheless where incompatibilities do occur they may involve potent drugs and failure to detect interactions may have serious clinical consequences.

Admixtures of Oral Liquids or the Addition of a Drug to an Oral Liquid

A gross incompatibility was reported by Gould and Brown[20] and discussed by Stenlake.[21] Immediate precipitation occurred in a prescribed admixture of equal volumes of Orbenin™ syrup (pH 5) and Phensedyl™ syrup (pH 1.8) due to a double-decomposition reaction between cloxacillin sodium (in Orbenin™) and any of the bases, codeine, ephedrine, and promethazine (in Phensedyl™). After 5 hours, 20% of the activity of cloxacillin was lost; after 5 days, the loss was 99%. Rapid degradation of the antibiotic was attributed to the low pH (3.5) of the admixture.

Formerly, a common incompatibility was the precipitation of unionised barbituric acids (often amylobarbitone or phenobarbitone) from aqueous solutions of their sodium salts in acidic vehicles. Prescriptions for such admixtures are now only encountered occasionally but incompatibility problems have been reported. A white sediment that was slowly formed in diphenhydramine hydrochloride elixir in which phenobarbitone sodium had been dissolved was identified by Dunker and Sirois[22] as an easily dissociated 1:1 complex or salt of phenobarbitone-diphenhydramine.

Precipitation in lithium citrate syrup when mixed with oral liquids that contained chlorpromazine hydrochloride, haloperidol lactate, thioridazine hydrochloride, or trifluoperazine hydrochloride was attributed by Theesen et al[23] to the salting-out of undissociated, solvated ion-pairs of the protonated neuroleptic bases and their respective anions.

A particular difficulty in dispensing admixtures of proprietary oral liquids is that, in general, the precise formula is not disclosed by the manufacturer. For example, prescriptions have been written for Stemetil™ syrup with added diamorphine hydrochloride (5 mg per 5 mL). According to the Data Sheet Compendium, Stemetil™ syrup contains prochlorperazine mesylate (5 mg per 5 mL), sugars (68% w/v), sodium sulphite, sodium metabisulphite, and sodium benzoate but the precise formula is not disclosed. Thus it is not possible to predict the solubility and stability of the diamorphine, prochlorperazine, or the excipients in the admixture; the microbiological stability of the admixture is not known, since the overall concentration of antimicrobial preservatives may be reduced to below an effective level. Similarly the stability of an admixture of paediatric paracetamol elixir and Phenergan™ elixir cannot be predicted; the proportion of cosolvents in paediatric paracetamol elixir is critical in maintaining the paracetamol in solution and, in addition, a reduction in pH can catalyse degradation of this drug. Another example is Ventolin™ syrup mixed with pholcodine linctus. Here, useful guidance is provided by the Data Sheet Compendium which states that Ventolin™ syrup should not be diluted with syrup or sorbitol solution because the cellulose thickening agent in Ventolin™ syrup may be precipitated.

Action by the Pharmacist. In prescriptions that require admixture of oral liquids or the addition of a drug to an oral liquid, there is always a possibility of incompatibility. In view of the complexity and large number of potential interactions and the limited interest of manufacturers of the constituent preparations in these problems, it is not surprising that there are virtually no published reports on the clinical significance or potential hazards of admixtures. The absence of pharmaceutical or clinical evidence means that only very cautious predictions can be made on the suitability of particular combinations of liquid medicines. The pharmacist should explain to the medical practitioner the nature of these problems, the possible hazards associated with dispensing admixtures and should strongly recommend that separate preparations be prescribed. In the absence of information on the chemical or microbiological stability of extemporaneous admixtures it is advisable to limit the shelf-life to 7 days.

Where there are special clinical reasons to justify prescribing admixtures in hospitals, experiments should be conducted in the laboratory to determine the suitability and safety of the preparation. Such experiments are usually time-consuming and costly.

Use of Preserved Syrup in Oral Liquids

Turbidity or precipitation has been observed in certain oral liquids prepared with or diluted with syrup preserved with hydroxybenzoates; this incompatibility is probably due to salting-out of the preservative. Examples include methadone linctus, methadone mixture 1 mg/mL, paediatric ferrous sulphate mixture, potassium citrate mixture, and paediatric opiate squill linctus. For other examples of incompatibility with *British Pharmacopoeia* and *British Pharmaceutical Codex* preparations see *Martindale: The Extra Pharmacopoeia.*[24] Unpreserved syrup should be used for preparing or diluting these liquids. Problems of dilution with syrup should be infrequent since the introduction of oral syringes to avoid dilution.

Incompatibilities in Topical Preparations

Incompatibilities in dermatological products can arise because of the number and variety of active ingredients and excipients and the complex physical structure of many vehicles. Interactions may result not only in adverse chemical, physical, or microbiological stability, but also in decreased clinical efficacy or increased irritant effects on the skin. Although, in general, anhydrous ointments and pastes present fewer incompatibility problems than other topical products, special care should be taken in dispensing those which contain water. The rapid inactivation of bacitracin in a base of macrogols and propylene glycol is associated with the presence of water in the base which is hygroscopic; stable ointments of bacitracin can be prepared with greasy bases.

In creams and lotions, ionic interactions can be particularly troublesome. Neomycin cracks emulsified products made with sodium lauryl sulphate and forms precipitates with anionic cellulose derivatives such as carmellose sodium; this antibiotic also becomes firmly bound to bentonite. Precipitation of unionised acids or bases may occur: for example, admixture of a proprietary cream of mafenide 8.5% as the acetate with an ointment of lignocaine 5% could result in the formation of crystals of unionised mafenide. The chemical stability of vitamin A or of neomycin is reduced in creams that are acidic. Degradation of benzoyl peroxide is accelerated by macrogols and propylene glycol in some products. Nonionic emulsifying agents in creams and lotions may inhibit the antimicrobial activity of phenols, sorbic acid, esters of *p*-hydroxybenzoic acid, benzalkonium chloride, and other preservatives. Gels made with carbomer (an anionic polymer) are incompatible with large cations such as chlorhexidine, neomycin, or amethocaine. Pectin gels which contain partially methoxylated polygalacturonic acids react similarly with cationic drugs and degrade by hydrolysis in the presence of acids or alkalis. Polyvinyl alcohol is precipitated by many inorganic salts, especially phosphates and sulphates. Another gelling agent, hydroxypropylcellulose, is salted-out by other dissolved salts. Further examples are given under Types of Physicochemical Incompatibility above.

Incompatibilities in Intravenous Infusions

Addition of intravenous injections to infusion fluids may result in physicochemical interactions with loss in potency, increase in toxicity, or other adverse changes. The greater the number of additives, the greater is the potential for interaction. Many examples of interactions in infusion fluids have been considered under Types of Physicochemical Incompatibility. These include specific examples of: precipitation of unionised acids or bases; precipitation of drugs from solutions which contain cosolvents; effects of infusion fluids on drug stability; the Maillard reaction between glucose and primary amines; and interactions (sorption and leaching) with plastic bags. It is important to avoid precipitation in intravenous infusions particularly where extravasation of drugs such as thiopentone sodium and many cytotoxics may result in necrosis or where diazepam may cause thrombophlebitis. Precipitation can also lead to blockages in administration sets.

Whole blood is incompatible with many drugs and no admixtures should be made. Fluids that contain amino acids, mannitol, or sodium bicarbonate frequently give rise to incompatibilities with added drugs. Admixture of beta-lactam antibiotics (semi-synthetic penicillins and cephalosporins) with proteinaceous materials is undesirable because of the possible formation of immunogenic and allergenic conjugates. Amphotericin (as a complex with sodium deoxycholate) is incompatible with a wide range of other drugs and the use of admixtures is inadvisable; simple infusions can be prepared in glucose infusion adjusted if necessary to pH 4.2 or above.

Amoxycillin is typical of drugs that degrade rapidly which should not be added to a large-volume fluid and given by continuous infusion; intermittent infusion in 100 mL of fluid over about 30 to 60 minutes is preferable. Intermittent infusion for 30 minutes can also be achieved by the 'piggy-back' technique in which the drug is added to a small secondary container connected to a Y-type injection site on the primary administration set. Unstable drugs are sometimes administered by direct bolus injection into a separate vein or via the drip tubing. Methods for the intravenous administration of drugs are described in greater detail in the chapter on Infusion Fluids: Admixtures and Administration.

Two examples are given to illustrate how incompatibilities can be predicted from a knowledge of the effects of pH on the solubility or stability of a drug.

Prediction of Precipitation of Unionised Acids and Bases

Changes in pH may result in precipitation of the unionised drug especially in infusions of relatively high buffer capacity, for example, those that contain acetates, bicarbonates, or lactates. Precipitation may occur in one batch of an infusion but not in another because of wide pH differences between batches.

Frusemide is a weak acid presented as an injection of the sodium salt (pH 8.0 to 9.3) equivalent to 10 mg of frusemide per mL. The pK_a of the acid is 3.9 and its aqueous solubility is 0.01 mg per mL. The pH *below* which precipitation will occur if the injection is diluted with an infusion fluid to a final concentration of 0.5 mg per mL can be calculated from the equation:

$$pH = pK_a + \log \left[\frac{S - S_0}{S_0} \right]$$

$$pH = 3.9 + \log \left[\frac{0.50 - 0.01}{0.01} \right]$$

$$= 3.9 + 1.7$$

$$= 5.6$$

For final concentrations of 0.25 mg per mL and 1.0 mg per mL, the critical pH values are 5.3 and 5.9, respectively. Therefore, glucose infusion is not a suitable vehicle for frusemide.

Prediction of Incompatibility from Kinetic Data

Incompatibilities in intravenous admixtures of one or more drugs in an infusion fluid may arise from unacceptable decomposition due to the unfavourable pH of the final solution. Stability problems causing incompatibilities are common with antibiotics, especially penicillins. Knowledge of the effects of pH on the kinetics of degradation of a medicinal substance in aqueous solution may enable incompatibility with an infusion fluid in the presence or absence of another active substance to be predicted. Since there may be batch variations in the pH of the infusion fluid or the drug in aqueous solution, it is usually necessary to measure the pH of the final solution.

To illustrate this approach consider the addition of benzylpenicillin or ampicillin to intravenous infusions. For these antibiotics, Lundgren and Landersjö[25] presented graphs of log $t_{10\%}$ against pH at 25°. For benzylpenicillin in aqueous solution, the $t_{10\%}$ is greater than 48 hours only if the final pH is 5.5 to 8.0; where the pH is less than 5.0 or greater than 9.1, the $t_{10\%}$ is less than 12 hours. Graphs for ampicillin sodium in aqueous solution show that the $t_{10\%}$ is greater than 24 hours at pH 3.1 to 8.9 and greater than 48 hours only at pH 3.5 to 8.0. The addition of ampicillin sodium to carbohydrate solutions usually produces alkaline solutions. A graph for solutions of ampicillin sodium in glucose 10% solution shows that the $t_{10\%}$ is less than 24 hours at pH 7.0 and less than 3 hours at pH 8.0 or above, in fructose 10% solu-

tion, the $t_{10\%}$ of ampicillin is less than 12 hours at pH 7.0 and less than 3 hours at pH 8.0 or above. Addition of a second drug to an infusion can lead to further problems. The effects of other active substances on the stability of benzylpencillin have been considered by Stella[26] who interpreted kinetic data published by several workers. For admixtures with metaraminol tartrate, pentobarbitone sodium and sodium bicarbonate, for instance, the measured first-order rate constant for degradation of benzylpenicillin was close to that predicted from a graph of the rate constant against pH; incompatibility with these substances appeared to be due simply to the unfavourable pH of the final solution. An exception was the incompatibility between benzylpenicillin and aminophylline where the final pH was 8.7. The measured $t_{10\%}$ of the antibiotic was only about 2.5 hours whereas the predicted $t_{10\%}$ was about 13 hours. This result suggests that the incompatibility is due to at least two factors, the alkaline shift in pH and the direct catalysis of degradation of benzylpenicillin by a component of aminophylline, probably ethylenediamine.

Further Information on Incompatibilities in Intravenous Infusions

Detailed information and guidance on incompatibilities of drugs in intravenous infusions is given by Neil[27] and Trissel.[28] The *British National Formulary* includes a useful appendix in which suitable infusion fluids are recommended for particular drug preparations together with suitable methods of administration and warnings of special precautions to be taken.

Incompatibilities are commonly encountered in infusions for total parenteral nutrition especially when the antibiotics or electrolytes are added to intravenous fat emulsions; fat globules may aggregate or coalesce and the phases of the emulsion may separate. Such incompatibilities are discussed in the chapter on Parenteral and Enteral Nutrition Fluids.

Incompatibilities of Diamorphine in Injections

Admixtures of diamorphine with anti-emetic drugs in plastic syringes are commonly administered subcutaneously during 10 to 24 hours using a syringe-driver. Allwood[29] reported that diamorphine hydrochloride (up to 50 mg per mL) was compatible with metoclopramide (2.5 mg per mL), haloperidol (0.75 mg per mL), hyoscine hydrobromide (0.03 mg per mL), prochlorperazine (0.625 mg per mL), cyclizine (2.5 mg per mL), and methotrimeprazine (2.5 mg per mL). There was no evidence of degradation of diamorphine after 24 hours in a dark place; degradation of the anti-emetic drugs was not measured. The statement in older reference books that diamorphine (free base) is precipitated from solutions of diamorphine hydrochloride in isotonic saline is misleading. Page and Hudson[30] showed that precipitation did not occur in unbuffered solutions of the drug (0.05 to 5.0%) in sodium chloride injection (of varying initial pH) when kept for several days. It appeared that addition of diamorphine hydrochloride to isotonic saline lowered the pH sufficiently to ensure that the drug ($pK_a = 7.6$, solubility of free base in water = 1 in 1700) remained in solution. Only in solutions buffered at pH 6.6 did precipitation occur; such buffered solutions are unlikely to be met in practice.

It should be borne in mind that precipitation or turbidity may occur during the storage of diamorphine hydrochloride in aqueous solution because of degradation to 6-monoacetylmorphine, morphine and possibly 3-monoacetylmorphine. Omar et al[31] reported that solutions that contained 1.56 to 25% of diamorphine hydrochloride became turbid or showed precipitation after two weeks storage at 21° or 37°; degradation was associated with a fall in pH and development of a strong odour characteristic of acetic acid. This work demonstrates the need for caution in the use of long-term continuous subcutaneous or spinal infusions of diamorphine hydrochloride because of the clinical hazards of precipitation and local irritation at the site of infusion.

REFERENCES

1. Stockley IH. Drug interactions. 2nd ed. Oxford: Blackwell, 1991.
2. Hansten PD, Horn JR. Drug interactions—updates. Philadelphia: Lea and Febiger, 1990.
3. Florence AT, Attwood D. Physicochemical principles of pharmacy. 2nd ed. London: Macmillan, 1988:139–47.
4. Florence AT, Attwood D. Physicochemical principles of pharmacy. 2nd ed. London: Macmillan, 1988:196–205 and 415–19.
5. El-Masry S, Khalil SAH. J Pharm Pharmacol 1974;26:243–8.
6. Butler LD, Munson JM, DeLuca PP. Am J Hosp Pharm 1980;37:935–41.
7. De Muynck C, De Vroe C, Remon JP, Colardyn F. J Clin Pharm Ther 1988;13:335–40.
8. Richards J, Gould K, Bain HH, Gardiner CA. Lancet 1988;2:1309–10.
9. Pitt AM. J Parenter Sci Technol 1987;41:110–13.
10. van der Oetelaar PJM, Mentink IM, Brinks GJ. Drug Dev Ind Pharm 1989;15:97–106.
11. Guilfoyle DE, Roos R, Carito SL. J Parenter Sci Technol 1990;44:314–19.
12. Wang YJ, Chien YW. Sterile pharmaceutical packaging: compatibility and stability. (Technical report No. 5). Philadelphia: Parenteral Drug Association, 1984.
13. Royce A, Sykes GJ. J Pharm Pharmacol 1957;9:814–823.
14. De Muynck C, Colardyn F, Remon JP. J Pharm Pharmacol 1991;43:601–4.
15. King RE, editor. Dispensing of medication. 9th ed. Easton: Mack, 1984.
16. Ford JL, Timmins P. Pharmaceutical thermal analysis: techniques and applications. Chichester: Ellis Horwood, 1989.
17. Monkhouse DC, Maderich A. Drug Dev Ind Pharm 1989;15:2115–30.
18. Leuenberger H, Becher W. Pharm Acta Helv 1975;50:88–91.
19. Davies PN, Storey DE, Worthington HEC. J Pharm Pharmacol 1987;39:86P.
20. Gould L, Brown MW. Pharm J 1974;212:276.
21. Stenlake JB. Pharm J 1975;215:533–40.
22. Dunker MFW, Sirois LM. J Pharm Sci 1982;71:962–3.
23. Theesen KA, Wilson JE, Newton DW, Ueda CT. Am J Hosp Pharm 1981;38:1750–3.
24. Reynolds JEF, editor. Martindale: The extra pharmacopoeia 29th ed. London: Pharmaceutical Press, 1989:1276.
25. Lundgren PG, Landersjö L. J Clin Hosp Pharm 1980;5:279–97.
26. Stella VJ. J Parenter Sci Technol 1986;40:142–63.
27. Neil JM. The prescribing and administration of IV additives to infusion fluids. Thetford: Travenol Laboratories, 1976.
28. Trissel LA, editor. Handbook on injectable drugs. 7th ed. Bethesda: American Society of Hospital Pharmacists, 1992.
29. Allwood MC. Br J Pharm Pract 1984;6:88–90.
30. Page J, Hudson SA. Pharm J 1982;228:238–9.
31. Omar OA, Hoskin PJ, Johnston A, Hanks GW, Turner P. J Pharm Pharmacol 1989;41:275–7.

FURTHER INFORMATION

Connors K, Amidon GL, Stella VJ. Chemical stability of pharmaceuticals: A handbook for pharmacists. 2nd ed. New York: John Wiley & Sons, 1986.

Monkhouse DC. Stability aspects of preformulation and formulation of solid pharmaceuticals. Drug Dev Ind Pharm 1984;10:1373–1412.

Monkhouse DC, Maderich A. Whither compatibility testing? Drug Dev Ind Pharm 1989;15:2115–30.

Rácz I. Drug formulation. Chichester: John Wiley & Sons, 1989:176–250.

Wang YJ, Chien YW. Sterile pharmaceutical packaging: compatibility and stability. (Technical report No. 5). Philadelphia: Parenteral Drug Association, 1984.

Pharmaceutical Packaging

Pharmaceutical materials must be contained, protected, and labelled from the point of manufacture to the final point of patient use. Protection is necessary against physical, climatic, chemical, and biological hazards. Product quality, safety, and stability must be maintained throughout.

The packaging must also be convenient in use in order to promote good patient compliance, that is, to encourage the patient to take their medication at the correct times. Containers should be easy to open and reclose, if required, especially if the medication is for an elderly or arthritic patient. However, some compromise in packaging design may be necessary in order to meet all requirements (for example, child-resistant closures, tamper-evident seals, low cost, and environmental considerations).

Sterile products require effective closure systems to preclude microbial contamination and the pack itself must be capable of withstanding any sterilisation process required. Careful consideration must also be applied to the choice of containers and closures, particularly if plastic or rubber materials are involved, because of the possibility of leaching or sorption. The antimicrobial activity of preservatives in some product formulations has been found to be compromised by leaching or sorption of the antimicrobial preservative to the container.

Manufacturers are responsible for presenting their commercial products in unit packages that will protect the products for their declared shelf-lives. They have to present large amounts of data to the registration authorities in order to obtain marketing authorisation. The data include stability information generated from tests undertaken using the packs intended to be used for sale. If subsequent repackaging occurs, the responsibility for determining the shelf-life of the product in the new pack lies with the person who performs the repackaging procedure. The American Society of Hospital Pharmacists has published guidance and recommendations for assigning expiry dates to repackaged bulk materials.[1]

Repackaging a pharmaceutical product from one type of container to another may alter the degree of protection afforded to the product in its original container. There are some situations where product protection requirements do not permit repackaging (for example, ampoules, owing to loss of sterility as soon as the seal is broken; or the transfer of glyceryl trinitrate tablets, owing to the potential loss of the volatile ingredient). It is possible that repackaging may occur several times during the life span of a product. A knowledge of packaging materials will ensure the adoption of a rational approach to the original choice of container and, if required, to the use of alternative packs, although stability requirements must always be considered (see chapters on Storage, and Stability of Medicinal Products).

Standards for the use and reuse of containers for dispensed medicines are included in the Royal Pharmaceutical Society *Code of Ethics*.[2] Specifications for dispensing containers are given in British Standard 1679:[3]

- Part 5: Eye dropper bottles
- Part 6: Specification for glass medicine bottles
- Part 7: Ribbed oval glass bottles
- Part 8: Specification for glass and plastics containers for solid dosage forms, semi-solids and powders

Containers for dispensing are discussed in the Dispensing Procedures and Practice-related Guidelines chapter.

Primary and Secondary Packaging

Primary (or immediate) packaging materials are those that are in direct contact with the product being packed; the container should not interact physically or chemically with the contents. **Secondary** packaging materials are those that are not in direct contact with the product.[4] Examples of primary and secondary materials are given in Table 1. It should be noted that each of the general material types listed can be subdivided into more specific identities, for example, plastic includes polyethylene—high density (HDPE) or low density (LDPE), polystyrene (PS), polyvinyl chloride (PVC), polypropylene (PP), and many other polymer materials. In the remainder of this chapter the main emphasis will be placed on the requirements of primary packaging materials; secondary packaging should also be functional and elegant in its appearance.

Table 1

Examples of general types of primary and secondary packaging materials and their uses

Material	Type	Use
Glass	primary	bottle, ampoule, vial containing solution or tablets
Plastic	primary	as for glass
	secondary	wrapper to contain multiple primary packs
Wool	primary	void filler
Metal	primary	aerosol container, closure material
Board	secondary	box to contain primary packs
Paper	secondary	patient leaflets, labels
Liners	primary	inside closures to give compression seal

Terminology

The *British Pharmacopoeia* (*BP*)[5] applies the following terms to the description of containers:

- **single-dose** containers hold a quantity of the preparation intended for total or partial use as a single administration
- **multidose** containers hold a quantity of the preparation suitable for two or more doses
- **well-closed** containers protect the contents from contamination with extraneous solids and liquids and from loss of contents under ordinary conditions of handling, storage, and transport
- **airtight** containers are impermeable to solids, liquids, and gases under ordinary conditions of handling, storage, and transport; if intended to be opened on more than one occasion, it must remain airtight after reclosure
- **sealed** containers are containers closed by fusion of the material of the container; an exception to this definition applies to a *British Pharmacopoeia* monograph for a Powder for Injection
- **tamper-evident** containers are closed containers fitted with a device that reveals irreversibly whether the container has been opened. A variety of tamper-evident systems are in use including the well established tear band lid, the break band, glue-end cartons, cellophane overwraps for cartons and shrink sleeves protecting the product from adulteration, contamination, or substitution.

Other types of containers include **light-resistant** containers, which protect the contents from the effects of radiation of wavelength between 290 nm and 450 nm, and **child-resistant** containers (CRCs), which are designed specifically to prevent children gaining access to potentially hazardous products. The requirements and testing procedures for reclosable child-resistant packaging are described in the British Standard EN28317:1993;[6] this supersedes British Standard 6652, which was withdrawn in May 1993. Child-resistant packaging must be treated as a complete system.

Special Types of Pack

Strip packs comprise one or more sealed pockets of material, each of which contains a single dose of the product. Although they are convenient to use, they tend to be bulky and they also require some form of individual labelling. Types of dosage form that may be presented in strip packs include tablets, capsules, granules, suppositories, eye drops, and (as larger sachets) liquid medicines. The pack is composed of two layers of film or laminate material; the layers can be the same (for example, an all aluminium pack) or dissimilar (for example, cellulose film and an aluminium layer). The nature and degree of protection required will influence the choice of layers. Cellulose film is clear and transparent conveying a bright appearance; however, it is subject to high moisture permeation. Aluminium is opaque, light-proof and provides good moisture protection but in thin films it is fragile. Paper has good mechanical strength. Polyvinyl chloride (PVC) gives reasonable protection from moisture; the level of protection can be improved by using a polyvinylidene chloride (PVDC) coating to provide a PVC/PVDC laminate—both give clear films. In all cases polyethylene may be laminated to the other film materials to make heat sealing easier.

Blister packs consist of a base layer which contains cavities containing pharmaceutical products, and a lid that is sealed by heat, pressure, or both. They are more rigid and less bulky than strip packs, and cannot be used for powders, semi-solids, or liquids. Blister packs are made on high speed machines and often form the basis of original packs (see below). Printing of blister packs with day and week identifiers to produce calendar packs aids patient compliance.

The base layer materials used in blister packs are similar to those used for strip packs, however, they must be able to withstand thermoformation; the most commonly used examples include aluminium, PVC, PVC/PVDC, polypropylene, and PVC/polymonochlorotrifluoroethylene (Aclar) which conveys greater protection against moisture vapour than PVC/PVDC. The extent of moisture protection afforded by the various materials used in blister packs can vary widely depending on the methods and equipment used, for example, intermittent or continuous motion machines, and vacuum, pressure, or plug assisted cavity formation. Environmental problems associated with PVC in recent years has promoted the case for research into the development of new laminate materials with similar thermoforming abilities; polypropylene (PP), a recent addition to materials used in this type of pharmaceutical packaging, has a narrow thermoforming temperature leading to difficulties during large-scale blister manufacturing (cooling times usually have to be increased thereby compromising speed).[7]

The material most commonly used for the 'lid' of a blister pack is aluminium, sometimes laminated on the outside with paper, but invariably either coated with a heat-seal lacquer or laminated with a thin polyethylene membrane on the inside to provide a sealing bond with the base material. Peelable adhesives can be used to facilitate easy removal of the product from the cavity if the dosage forms are likely to be damaged by the more normal pushthrough method of opening. Perforations between cavities are often present on packs with peelable lids and also on certain child-resistant blister packs.

Tropicalised packs are blister packs that have an additional aluminium membrane sealed over the polymer membrane to provide greater climatic protection against high humidity.

Pressurised packs expel the product through a valve mechanism, utilising the positive pressure of the propellant, a compressed or liquefied gas, which is contained in the pack (see Aerosols chapter). Pharmaceuticals packed in this way include some inhalations, local anaesthetics, foams, creams, spray-on bandages, and particularly, some treatments for asthma. The container used may be metal, plastic, or glass;[8] if glass, it will be further protected on the outside with a metal or plastic layer.

The aerosol canister is fitted with an actuator that when pressed allows the valve to open, releasing the contents through the valve/actuator assembly. This may contain a metering device to provide uniformity of dosage. Metered dose inhalers (see Inhalations chapter) are used to administer certain powder formulations by way of a pressurised system.[9] Bicompartmental aerosol cans utilise a 'bag-in-can' approach; the product is kept separate from the propellant and from the metal can.[10] There are two types of gas used to pressurise packs:

the liquefied gases (the chlorofluorohydrocarbons, CFCs, are still necessary for use in some medical aerosol sprays but research into new propellent gases should lead to the eventual removal of the environmentally unacceptable CFCs)[10] and the compressed gases (for example, nitrogen, carbon dioxide, argon). The product formulation and also the components of the container can influence the particle size distribution and spray pattern characteristics of the product being expelled through the valve; factors to be considered include the valve/actuator design, internal pressure, viscosity, and the physicochemical nature of the formulation materials.

Pressurised packs are costly to produce and disposal can be a problem; however, they do protect the product from moisture, light, and microbial contamination and they prevent the loss of volatile components. Preparations for external use can be applied evenly in thin layers without the need for rubbing, which may lead to irritation.

Original packs are commercially produced pharmaceutical packs for finite treatment periods that are intended to be dispensed in their original form. They are designed for dispensing directly to the patient, with the addition of a label by the pharmacist.[11] The batch number, expiry date, and other manufacturers' information is thus always provided on the dispensed product.

The primary container may be a bottle, a strip pack, a blister pack, or another form of pack. There is usually a space provided on the outer carton for the dispensing label; the packs usually contain a patient information leaflet. The use of patient leaflets is the subject of a European Community Directive[12] that will become effective in the UK by 1994.

The hospital 'unit-of-use' pack may be considered to be a special type of original pack.

Packaging Materials

Glass Containers

Glass containers are particularly useful for liquid preparations owing to their rigidity, their superior protective qualities, and their ability to allow easy inspection of the contents. Glass is impermeable to air and moisture, inert to most medicinal products, and can be coloured to protect the contents from light of certain wavelengths. Additionally, glass can be sterilised by heat and ampoules can be hermetically sealed by fusion.

Major disadvantages associated with the use of glass as a packaging material are its fragility, its weight, and, for certain types of glass, its ability to release alkali to aqueous contents, especially during heat sterilisation.

There are three main types of glass available for use with parenteral preparations and one for non-parenteral use.[13] Type I glass (commonly known as borosilicate or neutral glass), because of its method of manufacture, is chemically more inert than the other two types. Glass of Types II and III is made from soda glass and Type II receives a surface treatment to impart a higher hydrolytic resistance; the treatment offered by several glass manufacturers, known as sulphur treatment, involves exposing the glass to an atmosphere that includes acidic gases like sulphur dioxide at high temperature. The alkaline oxides on the surface of the glass are neutralised by the sulphur treatment rendering the glass more chemically resistant, however, a 'sulphate bloom' is left on the glass surface and this must be washed off before use. Type III glass offers only moderate resistance to leaching and should only be used for non-aqueous parenteral preparations or for powders for injection. Containers made from Type II or Type III glass should only be used once because of the possibility of breakdown of the surface layer. Solutions of alkali salts, particularly citrates, phosphates, and bicarbonates, can cause the detachment of flakes or spicules from soda glass into the product. General purpose soda glass which has an even lower hydrolytic resistance may be used for non-parenteral products.

Specifications for the technical requirements of glass containers, eye drop bottles, glass medicine bottles, and ribbed oval bottles are described in British Standard 1679:Parts 8, 5, 6, and 7, respectively.[3]

Plastic Containers

Plastic containers are now used for many different types of packs including rigid bottles for tablets and capsules, squeezable bottles for eye drops and nasal sprays, jars, flexible tubes, sachets, strip packs, and blister packs; plastic is a light, mouldable material which is usually very resistant to breakage.

The plastics used in containers consist of one or more polymers, together with certain additives (for example, plasticisers, resins, stabilisers, lubricants, anti-static agents, mould-release agents) if necessary. The nature of the additives is often dependent on the polymer composition and the method of manufacture of the plastic material. No component of the plastic should be capable of extraction into the contents of the container, nor should any of the contents be adsorbed onto the surface of the plastic or absorbed into the polymer matrix; these requirements are difficult to achieve. Opacifiers can also be added to provide protection from light.

Polymer materials used in pharmaceutical packaging include HDPE, LDPE, polypropylene, polystyrene, and poly(ethylene terephthalate) (PET). Type specifications for a number of the materials are given in the *European Pharmacopoeia*[14] and standards for plastic containers for tablets and ointments are given in British Standard 1679.[3] Typical properties of various types of plastic bottles are given in Table 2.

Table 2
Properties of various polymers when used in plastic bottles

Property	Low density polyethylene	High density polyethylene	Regular polypropylene	Polystyrene	Polyester
Resin density	0.91–0.925	0.94–0.965	0.89–0.91	1.0–1.1	1.35–1.40
Clarity	hazy but transparent	hazy but translucent	hazy but transparent	clear	clear
Barrier to:					
Water vapour	good	very good	very good		
Oxygen	poor	poor	poor	poor	moderate
Carbon dioxide	poor	poor	moderate	poor	good
Resistance to:					
Acids	fair to very good	fair to very good	fair to very good	fair to good	fair
Alcohol	good	good	good	fair	good
Alkalis	good to very good	good to very good	very good	good	poor to fair
Heat	fair	fair to good	good	good	poor to fair
Cold	very good	very good	poor to fair*	fair	good
Light (UV)	fair	fair	fair to good	poor	good
Stiffness	low	moderate	moderate to high	fair to poor	good
Resistance to impact	excellent	good to very good	poor to good[†]	moderate to high	moderate to high
				poor to good	good to excellent

For oriented polypropylene, * = very good, [†] = very good
Adapted from Paine FA. Packaging user's handbook. London: Blackie. 1991:320–1.

The thickness of the polymer material at its thinnest point will affect the barrier performance of the package during its shelf-life; during the formation of bottles and blister materials the plastic components will have both thin and thick spots depending on the method of manufacture (for example, a PVC film 200 micrometres thick may have thin spots of 60 micrometres after having been formed into a blister tray). Variation in the orientation of the molecules in a plastic can also impart widely different physicochemical characteristics to the end product; this is particularly relevant for blister-forming materials.

Additives included in polyethylene materials include antoxidants (for example, butylated hydroxytoluene) and antistatic agents (for example, macrogols). Polypropylene may contain some polyethylene to give it better resistance against impact at low temperatures. Containers made of PVC often have organo-metallic stabilisers, antoxidants, mould-releasing lubricants, and plasticisers incorporated to enable adequate processing and to yield a product with reasonable impact resistance. Polystyrene may contain various concentrations of rubber and acrylic compounds to improve impact strength and brittleness. Some drug regulatory bodies, during review of new drug applications, may require extensive information about polymer additive identification and investigation for possible product formulation-plastic component interactions.

Drug-plastic interactions may involve permeation, leaching, sorption, chemical reaction, or alteration of the physical characteristics of the polymer or the product. Permeation of gases or water vapour through a polymer material can have a marked effect on the stability of the product if the dosage form is susceptible to hydrolysis or oxidation. Conversely, if a product containing volatile ingredients is stored in plastic containers, loss of the volatile components may occur by permeation through the barrier material. Leaching of additives from the polymer into the dosage form can occur causing product contamination. When the dosage form is a solution, the addition of colouring agents to the polymer needs special consideration.

Factors that affect the absorption or adsorption of drug formulation components to the polymer layer include chemical structure, pH, concentration of ingredients, area of contact, time of contact, temperature, and the composition of the solvent system. Antimicrobial preservatives, present in formulations in low concentrations, may be effectively lost from a solution by adsorption onto plastic in sufficient concentration to render the product insufficiently protected against microbial growth.[16] Polymer material obtained from one manufacturer cannot readily be substituted with the same nominal material from another source. Each source will have its own range of additives and processing conditions for the basic plastic material; it is therefore important that, having established an acceptable source of polymer component, drug manufacturers insist that the blow-moulder or film-former does not alter the polymer formula or processing conditions. The polymer formulations may well be the subject of master files deposited with regulatory bodies to facilitate new drug applications from drug manufacturers.

Plastic tubes, made from polyethylene, polypropylene, or laminates (for example, ethylene/vinyl alcohol copolymer) offer considerable advantages over the use of metal tubes.[17, 18] A more distinctive style of presentation can be achieved with plastic tubes and the polymer material can be designed to provide a 'suck-back' feature if required. Co-extrusion structures have also been suggested for plastic containers used for intravenous solutions, thus providing a combination of advantages contributed by each of the various laminate layers.[19]

The large-scale manufacture of blister packs and strip packs is made on 'form-fill-seal' machinery using reel-fed polymer materials. 'Blow-fill-seal' machinery,[20] which also involves the use of reel-fed polymer materials, is used to produce certain eyecare products, inhalations, and intravenous solutions under aseptic manufacturing conditions at high output speeds.

Metal Containers

The collapsible metal tube, used for pharmaceutical ointments and creams, is made from aluminium, which, like the single laminate tubes, gives a 'deadfold' tube, where the tube remains collapsed as the product is removed.[17]

Rigid metal tubes, made from tinplate or aluminium, are mainly used in pressurised packs. The inner surface is coated with an epoxy resin or other suitable layer to provide product protection from the base metal. Anodising the aluminium cans counteracts the need for internal lacquering and renders the aluminium inert on exposure to certain formulations; it also prevents external scratching and scuffing.[21]

Aluminium foil, up to 0.05 mm thick, is used in strip and blister packaging. Laminates of aluminium foil with other film substrates adds strength to the relatively fragile aluminium component, which is used for its moisture barrier effect; the additional laminate will tend to block any pin-holing or perforations which may be found in thinner foil layers. The inner surface is bonded to a thin polyethylene membrane which 'melts' during heat sealing, or has a lacquer layer to provide a seal to another substrate; the value of aluminium as a moisture barrier is dependent on the adequacy of the seal obtained.

Closures

Provision of an effective seal is the fundamental requirement of any closure system. The product contents must be effectively contained and ingress of external substances, including gases, must be prevented. The adequacy of the seal has a material effect on the stability of the contents and depends on a number of variables, for example, the flatness of the sealing surfaces, the resilience of a liner if present, the tightness or torque applied to the closure, or the top pressure and dwell time in a pressure or heat sealing operation.

Closures for pharmaceuticals in bottles may take the form of threaded screw caps, which may be child resistant or tamper-evident, using either preformed caps or caps formed during application (for example, roll-on pilfer-proof aluminium caps). Preformed threaded screw caps may be made from tinplate or aluminium, in both cases they should have an inner lining material (for example, a lacquer or a more substantial liner); they may also be made from plastic, either a thermosetting or a thermoplastic material. The thermosetting plastic closures include those made from phenolic moulding compounds and those based on urea; these require the use of a liner and have now largely been replaced by the thermoplastic materials (for example, polyethylene and polypropylene), which may incorporate an integral flexible sealing strip, a pre-formed 'O' ring. Some closures have been specially produced with 'lugs' or 'ears' to give additional grip for use by arthritic or disabled patients.

A torque tester can be used to determine adequate closing tightness for screw cap closures to prevent either over- or under-tightening of the closure. Over-tightening makes cap removal difficult for the patient and may induce stresses in the closure components, whereas under-tightening will allow product leakage or contamination by external substances such as moisture vapour.

Push-on or plug type closures are usually formed from thermoplastic materials. They often have additional features to improve the closeness of the fit between the cap and the container, often providing a better overall seal against the entry of moisture vapour than the traditional screw cap closure.

A variant of the plug type closure is the rubber stopper used for multidose injection vials and for lyophilised preparations. The composition of this closure system is complex and hence closure-product interactions (leaching and sorption) can occur (see drug-plastic interactions discussed earlier under Plastic Containers). The main advantages of rubber are its ability to reseal itself after penetration by a needle and its ability to withstand heat sterilisation. Different colours can be used for the rubber closure and the aluminium overcap to aid product identification and security during manufacture of the sterile product. Automatic colour sensors can be incorporated into production lines to give 100% inspection for product verification. Rubber is also used in eye drop bottle closures and as a plunger in syringes. Different rubber compositions, for example, natural, butyl, and silicone, impart different physical characteristics to the end product thus influencing the stability of the pharmaceutical product.

Thermoplastic materials can also be sealed by applying heat to bond two surfaces together; this principle is applied when sealing ampoules and in strip and blister packing. Ultrasonic and impulse methods are also used for sealing or bonding plastic components. The effectiveness of a seal produced by bonding two materials together can be tested using destructive techniques involving either pressure or vacuum methods to confirm the seal integrity.

Alternative methods used to provide a tamper-evident secondary liner that seals to the bottle neck involve the application of pressure or induction heating on the closure system. The latter provides an even and controllable heat across the membrane to release it from its backing liner and to seal it to the container. The membrane material may be composed mainly of aluminium film to provide a moisture barrier, paper to give strength, or polystyrene foam.

Partial sleeves over the bottle neck and closure or full length sleeves over the majority of the container body and the closure provide a tamper-evident system.

Child-resistant containers are a professional requirement for dispensing solid dosage forms in the UK.[2] The types of CRCs most often used pharmaceutically include push-down and turn caps, squeeze and turn caps, and cap-bottle alignment systems. There are still problems with liquid medicines containing sugar which can cause crystallisation to build up around the mouth of the bottle making it difficult to remove the cap. Child-resistant containers can also be a serious problem for elderly, disabled, or arthritic patients, who may have poor manual dexterity.[22]

Metered-dose pump sprays are used for aerosols and for nasal sprays. The latter devices are typically based on plastic push-on or threaded screw closures. Aerosol closures will be crimped into place.

Labels and Leaflets

Labelling is a critical aspect of the packaging operation and constitutes one of the largest problem areas, as evidenced by the volume of product recalls associated with labelling errors.[23]

Overprinting of batch details and expiry information is now often done on-line using ink-jet or laser printing methods. The majority of labels used in pharmaceutical packaging are paper based. Vinyl labels are used for injectable products, enabling the contents to be seen through the label material. Some label adhesives are solvent based. Some printing inks are also solvent based, for example methylethyl ketone has been used for ink-jet printing where its rapid drying ability is a particular advantage. Organic solvents can migrate through plastic materials and the packaging technologist must always consider this possibility in instances where secondary packaging materials may be attached to the primary container.

As alternatives to the use of separate patient leaflets, patient support packs and complex multiform or 'piggyback' label systems have been introduced in recent years to provide additional information for the patient about their medicine. Both these advances enable the packaging production line to be simplified, and they may also reduce the amount of packaging waste per product (see below).

Critical print on labels, leaflets, and cartons can now be automatically checked on production lines using image scanning systems.[24] Other vision systems are used to detect faults on and off the production line, for example, missing labels or caps, underfilled bottles, empty blister cavity pockets, or the presence of particulates in injectables.

Testing of Components

Quality has to be built in to any product; this includes the packaging materials/components, both in the form of raw materials and as the finished product. Testing for compatibility between formulation ingredients and packaging components is fundamental to preformulation and stability investigations (see also Preformulation, and Incompatibility chapters).

Containers and closure systems should always meet a product purchasing and performance specification and should be formally tested against those specifications as part of good manufacturing practice.[25] Official compendia provide tests and standards for glass and plastic containers.[5,14,26] The United States Pharmacopeia[26] also specifies a standard for moisture vapour transmission.

The introduction of faster and more flexible packaging lines necessitates stringent controls on materials and specifications. Imaging techniques have been introduced to identify faulty components and materials. Dimensional tests for containers and closures to be used on automated packaging lines require close tolerances.

The testing of polymer and rubber materials for the presence of extractable products is particularly important for materials in contact with solutions and ointments. Testing of blister packing film materials for thickness and freedom from pinholes (in aluminium) is also essential. Torque testing of screw cap closures, and vacuum or pressure testing of blister and strip packs has been mentioned previously. Ampoules also require testing for adequacy of seal.

Environmental Concerns

Packaging has a positive role in protecting goods from the environment during storage and distribution, however, it also has a negative impact on the environment in that it utilises raw materials and energy and it ends up as waste, which requires disposal. The environmental impact of the manufacture and disposal of different packaging components has necessitated the application of life-cycle analysis to several materials. Life-cycle analysis is also known as eco-balance assessment, cradle-to-grave analysis, resource analysis, and environmental impact assessment.[27] The most important objective of these studies is probably to reduce the rate of fossil fuel depletion as such losses will be difficult, if not impossible, to reverse. The packaging life-cycle starts with the supply of the raw material and passes through pack manufacture, filling and packing, handling by intermediaries (wholesalers, retailers), and use by the consumer, before final disposal.[28] Recycling of paper- or board-based materials, glass, and aluminium has been possible for some time; recycling of plastic materials, however, is more difficult because the different types of plastic must initially be segregated; multi-layer laminates are not suitable for recycling. Due to the various additives used in making plastic primary container materials it is doubtful whether any recycled material will ever be used for primary pharmaceutical packs; the *British Pharmacopoeia*[5] and *European Pharmacopoeia*[14] specifically state that scrap material must not be used in manufacturing plastic medicine containers.

Germany has introduced legislation to reduce pollution and land-fill produced by packaging components (*The Avoidance of Refuse (Packaging) Ordinance*, adopted in April 1991). These 'take back' laws apply to manufacturers and retail outlets that issue goods in any kind of packaging (non-biodegradable or otherwise); they have to devise and provide systems for the return of all used packaging, packaging waste, or both, from the consumer or final user in order to channel it to the most appropriate and effective reuse or recovery programme. This type of legislation may well be extended to cover the rest of the European Community.

Separation of waste into different material types may facilitate recycling of, for example, paper, aluminium, metal, and some plastics. Life-cycle analysis may indicate potential uses for certain plastics, for example, during incineration some plastics may be used as components of the energy source for the incinerator to burn other non-recyclable material. The emission of gases and heat from the disposal plant itself may also be of use as a further energy source but consideration must be given to the possible emission of toxic gases (for example, during the incineration of PVC).[7] In addition to consideration of environmental pollution, concerns relating to the health and safety of personnel has led to the introduction of measures aimed at reducing or eliminating the use of volatile organic solvents in the manufacture of label adhesives and printing inks.

To facilitate recycling of plastic containers, new label substrate materials are being introduced where the label material used on a container will be the same plastic polymer as the container itself.

Recent Advances

The requirements of pharmaceutical packaging are becoming ever more sophisticated and diverse. A key factor is to meet the demands associated with the manufacture of higher specification products that are presented in a variety of dimensions and surface finishes. For example, laminate blister trays may be used as carriers for novel fast-dissolving dosage forms that are prepared using lyophilisation techniques; subsequently, the filled blister trays are sealed with a peelable lid material.[29]

Specially designed consumer wallets have been used for some commercially available products with the objective of aiding patient compliance. In effect, these tend to be extensions of the calendar blister pack concept. When used for short periods (for example, one week) compliance devices used for dispensed products should not, in general, compromise product stability.[30, 31]

Transdermal patches also require the use of sophisticated packs; the patch substrate material, which is in direct contact with the drug, is the primary packaging material. Transdermal patches often have multilaminate packaging constructions, including a pouch or overpouch, and both the formulator and the packaging technologist require considerable formulation skills.

Intravenous giving sets are available with a double chamber system that keeps two solutions separate until they are mixed immediately before use, thus eliminating any potential long-term incompatibility problems.

Bar codes aid stock inventory control. Two-dimensional bar code symbology[32] has the capacity to encode considerably more information than standard linear bar codes.

Caps that contain computer chips to record the opening times of medicine bottles have been introduced for use in clinical trials where the time of administration of the dose may be important.[33] A variation on this theme is now available where an electronic 'bleeper' can be incorporated into a pack to remind patients when to take their medication.[30, 31, 34, 35] Another example of an electronically active packaging device is the use of a flat piece of plastic that contains a silicon chip that is programmed to show whether the products (for example, certain vaccines) have been stored at the right temperature and are within their expiry dates.[34]

Thermochromic inks or label materials may be used on products that are to be sterilised by heat to indicate, by a change of colour, that the sterilisation temperature has been reached.

Holographic security labelling using embossed holographic images on a range of materials has been introduced into the pharmaceutical industry. The labels have a complex versatile design, which supposedly cannot be readily copied. It has been suggested that holograms may eventually replace bar codes as a source of pack information.[36]

Miniature tuned magnetic fields set up in thin printed metallic strips can be printed on packs or labels at the time of manufacture; the packs are activated when put on retail display and deactivated at the point of sale.[37]

The key issues of child resistance, tamper evidence, security, environmental considerations, and increasing legislation are at the forefront of current thinking and action in pharmaceutical packaging.

REFERENCES

1. Chaney RF, Summerfield MR. Am J Hosp Pharm 1984;41:1150–2.
2. Royal Pharmaceutical Society of Great Britain. Medicines, ethics and practice: a guide for pharmacists. Standards of good professional practice in medicines, ethics and practice. 1993;10:88.
3. British Standards Institution. British Standard 1679. Specifications for containers for pharmaceutical dispensing. Part 5: 1973, Part 6: 1984 (1991), Part 7: 1968 (1977) Part 8: 1992. London: The Institution.
4. Sharp J. Quality rules in packaging. Woodley: John Sharp, 1992.
5. British pharmacopoeia 1993. London: HMSO, 1993.
6. British Standards Institution. British Standard EN28317:1993. Child-resistant packaging—requirements and testing procedures for reclosable packages. London: The Institution, 1993.
7. Preker H. Mfg Chem 1992;63(5):33–5.
8. Ansel H, Popovich NG. Pharmaceutical dosage forms and drug delivery systems. 5th ed. Philadelphia: Lea and Febiger, 1990:390–405.
9. United States pharmacopeia XXII. National formulary XVII. Rockville: United States Pharmacopeial Convention Inc, 1990:1692.
10. Pidgeon R. Packaging Week 1992 Aug12:15–16.
11. Benoliel DM. Mfg Chem 1989;60(2):39–42.
12. Council Directive 92/27/EEC. On the labelling of medicinal products for human use and on package leaflets. Official Journal of the European Community 1992 April 30:L113.
13. Council of Europe. The European pharmacopoeia VI.2.1. Glass containers for pharmaceutical use. Luxembourg: EEC, 1991.
14. Council of Europe. The European pharmacopoeia VI.1. Materials used for the manufacture of containers, 1983. VI.2.2.1. Plastic containers and closures, 1991. Saint-Ruffine: Maisonneuve.
15. Paine FA. Packaging user's handbook. London: Blackie, 1991:320–1.
16. Ansel H, Popovich NG. Pharmaceutical dosage forms and drug delivery systems. 5th ed. Philadelphia: Lea and Febiger, 1990:116–29.
17. Mfg Chem 1987;58(6):45–7.
18. Mfg Chem 1988;59(6):61–3.
19. Lambert P. Pharmaceut Technol Int 1991;3(5):29–31.
20. Thorne A. Mfg Chem 1989;60(4):29–31.
21. Mfg Chem 1987;58(3):38–42.
22. Mfg Chem 1991;62(9):3, 49–51.
23. Greenburg EF. Mfg Chem 1990;61(1):29–31.
24. Orrell B. Mfg Chem 1991;62(9):24–7.
25. Commission of the European Communities. The rules governing medicinal products in the European Community, Vol IV: Good manufacturing practice for medicinal products. Luxembourg: The Commission, 1992.
26. United States pharmacopeia XXII. National formulary XVII. Containers, and containers—permeation. Rockville: United States Pharmacopeial Convention Inc, 1990:1570–6.
27. INCPEN Life Cycle Analysis—background. Panorama 1992;16(5):6–7.
28. Data collection for life cycle analysis, packaging and industrial film association. Packaging News 1992 October:45.
29. Virley P, Yarwood R. Mfg Chem 1990;61(2):36–7.
30. Walker R. Pharm J 1992;249:605–7.
31. Walker R. Pharm J 1992;248:124–6.
32. New Bar Code Symbology. Packaging Week 1991 June 26:46.
33. McNear M, Shaffer RE. Clinical supplies. In: Swarbrick J, Boylan JC, editors. Encyclopaedia of pharmaceutical technology. New York: Marcel Dekker 1990;3:1–19.
34. Packaging Week 1992 Jan 29:13.
35. Packaging News 1992 Jan:1.
36. Pitt P. Packaging Week 1992 Aug 12:9.
37. Goddard R. Packaging Week 1992 Oct 21:3.

FURTHER INFORMATION

Dean DA. Stability aspects of packaging. Drug Dev Ind Pharm 1984;10(8 and 9):1463–95.

Fischer A, Thomas RH. Packaging materials science. In: Lachman L, Lieberman HA, Kanig JL, editors. The theory and practice of industrial pharmacy. Philadelphia: Lea and Febiger, 1976:680–99.

Institute of Packaging. Dean DA. Packaging of pharmaceuticals—packages and closures. London: The Institute, 1992.

Hallworth GW. Pressurised packaging. Melton Mowbray: The Institute of Packaging, 1989.

Paine FA. Fundamentals of packaging. London: The Institute of Packaging, 1985.

Ross CF. Packaging of pharmaceuticals—products, sterilisation and safety. London: The Institute of Packaging, 1983.

Sciarra JJ, Cutie AJ. Aerosols. In: Gennaro AR, editor. Remington's pharmaceutical sciences. 18th ed. Easton: Mack, 1990:1694–712.

Storage

All medicinal products should be stored in such a way as to avoid contamination and, as far as possible, deterioration or degradation. Atmospheric gases, moisture, extremes of temperature, natural and artificial light, and prolonged storage time are all possible causes of deterioration or degradation and, during storage, precautions should be aimed at their elimination or reduction. Contamination of medicinal products can be limited by storage in suitably closed containers or packaging.

In their monographs the various pharmacopoeias specify, where appropriate, the precautions to be taken during storage of certain medicinal products. Additionally, general expressions are presented for storage temperatures, for containers, and for protection from moisture and light. The trend is away from vague expressions such as 'store in a cool place' (no longer in the *British Pharmacopoeia*) to more precisely defined conditions such as 'store at 8° to 15°'. In a monograph of the *United States Pharmacopeia*, if no directions for storage are included for a medicinal product, it is understood that the storage conditions will provide protection from light, moisture, excessive heat, and freezing. In other words, the medicinal product can be stored for a reasonable period of time at room temperature, in a normal atmosphere, and protected from light without adverse effects.

In contrast to the precise storage expressions found in the pharmacopoeias, the data sheets produced in Great Britain for individual medicinal products by manufacturers (in compliance with the requirements of the Medicines Act, 1968) use a large number of different expressions for storage conditions. Some conditions are very precise, for example, a definite temperature range may be stated. Other data sheets limit one extreme of storage condition but not the other, for example, 'not exceeding 25°'. Among the generally vague or nebulous expressions are 'store at room temperature', and 'store away from heat'.

The Royal Pharmaceutical Society in its *Guide to Good Dispensing Practice and Guide to Self Assessment of Professional Practice* states that all materials (defined as substances and products purchased for the purpose of dispensing, whether as received or as a component in a preparation to be dispensed) should be stored under suitable conditions, bearing in mind the nature of the material. Particular attention should be paid to protection from sunlight, atmospheric moisture, and adverse temperature. Toilet areas should not be used for the storage of stock. All containers of raw materials should be kept in a good, clean condition; they should be clearly labelled and marked with identifying reference characters, the manufacturer's name and, if appropriate, batch numbers and expiry dates. Where stock is transferred from one container to another, the label and identification particulars described above should be attached and the risks of contamination minimised. The guidelines advise pharmacists to exercise their full knowledge of the stability of materials and to be prepared to destroy any substances that have been in stock for unduly long periods, have deteriorated, or have passed their expiry date. It is especially important to ensure that drugs are stored and issued in chronological sequence.

It has been recommended that drugs should be stored according to a system that facilitates retrieval, preferably in alphabetical order. Only medicinal products which require special storage conditions, for example Controlled Drugs, potential fire hazards, and those kept between 2° and 8°, should be stored separately. In the ideal arrangement, working stock is removed from the front of the shelves and replenishment stock is refilled from behind.

STORAGE TEMPERATURES

Generally, a lower storage temperature decreases the rate of chemical and microbiological degradation of a medicinal product and so increases the shelf-life. However, reducing the temperature to below 0° may not extend the shelf-life of some medicinal products but cause physical damage. Examples of this effect at freezing temperatures are cracking in creams, and aggregation in insulin and some vaccines. Equally important are the medicinal products that must be kept warm or at room temperature; among these are soft gelatin capsules in which the gelatin shell may harden and crack if stored at a temperature lower than 15° or outside the ideal range of relative humidity (40% to 60%). When a monograph in a compendium does not state a storage temperature, it is assumed that the medicinal product may be satisfactorily stored at ambient room temperature. The meaning of 'room temperature' varies between compendia; the *European Pharmacopoeia* defines room temperature as 15° to 25°, but gives national authorities the right to decide 'in the light of desirable conditions of such storage and the seasonal climatic conditions of the country concerned'; the *United States Pharmacopeia XXII* states that room temperature is the temperature prevailing in a working area. Controlled room temperature is defined by the *United States Pharmacopeia XXII* as a temperature maintained thermostatically between 15° and 30°.

General terms for storage conditions and the relevant temperature ranges or limits of the *United States Pharmacopeia* and the *European Pharmacopoeia* appear in Table 1.

Table 1
Comparison of compendial storage terms and definitions

Term	United States (USP XXII)	Europe (Eur.Ph.)
In a freezer	between −20° and −10°	below −15°
In a refrigerator	between 2° and 8°	2° to 8°
Cold	not exceeding 8°	—
Cool	between 8° and 15°	—
Cold or cool	—	8° to 15°
Warm	between 30° and 40°	—
Excessive heat	above 40°	—

Storage Under Refrigerated Conditions

Many medicinal products are required to be stored in a refrigerator; for example insulin, certain vaccines, some cytotoxic injections, biologicals, diagnostic agents, chloramphenicol eye drops, liquid oral antibiotics, and other liquid preparations prepared by reconstitution.

In its *Code of Ethics*, The Royal Pharmaceutical Society of Great Britain states that the dispensary equipment should include a refrigerator equipped with a maximum/minimum thermometer and capable of storing products at temperatures between 2° and 8°. Most refrigerators are designed to maintain a temperature of 5° and pharmacists have been reminded by the Society that refrigerators should be defrosted at regular intervals to ensure efficiency. Dysfunction of a refrigerator will cause a rise in temperature which may approach room temperature (20°) within four hours. An instance is reported of 45-mL containers that were monitored for temperature during power loss. Although there was no change in temperature within 20 minutes of

power loss, containers reached 6° within 100 minutes and 9° to 10° within two hours. Factors which affect the rate of temperature increase include the refrigerator model, the density and type of insulation, the ambient temperature outside the refrigerator, and the load within the refrigerator.

In 1987, the Royal Pharmaceutical Society commended to its members the use of maximum/minimum thermometers in dispensary refrigerators because of the need to establish that storage conditions have at no time extended beyond the limits recommended by manufacturers for thermolabile products. However, a maximum/minimum thermometer may register a false high reading (which will show as a maximum) when the door of the refrigerator is opened. Certain maximum/minimum thermometers are designed to be read and re-set from outside the refrigerator; if a false high reading is to be avoided with such thermometers, it is essential to check the reading before opening the refrigerator door and to re-set the thermometer several minutes after closing the door. In more sophisticated equipment, temperature recording devices are situated outside the refrigerator and the temperature probe is located within. Such equipment can be pre-set to monitor the required high and low temperatures and linked to an audible alarm that sounds if the temperature within the refrigerator deviates from the set limits. A similar device can be used for monitoring temperatures during transport as well as during storage.

Within any refrigerator there will be a temperature gradient; the warmest area is usually at the top, but is dependent on the position of the cooling element. Materials stored near the cooling element may be exposed to cycles of freezing and thawing throughout any 24-hour period. Medicinal products such as bacterial vaccines and insulin injections are more likely to have their potency impaired by freezing than by storage at ambient temperatures. Vaccines and insulin injections damaged by freezing show increased rates of sedimentation and clumps of particles are evident on rotation of the vial. The increased vulnerability of vaccines and insulin to freezing is attributed to the adjuvants. In vaccines the adsorbents aluminium phosphate or aluminium hydroxide tend to be in the form of amorphous gels which rearrange on freezing as crystals that trap the antigen.

Medicinal products required to be stored under refrigerated conditions may on occasion be inadvertently stored at a higher, usually room, temperature. Such storage may adversely affect the medicinal product by either rendering it useless or shortening its shelf-life. Publications have appeared in which the shelf-life of preparations intended to be stored under refrigerated conditions are listed, together with their shortened shelf-life at room temperature.

Aseptically prepared infusion fluids may be stored in a refrigerator to increase their shelf-life. However, the intravenous administration of large volumes of cold fluids has been reported to produce cardiac and general hypothermia in patients. Thus, time should be allowed for an infusion fluid removed from a refrigerator to approach room temperature before administration. Investigations have shown that 500 mL of infusion fluid in either a polyvinyl chloride bag or glass bottle takes approximately three hours to reach ambient temperature. Infusion fluid emerging from a burette system and line may take up to 20 minutes to attain room temperature. A 30-mL volume of injection stored in a 60-mL plastic syringe attained room temperature within 90 minutes of removal from refrigerated conditions.

It is common practice to refrigerate partially used (that is, potentially contaminated) multidose vials of injections (which contain antimicrobial preservatives) on the assumption that such a procedure will inhibit bacterial proliferation. Experimental data have demonstrated that bacteria inoculated into insulin injection and four other injectables presented in multidose vials remained viable significantly longer under refrigeration than at room temperature. It has therefore been proposed that preserved sterile medicaments packaged in multidose vials are stored at room temperature after initial use (that is, after exposure to potential contamination) unless drug stability considerations dictate otherwise. These proposals are supported by early research on the influence of temperature on the activity of antimicrobial preservatives, which demonstrated that the activities of most preservatives increased as the temperature increased (but there are exceptions). The relationship between temperature and preservative activity can be expressed as:

$$\Theta (T_2 - T_1) = \frac{k_2}{k_1}$$

where Θ is the temperature coefficient of the preservative, k_1 is the death-rate constant at temperature T_1, and k_2 is the death-rate constant at temperature T_2.

Values for temperature coefficients vary according to the temperature range and the test organism; few values have been published. Therefore, although in theory it is possible to calculate the influence of temperature on preservative activity, in practice, each system must be experimentally tested.

Cold Chains

Medicinal products required to be stored under refrigerated conditions must be maintained between 2° and 8° during transit from manufacturer to user. Carriage may be by means of air, sea, or land transport and vigilance is required to ensure that refrigerated conditions are maintained at all times during such a distribution chain, that is, a cold chain. Manufacturers and distribution companies usually ensure suitable packaging for the journey. Specific standards are outlined in guidelines produced by WHO and UNICEF for the labelling and packaging of immunisation products for transportation to tropical climates. Although manufacturers normally deliver their products to some central point such as a regional centre or base hospital, the cold chain may have to be extended over many miles, possibly in hot conditions, to outlying clinics or vaccination centres. Special cooling systems, which ensure uninterrupted refrigeration temperatures both during storage and transport, have been developed in response to the WHO 'Extended Programme on Immunisation'. These cooling systems include:

- an ice lined refrigerator in which the ice lining safeguards the contents during electrical failure
- an ice pack freezer; this was developed for producing ice packs which are used during transport
- a vaccine refrigerator and ice pack freezer; these work on liquid petroleum gas
- a health centre refrigerator; a small cabinet refrigerator with thick insulation which works on liquid petroleum gas, kerosene, mains electricity or batteries
- insulated transport; a portable box with extremely thick insulation.

In addition the WHO has tested 27 insulated 'vaccine' boxes to assess their ability to maintain temperatures below 10°. In all instances ice packs were precooled to −20° and the tests carried out on fully loaded boxes. The tests have been criticised on the grounds that the container temperature rather than the product temperature was monitored and it was not determined whether product freezing had occurred. Product freezing would be detrimental to many vaccines including cholera, diphtheria, tetanus, measles, and typhoid.

Three insulated coolboxes (large, medium, and small capacity vaccine carriers) available in the United Kingdom have also been evaluated. Ice packs precooled to $-20°$ and used without insulation caused freezing of the contents of vaccine carriers. The findings led to the recommendation that in order to prevent the contents freezing and to extend the storage life of vaccines, the vaccine carrier itself should be precooled to $5°$ and the ice packs precooled to $-5°$. If longer transport times are necessary more ice packs should be included. However, it was stressed that each combination of vaccine, ice packs, and internal load requires validation if it is to be used in a cold chain.

Insulin-dependent diabetic patients, when travelling to warm climates, are recommended to carry their insulin injections in a polystyrene container or wide-necked vacuum flask. The container (not the insulin) should be precooled in a refrigerator before travelling and at hotels *en route*. Such patients are warned not to allow their insulin to freeze by inadvertent contact with frozen ice packs.

Storage at Freezer Temperatures

Storage of a medicinal product at freezer temperatures ($0°$ to $-21°$) is a means of extending its shelf-life beyond that expected at refrigerator or room temperatures. Medicinal products that may be suitable for storage at freezer temperatures are those that have very short shelf-lives at ambient temperatures and that need immediate compounding before use. Examples are injections admixed to infusion fluids and to parenteral nutrition solutions. Medicinal products unsuitable for freezing are emulsions, suspensions, insulin, and certain vaccines, where the formation of ice crystals during the freezing process would destroy the physical structure of the product.

Advantages of storing medicinal products at freezer temperatures are:

- the opportunity to implement prospective quality control
- the economic benefits associated with large-scale batch production as opposed to daily or individual compounding
- the convenience of 'off the shelf' availability.

However, considerable care must be exercised in choosing a freezer temperature and the method of freezing, since examples exist (amoxycillin sodium in water for injections) in which the apparently frozen system at $-20°$ showed little increased stability in comparison with the same system stored as a liquid above $0°$. If the eutectic temperature of the system is below that chosen as the freezer temperature, the apparently frozen product will contain vesicles of concentrated liquid solution in equilibrium with the frozen solvent. If the drug is unstable in aqueous solution the degradation rate may be increased in the liquid vesicles in the temperature range between $0°$ and the eutectic temperature.

Monitoring of temperatures at different levels within an upright freezer has shown that the temperature was not constant but fluctuated as the thermostat cut in and out. Fluctuation of temperature was of an unacceptable order when the freezer was empty; fluctuation decreased, but was still present, when the freezer was packed. Within the freezer, the temperature range was different for each compartment or shelf. Freezers used for storing injections should be run full, not empty, and temperature gradients should be mapped to ensure that all sections in freezers are suitable for storage.

Freeze-Microwave-Thaw Techniques

One major disadvantage of storage at freezer temperatures is the time taken to thaw the stored product before use. Intervals that have been reported range from 90 minutes for plastic minibags that contained 50 mL of infusion fluid to 8 to 10 hours for 3-litre bags of infusion fluids. More recently microwave ovens have been used to overcome the time constraints in the thawing process. Before instituting a microwave thaw system, it is essential to determine whether the microwave energy will increase the rate of degradation of the drug or will materially affect the container. The range of microwave wavelengths is defined as 0.01 to 10 cm but the energy produced by microwave radiation has only a very small potential for rupturing covalent bonds. In practice, when electromagnetic waves impinge upon molecules, energy transfer is distributed over several adjacent bonds thus diminishing the overall effect.

Microwave radiation is capable of affecting the stability of a drug molecule in solution by its potential for the formation of free radicals and for the evolution of heat. Peroxides, sulphides, disulphides, diazonium compounds, and halomethanes present as additives or contaminants in pharmaceutical solutions could produce free radicals during microwave irradiation. Extremely reactive free radicals are capable of disrupting covalent bonds within a drug molecule. However, pharmaceutical techniques used during the manufacture of intravenous solutions are designed to eliminate free radicals and free radical initiators. Thus the effects of microwave radiation on most intravenous solutions will be minimal.

During irradiation, 'hot spots' may occur in microwave ovens due to uneven radiation fields. Such 'hot spots' are a potential source of overheating of medicinal products and in consequence, extreme care must be taken when thermolabile drugs are thawed using microwaves. Concern has also been expressed that microwave thawing may overheat the contents of plastic infusion bags causing rupture and spillage. However, reports in the literature suggest that neither increased degradation nor container damage is a significant problem. Domestic microwave ovens with rotating carousels have been adapted successfully for thawing medicinal products but such equipment should include means for monitoring temperature to ensure that uniform exposure and safety from overheating are achieved. Additionally, an extended exposure time is required for the microwave thawing of more than one bag of injection/infusion fluid.

Storage of Medicinal Products at Temperatures other than those Recommended

Occasions arise when medicinal products are not stored at the recommended temperature or when it is not possible to attain the recommended temperature. For example, refrigeration units may fail, medicinal products may be left out of the refrigerator, or goods may be stored in transit at an undesirable temperature. Alternatively, it may be necessary to sterilise a medicinal product by autoclaving or to store it at freezer temperatures. Decisions must be made as to whether medicinal products are suitable for use after storage at a non-recommended temperature. Most monographs in the compendia only state the storage temperature or temperature range and the shelf-life under those conditions. For incorrectly stored medicinal products it is possible to quantitatively estimate the change in chemical stability due to temperature using the Q_{10} concept. A value for the effect of temperature on reaction rates is given by the Arrhenius equation:

$$k = A e^{-\left(\frac{E_a}{RT}\right)}$$

where k is the rate constant, A is the frequency factor, E_a is the activation energy (kJ/mol), R is the the gas constant and T is the temperature in degrees Kelvin.

The Arrhenius equation can be expressed in the logarithmic form as:

$$\ln k = \ln A - \frac{E_a}{RT}$$

or

$$\log k = \log A - \frac{E_a}{2.303RT}$$

A plot of $\log k$ versus $1/T$ produces a straight line with a slope of $-E_a/2.303R$ if the reaction is dependent on temperature. This linear relationship is used in isothermal stability testing to predict rate constants at unknown temperatures from rate constants determined at known temperatures. The predicted rate constants are utilised in the estimation of shelf-life. Since in practice the value of E_a is often unknown, a method has been developed which introduces approximations for E_a values into the calculations.

In the Q_{10} concept the temperature coefficient or Q_{10} is defined as follows:

$$Q_{10} = \frac{(K_T + 10)}{K_T} = e^{-\left(\left[\frac{E_a}{R}\right]\left[\frac{1}{(T+10)} - \frac{1}{T}\right]\right)}$$

Although Q_{10} is defined in terms of rate constant K_T, stability information on medicinal products in the literature is usually given in terms of shelf-life, for example, as $t_{10\%}$, $t_{50\%}$. Since $t_{10\%} = 0.105/k$ and $t_{50\%} = 0.693/k$ at all temperatures, it is possible to define Q_{10} in terms of shelf-life as follows:

$$Q_{10} = \frac{t_s^T}{t_s^{T+10}}$$

where t_s^T is shelf-life at temperature T and t_s^{T+10} is the shelf-life at a temperature 10° higher than T. The above equation can be further generalised for instances when the prediction of shelf-life is required for changes in temperature (ΔT) of more than 10°.

$$Q_{\Delta T} = Q_{10}^{\left(\frac{\Delta T}{10}\right)} = \frac{t_s^T}{t_s^{T+10}}$$

Where $Q_{\Delta T}$ is the average value of Q_{10} over the temperature range, $T + \Delta T$.

Rearrangement of the above equation can be expressed as:

$$t_s \text{ at } T \text{ unknown} = \frac{(t_s \text{ at } T \text{ known})}{Q_{10}^{\left(\frac{\Delta T}{10}\right)}}$$

where T unknown and T known are the temperatures in degrees Celsius of known and unknown values of shelf-life t_s, and ΔT is the difference between T unknown and T known.

The last equation can be used to estimate the remaining shelf-life of a medicinal product stored for a known time at a temperature different from that recommended, provided the shelf-life at the recommended storage temperature is known.

The value of Q_{10} is not constant for every $10°$ interval of temperature change, but decreases with increasing temperature and decreasing activation energy for all values of E_a. In most medicinal products the value of E_a will be unknown and so the value of Q_{10} has to be estimated. In practice the value of E_a for most drugs and medicinal products ranges from 50 to 125 kJ/mol, and so the value of Q_{10} near room temperature will be between the extreme values of 2 and 5. For the most conservative estimates of shelf-life using the Q_{10} concept, a value of $Q_{10} = 2$ would be chosen to predict the increase in shelf-life obtained by decreasing the storage temperatures, and a value of $Q_{10} = 5$ to predict the decrease in shelf-life expected by increasing the storage temperature.

An example of a shelf-life calculation based on the application of Q_{10} values of 2 and 4 appears in the chapter on Stability of Medicinal Products.

Whilst the Q_{10} concept is useful in estimating the shelf-life of medicinal products stored at temperatures other than that recommended, it is only valid if the order of the degradation reaction remains constant at the different temperatures and if the degradation reaction remains the same. For example, the Q_{10} concept is not valid if the degradation at a recommended storage temperature is caused by a hydrolytic reaction which at a different storage temperature is catalysed by another component present in the medicinal product, or if the order of the reaction changes with the change in temperature. Also, the Q_{10} concept cannot be applied to physical changes that may occur as a function of temperature, for example, if a suspending agent coagulates as temperature rises, or if rheological characteristics change, or if a drug crystallises from an aqueous solution due to a decrease in temperature.

Storage in Tropical Climates

Medicinal products stored and transported within countries with a tropical climate, unless kept in a controlled environment, will be exposed to high temperatures (exceeding $30°$ and up to $45°$ in summer) and in some areas to high relative humidity (RH). Such storage conditions provide a suitable environment for the degradation of thermolabile and moisture-sensitive medicinal products. In a worldwide classification four climatic zones have been specified: temperate ($21°$, 45% RH); Mediterranean and subtropical ($25°$, 60% RH); hot and dry ($31°$, 40% RH); and hot and humid ($31°$, 70% RH).

The stability of several medicinal products has been investigated during their transportation by sea from Europe to Sudan and during subsequent storage and transportation within Sudan. No significant degradation of the tested products was reported during transportation to Sudan, but significant degradation of three aqueous injections (lignocaine and adrenaline, suxamethonium chloride, and ergometrine maleate) occurred rapidly during storage in the tropical climate. In contrast, dry procaine penicillin powder for injection, which exhibited some degradation on storage, remained within the specified limits for total benzylpenicillin and procaine. The stability of this product was attributed to the absence of water in the drug molecule and to the type of packaging. In comparison, when stored under tropical climate conditions ampicillin trihydrate capsules initially underwent rapid hydrolytic degradation which slowed down until there was no further evidence of degradation. The presence of water in the drug molecule (as the trihydrate) was considered to be responsible for the hydrolytic degradation. Once the water had been used up in the hydrolytic reaction, no further degradation occurred. These experimental results indicate that most water-containing medicinal products stored under tropical conditions can be expected to deteriorate at a much higher rate than if stored in more temperate climates. Possible solutions to the problem could include the provision of separately packed dry powder and solvent in place of pre-prepared aqueous injections, anhydrous forms of a drug rather than the hydrate, better packaging, and pharmaceutical compounds with better stability profiles under hot and humid storage conditions.

Under artificially controlled tropical conditions, tablets prepared from lactose and rice or tapioca starch have been reported to spoil due to the growth of natural microbial contaminants. Tablets of lactose and potato starch inoculated with *Aspergillus niger* also spoiled but the addition of preservatives to tablets during manufacture prevented the growth of both *Aspergillus niger* and the natural contaminants. These findings led to a recommendation that preservatives should be added to all tablets destined to be stored under tropical conditions.

A publication of the industrial pharmacists section of the International Pharmaceutical Federation (FIP) states that it is vital that in tropical countries medicinal products should be kept in storerooms that are dry, adequately ventilated, shaded, and cool. In areas of constant sunshine, the roof should be well insulated and constructed so that sunlight cannot reach the floor area or foundations. With high external temperatures, it is essential to provide adequate ventilation and, if necessary, consideration should be given to a double or secondary roof such that wind can pass through the intermediate space. Walls with perforated or bored bricks allow air to circulate and limit the build-up of static, hot, and humid air in the storeroom. Theft and the ingress of children or rodents can be prevented by means of suitable grilles and security devices. The foundations should be as secure as possible against ground water and high enough to remain dry even under extreme rainfall and flood conditions.

STORAGE PERIODS

Excessive storage times may result in the development of ageing effects in a medicinal product. Ageing is a general term frequently used when the cause of deterioration cannot be readily identified. Examples of ageing effects after long storage include changes in the rheological properties of creams, emulsions, and ointments; changes in the polymorphic form of the drug; increases in the hardness and dissolution times of tablets; and changes in the colour, taste, or odour of a medicinal product.

STORAGE IN CONTAINERS

Storage of the medicinal product in the 'correct' container will prevent or reduce contamination and deterioration. Both the *United States Pharmacopeia XXII* and the *European Pharmacopoeia* emphasise that a container should not interact physically or chemically with its contents in any way that alters the strength, quality, and purity of the contents beyond the limits tolerated by official requirements.

The *British Pharmacopoeia* defines a 'well-closed container' as one that protects the contents from contamination with extraneous solids and liquids and from loss of contents under ordinary conditions of handling, storage, and transport. An 'airtight container' is impermeable to solids, liquids, and gases under ordinary conditions of handling, storage, and transport. If the container is intended to be opened on more than one occasion, it must be so designed that it remains airtight after closure. Definitions in the *United States Pharmacopeia* for 'well-closed' and 'tight' containers closely resemble those of their counterparts in the *British Pharmacopoeia*. However, the *United States Pharmacopeia* additionally applies a test for moisture permeation. See also the Pharmaceutical Packaging chapter.

Both 'well-closed' and 'airtight' containers are used when the medicinal product contains volatile constituents that may escape through an ill-fitting closure. Additionally, such containers reduce (to different degrees) the rate of ingress of moisture and atmospheric gases into the contents of the container.

Examples of volatile constituents lost from medicinal products because of ill-fitting closures include ethanol, which has been reported to evaporate during storage to form a concentration of the commercial product Nepenthe; other examples are methyl salicylate, camphor, menthol, and essential oils that have been lost from ointments and liniments. Inappropriate containers may adsorb or absorb substances from a medicinal product during storage. For example, methyl salicylate in ointments and liniments can act as a plasticiser and soften plastic containers, diazepam may be rapidly absorbed by flexible bags of polyvinyl chloride, certain preservatives in aqueous systems adsorb onto container surfaces, and volatile oils and flavourings may permeate polyethylene containers.

Conversely, the container may be the source of undesirable substances that enter medicinal products. Plasticisers may be leached from plastic containers and flakes of glass, or particles of rubber or metal from other containers may migrate from the surfaces of containers or closures into the medicinal product.

Protection from Light

Both natural and artificial light are known to cause deterioration of light-sensitive medicinal products during storage. Photo-induced decomposition may appear as colour development or colour fading or may not be visually evident. The effects of light depend on its source, the distance of the product from the source, the wavelength, and the light intensity. All light-sensitive products must be protected by enclosure in a light-resistant container, the definition of which is to be found in the chapter on Pharmaceutical Packaging. Light-resistant containers protect contents by virtue of their opacity, the presence of coloured metallic oxides, or incorporated ultraviolet light-absorbing substances. Alternatively, the container may be enclosed in an outer package which provides protection from light, or stored in a place from which light is excluded.

Protection from Humidity/Moisture

Effects of moisture and changes in humidity may be deleterious to medicinal products during storage. Water vapour may gain access to medicinal products through poorly-fitting closures, as a result of failure to re-apply closures or by direct permeation through the container walls. A low moisture content may be maintained within a container by the inclusion of desiccants provided that direct contact with the medicinal product is avoided. In such instances, care should be taken when the container is opened in a moist atmosphere.

Chemical reactions may be initiated in medicinal products during storage under moist conditions. For example, effervescent tablets and granules may react prematurely and drugs prone to hydrolysis may degrade. Exposure to excess moisture may induce visible physical changes in products such as hard gelatin capsules which become soft and tacky; changes in tablet hardness, disintegration, and dissolution characteristics are less obvious effects that may arise. Excess moisture may also cause corrosion of metal containers or closures. Conversely, under very dry storage conditions (low humidity) gelatin capsules become brittle, aqueous solutions and creams lose some of their moisture content, and plastic containers may develop an increase in electrostatic charge, which encourages particulate contamination.

Storage of Repackaged Products

The introduction of unit dose distribution systems into hospitals has led to pharmacists repackaging solid and liquid dosage forms obtained in bulk containers into single unit or unit dose packages.

Certain precautions need to be taken if the quality of the medicinal products repackaged by the pharmacist is to be maintained. The nature of the medicinal product repackaged, the characteristics (chemical and physical) of the package, the degree of protection needed or specified for the product, and the storage conditions to which the repackaged product may be subjected, should all be taken into account before instituting a repackaging service.

The American Society of Hospital Pharmacists has produced guidelines for repackaging, which recommend that all medicinal products should be packaged and stored in an environment of controlled temperature and humidity to minimise degradation caused by heat and moisture. A relative humidity of 75% at 23° should not be exceeded. Additionally, all packaging materials should be stored in accordance with the manufacturer's instructions.

Pharmacists may decide to dispense for individual patients, particularly in residential homes, sufficient for several days treatment of two or more prescribed medicinal products in a customised patient medication package (USA terminology) or a monitored dosage system (UK terminology). Such packages comprise a series of separate compartments, each of which is labelled with the day and time of day and contains the tablets/capsules to be taken by the patient at the specified times. Guidelines for customised patient medication packages are included in the *United States Pharmacopeia XXII*; they give details of labelling, packaging, and record-keeping requirements in addition to the pharmacists' responsibilities. An important requirement is that the container shall be either not reclosable or so designed as to show evidence of having been opened. Due account has to be taken of the physical, chemical, and therapeutic compatibilities of the dosage forms placed within each compartment.

Several reports describe the limited stability of liquid products (for example, gentamicin and dicloxacillin sodium) when repackaged and stored in clear and amber polypropylene oral dose syringes.

Storage of Parenterals and Admixtures in Administration Containers

Certain parenteral products may be packaged and stored in unit-of-use containers or sterile products may be admixed in such containers immediately before administration. Examples of unit-of-use containers are infusion bags with or without administration equipment, prefilled hypodermic syringes or reservoirs used with portable infusion pumps. Caution should be exercised when medicinal products are stored in administration containers because of possible stability problems. It has been reported that even during short storage periods, drugs may become sorbed onto infusion containers of polyvinyl chloride or polyolefins, as well as to components of administration sets. Water vapour may migrate through polyvinyl chloride infusion bags when stored without less permeable overwraps and from reservoirs used with portable infusion pumps.

In powders intended for reconstitution with unpreserved diluents, whatever the stringency of the controls applied to the aseptic transfer, the assurance of sterility of the product is recognised as being of a lower order than that of an injection subjected to a terminal sterilisation process. If reconstituted injections are not administered immediately, and if chemical stability allows, compendial and regulatory bodies have generally limited their storage to 24 hours under refrigeration. Recent advances in infusion technology and developments in home chemotherapy can require unpreserved injections, prefilled into syringes or into medication reservoirs, to be refrigerated for periods exceeding 24 hours before they are administered to patients (at 35° to 37°). Draft guidelines prepared for hospital pharmacists in the United States have recognised the need for longer storage periods and have classified sterile products at three levels of potential risk to patients. For products at Risk levels I and II, maximum storage times, storage temperatures, and administration periods are being assigned.

STORAGE OF MEDICINES IN RESIDENTIAL HOMES

Medicines stored in residential homes will include household remedies used to treat minor ailments, and prescribed medicines for individual residents. Some residents will be able to look after their own medicines and to take them correctly. In such instances each resident should be provided with a lockable drawer or cupboard for the safe keeping of personal medicines. All other medicines in the home are the responsibility of the officer in charge of the home; they should be stored in either a purpose-built and lockable medicines cupboard or a lockable medicines trolley.

Under ideal conditions, the medicines cupboard is suitably sited away from potential sources of heat or humidity; the medicines trolley is immobilised and secured to an immovable object when not in use. Both the medicines cupboard and the medicines trolley should be sited in a room not accessible to the general public. Nothing other than medicines should be kept in the medicines cupboard and trolley to avoid the need to unlock and open them except to administer medicines. On occasions when a medicine is required to be stored under refrigerated conditions, it is acceptable to store it in a separate closed plastic container in the domestic refrigerator belonging to the home.

Medicines prescribed on a continuous basis and which additionally need to be stored in a cool (but not refrigerated) place should not be received in quantities greater than one month's treatment. Such a limitation will reduce the extent of deterioration of the medicinal product if it can only be stored at room temperature.

Good housekeeping policies in the home in respect of the requisition and destruction of medicines will minimise the potential deterioration and wastage that result from inappropriate storage.

STORAGE OF MEDICINES ON WARDS

On hospital wards and in hospices, the responsibility for the safekeeping of medicines rests with the Appointed Nurse in charge. To accommodate different types of medicines, separate lockable enclosures are required as follows:

- a Controlled Drugs cabinet that complies with the Misuse of Drugs (Safe Custody) Regulations
- internal medicines cupboard (to British Standard 2881:1989)
- external medicines cupboard (to British Standard 2881:1989)
- a refrigerator/freezer for medicines.

Separate storage cupboards or spaces are required as follows for:

- diagnostic reagents, including urine testing equipment
- intravenous fluids and sterile topical fluids
- inflammable fluids and gases.

If a medicines trolley is used on the ward, it should be lockable and immobilised when not in use. Supplementary medicinal products that may be urgently required for clinical emergencies, for example cardiac arrest, should be held in boxes clearly marked 'for emergency use'. Although these boxes should be tamper-evident, they should not be stored in a locked cupboard but at a strategic and accessible site.

When patients self-administer medicines on the ward each patient involved should have access to a lockable receptacle, for example, a drawer that is not readily portable.

STORAGE OF MEDICINES IN CLINICS

In community or family planning clinics, medicines should be stored in lockable cupboards. When more than one type of clinic operates from the same building, the ideal circumstance is for each clinic to have a separate lockable cupboard. If this structure is unrealistic, medicines for each clinic should be stored in a separate area of the communal locked cupboard.

Urgent supplementary medicines for clinical emergencies should be held in tamper-evident boxes, clearly marked 'for emergency use only'. Such boxes should be stored in a strategic accessible place, not a locked cupboard.

Responsibility for the safe keeping of medicines in a clinic lies with the Designated Person (who is a professional) and who controls access to the medicines.

STORAGE AND CONTROL OF MEDICINES BY NURSING STAFF DURING DOMICILIARY VISITS

Once medicines are issued to nursing staff for use in the community, the medicines become the responsibility of the person to whom they are issued. Controlled Drugs in Schedule 2 which are issued to midwives must be kept in a locked receptacle. During visiting rounds, medicines should be kept out of sight in a locked car, except when carried on the person of the authorised community nurse. If it is necessary for nursing staff to keep medicines in their homes overnight, the medicines should be placed in a secure locked fixture under optimum conditions of temperature and light protection.

STORAGE OF MEDICINES IN AMBULANCES

Medicines are only carried on ambulances in extended training boxes, which additionally contain specialist kits of equipment. All kits are designed to be tamper-evident.

STORAGE OF MEDICINES IN THE HOME

It is a legal requirement in the United Kingdom that all dispensed medicines are labelled 'keep out of the reach of children'. As an added safeguard, it is a professional requirement that all oral solid dosage preparations are dispensed or packaged for sale either in reclosable child-resistant containers which comply with the relevant British Standard or in unit packaging of strip or blister type. Exceptions to the professional requirement apply when:

- the preparation is in a manufacturer's original pack so designed that transfer to a reclosable child-resistant container will be a retrograde or unnecessary procedure
- the patient is elderly or handicapped and will have difficulty in opening a child-resistant container, or

- the patient specifically asks that the product shall not be dispensed in a child-resistant container.

In the latter two instances, the pharmacist should make a particular point of advising that the medicines are kept well out of the reach of children.

Such professional and legal requirements emphasise the concern to reduce the accidental poisoning of young children by medicines. In 1987, a conservative estimate of the incidence of accidental poisoning of children from ingestion of plants, chemicals (household or garden), or medicinal products put the figure at 30 000 per annum in the United Kingdom.

Ideally, all medicines in the home should be stored in a purpose-built lockable medicine cabinet but in practice few homes possess such a cabinet. Surveys have shown that even in homes where a suitable cabinet is present, it may not be used for the storage of all medicines.

Data on accidental poisoning of children have shown that the kitchen is a comparatively safe place for the storage of medicines. Those medicines located in rooms other than the kitchen are more likely to be involved in child poisoning. A possible reason for the kitchen being a safer place is that the adult in charge of young children in the home is more likely to be located in that room than elsewhere and so is better able to supervise the access to medicines stored therein. However, because kitchens are more prone to high humidity and fluctuations in temperature than other rooms these adverse storage conditions must be weighed against the safety aspects.

A few medicines and in particular the liquid antibiotics, require storage under refrigerated conditions. Although the refrigerator has been shown to be comparatively unsafe as a storage place because of its easy accessibility to young children, child-resistant locks are available for domestic models and their use should be encouraged. In conclusion, it cannot be overstressed that all medicines in the home should be stored in a locked receptacle that is not accessible to young children.

FURTHER INFORMATION

Abu-Reid IO, El-Samani SA, Hag Omer AI, Khalil NY, Mahgoub KM, Everitt G et al. Stability of drugs in the tropics. A study in Sudan. Int Pharm J 1990;4(1):6–10.

Allwood MC. The effectiveness of preservatives in insulin injections. Pharm J 1982;229:340.

ASHP Draft guidelines on quality assurance for pharmacy-prepared sterile products. Am J Hosp Pharm 1992;49:407–17.

ASHP Guidelines for repackaging oral solids and liquids in single unit and unit dose packages. Am J Hosp Pharm 1983;40:451–2.

Ausman RK, Holmes CJ, Walter CW, Kundsin RB. The application of freeze-microwave thaw techniques to central admixture services. Drug Intell Clin Pharm 1980;14:284–7.

Bean HS. J Soc Cosmet Chem 1972;23:703–20.

Bos CE, van Doorne H, Lerk CF. Microbiological stability of tablets stored under tropical conditions. Int J Pharmaceutics 1989;55:175–83.

British Standards Institution. British Standard 2881: 1989. Specification for cupboards for the storage of medicines in health care premises. London: The Institution, 1989.

Brown DR, Sansum CJ. The transportation of vaccines: is the cold chain integrity maintained? Pharm J 1992;249:267–9.

Duthrie Report. Guidelines for the safe and secure handling of medicines. A report to the Secretary of State for Social Services, Department of Health 1988.

Elliott GT, McKenzie MW, Curry SH, Pieper JA, Quinn SL. Stability of cimetidine hydrochloride in admixtures after microwave thawing. Am J Hosp Pharm 1983;40:1002–6.

Hatton I, Christie G, Steventon S. Cost savings by freezing and re-issue of small volume infusions. Pharm J 1986;237:46–7.

Heath PE, Terry D, Wind KL [letter]. Monitoring freezer temperature. Pharm J 1987;239:708.

Hogerzeil HV, Battersby A, Srdanovic V, Sjernstrom NE. Stability of essential drugs during shipment to the tropics. Br Med J 1992;304:210–12.

Lehmann CR. Effect of refrigeration on bactericidal activity of four preserved multiple-dose injectable drug products. Am J Hosp Pharm 1977;34:1196–200.

Longland PW, Rowbotham PC. Stability at room temperature of medicines normally recommended for cold storage. Pharm J 1987;238:147–51.

Longland PW, Rowbotham PC. Room temperature stability of medicines recommended for cold storage. Pharm J 1989;243:589–95.

McDonald C, Sutherland VB, Lau H, Shija R. The stability of amoxycillin sodium in normal saline and glucose (5%) solutions in the liquid and frozen states. J Clin Pharm Ther 1989;14:45–52.

Miller LG, Loomis JH. Advice of manufacturers about effects of temperature on biologicals. Am J Hosp Pharm 1985;42:843–8.

Moles TH [letter]. Refrigerator thermometers. Pharm J 1987;239:254.

National Pharmaceutical Association. Information leaflet No 6. Storage of pharmaceutical preparations. St Albans: The Association, 1980.

Newton DW, Miller KW. Estimating shelf-life of drugs in solution. Am J Hosp Pharm 1987;44:1633.

Pharm Supplies Bull 1986;9(4):5 (42/86).

PMA's Joint QC-PDS Stability Committee. Room-temperature stability studies: storage conditions. Pharmaceut Technol Int 1991;3(10):48–51.

Prevention of infectious disease by immunisation [editorial]. Br J Pharm Pract 1982 Sept;4(6):35.

South Tees Health Authority Pharmaceutical Service. The Storage of drugs under controlled temperature conditions. 2nd ed. Middlesbrough: South Cleveland Hospital, 1975.

Sykes G. Disinfection and sterilization. London: E,F&N Spon Ltd, 1965.

Tarr MJ. Warming rates of refrigerated IV solutions. Pharm J 1987;238:623.

Thakker Y, Woods S. Storage of vaccines in the community: weak link in the cold chain? Br Med J 1992;304:756–8.

United States pharmacopeia XXII. National formulary XVII. Rockville: United States Pharmacopeial Convention Inc, 1990:1574.

West Berkshire Health Authority. Batch number identification directory. Reading: Battle Hospital, 1988.

Willan CE [letter]. 'Cool boxes' required. Pharm J 1987;238:293.

Wingfield J. Law and ethics bulletin. Pharm J 1988;240:28.

Wiseman HM, Guest K, Murray VSG, Volans, GN. Accidental poisoning in childhood; a multicentre survey 2. The role of packaging in accidents involving medications. Human Toxicol 1987;6:303–14.

Zeal S [letter]. Refrigerator thermometers. Pharm J 1987;239:254.

Pharmaceutical Aspects of Clinical Trials

Clinical trials are planned scientific investigations in groups of human subjects; they are designed to demonstrate the efficacy and safety of any medical treatment, procedure, or device intended for use in diagnosis, prophylaxis, or therapy. Most clinical trials, however, are for the evaluation of new drugs under development by pharmaceutical companies; such trials are commonly classified into four main stages which proceed through phases I to IV.

Phase I studies include the first trials in man and are primarily concerned with the safety, pharmacokinetics, and pharmacodynamics of the drug. The drug is initially given as a single, very low dose, then in gradually increasing amounts and, subsequently, in multiple doses. Radiolabelled compound of very low activity is also used at this stage to determine the metabolic fate of the compound. Phase I trials, each of which involve only small numbers of subjects, are generally conducted in normal volunteers unless ethical considerations dictate the use of patients, for example, in the testing of cytotoxic agents.

Phase II studies are carried out in patients to evaluate efficacy and to define both the therapeutic dose range and dosing regimen for a particular indication. The studies are designed to produce additional information on safety, pharmacokinetics, and pharmacodynamics in the presence of the disease process. Relatively small numbers of patients are studied, under close supervision, usually by highly qualified and specialised investigators.

Phase III studies are performed in considerably larger numbers of patients than in phase II and are frequently carried out on a multicentre basis. The principal aims are to demonstrate long-term safety and tolerance and to compare the new drug with existing standard treatments.

Phase IV studies are conducted after a product licence has been obtained and are frequently termed 'post-marketing surveillance'. They are generally large-scale, long-term trials, designed primarily to investigate the incidence of relatively rare adverse reactions. Additional comparative studies, for example against newly introduced competitor products, may also be carried out at this stage. Most phase IV studies are used to extend the range of approved indications.

There is a degree of overlap between the different phases, particularly phases I and II; each phase is not necessarily fully completed before the next is started. Clinical pharmacology studies of the phase I type may, for example, be carried out at late stages in the clinical testing programme. However, phase II studies only begin when adequate safety and pharmacokinetic data have been generated from phase I. Similarly, phase III studies are not initiated until efficacy and an acceptable risk profile have been established.

Administration of a new drug to man is preceded by extensive pre-clinical testing both *in vitro* and in *animals*. In the United Kingdom, before a supply of a new drug can be made available for a clinical trial in patients, approval must be obtained from the Medicines Control Agency (MCA). Although official permission is not required for trials in normal volunteers or in patient volunteers who are not expected to benefit from the proposed treatment, guidelines[1–3] on the conduct of such trials are essentially equivalent to the regulatory requirements for patient trials. In July 1993, an EC Directive was implemented which specifically addressed those manufacturing practices that may be different for investigational products that will be tested on human subjects, including volunteers; the Directive is intended as a reference point for member states, with the aim of developing common standards. Protocols for all trials, whether in volunteers or patients, must be approved on a local basis by independent ethical committees composed of clinicians and lay members.

The regulation of clinical trials was increased in 1990 when the Commission of the European Communities published guidelines on Good Clinical Practice for trials of medicinal products within member states as an addendum to the *Rules Governing Medicinal Products in the European Community*.[4] These guidelines set out the responsibilities of the sponsor of trials (usually a pharmaceutical company), the monitor (often an employee of the company or of a contract research organisation), and the clinical investigator.

The requirements of good clinical practice have been reviewed extensively[5] and should be familiar to anyone involved in clinical research.

Design of Trials

Whatever the design of trial chosen, it is essential that the protocol is written and finalised before the trial commences. A protocol must contain a full and detailed description of the objective of the trial, the patients to be included (and excluded), the medicine(s) to be administered, the tests to be performed, and the manner in which the data will be analysed. A protocol should contain sufficient information for the study to be repeated elsewhere without recourse to any other documents except easily accessible, medico-scientific literature.

Randomised, controlled trials are generally considered to be the most valid basic design. Randomisation of the allocation of treatments eliminates the possibility of bias in the selection of subjects. The inclusion of a control, which might be placebo, standard therapy, or no treatment at all, permits a valid comparison to be drawn. In any single study, more than one control can be used; for example, placebo and standard treatment. Similarly, more than one test group can be included within a given study; for example, in a comparison of different dosage regimens.

The most common designs are:

- **Parallel** where subjects are randomly allocated to either the new drug or control. A predetermined number of subjects are studied for a specified time and the results obtained in the groups are compared.

  A pre-treatment 'run-in' period, in which patients are untreated or receive placebo, is usually included to minimise any possible 'carry-over' effects of previous medication and to allow the stability of the disease condition to be assessed.

- **Cross over** where each subject receives both test drug and control therapy in a randomly-assigned sequence. Because each subject acts as his own control, cross over studies have the advantage over parallel studies that fewer subjects are required. However, cross over trials cannot be used when the treatment is curative, when the course of the disease is unstable with respect to time, or when treatment is required for long periods. Pre-treatment 'run-in' and between-treatment 'wash-out' periods are usually part of the trial protocol.

Other types of design employed include **sequential**, **factorial**, and **Latin square**. The most appropriate design is usually selected by the clinician initiating the study in consultation with a statistician. Statistical input is also required to estimate the number of subjects necessary to meet the trial objective and to determine and implement the optimum method of randomisation. Whatever the basic design chosen, a further decision must be made as to whether the trial should be open or blind.

Open studies are ones in which all the participants in the trial are aware of the identity of the treatment being administered.

Blind studies may be of two types:

- **Single blind** where the subject or the investigator is unaware of the identity of the treatment for a particular individual. A variation is to employ a 'blinded' third party, independent of the investigator, who may administer the doses or may act as the observer responsible for making the assessments in the study.

- **Double blind** where none of the trial participants is aware of the identity of the treatment for a particular subject.

The greater validity of double-blind studies is well recognised as they demonstrably eliminate any potential bias in both the management and the assessment of subjects. In double-blind studies, particularly those of the cross over type, all dosage forms used must be identical, not only in appearance, but also in other physical characteristics. Concerns have been expressed that differences were detectable between preparations in allegedly double-blind studies; the use of panels to assess matching has been suggested.[6-8]

Where exact matching of the dosage forms is not feasible or where the routes of administration of the products under comparison differ, the so-called 'double-dummy' technique can be employed to achieve double-blindness. As the name implies, this method requires matching placebos for each preparation. Thus for a trial of treatment A versus treatment B, each treatment would consist of either active A + placebo B or placebo A + active B.

It is essential in all double-blind trials that the investigator is provided with the treatment code for use in an emergency situation. A single sealed envelope is issued for each subject in the study, which contains only the treatment details for that particular subject. For hospital-based studies, a separate set of disclosure envelopes should also be supplied to the pharmacy department.

The use of double-blinding is always desirable but is sometimes neither practical nor ethical. Furthermore, where drugs produce characteristic effects or side-effects, their identification is frequently possible even in apparently double-blind studies.[9] In such situations, the use of alternative techniques, for example the blinded-observer method, is preferable.

Formulation of Clinical Supplies

One of the principal aims in the development of formulations for clinical trials is to produce, for use as early as possible in the clinical programme, a preparation that will subsequently be suitable for marketing. Changes in formulation not only involve additional stability studies, but may also necessitate further *animal* work and bioequivalence testing in human volunteers. For drugs with a high first-pass metabolism, the bioequivalence of different formulations can be difficult to establish because of large inter-subject variation. In such instances, it is particularly important to carry out all, or a major part, of the phase III programme with the final dosage form.

The main problems in achieving the desired final dosage form at an early stage are the almost inevitable shortage of active raw material available for formulation work, the difficulty in predicting the final human dose and, especially for capsules or tablets, the establishment of future marketing requirements.

In advance of any formulation work, the drug substance is subjected to a programme of preformulation studies (see Preformulation chapter). As well as providing essential data on physicochemical properties, these studies are directed to evaluating the compatibility and stability of the drug with potential excipients. A basis is thus obtained for a rational approach to the development of any formulation.

Important points to consider when formulating a product for international use are the availability and acceptability of excipients in different countries. The acceptability of dyes is an issue of special concern whether presented in a formulation or in a capsule shell.

For products intended to be administered orally as solid dosage forms, it is common to perform the early phase I studies using hard gelatin capsules, hand-filled with appropriate amounts of the drug substance alone. If the doses, which at this stage are usually tailored to the body-weight of the individual subjects, are too small to be weighed accurately, simple solutions or suspensions prepared by dilution may be provided. Drugs that are poorly soluble, however, may require formulation to optimise their bioavailability even at this stage

of the clinical programme; a possible approach to this situation has been outlined by Daniel *et al.*[10] In later phase I and phase II studies, hard gelatin capsules are still commonly employed to facilitate blinding when doses are different. However, the greater numbers of dosage forms now required necessitates the use of a formulation that can be filled on automatic or semi-automatic equipment. If a tablet is the intended commercial presentation, then tablets should be introduced in trials as soon as possible after the dose has been defined.

For products intended for non-oral routes of administration, it is usual to develop an initial formulation that will be suitable not only for toxicological testing but also, albeit with concentration changes, for clinical testing and for marketing. In such instances, input from marketing groups is usually limited to the type of packaging that will ultimately be required.

Methods of Blinding

Dosage Forms

Placebos. The preparation of matching placebos is usually straightforward unless the drug is coloured or has some other distinctive property, such as odour or taste. Even in these circumstances, adequate blinding of placebo and active capsule formulations can sometimes be achieved by the use of opaque, intensely-coloured capsule shells, possibly with banding to deter the inquisitive. Similarly, the application of a suitable coating to active and placebo tablets can be sufficient to mask colour and olfactory properties. However, there is always a risk that the subject, or indeed an investigator, may break open the dosage forms or that the subject may bite or chew the products.

Where colour is the problem, the inclusion of a permitted dye or colouring agent may be appropriate for oral or topical placebos, but the use of such additives in injections or ophthalmic products is not usually acceptable, if only for ethical reasons.

Comparator products. Alteration of a product made by a competitor company to effect blinding in a clinical trial is really only feasible for solid dosage forms. The blinding techniques used include the following:

- Encapsulation of the intact product. The comparator capsule or tablet is placed inside a hard gelatin capsule shell possibly with an inert filler such as lactose or starch to prevent audible movement. There are obvious limitations on the size of capsules or tablets which can be blinded in this way; for example, a size 0 capsule is generally regarded as the largest size that is clinically acceptable. Rice paper cachets have also been used in this manner as an alternative to capsules.

- Coating of tablets. Sugar, compression and, most commonly, film coating have been employed to blind both coated and uncoated tablets. The use of compression coating for this purpose is described by Hadfield *et al.*[11]
- Encapsulation/compression of a powder/granule blend obtained from the manufacturer of the comparator product.
- Grinding of comparator tablets followed by encapsulation or re-compression, with or without additional excipients.
- Milling of comparator capsules followed by re-encapsulation, with or without additional excipients.
- Formulation from the active raw material. This technique, which is only possible if patent protection is no longer an issue, is usually precluded by the resource implications.

Application of any of the above techniques of blinding must be accompanied by appropriate testing of the finished dosage form to show that bioavailability has not been altered. Disintegration and dissolution tests may be sufficient where no undue manipulation of the parent dosage form has occurred. However, when the comparator product has been substantially changed as in the last three methods above, *in-vivo* bioequivalence studies are also necessary if the validity of the subsequent clinical trial is not to be questioned.

If blinding of the comparator product cannot be accomplished, a supply of unmarked product with matching placebos can be requested from the manufacturer or, alternatively, provided that the product is no longer under patent protection, actives and placebos can be purchased from a generic supplier. In either instance, it will be necessary to use the double-dummy method of presentation to preserve the blinding of the trial.

Packaging

Packaging is an integral part of the blinding of the supplies for any study and may be the only method by which comparator products, which are not solid dosage forms, can be blinded. For example, colourless injections can be filled into ampoules identical to those used for the test products.

Packaging also assumes major importance in studies that involve variable dosage regimens, which compare treatments with different dosing schedules or which require double-dummy presentations. In order to maintain blindness and to avoid the use of multiple containers, which might lead to poor patient compliance, special packaging techniques are frequently adopted. A common method involves the production of daily or weekly dose cards comprising strip or blister-packed dosage forms. For example, in a trial of tablet A taken twice daily (at 11:00 and 23:00) versus capsule B administered three times daily (at 8:00, 16:00, and 23:00) a suitable daily card could be prepared by the attachment of four sachets, each labelled with the time of administration (see Fig. 1). The contents of the sachets would be as follows:

For treatment A:
  8:00, 16:00 — placebo B
  11:00 — active A
  23:00 — active A + placebo B

For treatment B:
  8:00, 16:00 — active B
  11:00 — placebo A
  23:00 — placebo A + active B

Similar schemes can be devised using folding stencilled cards in which blister packs are enclosed (see Fig. 2).

Manufacture of Clinical Supplies

All clinical supplies must be manufactured according to the requirements of good manufacturing practice (GMP). A manufacturing licence is not required, but if supplies are to be issued on a named-patient basis, then possession of a manufacturer's 'specials' licence is necessary. The granting and renewal of such a licence are dependent upon satisfactory audits by the Medicines Inspectorate of the Medicines Control Agency.

Safety of manufacturing personnel must also be a prime consideration because in the early stages of development, little information may be available on the potential hazards of handling the novel drug substance in bulk.

Most of the problems that arise in clinical manufacturing occur at early stages in the clinical trial programme and are frequently due to shortage of the active raw material for process development work. It is often the case that demands for the new compound for refinement, optimisation, and validation of manufacturing processes and for scale-up work must compete with other needs,

```
Study No: XXX/XXX100/GB      CT650      Patient No: _____
                                        Day No:     _____


INVESTIGATOR NAME:       _____
ADDRESS:                 _____

Directions: Take the contents of each sachet with water at
the time specified on the sachet, i.e. 08.00 h, 11.00 h,
16.00 h and 23.00 h.

        IT IS IMPORTANT THAT THE CORRECT SACHET IS OPENED
                    AT THE CORRECT TIME

   Protect from light and moisture.      Expiry date: _____


                    FOR CLINICAL TRIAL USE


    ┌──────────┐  ┌──────────┐  ┌──────────┐  ┌──────────┐
    │          │  │          │  │          │  │          │
    │  08.00   │  │  11.00   │  │  16.00   │  │  23.00   │
    │          │  │          │  │          │  │          │
    └──────────┘  └──────────┘  └──────────┘  └──────────┘


           Keep out of the reach of children
                [manufacturer, address]
```

Fig. 1
Strip-packed dosage forms presented on a daily dosing card.

such as those of toxicological and clinical studies. Control of product quality is usually demonstrated by detailed documentation and extensive testing during and at the end of processing; testing may be reduced with successive batches as further experience and information are obtained. The involvement and approval of quality assurance personnel at all stages is essential.

Stability Testing

At the start of the clinical programme, stability data generated from preformulation and formulation development work are usually only sufficient to justify a relatively short shelf-life for the product. As further data become available, the assigned shelf-life can be progressively lengthened. However, re-evaluation of the stability of supplies during a particular trial is frequently necessary.

Stability testing must be carried out on samples taken from the containers or packaging used for the clinical supplies, which are usually held under both stressed and normal storage conditions. Although it is not essential to carry out stability tests on every clinical batch produced, studies are required whenever a change in scale, equipment, or formulation is introduced. Similarly, additional stability studies are indicated when the synthesis of the actual drug substance is changed either in terms of scale or process. The possible effects on stability of such modifications are discussed by Lantz.[12]

During the course of any stability study, changes in appearance of the dosage form must be carefully monitored relative to its matching placebo or other comparative agent. For example, differential changes in colour which can occur on storage may compromise the blinding of a clinical trial.

Stability studies on comparator products are essential where the dosage form has been manipulated or repackaged for blinding purposes.

Packaging and Labelling

Although clinical trials can be successfully performed using dosage forms dispensed as required from bulk, the preferable approach is to pre-pack and label supplies ready for dispensing to individual patients. This approach permits all supplies for the study to be packaged simultaneously, thus reducing the margin for error; the use of containers in which the stability of the dosage form has been assessed is also ensured.

Study No: XXX/XXX100/GB   CT650   Patient No: _____
                                   Week No: _____

INVESTIGATOR NAME: _____
ADDRESS: _____
                   _____

Directions: Take the contents of each blister with water
at the time specified above each blister, i.e. 08.00 h,
11.00 h, 16.00 h, and 23.00 h.

   IT IS IMPORTANT THAT THE CORRECT BLISTER IS OPENED
              AT THE CORRECT TIME

Protect from light and moisture.   Expiry date: _____

FOR CLINICAL TRIAL USE

Fig. 2
Blister-packed dosage forms presented on a weekly dosing card.

As with manufacture, the procedures involved in packaging and labelling must comply with the requirements of good manufacturing practice. Essential elements in the prevention of mix-ups are the use of segregated work areas restricted to one product and one set of labels at any one time. The type of packaging selected will be dependent on the requirements of the trial protocol and is usually decided in consultation between pharmacists and clinicians. Child-resistant packaging is mandatory in the United Kingdom and is increasingly used in other countries.

Labelling must meet the regulatory requirements of the country in which the trial is to be performed and should be in the local language. For those countries that specify the inclusion of an expiry or retest date, it may be feasible to provide this information on a separate label which can be easily replaced as the stability of supplies is re-evaluated during the study. Appropriate storage directions, dosing instructions and, in the case of blinded studies, a means of identifying the contents of each pack by reference to the randomisation code or disclosure envelopes must be provided on the label. Identification is usually achieved by the use of a subject number, possibly in combination with a day, week, period, or phase number.

Whatever the type of packaging used, the importance of presentation cannot be over-emphasised. An elegant, clearly-labelled pack not only inspires confidence in both the investigator and the subject, but can also be expected to enhance compliance.

Compliance Monitoring

While imaginative packaging and labelling can considerably improve the level of compliance, it must be recognised that some subjects will fail to follow the prescribed drug regimen correctly. Non-compliant subjects can completely distort pharmacokinetic, efficacy, and safety data obtained in a clinical trial and the detection of such subjects is therefore of utmost importance.

The most common method of estimating compliance is by a combination of a personal interview and an assessment of the quantity of medication returned by each subject at the end of the dosing period. Assays of blood or urine for the drug or metabolite may be performed or the dosage form may include a marker such as a dye that can be detected in the urine. However, all these conventional methods tend to over-estimate compliance. Non-compliant subjects frequently follow the correct regimen for the few days preceding a clinic visit and may even discard unused doses. Incorporation of marker substances into the dosage form requires a change in formulation with all the attendant drawbacks.

Recently, compliance-monitoring containers fitted with microprocessors, have been introduced. The microprocessor records the date and time of each opening and closing of the container and the stored data are subsequently read by a computer.

Distribution of Clinical Supplies

An efficient and well-documented system for the distribution and receipt of clinical supplies is not only fundamental to the concept of good clinical research practice, but it also facilitates rapid recall of supplies. For studies that involve hospital patients or out-patients, supplies must always be despatched to the pharmacy department. To comply with the guidelines issued by the Royal Pharmaceutical Society of Great Britain,[13] information on the trial itself and on the medication should also be provided to the hospital pharmacy. Hospital pharmacists can contribute much to the successful conduct of a clinical trial. In addition to their role in ensuring proper storage and distribution of supplies, pharmacists should be involved at all stages from early planning through to the collection, return, or disposal of unused medication.

Transport of clinical supplies across national boundaries involves knowledge of the local legal requirements and appropriate customs procedures. For instance, before supplies can be shipped to the United States or Canada an Investigational New Drug Application must have been submitted for the study concerned. Other countries, for example, France, Holland, require that an import licence be obtained from the Health Authorities.

Although clinical supplies have no commercial value, the value assigned for customs purposes is of critical importance as it can affect the subsequent market price of the medication.

In July 1993, the EC published an annex to the EC *Guide to Good Manufacturing Practice* which specifically addresses those practices that may be different for investigational medicinal products. Guidance is also included on ordering, shipping, and returning supplies.

CONCLUSION

A trial should be a well thought and planned medico-scientific experiment. There are many individual elements that must be carefully considered before, during the study, and during the analysis of the trial. If the study has been well designed and executed, the results will be accepted by regulatory authorities. If not, the regulatory authorities may reject a product licence application because of the standard of the clinical data.

REFERENCES

1. Commission of the European Communities. Good manufacturing practice for investigational medicinal products. Annex to the EC guide to good manufacturing practice. Luxembourg: The Commission, 1993.
2. Association of the British Pharmaceutical Industry. Guidelines for medical experiments in non-patient human volunteers. London: ABPI, 1988.
3. Association of the British Pharmaceutical Industry. Guidelines on data needed to support the administration of new chemical entities to non-patient volunteers. London: ABPI, 1985.

4. Commission of the European Communities. The rules governing medicinal products in the European Community, Vol III, Addendum 1990: Guidelines on the quality, safety and efficacy of medicinal products for human use. Luxembourg: The Commission, 1990.
5. Spreit A, Dupin-Spreit T. Good practice of clinical drug trials. Basel: Karger, 1992.
6. Hill LE, Nunn AJ, Fox W. Lancet 1976;1:352–6.
7. Anderson TW, Ashley MJ, Clarke EA. Br Med J 1976;1:457–8.
8. Hill LE, Nunn AJ, Fox W. Br Med J 1976;1:710.
9. Huskisson EC, Scott J. Br J Clin Pharmacol 1976;3:331–2.
10. Daniel JE, Draper JR, Simon TH. Drug Dev Ind Pharm 1989;15:585–607.
11. Hadfield PJ, Holmes DS, Yarwood RJ. Drug Dev Ind Pharm 1987;13:1877–90.
12. Lantz RJ. Drug Dev Ind Pharm 1984;10:1425–32.
13. Pharm J 1989;242:105.

FURTHER INFORMATION

Principles and Practice of Clinical Trials. Association of the British Pharmaceutical Industry. Guidelines on good clinical research practice. London: ABPI, 1988.

Good CS, editor. The principles and practice of clinical trials. Edinburgh: Churchill Livingstone, 1976.

Medico-Pharmaceutical Forum. A report by the forum's working party on clinical trials. London: Medico-Pharmaceutical Forum, 1974.

Pocock Stuart J. Clinical trials. A practical approach. Chichester: John Wiley & Sons, 1983 [reprinted 1988].

Schwartz D, Flamant R, Lellouch J. Clinical trials. London: Academic Press, 1980.

Wessex Medico-Pharmaceutical Group. Clinical trial protocol notes. Wessex Medico-Pharmaceutical Group, 1987.

World Health Organization Technical Report Series No. 403. Principles for the clinical evaluation of drugs. Geneva: World Health Organization, 1968.

Ethics. Fried C. Medical Experimentation. Personal integrity and social policy. Amsterdam: North-Holland Publishing Co, 1974.

Manufacturing, Packaging, and Labelling. Drury M. Clinical trials of drugs in general practice. Prescribers' J 1993;33(1):8–15.

Macfarlane CB, Moonie LG. Clinical trials of drug substances. In: Lawson DH, Richards R, Michael E, editors. Clinical pharmacy and hospital drug management. London: Chapman and Hall, 1982.

Monkhouse DC. Dosage forms for clinical trials. Drug Dev Ind Pharm 1985;11:1729–55.

Statistics

Reviewers of the medical literature over the past 50 years found that about half the authors that use statistics do so incorrectly. These mistakes rarely involve advanced statistical theory, but are often quite basic misunderstandings. This causes concern as the application of statistics is an essential part of research, covering the design of experiments and surveys, data collection, analysis, and the drawing of conclusions from the results. This chapter will give a short overview of statistics and their applications in the pharmaceutical industry. It will emphasise how to apply statistics rather than how to calculate them, which is addressed in the books mentioned in the References section at the end of this chapter. An explanation of the different levels of measurement is followed by a section on how measurements vary and the use of statistics to summarise a group of measurements. This leads onto an explanation of the meaning of probability (P), sample size, and 'significance'. Only once these have been understood can the areas of hypothesis testing and regression be addressed; these complete the chapter.

Why use statistics? A well-designed experiment is still the most important part of research and a statistician should be consulted at the design stage, rather than later when trying to salvage something from an ill conceived data-collection exercise. There is a strong ethical case to support the use of good statistical practice as it leads to the efficient and effective use of resources. Mistakes can lead to the waste of time or money and, at worst, to poor treatments being promulgated or good treatments being ignored.

What is the alternative to statistics? The results of some experiments will be so clear that no tests are needed, for example, if two new drugs are tested and one kills all the test animals and the other kills none, then no test is needed; however, if one drug lowers blood pressure by an average of 5 mmHg and the other by an average of 8 mmHg, is one drug better than the other? Statistics will not give us a 'yes or no' answer to this question, but it will quantify our uncertainty and allow us, and others, to exercise judgement in the light of the information collected.

A great deal of statistics involves an understanding of 'variation'. If every tablet, mixture, or patient were identical then measurement of any one from each group would be sufficient to represent the whole. However, in practice, differences exist, so one measurement will not usually be sufficient. A pharmacist normally starts out wanting to know about everyone or everything in a very large group, which is called a **population**. The population may be all tablets produced, the bioavailability of a pharmaceutical formulation in all patients receiving it, or the behaviour of all patients prescribed a particular drug. It is clearly impractical to measure all the subjects, so a **sample** is selected that, it is hoped, is representative of the whole population. Having calculated the desired sample size (see under Hypothesis Testing) the subjects will be chosen, usually at random using random number tables. Once we have our sample, the two most common uses (and abuses) of statistics are to describe results succinctly ('descriptive statistics') and to test one idea (hypothesis) against another, so that we may find the likelihood that one is correct; this latter process falls into an area sometimes called 'inferential statistics'. These uses are covered by such a wide variety of measurements and tests that many people find it difficult to make the correct choice. The key to this problem is to understand which level of measurement has been used; this may seem an abstruse consideration, yet once the three levels of measurement below are understood, many of the common errors in statistics can be avoided.

LEVELS OF MEASUREMENT

Measurement is divided into three levels: nominal (based on name); ordinal (based on order); and interval/ratio (based on a known interval between measurements). Interval/ratio really incorporates two separate levels, but they can be treated in the same way for most statistical purposes.

Nominal

Nominal measurement is the most simple level and is so much a part of life we may not recognise it. It involves putting experimental values into named categories (it is called a 'categorical' level of measurement by some authors); common examples are alive/dead, whole/broken, male/female, pass/fail, tablet/capsule/injection. Note that symbols

(δ, $\circ$), letters, or numbers (such as a batch number) may be used. Each new measurement is allocated to its appropriate category; at the end of the study the number in each category is counted. These data are therefore usually a form of frequency data. The categories must be mutually exclusive and at this level of measurement it is assumed that all members of the same category are equal. For each new reading the decision to be taken is whether it is equal or not equal to the other members in each category; the fact that this only involves two mathematical operations ($=$, $\neq$) will be important later. It is sometimes useful to further subdivide the nominal level into measurements that fall into two categories (binomial) and those that involve more than two categories; this may allow more powerful analysis later.

Ordinal

Ordinal measurement is at a higher level as it allows categories to be arranged in some order. Examples are socioeconomic group; pain scores on a scale of 1 to 5; palatability of formulations on a scale of $+$, $++$, $+++$; or measurement of sedation as the distance from the right of a 100 mm visual analogue scale marked 'wide awake' at the right-hand end and 'nearly asleep' at the other. Not only can this information be categorised, as with the previous level of measurement, but the categories can now be related by putting them in order. This level of measurement is sometimes called a ranking scale. Although the categories can be put in order, the distance between them cannot be defined precisely. For example, it cannot be said that an increase in a pain score from 1 to 2 is the same 'aliquot of pain' as would raise the score from 4 to 5; nor can it be said that someone with a score of 4 is in twice as much pain as someone with a score of 2. Some scales produce a false impression of accuracy, for example, a reading of 40 mm on a visual analogue scale is exactly twice the distance of one of 20 mm, but the subject whose sedation is being judged from the scale could not measure their sedation to that accuracy. Any subjective measurement scale, where people rate themselves or others, must produce ordinal data. Expressed mathematically, the decisions made about a reading are whether it is equal, not equal, greater than or less than others ($=$, $\neq$, $>$, $<$).

Interval and Ratio

Height, weight, volume, temperature, concentration, pressure, and time are examples of interval/ratio data. Much more can be done with these data as the values are objective and have precise relationships: 4 kg is exactly twice as heavy as 2 kg; two 1 kg weights together weigh 2 kg. Often, readings can have any value and may be called continuous data. Mathematically, it can describe not only whether readings are equal to or greater than each other, but it also allows them to be added, subtracted, multiplied, and divided ($=$, $\neq$, $>$, $<$, $+$, $-$, $\times$, $\div$). If certain other assumptions are met then parametric statistical tests (explained below) can be used.

DESCRIPTIVE STATISTICS

Having chosen a sample from the population and measured it, it is necessary to be able to describe that sample as succinctly as possible. This description is provided by two figures: a 'typical' result, and one that gives an idea of the spread of the data. The 'typical' result is often called an average, although this term is discouraged as there are three to choose from, each with an associated measure of spread.

The **mode** is the result that occurs most frequently, that is, the most common result. It is the only method available for nominal data (as all that is needed in its calculation is $=$ and $\neq$), but the mode can also be used at higher levels of measurement. It ignores the size and relative position of all the other readings and therefore is not very representative. Its associated measure of spread is the range; this is the difference between the highest and lowest reading, although in practice the readings themselves are often quoted. Again, these will not be representative of the remaining readings.

The **median** is the midpoint when all the results have been ranked in ascending order. If there are 9 observations, then once they have been ranked from smallest to largest, the median will be the fifth observation. If there is an even number of points then the median is half way between the two middle points. The median can be used for ordinal or higher data (as the procedures in calculating it are $=$, $\neq$, $>$, $<$). It is useful as a description of data because half the results are above, and half below, the median. While it takes into account the relative size of the results, it is not sensitive to outlying points and so can be of use when there are extreme values or when some values are **censored** (that is, values are above or below a certain point, such as the sensitivity limit of an assay, but the exact value is not known). To describe the spread of the results, the ranked data are divided into quarters, each point that divides the quarters is called a quartile. The lowest is called the first quartile, the second quartile is the same as the median, and the highest is the third quartile. The difference between the first and third quartile is called the interquartile range, although it is more usual to give the median and quote the first and third quartiles. With large samples, centiles can be calculated. These divide the results into hundredths, for example the 5th and 95th centile would encompass 90% of the results.

The **mean** is calculated by adding the readings together and dividing by the number of readings. It can only be used on interval/ratio data (as it involves the operations +, ÷). It is very sensitive to the data; if any value is changed, then the mean will also change. To measure spread there are two quantities, the **variance** and the **standard deviation**. These are now on most scientific calculators and therefore seldom have to be calculated by hand, but it is worth understanding how they are derived. If each individual reading were subtracted from the mean and the differences added together, the answer would be zero, as half the values would be negative. Therefore, the difference between each value and the mean (in other words its deviation from the mean) is squared to make it positive. To get a 'typical' deviation, the mean of these squared deviations is calculated by adding them together and dividing by n, the number of readings. This value is the **variance** of the sample, but its units are still squared (for example, square minutes), so the square root is taken, and this gives the **standard deviation**. The standard deviation is usually denoted by SD, s, or σ (sigma), and the variance as s^2 or σ^2. The Greek letters refer to the population and Roman letters to the sample value. It is usual to cite the standard deviation of the population, rather than of our sample, so the sum of the squared differences is divided by $(n-1)$ rather than n.

If the results follow a Normal distribution (see below) then it is possible to begin to predict the likelihood of certain values occurring by using the values calculated for the mean and the standard deviation. However, if they follow a skewed distribution (which looks like a Normal distribution with one tail dragged out), then use of the mean and standard deviation is misleading (high or low values have an inordinately large effect on the mean). Salary is an example of a skewed distribution, for example, one person earning a million pounds per annum has the same effect on the mean as one hundred people earning £10 000 per annum. Results should always be graphed out, to enable assessment of the underlying shape of the distribution before choosing the statistics to describe them. When reading the literature, an indicator that researchers have inappropriately used the mean and standard deviation is that adding or subtracting two standard deviations from the mean produces an impossible result, such as a negative weight, or patient height of 30 mm. The standard deviation should not be confused with the standard error which is explained below.

THE NORMAL DISTRIBUTION

When many readings are taken of some characteristic that follows a Normal distribution (such as the weight of a sample of tablets) and graphed out as a histogram, as more readings are taken, the divisions of the histogram can be made smaller and smaller until they become infinitesimally small. At this point, the histogram becomes a smooth curve, shown on the inner axes of Fig.1. This is the familiar bell-shaped curve of a **Normal distribution** also called a **Gaussian distribution**. When data follows this distribution, a wide range of powerful and sophisticated tests become available for their analysis. The Normal distribution can be generalised (to a standard form with a mean of 0 and SD of 1) from a specific example: the x-axis is converted to a value known as Z, and the y-axis to a measure of the probability (the likelihood of that value occurring); these are shown on the outer axes of Fig.1.

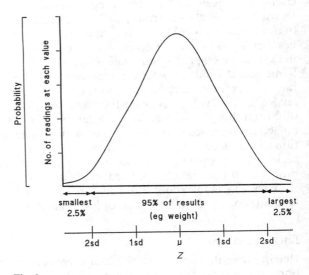

Fig. 1
Normal distribution.

When a variable follows the Normal distribution it is possible to calculate the likelihood of specific values occurring using the mean (sometimes signified by μ) and the standard deviation (σ). When all measurements have been collated, 68.3% of the results will be within one SD either side of the mean; for example, if a mean was 10 and SD = 1, then 68.3% of results would be between 9 and 11. Furthermore, 95.4% would be within 2 SD either side of the mean (8 to 12 in this example) and 99.7% within 3 SD either side of the mean. The probability that an individual result is more than 1.96 SD either side of the mean is $P = 0.05$. These figures are found from Z tables, normally headed 'cumulative normal frequency distribution'.

THE STANDARD ERROR

When a sample is taken from a population of a Normally distributed variable, the sample mean is unlikely to coincide with that of the population, so how representative of the population is it? If many random samples were taken from a population (replacing each sample after measuring it), then the means of each of the samples would themselves form a Normal distribution, which has the same mean as the population mean and a standard deviation of $\sigma/\sqrt{n}$, where σ is the SD of the population. The SD of these means is called the **standard error of the mean** (abbreviated to SEM or sometimes SE) and is used to calculate how the sample mean is related to the population mean. This is important in the calculation of confidence intervals (see below), but should not be used as a measure of spread of the sample (the SD should be used).

ONE OR TWO TAILS?

Another problem faced by researchers is whether to use a two-tailed or a one-tailed test. The tails can be thought of as the ends of a probability distribution. A two-tailed test will detect a difference in either direction (tail); for example an increase or a decrease in bioavailability. A one-tailed test would only allow the testing of, for example, an increase in bioavailability. Some researchers (but few statisticians) argue that if you predict the direction of change beforehand, then it is valid to use a one-tailed test. One suspects that the real reason is that a one-tailed test leads to an apparent halving of the P value, for example, $P = 0.08$ (two-tailed) becomes $P = 0.04$ (one-tailed). This is, to some extent, another aspect of the desire to attain 'significance'. Providing the Method section of a paper and also its Abstract clearly state that a one-tailed test was used, this need not be a pro-

blem for the reader, who can mentally double the P value. Some statisticians argue that a one-tailed test should only be used, for example to look for an increase, if a result in the opposite direction, such as a decrease, were impossible. It is prudent to use two-tailed tests unless a statistician recommends otherwise.

PARAMETRIC AND NON-PARAMETRIC STATISTICS

Statistics is often divided into two areas known as parametric and non-parametric statistics. These terms sometimes cause confusion, although they are easy to differentiate by using the level of measurement. In general, parametric statistics are used to analyse Normally distributed data measured at the interval/ratio level. Non-parametric statistics are used to analyse data at the nominal or ordinal level, or interval/ratio data that are not Normally distributed. Parametric statistics are so called because their foundations rely on assumptions, called parameters, about population values; if these assumptions are met then these techniques are more powerful and wide ranging than non-parametric techniques. Non-parametric techniques are also called distribution-free statistics as they make no assumptions about the shape of the population. Any form of data can be analysed by non-parametric means, if an appropriate test exists; however, if the use of a parametric test is valid, then it should be used, because of its greater power.

There are some situations in which the choice between parametric and non-parametric statistics becomes obscure. If interval/ratio data come from a non-Normal distribution, then the data can either be mathematically transformed to become a Normal distribution (for example by using the logarithm of each reading), or it can be analysed by using non-parametric statistics. Although transformation allows the use of parametric tests, it can be difficult to interpret the results. A number of non-parametric tests produce a test statistic that approximates to the Normal distribution with increasing sample size (for example $n > 30$) and parametric tests may be applicable to ordinal data when there is a large sample; Siegel and Castellan[1] give details. Under these circumstances the advice of a statistician should be sought.

HYPOTHESIS TESTING

Statistical testing often leads to a probability value, yet a dismally small proportion of researchers understand what the term 'probability' refers to. **Probability** is denoted by the letter P, for example:

$P = 1$ — certainty
$P = 0.5$ — a 1 in 2 probability
$P = 0.05$ — a 1 in 20 probability
$P = 0.01$ — a 1 in 100 probability.

When tossing a coin the chance of it coming down 'heads' could be expressed as $P = 0.5$. A P value is commonly quoted after testing an idea (hypothesis testing). It is important to understand exactly what is being tested and what the probability refers to. Two hypotheses should be formulated. Taking as an example the analysis of the bioavailability of two batches of tablets, then the first hypothesis would be that there is no difference between the population from which the two batches have been drawn; this is also called the **null hypothesis** (null = zero, so this is the hypothesis of zero difference); it is abbreviated as H_0. An alternative has also to be devised and must be mutually exclusive with H_0; this is called the **alternative hypothesis** (or H_1); in this example it would be that the batches of tablets were drawn from different populations (perhaps because of a different tableting machine, compression pressure, or formulation). Another example of H_1 would be that a new formulation of a soluble tablet decreases its dissolution time; H_0 is that it does not. Usually H_1 is derived from a research hypothesis. A statistical test will not tell us which is true, but it will give us the probability that one of them is wrong.

The P value is often misinterpreted, so it is important to understand what it represents. When a hypothesis test has been applied and a conclusion reached, the conclusion may be correct or one of two types of mistake could be made (Table 1):

- It is concluded that there is a difference (choose H_1), when in reality there is no difference (H_0 is true).
- It is concluded that there is no difference (choose H_0), when in reality there is a difference (H_1 is true).

The first of these is called a **Type 1 error**; the probability of it occurring is denoted by α and it is the probability value (P value) usually quoted in experimental work. The experimenter should set a level for α before the study. The second type of error is rarely considered and yet is even more disagreeable to the researcher; it occurs when H_1 is in fact true, but the results do not indicate that this is so. It is called a **Type 2 error**; the probability of it

Table 1

| | | Reality | |
		No difference	Difference exists
Findings	No difference	√	Type 2 error β
	Difference exists	Type 1 error α	√

√ indicates that the experimental results have led to the correct conclusions.

occurring is β. A statement that one formulation had better dissolution than another ($P = 0.05$), means there is a 1 in 20 chance that the statement is wrong, in other words, that H_0 was true and there was no difference between the formulations. It is good practice, when coming across a P value in a research paper, to say 'there is a 1 in x chance that this statement is untrue'. Considering the large number of published papers that make decisions at the $P < 0.05$ level, it is inevitable that quite a number (somewhere between 1 in 20 and 1 in 100, as $P = 0.01$ is the next level commonly reported) come to false conclusions.

The **power** of a test is its ability to detect a real difference and is therefore $1 - \beta$ (sometimes expressed as a percentage, for example, 90%). The value of β will also depend on the **sample size** (n) and the extent of the difference between the two groups. A large sample size will reduce the risk of making an error; similarly, for a given sample size a large difference will more likely be detected than a small difference. This interrelationship between α, β, n, and the size of the difference to be detected means that, given any three, the fourth can be calculated. This is the basis of sample size calculations. In addition, the standard deviation of the population is required. Altman[2] gives a nomogram and methods of calculating sample size for common situations; this can also be used to calculate the power of tests in published work. Formulae and tables are available as alternatives.

It is important to consider that there is always some risk of a Type 1 error where H_0 is rejected when it is in fact true; a one in a million chance ($P = 0.000\,001$) will happen exactly one in a million times even though the researcher may be amazed that it has happened to them. This emphasises the fact that one experiment is never enough and may also explain apparently contradictory findings in the literature.

A potentially misleading practice is to call values of $P < 0.05$ 'statistically significant' and those of $P < 0.01$ 'highly statistically significant' when describing results. It is important to separate the P value—the objective probability of a Type 1 error—from the subjective decision that the results have significance. To illustrate the difference, suppose someone were asked to play a game of squash and told that there was a 1 in 20 ($P = 0.05$) chance that they would be knocked by their opponent's racket. Most people consider this probability insignificant, however, a haemophiliac may consider the same probability highly significant; the probability is the same but the relevance different. Before making expensive changes to a production line it would be important to ensure that there was only a very small chance that H_1 had been accepted by mistake, therefore $P = 0.01$ or 0.001 may be chosen as a desirable value. One of the main consequences of linking significance and P values is that the opposite of 'significant' is 'insignificant', consequently experimenters with a P value of greater than 0.05 tend to consider that the experiment is a failure and that the results are of no interest. This is wrong for two main reasons. Firstly, it is just as important to know that a hypothesis is likely to be untrue as to know that it is likely to be true, however, there is a publication bias in the literature that leads to the under-reporting of 'negative' findings. To illustrate this problem with an extreme example, if twenty experimenters conducted the same experiment for which H_0 was true, by chance one may well get a result with $P = 0.05$; this may be published and all the others may be rejected or not submitted for publication. This also has implications for **meta-analysis**—the process by which studies that meet minimum design criteria are pooled and re- analysed to increase sample size and power. The second reason why the $P = 0.05$ watershed is inappropriate is that it focuses on one value, so that a result of $P = 0.049$ is treated differently to one of $P = 0.051$, yet the difference is only 2 in 1000. The convention of using $P = 0.05$ as a level at which to reject H_0 grew from early workers who were trying to balance the high costs of pursuing too many false hypotheses (which would happen if P was set at a higher level) and the costs of conducting large experiments in order to have a high level of certainty when rejecting H_0 and accepting H_1. Probabilities should be interpreted intelligently, according to the study.

Some statisticians think that there is an excessive use of hypothesis testing as it is beset by the problems discussed above and also because the acceptance or rejection of a hypothesis does not indicate the size of any difference; instead they prefer the use of confidence intervals (see below).

CONFIDENCE INTERVALS

The use of confidence intervals is growing in popularity as they can be a more informative alternative to hypothesis testing. The **confidence interval** of a sample is the range of values between which it is fairly certain that the true population mean lies. The uncertainty is quantified by choosing, for example, the 95% confidence intervals, between which we are 95% confident that the population mean lies; there is, therefore, a 1 in 20 chance that it lies outside those values. Consideration of a sample mean and its 95% confidence intervals provides a good indication of the true population. To illustrate how confidence intervals can be used as an alternative to a hypothesis test, consider the results of a study of the friability of two different tablet formulations. There would be measurements from two groups of samples. The null hypothesis is that both samples are drawn from the same population. If the 95% confidence intervals of the two groups overlap, then both of them could share the sample population mean and therefore be drawn from the same population; if they do not overlap, then it is reasonable to assume that the samples were drawn from different populations and to accept the alternative hypothesis (although there is still a small chance that the wrong decision will have been made). Non-parametric confidence intervals can be calculated in some circumstances.

TESTS FOR THE COMPARISON OF GROUPS

Most pharmacists who ask about statistics are only interested in which test they should use for the analysis of their data. This decision is relatively easy for most experiments as it depends on only three things: the level of measurement, the number of groups being tested, and whether the same subjects undergo each test condition. All tests are based on these assumptions and the data should be checked to see that they have been met; occasionally this is difficult to judge and statisticians may disagree which is the correct test to apply. Results that are presented as proportions and percentages should be converted back to their original values or have special tests applied. Details on how to perform the tests may be found in the books listed in the References section at the end of the chapter; alternatively, one of the many software packages now available may be used.

Of the three factors that determine the choice of test, the level of measurement has been dealt with above. The second, the number of groups being tested is important because tests designed for two groups should only be applied to two groups. If three or more groups are being studied, for example A, B, and C, it is wrong to compare A with B, B with C, and A with C using tests for two groups. If more than two groups are tested, a form of analysis of variance (often abbreviated to ANOVA) must be applied. The problem is that multiple testing of pairs of groups leads to 'false positives'; P values are then misleading, as the true probability of a Type 1 error is much higher. The only exception to this is if the **Bonferroni correction** is applied. Sometimes only one group is tested, against population data for example.

The third factor in choosing a test is, unfortunately, sometimes ignored. Studies in which subjects undergo all experimental conditions (for example each of two treatments), should be analysed differently to those in which a different group undergoes each treatment. It is to the researcher's advantage to use the correct test because experiments on the same subjects (such as in crossover studies) have less variation, and therefore more powerful tests can be applied to them.

For all tests on nominal data, the **Chi-squared** (χ^2) **test** can be used, irrespective of the number of groups. It can even be used to test against an expected frequency distribution, for example, that the number of failures on a production run are independent of the day of the week. If the data forms a 2×2 table (for example, two formulations and two outcomes), then the Chi-squared test should have **Yates' correction** applied. An alternative 2×2 test, which may be used on small numbers if the conditions for the Chi-squared test are not met, is **Fisher's exact test**. For larger tables, if the assumptions are not met, it may be necessary to merge categories until they are met.

Ordinal data from two groups can be compared using the **Mann-Whitney** U-test for independent samples, and the **Wilcoxon test** for samples undergoing all conditions. The Mann-Whitney U-test is now called the Mann-Whitney-Wilcoxon test by some authors, as all three researchers developed the test at about the same time. The results are pooled and put in rank order; special procedures should be followed if results in a group tie. An alternative to the Wilcoxon test is the **sign test**. These tests are powerful and easy to use.

The t-test (its full name is **Student's t-test**) is applied to two groups of small samples ($n < 30$) of data at the interval/ratio level that follows a Normal distribution. If the samples are independent, then the 'unpaired t-test' is used, if the samples undergo all conditions, then the 'paired t-test' is used. If there are more than about 30 samples in each group, it is usual to test using the Normal distribution Z statistic, this is sometimes called the Z-test. The t and Z values become very close at this point and in practice many people use the t-test for sample sizes larger than 30. For interval/ratio data that do not follow the Normal distribution, the above non-parametric tests can be used or it may be possible to transform the results (for example, by taking their logarithms) into a Normal distribution and to apply the t-test.

Analysis of Variance

This technique is used when more than two groups of observations are being compared. Measurement at the ordinal level is analysed by non-parametric analysis of variance; and measurement at the interval/ratio level (provided it is Normally distributed, or can be transformed to a Normal distribution) is by parametric analysis of variance. Analysis of variance is often shortened to 'ANOVA'.

The nomenclature in ANOVA is often confusing and is most suitably explained with an example. Imagine an experiment undertaken to identify the best cosolvent for a liquid formulation of a drug. Several batches using each cosolvent under test are made and the concentration of drug in solution is measured after a fixed time. The groups are classified by the type of cosolvent. There is, therefore, one classification—type of cosolvent. If we were also looking at different antibacterial preservatives in the same study, so each combination of cosolvent and antibacterial preservative was studied, there would be two classifications—cosolvent and antibacterial preservative. Because the first study has only been classified in one way, it is known as one-way ANOVA; the second study would be analysed by two-way ANOVA. Non-parametric tests cannot go above two-way ANOVA, but parametric tests can go to three-way, four-way, or n-way ANOVA, although such large studies are rarely performed. An example of a study suitable for analysis by non-parametric one-way ANOVA would be a tasting panel ranking the sweetness or palatability of different liquid formulations. The most common non-parametric tests of this type are the **Kruskal-Wallis one-way analysis of variance** and the **Friedman two-way analysis of variance**.

The principle of ANOVA is explained in its name; it analyses variation in the results. As it is a hypothesis test there are H_0 and H_1; H_0 is that all the samples are taken from the same population and H_1 is that samples are taken from different populations. Taking one-way ANOVA as the simplest case, using the example above, the type of cosolvent would either have no effect (H_0) on the drug concentration or it would have an effect (H_1). Firstly, the variation within each group is calculated. Then the variation between each group is calculated. A measurement called the 'mean square' is used to give the extent of variation in each group (remember that mean squared deviations were used in calculating variance and standard deviation). If all samples have been taken from the same population, the two mean squares will be similar. This is calculated by the **F-test** (named after RA Fisher who proposed the test in the 1920s):

$$F = \frac{\text{mean square between groups}}{\text{mean square within groups}}$$

The greater the value of F, the less likely it is that H_0 is true. Using tables of F values produces a P value to test the hypothesis. If there were only two groups, the P value would be the same as if the t-test had been performed. The F-test does not indicate where any differences are located, merely that all samples were not taken from the same population. Further testing is needed to find out where the differences lie. Examples are the **Scheffé test**, the t-test with Bonferroni correction, **Duncan's multiple range test**, and the **Newman Keuls method**. Snedecor and Cochran give details of these tests.[3] In order to avoid the problems of multiple testing, the above tests can be rather conservative (that is, they may not detect a true difference), and the statistician's art is in choosing the appropriate test for each study. The chances of finding a real effect are increased if there has been a good experimental design that specifies a limited number of comparisons, rather than comparing everything with everything else in the hope of a significant result. The results are only valid if the F-test has first been shown to be significant; it is incorrect, and may lead to false conclusions, to perform the other tests without a prior F-test.

Other assumptions important to ANOVA are that the sample size is the same in each group, as is the standard deviation. If these assumptions are not met then the data or calculations may have to be manipulated. If the SD of one group is quite different, it may be due to an outlier or extreme reading and the experimenter needs to decide whether to include the reading or not. This must be decided

in a formal manner; Snedecor and Cochran[3] give details on methods to deal with all these situations. In the earlier example, different cosolvents formed the classification, but some classifications are related to each other and can be put in order; for example, different concentrations of the same cosolvent, readings taken over time, or a range of temperatures. Under these circumstances the intention would be not to compare pairs of groups, but to look for a trend across the ordered groups. A test for linear trend produces an analysis of variance table in which the 'between groups' source of variation is split into linear and non-linear, each with its own F and P values. If both P values were significant, it would indicate that there was a significant linear trend, but also that there is a significant effect that is not linear.

The above examples deal with one model of one-way ANOVA, the fixed-effect model, so called because the experimenter chooses (fixes) the variables and the test reveals which variable is different to the others or exactly how something changes with time. In other circumstances the aim may be to ensure uniformity of something by testing random samples of it. This is called the random-effect model of one-way ANOVA and the F-test decides whether or not the samples come from the same population. For example, an international company may wish to confirm that the same instruments are behaving in the same way at different sites. A periodic test of a standard by a random sample of instruments can be analysed by one-way ANOVA to check if their performance is similar.

One-way ANOVA is the simplest model and far more complex models are possible. The next is two-way analysis of variance. This technique was developed in agricultural research in the 1920s as a method of conducting several experiments at once and consequently reducing the number of observations required. There are two classifications: one forming columns and the other forming rows. This produces a grid-like effect made of individual cells. As was seen for one-way ANOVA, there are two models: random and fixed effects. The random-effect model is sometimes known as the randomised-block design as the pioneers of the technique divided fields into treatment blocks at random. It can be seen as the equivalent of the paired t-test for more than two groups. The different treatments could form the columns and each patient (who would normally have been chosen at random) forms a row. Each cell may only have one reading in it or it may have several. Another application of the randomised-block design would be if each row were a sample of tablets taken at random from different batches.

The fixed-effect model is usually called a **factorial study**; for example, one factor may be type or concentration of cosolvent and the other may be the choice of antibacterial preservative or in a clinical study one factor may be the type of antihypertensive drug used and the other may be the clinical status of the patient, such as high or low renin status. Factorial experiments can be further subdivided into those where a classification consists of different variables, such as types of lubricant in a tablet formulation, and those where the same variable is studied at several levels, such as different concentrations of a substance or when readings are taken at different times. Frequently in pharmaceutics, the latter of these two types of design is of interest; it is known which compounds should be used, but the experimenter wishes to determine what happens when they are used together. For speed and economy it is usual to perform what is generally known as a 2^n factorial study. Each of 'n' classifications (or factors) is set at two levels, for example, two concentrations. A two-way ANOVA of this type is therefore known as a 2^2 factorial study and a three-way ANOVA as a 2^3 factorial study. When choosing the two levels of a factor, it is customary to take them as the first and third quartile of the range of values that are likely to occur.

The print-out from a two-way ANOVA test will show if there are significant differences between columns and between rows; it will also show if a significant interaction has occurred between the factors. How should these test results be interpreted? The answer is 'with care and common sense'. The figures in the ANOVA table should be studied carefully and the effects plotted as a graph before interpreting the results. Due care should be exercised if there are missing values, the definition of outliers must be correct, and problems may occur if the data is transformed. Snedecor and Cochran[3] and Armitage and Berry[4] provide advice in these situations. Analysis of variance is a special form of multiple regression (see below) and it may be possible to use multiple regression on data unsuitable for ANOVA.

CORRELATION

Given two sets of data, correlation will give an indication of the extent of their association. The measure, which tests for a linear relationship, is indicated by a value r, usually called the correlation coefficient, although its full title is **Pearson's product moment correlation coefficient**. Assuming the sets of variables are randomly sampled and Normally distributed, and that a scatter diagram of results shows a reasonable spread, an r value of $+1$ or -1 shows perfect correlation, 0 means no association has been shown. If one variable increases as the other does, then r is positive; if one decreases as the other increases then r is negative. It is useful to calculate a confidence interval for r and to perform a hypothesis test; the null hypothesis being no association between the two variables. Altman[2] gives a method for the former and a table of critical values for the latter. Calculation of the confidence intervals should be done routinely as they can be surprisingly wide, particularly for small samples. Another method that is useful in understanding the relationship between the two variables is to calculate $100\,r^2$. This value gives the percentage of the variability in the data that is explained by their association. An r value of 0.8 indicates that 64% of the variation originates from the association between the variables and, therefore, that 36% is from other sources.

If there is an association between two variables that is not linear (logarithmic, for example), then it may be possible to transform one of the variables to create a linear relationship and then calculate r. A powerful alternative, which can also be used if one or both of the variables are ordinal data, is to calculate the non-parametric rank correlation coefficient **Spearman's r** (also called Spearman's rho, ρ). **Kendall's tau**, τ, is an alternative, but it is more difficult to calculate.

If an association is found between two variables then one of several conclusions may be drawn: either one of the variables may influence the other, or both are influenced by another unmeasured variable, or there is no association and a very unlikely event has occurred. The chosen interpretation should be based on supporting evidence rather than hope. In addition, it should be remembered that association is not causation. The misuse and misinterpretation of correlation coefficients is so common that Altman[2] observes that 'some statisticians have wished that the method had never been devised'. His book gives some of the most common abuses.

REGRESSION

Like correlation, regression is concerned with the relationship between two variables, however, it provides much more information. It allows the prediction of the value of one variable when given the value of another. If the variables are plotted as the

x and y axes on a graph, the value of y can be predicted from a chosen value of x. The hardest part of understanding regression is understanding the terminology, which often seems arcane: x is called the independent or predictor variable, y is the dependent or outcome variable, and the way in which y changes as a result of changes in x is called the regression of y on x.

The most common use of regression occurs when the relationship between x and y is a straight line. When drawing a scatter diagram (a graph in which the two variables are plotted against each other and each individual point is shown), the points are unlikely to form a perfectly straight line as y should follow a Normal distribution for each value of x. Where should the straight line be placed amid the scatter of points? The best method (assuming y is Normally distributed and its standard deviation would be the same whatever the value of x) is the least squared vertical distance between the points and the line; the method is therefore known as the least squares method. This simple linear regression produces an equation for a straight line, usually noted in statistics as $y = a + bx$ (the regression equation) where y is predicted from x, a is the intercept and b, the gradient, is also known as the regression coefficient.

It was mentioned above that some assumptions must be met if the regression equation is to hold true. One way of visually checking these is to measure the vertical distance between each observed point and the regression line (this value is called the residual) and plot the residuals (positive and negative) against x, these should be evenly spread at all values of x. This quickly shows changes in variance and non-linearity.

The usual tests can be performed on b: a significance test (against a value of 0) and the 95% confidence intervals of the slope (if it includes 0 then it is possible that there is no relationship between x and y). It is also possible to calculate a confidence interval for the mean value of y for any value of x; this will be wider when x is large or small and narrowest at the mean value of x. If x and y do not have a linear relationship it may be possible to predict y by using **polynomial regression**, usually in the form of a quadratic curve with the equation:

$$y = a + bx + cx^2$$

An alternative presentation of the data is in an analysis of variance table. The P value will be that for the slope; the extent to which the model explains the data can be calculated from the regression sum of squares as a proportion of the total sum of squares. The proportion, expressed as a percentage or a decimal, is called R^2 and for simple linear regressions is the same as r^2. A value of 50% (or 0.50) would indicate that only half the variability in y is explained by variations in x.

One common use of regression and correlation in the laboratory is to compare two methods of measuring the same variable. However, it has been argued that there is a more informative alternative. If the mean of each pair of readings is taken and also the difference between the pair is calculated, a plot of mean value (x-axis) and difference (y-axis) should form a horizontal line if there is perfect agreement. In practice, the variations from this line give a better understanding of the relationship than a regression line alone.

Multiple Regression

In some circumstances, several variables may predict y. This relationship can be described using multiple regression, forming equations such as:

$$\text{Drug concentration} = a + (b \times \text{temperature})$$
$$+ (c \times \text{time})$$

The predictor variables such as temperature and time are known as covariates; b and c are partial regression coefficients.

Multiple regression is used in observational as well as experimental studies; ANOVA is a specialised form of it, designed for balanced experimental studies. Often, many variables, such as physicochemical parameters have been recorded and it is important to find out which ones determine a certain factor, such as solubility or stability. Computers calculate multiple regression equations with some or all the variables included; the model that gives the best fit is then determined by the proportion of total variation (measured as the sum of squares) that can be explained by the model; this proportion is called R^2 and is often expressed as a percentage. The greater the number of variables in the equation, the greater will be the value of R^2 but some of the variables may contribute a minuscule effect and could be safely ignored. There are several computer methods by which the most important subset of variables are selected. If y can only be one of two results a technique called **multiple logistic regression** should be applied.

Optimisation

Formulation is often concerned with achieving the best compromise between several factors. One way to attain this is by using 2^n factorial design, describing the results by multiple regression, and then applying a technique called optimisation. When a multiple regression equation has two predictor variables, the equation is of the type found in solid geometry and describes a surface called a response or regression surface. If the regression surface is thought of as a mountain top seen from the air, protruding through a layer of cloud, optimisation is an attempt to plant the flag on the top. The true relationship between the variables (rather than the relationship observed in the 2^2 study) is rarely known, so the results must always be tested in practice. The approaches to, and limitations of, optimisation are covered at length in Armstrong and James[5] and Bolton.[6]

REFERENCES

1. Siegel S, Castellan NJ. Non-parametric statistics for the behavioural sciences. 2nd ed. New York: McGraw-Hill, 1988.
2. Altman DG. Practical statistics for medical research. London: Chapman and Hall, 1991.
3. Snedecor GW, Cochran WG. Statistical methods. 7th ed. Iowa: Iowa State University Press, 1980.
4. Armitage P, Berry G. Statistical methods in medical research. 2nd ed. London: Blackwell, 1987.
5. Armstrong NA, James KC. Understanding experimental design and interpretation in pharmaceutics. London: Ellis Horwood, 1990.
6. Bolton S. Pharmaceutical statistics. New York: Marcel Dekker, 1990.

Section 3 Preparation and Supply of Medicines

Good Manufacturing Practice

Good manufacturing practice (GMP) comprises that part of quality assurance aimed at ensuring that a product is consistently manufactured to a quality appropriate to its intended use. GMP requires that the manufacturing process is fully defined before it is initiated and that all necessary facilities are provided. In practice, this means that personnel must be adequately trained, suitable premises and equipment used, correct materials used, approved procedures adopted, suitable storage and transport facilities available, and appropriate records made.

The quality of a pharmaceutical product depends on the degree of care taken in its preparation. Final checks carried out on the finished product are useful in confirming that the correct ingredients have been used and that the materials have been correctly processed. It is, however, essential that proper in-process control is exercised and that it is adequately documented to provide reli-

able evidence that the correct procedures have been followed. The essential components of GMP are summarised in Fig. 1.

Compliance with the principles of GMP is one of the major factors considered by the Licensing Authority when examining an application for a licence to manufacture under the Medicines Act 1968.

HISTORY

The term good manufacturing practice was introduced to regulate manufacturing and packaging operations in the pharmaceutical industry. Until the mid-1960s, operating procedures for the manufacture of pharmaceuticals consisted of formulae and the basic methods of making products. The written procedures were often concise and often relied on the individual operator's skill and experience in actually producing the product. As batches of pharmaceutical products increased in number

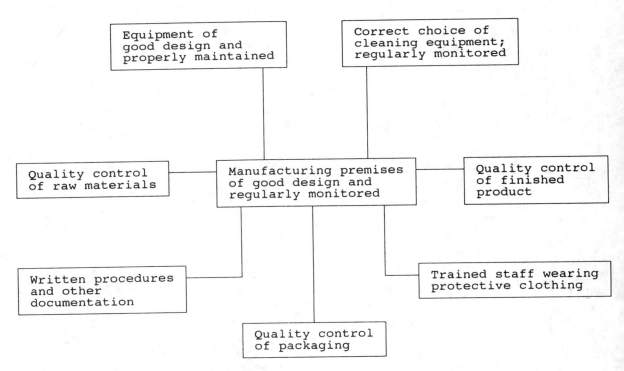

Fig. 1
Components of good manufacturing practice.

and size, it became apparent that the operating procedures were inadequate to produce consistent and reliable products. Much attention had focused on the purity of drug substances, particularly as many had been derived from natural products. Active ingredients with greater potencies were also being used in formulating new products. Pharmacopoeias and codices specified formulae for mixtures and other preparations, but gave little detailed information on the methods of preparation. The factors affecting processing and packaging procedures were becoming more apparent and the need for appropriate guidelines was evident.

The Medicines Inspectorate of the Department of Health and Social Security in consultation with other interested bodies compiled the *Guide to Good Manufacturing Practice* also known as the Orange Guide. The first edition was published in 1971, before any formal inspections of pharmaceutical manufacturers had been carried out under the Medicines Act. It was therefore written at a time when the nature, extent, and special problems of the manufacture of medicinal products were not completely known. Its purpose was to recommend steps that should be taken, as necessary and appropriate, by manufacturers of medicinal products with the object of ensuring that their products were of the nature and quality intended. The second guide was published in 1977, and the third and most recent edition in 1983.

In the USA, GMP regulations were developed by the Food and Drug Administration and issued in the US Code of Federal Regulations Chapter 21. The regulations were similar in concept to the Orange Guide, but were enforceable by law whereas the UK guide was advisory. The first GMP regulations were issued in 1963 and described the current good manufacturing practice to be followed in the manufacture, packaging, and storage of finished pharmaceutical products. The regulations were revised and updated in 1978 and became official in March 1979. These regulations present the minimum requirements to be met by industry for the manufacture, processing, packaging, and storage of human and veterinary drugs. Under the Federal Food, Drug and Cosmetic Act, a drug is considered to be adulterated unless the methods used in its manufacture, processing, packaging, and storage, as well as the facilities and controls used, conform to current good manufacturing practice. The drug should meet the safety requirements of the Act and should have the identity and strength to meet the quality and purity characteristics that it is represented to have.

In July 1978, the FDA issued regulations establishing similar good manufacturing practices for the manufacture, packaging, storage, and installation of medical devices. These were published following an amendment to the Food, Drug and Cosmetic Act of 1976, which provided the FDA with the authority to prescribe regulations for medical devices. In December 1978, regulations concerning good laboratory practices for the control and conduct of clinical studies were issued and for the first time came under FDA inspectional authority.

The FDA proposed, in 1978, regulations covering the GMPs relating to the manufacture and control of large volume parenteral products. These regulations, although never officially issued, have become the guideline used by the industry and FDA in the manufacture, control, and inspection of large volume parenteral production. Due to the similarity of the controls required for the production of small volume parenteral products, the guidelines also have been used to assess the adequacy of the manufacture and controls used with these products.

The need for GMP is recognised in many countries of the world. More than 20 countries have issued their own GMP guidelines. Within Europe several additional guidelines or monographs on GMP have been issued by organisations such as:

- The European Organization for Quality
- The Pharmaceutical Inspection Convention (PIC)
- The Pharmaceutical Quality Group (PQG) of the Institute of Quality Assurance
- The Parenteral Society of the UK.

The pharmaceutical industry in EEC member states encourages high standards of quality assurance in the development, manufacture, and control of medicinal products. A system of marketing authorisations issued by member states ensures that all medicinal products are assessed by a competent authority to ensure compliance with the contemporary standards of safety, quality, and efficacy. A system of manufacturing authorisations ensures that the licensed products are only manufactured by licensed manufacturers, whose activities are regularly inspected by the competent authorities. Manufacturing authorisations are required by all pharmaceutical manufacturers in the EEC whether the products are sold in the EEC or exported.

In order to further encourage the removal of barriers to trade in medicinal products and to promote uniformity in licensing decisions, the commission proposed, and member states agreed, that an EEC guide to good manufacturing practice for medicinal products should be prepared to provide a common, agreed basis throughout the EEC for maintaining good manufacturing practices in the pharmaceutical industry.

In 1992 the Commission of the European Communities published five volumes of *The Rules Governing Medicinal Products in the European Community*. Volume IV, entitled *Good Manufacturing Practice for Medicinal Products*, replaced national guidelines (for example, the Orange Guide) and other relevant GMP regulations. The Council of Ministers agreed that compliance with the principles of GMP should be compulsory throughout the EC with effect from 1 January 1992. All manufacturers should have a copy of the document in order to be able to comply with the EC law.

REQUIREMENTS OF GMP AND QUALITY MANAGEMENT

The holder of a manufacturing authorisation must produce medicinal products in a manner that ensures preparations are fit for their intended use, comply with the requirements of the marketing authorisation, and do not place patients at risk due to inadequate safety, quality, or efficacy. To achieve the quality objective reliably, there must be a comprehensively designed and correctly implemented system of quality assurance incorporating GMP and thus quality control. The basic concepts of quality assurance, GMP, and quality control are inter-related.

Quality assurance is a wide ranging concept that includes all matters that individually or jointly influence the quality of a product. It is the sum total of the organised arrangements made with the object of ensuring that medicinal products are of the quality required for their intended use. Therefore, quality assurance incorporates good manufacturing practice in addition to other factors. **Quality control** is that part of good manufacturing practice that is concerned with sampling, specifications, and testing and with the organisation, documentation, and release procedures that ensure that the necessary and relevant tests are actually carried out and that materials are not released for use, or products released for sale or supply until their quality has been judged to be satisfactory. **Validation** is the action of proving, in accordance with the principles of GMP, that

any procedure, process, equipment, material, activity, or system leads to the expected results.

In addition to being an essential component of quality assurance, good manufacturing practice is concerned with both production and quality control. The principal requirements of good manufacturing practice require that:

- manufacturing processes are defined and capable of producing products of suitable quality and specifications
- critical steps of manufacturing processes and significant changes to the process are validated
- necessary facilities are provided including qualified and trained personnel, adequate premises and space, correct materials, containers, and labels, approved procedures, and instructions, suitable storage areas, and transport
- instructions and procedures are clearly written
- operators are appropriately trained
- records are made demonstrating that all procedures and instructions were followed and that the quality and quantity of the product was as expected
- records of manufacture enabling the history of a batch to be traced should be retained
- distribution minimises any risk to product quality
- a system is available to recall any batch of product
- complaints about marketed products are examined and measures taken to prevent recurrences, if appropriate.

Initiating GMP, installing systems, training staff, and maintaining buildings and equipment is costly, but it should be considered a long-term investment. The cost may be negligible compared to anything other than strict adherence to GMP: regulatory authorities would not allow the product to be marketed, a defective product could have serious consequence for the patient receiving it, and the company may face serious repercussions. GMP in the pharmaceutical industry is an intrinsic part of technical strategy and business strategy.

GUIDE TO GOOD MANUFACTURING PRACTICE FOR MEDICINAL PRODUCTS

The following outline is consistent with *The Rules Governing Medicinal Products in the European Community*, Volume IV. *Good Manufacturing Practice for Medicinal Products*.

Personnel

The establishment and maintenance of a competent system of quality assurance and the correct manufacture of medicinal products relies upon personnel. There must be sufficient qualified personnel to carry out all the tasks that are the responsibility of the manufacturer. Individual responsibilities should be clearly understood by the individuals and recorded. All personnel should be aware of the principles of GMP that affect them and receive initial and continuing training, including hygiene instructions, relevant to their needs. Training records should be kept.

Three key personnel are specified: the head of production, the head of quality control, and the qualified person. The quality controller and the production manager must be different persons, acting independently, but jointly responsible for the quality of the products. The qualified person is responsible for the duties described in Article 22 of Directive 75/319/EEC if these are not performed by either the head of production or the head of quality control. These duties are to ensure that batches, including those imported from outside the European Community have been produced, tested, and checked in accordance with the Directives and Marketing Authorisation. The qualified person must also certify that each production batch satisfies the provisions of Article 22 as operations are carried out and before any release.

All personnel should have a medical examination on recruitment. Persons with potentially infectious diseases or open lesions on exposed surfaces should not be involved in the manufacture of medicinal products.

Appropriate protective garments should be worn in manufacturing areas. Care should be taken to avoid direct contact between the operator's hands and the exposed product, as well as any part of the equipment that comes into contact with the products. Eating, drinking, chewing, or smoking, the storage of food, drink, or smoking materials, or personal medication should be prohibited in the manufacturing area.

Premises and Equipment

The premises and equipment must be located, designed, constructed, adapted, and maintained to suit the operations to be carried out. The layout and design of premises and equipment should minimise the risks of errors and permit effective cleaning and maintenance in order to avoid cross-contamination, build up of dust or dirt and, in general, any adverse effect on the quality of products. Premises must be designed, built, and maintained to suit the operation being undertaken. The European Commission rules make recommendations on the design of the production areas, storage areas, quality control areas, and ancillary areas for rest and refreshment.

Equipment should be designed and installed to suit the process being carried out. It must be cleaned, maintained, and repaired without causing any contamination to materials or products.

Documentation

Good documentation is an essential requirement of the quality assurance system. Clearly written documentation avoids errors from spoken communication and allows tracing of batch history. Specifications, manufacturing formulae and instructions, procedures, and records must be free from errors and available in writing. The legibility of documents is important.

Documentation should be available to give details of:

- specification for starting materials, intermediate and bulk materials, finished products and packaging materials
- manufacturing formula, processing and packaging instructions
- procedures
- records.

All documentation should be unambiguous, regularly reviewed, and updated where necessary. Records must be completed at the time of action and kept until one year after the expiry of the final product.

When entries have to be altered, the alteration should be signed and dated and a reason given. The alteration should be made in such a way that the original entry is still legible.

When electronic data processing systems are used, access should be limited by a password or other means; only authorised persons should be able to enter or modify data. Electronically stored documentation must be readily available at all times, and be protected by a system of backup transfers. Records must be kept of changes to, or deletions from, electronically stored data.

Production

Production operations must follow clearly defined procedures. Operations must comply with the principles of GMP in order to produce products of the stipulated quality and be in accordance with their manufacturing and marketing authorisations.

The measures taken to prevent cross-contamination of starting materials and products should be regularly assessed. Validation studies should reinforce GMP and be conducted in accordance with defined procedures. Guidelines are given for the purchase, delivery, labelling, and storage of starting materials. The purchase, handling, and control of primary and printed packaging materials should be accorded attention similar to that given to starting materials. Processing and packaging operations should be conducted in accordance with the defined procedures. Finished products should be held in quarantine until their final release under conditions established by the manufacturer. Rejected materials and products should be clearly marked as such and stored separately in restricted areas. They should either be returned to the suppliers or, where appropriate, reprocessed or destroyed.

Quality Control

Quality control is concerned with sampling, specifications, and testing as well as the organisation, documentation, and release procedures that ensure that the appropriate tests are conducted, and that materials are not released for use, or products released for sale or supply, until their quality has been considered satisfactory. Each holder of a manufacturing authorisation should have a quality control department. Quality control is not confined to laboratory operations, but must be involved in all decisions that may affect the quality of the product. The independence of quality control from production is considered fundamental to the satisfactory operation of quality control. All quality control operations should be conducted in accordance with written procedures and, where necessary, recorded.

Sampling should be carried out in accordance with approved written procedures. Reference samples should be representative of the batch of materials or products from which they are taken and should be retained until one year after the expiry date. Samples of starting materials (other than solvents, gases, and water) should be retained for a minimum of two years. In Germany, France, and Greece such samples should be retained for as long as the corresponding product.

Methods of analysis should be validated and all testing operations should be undertaken according to the approved methods.

Contract Manufacture and Analysis

Contract manufacture and analysis must be suitably defined, agreed, and controlled in order to avoid misunderstandings that could result in a product or work of unsatisfactory quality. There must be a written contract between the contract giver and the contract recipient, which clearly establishes the duties of each participant. The contract must clearly state the way in which the qualified person releasing each batch of product for sale exercises his full responsibility. All arrangements for contract manufacture and analysis including any proposed changes in technical or other arrangements should be in accordance with the marketing authorisation for the product concerned.

Complaints and Product Recall

All complaints and other information regarding potentially defective products must be reviewed according to written procedures. In order to provide for all contingencies, and in accordance with Article 28 of Directive 75/319/EEC, a system should be designed to recall (if necessary) promptly and effectively, products known or suspected to be defective from the market.

A person should be designated, together with supporting staff, to deal with complaints. Where this person is not the qualified person (see Personnel above), the latter should be informed. The person responsible for quality control should also be involved in the study of any complaint or recall. Complaint records should be kept and regularly reviewed.

A person independent of sales and marketing should be designated, together with supporting staff, for execution and coordination of recalls. Where this person is not the qualified person (see Personnel above), the latter should be informed. Recalled products should be identified and stored separately in a secure area until a decision is made concerning their fate. The progress of the recall process should be recorded and a final report issued.

Self Inspection

Self inspection should be conducted at regular intervals in order to monitor the implementation and the regard for GMP and to propose necessary corrective measures. Competent persons from the company should be made responsible for self inspection, although independent audits by external experts may also be useful.

Manufacture of Sterile Medicinal Products

The European Community publication *Good Manufacturing Practice for Medicinal Products* provides supplementary guidelines on the manufacture of sterile medicinal products. These supplementary guidelines are not intended to take the place of the corresponding chapters of the guide, but only to stress specific points for the manufacture of sterile preparations.

Manufacture of sterile preparations needs special requirements to minimise risks of microbial contamination, and of particulate and pyrogen contamination. Much depends on the skill, training, and attitudes of the personnel involved. Quality assurance is of considerable importance. Manufacture must be in accordance with established and validated methods of preparation and procedures. The guidelines include information on air classification systems for manufacture of sterile products and sterilisation procedures.

Future Developments

It is the intention of the European Commission to publish further supplements on specific product groups and processes. These will include supplements on computerised systems, creams and ointments, sampling, and validation. The Orange Guide (1983) includes additional guidance on areas such as medical gases, manufacture of radio-pharmaceuticals, veterinary medicines, electronic data processing, and homoeopathic medicines.

The EC guide is not meant to place any restraint on the development of new technologies or new concepts, which have been validated and provide a level of quality assurance at least equivalent to those detailed in the guide. It is recognised that there are acceptable methods, other than those described in the EC guide, which are capable of achieving the principles of GMP.

FURTHER INFORMATION

Commission of the European Communities. The rules governing medicinal products in the European Community, Volume IV: Good manufacturing practice for medicinal products. Luxembourg: The Commission, 1992.

Department of Health and Social Security. Guide to good manufacturing practice. London: HMSO, 1983.

European Commission Directive 91/356/EEC, Laying down the principles and guidelines for good manufacturing practice for medicinal products for human use. Luxembourg: The Commission, 13 June 1991.

Good manufacturing practices (GMP). In: Goldberger F. Pharmaceutical Manufacturing: Quality management in the industry. Evreux: Ebur, 1991.

The Institute of Quality Assurance and The Pharmaceutical Quality Group. Bulk pharmaceutical chemicals. The Institute, 1992.

Late addition
Medicines Control Agency. Rules and guidance for pharmaceutical manufacturers. London, HMSO, 1993.
The publication contains the full text of the EC guide to GMP, together with its 14 annexes.

Licensing

The pharmaceutical and technical requirements for a marketing authorisation in the EC have developed from existing national systems, which were introduced largely as a response to the thalidomide disaster. New EC procedures for registering products have been set up alongside the existing systems in Member States. The Committee for Proprietary Medicinal Products (CPMP) has played an important role in appraising the different views of the Member States on particular products, and for developing the criteria that all EC Member States should embrace in relation to safety, quality, and efficacy of medicinal products.

This article should not be regarded as a complete or authoritative statement of current law.

HISTORY

In the UK, many of the present concepts of pharmaceutical regulation were included in the Therapeutic Substances Act of 1925, which applied mainly to vaccines and certain synthetic drugs. The Act provided for a licensing system administered by the Ministry of Health and for inspections of manufacturing premises. The Act also stipulated labelling requirements for the container, to identify the manufacturer and the batch. Records of sale had to be kept by manufacturers for each batch of controlled products. The system of batch release by an independent state laboratory is followed to this day in many EC countries.

CURRENT LEGISLATION IN THE UK

Licensing requirements that provide for product licences, manufacturers' licences, wholesale dealers' licences, clinical trial certificates, and animal test certificates are set out in Part II of the Medicines Act.

Licences are issued by the licensing authority, who may grant, refuse, review, suspend, revoke, or vary them. Licences expire at the end of five years or before if specified in the licence. If a licence, subsequent to its issue, contravenes any European Economic Community (EEC) obligation, a notice terminating the licence may be served on the holder. The licensing authority must send copies of licences to the appropriate Committee. When an application for a licence is refused, the licensing authority should specify to the applicant the reasons for refusal. A licence cannot be refused on any ground relating to the price of a product, and the licensing authority must consult the relevant Section 4 Committee on the Safety of Medicines or the Veterinary Products Committee before refusing an application on grounds of safety, quality, or efficacy.

If the Committee on the Safety of Medicines or the Veterinary Products Committee consider that they are unable to advise the granting of a licence, the applicant must be given the opportunity of appearing before the committee or of making representations in writing. If the committee still advise refusal, or advise the grant of a licence subject to specified conditions, notice of their reasons must be served on the applicant by the licensing authority. The applicant then has 28 days, or longer period as the authority may allow, to request an appeal be heard by the Commission or to submit a written representation to them. Subsequent to any response by the applicant, the Medicines Commission reports to the licensing authority. If the licensing authority considers any application in a way which differs from the advice given to them, the applicant must be notified of the reasons and must be given an opportunity to make written representations or to reappear before an independent person appointed by the authority. If the authority's objection to an application is based on grounds other than safety, quality, or efficacy, only the final stage of the procedure applies.

The licensing authority may suspend, revoke, or vary a licence for any of the reasons specified in the Act. These may include the giving of false or incorrect statements, contravention of the provisions of a licence, failure to comply with specified standards or to provide required information, or contravention of any regulations relating to EEC obligations as to labelling and marketing of containers and unit packages. These powers can also be applied when medicinal products are no longer regarded as safe or efficacious, or in respect of standards and specifications that are no longer satisfactory. There is also a similar procedure for representations to be made to the authority; details are given in Schedule 2 of the Act. Licences may also be varied on the application of the holder. The licensing authority makes the final decision on a licence application. Neither the validity of a licence nor any decision of the authority can be questioned in any legal proceedings. The applicant may, however, question its validity within three months of receiving notice of it. He may make an application to the High Court, but only on grounds that the decision is not within the powers of the Act, or that the requirements of the Act or regulations have not been complied with.

Manufacturer's Licence

A manufacturer's licence authorises the manufacture or assembly of medicinal products consistent with the licence holder's possession of appropriate and suitable facilities. The licence generally authorises the manufacture or assembly of a product only if the holder either holds the product licence (PL) for that product or is named as a manufacturer by the holder of the PL or if the product is exported. A **manufacturer's licence (assembly only)** permits the labelling, packaging, and boxing of the previously manufactured medicinal product. A **manufacturer's licence (specials)** permits the manufacture, assembly, or both, of a medicinal product for which no product licence exists. Manufacture in this way is subject to specific conditions and products can be supplied only in response to unsolicited orders received from doctors or dentists, and for use in hospitals, health centres, and registered pharmacies if under the supervision of a pharmacist.

Wholesale Dealer's Licence

A wholesale dealer's licence is required by any person who sells or offers for sale any medicinal products by way of wholesale dealing, or distributes, otherwise than by way of sale, any proprietary medicinal product which has been imported, but was not consigned from a Member State of the EEC. Sales made by the manufacturer of a product are excluded from the definition of wholesale dealing so that a licence is not required in order to sell the products. A further concession is provided in respect of wholesale sales made by a product licence holder who is not also the manufacturer, or by a person assembling to his order. Provided that the products do not leave the premises of the licenced manufacturer or licenced assembler until the actual sale, no wholesale dealer's licence is required.

Regulations exist requiring applicants for wholesale dealer's licences, which relate to products to which Chapter II to V of the 1965 Directive (65/65/EC) apply, to give the name and address of a responsible person who is to oversee wholesaling operations. Also required are details of an emergency plan for product recalls and arrangements for keeping records relating to products received or despatched.

Removal of Crown Immunity

The Royal Pharmaceutical Society and the Medicines Control Agency jointly issued guidance on the loss of Crown immunity, which stated that following 1 April 1991, the provisions of the Medicines Act 1968 should apply fully in relation to the marketing, manufacture, dispensing, sale, supply, and import of medicines by hospitals. The district health authority or, where appropriate, a trust, will constitute a business for registration or licensing purposes. However, Section 10 of the Medicines Act provides certain exemptions from licensing in connection with activities carried out in a hospital by, or under the supervision of, a pharmacist.

The guidance stated that as far as the licensing requirements under the Medicines Act 1968 are concerned, abolition of Crown immunity means that several options will be open to hospital pharmacy departments, the choice depending on the type of service provided. In practice, some departments may wish to seek the inclusion of their premises on the Society's register of premises, which will give them a degree of flexibility while avoiding expensive licensing procedures and fees. Larger departments engaged in small-scale manufacture may need a manufacturer's licence, while departments that distribute medicines across district health authority boundaries may need to acquire wholesale dealers' licences.

Product Licences

A substance or article is subject to licensing if it is manufactured, imported, or exported (there are exceptions) as a medicinal product. If it is not manufactured, imported, or exported as a medicinal product, but later becomes one, then it is subject to licensing when it is first sold or supplied as a medicinal product.

Subject to a number of exemptions, described later, a product licence for human use is required by any person who:

- imports, or procures the importation of, a medicinal product
- first sells or supplies a substance or article after it has become a medicinal product

- is responsible for the 'composition' of a medicinal product
- is responsible for placing on the market in the UK a 'proprietary medicinal product', that is a ready-prepared product under a special name and in a special pack. This does not include: vaccines, toxins, or serums; medicinal products based on human blood or blood constituents or radioactive isotopes; homoeopathic medicinal products; or veterinary drugs.

The holder of a product licence for a medicinal product may, in accordance with the licence:

- sell, supply, or export the product
- procure its sale, supply, or exportation
- procure its manufacture or assembly.

Applications must be made in the manner described in the regulations. Particulars required to be given in a full application include: the kind of activity to be undertaken; the pharmaceutical form of the product; its composition, physical characteristics and medicinal use; method of manufacture and assembly; quality control procedures; containers and labelling; reports of experimental and biological studies and of clinical trials and studies; and, where the product is made abroad, and documentary evidence of authorisation relating to manufacture and assembly. Abridged applications are permitted where the relevant data have been submitted in an earlier application, or data about the kind of product in question are well documented.

Standard provisions for licences are prescribed by regulations. These provisions are incorporated in a licence unless the applicant desires that any of them shall be excluded or modified in respect of the product and the request is granted.

The procedures that lead to the licensing of radiopharmaceuticals, medicated devices, and contact lens products are beyond the scope of this chapter. Specialist texts should be consulted.

Product Licences (Parallel Importing)

The importation from a Member State of the EC of a medicinal product that is a version of one already the subject of a UK product licence (PL) is known as parallel importing.

A modified form of licence application may be considered for such a product, subject to the following conditions:

- the imported product must be a 'proprietary medicinal product', which is not a vaccine, toxin, serum, or based on human blood, a blood constituent, or a radioactive isotope, or homoeopathic product
- it must be covered by a currently valid market authorisation granted by the regulatory body of an EC Member State
- the therapeutic effect should not differ from the product with the UK licence
- it must be made by, or under licence to, the UK manufacturer, or by a member of the same group of companies.

A licence granted in these circumstances is known as a Product Licence (Parallel Import)—PL(PI). A medicinal product for which a UK product licence has been granted must have the licence number on each pack. This will either be a PL or a PL(PI) number.

Clinical Trial and Animal Test Certificates

Subject to certain exemptions no person may sell or supply, procure the sale or supply of, procure the manufacture of, or assemble for the purpose of sale or supply a medicinal product for the purpose of a clinical trial or a medicinal test on animals unless the person is, or acts to the order of, the holder of a product licence which authorises the clinical trial, or unless a clinical trial certificate or animal test certificate, as appropriate, has been issued and is in force, and the trial or test is to be carried out in accordance with it.

Licences of Right

Licences of right were issued for medicinal products that were on the market in the UK before 1 September 1971 (the first appointed day), and about which information had been distributed. The licensing authority was obliged to issue licences of right as a matter of entitlement to those who fulfilled the required conditions. The Review of Medicines Committee was introduced to consider the safety, quality, and efficacy of these products.

Clinical trial certificates of right were also issued for trials that were in progress immediately before that date. A manufacturer could obtain a licence in respect of the manufacture or assembly of those medicinal products which he had been making or assembling in the 12 months before 1 September 1971.

Legislation in the EEC

The EC directives, the European guidelines on format of marketing authorisation applications and the content of the dossier, and the specific technical guidelines were all published in 1989 as a five volume set by the Office for Official Publications of the European Community in Luxembourg. The series title of all of the volumes is *The rules governing medicinal products in the European Community*. The individual volumes are as follows:

Volume I—*The rules governing medicinal products for human use in the European Community*
Volume II—*Notice to applicants for marketing authorisations for medicinal products for human use in the Member States of the European Community*
Volume III—*Guidelines on the quality, safety and efficacy of medicinal products for human use*
Volume IV—*Guide to good manufacturing practice for the manufacture of medicinal products*
Volume V—*The rules governing medicinal products for veterinary use in the European Community*.

In the EEC the Committee for Proprietary Medicinal Products (CPMP) is responsible for the procedures that enable companies to make multiple applications for marketing authorisations in other Member States once authorisation has been obtained in one. The following are within the jurisdiction of the CPMP:

- definition of proprietary medicinal products
- authorisation to place proprietary medicinal products on the market
- suspension and revocation of authorisation to market proprietary medicinal products
- labelling of proprietary medicinal products.

The work of the CPMP is concerned with the establishment of a foundation for achieving comparable standards of quality, safety, and efficacy in Member States, and with the establishment and implementation of procedures whereby a manufacturer who has received marketing approval in one country can apply for similar approval in at least five others. The general basis for comparable standards rests in the so-called 'norms and protocols' directive, which specifies in general terms the essential items of information that should normally be included in an application to market a medicinal product.

The directive (75/319/EEC) which sets up the CPMP also makes a number of other important provisions. It specifies that marketing applications are drawn up and signed by persons with the necessary technical or professional qualifications, defines the basis of their qualifications, and places certain obligations on such experts. It sets out a basis for the verification of particulars and quality control procedures, makes regulations for importation from non-Member States, and provides for the inspection of manufacturing premises.

The processing of marketing applications are subject to specific time limits as specified in Article 7 of Directive 65/65/EEC. These require that applications be processed within 120 days, but allow for an extension for a further 90 days in exceptional cases. If, however, the licensing authority requests further information in order to facilitate a decision, then there is provision for these time limits to be suspended while this information is awaited. The mechanism for processing multiple applications in more than one Member State requires that the State that has issued marketing authorisation submit a copy of the authorisation with all the manufacturer's application documents to the CPMP, for forwarding to the States named in the multiple application. Decisions to grant marketing authorisations must be reached and notified within 120 days. In the event of refusal, reasoned objections must, likewise, be lodged with the CPMP within 120 days.

The Single Market after 1992: New Directions

One of the provisions of the Single European Act, adopted in December 1985, was the adoption by the EC of the means to establish the Single Market by 31 December 1992. The Commission of the European Communities (CEC) announced that it would bring forward proposals on a future system for the authorisation of medicinal products.

Proposals for Procedures after 1992

The Commission issued an Explanatory Memorandum detailing three procedures as being available to the industry after 1992:

- a decentralised procedure
- a centralised procedure
- national procedures.

The function of the decentralised procedure should enable smaller companies to enter the pharmaceutical European market. It would probably be the most frequently used Community procedure, and any company that had obtained an authorisation in any one Member State could then apply for acceptance of the authorisation in one or more of the EC Member States. If the Member States concerned considered that they could not accept the authorisation, even after bilateral discussion and negotiation with the first country, the matter would then be referred to the CPMP for binding arbitration at Community level. The function of the centralised procedure would be to provide major innovative products with direct access to the whole European market. It is envisaged as being compulsory for biotechnology products, but optionally available to companies for new active substance products and also for some high technology products. National procedures should only be necessary for registering products in one country. Where products are traditionally marketed in several countries together such as the UK and Ireland, or the Benelux countries (Belgium, The Netherlands, and Luxembourg), it would involve the decentralised procedure.

Phasing and Transitional Arrangements for the New Procedures

National applications. Proposed transitional arrangements for national applications are envisaged as follows:

1993–96	Parallel applications in two or more Member States allowed, but if one or more Member States wishes to suspend its evaluation and wait for the other Member State to complete its assessment it can do so.
1996 onwards	Parallel applications not permitted after one Member State has authorised an application. After the first authorisation, all subsequent applications would be handled via the decentralised procedure.

Centralised applications. Transitional arrangements for a new active substance marketing authorisation application are envisaged as follows:

1993–99	Applications to be made either centrally or using the national/decentralised route at the choice of the company.
1999 onwards	The categories of product where applications would have to be made compulsorily via the centralised procedure would be reviewed. It seems likely, if the new European Medicines Agency is working well by this time, that the procedure would be extended to new active substance applications.

Products Authorised Nationally Before 1993

For products authorised nationally before 1993, the Member States would still be responsible for the management of the authorisations dealing with matters such as variations, renewals, suspensions, and revocations. However, reference may be made to the CPMP in cases where:

- Community interests are involved (Article 12 of Directive 75/319/EEC)
- divergent decisions have been made (Article 11 of Directive 75/319/EEC).

There will also need to be Community consideration of the pre-1993 products in relation to pharmacovigilance, defect reports, and proposals to revoke or suspend authorisations that exist in more than one Member State.

European Medicines Evaluation Agency (EMEA)

The draft regulation proposes the establishment of a new European Medicines Evaluation Agency, which would be responsible for both veterinary and human pharmaceutical products. The main responsibilities of the agency would be the coordination of the scientific and technical assessment of the quality, safety, and efficacy of medicinal products subject to EC procedures; and the presentation of assessment reports, summaries of product characteristics, labels, and patient and health-care professional information leaflets. It would be involved in the continued supervision of products authorised at a Community level, and in the coordination of manufacturing and testing requirements, enforcement, and inspection. It would promote cooperation with the European Pharmacopoeia Commission and would coordinate national pharmacovigilance reporting arrangements.

Summary of Product Characteristics

The decentralised registration system available for non-prescription medicines after 1992 is based on Member States accepting the Summary of Product Characteristics (SPC) issued by the first Member State. The SPC should specify the indications for which the product is to be marketed, the dosage form and route of administration, duration of use, and the contra-indications, side-effects, and warnings relevant to the product's intended use. The SPC is the basis for the production of consumer information on labels and leaflets of medicines, and for the control of advertising. The SPC issued in one Member State for a non-prescription medicine will become the passport allowing access to the internal market.

Since 1985 Member States have been required to prepare SPCs for each product that has been assessed and found satisfactory for marketing. Summaries have also been prepared for products on the market before 1985 as their marketing authorisations have been progressively reviewed or renewed.

The AESGP (European Proprietary Medicines Manufacturers' Association) is composed of national associations of groups of manufacturers and distributors of non-prescription medicines. The Association has developed SPCs and leaflets that serve as models for products containing these ingredients and for development of further SPCs for other key ingredients.

FURTHER INFORMATION

Appelbe GE, Wingfield J. Pharmacy law and ethics. 5th ed. London: Pharmaceutical Press, 1993.

Cartwright AC, Matthews BR, editors. Pharmaceutical product licensing: Requirements for Europe. New York: Ellis Horwood, 1991.

Commission of the European Communities. Future system for the free movement of medicinal products in the European Community. COM(90) 283 final-SYN 309 to 312. Luxembourg: The Commission, 14 November 1990.

Guidance to the NHS on the licensing requirement of the Medicines Act 1968. Medicines Control Agency, 1992.

Leach RH. NHS licensing requirements after Crown immunity removal. Pharm J 1992;249:739.

Lutener SJ. Guidance and advice on the removal of Crown immunity. Pharm J 1991;246:336–7.

Design Criteria for Production Facilities

The design of pharmaceutical production facilities and their environment can have a profound effect on product quality and cost. The importance of good design cannot be overemphasised in an industry where the procedures and methods of manufacture used determine the integrity of the products produced.

'Design' includes all aspects of process engineering, building, plant design, environmental services, and the validation of any new or modified facility. This chapter will identify the essential criteria that must be considered for a facility design to be acceptable in a pharmaceutical sense in order to conform to current good manufacturing practice (cGMP) and quality assurance (QA) requirements.

Many facilities are becoming increasingly complex; what was a labour intensive industry is becoming more capital intensive with new facilities incorporating computer controlled production processes, automated warehouses, and sophisticated handling systems. However, the fundamental design criteria are the same in terms of site selection, process definition, facility layout design, service requirements, and environmental factors.

OBJECTIVES

A key objective must be to design a facility that will incorporate all the essential criteria mentioned in the following paragraphs; in particular those criteria that allow the operational personnel to work comfortably, safely, and effectively.

Commonly available references such as the *Guide to Good Manufacturing Practice* ('Orange Guide'),[1] the US Food and Drug Administration (FDA) *Federal Code of Regulations*,[2] or the European Community (EC) Guide to Good Manufacturing Practice[3] offer clear advice on the overall objectives of good plant design, layout, and construction methods. By necessity, most of this advice has to be general in nature because of the wide variations encountered in production operations. However, current editions of these and other guides provide a firm foundation, upon which the more precise requirements of a particular plant, whatever its ultimate level of complexity or sophistication, can be established. Other recommended books on the subject of facility design are included under Further Information at the end of this chapter.

BASIC SITE REQUIREMENTS

Site requirements are essentially the same for any industry but the increasing importance of service, adaptability, and close proximity to the market are more significant influences in the choice of site location. The principal considerations are:

- ease of transportation to and from facilities (by road, rail, sea, and air)
- size and suitability of terrain for buildings and site services (and their expansion possibilities)
- ease of planning and building permission for the facility
- proximity to major clients and suppliers
- availability and cost of suitable labour and educational facilities for personnel and their families
- environmental restrictions and waste disposal (liquid effluent, gaseous/solvent emissions, reject product, and other forms of toxic or solid waste)
- noise and smell in relation to local housing and prevailing winds.

The layout of the site should ideally be as square and as level as possible with no unfavourable geological features, for example, old mine workings or marsh. The configuration of buildings and their proximity to one another is important to provide flexibility. Expansion possibilities for the buildings in two or more directions should exist at the outset. Main road access, the construction of single- or multi-storey buildings, and the siting of warehouses are vital considerations. These and other features have been discussed in detail.[4]

FACILITY PLANNING AND LAYOUT

The approach to the planning and design of the layout of the buildings should be systematic and must involve the client with the specialist engineers and architects. This stage in design is crucial. The main considerations are:

- capacity and growth expectations
- a complete process flow layout with material movements, people movements, and services flow requirements
- flexibility to modify and extend buildings and services

- building and maintenance costs
- time for construction
- any local knowledge or material availability for building purposes.

Some of these considerations will be discussed below.

An essential preliminary requirement in the establishment of a plant layout is the clear definition and understanding of the proposed operations to be undertaken within the facility. The pharmaceutical operations themselves and associated movements of both people and materials are the two most important considerations. Process flow charts and detailed 'write-ups' can be used to establish these variables quickly.

The next stage is to broaden the scope of the requirements definition, principally to include storage needs (initial, intermediate, final); materials handling (equipment, space, routes); process and packaging equipment needs and any related restrictions (sizes, access, services); support activities (laboratories, workshops, administration, cleaning); personnel areas (locker areas, changing rooms, toilets/showers); and services requirements (plant rooms, utilities, access, and escape routes). An assessment of longer term needs should also be included at this stage, ranging from future repairs and maintenance required through to potential changes of use or future expansion of activities.

The consideration of these and any additional aspects for a particular facility will enable the definition of both the physical sizes of, and the interrelationships between, the individual areas to be decided. The participation of actual or future users of the facility will help to transform ideas into firmer proposals for evaluation of feasibility, practicality, engineering, architectural, financial, and other considerations.

CONSTRUCTION AND FINISHES

Construction methods, materials, and finishes must be appropriate for protecting products from contamination; be easily cleaned and maintained; and prevent the accumulation of dust and dirt. Minimising the entry or harbouring of insects, birds, or rodents is a fundamental construction requirement. Smooth, non-porous surfaces free from crevices or ledges are more easily cleaned and maintained. Protection from accidental damage may be necessary in some instances.

Finishes for floors, walls, ceilings, doors, and windows should be impervious and unbroken to avoid accumulation or shedding of contamination. The choice of finishes should take account of cleaning and disinfection methods and frequencies. Fewer cupboards, shelves and surface-mounted equipment, fixtures, and fittings will reduce the build-up of contamination and allow for easier cleaning. The above criteria are equally relevant to sampling, testing, storage, and distribution areas as well as manufacturing or packaging zones. The actual materials of construction, style, and finishes, including doors and windows, will vary according to the intended use of each particular area; warehousing versus clean or sterile areas would represent the usual range encountered.

Floors and Walls

Floors should be hard, smooth and even, sealed, and unaffected by the cleaning materials and equipment to be used. The materials employed can vary from concrete in warehouse areas to epoxy resins, seam-welded polyvinyl chloride, or terrazzo in manufacturing areas. Integral smooth coving for the floor/wall intersection will facilitate cleaning.

Walls can be of solid masonry or hollow partition construction, with appropriate finishes applied, such as epoxy or polyester coating, welded polyvinyl chloride sheet or sprayed-on polymer with good flexibility and resistance to cleaning materials.

Various pre-fabricated panel systems are available for internal construction. These offer the advantages of speed, ease, and cleanliness of erection plus flexibility for future changes of use. These advantages should be assessed against the cost and the need to seal panels, windows, and doors according to intended use of the facility.

Ceilings

Ceilings may be of conventional board construction, with finishes such as those listed for walls. Suspended tile system ceilings need to be securely fitted, sealed against potential contamination from above, with a smooth surface for easy cleaning.

Integral coving between walls and ceiling will minimise cracking or opening of joints due to building movement as well as facilitating cleaning of the total surface.

Recessed lighting units are popular. Where surface mounted units are used, these must be easy to clean and maintain. Penetrations through ceilings by pipes and ducts should be avoided if possible, but in all cases these must be adequately sealed.

Doors and Windows

The use of smooth, hard, and impervious finishes for doors and windows are important for cleaning purposes. Resistance to damage and easy repair and restoration of finishes are especially important for doors. Windows and door frames should be installed flush with the adjacent walls.

In production areas, windows should be tightly sealed and must not be opened. Outside doors should also be well sealed and kept closed when not in use. Doors that link production areas to the outside of the building should be restricted to emergency exit use only and should otherwise be kept completely sealed.

SERVICES AND UTILITIES

All facilities require a basic package of services and utilities: heating, ventilation and air conditioning (HVAC); electricity; water; steam; compressed air; refrigeration or chilled water; drainage; and effluent treatment. The intended use of any particular facility will dictate whether any additional or specialised services will be required; for example, there may be a need for supplies of different qualities of water (purified water, water for injections), vacuum systems, clean steam, dust collection, and nitrogen or other gases.

Water

Incoming town or potable water is normally the source of water for drinking and hand-washing use, and is also the starting material for further purification treatments. Subject to its quality and reliability of supply, this water may also be used for some types of non-sterile products, if their formulations allow this. In such cases, the water should be used directly from the main supply, avoiding any intermediate storage. Whenever a storage tank is used in a water supply system, frequent and regular monitoring is necessary to avoid chemical and microbiological problems.

Purified water can be produced by deionisation, reverse osmosis, or distillation. Sampling, testing, and recording of chemical and microbiological quality is required, together with warning and action limits plus remedial procedures and responsibilities.

Circulation of purified water in any storage and distribution system is vastly preferable to the use of static storage tanks with long delivery deadlegs. Water quality can also be maintained at a high level by the use of stainless steel components and by using ultraviolet treatment lamps in the system or storing and circulating the water at high temperatures.

Water for injections can be produced by distillation, reverse osmosis, or ultra-filtration, according to the specifications of the various pharmacopoeias. The choice of technique is determined primarily by the intended use of the water and the regulations applying to that use in both the country of origin and the countries for which the final products are destined.

It is obvious that the quality demands for water for injections must be extremely stringent because of its use in preparing components and as an ingredient in injectable products. The design details, materials of construction, testing, and validation of the generating, storage, and distribution system should be carefully studied. The routine monitoring of an established system must include analysis for the presence of pyrogens as well as chemical and microbiological tests.

Water may also be required in some instances for cooling autoclave loads after sterilisation or for dye testing of glass containers to detect cracks. This water should also conform to water for injections standards and be monitored accordingly.

Electricity

The demand for electrical power and its distribution for pharmaceutical processes must be assessed and added to the total for site services and utilities. This can be derived from the earlier assessment of operations, equipment, and layouts. Critical areas and equipment should have back-up supplies with automatic changeover from normal mains to emergency supply to protect against the consequences of mains failure. The increasing use of sophisticated analytical instruments, microprocessors, and computer-based systems may require voltage stabilisation and protection equipment.

Steam

Within a pharmaceutical facility the requirements for steam range from its use in heating the environment, heating processes, cleaning, and particularly its use in sterilisation procedures. In instances where the steam may come into contact with products, components, or product contact surfaces, the feed water for its generation should be free from volatile additives. Steam that comes into contact with products should be frequently and regularly monitored. Filtration of the steam may be necessary in some systems or installations.

Steam used for product or component sterilisation should be generated from water for injections, and delivered to the point of application in a high quality system so that it arrives as clean or pure steam. The system must be monitored to check for continuing compliance.

Gases

A range of active and inert gases may be required in a facility for both production and laboratory use. Commonly used examples are compressed air, nitrogen, carbon dioxide, ethylene oxide for sterilisation, oxygen and inflammable gases for ampoule sealing, and aerosol propellants. If any form of pilot or full scale synthesis is included, additional reactive gases may also be required.

The gases that will come into contact with products or containers should be tested and formally released for use, as for any normal raw material. Drying and filtration at or before the point of use may be necessary.

Gases for use in processing sterile products must comply with both the microbiological and particulate standards for that environment. This is usually achieved by filtration, but regular quality checking should be implemented.

ENVIRONMENTAL CONSIDERATIONS

Heating and Ventilation

Production of pharmaceuticals must take place under conditions appropriate for their intended use. In the case of environmental requirements, as well as many other aspects, the most demanding conditions are those for sterile products, then oral and topical products, with warehousing areas at the further end of the spectrum.

The design of heating and ventilation systems must take account of several other factors. Geographical position, prevailing wind conditions, nearby industries or area infrastructure, as well as local legislation, are some of the considerations that can determine basic criteria for siting plant rooms, air intakes, and outlets.

Maintaining suitable personnel comfort levels, especially room temperature and humidity, will vary in complexity according to climatic conditions and their extremes, as well as the operations to be carried out and any specific clothing needs. Process requirements, such as very low humidities for some operations or heat generated by large equipment, may be in conflict with the maintenance of a comfortable environment.

The specification, design, and installation of heating and ventilation systems needs a great deal of expertise and input to ensure a cost effective solution, combining engineering feasibility with overall requirements.

Lighting

Lighting levels must be carefully selected to avoid the dangers of inadequate levels causing eye strain and fatigue, especially where detailed work is being undertaken. In addition, high levels can result in glare and dazzling, which may also be harmful to the eye. Daylight is preferable to artificial lighting where possible, but in most instances the use of artificial lighting is unavoidable. Therefore, careful consideration must be given to light intensity, positioning, and colour spectrum. Installation, operation, and maintenance costs should also be evaluated for the different alternatives available.

Noise

The adverse effects of noise as a part of the working environment are gaining increasing recognition. Long or continuous exposure to elevated noise levels will seriously affect personnel, often in an insidious manner. An upper limit of 80 dB is commonly quoted, but actual sound frequency and regularity can often cause greater distress than this single figure indicates. Reference to local or industrial codes of practice may give better guidance.

Reduction of noise can be achieved by a variety of different floor, wall and ceiling finishes, by detailed consideration of equipment installation, and by ensuring noise levels are included in machine specifications. Compliance with operator protection needs or legislation may ultimately mean providing suitable protective equipment.

Air Quality and Supply

Stringent standards are required for sterile operations, involving manufacture of eye or ear products, dressings, and sterile topicals as well as parenterals (see Cleanrooms for Pharmaceutical Production chapter). Assuming satisfactory attention to construction, finishes, services, and environmental factors discussed earlier, a major factor in achieving and maintaining a high quality environment for sterile operations is a satisfactory air system. Such areas should normally be supplied with at least 20 air changes per hour, although heat gain calculations often show a need for much more frequent air changes. The air supply should pass through High Efficiency Particulate Air

(HEPA) filters, preferably as close to the point of entry as possible, and be directed to the most critical zones first. In addition, these zones can be individually covered by independent HEPA filtered air supplies, to maximise product protection.

Conditions in cleanrooms are maintained by keeping them at a positive pressure to exclude contaminated outside air, with specially designed changing rooms for operator entry/exit. Monitoring of the physical parameters of the room (temperature, humidity, over-pressure) is necessary, together with checks on particulate and microbial contamination levels, especially in the critical zones. More guidance on the specification, construction, validation, and operation of controlled areas can be found in the British Standard 5295 and in Federal Standard 209 (FDA, current version).

The air conditions for the manufacture of oral liquids and topical products are generally less demanding than for sterile products. Incoming air is usually filtered, but not HEPA filtered, to reduce levels of particulate and microbial contaminants. The use of positive over-pressure for the air supplied to these areas also contributes to such a reduction. However, there is a growing consideration that the bioburden level for topical products should be minimised because of the potential for application to broken skin. In many cases, this is accomplished by the formulation and preservative systems used in the product, but future policies and restrictions may lead to the introduction of areas for the aseptic preparation of topical products. During the production of oral solid dosage forms, the major challenge to the maintenance of good air quality is contamination arising from the products themselves. The main requirements for the incoming air are a satisfactory level of filtration, volume, temperature, and humidity to suit the operational or product needs. It is then necessary to ensure the airflow is directed across the operating zone to minimise the effect of any airborne contamination on personnel and adjacent zones.

For dispensing operations, the requirements are broadly similar to those applied to solid dosage form production; there must be an adequate volume of suitably filtered and conditioned air directed to flow over the operations to maximise personnel protection and prevent or minimise cross-contamination.

Dust and Waste Control

Legislative measures, such as the UK Control of Substances Hazardous to Health (COSHH) have focused attention even more rigorously on the pro-

blems of dust and the potentially harmful effects of exposure.[5] In some instances, the apparent conflict between these measures and longer established GMP practices has forced a radical reconsideration of production practices, materials handling, cleaning methods, and waste handling.

The primary aim from an environmental point of view is the avoidance of dust generation, closely followed by containment. When these are not fully practicable, localised extraction must be used.[6] Reliance on the ventilation system for a given area to provide adequate control is not a viable solution. Systems that use a variety of techniques for measuring dust levels in an area are widely available and increasing in use. These may be supplemented by personnel monitoring in some instances, and further urine or blood level checks where specific hazards are involved.

Similarly, environmental legislation and greater public concern have directed attention to the handling of waste and effluent disposal from the pharmaceutical as well as other industries. Compliance with national and local requirements for land-fill, incineration, or discharge into rivers or the sea demands an increasing amount of expertise and familiarity with the ever-growing body of legislation. The same principles as those applied to dealing with bioburden or dust control also serve well in this particular area. Attention and effort should be directed firstly at eliminating the generation of hazardous waste, secondly at minimising the levels that are actually generated, and then at containment measures. The process can start at the product formulation stage, for example, replacement of mercurial preservatives, and extends across the spectrum of both production and laboratory practices to waste segregation and recycling measures.

EQUIPMENT

The Food and Drug Administration's *Code of Federal Regulations* at section 211.63 states that 'Equipment used in the manufacture, processing, packing, or holding of a drug product shall be of appropriate design, adequate size, and suitably located to facilitate operations for its intended use and for its cleaning and maintenance.' As the effectiveness of equipment, like the quality of a product, starts at the design stage, its specification and the criteria for its selection are important considerations.

Evaluation and Selection

The outcome of the selection process has a direct influence on the success of a production facility through reducing costs, improving safety and/or quality, or reducing environmental concerns. It is, therefore, worthy of a detailed approach to evaluation and selection.[7]

The principal considerations applied to the selection of equipment are:

- the operating criteria must be adequate for the process (for example, size, speed, effectiveness, and reliability in operation)
- the availability of spares and servicing
- the frequency and ease of maintenance, changeover, and cleaning
- the construction materials and design; particularly at points of product contact
- the cost
- any environmental issues like dust, noise generation, and energy consumption
- the availability of process controls, perhaps with automatic adjustment, for example, on tablet presses
- the degree of product containment required to ensure operator safety as well as to protect the environment and the product from contamination (for example, high activity drugs).

Equipment Cleaning and Maintenance

A design that permits a simple and effective cleaning and maintenance routine is the goal, with written procedures to describe the techniques. The means to validate such procedures and to calibrate the equipment should be established.

Clean in place (CIP) facilities are popular today, particularly for tanks and large vessels. The design and installation of such systems and suitable protocols for in-place cleaning have been reviewed.[8,9]

Automation and Computerisation

Adequate consideration must be given to the introduction of automated or computerised processes such that the scale of operation or capacity requirement justifies the high investment and effort required to establish more sophisticated processes; above all, their validation can be complicated and time consuming. The value of versatile, mobile, and easily changed equipment is often overlooked in the search for excellence.

PERSONNEL

The impact of design on the people who operate the facilities will be significant, and hence, their full involvement and contribution at the detailed stage of design is crucial. A full consideration of Health and Safety regulations and good manufacturing practice (GMP) requirements is necessary to ensure that the workplace layout is safe, well organised, and ergonomically efficient. A pleasant, open environment with good personnel and welfare facilities, effective communications, and good management will greatly enhance a production facility. Suitable facilities and well-qualified personnel to train operational staff in all aspects of their work are essential.

While the site should have a perimeter fence with suitable security arrangements, there should also be a personnel security system for company staff, visitors, and contractors.

Adequate communication facilities should be provided to ensure key personnel can be contacted routinely during normal working hours via a public address, bleeper, or transceiver system. Emergency contact or call-out arrangements should be established for 'out of hours' situations.

Of particular importance to the pharmaceutical industry are adequate cloakroom/toilet facilities and changing rooms (air-locked if necessary) that are readily accessible but separate from manufacturing areas. These should be regularly cleaned and sanitised. Guidelines exist for the provision of suitable protective clothing and footwear. Laundry facilities on site can be a useful addition to ensure containment of contamination.

Separate viewing facilities for visitors to the site are recommended where visits are part of a customer care programme or training programme for staff or key members of the general public.

FACILITIES FOR STORAGE AND HANDLING OF MATERIALS

Of increasing importance to the pharmaceutical industry today is the need for well designed and planned storage and materials handling facilities. Although the buildings used for these purposes are generally less sophisticated and less costly to construct than those used for production, the area/volume required and the cost of stock held at different stages can be significant.

Whereas GMP regulations dictate certain fundamental requirements for pharmaceutical warehousing, a professional approach to the study of storage needs, materials handling options, and their close integration with production departments will save operating time and costs.

The goods reception and dispatch areas are potential sources of dust and dirt, and possible sites for the ingress of pests; they may also be subject to adverse climatic conditions. Facilities to limit these factors, and to cope with a variety of vehicles (end-loaded, side-loaded, tankers, large and small), should be considered carefully in terms of yard access and the means of loading and unloading. Special facilities for the cleaning of tankers and for dealing with static electricity discharge when handling inflammable materials must not be overlooked.

Savings in time and quarantine space may be achieved by having an area reserved for quality control sampling of raw materials, and packaging components close to the point of arrival. A large separate area may not be necessary for the quarantine of all goods delivered if a secure system for location control of palletised loads is designed and adhered to in practice. Such a system of controlled location and release will have additional benefits for semi-finished batches if they are stored in the same facilities as it avoids the need for the creation of a separate store for approved and unapproved semi-finished batches.

Classification of the storage requirements for segregation of hazardous materials, controlled drugs, rejected materials, and the provision of suitable facilities for cool or refrigerated storage, printed packaging materials, and labels is clearly important at the preliminary design stage.

Advice should be sought on storage and handling in dispensing areas to ensure the provision of adequate dust extraction and weighing facilities (with automatic identity checking and labelling systems). The organisation and operation of a centralised raw materials management unit is beneficial.[10] The means of transporting materials to and from production departments should be considered from a safety and hygiene point of view. Further considerations include the provision of suitable containers and pallets, for which cleaning facilities should exist.

QUALITY ASSURANCE REQUIREMENTS

The subject of quality assurance (QA) and associated GMP requirements for documentation and validation of facilities is immense.

During the design of quality control (QC) laboratory facilities, the latest guidelines on good laboratory practice must be borne in mind. The range of requirements for analysis and testing require detailed consultation with the users. In particular, all hazards should be clearly identified and specialised construction facilities for sensitive electronic equipment and controlled environments should be specified.

While QC laboratory facilities should be close to the production area, they can be minimised by the provision of local in-process control facilities and by adopting a modern team approach to QC/QA. Instead of extracting laboratory samples during and/or after production, QA should be integrated into the process to provide 'closed-loop process control'. Together with engineering data, QA data from chemical testing can be used to control the manufacturing process.[11]

Secure storage of essential documentation, tapes, disks, and microfilm is necessary, with restricted access to personnel. Adequate back-up of such records is essential, in addition to the provision of effective fire protection.

CONCLUSION

This chapter can only serve as an introduction to the range of criteria that should be considered when designing a production facility. It must be stressed that the most practical and successful designs result from collaboration between teams of engineers and pharmacists, whose combined skills should embrace a high degree of creativity and imagination balanced by considerable experience, both of project work and day-to-day production operations.

REFERENCES

1. Department of Health and Social Security. Guide to good pharmaceutical manufacturing practice. 3rd ed. London: HMSO, 1985.
2. Code of Federal Regulations. Food and drugs 21. Washington: Office of Federal Register National Archives and Records Administration, 1992.
3. Commission of the European Communities. The rules governing medicinal products in the European Community, Volume IV: Good manufacturing practice for medicinal products. Luxembourg: The Commission, 1992.
4. Goldberger F. Pharmaceutical manufacturing: Quality management in the industry. Evreux: Ebur, 1992.
5. Association of the British Pharmaceutical Industry. Guidelines for the control of occupational exposure to therapeutic substances. 2nd ed. London: The Association, 1992.
6. Chambers D. Mfg Chem 1986 Oct;57:63–6.
7. Pack TM, Cunfer EA. Drug Dev Ind Pharm 1988;14:2687–703.
8. Myers T, Kasica T, Chrai S. J Parenter Sci Technol 1987;41(1):9–15.
9. Adams DG, Agarwal D. Pharm Engineering 1990;10(6):9–15.
10. Murthy KS, Onyiuke C, Skrilec M. Pharmaceut Technol Int 1991;3(8):28,30,32,34,38–9.
11. Meyhack U, Meyer D. Pharmaceut Technol Int 1992;4(7):18,19.

FURTHER INFORMATION

Cole GC. Pharmaceutical production facilities—design and applications. Chichester: Ellis Horwood, 1990.

DeSain C. Drug, device and diagnostic manufacturing—the ultimate resource handbook. USA: Interpharm Press, 1991.

EFTA Secretariat. Premises for pharmaceutical manufacture. Seminar papers Oslo, June 1985. Geneva: The Secretariat, 1985.

Falconer P, Drury J. Building and planning for industrial storage and distribution. London: Architectural Press, 1975.

Institute of Quality Assurance. Pharmaceutical premises and environment. The Institute, 1987.

Whyte W, editor. Cleanroom design. Chichester: John Wiley & Sons, 1991.

Willig SH, Stoker JR. Good manufacturing practices for pharmaceuticals. 3rd ed. New York: Marcel Dekker, 1992.

Process Development

No matter how elegant the formulation of a pharmaceutical product, it will be successful only if it can be manufactured reliably, economically, and safely. The transfer of a product from the formulation laboratory to the factory floor is known as 'process development' and includes activities such as validation and optimisation.

The process development requirements of a particular product depend upon a number of factors, including the nature of the dosage form, the characteristics of the active ingredients, the equipment available, and the location of the manufacturing site. For example, the preparation of a simple aqueous solution is likely to be similar for 1 litre or 1000 litres, but the development of a granulation process from bench-top to factory scale will probably involve a change of mixer design and the definition of mixing times and speeds to ensure that the granules have the correct characteristics for further processing. If a product is destined for manufacture at several sites with different equipment, it is essential that the process is robust enough to be transferred with minimal technical support if at all possible.

This need for 'transferability' is probably the main reason why pharmaceutical formulations have changed remarkably little over the years. Investment in machinery such as mixers, tablet machines, and capsule fillers represents substantial capital outlay and individual pieces of equipment usually must be suitable for the manufacture of several different products. Consequently, the tablet formulations of today are similar to those of 20 or even 50 years ago, and the unit processes are also similar although improved technology and the use of microprocessors and computers has allowed us to exert more control at each stage.

The formulations may have remained similar, but the development of a suitable manufacturing process has become increasingly critical as high-speed equipment has been introduced to allow greater manufacturing output. Processes must be well validated in order to avoid the wastage of valuable product through failure during manufacture.

SOLID DOSAGE FORMS

Solid dosage forms are the most common and perhaps the preferred presentation for most products and also for most patients. In this discussion, solid dosage forms for oral administration only will be considered, although sterile solid delivery systems for implantation are also available.

Tablets and capsules are often similar in their formulation and the early stages of their manufacture, particularly if they are 'simple' formulations for 'immediate' release. Modified-release dosage forms usually have a more complicated manufacturing process.

At their most simple, tablets and capsules are prepared by blending several powders together (for example, active ingredient, disintegrant, binder, lubricant) and then either compressing the powders into a tablet or filling them into a hard gelatin capsule shell (see Oral Solids chapter). Such a process can be performed in the simplest of equipment and appears to pose few scale-up problems. In many instances, this may well be the case and a smooth transition from 1 kg batches in a Kenwood mixer to 500 kg batches in a Fielder mixer may be achieved. However, the scale-up is more likely to identify weaknesses in the process and even if these are not obvious, considerable validation work will be required to verify that the process is under control.

Problems that may arise include: poor mixing of the powders on scale-up, poor weight control of tablet or capsule, or unacceptable physical parameters (particularly for tablets). The reasons for these problems are fairly obvious when the process is considered carefully, but are easily overlooked by an enthusiastic development scientist. Small quantities of powder are mixed easily in small planetary-type mixers. If the same type of mixer is used at larger scale, a longer mixing time may be needed to achieve the same degree of homogeneity. If the mixer type is changed, as it often is, to a high shear mixer such as Fielder or Diosna, the change in mixing action may result in rapid over-blending of the powders causing difficulties during compression or unacceptable physical characteristics (such as poor disintegration/dissolution, or soft tablets). Slow, small-scale compression or capsule-filling equipment may not be very sensitive to the flow characteristics of the powder blend, or if powder flow is poor, the operator may even occasionally 'encourage' it. When the process is scaled-up to high speed equipment, flow characteristics become a critical aspect of the operation and poor weight control will result if the powder flow is inadequate.

Granulation

The development of a process for a granulated product is complicated by the need to achieve a consistent degree of 'wetness' and then remove the granulating liquid to produce a granule with the desired particle size and handling characteristics. Attempts to simplify this scale-up operation have included the development, by equipment suppliers, of small, pilot-scale versions of their production equipment. It seems logical to assume that if a process works in a small model, it will also work in the full-size model. Sadly, this is not necessarily true and the process conditions for the larger batch size will have to be determined by controlled experimentation, from those established at small scale. For example, granules are often dried in a fluid bed drier, for speed and efficiency. The inter-particulate attrition may increase significantly with batch size and therefore, the granule may dry in the predicted time, but the particles will be smaller and more dusty than in the small-scale operation. This, in turn, may cause processing problems later, such as during compression.

Simple handling operations at small scale may become anything but simple on the factory floor and it is important, therefore, to consider the logistics of moving the ingredients and product, in process, from A to B. Granulation fluids are easily prepared in a beaker at laboratory scale and poured by hand into the mixer containing the powder blend. At full production scale, this may be impossible and the fluid may need to be pumped from the preparation tank to the mixer. Similar problems are encountered when sieving powders. Sieving serves two purposes: it breaks up aggregates of the material, thus facilitating the production of a homogeneous powder blend; it also removes foreign material such as pieces of packaging material. Sieving, when performed on large scale, requires either labour-intensive handling of bags of excipients, or a vacuum transfer system which sucks material out of one container into another.

Safety

Mass transfer of powders introduces a second problem which increases with scale, that is, safety. Dust explosions in the pharmaceutical industry are, fortunately, quite rare, due to the safety precautions observed by responsible manufacturers. These include earthing all equipment to prevent static discharge and, in some cases, blanketing the process mix with nitrogen. Incautious scale-up from small scale where such risks are not significant, could cause severe injury, or even death, not just a process failure.

Similar safety considerations should be borne in mind during the selection of materials, particularly liquids or solvents. It is sometimes possible to solve a formulation problem or to develop an elegant tablet coat, at small scale, by using solvents such as ethanol, propanol, or methylene chloride. The health and safety implications of such materials can be controlled quite simply by conducting the operation in a fume cupboard or in an area with good ventilation. This is much more difficult to achieve as the scale of operation increases and the use of organic solvents should be avoided whenever possible to minimise the risks of fire or toxic fumes.

LIQUID DOSAGE FORMS

After consideration of the potential pitfalls awaiting the manufacturer of solid dosage forms, it might appear relatively easy to develop a robust, reliable process for liquid manufacture. However, the process is not necessarily straightforward. Temperature and pH control are much easier to achieve at small scale and mixing efficiency is likely to decline markedly as the equipment evolves from beaker and stirrer to a tank containing several thousand litres. Further complications are introduced if the liquid is a suspension rather than a solution and if the rheological characteristics of the product are important.

Temperature

It is obvious that the larger the volume of liquid to be heated or cooled, the slower the process will be. This has implications in terms of scheduling (it may not be possible to complete the manufacture in one working day), quality (there may be more opportunity for microbial contamination and growth), and stability (ingredients may be exposed to high temperatures for much longer than they were previously during small-scale manufacture). Sensible process development will anticipate these problems and attempt to overcome them by, for example: heating only a portion of the total volume, sufficient to dissolve the particular ingredient; adding preservatives at the earliest possible stage and using low bioburden (see Sterilisation chapter) ingredients; and studying the stability profile of the active ingredients in advance to determine the effect, if any, of elevated temperatures during processing.

pH

The control of pH is closely linked with stirrer efficiency, particularly if pH adjustment is necessary as a part of the production process. If the bulk liquid is not kept well mixed while the adjusting solution is added, extreme pH values may be attained locally within the mixture. This might lead to the recording of an incorrect value for the pH of the bulk, or to local degradation of the active ingredient with consequent effects on product quality. Such problems should be avoided by knowledge of the product and defining acceptable ranges in advance. For example, it may be necessary to adjust the pH with a larger volume of more dilute acid or base, in order to minimise the effects of local extremes.

Suspensions

Large-scale production of suspensions can be difficult because of the need to disperse adequately the solid material and maintain the defined viscosity for the product. Suspending agents are notoriously sensitive to the effects of shear forces and therefore the design of mixers and pumps must be considered carefully and tested for their effect on the rheology of the product. Even if the formulation is robust and can withstand homogenisation to disperse the solid material, it may not be practical to do so at a larger scale for economic reasons and also because of restraints on time. It may be more appropriate to prepare a concentrated dispersion of the solid, which is then milled and added to the bulk. Each process has its own particular challenges and so the experienced process developer maintains an open mind and looks for alternative means of achieving the same end result.

SEMI-SOLID DOSAGE FORMS

In many ways, the problems associated with the manufacture of semi-solid preparations are similar to those for liquids, with extra consideration needed for the microbiological aspects of the process. Heat transfer is often of vital importance since it is frequently necessary to melt some of the fatty components of a cream or ointment. The rheology and even the stability of the final product may be dependent upon the cooling rate of the product. This is because the structure that forms as

the fatty materials solidify can vary considerably with the rate of heat transfer and also with stirring conditions. The droplet size in an emulsion or cream depends upon similar parameters. Consequently, a cream that is produced by a poorly controlled process may crack unexpectedly, or an ointment may be too soft or too stiff because the conditions under which it was produced resulted in the wrong internal structure of the molecules.

The presence of aqueous and organic phases in creams and emulsions make them particularly prone to microbial contamination. The extended heating and cooling times aggravate the problem by providing conditions conducive to growth for a longer period. Great care must be taken, therefore, to keep all vessels clean and to minimise the risk of contamination.

The development of transdermal patches has presented a new challenge in the development of semi-solids. The effective absorption of the active ingredient from these delivery systems is dependent upon maintaining saturation at the rate-determining membrane, thus ensuring constant delivery of the drug to the skin surface. Changes in the process conditions can result in a change of crystal form of the drug, in either size or structure, and can thus dramatically change the release rate from the patch. Simple parameters like heat exchange and mixing conditions are often responsible and problems can be avoided by studying the effect of changing these parameters before commencing the scale-up process.

STERILE PRODUCTS

Most sterile products are either liquid or are processed as liquids and then lyophilised. The processing of sterile solid dosage forms will not be considered here.

Many of the scale-up problems associated with sterile products are similar to those of any liquid product and have been discussed already in the section on Liquid Dosage Forms above. Of course, particular consideration must be given to microbial contamination; the bioburden must be kept as low as possible, even if the product is to be terminally sterilised. For this reason, all ingredients are normally 'sterile' before they are introduced into the production process. The main effect of scale-up is the extension of processing time and the implications of this towards the maintenance of a low bioburden. The time required for solution preparation may be extended if heating or cooling is required, but the filling of the product into ampoules or vials is likely to be the longest part of the process. If filling cannot be completed in one day, consideration must be given to the relative merits of reducing the batch size and thus perhaps running an autoclave or freeze-dryer only part-full, or of holding the bulk overnight to continue filling on a second day. This choice will be influenced by many factors and must be made on a product-by-product basis.

Sterilisation

The other major factor that can affect the product in different ways as a result of altering the scale of the operation is the sterilisation process. Unless the product is temperature sensitive, sterilisation is most often achieved by autoclaving. A wide range of time/temperature combinations can be used to achieve sterilisation, although it is usual to adopt a standard, pharmacopoeial cycle unless there are special reasons to do otherwise. Timing of the sterilisation process starts when the load achieves the target temperature. It is apparent that it will take longer to reach this temperature if the autoclave is full as opposed to containing a part-load, and also that the load will take longer to cool down at the end of the sterilisation cycle. This additional exposure to heat and pressure can increase the formation of degradation products and can also have deleterious effects on the container and closure. For example, leaching of materials from the glass or rubber stopper may be substantially increased. In some cases, cracking of the glass has occurred under the additional stress imposed by the scaled-up process.

Lyophilisation

Scale-up of lyophilisation (freeze-drying; see Parenterals chapter) may be less dramatic, but can be even more difficult since, by definition, such products are thermolabile. It is advisable to monitor closely each stage of the drying process to ensure that the heat input matches the drying rate and also that primary drying is complete before proceeding to secondary drying. Failure to check the drying process at regular intervals may result in loss of product due to melt-back or to high residual moisture at the end of the cycle. Cycle times may also vary considerably according to the condenser capacity of the equipment.

PLANNED PROCESS DEVELOPMENT

Process development is an integral part of the formulation development process and those responsible for process scale-up should work closely with the formulators and with the production staff who ultimately will be responsible for making the product for the market. Sometimes the same individuals are responsible for the formulation and development of product and process, from initiation through to transfer to factory-scale manufacture, and sometimes several different individuals have responsibility for defined stages of the process. Both systems have advantages and disadvantages but it is essential to maintain good communication and exchange of information between all those involved if the development is to be efficient. The development team also includes representatives from quality assurance and quality control analysts who conduct the tests on in-process and final product samples.

Process development and the ultimate need to be able to manufacture the product on commercial scale should be borne in mind even during the early stages of formulation. The use of unusual or expensive excipients should be avoided, particularly if they are poorly defined or available in limited quantities. Organic solvents should be avoided whenever possible, as discussed earlier, and the number of transfers from one piece of equipment to another should be minimised.

Equipment

Equipment selected for laboratory trials should have larger-scale equivalents. Some types of mill, for example, are suitable only for laboratory scale use and are either inefficient or do not comply with good manufacturing practice (GMP) at a larger scale. The need for compliance with GMP is crucial and is often overlooked at the laboratory formulation stage. Ball mills are useful laboratory tools but are not normally suitable for the manufacture of licensed pharmaceutical products. It is not advisable, therefore, to use such equipment to develop a formulation, only to find that it is impossible to achieve the same result using conventional pharmaceutical mills.

Validation

Process development and process validation are inextricably linked since successful process development depends upon the identification of the critical stages of the process and defining the means by which the correct result can be achieved. Process validation then confirms that the process variables are sufficiently well defined to ensure that the product is consistently manufactured to the specified standard (see Validation chapter).

Batch Records

It is essential to collect as much information as possible about both the process and the product during the manufacture of the early batches. Process conditions (such as mixing time/speed, temperature, particle size, pH, moisture content) should be recorded in the batch records, together with the details of all equipment used. This record will make it much easier to identify the reasons for a change in product characteristics if part of the process is changed, and will enable the critical process parameters to be identified for validation purposes. If the active ingredient is known to be sensitive to pH, temperature, or any other processing condition, analytical testing of samples from each stage of the process may be necessary to confirm that undue stress is not being imposed at any point. Stability testing of batches made by a significantly different process may be necessary also, since changes may take some time to become apparent.

Ingredients that may be varied in quantity according to the needs of the formulation (for example, granulating fluid) must be monitored carefully because they can be valuable indicators of a changing process. If additional granulating liquid is needed, when no other parameter has changed from the previous batch, a change in the specification of one of the ingredients may be suspected, or a fault in the mixing process.

If the problem is traced to the mixer, it suggests that the process is highly dependent upon mixing speed and conditions. This will make the transfer of the process to different sites, with different types of mixer, much more difficult. Process development, therefore, should aim to achieve a flexible process, which is not tied to a specific set of equipment and can be operated without the need for technical specialists. Sugar coating of tablets, a practice that is now on the decline, is an example of a process that was dependent upon experienced individuals who knew, almost instinctively, how much sugar solution to add at any given time and how to adjust the drying and tumbling conditions to achieve the desired result.

AIDS TO PROCESS DEVELOPMENT

Technological advances in the use of microprocessors and computerisation have given the process development scientist many tools to assist in the development of a rational manufacturing method. Instrumentation of mixers, granulators, dryers, and tablet and capsule machines enable data to be collected at every stage. In fact, there is a danger that more data can be collected than can be interpreted.

Instrumentation of both single punch and multiple punch rotary tablet presses is possible now and the information gained from experimentation can greatly assist the transfer of a formulation from small-scale manufacture on a single punch machine to pilot-scale or large-scale production on high-speed rotary equipment. The difference in compression action between the two types has always presented some difficulty in process transfer, but it is possible now to determine the optimum dwell time, compression pressure, and compression rate necessary to produce the 'ideal' tablet of a given formulation.

Compression simulators can be used to obtain this information. These machines allow individual compressions to be made under pre-defined conditions to mimic those that may be encountered on any type of compression equipment. They have the advantage of using limited amounts of material while allowing the effects of high-speed compression to be evaluated.

Similar advances have been made in the monitoring of conditions inside autoclaves, sterilising ovens, and freeze-dryers so that development of successful and reliable processes for sterile products is more efficient. However, mere collection of data is not enough and skilled interpretation is necessary to ensure that the information is used correctly. A crucial element in sterile processing, for example, is the correct placement and distribution of probes within the sterilising chamber. If this is not done correctly, the entire operation and the data generated will be meaningless.

REGULATORY ASPECTS OF PROCESS DEVELOPMENT

Although it is good economic and practical sense to develop products and processes that can be relied upon and can be transferred without difficulty to other manufacturing sites, it is also necessary to demonstrate to regulatory authorities that processes have been well thought out. The 'Development Pharmaceutics' section of a European marketing authorisation application will include a justification of the composition of the product and the reasons for the manufacturing process. Any critical aspects of the product such as particle size or viscosity that directly affect the safety or efficacy should be identified in this section, together with the means by which they are controlled. Reasons for selecting direct compression as opposed to wet granulation for the manufacture of a tablet would be given, as would the rationale for selecting a particular sterilisation cycle for an injectable product. This regulatory requirement to justify and explain critical processing choices helps to ensure that different options are considered and either adopted or rejected. In the United States, similar information is required by the Food and Drug Administration (FDA) during the conduct of pre-approval inspections, and should be documented in the development history of the product.

In-process Tests

Process development activities also should identify the key in-process checks that are needed to ensure that all is proceeding as intended. These in-process tests should be documented in the manufacturing records and in the regulatory commitments concerning the product. It is important to realise that in-process specifications are set by the manufacturer, to ensure that the final product will be of the required quality and to act as 'early warning' of process changes. They are not intended as hurdles or challenges for the production operators and should be set only if failure to meet them will affect the quality of the product.

Validation of Equipment

Another means of ensuring product quality through a well-controlled process is to validate all equipment used. Equipment validation should be performed regularly to confirm that it still performs to the expected standard. By this means, wear and tear (which can result in, for example, variable operating speed, poor temperature control, or inaccurate dosing) can be detected and corrected at an early stage before product quality is significantly affected. Food and Drug Administration inspectors, in particular, are examining qualification and verification of manufacturing equipment.

Definition of Batch Size

It should be noted that regulatory authorities increasingly require the batch size to be stated and the process to be validated for that scale of operation. Opportunities for unintentional process development should be eliminated as far as possible. For example, granulation operations are usually defined in terms of batch size by the capacity of the mixer-granulator. Mixing of the dried granule with the lubricant and other extra-granular excipients may be conducted in a tumble mixer of much greater capacity. In order to increase output and save time, it may be tempting to combine two granulations at the mixing stage. In theory this may not appear to be a problem, but the head space in the mixer will be substantially reduced, and hence the ability of the powders and granules to move and mix will also be reduced. The result may be a granule that does not compress well due to inefficient blending and hence inadequate lubrication. The opposite effect (over-lubrication) may result if the batch size is reduced for any reason. Process development, therefore, should define the limits of batch size for which the process may be expected to produce a satisfactory product.

PACKAGING

The concept of process development is frequently limited to the manufacturing process up to the production of bulk quantities of the final product. Apart from somewhat specialised pharmaceuticals such as injections and aerosols, where the packaging is an integral part of the product, packaging is sometimes regarded as an 'add-on' operation at the end (see Pharmaceutical Packaging chapter).

However, it is a fact that most product recalls are the result of packaging and labelling errors and so development of processes that ensure that the right product is packed in the right container with the correct label, is critical to the pharmaceutical industry. Modern technology that provides on-line monitoring of the packaging process can assist, but consideration must be given to how the product is handled during packaging. This can also help the formulation and process development operation by defining product characteristics. For example, tablets must be robust enough to withstand attrition on the packaging line, and liquids must not drip from filling nozzles and should not be adversely affected by shear forces during the filling operation.

Many solid dosage forms are packed in blister-strips and the blisters are usually thermo-sealed to the aluminium lidding foil. Process development studies should determine whether the product could be affected by the thermo-sealing and if so, determine the limits within which the process can be safely operated.

The manufacture of packaging components, particularly plastic components, is likely to become much more tightly controlled in the future as the importance of well-defined packaging becomes more widely appreciated. This means that pharmaceutical manufacturers may start to work much more closely with packaging manufacturers to develop processes and specifications that are acceptable to themselves and to regulatory authorities.

FUTURE DEVELOPMENTS

Although manufacturing processes for pharmaceutical products may have changed remarkably little over the years, our understanding of them has increased significantly. As a consequence, control of these processes to ensure the manufacture of satisfactory products has improved. As both understanding and control increases, by the sensible application of modern technology, the need for testing of samples of the finished product should decline. Quality will be assured because the critical aspects of the process are controlled and that control is documented.

If similar developments are applied to the manufacture of excipients and active ingredients, the traditional role of quality control analytical testing should decline and be replaced by in-process testing as a part of process development and process validation. This should improve the efficiency of the production operation and allow products to be released to the market more quickly.

The key to achieving this degree of confidence is cooperation and collaboration between formulators and analysts, and quality control, quality assurance, engineering, production, and validation personnel at all stages of the formulation, development, and manufacture of a pharmaceutical product.

FURTHER INFORMATION

Aulton ME, editor. Pharmaceutics. The science of dosage form design. Edinburgh: Churchill Livingstone, 1988.

Avis KE, Lachman L, Lieberman H, editors. Pharmaceutical dosage forms. Parenteral medications; vols 1 and 2. New York: Marcel Dekker, 1984.

Ridgway Watt P. Tablet machine instrumentation in pharmaceutics. Chichester: Ellis Horwood, 1988.

Validation

Definitions

Validation is a concept that has been evolving continuously since its first formal appearance in the United States in 1978. Because of this, it has an intangible quality that has led to confusion and controversy, resulting in a rash of different definitions.[1]

The definition most frequently encountered is that from the current US Food and Drug Administration (FDA) guideline:[2]

'Process validation is establishing documented evidence which provides a high degree of assurance that a specific process will consistently produce a product meeting its pre-determined specifications and quality characteristics.'

According to *The Rules Governing Medicinal Products in the European Community*,[3] validation is the:

'Action of proving, in accordance with the principles of good manufacturing practice, that any procedure, process, equipment, material, activity or system actually leads to the expected results.'

Further definitions are provided by the European Pharmaceutical Inspection Convention (PIC),[4,5] the Fédération Internationale Pharmaceutique (FIP),[6] and various guides issued at national level, for example the UK *Guide to Good Pharmaceutical Manufacturing Practice 1983* (Orange Guide).[7]

Reduced to its most basic form, validation is proving that a process works.

Regulatory Background

Validation is founded on, but not specifically prescribed by, regulatory requirements and is best viewed as an important and integral part of current good manufacturing practice (GMP). Validation is, therefore, one element of the quality assurance programme associated with a particular process. As processes differ so widely, there is no universal approach to validation, and regulatory bodies, such as the FDA and the EC authorities, have developed general, non-mandatory guidelines rather than attempting to provide detailed instructions.

The *United States Current Good Manufacturing Practices for Pharmaceuticals*, Part 211, Subpart F, Section 211.110, *Sampling and testing of in-process materials and drug products*[8] highlights the requirement for process validation. It does not, however, define what constitutes an acceptable level of validation. To rectify this, the FDA published a *Guideline on General Principles of Process Validation* in May 1987, following the circulation of several drafts for review and comment.[2] The guideline, which applies to medical devices as well as drug products, does not define a legal requirement, but is a formal description of what practices are acceptable to the FDA. Manufacturers of pharmaceutical products are not required to follow the guideline, but clearly would need to demonstrate, by equally convincing means, that the process is reproducible and in good control.

In the European Community, the regulatory basis of validation is enshrined in Directives 75/318/EEC and 75/319/EEC.[9] More recently, Directive 91/356/EEC *Laying Down the Principles and Guidelines for Good Manufacturing Practice for Medicinal Products for Human Use* was published.[10] This brief document describes the basic principles of GMP that manufacturers must comply with as a statutory requirement. To interpret these principles, reference must be made to the *Guide to Good Manufacturing Practice for Medicinal Products*, which includes a section on validation.[11]

From the European regulatory viewpoint, validation fits rather uncomfortably between the inspection programmes for compliance with current GMP and the information package required to secure a product marketing authorisation. This aspect is elaborated in *Development pharmaceutics and process validation*, included in *The Rules Governing Medicinal Products in the European Community, Volume III*.[12]

In the United States, process validation is not in principle a requirement for the approval of a New Drug Application (NDA) or an Abbreviated New Drug Application (ANDA), although it is helpful to include a validation commitment in the application. However, at the pre-approval inspection, the investigators will expect to see and review the proposed process validation documentation. The company cannot distribute the product until validation is complete and the FDA will make spot checks to ensure compliance with this condition. Any detected violations could result in seizure of the product and the company being refused future marketing approvals until validation is complete. Currently, process validation has to be completed before an FDA pre-approval inspection of a foreign (that is, not located in the USA) facility.

Although there is not always a clear distinction between regulations and non-mandatory guidelines, the situation in both the European Community and the United States is that a new product, or an old product manufactured using a modified process or facility, cannot be distributed for sale until the process has been adequately validated.

Scope of Validation

The concept of validation has expanded through the years to encompass a wide range of activities, from analytical methods used for the quality control of drug substances and drug products to equipment, facilities, and processes for the manufacture of drug substances and drug products, to computerised systems for clinical trial labelling or process control. Any piece of equipment, facility, or process operated under current GMP should be validated and this includes manufacturing and packaging operations for clinical trial materials, storage stability studies, as well as those involving products for distribution and sale.

Hierarchy of Validation

Process validation as previously defined is a component of GMP. It is complementary to and not a replacement for other aspects of GMP, such as personnel training records, standard operating procedures, adequate batch documentation, and good quality management systems. Before a process can be properly validated, the equipment, facilities, and services used in the process must themselves be validated. Such an operation is often called **qualification.** Qualification is, therefore, an integral part of process validation which, in turn, is part of GMP.

Application of Validation

By definition, validation requires the accumulation of documentary evidence relating to a process, item of equipment, or facility. This is achieved by means of a **validation protocol** which details the tests to be carried out, the frequency of testing, and the results expected (**the acceptance criteria**).

If the validation programme is designed, and the protocol issued, before the equipment or facility comes on stream or before the product manufactured by the process being validated is distributed, then this constitutes **prospective validation**. Sometimes, however, systems or processes are in place that have not previously been validated, but are functioning well and consistently producing good products, already in distribution. Validation of such facilities or processes is called **retrospective validation** and is achieved by the review of historical manufacturing and testing data.

Prospective and retrospective validation may be combined advantageously in sequence to provide a higher level of assurance than is given by the pre-marketing prospective validation alone. **Concurrent validation** is a newer term that has led to some confusion. It is applied either to ongoing prospective validation or to the ongoing review and evaluation of historical data associated with retrospective validation. **Revalidation** is the act of repeating all or a portion of the validation as a result of any modification to the process or facilities that may lead to changes in the quality or reproducibility of the product. Revalidation may be triggered by the operation of an established **change control system.** It can also refer to the regular, planned repetition of validation steps for equipment or processes where performance may change with time.

Companies with a roster of ageing products manufactured by non-validated processes, or who are commissioning new or modified facilities, will have a backlog of validation work to do. This should be tackled in order of priority; those products with potential safety or quality problems, if they are not manufactured by properly controlled processes, should be at the top of the list.[13] However, it is important that enough resource is allocated to complete all the validation backlog in a reasonable time. It is not sufficient to validate only the most vulnerable products.

Validation in Pharmaceutical Development

Good manufacturing practice is required at the stage in development of a pharmaceutical product where supplies are manufactured and packaged for clinical trials. Storage stability samples prepared to support clinical trials and provide data for marketing authorisation applications should also be produced to standards of GMP. It follows that, as validation is an important part of GMP, such drug products should be manufactured using validated processes.[14, 15] This is made clear in a guideline issued by the FDA in March 1991.[16]

The FIP guideline[6] also states that validation is important for the development phase as well as for the manufacture and quality control of medicaments.

Clearly, the drug product must be manufactured and packed using qualified equipment in qualified facilities, but it is less obvious to what extent process validation is required, considering that marketing authorisation in the USA may in principle be granted before process validation is started.

Many companies start phase I clinical trials with an initial dosage unit, for example, pure drug or a simple formulation filled into capsules for an oral presentation. As experience is gained, the formulation is refined and the dosage form may even be changed. Detailed process validation studies are not appropriate for a rapidly evolving formulation, although in-process controls and final product testing should be adequate to ensure the quality of each batch produced. The manufacturing process should be demonstrated to be reproducible and in good control for the pivotal clinical trials in which bioavailability and efficacy are to be established. This is particularly important in the case of sterile products.[17]

Process validation is simplified by good formulation design and optimisation. A robust formulation in which the critical process variables have been identified and explored as part of the development pharmaceutics will be easier to scale-up and validate.

Benefits of Validation

The conscientious validation of facilities and processes consumes significant resources. However, there are substantial benefits. Processes consistently under control require less process support, will have less down time, fewer batch failures, and may operate more efficiently, with greater output. In addition, timely and appropriate validation studies will transmit a commitment to product quality, which may facilitate pre-approval inspections and expedite the granting of marketing authorisations. Validation makes good business sense.

Facilities, Equipment, and Services Validation

Definitions

The validation of facilities, equipment, and services is commonly called qualification.[18-20] Qualification is usually divided into installation qualification (IQ) and operational qualification (OQ).

An **installation qualification** (see below) documents specific static attributes of a facility or item of equipment to prove that the installation of the unit has been correctly performed and that the installation specifications of the manufacturer have been met. An **operational qualification** (see below) documents specific dynamic attributes of a facility or item of equipment to prove that it operates as expected throughout its operating range, including 'worst case' conditions. The qualification programme is co-ordinated by means of a written general plan, called a **validation master plan** (see below) or **master qualification plan**.

The administration of the qualification programme is normally by means of a **validation committee**, comprised of representatives of the different disciplines involved with the programme. Typically, these representatives may be from departments such as pharmaceutical production or operations, quality assurance, microbiological quality control, analytical quality control, pharmaceutical development, engineering, and maintenance. The committee approves and issues written protocols, and reviews the data obtained against the results expected, that is, the acceptance criteria, to approve or reject the qualification or validation.

Validation Master Plan

The validation master plan (VMP) complements the facilities master file and is usually the first document to be reviewed during an inspection by a regulatory authority. It reinforces the commitment of the company to GMP and should provide a clear overview of the validation programme, including schedules and responsibilities. It must also direct an inspector to the more specific, detailed documents, such as qualification protocols, standard operating procedures, and personnel training records.

The VMP is also a convenient guide for the validation committee and those performing the qualifications. Because new equipment or facilities may enter the validation programme from time to time, the VMP is best considered as a live document, most conveniently contained in a ring binder, to which supplementary (dated) pages may be added as required. The VMP should be concise so that it can be easily read in one sitting and may typically include the following:

- table of contents
- introduction and objectives
- description of facilities, including plans
- constitution of validation committee
- glossary of terms

- description and history of equipment
- construction documentation
- description and listing of protocols
- list of standard operating procedures
- preventative maintenance programme
- personnel training programme
- storage documentation
- examples of protocols
- examples of standard operating procedures
- approvals.

Installation Qualification

The installation qualification (IQ) of a facility or item of equipment is documented by means of an **installation qualification protocol** and where necessary, addenda such as drawings, chart recorder traces, and print-outs. The IQ protocol should be numbered and dated, and approved for issue by appropriately authorised personnel. The document may include:

- introduction and objectives
- identification information, including plant inventory number and standard operating procedure (SOP) number
- purpose of the facility or equipment
- design and construction details
- details of services, required and provided
- acceptance criteria.

When the IQ is complete, the data should be reviewed, and the protocol approved and signed before work starts on the operational qualification.

Operational Qualification

The operational qualification (OQ) of a facility or item of equipment is documented by means of an **operational qualification protocol**, together, if necessary, with a compilation of test results. As with the IQ protocol, the OQ protocol should be numbered and dated, and approved for issue. The contents of an OQ protocol will be specific to the facility or item of equipment. The tests should be designed to demonstrate that the unit performs properly at the limits of its operating conditions, as well as within the normal range that will be used. If measurements are made on a statistical basis, then this must be fully described in the protocol. In addition to the operational tests, an OQ protocol may typically include:

- introduction and objectives
- brief identification information
- visual inspection (for example, damage to exterior, obstructions to filter panels, fit of gaskets and doors)

- functioning of switches and indicator lights
- check and calibration of sensors, probes, gauges, recorders, air flow rates, directions, pressures, and temperatures
- filter integrity and efficiency tests
- cleaning procedures
- details of qualification instrumentation used
- acceptance criteria
- actions resulting from the OQ—what to do if one or more of the parameters are not satisfactory
- requalification—timescales and triggering factors.

When the OQ is completed, the data should normally be reviewed and the protocol approved and signed before the validation of processes using the equipment or facility can commence. For some facilities, utilities, and items of equipment, performance data may be gathered over a long period of time. Under these circumstances it is difficult to 'sign off' the OQ as complete. One solution is to define and approve the OQ at a single time point and to create another protocol (sometimes called a **performance qualification protocol**) as a vehicle to amass the ongoing data. A completed and approved OQ is then quickly available for presentation to regulatory authorities.

Sterile Facility and Equipment Qualification

The application of qualification procedures is especially important for facilities, services, and items of equipment that are used in the manufacture of sterile products. The most critical aspects are:

- heating, ventilation, and air conditioning (HVAC) of the sterile facility[21]
- pure water supply (water for injections)[22]
- sterilisation equipment[23,24]
- filling and sealing equipment for aseptic processes
- cleaning and sanitation.

Air quality requirements for sterile areas are well established, defining a cascade of cleanroom classifications.[25] Standards are given in British Standard 5295:Part 1:1989 and in US Federal Standard 209E (see also the Cleanrooms for Pharmaceutical Production chapter). The standards are determined largely by the effectiveness of the air filtration systems, and the qualification of a sterile facility starts by checking the pre-filter and HEPA filters for leaks, particle penetration, and air velocity at the filter face. Other HVAC parameters that should be monitored and challenged include temperature, humidity, and pressure differentials and air movement patterns, to identify dead spots.

Microbiological qualification requires that particle counts should be performed and the time for each room to recover to within its classification standard from a state where it contains a known level of particulates (the clean-down time) should also be determined. The definition of cleaning regimens and the evaluation of swab samples, settle plates, and Biostat™ strips is also necessary. All the tests should be undertaken when the facility is both empty and fully populated.

Sterilisation equipment qualification is of fundamental importance and is often undertaken concurrently with process validation.

Firstly, the usual checks and calibration of sensors, timers, gauges, couplings, and seals are made and the quality of services to the steriliser is established. Then, the distribution of heat throughout the chamber, with and without a load, is measured using at least three layers of thermocouples. This reveals the coolest positions within the chamber. At the coolest location, the profile of heat penetration into a container or item of equipment should be determined. The objective is to prove and document that the coolest part of an item, in the coolest position, reproducibly reaches at least the prescribed temperature for the prescribed time, thereby ensuring an acceptable sterility assurance level (SAL; see also the Sterilisation chapter). The SAL is the probability that a product following sterilisation may contain viable organisms. For terminally sterilised products, an SAL of 10^{-6} or better is expected.

Process Validation

When qualification is complete, **process validation** (PV) can begin.[26] In some cases, PV may be conducted concurrently with IQ, for example, where an item of equipment is dedicated to one process, producing one product. Process validation is organised and administered in the same way as qualification, by the writing and issuing of **process validation protocols** and the accumulation and review of data against agreed acceptance criteria.

Validation of Non-sterile Products

Non-sterile products range from simple topical solutions to sophisticated solid oral dosage products and the level of validation should reflect the complexity of the process.[12, 27–31] Although it may be superficially impressive to gather vast amounts of validation data, it is more effective to identify the critical process parameters and design

the validation protocol to properly challenge and explore them. The critical process parameters should be defined during the course of preformulation, pharmaceutical development, and scale-up studies.

For a simple topical or oral solution, critical parameters could be:

- order or rate of addition of ingredients
- pH
- mixing time and geometry
- light sensitivity during processing
- time between manufacture and filling.

In the case of an oral tablet manufactured by granulation and compression, the critical process parameters may include:

- particle size distribution of the drug
- blending time of the powder
- granulating time and speed
- amount of granulating fluid—binder concentration
- drying time—final moisture content
- granule particle size distribution
- granule drug content and homogeneity
- blending time of external phase
- tablet hardness with respect to water content, friability, disintegration, and dissolution
- lubrication level with respect to tablet hardness, disintegration, dissolution, and die-ejection force
- tablet weight and thickness control
- tablet drug content uniformity.

If the tablet is then film coated, additional parameters may require evaluation, for example:

- spray rate of film coating solution
- inlet and outlet air temperatures
- coating weight of polymer with respect to tablet appearance, friability, disintegration, and dissolution.

The above critical parameters are given by way of example only. More complex presentations, for example, modified-release or multilayer tablets, may require the control of different or additional aspects of the process to ensure that the product is manufactured to consistently meet the appropriate specifications.

The second stage of process validation is to manufacture batches of product, controlling the critical parameters identified in the first stage and thoroughly testing for compliance to specifications throughout the process. There is a general consensus that three satisfactory batches, properly

documented are an acceptable minimum requirement for a successful PV.

Validation of Sterile Products

The general pattern of process validation is the
same as for non-sterile products and similar critical process parameters need to be defined and controlled.[32, 33] The key additional requirement is the
complete absence of microbial contamination;
this necessitates validation of the sterilisation process for terminally sterilised products, or of the
sterilisation, filling, and sealing processes for aseptically filled products.

Terminally Sterilised Products. The bioburden
before sterilisation should be demonstrated to be
reproducibly low. The subsequent course of validation depends on the sterilisation process. Steam
sterilisation using an autoclave is the most common, being particularly suited to ampoule and bottle presentations where the drug product is not
degraded by heat.[23]

Assuming a properly qualified area and steriliser,
process validation involves repetition of the heat
distribution and profile studies, with the product
in question, using thermocouples calibrated immediately before and after the measurements. If the
product is presented in a range of container sizes,
then the largest and smallest should be validated.
The effects of half and minimum chamber loadings
should also be explored. A minimum of three
batches of each size at each loading condition
must be documented.

An appropriate biological indicator, inoculated
into the product, can provide additional assurance
of an adequate SAL. However, many companies
are wary of introducing viable organisms into
their sterile facilities and therefore rely on accurate
temperature mapping and overkill conditions.

Aseptically Filled Products.[34-36] Because of the
lower achievable SAL (typically 10^{-3} compared
to 10^{-6}), the FDA have proposed that aseptic filling can only be used if terminal sterilisation is
shown to affect the drug product.[37] Assuming
that the facility, both inside and outside the aseptic
area, is qualified to the appropriate classification
standards, process validation requires assurance
that the drug product and packaging components
are sterile and that the filling and closing operations do not introduce any contamination.
Solution products are often sterilised by filtration
'through the wall' into the aseptic area. The filter
effectiveness should be validated for the product

by means of appropriate tests, for example, forward flow rate for cartridge filters or a bubble
point test for membrane filters, using at least three
batches of product. These validation studies can be
performed as a service by the filter manufacturer
and should be supplemented by the routine determination of pressure drop, stability time, pressure
hold time, and pressure decay, before and after
each production run.

Packaging components may be passed through a
tunnel steriliser into the aseptic area. The validation of tunnels is more complicated than dry heat
ovens because of the additional variables of belt
speed, air flow patterns and speeds, and HEPA filter integrity. As the tunnels invariably have to be
validated for reduction and elimination of endotoxins, this provides a satisfactory means of establishing an acceptable SAL as the conditions
required for endotoxin reduction are far more
severe than those for sterility.

An acceptable way of validating the entire manufacturing, filtration, filling, and closing process is
by means of a minimum of three media (or broth)
runs.[38] These should be repeated on a regular basis
and also if there is any change to the process or personnel. The validation of aseptic drug powder filling processes is accomplished in a similar way. A
liquid or a dry powder medium can be used, but
neither is a true process simulation test.[39, 40] More
complicated aseptic processes, such as form-fill
sealing[1] and lyophilisation[17, 41-43] may require
additional levels of validation.

Raw Materials Validation

Active Materials from Primary Manufacture

For a drug substance, the active structure is
assembled and its purity defined and refined during the stages of its synthesis. Subsequent formulation into a drug product cannot improve on this
intrinsic quality, and therefore reproducible manufacture of the drug substance to consistently meet
an agreed specification contributes significantly to
the overall quality of the drug product. It follows
that the principles of qualification of plant and services, and process validation should be applied to
the drug substance manufacturing process. Particular attention must be paid to the validation of
quality-critical steps in the synthetic route, and of
the final manufacturing stages, in which the drug
substance is formed, isolated, and purified.
Critical parameters that may be explored during
process validation studies include, for a non-sterile
solution product:

- yields at each stage and overall
- impurity profile and residual solvents
- colour
- absence of particulate contamination
- satisfactory microbiological profile.

For a non-sterile solid dosage product, the following may be added to the list:

- polymorphism and crystal habit
- particle size distribution
- bulk density.

For a sterile product, a low level of endotoxins is also a critical requirement.

Particularly rigorous plant qualification and process validation is necessary for the manufacture of sterile solids, for example, by aseptic crystallisation.

Active and Inactive Materials (Excipients) from Third Parties

The validation of purchased active materials and excipients is sometimes considered to be a separate issue, but it is probably best regarded as an integral part of the pharmaceutical development and process validation of a product.[44] During these steps any critical parameters will be defined and appropriate control measures instigated. The materials should be obtained from audited suppliers to agreed specifications and be subject to the usual quality control checks. Where a particular excipient, or grade of excipient, is identified as having a critical effect on the quality or reproducibility of a drug product, at least three batches of the excipient should be evaluated as part of the process validation studies.

Cleaning Validation

The validation of cleaning methods is an important element of both qualification and process validation for drug substance and drug product manufacture.[45] The objective is to minimise the possibility of significant cross-contamination. The difficulty is in knowing what level is significant and how this relates to amounts that may be detected on equipment or facilities.

The regulatory authorities have not issued formal guidelines on cleaning validation; however, an FDA inspection guide has recently become available.[46] Although each situation requires assessment, it is often considered that a cleaning procedure that consistently reduces the contaminant to a level not exceeding one-thousandth of its lowest daily therapeutic dose in the highest daily therapeutic dose of the product, can be regarded as validated.

Three sampling methods are in general use: swabs, rinses, and placebos. Swab samples are usually taken from an area of 100 cm^2 (approximating to the size of the hand) at positions likely to be contaminated or where the presence of contamination would be critical. A suitable solvent for the drug must be used. Rinse samples are taken from the final wash solution for the item of equipment or facility. Placebo samples are taken from a placebo run in the equipment after cleaning. This method is closest to the real situation; however, there is some concern that such placebo samples may not be sufficiently discriminating and may miss small pockets of contamination. The current view is that this method, if used, should be supplemented by the analysis of swab or rinse solution samples.

The establishment of acceptance criteria for contaminant levels in the samples is a difficult task. The limits should be practical and achievable. With the ever increasing sensitivity of analytical methodology, residues will always be found. Common sense and good judgement are required, taking into consideration the properties of the contaminant, the position from which the sample was taken, and the potential dilution effects. The rationale for establishing limits may be reviewed during an inspection by a regulatory authority.

A simple and practical assessment method that should not be overlooked is the visual and tactile inspection. Except for very potent or toxic drugs, the amounts of residues that are likely to result in significant contamination can usually be seen or detected by touch.

Residues from the cleaning agents used do not at present have to be determined as part of the validation. Such materials should be of pharmaceutical or food grade quality and, since only very low residual levels would be expected, the safety risk should be negligible.

Many companies are adopting a 'modelling concept' in which representative products, comprising the most difficult to clean water-soluble and water-insoluble drug substances, are selected for cleaning validation. This is the 'worst case' situation, the implication being that cleaning procedures validated using these compounds will also encompass the more easily cleaned products. A similar modelling procedure can be applied to equipment and facilities where justifiable comparisons can be made.

Cleaning validation can be documented either as part of an OQ or PV protocol, or separately, if appropriate. Whatever the format, the document should include a detailed cleaning procedure (or refer to an SOP in which it is described), sampling plan, analytical methods, acceptance criteria, and revalidation rationale.

The validation of cleaning methods is only meaningful if the written cleaning procedures on which the validation is based are always meticulously followed.

Change Control

Once the qualification of a facility or item of equipment, or the validation of a process, has been achieved, it has to be maintained. A change control system (described by an SOP) should be in place so that any alterations to facilities, equipment, materials, processes, or documentation can be identified.[2] An assessment of the significance of the change can then be made, most appropriately by the validation committee, who can decide if the change affects product quality. If it does, then further validation work (revalidation) is required before the products impacted by the change can be distributed and sold. Preferably, the change control system should operate prospectively, with the effects of proposed changes being evaluated before they are authorised. All aspects of the change control system should be documented as part of the overall validation programme.

Further Validations

Analytical Methods Validation

Reproducible and accurate analytical results are a prerequisite throughout pharmaceutical development and manufacturing.[47, 48] Achieving these depends on the use of valid, robust methods. Validation of the analytical methods used is required in most sophisticated territories and is covered by several guidelines. Critical factors that should be evaluated include: accuracy (as evidenced by selectivity, specificity, and lack of bias), precision, recovery, linearity, and system suitability for chromatographic determinations. The method may or may not be stability indicating.

The validated analytical methods should be documented in sufficient detail to facilitate their evaluation and repetition by skilled staff from a regulatory laboratory, or their transfer to another laboratory within the company. Such technology transfers, often exemplified by a change from analytical development to quality control as products progress towards the market place, may require additional validation or revalidation studies if equipment is different in the two laboratories.

Packaging Components Validation

For either sterile or non-sterile products, packaging materials should be evaluated and selected throughout the course of the pharmaceutical development to provide the required properties of compatibility, stability, security, and sterility. Their validation should be considered as part of the process validation for the product. The impact of critical packaging material parameters on the quality of the product should be explored, and the established quality and change control systems used to ensure that no batches of the packaging components are likely to have a deleterious effect on product quality.

Medical Device Validation

The FDA guideline[2] applies equally to medical devices and to conventional drug products, and the need for qualification and validation studies is similar, but also encompasses design.[19, 49]

Computer Systems Validation

This is an area that has expanded rapidly over the last few years, reflecting the ever increasing impact of computerisation on pharmaceutical processes.[50–57] Computer systems range from standard wordprocessing software and personal computers used to produce documentation and labels for clinical trials, through dispensing and stock-keeping systems, to full auto-control 'lights out' operation of complete plants. Assurance of reproducible, accurate performance is essential, as is a secure system of change control to cope with software and hardware updates and modifications.

REFERENCES

1. Sharp JR. Mfg Chem 1988;59(2):22-3,27,55.
2. Food and Drug Administration. Guideline on general principles of process validation. Rockville, MD: The Administration, 1987.
3. Commission of the European Communities. The rules governing medicinal products in the European community, Vol IV. Good manufacturing practice for medicinal products. Luxembourg: The Commission, 1992:162.
4. EFTA Secretariat. Basic standards of good manufacturing practices for pharmaceutical products. Geneva: The Secretariat, March 1983.
5. EFTA Secretariat. Guidelines for the manufacture of sterile products. Geneva: The Secretariat, May 1981.
6. Joint FIP. Int J Pharm Tech Prod Mfr 1983;4:45.
7. Sharp JR, editor. Guide to good pharmaceutical manufacturing practice 1983. London: HMSO, 1983.
8. United States Current Good Manufacturing Practices (GMP) for Pharmaceuticals 21 CFR Ch.1 (4-1-90 ed.) Section 211.110.
9. European Commission Directives 75/318/EEC, 75/319/EEC. Luxembourg: The Commission, 20 May 1975.
10. European Commission Directive 91/356/EEC. Luxembourg: The Commission, 13 June 1991.

11. Commission of the European Communities. The rules governing medicinal products in the European community, Vol IV. Good manufacturing practice for medicinal products. Luxembourg: The Commission, 1992:46.

12. Commission of the European Communities. The rules governing medicinal products in the European community, Vol III. Guidelines on the quality, safety and efficacy of medicinal products for human use. Luxembourg: The Commission, 1989:10.

13. Arambulo AS. Drug Dev Ind Pharm 1979;5:523–43.

14. Lignau J. Drug Dev Ind Pharm 1989;15:1029–46.

15. Morris JM. Drug Dev Ind Pharm 1990;16:1749–59.

16. Food and Drug Administration. Guideline on the preparation of investigational new products. Rockville, MD: The Administration, 1991.

17. Levchuk JW. J Parenter Sci Technol 1991;45(3):152–5.

18. Bastow R. Mfg Chem 1985;56(2):55, 57.

19. De Sain C. Drug, device and diagnostic manufacturing. Buffalo Grove, IL: Interpharm Press, 1990.

20. Cole G. Pharmaceutical production facilities, design and applications. Chichester: Ellis Horwood, 1990:237–65.

21. Panezai AK. Mfg Chem 1987;58(7):34–5,37.

22. Parenteral Drug Association. Design concepts for the validation of a water for injection system. Technical Report No.4. Philadelphia, PA: The Association, 1983.

23. Parenteral Drug Association. Validation of steam sterilization cycles. Technical Monograph No.1. Philadelphia, PA: The Association, 1978.

24. Parenteral Drug Association. Validation of dry heat processes used for sterilization and depyrogenation. Technical Report No.3. Philadelphia, PA: The Association, 1981.

25. Cole G. Pharmaceutical production facilities, design and applications. Chichester: Ellis Horwood, 1990:90.

26. Berry IR, Nash RA, editors. Drugs and the pharmaceutical sciences; vol 57. Pharmaceutical process validation. New York: Marcel Dekker, 1993.

27. Edwards CM. Drug Dev Ind Pharm 1989;15:1119–33.

28. Berry IR. Drug Dev Ind Pharm 1988;14:377–89.

29. Lewis A, Simpkin GT, O'Reilly A, Thomas RD. Mfg Chem 1987; 58(6):31–2,35,43.

30. Colombo P. Drug Dev Ind Pharm 1989;15:1047–58.

31. Rudolph JS. In: Berry IR, Nash RA, editors. Drugs and the pharmaceutical sciences; vol 57. Pharmaceutical process validation. New York: Marcel Dekker, 1993;167–88.

32. Akers MJ, Anderson NR, Hofmann KL. Both in: Berry IR, Nash RA, editors. Drugs and the pharmaceutical sciences; vol 57. Pharmaceutical process validation. New York: Marcel Dekker, 1993;25–87,89–166.

33. Begg D. In: Greenshields R, editor. Biomedical technology. Hong Kong: Century Press, 1992;273–4,276,278.

34. Olson WP and Groves MJ, editors. Aseptic pharmaceutical manufacturing technology for the 1990's. Buffalo Grove, IL: Interpharm Press, 1987.

35. Food and Drug Administration. Guideline on sterile drug products produced by aseptic processing. Rockville, Maryland: The Administration, 1987.

36. Parenteral Drug Association. Validation of aseptic filling for solution drug products. Technical Monograph No.2. Philadelphia, PA: The Association, 1980.

37. Federal register; vol 56, No.198 Friday Oct. 11, 1991; 51354–8.

38. Parenteral Society. The use of media fills in process simulation testing. Monograph No.4. Swindon: The Society (in preparation).

39. Parenteral Drug Association. Validation of aseptic drug powder filling processes. Technical Report No.6. Philadelphia, PA: The Association, 1984.

40. Prout G. J Parenter Sci Technol 1982;36(5):199.

41. Avallone HL, Wolk AE. J Parenter Sci Technol 1986;40:81–2.

42. Avallone HL., J Parenter Sci Technol 1990:44:228–30.

43. Trappler EH. Pharmaceut Technol 1989;13(1):56,58,60.

44. Berry IR. In: Berry IR, Nash RA, editors. Drugs and the pharmaceutical sciences; vol 57. Pharmaceutical process validation. New York: Marcel Dekker, 1993;369–410.

45. Mendenhall DW. Drug Dev Ind Pharm 1989;15:2105–14.

46. Avallone HL, Davis RJ, D'Eramo PN, Phillips JX. Food and Drug Administration. Mid Atlantic Region Inspection Guide. The Administration, 28 July, 1992.

47. Commission of the European Communities. The rules governing medicinal products in the European community, Vol III. Addendum. Note for guidance; analytical validation, July 1989. Luxembourg: The Commission, 1990.

48. Pasteelnick LA. In: Berry IR, Nash RA, editors. Drugs and the pharmaceutical sciences; vol 57. Pharmaceutical process validation. New York: Marcel Dekker, 1993;411–428.

49. Campbell I, Corby GE, Hoxey E. In: Proceedings of the medical device conference, Cologne:1990. Chester: Aster Publishing Corporation, 1990.

50. Chapman KG, Harris JR et al. Pharmaceut Technol Int 1989;1(5):54–8.

51. Trill AJ. Pharmaceut Technol Int 1993;5(2):12–26;5(3): 49,50,52,54,56,58,60,62;5(5):17–18,20,22,24,26,28,30.

52. Alford JS, Cline FL et al. Pharmaceut Technol 1990;14(9):88,90,92,94,96,98,100,102.

53. Agalloco J et al. Pharmaceut Technol 1990;14(1):20–1,24,26,28,32,34,36,40,75.

54. Bluhm AR. Pharmaceut Technol 1989;13(11):32,34,36,40.

55. Clark AS. Pharmaceut Technol 1988;12(1):60,62,64–6.

56. Commission of the European Communities. The rules governing medicinal products in the European community, Vol IV. Good manufacturing practice for medicinal products. Luxembourg: The Commission, 1992:Annex 11, 139.

57. Chamberlain R. Computer systems validation for the pharmaceutical and medical device industries. Libertyville, IL: Alaren Press, 1991.

Dispensing Procedures and Practice-related Guidelines

The profession of pharmacy is concerned with all aspects of medicines, from the synthesis or isolation of drug molecules to the manufacture, control, distribution, and use of the formulated product. Pharmacists have traditionally been concerned with the preparation and dispensing of prescriptions, although the profession now encompasses other activities. Pharmacists provide an advisory role on a range of health-care matters, particularly in treating minor self-limiting conditions, and many offer domiciliary and diagnostic services. However, the practice of dispensing remains central to the professional role of the pharmacist.

Dispensing includes all of the activities that occur from the prescription being handed in at the pharmacy, to the medicine or other prescribed items being collected. In the hospital service, dispensing includes supplies of medicines for patients on the wards. Furthermore, pharmacists must ensure that patients understand exactly how their medicines should be taken and for how long.

This chapter is intended to be read in conjunction with Standards of Good Professional Practice, which is published as part of the Royal Pharmaceutical Society Code of Ethics. The legal aspects of dispensing are comprehensively covered in *Medicines, Ethics and Practice: A Guide for Pharmacists*, which is published every six months, and *Pharmacy Law and Ethics* (Appelbe and Wingfield).

THE PREPARATION OF MEDICINES

Medicines may be manufactured on a large-scale or on a small-scale basis. The pharmaceutical industry undertakes large-scale manufacture whereas small-scale manufacture is carried out mainly in hospital practice, but also to some extent in community pharmacy. These activities must be undertaken by trained and qualified personnel in suitable premises and with appropriate equipment. All products must be manufactured in accordance with good manufacturing practice. Control procedures are necessary at every stage from receipt of raw materials to distribution of the finished products. Certain of these procedures are controlled under the Medicines Act 1968, while others are the result of experience and constitute good pharmaceutical practice in both the technical and professional sense.

PRESCRIPTIONS

The authority to write prescriptions for medicines and the information which must be given on them are the subject of legislation under the UK Medicines Act 1968. Records of dispensing transactions are also necessary for medicines restricted by legislation to be supplied only on the authority of a prescription and not supplied on an NHS prescription. Such records may be subject to inspection by appropriately authorised persons under the Act.

The traditional format of prescriptions has undergone modification in both hospital and general practice. In hospital the prescription is usually written on highly stylised forms in order to avoid ambiguity, while the way in which prescriptions are written outside hospital may follow the traditional pattern. Legislation dictates, in many cases, precisely what information the prescription must contain in order to be legally valid.

Prescriptions for medicines may be written by doctors, dentists, veterinary surgeons, or veterinary practitioners. Comprehensive guidance on both prescribing and prescription writing is given in the *British National Formulary*, a joint publication of the British Medical Association and The Royal Pharmaceutical Society, and in *Medicines, Ethics and Practice: A Guide for Pharmacists*.

A well written prescription should contain the following information:

- Name and address of a patient (or keeper of animals for veterinary work) and the age if for a child under the age of 12.
- Name, strength, quantity or number of dose units or the name of individual ingredients to be compounded into a medicine and the quantities to be used. The type of pharmaceutical preparation required (for example, a mixture, suppository, lotion) may also be specified, but this is often omitted and taken as understood.

- The directions to be included on the label of the medicine to enable the patient to use the medicine correctly. Directions should preferably be in English without abbreviation, but it is recognised that some Latin abbreviations are still used. For a list of abbreviations used in prescriptions see Miscellaneous Data.
- Any instructions on the number of times the prescription may be repeated. Repeats are not allowed in certain circumstances (for example, NHS prescriptions).
- Prescriptions that are intended to be dispensed in instalments to drug misusers, must specify the amount of each instalment, the total amount to be dispensed, and the intervals to be observed between instalments.
- The signature (address and qualifications are sometimes required) of the person who wrote the prescription and the date on which it was written.
- For controlled drugs the quantity should be written in words and figures, and the prescription should be in the practitioner's own handwriting unless exempted. In addition, the pharmaceutical form of the preparation must be specified.

Forged Prescriptions

The pharmacist should be aware of the lengths to which drug misusers may go to obtain supplies. Although it can be difficult to detect a forged prescription, every pharmacist should be alert to the possibility that any prescription calling for a preparation liable to misuse could be a forgery.

If the prescriber's signature is known, but the patient has not previously visited the pharmacy, or is not known to be suffering from a condition that requires the medicinal product prescribed, the signature should be carefully examined and, if possible, checked against an example on another prescription known to be authentic. Large doses or quantities should be checked with the prescriber in order to detect alterations to previously valid prescriptions.

If the prescriber's signature is not known, the prescriber must be contacted and asked to confirm that the prescription is genuine. The prescriber's telephone number must be obtained from the telephone directory, or from directory enquiries, not from the headed notepaper, as forgers may use false letter headings.

Factors that should alert a pharmacist to the possibility of a forgery include:

- unknown prescriber
- new patient
- excessive quantities
- uncharacteristic prescribing or method of prescription writing by a known doctor
- letter heading compiled using Letraset or by similar methods
- 'Dr' before or after prescriber's signature.

These precautions should be applied to all prescriptions for drugs liable to misuse, and not only for controlled drugs.

Prescription Collection and Delivery

For those patients who have difficulty collecting repeat prescriptions from the surgery and medicines from the pharmacy, many community pharmacists provide a prescription collection and delivery service. As long as the service is provided at the request of the patient, there is no conflict with the Code of Ethics.

The patient must always make the request for a repeat prescription, and this request will normally be direct to the surgery. The patient will usually indicate, when requesting a repeat prescription from the surgery, which pharmacy will collect the prescription. In other cases, it may be appropriate to introduce a consent form, which will be held at the surgery, naming the pharmacy that will collect. Any written consent of this kind should be reconfirmed from time to time.

When delivering medicines, it is important that any advice the patient would have received on collecting the medicines at the pharmacy should be conveyed to the patient by whoever is delivering the medicine. Arrangements should be made with the patient as to what will be done if no-one is at home to take delivery of the medicine. Under no circumstances should controlled drugs be delivered to anyone other than the patient or someone who has care of the patient. Dispensed medicines should not be left with young children or in any place where children or unauthorised persons will have access to them.

THE DISPENSING OF MEDICINES

A dispensed medicinal product includes a medicinal product prepared or dispensed by a practitioner (doctor, dentist, or veterinarian) or prepared or dispensed in accordance with a prescription given by a practitioner; and a medicinal product prepared or dispensed in a registered pharmacy by or under the supervision of a pharmacist, either in accordance with a specification furnished by the purchaser (for example, a customer's recipe) or in accordance with the pharmacist's own judgment as to the treatment required for a person present in the pharmacy (that is, a counter prescribed preparation).

A dispensed medicine is supplied for the treatment of an individual patient or an animal or herd of animals. In general, dispensing involves the selection of a medicine in a dosage form already prepared by the pharmaceutical industry, but it may sometimes necessitate the extemporaneous preparation of a product from several ingredients.

Pharmacists preparing or dispensing a medicinal product in accordance with a prescription given by a practitioner or preparing a stock of medicinal products for this purpose are exempt from licensing under the Medicines Act 1968 for work undertaken in a registered pharmacy.

The control procedures required in dispensing differ in kind from those necessary in the manufacture of medicines, but they are no less important. Quality is dependent on in-process control exercised by the pharmacist who must personally carry out all operations or maintain a close scrutiny and be satisfied that, before the medicine is released, the prescription has been correctly interpreted and that procedures have been carried out by trained staff. An appendix to the Royal Pharmaceutical Society's Code of Ethics includes standards for premises, dispensary design and equipment, procurement and sources for materials, and dispensing procedures (see below). Dispensaries should be kept as free from disturbance as possible and benches clear from all apparatus and materials other than those necessary for the operations being carried out. When the dispensing of a prescription has to be interrupted, a clear sequence of events should be established to prevent the possibility of duplication or omission. In larger dispensaries, where many operations are going on simultaneously, special vigilance is needed to ensure that no mix-up can occur in labelling medicines or in identification of patients. The pharmacist should establish that the recipient is aware of the correct use of the medicine and ensure that there are no inadvertent hazards introduced by the supply of the medicine.

The dispensing of prescriptions for medicines involves both interpretation of the prescriber's instructions and the technical knowledge required to carry out these instructions with accuracy and safety to the patient. An appendix to the Royal Pharmaceutical Society's Code of Ethics includes standards for dispensing procedures.

There is a considerable variety of factors that require close attention in dispensing, and proficiency requires the establishment of a routine system which can be followed safely even under stress. The pharmacist should be satisfied that the product, dosage, and directions convey the intentions of the prescriber.

Individuals frequently evolve their own routine methods but the following may prove a useful basis for the development of a satisfactory routine:

- On receiving the prescription the pharmacist should verify that the name and address of the patient are correct, the prescription is legally valid, and is correctly written.
- The interpretation of the prescriber's instructions should be checked. This includes checking that the dosage regimen is within normal limits and is commensurate with the apparent therapeutic use of the medicine as far as can be ascertained by reference to the pharmacological class of the drug. Any apparent anomalies should be checked with the prescriber. The keeping of patient medication records (PMRs) (see below) is of value, especially for repeat prescriptions.
- An appropriate label should be prepared, containing all the necessary directions and complying with legal requirements.
- It should be ascertained whether any additional labelling is required. This may be a legal obligation or professional compliance with good pharmaceutical practice. Dilutions of standard preparations are sometimes required and such preparations then have a limited shelf-life. An expiry date for the product should be included in the labelling. Mixtures required to be freshly or recently prepared should also be labelled with an expiry date.
- An appropriate container and closure should be selected.
- The medicines should be selected from stock and, if in unit dose form such as capsules or tablets, the correct number should be counted and filled into the previously selected container. If extemporaneous preparation of the medicine is necessary, the required drugs should be selected from stock, the ingredients weighed or measured, and the preparation compounded.

- The labels of all containers of stock drugs, whether for extemporaneous preparation or not, should be checked when selected from and replaced in stock, as well as at the time of actual dispensing, making three checks in all.
- The appearance of the medicine, the prescription, and the labels should be rechecked. The label(s) should be affixed to the container, the surface of which, if a bottle, should be clean and polished.
- It should be determined whether the patient will require additional counselling on the correct use of the medicine or on precautions that should be taken.
- The medicine(s) should be packaged and the outside labelled appropriately to avoid possible confusion with any other medicine awaiting collection.
- All records should be completed, including those required by good pharmaceutical practice as well as those required by legislation.
- The pharmacist should never hesitate to seek the advice or help of another individual in case of doubt. The pharmacist's attitude and care in the final presentation and delivery of the medicine is important to maintain an appropriate professional image.

The technical aspects of dispensing (such as counting tablets, pouring liquids, and labelling containers) can properly be conducted by trained support staff under supervision. However, there is no alternative to the direct involvement of the pharmacist in assessment of the prescription and to ensure that all necessary information is provided to the carer or patient to achieve maximum therapeutic benefit.

Oral Syringes

When the dose of an oral liquid is not 5 mL or a multiple of 5 mL, and an appropriate measuring device is not supplied by the manufacturer, a 5 mL plastic oral syringe should be provided along with a bottle adaptor and an instruction leaflet (which is available in several languages). The oral syringe should comply with British Standard 3221:Part 7:1986 or an equivalent European standard. The syringes are graduated at intervals of 0.5 mL and numbered at intervals of 1 mL.

The 5-mL spoon remains in use for doses of 5 mL (or multiples thereof). The previous convention of diluting oral liquids had the potential to adversely affect the stability of liquid medicines.

LABELLING OF DISPENSED MEDICINES

The primary function of a label is that of accurately directing the patient how and when the medicine should be taken or used.

Legal Requirements

Legal labelling requirements for dispensed medicines differ from those for products sold over-the-counter. Legal requirements for the labelling of medicines in Great Britain are explained in *Medicines, Ethics and Practice: A Guide for Pharmacists*. The label is an important factor in the appearance of the final medicine and a high standard in label presentation will do much to maintain the confidence of the patient. Labels should be legible and clear, and lettering should be mechanically produced. The style of the label should be appropriate to the preparation and the size of label should match the container. The main label should clearly state:

- the name and strength of the preparation unless otherwise directed
- the total quantity of the product dispensed in the container to which the label refers
- precise instructions for use by the patient
- the date of dispensing
- the name of the patient
- the name and address of the pharmacy
- 'Keep out of the reach of children'
- a reference number (private prescriptions).

Where appropriate:

- 'For external use only'
- 'Not to be used for babies' (preparations containing hexachlorophane)
- Cautionary and advisory labels (*BNF*: Appendix 9).

Dose-volume Expressions

In Great Britain, a 5-mL spoon is used as a standard measure for liquid oral medicines and the use in labelling instructions of such terms as 'teaspoonful', 'dessertspoonful', and 'tablespoonful' has been abandoned.

In labelling such medicines the pharmacist must adopt the following style of wording for linctuses, elixirs, and syrups: '...5-mL spoonful(s) to be taken...', and for mixtures: '...5-mL spoonfuls to be taken...in water'.

When fractional doses of a medicine are prescribed, requiring the supply of an oral syringe (see above), the medicine must be labelled appropriately; care must be taken to avoid ambiguity.

Table 1
Auxiliary labelling

Auxiliary label	Circumstances in which label is used	Examples of preparations
Shake the Bottle	Liquid preparations which are disperse systems. Liquid preparations where precipitation or separation is considered possible	emulsions; suspensions
For External Use Only	Liquid preparations or gels for external application (legal requirement in Great Britain if preparation is not on a general sale list); dusting-powders	applications; embrocations; liniments; lotions; skin paints; creams; ointments
Not to be Taken	Liquid preparations that are not administered orally and that are applied to a skin surface	ear drops; eye lotions; eye drops; inhalations; nasal drops; enemas
	Solid dosage forms that might inadvertently be administered by the oral route ('Not to be taken by mouth' is a possible alternative)	inhalation capsules; pessaries; some solution-tablets; suppositories
Keep Out of the Reach of Children	All dispensed medicines	

Table 2
Other labelling instructions

Instructions explaining use and administration	
To be added to hot, but not boiling, water and the vapour inhaled for 5 to 10 minutes	inhalations (unless otherwise directed)
Not to be swallowed in large quantities	throat paints
Not to be swallowed	gargles (unless otherwise directed); mouthwashes
Not to be applied to open wounds or to raw surfaces of large area	dusting-powders
Warm to body temperature before use	enemas (large volume)
Sip and swallow slowly without the addition of water	linctuses
Instructions emphasising correct storage conditions	
Do not use [this medicine] after . . .	liquid medicines; recently or freshly prepared medicines; eye lotions
Store in a dark place	preparations where exposure to light would accelerate deterioration
Store in a cool place	capsules; creams; antibiotic mixtures; ointments; pessaries; suppositories

Auxiliary Labels

For some preparations, instructions that are not specifically detailed on the prescription must be given on the container (Table 1). Such instructions serve to amplify how the medicine is to be used or to guide the patient regarding the best storage conditions. Other labelling instructions may also form the basis of additional labels (Table 2).

Numbers following the preparation entries in the *British National Formulary* correspond to the code numbers of the cautionary labels that should be added when dispensing. A monthly update of additions to the list is published in *The Pharmaceutical Journal*. Many preparations are now dispensed in unbroken original packs that bear complete instructions for the patient or provide a leaflet addressed to the patient.

It is recognised that there may be occasions when pharmacists will use their knowledge and professional discretion, and decide to omit one or more of the recommended labels for a particular patient. In such cases, counselling is of utmost importance. In some instances, the prescriber may indicate that additional cautionary labels should not be used; the exact wording that is required instead should be specified on the prescription.

Veterinary Dispensed Medicines

A prescription for a medicine for veterinary use must carry a declaration by the veterinarian giving it that the medicine is prescribed for an animal or herd under his or her care. The label must comply with the legal requirements for a dispensed medicine and, also, should provide the following information:

- The name of the person having possession or control of the animal or herd and the address of the premises where the animal or herd is kept, or the address of one such premises.
- If the drug contains hexachlorophane and is for oral administration for the prevention or treatment of fluke disease in cattle, a warning that:
  (a) the product is not for use in lactating cattle
  (b) protective clothing must be worn by the operator when the product is being administered.

CONTAINERS FOR DISPENSING

The container must be appropriate for the product dispensed, bearing in mind the need to protect the product from moisture and light as well as from mechanical stresses imparted by transport and use of the product. All containers intended for medicinal products must be protected and kept free from contamination.

All solid dose oral preparations must be dispensed in either a reclosable child-resistant container or in unit packaging of strip or blister type unless:

- the original is such as to make this inadvisable
- the patient is elderly or handicapped and will have difficulty in opening a child-resistant container
- a specific request is made that the product shall not be dispensed in a child-resistant container.

In the above cases, advice must be given to keep all medicines out of the reach of children.

Reuse of Containers

Plastic containers and closures must not be reused as satisfactory cleaning cannot be ensured. Under no circumstances should reclosable child-resistant closures be used more than once, as continued use affects the child-resistant properties of the closure.

Glass containers are capable of being reused only after satisfactory cleaning and drying. High standards must be maintained, which may make reuse uneconomical.

Compliance Devices

A medication compliance device is a container or device that is designed to hold solid oral dosage forms for a defined period. It serves to remind a patient to take their medication, reduces dose schedule or timing errors, and facilitates self-monitoring of medication intake. Ideally, a compliance device should be filled by the pharmacist, but in some cases this may be carried out by the patient or a carer.

Pharmacists should exercise professional judgement when products marketed as daily dose reminders are supplied.

The use of factory-filled special packaging, such as a calendar pack (see Pharmaceutical Packaging chapter), to improve compliance may be a useful, and relatively inexpensive, option. However, despite their widespread use, there is little evidence for their effectiveness as a sole intervention, and it has been suggested that elderly patients may find them difficult to understand and use.

Compliance devices can be useful in a small group of patients. Common problems with all such devices include a lack of child resistance and the inability of the containers to contain liquids and environmentally-sensitive dosage forms. Other possible limitations on the use of compliance aids are described under Monitored Dosage Systems, below. Refilling is also a problem, particularly if carried out by the patient or a carer.

It is illegal to dispense prescribed dosage forms directly into a daily dose reminder if the labelling regulations cannot be fulfilled. If a pharmacist loads a daily dose reminder, he should do so from the container of the patient's dispensed medicine which bears the legally required label; in addition, the pharmacist should stress that the device should be kept out of the reach of children.

Commercially available multicompartment containers or compliance aids generally hold seven days supply.

Monitored Dosage Systems

Many pharmacists are now using monitored dosage systems for medication intended for patients in residential or long-term care. The labelling regulations of 1976 do not cover the position of monitored dosage systems. However, the labelling regulations do require that dispensed medicines shall bear, as a minimum, the name of the patient, the name and address of the supplier, the date of dispensing, and the words 'Keep out of the reach of children' (or similar wording). In almost every case, directions for use will also be required.

The Council of the Royal Pharmaceutical Society has approved guidelines for the profession on the use of monitored dosage systems. The guidelines are summarised below, and are presented in full in *Medicines, Ethics and Practice: A Guide for Pharmacists*.

- Monitored dosage systems must be filled under the supervision of a pharmacist.
- Medicines should not be left in sealed monitored dosage systems for longer than eight weeks.
- Changes to medications in monitored dosage systems must be done under the supervision of a pharmacist.
- Tablets or capsules that cannot be identified and readily distinguished from each other should not be placed in the monitored dosage system. Labelling should enable identification of individual medicinal products.

- If it is necessary to place 'PRN' medication in monitored dosage systems, guidance must be given by the pharmacist on how to administer such medication.
- Certain medication should not be placed in monitored dosage systems (for example effervescent tablets, dispersible tablets, buccal tablets, sublingual tablets, and significantly hygroscopic preparations).
- Uncoated tablets should not be placed in the same section as other uncoated tablets.
- In filling monitored dosage systems the requirements set out in 'Standards of Good Professional Practice' must be adhered to.
- After filling, the monitored dosage systems should be protected from light and stored in a cool dry place.
- If the monitored dosage system has to be delivered to the patient, the requirements for the delivery of medicines set out in the Code of Ethics should be met.
- Pharmacists should advise the establishment receiving the monitored dosage system of the procedures to be followed regarding storage, record keeping, and related factors.
- Any unwanted medicines from the monitored dosage systems should be returned to the pharmacy and not reused.

Most of the problems associated with monitored dosage systems also apply to compliance devices. Limitations include: mixing in the same compartment of dosage forms with different routes of administration; mixing of dosage forms to be taken with or after food, and those to be taken before meals; and removal of tablets or capsules from blister or foil packs. Many products are unsuitable for monitored dosage form and compliance packaging (see above).

Where the system involves reuse of the tray or compartments, great care should be taken to remove all traces of the previous supply of tablets or capsules. Any liquids should be supplied in traditional screw-top bottles, and carers should be advised not to prepare individual cups more than one day in advance.

COMMUNICATION

In addition to providing a clearly produced label, the pharmacist must ensure that the patient fully understands how to use the medicine. Written information, such as advisory leaflets and treatment cards and booklets (for example, for patients receiving anticoagulants, MAOIs, lithium, or steroids) may be used to supplement oral communication, as appropriate.

Labels in braille and produced with large print are available for the visually impaired but it is important, when using these, to ensure that the statutory requirements for labelling dispensed medicines are observed. In providing help for patients for whom English is not their first language the pharmacist must comply with the requirement of the Medicines Act 1968 that all particulars on dispensing labels are written in English. In this particular situation the use of pictographs and leaflets in various languages can provide help for patients. Patient information leaflets are produced by some pharmacy computer systems and are given to the patient. As from 31 December 1993, manufacturers are required to introduce patient-orientated information leaflets to comply with a European Community Directive. The pharmacist should be prepared to explain the contents of such leaflets to the patient.

Patient information leaflets, issued by pharmacists or included by manufacturers in proprietary medicine packs, assist patients in the use of their medicines. Where these incorporate visual information, as with pictographs, the particular needs of the illiterate and others with language difficulties may be addressed.

European Community regulations on the content of package leaflets apply to medicines for which product licences are granted or renewed on or after 1 January 1994. The legislation implements parts of the EC Directive 92/27/EEC, which aims to improve and harmonise the provision of information about medicines for human use. The new leaflet regulations set out the particulars to be included on any medicines package leaflet. They also specify the order in which the information must appear.

PHARMACY COMPUTER SYSTEMS

Computers in pharmacies are mostly used for labelling medicines, but also increasingly for monitoring drug interactions and keeping patient medication records. Newer applications include electronic point of sale (EPoS) systems, computer-generated patient information leaflets, and automated prescription endorsement.

Labelling Systems

A comprehensive and regularly updated drug directory is essential in order to ensure that information is maintained on cautionary labels and interactions. All cautionary and advisory labels must follow the advice given in the *British National Formulary*. If additional counselling is necessary, this should also be indicated. In order to avoid obsolete software which can lead to serious problems, a supplier should be chosen who provides regular software updates.

Drug interactions information should be obtained from a reliable source and should be regularly updated. However, pharmacists must always be alert for other possible interactions that would require some intervention. The commonest type of drug interaction is where two drugs are given with the same actions or same adverse effects. All drug interactions should be stored on the computer; however, the pharmacist should exercise professional judgement when providing the patient with information about potential interactions.

Ideally, the computer system should highlight changes in, for example, legal requirements. A feature to detect overdoses is desirable, but would require access to up-to-date drug information. Such a feature would not detect all overdoses, but would bring to the pharmacist's attention those cases of gross overdosage with drugs of a narrow therapeutic index.

Patient Medication Records

Patient medication records (PMRs) have many applications and may be used to ensure that a prescribed medicine does not interact with other medications and is consistent with a continuing therapy.

The information held in patient records should include: full name, address, telephone number, National Health Service Number, sex, date of birth, name of general practitioner, drug sensitivities, allergies, chronic conditions, medicines purchased, and a section in which notes can be made. Separate fields should be provided for each section of the patient's name and address. The database should be capable of being searched by name or part name. The computer should generate its own unique number for each patient if no external identifying number such as the patient's National Health Service number is available. Patients should be given a card to remind them that a particular pharmacy is keeping a record of their medication and is able to give advice on any past or new medication, including over-the-counter remedies.

The following details should be held in medication records from each prescription: date, quantity of medicine dispensed, name of product, form, and dose. It is desirable that any system should be capable of retaining information on the batch number and manufacturer for product liability purposes. The minimum period for searching information for drug interactions with previously dispensed medicines should be three months, but for elderly and confused patients this should be extended to two years as they are likely to be taking a number of medicines, some of them on a long-term basis. When updating a patient's record, the information should be transferred immediately to disk and not held solely in memory. A pharmacist must respect the confidentiality of information acquired in the course of his professional practice relating to a patient and the patient's family. Such information must not be disclosed to anyone without the consent of the patient or appropriate guardian unless the interest of the patient or the public requires such disclosure.

Data Protection Act

Patients or their authorised representatives may be given a printed copy of the material to which they have legal access. It is permitted to withhold health data that is likely to cause serious harm to the physical or mental health of the patient. However, in most cases any information will have been provided by the patient themselves.

Retention of Records

Archive material should be held for ten years to comply with the requirements of the Consumer Protection Act. It is important to establish ease of access to archive material, and the method of achieving this. The ability to use a tape-streamer to accelerate transfer of data to storage would be advantageous.

Records subject to a payment by the Department of Health should be held on the computer for at least one, but preferably two years. Pharmacists may decide to keep all records for this length of time.

BASIC TECHNIQUES OF EXTEMPORANEOUS COMPOUNDING

Mixing

Efficient mixing of the ingredients is essential in any pharmaceutical preparation, liquid or solid, in order to ensure uniformity of dosage. Ideally, any fraction of the mixture should be of the same composition as the bulk material. Further, where colouring or flavouring is added, uniform dispersion is required in order to ensure perfect blending and good appearance of the product.

Mixing of Liquids

Since liquids are, by definition, homogeneous systems, two or more miscible liquid phases will eventually produce a completely homogeneous mixture by diffusion. The aim of the mixing operation is therefore to speed this process.

Simple stirring or shaking is often sufficient to produce a good liquid mix but, in many cases, the effort involved may be considerable, especially where the liquids differ greatly in density or viscosity, or where the degree of miscibility is small. In these cases, mechanical stirring is necessary and a useful aid is the simple laboratory stirrer consisting of a variable speed motor to which various types of paddle can be attached.

Mixing of Solids with Liquids

Similar considerations to those involved in liquid mixing also apply here, the solubility of the solid having an important effect. Mixing devices which can again be employed use the principle of a rapidly moving paddle immersed in the suspension.

Mixing of Solids

Mixing depends on the movement of the different types of particle relative to one another and it follows that any mixing device must allow sufficient space for adequate movement to occur; it must not be overfilled. Secondly, the only force that will produce relative particle movement is one of shear, and the mixing process used must therefore produce movement in all directions.

Where small quantities of powders are to be mixed in approximately equal proportions, mixing can be effected by simple rotation or shaking in a jar.

Where a small quantity of medicament is to be incorporated in a large bulk of powder—often necessary for individual powders containing potent drugs—this is best carried out using a pestle and mortar. The medicament is first mixed with an equal weight of diluent, a further quantity of diluent equal in weight to the mixture in the mortar is then incorporated, and the process is repeated until all the diluent has been added. This is known as mixing by geometric dilution.

It is important to select a mortar of suitable size so that overfilling does not occur. Glass pestles and mortars should be used for small quantities of fine powders and for incorporation of substances that are absorbed by and stain the composition or porcelain type (for example, iodine and dyes).

For larger quantities, these are slow processes, since there is little expansion of the powder mass. Cone or cube mixers give a continual tumbling action and are useful for the preparation of moderately sized batches of bulk powders.

Mixing of Semi-solids

It is often necessary to incorporate a medicament in a semi-solid basis, or to produce a compound basis from semi-solid components, as in the preparation of pastes and ointments, suppositories, and pessaries.

The most convenient method is by fusion of the semi-solid ingredients on a water-bath to produce a liquid mass. Overheating may cause physical or chemical changes in some materials and the traditional fusion method was to heat in order of decreasing melting point. It has been shown, however, that this has little advantage over simple melting of the ingredients all together, although the temperature should be kept as low as possible. The mixture is then stirred continuously until cold in order to avoid segregation of the components as setting occurs. Any insoluble medicaments to be incorporated must be in fine powder form and, to ensure even dispersion, it is advisable to levigate with a little of the melted basis on a tile, if the quantities are small, or in a warmed mortar. The remainder of the melted basis may then be added and the mixture stirred until cold. Unless stirring is continued at least until setting begins, sedimentation of the insoluble solid will occur in the liquid mass with consequent uneven dispersion.

Clarification

It is occasionally necessary to separate solid particles from a suspension, either to produce a clear liquid as the final product or to recover the solid, or both.

Decantation

A high degree of separation can often be effected by allowing the suspension to stand, when the heavier solid settles and the clear liquid can be poured or siphoned off. This process of decantation, however, has severe limitations. If the solid is in fine particle form, the supernatant liquid may remain cloudy and complete separation is impossible. Further, it is never possible to recover all the liquid.

Filtration

Filtration can be used to remove very fine particles, provided that a suitable filter medium is chosen.

Filter paper is suitable for general clarification purposes but tends to yield fibres to the filtrate and may adsorb significant amounts of medicament from dilute solutions. Paper is available in many different grades, giving different filtration speeds and having different particle-retaining qualities. Other grades are treated to give acid or alkali resistance, while resin-bonded paper reduces fibre shedding.

Sintered glass fibres of grade 3 (pore size 15 to 40 micrometres) produce a clean filtrate for general clarification purposes and most solutions will pass by gravity. Large volumes may, however, take a long time and assistance by the application of vacuum to the receiver may be necessary. Grade 4 (pore size 5 to 15 micrometres) is too slow for gravity filtration.

Glass filters do not shed fibres and are easy to clean. Material retained within the pores of the filter can be removed by washing with acid and/or alkali and then with purified water until neutral.

Size Reduction

Size reduction or comminution of solid materials to produce a fine powder may be necessary in order that the substance may be more easily administered or more rapidly dissolved in a liquid solvent. A more uniform distribution is obtained in the mixing of several substances in dry form if each of the substances is in fine powder and approximately of the same degree of fineness.

The use of the pestle and mortar is familiar, but the choice of a suitable type deserves consideration. For the grinding of dry powders, a flat-bottomed mortar with a flat-ended pestle is most efficient, giving a maximum area of contact between the two surfaces. The use of a rounded pestle in a flat-bottomed mortar or vice versa is a waste of labour.

For levigation purposes (the grinding of a solid in the presence of a liquid), it is again important to use matching pestles and mortars. Frequent scraping down of the sides of the mortar and of the pestle is essential for all materials, to keep all particles within the grinding area.

Glass pestles and mortars are not suitable for size reduction purposes, except for friable materials such as crystals, but are useful when dissolving small quantities of medicaments or for the incorporation of substances such as iodine or dyes which are absorbed by and stain mortars of the composition or porcelain type.

Pestles and mortars are also commonly used for the preparation of emulsions, a process involving the size reduction of liquid globules constituting the disperse phase, but electric mixers and hand (or powered) homogenisers are now readily available, removing much of the labour from emulsion making. Homogenisation is a process in which the mixed phases are caused to pass through a fine orifice valve under high pressure. Atomisation occurs, assisted by impact received by the mixture as it strikes the valve head. A homogeniser may be used as the sole emulsification process after rough mixing of the ingredients, or for improving an existing emulsion prepared by other means. Inexpensive hand homogenisers are available, suitable for the processing of about 500 mL of emulsion at one filling, while for larger quantities there is a wide range of electrically powered machines.

HOMOEOPATHIC PHARMACY

The homoeopathic system of medicine was founded and developed by Samuel Hahnemann a German chemist and physician born in 1755. The system is based on a doctrine that Hahnemann called the Law of Similars: '*similia similibus curentur*' or 'like may be cured by like'. Hahnemann developed this law from his discovery that if cinchona bark was given to a healthy person, it tended to produce symptoms similar to those of malaria, the disease that it was used to treat. To validate his hypothesis Hahnemann systematically studied the effect of drugs given to healthy volunteers. The effects of these 'provings' were observed and recorded. The pattern of symptoms that any medicinal substance could cause was called the 'drug picture', whereas the symptoms of an illness was called the 'disease picture'. Hahnemann discovered that the closer the symptoms in these two pictures could be matched, the more effective was the homoeopathic remedy. The remedy is believed to stimulate an individual's reaction to a specific disease state. All these results have been collated, documented, and published in homoeopathic materia medica books.

Therefore, a homoeopathic remedy is one that produces symptoms similar to those experienced by the sick person and in so doing it is believed to stimulate the body's own mechanism to deal with the underlying cause of the symptoms. This therapeutic approach differs from orthodox or allopathic treatment where drugs are most commonly used to suppress symptoms or to remove an individual's innate response to the underlying cause of those symptoms. Nevertheless, allopathic medicines may also be prescribed if necessary.

The skill of the homoeopathic practitioner is associated with the ability to match a range of symptoms presented by a patient to a remedy that provings have demonstrated to have similar effects in a healthy volunteer. This establishes the first of Hahnemann's three principles:

- a medicine which in large doses produces the symptoms of a disease will, in small doses, cure that disease.

Hahnemann claimed that diluting the remedies increased their efficacy and reduced harmful side-effects. This was the basis of his second principle:

- by extreme dilution the curative properties of the medicine are enhanced and the poisonous or undesirable side-effects are lost.

Hahnemann's third principle is based on the holistic approach:

- homoeopathic medicines are prescribed individually by the study of the whole person according to the basic temperament and response of the patient.

The aim is to treat the 'whole person', which requires a detailed evaluation of the physical, mental, and emotional state of the patient. Two patients ostensibly suffering from the same complaint may be treated with totally different remedies to achieve a better matching of the drug/disease symptom picture.

The substances that were initially proved and used in practice were the drugs of Hahnemann's day. These are still widely used as they are well understood and documented. However, the range of remedies used today is much greater and may come from any source, whether animal, vegetable, or mineral. When the remedy is sourced from diseased tissue it is called a 'nosode'.

Homoeopathic Medications

The pharmacist may not be directly concerned with the theory and practice of homoeopathy, but may be called upon to dispense the prescriptions of a practitioner of homoeopathy. Therefore, a knowledge of the elements of homoeopathic pharmacy is essential. Counter prescribing homoeopathic medicines requires considerable knowledge and should not be undertaken lightly.

The starting point for the production of homoeopathic remedies is a Mother Tincture (ϕ or TM). This is the alcoholic solution or extract of the original material in alcohol, usually prepared by maceration of the vegetable material and subsequent filtration. The ratio of plant material to alcohol varies depending on the homoeopathic pharmacopoeia in use; essentially it is 1:3 for German and British methods of production and 1:10 in the French pharmacopoeia. The ethanolic content of the alcohol in the cosolvent varies depending on the water content of the plant material. These processes must be undertaken in accordance with the standards of the British Homoeopathic Manufacturers Association.

Liquid attenuations are made from the Mother Tincture. The remedy is attenuated by a process involving successive dilutions and succussions (that is, each dilution is subjected to extremely vigorous shaking before proceeding to the next dilution). The resulting attenuations of the remedy are called potencies. One part of Mother Tincture is diluted with 99 parts of an alcohol/water mixture and then succussed. This centesimal attenuation gives a potency of 1c. The dilution process is repeated and there is no limit to the number of times that successive dilutions may be carried out. The most common potencies are:

$$\text{low potency} \xleftarrow{\quad 6c, 12c, 30c, 200c, 1m, 10m \quad} \text{high potency}$$

(m = 1000c dilution)

Trituration

Insoluble substances such as minerals are triturated with lactose; the dilution scale is 1:100. Trituration continues to the third centesimal dilution (1 ppm), after which the remedy is considered, in homoeopathic terms, to be soluble. Subsequent dilutions are made in alcohol. The 'potentisation' process includes a succussion phase at each stage of dilution; the 99 parts of lactose are divided into 3 aliquot parts, each of which is triturated for 20 minutes.

In the UK, the centesimal scale is used: 6c, 30c, 200c; if the number appears on its own (6, 30) the c is assumed. In France the centesimal scale is represented by cH, and the potencies most often used are 5cH, 9cH, and 15cH. To a lesser extent a decimal scale of attenuation is used, that is, 1 part of Mother Tincture is succussed with 9 parts of diluent. This is represented by a prefix D or suffix X; D6 = 6X.

Dispensing Forms

The remedy at the chosen potency may be used to 'potentise' a variety of unmedicated products. Solid dosage forms include tablets (lactose), pilules (sucrose), granules (sucrose), and powders (lactose). The unmedicated dosage forms are medicated with the homoeopathic remedy in 95% alcohol solution, which is dropped onto the dosage form in the final glass container. The alcohol is allowed to evaporate before the closure is applied. A liquid potency (LP) is prepared by adding drops of the 95% alcoholic solution to a 30% alcoholic solution. External preparations are usually made by incorporating 5% of a Mother Tincture into a suitable basis for lotions, ointments, and creams.

Pack Size

The quantity of the remedy to be supplied is often specified on prescriptions as 1 g, 2.5 g, 7 g, 14 g, or 25 g. The corresponding quantity of tablets, pilules, or granules intended is:

      1 g = 10 tablets
    2.5 g = 18 tablets
      7 g = 50 tablets (approximately)
     14 g = 100 tablets
     25 g = 200 tablets

Containers

All containers should be made of glass; 1 g and 2.5 g vials are closed with a small cork and all other containers are sealed with a plastic screw cap.

Shelf-life/Storage

Storage conditions are critical. Remedies should be kept in the original well-closed container, and kept away from heat, light, and substances with strong odours such as camphor and menthol.

Guidance for the Pharmacist

It is claimed that homoeopathic remedies have no side-effects. However, they can promote an aggravation of symptoms before improvement is apparent. The remedy is considered to act by a primary and a secondary response. The primary response is the action of the homoeopathic remedy on the body and is generally unnoticed. The secondary response is the innate response of the body to the remedy; this is the healing response and it occurs if the remedy is homoeopathic or produces an effect similar to the patient's symptoms. If the secondary response is very large an aggravation may occur, which is defined as an exacerbation of the existing symptoms; no new symptoms are apparent. Thus, in homoeopathy, an aggravation is viewed as a positive indication of the healing response to the remedy.

The direction in which the remedy works is defined by Hering's Law, which states that symptoms will improve from above – downwards, from within – outwards, from a more vital to a less important organ, and in the reverse order to which the symptoms were acquired. This is a cathartic process which in practice may result in the recurrence of older pathology during the healing phase, for example, a chronic internal complaint may manifest an old skin eruption during the healing process. This should not be suppressed by an external application as this would reverse the healing direction.

Pharmacists should ensure that patients using high potencies have either had the remedy prescribed by a homoeopathic practitioner or have an understanding of the principles of homoeopathy. The important factor to consider is that of the frequency of administration of the remedy. The homoeopathic remedy is a stimulus and as such should only be used until it achieves the desired response. Further administration is not helpful and may result in the occurrence of a 'proving'. Potencies of 200c and higher should only be prescribed by people who are experienced in homoeopathy.

Frequency of Administration

The frequency of administration of a homoeopathic preparation is usually indicated by the prescriber and is based on the case study of the patient, but under circumstances of self administration, when the pharmacist's advice is sought, an approximate guide is as follows:

Acute complaint. One dose every 2 hours up to a maximum of six doses in 24 hours, then one dose 3 times daily for a further few days.

Chronic complaint. One dose 2 or 3 times daily, in low potency.

Single day regimens. These are usually supplied in three equal parts to be taken at 12-hourly intervals (that is, at 0, 12, and 24 hours). Such regimens have been referred to as 'single dose regimens'.

Nomenclature and Interpretation of Prescriptions

Homoeopathic physicians adopt a particular form of nomenclature based on original drug names; thus they prescribe potencies of, for example, potassium iodide, sodium carbonate, and mercuric chloride as Kali iod., Natr. carb., and Merc. corr., respectively. There are over 2000 remedies, approximately 200 are in common use.

Homoeopathic prescriptions may call for 2 or 3 active dose forms followed by several weeks supply of unmedicated dose forms to be taken afterwards, for example:

Bryonia 10M 1–3
S.L. 56 n and m

This requires Bryonia 10M on Saccharum Lactis (lactose powder) in individually packed powders numbered 1, 2, and 3 and Saccharum Lactis in unmedicated powders numbered 4 to 56. One powder is to be taken on the tongue each night and morning in the order numbered.

Instructions to the Patient

During the dispensing of a homoeopathic preparation, the following information should be conveyed:

- The remedies should be sucked or chewed (powders should be placed directly onto the tongue). The mouth should be clean and remedies should not be taken within 15 minutes of the ingestion of food or drinks, smoking tobacco, or using toothpaste.
- The remedies should be kept in the glass container in which they were supplied; the container should be well-closed.
- Preparations should be kept away from strong smelling substances and direct sunlight.
- The remedies should not be handled, they should be placed on a clean metal spoon or on the lid of the container and then transferred directly into the mouth.
- When a response is obtained the patient should stop taking the remedy.

UK Legal Status

Homoeopathic medicines are subject to the requirements of the Medicines Act 1968, and are classified depending on their strength (in orthodox terms), for example:

Belladonna ϕ—P
Belladonna 6x—GSL
Belladonna 6c—GSL

EC Legislation

In September 1991 the European Commission proposed a Directive extending the scope of the 1965 and 1975 Directives on the distribution of pharmaceuticals to make provision for homoeopathic medicines, both for humans and for animals. After consultation 17 amendments were accepted, and two Directives were published in October 1992, one for human medicines and the other for veterinary medicines. These Directives granted the registration of some products under a simplified system that did not require demonstration of the efficacy of the product. For products not appropriate to the simplified system, proof of therapeutic effect will be required 'in accordance with homoeopathic principles'.

FURTHER INFORMATION

Appelbe GE, Wingfield J. Pharmacy law and ethics. 5th ed. London: Pharmaceutical Press, 1993.

Phillips SA, Temple DJ. Quality assurance and professional audit in community pharmacy. Pharm J 1992;249:208–9.

Royal Pharmaceutical Society of Great Britain. Medicines, ethics and practice: A guide for pharmacists. London: Pharmaceutical Press.

Standards of Good Professional Practice; published as part of the Royal Pharmaceutical Society Code of Ethics.

Walker R. Stability of medicinal products in compliance devices. Pharm J 1992:248:124–6.

Walker R. Which medication compliance device? Pharm J 1992;249:605–6.

Homoeopathy. Beneviste J, Davenas E, Beauvais J *et al.* Human basophil degranulation triggered by very dilute antiserum against IgE. Nature 1988;333:816–18.

Boyd HW. Introduction to homoeopathic medicine. 2nd ed. Beaconsfield: Beaconsfield Publishers, 1989.

Gibson RG, Gibson LM, MacNeill AD, Watson Buchanan W. Homoeopathic therapy in rheumatoid arthritis: Evaluation by double-blind clinical therapeutic trial. Br J Clin Pharmacol 1980;9:453–9.

Hill C, Doyon F. Review of randomized trials of homoeopathy. Rev Epidemiol Sante Publique 1990;38:138–47.

Kane SB. Homoeopathy—demand and scepticism. Pharm J 1991;247:602–4.

Kleijnen J, Knipschild P, ter Riet G. Clinical trials of homoeopathy. Br Med J 1991;302:316–23.

Lockie A. The family guide to homoeopathy: the safe form of medicine for the future. London: Elm Tree, 1989.

Pratt NJ. Homoeopathic prescribing. Revised ed. Beaconsfield: Beaconsfield Publishers, 1985.

Reilly DT, Taylor MA, McSharry C, Aitchison T. Is homoeopathy a placebo response? Controlled trial of homoeopathic potency, with pollen in hayfever as model. Lancet 1986;2:881–5.

Weighing, Measuring, and Counting

BALANCES AND BEAM SCALES

The essential qualities of any weighing instrument used in dispensing are sensitivity, accuracy, stability, and durability, over a range of loads up to the maximum capacity of the instrument. To ensure a high degree of accuracy, it is important to maintain the instrument in good mechanical condition and to ensure that the correct weighing techniques are employed.

Until the end of 1992, non-automatic weighing instruments used in Great Britain for certain retail transactions were subject to the provision of the Weights and Measures Act 1985 and the Measuring Instruments (EEC Requirements) Regulations 1988.

In order to implement a Council Directive 90/384/EEC on the harmonisation of the laws of the member states which relate to non-automatic weighing instruments, further regulations have been introduced. In July 1992 the Weighing Equipment (Non-automatic Weighing Machines) (Amendment) Regulations 1992 (EEC Requirements) were published; these became effective on 1 January 1993. The Directive allows for an eight-year transitional period (until January 2000) for manufacturers and suppliers of weighing equipment to introduce procedures that will ensure conformity with these Regulations; after eight years, national provisions will be replaced in their entirety.

Under the 1985 Act and 1988 Regulations in force in Great Britain, weighing instruments used for certain retail transactions are controlled in terms of design, construction, and performance; they are classified into four types: Class I, Class II, Class III, and Class IIII. A certificate is issued after the Department for Trade and Industry has been satisfied that the instrument conforms to the regulations and each balance manufactured must carry this certificate number.

In Great Britain, weighing instruments for trade use must be stamped by an Inspector of Weights and Measures. Each machine submitted for stamping is fully inspected for compliance with the certification and given operational tests, which include tilt testing, error testing, maximum and minimum load testing, and eccentric load tests. The Class II instruments used for dispensing and retail transactions involving drugs are similar to the old 'Class B' balances, but in addition to being required to display a maximum weight they must now display a minimum weight together with the verification scale interval 'e'. Since 1 January 1993, it has been illegal to weigh less than the stated minima on these balances.

The calculation that is applied to determine the minimum weight that a balance can meet is:

$$\frac{\text{maximum weight}}{2000} \times 10$$

Thus, a Class II balance stamped with a maximum operating weight of 100 g is stamped with a minimum operating weight of 500 mg; for a 60 g maximum the minimum is 300 mg. Because these lower limits are too high for many pharmaceutical dispensing operations, Class II dispensing balances are under development which have an operating range of 25 g to 125 mg. The National Weights and Measures Laboratory has granted dispensations for certain Class II machines, marked with maximum weight 100 g, which may be used to weigh down to 250 mg instead of the stamped 500 mg.

For accurate weighing of smaller quantities a Class I balance should be used.

The EC Directive 90/384/EEC on the harmonisation of laws relating to non-automatic weighing instruments describes the accuracy of classes of instruments as being; I (special), II (high), III (medium), and IIII (ordinary).

Weights

The Weights and Measures Act and its regulations specify the shape of weights, the material from which they are to be made, and permitted errors in excess or deficiency on verification or inspection. Weights are an important part of a pharmacist's dispensing equipment and require care in handling and use. In pharmaceutical general practice stamped weights must be used for dispensing. It is unlawful in Britain to use apothecary weights. Specifications for weights to be used in testing instruments appear in the Weighing Equipment (Non-automatic Weighing Machines) Regulations 1992 (EEC Requirements).

Rules for the Use of Dispensing Scales

1. Check the instrument for inaccurate adjustment and sticking by releasing the beam on a trial swing and observing the movement of the pointer over the calibrated scale.
2. Place the instrument in a position on the bench which permits a comfortable weighing action and is free from draughts. The calibrated scale, pointer, and spirit level should be clearly observed.
3. In the case of a magnetically damped instrument, adjust the levelling feet until the spirit level is centred and the pointer is exactly opposite the null-point.
4. A sheet of paper, appropriately cut to size and placed under the scale-pans, will help to protect the balance casing when drugs are accidentally spilt.
5. Keep the weight drawer closed during weighing to exclude dust and drugs. Otherwise weights will become contaminated and inaccurate.
6. Weighings in excess of the stated maximum capacity of the instrument should not be attempted.
7. Do not tap the glass scale-pan against the side of a mortar or measure—the pan may be damaged and this will lead to significant errors during subsequent weighings. The shedding of glass spicules from the pan into the preparation is obviously unacceptable.
8. Greasy and semi-solid materials should be weighed on counter-balanced parchment or waxed paper.
9. Loss of solid material on transference from a scale-pan is usually slight and varies from drug to drug according to the physical nature of the drug and the surfaces involved. If the drug is to be made into a solution or suspension it may be washed from the scale-pan with the appropriate liquid vehicle.
10. Certain drugs react with metal and, in such cases, metal scale-pans and spatulas must be avoided (for example, with chlorinated lime, iodine, and phenylmercuric salts).
11. Wipe the scale-pan clean after the completion of each weighing and never weigh a second material on top of the remains of the first.

Electronic Balances

European Community regulations require that electronic balances should not be affected by minor changes in their environment; any fault in the instrument should be detected automatically. A visible or audible alarm should indicate any fault and should continue to do so until the fault is remedied.

All weighing instruments are required to be properly installed in a suitable environment and must remain accurate in use.

MEASURES

Dispensing measures are conical or beaker-shaped as specified by the British Standard 1922:1987, Specification for glass dispensing measures for pharmaceutical purposes. Dispensing measures, of either shape, are required to be tested, passed for use in trade, and stamped by an Inspector of Weights and Measures.

Limits of error specified in the Standard vary with capacity and shape for both types of measures but limits for the two beakers of 500 mL and 1000 mL capacity are less stringent than those for conical measures at similar capacity levels.

Dispensing measures are permanently marked with unnumbered levelling lines on the opposite side to, and at the same level as, the top and other specified graduation lines.

Graduated glass measuring cylinders to British Standard 604:1982 (1988) (ISO 4788—1980) are intended for general laboratory purposes; they do not have levelling lines. Their accuracy (except at the 5 mL and 10 mL graduation lines) is less than that of conical dispensing measures to British Standard 1922; often, accuracy is also less than that of volumetric glassware intended for analytical use.

Rules for the Use of Measures

1. Choose a measure appropriate to the liquid requiring measurement and of appropriate capacity, to minimise errors in judging the position of the liquid meniscus in relation to the graduation mark.
2. The measure should be held at eye level, with front and rear graduations in alignment. The bottom of the liquid meniscus must be on the graduation mark. Under the condition of a bright and uniformly coloured background, difficulty may be experienced in locating the true meniscus. A finger or strip of dark paper held at the back of the measure and just below the liquid surface will provide conditions necessary to establish clearly the true meniscus.
3. During the measurement of a liquid the bottle should be held in a position that enables the full label to be seen throughout. Such a

precaution will also ensure that liquid cannot run down the label and disfigure it.

4. In the measurement of viscous liquids, care must be taken to ensure that the measured quantity is actually delivered to the preparation. Where possible, the liquid should be washed out of the measure. Alternatively, the liquid can be measured by difference.

5. In the measurement of the 'non-rounded' volumes such as are required in the reconstitution of antibiotic mixtures it may be necessary to make two measurements rather than to attempt to measure, for example, 61 mL or 89 mL in a 100 mL measure.

PIPETTES

The accurate measurement of mobile liquids in quantities of less than 5mL requires the use of pipettes. In pharmaceutical general practice, stamped pipettes must be used for dispensing.

Rules for the Use of Pipettes

1. Select an adequately graduated pipette whose capacity is appropriate to the volume of liquid requiring measurement.
2. Determine whether the pipette is of the 'drainage' or 'blow out' type, and accordingly adopt the appropriate method in practice.
3. For corrosive and toxic liquids, attach a rubber bulb to the stem of the pipette. Under no circumstances should mouth suction be used.

COUNTING DEVICES

A very high proportion of dispensed medicines consists of tablets or capsules and the methods used for counting them vary from purely manual to the use of a counting triangle, a perforated counting tray, or an electronic counting device.

The simplest manual method is to place the products on white demy paper which overlaps a second piece of white demy paper. The products are counted by tens using a spatula and transferred across to the second piece of paper which is then formed into a trough or funnel to transfer the dosage forms into a container.

Counting triangles and perforated counting trays enable more rapid counts than the manual method. Both types are easily cleaned but counting trays may need plate changes to accommodate products of marked size difference. In 1978 the triangle was reported to be the most accurate counting method, followed by manual counting, and the use of perforated trays. Machine counting

was the most frequently inaccurate; counts tended to err on the side of small excesses.

Electronic Counting Systems

The operating principles embodied in the currently available commercial equipment for counting tablets or capsules depend on either the weighing of a reference sample of dosage forms on a computerised balance or the direct counting of objects as they pass between a light source and a photo-electric sensor.

Electronic Balances

Most devices of this type require that there is consistent uniformity of tablet weight. From the weight of a reference sample of between 5 and 20 dosage forms a microprocessor computes the total number as further dosage forms are added to the balance pan or scoop.

Between counts of different dosage forms, balances may need resetting; balances tend to be sensitive to vibration and air movement. Cleaning of those parts in contact with the dosage forms is usually quick and simple. Accuracy of counts is subject to weight uniformity and may be compromised slightly when sugar coated tablets or very small tablets are being counted.

Photo-electric Counters

By means of a turntable with a guide channel, or by passage through a multi-channel hopper, dosage forms are separated into single lines which interrupt a light beam impinging on a photocell linked to an electronic counter.

Counting speeds vary between devices, from a claimed 100 tablets in 5 seconds through a hopper device, to a slower rate with a turntable counter. Adjustment of guide rails may also be necessary when dosage forms are changed on turntable counters. Limitations of most photo-electric counters are their failure to discriminate between whole and fragmented tablets, their inaccuracy when counting transparent capsules such as Atromid-S, and their complex surfaces which can make cleaning a time-consuming activity.

Visual checks of the identity and the physical state of the dosage forms being counted are less readily made in hopper-fed than in turntable-fed counters. Whereas no specific prediction is offered for the accuracy overall of a turntable-fed counter, a value of 0.5% is claimed by the manufacturer of a hopper-fed counter.

The Council of the Royal Pharmaceutical Society has issued the following advice on the use of tablet counters:

'Severe allergic reactions can be initiated in previously sensitised persons by very small amounts of certain drugs and of excipients and other materials used in the manufacture of tablets and capsules. In order to minimise that risk, counting devices should be carefully cleaned after each dispensing operation involving any uncoated tablet, or any coated tablet or capsule from a bulk container holding damaged contents. As cross-contamination with the penicillins is particularly serious, special care should be taken when dispensing products containing those drugs.'

Most electronic counting machines are difficult to clean adequately and it is therefore recommended that such machines are used only for coated tablets or capsules, or for pre-packing operations.

Infusion Fluids: Admixtures and Administration

The first recorded use of infusion fluids was by Dr Thomas Latto of Edinburgh in 1832 when a solution of salts was administered to treat the symptoms of cholera. The treatment was nonsterile, chemically impure, and hypotonic. It was many decades before this rationally based therapy was scientifically confirmed and exploited.

INTRAVENOUS ADMINISTRATION

The intravenous route of administration is now a well established route of drug delivery and is indicated in situations where:

- the drug is not absorbed orally
- there is erratic absorption after intramuscular injection
- the drug is inactivated in the gastro-intestinal tract
- a rapid response is required
- the patient is unable to tolerate drugs or fluids orally
- the intramuscular or subcutaneous route is not practicable
- the drug must be well diluted or requires a carrier fluid
- the drug has a very short half-life and must be continuously infused
- correction of fluid and electrolyte imbalances is required
- the drug is only active by the intravenous route.

Complications of Intravenous Drug Delivery

Despite the many indications and advantages of intravenous therapy it may also cause complications such as:

- air emboli
- drug incompatibilities
- hypersensitivity
- infiltration or extravasation
- sepsis
- thrombosis or phlebitis.

CENTRALISED INTRAVENOUS ADDITIVE SERVICE (CIVAS)

In order to reduce some of the hazards associated with intravenous drug therapy the **Centralised Intravenous Additive Service (CIVAS)** was developed in the United Kingdom in the mid to late 1960s.[1]

The problems of adding drugs to intravenous solutions were highlighted in the report *Addition of Drugs to Intravenous Infusion Fluids* published by the Department of Health as Health Circular (76) 9 (March 1976). The report describes a rational approach to intravenous drug administration and identifies the responsibilities of the doctor, nurse, and pharmacist. A principal conclusion was that wherever possible, drug infusion mixtures should be provided from the pharmacy.

Centralised intravenous additive services usually include reconstitution of drugs such as antibiotics for bolus or short duration infusion; reconstitution of cytotoxic agents; and preparation of individualised prescriptions for total parenteral nutrition (TPN). The finished products may be in bags, vials, or preloaded into syringes. Some components may have been prepared in advance and stored, for example, standard formulations of TPN fluids before being modified in the CIVAS unit to suit individual patient electrolyte and vitamin needs.

Most hospitals now have a centralised intravenous additive service managed by pharmacists and some have established specialist satellite dispensing units (for example, in intensive care units) under pharmacy control. Satellite units are able to respond to local demands but are expensive to operate and require duplicate drug and fluid stocks. It may be difficult to maintain adequate staff cover during times of holidays and sickness when compared with a central pharmacy based unit.

The advantages of centralisation of dispensing services include savings in nurses' and junior doctors' time, efficient use of drug vial contents, reduction in ward stock holding, the implementation of controlled training procedures, and improved safety and facility monitoring. The disadvantages include problems arising from poor communication between ward and dispensary when doses are prepared and treatment has stopped, removal of a traditional nurse role, and incomplete cover from pharmacies such as the inability to provide a weekend service.

LICENSING REQUIREMENTS FOR ASEPTIC PREPARATION

The removal of Crown Immunity in 1991 has led to a differentiation between 'dispensing' and 'manufacturing', since manufacturing activity must only occur in premises licensed by the Medicines Inspectorate of the Medicines Control Agency (MCA). Guidance issued by the MCA[2] in 1992 can be summarised as follows:

'Aseptic preparation for stock should be avoided wherever possible. Products for stock should be manufactured in licensed manufacturing units. In general, it is desirable for aseptically prepared products to be dispensed for individual patients, as and when required. However, it is recognised that preparation for stock in an aseptic dispensary might be helpful in maintaining controlled supplies to patients, particularly over weekends and holiday periods. The following guidance has been issued to cover these circumstances.'

If aseptic preparation has to take place outside licensed facilities, a manufacturer's licence will not be required provided the following conditions apply:

- preparation is by or under the supervision of a pharmacist
- preparation takes place using closed systems
- all ingredients should be licensed medicinal products or prepared in licensed facilities
- products will be given a maximum expiry date of one week; the shelf-life should be supported by stability data
- all activities should be in accordance with recommended guidelines.

Most hospitals operate dispensing activity within these guidelines and do not require a manufacturing licence. Units that manufacture long-life products (for example, total parenteral nutrition mixtures with a 90-day shelf-life) must hold a 'Specials' manufacturing licence.

STORAGE AND STABILITY

Although preparation for stock in aseptic dispensaries should be kept to a minimum and comply with the criteria listed above, it would be a clear advantage if reconstituted drugs could be stored without loss of potency and be immediately available for patient use.

Preparation in licensed facilities with subsequent freezing and cold storage would provide pharmacies with much greater flexibility in providing an all-year-round reconstituted drug service, even in units not capable of providing any aseptic dispensing service. Drugs could be stored in the pharmacy or on the ward and rapidly thawed immediately before use.[3–6] Tredree[3] describes the freezing of intravenous admixtures and subsequent thawing using a microwave warmer. The dangers of instability in slow freezing and the formation of eutectic mixtures, and the possibility of decomposition through hot-spot overheating during microwave warming are described. Rapid freezing and storage at $-20°$ to $-25°$ and the use of specially designed microwave warmers can overcome most of these problems. All formulations that are dispensed for storage, however short or long, should have their chemical and microbiological stability assessed by a quality assurance laboratory for the specified storage period. The *Handbook on Injectable Drugs* (Trissel LA, 1992) is an essential reference and gives comprehensive data on incompatibility and stability of a wide range of drugs. Table 1 provides references to instability data covering the period 1990 to 1992. Vapour transfer from bag or preloaded syringe is unlikely to be a problem with short-life dispensed products, but may need to be considered for items manufactured in a licensed 'specials unit'.

STERILITY ASSURANCE

The aseptic technique of staff involved in sterile dispensing must be regularly validated. Confidence levels could be increased further by carrying out sterility tests on dispensing vial residues or surplus product. **Environmental monitoring** of the dispensing unit is essential and should include settle plate sampling, air sampling and air flow monitoring, finger dabs, surface sampling, and clean air cabinet testing. For further information see the chapter entitled Cleanrooms for Pharmaceutical Production. Rules concerning **personal hygiene** and the wearing of make-up and jewellery should be incorporated into the dispensing procedure manual along with the specification for low-lint cover-all garments. Further guidance for aseptic dispensary operation are given in notes prepared by the Regional quality control pharmacists.[7]

Aseptic Dispensing

Safe aseptic dispensing can be achieved with the simple equipment of syringe and needle, if pressure equalisation techniques are used when adding fluid to a closed vial. However, the increasing demand placed upon aseptic dispensaries means

Table 1

Centralised Intravenous Additive Service (CIVAS) literature references (1990–92). Stability data collated by Dr Frank Haines-Nutt, Truro Hospital Pharmacy.

Product	Container	Shelf-life	Reference
Amiloride HCl 0.001M NaCl 0.9%	syringe	30 days at 4°	Pharm J 1992;248(Suppl):HS40–1
Aminophylline 250 mg/50 mL NaCl 0.9%	syringe	No significant loss after 6 weeks at 4° and RT	Pharm J 1992;248(Suppl): HS24–6
Amiodarone NaCl 0.9%	bag	Precipitate in 24 h	Am J Hosp Pharm 1985;42:2679–82
Amiodarone glucose 5%	bag	10% loss in 3 h due to adsorption	Am J Hosp Pharm 1985;42:2679–82
Amphotericin 5 mg/50 mL glucose 5%	bag	Stable for 24 h 25° (no significant loss)	Am J Hosp Pharm 1991;48:2430–3
Amphotericin 60, 80, and 100 mg/50 mL glucose 5%	bag	>36 h at 6° and 25°	Am J Hosp Pharm 1991;48:283–5
Amphotericin 5 mg/50 mL glucose 10%	bag	Stable for 24 h 25° (no significant loss)	Am J Hosp Pharm 1991;48:2430–3
Amphotericin 5 mg/50 mL glucose 15%	bag	Stable for 24 h 25° (no significant loss)	Am J Hosp Pharm 1991;48:2430–3
Amphotericin 5 mg/50 mL glucose 20%	bag	Stable for 24 h 25° (no significant loss)	Am J Hosp Pharm 1991;48:2430–3
Ampicillin 250 mg/1.8 mL WFI 0.2 mL/syr	syringe	Not recommended 36% loss in 48 h in fridge	Hosp Pharm Prac 1992;2:285–9
Atracurium 25 mg/2.5 mL	syringe	No significant loss after 21 days at 4°	Pharm J 1992;248(Suppl):HS24–6
Atropine 0.6 mg/mL	syringe	No significant loss after 21 days at 4°	Pharm J 1992;248(Suppl):HS24–6
Azlocillin 5 g NaCl 0.9% 100 mL	bag	6 days in a fridge use within 3 days at RT	Pharm J 1992;248(Suppl):HS40–1
Baclofen 50 micrograms/mL NaCl 0.9%	syringe	2 months at RT and 4°	Pharm J 1992;248(Suppl):HS40–1
Benzylpenicillin 600 mg/4 mL WFI	syringe	Stable for 8 days in fridge	Hosp Pharm Prac 1991;1:243–52
Bleomycin 0.3 units/mL NaCl 0.9%	bag	<1% loss in 24 h at 20°	Am J Hosp Pharm 1990;47:2528–9
Bleomycin 0.3 units/mL NaCl 0.9%	vial	<1% loss in 24 h at 20°	Am J Hosp Pharm 1990;47:2528–9
Bleomycin 0.3 units/mL glucose 5%	bag	10% loss in 8 h, 12% in 24 h at 20°	Am J Hosp Pharm 1990;47:2528–9
Bleomycin 0.3 units/mL glucose 5%	vial	10% loss in 9 h, 14% in 25 h	Am J Hosp Pharm 1990;47:2528–9
Bleomycin 3 units/mL NaCl 0.9%	bag	5% loss in 24 h at 20°	Am J Hosp Pharm 1990;47:2528–9
Bleomycin 3 units/mL NaCl 0.9%	vial	2% loss in 24 h at 20°	Am J Hosp Pharm 1990;47:2528–9
Bleomycin 3 units/mL glucose 5%	bag	9% loss in 7 h,11% in 24 h at 20°	Am J Hosp Pharm 1990;47:2528–9
Bleomycin 3 units/mL glucose 5%	vial	8% loss in 9 h, 16% in 25 h	Am J Hosp Pharm 1990;47:2528–9
Bupivacaine 0.125% and iohexol 300 mg		No loss in 24 h at RT	Pharm Week Sci Ed 1991;13(6):254
Bupivacaine 0.25% and iohexol 300 mg		No loss in 24 h at RT	Pharm Week Sci Ed 1991;13(6):254
Cefotaxime 1 g/3.4 mL WFI 0.18 mL/syr	syringe	7 days in fridge but increased coloration	Hosp Pharm Prac 1992;2:285–9
Ceftazidime 500 mg/4.5 mL WFI 0.4 mL/syr	syringe	7 days in fridge but increased coloration	Hosp Pharm Prac 1992;2:285–9
Cefuroxime 250 mg/1.8 mL WFI 0.2 mL/syr	syringe	7 days in fridge but increased coloration	Hosp Pharm Prac 1992;2:285–9
Cefuroxime 750 mg and 1.5 g in 50 mL NaCl 0.9%	bag	20 days at 4°, use within 24 h atRT	Pharm J 1992;248(Suppl):HS40–1
Cefuroxime 750 mg and 1.5 g in 50 mL glucose 5%	bag	20 days at 4°, use within 24 h at RT	Pharm J 1992;248(Suppl):HS40–1
Ciprofloxacin 200 mg/100 mL NaCl 0.9%	bag	>2 days at 25°	Am J Hosp Pharm 1991;48:2166–71
Ciprofloxacin 200 mg/100 mL glucose 5%	bag	>2 days at 25°	Am J Hosp Pharm 1991;48:2166–71

Table 1—*Continued*

Product	Container	Shelf-life	Reference
Ciprofloxacin 200 mg/100 mL metronidizole 0.5%	bag	>2 days at 25°	Am J Hosp Pharm 1991;48:2166–71
Clindamycin 750 mg/mL glucose 5%	bag	30 days frozen and 14 days in fridge	Am J Hosp Pharm 1991;48:2184–6
Cytarabine 1.25 and 25 mg/mL NaCl 0.9%	pump res	28 days at 4–22° and 7 days at 35°	Am J Hosp Pharm 1992;49:619–23
Cytarabine 1.25 and 25 mg/mL glucose 5%	pump res	28 days at 4–22° and 7 days at 35°	Am J Hosp Pharm 1992;49:619–23
Diamorphine 1 and 20 mg/mL NaCl 0.9%	infusor	15 days at 4, 20 and 31°	Am J Hosp Pharm 1990;47:377–81
Diamorphine 1 and 20 mg/mL in NaCl 0.9%	bag	15 days at 4 and 20°	Am J Hosp Pharm 1990;47:377–81
Diamorphine 400 mg and chlorpromazine 25 mg/mL 3 mL WFI	syringe	9% degrad of diamorphine after 9 days, No degrad of chlorpromazine	Pharm J 1992;248(Suppl):HS24–6
Diethanolamine fusidate 580 mg/250 mL glucose 5%	bag	10% degrad after 2 days at 37°, 10 days at 25°, and >162 days at 4°	Hosp Pharm Prac 1992;1:59–62
Diethanolamine fusidate 580 mg/500 mL glucose 5%	bag	10% degrad after 2 days at 37°, 10 days at 25°, and >162 days at 4°	Hosp Pharm Prac 1992;1:59–62
Dobutamine 250 and 500 mg/50 mL NaCl 0.9%	syringe	No significant degrad after 4 weeks at 4°	Hosp Pharm Prac 1991;5:255–6
Dobutamine 250 and 500 mg/50 mL glucose 5%	syringe	No significant degrad after 4 weeks at 4°	Hosp Pharm Prac 1991;5:255–6
Dopamine 0.3 and 1 mg/mL glucose 10%/NaCl 0.18%	bag	No loss over 48 h	Pharm J 1991;246:220
Dopamine 0.3 and 1 mg/mL glucose 10%	bag	No loss over 48 h	Pharm J 1991;246:220
Doxorubicin 1.25 and 0.5 mg/mL NaCl 0.9%	pump res	14 days at 4–22° and 7 days at 35°	Am J Hosp Pharm 1992;49:619–23
Doxorubicin 1.25 and 0.5 mg/mL glucose 5%	pump res	14 days at 4–22° and 7 days at 35°	Am J Hosp Pharm 1992;49:619–23
Doxorubicin 2 mg/mL NaCl 0.9%	cassette	>30 days at 30°	Am J Hosp Pharm 1991;48:1976–7
Famotidine 2 mg/mL NaCl 0.9%	syringe	Stable for 8 weeks at −20°	Am J Hosp Pharm 1990;47:2073–4
Famotidine 2 mg/mL glucose 5%	syringe	Stable for 3 weeks at −20°	Am J Hosp Pharm 1990;47:2073–4
Fentanyl 20 micrograms/mL in NaCl 0.9%	pump	>30 days at RT and 3°	Am J Hosp Pharm 1990;47:1572–4
Fentanyl 500 micrograms/100 mL NaCl 0.9%	bag	>97.8% remaining after 48 h at RT	Am J Hosp Pharm 1990;47:1584–7
Fentanyl 500 micrograms/100 mL glucose 5%	bag	>97.8% remaining after 48 h at RT	Am J Hosp Pharm 1990;47:1584–7
Fentanyl and bupivacaine NaCl 0.9%	cassette	30 days at 23°	Am J Hosp Pharm 1990;47:2037–40
Flucloxacillin 250 mg/1.8 mL WFI 0.16 mL	syringe	7 days in fridge	Hosp Pharm Prac 1992;2:285–9
Fluorouracil 10 and 50 mg/mL NaCl 0.9%	pump res	28 days at 4–35°	Am J Hosp Pharm 1992;49:619–23
Fluorouracil 10 and 50 mg/mL glucose 5%	pump res	28 days at 4–35°	Am J Hosp Pharm 1992;49:619–23
Frusemide 10 mg/mL	syringe	,2 months at RT and 4°	Pharm J 1992;248(Suppl):HS40–1
Frusemide 2 mg/mL in glucose 5% and 10%	bag	24 h (no chemical degradation)	Hosp Pharm Prac 1991;1:191–5
Ganciclovir 100 mg/100 mL NaCl 0.9%	bag	Stable for 35 days at 5° and 25°	Am J Hosp Pharm 1992;49:116–8
Ganciclovir 100 mg/100 mL glucose 5% 100 mL	bag	Stable for 35 days at 5° and 25°	Am J Hosp Pharm 1992;49:116–8
Ganciclovir 2 and 4 mg/mL NaCl 0.9% 100 mL	bag	5 weeks at 4°	Pharm J 1992;248(Suppl):HS40–1
Ganciclovir 500 mg/100 mL NaCl 0.9%	bag	Stable for 35 days at 5° and 25°	Am J Hosp Pharm 1992;49:116–8
Ganciclovir 500 mg/100 mL glucose 5%	bag	Stable for 35 days at 5° and 25°	Am J Hosp Pharm 1992;49:116–8

Table 1—*Continued*

Product	Container	Shelf-life	Reference
Gentamicin 10 mg/mL 0.15 and 0.75 mL	syringe	Stable for 7 days	Hosp Pharm Prac 1991;1:243–52
Glyceryl trinitrate 25 mg/25 mL NaCl 0.9%	syringe	5% in 7 days, 10% in 3 weeks at 4°, 10% in 7 days and 15% in 3 weeks at RT	Hosp Pharm Prac 1992;2:137–41
Glyceryl trinitrate 25 mg/25 mL glucose 5%	syringe	5% in 7 days, 10% in 3 wks at 4°, 8% in 7 days, and 10% in 2 wks at RT	Hosp Pharm Prac 1992;2:137–141
Hydrocortisone sod succ 100 mg/100 mL NaCl	bag	10% degradation after 3 days at RT and 26 days at 4°	Pharm J 1992;248(Suppl):HS40–1
Hydrocortisone Sod succ 100 mg/100 mL glucose 5%	bag	10% degradation after 3 days at RT and 56 days at 4°	Pharm J 1992;248(Suppl):HS40–1
Hydrocortisone sod succ 100 mg/2 mL WFI	syringe	10% degradation after 3 days at RT and 42 days at 4°	Pharm J 1992;248(Suppl):HS40–41
Ifosfamide 10–80 mg/mL NaCl 0.9%	cassette	8 days at RT	Am J Hosp Pharm 1992;49:1137–9
Ifosfamide 50 mg mesna 40 mg/mL NaCl 0.9%	syringe	21 days at 4° and RT	Pharm J 1992;248(Suppl):HS40–41
Isosorbide dinitrate 40 mg/540 mL NaCl 0.9%	bag	>70% loss in 15–30 min due to adsorption	J Clin Hosp Pharm 1981;6:209
Metronidazole 25 mg/5 mL	syringe	Stable for 3 months in fridge	Hosp Pharm Prac 1991;1:243–52
Metronidazole 5 mg/5 mL glucose 5%	syringe	Stable for 3 months in fridge	Hosp Pharm Prac 1991;1:243–52
Mitozantrone 0.05 mg and etoposide 0.5 mg/mL NaCl 0.9%		No loss in 24 h at RT in dark	Acta Pharm Nord 1991;3(4):251
Mitozantrone 0.1 mg and etoposide 1 mg		No loss in 24 h at RT in dark	Acta Pharm Nord 1991;3(4):251
Morphine 100 mg/50 mL NaCl 0.9%	syringe	Stable for 6 weeks at RT	Pharm J 1992;248(Suppl):HS24–6
Morphine 100 mg/50 mL NaCl 0.9%	syringe	With sodium metabisulphite (0.1%) 15% degrad in 6 weeks	Pharm J 1992;248(Suppl):HS24–6
Morphine 0.5–60 mg/mL NaCl 0.9%	bag	14 days at 5° and 37° 60 mg/mL at 37° but not 5°	Am J Hosp Pharm 1990;47:2040–2
Morphine sulphate 2 and 15 mg/mL WFI	bag	>12 days at 2° and RT	Am J Hosp Pharm 1990;47:143–6
Morphine sulphate 2 and 15 mg/mL WFI	infusor	>12 days at 2°, RT, and 31°	Am J Hosp Pharm 1990;47:143–6
Netilmicin 15 mg/1.5 mL	syringe	30 days at 4°	Pharm J 1992;248(Suppl):HS40–1
Oxytocin 10 units/mL	syringe	$t_{5\%} = 10$ days at 4°	Pharm J 1992;248(Suppl):HS24–6
Papaverine 12 mg/mL NaCl 0.9%	syringe	3 months at 5°	Hosp Pharm Prac 1992;2:361–2
Papaverine 1 mg/mL NaCl 0.9%	syringe	6 months in fridge	Hosp Pharm Prac 1992;2:361–2
Papaverine 40 mg/mL NaCl 0.9%	syringe	Precipitation after 1 month at 5°	Hosp Pharm Prac 1992;2:361–2
Pethidine 600 mg/60 mL NaCl 0.9%	syringe	No degrad after 16 days at RT in light	Pharm J 1992;248(Suppl):HS24–6
Phenylephrine 0.005% NaCl 0.9%	syringe	No degrad after 7 days at 4°, <5% at RT and 40°	Pharm J 1992;248(Suppl):HS24–6
Piperacillin 450 mg/mL glucose 5%	bag	30 days frozen and 7 days in fridge	Am J Hosp Pharm 1991;48:2184–6
Procainamide 0.4 and 0.8% glucose 5%	bag	0.4% 6 h at RT, 12 h at 5°; 8% 6–12 h at RT, 24 h at 5°	Am J Hosp Pharm 1988;45:2513–7
Ranitidine 0.05 mg/mL glucose 5%	bag	5% loss in 2 days, 7% in 7 days at RT	Am J Hosp Pharm 1990;47:1580–4
Ranitidine 0.5–2 mg/mL glucose 5% (500 mL)	bag	5% loss in 7 days at RT, about 2% after 30 days at 4°	Am J Hosp Pharm 1990;47:2043–6
Ranitidine 1.8 mg/mL glucose 5%	bag	2% loss in 7 days, about 5% in 28 days at RT	Am J Hosp Pharm 1990;47:1580–4
Ranitidine 350 mg/mL in glucose 5%	bag	30 days frozen and 10 days in fridge	Am J Hosp Pharm 1991;48:2184–6
Ranitidine 50 mg/mL in glucose 5%	bag	92 days at 4°	Can J Hosp Pharm 1988;41:105–8

Table 1—*Continued*

Product	Container	Shelf-life	Reference
Ranitidine 0.05 mg/mL glucose 10%	bag	6.5% loss in 2 days, 11% in 7 days at RT	Am J Hosp Pharm 1990;47:1580–4
Ranitidine 0.5–2 mg/mL glucose 10% (500 mL)	bag	About 3% loss in 7 days at RT, about 2–6% after 30 days at 4°	Am J Hosp Pharm 1990;47:2043–6
Ranitidine 0.05 mg/mL NaCl 0.9%	bag	2% loss in 7 days, 3% in 28 days at RT	Am J Hosp Pharm 1990;47:1580–4
Ranitidine 0.5 mg/mL NaCl 0.9%	bag	No significant loss in 28 days at RT at >0.44 mg/mL	Am J Hosp Pharm 1990;47:1580–4
Ranitidine 0.5–2 mg/mL NaCl 0.9% (500mL)	bag	No loss in 7 days at RT, 30 days at 4°, 60 days at −20°	Am J Hosp Pharm 1990;47:2043–6
Ranitidine 0.05 mg/mL glucose 5%/NaCl 0.45%	bag	5% loss in 2 days, 8% in 7 days at RT	Am J Hosp Pharm 1990;47:1580–4
Ranitidine 0.5–2 mg/mL glucose 5%/NaCl 0.45% 500 mL	bag	About 3–5% in 7 days at RT, about 0–8% after 30 days at 4°	Am J Hosp Pharm 1990;47:2043–6
Ranitidine 0.5–2 mg/mL glucose 5%/Lac Ringers	bag	About 5% loss in 7 days at RT, about 0–8% after 30 days at 4°	Am J Hosp Pharm 1990;47:2043–6
Ranitidine 0.05 mg/mL glucose 5%/Lac Ringer	bag	14% loss in 2 days, 20% in 7 days at RT	Am J Hosp Pharm 1990;47:1580–4
Tauromustine NaCl 0.9%	bag	$t_{50\%}$ = 105.9 h	Int J Pharm 1989;56:37–41
Tolazoline 8 mg and dopamine 1 mg/mL glucose 10%	infusion	<5% degrad dopamine, no loss of tolazoline in 24 h at RT	Hosp Pharm Prac 1992;3:205–10
Tolazoline 8 mg and dopamine 1 mg/mL glucose 10%/NaCl 0.18%	infusion	<7% degrad dopamine, no loss of tolazoline in 24 h at RT	Hosp Pharm Prac 1992;3:205–10
Vancomycin 1000 mg/250 mL glucose 5%	bag	9% loss in 30 days at 4°, about 8% in 17 days at RT	Can J Hosp Pharm 1988;41:233–8
Vancomycin 1000 mg/250 mL NaCl 0.9%	bag	5% loss in 30 days at 4°, 10% in 24 days at RT	Can J Hosp Pharm 1988;41:233–8
Vancomycin 500 mg/100 mL NaCl 0.9%	bag	5% loss in 30 days at 4°, about 8.5% in 24 days at RT	Can J Hosp Pharm 1988;41:233–8
Vancomycin 500 mg/100 mL glucose 5%	bag	9% loss in 30 days at 4°, about 8% in 17 days at RT	Can J Hosp Pharm 1988;41:233–8
Vinblastine 10 mg/250 mL NaCl 0.9%	bag	Stable for 7 days at 4°	Int J Pharm 1991;77:279–85
Vinblastine 10 mg/250 mL glucose 5%	bag	Stable for 7 days at 4°	Int J Pharm 1991;77:279–85
Vincristine 2 mg/250 mL NaCl 0.9%	bag	Stable for 7 days at 4°	Int J Pharm 1991;77:279–85
Vincristine 2 mg/250 mL glucose 5%	bag	Stable for 7 days at 4°	Int J Pharm 1991;77:279–85
Vincristine 1.6 mg and mitozantrone 16 mg/mL NaCl 0.9% 100 mL	cassette	4 days at RT	Pharm J 1992;248(Suppl):HS40–41
Vindesine 4 mg/250 mL NaCl 0.9%	bag	Stable for 7 days at 4°	Int J Pharm 1991;77:279–85
Vindesine 4 mg/250 mL glucose 5%	bag	Stable for 7 days at 4°	Int J Pharm 1991;77:279–85
Vinorelbine 50 mg/250 mL NaCl 0.9%	bag	Stable for 3 days not 7 at 4°	Int J Pharm 1991;77:279–85
Vinorelbine 50 mg/250 mL glucose 5%	bag	Stable for 7 days at 4°	Int J Pharm 1991;77:279–85
Zidovudine 4 mg/mL NaCl 0.9%	bag	98% remaining after 8 days at RT and fridge	Am J Hosp Pharm 1991;48:280–2
Zidovudine 4 mg/mL glucose 5%	bag	98% remaining after 8 days at RT and fridge	Am J Hosp Pharm 1991;48:280–2

Lac Ringer = Lactated Ringer's Injection
NaCl 0.9% = sodium chloride 0.9% intravenous infusion
RT = room temperature
WFI = water for injections

that speed is an important issue. A vast range of 'dispensing aids' are marketed, which are designed to speed the dispensing process and give greater assurance of sterility. The more important aids are those that reduce the potential for aerosol release of toxic drug by safely venting vials when fluid is added. Most of these consist of a double-lumen plastic needle, one lumen forming the fluid pathway and the other the air venting pathway terminated by a 0.22 micrometre porosity hydrophobic (non-wetting) membrane filter. Other aids include plastic quills for rapidly drawing fluids from ampoules, double-ended needles for rapid transfer of fluid from vehicle vial to powder vial, and small membrane or sintered steel filter units for removal of particles (5 micrometres pore size) or sterilisation of the product (0.22 micrometre pore size). All these aids are presterilised by gamma irradiation or ethylene oxide gas. Dispensing aids and syringes with Luer-lock rather than Luer-slip connections provide greater security and reduce the risk of leakage or spillage of toxic or expensive drugs.

More complex devices include spring-loaded syringes with a three-way valve system and tubing, which connects to a vehicle reservoir (bottle or bag), the syringe, and a filling needle or quill. As the syringe fills, the valve attached to the needle line is closed; as the syringe empties, the valve to the reservoir is closed. There is usually an adjustable stop on the plunger that allows repetitive aliquots to be dispensed accurately. These repetitive dispensing syringes can also be motorised with a foot-operated control for automatic or semi-automatic filling. Blind hubs for sealing preloaded syringes and sterile plastic cases for holding loaded syringes for transportation to wards are other important dispensing aids.

Reconstitution

Many drugs for intravenous injection are supplied in vials as a sterile lyophilised powder, which must be dissolved in a suitable vehicle before injection or further processing. The number of drugs offered in solution form in vials is increasing since manufacturers recognise the practical advantages in reducing manipulations carried out by pharmacists or others who prepare the product for injection. Despite this, there are still a substantial number of products presented in the dry powder state that require reconstitution by adding an appropriate volume of water for injections or sodium chloride 0.9% injection. Some products require reconstitution with a particular solvent before dilu-

tion (for example, carmustine, amsacrine, and melphalan). Bacteriostatic solvents must never be used to prepare intrathecal injections. The choice of diluent depends upon factors such as: the compatibility of the drug with the diluent, the osmolality of the diluted formulation, and the patient's ability to tolerate the chosen fluid. Guidance concerning reconstitution often appears in the manufacturer's data sheet, but there are instances where this may not be the optimum procedure. These include consideration of the displacement value (stated in most data sheets) of the dry powder when reconstituting doses for use in neonates and children or the preparation of more concentrated solutions for use in fluid-restricted patients. It is always important to ensure the powder has been dissolved, by shaking or swirling the vial. Some therapeutic agents should not be shaken too vigorously either because of froth formation (for example, ceftazidime and asparaginase) or because the product may be denatured (for example, interferons and interleukins).

Withdrawal

Although using the pressure equalisation technique is a cost effective and efficient method of loading the syringe, the use of vented spikes (dispensing pins) permits easy withdrawal of a number of doses at any one session and offers the advantage of being able to place a sealing cap over the vial closure for further use at some other time within the stability period of the reconstituted product. For batch reconstitution and withdrawal there are various automated syringe pumps available (see Aseptic Dispensing above).

The hazards associated with the infusion of particles in intravenous fluids are well known;[8] and for this reason the majority of pharmacy-controlled intravenous additive units employ filter needles or filter straws to a greater or lesser extent depending upon the number of glass ampoules opened and the drug or solvent employed.[9, 10]

Measurement of Doses

Syringes manufactured to British Standard specification British Standard 5081:Parts 1–2:1987 have markings that are satisfactory for accurate dose measurement (see Syringes, Needles, Cannulae, and Catheters below).

If a drug dose, or the volume of drug available, is very small and cannot be accurately measured by a syringe (less than 0.2 mL) a suitable drug dilution must be prepared. Drawing up small volumes of drug solution into a syringe, which are then diluted by drawing up dilution fluid into the same syringe, may lead to errors due to the dead-space in the hub of the syringe. In these circumstances the drug should be drawn up in an appropriately-sized syringe and a measured volume then injected into another empty syringe which may then be used to draw up the dilution fluid to the correct volume. If the volume of diluting fluid is also very small, both drug and diluent should be drawn up separately. When preparing doses for neonates, the dose required may be so small relative to the concentration of the standard presentation that a double dilution may have to be performed.

Administration of very small doses to neonates may require the use of primed needles. This is achieved by drawing up into the syringe slightly more drug solution than is required and then expressing the excess drug through the attached needle. It is not necessary to consider the dead-space in the hub of the syringe as this is already accounted for on calibration.

Factors to be considered when preloading drugs into syringes include the stability of the drug in the syringe for the storage time required (see Storage and Stability above), the matching of syringe to syringe pump, and the method of capping the syringe hub. For storage and distribution the syringe should be capped with a blind hub, not a needle.

Addition of Drugs to Infusion Fluids

Some drugs must be administered as an intermittent or continuous infusion rather than a bolus dose from the syringe. In this case the reconstituted drug must be transferred to the bag or bottle containing the infusion fluid. Factors to consider must include: compatibility of the drug with the infusion fluid, container, and any concurrent additives; stability of the drug at that concentration; and the ability of the patient to tolerate the type and volume of fluid employed. If the concentration of drug is critical, the infusion volume should be measured. This only applies to drugs prescribed in milligrams or micrograms per hour or minute, and for most of these agents, such as dopamine, dobutamine, and glyceryl trinitrate, the infusion rate is titrated to patient response.

As a general rule, up to 10% of the nominal volume of the infusion bag or bottle may be added without overfilling the container. If larger volumes of drug solution are to be added to an infusion then fluid should be removed from the bag before addition. This practice may also be preferable if the infusion is administered over a precise time scale and may

prevent unwittingly discarding any active treatment. It is essential to ensure thorough mixing of all additives to infusion fluids in order to avoid the danger of a patient receiving a potentially fatal bolus dose of a medication that is intended to be administered well-diluted over a protracted period. Potassium chloride is a particular problem in this respect, but the widespread manufacture of infusions already containing the electrolyte have largely removed this hazard. Complete mixing is mandatory between each addition when making multiple additions to one bag to prevent incompatibility problems arising (for example, calcium and phosphate additions). Once the additive process is complete, it is advisable to place a sealing cap over the additive port on the infusion bag to prevent further additions at ward level that may not be compatible.

INTRAVENOUS DRUG DELIVERY

Adult Patients

In the majority of adult patients requiring intravenous therapy, the medication is administered either by bolus injection directly into the vein, by bolus injection via the additive port of an established intravenous line, or by intermittent infusion using a 'piggyback' system. Critically ill patients frequently require intravenous medication as a continuous infusion where flow control is achieved by use of infusion pumps. Many of these are potent cardiac drugs and their use must be individualised in respect of patient body-weight, dose rate, and method of infusion. Standardised charts can be constructed for drugs such as dopamine, dobutamine, and glyceryl trinitrate to facilitate rapid, easy, and accurate dosage calculations (see Table 2).

Table 2

Dopamine hydrochloride 800 mg/500 mL [as Intropin^{TM}] infusion rate (microdrops/minute); 60 paediatric microdrops/minute = 15 standard drops/minute = 1 mL/minute

		Body-weight (kg)								
		30	40	50	60	70	80	90	100	110	120
Dosage µg/kg/min	2	2	3	4	5	5	6	7	8	9	9
	5	6	8	10	12	14	16	18	20	21	23
	10	12	16	20	23	27	31	35	39	43	47
	15	18	23	29	35	41	47	53	58	64	70
	20	23	31	39	47	55	62	70	78	86	94
	25	29	39	49	58	68	78	88	97	107	117
	30	35	47	58	70	82	94	105	117		
	35	41	55	68	82	96	109				
	40	47	62	78	94	109					
	45	53	70	88	105	Use a more concentrated solution					
	50	59	78	97	117	(for example, 1600 mg/500 mL)					

Paediatric and Neonatal Patients

The administration of small volumes of intravenous drugs to neonates and children poses particular problems. The principal difficulty is that of ensuring that the patient actually receives the entire dose prescribed. The injection system may trap a substantial proportion of the drug, thus resulting in underdosing. In order to overcome this problem many units institute flushing procedures but this can result in the patient being administered large amounts of additional, often unprescribed, fluid. The use of injection ports with minimal dead-space is an important factor in reducing the need for flushing procedures.

Extension sets added to existing intravenous lines for the administration of intermittent infusions may require priming to ensure accurate dosing. This is standard practice in many neonatal units particularly for constant 24-hour infusions, where the syringe driver can be programmed to deliver a precise dose. If the extension set has been primed, it must be removed after the infusion of each drug to ensure that no extra drug is inadvertently administered. The use of primed needles for the administration of very small doses to neonates is described under Measurement of Doses above.

There is a perception that doses of intravenous drugs injected via the additive port or extension set enter the patient's circulation rapidly. However, the time before the patient actually receives the drug may be delayed, particularly in neonates and children. This time is determined by the distance between the drug injection site and the patient, the diameter of the tubing, the base infusion rate, and the volume of injected drug.

Infusion Administration

There is a vast array of administration sets available for use in special circumstances, but the majority of crystalloid fluids are administered through a **standard infusion set** specified in British Standard 2463:Part 2:1989. This consists of a hard plastic spike for introducing into the fluid container, the semi-rigid drip chamber that provides a standard drop size (20 drops/mL for adult sets and 60 drops/mL for paediatric sets) and aids visible flow rate monitoring, and a flexible polyvinyl chloride delivery tube to the patient that incorporates a resealing injection 'flash' or sleeve for bolus drug dosing. Some chambers have an integral 15 micrometre membrane filter. Flow is controlled manually using a roller clamp in the patient line but manufacturers market sets with a wide variety of sophis-

ticated flow restrictors in an attempt to give consistent flow during the whole period of administration. Since flow rate can be greatly influenced by viscosity, temperature, and fluid pressure (height above the patient) with these systems, investment in a low-cost peristaltic pump using standard sets is likely to give better flow control for a wider range of fluids.

Another commonly used set consists of two spikes and drip chambers with independent flow controllers, connected to a single patient line and known as a **Y-set**. These are principally used for 'piggybacking' small volume (50 to 100 mL) intermittent infusions of antibiotics or drugs requiring similar small-volume administration.

In paediatric practice, **volumetric sets** are used that incorporate a graduated 100mL to 200mL vented reservoir between the spike and the 60 drops/mL drip chamber. This allows the reservoir to be filled with a precise measure from the bulk infusion bag, which can then be clamped off but recharged as required. The reservoir can be used for mixing and delivering intermittent drug doses.

In-line Filtration

Filters of various sizes (0.22 to 5.0 micrometres pore size) have been attached to administration sets to reduce the risk of particulate contamination and subsequent embolus formation or thrombophlebitis.[10] It has been argued that adding a 0.22 micrometre membrane filter to high-cost cassette pump administration sets (see below) can safely extend their useful life from 24 to 72 hours.

Infusion Control

For simple gravity flow systems, flow rate depends upon the physical characteristics of fluid and administration set and any in-line flow control device such as a roller or screw clamp. In terms of volume, most fluids used in hospitals are simple, low-viscosity solutions for salt and water replacement and the standard intravenous administration set with in-line manually operated clamp provides adequate flow control.

There are, however, some situations that do require precise control of fluid or drug delivery, for example, in intensive care, neonatology, surgery, and oncology. In these circumstances, there is a vast array of electromechanical pumps, controllers, and syringe drivers available and selection depends on the complexity of control required and the volume to be delivered. A range of currently available high technology infusion devices have been described.[11–13] Detailed evaluations of this type of equipment have also been carried out by the Department of Health, Medical Devices Directorate.[14]

High technology, high-cost flow-control devices are often used when low technology, low-cost equipment would have satisfied the application criteria. It is, therefore, important that audit systems are established to monitor device selection and use, in order to avoid unnecessary capital investment or waste in customised administration sets.

Devices for controlling large volume infusions are usually designed to deliver 1 to 9999 mL at flow rates of 1 to 999 mL/hour. Large volume devices for paediatric use usually deliver 0.1 to 999.9 mL at 0.1 to 99.9 mL/hour.

The **infusion controller** is the simplest device and relies on gravity for fluid movement, but applies variable constriction to an administration set depending on a preselected drop rate. Ideally, such devices should accept a standard fluid administration set and have the drop rate control calibrated in volume per hour. Drop rate is monitored by a photo-electric mechanism across the administration set drop chamber and translated into a mechanical restriction via an electronically controlled solenoid or screw. Flow rate is dependent on fluid height and viscosity.

Infusion pumps (see Fig. 1) can be divided into two categories: those that move fluid by rotary or linear peristalsis and those that move fluid by a piston and valve mechanism (cassette pump). Flow rates are not dependent on fluid height or viscosity and these devices are generally used for drug delivery or parenteral nutrition.

Rotary peristaltic pumps propel the fluid by a rotary cam pressing along a resilient rubber (usually silicone) or plastic tube. The **linear peristaltic pump** has finger-like projections arranged in a straight line pressing sequentially along a similar length of resilient tube. Standard sets can be used with some peristaltic pumps but many require specially designed sets. Most of these pumps also monitor drop rate. The **cassette pump** uses an elaborate disposable unit consisting of a small piston and a chamber that fills and empties sequentially, thereby delivering a precise volume of fluid. All these pumps have microchip electronics and the most sophisticated can be programmed to control several infusions at different rates, to increase or decrease (ramping) the infusion rate, and to provide

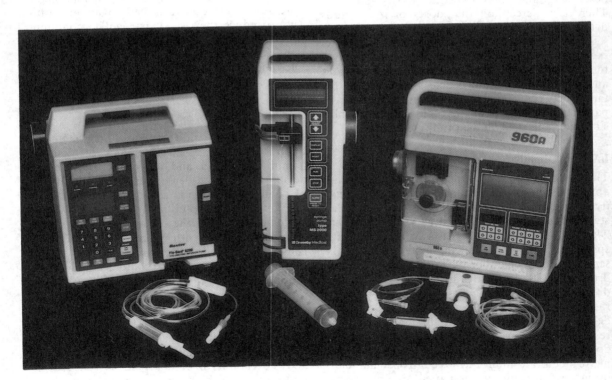

Fig. 1
Infusion controllers: left, peristaltic pump; centre, syringe driver; right, cassette type pump.

Table 3
General features of infusion controllers and pumps

Power supply	Mains and rechargeable battery backup
Low risk infusion devices	Usually controllers and some linear peristaltic pumps. Should accept a standard infusion set (adult 20 drops/mL, paediatric 60 drops/mL)
High risk infusion devices	Usually peristaltic or cassette pumps with greater precision and complex programming capacity
Alarms	A comprehensive range of alarms including set incorrectly loaded, drop detector failure, occlusion, air in line, equipment malfunction, end of infusion, pump on hold, low battery. Alarms should be visual and audible
Display	LED or back-lit LCD with memory. Displays may provide complex descriptive alarm messages and include volume to be infused, volume infused, and flow rate
Flow rates	0.1 to 99.9 mL/hour (paediatric) 1 to 999 mL/hour (adult)
Volume to be infused	0.1 to 999.9 mL (paediatric) 1 to 9999 mL (adult)
Administration sets	Standard or specific to pump
Pole mounted	
Standards	Should comply with BS5724 for electrical safety

Table 4
General features of syringe drivers

Power supply	Mains and rechargeable battery backup
Alarms	A comprehensive range of alarms including empty syringe, end of timed infusion, equipment malfunction, occlusion, pump switched off or rate changed during infusion, mains off, low battery. Alarms should be visual and audible.
Display	LED or back-lit LCD with memory
Syringes accepted	Various sizes of British Standard design
Flow rate indicator	0.1 to 99.9 mL
Volume to be infused indicator	0.1 to 99.9 mL
Volume infused indicator	0.1 to 99.9 mL
Stated occlusion pressure	Specified by manufacturer (in mmHg)
Pole or bench mounting facility	Very small volume battery operated devices can be strapped to the patient
Standards	Should comply with BS5724 for electrical safety

intermittent dose delivery. The cost of the disposable components should be carefully considered when selecting such pumps. Table 3 lists the general features of large-volume controllers and pumps.

Devices for controlling small volume infusions are usually designed to deliver 0.1 to 99.9 mL at flow rates of 0.1 to 99.9 mL/hour. The **syringe driver** (see Fig.1) is the most commonly used small volume infusion controller. Ideally, they should accept any disposable syringe manufactured to British Standard 5081:Part 1:1987. The syringe plunger is moved by a motor driven screw, the motor speed determining the rate of infusion. The majority are mains or battery operated, but small clockwork syringe drivers are available for low risk applications. Some syringe drivers can be controlled by the patient to deliver intermittent doses (prescriber controlled bolus and fixed infusion period) of opioid analgesics; this is often referred to as patient controlled analgesia (PCA). Battery driven pocket-sized peristaltic pumps are available, which utilise pharmacy-filled disposable cassettes as the drug reservoir. The main features of syringe drivers are listed in Table 4.

The **elastomeric infusion system** (see Fig. 2) is a sterile, single-use device consisting of a rigid plastic vessel housing an elastomeric sack or balloon. When filled, the elasticity of the reservoir exerts a constant pressure and forces the medication through a fixed-orifice flow restrictor that controls flow rate. Since the exerted pressure is relatively low, fluid viscosity and temperature may affect flow rate. A 1.2 micrometre membrane filter is usually incorporated into the delivery line, which connects to the percutaneous catheter. Systems are available with reservoir volumes of 50 to 200 mL and flow rates of 50 to 200 mL/hour. The units are small and completely portable and do not require a power source. The reservoirs are filled aseptically. The major advantages of these systems are their simplicity and suitability for home care where they can be connected intermittently to an indwelling cannula for administration of antibiotics or chemotherapy. Manufacturers supply drug compatibility details with their products.

Novel infusion control devices currently under investigation include implantable devices capable of delivering drugs at rates from 0.001 to 10 mL/hour. Pumps are of similar size to, or smaller than, cardiac pacemakers and use either battery-powered peristaltic action, evaporation and condensation of a volatile gas, or pressure exerted by osmosis through a semi-permeable membrane as the drug delivery driving force. The more sophisticated devices can be programmed to change flow rate using magnetic field telemetry, via a telephone link.

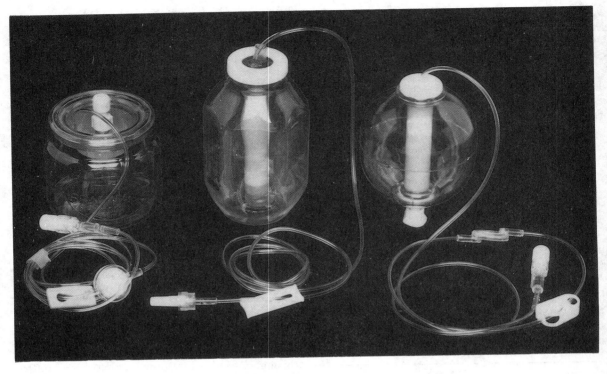

Fig. 2
Elastomeric infusion devices: left, Imed-Kabi; centre, Baxter Healthcare; right, Block-Fresenius.

Most devices are being used experimentally and applications in regional drug delivery are being increasingly identified.[15] Recharging with drug can be carried out through an implanted port and driving power can be available for more than twelve months. The continuing developments in microprocessor research ensure the continuing miniaturisation of drug delivery systems.[16, 17]

Syringes, Needles, Cannulae, and Catheters

Disposable hypodermic syringes, needles, cannulae, and catheters are constructed from physiologically inert materials, which may be radio-opaque in the case of cannulae and catheters, generally to specifications described in the appropriate British Standards. The dimensions and colour codes of commonly used needles, cannulae, and catheters are provided in Table 5. They are usually sterilised in the final packaging by gamma-irradiation, or with ethylene oxide gas.

Manufacturers should comply with good manufacturing practice for sterile medical devices and surgical products.[18]

The construction and performance of hypodermic **syringes** is described in British Standard 5081:Part 1:1987. They consist of a polypropylene barrel and a rubber piston attached to a plunger (three parts). Other suitable materials may be used for construction and should be compatible with most drug formulations. Two-part syringes are available where the piston and plunger are moulded as an integral unit from the same material. Amber coloured syringes that block more than 90% light transmission are also available. Common sizes are 2 mL, 5 mL, 10 mL, 20 mL, 30 mL, 50 mL, and 60 mL. Graduation marks should not be removed by spirit-based disinfectants.

Most hypodermic **needles** are of the single-use type (disposable) and are widely used for injection and aseptic manipulation. Needles are manufactured from a thin-walled stainless steel tube with moulded plastic hub and comply with British Standard 5081:Part 2:1987. Needles generally have a double bevel point, the longest bevel being 12°. Hubs are Luer fitting and are described in British Standard 3930:Part 1:1987 with a 6% taper. They are commonly referred to by gauge size, but package labels should indicate the wire gauge and length (Imperial) and metric dimensions with a colour coded flash defined in British Standard 7128:1989.

Table 5
Commonly used needles, cannulae, and catheters

SWG* Number	Nominal dimensions (external) mm	Nominal dimensions (length) mm	Colour code[†]	Usual use
Needles				
19G	1.0	40	cream	transfer needle
20G	0.9	25, 40	yellow	IV
21G	0.8	25, 40, 50	green	IM, blood collection
22G	0.7	25, 30, 40	black	IV
23G	0.6	25, 30	blue	IV, IM children
25G	0.5	12, 16	orange	SC, IM children
26G	0.45	12	brown	SC
IV cannulae				
14G	2.0	50		
16G	1.6	50		} adult
18G	1.2	45		
20G	0.9	30		
22G	0.7	25		} paediatric
24G	0.55	20		
IV catheters				
14G	2.0	150, 180, 200, 250, 300		
16G	1.6	150, 180, 200, 250, 300		} adult
17G	1.4	250		
18G	1.2	180, 250		} paediatric
20G	0.9	80		

*SWG = Standard Wire Gauge
[†]Cannulae and catheter hubs are colour coded according to external diameter but may not follow the convention in BS7128 for needles.

Intravenous **cannulae** are constructed from poly(tetrafluoroethylene), ethylene tetrafluoroethylene copolymer, polyurethane, or similar inert extruded tube with a steel needle introducer that is removed once the cannula is in place. They are used to provide access to the vascular system for up to several days. The Luer-lock connection can have moulded plastic butterfly wings that aid placement and assist anchorage. Cannulae can be straight or ported, incorporating a side arm access consisting of a self-seal rubber diaphragm through which bolus doses of intravenous preparations can be administered. Construction and performance tests are specified in British Standard 4843:1987.

Catheters are of similar construction to cannulae, but are longer and may have more than one lumen allowing multiple drug or fluid delivery with pressure monitoring, which is often required in intensive care units. Catheters are used for long-term vascular access or delivering fluids to the large (non-peripheral) vessels. They may incorporate a guide wire, ultimately withdrawn, to assist placement of the catheter in the large vessels. Details of these catheters are described in British Standard 7174:Parts 1–3:1990.

Introducer needles are never reintro[duced while a] cannula or catheter is in place or p[...] since cannulae have been severed [...] hazardous loss of plastic into the [...] Short steel cannulae scalp vein set[s...nee]dles with a butterfly anchor on the hub and a l[ength] of fine-bore, plastic tube) are frequently used for short duration access in anaesthetics, dialysis, and chemotherapy. Consideration of the 'dead space' may be important with cannulae and catheters when very small volumes of drug are being administered and flushing is inappropriate. Selection of cannulae or catheter size depends on the size of the vein, and the required flow rates and viscosity of the fluid. The larger the diameter the greater the flow.

Novel presentations are available whereby needles or cannulae are resheathed automatically as the product is withdrawn from the injection site. These are designed to prevent needle-stick injuries and are advocated for use where infection risk is high.

The **'jet injector'** is a needleless gun-like device that uses compressed air to 'fire' a metered-dose of drug from a high pressure nozzle positioned on the skin at the point of injection. The drug reservoir is usually a multidose vial. They are used for mass vaccination programmes.

CHARACTERISTICS OF INFUSION FLUIDS

The main physicochemical characteristics of commonly used intravenous infusion solutions are summarised in Tables 6 and 7. Probably the most commonly used, and clinically relevant, parameter is that of osmotic activity. This is described by the terms osmolality, osmolarity, and isotonicity.

The concentrations of solute are most commonly expressed in terms of osmoles (osmol) or milliosmoles (mosmol). An osmole is equal to a mole of osmotically active particles, a milliosmole is one thousandth of this amount. The osmotic activity of a substance in solution depends only on the number of discrete particles dissolved. A millimole of sodium chloride that is nearly completely dissociated into sodium and chloride ions contributes 2 mosmol whereas for an unionised substance, such as glucose, 1 mmol is equal to 1 mosmol of the substance.

The **osmolality** of a solution is the number of osmoles of solute per kilogram of solvent. It is most often expressed as milliosmoles per kg when referring to body fluids. The **osmolarity** of a solution is the number of osmoles of solute per litre

Table 6
Physicochemical properties of commonly used intravenous fluids

Solution	pH (approx)	Osmolarity (mosmol/litre) (approx)	Indication	Caution
Compound Sodium Lactate Intravenous Infusion BP (Hartmann's Solution; Ringer-Lactate Solution)	6	278	Replacement of extracellular fluid volume. Lactate is converted to bicarbonate in the blood; has a limited value in restoration of the body's buffering capacity	Patients with impairment of lactate utilisation eg severe liver damage or respiratory alkalosis As for sodium infusions
Glucose Intravenous Infusion BP 5%	4	278	Replacement of water loss	Excessive infusion may lead to water intoxication
Glucose Intravenous Infusion BP 10% 15% 20% 30% 40%	4 4 4 4 4	555 833 1110 1665 2220	Hypoglycaemic coma, energy supplementation and parenteral nutrition	Glucose intolerance, hypertonic solutions may cause vein irritation and thrombophlebitis
Mannitol Intravenous Infusion BP 10% 20%	6 6	549 1098	Produces an osmotic diuresis which may be used in the treatment of conditions such as: oliguric phase of acute renal failure; raised intracranial pressure and cerebral oedema; elevated intraocular pressure	In patients with anuria, pulmonary oedema or congestion, dehydration, cardiac failure
Potassium Chloride 0.15% or 0.3% and Glucose 5% Intravenous Infusion BP	4.5 4.5	318 358	Replacement of water and potassium loss or prevention of potassium deficiency	Hyperkalaemia, renal impairment, glucose intolerance
Potassium Chloride 0.15% or 0.3% and Sodium Chloride 0.9% Intravenous Infusion BP	5.5 5.5	350 390	Replacement of fluid and electrolytes	Patient with cardiac failure, renal impairment, sodium retaining conditions and conditions when hyperkalaemia may be present
Potassium Chloride 0.15%, Sodium Chloride 0.18% and Glucose 4% Intravenous Infusion BP	4.5	322	As above with the addition of prevention or treatment of potassium deficiency	As for sodium glucose and and potassium infusions

Table 6—*Continued*

Solution	pH (approx)	Osmolarity (mosmol/litre) (approx)	Indication	Caution
Sodium Bicarbonate Intravenous Infusion BP 1.26% 1.45% 4.2% 8.4%		300 345 1000 2000	Metabolic acidosis correction	Sodium bicarbonate 4.2% and 8.4% are hypertonic and may cause vein damage and thrombophlebitis at the site of infusion
Sodium Chloride Intravenous Infusion BP 0.9%	5.5	308	Maintenance of ECF volume, replacement of ECF fluid loss	In patients with cardiac failure, renal impairment or other sodium-retaining conditions, prolonged infusion may lead to hyperchloraemic acidosis
Sodium Chloride Intravenous Infusion BP 0.45%	5.5	154	Hyperosmolar states, for example, hyperosmolar hyperglycaemic coma	Hypotonic solution
Sodium Chloride 0.18% and Glucose 4% Intravenous Infusion BP	4.5	284	Replacement of fluid and sodium where water exceeds sodium loss, or patient cannot tolerate sodium chloride 0.9% intravenous	As for sodium and glucose infusions
Sodium Chloride 0.45% and Glucose 2.5% Intravenous Infusion BP	4.5	293	Hydration regimens	As for sodium or glucose infusions
Sodium Chloride 0.45% and Glucose 5% Intravenous Infusion BP	4.5	432	Pyloric stenosis	

of solution and is, therefore, temperature dependent. This is expressed as milliosmoles per litre. Osmolality is approximately equal to osmolarity when considering dilute solutions but in concentrated solutions the solute mass may reach significance. Normal plasma osmolality is 280 to 295 mosmol/kg.

Tonicity refers to the tone of a living cell. A solution that is isotonic causes the cell to undergo neither a net gain nor loss of water. Hypertonicity is a consequence of an increased concentration of impermeable solutes resulting in movement of water from the cell causing cellular dehydration. Hypotonicity ensues from a decreased concentration of impermeable solutes resulting in movement of water into the cell causing cell swelling.

The terms isotonic and iso-osmotic are often used interchangeably although they are not synonymous. An iso-osmotic solution is one that has an osmolality equal to that of plasma, 280 to 295 mosmol/kg, hyperosmolality and hypo-osmolality having greater and lesser osmolality, respectively. It is possible to have hyperosmolality without hypertonicity in a patient with elevated blood urea.

The properties of isotonic and iso-osmotic solutions are covered in more detail in the Solution Properties chapter.

Clinical Aspects

Osmolality and tonicity assume great importance when considering intravenous infusion therapy.

Table 7
Formulation of commonly used intravenous fluids

Solution	Na^+	K^+	Ca^{2+}	Cl^-	HCO_3^-	glucose	
		(mmol/L)			g/L	kcal	
Compound Sodium Chloride (Ringer's)	147.5	4	2	156		—	—
Compound Sodium Lactate Intravenous Infusion BP (Hartmann's Solution, Ringer Lactate)	131	5	2	111	29*	—	—
Glucose Intravenous Infusion BP 5%	—	—	—	—	—	50	200
10%	—	—	—	—	—	100	400
15%	—	—	—	—	—	150	600
20%	—	—	—	—	—	200	800
30%	—	—	—	—	—	300	1200
40%	—	—	—	—	—	400	1600
50%	—	—	—	—	—	500	2000
Glucose 4% and Sodium Chloride 0.18% Intravenous Infusion BP	30	—	—	30	—	40	160
Potassium Chloride 0.15% and Glucose 5% Intravenous Infusion BP	—	20	—	20	—	50	200
Potassium Chloride 0.3% and Glucose 5% Intravenous Infusion BP	—	40	—	40	—	50	200
Potassium Chloride 0.15% and Sodium Chloride 0.9% Intravenous Infusion BP	150	20	—	170	—	—	—
Potassium Chloride 0.3% and Sodium Chloride 0.9% Intravenous Infusion BP	150	40	—	190	—	—	—
Potassium Chloride 0.15% or 0.3%, Sodium Chloride 0.18%, and Glucose 4% Intravenous Infusion BP	30	20	—	50	—	40	160
	30	40	—	70	—	40	160
Sodium Bicarbonate Intravenous Infusion BP 1.26%	150	—	—	—	150	—	—
1.4%	167	—	—	—	167	—	—
4.2%	500	—	—	—	500	—	—
8.4%	1000	—	—	—	1000	—	—
Sodium Chloride 0.9% Intravenous Infusion BP	150	—	—	150	—	—	—
Sodium Chloride 0.45% Intravenous Infusion BP	75	—	—	75	—	—	—
Sodium Chloride 0.45% and Glucose 2.5% Intravenous Infusion BP	75	—	—	75	—	25	100
Sodium Chloride 0.45% Glucose 5% Intravenous Infusion BP	75	—	—	75	—	50	200

*as lactate

Isotonic infusions include sodium chloride 0.9%, glucose 5%, and sodium chloride 0.18% and glucose 4%. These solutions are ideal for the peripheral route, although excessive infusion of iso-osmotic sodium chloride 0.9% may lead to increases in extracellular fluid volume causing circulatory overload in vulnerable groups of patients such as the elderly and the very young.

Hypotonic large volume parenteral solutions usually have their tonicity adjusted by the addition of sodium chloride or glucose to achieve an intravenous infusion fluid approximating to isotonicity. There are exceptions, for example, sodium chloride 0.45% (154 mosmol), a solution that is used for the treatment of dehydration especially in diabetic patients. If excessive amounts of hypotonic fluids are administered then swelling and haemolysis of erythrocytes may occur as well as water intoxication resulting in convulsions and oedema (particularly pulmonary oedema).

Infusion of hypertonic or hyperosmolar fluids can cause tissue irritation, pain on injection, phlebitis, and even necrosis if administered via the peripheral route. Historically, the general rule has been that any solution with an osmolarity greater than 800 mosmol should be administered via a central line where the blood flow is fast enough to ensure rapid dilution of the infused solution. Perhaps the most common example of hyperosmolar solutions being administered to patients is that of total parenteral nutrition (TPN). Because of the need for surgical placement of central catheters and the associated risk of infection, these hyperosmolar solutions are being given more frequently via a peripheral vein. The risks of phlebitis or local vein damage may be reduced by the addition of heparin and hydrocortisone to the TPN bag and by placing glyceryl trinitrate patches distal to the administration site. There is, however, controversy surrounding the addition of heparin and the destabilisation of the lipid emulsion in amino acid and fat mixtures.

Hyperosmotic fluids, such as sodium bicarbonate 8.4%, should ideally be diluted before administration and infused slowly to prevent thrombophlebitis, cellular dehydration, and crenation of erythrocytes. It is vital to ensure that infiltration does not occur as this will cause trauma and possibly tissue necrosis. It is now more common to use sodium bicarbonate 4.2% injection to treat metabolic acidosis.

REFERENCES

1. Hetherington C. Pharm J 1971;206:267–8.
2. Medicines Control Agency. Guidance to the NHS on the licensing requirements of the Medicines Act 1968. The Agency, 1992 Sept.
3. Tredree RL. Proc Guild Hosp Pharm 1982;15:20–37.
4. Brown AF, Harvey DA, Hoddinnott DJ, Britton KJ. Br J Parenter Ther 1986;7(2)42–4.

5. Hatton I, Christie G, Steventon S. Pharm J 1986;237:46–7.

6. Sewell GJ, Palmer AJ, Tidy PJ. Int J Pharmaceutics 1991;70:119–27.

7. Lee MG, Munton T, Haines-Nutt F, Thorn E, Jones K, Fenton-May V. Pharm J 1992;248(Suppl):HS36–9.

8. Longe RL. Canad Anaesth Soc J 1980;27(1):62–4.

9. Evans WE, Barker LF, Simone JV. Am J Hosp Pharm 1976;33:1160–3.

10. Allcutt DA, Lort D, McCollum CN. Br J Surg 1983;70:111–13.

11. Kwan JW. Am J Hosp Pharm 1989;46:320–35.

12. Kwan JW. Am J Hosp Pharm 1990;47(Suppl 1):S18–S23.

13. Kwan JW. Am J Hosp Pharm 1991;48(Suppl 1):S36–S51.

14. Department of Health and Social Security. Medical Devices Directorate. Evaluations. London: HMSO, 1992 March.

15. Selam JL. Hormone Metabolism Research 1990;24(Suppl):144–54.

16. Damascelli B, Bonalumi MG, Marchiano A, Spreafico C, Garbagnati F, Amadeo A et al. Eur J Radiol 1991;12:191–4.

17. Buchwald H, Rhode TD. Am Soc Artificial Int Org J 1992;38(Pt 4):772–8.

18. Department of Health and Social Security. Quality systems for sterile medical devices and surgical products—good manufacturing practice. London: HMSO, 1990.

FURTHER INFORMATION

Allwood M, Wright P, editors. The cytotoxics handbook. Oxford: Radcliffe Medical Press, 1990.

British Standards Institution. British Standard 7174:1990. Sterile intravascular catheters and ancillary devices for single use. Parts 1, 2, 3. London: The Institution, 1990.

British Standards Institution. British Standard 4843:1987. Sterile intravascular cannula units for single use. London: The Institution, 1987.

British Standards Institution. British Standard 2463:1989. Transfusion equipment for medical use. Parts 1, 2. London: The Institution, 1989.

British Standards Institution. British Standard 3930:1987. Conical fittings with a 6% (Luer) taper for syringes, needles and other medical equipment. Parts 1, 2. London: The Institution, 1987.

British Standards Institution. British Standard 5081:1987. Sterile hypodermic syringes and needles. Parts 1, 2. London: The Institution, 1987.

British Standards Institution. British Standard 7128:1989. Colour coding of hypodermic needles for single use. London: The Institution, 1989.

Trissel LA, editor. Handbook on injectable drugs. 7th ed. Bethesda: American Society of Hospital Pharmacists, 1992.

The stability of drugs in syringes and bags: a collaborative study by hospital quality control staff. Pharm J 1992;249(Suppl):HS20–21.

Paediatric Preparations

Specialised paediatric preparations are often required because of the problems encountered in the treatment of children. Children require their medicines to be palatable and in a form that they can readily accept. In addition, there are pharmacokinetic considerations: children, and neonates especially, absorb, distribute, metabolise, and eliminate drugs at different rates and by different pathways from those in adults. Doses of drugs required by children can vary over a wide range.

It is intended that this chapter should serve as a guide to the special problems associated with the formulation and presentation of medicines for children.

Dosage Forms used in Paediatric Medicine

Drugs may be administered to children using most of the dosage forms employed in adult therapeutics. The choice of dosage form is, however, dependent on the age and size of the child, as well as pharmaceutical factors.

Oral liquids are the most common dosage forms used in paediatrics because of their palatability and ease of administration. When a commercial preparation of the prescribed drug is not available, pharmacists are frequently called upon to prepare oral liquids extemporaneously. However, even when a suitable formulation has been developed, extemporaneous preparation is time-consuming and expensive, and consideration should be given to whether an alternative dosage form could be used. Solid oral dosage forms may be accepted by some children, particularly if **tablets** are crushed, or **capsules** are opened, and mixed with a pleasantly flavoured food or drink. Jam, honey, apple sauce, ice cream, and fruit juice have all been used with success. Some parenteral preparations may also be suitable for administration by the oral route. However, it is important that modified-release tablets should not be crushed.

Formulation

The formulation of preparations for paediatric use is complicated by the low doses required and by the greater need for patient acceptability. In addition, concern about the inclusion of additives in medicines imposes further constraints on the development of formulations. For a detailed discussion of the formulation of specific dosage forms, see the relevant chapters.

Excipients

An increased awareness, among members of the medical and allied professions and the general public, of the undesirable properties of certain excipients has resulted in a reduction in their use in paediatric medicines. Azo dyes, benzyl alcohol, chloroform, ethanol, lactose, propylene glycol, saccharin, sucrose, and sulphites have all been the subject of much criticism. The American Academy of Pediatrics have considered the safety of excipients in medicines.[1]

Colouring Agents. Although the correlation of the inclusion of azo dyes in preparations with the onset of hyperactivity in children is unproven, these substances should be avoided if at all possible. There are several natural colouring agents available and the suitability of these should be assessed before considering the use of an azo dye. Oral liquid preparations in the *British Pharmacopoeia* have been amended to 'open formulae', thus allowing the omission of tartrazine if required. For further information on colouring agents, see the Oral Liquids chapter.

Ethanol. It is desirable to reduce the ingestion of ethanol by children to a minimum. Any ethanol that is not required for the maintenance of the chemical or physical stability of a product should be omitted. It should not be necessary to include ethanol as a preservative in any system, as more acceptable and effective preservatives are available. However, paediatric mixtures do exist in which the inclusion of ethanol is essential; for example, Phenobarbitone Elixir BP, in which ethanol is included because of the poor water solubility of phenobarbitone. Many hospital pharmacies produce ethanol-free phenobarbitone mixtures but the long-term stability of these products is poor.

Chloroform. The Medicines (Chloroform Prohibition) Order 1979. SI1979 No382 imposed a general restriction on the sale or supply of medicinal products (for internal human use) that contain chloroform at a concentration greater than 0.5%, the intention being to confine chloroform use solely to that of a preservative. This action followed the presentation of evidence that suggested that chloroform may be carcinogenic.

The decision as to whether chloroform is suitable for use in oral products for children and neonates rests with the formulator who must consider the circumstances in which the preparation will be administered. Factors to consider are the dose to be given, the frequency of administration, and the condition of the patient. Preservatives, other than chloroform, suitable for oral ingestion are discussed in the chapters entitled Control of Microbial Contamination and the Preservation of Medicines, and Oral Liquids.

Sugars. Syrup *BP*, containing sucrose, is one of the most widely used diluents for oral liquid formulations; it is used to increase palatability, to aid formulation, and (to a limited extent) to minimise microbial contamination. However, sugar in medicines has been implicated as a causative factor in dental caries and considerable pressure has been brought to bear on the pharmaceutical industry to produce **sugar-free** medicines. Paediatric preparations should contain as little sugar as possible; this is particularly important with medicines that are to be taken over a prolonged period. Alternatives to sucrose do exist but they have disadvantages. Glucose, fructose, and lactose are fermentable and thus could also cause caries. Sorbitol and mannitol are expensive and may cause diarrhoea. Saccharin is used occasionally but it leaves a bitter aftertaste and concern has been expressed about its safety after reports of carcinogenicity in animal tests. However, it is generally accepted that this is not applicable to saccharin used as a sweetener in man. Aspartame has gained acceptance by the food industry, but information on its use in pharmaceuticals is not readily available. Other sweeteners that have been tried but rejected for various reasons are cyclamates, dulcin, protein sweeteners, and ammonium glycyrrhizinate. Clinical trials of the natural substance xylitol have shown that ingestion of relatively small quantities (7 to 10 g in chewing gum; additional to the normal diet) each day, reduces the incidence of dental caries in children. Xylitol inhibits the growth of *Streptococcus mutans*, one of the main organisms that cause acid attack. Xylitol is not fermented by micro-organisms and does not give rise to acid formation. Xylitol also reduces the amount of plaque formed and is thought to aid remineralisation of teeth by increasing the production of saliva. The full benefit of the protective effects of xylitol are only obtained when it is in contact with the teeth over a prolonged period; this would not occur if xylitol was included as a sweetening agent in a paediatric preparation. Xylitol, although an effective sweetener, is expensive and unlikely, at least in the near future, to be a viable alternative to sucrose. A more detailed discussion of sweetening agents is given in the Oral Liquids chapter.

Lactose. Lactose is used as a diluent or filler in tablets and capsules and as a bulking agent for powders. Lactose should be excluded from any formulation intended for administration to children with lactase deficiency.

Formulations for Neonates

Excipients should be used cautiously in medicines for neonates, particularly premature babies. Ideally, preparations should be free of preservatives; this is especially important when large or frequent doses are to be administered. It may be necessary to prepare the medicine as sterilised unit doses. Flavouring agents may not be necessary, as the sense of taste is not fully developed at birth, and colouring agents have little influence on neonates and should be excluded.

Osmolality of Paediatric Preparations

Hypertonic oral and injectable preparations can produce side-effects in young children. It has been reported that a preterm infant developed necrotising enterocolitis after the administration of an oral calcium supplement with an osmolality of 2000 mosmol/kg.[2] Pain and phlebitis have been reported after injection of products with an osmolality greater than 600 mosmol/kg.[3] According to Leff and Roberts,[4] oral mixtures for administration to the newborn should have an osmolality not exceeding 460 mosmol/kg and injectable preparations should have an osmolality not exceeding 600 mosmol/kg. Preparations of high osmolality should be diluted before being administered to neonates and should be labelled accordingly. A more detailed discussion of osmolality is given in the Solution Properties chapter.

Preparation of Paediatric Medicines

Frequently, the only source of a drug is a proprietary preparation intended for administration to adults. Points to be considered when using these preparations to produce paediatric medicines include the following:

- In the absence of solubility and stability data, risks are taken when commercially available solid dosage forms are used to formulate liquid medicines.

- The concentration of active ingredient in a liquid-filled capsule is unpredictable, owing to migration of the vehicle or the active ingredients through the capsule shell.
- Most dry powder injections are formulated such that on reconstitution an adult dose is contained in the vial. Errors can occur if due attention is not given to the displacement volume of the powder[1,2] when calculating the volume of diluent to add when preparing a paediatric dose.

Displacement values and information on reconstitution of a range of powder injections are listed in the Miscellaneous Data chapter.

Several official paediatric preparations exist. In addition, formularies are published by children's hospitals in the United Kingdom and elsewhere giving details of formulations developed and used in these hospitals. The amount of stability data available for these formulations varies considerably. Details of several hospital formularies are given in the Further Information section at the end of this chapter. Many manufacturers are prepared to produce paediatric preparations as special orders.

Presentation and Labelling

It is desirable that the label should state that the product is for paediatric use.

Comments have appeared in the literature concerning the lack of information provided on labels about the reconstitution of dry powder formulations. It is desirable that full instructions on reconstitution for a wide dosage range be available. The availability of such information enables drugs to be administered to children more safely.

Extemporaneously prepared oral medicines should be packaged in amber glass bottles and labelled 'Store in a refrigerator', unless stability studies indicate otherwise. A conservative expiry date should be assigned. Suspensions must be well shaken before removal of each dose and should be labelled accordingly.

Administration of Oral Medicines to Children

When the dose of an oral liquid medicine is not 5 mL, or a multiple of 5 mL, and an appropriate measuring device is not supplied by the manufacturer, a 5-mL plastic oral syringe should be provided along with a bottle adaptor and an instruction leaflet. This policy was introduced following the abolition of the dilution convention in July 1992. The convention was abandoned for three main reasons:

- the increased incidence of dental caries in children on long-term medication
- the problems associated with the administration of relatively large volumes of oral liquids to neonates
- the reduced physicochemical stability of diluted oral liquid medicines.

Oral syringes should comply with British Standard 3221:Part 7:1986, or an equivalent European standard. The syringes are graduated at intervals of 0.5 mL and numbered at intervals of 1 mL. The leaflet issued with the oral syringe gives instruction on measuring and administering the dose, and on dismantling and washing the syringe and bottle adaptor.

Unpalatable medicines may be mixed with a favourite food or drink to render them more acceptable, but this should only be done immediately before administration.

Paediatric Dosage Calculation

Ideally, children's doses should be determined after extensive clinical studies; however, because of ethical difficulties, this is rarely possible.

Children cannot be thought of merely as small adults: they absorb, distribute, metabolise, and eliminate drugs differently at the various stages in their development. Concurrent disease processes may also affect the dose of a drug required to attain a therapeutic effect.

In the absence of clinical data, formulae exist for estimating a child's dose from the adult dose. Three of the most widely used formulae have been:

Young's rule

$$\text{Child's dose} = \frac{\text{age}}{\text{age} + 12} \times \text{adult dose}$$

Clark's rule

$$\text{Child's dose} = \frac{\text{weight (kg)}}{70} \times \text{adult dose}$$

Dilling's rule

$$\text{Child's dose} = \frac{\text{age}}{20} \times \text{adult dose}$$

However, it is recognised that a more accurate assessment of drug dosage can be made by using the surface area of the child in the calculation:

$$\text{Child's dose} = \frac{\text{surface area (m}^2)}{\text{surface area of adult}} \times \text{adult dose}$$
$$(1.8\,\text{m}^2)$$

To use this formula a knowledge of the child's weight and height is required; Catzel and Oliver[5] produced a table that gives the percentage of the adult dose required over a range of ages and weights. These figures are based on children of average height and weight.

The percentage method given by the *British National Formulary* may be used to calculate paediatric doses of commonly prescribed drugs that have a wide margin between the therapeutic and toxic dose.

Table 1
The percentage method for the calculation of paediatric doses

Age	Ideal body-weight kg	lb	Height cm	in	Body-surface m^2	Percentage of adult dose
Newborn*	3.4	7.5	50	20	0.23	12.5
1 month*	4.2	9	55	22	0.26	14.5
3 months*	5.6	12	59	23	0.32	18
6 months	7.7	17	67	26	0.40	22
1 year	10	22	76	30	0.47	25
3 years	14	31	94	37	0.62	33
5 years	18	40	108	42	0.73	40
7 years	23	51	120	47	0.88	50
12 years	37	81	148	58	1.25	75
Adult						
Male	68	150	173	68	1.8	100
Female	56	123	163	64	1.6	100

*The figures relate to full term and not preterm infants who may need reduced dosage according to their clinical condition.

If the dose of a drug is calculated by each of the above formulae, considerable differences will be found. It is for the prescriber to decide which to use and for the pharmacist to be aware that any of the formulae may have been used. Whichever method is employed, the need to modify the dose as response and blood-drug concentrations are monitored should be recognised.

Several paediatric dosage guides exist and these are an invaluable aid for the pharmacist. A list is given below in the Further Information section.

REFERENCES

1. American Academy of Pediatrics. Committee on Drugs. Pediatrics 1985;76:635.
2. Congdon PJ, Lloyd CA, Lindsay P, Cooke J. J Clin Hosp Pharm 1982;7:127–30.
3. Leff RD, Roberts RJ. Am J Hosp Pharm 1982;39:468.
4. Leff RD, Roberts RJ. Am J Hosp Pharm 1987;44:865–70.
5. Catzel P, Oliver R. The paediatric prescriber. 5th ed. Oxford: Blackwell, 1981:8.

FURTHER INFORMATION

Anderson SA. A formulary of paediatric preparations. London: Guild of Hospital Pharmacists/ASTMS, 1978.

Caro J, Dombrowski SR, Elliot S, editors. Handbook on extemporaneous formulations. Bethesda: American Society of Hospital Pharmacists, 1987.

Evans K. Paediatric radiopharmacy. In: Sampson CB, editor. Textbook of radiopharmacy. Theory and practice. New York: Gordon and Breach, 1990:347–61.

Green M, editor. Harriet Lane handbook. 12th ed. Chicago: Year Book Medical, 1990.

Insley J, Wood B, editors. Paediatric vade-mecum. 12th ed. London: Lloyd Luke, 1990.

Intravenous preparations. In: Ford DC, Leist ER, Phelps SJ. Guidelines for the administration of intravenous medications to pediatric patients. 3rd ed. American Society of Hospital Pharmacists, 1988.

McCrea J, Rappaport P, Stansfield S, Baker D, Lee Dupuis L, James G. Extemporaneous oral liquid dosage preparations. Toronto: Canadian Society of Hospital Pharmacists, 1988.

Milap C, Nahata C, Hipple TF. Pediatric drug formulations. Cincinnati: Harvey Whitney, 1990.

Paediatric formulary. 2nd ed. Lewisham and North Southwark Health Authority, 1990.

Radiopharmaceuticals

Radiopharmaceuticals are medicinal products that are radioactive. They are used for both diagnosis and therapy, principally in the branch of medicine known as Nuclear Medicine. Radiopharmaceuticals vary from inorganic salts to large organic molecules and complexes, and are prepared in a variety of presentations which include intravenous injections, gases, aerosols, oral solutions and capsules. Radiopharmaceuticals which contain radionuclides with long half-lives are obtained from commercial suppliers. However, as the majority of radiopharmaceuticals in clinical use contain radionuclides with short half-lives, commercial supply is often impractical and such products are prepared in hospital radiopharmacies. The content of this chapter reflects the fact that this represents the largest area of radiopharmaceutical work.

RADIATION PHYSICS

Structure of the Atom

An atom comprises a central nucleus surrounded by a number of negatively charged electrons spinning in orbits. Most of the naturally occurring elements have a stable nucleus which consists of protons and neutrons in about equal numbers. Each proton has a mass of one atomic unit and a positive charge equal but opposite to that on an electron. Neutrons also have a mass of one atomic unit but no charge. In a neutral atom, the number of electrons is equal to the number of protons. The mass of the electron is approximately 1/2000 part of that of either the proton or neutron; the major part of the mass of the atom is therefore in the nucleus.

The chemical identity of an atom is determined by the number of protons in the nucleus; this provides the **atomic number** (Z). The mass of an atom is the sum of the number of protons and neutrons in the nucleus and is termed the **mass number** (A). To describe a nuclide the nomenclature used is $^A_Z E$, where E is the chemical symbol. In practice, when referring to a radionuclide, the atomic number (Z) is not shown.

While the number of protons in the nuclei of all atoms of an element is identical, the number of neutrons varies. In nature, elements mostly occur as constant mixtures of atoms with various configurations. Thus, although the atomic mass of any atom must be a whole number, this proviso need not apply to the atomic mass (average) of an element. These different nuclear arrangements of an element are known as **isotopes**. All isotopic forms of an element (including the radioactive ones) are chemically undistinguishable, and the nuclear radiation from each radionuclide has characteristic properties.

Nuclei of an isotope which contain fewer or more neutrons than protons may be unstable. An isotope with unstable nuclei is known as a radioisotope. Since each atomic species is a nuclide, radioactive atomic species are known as radionuclides. Any radionuclide tends to change into a more stable configuration by the process known as radioactive decay. In order to assume a stable state, the nucleus of the radionuclide must either capture an orbital electron and lose its excess energy or lose a charged particle. The charged particles and the energy emitted by a nucleus undergoing transformation are termed nuclear radiation. The resulting nucleus has a lower energy content than that of its parent (radioactive) nucleus. Energy lost from the nucleus appears as the energy of the emitted radiation.

Radioactive Decay

Radionuclides decay in various ways which depend on their initial structure. Whatever its structure any given radionuclide disintegrates at a constant rate and the time taken for conversion of one half of the number of atoms originally present is known as the physical half-life ($t_{1/2}$). Each radionuclide has a characteristic physical half-life which can range in value from fractions of a second to many years. Most radionuclides used in medicine have half-lives in the range of minutes to months.

Certain radionuclides of high mass number decay by emission of alpha particles (α). These particles consist of two neutrons and two protons and hence have a mass of four atomic units and carry two units of positive charge. The alpha particle is identical to the nucleus of the helium atom. Following decay by alpha emission, the atomic number of an atom is reduced by 2 and the mass number by 4.

Many radionuclides decay by emission of beta particles (β). Each particle carries a single unit of charge of either sign and has a mass equal to that of an electron. A negative beta particle, denoted by the symbol β^-, is therefore identical to the electron. The positive beta particle, known as the positron, is denoted by the symbol β^+ Normally, negative beta decay occurs in atoms with an excess of neutrons and results in the conversion of a neutron into a proton. The atomic number of the atom is therefore increased by 1 while the mass number remains unchanged. Positive beta decay normally occurs when there is an excess of protons in the nucleus and a proton is effectively converted into a neutron. In this instance, the atomic number of the atom is reduced by 1 while the mass number remains unchanged.

Some radionuclides with nuclei which contain an excess of protons decay by electron capture. An electron from the innermost shell (the K shell) is captured by the nucleus where a proton is converted into a neutron. When the missing K-shell electron is subsequently replaced by a free electron, the energy loss due to this action results in the emission of an X-ray which is characteristic of the product atom.

Radioactive decay is frequently accompanied by the emission from the nucleus of electromagnetic radiation which carries away the excess energy that has not been removed by the particulate radiation. These emissions are known as gamma rays (γ). A metastable radionuclide (designated by m either after the mass number or to the top right of the chemical symbol) differs from a more stable state only in having a slight excess of energy; it decays by the emission of a gamma ray.

The most common example of a metastable radionuclide is technetium-99m (^{99m}Tc) which decays to ^{99}Tc. This decay process is called isomeric transition.

Nuclear Radiations

Alpha radiation consists of alpha particles. As a result of their relatively large charge and mass, alpha particles have very limited penetrating power. The dense ionisation that they produce results in a high rate of tissue damage; alpha-emitters are not used routinely in radiopharmaceuticals.

Beta radiation consists of beta particles. Beta radiation is more penetrating than alpha radiation but its range is relatively short. A high energy β^- particle such as that from phosphorus-32 (^{32}P), with an energy of 1.7 MeV, has a range in water of 7 mm, while in contrast, a tritium (^{3}H) β^- particle with an energy of 18 keV has a range of only

0.007 mm. When a β^- particle comes to rest, it becomes a free electron and joins the population of free electrons in the same region. However, as a positron (β^+) comes to rest, it unites with a free negative electron and both particles are destroyed to produce two gamma ray quanta of equal energy emitted in opposite directions. This process is known as annihilation and the gamma rays are known as annihilation radiation. Because positron emitters all have annihilation energy photons of 511 keV in their emissions this property is used in a specialised imaging technique known as positron emission tomography (PET). Radiopharmaceuticals which contain beta (β^-)-emitting radionuclides such as iodine-131 (^{131}I) are used commonly in radiotherapy whereas radiopharmaceuticals containing positron-emitting radionuclides such as fluorine-18 (^{18}F) are used predominantly in imaging procedures.

Gamma radiation consists of quanta of electromagnetic radiation known as photons whose energy is characteristic of their radionuclidic source. Photons are uncharged and can be highly penetrating. Radiopharmaceuticals containing gamma-emitting radionuclides such as ^{99m}Tc are most commonly used in imaging procedures.

X-rays are physically identical to gamma rays, the only distinction being that gamma rays emanate from a nucleus which is undergoing a transformation whereas X-rays are produced either as a result of the replacement of inner shell electrons or, as in the case of an X-ray machine, by causing a beam of electrons to strike a target. Thallium-201 (^{201}Tl) is a radionuclide which emits X-rays and which is incorporated in a radiopharmaceutical.

Radiation Units and Definitions

Activity

The activity of a radioactive source is the number of nuclear transformations per unit time. The unit of activity is the becquerel (Bq) which is one nuclear transformation per second. Radiopharmaceuticals tend to have activities which are measured in kilobecquerels (kBq) or megabecquerels (MBq). Since radioactive materials undergo continuous decay, it is necessary to state the time at which activity is measured and to recognise that the shorter the half-life of the radionuclide, the more accurately the time should be specified. The activity at any given time can be calculated from the expression:

$$A = A_0 e^{-0.693 t / t_{1/2}}$$

where A is the activity at time t, A_0 is the initial activity, t is the elapsed time, $t_{1/2}$ is the half-life.

Specific Activity

The specific activity of a preparation of a radioactive material is the activity of the particular radionuclide per unit mass of the element or compound; it is usually expressed as the activity per gram.

Radioactive Concentration

The radioactive concentration of a solution is the activity of the particular radionuclide in a unit volume.

Electron Volt

Ionising radiation is a form of energy. The unit of energy is the electron volt (eV) which is the kinetic energy acquired by an electron when it is accelerated through a potential difference of 1 volt. The energy of nuclear radiations is measured in kilo electron volts (keV) and mega electron volts (MeV).

Absorbed Dose

Absorbed dose is the energy deposited per unit mass of material. The unit of absorbed dose is the gray (Gy) which corresponds to 1 joule per kilogram.

Dose Equivalent

Biological effects depend not only on absorbed dose but also on the type of ionising radiation to which a tissue is exposed. Dose equivalent takes into account the variation in biological effectiveness of different radiations. It is calculated as the product of absorbed dose and a quality factor for the particular ionising radiation. The unit of dose equivalent is the sievert (Sv). For the gamma and beta radiations emitted by radiopharmaceuticals the quality factor is 1; values of dose equivalent and absorbed dose are therefore identical.

Detection of Radiation

Various effects which arise from the interaction of matter with beta and gamma radiation can be used for the detection and measurement of radiation. The most important interactions are the ionisation of gases and scintillation effects. Three types of detector are used routinely in radiopharmacy.

The Ionisation Chamber. When beta or gamma rays pass through a gas, some atoms of gas are ionised. If a voltage is applied between two electrodes placed in the gas, the gas ions move to the electrodes and produce an electric current which is pro-

portional to the intensity of the radiation. This phenomenon is the basis for the instrument known as the ionisation chamber. The most common use of the ionisation chamber in radiopharmacy is in radionuclide calibrators. These latter instruments which measure the activity of radioactive sources are available commercially from several manufacturers. The instrument consists of a well-type ionisation chamber coupled to an electrometer. The electrometer is fitted with means for specifying the radionuclide to be measured; this may take the form of either a continuously variable dial set by the operator to a particular calibration factor for each radionuclide or precalibrated push-buttons each of which is allocated to a commonly used radionuclide. Depressing a push-button results in the appropriate calibration factor being used. Push-button instruments also tend to be fitted with a continuously variable dial to permit the measurement of radionuclides other than those to which buttons have been allocated. When a radioactive source is placed in the well and the appropriate calibration factor is selected, the activity of the source is shown on a digital display on the electrometer. Radionuclide calibrators are capable of measuring activity at levels ranging from a few kilobecquerels to tens of gigabecquerels. When using a radionuclide calibrator, care must be taken to ensure that the activity reading is not adversely affected by either the type of vial used to contain the radiopharmaceutical or the volume of solution it contains. The calibration factors provided by the manufacturer of the instrument are for radionuclides contained in a specific volume of liquid in a specific container. Measurement of a radionuclide in a different container or volume cannot be guaranteed to result in an accurate measurement of activity. It is therefore essential for the user to determine the appropriate calibration factors for the containers and volumes used routinely in the radiopharmacy.

In practice, the radionuclide calibrator can be interfaced to a computer to allow automatic transfer of the activity measured by the calibrator to a label which is printed for the radiopharmaceutical.[1]

The Geiger Counter. This instrument is similar to the ionisation chamber but the intensity of its electric field is increased so that the ions produced are accelerated and a cascade of secondary ionisation is generated. The result is a breakdown of the insulation of the gas and the generation of an electric pulse which can be detected. As with the ionisation chamber, the Geiger counter measures the intensity of the radiation but not the energy. Geiger counters are most efficient for the detection of beta radiation. As detectors of gamma radiation they are extremely inefficient. The principal use of the Geiger counter is in radiation protection where it is used to monitor contamination on hands, clothing, benches, and other equipment. Certain personal electronic dosimeters, which are also used in radiation protection work, incorporate a Geiger counter as the radiation detector.

The Scintillation Detector. This detector device depends upon the emission of a weak flash of visible light by certain phosphors when they are exposed to radiation. These flashes of light, known as scintillations, are detected and converted into electrical pulses by a photomultiplier tube. After amplification, the pulses are counted and their amplitudes are measured. Because the amplitude is proportional to the energy of the radiation detected, the energy spectrum of the radiation emitted from a radioactive source can be recorded by a pulse height analyser.

There are two main types of scintillation detector. In the first, the phosphor is usually a thallium-activated sodium iodide crystal which is contained in an aluminium can with a glass window on the face adjacent to the photomultiplier. The photomultiplier is contained in a light-tight assembly. This type of detector is used for the detection of gamma radiation and is of no value in the detection of beta radiation. Beta particles have insufficient energy to pass through the aluminium can in which the crystal is housed and are therefore unable to interact with the sodium iodide to produce scintillation. In the second type, which is used to detect beta radiation, the beta emitter is added to a transparent glass or plastic vial containing a solution of a phosphor. The scintillations produced in the solution are then detected with one or more photomultipliers positioned outside the vial. This technique is known as liquid scintillation counting and is one of the most sensitive techniques for measuring the activity of beta-emitting radionuclides.

The scintillation detector is widely used in radiopharmacy and in nuclear medicine. It is used in many pieces of equipment such as sample counters, chromatography detectors, organ uptake counters, whole body monitors and gamma cameras. The ubiquitous gamma camera is the instrument used for the majority of radionuclide-imaging procedures performed on patients. The detector on a typical gamma camera contains a sodium iodide crystal which is approximately 15 mm thick and may be over 40 cm in diameter. Following administration of the radiopharmaceutical and its localisation in the organ under investigation, the detector of the gamma camera is positioned to record the gamma rays being emitted from the organ. Over a period of time, which is typically a few minutes, an image is built up of the distribution of the radiopharmaceutical in the organ. This image can be displayed on photographic film or recorded in a computer for analysis at a later time.

More advanced imaging techniques involve the use of single photon emission computed tomography (SPECT) and positron emission tomography (PET). These techniques provide images of 'slices' through the body. SPECT is performed with standard radiopharmaceuticals such as the ^{99m}Tc agents and is in widespread use. As its name implies, PET is used in conjunction with positron-emitting radiopharmaceuticals which contain radionuclides such as nitrogen-13 ($t_{1/2} = 10$ minutes), oxygen-15 ($t_{1/2} = 2$ minutes), fluorine-18 ($t_{1/2} = 1.8$ hours), bromine-77 ($t_{1/2} = 56$ hours) and gallium-68 ($t_{1/2} = 1.1$ hours). In the PET technique, the 511 keV annihilation gamma rays are detected. Except when used with the ^{77}Br radiopharmaceuticals, PET requires that the imaging equipment is close to a cyclotron in which the short half-life radionuclides can be produced. The exceptionally high cost of the equipment to perform PET means that it is not a widely available technique but is restricted to research institutions.

PRODUCTION OF RADIONUCLIDES

The radionuclides incorporated into radiopharmaceuticals and in radionuclide generators are produced either as a result of nuclear fission of heavy nuclides such as uranium-235 or of the bombardment of a stable target nuclide with particles such as neutrons or protons. The nomenclature used to describe the route of production is A(x,y)B where: A is the target nuclide; B is the radionuclide produced; x is the particle used to bombard the target nuclide (x = n if neutrons are used, or p if protons are used); and y is the response to the capture of the bombarding particle (y = γ if gamma radiation is emitted, or f if the target nuclide undergoes fission). In choosing a production route, the manufacturer considers factors such as the yield, the radionuclidic purity of the product and whether the outcome of the process is a carrier-free radionuclide. A radionuclide is described as 'carrier-free' when every atom of the element is present as the radionuclide and therefore no other isotopes of the element are present. The carrier-free state can only be achieved when the production process leads to the formation of a new element. By the use of a carrier-free radionuclide only a trace amount of the element is administered to the patient. Freedom from carrier is particularly important in radiopharmaceuticals which contain toxic elements such as the ^{201}Tl isotope of thallium and the ^{67}Ga isotope of gallium. In the synthesis of a radiolabelled compound, the success of the labelling reaction may depend upon the radionuclide being in a carrier-free state.

Radionuclides Produced in a Reactor

Most of the radionuclides used in nuclear medicine are produced in a nuclear reactor. In this process, a target element is inserted into the core of the reactor where it is bombarded by neutrons. When a neutron enters the nucleus of a target atom, the nucleus undergoes a rearrangement and a new isotope of the target element is produced. In the most common reaction of this type, the capture of the neutron is accompanied by the emission of a gamma-ray. This process, known as the (n, γ) reaction, is the route by which most reactor-produced radionuclides are prepared and results in the formation of radionuclides with an excess of neutrons. An example of the reaction is the production of chromium-51 (^{51}Cr) wherein a target which contains chromium, either of natural isotopic composition or enriched in chromium-50, is inserted into a reactor. When the nucleus of a ^{50}Cr atom captures a neutron, ^{51}Cr is formed and a gamma ray is emitted. The reaction is therefore described as ^{50}Cr(n, γ)^{51}Cr. As this type of reaction is not 100% efficient, the product contains both ^{50}Cr and ^{51}Cr. Chemical separation of these isotopes is not possible and therefore ^{51}Cr cannot be obtained as a carrier-free product when prepared by this route. Other important radionuclides produced by this reaction are ^{32}P, ^{59}Fe, ^{75}Se, ^{113}Sn and ^{198}Au.

A variation of the (n, γ) reaction occurs when the radionuclide produced decays to a daughter radionuclide. The reaction is an important means for the production of ^{131}I. A tellurium target is irradiated in the reactor to form ^{131}Te which disintegrates by β^- emission ($t_{\frac{1}{2}} = 25$ minutes) to yield ^{131}I; the reaction is described by the equation:

$$^{130}\text{Te(n, }\gamma)^{131}\text{Te} \rightarrow ^{131}\text{I}$$

Finally, the iodine is chemically separated from the target material to produce carrier-free ^{131}I.

The other important method of obtaining radionuclides from a reactor is by bombarding a uranium target with neutrons. When the nucleus of an atom of uranium-235 captures a neutron, it undergoes fission to produce a wide variety of nuclides, many of which are radioactive. Being fission products, the radionuclides are carrier-free and can be recovered from the target material by chemical separation. This is the principal production route of molybdenum-99 (^{99}Mo), probably the most important radionuclide for nuclear medicine since it is the parent radionuclide in the ^{99m}Tc generator. In addition to its preparation by the (n, γ) reaction, ^{131}I can also be obtained as a product of uranium fission.

Radionuclides Produced in a Cyclotron

In a cyclotron, positively charged particles such as protons, alpha particles or deuterons ($^2_1$H nuclei) are accelerated to a high energy and then directed onto a target. The products are nuclides which are deficient in neutrons and which can be recovered from the target by chemical separation. Several medically useful radionuclides are prepared in this way; examples are indium-111 by ^{111}Cd(p, n)^{111}In, gallium-67 by ^{68}Zn(p, 2n)^{67}Ga and cobalt-57 by ^{56}Fe(d,n)^{57}Co. Useful radionuclides are also obtained following decay of the primary product; among these are iodine-123 by ^{127}I(p, 5n)^{123}Xe $\rightarrow ^{123}$I and thallium-201 by ^{203}Tl(p, 3n)^{201}Pb $\rightarrow ^{201}$Tl. An important aspect of cyclotron production is that the target material is converted to a different element and therefore the radionuclides produced are carrier-free.

Radionuclide Generators

One of the principal reasons for the growth of nuclear medicine was the development of the technetium-99m (^{99m}Tc) generator during the 1960s. This device is a relatively inexpensive and easily transportable source of an extremely useful radionuclide with a short half-life.

Production of a short half-life radionuclide by means of a radionuclide generator is only feasible if a parent radionuclide of relatively long half-life decays into the daughter radionuclide of interest, and the daughter can also be separated easily from the parent. Separation is most commonly achieved by employing an adsorbent for which the parent has a high affinity and the daughter has no affinity. The adsorbent is packed into a short glass column and when the parent is applied

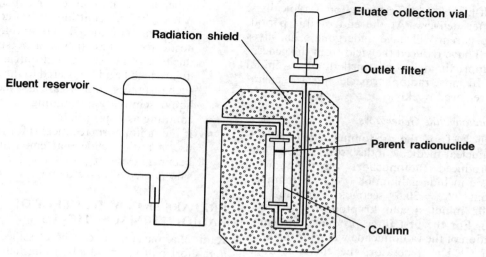

Fig. 1
Radionuclide generator.

it becomes bound to the upper levels. To recover the daughter, produced as a result of decay of the parent, a suitable eluting solvent, is passed through the column and collected at the outlet. This solution which contains the daughter radionuclide is known as the eluate. A radionuclide generator is shown schematically in Fig. 1. The principal radionuclide generators that are of interest in nuclear medicine are listed in Table 1. The radionuclide ^{68}Ga is positron emitting and although the ^{68}Ge/^{68}Ga generator is not widely used at present it may become more common as positron emission tomography becomes more widely available. Similarly, the ^{90}Sr/^{90}Y generator currently has limited application but may become an important source of ^{90}Y for incorporation into therapeutic radiopharmaceuticals.

Table 1
Radionuclide generator systems

Parent	(half-life)		Daughter	(half-life)
^{68}Ge	(288 days)	$\longrightarrow$	^{68}Ga	(1.1 hours)
^{81}Rb	(4.6 hours)	$\longrightarrow$	^{81m}Kr	(13 seconds)
^{90}Sr	(28 years)	$\longrightarrow$	^{90}Y	(2.7 days)
^{99}Mo	(2.8 days)	$\longrightarrow$	^{99m}Tc	(6 hours)
^{113}Sn	(115 days)	$\longrightarrow$	^{113m}In	(1.7 hours)
^{195m}Hg	(1.7 days)	$\longrightarrow$	^{195m}Au	(31 seconds)

^{99m}Tc Generator

Of the radionuclide generators used in radiopharmacy the ^{99m}Tc generator is the most impor-

tant. The parent of ^{99m}Tc is ^{99}Mo which has a half-life of 66.2 hours; ^{99}Mo is obtained either from the products of uranium fission or by the irradiation of molybdenum with neutrons in a reactor. The adsorbent used in the column of the generator is alumina and the eluent is sodium chloride injection. Because of the high activity of ^{99}Mo and the high energies of the gamma radiation emitted, extensive shielding is required to be incorporated into the generator. Shielding is normally constructed from lead but in high activity generators, the amount of lead required for adequate shielding makes them too heavy for safe handling. In such generators, the lead can be replaced by depleted uranium which is a more efficient material for shielding. Depleted uranium is not used in all generators because of its high cost.

The product obtained from a ^{99m}Tc generator is Sodium Pertechnetate [^{99m}Tc] Injection BP which is a sterile solution of sodium pertechnetate in sodium chloride injection. Sterility of the generator eluate is essential since it is administered intravenously or used in the preparation of radiopharmaceuticals for intravenous administration. The generator is therefore supplied by the manufacturer as a sterile appliance and must be handled using aseptic technique to preserve its sterility. Elution is most commonly achieved by using an evacuated sterile multidose vial to draw the ^{99m}Tc solution from the generator. Eluate volumes are typically in the range 5 to 20 mL.

The shelf-life of a ^{99m}Tc generator is typically 2 weeks after delivery. At the end of this period, the ^{99}Mo parent will have undergone 5 half-lives which will have reduced the yield from the generator to approximately one thirtieth of its initial activity. In most radiopharmacies, ^{99m}Tc generators are replaced weekly.

Other Radionuclide Generators

Although ^{99m}Tc is the predominant radionuclide used in nuclear medicine today, several other generator-produced radionuclides have important uses; these include gallium-68 ($t_{1/2} = 68$ minutes), gold-195m ($t_{1/2} = 30.5$ seconds), indium-113m ($t_{1/2} = 102$ minutes) and krypton-81m ($t_{1/2} = 13$ seconds). For the first three products, the eluate is a solution of the radionuclide while for the krypton-81m (^{81m}Kr) generator, the eluate is a gas which the patient breathes directly from the generator.

Choice of Radionuclide

When selecting a radionuclide for use in a radiopharmaceutical several factors must be considered. These include the following:

- The radionuclide should be readily available; to be of practical value, a short half-life radionuclide ($t_{1/2} < 12$ hours) must be available from a radionuclide generator.
- If the radiopharmaceutical is for diagnostic use, the half-life of the radionuclide should not be unduly long as this will lead to unnecessary irradiation of the patient. Ideally, the effective half-life of a radiopharmaceutical (a combination of the physical half-life of the radionuclide and the biological half-life of the radiopharmaceutical) should not be longer than the time required to perform the study.
- A radiopharmaceutical for diagnostic use which is to be detected from outside the patient's body, must incorporate a gamma-emitting radionuclide. Ideally, the radionuclide should not emit alpha or beta particles as these lead to unnecessary irradiation of the patient. If a gamma camera is to be used, the energy of the gamma rays should be between 100 and 250 keV; this is the range in which the detector of the gamma camera operates most efficiently.
- If the investigation involves measurement of the activity in samples of body fluids such as plasma or urine, the radionuclide may be either a gamma emitter or a beta emitter. Although beta-emitting radionuclides are, in general, considered undesirable for diagnostic techniques, they can be suitable for this type of investigation if only a low activity needs to be administered to the patient. In such instances, samples are assayed either by liquid scintillation counting or by gamma counting as appropriate.
- If the radiopharmaceutical is for therapeutic use, a radionuclide that emits high energy beta particles is required to induce the necessary degree of tissue damage.

PREPARATION AND SUPPLY OF RADIOPHARMACEUTICALS

Radiopharmaceuticals can be classified into long and short half-life products. Long half-life radiopharmaceuticals are those which contain a radionuclide with a half-life of greater than 12 hours. Such radiopharmaceuticals are usually manufactured commercially and supplied to the user as finished products. The radionuclides in these products include indium-111 (^{111}In), gallium-67 (^{67}Ga), thallium-201 (^{201}Tl), iodine-125 (^{125}I) and iodine-131 (^{131}I). Short half-life radiopharmaceuticals are those in which the radionuclide has a half-life of less than 12 hours; these include technetium-99m (^{99m}Tc) and indium-113m (^{113m}In). The supply of short half-life radiopharmaceuticals directly from a manufacturer is difficult to achieve due to the rapid decay of the radionuclide. Short half-life radiopharmaceuticals are therefore prepared in hospital radiopharmacies using radionuclides obtained from commercially manufactured generators. The preparation of these products constitutes a large proportion of the workload in hospital radiopharmacies.

Sterile Radiopharmaceuticals

Most radiopharmaceuticals are administered by the intravenous route and are therefore prepared as sterile products. Terminal sterilisation is not usually feasible due to the short half-life of the radionuclide and reliance must be placed on preparation by aseptic manipulations. Most products of this type are prepared using a closed procedure technique. This is defined as 'a procedure whereby a sterile radiopharmaceutical is prepared by the addition of sterile ingredients to a pre-sterilised closed container via a system closed to the atmosphere'.[2] In contrast, an open procedure is defined as 'a procedure during which the ingredient or semi-finished product is at some stage after sterilisation open to the atmosphere, that is, not closed in a vial, syringe, generator or other sealed container'. The hazards to both product and operator are greater with open procedures and such procedures should be avoided whenever possible.

Technetium-99m Radiopharmaceuticals

Typically, more than 80% of the radiopharmaceuticals prepared in hospital radiopharmacies are ^{99m}Tc-containing products for administration by the intravenous route. The first step in the preparation of a ^{99m}Tc radiopharmaceutical is elution of the ^{99m}Tc generator. The activity of ^{99m}Tc obtained from the generator is influenced by the age of the generator and the time since the previous elution. To obtain the maximum activity, at least 24 hours must elapse between elutions. During a working day, a generator may be eluted on more than one occasion but the yield of ^{99m}Tc will be low if only a few hours have elapsed since the previous elution. After elution, the activity of the eluate is measured in a radionuclide calibrator and the radioactive concentration determined. The volume of generator eluate required for each radiopharmaceutical to be prepared is then calculated. Since administration to the patient is likely to take place some time after preparation, the activity dispensed must incorporate an allowance for the radioactive decay that occurs between preparation and administration.

Sodium pertechnetate [^{99m}Tc] injection is prepared by aseptically transferring the required volume of generator eluate to a sterile vial. Sodium chloride injection may also be injected into the vial to produce an injection of the desired radioactive concentration. All other ^{99m}Tc radiopharmaceuticals involve 'labelling' the ^{99m}Tc to a molecule, particle or other moiety to achieve the required biological distribution after administration. Most labelling procedures are accomplished through the use of a radiopharmaceutical kit which contains all the ingredients required for the preparation of a radiopharmaceutical with the exception of the radionuclide. Kits are commercially manufactured, and comprise a vial containing sterile lyophilised powder which may be sufficient for the preparation of several patient doses. To prepare a radiopharmaceutical from a kit, the required volume of sodium pertechnetate [^{99m}Tc] injection is withdrawn from the vial of generator eluate and injected into the kit. If necessary, sodium chloride injection may be used to dilute the generator eluate to a lower radioactive concentration before it is used. The reconstitution volume for kits is typically 1 to 10 mL. After reconstitution, the vial is usually shaken and allowed to incubate at room temperature for a few minutes during which the ^{99m}Tc complex is formed; with certain kits, boiling or treatment in an ultrasonic bath may be required. Close attention must be paid to the manufacturer's instructions for reconstitution, particularly with regard to the maximum activity and volume that can be added. A reconstituted kit may be issued either as a multidose container or subdivided into individual patient doses. Kits have long shelf-lives and are fully tested by the manufacturers to ensure that a product of high radiochemical purity is obtained upon reconstitution. Reconstituted kits may be stable for up to 8 hours although some may only be stable for shorter periods. If the manufacturer's instructions are closely followed, the final product should exhibit the expected biodistribution and have the desired diagnostic effectiveness.

Long Half-life Radiopharmaceuticals

Many of the radiopharmaceuticals that contain long half-life radionuclides are commercially available as single doses; these are ready for administration to the patient and require no manipulation in the radiopharmacy. However, it is also common practice to purchase long half-life radiopharmaceuticals in multidose containers. In the hospital radiopharmacy, the handling of long half-life products is restricted to the dispensing of individual patient doses from a stock container. Dispensing may involve dilution of the product to a radioactive concentration at which the volume required for a patient dose can be measured accurately. Radiopharmaceuticals that are supplied as multidose preparations may contain an antimicrobial preservative. When dilution is performed, the diluent should contain the antimicrobial preservative at the same concentration as the original preparation if the antimicrobial activity is to be maintained. Of the antimicrobial preservatives used in injections many are broken down by radiation, sometimes with deleterious effects on the preparation; that most commonly used is benzyl alcohol (0.9% v/v).

It is essential that the diluent is also compatible with the radiopharmaceutical. For example, precipitation occurs in products such as gallium [^{67}Ga] citrate injection and ferric [^{59}Fe] citrate injection if an inappropriate diluent is used. Information on the most appropriate diluent is often available from the manufacturer of the radiopharmaceutical.

Oral Preparations

The oral route can be used for the administration of certain radiopharmaceuticals. The most common example is sodium iodide [^{131}I] solution for the treatment of thyroid disorders. Solution of high activity can be purchased in multidose vials from which small volumes are dispensed for individual patients. Due to its hazardous nature, the solution should be dispensed into closed vials similar to those used for sterile preparations. Alternatively, sodium iodide [^{131}I] capsules can be purchased for individual patients.

Other radiopharmaceuticals that are prepared for administration by the oral route include tritiated [^{3}H] water, para-aminobenzoic acid [^{14}C] solution and cyanocobalamin [^{57}Co] and [^{58}Co] oral solutions.

Radioactive Gases and Aerosols

The radioactive gases xenon-127 (^{127}Xe) and xenon-133 (^{133}Xe) are supplied in a variety of ways for example, in ampoules or vials and in solution in multidose and single dose cartridges. One of the most common presentations of ^{133}Xe is a multidose container which contains a collapsible bag fitted with a rubber septum. A hypodermic needle and syringe are used to remove individual patient doses as required. Both ^{127}Xe and ^{133}Xe are also available in gas-tight rubber-capped vials which are used in conjunction with a gas dispenser provided by the supplier of the gases.

A radionuclide generator is available for the production of ^{81m}Kr. The short half-life of ^{81m}Kr (13 seconds) requires that the patient inhales directly from the generator which must be sited next to the gamma camera. The generator has a useful life of only one day due to the short half-life of the rubidium-81 parent (4.6 hours).

An aerosol of ^{99m}Tc is an alternative to the radioactive gases. Aerosols are created by means of a nebuliser attached to a delivery system from which the patient breathes. More recently, equipment has become available for the preparation of ^{99m}Tc as a 'pseudo-gas';[3] this is a dispersion of ^{99m}Tc-labelled carbon particles with a diameter of 20 nm. The patient breathes the 'pseudo-gas' directly from the equipment in which it is created.

Radiolabelled Blood Cells

Autologous erythrocytes, leucocytes and platelets are radiolabelled and used routinely as diagnostic agents in nuclear medicine. In the preparation of these agents, in-vitro isolation of the cells to be radiolabelled is often necessary. Isolation techniques include differential sedimentation, centrifugation and the use of density gradients; they are invariably carried out as 'open' procedures. With the increasing incidence of blood-borne infectious material such as the human immunodeficiency virus (HIV) and the hepatitis B virus, the handling of blood is an additional hazard to the operator and all blood samples should be treated as being potentially contaminated.

Erythrocytes are radiolabelled with ^{51}Cr using an in-vitro technique which involves the incubation of packed erythrocytes with sodium chromate [^{51}Cr] solution.

For radiolabelling of erythrocytes with ^{99m}Tc, two principal techniques are available. The in-vivo technique involves the intravenous injection of a stannous-containing agent such as stannous pyrophosphate into the patient. Thirty minutes later, when sodium pertechnetate [^{99m}Tc] injection is administered intravenously the ^{99m}Tc labels to the erythrocytes in vivo.[4] By the in-vivo/in-vitro technique, the stannous agent is injected into the patient as above but 30 minutes later, a sample of blood is withdrawn and incubated with sodium pertechnetate [^{99m}Tc] injection in a syringe before being re-injected.[5] This latter technique results in more efficient radiolabelling but involves more handling of blood and therefore constitutes a greater risk.

Granulocytes and mixed leucocytes can be radiolabelled in vitro with ^{111}In using indium [^{111}In] oxine solution[6] or indium [^{111}In] tropolone solution.[7] More recently, a technique which uses technetium [^{99m}Tc] exametazime to radiolabel leucocytes with ^{99m}Tc has become increasingly popular.[8]

'In-house' Preparations and Radiolabelled Antibodies

New and rarely used radiopharmaceuticals are not always available from commercial sources and must therefore be prepared by 'in-house' techniques. 'Open' procedures may be required which involve the weighing of raw materials, preparation of solutions, radiolabelling, purification and sterilisation. In-process testing is an essential part of this type of procedure. In addition, the final product should be tested for radiochemical purity and any other relevant parameters before it is released for administration to the patient. If the procedure is lengthy, a degree of operator protection greater than usual may be necessary to limit radiation exposure.

Radiolabelling of 'in-house' products invariably involves the use of carrier-free radionuclides. Methods of labelling with the radioisotopes of iodine (^{123}I, ^{125}I and ^{131}I) include oxidation and isotopic exchange. Oxidation methods are the most common and are used to label iodine to tyrosine in peptides and proteins by the action of oxidising agents such as chloramine-T[9] and iodogen.[10] Isotopic exchange labelling is normally used for relatively small molecules such as iodohippuric acid which already contain iodine atoms.[11] Proteins can also be radiolabelled with metallic radionuclides such as yttrium-90 (^{90}Y), technetium-99m (^{99m}Tc) and indium-111 (^{111}In). Firm attachment of these radionuclides to proteins is achieved through an intermediate linking molecule known as a bifunctional chelating agent. At one end of this molecule is a reactive group that binds to the protein and at the other end is a group which chelates the radionuclide. A number of these bifunctional chelating systems have been described. The one used most commonly is the cyclic anhydride of diethylenetriaminepentaacetic acid (DTPA).[12]

In an attempt to improve the specificity of radiopharmaceuticals, antibodies and antibody fragments have been developed as carriers of radionuclides. When radiolabelled with ^{99m}Tc, ^{111}In, ^{123}I and ^{131}I antibodies have been used as diagnostic agents whereas antibodies radiolabelled with ^{90}Y and ^{131}I have been used therapeutically. A few radiolabelled antibodies are available commercially as finished products and several commercial kits for antibody labelling are available for processing in the radiopharmacy. However most radiolabelled antibodies are prepared by 'open' procedures using 'in-house' formulations. Examples of techniques commonly used are column chromatography for purification of the labelled product and sterilisation by filtration. Consideration should be given to the possibility that these techniques could result in a high radiation dose to the operator.

Containers

Whether radiopharmaceuticals are supplied as single dose or multidose preparations, the most common container is the 10 mL rubber-capped multidose vial. Because most ^{99m}Tc radiopharmaceuticals are susceptible to oxidation, multidose vials containing such products should have a nitrogen-filled headspace.

Although glass ampoules are regarded as ideal containers for single dose non-radioactive injections, they are not considered ideal for radiopharmaceu-

ticals due to the potential for radioactive contamination should they break while being opened. One inviolable exception to this proviso is in the supply of radiopharmaceuticals for intrathecal, intracisternal or peridural injection. Such injections, for example, indium [^{111}In] pentetate injection, must be supplied in ampoules; after administration, any residue must be discarded.

In some situations, it may be convenient to supply radiopharmaceuticals in single-dose syringes. If this practice is adopted, Luer-lock syringes should be used to minimise the possibility of the hypodermic needle or cap falling off while the syringe is in transit.

Labelling of Containers

The label for a radiopharmaceutical should state:

- the name of the radiopharmaceutical
- the route of administration
- the activity in the container
- the time and date at which the radiopharmaceutical will have the stated activity
- the volume, if the radiopharmaceutical is in liquid form
- the lot number
- the expiry time and date
- the name and concentration of any added substances
- any special instructions such as 'Shake well before use'
- any special storage conditions
- the name of the supplier
- that the preparation is radioactive.

When the container is supplied in a shield, identical labels should be placed on both the container and the shield.

FACILITIES

In the design of a radiopharmacy, both pharmaceutical and radiological factors must be considered together with any relevant legislation. The majority of radioactive sources used in radiopharmacy are unsealed and the areas in which they are handled must be suitable for safe working. The design should therefore be drawn up in consultation with the local advisor on radiation protection. Facilities should also be planned and equipped to carry out the appropriate pharmaceutical procedures, in particular, the preparation of sterile products.

General guidance on pharmaceutical aspects of design is contained in the *Guide to Good Pharmaceutical Manufacturing Practice*[13] and *The Rules*

Governing Medicinal Products in the European Community, Volume IV: Good Manufacturing Practice for Medicinal Products.[14] More specific advice is contained in the *Guidance notes for hospital, premises and environment for the preparation of radiopharmaceuticals.*[2] The requirements for good radiological practice are contained in the Ionising Radiations Regulations 1988,[15] its Code of Practice[16] and in the Guidance notes for the protection of persons against ionising radiation arising from medical and dental use.[17]

Radiopharmacy Design

In designing a radiopharmacy, the overall aims should be:

- to protect the product from its environment and the operator
- to protect the operator from exposure to radiation and hazardous materials, and
- to protect the environment from hazards associated with the product.

To achieve these aims, careful consideration must be given to the nature of surfaces within the radiopharmacy, including walls, floors, ceilings, work benches and workstation interiors. All surfaces should be made from materials which do not shed or absorb particles which may be either radioactive or contaminated with micro-organisms. Additionally, surfaces must withstand regular cleaning with disinfectants and be strong enough to resist wear and tear and the actions of radiochemical decontamination liquids. Bench surfaces are coved to the walls and raised at the edges to contain any spillage of radioactive liquids. Floor coverings should be non-absorbent, laid in a continuous sheet and coved to the walls.

Floors and benches must be strong enough to support the weight of any shielding that may be required. All surfaces should be easily accessible for cleaning. Ledges and places where dust and particles can accumulate should be avoided.

Cleanrooms in the radiopharmacy should be entered through a changing room and should be maintained at a pressure that is higher than that in the surrounding areas. This pressure differential limits the ingress of particulate and microbial contamination into the cleanroom. Double-ended interlocking hatches should be installed to enable items to be passed into and out of cleanrooms without loss of overpressure. Cleanrooms should not contain sinks although hand washing facilities are required in changing rooms. The use of sinks in other areas will be essential, for example, for the disposal of radioactive waste.

Any work which is liable to cause the release of airborne radioactive contamination should be performed under conditions which contain the contamination and eliminate any hazard to the surroundings and personnel. Attainment of these conditions may require the inclusion of ventilation exhaust systems in the design, or the use of contained workstations.

To protect the operator from accidental spillage of the product and also the product from contamination by the operator, protective clothing should be worn when radiopharmaceuticals are being prepared.

Dispensing Areas

Most radiopharmaceuticals are administered by the intravenous route and are prepared by aseptic manipulations. The aseptic procedures should be carried out in a contained workstation which is sited in a pharmaceutical cleanroom. Radionuclide generators are stored and eluted in a contained workstation that is set aside specifically for this purpose. If the radiopharmacy undertakes only the preparation of short half-life radiopharmaceuticals from kits using closed procedures, and these products are used within one working day, the contained workstation may be located in a room with a good standard of hygiene.

Radiopharmaceuticals intended for oral administration should be prepared in a room with a good standard of hygiene. For those that are potentially volatile preparation should be in a workstation that provides operator protection and discharges its exhaust outside the building. Discharge may be achieved by means of either a contained workstation with a total exhaustion system or a fume cupboard.

Radiolabelling of autologous blood cells should be undertaken in facilities similar to those described for the preparation of radiopharmaceuticals by aseptic manipulation. To avoid cross-contamination between blood products and conventional radiopharmaceuticals, it is desirable that the handling of blood is carried out in a room set aside for this purpose.

The standards to which cleanrooms, workstations and clean air devices must operate to achieve certain levels of cleanliness are contained in British Standard 5295.[18] See also the chapter on Cleanrooms for Pharmaceutical Production.

Contained Workstations

Contained workstations for radiopharmaceutical manipulations afford protection for both product and operator. Product protection is achieved by the provision of a work space which is flushed with a downward flow of laminar, filtered air. Typically, the contained workstations used in radiopharmacy are of the recirculating type in which the air is circulated and is mostly retained within the equipment. Approximately 10 to 20% of the air is exhausted from the workstation either into the room or outside the building. The exhausted air is replaced by an inward air flow through the working aperture at the front of the workstation. It is this inward flow which provides the operator protection by preventing the escape of aerosols or gases generated during the handling of materials. A specification for operator protection is contained in British Standard 5726.[19]

Enclosed Workstations/Isolators

Isolator technology provides an alternative to the use of conventional aseptic suites for the preparation of radiopharmaceuticals. Isolators are microbiological safety cabinets with a filtered air supply which complies with the highest standards. These enclosures are designed to operate in domestically clean rooms rather than in pharmaceutical clean rooms as in the case of contained (downdraught) workstations. In isolators, manipulations are carried out via glove ports; the integrity of the gloves is therefore critical. An isolator can provide an environment of high quality for pharmaceutical manipulations with excellent operator protection. Isolators specifically used for the handling of radiopharmaceuticals should incorporate shielding and operate under negative pressure. If appropriate, the processing chamber of an isolator can be equipped with a centrifuge and radionuclide calibrator.

Advantages of an isolator over a conventional aseptic suite are lower operating costs due to the lower power consumption and reduced expenditure on cleanroom clothing and associated laundry charges. Time spent on changing clothing and on the cleaning and maintenance of an aseptic suite is eliminated. The operator protection factor provided by an isolator is considerably greater than that provided by downdraught workstations. Since the isolator is totally enclosed and operates under negative pressure, the risk of radioactive material escaping from the unit is small. However, repeated use of the gloves in this type of cabinet may permit the diffusion of toxic material.

Disadvantages are that when it is necessary to perform a novel activity as part of a production or dispensing process, an isolator does not have the flexibility of a cleanroom. It is not possible to insert bulky items of specialised equipment into the unit and expensive modifications may be required to accommodate such changes. Aseptic manipulations in an isolator are more cumbersome and time consuming, making them unsuitable for departments with a high workload. Isolators are best suited to departments with a small workload and to situations where potentially hazardous materials are handled such as during the radiolabelling of autologous blood cells.

QUALITY ASSURANCE

Radiopharmaceuticals intended for clinical use must be of the desired quality. Unlike most pharmaceutical preparations, many radiopharmaceuticals have a very short useful life after preparation and must therefore be administered to patients before the results of quality assurance tests are known. In the assurance of final product quality, great emphasis must be placed on the procedures used to prepare radiopharmaceuticals and the in-process controls that are undertaken. The outcome of this combined system of procedures and controls should be monitored by a programme of retrospective tests on final products.

Environmental and Process Controls

Documentation

If radiopharmaceuticals of a consistently high quality are to be prepared, it is essential that standard procedures are used. The first aim of any system of documentation is to describe the standard procedures for all aspects of work undertaken in the radiopharmacy. This need for description applies not only to preparative procedures but also to activities such as the testing of raw materials and finished products, environmental monitoring, and the calibration and maintenance of equipment. The documentation system should allow the complete history of a product to be traced. Essential to the documentation are work sheets and a system of batch numbering of products such as that outlined in the *Guide to Good Pharmaceutical Manufacturing Practice*.[13] A specification should be drawn up for each radiopharmaceutical that is prepared in the radiopharmacy; there should also be a formal system for releasing each finished product against its specification.

Purchase of Radiopharmaceuticals and Raw Materials

On arrival all goods received should be carefully inspected with attention given to labelling and the integrity of the packaging. Records should be kept of batch numbers and quantities received. When a national system of product licensing exists, licensed products should be used whenever possible. If non-licensed products are purchased a certificate of analysis should be obtained from the manufacturer. In addition, the full range of relevant analytical tests should be performed on each batch of unlicensed material before administration of the material to the patient. Where radiopharmaceuticals are prepared 'in house', all starting materials should be processed in accordance with the *Guide to Good Pharmaceutical Manufacturing Practice*.[13] Radionuclides purchased for incorporation into radiopharmaceuticals should be assessed for radionuclidic identity and purity.

Radionuclide Calibrator Performance

The following checks on radionuclide calibrators should be performed on a regular basis:

- stability check against long half-life reference sources
- assessment of assay accuracy
- assessment of variations with sample geometry
- assessment of linearity of response.

Guidance on procedures and the frequency of these tests is available.[20]

Validation of Operator Technique

A programme of broth transfer testing can be adopted to demonstrate that the techniques used in the radiopharmacy result in sterile products. In such tests, all procedures employed in the preparation of radiopharmaceuticals are mimicked using sterile nutrient broth in place of the normal solutions. Incubation of the broth provides a measure of both operator technique and the adequacy of the environment. An operator who is new to the radiopharmacy should not be authorised to prepare radiopharmaceuticals until satisfactory trials have been carried out.

Environmental Monitoring

A programme of monitoring should be undertaken to demonstrate that the environment meets the required standards for the procedures being carried out.[15,18,19] This programme should include monitoring of the following factors:

Overpressures in Aseptic Suites. The air pressure should be highest where the product is at greatest risk of contamination. Overpressures are dependent on the rate at which air enters the area relative to its surroundings and should be such that pressure differentials between rooms are at least 15 Pa. Differentials are most conveniently monitored on a continuous basis by installation of suitably placed manometers.

Particulate Contamination of the Environment. Within contained workstations and cleanrooms contamination is most commonly determined using an instrument which measures the scattering of a beam of light due to the passage of particles. The instrument is calibrated to measure particles of a given size range and by sampling a known volume of air it is possible to calculate the number of particles per cubic metre of air.

Air Flow Rates within Contained Workstations and Air Change Rates in Cleanrooms. Measurements are made using an anemometer.

Efficiency of Filters in Contained Work Stations and Supply Inlets to Cleanrooms. Efficiency is measured by challenge testing using an aerosol photometer, for example, by the dioctyl phthalate (DOP) test. In this technique, a fine stream of DOP particles, 0.3 micrometre in diameter, is generated on the inlet side of the filter. A photometer positioned on the outlet side gives a measure of filter efficiency by detecting DOP that has not been arrested.

Protection Factor afforded by Contained Workstations. Operator protection should be tested using a technique such as the potassium iodide disc method described in British Standard 5276.[19]

Microbial Contamination of the Environment. Evaluation is commonly carried out using settle plates containing nutrient agar which are exposed to the atmosphere at critical sites in the working environment. After incubation, the plates are inspected for microbial growth. A more accurate way of quantifying contamination requires the use of either a slit air sampler or a centrifugal sampler. With these instruments, a known volume of air is directed onto a solid culture medium strip and any microorganisms in the air sample are detected after incubation of the strip. Microbial contamination of work surfaces can be assessed by use of contact plates. This test involves bringing an appropriate solid culture medium into contact with the surface to be examined. Any micro-organisms present adhere to the medium and can be detected after incubation. After such a test, thorough cleaning of the work surface must be carried out to remove all traces of culture medium.

Radioactive Contamination of Surfaces. The locations of particular relevance are the internal surfaces of workstations in which radiopharmaceuticals are manipulated. Assessment can be performed either by direct monitoring using a suitable instrument or by a wipe test in which the surface is swabbed followed by monitoring of the swab for radionuclides.

Tests on Starting Materials and on the Final Product

The quality of long half-life radiopharmaceuticals from commercial sources is the responsibility of the manufacturer who will perform the appropriate tests before the product is released for sale. In the instance of radiopharmaceuticals which are prepared in hospitals, product quality is the responsibility of the person in charge of the radiopharmacy. Monographs which include final product specifications for many radiopharmaceuticals are published in the *British Pharmacopoeia* and in the *European Pharmacopoeia*.[21,22]

Measurement of Activity

The activity of each radiopharmaceutical prepared in the radiopharmacy should be measured in a radionuclide calibrator to ensure that it meets the appropriate specification.

Radionuclidic Identity

The identity of a radionuclide may be established by determination of its half-life, by characterisation of the radiations emitted, or by a combination of the two techniques. Each radionuclide has a gamma ray spectrum which is unique and can be established by means of gamma ray spectrometry.

Radionuclidic Purity

In the *British Pharmacopoeia*, radionuclidic purity is defined as 'the ratio, expressed as a percentage, of the radioactivity of the radionuclide concerned to the total radioactivity of the source'.[21] Radionuclidic purity is determined by the technique of gamma ray spectrometry. For generator-produced radionuclides of short half-life, the manufacturer can check the radionuclidic purity of eluates before the dispatch of generators, but he cannot be held responsible for misuse or damage in transit. Control of radionuclidic impurities is necessary to protect the patient from unnecessary irradiation. The most probable source of a radionuclidic impurity is the parent nuclide 'breaking through' into the eluate and it is essential to measure the level of this impurity to ensure that it falls within acceptable limits. Impurity concentration should be measured in the first eluate from each new generator and on a regular basis thereafter. An example is the determination of ^{99}Mo in the eluate from a ^{99m}Tc generator.

Activity of the eluate is first determined in a radionuclide calibrator, using the calibration factor for ^{99m}Tc. The vial of eluate is then placed inside a 6 mm lead shield which is inserted into the radionuclide calibrator and remeasured using a calibration factor for ^{99}Mo. The lead container is sufficiently thick to attenuate virtually all the 140 keV gamma rays of ^{99m}Tc but it still allows the higher energy 740 keV and 780 keV gamma rays of the parent ^{99}Mo to be measured. The extent of breakthrough of the parent is quantified by expressing the ^{99}Mo activity as a percentage of the ^{99m}Tc activity.

Radiochemical Purity

A compendial definition is 'the ratio, expressed as a percentage, of the radioactivity of the radionuclide concerned that is present in the source in the chemical form declared to the total radioactivity of that radionuclide present in the source'.[21] Radiochemical purity is required to be high if the radiopharmaceutical is to have the desired *in-vivo* behaviour. The presence of radiochemical impurities can be detected by separation techniques such as paper and thin layer chromatography, electrophoresis and gel filtration. Thin layer chromatography techniques which use rapid miniaturised methods have been specifically devised for the analysis of technetium preparations and other radiopharmaceuticals.[23-25] Although more costly and time consuming, high performance liquid chromatography (HPLC) has a place in radiopharmaceutical development and quality control. Separation of most, if not all, impurities and degradation products is obtained by HPLC and it may be used to measure the radiochemical purity and stability of developed products.[26] Chromatographic and other separation techniques for radiochemical purity determinations have been extensively reviewed by Wieland *et al.*[27]

The radiochemical purity of ^{99m}Tc radiopharmaceuticals prepared from kits should be measured each time a new batch of kits is put into use. As many seemingly innocuous factors are known to have deleterious effects on the radiochemical purity of ^{99m}Tc radiopharmaceuticals,[28-31] the effect of any change to a preparative procedure must be assessed. Non-licensed products and 'in-house' preparations should be subjected to a more intensive programme of radiochemical purity checks.

Chemical Purity

Chemical purity is defined as 'the ratio, expressed as a percentage, of the mass of substance present in the declared chemical form to the total mass contained in the source, disregarding any excipients or solvents'.[21] A chemical impurity that can be encountered in hospital practice is the presence of aluminium in the eluate from a ^{99m}Tc generator. Aluminium may be determined by a technique described in the *British Pharmacopoeia* which uses the dye chrome azurol S. The colour produced when this dye is mixed with the eluate under test must be less than that of a standard solution which contains 2 parts per million of aluminium.

Absence of Foreign Particulate Matter

Products for parenteral administration should be free of gross particulate contamination. Visual examination of the product using a lead glass screen for protection of the eyes, or examination with the aid of a mirror, gives adequate control when dealing with small volume radiopharmaceuticals. Polarised light may make visualisation of particles easier. Products found to contain particulate contamination must be filtered or discarded.

Particle Size

Some radiopharmaceuticals are particulate in nature, for example, colloids and macroaggregates of albumin. Variations in particle size may give rise to differences in the biological distribution of the preparations. In view of the large range of particle sizes encountered, several methods are used to determine particle size; these include membrane filtration, photon correlation spectroscopy and microscopy.

Sterility

As a consequence of their radioactive nature, batches of most radiopharmaceuticals cannot be tested for sterility before they are released for use. Retrospective testing may be performed as a method of assessing preparative procedures. A method that is employed widely is that of performing a sterility test on a short half-life radiopharmaceutical after its activity has decayed to an insignificant level. However, the value of this technique has been questioned as it has been shown that micro-organisms may not survive in radio-

pharmaceuticals because of their poor nutritional value and the degree of radiation damage incurred.[32] It is therefore recommended that reliance should be placed on validation methods such as broth transfer trials.

Pyrogens

It is not normally necessary to carry out pyrogen tests on radiopharmaceuticals in view of the small volumes usually administered. If, however, pyrogen testing is thought desirable, the rabbit test may be supplemented by the limulus amoebocyte lysate test for bacterial endotoxin. Because this test is more rapid and can be completed before the product is administered to the patient it is of most benefit for testing radiopharmaceuticals intended for administration by any route that gives access to the cerebrospinal fluid.

Biological Distribution

The ultimate test of the efficacy of a diagnostic radiopharmaceutical is its biodistribution and the quality of information that is generated. Continued evaluation of clinical images is therefore a valuable method of ensuring the continued acceptability of a product.

RADIATION PROTECTION

Radiopharmaceuticals are unsealed radioactive sources which constitute a radiation hazard. Handling procedures which minimise this hazard must therefore be adopted. In any department in which radioactive materials are handled, a member of staff should be designated as being responsible for supervising all aspects of radiation safety. These responsibilities will include the monitoring of radiation doses received by members of staff, handling procedures, training in radiation protection, disposal of waste and the transport of radioactive materials.

Radiation Dose Limits

Exposure to ionising radiation causes damage in living cells, the extent of damage being dependent on the dose of radiation to which tissues are exposed. Persons who handle radioactive materials in the course of their work must therefore be protected from the harmful effects of radiation. To this end, the International Commission on Radiological Protection (ICRP) has recommended maximum annual dose equivalents for both radiation workers and members of the public.[33] The recommendations of the ICRP are used by countries worldwide as the basis for their legislation concerning radiation exposure. In the UK, the relevant legislation is The Ionising Radiations Regulations 1985.[15] These regulations were based on earlier recommendations and, over the next few years, will undergo revision to take account of the lower dose limits set out in the most recent ICRP recommendations. Associated with these regulations is an Approved Code of Practice which provides an interpretation of the regulations[16] and a set of guidance notes.[17] However, it is not sufficient to keep doses within the prescribed limits. An employer must keep radiation exposure to as low a level as is reasonably achievable, when economic and social factors are taken into account. This objective is often referred to as the ALARA principle, that is, As Low As Reasonably Achievable.

Minimisation of Exposure

The work of a radiopharmacy is concerned principally with the handling of high activity radiation sources in liquid form. Exposure of members of staff can arise from either irradiation from an external source or irradiation of internal organs following ingestion or inhalation of a radionuclide. To minimise radiation exposure, the following precautions should be observed:

- Procedures should be performed as quickly as possible to minimise exposure time.
- The distance between operator and source should be maximised.
- Among the simple yet effective techniques applied to extend the distance are: radioactive sources should be handled with forceps rather than the fingers; when using a syringe to handle a radioactive solution, it should be less than half full in order to keep the fingers several centimetres from the radioactive liquid; radionuclide generators should be sited away from the main work area; in situations where exceptionally high activities of radioactive materials are handled, the use of remotely controlled automatic equipment might be considered.
- Appropriate shielding should be placed between operator and source to reduce radiation exposure.

In its passage through an absorbing material, the intensity of radiation falls exponentially with distance, that is equal thicknesses of material reduce the intensity by equal fractions. A useful parameter that is used to measure absorption is the thickness of material that is required to reduce the intensity of the radiation to one half of its initial value; this is called the half thickness or half value layer. Gamma-emitting sources should be stored in lead containers of sufficient thickness to reduce the external dose-rate to an acceptable level. Most manufacturers of radionuclide generators can supply additional shielding to supplement the shield that is contained in the generator. Lead-impregnated glass or acrylic sheet can be used to provide an effective shield behind which radioactive sources can be handled, thus confining exposure to the hands. Shielding of this type is most appropriate for low energy gamma-emitting radionuclides such as ^{99m}Tc which require only a few centimetres to be effectively shielded. The use of shields on syringes reduces exposure of the hands. Such shields are commonly made from tungsten which is less easily deformed than lead; they incorporate either a slit or a lead glass window through which the graduations on the barrel of the syringe can be viewed.

- Protective clothing and disposable gloves should be worn to prevent irradiation due to accidental contamination of the skin.
- Handling of radioactive solutions should be performed over a tray to prevent the spread of accidental spillage.
- Handling of gaseous or volatile radionuclides should be undertaken in a fume cupboard.
- Preparation of radiopharmaceuticals by aseptic technique should be undertaken in a contained workstation which provides operator protection.
- Eating, drinking, smoking and the application of cosmetics should be forbidden in areas where radioactive materials are handled.
- Work surfaces, floors and walls of rooms should be smooth and non-absorbent to permit easy cleaning and decontamination. Bench surfaces should be coved against walls and lipped at the edges.
- Hands, worktops, door handles, telephones and other hand-held equipment should be monitored regularly for radioactive contamination.

Measurement of Radiation Dose

Measurement of the whole body dose from external irradiation is normally by means of a film badge worn on the trunk at chest or waist height. The film badge consists of a piece of photographic film sealed in a light-tight envelope which is mounted in a holder. After having been worn for the period of monitoring, the film is developed. From the degree of exposure the radiation dose to which the film and therefore the wearer has been exposed can be calculated. A member of staff who is issued with a film badge should wear it at all times while at work. Care should be taken to prevent the film badge from becoming contaminated or being inadvertently exposed to radiation while not being worn. Each film badge is normally worn for one month.

Whole body dose can also be measured by means of a pocket-sized electronic dosimeter. These instruments show the cumulative dose on a digital display and are useful for assessing the dose received over a short period of time, for example, that resulting from a particular procedure. Electronic dosimeters often incorporate an audible alarm which can be set to sound at particular dose-rates. In the radiopharmacy, the most significant dose is likely to be that received by the hands of members of staff involved in the manipulation of radioactive solutions in syringes. These doses can be measured by thermoluminescent dosimeters worn either in a finger stall or as a ring at the base of a finger.

Disposal of Radioactive Waste

The three principal routes of disposal for radioactive waste are discharge into the drains, incineration and special collection. For disposal by each route it is likely that authorisation will be necessary and that a record of the disposal will be required. In the case of short half-life waste, a most convenient means of disposal is to store the waste until it has decayed to an insignificant activity and then dispose of it as non-radioactive waste.

Transport of Radioactive Materials

In 1985, the International Atomic Energy Agency (IAEA) published Regulations for the Safe Transport of Radioactive Materials. The regulations underwent minor amendment in 1990.[34] These recommendations are used as the basis for legislation in individual countries to control the transport of radioactive materials. The United Kingdom legislation which governs the transport of radioactive substances by road is the Radioactive Substances (Carriage by Road) (Great Britain) (Amendment) Regulations 1985,[35] although new regulations are under preparation. In these regulations are specified details such as the design

and labelling of packages, the documentation which must accompany packages while in transit, the permissible dose-rates from packages, the placarding of vehicles and the action to be taken in the event of an accident. Transport of radiopharmaceuticals between manufacturer and user and between central hospital radiopharmacies and outlying hospitals must be undertaken in accordance with these regulations.

CLINICAL USES OF RADIOPHARMACEUTICALS

Radiopharmaceuticals have a well-established role in the investigation of a wide range of clinical conditions and are used as sources of radiation for therapeutic purposes. The principal radiopharmaceuticals and their indications are summarised in Tables 2 to 5. The types of investigations in which radiopharmaceuticals are used can be classified as follows:

- **Static imaging procedures** which provide essentially structural information, although the way in which the radiopharmaceutical is handled by the organ under investigation may give an indication of its functional state. Radiopharmaceuticals for static imaging provide information in one of two ways. Some types function by being concentrated only in the normal tissue of the organ, in which case the diseased tissue appears on the image as an area of reduced activity, sometimes referred to as a 'cold' area. Other types become concentrated selectively in the diseased tissue which appears on the image as an area of increased activity, sometimes referred to as a 'hot' area.

- **Dynamic imaging procedures** which provide information about the function of an organ by demonstrating the way in which a radiopharmaceutical is handled by the organ over a period of time.

- **Uptake and retention measurements** which are performed using external counting equipment to measure the ability of an organ or the whole body to concentrate and retain a radiopharmaceutical.

- **Clearance measurements** which are usually performed by measuring the rate at which a radiopharmaceutical clears from the blood stream.

- **Dilution techniques** in which the total volume of a body fluid is determined by measuring the dilution of a radiopharmaceutical following administration to the patient.

● **Therapy procedures** in which a radiopharmaceutical is administered to the patient and the radiation emitted has a therapeutic effect by causing the destruction of diseased tissue.

Table 2
Common technetium-99m radiopharmaceuticals for imaging procedures

Radiopharmaceutical	For imaging of:
^{99m}Tc-aerosol	lung ventilation
^{99m}Tc-albumin	cardiac function
^{99m}Tc-colloids	liver
	spleen
	bone marrow
^{99m}Tc-denatured erythrocytes	spleen
^{99m}Tc-disofenin	gall bladder
^{99m}Tc-erythrocytes	cardiac function
^{99m}Tc-exametazime	brain
^{99m}Tc-glucoheptonate	brain
	kidney
^{99m}Tc-leucocytes	sites of inflammation
^{99m}Tc-macrosalb	lung perfusion
^{99m}Tc-medronate	bone
^{99m}Tc-mercaptoacetyltriglycine (MAG3)	kidney function
^{99m}Tc-pentetate	brain
	kidney function
^{99m}Tc-pyrophosphate (PYP)	myocardial infarct
^{99m}Tc-sestamibi	myocardial perfusion
^{99m}Tc-sodium pertechnetate	brain
	Meckel's diverticulum
	thyroid
^{99m}Tc-succimer	kidney

Table 3
Common long half-life radiopharmaceuticals for imaging procedures

Radiopharmaceutical	For imaging of:
^{67}Ga-gallium citrate	tumours
	sites of inflammation
^{111}In-pentetate	cerebrospinal fluid kinetics
^{111}In-leucocytes	sites of inflammation
^{123}I-sodium iodide	thyroid
^{123}I- and ^{131}I-meta-iodobenzyl-guanidine (MIBG)	phaeochromocytoma
	neuroblastoma
^{123}I-sodium iodohippurate	kidney function
^{75}Se-methylselenomethyl-norcholestenol	adrenal glands
^{201}Tl-thallous chloride	myocardial perfusion
^{127}Xe- and ^{133}Xe-gas	lung ventilation

Table 4
Common radiopharmaceuticals for non-imaging procedures

Radiopharmaceutical	For measurement of:
^{57}Co- and ^{58}Co-cyanocobalamin	vitamin B_{12} absorption
^{51}Cr-edetate	glomerular filtration rate
^{51}Cr-erythrocytes	red cell volume
^{59}Fe-ferric citrate	iron metabolism and absorption
^{3}H-tritiated water	total body water
^{125}I-albumin	plasma volume
^{125}I- and ^{131}I-sodium iodide	thyroidal iodine uptake
^{125}I- and ^{131}I-sodium iodohippurate	effective renal plasma flow
^{125}I-sodium iothalamate	glomerular filtration rate
^{75}Se-tauroselcholic acid	bile acid pool loss

Table 5
Common radiopharmaceuticals for therapy

Radiopharmaceutical	For treatment of:
^{131}I-meta-iodobenzylguanidine (MIBG)	phaeochromocytoma
	neuroblastoma
^{131}I-sodium iodide	thyrotoxicosis
	carcinoma of the thyroid
^{32}P-sodium phosphate	polycythaemia vera
^{89}Sr-strontium chloride	pain from bone metastases
^{90}Y-colloidal yttrium silicate	malignant disease
	arthritic joints

Diagnostic Procedures

Adrenal

Adrenal imaging using ^{75}Se-methylselenomethyl-norcholestenol is performed to distinguish bilateral hyperplasia from unilateral adenoma. Normal or hyperplastic adrenals take up a small amount of the radiopharmaceutical whereas an adenoma shows a higher uptake with little or no activity in the normal gland.

Functional tumours of the adrenal medulla (phaeochromocytomas) are detected by imaging with metaiodobenzylguanidine (MIBG) radiolabelled with ^{131}I or ^{123}I.[36] The normal adrenal medulla is not visualised but the tumour appears as an area of increased activity. When an ectopic phaeochromocytoma is suspected, whole body imaging is performed. Uptake of the radiopharmaceutical may be inhibited by drugs such as cimetidine and the tricyclic antidepressants. Such drugs should therefore be discontinued before radiolabelled MIBG is administered.

Blood

Measurement of erythrocyte volume is carried out in conjunction with measurement of plasma volume in the determination of blood volume and is valuable in the diagnosis of polycythaemia. Measurement of the erythrocyte volume is dependent on the dilution principle. The erythrocytes in a sample of the patient's blood are labelled with a known activity of ^{51}Cr-sodium chromate and re-injected. After radiolabelled erythrocytes have been allowed to mix with the circulating blood a blood sample is taken and the concentration of ^{51}Cr in the blood is measured. From the dilution of the ^{51}Cr the erythrocyte volume is calculated. The erythrocyte volume is increased in patients with polycythaemia and decreased in those with anaemia. Measurement of plasma volume also depends on the dilution principle and is performed with ^{125}I-albumin. Knowledge of the plasma volume helps to differentiate those patients with true polycythaemia from those with apparent polycythaemia due to contraction of the plasma volume.

^{57}Co-cyanocobalamin and ^{58}Co-cyanocobalamin are both used to measure the absorption of vitamin B_{12} from the gastro-intestinal tract. The radiopharmaceutical is administered by mouth either in the form of a liquid or as a capsule. In the Schilling's test, an intramuscular injection of vitamin B_{12} is administered at the same time as the radiopharmaceutical to saturate non-specific binding sites with vitamin B_{12}. Any absorbed radioactive vitamin B_{12} is not therefore retained in the body but is excreted in the urine which is collected for 24 hours and then counted for the presence of the radionuclide. The radionuclide appears in the urine only if it has been absorbed from the gastro-intestinal tract. When very little, or no radionuclide is detected in the urine, the procedure is repeated and intrinsic factor is administered together with the radiopharmaceutical. In pernicious anaemia, absorption only occurs in the study which includes intrinsic factor. In a refinement of this technique, both parts of the study are performed simultaneously by using ^{58}Co-cyanocobalamin together with a complex of ^{57}Co-cyanocobalamin bound to intrinsic factor. The difference in energy of the radiation emitted by the two isotopes of cobalt allows both to be measured simultaneously in the 24 hour-urine collection. An alternative to these tests is the measurement of whole body retention of radiolabelled cyanocobalamin. This determination is performed one week after administration of the radiopharmaceutical. Retention of the radionuclide occurs only if the radiopharmaceutical has been absorbed. However, this technique requires the use of a whole body monitor.

Bone

Bone imaging is performed using one of the ^{99m}Tc-diphosphonates, such as ^{99m}Tc-medronate, which show good sensitivity for skeletal abnormalities. These radiopharmaceuticals are adsorbed onto hydroxyapatite crystals in bone and the degree of their uptake is related to the rate at which new bone is being formed and the blood flow to the area. Bone imaging is the most frequently performed investigation in nuclear medicine. A common application is in the screening of patients with malignant disease for bone metastases. Abnormalities on a bone scan usually appear as areas of increased activity as a result of increased bone formation in the diseased sites. Occasionally however, 'cold' areas may be seen if the bone is avascular or if bone destruction is occurring. Bone imaging is also of value in the investigation of metabolic bone diseases such as Paget's disease.

Brain

Three radiopharmaceuticals ^{99m}Tc-sodium pertechnetate, ^{99m}Tc-glucoheptonate and ^{99m}Tc-pentetate are used in brain imaging. Under normal circumstances these radiopharmaceuticals do not cross the blood-brain barrier and the brain therefore appears to be 'cold' on the image. When there is cerebral pathology, capillaries which are more permeable than normal are usually found in the abnormal area; these allow the radiopharmaceutical to accumulate at the site which then appears as a hot spot on the image. In recent years, X-ray computed tomography of the brain has largely replaced this type of radionuclide investigation. More recently, ^{99m}Tc-exametazime has been developed for imaging the distribution of blood flow in the brain.[37] It is a lipophilic compound which crosses the blood-brain barrier and is retained in the brain, its deposition being related to blood flow. Imaging by SPECT is of high resolution and represents a 'map' of blood flow in a section through the brain.

Gall Bladder

Hepatobiliary imaging with one of the ^{99m}Tc-iminodiacetate compounds such as ^{99m}Tc-disofenin provides information about the biliary tree and bile outflow. These radiopharmaceuticals are actively transported into the polygonal cells of the liver before excretion via the biliary system into the duodenum. Delay in the appearance of activity in the biliary tract, non-visualisation of the gall bladder, and reduced rate of liver clearance are all indications of abnormality.

Gastro-intestinal Tract

Detection of Meckel's diverticulum is performed after administration of ^{99m}Tc-sodium pertechnetate which is taken up by cells of the gastric mucosa. The presence of the radiopharmaceutical in these cells in a Meckel's diverticulum allows its detection by imaging.

Measurement of the rate of gastric emptying is performed after administration of a radioactive meal. The radiopharmaceuticals ingested during this technique must not be absorbed from the gastro-intestinal tract. Technetium-99m is normally incorporated into the solid phase of the meal while indium-113m or indium-111 is added to the liquid phase. A wide range of solid phases is used such as cornflakes, cooked egg, pancakes, chicken liver pâté and bran. Simultaneous imaging of the two radionuclides over a period of time allows calculation of the rate of emptying of each phase from the stomach. The principal uses of the technique are in the investigation of patients with diarrhoea and in the evaluation of the outcome of gastric surgery.

When ^{99m}Tc-labelled erythrocytes are used in the localisation of sites of gastric bleeding frequent abdominal images are recorded to establish the bleeding site which appears as an area of increased activity due to the collection of blood. Erythrocytes labelled with ^{51}Cr are used to quantify gastrointestinal bleeding by measuring their excretion in the stools.

Loss of protein from the blood into the gastrointestinal tract is measured using ^{51}Cr-chromic chloride. After intravenous injection, the ^{51}Cr becomes bound to plasma proteins. If protein is being lost from the plasma, ^{51}Cr is detectable in the stools.

To investigate bile salt absorption, a capsule which contains ^{75}Se-tauroselcholic acid (^{75}SeHCAT) is administered orally. The activity of ^{75}Se in the patient is measured in a whole body counter immediately after the radiopharmaceutical is ingested and after an interval of seven days. The percentage of retained bile salt can then be calculated. In patients with diseases of the terminal ileum such as Crohn's disease, most of the ^{75}SeHCAT is excreted in the faeces due to malabsorption of the bile salt.

Carbon-14 [^{14}C] urea is used in a breath test to detect the colonisation of the stomach by *Helicobacter pylori*, an organism high in urease activity. In the presence of this organism, orally-administered ^{14}C-urea is broken down and the released ^{14}C is exhaled as carbon dioxide. Detection of ^{14}C in the breath confirms the infection which is thought to be implicated in peptic ulceration. Relapse of duodenal ulcer can be prevented by treatment which eradicates the bacterial infection.

Heart

Labelled ^{99m}Tc-erythrocytes and ^{99m}Tc-albumin remain in the blood stream after intravenous injection and are therefore used in dynamic imaging of the cardiac blood pool. In this technique, the patient's electrocardiogram and a sequence of images of the heart throughout the cardiac cycle are recorded simultaneously in a nuclear medicine computer. From this information, the ejection fraction and other details of left ventricular function can be calculated.

Myocardial perfusion imaging provides information about blood flow to the different parts of the myocardium and is invaluable in assessing patients with ischaemic heart disease. Imaging is performed after administration of ^{201}Tl-thallous chloride which becomes distributed in the myocardium in relation to blood flow. Poorly perfused myocardium appears as a cold area on the image. The physical properties of ^{201}Tl are less than ideal for imaging and recently, ^{99m}Tc-isonitriles such as ^{99m}Tc-sestamibi[38] have become available as replacements for ^{201}Tl.

Because ^{99m}Tc-pyrophosphate is concentrated by infarcted tissue it is used to image myocardial infarcts. Although the diagnosis of myocardial infarction is relatively straightforward from electrocardiogram disturbance and the release of enzymes from the damaged myocardium, imaging can be of value in certain patients in whom these changes are equivocal.

Recently, a new radiopharmaceutical containing antibodies directed against cardiac myosin and labelled with indium-111 has been developed for imaging infarcted myocardium directly.[39] The method may offer several advantages over nondirect methods.

Infection/inflammation

Radiolabelled autologous leucocytes are widely used to localise occult sites of infection and diagnose the extent of inflammatory bowel disease. To perform these investigations, blood is withdrawn from the patient, the leucocytes are separated and then radiolabelled with ^{99m}Tc using ^{99m}Tc-exametazime or with ^{111}In using ^{111}In-oxine. After re-injection into the patient, a proportion of the radiolabelled cells migrate to the site of infection or inflammation which is then detected by imaging. A ^{99m}Tc kit for the preparation of ^{99m}Tc-human immunoglobulin (HIG) has recently been introduced as a convenient radiopharmaceutical for the detection of sites of infection.[40] The product has a major advantage in not requiring the handling of blood. At present, the indications for this radiopharmaceutical have not been established definitively; they appear to be restricted to the detection of infection in bone.

^{67}Ga-gallium citrate is also used in the imaging of sites of infection. A disadvantage of this radiopharmaceutical is its non-specific mode of action which also leads to uptake in other areas of inflammation and to certain tumours.

Kidneys

Uptake of ^{99m}Tc-succimer by the renal parenchyma allows static imaging of the kidneys to demonstrate kidney size, position and morphology. Lesions in the kidney appear as cold areas on the image. The percentage of uptake in each kidney provides a measure of relative kidney function.

After intravenous injection, ^{123}I-sodium iodohippurate is cleared from the blood stream by tubular secretion in the kidneys. Dynamic imaging of the kidneys after administration of this radiopharmaceutical is used to produce an activity/time curve, also known as a renogram, for each kidney. The shape of this curve is indicative of kidney disorders such as renal artery stenosis and urinary tract obstruction. ^{99m}Tc-mercaptoacetyltriglycine (MAG3) has a similar excretion pattern to iodohippurate and due to advantages of cost and convenience is used as an alternative.[41] ^{99m}Tc-pentetate is also widely used for dynamic renal imaging. Because this compound is excreted by glomerular filtration, excretion occurs much more slowly than with ^{123}I-iodohippurate or ^{99m}Tc-MAG3. Studies therefore take much longer to perform and the curves are much flatter, making their interpretation more difficult.

Non-imaging techniques are also used to investigate renal function. The degree of renal impairment in patients with renal disease can be determined by measuring glomerular filtration rate (GFR). In this technique, a known activity of ^{51}Cr-edetate is injected intravenously into the patient. Blood samples are withdrawn at time intervals after injection and assayed for ^{51}Cr. From the rate of clearance of the ^{51}Cr from the blood stream, the GFR is calculated.

Liver, Spleen, and Bone Marrow

Reticuloendothelial cells found throughout the liver, spleen and bone marrow have the ability to remove particles from the blood stream by phagocytosis. Colloids labelled with ^{99m}Tc are rapidly cleared from the blood stream following intravenous injection; the greatest proportion appear in the liver, most of the remainder in the spleen, and a small proportion in the bone marrow. Colloids with particle sizes ranging from a few nanometres to a few micrometres are used. The relative uptake of the colloids by the liver, spleen or bone marrow is determined by their particle size. The main clinical application of colloid imaging is in non-invasive detection of mass lesions in the liver. Where there is focal liver pathology, abnormalities

appear as cold defects. In the presence of diffuse liver disease such as cirrhosis, there may be very poor uptake by the liver whereas the spleen and bone marrow show higher than normal uptake of the radiopharmaceutical. This type of investigation has now largely been replaced by imaging with ultrasound which does not subject the patient to ionising radiation.

By using a colloid at the lower end of the size range, a greater proportion of the radiopharmaceutical is taken up by the bone marrow. Imaging techniques using small colloids are used to demonstrate the distribution of marrow. Cold defects are seen in patients with tumour deposits.

Spleen imaging is performed using ^{99m}Tc-denatured erythrocytes. After a blood sample is withdrawn from the patient the erythrocytes are labelled with ^{99m}Tc in vitro; the labelled cells are then denatured by heating at 49.5° for 15 minutes. Following re-injection into the patient, the cells are taken up by the spleen. Imaging with ^{99m}Tc-denatured erythrocytes is used to detect splenunculus.

Lungs

Lung imaging is usually performed as two procedures; perfusion imaging to depict the distribution of blood flow in the lungs, and ventilation imaging to delineate the areas of ventilated lung. It is often necessary to compare the patterns of perfusion and ventilation to reach a diagnosis.

Perfusion images are obtained following intravenous injection of ^{99m}Tc-macrosalb. This radiopharmaceutical contains macroaggregates of human albumin in the size range 10 to 100 micrometres. After intravenous injection, the radiolabelled particles lodge in the first capillary bed that they encounter, that is, in the lungs, thus allowing images of the lungs to be recorded by gamma camera. The technique reveals obstructions to the circulation from pulmonary emboli or early bronchial carcinoma when the chest X-rays are normal.

Xenon-133 (^{133}Xe) is the most widely used gas for ventilation imaging. Although ^{127}Xe and ^{81m}Kr have better physical properties for imaging they are less readily available. To obtain the ventilation image, the patient is positioned in front of the gamma camera before starting to breathe the radioactive gas from a closed system or from a generator in the case of ^{81m}Kr. Depending on the radiopharmaceutical used, ventilation imaging is performed either before or after the perfusion study. In patients with pulmonary emboli, the perfusion image reveals multiple segmental cold defects while the ventilation image is normal.

As an alternative to the radioactive gases, a ^{99m}Tc-aerosol can be used for ventilation imaging. Aerosols tend to be cheaper and more readily available than gases. An additional advantage is that once inhaled, the ^{99m}Tc becomes localised in the lungs thus allowing multiple images to be obtained in different projections. The technique has the disadvantage, however, of using the same radionuclide as is used for the perfusion imaging.

In normal patients, the distribution of ventilation matches that of perfusion. Defective ventilation with normal perfusion occurs in acute airways disease and lung infection. Defects of both perfusion and ventilation are seen in patients with bullous emphysema and carcinoma of the bronchus.

Thyroid

Iodine is taken up selectively by the thyroid gland for incorporation into the thyroid hormones. Studies of the thyroid are therefore carried out with radioisotopes of iodine. ^{123}I-sodium iodide is used in imaging since it has ideal physical characteristics and results in a much lower radiation dose to the patient than other radio-iodines. However, being a cyclotron-produced radionuclide with a relatively short half-life (13.2 hours), it is not readily available. More commonly used for thyroid imaging since it is readily available is ^{99m}Tc-sodium pertechnetate which is also trapped by the thyroid gland although not incorporated into the thyroid hormones. Symmetrical uptake of the radiopharmaceutical throughout the gland is observed in normal individuals. Functional defects are seen as areas of increased uptake whereas non-functioning nodules appear as cold spots. In individuals with cancer of the thyroid it is necessary to perform whole body imaging. Ectopic thyroid tissue or functioning metastases appear as areas of increased uptake.

Radioisotopes of iodine are also used to quantify thyroid activity. Measurement of thyroidal uptake of radio-iodine is used to differentiate thyrotoxicosis in which uptake is high, from thyroiditis in which uptake is low. Uptake measurements are also used to assess thyrotoxic patients before treatment with ^{131}I-sodium iodide.

Tumours

Traditional approaches to imaging cancer have relied on non-specific alterations in function or metabolism of surrounding tissue such as the osteoblastic response of bone, the loss of liver Kupffer cells or the alteration of the blood-brain barrier. Imaging with ^{67}Ga-gallium citrate, for example, relies upon its non-specific uptake by tumour tissue but it is also taken up in other inflammatory conditions. However, despite its non-specific mode of action, this radiopharmaceutical is useful in the detection of primary liver tumours and in the assessment of the extent of lymphomas.

Several radiopharmaceuticals with more specific modes of action are used to identify suspected tumours. The use of radioactive iodine in imaging thyroid cancer has been discussed. In addition to its use in imaging phaeochromocytoma, radiolabelled MIBG is also taken up specifically by neuroblastoma and medullary carcinoma of the thyroid. ^{99m}Tc-pentavalent dimercaptosuccinic acid (^{99m}Tc(V)DMSA) has also been found useful for imaging of medullary thyroid carcinoma.[42] However, the greatest efforts in tumour imaging have been directed towards the development of radiopharmaceuticals based on monoclonal antibodies.

In recent years, significant advances have been made in the isolation of tumour-specific antigens and in the development of monoclonal antibodies to these antigens. Radioimmunoscintigraphy (RIS) is the term used to describe the *in-vivo* use of radiolabelled antibodies to detect tumour sites by imaging with a gamma camera. There are many factors which affect the localisation of a radiolabelled monoclonal antibody in a tumour.[43] At the present time, the majority of antibodies in clinical use are directed against tumour-associated antigens. A few have become available through commercial sources, for example, antibodies to carcinoembryonic and melanoma-associated antigens. These radiopharmaceuticals are available either prelabelled with ^{131}I or ^{111}In or as kits for 'in-house' labelling with the latter radionuclides or with ^{99m}Tc.[44] At present, the role of RIS in primary diagnosis remains limited for most tumour types due to the relatively low sensitivity and specificity of the radiolabelled antibodies. However, encouraging results are being reported[45] and whilst it is clear that radiolabelled monoclonal antibodies have not yet fulfilled their theoretical potential, they do have a useful role. The selective uptake of radiolabelled antibodies in cancer tissue carries with it the hope of selective therapy.

In addition to their use in the diagnosis of cancer, several commercial radiolabelled antibodies are available for use in other areas of diagnosis; examples are antibodies to cardiac myosin for the investigation of myocardial infarction and antibodies to fibrin which are used to detect deep vein thrombosis (DVT).

Therapeutic Procedures

Blood

Polycythaemia vera is treated with ^{32}P-sodium phosphate. Following intravenous injection, the ^{32}P is taken up into bone where irradiation of the haematopoietic red marrow by beta radiation from ^{32}P causes a reduction in the formation of erythrocytes.

Bone

Palliation of pain from skeletal metastases can be achieved by treatment with ^{89}Sr-strontium chloride. When administered by the intravenous route, strontium is taken up by both the normal skeleton and, to a greater extent, skeletal metastases. Irradiation of the tumour deposits by the ^{89}Sr induces pain relief.

Joints

Yttrium-90 in the form of ^{90}Y-colloidal yttrium silicate is injected into joints for the treatment of chronic synovitis and effusions. It is particularly useful in the treatment of rheumatic conditions of the knee. The beta particles from the ^{90}Y bring about a partial radiation synovectomy which restores a degree of mobility to the joint.

Thyroid

As discussed previously, iodine is taken up by the thyroid gland. Activities of ^{131}I-sodium iodide far higher than those used diagnostically are used for the treatment of thyrotoxicosis and thyroid tumours. In these treatments, the radiopharmaceutical is normally administered by mouth, either as a liquid or in a capsule.

The radiopharmaceuticals used in the treatments described above are simple inorganic compounds and have been in clinical use for several decades. Over the last 10 years, targeted radiotherapy using radiopharmaceuticals has become increasingly popular, particularly in the fields of oncology and endocrinology. This development is due, in part, to the expanding availability of suitable radiopharmaceuticals and the recognition of new indications, and, in part, due to the fact that old therapies are being rediscovered such as the use of ^{89}Sr for metastatic bone pain.[46]

When using therapeutic radiopharmaceuticals, the uptake in critical organs and the radiation dose to tissues around the target area pose a considerable problem. The introduction of tumour-seeking carriers such as MIBG[47] and monoclonal antibodies[48] has greatly increased the potential to deliver a therapeutic radionuclide to its target. Future developments could also see the replacement of the traditional ^{131}I 'warhead' with more lethal radionuclides. High energy beta emitters such as yttrium-90 and short half-life alpha emitters such as astatine-211 can deliver a greater radiation dose than iodine-131, further improving radiotoxicity to the target cells.

Other attempts to increase the radiation dose to the target tissue include the use of more direct routes of administration. The intra-arterial route has been used to deliver formulations which preferentially lodge in the arterioles and capillaries of the tumour. Treatment of liver tumours by the intra-arterial administration of ^{90}Y-labelled microspheres is a typical development. Localised treatment of tumours that are spread over the linings of cavities and of tumour cells present in malignant effusions can be achieved by injecting the radiopharmaceutical into these cavities. An example of this approach is the intraperitoneal administration of colloids and antibodies labelled with ^{90}Y or ^{131}I for adjuvant therapy of ovarian carcinoma. Together with chemotherapy and external beam radiation, the use of radionuclide therapy offers a realistic additional mode of treatment for the management of malignant disease.[49]

Factors Affecting the Biodistribution of Radiopharmaceuticals

The biodistribution of radiopharmaceuticals is known to be affected by many factors. Altered biodistribution may lead to poor visualisation of an area of interest, misleading results from quantitative investigations or unnecessary irradiation of the patient. Radiochemical purity has an effect on the diagnostic or therapeutic outcome of a procedure, and can be adversely affected by the introduction of small amounts of contaminants during preparation.[50] There are many reports of concomitant drug therapy interfering with the biodistribution of radiopharmaceuticals and these have been reviewed extensively.[51] The most common of these effects have been published in tabular form for ease of reference.[52]

Conversely, some drugs are useful in enhancing the diagnostic value of nuclear medicine investigations, for example, the use of dipyridamole in cardiac imaging with ^{201}Tl and the use of diuretics in dynamic imaging of the kidneys with ^{123}I-iodohippurate and ^{99m}Tc-MAG3. Other drugs are used to reduce the radiation dose to particular organs by blocking uptake or increasing the rate of excretion; a well-known example is the use of iodide or perchlorate to block the uptake of radioisotopes of iodine into the thyroid.

Adverse Reactions

Although the chemical content of most radiopharmaceuticals is very small, adverse reactions are reported occasionally. The majority of reactions are mild, transient and require little or no treatment; the usual types are allergic, anaphylactic and vasovagal. However, serious reactions such as cardiorespiratory arrest, tachycardia, dyspnoea and hypotension have been reported occasionally. In the United Kingdom, a system for reporting adverse reactions is run by the British Institute of Radiology.[53]

REFERENCES

1. Millar AM, Macleod I, Marshall I. Pharm J 1990;245 (Hosp Pharm Suppl):9–11.
2. Department of Health and Social Security. Guidance notes for hospitals: premises and environment for the preparation of radiopharmaceuticals. London: HMSO, 1982.
3. Burch WM, Sullivan PJ, McLaren CJ. Nucl Med Commun 1986;7:865–71.
4. Pavel DG, Zimmer AM, Patterson VN. J Nucl Med 1977;18:305–8.
5. Callahan RJ, Froelich JW, McKusick KA, Leppo J, Strauss HW. J Nucl Med 1982;23 315–18.
6. Segal AW, Thakur ML, Arnot RN. Lancet 1976;2:1056–8.
7. Danpure HJ, Osman S, Brady F. Br J Radiol 1982;55:247–9.
8. Peters AM, Henderson BL, Kelly JD, Danpure HJ, Hawker RJ, Osman S et al. Lancet 1986;2:946–9.
9. Hunter WM, Greenwood FC. Nature 1962;194:495–6.
10. Fraker PJ, Speck Jr JC. Biochem Biophys Res Commun 1978 80:849–57.
11. Hawkins LA, Elliott AT, Shields R et al. Eur J Nucl Med 1982;7:58–61.
12. Hnatowich DJ, Layne WW, Childs RL et al. Science 1983;220:613–15.
13. Department of Health and Social Security. Guide to good pharmaceutical manufacturing practice. 3rd ed. London: HMSO, 1983.
14. Commission of the European Communities. The rules governing medicinal products in the European Community, Volume IV: Good manufacturing practice for medicinal products. Luxembourg: The Commission, 1992.
15. Ionising Radiations Regulations (S.I. 1985 No. 1333). London: HMSO, 1985.
16. Approved Code of Practice. The protection of persons against ionising radiation arising from any work activity. The Ionising Radiations Regulations 1985. London: HMSO, 1985.
17. National Radiological Protection Board. Guidance notes for the protection of persons against ionising radiations arising from medical and dental use. Oxford: NRPB, 1988.
18. British Standard Institution. British Standard 5295:1989. Environmental cleanliness in enclosed spaces. Parts 1, 2, 3. London: The Institution, 1989.
19. British Standard Institution. British Standard 5726:1979. Specification for microbiological safety cabinets. London: The Institution, 1979.
20. The Institute of Physical Sciences in Medicine. Report No 65–Calibration and quality control of medical radionuclide calibrators. York: The Institute, 1992.
21. British pharmacopoeia 1993. London: HMSO, 1993.
22. Council of Europe. The European pharmacopoeia. 2nd ed. Saint-Ruffine: Maisonneuve.
23. Zimmer AM, Pavel DG. J Nucl Med 1977;18:1230–3.
24. Zimmer AM, Pavel DG. Am J Hosp Pharm 1978;35:426–8.
25. Robbins PJ. Chromatography of technetium-99m radiopharmaceuticals — a practical guide. New York: The Society of Nuclear Medicine, 1984.
26. De Groot GJ, Das HA, de Ligny CL. Int J Appl Radiat Isot 1988;36:349–55.
27. Wieland DM, Tobes MC, Manger TJ, editors. Analytical and chromatographic techniques in radiopharmaceutical chemistry. New York: Springer-Verlag, 1986.
28. Slater DM, Anderson M, Garvie NW. Lancet 1983;2:1431–2.
29. Sampson CB, Keegan J. Nucl Med Commun 1985;6:313–18.
30. Murray T, Hilditch TE, Whateley TL, Elliott AT. Nucl Med Commun 1986;7:505–10.
31. Hilditch TE, Elliott AT, Murray T, Whateley TL. Nucl Med Commun 1986;7:845–50.
32. Brown S, Baker MH. Nucl Med Commun 1986;7:327–36.
33. International Commission on Radiological Protection. Publication 26–Recommendations of the International Commission on Radiological Protection, 1977. Annals of the ICRP 1977; 1 and subsequent statements 1978–85; 2(1), 4(3/4), 14(1), 14(2), 15(3). Oxford: Pergamon.
34. International Atomic Energy Agency. Regulations for the safe transport of radioactive material, Safety series no. 6. Vienna: The Agency, 1985 (as amended 1990).
35. The Radioactive Substances (Carriage by road) (Great Britain) (Amendment) Regulations 1985 (S.I. 1985 No. 1729). London: HMSO, 1985.
36. Wieland DM, Wu J, Brown LE, Manger TJ, Swanson DP, Beierwaltes WH. J Nucl Med 1980;21:349–53.
37. Nowotnik DP, Canning LR, Cumming SA et al. Nucl Med Commun 1985;6:499–506.
38. Holman BL, Jones AG, Lister-James J et al. J Nucl Med 1984;25:1350–5.
39. Khaw BA, Gold HK, Yasuda T et al. Circulation 1986;74:501–8.
40. Buscombe J R, Lui D, Ensing G et al. Nucl Med 1990;16:649–55.
41. Fritzberg AR, Sudhakar K, Eshima D, Johnson DL. J Nucl Med 1986;27:111–16.
42. Ohta H, Kazutaka Y, Endo K et al. J Nucl Med 1984;25:323–5.
43. Goodwin DA. J Nucl Med 1987;28:1358–62.
44. Britton KE, Granowska M, Mather SJ. Nucl Med Commun 1991;12:65–76.
45. Granowska M, Britton KE. Nucl Med Commun 1991;12:83–98.
46. Robinson RG, Blake GM, Preston DF et al. RadioGraphics 1989;9:271–81.
47. Sisson JC, Shapiro B. J Nucl Med 1984;24:197–206.
48. Britton KE, Mather SJ, Granowska M. Nucl Med Commun 1991;12:333–47.

49. Hoefnagel CA. Eur J Nucl Med 1991;408–31
50. Kristensen K. Factors which affect the integrity of radio-pharmaceuticals. In: Sampson CB, editor. Textbook of radiopharmacy–theory and practice. London: Gordon and Breach Science, 1991:319–28.
51. Sampson CB, Hesslewood SR. Adverse reactions to and drug incompatibilities with radiopharmaceuticals. In: Theobald AE, editor. Radiopharmaceuticals–using radio-active compounds in pharmaceutics and medicine. Chichester: Ellis Horwood, 1989:132–48.
52. Leung E, Hesslewood SR. Pharm J 1992;248:47–9.
53. Keeling DH. Nucl Med Commun 1988; 9: 259–61.

FURTHER INFORMATION

Frier M, Hardy JG, Hesslewood SR, Lawrence R. Hospital radiopharmacy: principles and practice. York: The Institute of Physical Sciences in Medicine, 1988.
Frier M, Hesslewood SR, editors. Quality assurance of radiopharmaceuticals: a guide to hospital practice. London: Chapman and Hall, 1980.
Fogelman I, Maisey M. An atlas of clinical nuclear medicine. London: Dunitz, 1988.
Maisey M, Britton KE, Gilday DL, editors. Clinical nuclear medicine, 2nd ed. London: Chapman and Hall, 1991.
Parker RP, Smith PHS, Taylor DM. Basic science of nuclear medicine. Edinburgh: Churchill Livingstone, 1978.
Perkins AC, Pimm MV. Immunoscintigraphy: practical aspects and clinical applications. New York: Wiley-Liss, 1991.
Saha G. Fundamentals of nuclear pharmacy. 2nd ed. New York: Springer-Verlag, 1985.
Sampson CB, editor. Textbook of radiopharmacy: theory and practice. New York: Gordon and Breach, 1990.
Theobald AE, editor. Radiopharmaceuticals: using radioactive compounds in pharmaceutics and medicine. Chichester: Ellis Horwood, 1989.
Wieland DM, Tubes MC, Manger TJ, editors. Analytical and chromatographic techniques in radiopharmaceutical chemistry. London: Springer-Verlag, 1986.

Cytotoxic Drugs: Handling Precautions

In recent years, advances in the specialities of surgery, radiotherapy, and chemotherapy have improved the prognosis for the cancer patient. With respect to the last aggressive form of treatment, the possibility of irreversible damage being incurred by normal tissue is a well recognised danger of cytotoxic drug therapy. Consequently, there is concern about the potential risk to staff who regularly handle these agents as traces of cytotoxic drugs may gain access to the body via inhalation, ingestion, or contact with skin. In an attempt to minimise this hazard to personnel, various organisations have published guidelines which detail the procedures to be followed when handling cytotoxic drugs.[1-4]

In 1983, the Pharmaceutical Society of Great Britain published guidelines, drawn up by a working party, for pharmacists, nurses, physicians, and other workers involved with the handling of cytotoxic drugs.[1] As the majority of information included in these guidelines is still relevant, the guidelines are presented as the main framework of this chapter (indented), supported by additional information on more recent progress in this field.

1. INTRODUCTION

Certain cytotoxic drugs have been shown to have mutagenic, carcinogenic, and teratogenic effects both in animals and man. There is, however, little evidence to show that cytotoxic drugs are mutagenic in man at the level of exposure that arises when they are prepared for injection and administered under suitable conditions and with reasonable care. In addition, many cytotoxic drugs and their preparations have properties that cause contact damage to the skin, eyes, and mucous membranes and precautions are required for their safe handling. It is, in the view of the working party, prudent to extend and develop such precautions to cover all cytotoxic drugs.

The following guidelines are intended to prevent, as far as possible, risks to all persons coming into contact with such drugs, both in their preparation and on their administration, while simultaneously helping to maintain a high standard of product.

Sections 2 to 6 are intended to provide the guidelines for the handling of injections and irrigations, and Section 7 gives additional consideration to oral dosage forms.

2. PERSONNEL AND LOCATION

2.1 Cytotoxic injections should be prepared in designated areas by nominated personnel.

2.2 Specific attention should be paid to the pharmaceutical requirements of each product, for example, diluent, reconstitution, storage, and labelling.

2.3 It is desirable that the preparation of these products should, where possible, be centralised so that expertise in handling may be built up, and so that any hazards are restricted to a single area.

The merits of a centralised reconstitution service in comparison to a decentralised system were examined from financial, safety, and time management viewpoints by Oakley and Reeves.[5]

The Aseptic Area

2.4 (i) The aseptic unit of a pharmacy department is suggested as the most appropriate place in a hospital, in which case the preparation should be under the control of a pharmacist.

(ii) Where such an aseptic unit is used the laminar flow cabinet should conform to British Standard 5726,[6] which will ensure adequate operator protection, and to British Standard 5295,[7] which provides product protection. Most Class II microbiological safety cabinets conform with both those standards and some have additional safety features for the aseptic preparation of cytotoxic products. Horizontal laminar flow cabinets should not be used for the preparation of cytotoxic substances.

(iii) Where a laminar flow cabinet is used it is preferable that it should be reserved solely for cytotoxic preparations.

Safety cabinets should preferably be vented to the outside environment (Class II, Type B).[3,4,8-10] The cabinets should be well-maintained and cleaned, disinfected, and decontaminated regularly.[3] Certification of biological safety cabinets

461

on installation, on physical movement, and at regular intervals during routine use is a further requirement.[3, 4, 8]

Alternative Area

2.5 (i) If aseptic facilities are not available or the workload is too small, preparation may be undertaken locally in a designated side room of a ward or clinic.

(ii) The side room should be away from ward traffic and food areas. The windows and doors should be closed to eliminate draughts and steps taken to ensure that the room is not used for other purposes while the preparation is being carried out.

(iii) The side room should be equipped with a work top or a table which has a laminate or stainless steel surface and intact edges. A sink and running water should be available.

(iv) If it is essential that a side room is used, consideration should be given to the local preparation or purchase of specific clothing or equipment packs which would facilitate a safe procedure. Such packs would be particularly relevant when the injections are to be administered in the community.

Negative pressure, unidirectional airflow isolators have been designed for use in the preparation of (parenteral) cytotoxic drugs. A detailed description of several designs of isolator can be found in *The Cytotoxics Handbook* (see Further Information). The development and practical use of one such system was described by Moore and Simpson.[11] The installation and operating costs of the isolator were relatively low. Levels of microbial and particulate contamination were monitored and operating procedures ensured protection of the product from microbial attack. The system was popular with staff because of its ease of use and the high degree of protection provided (due to the existence of a 'physical barrier' between the cytotoxic drug and the operator). Isolators are particularly suitable for small-scale operations.

Procedures and Training

2.6 (i) Detailed, agreed, written policies and procedures should be prepared locally for the preparation and administration of cytotoxic drugs which will cover practice both in the hospital and the community.

(ii) All personnel concerned should be instructed and trained in the precautions and techniques involved in conjunction with the written policies and procedures.

(iii) Local policies should identify persons who are responsible for supervising training and the operation of these policies.

A variety of methods are now employed to monitor personnel who are exposed to cytotoxic agents. Kaijser *et al*[12] published a comprehensive review of the biological and physical/chemical tests undertaken on the urine or blood of at-risk staff; these included tests on urine mutagenicity, cytogenetic methods, tests on immunological function, and spectrophotometric and chromatographic assays (on plasma, blood, and urine). However, the reliability and accuracy of the techniques currently applied are debatable.

The merits of applying a surveillance programme to staff who handle cytotoxic drugs were discussed by McDiarmid.[13] The approaches appropriate to such a scheme include: keeping a record of the time of exposure, protective clothing worn, spillages, accidents, and any symptoms reported which may be attributed to the agent concerned; physical examinations; laboratory studies; biological monitoring; and efficient record keeping.

3. TECHNIQUES AND PRECAUTIONS

Protective Clothing

3.1 The following protective items should be worn during the handling of all cytotoxic products:

Amendment (1987)

3.1 (i) Disposable gloves of surgical latex or polyvinyl chloride should be worn. Neither latex nor polyvinyl chloride are absolute barriers to all cytotoxic agents and a specification for the type of glove which affords best protection may appear in the manufacturer's data sheet for the particular cytotoxic product. In the absence of a definitive recommendation it would appear that, in general, latex gloves provide better protection than polyvinyl chloride.

Permeation of cytotoxic agents varies in rate and extent between gloves of the same material and within individual gloves; it can be reduced by wearing two pairs of gloves.

Because glove permeability increases with time, periods of continuous wear should not exceed one hour. Gloves should be discarded after use or immediately if punctured.

It is now widely accepted that the permeability of disposable gloves to cytotoxic drugs is related to glove thickness;[14–16] the lag time before penetration increases with increasing thickness. It is recognised that dexterity is compromised when operators wear two pairs of gloves and therefore this approach is not always suitable.[17] However, when dealing with spillages of particularly hazardous agents (for example, mustine) double gloving should be considered.

Some organisations recommend that only powder-free gloves should be used, however, due to the nature of the material and the moulding techniques used during their manufacture, few latex gloves can be classified as absolutely powder free.[18] Manufacturers should be responsible for testing the leakage rate of gloves to cytotoxic agents.[18]

Mader and co-workers[19] assessed the permeability of thick latex gloves (Sempermed Protector™, Semperit, Austria) produced for the handling of cytotoxic agents. The twelve drugs tested were classified into three groups according to their rate of diffusion (ranging from 15 minutes to over 4 hours). Diffusion through the latex membrane was parallelled with diffusion through biological membranes, the rate being a function of pH, lipophilicity, and molecular weight.

(ii) Surgical face mask of good quality.

(iii) Protective goggles or glasses, which should conform to British Standard 2092[20] and which should be washed thoroughly with water after use.

(iv) Disposable apron.

In aseptic rooms other suitable clothing will be required.

3.2 Adequate washing facilities and suitable eye wash should be easily available for immediate use in the event of contamination of the eyes, mucous membranes, or skin. Copious amounts of tap water should be used if eye wash is for any reason not available [See 6.1 (iv)].

Protective clothing must be removed before leaving the work area.[8]

For the handling of cytotoxic drugs in the domestic environment, the provision of packs which contain appropriate protective clothing and facilities for disposal of contaminated waste is recommended. In a programme introduced to provide ambulatory patients with home-based cytotoxic infusion therapy[21] patients were supplied with latex gloves (for syringe changes) and a 'burn bin', in addition to their drug supply. Participants were educated on the use of their infusion pump, the correct storage conditions for their cytotoxic drugs (supplied as prefilled syringes), and the safe disposal of contaminated waste. The importance of providing suitable guidelines on the handling of cytotoxic agents to home-based patients and their families and physicians is self-evident. A letter or instruction sheet proves beneficial in supporting information given verbally.[9, 22]

Preparation

3.3 (i) Spillage should be contained by a broad-edged tray when no other facility is available. The tray should contain a suitable vessel and/or non-fibrous gauze for aspiration of air and excessive drug volume.

(ii) For vials, techniques should be used to prevent pressure differentials between the inside and outside.

(iii) Ampoules should be held away from the face and covered with sterile, non-fibrous gauze when opened. Liquid-filled ampoules can produce aerosols during opening. Powders in ampoules are considered especially hazardous, as particles of drug can be liberated during opening.

(iv) Diluent should be slowly introduced down the wall of the vial or ampoule to ensure that the powder is thoroughly wet before agitation.

(v) If air is to be expelled when filling syringes, the top of the needle should be covered with sterile, non-fibrous gauze or the air expelled into a suitable vessel.

(vi) Luer-lock syringes and fittings should always be used to ensure that needles are firmly attached to syringes at all times.

The use of Luer-lock fittings is favoured over the use of friction fittings or push connections on syringes, tubing, and giving sets.[2, 3]

Various venting devices are available which help to minimise aerosol production when handling vials.[2, 3, 8]

The use of polypropylene syringes is recommended. Drug volumes contained within syringes should be considerably less than their full capacity.[3, 4]

4. LABELLING, PACKAGING, AND DISTRIBUTION

This section is particularly relevant where injections are prepared centrally for distribution to the wards or community.

4.1 Labels should be specifically designed and should state that there is a cytotoxic substance in the preparation.

4.2 The label should also state the total amount and volume of the preparation, the time and date after which it should not be used, and storage recommendations.

4.3 Procedures should be developed locally for the safe transport of cytotoxic preparations and may include specifically designed packs to avoid and contain spillage. A recording procedure for their issue and receipt should be considered.

In addition to attaching warning labels to all containers that hold cytotoxic preparations, there is merit in similarly labelling shelves on which these products are stored and also disposal bins.[3]

The value of including information in package inserts on suitable facilities for the preparation and disposal of cytotoxic drug products was discussed by Colls.[23] In 1986, the Committee on the Review of Medicines compiled a set of guidelines on information that should be included on data sheets and package inserts.[24]

After preparation, cytotoxic products should be packaged in sealed containers that allow immediate identification of any damage to its contents or signs of leakage.[3,8]

Refrigerated, padded, and locked boxes have been found to be suitable for the protection of products during transport off-site.[3] More detailed information on the labelling, packaging, and distribution of cytotoxic products is given in *The Cytotoxics Handbook* (see Further Information).

5. ADMINISTRATION

5.1 Strict observance of the normal procedures for administration of parenteral solutions is essential.

5.2 Although every precaution should be taken to avoid unnecessary risk, care should be taken to ensure that the patient is not made unduly anxious by the procedures used.

5.3 Intravenous infusion sets and containers should be assembled to avoid leakage. The patient's eyes, skin, and mucous membranes should be protected from contact with the drug. The patient's clothing, body, and bedding should be protected by the use of a waterproof layer with an absorbent disposable layer on top.

5.4 Needles must be changed between preparations and administration to avoid trailing solutions on the needle. New syringes and needles should be used on every occasion.

5.5 All personnel involved in administration of cytotoxic drugs should be trained in the identification of extravasation and the immediate action to be taken according to locally agreed policies.

During the selection of intravenous administration sets and infusion devices, consideration must be given to the particular cytotoxic preparation that is to be administered.[3] Again, the use of Luer-lock fittings is recommended.[3,4,8] Administration equipment should be monitored for signs of leakage.[3,4,10]

Special care must be applied to the priming of intravenous sets, irrespective of the method used for this procedure.

6. SPILLAGE AND DISPOSAL

Spillage

6.1 (i) Any spillage should be dealt with immediately or as soon as a procedure is completed. Protective clothing as for the preparation of cytotoxic products should be worn [See Section 3.1].

(ii) The spillage should be wiped up with damp, disposable paper towels and these placed in a high-risk, waste-disposal bag. The containers and bags used should be those specified in *Safe Disposal of Clinical Waste*, Health and Safety Commission, Health and Safety Advisory Committee, HMSO, 1982.[25]

(iii) Contaminated surfaces should be washed with copious amounts of water.

(iv) If spillage is on the skin, soap and cold water should be used. If the eyes are contaminated, immediate irrigation with sodium chloride eye wash should be carried out, and medical help sought.

It has been suggested that personnel should be given training on the management and clean-up of spillages.[3] In order to protect personnel working in the vicinity of a spill, the use of warning signs to identify the contaminated area has been recommended.[4] It is also good practice to record details pertaining to the cause and management of a spill along with a note of all staff exposed during the incident.[3]

Spill-kits for the rapid and efficient management of spillages should be readily available in all areas where cytotoxic drugs are being handled (including the domestic environment).[3,4,26] Batty and Plumridge[26] designed a cytotoxic spill-kit and detailed procedures to be followed during its use;

in addition to the standard contents of each kit, those situated in areas distant to the central cytotoxic preparation area were supplemented with gowns and overshoes.

Spill-kits are also recommended[3] for the containment of spills of volume greater than 150 mL or the contents of one drug ampoule or vial that occur within the biological safety cabinet; the need to decontaminate the cabinet should also be assessed. If the spillage is within the hood, involving contamination of the HEPA filter, the filter may have to be replaced.[4]

Large spillages should be contained by the use of absorbent materials of adequate capacity;[4] powder spills should be covered with damp cloths before clean-up and a respirator should be worn if airborne particles are present.

Johnson and Janosik[27] examined the section entitled 'Spill, Leak and Disposal Procedures' in Material Safety Data Sheets produced by the manufacturers of 22 injectable cytotoxic agents in the USA. The five most commonly recommended neutralising agents for spillage control were sodium hypochlorite, sodium hydroxide, potassium permanganate, trisodium phosphate, and sulphuric acid. Individual agents recommended for each cytotoxic preparation were tabulated. However, of all the methods mentioned in the above survey for the management of spills, Lunn and Sansone[28] were aware of only two that had actually been validated.

Wren et al[29] also identified the apparent lack of information available on the validation of clean-up procedures; they commented on the potential application of bioluminescent methods to validate inactivation of cytotoxics by decontaminating agents.

Disposal

6.2 (i) Disposal of dry waste, intravenous administration sets, and other contaminated materials should be in high-risk, waste-disposal bags.

(ii) Disposal of sharp objects, for example needles, syringes, vials, ampoules, should be in suitable rigid containers labelled with a hazard warning seal.

(iii) Arrangements should be made for collection and disposal of waste materials, ensuring that the personnel concerned are aware of the hazards involved. The material should be destroyed by incineration.

(iv) Cytotoxic drugs and their metabolites are excreted in urine and faeces. Patients should

be warned of the possible hazard and instructed in personal toilet care and washing. Cleaning staff within the cytotoxic preparation area should be informed of the need to handle cytotoxic waste (conspicuously labelled) with care; they must also wear suitable protective garments.[4] The requirement to provide adequate containers for waste products generated in the domestic environment should also be emphasised.[3]

Cytotoxic drugs should not be included in consignments of waste pharmaceuticals.

National (and in some cases international) and local regulations governing the procedures to be followed for the disposal of cytotoxic waste must be followed.

The Health and Safety Commission published guidelines on the safe disposal of clinical waste, including unwanted pharmaceuticals and soiled syringes and needles. The guidelines include information on compliance with the Control of Substances Hazardous to Health Regulations 1988 (COSHH) and other health and safety requirements.

During transportation, cytotoxic waste should be contained within spill-resistant receptacles and high levels of security must be maintained.[3]

Incineration is the preferred method for the disposal of cytotoxic waste, however the temperature at which the incinerator should be operated is the subject of much controversy as recommended temperatures are often in excess of those at which hospital incinerators function. Possible alternative disposal methods include land interment (at authorised sites) and chemical inactivation.

Garner et al[30] consulted manufacturers of cytotoxic drugs in the UK for advice on disposal procedures for their products. Recommendations for the disposal of both reconstituted material and unopened vials were tabulated.

In 1984, workers in the USA[31] drew up suggested procedures to be followed in National Institutes of Health when disposing of cytotoxic waste. Laws enforced by federal, state, and local regulatory bodies were outlined. Waste cytotoxic products and equipment or clothing contaminated with these agents were designated either as 'trace-contaminated' or 'bulk-contaminated' material; disposal of the former was by incineration and of the latter was by land interment or off-site incineration at Environmental Protection Agency approved sites. The options available to healthcare organisations involved with disposal of cytotoxic waste products were tabulated.

In 1983, Wilson[32] summarised information from manufacturers that related to the safe disposal of their injectable cytotoxic products. The methods examined were chemical neutralisation, incineration, and a third option of a return service for unused, expired products.

Lunn *et al*[33] reported in detail their 'Recommended Procedures' for the chemical degradation of several cytotoxic drugs with the aim of producing non-mutagenic products. The report concluded that the methods described were safe and effective for disposal of nitrosourea drugs and were suitable for degrading bulk quantities of unused drug and expired pharmaceutical preparations.

7. ORAL DOSAGE FORMS

Tablets and Capsules

7.1 (i) Many tablets, particularly the alkylating agents, either have an outer compression coating with the drug in an inner core, or are film coated. Therefore, there is no handling risk if the coatings are not broken down.

(ii) A small number of tablets are simply compressed powders. Where these are free from any loose powder there is no appreciable risk to the handler.

(iii) Capsules, whether hard or soft gelatin, are free from risk unless they are opened or have broken or leaked. Capsules should not be opened or crushed. In the event of spillage, precautions similar to those previously described under the handling and spillage of injections should be taken [See Section 6.1].

(iv) Personnel dispensing tablets and capsules should not touch them at any stage.

(v) Automatic counters should not be used unless cleaned after use. In most instances clean tablet counting triangles are suitable.

Suspensions

7.2 (i) Where a paediatric dosage is required a suspension is preferable to powders, which would be of greater risk to handlers.

(ii) Some formulations have been developed at paediatric oncology centres in conjunction with the pharmaceutical industry to meet existing needs. However, there are little stability data on these at the present time.

(iii) Where possible the preparation of such formulations should be restricted to oncology centres. The precautions and equipment necessary to protect the formulator would

be as previously described under injections [See Sections 2 and 3].

Advice to Patients and Their Relatives

7.3 Where an extemporaneous formulation is to be used the patient or relative (often the parent) should be counselled so as to protect individuals in the home from unnecessary exposure to the drug, and be given a verbal reminder to keep the preparation away from children. Discretion should be exercised on this matter so that no undue alarm is caused.

It has been recommended[3] that gloves should be worn for the routine handling of non-injectable hazardous drugs and also that only clean equipment reserved for work with these drugs be used. Protective garments should be worn during extemporaneous dispensing of preparations and this activity should be undertaken in a designated area. The varying levels of care required when dispensing uncoated, cored, or coated tablets and capsules were observed by Morris.[34] The potential for dust generation when crushing tablets was emphasised.

CONCLUSIONS

1. The guidelines give the general procedures that should be followed by medical, nursing, and pharmaceutical staff when handling cytotoxic drugs. Such general guidelines may require supplementation to take into account local conditions and practices.

2. All personnel handling cytotoxic drugs should undergo thorough training, which should be on a continuing basis. Personnel should be encouraged to report any difficulties they encounter in handling cytotoxic drugs and any adverse effects they experience that are considered to be due to such drugs. The administration of cytotoxic drugs by community nurses is increasing and the working party considers it important that such nurses should be trained in this work and provided with suitable equipment to enable them to handle cytotoxic drugs safely.

3. It is the view of the working party that the keeping of records of the handling of cytotoxic drugs by individuals has little immediate value. However, provided all essential information is recorded and there are suitable resources for retrieval and analysis, such records may be of value in the long term for retrospective studies.

4. There appears to be little basis for limiting the period in which an individual is involved in the handling of cytotoxic drugs. Evidence is not available on the effect of the handling of cytotoxic drugs on women with suspected or confirmed pregnancy and, therefore, firm guidance cannot be given. However, all female staff with suspected or confirmed pregnancy should immediately notify the appropriate responsible person so that their involvement in the handling of cytotoxic drugs can be considered.

5. Medical screening tests currently used or proposed give little relevant information of the possible hazard. However, the working party considers it important that studies are carried out on personnel in an attempt to assess the degree of hazard involved in the handling of cytotoxic drugs in accordance with these guidelines.

6. The working party recommends that manufacturers should consider improving the packaging of cytotoxic drugs to minimise the main hazards of their handling, which are the liberation of powder and aerosol formation. It may be, for example, that in some instances packaging in vials is to be preferred to ampoules and that certain injections could be available in unit-dose syringes. Manufacturers should also consider if any additional warning labelling is required for cytotoxic drugs. All solid dosage forms should be strip or blister packed.

7. Consideration should be given to the design of a suitable hazard symbol for cytotoxic preparations.

REFERENCES

1. Pharmaceutical Society Working Party Report. Guidelines for the handling of cytotoxic drugs. Pharm J 1983;230:230–1.
2. Health and Safety Executive. Guidance note MS 21: Precautions for the safe handling of cytotoxic drugs. London: HMSO, 1983.
3. American Society of Hospital Pharmacists. Technical assistance bulletin on handling cytotoxic and hazardous drugs. Am J Hosp Pharm 1990;47:1033–49.
4. Occupational Safety and Health Administration. OSHA work-practice guidelines for personnel dealing with cytotoxic (antineoplastic) drugs. Am J Hosp Pharm 1986;43:1193–204.
5. Oakley PA, Reeves E. Pharm J 1984;232:391–2.
6. British Standards Institution. British Standard 5726:1979 (1990). Specification for microbiological safety cabinets. London: The Institution, 1979.
7. British Standards Institution. British Standard 5295. Environmental cleanliness in enclosed spaces. London: The Institution, 1989.
8. National Study Commission on Cytotoxic Exposure. Recommendations for handling cytotoxic agents. Boston: The Commission, 1987.
9. Kaijser GP, Underberg WJM, Beijnen JH. Pharm Weekbl (Sci) 1990;12(6):228–35.
10. Zimmerman PF, Larsen RK, Barkley EW, Gallelli JF. Am J Hosp Pharm 1981;38:1693–5.
11. Moore AC, Simpson C. Pharm J 1989;242(Hosp Suppl):HS12–HS15.
12. Kaijser GP, Underberg WJM, Beijnen JH. Pharm Weekbl (Sci) 1990;12(6):217–27.
13. McDiarmid MA. Am J Hosp Pharm 1990;47:1061–6.
14. Laidlaw JL, Connor TH, Theiss JC, Anderson RW, Matney TS. Am J Hosp Pharm 1984;41:2618–23.
15. Thomas PH, Fenton-May V. Pharm J 1987;238:775–7.
16. Oldcorne MA, Taylor PA, White PJP [letter]. Pharm J 1987;238:488.
17. Horry JM. Pharm J 1987;238:501–2.
18. Wong RJ [letter]. Am J Hosp Pharm 1990;47:2459.
19. Mader RM, Rizovski B, Steger GG, Moser K, Rainer H, Dittrich C. Int J Pharmaceutics 1991;68:151–6.
20. British Standards Institution. British Standard 2092:1987. Specification for eye-protectors for industrial and non-industrial uses. London: The Institution, 1987.
21. Sewell GJ, Bradford E, Rowland CG. Pharm J 1989;243:139–41.
22. Begg S [letter]. Am J Hosp Pharm 1987;44:1024.
23. Colls BM. Br Med J 1985;291:1318–19.
24. Asscher W [letter]. Br Med J 1986;292:59.
25. Health and Safety Commission. Safe disposal of clinical waste. London: HMSO, 1982.
26. Batty KT, Plumridge RJ. Am J Hosp Pharm 1986;43:2235–6.
27. Johnson EG, Janosik JE. Am J Hosp Pharm 1989;46:318–19.
28. Lunn G, Sansone EB [letter]. Am J Hosp Pharm 1989;46:1131.
29. Wren AE, Denyer SP, Melia CD, Kendall J, Wilson JV, Garner ST. Int Pharm J 1991;5(3):119.
30. Garner S, Ross M, Wilson J. Pharm J 1988;241(Hosp Suppl):HS32.
31. Vaccari PL, Tonat K, De Christoforo R, Gallelli JF, Zimmerman PF. Am J Hosp Pharm 1984;41:87–93.
32. Wilson SJ. J Clin Hosp Pharm 1983;8:295–9.
33. Lunn G, Sansone EB, Andrews AW, Hellwig LC. J Pharm Sci 1989;78(8):652–9.
34. Morris JT [letter]. Pharm J 1988;240:171.

FURTHER INFORMATION

Allwood M, Wright P, editors. The cytotoxics handbook. Oxford: Radcliffe Medical Press, 1990.
Barcon DL, Presant CA, Melville J. Purging procedure eliminates antineoplastic drug solution spillage. Am J Hosp Pharm 1987;44:2254.
Bayhan A, Burgaz S, Karakaya AE. Urinary thioether excretion in nurses at an oncologic department. J Clin Pharm Ther 1987;12:303–6.
Castegnaro M, Adams J, Armour MA et al, editors. Laboratory decontamination and destruction of carcinogens in laboratory wastes: some antineoplastic agents. London: International Agency for Research of Cancer, 1985.
Clinical Oncology Society of Australia. Guidelines and recommendations for safe handling of antineoplastic agents. Med J Aust 1983;1:426–8.

Cohen IA, Newland SJ, Kirking DM. Injectable-antineoplastic-drug practices in Michigan hospitals [assessment of compliance with American Society of Hospital Pharmacists and Occupational Safety and Health Administration recommendations]. Am J Hosp Pharm 1987;44:1096–105.

Cooke J. Cytotoxic drugs: handle with care. Chemist Drugg 1987;2:884.

Cooke J, Williams J, Morgan RJ, Calvert RT. Environmental monitoring of personnel who handle cytotoxic drugs. Pharm J 1987(Suppl);239:R2.

Council on Scientific Affairs of the American Medical Association. Guidelines for handling parenteral antineoplastics. JAMA 1985;253:1590–2.

Dinter-Heidorn H, Carstens G. Comparative study on protective gloves for handling cytotoxic medicines: a model study with carmustine. Pharm Weekbl (Sci) 1992;14(4):180–4.

Gregoire RE, Segal R, Hale KM. Handling antineoplastic-drug admixtures at cancer centers: practices and pharmacist attitudes. Am J Hosp Pharm 1987;44:1090–5.

Guidance on cytotoxic services [contributed]. Pharm J 1988;241:751–2.

Health and Safety Commission. Safe disposal of clinical waste. London: HMSO, 1992.

Jones P. Disposal of waste cytotoxics [letter]. Pharm J 1989;242:56.

Laidlaw JL, Connor TH, Theiss JC, Anderson RW, Matney TS. Permeability of four disposable protective-clothing materials to seven antineoplastic drugs. Am J Hosp Pharm 1985;42:2449–54.

Larrouturou P, Huchet J, Taugourdeau MC. Centralized preparation of hazardous drugs. A choice between isolator and laminar airflow. Pharm Weekbl (Sci) 1992;14(3):88–92.

Melamed AJ, Kleinberg ML. Bibliography: handling considerations for cancer chemotherapeutic agents. Drug Intell Clin Pharm 1988;22:247–50.

Oakley PA, Reeves E. Setting up a centralised reconstitution service. Pharm J;1984;232:739–40.

Power LA, Anderson RW, Cortopassi R, Gera JR, Lewis RM. Uptake on safe handling of hazardous drugs: the advice of experts. Am J Hosp Pharm 1990;47:1050–60.

Sessink PJM, Anzion RB, Van den Broek PHH, Bos RP. Detection of contamination with antineoplastic agents in a hospital pharmacy department. Pharm Weekbl (Sci) 1992;14(1):16–22.

Van Raalte J, Rice C, Moss CE. Visible-light system for detecting doxorubicin contamination on skin surfaces. Am J Hosp Pharm 1990;47:1067–74.

Venitt S, Crofton-Sleigh C, Hunt J, Speechley V, Briggs K. Monitoring exposure of nursing and pharmacy personnel to cytotoxic drugs: urinary mutation assays and urinary platinum as markers of absorption. Lancet 1984;1:74–7.

de Werk NA, Wadden RA, Chiou WL. Exposure of hospital workers to airborne antineoplastic agents. Am J Hosp Pharm 1983;40:597–601.

Medical Gases

Carbon dioxide, nitrous oxide and oxygen are the gases recognised in the *British Pharmacopoeia*. However, the gases most commonly used in hospital practice that will be the main subject matter of this chapter, are carbon dioxide, oxygen, nitrous oxide, and the combination of the two latter gases, which is known as Entonox. Compressed air and vacuum are also considered because in piped systems they present similar problems to medical gases.

METHODS OF SUPPLY AND STORAGE

By their very nature, medical gases present more problems with regard to supply and storage than most other types of medicinal product.

Hospital Supplies

When a hospital uses large quantities of a gas, it becomes cost-effective to supply individual treatment points by means of a pipeline network from a central storage point. Gases which may be distributed in this manner are oxygen, nitrous oxide, Entonox, and air. A typical supply system comprises a central source, a distribution network, outlets at each point of use, and an alarm system. Installation and maintenance of such systems are rigidly controlled to ensure that continuous, safe, and trouble-free supplies of gas are available.

Central Source

Oxygen may be supplied from either a manifold or a liquid oxygen storage vessel depending on the size and type of hospital and the consequent demand for gas. A manifold comprises a collection of cylinders situated at a central point in the hospital in an area designated for cylinder storage. There are normally two separate banks of cylinders, which each carry two days supply; both are connected to the pipeline. The bank carrying the supply currently in use is known as the 'duty bank'. When the duty bank is about 95% depleted supply is switched automatically through a pneumatic changeover valve to the second or 'reserve' bank. The cylinders in the used bank are replaced manually. An additional separate manifold is kept as an emergency supply.

A liquid oxygen supply is more economical when weekly consumption exceeds 100 cubic metres. Liquid oxygen is stored in a stainless steel pressure vessel which may be thermally insulated by means of a combination of expanded perlite and a vacuum within a carbon steel outer shell. Such an installation is known as a vacuum insulated evaporator (VIE). The size of the storage vessel should be sufficient to hold a six-day supply for the hospital. Liquid oxygen flows from the storage vessel into a pressure-raising evaporator and then to a superheater that brings the gas up to ambient temperature. Various safety factors are incorporated in the system so that when there is no demand for gas, the oxygen that evaporates by ambient heat can be vented through a relief valve. A small manifold with two banks of five (J-size) cylinders is provided for emergencies.

Nitrous oxide and **Entonox** may be supplied directly from cylinders, but in large operating areas a manifold system is usually installed. The manifold is similar to that used for oxygen except that an automatic heater is included to overcome the problem of rapid cooling which occurs as the liquid nitrous oxide evaporates.

For **medical air**, a manifold system is acceptable when demand is small, but in larger hospitals a central compressor unit may be a more efficient method of supply. There are normally two identical compressors (duty and stand by). Air that is drawn in from the surroundings is filtered, compressed, cooled, and stored at pressures of between 930 and 1030 kPa in a welded steel receiver. As the air leaves the receiver it is further purified by the removal of oil before passage through two desiccant columns. The dried air is subjected to further filtration followed by pressure regulation to either 720 kPa (7 bar) for driving tools or 410 kPa (4 bar) for ward use.

Although not a gas, **vacuum** is subject to installation, monitoring, and service procedures similar to medical gases. A typical system consists of two identical pumps operating intermittently to provide a level of vacuum of not less than 53.3 kPa (400 mm mercury). Separators or traps are fitted in-line to prevent damage to the pumps; bacterial filters are also an in-line feature.

Distribution System

Gases are distributed by a network of piping from the source to the point of use within the hospital.

Copper pipes of a diameter calculated from a knowledge of the expected flow rates are used. Pipes should be laid or supported in such a way that they are protected from outside influences; special cladding is required when the supply is laid below a road surface. To join sections of pipe 'fluxless brazing' is the recommended technique;[1] this employs carbon dioxide or nitrogen as a shield gas and obviates the need to use flux.

A standard system for the identification of pipelines[2] is employed, by which identity marks are repeated at intervals of 2 to 4 metres along the length of the pipe, and before and after the pipe passes through a partition.

Outlets

The point in a ward or theatre at which clinical apparatus is connected to the gas supply is known as a **terminal unit**. Terminal units are designed to be gas-specific to minimise the risk of cross-connection of clinical equipment (and the patient) to the wrong gas. New terminal units must comply to British Standard 5682,[3] but non-standard systems can still be found in use in some British hospitals. In wards, terminal units are wall-mounted, but in theatres the feeder lines may be flexible pendant hoses or fixed boom pendants.

Where several gas outlets are closely adjoined the following positional order is recommended as a standard: oxygen; nitrous oxide; Entonox; air 4 bar; air 7 bar; vacuum.

Alarm Systems

Pipeline services are required to have a low pressure detector fitted to the main pipe leading from the central source. If the pressure drops to a preset level below the normal working value, visual and audible alarms are activated. So that immediate remedial action can be implemented, alarm panels are situated at key points, for example adjacent to operating areas and in a constantly manned area of the hospital such as the switchboard.

Domestic Supplies

The most common gas supplied to patients at home is oxygen. Depending on demand, the gas may be generated from an oxygen concentrator or supplied from cylinders.

Oxygen Concentrators

Of the two types of oxygen concentrators the most widely used operates on the principle of a molecular sieve. Oxygen and nitrogen are separated from ambient air; the nitrogen is vented to leave a gas mixture rich in oxygen that also contains inert gases. Depending on flow rate, it is possible to achieve oxygen concentrations of 95%.

Only certain patients are suitable for treatment with oxygen concentrators. In terms of cost-effectiveness, a concentrator would be considered for a patient who requires more than eight hours therapy daily.[4] The needs of patients on short-term therapy are usually met by cylinders. Referral to a consultant is necessary before a concentrator is installed.[5] To allow the patient freedom of movement in the home, oxygen is distributed from the concentrator to other rooms by means of plastic tubing. The patient is also supplied with a back-up cylinder for emergency use. Oxygen concentrators have also been considered for use in hospitals.[6,7]

Cylinders

Cylinders are supplied to a patient's home by a pharmacist contractor who is registered with the Family Health Services Authority (FHSA) to supply domiciliary oxygen. A disposable plastic face-mask, tubing, and a control valve are also provided. A size F cylinder contains 1360 litres of oxygen. A patient receiving 15 hours therapy daily would require 15 such cylinders each week. Small portable cylinders are available with capacities of 230 litres of oxygen (sufficient for two hours). Cylinders that can be filled from a larger cylinder in the patient's home provide sufficient gas to allow for short journeys away from home.

Oxygen maintained in a liquid state at low temperature is available for home use in the USA, but is not currently supplied in the UK.

IDENTIFICATION AND LABELLING OF CYLINDERS

Most medical gases are the subject of pharmacopoeial monographs and in addition cylinders, valves, and couplings associated with such gases are specified in British Standard 1319.[8] An appendix makes recommendations for the care and handling of anaesthetic equipment. Cylinders for individual gases are identifiable by standard combinations of colour and markings depicted on a BS chart[9] (see Table 1). The name of the gas or chemical symbol is stencilled in paint on the shoulder of the cylinder and should be clearly and indelibly stamped on the cylinder valve.

Regulatory Requirements for Markings, Labels, and Information

Cylinders must be painted in accordance with the colour code in BS 1319C; cylinders of liquefiable

Table 1
Medical gas cylinders: identification

Name of gas	Symbol	Colour of cylinder body	Colour of valve end where different from body
Oxygen	O_2	black	white
Nitrous oxide	N_2O	blue	–
Cyclopropane*	C_3H_6	orange	–
Carbon dioxide	CO_2	grey	–
Ethylene	C_2H_4	violet	–
Helium	He	brown	–
Nitrogen	N_2	grey	–
Oxygen and carbon dioxide mixture	$O_2 + CO_2$	black	black
Oxygen and helium mixture	$O_2 + He$	black	white and grey
Oxygen and nitrous oxide mixture	$O_2 + N_2O$	blue	white and brown
Air (medical)	AIR	grey	blue and white
			white and black

*Cyclopropane is no longer manufactured in the UK.

gases are stamped on the valve with the empty (tare) weight.

Current regulations[10] require the following information to appear on the cylinder label:

- chemical name and symbol of product
- cylinder size (letter code)
- nominal contents in litres
- nominal pressure in bars
- hazard warning sign and number
- specific product and cylinder handling precautions
- instructions for use.

A safety data sheet is supplied to each user so that the risks to staff involved in handling the cylinder and its contents may be assessed.[11]

Cylinder Valves

Pin-index valves have been designed to eliminate the possibility of the wrong equipment being connected to a cylinder. The pin position on the cylinder valve is dimensionally related to the gas outlet: pin positions are unique for each gas. If an attempt is made to connect a cylinder to the wrong equipment, the pins will not fit and a gas-tight connection cannot be made. The relative pin positions on oxygen cylinders and nitrous oxide cylinders are shown in Fig. 1. Pin-index valves that have the opening spindle on top are fitted on all cylinders up to size E and on Entonox cylinders of sizes F and G. Pin-index valves with a spindle at the side are fitted to J-size cylinders of oxygen and air. Nitrous oxide cylinders of sizes F and G and carbon dioxide cylinders of size F are fitted with a hand-wheel valve. All other cylinders are fitted with a bullnose top outlet valve; among these are the oxygen cylinders prescribed for domiciliary use (size F). The bullnose valve is not gas specific

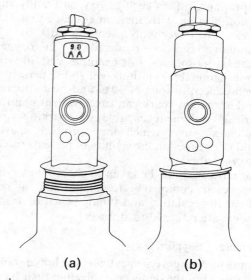

(a)   **(b)**

Fig. 1
Relative pin positions of (a) oxygen and (b) nitrous oxide cylinders.

and, therefore, extra vigilance is essential in confirming the identity of the cylinder.

SAFETY ASPECTS

Storage

Where it is necessary to keep large quantities of cylinders of different gases, the guidelines on the design and maintenance of separate stores should be closely followed. Generally, the rules of good storekeeping apply, with the additional requirements that oxidising and inflammable gases should be segregated and that there should be clearly defined 'full' and 'empty' areas. Cylinders should be stored vertically or horizontally according to size (except Entonox) and held securely to prevent them from falling. Entonox cylinders must always be stored horizontally. When cylinders of Entonox have been stored at temperatures below 5°, there is a possibility that the contents may have separated into the two constituent phases; cylinders subjected to such temperatures should be allowed to reach room temperature before use. Stores should be kept clean and free from extraneous material. The relevant fire and security services should be familiar with the locations of the stores.

Fire Precautions

While some gases are inflammable, for example cyclopropane, others such as oxygen readily support combustion with the consequence that substances not normally considered to be inflammable can be rendered so in oxygen-enriched atmospheres. For example, certain types of 'non-flammable' clothing will burn fiercely in oxygen concentrations of 30% and over. Because even the smallest spark can cause violent ignition, electrical equipment capable of sparking (and even certain toys which may produce sparks) should not be used in the vicinity of patients receiving oxygen therapy.

Particular care must be taken to ensure that cylinder valves are completely closed, and that any residual gas in regulators and tubing is vented before cylinders are returned to storage.

Domiciliary Supplies

Patients receiving oxygen cylinders at home should be informed of the dangers involved in their handling and use. Counselling and an information leaflet should be provided by the pharmacist contractor who supplies the cylinders.

Anaesthetic Gases

Heavy or prolonged exposure to nitrous oxide has been shown to be associated with neurological problems.[12] The gas may induce adverse haematological effects due to an interaction with vitamin B_{12}.[13] A survey among nursing staff working in a theatre showed that exposure levels of nitrous oxide reached 360 ppm and averaged 100 ppm;[14] a proposed Occupational Exposure Standard for nitrous oxide is 100 ppm.[15] In order to achieve occupational levels that are as low as possible, waste gas disposal systems (scavenging units) are installed in operating theatres. Passive disposal systems vent the waste gas to a wall terminal unit or make use of extraction via the room ventilation system. Active systems consist of a vacuum pump that draws the waste gas to the atmosphere through a separate terminal unit situated close to the operating point; a usual location is on the fixed boom pendant that supplies the other medical gases. Since patients recovering from anaesthesia continue to exhale anaesthetic gases, scavenging units often have wall terminal units in recovery rooms.

Decanting

Decanting involves the transfer of gas (oxygen only) from one cylinder to another smaller cylinder. The process should be strictly controlled and only carried out by properly trained personnel. Oxygen is a licensed medicinal product and decanting could therefore be classed as an assembly operation; relevant documentation should be available.

QUALITY AND PURITY

Pipeline Systems

The responsibility for assuring the quality of gas issuing from a pipeline system is held jointly by the hospital engineer and the pharmacist. Physical or chemical testing of the gas is normally only necessary after the installation of a new system or the repair or upgrading of an existing system. An evaluation of the level of hazard is necessary when there is a possibility that the quality of the gas supply may have been compromised as a result of the work carried out. No work should be undertaken on any part of an installation without the knowledge and approval of medical, nursing, and pharmacy staff who may be affected. A pharmacist designated as the 'suitably qualified person' is responsible for confirming the identity and purity of the gas.

Contaminants

Contaminants in medical gases can be divided into two main categories: those due to the nature of the gas itself and those that occur as a result of the method of supply.

Contaminants directly associated with the gas are the pharmacopoeial impurities for which limits are stated in the official monograph. Since the gases in use are licensed medicinal products of a high purity, it is unlikely that such impurities will be present. It is more likely that any impurities found will be a result of the means by which the gas is processed, supplied, or circulated throughout the distribution network.

Particles. Particulate contamination can be present in the form of copper oxide (from pipework brazing), metal particles, and general dirt and grime. Following the introduction in 1982 of 'fluxless brazing', pipeline joints are much cleaner with virtually no oxide formation; it is therefore only in older installations (pre-1982) that particulate contamination presents a serious problem.

Shield Gases. Inert gases such as carbon dioxide or nitrogen are introduced into pipelines during fluxless brazing. If not adequately purged from the system, residues can travel throughout the length of the pipeline system eventually emerging from a terminal unit.

Medical Air

While there is no official monograph for medical breathing air, recommendations on limits of impurities are available.[16, 17] The contaminants found are those present in normal breathing air and those likely to be contributed during processing. Oil may be present as droplets or vapour. Water may be detected where driers are faulty or when poor design of the pipeline system permits the presence of 'dead legs' in which condensation may occur. The presence of moisture in piped air may cause damage to the delicate mechanisms of air-driven tools.

Bacterial contamination of air supplies has been reported;[18] *Penicillium* and *Aspergillus* species were detected. It is considered that organisms such as *Pseudomonas* would not survive in dry air, but could present problems where driers were not functioning efficiently.

Test Methods

Identity

In order to ensure that there has been no cross-connection of pipelines during work on the system, a test to confirm the identity of the gas issuing from a pipeline is of paramount importance. The most common method is to analyse the oxygen content of the gas using a paramagnetic oxygen analyser, which is specific for oxygen in the presence of the gases normally found in hospital systems. The expected oxygen and nitrous oxide contents of medical gases is shown in Table 2. Nitrous oxide content may be measured by means of a thermal conductivity detector. Alternatively, a simple gas differentiator may be used to indicate the identity of the gas. Instruments that operate by measuring thermal conductivity or capacity have the disadvantage that nitrous oxide and carbon

Table 2
Typical contents of piped gases

Piped gas	Oxygen concentration (%v/v)	Nitrous oxide concentration (%v/v)
Oxygen	not less than 99	
Nitrous oxide	–	not less than 97
Entonox	48–52	48–52
Air	20–22	–

dioxide cannot be differentiated. Therefore, a further qualitative test for the presence of carbon dioxide is necessary when testing nitrous oxide pipelines. The presence of vacuum is confirmed by measuring the level of vacuum drawn through the relevant outlets.

Purity

Particulate Contamination. The most common technique used for the detection of particles is to pass a known volume of gas through a membrane filter. No solid particles should be visible. If particles are present the line is purged by venting a quantity of gas (taking care to discharge safely to protect operators) and the test is repeated.

Specific Contaminants. Gas detector tubes are available in a wide range. The tubes contain reagents that change colour in the presence of specific contaminants. They provide a quantitative indication of the amount of contaminant present and are used to detect such impurities as water, carbon monoxide, carbon dioxide, and a range of other substances that are mentioned in the pharmacopoeial monographs.

Non-specific Contaminants. An indication of the presence of impurities such as welding gases may be obtained using a non-specific indicator tube (for example, Polytest™).

Oil. The presence of oil may be detected by passing a known volume of gas over the surface of a membrane filter. Any oil present appears as translucent spots on the filter surface.

ANCILLARY EQUIPMENT

The safe delivery of gas to a patient is dependent on the correct selection of pressure regulators and flowmeters and the appropriate types of tubing and face-pieces.

Domestic Supplies

A pharmacist contractor who provides oxygen to a home patient will also supply the necessary control and delivery equipment.

Hospital Supplies

Delivery of gas to a patient is by means of a probe which fits the terminal unit and is connected to a flowmeter, tubing, and, if the gas is oxygen, a mask. Anaesthetic gases may be further by-passed through a variety of anaesthetic equipment.

Probes

A probe connects with a terminal unit and is rendered gas-specific by means of a collar which is designed to fit only the terminal unit of the required gas.[19]

Flowmeters

Flowmeters allow regulation of the velocity of gas and are available for air or oxygen although the two types should not be interchanged.

Humidifiers

If required for long-term therapy an external water humidifier or nebuliser may be fitted downstream of the flowmeter.

Anaesthetic Equipment

During the course of anaesthesia, a number of different gases may be administered. Volatile liquid anaesthetics are often employed and all are mixed with oxygen before administration. Most anaesthetists use a trolley that supplies the necessary gases, either from cylinders or from the pipeline system. The cylinders are attached by means of pin-indexed yokes that prevent inadvertent cross-connection of the wrong gas. Volatile liquids are vapourised and all gases are passed through flowmeters. An absorber is used to remove carbon dioxide from exhaled gas, which is then passed back to the patient mixed with additional oxygen.

Ventilators and Resuscitators

Both ventilators and resuscitators are used mechanically to assist ventilation either during anaesthesia or to patients in intensive care areas. Resuscitators are simple, lightweight, and portable instruments intended for short-term emergency use; they may be operated manually.

Ventilators are designed for longer use and are more sophisticated. Most commonly, ventilators operate under positive pressure to maintain tidal volume in patients with reasonable consistency. Certain types used in intensive care areas have patient triggering devices that deliver air when the patient attempts to inhale.[20]

SPECIAL APPLICATIONS

Hyperbaric Oxygen

Oxygen at 2.5 times atmospheric pressure is used in the treatment of carbon monoxide poisoning. Treatment involves placing the patient in a special high-pressure chamber, of which few are currently available. The time taken to eliminate the carbon monoxide bound to haemoglobin is reduced and it has been shown that later complications are prevented.[21] Hyperbaric oxygen has been used to enhance the effectiveness of the irradiation of tumours of head and neck, and as an adjunct to treatment of gas gangrene.

Liquid Gases

Liquid carbon dioxide is required for the operation of certain types of lasers used in surgery.

REFERENCES

1. Department of Health and Social Security. Introduction of new jointing methods for the installation of medical gas pipelines. WKO(72)1. London: HMSO, 1982 January.
2. Department of Health and Social Security. Health Technical Memorandum No.22. Piped medical gases, medical compressed air and medical vacuum installations. London: HMSO, 1977 March:(Appendix 4)44.
3. British Standards Institution. British Standard 5682:1984. Medical gas pipeline systems: terminal units, hose assemblies and connections to medical equipment. London: The Institution, 1984:5.
4. Axon S. Pharm J 1987;239:733–4,776–7.
5. Flenley DC. Pharm J 1984;233:145.
6. Houldsworth HB, O'Sullivan J, Smith M. HSE Bulletin 1987;60:15–18.
7. Arrowsmith LWH. HSE Bulletin 1988;61:62–5.
8. British Standards Institution. British Standard 1319:1976. Medical gas cylinders, valves and yoke connections. London: The Institution, 1976.
9. British Standards Institution. British Standard 1319C:1976. Chart of colours for identification of the contents of medical gas cylinders. London: The Institution, 1976.
10. Health and Safety Executive HS(R)22. A guide to the classification, packaging and labelling of dangerous substances regulations 1984. London: HMSO, 1986:27.
11. Control of substances hazardous to health regulations. London: HMSO, 1988.
12. Layzer RB. Lancet 1978;2:1227.
13. Nunn JF. Br J Anaesthesia 1987;59:3–13.
14. Manley AJ. Br Med J 1986;293:1063,1280.
15. Health and Safety Executive EH 40/93. Occupational exposure limits 1993. London: HMSO, 1993:28.
16. Department of Health and Social Security. Health Technical Memorandum No.22. Piped medical gases, medical compressed air and medical vacuum installations. London: HMSO, 1978 March:20.
17. British Standards Institution. British Standard 4275:1974. Recommendations for the selection, use and maintenance of respiratory protective equipment. London: The Institution, 1974:12.

18. Warren RE, Newson SWB, Matthews JA, Arrowsmith LWH. Lancet 1986;1:1438.
19. British Standards Institution. British Standard 5682:1984. Specification for medical gas pipeline systems: terminal units, hose assemblies and connections to medical equipment. London: The Institution, 1984:9.
20. Barbarash RA, Smith LA, Godwin JE, Sahn SA. DICP Ann Pharmacother 1990;24:259–70.
21. Hyperbaric oxygen. Drug Ther Bull 1988;26(20):77–8.

FURTHER INFORMATION

Installation and Maintenance of Pipeline Systems. Department of Health and Social Security. Health Technical Memorandum No.22: Piped medical gases, medical compressed air and medical vacuum installations. London: HMSO, 1977 March.

National Health Service Model Engineering Specifications C11: Medical gases. Wessex Regional Health Authority, 1990 January.

Domestic Supplies. Domestic Oxygen Supplies. Drug Ther Bull 1990;28(25):99–100.

Evans TW, Waterhouse J, Howard P. Clinical experience with the oxygen concentrator. Br Med J 1983;287:459.

Harman RJ. Oxygen therapy. In: Patient care in community practice. A handbook of non-medicinal health care. London: The Pharmaceutical Press, 1989:139–56.

Safety. Department of Health and Social Security. Health Equipment Information 163. Code of practice—safety and care in the storage, handling and use of medical gas cylinders on health authority premises. London: HMSO, 1987.

Quality and Purity. Department of Health and Social Security. Health Technical Memorandum No.22 Supplement. Permit to work system for piped medical gases, medical compressed air and medical vacuum installations. London: HMSO, 1977 March.

Ancillary Equipment. Jones HA, Turner SL, Hughes JMB. Performance of the large reservoir oxygen mask (Venti-mask). Lancet 1984;1:1427.

Worby RG. Oxygen for use in the home. Chemist Drugg 1991;236:380–3.

Immunological Products

IMMUNOLOGY

In mammalian tissues, complex systems exist for the recognition, neutralisation, and removal of foreign particles (for example, micro-organisms and foreign proteins) that may gain entry to the body. These defence mechanisms may be specific or non-specific. Specific defence mechanisms, such as the reaction of antibody with antigen, operate only when a person has been previously exposed to a particular antigenic substance. Non-specific mechanisms do not depend on previous exposure to foreign substances; they include phagocytosis by macrophages and the presence of antimicrobial substances in body secretions (for example, lysozyme in tears). In cell-mediated (non-specific) immunity the cells react in the same way to every antigen and do not distinguish between antigens. Humoral (specific) immunity is a property of lymphocytes.

Lymphocytes

Lymphocytes are the principal cells involved in immunological reactions. There are two major types of lymphocyte known as T-cells and B-cells. Both types appear to arise from a primitive stem cell in bone marrow. The immature T-cells migrate to the thymus where they mature. Various subpopulations of T-cells are produced, which differ in certain aspects (for example, functional capacity, surface receptors). B-cells were so named because in birds they were found to be processed in the Bursa of Fabricius. After stimulation by antigen, B-cells differentiate into plasma cells and secrete specific antibodies.

Antigens

Substances capable of stimulating an immunological response, such as the formation of antibodies, are known as antigens or immunogens. Antigenic substances may be proteins, polysaccharides, or complex lipids (for example, bacterial cell walls, the surface of erythrocytes, the protein capsule of viruses, the exotoxins and endotoxins of bacteria). The ability to stimulate an immune response usually resides in a part of the molecule that is called the determinant group.

Some molecules, including common chemicals and drugs, which are not antigenic by themselves may become antigenic when attached to other larger molecules called haptens. Penicillin is a hapten that becomes antigenic when attached to certain proteins in the skin. Other haptens, including benzodiazepines and oral hypoglycaemics, are activated by ultraviolet irradiation and are known as photosensitisers.

Histocompatibility Antigens

Histocompatibility or transplantation antigens are genetically determined antigens that are present on the surface of various cells. In man, the major histocompatibility system is known as HLA (human lymphocyte antigen). These antigens are found on most tissues but differ in distribution on these tissues. They are present on leucocytes and platelets but not on erythrocytes. They can be detected by serological techniques (HLA-A, HLA-B, HLA-C series) or in lymphocyte culture (HLA-D).

The HLA antigens are responsible for rejection of skin grafts and kidney transplants. Grafts from a genetically different donor will contain foreign antigens. Although the graft may vascularise and appear healthy for some time, rejection may eventually occur with inflammation and necrosis owing to the reaction of lymphocytes to the foreign antigens. Immunological tolerance to the body's own antigens develops during foetal life. In abnormal situations where an immune reaction does occur to a component of the body's own tissue, the reaction is known as an auto-immune reaction.

Antibodies

Antibodies or immunoglobulins are proteins that are found in association with the gamma globulin fraction of plasma. The antibody molecule comprises four polypeptide chains: two identical heavy chains and two identical light chains joined by disulphide bridges. There are two types of light chain, which are called kappa and lambda, and each antibody has either two kappa or two lambda chains. Each light chain has a constant portion, which is the same for each type of chain, and a variable portion which is responsible for antibody specificity. The heavy chains also contain a constant and a variable portion. The variable portion contributes to antibody specificity. The rest of the heavy chain is constant for any given type of antibody and antibodies can be classified according to this constant portion into five types:

- **Immunoglobulin M (IgM)**, the largest antibody, is concerned with complement fixation, agglutination, and opsonisation. It is formed early in an immune response and declines rapidly, and because of its large size does not leave the blood vessels or cross the placenta. The isoagglutinins of blood groups A and B belong to this group.

- **Immunoglobulin G (IgG)** is the most abundant of antibody molecules. It is formed later than IgM and is concerned with precipitation, complement fixation, and antitoxic activity. Antibodies to most viruses, bacteria, and bacterial toxins belong to this group. Immunoglobulin G antibodies can cross the placenta and confer passive immunity on the infant for the first few months of life.

- **Immunoglobulin A (IgA)** is concerned with the protection of surfaces such as nasal, buccal, and gastric mucosa.

- **Immunoglobulin D (IgD)** is present in trace amounts in plasma. Its precise function is not yet clear, but it is believed to be involved in lymphocyte differentiation.

- **Immunoglobulin E (IgE)** is present in trace amounts in plasma. It binds specifically to mast cells and basophils. Combination of specific antigen with the IgE antibodies on mast cells initiates a series of events that leads to release of substances such as histamine and SRSA (slow reacting substance of anaphylaxis) from the mast cells causing degranulation of mast cells, and thus the symptoms of anaphylaxis and allergy.

COMPLEMENT

The complement system consists of nine proteins or components that are present in plasma in non-activated forms. Activation is effected by antigen-antibody reaction (IgG or IgM), by fungal or bacterial products, or by trypsin. Activation of the complement system leads to sequential activation of individual complement components (cascade). Complexes and enzymes are generated that have diverse biological activities ranging from cell lysis to recruitment of the essential ingredients of an inflammatory response. Although specific activation of the complement system benefits the host in terms of resistance to infectious organisms, certain diseases and clinical disorders are associated with abnormalities of the complement system. Genetic deficiency of either the components or inhibitors of the complement system may result in either incomplete activation (recurrent bacterial infection) or excessive activation (hereditary angioneurotic oedema).

Antigen-Antibody Reactions

If antigens and their specific antibodies are mixed *in vitro*, the observable reactions that take place depend more on the form of the antigen and the presence of other substances than on the nature of the antibody. The visible reactions are:

- precipitation, where the antigen is in a soluble form (for example, toxin solutions) and electrolytes are present
- agglutination, where the antigen forms part of a whole cell (for example, bacterial suspensions)
- opsonisation, where the antigen forms part of an intact cell and the antibody sensitises the cell to ingestion by phagocytes (for example, phagocytosis of virulent bacteria)
- lysis, where the antigen-containing intact cell is sensitised by the antibody to the lytic action of complement.

One reaction that is not visible *in vitro* and requires tests on animals *in vivo* is the neutralisation reaction. This includes neutralisation of a toxin by its antitoxin and neutralisation of a virus by its antiserum in cell culture.

It is generally considered that any antibody is capable of producing any of these reactions with its specific antigen if the conditions are right.

Immune Responses

There are two basic types of immune mechanism: humoral and cell-mediated immunity. In humoral immunity, antibodies are formed by plasma cells derived from B-cells. The antibody is released into the circulation and it is this antibody that reacts with the antigen.

In cell-mediated immunity, T-lymphocytes sensitised to specific antigens react directly with these antigens without the presence of free antibody. T-cells have surface receptors for specific antigens and can destroy the antigen directly or can promote macrophage activity.

Immunity

If an animal possesses humoral (or circulating) antibodies against a particular bacterium or virus, it is said to be immune. The immunity may be acquired by a number of methods, most notably after recovery from an infection (natural active immunity), after injection with vaccines (artificial active immunity), or after injection of preformed antibodies derived from another immune animal (artificial passive immunity). Infants possess antibodies derived from the mother via the placenta before birth and in breast milk after birth, and these confer immunity for the first few months of life (natural passive immunity).

A state of immunity to a particular infection is rarely permanent, its duration depending on the type of organism from which the antigens were derived and the way in which the immunity arises. For example, immunity to viral infections generally lasts longer than that to bacterial infections. Immunity acquired by infection is longer-lived than that acquired by artificial means and active immunity is much more durable than passive immunity. There are a number of exceptions to these generalisations, for example, immunity to the common cold virus appears to be short lived.

After the introduction of antigens into the body, time is required for antibodies to appear in the blood in detectable quantities. The quantity of antibody per unit volume of blood (or titre) rises to a maximum over a fairly short period of time and then declines at a rate depending on the particular type of antigen. In vaccine administration, the dose is usually repeated while the antibody concentration is rising and this causes a considerable increase in the final titre obtained. When this has finally declined to negligible levels, a further 'booster' dose is given which results in a much more rapid and copious response than the same dose given to a non-immunised animal. The ability to respond in this way to subsequent doses of the same antigen depends on the 'memory cells' of the lymphatic system. These are certain lymphocytes that act as specific antigen detectors and which stimulate the appropriate specific plasma cells to produce the complementary antibody.

The body can respond to more than one antigen at a time but as the number of antigens in a mixed dose increases there is a falling-off in the response to each antigen compared to that produced by the same antigen given by itself.

When preformed antibodies (for example, antitoxins, antivenins, or antisera) are injected, they are utilised by the body at the same rate as normal plasma protein and hence disappear fairly rapidly. Therefore, it is necessary to give repeated doses during an infection and this immunity quickly declines after doses are withdrawn. The proteins may themselves act as antigens and the resulting antigen-antibody reaction may lead to anaphylactic shock or serum sickness. This is minimised by the use of purified globulin preparations and by limiting the amount administered and is now fortunately rare.

Allergy

Allergic or anaphylactic reactions (immediate hypersensitivity) are caused by antigen-antibody reactions on the surface of mast cells initiating a series of events leading to release of histamine and other agents from the mast cells. Relatively mild symptoms occur if the antigen-antibody reaction occurs at the nasal mucosa (hay fever or allergic rhinitis), whereas intense bronchospasm may occur as a result of inhalation of antigens (asthma). These reactions occur most commonly to pollen, dust, and animal dander. If the antigen is injected, as in the case of foreign sera, penicillin, or insect sting, the systemic anaphylaxis may occur; this is a potentially fatal condition. Urticaria can develop as a result of absorption of antigen from the gastro-intestinal tract. Antigens are commonly present in strawberries, nuts, eggs, and shellfish.

The antigens responsible for initiating allergic reactions are usually called allergens.

VACCINES

Vaccines are preparations of antigenic material that are administered with the object of inducing, in the recipient, a specific active immunity to infection or intoxication by the corresponding infecting agents. They are prepared from bacteria, rickettsiae, or viruses and may be suspensions of the living or inactivated organisms, or fractions thereof, or toxoids. Where antigens cannot conveniently be separated from bacterial cells (for example, endotoxins) and are of comparatively low toxicity, suspensions of intact bacterial cells may be used. Vaccines may be simple (prepared from one species only) or mixed (prepared from two or more vaccines). Where there is antigenic variation between strains within a single species, the final suspension may be a mixture of strains exhibiting the major antigens of the species (for example, cholera vaccine).

The methods of preparation are designed to ensure that the identity of specific antigens is maintained and that no microbial contaminants are introduced. Injectable products are distributed under aseptic conditions into sterile tamper-evident containers which are then sealed to exclude extraneous micro-organisms. Oral vaccines may be presented as suspensions of live attenuated virus (Poliomyelitis Vaccine, Live (Oral) BP) or in enteric-coated capsules (Typhoid Vaccine, Live (Oral)). Alternatively, the products may be lyophilised by a procedure that reduces the water content of the final product to not more than 2% w/w unless otherwise stated in the official monograph. The containers may then be sealed under vacuum or they may be filled with oxygen-free nitrogen or another suitable inert gas before being sealed. All products, with the exception of certain living vaccines, must comply with the *European Pharmacopoeia* test for sterility.

Inactivated Bacterial Vaccines

These are usually prepared from killed cells. They may be prepared from one species only or may contain two or more different species or varieties. Each culture used for the preparation of bacterial vaccines is carefully examined for its identity, antigenic properties, and purity. The culture is grown on a suitable solid medium under appropriate conditions and is then washed off with sodium chloride 0.9% injection or other suitable solution; alternatively, it is grown in a fluid medium. The whole culture, or an extract or derivative of the culture, may be used for preparing the vaccine. The bacteria are killed in such a manner that the antigenic potency of the vaccine is not impaired. Methods used include minimal heat (about 56°) or exposure to bactericides (for example, formaldehyde). A suitable antibacterial substance, in a concentration sufficient to prevent the growth of micro-organisms, may be added to sterile bacterial vaccines that are issued in multidose containers. The final vaccines are suspensions of varying opacity, usually white, in colourless or slightly coloured liquids. They may be standardised by determining the number of bacteria per millilitre, either by direct counting in a counting chamber or by comparison of the opacity of the suspension with that of a preparation of standard opacity.

OFFICIAL EXAMPLES:
    Cholera Vaccine BP
    Meningococcal Polysaccharide Vaccine BP
    Pertussis Vaccine BP
    Typhoid Vaccine BP

Living Bacterial Vaccines

In some cases, adequate antigenic stimulus cannot be achieved with killed bacteria. It is then necessary to infect the recipient with a preparation of a selected live strain of the bacterium that produces the same antigens but is of negligible virulence (attenuated strain).

OFFICIAL EXAMPLES:
    Bacillus Calmette-Guérin Vaccine BP (BCG Vaccine)
    Percutaneous Bacillus Calmette-Guérin Vaccine BP (Percut. BCG Vaccine)

Bacterial Toxoids

With many exotoxin-producing bacteria, the physiological and clinical symptoms of infection are due almost entirely to these exotoxins. In such cases, solutions of exotoxins freed from the bacterial cells can be used as antigens. Bacterial toxoids are prepared from toxins by diminishing their toxicity to a non-detectable level or by completely eliminating it, without destroying their immunogenicity, by methods that avoid the reversion of toxoid to toxin. Usually, the toxic activity can be reduced to negligible levels by treatment with formaldehyde, which does not significantly affect the antigenic activity. These are called formol toxoids or anatoxins.

Formol toxoids can be further freed from other non-specific matter by adsorption on aluminium hydroxide, hydrated aluminium phosphate, or other suitable substances. The precipitate may be separated, washed, and suspended in sodium chloride 0.9% injection or other appropriate solution isotonic with blood. Bacterial toxoids are clear colourless or yellow liquids, or if adsorbed they consist of white or grey particles in colourless or pale yellow liquids. They comply with tests for minimum potency as immunising antigens. Adsorbed toxoids provide more concentrated and purer preparations having an additional depot effect on injection.

OFFICIAL EXAMPLES:
    Adsorbed Diphtheria Vaccine BP
    Tetanus Vaccine BP
    Adsorbed Tetanus Vaccine BP

Viral and Rickettsial Vaccines

These are prepared by culture in embryonated eggs, or from cell or tissue cultures. After harvesting, they are freed from tissue debris as far as possible. Virulent viruses and rickettsiae are inactivated chemically, whereas active attenuated types are carefully preserved, often by freezing or lyophilisation. A suitable antibacterial substance may be added to inactivated or living viral or rickettsial vaccines provided that it has no action against the specific organisms. Viral and rickettsial vaccines vary in appearance from clear colourless liquids to suspensions of varying opacity and colour. Like the bacterial vaccines, the final preparation may consist of mixed antigenic strains (for example, poliomyelitis vaccine). In general, the use of vaccines prepared from active attenuated viruses is preferred as they give higher antibody concentrations and longer-lasting immunity than vaccines prepared from inactivated virulent viruses.

OFFICIAL EXAMPLES:
Inactivated vaccines:
  Inactivated Influenza Vaccine (Whole Virion) BP
  Inactivated Influenza Vaccine (Split Virion) BP
  Inactivated Influenza Vaccine (Surface Antigen) BP
  Inactivated Poliomyelitis Vaccine BP
  Rabies Vaccines BP
  Typhus Vaccine BP

'Living' vaccines:
  Measles Vaccine, Live BP
  Mumps Vaccine, Live BP
  Poliomyelitis Vaccine, Live (Oral) BP
  Rubella Vaccine, Live BP
  Yellow Fever Vaccine, Live BP

Mixed Vaccines

To reduce the frequency of injection in the mass immunisation of children or in the immunisation of travellers, where immunity to several diseases is required, mixed vaccines can be used. These are mixtures of sterile bacterial vaccines, bacterial toxoids, and inactivated viral vaccines in a variety of combinations. They are clear liquids or suspensions of varying opacity, usually white, in colourless or slightly coloured liquids.

OFFICIAL EXAMPLES:
  Adsorbed Diphtheria and Tetanus Vaccine BP
  Adsorbed Diphtheria, Tetanus and Pertussis Vaccine BP
  Measles, Mumps and Rubella Vaccine, Live BP
  Typhoid and Tetanus Vaccine BP

ANTISERA

Antisera are sterile preparations containing the specific immunoglobulins obtained from serum of animals by purification. Antisera have the specific power of combining with venins or with the toxins formed by bacteria, or of combining with the bacterium, virus, or other antigen used for their preparation.

Antitoxic Sera

These are antisera prepared against bacterial toxoids or toxins. Susceptible animals, usually horses, are given repeated injections of toxoid, toxin preparations, or both, over a long period. When the antibody titre of the serum reaches a maximum, the animal is bled, the erythrocytes and fibrin clot removed, and the separated serum sterilised by filtration. The serum may then be assayed and standardised to contain a specified number of units per millilitre. This is native (unconcentrated) serum and it contains much non-specific protein. The latter can be removed and the globulins concentrated by selective enzymatic digestion with pepsin or by fractional precipitation with salts such as ammonium sulphate. This is refined (concentrated) serum and a serum of this type is preferred to native serum because it minimises the possibility of serum sickness. The injection of animal protein may be avoided by the use of the appropriate human immunoglobulin (if available) in place of antiserum.

OFFICIAL EXAMPLES:
  Botulinum Antitoxin BP
  Diphtheria Antitoxin BP
  Gas-gangrene Antitoxin (Novyi) BP
  Gas-gangrene Antitoxin (Perfringens) BP
  Gas-gangrene Antitoxin (Septicum) BP
  Mixed Gas-gangrene Antitoxin BP
  Tetanus Antitoxin BP

Antivenins

Antivenins are prepared in a similar fashion to antitoxic sera by using preparations of specific snake or scorpion toxins, either as formolised venoms (anavenoms) or as unmodified venoms. They may be presented as monovalent preparations containing one specific antivenin or polyvalent preparations containing a mixture of different antivenins. The constitution of the latter varies in different countries according to the range of indigenous snakes.

OFFICIAL EXAMPLES:
  European Viper Venom Antiserum BP
  Scorpion Venom Antiserum BP

Antiviral Sera

These are usually obtained from the blood of patients recovering from a specific viral infection (convalescent sera) or from artificially immunised adults (hyperimmune sera) or from adults with naturally acquired immunity (adult sera). As viruses are species-specific in their attack, it is not usually possible to find susceptible animals capable of providing viral antisera by the traditional methods.

Antisera issued in liquid form are distributed under aseptic conditions into sterile containers, which are then sealed to exclude micro-organisms. A suitable antibacterial substance, in a concentration sufficient to prevent the growth of micro-organisms, is usually added; this is essential when antisera are issued in multidose containers.

IMMUNOGLOBULINS

Immunoglobulins are preparations of antibodies usually derived from human plasma or serum. Normal immunoglobulin contains several antibodies against infectious diseases and is prepared from material from blood donors. Specific immunoglobulins contain specified levels of one type of antibody. Antibodies may also be prepared by genetic engineering techniques. The use of immunoglobulins to confer passive immunity has generally replaced the use of antisera, because of serum sickness and other allergic type reactions that have occurred following injection of the latter.

The final products are distributed under aseptic conditions into sterile containers. Immunoglobulin preparations may be lyophilised.

OFFICIAL EXAMPLES:

Anti-D (Rh$_0$) Immunoglobulin BP
Hepatitis B Immunoglobulin BP
Measles Immunoglobulin BP
Normal Immunoglobulin BP
Rabies Immunoglobulin BP
Tetanus Immunoglobulin BP

MONOCLONAL ANTIBODIES

Nebacumab (HA-1A) is a human IgM monoclonal antibody that has been used for the treatment of Gram-negative sepsis and septic shock. It is thought to bind specifically to the lipid A moiety of endotoxin, thus inhibiting the release of tumour-necrosis factor and other mediators of shock and tissue damage. The cell line used to produce the human monoclonal antibody HA-1A was prepared from cells derived from a patient immunised with a heat-inactivated J5 mutant *Escherichia coli* 0111:B4 vaccine. The product has now been withdrawn from use.

STORAGE AND DEGRADATION

Vaccines and antisera should be protected from light. Unless otherwise stated by the manufacturer, preparations should be stored at a temperature of 2° to 8° and should not be allowed to freeze. Liquid immunoglobulin preparations should be stored, protected from light, in sealed colourless, glass containers at a temperature of 2° to 8°. Lyophilised immunoglobulin preparations should be stored similarly, but either under vacuum or under an inert gas. Under these conditions, liquid immunoglobulin preparations may be expected to retain their potency for three years and the lyophilised preparations for five years.

For native antisera, solutions of globulins, and liquid preparations obtained by simple fractionation with salts, the rate of deterioration during storage at 0° is negligible for five years and at 5° does not exceed in each year 5% of the previous year's activity. At higher temperatures the annual rate of deterioration is greater; at 15° it may be about 10%, at 20° it may approach 20%, and at 37° preparations may lose 25% to 50% of their activity in a year. With enzyme-treated antisera the rate of deterioration is usually less; they are most stable at pH 5.0 to 6.5, when the rate of deterioration at 0° to 5° is negligible; up to 15° it does not exceed 3%, and at 20°, 5%; at 37° preparations may lose 10% to 20% of their activity in a year.

DIAGNOSTIC BACTERIAL PRODUCTS

These may be toxins, which are used to determine if the person under test possesses an adequate level of active immunity, or extracts of micro-organisms such as the tuberculins, containing substances that produce a reaction in persons infected with the same species of micro-organisms. They are standardised to contain a specific amount of activity in a test dose and they are administered intradermally to elicit a characteristic localised skin reaction.

Schick Test Toxin is used in the Schick test to determine susceptibility to diphtheria. It is prepared from a sterile filtrate of a culture of *Corynebacterium diphtheriae*. In immune subjects, the circulating antibody combines with and neutralises the toxin and no reaction is produced. Schick Control, which is administered at the same time, is Schick Test Toxin heated to destroy the specific toxin. The control injection detects skin reactions due solely to non-specific substances in the Test Toxin solution. The positive Schick reaction thus indicates susceptibility to diphtheria and the negative Schick reaction indicates some degree of immunity.

Tuberculins are preparations of the protein sensitising agents produced by cultures of *Mycobacterium tuberculosis*. They can be presented in the impure form (concentrated broth filtrates) as Old Tuberculin BP, or in the purified form (separated protein) as Tuberculin Purified Protein Derivative BP. Patients infected with active or inactive tubercle bacilli develop a specific skin sensitivity to these proteins. Intradermal injection of the tuberculin then causes swelling and sometimes a red weal to develop at the site of injection. A positive tuberculin reaction indicates infection with the tubercle bacillus at some stage and a negative tuberculin reaction indicates an absence of infection. The latter can be used to show the suitability of a subject for immunisation with BCG vaccine.

FURTHER INFORMATION

Department of Health. Immunisation against infectious disease. London: HMSO, 1992.
Reynolds JEF, editor. Martindale: The extra pharmacopoeia. 30th ed. London: Pharmaceutical Press, 1993.

Section 4 Pharmaceutical Microbiology, Sterile Processing, and Contamination Control

Pharmaceutical Microbiology

Organisms can be broadly classified into three groups according to their degree of organisation and the type of cell of which they are composed. The **eukaryotic** cell possesses deoxyribonucleic acid (DNA) in a clearly defined nucleus with chromosomes as the structural subunit and some cells have a characteristic wall. A number of discrete organelles, for example, mitochondria, may be found in the cytoplasm. Organisms having this type of cell structure comprise the kingdoms of animals, plants, and the **protists**. The latter comprise the protozoa, the fungi, and the algae.

The **prokaryotic** cell possesses no clearly defined nucleus and the DNA probably exists as a single continuous loop, single or double stranded according to the stage of reproduction. Most possess a distinct cell wall whose structure differs from that of eukaryotes and have no specific organelles in the cytoplasm except for the ribosomes. The only membrane present is the cytoplasmic membrane which is the site of much enzymatic activity. This group comprises those organisms now known as the bacteria, a diverse and extensive kingdom including the Gram-positive and Gram-negative bacteria, the spirochaetes, the actinomycetes, the rickettsias, and the mycoplasmas.

Viruses form a separate class altogether, being sharply differentiated from any cellular organism. They could be regarded as a link between complex macromolecules and the simplest form of prokaryotic cell.

BACTERIA

Bacteria are organisms of highly complex enzymatic structure. This enables them to adapt themselves to a wide variety of environments. They are universally distributed in nature, being found in soil, in fresh and sea water, at all levels of the atmosphere, on and in animals and vegetation.

Morphology and Cytology

Bacteria have three basic shapes: spherical or ovoid (coccus), cylindrical (rod), or helical (spirillum).

In size, the cocci range from 0.75 to 1.25 micrometres in diameter and the rods from 0.7 to 8.0 micrometres in length. The spirillar forms are very variable, from the smallest vibrio of 1 micrometre in length to multiple coiled types 18 to 20 micrometres long, or even more among the spirochaetes.

Most bacteria reproduce by simple binary fission, the daughter cells separating after completion. If cells remain attached through several generations, typical cell aggregates may be formed. Cocci form chains, platelets, packets, or irregular masses. The rod forms may produce chains, though this is only typical of certain groups. Some bacteria can reproduce by budding, and the actinomycetes by characteristic mycelial growth similar to fungi. When growing in a mass on solid media, they produce colonies whose shape may be typical for that bacterium.

Basic Structure

There are three main parts to the bacterial cell:

- The exterior cell wall: a rigid slightly elastic structure of considerable strength, defining the cell shape. It contains a mucocomplex substance which is responsible for its strength, but other components differ in Gram-negative and Gram-positive bacteria.
- The inner cytoplasmic membrane: an area of intense enzymatic activity immediately beneath the cell wall, composed of surface-active materials, lipids, and lipoproteins. It controls the passage of substances into the cell and may be the site of respiratory activity. The cell wall and the cytoplasmic membrane together are known as the cell envelope.
- The protoplast: the interior cytoplasm of the cell.

Cytoplasmic Contents and Appendages

The protoplast consists of the nuclear material, with the DNA as a single molecular loop in the form of a folded helix in a loosely defined area, and the ground cytoplasm filled with ribosomes, the sites of protein synthesis. Bacteria may also contain transient granules of cellular reserve materials, for example, volutin granules, polysaccharide granules such as glycogen, fat droplets, and, in the sulphur bacteria, elemental sulphur.

Spores. Bacteria of the genera *Bacillus* and *Clostridium* (among others) typically produce endospores within the vegetative cell. Bacterial spores are characterised by a thick spore coat, high refractility, high calcium content, low free moisture content, and the possession of unusual small molecules, for example, dipicolinic acid and sometimes sulpholactic acid. The dehydrated nature of the protoplast renders the enzymes and DNA that it contains highly resistant to heat, chemical disinfectants, and radiation. Enzymatically, antigenically, and physiologically, it is quite different from the vegetative cell (sporangium) in which it is formed.

Capsules. Some bacteria secrete complex polymers around the outside of the cell wall. When this layer is small and well defined, it is known as a capsule. When it is diffuse and thick, it is known as a slime layer. These polymers are generally polysaccharides although some species of *Bacillus* secrete polypeptides. Bacteria capable of producing capsules, only do so in the correct environment. Some, for example, *Klebsiella*, are capsulate in simple bacteriological media, while others, for example, the pneumococci, may require cultivation in living animal tissue, the capsule being lost in artificial media. The capsule may contain toxins which can be responsible for the virulence of the organism.

Flagella and fimbriae. Some bacteria are motile by means of flagella. These are very fine hair-like processes of a wavy form composed of a specific protein and originating from a granule in the cell envelope. They are often longer than the organism and the arrangement of the flagella may be peritrichous, or lateral, when they originate from the sides of the cell, or polar, when they originate from one or both ends. The flagella rotate rapidly about their long axis thus driving the cell through fluids. They are antigenically distinct from the remainder of the cell and can be lost by mutation. The surface of some bacteria is covered with thicker, shorter threads called fimbriae or pili. They are not concerned with motility. There is evidence that fimbriae may function as organs of adhesion.

Reproduction in Bacteria

True bacteria (or eubacteria) reproduce by simple binary fission. The cell first enlarges to about twice its normal size with an increase in cytoplasmic contents and the unfolded DNA molecule becomes attached to a mesosome formed by the cytoplasmic membrane. Here the DNA replicates and the daughter chromosomes are separated. A transverse septum is then formed by the ingrowth of the cytoplasmic membrane separating the cytoplasm into two equal parts including the DNA. The septum thickens and a transverse fissure develops along the same line while new cell wall material is laid down separating the two daughter cells. These may eventually part or may remain attached through several succeeding generations, giving aggregates. Reproduction is thus asexual. There is evidence of sexuality among some of the bacteria, for example, *Escherichia coli*, but this is more concerned with the one-way transfer of genetic material than with a sexual type of reproduction. It is doubtful if spore formation among bacteria can be regarded as reproduction as there is no increase in numbers, although it may represent an unusual modification of binary fission. *Nitrobacter* reproduce by budding, similarly to the yeasts, while the actinomycetes produce single cells by fragmentation of their mycelia. The latter are capable of forming new mycelia from each cell.

Actinomycetes

The actinomycetes comprise two groups of bacteria, the proactinomycetes and the euactinomycetes. The proactinomycetes are closely related in form to the Gram-positive rod-shaped bacteria but have a transitory mycelial type of growth resembling the fungi. The cells are narrow, about one micrometre in diameter, and are non-chitinous. The more primitive forms are acid-fast. Soil or water is their primary habitat but some are parasitic on man and animals.

Mycobacteria are typically acid-fast, non-motile, usually non-sporing, rod-shaped cells showing true branching only in the early stages of growth. Growth is generally slow on laboratory media and some are obligate parasites, for example, *Mycobacterium leprae*. They are aerobes and may be capable of intracellular growth. They are considered to be the most primitive of the actinomycetes, and those of chief interest in medicine are *M. tuberculosis* (the human tubercle bacillus), *M. bovis* (the bovine tubercle bacillus) and *M. leprae* (the leprosy bacillus).

The genera *Nocardia* and *Actinomyces* show more typical mycelial form, and at a late stage in growth fragment into short cells similar to bacteria. The aerobic *Nocardia* are mainly soil organisms although some species are pathogens. Of the anaerobic *Actinomyces*, *A. bovis* (causing 'lumpy jaw' in cattle) and *A. israelii* (actinomycosis in man) are of medical interest. Some genera, for example, *Thermoactinomyces*, produce true bacterial endospores.

The genera showing the closest structural resemblance to the fungi are the euactinomycetes, for example, *Streptomyces* and *Micromonospora*. These form a typical and dense mycelial growth, producing conidia from the tips of developing hyphae. They are soil and water organisms and it is among *Streptomyces* species that the majority of the antibiotic producers are found.

Mycoplasmas

Mycoplasmas are very small Gram-negative bacteria, devoid of a true cell wall but surrounded solely by a triple-layered membrane. They vary in shape from the coccoid to the filamentous and form minute 'fried egg' colonies on solid bacteriological media. Their mode of reproduction is in doubt but may include the formation of coccoid structures within the filaments (elementary bodies), which are then released, and perhaps also by the process of budding.

Mycoplasmas are widely distributed in nature and have been found in man, animals, and plants, and in sources such as soil and sewage. They are saprophytic, parasitic, and/or pathogenic, and are penicillin resistant. They are the cause of a number of animal and plant diseases including pleuropneumonia and possibly some forms of arthritis.

Rickettsias

Rickettsias are among the smallest prokaryotic cells known. They may assume a variety of shapes (including coccal forms, rod forms), the 'elementary' bodies being the smallest (about 0.3 micrometre) but larger 'initial' forms may develop as inclusions in the host cell. The majority are obligatory intracellular parasites.

It is now clear that they are bacteria in that they reproduce by binary fission, they have a cell wall containing two amino sugars, glucosamine and muramic acid, and possess both DNA and RNA. In addition, they are sensitive to antibiotics, which argues extensive enzyme systems within the cell. This serves to distinguish them clearly from the larger viruses which they resemble superficially. Like the viruses, many can only be cultivated in the embryonic tissue or the yolk sacs of fertile chick eggs.

Rickettsias are normally obligate parasites of the alimentary tract of arthropod hosts, particularly lice, fleas, and ticks, but are non-pathogenic in their primary host. When transmitted to man by bites, they may produce diseases of which the various forms of typhus, caused by species of *Rickettsia*, are best known.

Apart from the rickettsias, other related but distinct organisms in this group include *Coxiella*, *Chlamydia*, and *Bartonella*, species of which are the causative organisms respectively of Q fever, trachoma and psittacosis, and Oroya fever.

Spirochaetes

Spirochaetes are organisms of unusual structure, slender, helical cells, between 4 and 500 micrometres in length, the coils being flexuous, unlike the spirillar bacteria. Some forms have an axial filament traversing the cell, which is anchored at each end of the cytoplasm. In others, this is reduced to a simple exterior ridge. All are motile without the aid of demonstrable flagella, and movement is accompanied both by expansion and contraction of the spirals and rotation about the long axis. Many do not take the normal bacteriological stains. Larger spirochaetes can be seen easily in films stained by Giemsa or silver staining techniques. Thin spirochaetes are best demonstrated by dark field microscopy in wet preparations. Some have not been grown under laboratory culture, and, of those that have, most require living tissue in the medium together with anaerobic or micro-aerophilic conditions. Spirochaetes are sensitive to heat, drying, changes in pH, and inhibitory chemicals, for example, antibiotics. They reproduce by binary fission. The larger forms comprise two genera, *Spirochaeta* and *Cristispira*, which are either free-living aquatic types or parasites on molluscs.

The shorter forms (3 to 20 micrometres) contain genera of medical importance. The majority of these are parasites and many are pathogens. A number of the genus *Borrelia* are responsible for the different types of relapsing fever in man, being transmitted by arthropod vectors, particularly the human body-louse and ticks. Of the genus *Treponema*, *T. pallidum* (causing syphilis) and *T. pertenue* (causing yaws or framboesia) are the organisms of main interest. Both are transmitted by contact. The many serotypes of the genus *Leptospira* are responsible for leptospirosis, notably *L. icterohaemorrhagiae* (Weil's disease or spirochaetal jaundice). These are unusual in being transmitted via the skin after contact with water into which they have been excreted by infected animals. Rodents, particularly *rats* and *mice*, are often implicated as reservoirs of infection.

Bacterial Metabolism

All bacteria require a source of water, nitrogen, and carbon in relatively large quantities and phosphorus and sulphur in smaller amounts. In addition, many inorganic ions may be needed, for example, potassium, calcium, magnesium, iron, and heavy metal trace elements, for example, cobalt and copper. Utilisable sources of these elements range from the simplest inorganic chemicals, for example, carbon dioxide, ammonium salts, nitrates, and even nitrogen, to carbohydrates, amino acids, and proteins.

Non-exacting organisms have complex enzyme systems and can use the simplest substrates for synthesis and as energy sources. Those requiring some cell components partially or entirely presynthesised are said to be exacting for that compound, for example, the 'bacterial vitamins' or accessory growth factors. These bacteria usually show some degree of parasitism.

A few soil organisms (the phototrophic bacteria) contain specific chlorophylls and can thus obtain their energy from sunlight, but the majority rely on oxidation-reduction reactions particularly from carbon-containing substrates.

Micro-organisms obtaining their nutrients from a host are called parasites, either as commensals (where they cause no detriment to the host) or pathogens (where the host suffers from the parasitism). Potential pathogens are those bacteria that can parasitise one site in the host as commensals, for example, *Escherichia coli* in the mammalian gut, but with a change of site or conditions become pathogenic, for example, causing peritonitis or coliform infections of the bladder.

Pathogens often form toxins which poison the host. Exotoxins are usually heat-labile proteins of great toxicity with highly specific physiological action which diffuse rapidly from the site of infection; and are typically formed by Gram-positive organisms. Endotoxins are usually heat stable lipopolysaccharide-protein complexes of much lower toxicity. Their rate of diffusion is also slower and the physiological reaction of the host is non-specific, that is the reaction to one endotoxin is similar to the reaction to a different endotoxin. They are typically formed by Gram-negative organisms, for example, the endotoxins of the coliform bacteria.

Factors which affect Metabolism

Temperature. Every bacterium has a series of temperature ranges which are optimum for certain metabolic activities. For growth and reproduction, bacteria can be roughly divided into three classes:

- Psychrophiles: optimum temperature range below $20°$

- Mesophiles: optimum temperature range between $20°$ and $45°$
- Thermophiles: optimum temperature range above $45°$.

Most animal pathogens have an optimum growth temperature range of about $35°$ to $38°$, but with other types great variations occur. For the recovery of bacteria shocked by sublethal amounts of heat, chemicals, or radiation, temperatures different from their normal optima must be used. In some cases this may be $10°$ below the normal, but the type of bacteria and mechanism of shocking can affect this.

In addition, each bacterium has a much wider range of temperature within which growth is possible. When cooled below this range, many micro-organisms can survive for long periods, although a proportion may die from cold shock. In the frozen state, the survivors can exist for long periods provided that the cells are undamaged by ice crystal formation. Above this range, bacteria are quickly killed except for the thermoduric organisms, which can withstand temperatures much above the maximum for growth. The latter are usually spore-formers but are not necessarily thermophilic.

pH. Bacteria also have optimum pH ranges for growth. For most pathogens this is pH 7.2 to 7.6, with a possible growth range from about pH 5.0 to 8.0. There are, however, many exceptions to this. Bacteria which can grow in acid solutions are called aciduric organisms, for example, the lactobacilli, and those able to withstand alkaline conditions, alkaliduric, for example, *Vibrio cholerae*. A few bacteria can withstand both conditions, for example, the enterococci.

The inhibitory effects of changes of pH from the optimum appear to be due more to the formation of undissociated molecules of weak acids or bases in the environment than to the increase in hydrogen or hydroxyl ion content.

Osmotic Pressure. Most bacteria are unaffected by relatively large changes in osmotic pressure owing to the strength of their cell walls. In hypertonic solutions, partial dehydration of the substrate may occur and this may inhibit growth but very high pressures are needed before plasmolysis is seen. Even in grossly hypertonic solutions normal metabolism continues. The inhibitory activity of salts is due more to the toxicity of their ions than to their effect on the osmotic pressure. In grossly hypotonic solutions some sensitive vegetative bacteria may suffer osmotic shock and lysis may occur depending on the state of the cell wall.

Oxygen. Bacteria can be divided into four classes on the basis of their behaviour towards molecular oxygen.

- Obligate (strict) aerobes, for example, *Mycobacterium tuberculosis* require a high oxygen tension for growth or even survival. They cannot grow anaerobically.
- Obligate (strict) anaerobes, for example, *Clostridium* species require a complete absence of oxygen for growth. Even small quantities may prove toxic, but they can be protected from this effect by the inclusion of strong reducing agents in the medium. Compounds containing sulphydryl groups (-SH) are particularly successful, for example, sodium thioglycollate, as their toxicity is usually low. Such compounds are often included in anaerobic media.
- Facultative anaerobes, for example, *Staphylococcus* and *Escherichia* species constitute the majority of bacteria which can use either aerobic respiration or anaerobic fermentation as a means of obtaining energy. As respiration is a more efficient method, these organisms usually grow more rapidly in oxidative conditions.
- Microaerophiles, for example, *Hydrogenomonas* species are obligate aerobes which are sensitive to the very high oxygen tensions found in normal air. They can only be cultivated at much reduced oxygen concentrations.

These divisions mainly represent the response of the energy-releasing enzymes to the redox potential of the growth medium.

Carbon Dioxide. Apart from its role as a main carbon source for autotrophic bacteria, carbon dioxide has a stimulatory action on the growth or toxin production of many heterotrophic organisms, for example, growth of *Escherichia coli* and toxin production in *Corynebacterium diphtheriae*. In some cases it appears to be an essential nutrient for the growth of a number of organisms including anaerobes. Concentrations of up to 10% may be needed in the environmental atmosphere before optimum growth or metabolic activity can occur.

Radiation. Visible light (400 to 760 nm) has little if any inhibitory effect on bacteria, and the photosynthetic types utilise light energy in this region. Infra-red radiation (760 nm to 50 micrometres) has no effect *per se* but can kill bacteria by its heating effect. In this it is no different from other sources of heat. A similar action is shown by microwaves (2 to 12 cm). Ultraviolet light between 240 and 280 nm may be used to reduce bacterial contamination of air, but is only active at a relatively short distance from the source. Bacteria and mould spores may be resistant to such treatment. Ultraviolet light is used for water disinfection. Ionising radiations, such as high speed electrons, X-rays 5×10^{-2} to 10 nm, and gamma-rays less than 5×10^{-2} nm are lethal to all cells, their activity increasing with decreasing wavelength. They act by producing excited molecules and free radicals which disrupt the normal function of cell enzymes and damage the DNA. The latter damage may be repairable by cell enzymes. Gamma rays from a radioisotope (for example, Cobalt-60) or high energy electrons from an electron accelerator are used mainly for the sterilisation of heat-sensitive materials and products. Ultraviolet irradiation is not effective.

Cultivation of Bacteria

In order to detect, isolate, and identify bacteria, it is necessary to grow them in conditions free from all possible natural contaminants. To this end all apparatus and media used must be sterilised and all transferences carried out with the correct technique and in a clean atmosphere to reduce the probability of contamination to a minimum.

The commonest tools for the handling and transference of bacterial cultures are the bacteriological loop, Pasteur pipettes, graduated pipettes, and 'pipettors'. The bacteriological loop is a length of 23 or 24 SWG platinum or Nichrome wire, with one end formed into a flat closed loop of about 2 mm diameter and the other set in a special metal handle or fused into the tip of a glass rod. The wire can be sterilised by heating it red-hot in a Bunsen flame. It is used for handling a drop of fluid culture or removing surface culture from solid media. Pasteur pipettes are lengths of soft glass tubing with one end drawn out into a capillary and the other plugged with non-absorbent cotton wool. They are sterilised by dry heat and a rubber teat is fitted over the plugged end for use. Pasteur pipettes may be purchased ready-made where large numbers are required. They are used for handling fluid cultures where the quantities to be transferred are greater than can be handled with the loop. Graduated straight-side pipettes are used for handling 1 to 10 mL volumes. They are plugged with non-absorbent cotton wool at the suction end, packed in aluminium boxes, and sterilised by heat. They are used with rubber teats and pipetting devices. Sterile disposable 1- and 10-mL graduated pipettes are available commercially. 'Pipettors' include rubber bulbs with valves, syringe-like attachments, electrically operated pumps with flexible tubes for insertion of pipettes, and mechanical plungers for use with sterile, plastic pipette tips.

Culture Media

Media for the cultivation of bacteria must be capable of satisfying all their nutritional requirements as outlined under Bacterial Metabolism.

Synthetic or **defined media** are prepared entirely from pure inorganic or organic chemicals such that the exact composition of the medium is known and can be reproduced with precision on different occasions. They are mainly used for research purposes and in the preparation of bacterial products, for example, toxins.

Routine media are prepared from a mixture of digested or extracted animal or plant protein, for example, beef or soya bean, sometimes supplemented with accessory growth factors, for example, yeast extract, in aqueous solution. They are used for the routine growth of many bacteria, commensals or pathogens, and their composition is only approximately known. For the growth of these organisms the pH of the media should be about 7.2 (approximate to that of tissues and body fluids).

Enriched media are routine media supplemented with additional stimulatory substances (for example, whole blood, serum, ascitic fluid, additional sugars) for the growth of more exacting organisms, for example, *Bordetella* and *Streptococcus* species.

Selective media are routine media to which have been added selectively inhibitory chemicals that suppress or kill all but a few types of organism. They are used to aid in the isolation of specific bacteria from mixed inocula, for example, from throat swabs or pus samples.

Indicator media are routine media containing added specific substrates or indicators. The attack on the substrate by a particular organism results in a change in appearance of the medium, or of the pH, or of the redox potential in the area of growth, for example, haemolysis of erythrocytes by haemolytic bacteria.

Many diagnostic media in regular use are combinations of the above media. Examples of all types are given under Culture Media later in this chapter.

Media can be used in either of two forms, liquid and solid. The latter are usually prepared from liquid media by the addition of agar in concentrations of 1% to 4% depending on the gelling power of the agar. Gelatin is now reserved as a test for gelatinase activity. Liquid media, or 'broths', are used for the routine cultivation of pure cultures, sterility testing, and anaerobic culture. However, mixed cultures cannot be separated in them unless the media are highly selective. Also, organisms tend not to produce distinguishable growth patterns. However, they do allow the addition of fairly large volumes of liquid without seriously interfering with their properties, as in sterility testing and the bacteriological examination of water and milk.

Solid media permit the separation of mixed cultures into isolated colonies and the growth of heavy concentrations of bacteria for harvesting, for example, in vaccine production and the preparation of spore suspensions. Agar does not have any nutritive properties for the majority of organisms. It requires heating to about 95° to dissolve it, or to melt prepared media, but once melted it must be cooled to about 42° before the gel reforms. This permits the addition of thermolabile additives, for example, whole blood, serum, or antibiotics, to the liquefied medium at low temperatures (about 45°).

Containers for Culture Media

Liquid media are generally stored in rimless conical flasks, rimless hard-glass test-tubes, or aluminium screw-capped flint-glass bottles. Tubes or flasks are most conveniently closed with aluminium or stainless steel slip-on caps. The latter can be obtained with spring grips that ensure a tight fit, but both types are suitable only for relatively short periods of storage of sterile media or cultures. Long staple non-absorbent cotton wool plugs can also be used as closures although their manipulation is not as easy as the metal caps. They may be replaced by preformed silicone rubber foam plugs which are easy to handle, clean, and sterilise. Screw-capped bottles are suitable for prolonged storage of sterile media or cultures provided they are fitted with thick rubber liners.

Solid media are best stored in screw-capped bottles that will withstand autoclaving. For use, the melted medium, at about 50°, is poured aseptically into sterile glass or disposable polystyrene Petri dishes (or plates) in a thin layer and allowed to set. Where isolated colonies are not required, cultures can be propagated and stored on 'slopes' or 'slants'. These are prepared by sterilising small volumes of solid medium in test-tubes or screw-capped bottles and allowing the medium to set while the container is held at an angle. When set, the containers are stored vertically to allow the 'water of condensation' to remain in the base. Alternatively 'stab cultures' may be used. Here a tube of solid medium is inoculated by stabbing into its depths a straight wire infected with the bacterium, and incubating. Some organisms survive storage for longer periods at low temperatures by this method than with surface inoculation.

The foregoing is only an outline of the methods available. For a detailed account a standard reference work should be consulted.

Classification of Bacteria

There is at present no single internationally accepted method of classification of bacteria. In structurally complex organisms like plants and animals, the differences between types are fairly clear-cut, relatively stable, and often visible to the naked eye. In addition, fossil evidence of common ancestry is available. With bacteria, the reverse is true, and generally they are better defined by their activities than their appearance as this provides a better estimate of their genetic relationships. In the absence of any completely satisfactory system, which is probably impossible, two main types of classification are in use, the 'natural' and the 'numerical'.

The 'natural' classification is based on a combination of morphological and physiological characters, for example, shape, motility, distribution of flagella, and formation of spores. Some characteristics are given more weight than others in grouping the bacteria into classes, orders, families, genera, and species. The inclusion of an organism in any of these depends on the presence or absence of certain key characters which are considered of major importance. The taxonomic unit of this system is the species and it is essentially a modified form of the classical botanical and zoological classification method. However, the extreme diversity of the bacterial kingdom does not lend itself to a rigid hierarchical classification.

The classification set out in *Bergey's Manual of Determinative Bacteriology*, which has been considerably modified since it was first published in 1923, is an extremely useful and complete reference work for the identification of all bacteria.

The 'numerical' classification is sometimes known as the 'Adansonian' classification. Here the basic taxonomic unit is the strain, defined as a pure culture of a bacterium from a single isolation. As many characteristics as possible are determined for each unit, but no weighting is applied to any of them. Organisms are then grouped into 'phenons' according to the extent to which they share characteristics. Thus there may be 90% phenons or 80% phenons, roughly analogous to the groupings in the natural classifications. This system lends itself to computer analysis and in the cases where it has been used has shown some unexpected relationships between organisms, hitherto unsuspected.

Nomenclature

It is traditional to retain the Linnaean binomial system of nomenclature for bacteria. The generic name is given first and is always capitalised, for example, *Clostridium*, and the species name second but it is never capitalised, for example, *Clostridium perfringens*.

Since much variation can occur within species, the following terms are used to describe these variant types:

Strain:	a pure culture of a bacterium from a single isolation
Serotype:	a class having similar antigenic characters
Morphotype:	a class having similar morphological characters
Phagotype:	a class having similar phage sensitivity
Group:	a class having similar general characters
Phase:	alternative immunological states in a species
Form:	a subdivision of a species with adaption to a particular host
Variant:	an organism showing some variation from the parent culture.

These terms are often used in conjunction with the name of the organism to particularise it more precisely.

Identification of Bacteria

It is first necessary to isolate the bacterium in pure culture before carrying out identification tests. This is most usually achieved by streaking or spreading on the surface of solid selective media to produce isolated colonies of the desired organism. A colony is then picked off and may require subculturing in routine or enriched media to restore normal growth before examination.

If a natural classification system is to be followed, the process of identification is often carried out in the following order.

Morphology. Stained microscopic mounts are examined for size, shape, cell aggregates, and the presence of spores. Hanging-drop mounts of the living organism are examined for motility, preferably by phase-contrast microscopy. Special examination for capsules and flagella are normally only used for confirmation purposes.

Staining Reactions. The Gram stain is the most important of the staining reactions and, in conjunction with the morphological details, is often enough to narrow the field considerably. Acid-fast staining by the Ziehl-Neelsen technique is performed if *Mycobacterium* or *Nocardia* is suspected.

Cultural Characteristics. The shape, size, and colour of colonies on solid media are sometimes helpful in diagnosis, but generally the appearance on solid or liquid media is not stable enough to be of routine value. The ability of the organism to grow on different basal media including the stimulatory effects of added substances such as glucose, whole blood, or serum is studied along with the observation of the optimum temperature and pH ranges for growth and the appearance of any pigment formed. Gaseous requirements, aerobic or anaerobic, are determined, and the reaction of the organism to selective inhibitors such as antibiotics, bile salts, and high salt concentrations is examined.

Biochemical Reactions. The ability of the bacterium to utilise particular substrates, for example, bacteriological sugars, with the formation of detectable end-products is determined. A wide range of these biochemical tests are available (for example, fermentation patterns, catalase and oxidase production, nitrate reduction), and these are perhaps the most useful aids to identification. Ready prepared kits for multiple biochemical analysis systems are now available commercially. Currently, these kits do not identify all bacteria but do have the advantage of savings in media preparation, equipment, and labour. There is increasing potential for automation using robotisation and knowledge-based computer systems. All help to build up a pattern of the metabolic activity of the organism which, with the information gained from microscopical and cultural examination, may be sufficient to identify the bacterium.

Serological and Phage Typing. It is often possible to identify bacteria by determining their antigenic composition. Replicate suspensions of the organism are mixed, *in vitro*, with a series of different standardised solutions of purified antibodies.

In cases where a reaction such as agglutination takes place, it can be inferred that the organism possesses the specific antigen against which that antibody was originally prepared. In this way a picture of the antigenic structure can be built up rapidly and the results compared with those of known bacteria. Antigenic variants within some species can be identified in this way.

Bacteriophages are also highly specific in their lytic action on bacteria. Stock preparations of known phages can thus be used in a similar way to antisera and sometimes allow precise identification of variants within species, for example, phage typing of staphylococci and the coliforms.

Animal Tests. Although *in-vitro* methods often give more reproducible results, some animal experiments are essential as certain tests depend on physiological interaction of organs in the animal. The identification of pathogenic organisms may require the use of animal inoculation as a final test. This is only of value where the bacterium produces specific symptoms or lesions in sensitive laboratory animals. The test is therefore usually limited to the Gram-positive toxin producers or the mycobacteria, for example, *Mycobacterium tuberculosis*. Animal inoculation is often combined with the simultaneous administration of specific antisera to demonstrate that in their presence the symptoms or lesions are not produced, thus eliminating non-specific reactions. A licence from the Home Office is required for all animal experiments.

Counting Bacteria

It is often necessary to know the number of bacterial cells in a suspension for the purpose of standardisation, for example, in the preparation of vaccines. Sometimes only the total count of cells (living and dead) is required, for example, with killed vaccines, but in other cases, the number of living cells (or viable count) is of the greatest importance, for example, in milk and water testing, and in experimental work.

Total Counting Methods

The basis of all total counting methods is the direct enumeration of the cells, usually by microscopic count with a haemocytometer. Here the cell suspension, suitably diluted and treated with formaldehyde, is examined in a slide counting chamber

(Thoma ruling) by phase contrast or dark-ground illumination. Bacteria lying in the squares engraved on the base of the chamber are counted and an average number of cells per square is calculated. Not less than 300 squares must be examined and the mean value calculated. As the volume of cell suspension lying over each square is known (5×10^{-8} mL) the total count of the original suspension can be deduced.

Counting errors may be minimised by counting as many squares as possible and performing replicate counts on the same suspension. The human error implicit in the haemocytometer method can be eliminated by substituting mechanical counters, for example, by Coulter counter techniques.

As the opacity of the suspension varies with the total number of cells that it contains, use can be made of this fact to obtain rapid estimates of the total count. Absorptiometer techniques enable this to be done. These require preliminary calibration by direct counting methods.

Viable Counts

Owing to the difficulty of determining whether an individual cell is alive or dead, it is usual to define 'viable' as meaning 'capable of reproduction at least through several generations'. Viable counts may be performed by adding to the cell suspension substances capable of being utilised by the living cells only, to produce a coloured compound. The mixture is incubated for a period of time, followed by a haemocytometer count of the coloured cells. Tetrazolium salts and neutral red have been used for this.

More usually, aliquot portions of the suitably diluted suspension are placed in or on the surface of a solid nutrient medium and incubated at the optimum recovery temperature for the bacterium. Developing colonies can be counted visually and it is assumed that one organism or aggregate of organisms gives rise to one colony. Again, a number of replicates are necessary to minimise errors.

In the 'pour plate' method, the aliquot (about 1.0 mL) is mixed with the molten agar medium cooled to 45° to 50° in a Petri dish. After setting and incubation, the number of colony forming units (cfu) is counted with the aid of a colony counter that uses combined reflected and obliquely transmitted artificial light against a dark background. Counts are made on plates yielding between 50 cfu and 500 cfu (ideally 200 cfu to 400 cfu). A mark is made on the base of the Petri dish for each cfu. To obtain the number of cfu per mL or per gram of sample, the average number per plate is multiplied by the dilution factor. When viable counts are performed it is essential to include positive and negative controls. However, viable count methods are not very accurate and a strict viable count limit should not be adopted.

Another method is the 'surface' or 'spread' plate technique in which the aliquot (for example, 0.2 to 0.5 mL, accurately measured) is spread evenly over the surface of a plate of medium. Prior to inoculation, the plate of medium is dried for at least two hours at 37° or for 10 to 15 minutes at 50° with the lid ajar. The fluid is absorbed by the medium so that all colonies develop in similar conditions on the surface and are easily counted.

To reduce the amount of medium and plates necessary, the technique of Miles and Misra can be used. Drops of diluted suspension (0.02 mL) from a calibrated dropping pipette are allowed to fall from a height of 2.5 cm onto different positions on the surface of the medium. Colony forming units then develop only in the area of the drop, thus allowing a large number of replicates to be performed within a small area. Due to the small volumes employed, this method tends to have a greater general error than the spread plate technique.

A modification of the 'pour plate' method is the use of roll tubes. Small volumes of melted medium and diluted suspension are mixed and spun into a thin shell over the inside of special bottles until set. Colonies then develop as in the pour plate technique. The Astell Roll Tube apparatus has been developed to facilitate the spinning of the tubes.

Where the number of bacteria present in the original suspension is too low to allow the above methods to be used (for example, in water testing or, sterility testing), filtration through sterile cellulose membrane filters (pore size 0.2 micrometres) is useful. Organisms from large volumes of suspension can be collected on the membrane, which is then placed on a supporting cellulose pad soaked in a nutrient medium and incubated. Due to the high porosity of the membrane, bacteria on its surface can obtain nutrients through it without disturbance, and develop into discrete colonies which may be counted. The method is also of value where the original suspension contains inhibitory agents, for example, antibiotics, preservatives, or disinfectants, which may be washed away from the bacteria with sterile solvents. It is essential to ensure that the type of membrane used is suitable for the organism under test as membranes vary in their ability to support maximum growth.

Although the 'most probable number' (MPN) technique is seldom used for counting organisms in pharmaceuticals, it is used extensively in the dairy and water industries for the detection of coliforms. In this method, known amounts of sample or diluted sample are inoculated into a series of tubes, containing 9 or 10 mL broth medium. After incubation, the number of tubes producing growth is recorded. The MPN is estimated by reference to statistical tables. Dip-type samplers, for example, Millipore™, may be used for monitoring areas and critical control points in manufacturing areas. The sampler contains a membrane filter (0.45 micrometre) and an absorbent pad containing nutrient in a transparent plastic case. After immersion in the sample, the pad is returned to its case for incubation.

Rapid Evaluation Techniques in Microbiology

Traditional methods described for identifying and counting bacteria are demanding in operator skills, in setting up the procedures, and in interpreting the results. In addition, the incubation time required for bacterial growth may extend over several days.

In recent years, methods have been developed which enable the rapid detection of bacterial growth and, in some cases, the identification and quantification of the organisms involved. In general, some early index of the presence or development of organisms, which can be detected by various analytical techniques and instruments, is utilised.

Rapid identification may be facilitated in various ways including the use of deoxyribonucleic acid probes and enzyme-linked immunosorbent assays. Gas chromatography is used to separate and identify bacterial fatty acids, which are species characteristic. Electrophoresis of radiolabelled proteins from bacteria, grown on media containing radioactive tracers, produces species-distinct patterns. **Direct counting** is rapidly achieved using electronic particle size analysers or by a direct epifluorescent filter technique (DEFT) in which bacteria are stained with a fluorescent dye and counted under a fluorescence microscope. **Early detection** of bacterial contamination is important in the microbial quality assurance of pharmaceuticals, foods, and cosmetics. Heat or light generated by growing organisms or the increase in optical density accompanying cell multiplication can all be detected, using appropriate instruments, much sooner than visible growth. Other early changes accompanying growth are conductance and impedance, which can be measured, and redox changes, detected by the use of dyes or electrochemical measurements.

Rapid measurement techniques require sophisticated equipment and may be rendered difficult by complex or viscous formulations. Nevertheless, they can provide results in minutes rather than days and allow automation for ease of data handling.

FUNGI

The majority of **fungi** are filamentous, although a few are unicellular. The unit of vegetative growth is the hypha, a single, elongated, much branched tube with a partly chitinous cell wall. Hyphae are rigid and extensively branched, forming a tangled mat visible to the naked eye and called the mycelium.

Growth proceeds rapidly from the tip of the hypha and can continue almost indefinitely, limited only by the supply of nutrients. Fungi are heterotrophic and these nutrients are obtained by penetration of the substrate by submerged hyphae, which are often thicker and shorter than the surface hyphae, which form the major part of the mycelium. The cell wall is mainly composed of the polysaccharide chitin.

The unit of reproduction is the spore, which may be produced asexually or sexually and may be uninucleate or multinucleate. Asexual spores are produced by abscission of the tips of the hyphae, most often from specialised spore-bearing structures distinguishable from the basic hyphae. The sexual spore is formed by the fusion of two specialised cells from different hyphae and the transference of their nuclear material. The resulting nuclei may be finally diploid or haploid.

Like bacteria, fungi can only absorb nutrients in solution, although most requirements are satisfied by the simplest sources. As they are non-photosynthetic they cannot utilise carbon dioxide and require a more complex carbon source, for example, glucose. Fungi prefer a lower pH (5.5 to 6.0) and temperature (20° to 30°) than most bacteria for optimum growth. They are obligate aerobes, a very few being capable of micro-aerophilic growth. They are often very resistant to high osmotic pressures and low pH values. For example, aspergilli and penicillia can grow at pH 1.5 to 2.0 and some of the *Aspergillus glaucus* group can grow on jams and syrups.

Classification

Fungi can be divided into three main groups, the Zygomycetes, the Ascomycetes, and the Basidiomycetes, according to the septation of their hyphae and the type of spore formation.

Zygomycota

Zygomycetes are primitive fungi; most are found in soil although some are parasites of plants or insects. The majority are coenocytic, that is, have non-septate mycelia, and produce endogenous asexual spores (sporangiospores) within a sac called a sporangium. Their sexual reproduction involves the production of thick-walled structures called zygosporangia. Examples from this group include *Rhizopus*, the common bread mould, and *Mucor*, which are frequently found as aerial contaminants. About 765 species of zygomycetes are thought to exist.

Ascomycota

Ascomycetes are higher fungi whose habitat is primarily the soil. They possess septate mycelia although these septa are perforated so that the cytoplasm is continuous throughout the mycelium. Their asexual spores (conidia) are exogenous, being produced by specialised (conidiogenous) cells in various ways. These cells are borne on fruiting structures (conidiophore) that have a wide diversity of shapes. The sexual spores (ascospores) are produced endogenously in a sac called an ascus which in turn may be enclosed within an ascoma, a complex structure comprising tightly interwoven hyphae. There are three types of ascoma: the cup-shaped apothecium; the closed and spherical cleistothecium; and the spherical or flask-shaped perithecium.

This group includes the edible morels and truffles and many spoilage organisms; *Chaetomium* (paper spoilage), *Neurospora* (red bread mould), and some of the aspergilli and penicillia are examples of the latter. Many ascomycetes are plant pathogens. Approximately 30 000 species of ascomycetes have been described.

Yeasts. Yeasts are primarily unicellular ascomycetes. This restricted unicellular growth form is observed in some members of all three divisions of fungi and at least 25% of the genera of yeasts belong to the basidiomycetes (see below).

The typical yeast cell is spherical, ovoid, or, in a few cases, rod-shaped. Reproduction may involve several different mechanisms; however most yeast cells multiply vegetatively by some form of budding. Some yeasts exhibit hyphal growth, others exist in unicellular form under all conditions.

Examples of yeasts include the various strains of *Saccharomyces cerevisiae*, which are used in the production of alcohol and bread; and the pathogenic yeasts *Candida albicans* and *Cryptococcus neoformans*, which are capable of producing superficial and deep-seated infections.

There are about 500 known species of yeasts.

Deuteromycota. Often referred to as 'Fungi Imperfecti', the deuteromycetes (or conidial fungi) are a mixed collection of approximately 17 000 species of fungi for which details of reproduction mechanisms are either unknown or not used as the basis of classification. Examples of species belonging to the deuteromycete genera include *Aspergillus* and *Penicillium*. Most deuteromycota are ascomycetes, although some are basidiomycetes (see below).

Lichens. Lichens are mutualistic symbiotic associations between ascomycetes and certain genera of green algae or cyanobacteria.

Basidiomycota

Basidiomycetes are similar in many ways to the ascomycetes but differ in the mode of formation of the sexual spore. The zygote is formed in a characteristic club-shaped cell called a basidium, on the surface of which develop slender sterigmata. The basidiospore is formed on the sterigma, from which the mature spore is released, sometimes vigorously.

The fleshy, spore producing bodies are called basidiomata (singular: basidioma). These are produced by dikaryotic mycelia.

The basidiomycetes can be divided into three classes. The **Hymenomycetes** produce basidiospores exposed early *on* a basidioma; examples include mushrooms and shelf fungi. In the **Gasteromycetes** class, spores are formed enclosed *in* a basidioma; examples include puffballs. The **Teliomycetes** do not form a basidioma, but produce spores in their masses; these are the rusts and smuts.

There are about 16 000 species of basidiomycota.

PROTOZOA

The protozoa are large, non-photosynthetic unicellular organisms; a few are colonial. The majority of protozoa parasitic in humans are less than 50 micrometres in size. The smallest are 1 to 10 micrometres; larger protozoa may measure 100 to 150 micrometres. From an evolutionary point of view they appear to be derived from the unicellular algae, losing photosynthetic capacity in the process. Protozoa are eukaryotic protists with a thin, flexible, outer pellicle and are often motile by means of amoeboid movements or by flagella. Some have external structure, such as undulating membranes or cilia, and internal organelles of a variety of types.

The protozoa are classified into several phyla, based mainly on their morphology, mechanism of motility, and life-cycles. The phyla of protozoa comprise the **Sarcomastigophora** (subphyla Sarcodina and Mastigophora), **Labyrinthomorpha**, **Apicomplexa**, **Microspora**, **Myxozoa**, and **Ciliophora**. A list of pathogenic protozoa is given under Microorganisms Pathogenic to Man (Protozoa).

VIRUSES

The viruses are very small pathogenic structures which are clearly differentiated from all other forms of cellular life. It seems doubtful if they are 'living' in the classical sense of the term. There are four main groups:

- the animal viruses
- the bacterial viruses (bacteriophages or phages)
- the invertebrate and insect viruses, and
- the plant viruses.

They are all host-specific within these groups.

In all cases, the basic infective particle is the virion, which consists of a central core of nucleic acid (the nucleoid) surrounded by a coat (the capsid) composed of regularly shaped blocks of protein (the capsomeres). Some animal viruses may be enclosed in an envelope. The nucleic acid may be either deoxyribonucleic acid (DNA) or ribonucleic acid (RNA), but not both, and this may be coiled in helical strands. Generally, the bacteriophages contain DNA, the plant viruses RNA, and the animal viruses either DNA or RNA. The shape of the individual capsomeres determines the final shape of the virion, which may be polyhedral (for example, poliomyelitis virus) or helical (for example, the influenza virus).

Larger viruses may possess additional structures, such as a lipoidal surrounding membrane, and a very few may have enzymes and coenzymes, although these may derive from the host cell. In general, the viruses are devoid of enzymes.

The bacteriophages are unique in that they may have a complex structure. Tailed phages (or T-phages) are shaped like a spermatozoon with a polyhedral head containing DNA, a hollow tail surrounded by a contractile sheath of helically arranged protein, and slender protein fibres attached to the tip of the tail.

In general, the nucleoid is the infective unit of the virion while the capsid appears to confer stability on the whole structure and may assist in the penetration of the host cell.

Viruses vary in their sensitivity to variations from the optimum in temperature, pH, and moisture content. Normally, their resistance to change is similar to that of vegetative bacteria, although some are very labile (for example, influenza virus). Viruses are resistant to very low temperatures and most can be preserved by deep freezing ($-35°$ to $-70°$) or by freeze-drying. Those which contain lipids are sensitive to fat solvents (for example, ether) or surfactants, but all are sensitive to oxidising agents such as hydrogen peroxide, hypochlorites, and permanganates. Unlike bacteria, most viruses tend to be resistant to phenolic disinfectants and are insensitive to antibiotics.

Viruses are often specific toward their host, both as regards species and the tissues or organs within which replication can occur. They are strict intracellular parasites and cannot be cultivated on artificial media because of their mode of replication.

Viral Replication

Being non-motile, the virion makes contact with the susceptible cell by chance and is adsorbed on to the surface membrane through which it passes. With the animal viruses, the mechanism of penetration is probably by pinocytosis similar to ingestion of droplets by phagocytes.

Within the cell, the virion dissociates (eclipse phase), the viral nucleic acid is released into the cytoplasm, and, after a period of time, viral DNA or RNA is elaborated close to the nucleus. Viral protein is formed separately in the cytoplasm, and the new virions are then assembled, often close to the cell membrane. During the latter phase the typical 'inclusion bodies' may appear in the cell and these may be diagnostic for some virus infections. The assembly of the new virion from its constituent parts appears to be automatic.

Finally, the host cell may disintegrate (burst phase) to liberate the new virus particles which then infect other susceptible cells in the area. In some cases (for example, influenza) the host cell may not disintegrate but allow the new virions to emerge over a period of time without substantial cell damage.

Viruses are capable of varying their genetic structure by spontaneous mutation and by this method variants of known strains and even new viruses may arise. This may result in an increase or decrease in the virulence of known virus infections (for example, influenza type A) and is in part responsible for cyclic pandemics of this type of infection. Recombination of genetic material from two different viruses may also occur to produce new viral types.

Viral Cultivation

Many viruses can be cultivated in the laboratory by using susceptible animals or by replication in fertile chick eggs or in tissue culture. Sites of egg inoculation are the yolk sac, the chorio-allantoic cavity, the allantoic membrane, and the amniotic cavity. The site selected depends on the type of virus. Isolated tissue culture is generally preferred where possible because of the absence of unwanted structures. The tissues used may be from the liver, kidney, muscle, cornea, or from human carcinomas. The initial living tissue is finely minced, separated into individual cells by treatment with trypsin or disodium edetate, and gently centrifuged to separate the detached cells. These can then be cultivated in flasks or bottles by incubation with a suitable growth medium containing a variety of salts, glucose, and biological extracts (for example, serum, amniotic fluid, embryonic extracts). The cells adhere to the glass in a monolayer on which they grow as a cell sheet. An advantage of this method is that the cells are capable of microscopic examination without disturbance, both before and after the addition of the viral suspension. The effect of viral reproduction on the appearance of the tissue cells is often typical and can be used as an aid to diagnosis.

Viral Groups

The main viral families of importance in man are as follows.

Adenoviridae. Polyhedral DNA-containing viruses (60 to 85 nm) characterised by an affinity for mucous membranes, particularly adenoidal and tonsillar tissue.

Arenaviridae. Polyhedral enveloped RNA-containing viruses (approximately 100 nm) having rodent reservoirs. It includes the Arenavirus group and Lassa virus.

Calciviridae. Includes the Calciviruses and Astroviruses, which are non-enveloped, RNA-containing viruses (28 to 30 nm) and have been associated with gastroenteritis.

Coronaviridae. Enveloped RNA-containing viruses (80 to 160 nm) showing replication in the cytoplasm of the cell.

Herpesviridae. Polyhedral enveloped DNA-containing viruses (100 to 180 nm) characterised by intranuclear replication in the host cell and an affinity for skin and mucous membranes.

Orthomyxoviridae. Helical or filamentous enveloped RNA-containing viruses (60 to 200 nm) having an affinity for mucous and respiratory epithelium and showing intranuclear replication.

Papovaviridae. Polyhedral DNA-containing viruses (mostly 50 to 60 nm) characterised by the formation of papillomata.

Paramyxoviridae. Similar to Orthomyxoviruses but showing replication in the cytoplasm of the cell.

Parvoviridae. Non-enveloped DNA-containing viruses, which include human parvovirus B-19.

Picornaviridae. Very small polyhedral RNA-containing viruses (mostly 25 to 33 nm). Genera include Enterovirus and Rhinovirus.

Poxviridae. Large polyhedral DNA-containing viruses (200 to 300 nm) which cause pustules and vesicles on the skin, which may leave pocks on healing.

Reoviridae. Polyhedral RNA-containing viruses (about 70 nm) found in respiratory and enteric epithelia, including Rotavirus and Reovirus.

Retroviridae. Enveloped (approximately 100 nm). The group includes HIV, responsible for AIDS (acquired immune deficiency syndrome), which specifically targets the immune system, fatally enhancing susceptibility to opportunistic infections, and the human T-cell leukaemia virus.

Rhabdoviridae. Helically coiled enveloped RNA-containing viruses (approximately 180 nm) having a strong affinity for the CNS.

Togaviridae. Pleomorphic, enveloped, single stranded RNA-containing viruses (50 to 60 nm). Genera include Alphavirus, Flavivirus, and Rubivirus.

Other viruses of importance to man are also known but are excluded from the above groups on the grounds of insufficient information being available or significant differences in characteristics being known. In addition, a number of different viruses have been shown to be **oncogenic** or tumour-producing in animals and to produce transformation in tissue-culture cells.

For examples of virus infections caused by agents within these groups see under Micro-organisms Pathogenic to Man (Viruses).

STAINS AND STAINING

One of the aids to the identification of bacteria is their reaction towards certain stains, which usually consist of solutions of aniline dyes. The most important is the Gram stain which can be used to divide all bacteria into two classes, those which retain the stain and those which do not. Reaction to the Gram stain reflects a fundamental difference in the cell-wall structure of the two groups. Those retaining the stain are called Gram-positive and those which do not are Gram-negative. This is the first identification staining reaction which should be performed, and should be followed by special staining methods which will give further information.

There are special stains which are used for the detection of spores, capsules, flagella, and volutin granules. One class of bacteria is termed acid-fast, because, if stained with carbol-fuchsine, they retain it when immersed in 20% sulphuric acid. Other stains are Loeffler's methylene blue, which is used for the simple observation of all organisms, and dilute carbol-fuchsine which is used as a counterstain in Gram's stain (a differential method).

Preparation of Stained Films or Smears

In the centre of a clean, grease-free, microscope slide place one or two drops of filtered sterile water. Using a sterilised bacteriological loop, remove a very little of the colony to be examined (if on solid media) or one or two loopfuls (if from a broth culture). In the latter case the water can often be omitted.

Emulsify the growth in the water until a smooth homogeneous suspension is obtained. Spread this over the central portion of the slide until a thin film is formed. Allow to dry completely, in air. Fix the organisms by passing the slide twice through a Bunsen flame and place it to cool on a staining rack over a sink or tray.

When cool, flood the whole of the slide with the stain, preferably filtered beforehand, and leave in contact for the specified length of time. After treatment wash carefully with water and blot dry with fluffless blotting paper. Allow to dry completely before examination. It will now be ready for observation, first under a low power objective (to select a suitable field) and then under the oil-immersion (2 mm) objective. This process is for temporary mounts only.

Composition and Use of Stains

Simple Stains

For simple observation of bacteria the following are suitable.

Loeffler's Methylene Blue.

Methylene blue, saturated solution in alcohol	30 mL
Potassium hydroxide solution, 1%	1 mL
Water	100 mL

Stain for five minutes and wash off with water

Dilute Carbol-fuchsine. Dilute Ziehl-Neelsen carbol-fuchsine 1 in 15 with water immediately before use. Stain for 30 seconds only and wash well with water.

Crystal Violet. A 0.5% solution in water. Stain for one minute and wash well with water.

Differential Stains

Gram's Stain Preston and Morell's Modification. Reagents required
(1) Ammonium oxalate-crystal violet

Crystal violet	20 g
Methylated spirit (64 O.P.)	200 mL
Ammonium oxalate, 1% aqueous solution	800 mL

(2) Lugol's iodine

Iodine	10 g
Potassium iodide	20 g
Water	1000 mL

(3) Iodine-acetone

Strong Solution of Iodine (BP 1958)	35 mL
Acetone	965 mL

Flood the fixed film with ammonium oxalate-crystal violet and allow to act for 30 seconds. Pour off and wash well with Lugol's iodine. Cover with fresh Lugol's iodine and allow to act for 30 seconds. Pour off Lugol's iodine and wash well with iodine-acetone. Cover with fresh iodine-acetone and allow to act for 30 seconds. Wash well with water. Counterstain with dilute carbol-fuchsine (see above) for 30 seconds. Wash with water and blot dry. Gram-positive bacteria stain deep purple; Gram-negative bacteria stain cherry-red to pink. The method can be recommended as reliable, but caution is needed as the vapour from iodine-acetone is irritant to the eyes.

Spore Stain. Thin films must be used, fixed with the minimum of heat. Filter strong carbol-fuchsine (below) on to the slide until completely flooded and warm gently over a small flame until steam rises. Continue the heating for 3 to 5 minutes, making up evaporation losses with freshly filtered stain solution from time to time. Do not boil. Wash off with water and dip the slide rapidly in a 2% solution of nitric acid in absolute alcohol. Immediately wash in water. Counter-stain with Loeffler's methylene blue for one minute. Wash briefly in water, and blot dry. Spores stain cherry-red and the sporangium blue.

Some spores are more rapidly decolorised than others, and if the above process results in unstained spores, it may be necessary to substitute

Table 1
Gram-positive and Gram-negative bacteria

Genus	Type species	Character of genus	
Gram-positive bacteria			
Micrococcus	M. luteus	irregularly arranged	non-motile cocci
Staphylococcus	Staph. aureus	irregularly arranged, catalase positive	
Streptococcus	S. pyogenes	cell in chains, catalase negative	
Corynebacterium	C. diphtheriae	oxidative	non-motile straight rods
Lactobacillus	L. delbrueckii	lactic acid from sugars	
Bacillus	B. subtilis	aerobic or facultatively anaerobic	motile, sporing straight rods, with peritrichous flagella
Clostridium	Cl. butyricum	anaerobic	motile or non-motile sporing straight rods
Gram-negative bacteria			
Brucella	Br. melitensis		non-motile cocci (some cocco-bacilli)
Haemophilus	H. influenzae		
Neisseria	N.gonorrhoeae	aerobic	
Yersinia	Y. pestis	bipolar staining	
Escherichia	E. coli	lactose fermenter	motile, straight rods, with peritrichous flagella (some non-motile), facultative anaerobes
Klebsiella	Kleb. pneumoniae	non-motile	
Proteus	Pr. vulgaris	non-lactose fermenter	
Salmonella	S. choleraesuis	non-lactose fermenter	
Serratia	S. marcescens	pigment producer	
Shigella	Sh. dysenteriae	non-motile	
Acetobacter	A. aceti	acetic acid from ethanol	motile or non-motile rods, aerobic
Pseudomonas	Ps. aeruginosa	yellow-green pigment	motile rods, aerobic
Bacteroides	B. fragilis	anaerobic	motile or non-motile rods
Spirillum	S. undula	rigid helical cells, microaerophilic	motile, bipolar
Vibrio	V. cholerae	straight or curved rods, facultative anaerobe	motile, polar

0.5% sulphuric acid for the solution of nitric acid in absolute alcohol and to prolong the treatment to 1 or 2 minutes.

Ziehl-Neelsen Method. For differential staining of the tubercle bacillus and other acid-fast organisms.
Reagents required
(1) Strong carbol-fuchsine

Basic fuchsine (powder)	10 g
Phenol crystals	50 g
Alcohol (95% or absolute)	100 mL
Water	1000 mL

Place the basic fuchsine and the phenol in a large flask and heat in a boiling water-bath for five minutes, with shaking, until dissolved. Add the alcohol and mix. Add the water in one portion, mixing well during addition.
This solution precipitates on standing and must be filtered immediately before use.
(2) 20% sulphuric acid solution
(3) 95% ethanol
Flood the slide with filtered strong carbol-fuchsine and heat until steam rises. Maintain the heat for five minutes making up any losses through eva-

poration with freshly filtered stain. Wash with water. Cover the slide with 20% sulphuric acid and allow to act for about one minute. Pour off the acid, wash with water, and flood with fresh acid. This decolorisation process should be repeated until the film is a pale pink. Finally, wash well with water, then treat with 95% ethanol for about two minutes. Wash with water. Counter-stain with Loeffler's methylene blue for 30 seconds, wash with water, and dry.
Bacteria that are both acid-fast and alcohol-fast stain cherry-red and all other structures blue. If it is only required to know if the organism is acid-fast, the alcohol treatment may be omitted.

Albert's Method. For the diphtheria bacillus and other volutin-containing organisms.
Reagents required
(1) Albert's stain

Toluidine blue	1.5 g
Malachite green	2.0 g
Acetic acid (glacial)	10 mL
Ethanol (95%)	20 mL
Water	1000 mL

Dissolve the toluidine blue and the malachite green completely in the ethanol. Mix the acetic acid with the water and add the dye solution gradually with continuous mixing. Allow to stand for 24 hours and filter.

(2) Lugol's iodine

Flood the slide with Albert's stain and allow to act for five minutes. Wash in water and blot dry. Flood with Lugol's iodine and allow to act for one minute. Wash with water and blot dry.

Volutin granules stain bluish-black and the cytoplasm of the organism green.

Muir's Method. For the differential staining of capsulate organisms.

Reagents required

(1) Strong Carbol-fuchsine

(2) Muir's Mordant

Tannic acid solution, 20%	2 parts
Mercuric chloride solution (saturated)	2 parts
Potash alum solution (saturated)	5 parts

Flood the thin film with filtered strong carbol-fuchsine and heat gently for one minute. Pour off the stain, rinse rapidly with ethanol and immediately wash well with water. Flood with Muir's mordant and allow to act for 30 seconds. Pour off and wash well with water, followed by treatment with alcohol for about 30 seconds until the film is pale pink. Wash with water. Counterstain with Loeffler's methylene blue for 30 to 60 seconds. Wash briefly with water, blot, and dry.

Capsules appear as a blue area surrounding a dark red organism.

Some practice is needed to achieve satisfactory results with this method. Better results are often obtained with the wet-film India ink method, which also requires practice.

Preparation of Unstained or Stained Material for the Identification of Fungi

Microscopic examination of unstained or stained specimens from the patient and from the resultant cultures are often the only tests performed in the identification of fungi. Specimens of skin scales, hair or nail clippings are first rendered transparent. Fragments of the specimen are placed on a glass slide and covered with 20% sodium hydroxide or potassium hydroxide solution. The slide is left at room temperature to allow the keratin to partially dissolve (skin scales clear in 5 to 10 minutes; nail may take 1 to 2 hours at 37°). A coverslip is applied and the film examined under the dry objectives. If necessary, cleared preparations may be stained by adding lactophenol cotton blue staining solution.

Gram's staining method is also used in the diagnosis of fungal infections, for example, in *Candida* infections.

Motility

Wet Films. The microscopic examination of unstained living organisms in wet films is often carried out to determine whether the organism belongs to a species that is motile. The specimen may be a liquid culture or a suspension in saline prepared from a liquid or solid culture.

A wet film is prepared between a slide and a coverslip. When examining the film it is necessary to defocus the microscope condenser to maximise the contrast between the organism and its background. Also, it is essential to distinguish true motility (where the organisms move in different directions) from passive drifting (organisms move in the same direction) and Brownian movement (organisms oscillate around an almost fixed point).

Craigie Tube Method. The motility of organisms may also be demonstrated by the Craigie tube method. Broth containing 0.1% to 0.2% agar allows the migration of motile cells. This allows motile organisms to be separated from non-motile organisms in the Craigie tube.

CULTURE MEDIA

Only the highest quality materials should be used in the preparation of media. Where agar is included in the formula the use of a preclarified grade is advisable to avoid the necessity of filtering the final medium. Deionised or distilled water, free from bactericidal and inhibitory properties, is used for media preparation. The pH of media should be checked after autoclaving to ensure compliance with recommended pH limits. Additionally, sterility and growth checks, using working standards of known organisms, should be carried out on each batch of medium. Guidance on storage times of culture media can be found in British Standard 5763:Part 0.

Liquid Media

Heat-stable ingredients are dissolved in the bulk of the water with the aid of gentle heat. If absolute clarity is necessary, adjust the pH to 8.0, heat at 100° for 30 minutes, and filter off the precipitate of phosphates. Cool, adjust to the final pH required, and make up to volume. Sterilise on the day of preparation.

Heat-labile ingredients are best sterilised separately by filtration in a concentrated form and an aliquot added aseptically to the sterilised medium basis immediately before use.

Solid Media

For standard agar media, 1% to 2% (according to grade) of preclarified agar is added to the liquid medium basis, allowed to hydrate at room temperature for 15 minutes, and dissolved by steaming at 100° or by autoclaving. The medium can often be sterilised and the agar dissolved at the same time, provided that it is adequately mixed after sterilisation and before it sets.

Agar media, once set, need to be held at 98° to 100° before they will melt. Once melted they can be cooled to about 45° to 48° before setting again.

Many complete media are now available in a convenient dehydrated form as granules or tablets, requiring only solution and sterilisation before use. They can be recommended for general use.

Aminobenzoic Acid Media

Add 5 to 10 mg of *p*-aminobenzoic acid to 100 mL of medium (any type), check the pH, and adjust if necessary to the correct pH of the medium. Sterilise at the appropriate temperature. Aminobenzoic acid media are used as inactivators for sulphonamides in sterility testing and blood culture and in the isolation of pathogenic cocci.

Blood Agar

Add aseptically 5% to 10% of sterile human or horse blood to sterile nutrient agar, melted and cooled to 50°. Mix gently, avoiding the formation of air bubbles, and slope or pour plates. Blood agar is used for the growth of delicate pathogens and for showing the haemolytic properties of bacteria, for example, *Streptococcus pyogenes*.

Blood Broth

Add aseptically 5% to 10% of sterile human or horse blood to sterile nutrient broth and mix. Blood broth is used for the growth of delicate pathogens.

Chocolate Agar

Chocolate agar is prepared by heating 10% of sterile human or horse blood in sterile nutrient agar. Melt the agar and cool it in a waterbath to 75°. Add the blood and mix gently. Allow the medium to remain at 75° until 'chocolating' has occurred, within 10 minutes. Pour as slopes or plates. Chocolate agar is used for the growth of *Haemophilus* and *Streptococcus* species and other fastidious organisms.

Cooked Meat Medium

Squeeze dry meat residue from meat infusion broth. Rinse in acetone, strain off through muslin, and dry thoroughly on filter paper in air. Place enough dried meat in tubes or bottles to give a layer 1 cm deep and add sufficient nutrient, meat infusion, or digest broth to give a layer at least 5 cm deep. Close the container and sterilise at 121° for 15 minutes. It should be heated at 98° to 100° for 5 to 10 minutes before use to drive off oxygen. Cooked meat medium is used as a general purpose medium for anaerobes and as a good maintenance medium for aerobic and anaerobic bacteria. If 10% sodium chloride is added to the broth, the medium can be used for the isolation of staphylococci from grossly contaminated samples.

Dorset's Egg Medium

Scrub 2 to 4 whole fresh eggs in soap and warm water, rinse thoroughly in running water, and immerse in alcohol for five minutes. Remove, cover, and dry. Crack the eggs into a sterile beaker, beat with a sterile whisk, and measure the volume in a sterile cylinder. To each 75 mL of egg add 25 mL of sterile nutrient broth and mix. Distribute aseptically 5-mL amounts in sterile McCartney bottles. Slope and heat in the inspissator at 75° to 80° for one hour. Can be kept in the cold for not more than one month. Dorset's egg medium is used for isolation and growth of tubercle bacilli. If used for isolation of tubercle bacilli, 1.25 mL of 2% aqueous malachite green solution should be added before distributing.

Fluid Thioglycollate Medium

L-Cystine	0.5 g
Agar	0.75 g
Sodium chloride	2.5 g
Glucose	5.5 g
Yeast extract	5.0 g
Pancreatic digest of casein	15.0 g
Sodium thioglycollate	0.5 g
or thioglycollic acid	0.3 mL
Resazurin sodium solution (0.1%, freshly prepared)	1.0 mL
Water	1000 mL

Mix all ingredients except the thioglycollate and the resazurin solution with 1000 mL of water and heat to dissolve. Add sodium thioglycollate (or thioglycollic acid) and adjust pH to 7.0 to 7.2. If cloudy, reheat (do not boil), and filter through filter paper. Add the resazurin solution, mix, and distribute at once in suitable amounts into final containers. Sterilise at 121° for 20 minutes, once only. Store in the dark between 20° and 30°. If more than the upper third of the medium becomes pink, heat to 98° to 100° for 5 to 10 minutes before use. This heating must not be repeated. Fluid thioglycollate medium is used for the cultivation of anaerobes; general purpose medium for sterility testing.

Glucose Agar

Add aseptically 0.5 to 1.0 mL of a sterile 10% solution of glucose to each 10 mL of sterile melted nutrient agar. Mix and slope or pour plates. Glucose agar is used as an enrichment medium for many bacteria and as an enriched base for blood agar.

Glucose Broth

Prepare as glucose agar using sterile nutrient broth. Mix. Glucose broth is used as an enrichment medium for bacteria.

Loeffler's Serum Medium

Add aseptically 10 mL of sterile 1% glucose broth to 30 mL of sterile serum (*horse*, *ox*, or *sheep*) and mix. Tube or bottle aseptically in suitable amounts, for example, 2.5 mL in screw-capped Bijou bottles. Slope, and heat slowly to 80° to 85° and maintain for two hours until coagulated. Avoid rapid heating and formation of air bubbles. Loeffler's serum medium is used for the cultivation of diphtheria bacilli and to demonstrate proteolytic activity of clostridia.

MacConkey's Agar

Peptone	20 g
Sodium taurocholate	5 g
Agar	20 g
Neutral red solution (2% in 50% ethanol)	3.5 mL
Lactose (10% aqueous solutions)	100 mL
Water	1000 mL

Dissolve the peptone and taurocholate in the water with heat. Add agar, hydrate, and dissolve by autoclaving. Cool to 55° and adjust to pH 7.5. Add the lactose and neutral red solution and mix. Heat at 98° to 100° for one hour in steam, then sterilise at 115° for 15 minutes. The medium should be reddish-brown. If pink, it has become acid. If the medium is to be stored, omit neutral red and add it aseptically to the melted medium at 55° immediately before pouring plates. MacConkey's agar is used for the cultivation, isolation, and identification of enteric bacteria; colonies of lactose fermenters are pink, non-lactose fermenters are colourless. Many modifications of MacConkey's agar are available.

Malt Extract Agar

Malt extract	40 g
Agar	20 g
Water	1000 mL

Dissolve the malt extract in 500 mL of water. Autoclave at 115° for 10 minutes. Filter hot through paper, cool, and add 400 mL of water. Adjust to pH 5.4 with 10% lactic acid and add the remainder of the water. Add agar, hydrate, and sterilise at 115° for 15 minutes. It is not advisable to repeat sterilisation more than once. If desired, 5 g of mycological peptone can be added as enrichment. To inhibit bacterial growth, add aseptically 1.8 mL of sterile 2% potassium tellurite solution to melted medium at 55° before sloping or pouring. Malt extract agar is used as a general purpose medium for cultivation of fungi.

Malt Extract Broth

Prepare as for malt extract agar, omitting agar. Malt extract broth is used as a general purpose medium for cultivation of fungi.

Meat Infusion Broth

Lean meat (beef or ox heart)	500 g
Peptone	10 g
Sodium chloride	5 g
Water	1000 mL

Carefully remove all fat from fresh meat, mince the meat finely, and add to water. Refrigerate for 24 hours. Strain off meat through muslin and express residue. Remove any fat from surface of liquor and heat at 100° for two hours. Filter hot through a hardened filter paper to give a clear, light-yellow filtrate. Add the peptone and salt, dissolve, and cool. Adjust to pH 7.5 with sodium hydroxide solution. Tube or bottle, and sterilise at 121° for 15 minutes. Meat infusion broth is used as a general purpose broth.

Milk Agar

Defatted milk powder or granules	10 g
Agar	2 g
Water	100 mL

Disperse milk powder completely in 50 mL of water. Autoclave at 115° for five minutes and cool rapidly. Dissolve the agar in 50 mL of water and sterilise at 121° for 15 minutes. Immediately before use mix equal volumes of sterile milk solution and melted agar solution at 60° and pour thin (15mL) plates. Commercial domestic defatted milk granules are very suitable for this medium. They must not be overheated. Milk agar is used for the rapid identification of *Pseudomonas aeruginosa* (green pigment and zones of casein lysis formed in 24 to 48 hours at 35°).

Nutrient Broth (Meat Extract or Lemco Broth)

Peptone	10 g
Meat extract (Lab-Lemco)	10 g
Sodium chloride	5 g
Water	1000 mL

Mix all ingredients, dissolve with gentle heat, cool, and adjust to pH 7.5 to 7.6 with sodium hydroxide solution. Filter, tube or bottle, and sterilise at 121° for 15 minutes. Nutrient broth is used as a general purpose broth. Many modifications of this broth are available.

Nutrient Gelatin

Add 150 g of gelatin to 1000 mL of broth (any general purpose type). Allow to soak overnight in the refrigerator. Warm to 45° to dissolve, adjust to pH 8.4, and steam at 100° for 10 minutes. Cool rapidly to 45°, add beaten whites of two eggs, mix, and steam at 100° for 30 minutes with occasional stirring. Filter hot through paper pulp. Check the pH and adjust to pH 7.6. Tube or bottle and sterilise, first at 100° for 10 minutes and then at 115° for 10 minutes. Cool rapidly and keep cold. If absolute clarity is not required, use a high-grade gelatin and omit the clarification with egg-white, from 'add beaten...' to '...paper pulp'. Nutrient gelatin is used in tests for gelatinase activity of proteolytic bacteria by stab culture.

Peptone Water

Peptone	10 g
Sodium chloride	5 g
Water	1000 mL

Dissolve the peptone and sodium chloride, adjust to pH 7.4 to 7.5, filter and bottle as required. Sterilise at 121° for 15 minutes. If used as a base for sugar fermentation media, add aseptically sterile concentrated sugar solutions to give a final concentration of 0.5% to 1.0% of sugar in medium. Indicators for acid production are usually best added after growth and fermentation have occurred. Peptone water is used as a growth medium for non-exacting bacteria; base for sugar fermentation media and as a medium for testing for indole formation.

Sabouraud's Glucose Agar

Glucose	40 g
Peptone (mycological)	10 g
Agar	20 g
Water	1000 mL

Dissolve the glucose and peptone in water with heat. Cool, adjust to pH 5.4 with 10% lactic acid, and filter. Add agar, hydrate, dissolve, and sterilise at 115° for 15 minutes. This medium should not be repeatedly heated. Sabouraud's glucose agar is used for the isolation of fungi.

Sabouraud's Glucose Broth

Prepare as Sabouraud's glucose agar omitting agar. Sabouraud's glucose broth is used for the isolation of fungi and as a fungal medium for sterility testing.

Serum Agar

Prepare as blood agar using 10% of human or *horse* serum. Serum agar is a clear medium for cultivation of delicate pathogens.

Serum Broth

Prepare as blood broth using 10% of human or *horse* serum. Serum broth is a clear medium for cultivation of delicate pathogens.

Teepol-lactose Agar

Peptone	20 g
Lactose	10 g
Sodium chloride	5 g
Teepol (*Shell Chemicals Ltd*)	1 g
Bromothymol blue (0.2% solution)	25 mL
Agar (deionised grade)	9 g
Water	1000 mL

Dissolve all ingredients except the agar in the water, and adjust to pH 7.5. Add agar, hydrate, and sterilise at 115° for 15 minutes. Teepol-lactose agar is used as a standardised substitute for MacConkey's agar (lactose fermenters form pale cream colonies; non-lactose fermenters form pale green colonies).

Tryptic Digest Broth (Hartley's Digest Broth)

(1) Preparation of pancreatic extract

Fresh pig pancreas	500 g	
Water	1500 mL	
Absolute alcohol or methylated spirit	500 mL	
Concentrated hydrochloric acid about	2 mL	

Remove fat from pancreas, mince, and mix with the water and alcohol in a large stoppered bottle.

Shake thoroughly and allow to stand for three days at room temperature with occasional shaking. Strain through muslin, then through filter paper. Measure the filtrate and add 0.1% of hydrochloric acid. Allow to settle in the cold and filter. Can be stored in the refrigerator for not more than two months.

(2) Preparation of medium

Lean meat (beef or ox-heart)	500 g
Sodium carbonate (0.8% solution)	2500 mL
Pancreatic extract	50 mL
Chloroform	50 mL
Concentrated hydrochloric acid	40 mL
Water	2500 mL

Mince the meat and mix with the water. Heat in steam to 80°, add the sodium carbonate solution, and cool to 45°. Add the pancreatic extract and chloroform and incubate at 37° for six hours or 45° for three hours with frequent stirring. Add the acid, steam at 100° for 30 minutes, strain, and filter. Bottle, add 0.25% chloroform, and keep in a cool dark place for two to three days, shaking frequently. Store in a cool dark place. For use, adjust to pH 8.0, steam at 100° for one hour, and filter hot. Cool, adjust to pH 7.6, distribute, and sterilise at 115° for 20 minutes. Tryptic digest broth is used as a complete general purpose medium giving luxuriant growth of most exacting bacteria; not to be used as a maintenance medium.

Tryptone Soy Agar

Tryptone	15 g
Soy peptone	5 g
Sodium chloride	5 g
Agar	12 g
Water	1000 mL

Dissolve all the ingredients except the agar in the water and adjust to pH 7.4. Add agar, hydrate, and sterilise at 121° for 15 minutes. Tryptone soy agar is used as a stimulatory general purpose medium for bacteria and fungi and as a blood agar base.

Tryptone Soy Broth

Tryptone	17 g
Soy peptone	3 g
Sodium chloride	5 g
Dipotassium phosphate	2.5 g
Glucose	2.5 g
Water	1000 mL

Dissolve all the ingredients and adjust to pH 7.2. Tube and sterilise at 121° for not more than 15 minutes. Cool rapidly. This medium should not be overheated and the phosphate can be omitted if necessary. Tryptone Soy Broth is used as a stimulatory general purpose medium for bacteria and fungi, for sterility testing, and for antibiotic sensitivity tests.

Yeast Extract Agar

Yeast extract	2 g
Peptone	5 g
Agar	15 g
Water	1000 mL

Dissolve peptone and yeast extract in the water with heat. Cool and adjust to pH 7.4. Add agar, hydrate, dissolve, and sterilise at 121° for 20 minutes. If absolute clarity is required, filter hot through paper pulp and adjust pH of filtrate to 7.0 at 50°. Distribute and sterilise at 121° for 20 minutes. If testing milk supplies or rinse-water from utensils, add 10 mL of fresh or spray-dried, skimmed, or whole milk per litre of medium during preparation. Yeast extract agar is used for plate counts of viable bacteria in drinking water and for the cultivation of non-exacting bacteria.

MICRO-ORGANISMS PATHOGENIC TO MAN

The following lists of micro-organisms and associated diseases are not comprehensive but include the principal pathogens and other micro-organisms of medical interest.

BACTERIA

Families	Genera
Spirochaetes	
Spirochaetaceae	*Treponema; Borrelia; Leptospira*
Spiral and curved bacteria	
Spirillaceae	*Spirillum*
Gram-negative aerobic rods and cocci	
Pseudomonadaceae	*Pseudomonas*
Uncertain affiliation	*Brucella; Bordetella; Francisella*
Gram-negative facultatively anaerobic rods	
Enterobacteriaceae	*Escherichia; Salmonella; Shigella; Klebsiella; Proteus; Yersinia*
Vibrionaceae	*Vibrio*
Uncertain affiliation	*Cardiobacterium; Calymmatobacterium; Haemophilus; Pasteurella; Streptobacillus*

Gram-negative anaerobic bacteria
  Bacteroidaceae   *Bacteroides;*
                          Fusobacterium
Gram-negative aerobic cocci
and coccobacilli
  Neisseriaceae   *Moraxella; Neisseria*
Gram-positive cocci
  Micrococcaceae   *Micrococcus;*
                          Staphylococcus
  Streptococcaceae   *Streptococcus*
Endospore-forming rods and cocci
  Bacillaceae   *Bacillus; Clostridium*
Gram-positive non-sporing rod-
shaped bacteria
  Lactobacillaceae   *Lactobacillus*
  Uncertain affiliation   *Listeria; Erysipelothrix*
Actinomycetes and related organisms
  Coryneform group   *Cornyebacterium*
  Actinomycetaceae   *Actinomyces*
  Mycobacteriaceae   *Mycobacterium*
  Nocardiaceae   *Nocardia*
Rickettsias
  Rickettsiaceae   *Rickettsia; Rochalimaea;*
                          Coxiella
  Bartonellaceae   *Bartonella*
  Chlamydiaceae   *Chlamydia*
Mycoplasmas
  Mycoplasmataceae   *Mycoplasma*

Actinobacillus actinomycetemcomitans: a cause of infection in the jaw and in endocarditis
Actinomyces israelii: the cause of actinomycosis in man
Bacillus anthracis: the cause of anthrax
Bacillus cereus: one cause of enterotoxic food poisoning, particularly associated with cooked rice
Bacteroides fragilis: a very common anaerobic isolate from human soft-tissue infections; other species of Bacteroides are commonly associated with many infected lesions in man
Bartonella bacilliformis: the probable cause of Oroya fever and Verruga peruana
Bordetella bronchiseptica (*Syn. Haemophilus bronchisepticus*): associated with bronchopneumonia in rodents, a secondary infection in canine distemper, and, occasionally, a form of whooping cough in man
Bordetella parapertussis (*Syn. Haemophilus parapertussis*): an occasional cause of a mild form of whooping cough
Bordetella pertussis (*Syn. Haemophilus pertussis*): the principal cause of whooping cough

Borrelia recurrentis: the cause of European relapsing fever. Other *Borrelia* species have been reported as causing relapsing fever in various parts of the world
Borrelia vincentii: associated with a fusiform bacillus in Vincent's angina and in other necrotic inflammatory conditions of the mouth (for example, gingivitis, stomatitis) and elsewhere in the body
Boyd's dysentery bacillus—see *Shigella boydii*
Brucella abortus: causes contagious abortion in cattle; one cause of brucellosis in man
Brucella melitensis (*Syn. Micrococcus melitensis*): Brucella infection of goats and sheep; one cause of brucellosis in man
Brucella suis: Brucella infection of swine; one cause of brucellosis in man
Brucella tularensis—see *Francisella tularensis*
Calymmatobacterium granulomatis (*Syn. Donovania granulomatis*): a cause of inguinal and other granulomas
Cardiobacterium hominis: one cause of bacterial endocarditis
Chlamydia pneumoniae: a cause of upper and lower respiratory tract infection including pneumonia
Chlamydia psittaci: the cause of psittacosis (*Syn.* ornithosis)
Chlamydia trachomatis: the cause of trachoma, lymphogranuloma venereum, and associated infections
Clostridium botulinum: the cause of botulism
Clostridium difficile: a cause of pseudomembranous colitis
Clostridium novyi (*Syn. Cl.oedematiens*): one cause of gas gangrene
Clostridium oedematiens—see *Clostridium novyi*
Clostridium perfringens (*Syn. Cl. welchii*): the principal cause of gas gangrene
Clostridium septicum (*Syn. Vibrion septique*): one cause of gas gangrene
Clostridium tetani: the cause of tetanus
Clostridium welchii—see *Clostridium perfringens*
Comma bacillus—see *Vibrio cholerae*
Corynebacterium diphtheriae (*Syn.* Klebs-Loeffler bacillus): the cause of diphtheria
Coxiella burnetii (*Syn. Rickettsia burneti, Rickettsia diaporica*): the cause of Q fever
Diplococcus pneumoniae—see *Streptococcus pneumoniae*
Donovania granulomatis—see *Calymmatobacterium granulomatis*
Ducrey's bacillus—see *Haemophilus ducreyi*
Enterobacter species: widely distributed in nature and common in man and animals; some species,

for example, *E. aerogenes*, *E. agglomerans*, *E. cloacae*, and *E. sakazakii*, can behave as opportunistic pathogens

Enterococcus faecalis: found in some non-sterile foods and pharmaceuticals but presence not often due to faecal contamination; a cause of urinary tract infection, also subacute endocarditis

Erysipelothrix insidiosa—see *Erysipelothrix rhusiopathiae*

Erysipelothrix monocytogenes—see *Listeria monocytogenes*

Erysipelothrix murisepticus—see *Erysipelothrix rhusiopathiae*

Erysipelothrix rhusiopathiae (*Syn*. *E. insidiosa*, *E. murisepticus*): causes erysipelas in swine and erysipeloid in man

Escherichia coli: a cause of local inflammation (cholecystitis, cystitis, pyelitis); found occasionally in septicaemia; a few strains are associated with infantile enteric infections

Flexner's dysentery bacillus—see *Shigella flexneri*

Francisella tularensis (*Syn*. *Brucella tularensis*, *Pasteurella tularensis*): the cause of tularaemia

Friedländer's bacillus—see *Klebsiella pneumoniae*

Fusiformis fusiformis—see *Fusobacterium nucleatum*

Fusobacterium nucleatum (*Syn*. *Fusiformis fusiformis*)—see under *Borrelia vincentii*

Gardnerella vaginalis (*Syn*. *Haemophilus vaginalis*): one cause of 'non-specific' vaginitis and urethritis

Gonococcus - see *Neisseria gonorrhoeae*

Haemophilus bronchisepticus—see *Bordetella bronchiseptica*

Haemophilus ducreyi (*Syn*. Ducrey's bacillus): associated with chancroid or soft chancre

Haemophilus influenzae (*Syn*. Pfeiffer's bacillus): associated with acute and chronic infections of the respiratory tract and with pyogenic meningitis

Haemophilus parapertussis—see *Bordetella parapertussis*

Haemophilus pertussis—see *Bordetella pertussis*

Haemophilus vaginalis —see *Gardnerella vaginalis*

Helicobacter pylori (*Syn*. *Campylobacter pylori*): associated with diarrhoea and chronic gastritis

Klebs-Loeffler bacillus—see *Corynebacterium diphtheriae*

Klebsiella ozaenae: frequently associated with ozaena and with atrophic rhinitis

Klebsiella pneumoniae (*Syn*. Friedländer's bacillus, pneumobacillus): associated with some bacterial pneumonias and inflammations of the respiratory tract

Klebsiella rhinoscleromatis: associated with rhinoscleroma

Legionella pneumophila: ('Legionnaire's agent') a Gram-negative bacillus, which is the cause of Legionnaire's disease, an acute respiratory infection

Leptospira canicola: a common cause of leptospiral infection in dogs and, occasionally, in man ('canicola fever')

Leptospira icterohaemorrhagiae: cause of haemorrhagic (spirochaetal) jaundice (*Syn*. Weil's disease)

Listeria monocytogenes (*Syn*. *Erysipelothrix monocytogenes*): a cause of meningo-encephalitis, endocarditis, and granulomatosis infantiseptica

Loefflerella pseudomallei—see *Pseudomonas pseudomallei*

Meningococcus—see *Neisseria meningitidis*

Micrococcus melitensis—see *Brucella melitensis*

Micrococcus pyogenes—see *Staphylococcus aureus*

Morax-Axenfeld bacillus—see *Moraxella lacunata*

Moraxella lacunata (*Syn*. Morax-Axenfeld bacillus): associated with subacute or chronic conjunctivitis

Moraxella catarrhalis (*Syn*. *Branhamella catarrhalis*, *Neisseria catarrhalis*): a cause of respiratory disease and otitis media

Mycobacterium leprae: the cause of leprosy

Mycobacterium marinum (*Syn*. *Mycobacterium balnei*): associated with skin lesions in man resulting from abrasions occurring in swimming pools, aquariums (swimming pool granuloma)

Mycobacterium tuberculosis (*Syn*. tubercle bacillus): the cause of tuberculosis of lungs and other organs; other species of *Mycobacterium* can also cause tuberculosis in man

Mycobacterium ulcerans: a cause of skin ulcers

Mycoplasma species (*Syn*. PPLO, Pleuropneumonia-like organisms): a cause of primary atypical pneumonias in man

Neisseria gonorrhoeae (*Syn*. gonococcus): the cause of gonorrhoea

Neisseria meningitidis (*Syn*. meningococcus): the cause of cerebrospinal meningitis and a cause of septicaemia

Nocardia species: causes of nocardiosis including mycetoma

PPLO—see *Mycoplasma* species

Paratyphoid A bacillus—see *Salmonella paratyphi-A*

Paratyphoid B bacillus—see *Salmonella schottmuelleri*

Paratyphoid C bacillus—see *Salmonella hirschfeldii*

Pasteurella pestis—see *Yersinia pestis*

Pasteurella tularensis—see *Francisella tularensis*

Pfeiffer's bacillus—see *Haemophilus influenzae*

Pleuropneumonia-like organisms (PPLO)—see *Mycoplasma* species

Pneumobacillus—see *Klebsiella pneumoniae*

Pneumococcus—see *Streptococcus pneumoniae*

Proteus species: associated with infections of the urinary tract and of wounds

Pseudomonas aeruginosa (*Syn. Ps. pyocyanea*): found in urinary infections, secondary infections of wounds, burns, and the epithelia of the ear and eye, and generalised infection in infants and the debilitated

Pseudomonas cepacia: very occasionally isolated from clinical specimens and non-sterile pharmaceuticals; opportunistic human pathogen, also associated with infections of nosocomial origin

Pseudomonas pseudomallei (*Syn. Loefflerella pseudomallei*): the cause of melioidosis

Pseudomonas pyocyanea—see *Pseudomonas aeruginosa*

Rickettsia akamushi—see *Rickettsia tsutsugamushi*

Rickettsia akari: a cause of mite-borne typhus—rickettsialpox

Rickettsia burneti—see *Coxiella burnetii*

Rickettsia conorii: a cause of tick-borne typhus, boutonneuse fever (*Syn.* Mediterranean fever), also tick-bite fevers of the southern hemisphere

Rickettsia diaporica—see *Coxiella burnetii*

Rickettsia mooseri—see *Rickettsia typhi*

Rickettsia prowazekii: a cause of louse-borne typhus—(1) epidemic typhus (2) recrudescent typhus (*Syn.* Brill's disease)

Rickettsia quintana—see *Rochalimaea quintana*

Rickettsia rickettsii: a cause of tick-borne typhus—Rocky Mountain spotted fever

Rickettsia tsutsugamushi (*Syn. R. akamushi*) a cause of mite-borne typhus-scrub typhus (*Syn.* tsutsugamushi fever)

Rickettsia typhi (*Syn. R. mooseri*): a cause of flea-borne typhus-murine endemic typhus (*Syn.* tabardillo)

Rickettsia wolhynica—see *Rochalimaea quintana*

Rochalimaea quintana (*Syn. Rickettsia quintana, Rickettsia wolhynica*): a cause of louse-borne typhus-trench fever (*Syn.* quintan fever)

Salmonella hirschfeldii (*Syn. S. paratyphoid*-C, the paratyphoid C bacillus): a cause of paratyphoid fever

Salmonella paratyphi-A (*Syn.* the paratyphoid A bacillus) a cause of paratyphoid fever

Salmonella paratyphoid B—see *Salmonella schottmuelleri*

Salmonella paratyphoid C—see *Salmonella hirschfeldii*

Salmonella schottmuelleri (*Syn. S.* paratyphoid B, the paratyphoid B bacillus): a cause of paratyphoid fever

Salmonella serotypes: several hundred other *Salmonella* serotypes have been distinguished which may be responsible for food poisoning in man

Salmonella typhi (*Syn.* typhoid bacillus): the cause of typhoid fever

Shiga's dysentery bacillus—see *Shigella dysenteriae*

Shigella boydii (*Syn.* Boyd's dysentery bacillus): a cause of bacillary dysentery (uncommon outside India)

Shigella dysenteriae (*Syn.* Shiga's dysentery bacillus, *Sh. shigae*): a cause of bacillary dysentery (acute, severe)

Shigella flexneri (*Syn.* Flexner's dysentery bacillus, *Sh. paradysenteriae*): a cause of bacillary dysentery (one of the common forms)

Shigella paradysenteriae—see *Shigella flexneri*

Shigella shigae—see *Shigella dysenteriae*

Shigella sonnei (*Syn.* Sonne's dysentery bacillus): a cause of bacillary or Sonne dysentery (mild; one of the common forms)

Sonne's dysentery bacillus—see *Shigella sonnei*

Spirillum minor: one cause of rat-bite fever

Staphylococcus aureus (*Syn. Micrococcus pyogenes, Staph. pyogenes*): a common cause of suppuration; found in furunculitis, folliculitis, mastitis, pyaemia, and osteomyelitis

Staphylococcus pyogenes—see *Staphylococcus aureus*

Streptobacillus moniliformis: one cause of rat-bite fever

Streptococcus erysipelatos—see *Streptococcus pyogenes*

Streptococcus haemolyticus—see *Streptococcus pyogenes*

Streptococcus pneumoniae (*Syn. Diplococcus pneumoniae,* pneumococcus): a cause of lobar pneumonia; associated with other acute and chronic infections

Streptococcus pyogenes (*Syn. S. erysipelatos, S. haemolyticus, S. scarlatinae*): a cause of local abscesses, erysipelas, impetigo, puerperal sepsis, scarlet fever, tonsilitis, and septicaemia

Streptococcus scarlatinae—see *Streptococcus pyogenes*

Streptococcus species (*Syn. S. viridans*): α-haemolytic strains of streptococci are associated with subacute bacterial endocarditis and with urinary-tract infections

Streptococcus viridans—see *Streptococcus* species

Treponema carateum (*Syn. T. herrejoni*): the cause of pinta (*Syn.* carate)

Treponema herrejoni—see *Treponema carateum*

Treponema pallidum: the cause of syphilis

Treponema pertenue: the cause of yaws (*Syn.* framboesia)

Tubercle bacillus—see *Mycobacterium tuberculosis*

Typhoid bacillus—see *Salmonella typhi*

Vibrio cholerae (*Syn.* comma bacillus, *V. cholerae-asiaticae*, *V. comma*) the cause of Asiatic cholera

Vibrio cholerae-asiaticae—see *Vibrio cholerae*

Vibrio comma—see *Vibrio cholerae*

Vibrion septique—see *Clostridium septicum*

Yersinia pestis (*Syn. Pasteurella pestis*): the cause of bubonic and pneumonic plague

FUNGI

Allescheria boydii—see *Petriellidium boydii*

Aspergillus species: cause of aspergillosis, otomycosis, and tinea unguium (*Syn.* onychomycosis, ringworm of nails)

Blastomyces brasiliensis—see *Paracoccidioides brasiliensis*

Blastomyces dermatitidis: the cause of North American blastomycosis

Candida albicans (*Syn. Monilia albicans, Monilia pinoyi, Oidium albicans*): a cause of candidiasis (*Syn.* moniliasis, candidosis)

Cephalosporium falciforme: a cause of mycetoma

Cladosporium carrionii: a cause of chromomycosis (*Syn.* chromoblastomycosis)

Coccidioides immitis: the cause of coccidioidomycosis (*Syn.* desert rheumatism, valley fever)

Cryptococcus neoformans: the cause of cryptococcosis (*Syn.* torulosis)

Epidermophyton cruris—see *Epidermophyton floccosum*

Epidermophyton floccosum (*Syn. E. cruris, E. inguinale*): a cause of tinea (*Syn.* ringworm)

Epidermophyton inguinale—see *Epidermophyton floccosum*

Exophiala werneckii: the cause of 'tinea nigra'

Geotrichum candidum: the cause of geotrichosis

Histoplasma capsulatum: the cause of histoplasmosis

Madurella grisea: a cause of mycetoma

Madurella mycetomatis (*Syn. Madurella tozeuri*): a cause of mycetoma

Madurella tozeuri—see *Madurella mycetomatis*

Microsporum species: a cause of tinea (*Syn.* ringworm)

Monilia albicans—see *Candida albicans*

Monilia pinoyi—see *Candida albicans*

Oidium albicans—see *Candida albicans*

Paracoccidioides brasiliensis (*Syn. Blastomyces brasiliensis*): the cause of paracoccidioidomycosis (*Syn.* South American blastomycosis, paracoccidioidal granuloma)

Petriellidium boydii (*Syn. Allescheria boydii*): a cause of mycetoma

Phialophora vernicosa: a cause of chromoblastomycosis

Sporothrix schenckii: the cause of sporotrichosis

Trichophyton schoenleinii: the cause of human favus

Trichophyton species: a cause of tinea (*Syn.* ringworm)

PROTOZOA

Acanthamoeba species: a cause of keratitis in contact lens wearers

Balantidium coli: a cause of balantidiasis (*Syn.* balantidial dysentery)

Entamoeba histolytica: the cause of amoebiasis (*Syn.* amoebic dysentery)

Giardia intestinalis (*Syn. G. lamblia*): the cause of giardiasis (*Syn.* lambliasis)

Giardia lamblia—see *Giardia intestinalis*

Leishmania brasiliensis: the cause of South American mucocutaneous leishmaniasis (*Syn.* espundia, forest yaws)

Leishmania donovani: the cause of visceral leishmaniasis (*Syn.* kala-azar)

Leishmania tropica: the cause of cutaneous leishmaniasis (*Syn.* oriental or tropical sore)

Naegleria species: a cause of meningo-encephalitis

Plasmodium falciparum: the cause of malignant tertian malaria

Plasmodium malariae: the cause of quartan malaria

Plasmodium ovale: the cause of ovale malaria

Plasmodium vivax: the cause of benign tertian malaria

Pneumocystis carinii: a cause of epidemic interstitial plasma cell pneumonia, occurring in immunosuppressed or severely debilitated patients

Schizotrypanum cruzi—see *Trypanosoma cruzi*

Toxoplasma gondii: the cause of toxoplasmosis of the reticulo-endothelial system

Trichomonas vaginalis: a cause of vaginitis and urethritis

Trypanosoma cruzi (*Syn. Schizotrypanum cruzi*): the cause of American (Brazilian) trypanosomiasis (*Syn.* Chagas' disease)

Trypanosoma gambiense: a cause of African trypanosomiasis (*Syn.* African sleeping sickness)

Trypanosoma rhodesiense: a cause of African trypanosomiasis (*Syn.* African sleeping sickness)

VIRUSES

The following list outlines the main groups and their associated diseases.

Adenoviruses: the causative agents of some virus infections involving the respiratory tract and the conjunctiva in man

Arboviruses: including the causative agents of yellow fever, dengue fever, sandfly fever, Rift Valley fever, and a variety of tick-borne encephalitic infections in many parts of the world

Arenaviruses: including the causative agents of lymphocytic choriomeningitis and Lassa fever

Coronaviruses: the causative agents of some respiratory and gastro-intestinal infections in man and animals

Hepatitis viruses: the five forms of acute viral hepatitis are similar clinically, but the agents that cause them are quite distinct

Herpesviruses: including the causative agents of herpes simplex (cold sore), chickenpox and shingles (varicella-zoster virus), infectious mononucleosis, and cytomegalic inclusion disease. Various animal virus infections, some transmissible to man by contact

Orthomyxoviruses (myxoviruses): the causative agents of influenza (Types A, B, and C)

Papovaviruses: including the causative agents of papilloma (warts and verruca) in man and animals

Paramyxoviruses: including the causative agents of mumps (epidemic parotitis), Newcastle disease, and measles. Also respiratory infections associated with 'para-influenza' viruses (including Sendai, croup, and haemadsorption viruses, various animal influenzas, distempers, and viral tumours)

Picornaviruses: a large group including the causative agents of (1) poliomyelitis, (2) herpangina, epidemic myalgia (pleurodynia, Bornholm disease) due to Coxsackie viruses, (3) aseptic meningitis and other infections due to ECHO viruses, (4) the common cold due to rhinoviruses and others, and (5) foot-and-mouth disease in domestic animals

Poxviruses: including the causative agents of variola major (smallpox), variola minor (alastrim), vaccinia, and molluscum contagiosum in man; also a variety of animal pox diseases

Reoviruses: associated with some types of respiratory infection and diarrhoea in children

Retroviruses: includes the causative agent of AIDS (human immunodeficiency virus (HIV)) and the human T-cell leukaemia virus (HTLV) types

Rhabdoviruses: including the causative agent of rabies

Togaviruses: including the causative agents of yellow fever and rubella.

Other viruses including the causative agents of Marburg disease, hepatitis A and B, and some tumour viruses

FURTHER INFORMATION

Bloomfield SF, Baird R, Leak RE, Leech R, editors. Microbial quality assurance in pharmaceuticals, cosmetics and toiletries. Chichester: Ellis Horwood, 1988.

British Standards Institution. British Standard 5763. Methods for microbiological examination of food and animal feeding stuffs. Part 0. General laboratory practices. London: The Institution, 1986.

Central Public Health Laboratory. Catalogues of the National Collection of type cultures and pathogenic fungi. London: The Laboratory, 1989.

Collee JG, Duguid JP, Fraser AG, Marmion BP, editors. Mackie and McCartney practical medical microbiology. 13th ed. London: Churchill Livingstone, 1989.

Collins CH, Lyne PM, Grange JM. Microbiological methods. 6th ed. London: Butterworths, 1989.

Denyer S, Baird R, editors. Guide to microbiological control in pharmaceutics. Chichester: Ellis Horwood, 1990.

Duerden BI, Draser BS, editors. Anaerobes in human disease. London: Edward Arnold, 1991.

Greenwood D, Slack RCB, Peutherer JF, editors. Medical microbiology. A guide to microbial infection. 14th ed. London: Churchill Livingstone, 1992.

HMSO Categorisation of pathogens according to hazard and categories of containment. 2nd ed. London: HMSO, 1990.

Hugo WB, Russell AD, editors. Pharmaceutical microbiology. 5th ed. London: Blackwell, 1992.

Krieg NR, Holt JG, editors. Bergey's manual of systematic bacteriology; vol 1. London: Williams and Wilkins, 1984.

Lederberg J, editor. Encyclopedia of microbiology; vol 2. San Diego: Academic Press Inc, 1992.

Lillie RD, editor. Conn's biological stains. 9th ed. Baltimore: Williams and Wilkins, 1977. Reprinted by Sigma Chemical Company, 1990.

Onions AHS, Allsop D, Eggins HOW, editors. Smiths introduction to industrial mycology. 7th ed. London: Edward Arnold, 1981.

Raven PH, Evert RF, Eichhorn SE. Biology of plants. 5th ed. New York: Worth, 1992:208-43.

Smith JE, Moss MO. Mycotoxins, formation, analysis and significance. Chichester: John Wiley & Sons, 1985.

Sneath PHA, Mair NS, Sharpe ME, Holt JG, editors. Bergey's manual of systematic bacteriology; vol 2. London: Williams and Wilkins, 1986.

The National Collections of Industrial and Marine Bacteria Ltd. Catalogue of Strains. Aberdeen: The National Collection, 1990.

Control of Microbial Contamination and the Preservation of Medicines

From a microbiological viewpoint, only two types of medicinal product exist: those that are sterile and contain no viable micro-organisms and those that are non-sterile and contain viable micro-organisms. The latter category represents the majority of pharmaceutical formulations.

Although **non-sterile products** contain micro-organisms, they should not produce injurious effects or degrade because of this contamination. **Sterile products** that are for single use should not present a microbiological problem to the consumer; however certain multi-use sterile preparations (for example, eye drops) have the potential to become contaminated in use and can cause problems. Consequently, non-sterile and multi-use sterile products contain preservatives that are designed to kill or limit the growth of any micro-organism that may gain entry. There must, however, be a balance between the presence of micro-organisms and the possible toxicity of the preservative. The choice of preservative for any one particular product is an important and complex feature in formulation and product performance. Linked to this is the need to manufacture non-sterile products in a reproducible manner with an acceptably low level of microbial contamination.

EFFECTS OF MICROBIAL CONTAMINATION

The presence of micro-organisms leads to two possible problems: one is spoilage and the other is transmission of disease to the user. **Spoilage** renders a product unfit for its intended use and occurs when the contaminating micro-organism uses the product as a growth medium. Viable cells excrete enzymes into their environment to break down complex macromolecules into easily assimilated nutrients: for example, starch is broken down to sugars by amylase (present in many fungi and bacteria). The excipients, and sometimes the drug, may be destroyed and consequently the formulation breaks down. This, together with the presence of large numbers of micro-organisms, produces visible, olfactory, taste or tactile changes in the pro-

duct, which should alert the consumer to the need to discard it.

The micro-organisms present in a pharmaceutical preparation may also induce **disease** in the consumer without necessarily producing spoilage of the product.[1] There are two possible mechanisms: either infection, if the organism is pathogenic; or through toxins excreted into the product. The risk of micro-organisms producing an **infection** is difficult to assess and depends upon the species, dose administered (number of viable cells), route of administration, and susceptibility of the host. For example, it has been reported that a dose of around 10^6 cells of *Salmonella anatum* or *S. meleagridis* produces symptoms in healthy volunteers,[2] but only 50 cells of *S. napoli* are required to produce an effect.[3] There are many examples of pathogenic micro-organisms contaminating medicinal products and inducing disease (see Table 1).

Table 1
Examples of reported contamination of pharmaceutical products

Year	Product	Contaminant
1943	Fluorescein eye drops	*Pseudomonas aeruginosa*
1966	Thyroid tablets	*Salmonella muenchen*
1970	Chlorhexidine-cetrimide solution	*Pseudomonas cepacia*
1981	Surgical dressing	*Clostridium* species
1986	Mouthwashes	Coliforms

Microbial metabolites excreted into a pharmaceutical preparation may produce toxicity and will remain in the product even after the micro-organisms have died. In parenteral products, the hazards of contaminating pyrogens (Gram-negative lipopolysaccharides) are well documented and techniques are available to monitor and avoid this problem. There is evidence that the contamination of foodstuffs with microbial toxins constitutes a health hazard;[4] it is possible that a similar risk exists with non-sterile pharmaceutical products, although no examples have been reported.

In addition to the risk to health, spoilage and disease transmission represent a financial loss to the consumer and producer, through the cost of replacement, lost sales, or litigation.

ASSESSMENT OF MICROBIAL CONTAMINATION

Sterile products must contain no viable micro-organisms, as demonstrated either by a sterility test or by validation of the sterilisation process (see Sterilisation chapter). For non-sterile products, two features of contamination are recognised: the total number and the types of micro-organism present. In the latter case, pathogenic or potentially pathogenic micro-organisms should be absent. The organisms *Salmonella* species, *Escherichia coli*, *Pseudomonas* species, and *Staphylococcus aureus* are recognised pathogens, opportunist pathogens, or indicator organisms whose presence suggests other pathogenic contaminants. The *British Pharmacopoeia* (*BP*) and the *United States Pharmacopeia* (*USP*) include tests for the absence of certain organisms in specified raw materials (see Table 2). Additionally, the *European Pharmacopoeia* and the *United States Pharmacopeia* include a test for the **total viable count** (colony forming units, cfu, per gram or millilitre), irrespective of species, in selected raw materials. The risk to the consumer is directly related to the number of organisms in the product, and the total viable count is a measure of the overall cleanliness of the material. The *United States Pharmacopeia* and other published guidelines employ similar criteria for the microbial contamination of finished products (see Table 3).

The guidelines for microbial contamination are based on the potential risk to the user and historical data indicating that certain raw materials or products are prone to contamination. Unfortunately, the requirements of the various pharmacopoeias differ (see Table 2), and there is no single standard applicable to either raw materials or finished products. Additional 'in-house' or other published limits are normally applied by manufacturers (see Table 3) to supplement official guidelines. For example, topical preparations are tested for the absence of *Clostridium* species since these organisms usually infect by the topical route. The absence of other organisms must also be determined, depending upon the route of administration of the product.[5] The limits applied 'in house' are usually a compilation of official criteria, allowing the product to comply with as many specifications as possible. To meet these limits requires a combination of quality control, good manufacturing practice, formulation design, raw material selection, and package design.

SOURCES OF MICROBIAL CONTAMINATION

The microbiological fauna of a product is derived from all its constituent materials, the processing equipment, and the environments with which it comes into contact during its manufacture, packaging, and storage. This provides scope for the introduction into a product of a wide range of micro-organisms at differing levels. The individual sources vary in importance but the primary emphasis during formulation and manufacture should be to reduce the overall contamination. This may be achieved by examining each raw material and processing stage individually for its contribution to contamination. This process is taken to extremes in the manufacture of sterile products. For non-sterile products, a balance must be struck between the costs of reducing contamination and the possible risks to the product and consumer. Some of the major sources of contamination and the types of organisms that may be introduced are discussed below.

Water

Water is a ubiquitous material and a pharmaceutical product will either contain water, utilise water during processing, or come into contact with surfaces cleaned using aqueous solutions. Since micro-organisms are essentially aquatic, water is the ideal vehicle for supporting and transferring contamination. Gram-negative rods can grow rapidly in water to 10^5 to 10^6 cfu/mL under ambient conditions and this contamination level will not be visible to the naked eye. Different standards for the microbiological quality of water may be employed during manufacture depending on the extent of control required. Three types of water are generally utilised in the pharmaceutical industry: these are potable water, purified water, and water for injections[6] (see also the Oral Liquids chapter).

Potable or drinking water must pass tests for freedom from contamination with faecal coliforms, and is adequate for some products, but has the disadvantage that its chemical purity may vary with time and location. Normally, therefore, it is only used as a feed stock for the production of other grades of water.

Purified water is water obtained by distillation, ion-exchange, reverse osmosis, or other suitable process; it contains no added substances. This grade of water is normally used for the manufacture of tablets, syrups, suspensions, and other non-sterile products, and for the cleaning of equipment.

Table 2

Pharmacopoeial limits for microbial contamination of selected raw materials; for complete specifications, consult individual pharmacopoeial monographs

| Raw material | British and European Pharmacopoeias | | United States Pharmacopeia | |
	Absence of*	Total viable count[†] (cfu/g or cfu/mL)	Absence of	Total viable count (cfu/g or cfu/mL)
Acacia	*Escherichia coli* in 1 g	$< 10^4$		
Aluminium hydroxide	*Escherichia coli* in 1 g[‡]	$< 10^3$	*Salmonella* species in 10 g	
Prepared digitalis	*Escherichia coli* in 1 g, *Salmonella* species in 10 g		*Salmonella* species in 10 g	
Gelatin	*Escherichia coli* in 1 g, *Salmonella* species in 10 g	$< 10^3$	*Escherichia coli* in 10 g, *Salmonella* species in 10 g	$< 10^3$
Starches	*Escherichia coli* in 1 g	$< 10^3$ bacteria, $< 10^2$ fungi	*Escherichia coli* in 10 g, *Salmonella* species in 10 g	
Tragacanth	*Escherichia coli* in 1 g, *Salmonella* species in 10 g	$< 10^4$	*Escherichia coli* in 10 g, *Salmonella* species in 10 g	

*British Pharmacopoeia requirement.
[†]Applicable to the *European Pharmacopoeia* only.
[‡]Freedom from Gram-negative bacteria in 1 g(see monograph for full details).

Table 3

Limits for microbial contamination of pharmaceutical products (compiled from several sources)

	Total viable count (cfu/g or cfu/mL)	Objectionable micro-organisms
Sterile products*	0	All micro-organisms and pyrogens
Non-sterile products		
Oral preparations	$< 10^3$ to 10^4 bacteria, $< 10^2$ fungi	All enteric pathogens (for example, *Salmonella* species), *E. coli, Enterobacter* species, *Citrobacter* species, *Clostridium* species, *Pseudomonas* species, pathogenic yeasts (for example, *Candida albicans*), and mycotoxin-producing fungi
Oral preparations *USP*[†]	$< 10^2$	*E. coli* and *Salmonella* species
Topical preparations	$< 10^2$ bacteria, $< 10^2$ fungi	*Ps. aeruginosa, Ps. putida, Ps. multivorans, Clostridium perfringens, Cl. tetani, Cl. novyi, Staphylococcus aureus, Serratia marcescens, Ser. liquifacens,* and *Klebsiella* species
Topical preparations *USP*[†]	$< 10^2$	*Staph. aureus* and *Ps. aeruginosa*

*Consult the requirements of the sterility test for full details.
[†]Consult individual product monographs for complete information.

The microbiological quality of purified water varies with the production method. Deionisation is the commonest treatment but has the highest potential for microbiological contamination; water-softening units and filters in the system can become heavily contaminated with micro-organisms which will be released into the water. Species of *Alcaligenes, Acinetobacter,* and *Pseudomonas* are the main contaminants but Gram-positive rods and cocci may also be present. Ion-exchange resins are treated with strong acids and alkalis during regeneration, which destroys any contamination present in the resin bed.

Distilled and reverse-osmosis water are sterile immediately after production, the former because of the boiling and entrainment requirements, and the latter because it is forced through a membrane with a pore size equivalent to a molecular weight of 200 to 300. In practice, these two production methods are too expensive for the manufacture of non-sterile products unless specialised requirements dictate.

After production, purified water is usually treated either by exposure to ultraviolet light or by filtration through a bacteria-proof membrane to ensure a low level of microbial contamination. To minimise microbial adhesion to pipework and subsequent sessile growth of a biofilm, the distribution system must re-circulate the water at speeds in excess of 1 to 2 m/s. Precautions must be taken to avoid dead-legs in the system and air vents should be protected with suitable filters to prevent microbial ingress. In all cases, microbiological quality will depend heavily upon the design of the water treatment and distribution system, its operation, its maintenance, and the control procedures applied. **Water for injections** may be produced by distillation or reverse osmosis followed by aseptic storage and handling, which is achieved by maintaining a temperature of around 80°. Under these conditions any vegetative organisms that may be introduced will be rapidly killed and sterility maintained. Pharmacopoeial limits are specified for microbial and pyrogenic (endotoxin) contamination. Water for injections is essential for sterile products, but is too expensive for the manufacture of non-sterile pharmaceuticals unless special conditions necessitate its use. Topical steroid creams, for example, may be manufactured using water of high microbial quality as a precaution against contamination.

Raw Materials

The range of raw materials used in the manufacture of medicinal products is extremely large. There are four considerations that are important in evaluating the risk of microbial contamination from a particular material:

- is the material of natural origin?
- is it of synthetic origin?
- is it processed during manufacture by methods likely to increase or decrease the number of micro-organisms present?
- will it support the growth of micro-organisms?

Natural raw materials such as plant or animal extracts (for example, belladonna or thyroid, respectively) or minerals (for example, talc) are normally heavily contaminated with micro-organisms, with the species present reflecting the source of the material. Powdered plant material may contain up to 10^4 cfu/g of fungi and 10^5 cfu/g of bacteria: the fungi would include species of *Aspergillus*, *Penicillium*, *Mucor*, *Cladosporium*, and *Rhizopus*; the bacteria would be mainly spore-forming Gram-positive *Bacillus* species, with micrococci and staphylococci occasionally present. The majority of natural materials are reported to be contaminated with the Enterobacteriaceae, especially if no processing has been applied. Natural materials, because of their complex nature, are also subject to microbial colonisation if not stored properly. These ingredients must be considered a potential source of contamination and should be subjected to critical microbiological examination before inclusion.

Semi-synthetic and **synthetic materials** are normally manufactured by processes that are injurious to micro-organisms, such as heating under pressure or extremes of pH. Their microbiological content is therefore low, and derived from the environment in which they are handled and stored after production. For example, paracetamol-povidone mixtures have been reported, on average, to contain less than 10 cfu/g. Exceptions can arise if the material has been treated with water of poor microbiological quality after processing. Synthetic and semi-synthetic materials generally have a low potential for microbial colonisation but growth may occur in certain circumstances, if storage conditions are inadequate.

All unsterilised raw materials will be contaminated to some extent and the manufacturer should examine them microbiologically before use. The extent and frequency of testing will depend on the material's quality, the risk to the consumer, and the experience of the manufacturer with the supplier and raw material. Any material that is stored or handled improperly can easily become contaminated and provide a suitable growth medium for micro-organisms, thus rendering any previous testing invalid.

Reduction or Elimination of Contamination in Raw Materials

Various techniques are available for reducing or eliminating unacceptably high levels of contamination in raw materials. The methods available are based on sterilisation processes, but the conditions normally employed are not as severe (see Sterilisation chapter for more information). The particular process and extent of application will depend on the raw material and the perceived risk from the contamination to the product and consumer.

Gamma-irradiation. Gamma radiation will effectively kill both spores and vegetative micro-organisms. It has a high penetration capacity, can be used to treat a variety of dry materials and will kill organisms both on the surface and within the material. The reduction in total viable count is proportional to the dose and may be titrated to achieve a desired reduction in contamination. A dose of 25 kGy is recommended for sterilisation but lower values of 5 to 10 kGy may be used for decontamination. Depending on the strength of the source employed (Cobalt-60 or Caesium-137) this can take up to twenty hours, in either a continuous or a batch operation.

Since gamma-irradiation is capable of chemically damaging materials or products, validation is required to ensure no deleterious effects are produced by this treatment. Powdered beta-lactam antibiotics and neomycin, for example, are stable to gamma-irradiation: benzylpenicillin degrades by 0.6%/10 kGy.[7] Solutions of preservatives and polymeric materials are degraded by exposure to gamma radiation and in the latter case this will affect product viscosity.

An alternative to gamma-irradiation is the use of **electron beams**, generated by accelerating and focusing a beam of electrons to an energy of around 10 MeV. In contrast to gamma-irradiation the exposure time is very short and material is normally passed under the beam on a conveyor belt. The penetrative capacity of the beam is low and is influenced by the density of the material.

Ultraviolet Radiation. Ultraviolet (UV) light at a wavelength of 190 to 370 nm may be used to reduce contamination but it has a low energy, low penetrative power, and low killing efficiency. Normally, a mercury source is used, which emits light at 254 nm; this is close to the absorption maximum of DNA, the putative target for this method. Ultraviolet light will not kill spores and the sensitivity of viable bacteria varies markedly; most organisms possess enzymes capable of repairing UV-induced damage. It is only effective on surfaces directly exposed to the light, and organisms can be protected by dirt or remain unaffected in the core of the material. Ultraviolet radiation is only used, therefore, for the treatment of air or water; in the latter instance, the light can penetrate to a depth of 2 cm and water should be re-circulated around the source to ensure even exposure.

Ethylene Oxide. Ethylene oxide is a reactive chemical that alkylates essential macromolecules in the micro-organism, thus reducing metabolic capacity and ultimately causing death. It is equally active against both spores and vegetative cells but requires an increased temperature and humidity to be fully effective. It is used in the form of a gas, and penetration into all parts of the load must be ensured to achieve killing throughout the material. Its antimicrobial activity is dependent on the inter-related parameters of ethylene oxide concentration, temperature, relative humidity, exposure time, and material to be treated. Typical conditions require a temperature of 30° to 65°, a humidity of 30% to 90%, and a gas concentration of 250 mg/L to 1500 mg/L, with treatment times up to 24 hours. Ethylene oxide may also react with the material, and measures must be taken to ensure that no deleterious effects are produced. For example, neomycin sulphate is chemically and visibly changed after exposure to ethylene oxide.[8] Additionally, ethylene oxide is toxic to humans; tests must be performed to ensure that no residues or toxic breakdown products such as ethylene chlorohydrin remain after treatment. Ethylene oxide treatment is normally used for crude drugs and powders and is not applicable to solutions of materials.

Other Methods. If the material is thermostable, sterilisation methods such as autoclaving or dry heat may be employed; if it is liquid, filtration may be used. Simple storage of the material under conditions that are injurious or do not allow the multiplication of micro-organisms will gradually reduce the contamination level. A dry atmosphere with an elevated temperature will reduce the total viable count; most human pathogens, for example, are killed by temperatures of around 60°. This will reduce the number of vegetative organisms but is unlikely to affect any bacterial or mould spores that may be present; these are mainly a problem because of their potential for spoilage. When raw materials carry a risk of contamination and they are to be used in situations that favour infection, the only safe method is to sterilise the material. To reduce contamination problems, materials should be obtained from a reputable supplier who is audited and aware of the microbiological requirements for the material.

Personnel

Modern processing equipment is generally automated but human intervention is normally required during the manufacturing process. Operators represent a significant risk of contamination since humans possess a microbiological fauna on the skin and in body secretions. Around 10^4 skin squames per minute are shed continually, and a high proportion of these will be contaminated with non-pathogenic micrococci, diphtheroids, staphylococci, and occasionally *Staphylococcus aureus*. Transient skin contamination with Enterobacteriaceae may occur if poor hygiene practices are employed. These micro-organisms may enter the product by direct contact, or via skin squames or body secretions. Personnel suffering from infectious or other medical conditions that would increase the risk of contamination should be excluded from production areas. Operator clothing should also be considered as a possible source of contamination and adequate clean protective clothing should be supplied by the manufacturer.

One means of limiting personnel contamination that might be overlooked is training: operators should be aware of the risk they present to the product and how to reduce this by following correct procedures, for example, by wearing gloves or hair-covers. For contamination to spread, a non-contaminated and a contaminated material must come into contact, a process usually aided by human intervention. Operator training and operating procedures should be aimed at the prevention of this situation, supported by continual vigilance and reinforcement by quality assurance staff.

Environment

A factory contains different locations that require varying environmental provisions, such as temperature, humidity control, or air extraction facilities. This can be extended to microbiological control and is taken to extremes in sterile production facilities where highly controlled environments are utilised (see Cleanrooms for Pharmaceutical Production chapter). Non-sterile medicinal products are normally produced under hygienic conditions in an environment that will contain micro-organisms derived from the personnel and outside sources; the level of contamination tolerated will depend on the operations and types of products handled in that area.

The plant layout should be designed to provide a unidirectional flow of materials within a construction that is easy to clean and maintain. A goods receiving area, for example, may be exposed to the outside, and airborne contamination will be present along with organisms derived from external packaging. This contamination will be mainly spore-forming bacteria or fungi such as species of *Bacillus*, *Penicillium*, and *Aspergillus*. In a dispensary area, external packaging (particularly wood and straw) should be removed, along with any extraneous dirt; disinfection may be required before the goods are transferred to production zones. Similar restrictions should be applied to personnel in the form of changing and clothing requirements for entry into manufacturing areas. Contamination in areas where dry products such as tablets are manufactured will probably be derived from the operator's skin, along with spores from the environment; this does not normally represent a significant risk to these formulations. Products containing water, such as creams and liquids, are at a greater risk of microbial contamination from the production environment. The greatest risk is from Gram-negative bacteria (especially pseudomonads), which will be present in wet locations and may be introduced by personnel, equipment, or cleaning fluids. Good manufacturing practices

and microbiological control are important in preventing this type of contamination.[9] Increased microbiological control may be necessary for some high-risk non-sterile products, even to the extent of utilising controlled environments such as Class J or K cleanrooms (see the Cleanrooms for Pharmaceutical Production chapter).

Equipment

The manufacturing equipment used should not add to the contamination; the ideal machine is smooth, crevice-free, accessible, and easily cleaned, drained, and dried. Modern processing equipment is, however, intricate and cleaning creates the potential for contamination by a variety of routes. The microbiological quality of the cleaning fluid should be considered, as contamination of this material will inevitably lead to equipment contamination. Inadequate cleaning may leave product residues in crevices, which may act as a growth medium and a reservoir of contamination for subsequent batches. Residues containing diluted products, and therefore diluted preservative systems, may foster the growth of preservative-resistant strains of micro-organisms. If the equipment (or production area) cannot be completely dried, and water remains, then the growth of Gram-negative bacteria must be expected. These problems can be minimised by the correct design of equipment and the utilisation of validated, documented cleaning procedures. Designs should eliminate long pipe runs, dead-legs, and U-bends where accumulation can occur. Certain types of equipment that utilise compressed air can be at risk of contamination from condensed water droplets containing Gram-negative organisms; this can be eliminated by an air filter. Other problems exist with equipment that consumes large volumes of air, such as fluid bed dryers, and the effect this will have on the airflow in the locale should be considered.

GROWTH OF MICRO-ORGANISMS IN MEDICINAL PRODUCTS

In order to grow, a micro-organism must be able to obtain from the product all the nutrients that it requires for the synthesis of cellular constituents and the generation of energy. Additionally, factors that would inhibit growth must be absent. It is difficult to predict when colonisation will occur but certain species of micro-organisms that are metabolically versatile (for example, pseudomonads) are frequently involved. Gram-negative organisms easily colonise aqueous infusion fluids to a level of 10^6 cfu/mL, while Gram-positive cocci either die or their numbers remain stationary.[10]

A wide range of products have been shown to suffer from degradative changes after microbial contamination. Growth does not have to occur throughout the entire product but can be limited to one or several foci of contamination. These locations may provide conditions that are suitable for growth but are different from the bulk of the material. Failure to sample these areas properly will lead to misleading estimates of the product's contamination and ability to support growth. Small pockets of water in oil-based products or condensates in syrups, for example, can allow microbial growth in these materials.

For all products it is probably safe to assume that colonisation will occur, given an appropriate micro-organism and the correct conditions. It should be noted that an organism does not need to proliferate in the product in order to transmit disease; it just needs to survive. Spores, for example, will not germinate until favourable growth conditions occur and may lie dormant in a product for prolonged periods.

PRINCIPLES OF PRESERVATION

Most pharmaceutical products contain a preservative system to prevent the survival and growth of micro-organisms. The preservative's function is to prevent product contamination and colonisation after production, and not to cover for poor manufacturing or control techniques. The antimicrobial activity required of a preservative depends on the type of product in which it will be used: sterile products must be capable of self-sterilisation, but microbial reduction or stasis would be sufficient in an oral liquid. The ideal properties of a preservative are listed in Table 4. An appreciation of these is crucial in choosing an agent for a formulation. It is recognised, however, that no single agent completely meets these requirements.

Two basic types of preservative system exist: chemical agents, of either natural or synthetic origin; and approaches based on altering the product's physical conditions to limit microbial growth. Combinations of these systems can be utilised to maximise product protection.

Physical Preservative Systems

Micro-organisms require certain physical conditions to survive; the deliberate adjustment of these to kill or suppress micro-organisms is one of the oldest known forms of preservation.

Table 4
Ideal properties of an antimicrobial preservative

Property	Comments
Broad spectrum of antimicrobial activity	The agent should be active against all basic groups of micro-organisms such as Gram-positive and Gram-negative bacteria, yeasts, and moulds
Rapid antimicrobial action	Rapid antimicrobial activity reduces the risk of adaptation and the development of resistance
Chemically stable and microbiologically effective under all pH conditions	The agent should be able to function effectively at product pH and should be chemically stable without loss of activity over the shelf-life
Compatible with excipients and packing materials	The agent's activity should not be reduced by interaction with the excipients or packaging
Physically undetectable	The agent should not alter the physical properties of the product, such as colour, taste, or viscosity
Safe to use	The agent should possess a toxicity profile acceptable to regulatory authorities and be safe to handle during manufacture and packaging, and in use
Cost effective	The cost of the agent should not constitute a large portion of the product's cost

Available Water

Most organisms require over 70% water to grow, so dry products (such as powders and tablets) are unlikely to suffer colonisation unless water is added. Products containing large amounts of water (for example, suspensions and mixtures) must be considered at risk from colonisation.

The amount of water that is available to an organism in a product is given by:

$$A_w = \frac{\text{Vapour pressure of product}}{\text{Vapour pressure of water}}$$

(at constant temperature).

This value is always less than one, owing to hydrogen bonding of the water in the product. Certain organisms will only survive and grow at specific A_w levels (see Table 5); if the A_w is lowered by adding solutes, microbial growth can be prevented. A product with an A_w value of 0.9 is unlikely to be affected by *Pseudomonas* species but could be colonised by other bacteria, or fungi and moulds. A variable level of preservation can therefore be achieved by simple manipulation of a product's A_w value. Syrup BP, for example, contains 66.7 % w/w of dissolved sucrose, and has an A_w value of 0.86, but can be colonised by osmophilic yeasts and moulds that can grow at A_w values as low as

Table 5
Limits of available water (A_w) at which microbial growth can occur

Micro-organism	A_w (lower limit for growth)
Pseudomonas species	0.96
Gram-negative rods	0.95
Staphylococcus aureus	0.90
Gram-positive bacteria	0.90
Moulds and yeasts	0.85
Osmotolerant yeasts	0.70
Aspergillus glaucus	0.61

0.6. Some other products (such as toothpaste) are preserved in a similar fashion, but the scope of this technique is limited by the large quantities of solute required to reduce A_w sufficiently.

pH Value

The majority of micro-organisms grow best at a pH of about 7 but survival is known at pH values from 3 to 11. Lowering or raising the product pH from neutrality provides a degree of preservation; however, the scope for pH variation in pharmaceutical products is limited by physiological acceptability and formulation stability. Values of pH below 5.5 can be utilised along with certain organic acids (for example, benzoic acid) to preserve products from bacterial colonisation, although these lower pH values favour the growth of moulds and fungi.

Temperature

The correct temperature is a prerequisite for microbial growth and the majority of contaminants in pharmaceutical products are mesophilic organisms that grow best at ambient temperatures (15° to 45°). A reduced storage temperature can therefore be used as a means of inhibiting growth, but has the disadvantage that the conditions are not integral to the product and depend upon the user or distributor. Pharmaceuticals are normally stored at a reduced temperature to improve chemical stability, and any antimicrobial effect is secondary.

Chemical Preservative Systems

The earliest applications of preservation employed natural substances such as essential oils or perfumes; these materials are, however, complicated mixtures and therefore difficult to control. Modern preservatives are normally synthetic, chemically defined entities. In pharmaceutical products, synthetic preservatives are used almost exclusively, owing to the demands of quality control. However, natural preservatives are being re-investigated, in view of consumer pressure to eliminate synthetic additives.

Natural Preservative Agents

Essential Oils. The antimicrobial properties of essential oils and perfumes can be ascribed to their chemical constituents, which are a blend of alcohols, aldehydes, esters, ketones, and terpenes. Many of these have been investigated or the constituents separated and tested individually. Sage oil, for example, is bactericidal and fungicidal; thyme oil, which has been used as an antimicrobial, contains 40% of phenolic compounds. A major restriction on the use of essential oils is the high concentrations required for activity, which impart unusual organoleptic properties to the product. The antimicrobial activity may be beneficial in perfumed cosmetic products where the olfactory properties are also desirable. Essential oils may possess other biological activities and are normally expensive, both features that mitigate against their use.

Enzymes and Proteins. The iron-binding proteins lactoferrin and ovotransferrin reduce free iron concentrations to around 10^{-18} M, which inhibits the growth of many organisms, with exceptions such as *Pseudomonas aeruginosa*.[11] Enzymes such as lysozyme act to hydrolyse β(1-4) glycosidic bonds between *N*-acetyl glucosamine and *N*-acetyl muramic acid in the bacterial cell wall. Lysozyme is active against a range of organisms but resistance has been demonstrated especially in Gram-negative bacteria. The peptide antibiotics Pep5 and nisin have also been examined but are only active against Gram-positive bacteria. These types of agent have been used primarily in the food industry and have not found common use in pharmaceuticals. Their protein nature precludes them from use in parenteral products.

Synthetic Preservatives

Synthetic preservatives constitute the biggest and most commonly used group in the preservation of pharmaceutical products. They are normally classified on the basis of their chemical structure, which provides only limited information on their activity and applicability. There is no common pathway by which they exert their effect, and for some agents it is difficult to ascertain the site of action. Also, the site of action and degree or extent of antimicrobial activity can be concentration-dependent. Some agents are bacteriostatic at low concentrations, whereas higher concentrations produce bactericidal effects. Within an individual chemical group several agents may be used as preservatives at low concentrations and as disinfectants or antiseptics at higher concentrations. The chemical classification is useful, however, as agents from within a group will behave similarly when exposed to equivalent conditions. Examples of the various groups are discussed below and further details of their properties and uses are given in Tables 6 to 8. Further details of some of these compounds can be found in the Disinfectants and Antiseptics chapter.

Acids and Salts. Weak carboxylic acids such as benzoic or sorbic acids possess useful antimicrobial activity. **Benzoic acid** has a pK_a of 4.2 and **sorbic acid** has a pK_a of 4.8, and only the acid form is antimicrobial; their activity is therefore greatest at acid pH values.[12] The use of these preservatives is restricted to products with a pH of less than 5. Benzoic acid is chemically stable but sorbic acid is sensitive to light and air, and may require the addition of an antoxidant, or refrigerated storage, to increase its stability.

Sulphites and **metabisulphites** are normally used as antoxidants, but they also possess antimicrobial activity that may be a useful adjunct in a formulation.[13] This activity is greatest at low pH values that promote the release of sulphur dioxide (which is antimicrobial).

Alcohols. Although many members of the alcohol series possess antimicrobial activity, only the arylalkyl and highly substituted aliphatic alcohols are used as preservatives. **Benzyl alcohol**[14] slowly oxidises to benzaldehyde and benzoic acid in the presence of air but is thermostable.

Table 6

Antimicrobial activity of selected preservatives and possible sites of action (1, highly active; 2, moderately active; 3, weakly active)

| Agent | Basic microbial classification and activity | | | | Possible sites of action |
| | Bacteria | | Moulds | Yeasts | |
	Gram-positive*	Gram-negative			
Acids and salts					
Benzoic acid	1	2[†]	3	3	cytoplasmic membrane permeability
Sorbic acid	2	2	2	1	cytoplasmic membrane permeability
Sulphites	3	3	2	2	enzyme/protein thiol and amino groups
Alcohols					
Benzyl alcohol	1	3	3	3	cytoplasmic membrane permeability
Bronopol	2	1	3	3	enzyme/protein thiol groups
Chlorbutol	1	1	3	2	cytoplasmic membrane permeability
Ethanol	1	1	2	2	cytoplasmic membrane permeability
Phenoxyethanol	2	1	3	3	cytoplasmic membrane permeability
Phenylethanol	2	1	3	3	cytoplasmic membrane permeability
Biguanides					
Chlorhexidine salts	1	1[†]	3	2	cytoplasmic membrane permeability, cytoplasmic coagulation
Hydroxybenzoates					
All members of the series and salts	1	3[†]	2	2	cytoplasmic membrane permeability, nucleic acid synthesis
Mercurials					
Phenylmercuric salt	1	1	2	2	cell wall, enzyme/protein thiol groups, cytoplasmic coagulation (high concentrations)
Thiomersal	1	2	3	2	cell wall, enzyme/protein thiol groups, cytoplasmic coagulation (high concentrations)
Phenols					
Chlorocresol	1	2	3	3	cell wall, cytoplasmic membrane permeability
Cresol	2	3	3	3	cell wall, cytoplasmic membrane permeability
Phenol	2	3	3	3	cell wall, cytoplasmic membrane permeability
Quaternary ammonium compounds					
Benzalkonium chloride	1	2[†]	3	2	cytoplasmic membrane permeability
Cetrimide	1	2[†]	3	2	cytoplasmic membrane permeability

*Activity against spores not considered.
[†]Poor activity against *Pseudomonas* species.

Table 7
Microbiological and physicochemical properties of selected antimicrobial preservatives

Agent	In-use concentration (%w/v)	Concentration exponent* (η)	Property Temperature coefficient (Q_{10})	Optimal pH range	Water solubility	Oil-water partition coefficient
Acids and salts						
Benzoic acid	0.1	3.5Y		2–5	1 in 350 (sodium salt 1 in 2)	3–6
Sorbic acid	0.2	3.1	2.3	≤ 6.5	1 in 700 (salts more soluble)	3.5
Sulphites	0.1	1.3, 1.6Y, 1.8M		≤ 4	1 in 2	
Alcohols						
Benzyl alcohol	1.0	6.6, 4Y, 2M	2.3–7.2	≤ 5	1 in 25	1.3
Bronopol	0.01–0.1	0.9	2.9	5–7	1 in 4	0.11
Chlorbutol	0.3–0.5	2		≤ 4	1 in 130	
Ethanol	20–70	4.5, 5.7Y, 3M	45		miscible	
Phenoxyethanol	1.0	9		broad	1 in 43	
Phenylethanol	0.25–0.5	5.6		≤ 7	1 in 50	
Biguanides						
Chlorhexidine salts	0.01–0.1	1.9	3–16	5–8	acetate 1 in 55 gluconate 1 in 5	0.04
Hydroxybenzoates						
All members of the series and salts	0.4–0.8 acid	2.5		3.0–9.5	methyl 1 in 500 ethyl 1 in 1300 propyl 1 in 2500 butyl 1 in 6500 benzyl 1 in 10 000	methyl 7.5 propyl 80 butyl 280
Mercurials						
Phenylmercuric salts	0.001–0.002	1		6–8	acetate 1 in 600 nitrate 1 in 1500	< 1
Thiomersal	0.002–0.01	1		7–8	1 in 1	
Phenols						
Chlorocresol	0.1	8.3	3–5	≤ 8.5	1 in 260	117–190
Cresol	0.3	8	3–5	≤ 9	1 in 50	
Phenol	0.25–0.5	5.8, 4Y, 4.3M	5	≤ 9	1 in 15	
Quaternary ammonium compounds						
Benzalkonium chloride	0.01–0.25	3.5, 1.8Y, 9M	2.9–5.8	4–10	very soluble	< 1
Cetrimide	0.01–0.1	1		4-10	1 in 2	< 1

*Value for bacteria unless stated (Y, yeasts; M, moulds).

Phenoxyethanol and **phenylethanol** are more active against Gram-negative than Gram-positive bacteria; phenoxyethanol is highly active against *Pseudomonas aeruginosa*. They are normally used in combination with other preservatives (for example, phenoxyethanol with hydroxybenzoates and phenylethanol with benzalkonium chloride) and both are thermostable but phenylethanol is susceptible to oxidation.

Chlorbutol is a highly substituted aliphatic alcohol that is unstable in alkaline solutions but stable in acid conditions at ambient temperatures, although it degrades rapidly on heating. The concentration of chlorbutol used as a preservative is close to its saturation solubility at low temperatures; crystallisation may therefore be a problem.

Bronopol is active against *Pseudomonas aeruginosa* and is widely used in both pharmaceutical and cosmetic products. It is stable in aqueous solutions at acid pH values but degrades rapidly under alkaline conditions (with the generation of formaldehyde), especially at elevated temperatures.

Ethanol, which could be considered a natural agent, is not normally used as a preservative, because of the high concentrations required (at least 15% to 20% v/v).[13] However, if ethanol is present as an excipient in a formulation, it may provide a useful adjunct to antimicrobial activity.

Hydroxybenzoates. The esters of *p*-hydroxybenzoic acid (**hydroxybenzoates**, or **parabens**) and their salts are useful preservatives in pharmaceuticals and cosmetics with a wide spectrum of antimicrobial activity. There are several members of the series, with different alcohols esterified to the benzoic acid: methyl, ethyl, propyl, butyl, and benzyl derivatives

Table 8
Selected preservatives used in pharmaceutical formulations

Agent	Formulation type
Acids and salts	
Benzoic acid	oral, topical
Sorbic acid	oral, topical
Sulphites	parenteral
Alcohols	
Benzyl alcohol	parenteral, topical
Bronopol*	oral, topical
Chlorbutol	parenteral, ophthalmic
Ethanol	oral
Phenoxyethanol	topical
Phenylethanol	parenteral, ophthalmic
Biguanides	
Chlorhexidine salts	ophthalmic, topical
Hydroxybenzoates	
All members of the	oral, topical, parenteral[†],
series and salts	ophthalmic[†]
Mercurials	
Phenylmercuric salts	ophthalmic
Thiomersal	parenteral, ophthalmic
Phenols	
Chlorocresol	parenteral, topical
Cresol	parenteral, topical
Phenol	parenteral, topical
Quaternary ammonium compounds	
Benzalkonium chloride	parenteral, ophthalmic, topical
Cetrimide	ophthalmic, topical

*Some countries do not allow the use of bronopol in medicinal products.
[†] Use in these formulations is not ideal.

are available. Water solubility is related to the size of the ester group; the methyl derivative being the most soluble. The higher members of the group have saturation solubilities only slightly greater than the concentrations needed for preservative effect; the sodium salts of the esters have a higher solubility than the free acids. Unlike benzoic acid, the hydroxybenzoates retain their antimicrobial activity at raised pH values (pH 7 to 9). They are chemically stable in acid conditions and will withstand heating, but hydrolysis will occur as the pH increases; strongly alkaline solutions undergo rapid degradation at elevated temperatures. The higher esters exhibit the greatest antimicrobial activity but this is offset by a lower solubility. To achieve maximal activity, the hydroxybenzoates are normally used as mixtures of two or more esters to provide a higher total concentration in solution.

Mercurials. Organomercurial compounds have been utilised in pharmaceutical products for many years, but their use is declining, owing to concerns about their toxicity and effects on the environment. The phenylmercuric salts (**phenylmercuric acetate**, **nitrate**, and **borate**) and **thiomer-**

sal are the most commonly used members of this series. The antimicrobial activity of the organomercurials is not greatly affected by changes in pH. They are thermostable and will withstand autoclaving but are sensitive to light and exposure to air. The agents are incompatible with sulphides, thiol-containing compounds, halides, aluminium, and other metals. Because of the toxicity of mercury, they are not recommended in situations where prolonged administration is necessary.

Phenols. **Phenol** was the first antimicrobial agent, and is still in use along with phenolic derivatives such as cresol and chlorocresol.[15] **Cresol** is a mixture of isomers with the *meta* form (3-methylphenol) predominating; similarly, **chlorocresol** is mainly 4-chloro-3-methylphenol. The antimicrobial activity of the phenolic agents is pH-dependent and is greatest below pH 9. The compounds are thermostable and can be autoclaved or sterilised by dry heat but they are sensitive to light and air, and they interact with iron.

Quaternary Ammonium Compounds. Several chemical structures based around the quaternary ammonium ion linked to a long-chain hydrocarbon have found use as preservatives and disinfectants. The two most frequently used are benzalkonium chloride[16] and cetrimide. **Benzalkonium chloride** is a mixture of alkylbenzyldimethylammonium chlorides with a variable alkyl chain length ranging from C_8 to C_{18}, and with C_{12} and C_{14} as the principal chain lengths. Antimicrobial activity is most potent with the C_{14} member of the series. **Cetrimide** is tetradecyltrimethylammonium bromide with small amounts of the dodecyl and hexadecyl derivatives. All these agents have almost no activity against *Pseudomonas aeruginosa*; indeed, solid nutrient media containing cetrimide can be used to isolate and culture this organism. Both benzalkonium chloride and cetrimide are chemically stable in aqueous solutions and will withstand autoclaving, but are incompatible with heavy metals, alkalis, oxidants, soaps, and anionic surfactants.

Biguanides. The only agent in this series is **chlorhexidine** which is a symmetrical molecule with a hexamethylene chain linking two *p*-chlorophenyl-substituted biguanide groups. Chlorhexidine is normally used as either the diacetate, the digluconate, or the dihydrochloride salt. It is most active in the pH range 5 to 8 but has poor activity against *Pseudomonas aeruginosa*. It is generally stable in aqueous solutions but breaks down at raised temperatures to produce 4-chloroaniline, especially in alkaline conditions. The acetate and gluconate salts can be autoclaved at 115° for 30 minutes. Chlorhexidine is incompatible with borates, bicarbonates, chlorides, citrates, phosphates, sulphates, and anionic surfactants.

Other Agents. A diverse collection of agents have found use as preservatives, ranging from compounds such as hydroxymethylhydantoin (which acts by slowly releasing formaldehyde) to hexetidine, hexamidine, zinc pyrithione, and triclosan. The latter two agents are effective antimicrobials and are included in medicated shampoos as active ingredients.

REGULATORY REQUIREMENTS FOR PRESERVATIVE SYSTEMS

The regulatory authorities influence the choice of preservative systems through two mechanisms: firstly, the available agents are limited by statute, and secondly, minimum preservative and stability standards are required in various types of product. These requirements vary with time and published pharmacopoeial standards may not reflect the current situation.

The permitted agents are normally listed in national pharmacopoeias or other statutes but there is no international coherence and approved lists vary from country to country. Before formulation development, the current guidelines in proposed markets should be checked to determine which preservatives are permitted. The route of administration and frequency of the product's use should be considered, as well as the toxicity profile of the preservative. The current approach in the United Kingdom is to remove artificial preservatives from medicines as far as possible to reduce the potential for adverse reactions.

If an established preservative system is utilised, testing will only have to demonstrate that its activity is as expected and that nothing unanticipated occurs with this formulation. Novel systems or agents will require increased testing; the extreme is represented by a new chemical entity, which will need a complete safety and efficacy study.

Challenge Testing

Performance is measured by the product's antimicrobial activity and cannot be predicted from a simple chemical concentration. Antimicrobial activity is measured by a challenge test, based on the ability of the preservative system to kill or prevent the proliferation of specified micro-organisms that are deliberately introduced into the product

(see Table 9). Sterile products have the strictest requirements in terms of microbial kill and continued suppression of growth; the demands are not so severe for non-sterile products. The test is designed to demonstrate the survival and growth of micro-organisms in a product if it is inadequately preserved. The product must be tested in its final container, if possible, and is required to meet the test standards at all times during its proposed shelf-life. Failure of preservation during storage is considered as significant as degradation of the active ingredient.

Test Organisms

The test organisms specified by the pharmacopoeias represent the major microbiological groups: that is, Gram-positive and Gram-negative bacteria, yeasts, and moulds. The organisms are typical of those that the product might encounter in raw materials, and from the environment during manufacture and in use. *Pseudomonas aeruginosa* is chosen for the aforementioned reasons and because it is recognised to represent a profound challenge to preservation. Manufacturers may challenge the product with other organisms found in the production environment or raw materials. Additional challenge organisms may be those that would use the product as a route of infection or those that are liable to colonise the product because of its formulation. A product with a low A_w value, for example, may be challenged with an osmophilic yeast (*Zygosaccharomyces rouxii*), which would selectively colonise this type of product. Supplementary challenge testing can be carried to extremes, and a balance must be struck between possible risk to the patient and excessive testing requirements.

The product is tested individually against each organism by introducing a challenge of 10^5 to 10^6 cfu per mL or per gram of product. The inoculated product is then stored at a defined temperature (20° to 25°) and sampled using a plate-counting technique for the presence of viable micro-organisms. The samples are taken at defined time intervals up to a period of 28 days and activity is assessed by the reduction in viable count with respect to a control sample. As yet there is no single international specification and the requirements of the national pharmacopoeias differ (see Table 9). It has also been recognised that the requirements of pharmacopoeial challenge tests may be excessive in relation to possible levels of contamination; for some categories of product, there has been a change in the performance levels required.

Table 9

Pharmacopoeial limits for preservative challenge testing

(NR, no recovery; NI, no increase in viable count thereafter; h, hours; d, days). The starting concentration of micro-organisms is 10^6 cfu/g or mL for the *BP* test and 10^5 to 10^6 cfu/g or mL for the *USP*. The *USP* makes no recommendations for the preservative challenge testing of topical or oral products.

Product	Test organism		Log reduction in viable count at time point					
			6 h	24 h	48 h	7 d	14 d	28 d
British Pharmacopoeia								
Parenteral and ophthalmic	Pseudomonas aeruginosa and Staphylococcus aureus	A*	2	3	—	—	—	NR
		B*	—	1	—	3	—	NI
	Candida albicans and Aspergillus niger	A	—	—	—	2	—	NI
		B	—	—	—	—	1	NI
Topical	Pseudomonas aeruginosa and Staphylococcus aureus		—	—	3	NR	NR	NR
Oral liquids	Candida albicans and Aspergillus niger		—	—	—	—	2	NI
	Pseudomonas aeruginosa, Staphylococcus aureus, and Escherichia coli		—	—	—	—	3	NI
	Candida albicans, Aspergillus niger, and Zygosaccharomyces rouxii†		—	—	—	—	1	NI
Ear	Pseudomonas aeruginosa and Staphylococcus aureus		2	3	—	—	—	NR
	Candida albicans and Aspergillus niger		—	—	—	2	—	NI
United States Pharmacopeia								
Parenteral and ophthalmic	Pseudomonas aeruginosa, Staphylococcus aureus and Escherichia coli		—	—	—	—	3	NI
	Candida albicans and Aspergillus niger		—	—	—	—	NI	NI

*The A criteria express the recommended efficacy to be achieved. In justified cases where the A criteria cannot be attained, for example, for reasons of increased risk of adverse reactions, the B criteria must be satisfied.

†*Zygosaccharomyces rouxii* is included for oral preparations containing a high concentration of sugar.

Validation

Validation studies must be conducted to ensure that the activity measured in a challenge test is due to the preservative system and not the test method. Two practical features are important in this respect, sampling the micro-organism from the product and removing the residual preservative activity of the sample. It is easy to recover micro-organisms from liquid products but biphasic systems (such as creams) can present difficulties, since solubilisation may be necessary for sampling. The technique chosen should not affect the microbial count and should allow representative samples to be taken. The sample of product will contain preservative and this must be neutralised to allow unhindered microbial growth. Three techniques are available: the recommended method is filtration, but dilution, chemical neutralisation, or both, may be employed. Filtering the sample through a membrane with a 0.45 micrometre pore size will retain the micro-organisms and allow the physical removal of preservative by washing. It also ensures that sampling is more efficient as the complete sample is passed through the filter rather than an aliquot added to a growth medium. This increases the probability of detecting small numbers of micro-organisms, although it does create problems when semi-solid and solid preparations are sampled. After filtration, the membrane is placed on a solid growth medium to determine a viable count. An alternative method of removing residual antimicrobial activity is to add specific chemical inactivating agents to the diluent and media; a third technique is to use large dilutions to reduce the concentration of preservative. All challenge testing must be carried out under aseptic conditions to prevent ingress of extraneous micro-organisms.

D-values

Other methods of preservative evaluation have been proposed on the basis of the logarithmic or linear killing of micro-organisms by a chemical under certain conditions. This allows the determination of a decimal reduction value (D-value) for the combination of preservative and micro-organism at their respective concentrations in that product. The technique is comparable to the use of D-values in heat or radiation sterilisation (see Sterilisation chapter), and a D-value will have to be determined for each micro-organism and preservative system. To calculate a value requires significant numbers of micro-organisms in order to measure cell death over at least one log cycle. The D-value can then be applied to calculate the time required to reduce microbial contamination to a desired level. However, in many cases, microbial death is not logarithmic or linear, owing to the chemical acting on multiple target sites and the re-growth or selection of resistant organisms. Also the action of several preservatives is not logarithmic over the 28-day period required by pharmacopoeial tests. D-value testing is extensively used in the formulation of cosmetics but is not included in the challenge tests described in national pharmacopoeias.

To conduct a pharmacopoeial challenge test on a product requires the use of at least four organisms and up to five samples over a 28-day period, that is 20 samples in all. Because of the problems involved in microbial counting, the test will be performed at least in duplicate. The development of a preservative system may involve testing different agents at varying concentrations in a product, and can therefore be time consuming and costly. To alleviate this problem the D-value method can be employed to screen putative preservative systems over shorter time periods (24 hours) with fewer samples. From the calculated D-values, the most appropriate preservative system for use in that particular product can be ascertained and then subjected to a full pharmacopoeial test.

SELECTION OF AN ANTIMICROBIAL PRESERVATIVE SYSTEM

The selection of a preservative system should be based on the ideal characteristics listed in Table 4, and should permit the product to pass the appropriate pharmacopoeial challenge test. The preservative system must also be acceptable in terms of its toxicity profile for the intended route of administration (see Table 8). Formulations for parenteral, oral, or topical use have different challenge test and toxicity requirements. Additional restrictions are imposed by the physical and chemical nature of the formulation; the preservative system required for a solution will be very different from that for an emulsion, irrespective of the route of administration. The choice of preservative must be a compromise between the microbiological activity of the agent and its physicochemical compatibility with the formulation.

Microbiological Considerations

The antimicrobial activity of a preservative is dependent upon a chemical reaction between the agent and receptor molecule(s) in or on the organism. The chemical reaction is affected by concentration and temperature; irrespective of the organism

used, these two parameters are important in controlling the activity of any antimicrobial chemical.

Effect of Concentration

The simplest measure of antimicrobial activity is the minimum inhibitory concentration (MIC) or lowest concentration required to inhibit the growth of a micro-organism. For a single agent, this varies with the test organism, and there is a large variation between agents for the same organism. The MIC only provides information about the bacteriostatic properties of a preservative, but challenge tests generally require bactericidal activity to be demonstrated (see Table 9). Bactericidal effects occur at concentrations higher than the MIC and the relationship of concentration to bactericidal efficacy is measured by the concentration exponent (η). This is described by the following equation:

$$C_1{}^{\eta}t_1 = C_2{}^{\eta}t_2$$

where, C_1 and C_2 represent two concentrations of the agent, and t_1 and t_2 the times required at these concentrations to provide the same degree of microbial killing. The equation is linear when η is equal to 1 but for most agents, it follows an exponential relationship as η is greater than 1 (see Table 7). If η has a value of 1, halving the concentration halves the antimicrobial activity and doubles the time required to achieve the same degree of cell death. If η is greater than 1, halving the concentration reduces the activity to $(\frac{1}{2})^{\eta}$ and provides a 2^{η} increase in the time required for microbial killing. For example, with phenol ($\eta = 6$) halving the concentration produces a reduction in activity to 1/64 and a 64-fold increase in the time required to produce the same degree of cell death. Preservatives with high η values are therefore sensitive to even small reductions in concentration and are easily diluted to the point at which antimicrobial efficacy is lost. Small reductions in concentration can occur through chemical degradation or physical loss; this feature must be taken into account when deciding the concentration to be used, and for high η value agents, it necessitates careful consideration.

Effect of Temperature

The basic antimicrobial activity of chemicals is controlled by the temperature at which the organism and agent are incubated. The effect of increasing temperature is to increase antimicrobial activity, which is measured by the temperature coefficient (Q_{10}), normally reported for a 10°

change in temperature. This is described by the following equation:

$$Q_{10} = \frac{t_T}{t_{(T+10°)}}$$

where, t_T and $t_{(T+10°)}$ represent the times required to produce the same degree of microbial killing at two temperatures, T and T + 10°. Different preservatives have varying Q_{10} values (see Table 7), which depend on the temperature of measurement and the micro-organism used. This value is important in extrapolating results from experiments conducted at room temperature to the recommended storage temperature, and should always be considered for pharmaceutical products that may be refrigerated.

Preservative Combinations

An important feature of an antimicrobial agent is its intrinsic activity and its ability to kill a wide range of micro-organisms. Most agents have useful activity against selected groups of organisms but do not completely cover the spectrum required by challenge tests (see Table 6). In order to broaden the activity spectrum provided by a single agent, combinations may be used. The use of benzalkonium chloride with chlorhexidine gluconate is an example of this approach. The choice of combination must be carefully considered to ensure that no gaps exist in the spectrum of activity and that antagonistic effects do not occur. This situation has led to the widespread use of combinations of agents with complementary activities, although not necessarily synergistic effects (see Table 10). True synergistic interactions between preservatives are difficult to prove but are widely claimed in the literature,[17] for example, cresol and phenylmercuric salts. Also an agent with a weak or negligible antimicrobial activity may potentiate the effects of another. The activity of several preservatives, especially against *Pseudomonas aeruginosa*, is increased by edetic acid. These agents include: benzalkonium chloride, bronopol, cetrimide, chlorhexidine, hydroxybenzoates, phenol, phenylethanol, and sorbic acid. Edetic acid is a chelator of divalent cations and helps disrupt the lipopolysaccharide membrane of micro-organisms by removing essential cross-linking magnesium ions; this sensitises the cell to the action of the other agent. Both types of effect can be produced by other excipients (such as alcohols or reducing agents) and should be used to advantage in product formulation. Combination systems will only perform optimally when the concentrations of both agents lie within defined limits. It is necessary, therefore, to examine the physicochemical properties of these systems to ensure that the agents remain stable and effective over the shelf-life of the product.

Microbial Resistance

The activity of an agent will depend upon it reaching its target site and the ability of the micro-organism to mitigate against its effect. Bacteria possess a cell envelope that functions as a homoeostatic barrier between the organism and its environment. The outer layer is the capsule or extracellular slime layer, composed of cross-linked carbohydrate, which allows cells to aggregate as a biofilm. Preservatives must diffuse through the biofilm before they can reach the outer membranes of the cell. The contribution of biofilm formation to resistance is well documented for production equipment but has not been studied in products. Gram-negative organisms have an extra external lipopolysaccharide membrane which provides intrinsic resistance to hydrophilic preservatives by limiting their entry to the cell. The MIC of chlorhexidine, for example, is 0.3 microgram/mL against *Staphylococcus aureus* but 1.2 micrograms/mL against *Escherichia coli*. Owing to these cytological differences, the organisms providing the greatest resistance problems to preservatives are normally Gram-negative.[18] Micro-organisms are able to alter their outer membrane permeability to small molecules (such as preservatives) and the number of target sites present, depending upon their metabolic state. These changes are well documented but difficult to predict but, in general, organisms with low growth rates are more resistant. There is a large difference, therefore, between the challenge organisms cultured in nutrient broth and those that may contaminate the product and which are derived from natural environments. Micro-organisms also alter their metabolism depending on the substrates present in the growth medium, and this can lead to adaptation, and resistance via metabolism of the

Table 10

Examples of combinations of preservative agents and their effect on antimicrobial activity

| | Interacting agent and type of interaction | | |
Agent	Synergism	Potentiation	Antagonism
Benzoic acid	Dehydroacetic acid	Hydroxybenzoate	Boric acid
Chlorhexidine	Phenylethanol	—	—
Chlorbutol	Phenylethanol	—	Edetic acid
Hydroxybenzoates	Phenylethanol	Benzoic acid	Boric acid

preservative. For example, it has been demonstrated that *Pseudomonas cepacia* can utilise hydroxybenzoate preservatives as a source of carbon and energy.[19] Metabolism of the preservative reduces its concentration, so that other micro-organisms may be able to colonise the product. This is an insidious process that only appears during product storage, or in use; challenge tests are not conducted over a long enough time-scale to demonstrate this problem.

Physicochemical Considerations

Preservative choice is also controlled by the physicochemical properties of the formulation and the processes involved during manufacture. Since micro-organisms are aquatic the aim must be to achieve an adequate preservative concentration in the aqueous phase of the product. Moreover, the preservative must be free and in the correct form to interact with its target site on the organism. Physicochemical features that control preservative distribution, chemical form, and stability in the product must, therefore, be examined closely.

Chemical Stability of the Preservative

The preservative must be chemically stable in the product and able to withstand the processing techniques used during manufacture, such as application of heat. The nature of the product determines the degree of chemical stability required from the preservative. Degradation of even a small percentage of the preservative may be critical if it has a high η value or is being used in a combination.

pH of the Product

The pH of the aqueous phase of the formulation controls the extent of ionisation of the preservative and the micro-organism receptor sites. Preservatives have optimal activity at specific pH ranges (see Table 7) and the agent must be chosen with reference to the pH of the formulation. The pH also has physicochemical effects; preservative solubility, stability, or both, may be pH-dependent (for example, benzoic acid).

Partitioning of the Preservative

In biphasic formulations, the preservative may partition from the aqueous phase, thus reducing its free concentration and antimicrobial activity. In emulsions, partitioning into oil or micellar phases may occur; in suspensions, adsorption onto surfaces may take place. The activity of preservatives in oil-in-water systems has been correlated to the free aqueous phase preservative concentration (C_w) at equilibrium. This can be shown mathematically by the following relationship:

$$C_w = \frac{C(\phi + 1)}{(K_o \phi + R)}$$

where, C is the total preservative concentration; ϕ, the oil-to-water ratio; K_o, the preservative partition coefficient; and R, the ratio of total preservative to free aqueous phase preservative in the presence of a nonionic surfactant. The relationship demonstrates that the higher K_o, R, and ϕ are for any system, the lower will be C_w. If the preservative is a weak acid or base, partitioning will also be affected by the pH of the aqueous phase.

Solid phases such as suspensions can also influence preservative activity, either by adsorbing the agent to reduce its concentration in the aqueous phase or by acting as a solid phase for sessile microbial growth. The interaction between preservative and solid phase is dependent upon the physical conditions and cannot be quantitatively described. Kaolin, talc, and magnesium trisilicate adsorb chlorhexidine, chlorocresol, and benzalkonium chloride to a greater extent than benzyl alcohol or sorbic acid[20]. Other quaternary ammonium compounds are also adsorbed by kaolin and this effect depends upon the concentration of suspended solid.

Sorption of the Preservative to Packaging

Similar partitioning of preservatives can occur from the formulation into rubber or plastic packaging materials. For example, hydroxybenzoates (see Table 11), benzyl alcohol, and phenol interact with olefin-based plastics such as polyethylene and polypropylene,[21] whereas organomercurials sorb to certain types of rubber. These interactions can significantly reduce free preservative concentration in a product. It is difficult to determine quantitative relationships for this process and individual studies must be conducted during formulation.

Interactions Between the Preservative and other Ingredients

An additional physicochemical process is the possible interaction between the preservative and other excipients or active agents present in the formulation. Few systematic studies have been conducted on the interaction of preservatives with active pharmacological agents. It has been reported that the activity of benzalkonium chloride is reported to be greater in the presence of pilocarpine or physostigmine than atropine.[22] Other studies with eye

Table 11
Interaction of hydroxybenzoate preservatives with plastics (initial solution strength $3 \times 10^{-5} M$)

Hydroxybenzoate		Percentage adsorption per gram of plastic			
	High density polyethylene	Polypropylene	Polycarbonate	Polymethacrylate	Polystyrene
Methyl	0.6	0.4	4.8	1.0	0.0
Ethyl	1.2	0.2	5.9	0.8	0.3
Propyl	1.5	2.4	1.4	2.9	2.8
Butyl	6.6	5.7	7.8	6.5	2.1

drop formulations have failed to find a correlation between preservative activity and active ingredient.[23] The excipients present in a formulation may have a definite effect on preservative activity. Surfactants that are present in concentrations above their critical micelle concentration can solubilise lipophilic preservatives, resulting in a reduced free aqueous concentration and reduced antimicrobial activity. Large macromolecular compounds such as tragacanth or hypromellose can complex with preservatives such as benzalkonium chloride to reduce activity. Smaller molecules like cyclodextrins form inclusion complexes with hydroxybenzoates with consequent reduction of activity.[24] Other excipients may directly antagonise the preservative system; for example, divalent cations such as calcium or magnesium will reduce the effectiveness of edetic acid-based combinations. These interactions are difficult to predict, but can be used to neutralise preservative activity during testing.

The problems outlined above can be circumvented either by increasing the concentration of preservative or by judicious choice of the preservative system and formulation excipients. The former solution can lead to excessively high preservative concentrations that may contravene regulatory requirements. Preservative choice may also be limited by the formulation parameters and the formulator will have to seek the optimum system. The excipients chosen should posses weak antimicrobial activity, be resistant to microbial degradation, and be inherently free from microbial contamination.

Problem Products

Some formulations are notoriously difficult to preserve; such products usually possess one or two features that act against preservation and for microbial growth. Antacid suspensions, for example, have a high A_w, a pH around neutral, and contain suspended solids with a large surface area for adsorption; ingredients such as concentrated peppermint water are often contaminated and may support microbial growth. Studies have demonstrated the inability of some marketed antacid suspensions to meet challenge test requirements;[25] failure was primarily due to inappropriate choice of preservative with respect to formulation pH, but adsorption onto solids may also have been a feature. Formulations that contain large quantities of surfactants, cosolvents, or oils can also present preservation problems. These systems are formulated around neutral pH and with high proportions of surfactants and oil, so that preservatives are likely to partition from the aqueous phase or at least suffer interference from the surfactants. The oil phase also provides a carbon-based energy source that may be utilised by colonising micro-organisms. Careful choice of preservative is required to ensure that adequate concentrations remain in the product's aqueous phase.

IN-USE CONTAMINATION

Once manufactured, packaged, and sold the product is no longer controlled by the producer and may be exposed to a variety of conditions in use that can lead to microbial contamination and colonisation. The producer must take all reasonable steps to reduce this possibility and it has been suggested that products should be 'effectively preserved', which takes into account in-use contamination. In normal use, some products will be repeatedly contaminated, owing to their method of delivery and mode of use. Semi-solid preparations packed in tubs will be contaminated by repeated finger insertions to remove the product. The use of tubes will reduce but not eliminate this problem; however, a build-up of residue around the nozzle may allow microbial adaptation to the product and subsequent contamination. Other products (such as nasal sprays) may suffer inadvertent dilution or contamination with water or body fluids, which will also allow adaptation and possible colonisation of the product. Storage in less-than-ideal situations and for prolonged periods will also promote the growth of contaminants. In-use contamination can be eliminated by packaging the product as a unit dose that is opened, used once, and the remainder discarded; however, this relies on the consumer following instructions. Experience of the performance of preservative systems in use over a prolonged period will provide a knowledge base that may be used in assessing the suitability of preservatives in new products.

SUMMARY

Owing to the expense required to demonstrate safety, few new antimicrobial preservatives are likely to be available in the future. This, combined with increasing concerns about adverse reactions to preservatives,[26] and the move towards additive-free products, creates problems for the formulator. Improvements are still possible with existing preservatives and there is increasing use of combinations to obtain broad spectra of activity and synergy. Natural preservative systems can be utilised or the product itself formulated to be antimicrobial, although both of these methods are highly product-dependent and not always possible. Studies suggest that microbial contamination during manufacture is no longer a major problem. This can be reduced further by increasing emphasis on quality control during manufacture. Contamination in use can be prevented by using unit-dose packaging which reduces the requirements for preservation and possible challenges to the preservative system.

No one preservative system is suitable for all products or even different formulations within a product group. Choice is based on a complex consideration of product type, excipients, container, shelf-life required, and the formulator's experience. The eventual decision will be the best compromise available and should be rigorously tested before final release to the consumer. Even if all possible contamination testing scenarios are covered, there will still be occasions when a micro-organism will overcome the product's defences. The application of formulation design, good manufacturing practice, quality control, and an adequate preservative system will reduce the incidence of these problems but will not completely eliminate them. This fact argues for continued vigilance by the formulator and manufacturer of non-sterile medicinal products, coupled with an appreciation of product susceptibility and microbial adaptability.

REFERENCES

1. Ringertz O, Ringertz S. Adv Pharm Sci 1982;1:201–25.
2. McCullough NB, Eisele CW. J Infect Dis 1951;88:278–9.
3. Greenwood MJ, Hooper WL. Br Med J 1983;286:1394.
4. Jarvis B. Mycotoxins in food. In: Skinner SA, Carr JG, editors. Microbiology in agriculture, fisheries and food. London: Academic Press, 1976:251–67.
5. Bruch CW. Drug Cosmet Ind 1972;111:51–4,151–6.
6. Meltzer TH. Pharmaceutical water: generation, storage, distribution, and quality testing. In: Groves MJ, Olson WP, Anisfeld MH, editors. Sterile pharmaceutical manufacturing applications for the 1990's; vol 1. Buffalo: Interpharm Press, 1991:109–221.
7. Tsuji K, Rahn PD, Steindler KA. J Pharm Sci 1983;72:23–6.
8. Gopal NGS, Rajagopalan S. Int J Pharmaceutics 1981;9:359–60.
9. Maurer IM. Hospital hygiene. 3rd ed. London: Edward Arnold, 1985.
10. Maki DG. Growth properties of micro-organisms in infusion fluids and methods of detection. In: Phillips I, Meers PD, D'Arcy PF, editors. Microbiological hazards of infusion therapy. Lancaster: MTP Press, 1976:13–48.
11. Griffith E. Iron and biological defense mechanisms. In: Gould GW, Rhodes-Roberts ME, Charnley AK, Cooper RM, Board RG, editors. Natural antimicrobial systems. Bath: Bath University Press, 1986:56–71.
12. Hurwitz SJ, McCarthy TJ. J Clin Pharm Ther 1987;12:107–15.
13. Karabit MS, Juneskans OT, Lundgren P. Int J Pharmaceutics 1989;54:51–6.
14. Karabit MS, Juneskans OT, Lundgren P. J Clin Hosp Pharm 1986;11:281–9.
15. Karabit MS. Int J Pharmaceutics 1990;60:147–50.
16. Karabit MS, Juneskans OT, Lundgren P. Int J Pharmaceutics 1988;46:141–7.
17. Denyer SP, Hugo WB, Harding VD. Int J Pharmaceutics 1985;25:245–53.
18. Richards RME, Richards JM. J Pharm Sci 1979;68:1436–8.
19. Close J, Nielson PA. Appl Environ Microbiol 1976;31:718–22.
20. McCarthy TJ. J Mond Pharm 1969;12:321–9.
21. Autian J. Bull Parenter Drug Assoc 1968;22:276–88.
22. Richards RME, McBride JR. J Pharm Pharmacol 1972;24:145–8.
23. Tromp TFJ, Nusman-Schoterman Z, Snippe H, Huizinga T. Pharm Weekbl 1977;112:461–6.
24. Lach JL, Cohen J. J Pharm Sci 1963;52:137–42.
25. Vanhaecke E, Remon JP, Pijck J, Aerts R, Herman J. Drug Dev Ind Pharm 1987;13:1429–46.
26. D'Arcy PF. Adverse reactions to excipients in pharmaceutical formulations. In: Florence AT, Salole EG, editors. Formulation factors in adverse reactions. London: Wright, 1990:1–22.

FURTHER INFORMATION

Bloomfield SF, Baird R, Leak RE, Leech R, editors. Microbial quality assurance in pharmaceuticals, cosmetics and toiletries. Chichester: Ellis Horwood, 1988.

Denyer SP, Baird R, editors. Guide to microbiological control in pharmaceuticals. Chichester: Ellis Horwood, 1990.

Hugo WB, Russell AD, editors. Pharmaceutical microbiology. 5th ed. London: Blackwell, 1992.

Kabara JJ, editor. Cosmetic and drug preservation, principles and practice. New York: Marcel Dekker, 1984.

Pyrogens

The terms 'pyrogen' and 'pyrogenic substance' were coined in the late 19th century. As early as 1876, in his studies on the process of fever, Burdon-Sanderson theorised that bacteria were implicated in the process and that substances secreted by the host cells were also involved.[1]

The association between the intravenous injection of pharmaceuticals and pyrogenic reactions was discovered in the early 1900s; the terms 'injection fever', 'Salvarsan fever', or 'salt fever' being variously applied to the reaction.

Physiological Effects

In humans, a pyrogenic reaction to an intravenous injection occurs approximately 1 to 2 hours after the administration of the substance.[2] The characteristic signs are: rapid rise in temperature with a sensation of chill, shivering, vasoconstriction, pupillary dilatation, respiratory depression, and an increase in arterial blood pressure. In addition there may be pain in the joints and back, headache, nausea, and a general feeling of malaise. The chill may last for about 20 minutes, and the fever normally reaches a peak after approximately 3 hours. These symptoms may have dangerous clinical implications in seriously ill patients who are receiving large volume parenteral fluids.

PHYSICOCHEMICAL PROPERTIES OF PYROGENS

There are two main classes of pyrogens—endogenous and exogenous. **Endogenous** pyrogen is a substance that is produced by the host following the administration of an **exogenous** pyrogen. This response is considered to be the prime mediator in the fever process.

Exogenous pyrogens are substances which, on administration to humans and animals, result in an elevation of temperature. Many substances are known to cause this reaction; examples include some steroids, viruses, certain chemicals, and drugs. However, as far as the pharmaceutical industry is concerned, the most important exogenous pyrogen is the endotoxin produced from the outer cell walls of certain Gram-negative bacteria. **Bacterial endotoxin** from Gram-negative bacteria is a lipopolysaccharide made up of three main parts: the innermost part (Lipid A—a disaccharide of glucosamine) linked to a central core (a polysaccharide) linked to an outer O antigenic side-chain the composition of which is specific to the type of bacteria. Pyrogenic activity is associated with the Lipid A portion of the molecule.

Endotoxins have a high molecular weight. They can exist in various aggregation states; the level of aggregation has a significant effect on biological activity.[3] Endotoxins are water-soluble, heat-stable, non-volatile substances; particle size and mass are affected by the presence of ions such as calcium or magnesium, and by other substances such as detergents.[4] Many pyrogens withstand autoclaving, and can pass through filters of 0.2 micrometre pore size that are normally used for terminal sterilisation.

The physicochemical properties of endotoxins have been utilised in the development of various industrial depyrogenating processes (see below).

Sources of Contamination

It is difficult to prevent the contamination of a product by pyrogenic substances as this can occur at any stage during manufacture. They may be present in starting materials (most commonly raw water), containers, or in the manufacturing equipment itself.[5] Since endotoxin is shed by bacteria during metabolism or autolysis, it will remain even after the source bacteria have been destroyed by sterilisation.

Depyrogenation

Depyrogenation of materials, apparatus, and containers used in pharmaceutical production may be effected by either inactivation or removal.

Inactivation

Inactivation tends to involve some form of chemical reaction (for example, oxidation, alkylation, or hydrolysis of the endotoxins). Such methods have limited use in the treatment of raw materials and water. Careful consideration of the chemical composition of the ingredients is necessary to ensure that any chemicals used in treatment have no adverse effects.

Moist heat at $80°$ to $90°$ or autoclaving at $121°$ have shown some promise in the inactivation of pyrogens but the necessary pH adjustment limits the use of this method.[6]

Inactivation by incineration, that is subjecting the material to dry heat, is an effective method of treating glassware and heat-stable oils and powders. Suggested operating temperatures for the incinerator range from 170° to 350°.[7] The most commonly used temperature is 250° for a duration of 30 minutes. Lower temperatures require heating times in the region of 10 to 12 hours.[8]

Removal

Removal of pyrogens by physical means has the advantage that no additional chemicals are involved.

Rinsing/dilution with pyrogen-free water is a simple and effective way of treating containers and closures.[9] **Distillation** is a common method used for the treatment of raw water as pyrogens are nonvolatile and are therefore not present in the distillate. **Ultrafiltration** is a separation technique based on the size of the endotoxin molecule. Biologically active endotoxin exists as aggregates of molecular weights in excess of 10 000. A combination of an ultrafilter of pore size 0.1 micrometre with a sterilising filter (0.2 micrometre) is used to process large volumes of parenteral solutions.[10] The use of **depth filters** involves passing the solution through a cartridge or pad composed of kaolin, aluminium oxide, or kieselguhr.[11]

Endotoxin is removed either by electrostatic absorption or by mechanical obstruction. More recently, charge-modified filters have been developed in which the filter medium has been altered to enable it to carry a positive charge thus increasing the attraction for the (negatively charged) endotoxin.[12, 13] **Adsorption** to charcoal has been used but this material is strongly adsorbent to many drugs, particularly in dilute solutions, and is inherently difficult to remove from the final solution. Adsorption to barium sulphate suspensions is a possible alternative.[6] **Reverse osmosis** followed by continuous deionisation has been found to successfully remove many contaminants, including endotoxins, from raw water.[14] **Ion-exchange resins** and **gamma irradiation** are two further methods that have been used for the removal of endotoxins from parenterals.

DETECTION AND QUANTIFICATION

The *British Pharmacopoeia*[15] includes detailed procedures and specifications for both a Test for Pyrogens and a Test for Bacterial Endotoxins.

Rabbits are used for the Test for Pyrogens; it involves measurement of the increase in body temperature of the test animals following the intravenous injection of a sterile solution of the test substance. *Rabbits* are used because their febrile response closely resembles that of humans. The *British Pharmacopoeia* specifies that, where no test for bacterial endotoxins is prescribed or authorised, the test should be performed on all parenteral fluids where the volume administered in a single dose is 15 mL or more.

Disadvantages of the '*rabbit*' test are that it is expensive and time-consuming; it cannot be quantified; and certain parenteral solutions (for example, those containing phosphate or high levels of potassium) will elicit a pyrogenic response.

The Test for Bacterial Endotoxins, also known as the Limulus Amoebocyte Lysate (LAL) test, is widely used in industry where quantitative estimation is required. The basis of the test is that a lysate of amoebocytes from the blood of the Horseshoe Crab (*Limulus polyphemus*), on addition of endotoxin, undergoes clotting (gelation), turbidity, or precipitation.[15, 16]

The LAL test has proved so successful that a number of commercial companies now supply test kits for the rapid identification of endotoxin contamination. These are widely used to monitor process water[17] and for the end-process testing of parenterals, radiopharmaceuticals,[18] and medical devices.[19] While the gel-clot end-point serves as the basis for many commercial test kits, further refinement has allowed for detection of the endpoint by turbidimetric, colorimetric, nephelometric, and chromogenic-substrate reactions.[20]

However, there are disadvantages associated with the LAL test. A number of factors can affect the outcome of the test:[21, 22] pH of test solution, source of reagents used, concentration of cations (calcium or magnesium) in the test solution, and aggregation state of the endotoxin can all affect the end-point. Simple factors such as storage conditions and degree of agitation of vials[23] may cause variable results due to adsorption of endotoxin to the surface of the container.[24] It has also been shown[25] that the LAL test does not detect endotoxin from Gram-positive cocci (which have no lipopolysaccharide-containing outer membrane). The advantages of the LAL test are that it is quick, relatively inexpensive, simple to use, and quantifiable. Results of a multicentre study[25] have shown that, whereas the LAL and *rabbit* tests are of equivalent sensitivity when there are high levels of endotoxin, the LAL test is much more sensitive at low endotoxin concentrations; it is in fact capable of detecting endotoxins at concentrations below those which produce a pyrogenic response in humans. For this reason this method finds use in process testing and for monitoring the effectiveness of cleaning procedures.

Bioluminescence, radioimmunoassay, and immunoelectrophoresis are among other techniques which have been investigated for the detection of pyrogen.

REFERENCES

1. Burdon-Sanderson J. Practitioner. 1876;417–19.
2. Hugo WB, Russell AD. Pharmaceutical microbiology. 4th ed. Oxford: Blackwell, 1987.
3. Ribi E, Anacker RL, Brown R *et al.* J Bacteriol 1966;92:1413–509.
4. Baggerman C, Pathmamanharan C, Spies F *et al.* J Pharm Pharmacol 1985;37:521–7.
5. Stansfield SA, Lee-Ford Jones E. Can J Hosp Pharm 1983;36(1):21–8.
6. Mosier LD, Bosworth ME, Jurgens RW *et al.* J Parenter Sci Technol 1987;41(1):21–5.
7. Ludwig JD, Avis KE. J Parenter Sci Technol 1988;42(1):9–14.
8. Ludwig JD, Avis KE. J Parenter Sci Technol 1990;44(1):4–12.
9. Berman D, Kasica T, Myers T, Chrai S. J Parenter Sci Technol 1987;41(5):158–63.
10. Cradock JC, Guder LA, Francis DL, Morgan SL. J Pharm Pharmacol 1978;30:198–9.
11. Baggerman C, Brandesma C, Humer M, Visser J. J Pharm Pharmacol 1981;33:685–91.
12. Gerba CP, Hou KC, Babineau RA, Fiori JV. Pharmaceut Technol 1980;4:83–9.
13. Hou KC, Zaniewski R. J Parenter Sci Technol 1990;44(4):204–9.
14. Ganzi GC, Parise PC. J Parenter Sci Technol 1990;44(4):231–41.
15. British pharmacopoeia 1993. London: HMSO, 1993.
16. European Pharmacopoeia Commission: LAL Test for Bacterial Endotoxin: PA/PH/EXP1L/T(86)4: 3rd April 1986.
17. Weary M. Pharm Int 1986;7(4):99–102.
18. Twohy CW, Duran AP, Munson TE. J Parenter Sci Technol 1984;38(5):190–201.
19. Twohy CW, Duran AP, Peeler JT. J Parenter Sci Technol 1986;40(6):287–91.
20. Pearson FC. Pyrogens: endotoxins, LAL testing and depyrogenation. In: Robinson JR, editor. Advances in parenteral sciences; vol 2. New York: Marcel Dekker, 1985:119–47.
21. McCullough KZ. J Parenter Sci Technol 1990;44(1):19–21.
22. Cooper JF. J Parenter Sci Technol 1990;44(1):13–15.
23. Guilfoyle DE, Yager JF, Carito SL. J Parenter Sci Technol 1989;43(4):183–7.
24. Novitsky TJ, Schmidt-Gengenbach J, Remillard JF. J Parenter Sci Technol 1986;40(6):284–6.
25. Pearson FC. Pyrogens: endotoxins, LAL testing and depyrogenation. In: Robinson JR, editor. Advances in parenteral sciences; vol 2. New York: Marcel Dekker, 1985:152–5.

Particulate Contamination

Particulate contamination may be defined as the presence of visible and/or subvisible extraneous particulate matter in parenteral systems. Foreign particulate matter has been defined by Krueger and Riggs[1] as 'mobile undissolved substances unintentionally present in parenteral solutions'. Akers[2] stated that a lack of particulate matter produces a clean, quality product, indicative of the standards employed by the manufacturer. There are three major reasons for monitoring the levels of particulate contamination in parenteral products. Firstly, as a guide to product quality; secondly, to alleviate safety concerns for the patient; and thirdly, the requirement to comply with compendial and regulatory standards.

Hazards of Particulate Contamination

Before the classical work of Garvan and Gunner[3,4] there had been few reports in the literature about the potentially harmful effects of particulate matter present in parenteral solutions. However, Konwaler[5] found that cotton fibres could cause pulmonary emboli and granulomas, and Wartmann, Hudson, and Jennings[6] reported similar findings with cellulose fibres from filter papers. Garvan and Gunner demonstrated that foreign body granulomas could be produced experimentally in the lungs of *rabbits* following the intravenous administration of sodium chloride 0.9% containing visible particles. Post-mortem examinations revealed similar granulomas in the lungs of premature infants who had received large quantities of intravenous solutions. Garvan and Gunner reported the presence of visible particulate material in all test samples of commercially manufactured intravenous solutions; the particles were thought to have been generated from rubber closures. Although these closures are undoubtedly a contributing factor, there are many other possible sources of particles in parenterals (see Sources of Particulate Contamination below). The publication of these reports[3–6] stimulated many other investigations, which have been reviewed by Turco and Davis,[7] Akers,[2] and Groves.[8] The physiological and clinical effects and the pathological conditions that can be initiated by the presence of particulate matter are still controversial subjects. *Animal* studies have provided many positive indications of harmful effects but, in the absence of controlled studies, the clinical significance in humans is largely circumstantial. The main evidence for the harmful effects of particulate contamination in humans can be found in the literature on drug abuse,[9–15] which illustrates that the use of crushed solid dosage forms in aqueous media as injectable material has often resulted in serious consequences including pulmonary emboli, granulomas, and abnormal pulmonary function. These events and numerous *animal* studies have been reviewed by Borchert et al.[16]

There is evidence that particles can pass through the pulmonary capillary bed and enter the systemic circulation. Schroeder et al[17] and Kanke et al[18] followed the route of radio-labelled divinylbenzene microspheres of diameter 3, 8, 15, and 25 micrometres injected intravenously into *dogs*. They found that particles of diameter greater than 8 micrometres were retained in the lung whereas smaller particles were deposited in various organs of the body. Particles of 3 and 5 micrometres diameter may reach the spleen and liver by transport via the reticuloendothelial system but there appears to be an upper size limit where phagocytosis does not occur. Illum and Davis[19] demonstrated that, in addition to their size, the surface properties of particles were important in determining whether or not phagocytosis occurs.

Kirkpatrick[20] reviewed the evidence for particulate matter being a primary causative factor in adult respiratory distress syndrome (ARDS), which plays an important role in multiple organ failure (MOF). Adult respiratory distress syndrome has been described in detail by Pepe et al[21] and multiple organ failure has been discussed by Parillo et al.[22] Kirkpatrick put forward the hypothesis that foreign particulate matter could play a pathogenetic role in the development of adult respiratory distress syndrome; he supported this with evidence generated by other workers. Walpot et al[23] demonstrated, using Scanning Electron Microscopy/Energy Dispersive Analysis by X-ray (SEM/EDAX), that in patients suffering from adult respiratory distress syndrome particles of diameter less than 2 micrometers represented the major component of particle loading in the pulmonary microcirculation. They identified most of the particles as glass, rubber, or latex. Kirkpatrick also stated that foreign surfaces have the ability to activate the coagulation Factor XII in the plasma and therefore can form the foci for thrombi. This has been demonstrated *in vivo* by Steffens.[24] In addition, Steffens presented a histological section from the myocardium of a patient who had died from multiple organ failure where a thrombus located in the coronary artery was associated with polymeric material. The conclusions drawn from these studies indicate that particle loading of the microcirculation during intravenous therapy can have adverse effects on the course of adult respiratory distress syndrome and multiple organ failure. According to Turco,[25] the potentially harmful effects of the presence of particles in parenterals were that particles could produce:

- physical occlusion
- inflammatory reactions
- neoplastic responses
- antigenic responses.

These effects have, with the possible exception of neoplastic responses, been verified by a number of workers. It is, therefore, reasonable to conclude that the presence of particulate material in intravenous systems is at least undesirable and at worst dangerous.

Sources of Particulate Contamination

Groves[26] classified the origins of particulate contamination into two main categories, intrinsic and extrinsic. **Intrinsic** contamination comes from the raw materials and packaging components used in the production of parenteral fluids and equipment; it is not removed during manufacturing processes. It is difficult to define the extent of extrinsic contamination in a parenteral product as the particles involved are below the limits of visual detection. **Extrinsic** contamination is generated mainly from environmental contaminants, processing equipment, and operators. For example, extrinsic contamination occurs when an ampoule is opened or when an injection vial is pierced with a needle. The types of particles that have been identified in parenterals have been described by many workers including Groves,[26] Draftz and Graf,[27] and Whyte.[28] The sources of particles may often be traced by microscopic and analytical methods and by reference to the Particle Atlas,[29] which is a compilation of particle properties and information on identification procedures. DeLuca *et al*[30] published guidelines for the identification of parti-

culate matter in parenterals; the guidelines included methods of sampling, isolation, and measurement.

Particulate Matter Standards

The history of the development of standards for the limitation of particulate matter in parenteral fluids has been discussed by Akers.[2] The *British Pharmacopoeia* and the *European Pharmacopoeia* specify standards for visible particles in all parenterals, and for subvisible particles in large volume parenterals. The *United States Pharmacopeia* specifies standards for visible and subvisible particulate matter in large and small volume parenterals. However, the requirements specified and the methods of determination applied do vary among the different compendia.

Inspection and Counting Methods

Visual Inspection

The use of visual tests for the presence of particulate material in parenterals has always produced problems, essentially because they are reliant on subjective judgement, normally under ill-defined conditions of inspection, and certainly with undefined qualities of human visual acuity. Additional problems are posed by the selection of appropriate criteria for the rejection of an injection (the sizes of the particles that can be discerned by the unaided eye have a lower limit of approximately 50 micrometres and the number of particles of that size, or greater, in parenteral products is small).

Although the *British Pharmacopoeia* and the *European Pharmacopoeia* do not specify the requirement for 100% inspection of injectable preparations, current Good Manufacturing Practices (cGMP) demand that every container in a batch should be visually inspected by trained individuals under appropriate viewing conditions. The methods used for the detection of visible particles fall into two distinct categories: one is the use of people and the other is the use of machines. It could be argued that the latter does not conform with the requirements of the compendia, but properly validated machine methods are consistent and swift, with acceptance parameters that can be adjusted to equate with previously accepted manual procedures.

Manual Methods. Examination of manual procedures reveals that there is no standardisation for the visual inspection method either within a particular pharmacopoeial requirement or among pharmacopoeias. The areas in which inspections are carried out, the construction of viewing equipment, the type of light source used, and the criteria for selection and training of operators are all major variables associated with the visual method. These variables and others such as visual acuity, aptitude, operator fatigue, environment, and inspection speed have been discussed by Hodgson.[31] Standardisation of the visual method is therefore essential, and future proposals, assuming that total inspection takes place and therefore the need for sampling is avoided, should address the factors listed above. In addition, the procedure for manual inspection, the acceptance criteria, and training programmes for operators should also be standardised.

A basic procedure for manual inspection has been proposed by Akers.[2] The method involves the removal of all labels followed by the cleaning of the containers with non-linting cloths or sponges, the contents of the container are swirled while being in a vertical plane. Examination for particles is achieved by holding the container in a horizontal plane four inches below a light source against a black and white background. If no particles are seen, the container is inverted slowly and scrutinised for the presence of large particles. Containers are rejected if any visible particles are observed at any time during the inspection process. Akers also noted that the Standard Operating Procedures (SOP) for inspection will differ depending on the type of parenteral being inspected, the volume of the product, and the type of ampoule, vial, plastic container, or glass container being used. The time of examination should be specified in the Standard Operating Procedure for every product.

The manual inspection procedure, which is a subjective judgement on the part of the observer, has been investigated extensively to ascertain whether it is a deterministic or probabilistic procedure. In a deterministic process, if the same set of containers is examined under the same conditions several times, the same containers would be rejected each time. The rejection probability is either 0 for good containers or 1 for those containing particles. In a probabilistic process, each container has a rejection probability associated with it, with rejection probabilities ranging between 0 and 1. This concept has been reviewed in detail by Borchert et al.[16] The relationships between particle sizes and rejection probability and information on the detection limits for visual methods have been discussed by Knapp and co-workers.[32–35] The reproducibility of human visual inspection systems is moderate. Knapp et al demonstrated that performance varied among different inspectors and that, over a period of time, the performance of each individual inspector was also variable. Adequate training methods including the detection of particles of different sizes improves performance. Borchert et al[36] demonstrated a suitable training method using known sizes and distributions of particles.

Automatic Methods. The alternative to manual visual examination is machine-based inspection. The design of machines may be based on a variety of different principles ranging from **semi-automatic** systems such as the Brevetti device described by Wynn;[37] the Strunck and RCA machines, in which the ampoules or containers are spun and then presented to an observer via an illuminated viewing window, have been described by Martyn[38] and by Levine,[39] respectively. The observer inspects the contents and accepts or rejects the container. Groves[26] examined these systems and noted that they are still subjective methods and become less effective as the operator becomes fatigued. He further commented that two inspectors would be unlikely to agree entirely on which containers should be rejected from the same batch. Consequently, re-examination, a common industrial practice, could mean that unsatisfactory containers may be accepted.

Instruments used for **automatic** inspection, sometimes referred to as video inspection, use one of two basic mechanisms for the automated inspection of parenteral containers; these have been described by Kaye[40]. One system, the Autoskan™, spins the containers at a predetermined speed that is capable of producing vortexing of the liquid and suspension of any particulate material present. The container is illuminated from below with a white light source and when presented to the video lens a number of images of the container are recorded and compared with a 'master image'. Using preset upper and lower liquid levels in the master image, an error message can be generated for underfilled, overfilled, and empty containers, which are then rejected by the machine. Acceptance at this level means that any other image differences are caused by the scattering of light from suspended particulate matter. Akers[2] stated that up to 4500 containers per hour can be inspected in this way and Louer et al[41] demonstrated that the machine was capable of rejecting 93% of control substandard ampoules, whereas manual visual inspection rejected only 54%.

A widely used automatic method is the EISAI™ system, which also uses white light but employs light blockage as the detecting mechanism rather than the scattering theory applied with the Autoskan™. The threshold levels for detection of images are preset and if that level is exceeded the container is rejected. Additional refinements are that the machine can be adjusted for differences in container size and colour, and for the viscosity of the liquid contents. Like the Autoskan™, it can also reject improperly filled containers. Detailed assessments of these instruments have been written by Akers[2] and by Borchert et al.[16]

Subvisible Particulate Matter

The presence of subvisible particulate matter in parenteral systems is known to be undesirable (see Hazards of Particulate Contamination above). It is therefore necessary to detect and measure such particles. The methods employed were reviewed at an International Conference on Liquid Borne Particle Inspection and Metrology held by the Parenteral Drug Association in 1987[42] and more recently by Groves.[43] This brief account will refer to those methods that are used as compendial methods in the British Pharmacopoeia, the United States Pharmacopeia, and the European Pharmacopoeia, with comment on their various advantages and disadvantages. The detailed methodology for each method is not described as this is given in the relevant compendia.

Optical Microscopy

In 1975, the First Supplement to the United States Pharmacopeia XIX introduced a microscopic method for the examination of particulate matter in large volume parenterals. Twenty-five millilitres of the solution is filtered under ultraclean conditions using a membrane filter (1.2 micrometres) and the particles on the surface of the filter are observed and counted by using 100× magnification with an incident light source. Those particles with effective linear diameters exceeding 10 micrometres and 25 micrometres are counted and blank counts from the membrane only are subtracted.

The main disadvantages of the method are that relatively small samples are used, and the method is tedious, time-consuming, and requires skilled observers. Groves[43] noted that, in addition to the difficulties involved in counting the amorphous particles that occur in glucose solutions, oil droplets are absorbed onto the surface material of the membrane and are not detected, although they are classified as particulate contaminants.

Electrical Sensing Zone Method (Coulter Principle)

This method has been in the British Pharmacopoeia since 1973 and is currently one of two official methods used for the estimation of the degree of particulate contamination in large volume parenterals, the other being light blockage (see below). The equipment is described in British Standard 3406:Part 5:1983(1991) and in many papers in the literature.[44-46] The application of this method for the determination of particulate contamination was described critically by Barnett.[47] The disadvantages of the method are that small samples are used, the solutions must be electrolytes with sufficiently high conductivities, and the data generated is in the form of equivalent sphere diameters and hence no indication of the fibrous nature of any contaminating particulate matter will be perceived. The presence of air bubbles may also adversely affect the true particulate count and this must be taken into account during the preparation of samples. The advantages of this method are that it is not dependent on operator technique, it is reproducible and reliable, and it easily detects particles at the specified pharmacopoeial levels of 2 micrometres and 5 micrometres.

The Light Blockage Method

This method has been variously referred to as light blockage, light extinction, or light obscuration. It involves passing particles suspended in a fluid through a small rectangular cell across which a collimated beam of light (tungsten or laser) is passed to impinge directly onto a photodiode. When no particles are present the intensity of light received by the photodiode is constant; however, when a particle interacts with the light beam a reduction of the light intensity falling on the photodiode results, with the decrease being proportional to the cross-sectional area of the particle that is presented to the beam. The instrument is calibrated using a series of spheres of known size and hence the method measures the equivalent circle diameter of the particle. There are a number of instruments commercially available that are based on the light blockage principle but it must be emphasised that they are not all equivalent in their perception and measurement of dispersed particulate material. These differences are caused by variations in optical construction, sensor resolution, flow rates, sample volume accuracy, and calibration methodology. These factors have been considered in detail by Groves[43] and Barber.[48] Barnett et al[49] have examined other problems inherent in the method: the refractive index differences between the particles and the suspending liquid, and the sensitivity of the sensor to particle shape. The validation of light blockage instruments has been described by Lieberman.[50] The *United States Pharmacopeia XXII* includes procedures for the determination of sensor resolution and sample volume accuracy, and instrument calibration.

Light blockage is given as an alternative method for the analysis of large volume parenterals in the *British Pharmacopoeia 1993* and will be the compendial method for the detection of particulate contamination in Europe for large volume parenterals following the publication of the definitive standard in the *European Pharmacopoeia* in 1994. Neither the *British Pharmacopoeia* nor the *European Pharmacopoeia* has an instrumental method for the detection of particulate contamination in small volume parenterals, but this situation should be rectified in the near future.

Particulate Contamination in Administration Systems

Particulate contamination is present in intravenous administration sets, in syringes (both plastic and glass), in cannulae, and in the empty containers used for the extemporaneous preparation of intravenous admixtures. Currently, no standards exist for the limitation of particulate contamination in such systems, although the methodology for such determinations has been described by Williams and Barnett.[51] If the premise that particulate contamination is a potential hazard to the patient is accepted, as it appears to be, then attention to the introduction of limitation standards in these systems is imperative.

REFERENCES

1. Krueger EO, Riggs TH. Bull Parenter Drug Assoc 1968;22:99.
2. Akers MJ. Parenteral quality control. New York: Marcel Dekker, 1985.
3. Garvan JM, Gunner BW. Med J Aust 1963;2:140.
4. Garvan JM, Gunner BW. Med J Aust 1964;2:1.
5. Konwaler BE. Am J Clin Pathol 1950;20:385.
6. Wartmann WB, Hudson B, Jennings RB. Circulation 1951;4:756.
7. Turco S, Davis NM. Hosp Pharm 1973;8:5.
8. Groves MJ. Proc Soc Anal Chem 1971;8:271.
9. Atlee WE. J Am Med Assoc 1972;219:49.
10. Richman S, Harris RD. Radiology 1972;103:57.
11. Butz WC. J Forensic Sci 1969;14:317.
12. Douglas FG. Ann Intern Med 1971;75:865.
13. Hopkins GB. J Am Med Assoc 1972;211:909.
14. Burton JF, Zwadzki ES, Wetherell HR, Moy TW. J Forensic Sci 1965;10:466.
15. Johnston WH, Waisman J. Arch Pathol 1971;92:196.
16. Borchert SJ, Abe A, Aldrich DS *et al*. J Parenter Sci Technol 1982;40:212–41.
17. Schroeder HG, Bivins BA, Sherman GP, DeLuca PP. J Pharm Sci 1978;67:508.
18. Kanke M, Simmons GH, Wiess DL, Bivins BA, DeLuca PP. J Pharm Sci 1980;69:755.
19. Illum L, Davis SS. J Pharm Sci 1983;72:1086.
20. Kirkpatrick CJ. In: Lee HA, Barnett MI, editors. Managing complications of intravenous therapy. Portsmouth: Pall Biomedical, 1993:5–11.
21. Pepe P, Potkin RJ, Holtman-Reus *et al*. Am J Surg 1982;144:1243.
22. Parillo JE, Parker MM, Natanson C *et al*. Ann Intern Med 1990;113:227.
23. Walpot H, Franke RP, Burchard WG *et al*. Ruckstreu-Anaathetist 1989;38:544.
24. Steffens K-J. Pharm Ind 1989;51:799.
25. Turco SJ. The clinical effects of particulate matter. Philadelphia: Burron Medical, 1978.
26. Groves MJ. Parenteral products. London: Heinneman, 1973.
27. Draftz RG, Graf J. Bull Parenter Drug Assoc 1974;28:35.
28. Whyte W. In: Proceedings PDA international conference on liquid borne particle inspection and metrology. Philadelphia: Parenteral Drug Association, 1987:75.
29. McCrone WC, Delly JG. The particle atlas; vols 1-6. Ann Arbor: Ann Arbor Science Publishers, 1980.
30. DeLuca PP, Baddapati S, Sophann I. FDA guidelines 1980;10(3):111–65.
31. Hodgson I. Mfg Chem 1985;56(2):29.
32. Knapp JZ, Kushner HK. J Parenter Drug Assoc 1980;34:14.
33. Knapp JZ, Kushner HK, Abramson LR. J Parenter Sci Technol 1981;35:21.
34. Knapp JZ, Kushner HK, Abramson LR. J Parenter Sci Technol 1981;35:176.
35. Knapp JZ, Kushner HK. J Parenter Sci Technol 1982;36:121.
36. Borchert SJ, Maxwell RJ, Davison RL, Aldrich DS. J Parenter Sci Technol 1986;40:265.
37. Wynn JB. Bull Parenter Drug Assoc 1968;22:13.
38. Martyn GW. Bull Parenter Drug Assoc 1970;24:281.
39. Levine S. Bull Parenter Drug Assoc 1966;20:33.
40. Kaye BH. Bull Parenter Drug Assoc 1979;33:239.
41. Louer RC, Russoman JA, Rasanen PR. Bull Parenter Drug Assoc 1971;25:54.
42. Parenteral Drug Association. Proceedings PDA international conference on liquid borne particle inspection and metrology. Philadelphia: The Association, 1987.
43. Groves MJ. Particle size distribution.II. In: Provder E, editor. Assessment and characterisation. Washington: American Chemical Society, 1991:123.
44. Allen T. Particle size measurement. London: Chapman and Hall 1981:392.
45. Lines RW. Anal Proc 1981;18:514.
46. Taylor SA, Spence J. J Pharm Pharmacol 1983;35:769.
47. Barnett MI. In: Proceedings PDA international conference on liquid borne particle inspection and metrology. Philadelphia: Parenteral Drug Association, 1987:222.
48. Barber TA. Pharmaceut Technol 1988;12:34.
49. Barnett MI, Nystrom CC, Engvall H. Int J Pharmaceutics 1980;6:131.
50. Lieberman A. Pharm Manufact 1985;2:11.
51. Williams A, Barnett MI. Pharm J 1973;211:190.

Sterilisation

Sterility is defined as the absolute freedom from all viable forms of life and **sterilisation** is the process of producing a condition of sterility. In the context of pharmaceutical products and medical devices, sterility is generally interpreted as the absence of viable micro-organisms. Sterility is therefore an absolute condition and degrees of sterility are not possible. While it is easy to define sterility, there are serious practical problems both in achieving the condition and in demonstrating that such a condition has been achieved.

The major problem in achieving sterility is that when homogeneous populations of organisms are exposed to a lethal agent, they do not all die at the same time. In general, a constant proportion of the surviving population is inactivated for each increment of exposure, that is, the number of organisms decreases exponentially with the extent of exposure (see Microbial Inactivation below). Survival levels below one organism are described as probability functions, for example, a survival level of 10^{-2} is described as a 1 in 100 probability of finding one surviving organism. Because microbial inactivation is exponential, there will always be a finite probability that an organism will survive and although this probability decreases with increasing exposure to the lethal agent it never reaches zero. Sterility, the absence of all viable micro-organisms, is therefore a condition that cannot be practically attained.

Populations of micro-organisms larger than around five organisms can be counted directly by their ability to form colonies on the surface of solid nutrient medium. Survival levels down to 10^{-2} can be determined by the ability of the organism to produce growth, in the form of turbidity in liquid nutrient medium, and the application of Most Probable Number analysis. It should be noted that in both of these enumeration systems, a single organism must be capable of proliferating through many generations to be detected and if it is only able to reproduce through a few generations, it would be classified as non-viable. Below a survival level of 10^{-2}, it is not possible to differentiate between different survival levels since all will result in no visible growth, or apparent total kill. Consequently, even if it was theoretically possible to achieve a condition of sterility, it would not be possible to demonstrate its achievement by practical means.

The problems that are inherent in the strict definition of sterility have led to the development of practical or process definitions of sterility as the probability of a product containing surviving micro-organisms after exposure to a sterilisation process. For a pharmaceutical product or a medical device to be labelled 'sterile', it is generally considered that, on completion of the sterilisation process, the theoretical probability of there being one viable micro-organism present shall be equal to or less than 1 in 10^6 processed items. This is expressed as a **probability of a survivor per item (PSI)**, or more usually as a **sterility assurance level (SAL)**, of equal to or better than 1×10^{-6}. It must be understood that this does not infer that 1 in 10^6 products is allowed to be non-sterile.

The achievement of a defined sterility assurance level is determined by the initial population of micro-organisms (**bioburden**), their resistance to the lethal agent, and the extent of exposure to the lethal agent during the sterilisation process. Factors that influence the resistance of micro-organisms are discussed later in this chapter. Control of materials and processing factors to maintain a very low bioburden on or in the product before sterilisation not only increases the sterility assurance level of the process but also ensures low particulate levels and low endotoxin levels in the sterilised product. Properly conducted and validated terminal sterilisation, where the product in its final sealed container is subjected to a sterilisation process, can achieve a sterility assurance level of equal to or better than 1×10^{-6}. In contrast aseptic processing methods usually provide a sterility assurance level of 1×10^{-3} to 5×10^{-4} as demonstrated by media fill validation studies (see Validation chapter; validation of sterile products). Two approaches have been used to achieve satisfactory sterilisation cycles, the overkill method and the bioburden method. These methods are also used in the validation of sterilisation processes. The **overkill** method designs sterilisation cycles on the basis of the inactivation of a microbial challenge that is greater in numbers and resistance than the natural bioburden of the product. The method may require experimental determination of the decimal reduction time or D-value (see below) of resistant spores in the product, or may be based on a stipulated minimum D-value. A minimum sterility assurance level or, alternatively, a minimum lethality input, for example 6 D or 12 D, for the process is defined and the required sterilisation cycle determined. Compendial sterilisation cycles have been devised using overkill methods. Problems with product stability are often encountered with sterilisation cycles determined by this method.

The **bioburden** method designs sterilisation cycles on the basis of the number and resistance of micro-organisms on or in the product before sterilisation. The maximum bioburden is determined together with the D-value, in the product, of the most resistant bioburden isolate. These data are used, with a suitable safety factor, to determine the sterilisation cycle required to achieve a defined sterility assurance level for the product.

In both methods, D-values are determined from sub-lethal incremental exposures to the sterilisation process and either direct enumeration of survivors and construction of survivor curves or Most Probable Number analysis of fraction-negative data. With sterilisation processes where it is not possible to generate reliable D-values in the steriliser, for example in some ethylene oxide systems, the minimum exposure at which there are no survivors is determined and the cycle is defined as at least double this minimum exposure. This is known as the half-cycle method for sterilisation cycle development. International and European Standards for estimation of bioburden (ISO 11737 and EN 1174) are in preparation.

The physical and chemical agents that are used in sterilisation induce irreparable damage to essential molecules in organisms. There is always the potential for similar reactions to occur in materials subjected to a sterilisation process. These reactions can result in damage to the product or its packaging and may render it unsuitable for its intended purpose. Sterilisation processes are therefore a compromise between the maximum acceptable risk of failing to achieve sterility assurance and the maximum level of product damage that is considered acceptable. The application of bioburden methods and concepts such as F_0 (see below) have led to the development of sterilisation cycles that achieve acceptable sterility assurance levels with minimal product deterioration. Consequently, in the preparation of sterile pharmaceutical products and medical devices, terminal sterilisation is preferred and aseptic processing should only be used if terminal sterilisation compromises product integrity.

KINETICS OF MICROBIAL INACTIVATION

The design of sterilisation processes requires not only a knowledge of the type and initial number of micro-organisms in the material being processed but also an understanding of the kinetics of inactivation of the micro-organisms when exposed to the sterilant and the terms that have been derived to describe microbial inactivation. An appreciation of the factors that influence the resistance of organisms to the sterilant is also necessary.

Microbial Inactivation

When a population of micro-organisms is exposed to a lethal agent the number of surviving cells decreases exponentially with extent of exposure, independent of the initial number of organisms, until viable organisms can no longer be detected. In each equal successive exposure interval the same fraction of remaining survivors is inactivated. When this holds true for the whole of the exposure the '**survivor curve**', that is the plot of logarithm of the number of survivors against exposure time or dose, is linear.

With some organisms there may be an initial lag in killing with extent of exposure before the survivor curve begins to decrease exponentially. This produces a shoulder to the curve which may thereafter be linear. During heat treatment of certain bacterial spores an activation phase representing an initial increase in viable count may be observed. With other organisms the initial portion of the curve may be very steep and non-exponential before it becomes linear, or the survivor curve may begin in a linear fashion but after a certain exposure shows a slowing in the rate of kill known as tailing. In all cases the slope of the linear portion of the survivor curve varies in response to many factors including the severity of the lethal treatment and the presence of protective agents.

Microbial Inactivation Rate Constant (k). A process where microbial inactivation is exponential with respect to time of exposure to the lethal agent can be described by the equation:

$$N_t = N_0 \, e^{-kt}$$

where N_t is the number of surviving organisms after exposure time t, N_0 is the number of viable organisms at time zero and k is the microbial inactivation rate constant. A plot of the logarithm of the fraction of survivors (N_t/N_0) against exposure time will yield a survivor curve which is linear with a negative slope equal to k/2.303, from which k can be calculated. Where ionising radiation is the lethal agent the absorbed dose is substituted for exposure time in the equation.

Decimal Reduction Time (D-value). It is often more convenient to use the **D-value** instead of k as a measure of the rate of microbial inactivation. This is the value of the appropriate parameter of the lethal process (exposure time on absorbed dose) required to reduce the number of viable micro-organisms by 90%, that is, to 10% of the original number. This corresponds to a one log cycle decrease in the survivor curve. For a linear survivor curve the D-value is equal to 2.303/k. D-value and k are measures of the resistance of a micro-organism to a lethal agent and, when reported, the conditions under which they are determined must be precisely defined and quoted. For heat inactivation the D-value is expressed as time in minutes at a defined temperature and the temperature is shown as a subscript, for example, D_{121}. For ionising radiation the D-value is expressed as absorbed dose in kGy, and for gaseous agents it is expressed as time in minutes. Since the calculation of the D-value assumes a linear survivor curve, a correction must be applied where deviations from linearity are observed.

Inactivation Factor (IF). The total microbial inactivation produced by a lethal process can be described by the **inactivation factor (IF)** which is defined as the reduction in the number of viable organisms brought about by the process. The inactivation factor is expressed in terms of the D-value as equal to $10^{t/D}$ where t is the exposure time (or absorbed dose) and D is the D-value for the micro-organism under the specified exposure conditions.

Factors Affecting Microbial Resistance to Inactivation

Resistance to inactivation by physical and chemical agents used in sterilisation processes is a genetically determined characteristic of an organism. Although there are considerable differences in degrees of resistance between different general species and strains of organisms the general pattern of resistance is similar for each type of lethal agent. Unicellular organisms are typically more resistant to inactivation than multicellular organisms. Of the unicellular organisms, non-sporing bacteria

are the most sensitive to inactivation; the psychrophilic bacteria are particularly sensitive. Protozoa and algae, the vegetative forms of yeasts and moulds, and the larger viruses (in particular the non-enveloped viruses) exhibit similar resistance to vegetative bacteria. Acid-fast bacteria are usually more resistant than other vegetative bacteria, especially to inactivation by chemical agents. Bacterial endospores are generally considered to be the most resistant entities to inactivation by physical and chemical agents although there are exceptions, for example, the non-sporing bacterium *Deinococcus radiodurans* is more resistant to ionising radiation. There is also evidence that some of the causative agents of the transmissable degenerative encephalopathies (TDE) exhibit extremely high resistance to lethal agents. Yeast and mould spores are usually less resistant to inactivation than bacterial spores and may be no more resistant than the vegetative forms from which they are derived. Small viruses, in particular the enveloped viruses, exhibit resistance intermediate between that of non-sporing bacteria and bacterial spores.

A criterion of the efficiency of a sterilisation process is its ability to kill high concentrations of resistant bacterial spores. Spores of different bacterial species differ widely in their resistance to a given lethal agent and the resistance of a particular species varies with different lethal agents. For this reason the reference organisms used for testing the efficiency of a particular sterilisation process are spores of a defined species, for example, *Bacillus stearothermophilus* for moist heat, *Bacillus subtilis* for dry heat and ethylene oxide, and *Bacillus pumilus* for ionising radiation. The strain of the organism is also defined since there is considerable genetic variation in the resistance to a specific lethal agent between different strains of the same species.

The apparent resistance of an organism to a specific lethal agent is markedly influenced by environmental factors operating during growth of the organism, during exposure of the organisms to the lethal agent, and during post-exposure recovery of the organism.

The degree of resistance shown by non-sporing organisms may be influenced by their growth phase and age; organisms in the logarithmic phase of growth are generally less resistant than organisms in the stationary phase of growth. The growth temperature, nutrient composition and pH of the growth medium, and availability of gaseous nutrients also influence the resistance of the organisms. Environmental influences during growth of organisms are particularly important where specific resistant isolates from a product are used as reference organisms for a sterilisation process. When the isolates are cultured under laboratory conditions their resistance to lethal agents is invariably reduced.

Resistance of bacterial spores is influenced by the composition of the sporulation medium and the sporulation temperature and may be affected by the techniques used to harvest and clean the spores and by the conditions under which the spores are stored. In the production of bacterial spores for use as reference organisms it is often necessary to use chemically defined sporulation media and standardised growth, harvesting, cleaning, and storage procedures in order to obtain batches of spores with reproducible resistance to a specific lethal agent.

A pharmaceutical formulation may present many factors that are influential during exposure to the lethal agent and can therefore modify the resistance of contaminating micro-organisms. Many organisms in aqueous suspension are more resistant at a neutral pH and the efficiency of a lethal process will therefore be greater with acid or alkaline formulations. Buffer components, ionic strength, and the presence of organic solvents and cosolvents also influence resistance. Carbohydrates, proteins, and lipids have a protective effect on organisms, particularly against heat inactivation. The presence of soluble organic and inorganic compounds can also modify the resistance of organisms to lethal agents.

In general, the presence of moisture and oxygen increases the efficiency of lethal agents although there may be critical ranges of relative humidity for activity of some agents, for example, bactericidal gases. Differences in degrees of resistance, particularly to heat, of bacterial spores on different materials have been attributed to differences in the water activity of the micro-environment of the spores during exposure to the lethal agent. Because microbial resistance is affected by environmental influences during exposure to the lethal agent caution must be exercised in attempting to predict the resistance of organisms in complex pharmaceutical formulations from experimental data obtained in simple solutions. In the design of sterilisation protocols it is necessary to determine the resistance of the reference organism in the product to be processed.

After exposure to the lethal agent an organism must be able to reproduce to the point where it can be detected visually, for example, as a colony on the surface of solid nutrient medium or turbidity in liquid nutrient medium, in order to be classified as a survivor. Suitable conditions for repair of damage and in the case of spores, for activation, germination, and outgrowth, must be available. The recovery conditions that are available to the organisms after exposure to the lethal agent will therefore influence their apparent resistance. Damaged organisms may require longer incubation times than undamaged organisms and the optimum incubation temperature for recovery may be lower than the optimum growth temperature. Damaged organisms are sometimes more exacting in their growth requirements than undamaged organisms and the composition of the recovery medium may thus influence their apparent resistance. In the design of sterilisation protocols the determination of the resistance of the reference organism requires that the recovery conditions must be carefully defined.

METHODS OF STERILISATION

Heat Sterilisation

Of the methods available for sterilisation, heat is the most reliable, versatile, and universally used. Heat is a non-quantised form of energy and therefore its lethal effect on cells is more likely to be due to an accumulation of irreparable damage resulting from generalised chemical reactions within the cell than to destruction of a specific target molecule. The lethal chemical reactions occur more readily in the presence of water and consequently much lower time-temperature exposures are required to kill micro-organisms in the hydrated state than in the dry state. In the hydrated cell, heat inactivation is generally considered to result from irreversible denaturation and coagulation of enzymes and structural proteins, probably by hydrolytic processes, whereas in the dehydrated cell, heat inactivation is primarily the result of oxidative processes. Both types of heat are used for sterilisation; moist heat, usually in the form of saturated steam, at temperatures above $100°$; and dry heat, in the form of hot air, at temperatures above $140°$.

Effect of Temperature on Microbial Resistance

In the design of heat sterilisation processes it is necessary to quantify the effect of temperature changes on the thermal resistance of micro-organisms.

Z-value. When a thermal resistance curve is constructed by plotting the logarithm of the D-value against temperature, a linear relationship is observed. The negative reciprocal of this line is the **Z-value** and represents the increase in temperature that is required to reduce the D-value by 90% or to produce a one log-cycle decrease in the thermal resistance curve. The Z-value is a fundamental characteristic of a micro-organism. For practical purposes it is constant over the small temperature ranges used in heat sterilisation, for example, 115° to 135° for moist heat and 170° to 190° for dry heat.

Q₁₀ Value. The **Q₁₀ value** or temperature coefficient is also a measure of the effect of temperature on microbial resistance and is defined as the change in the microbial inactivation rate constant for a change in temperature of 10°.

Activation Energy for Microbial Inactivation (E). During the heat inactivation of micro-organisms an increase in temperature results in an increase in the microbial inactivation rate constant. The Arrhenius rate theory used in chemical reaction kinetics can also be used to estimate the activation energy for microbial inactivation. If the logarithm of the microbial inactivation rate constant is plotted against the reciprocal of absolute temperature a linear relationship is obtained where the slope of the line is equal to $-E/2.303R$ where R is the universal gas constant. Over the temperature ranges normally used for heat sterilisation there is general compliance with the Arrhenius relationship but caution must be exercised if microbial inactivation data obtained at low temperatures are used to predict the lethal effects of high temperature.

Measures of Heat Sterilisation Efficiency

For heat sterilisation processes a series of time at temperature relationships has become accepted as providing satisfactory sterilisation conditions. These relationships have evolved through a long history of successful use rather than from the application of scientific principle. The currently adopted approach is to design sterilisation protocols with reference to experimentally determined microbial inactivation data and to define the equivalence of different sterilisation processes with respect to the lethality that they impart to specific micro-organisms. The following terms have been derived as measures of heat sterilisation efficiency.

F-value. The **F-value** is a 'unit of lethality' and equates heat treatment at any temperature with the time in minutes at a designated reference temperature with respect to its capacity to destroy spores or vegetative cells of a particular reference organism of stated Z-value. For moist heat at a reference temperature of 121° and a Z-value of 10° the F-value is referred to as F_0, the 'reference unit of lethality'. If a process has an F_0 of 8 the total of all lethal effects of the process on the reference organism is equivalent to 8 minutes at 121°. F_0 can be determined from the following equation:

$$F_0 = D_{121}(\log N_0 - \log N) = D_{121} \log IF$$

where D_{121} is the D-value at 121° for the reference organism, N_0 and N are the initial and final numbers of viable reference organisms respectively and IF is the inactivation factor.

In pharmaceutical applications of moist heat sterilisation the reference organism is usually spores of *Bacillus stearothermophilus* with assumed Z-value of 10° and D_{121} of 1.5 minutes in aqueous systems. Since formulation components can influence the heat resistance of micro-organisms it would be necessary in practice to determine the D_{121} of the reference spores in the product that is being processed. Sterilisation cycles would then be designed on the basis of the F_0 value delivered to the product in its final container located in the slowest heating zone of the steriliser.

The *British Pharmacopoeia 1993* states that 'in general for aqueous preparations a microbiologically validated steam sterilisation process that delivers, in total, an F_0 value of not less than 8 to every container in the load is considered satisfactory. In certain circumstances, however, use of a steam sterilisation process that delivers, in total, an F_0 of less than 8 may be considered justifiable, for example where the product is especially heat sensitive'. For processes that deliver an F_0 of less than 8 the number and resistance of micro-organisms in the product immediately before sterilisation must be known and closely monitored.

The F concept has been applied to dry heat sterilisation using 170° as the reference temperature and spores of *Bacillus subtilis* var. *niger* with Z-value of 20° and D_{170} of 3.2 minutes as the reference organism. It has also been applied to the dry heat destruction of *Escherichia coli* endotoxin using 170° as the reference temperature and a Z-value of 54°.

Lethality Factor (F_i). For moist heat this is the time at any temperature equivalent, in terms of lethality to a particular reference organism of stated Z-value, to one minute at 121°. For a reference organism with a Z-value of $10°$, F_i is equal to the reciprocal of F_0.

Lethality Coefficient (L). The **lethality coefficient** or lethal rate is the rate of microbial inactivation at any process temperature expressed in terms of that at a reference temperature, that is, minutes at the reference temperature per minute at the process temperature. The lethality coefficient is therefore a function of the difference between the process temperature and the reference temperature and the Z-value of the reference organism. For a process temperature T, if the reference temperature is $121°$ and the Z-value of the reference organisms is $10°$, the lethality coefficient is:

$$L = 10^{\frac{(T-121)}{Z}}$$

Integrated Lethality. Heat sterilisation protocols define a holding time at a selected temperature and take no account of the heating-up and cooling-down stages of the sterilisation cycle. Where the bulk and thermal capacity of the load is large, the heating-up and cooling-down stages can be prolonged resulting in significant overheating and product degradation. Moist heat above $100°$ is lethal to bacterial spores and thus during sterilisation the heat imparted during heating-up from $100°$ to the selected temperature and in cooling-down from that temperature to $100°$ will contribute to the overall lethality of the process. The lethality coefficient and the F_0 concept enable integration of the lethality of the total sterilisation process with consequent reduction in processing time and product degradation.

Accurate temperature-time data are required for the product in the slowest heating zone of the steriliser. The temperature at discrete time intervals can then be equated to minutes at $121°$ using the lethality coefficient. The F_0 for the total process is the summation of the lethality coefficients (ΣL) multiplied by the time interval (Δt), that is:

$$F_0 = \Delta t \Sigma L$$

Alternatively, if the lethality coefficients are plotted on a linear scale against time, the F_0 for the process can be obtained from the area under the curve. Computer programs are available that enable the F_0 value to be determined directly and continuously from temperature-time data and are the basis for micro-processor controllers for moist heat sterilisers.

Moist Heat Sterilisation

Moist heat is heat derived from water either as a liquid or as steam under pressure. Moist heat sterilisation usually involves the use of saturated steam under pressure. **Dry saturated steam** is defined as water vapour at a temperature corresponding to the boiling point of the source liquid appropriate to its pressure. Approximately 80% of the heat energy in saturated steam is in the form of latent heat and this is released when the steam contacts a cooler surface and condenses. Condensation is accompanied by an instantaneous contraction of the steam, creating a low pressure region into which more steam flows. The result is rapid penetration of the steam into articles being sterilised together with rapid heating and moisture input.

Dry saturated steam is used as a heat transfer medium, for example, to raise the temperature of fluids in containers to the selected temperature or as a direct contact sterilant, for example, in porous load sterilisers. When used as a direct contact sterilant, the quality of the steam is of paramount importance.

If the temperature of dry saturated steam is raised, at constant pressure, or if the pressure is reduced at constant temperature, the degree of saturation is reduced and the steam becomes superheated. **Superheated steam** condenses less readily than dry saturated steam and, since the heat transfer will be the same as that of hot air, it is a less effective sterilant. Superheat can arise from adiabatic expansion as a result of excessive reduction in pressure through reducing valves, from evolution of heat of hydration from very dry cotton textiles, or from the steriliser jacket being maintained at a higher temperature than the chamber. Non-condensable gases in the steam supply may also produce superheat, in addition to restricting steam penetration.

Wet steam must also be avoided since this will result in reduced penetration of steam in materials and wet loads at the end of the sterilisation process. A maximum concentration of entrained moisture of 5% by weight is recommended.

The holding time-temperature relationships for moist heat sterilisation are shown in Table 1.

Table 1
Holding time-temperature relationships for moist heat sterilisation

Temperature range (°C)	Minimum holding time at temperature (minutes)	F_0 value (minutes)
115–118	30	7.5–15
121–124	15	15–30
126–129	10	32–63
134–138	3	60–150

It is apparent from observing the F_0 delivered by these protocols that they are not comparable in terms of the microbial lethality that they produce. The application of the F_0 concept to moist heat sterilisation has facilitated a more rational approach to the design of sterilisation protocols. An understanding of the activation energies for microbial inactivation and product degradation has led to the design of optimum time-temperature relationships for particular applications that ensure maximum microbial inactivation with minimum damage to the product. The activation energy for microbial inactivation is of the order of 270 to 300 kJ per organism for bacterial spores whereas the activation energy for hydrolytic or oxidative chemical degradation in aqueous solution is of the order of 70 to 100 kJ/mol. These differences mean that a short time-high temperature sterilisation cycle that will deliver the same microbial lethality or F_0 as a long time-low temperature cycle will result in significantly less product deterioration.

Moist heat sterilisation is the method of choice for sterilising aqueous pharmaceutical preparations and surgical materials. It is not suitable for materials that are temperature, pressure, or moisture sensitive. Thermostable aqueous solutions presented as small volume injections (1 to 50 mL) in glass ampoules, as large volume injections (greater than 100 mL) in glass or plastic containers, or as ophthalmic preparations and irrigation solutions can be sterilised by moist heat. Thermostable aqueous suspensions and oil-in-water emulsions used in parenteral nutrition can also be sterilised by this method. Moist heat sterilisation is also applied to plastic and glass containers, to elastomeric closures, and to polymeric membrane filters. Polycarbonate, polypropylene, some polyurethanes and polysulphones are particularly suited to moist heat processing. Preparation of sterile culture media and decontamination of contaminated materials is also carried out using moist heat.

Moist heat is used in porous load sterilisers to process rubber gloves, rubber sheets and tubing, surgical gowns and drapes, and surgical dressings composed of cotton, rayon or other cellulose material. In these situations it is essential that the packaging material must be permeable to air and steam and must maintain resistance to heat and damage particularly when wet. European Standards for packaging materials for sterilisation of wrapped goods are in preparation. A number of complex medical devices such as dialysers, extracorporeal blood circuit devices and fistula cannulae are also available as moist-heat sterilised items. Caution must be exercised in heat sterilising items made up of a combination of materials where differential expansion on heating can lead to breakage.

Bench Sterilisers

The simplest design of steam steriliser or autoclave is the bench or laboratory steriliser. This is usually a non-jacketed upright vessel of about 15 litres capacity generating its own steam from water in the base of the steriliser chamber by external (gas) heating or internal (electric immersion or steam coil) heating. The chamber temperature is generally controlled by a bimetallic thermostat regulating the heating system. It is equipped with an air and steam discharge valve, a pressure gauge, a thermometer or thermocouple and an adjustable safety valve.

In operation, preparations in their final sealed containers are placed in the cold chamber and the lid sealed. Air is vented from the chamber by means of the air and steam discharge valve during the initial heating-up and boiling period. When steam has issued freely from the discharge valve for 3 to 5 minutes, most of the air capable of being displaced by this method will have been dispersed. The discharge valve is then closed and the temperature of the chamber allowed to rise until a preselected sterilisation temperature is reached. The thermostat which is preset to operate at the chosen temperature then maintains the correct conditions until the end of the sterilising period. The heat is then turned off and the steriliser allowed to cool, without releasing the pressure, until zero gauge pressure (atmospheric pressure) is reached. The discharge valve is opened to avoid the creation of a partial vacuum and the load allowed to cool until any fluids are below 80°.

Some older bench sterilisers operate in the same way as domestic pressure cookers and are controlled by regulating the steam pressure rather than the temperature. In general, it is unwise to rely on any bench steriliser not fitted with an adjustable thermostat and depending on pressure regulation alone to control the temperature.

Due to the ejection of water droplets from the surface of the boiling water, the bench steriliser is only suitable for bottled fluids. It may be used for laboratory work and small-scale production of materials such as culture media. Other materials, for example apparatus or dressings, including their wrappings, will become soaked with water during sterilisation. This may be deleterious to them and can result in their recontamination after removal into a non-sterile atmosphere unless they are immediately subjected to a drying process.

Transportable Steam Steriliser

This is a small electrically heated bench-top steam steriliser designed for the sterilisation of unwrapped instruments and utensils. In order to provide a rapid cycle they are non-jacketed. Steam is generated as in the bench steriliser by boiling water in the chamber. Air within the chamber is removed through the discharge valve by turbulent mixing of the steam and the air. The requirements for this type of steriliser are detailed in British Standard 3970:Part 4:1990 and in Health Equipment Information (HEI) 185(1988) and 196(1990). The standard covers machines that provide a single operating cycle at the preferred sterilisation temperature of 134° to 138°. To prevent the selection of inappropriate conditions for the cycle, the operation of the cycle is controlled by an automatic controller with the conditions preset within the controller. Temperature measurement is either in the coolest part of the steriliser chamber or in the discharge valve; separate systems for indication and control of temperature are required. Instrumentation to indicate pressure within the chamber and a system to indicate the stage of the sterilisation cycle are also provided. In the event of appropriate conditions not being maintained during the sterilisation cycle, a fault indication is displayed. In this situation it is not possible to open the door in the same manner as after a satisfactory cycle, thus preventing the inadvertent use of instruments processed in an unsatisfactory cycle. Transportable steam sterilisers are designed to process unwrapped goods for immediate use. The attainment of sterilisation is dependent upon intimate contact between saturated steam and the surface of the instruments to be sterilised and requires effective removal of air from the steriliser and its replacement with steam. Air removal from this type of steriliser is inefficient and consequently these sterilisers are not suitable for processing wrapped goods or porous loads since they do not incorporate features to adequately remove air from such loads. Furthermore, although some transportable steam sterilisers incorporate 'drying' in the operating cycle, the lack of a suitable vacuum drying stage means that the majority of such loads would be wet at the end of the cycle and prone to recontamination. Transportable steam sterilisers are also unsuitable for processing fluids in sealed containers.

Downward Displacement Steriliser

The downward or gravity displacement steriliser consists of a sterilising chamber, usually horizontal, fed from an external steam source via a separator which removes water droplets from the steam. The steam is admitted to the top of the chamber by means of a baffle. As the steam entering the chamber is at a lower density than air at the same temperature, the latter is displaced in a downward direction and is vented through a drain in the lowest point of the chamber. Condensation of steam occurs on the cooler surfaces within the chamber and the condensate will also be vented through the drain. The venting continues throughout the sterilising cycle as condensate is formed and air flows out of the load, and the drain line must therefore be fitted with an automatic near-to-steam trap which discharges air and condensate while retaining saturated steam in the chamber. The drain is sited so as to prevent back-syphoning of contaminated water into the steriliser chamber.

Temperature is monitored by thermocouples placed in the load which record externally and by a thermocouple located in the drain line. Temperature control is by regulation of the steam pressure from a high pressure steam line via reducing valves. The provision of dry saturated steam and the control of steam quality are therefore important. British Standard 3970:Part 2:1991 outlines the detailed requirements for this type of steriliser. The chamber is loaded, adequate spaces being allowed between the items comprising the load so that air can escape in a downward direction and pockets of trapped air are avoided. This also applies to the arrangement of separate articles inside wrapped packages. The chamber is then closed and steam is admitted. The timing of the sterilising cycle commences when the load thermocouple indicates that the chosen temperature has been reached. This is then usually maintained by the automatic operation of the reducing valve in the main steam line.

The cooling phase of the cycle depends upon the nature of the material being sterilised. With packages, rapid exhaust is normally used to eject the steam as rapidly as possible from the chamber to flash-dry the contents. Bottled fluids must be subjected to slow reduction of chamber pressure due to the high internal pressure in the container. These are allowed to cool in the chamber until zero gauge pressure is reached, and a further cooling period allowed until the contents of all containers are below 80°. A door interlock operating through a load simulator is fitted to prevent premature opening of the steriliser, since explosions have resulted from the transfer of loads of hot bottled fluids from sterilisers into areas at ambient temperature.

The cooling time for a large load of bottled fluids to cool to 80° can be extremely long due to the large heat capacity and the slow rate of heat transfer through and from the glass walls. To minimise thermal degradation of the product and at the same time reduce process time, it may be necessary to achieve cooling as rapidly as possible. This may be achieved by water-spray cooling. The water used for the purpose is usually sterile. The chamber must be pressurised with air, before the start of the water spray, to compensate for the reduction in pressure produced when the steam is rapidly condensed. At the end of the sterilising cycle, filtered compressed air is admitted to the chamber and after the pressure has stabilised, water-spray cooling is initiated.

Steam-Air Overpressure Steriliser

Flexible plastic containers have largely replaced glass containers for the packaging of sterile fluids, particularly intravenous fluids. The internal pressure that develops in these containers during the sterilisation cycle can cause them to burst. It is therefore necessary to provide an overpressure greater than the corresponding saturated steam pressure by maintaining a proportion of air within the steriliser chamber. The extent of the overpressure will depend upon the type and design of the container and the amount of airspace above the fluid.

In steam-air overpressure sterilisers, air removal is unnecessary. Steam is admitted to the chamber and a circulating fan system is used to ensure good circulation and mixing of the steam and air. The chamber temperature is maintained by incremental addition of steam and the chamber pressure is controlled by venting or introduction of filtered compressed air. At the end of the sterilising cycle the steam input is stopped but the chamber pressure is maintained until the load has cooled to a temperature sufficient to permit the overpressure to be reduced. Water-spray cooling may be incorporated to accelerate the cooling stage of the cycle.

Water Spray-Air Overpressure Steriliser

This type of steriliser is designed for the processing of fluids packaged in flexible plastic containers. Since in this process the heat transfer medium is superheated water, loading of the chamber must ensure that the water contacts all containers.

Water in the chamber is heated in a heat exchanger or by steam injection and continuously circulated and sprayed into the chamber to ensure uniform heating of the product. Chamber pressure is controlled by the addition of filtered compressed air to obtain the required overpressure. At the end of the sterilising cycle, heat input is stopped but the air overpressure and the water spray are maintained. The water is cooled in an external heat exchanger to accelerate cooling of the load to the temperature at which the chamber pressure can be reduced to atmospheric pressure without causing the containers to burst.

Porous Load Steriliser

Sterilisation of porous loads in a downward displacement steriliser presents serious problems concerning removal of air from the load and drying of the load at the end of the sterilisation cycle. These problems have been overcome with the development of porous load or high-vacuum sterilisers. These consist of a jacketed chamber capable of being evacuated to a low residual pressure by means of oil-sealed or water ring pumps backed by cold condensers. Detailed requirements for this type of steriliser are outlined in British Standard 3970:Part 3:1990.

Unlike the downward displacement steriliser, the porous load steriliser functions best with a full load. Air and non-condensable gases are removed in the first part of the cycle, the pre-vacuum stage, where the chamber pressure is reduced to about 2.5 kPa absolute pressure. This is followed by alternate steam injection and evacuation (pulsing) and further evacuation to dilute and remove traces of residual air. When the latter is at a negligible level, steam is admitted rapidly to operating pressure and temperature. During the sterilising stage of the cycle the chamber temperature is maintained at the process temperature, usually 134°, by controlled steam input.

The post-vacuum stage follows involving very rapid evacuation to 6.7 kPa absolute pressure or less to remove the steam and flash-dry the chamber contents. If this evacuation is rapid, no holding time is necessary with loosely packed items as all condensate and retained moisture boils off almost instantly. With tightly packed dressings or apparatus such as tubing or pipettes, prolongation of this drying cycle may be necessary according to the permeability of the load. Air is then admitted to the chamber through a bacteria-proof filter until atmospheric pressure is reached.

Operation of the steriliser is under automatic control and the total cycle time from loading to unloading should not exceed 35 minutes. Leak detection devices are fitted to the steriliser to test the integrity of the chamber and air detectors are incorporated to ensure that adequate air removal is achieved. The Bowie Dick Test (see below) is the standard test for steam penetration and is performed on porous load sterilisers on each day of operation.

Continuous Steriliser

Industrial requirements for the production of large batches of sterile fluids have led to the development of continuous sterilisers. These consist of a tower approximately 17 m high containing three interconnecting chambers; a water-filled preheating column, a central steam-filled sterilising column, and a water-filled cooling column. The hydrostatic pressure in the pre-heating and cooling columns seals and counterbalances the pressure of steam in the sterilising column. The sterilising temperature in the continuous steriliser is therefore infinitely variable. Containers are moved through the columns on an ascending and descending conveyor belt, the holding time in each column being governed by the conveyor belt speed. Additional sequential spray-cooling and drying sections may be incorporated in the steriliser.

Steam Sterilisation-in-place

Steam sterilisation-in-place (SIP) is being used in the pharmaceutical and biotechnology industries to provide enhanced sterility assurance for processes such as aseptic filling. With SIP a complete system of holding tanks, product transfer lines, and filling lines can be sterilised as a unit thereby reducing the amount of aseptic assembly required. Initial removal of air is crucial to ensure that dry saturated steam is used in the sterilisation process. Evacuation systems are not usually practicable and air removal must be via carefully positioned bleed valves. Since SIP systems are not usually jacketed or insulated they will produce large amounts of condensate. Condensate removal via near-to-steam traps must be provided in all horizontal legs and at all low parts in the system and, where possible, pipework is angled to improve drainage. The process can be automatically controlled to maintain sterilising conditions as monitored at the lowest temperature region of the system, usually the condensate drain line, to attain a pre-designated F_0 value.

At the end of the steam sterilising period, air or nitrogen is introduced through a bacteria-proof filter and the system purged of residual steam and condensate. A flow of pressurised gas is maintained to dry the system which is then kept under positive pressure to maintain sterility before use. Care must be taken in the design of SIP systems to ensure that the integrity of components, particularly filters, is maintained.

Dry Heat Sterilisation

Holding time-temperature relationships for dry heat sterilisation are given in Table 2.

Table 2
Holding time-temperature relationships for dry heat sterilisation

Temperature (°C)	Minimum holding time at temperature (minutes)
160	120
170	60
180	30

The *British Pharmacopoeia 1993*, in recommending these protocols, accepts other holding time-temperature relationships, for example some oils require lower temperatures.

Dry heat sterilisation is used for items that are thermostable but are either moisture sensitive or impermeable to steam. It is used for the sterilisation of dry powdered drugs and for suspensions of drugs in non-aqueous solvents. Oils, fats, waxes, liquid, soft and hard paraffin, and lubricants such as silicones can also be sterilised by dry heat. The process is applicable to oily injections, implants, and ophthalmic ointment bases and to certain surgical dressings, for example paraffin gauze dressing and absorbable gelatin sponge. Glass and metal containers and surgical instruments are also sterilised by dry heat. At temperatures above 250° dry heat is used to both sterilise and depyrogenate glassware.

Hot Air Oven

The hot air oven comprises an electrically heated, insulated chamber fitted with an insulated door. The chamber is usually of stainless steel construction and the inner surfaces are polished to minimise heat loss. Heating elements are arranged around the chamber walls in a manner that prevents localised heating within the chamber. Heat is delivered to the load primarily by convection and radiation and, since the rate of diffusion and penetration by these methods is low, a fan or turbo blower must be fitted for efficient air circulation and heat distribution within the oven. Shelves within the chamber are perforated or of mesh construction to allow the free circulation of air. Temperature is controlled by a bimetallic thermostat and thermocouples are used to monitor the temperature in the chamber and in the load. Hot air ovens must be fitted with door interlocks to prevent opening during the sterilisation cycle and should be automatically controlled. A British Standard defining the requirements for hot air ovens for sterilisation (replacing British Standard 3241:1961), is in preparation. The oven should be pre-heated to the temperature of operation before loading to minimise heating-up time. Individual items in the load should be positioned to allow plenty of air space and good air flow between them and to prevent contact with the sides of the chamber. Wrapping and containers should be composed of suitable materials and should be of adequate thickness to provide good heat conduction. Paper and cardboard are suitable but may char at high temperatures, therefore aluminium foil and metal containers are usually used. Metal containers are best anodised black to accelerate heat absorption. Container geometry should be such as to maximise heat penetration. As the variation in heating lag can be considerable for different objects, it is advisable to avoid loads of mixed type. The heating-up time for a given load can also be very variable and should be determined for each load.

The load is maintained at the sterilising temperature for a period long enough to ensure that the whole has been subjected to the correct temperature for the correct time. The temperature variation in the loaded oven should not exceed ±5° of the sterilisation temperature during the hold period. The load is then allowed to cool in the oven to around 40° before removal.

Poor heat conduction of materials can necessitate extended heating-up times and this, together with the long exposure times required for dry heat sterilisation and subsequent slow cooling of the product, results in long process times. Reductions in total process time have been achieved by the use of forced cooling and the introduction of sterile air to the chamber at the end of the hold period.

Infrared Conveyor Oven

As batch sterilisation in a hot air oven has a prolonged cycle time, other dry heat methods have been evolved to increase efficiency. For continuous production of large numbers of sterile items, infrared heated ovens have been devised, equipped with conveyor belts. Infrared heaters are usually spiral wound nickel chrome elements enclosed in quartz envelopes. Infrared radiation transmits heat directly to surfaces that absorb it. Subsequent heat penetration is by conduction and is very slow. Loading of the steriliser must ensure that no part of the load is occluded from direct contact with the radiation. This type of dry heat steriliser was originally designed for use with glass syringes but with the introduction of disposable plastic syringes is no longer widely used.

A high speed infrared oven operating *in vacuo* has been designed for sterilisation of surgical instruments. This functions at 280° in high vacuum and the vacuum break is achieved with sterile nitrogen to avoid oxidation of the cutting edges. The total cycle time is about 15 minutes.

Sterilisation and Depyrogenation Tunnels

The industrial production of aseptically prepared parenteral products requires the provision of containers that are clean, sterile, pyrogen-free, and protected from subsequent contamination before filling and closure. Pyrogens of bacterial origin (endotoxins) are highly resistant to physical and chemical inactivation (see Pyrogens chapter). The method of choice for inactivation of heat-resistant material such as glass and metal has been exposure to dry heat at temperatures above 250° for not less than 30 minutes. These conditions provide a combined sterilisation and depyrogenation process.

Continuous sterilisation and depyrogenation tunnels have been developed to satisfy the demands of modern high-speed filling lines. In these tunnels, air is heated and passed through HEPA filters (see below) in a vertical downward direction. The hot laminar flow air is a more efficient heat transfer medium than conventional hot air and also prevents particulate contamination. A conveyor belt transports the containers through the tunnel where they are exposed to a short time-high temperature protocol and then cooled rapidly in HEPA filtered laminar flow air.

An alternative design utilises the infrared conveyor oven in combination with HEPA filtered air in the cooling zone of the tunnel. A system of fans and air curtains uses the HEPA filtered air in the cooling zone to generate a horizontal laminar flow of clean air in the heating zone moving towards the tunnel entrance (counter flow).

Radiation Sterilisation

Radiation sterilisation is the method of choice for heat sensitive materials that are able to withstand the high radiation levels employed in the process. Two types of radiation are used in sterilisation: electromagnetic (for example, gamma-rays, X-rays, and ultraviolet light) and particulate (for example, high energy electrons).

Gamma Radiation

Gamma-rays are high energy electromagnetic emanations with a wavelength in the range of 1 to 10^{-4} nm and energy values of 10^6 to 10^9 eV. When absorbed within the cell, they cause ionisation of the cell contents, free radical formation and excited molecules leading to disorganisation of enzymes and DNA and cell death. Resistance to radiation is related to the extent of cell damage necessary to cause death and the capacity of the organism to effectively repair the damage. Unlike heat, the effect of gamma radiation is cumulative, divided doses being as effective as a single dose of the same total magnitude. It is highly penetrative, produces a negligible temperature rise in the irradiated object at normal dose rates, and does not induce radioactivity.

The usual source of gamma radiation for sterilisation is Cobalt-60 which emits radiation consisting of two photons of 1.33 MeV and 1.17 MeV, respectively, and has a half-life of 5.25 years. Some smaller radiation plants use Caesium-137 which emits radiation consisting of a single photon at 1.61 MeV and has a half-life of around 30 years. Gamma radiation plants usually contain 1×10^{16} to 4×10^{16} Bq of activity. Emission of gamma-rays from the source is continuous and elaborate housing and safety precautions are required to protect the environment and the operators from radiation effects. The source in the form of an array of rods is housed in a reinforced concrete building and when not in use is submerged in water to provide both shielding and cooling.

Radiation sterilisation is performed either as a batch or as a continuous process. In a batch process the load is placed in a static position in the irradiation chamber, close to the source. Variation in the dose absorbed by items within the load can occur and to overcome this a system may be employed to change the position of the load at regular intervals. In the continuous process the load is passed through the irradiation chamber on a conveyor system in a manner that ensures that all parts of the load receive an equal dose.

The dose delivered to the load is dependent upon the source strength, the distance of the load from the source, the density of the material between the load and the source, and the exposure time, which may be up to 18 hours. The exposure time must be corrected to take into account the decay of the source. In the UK and most of Europe a minimum absorbed dose of 25 kGy has normally been required for radiation sterilisation. In Scandinavia doses of up to 35 kGy have been specified. In order to obtain an adequate assurance of sterility with minimum product damage the Association for the Advancement of Medical Instrumentation (AAMI) in the USA has developed dose-setting guidelines, based on the radiation resistance and numbers of the bioburden, to determine the minimum acceptable dose. These methods are based on determining the radiation dose that yields a sterility assurance level of 10^{-2} and using a dose-setting multiplier to extrapolate to a sterility assurance level of 10^{-6}. International and European Standards in press (ISO 11137 and EN 552), allow both the overkill (defined minimum dose) approach and the bioburden approach to be taken when establishing the sterilising dose.

The efficiency of gamma radiation is markedly affected by environmental factors. The presence of oxygen increases the sensitivity of organisms to ionising radiation due to the formation of hydroperoxyl radicals. Organisms are more sensitive to radiation in the fully hydrated state due to the additional lethality induced by the radiolysis products of water. Protective agents such as sulphydryl-containing compounds, ascorbates, and glycerol increase resistance.

Some materials such as natural rubber, acrylonitrile butadiene styrene (ABS), styrene, polyethylene, polycarbonate, polysulphones, silicones, cellulosics, and nylon exhibit few if any changes after gamma irradiation. However, the radiation doses used in sterilisation can adversely affect many materials. Discoloration may occur during irradiation with some glass and plastics such as polyvinyl chloride, polytetrafluoroethylene, and polypropylene and may continue after irradiation. Liberation of gas may occur (for example, hydrogen chloride from polyvinyl chloride) and alterations in mechanical properties such as brittleness and hardness may be observed. Radiation-induced degradation of materials is greatest in the presence of water and this limits the use of gamma radiation for sterilisation of aqueous drug solutions.

Gamma radiation has been successfully used for the sterilisation of a broad range of pharmaceutical materials including enzymes, vitamins, minerals, antibiotics, monoclonal antibodies, and peptides. It is also used to sterilise containers and closures and cleanroom consumables. Plasma, tissue, and bone grafts can be sterilised by gamma radiation. A major use of gamma radiation is for the sterilisation of medical devices including surgical gowns, hoods and masks, dressings, plastic disposable equipment (for example, petri dishes, catheters and syringes), needles, surgical blades, prosthetic implants, blood dialysis devices, and oxygenators.

High Energy Electrons

These are β-particles, accelerated to a high energy level by the application of high voltage potentials, with which the articles to be sterilised are bombarded. Generation of accelerated electrons can be discontinuous and does not require radioactive materials. In the van de Graaff accelerator a high energy electron beam is generated by accelerating electrons from a hot filament down an evacuated tube under high potential difference. Electrons with energies up to 5 MeV are produced in this type of accelerator. In the microwave linear accelerator a synchronised travelling microwave is used to impart additional energy to the electron beam to produce a pulsed beam of accelerated electrons with a maximum energy of 10 MeV. A maximum energy of 10 MeV is used to minimise induced radioactivity in the product.

Since accelerated electrons can generate X-rays the environment and personnel must be protected by concrete shielding. Products are passed through the electron beam steriliser on a conveyor system that is designed to ensure that the containers are irradiated from two opposing sides. The electron beam is of small dimensions and is therefore magnetically scanned over the surface of the container. Absorbed dose is determined by the speed of the conveyor and the scan speed of the electron beam.

A major restriction to the use of high energy electrons is their low penetrative power compared to gamma-rays. Penetration is a function of the energy of the electrons and the density of the material being irradiated. Products consisting of components of differing densities can present serious problems. Orientation of items in the container and of the container with respect to the electron beam can also affect the absorbed dose. The high dose rates, of the order of 2 kGy/s, that can be obtained with high energy electrons mean that the minimum absorbed dose of 25 kGy can be achieved very rapidly. A further consequence of a high dose rate is that less damage may be induced in products during irradiation. A slight but significant increase in the product temperature can occur after exposure to a high electron beam dose rate. High energy electrons are used as an alternative to gamma radiation in the industrial sterilisation of single-use health-care products. The development of accelerators that can achieve powers of up to 100 kW at energies of 5 MeV to 10 MeV could enable the construction of plants that could operate in dual-mode as X-ray or electron beam sterilisers.

Machine-generated X-radiation

The generation of electromagnetic radiation with high penetrative power, discontinuously and without the use of radioactive materials, has potential advantage in sterilisation applications and has led to current investigations into the use of machine generated X-rays as a sterilant. X-rays are produced as secondary radiation by the bombardment of a heavy metal target with a beam of high energy electrons from a linear accelerator. There are problems in establishing dosimetry and in dissipating the large amount of heat produced by the process. Since only a small percentage of the electrons are converted into X-rays, utilisation of input energy in the process is low and machine-generated X-radiation is consequently very expensive.

Ultraviolet Light

Ultraviolet (UV) radiation has a wavelength range between 210 nm and 328 nm. Maximum bactericidal activity is shown at 253.7 nm. This is the absorption peak for DNA which is the major target site for ultraviolet radiation. Ultraviolet radiation is normally produced by low pressure, hot cathode mercury vapour lamps designed to operate at an ambient temperature of about 30° to 40°. Their efficiency is seriously affected by dust, a decrease in the ambient temperature and the ageing of the lamp.

Ultraviolet radiation is low energy (around 10^2 eV) and is non-ionising, producing only increased excitation of molecules. Only micro-organisms directly exposed to the radiation will be affected by it. Furthermore, most organisms possess enzymatic processes that are capable of repairing damage induced by ultraviolet radiation. Radiation of this type has poor penetrating power and is extensively absorbed by glass, plastics, and turbid liquids. It is therefore only suitable for the sterilisation of air and water in thin layers and of hard impermeable surfaces; it is not recommended for product sterilisation. The synergy that has been observed between ultraviolet radiation and hydrogen peroxide may provide the basis for a more efficient sterilisation process. Operators need protection from the effects of ultraviolet radiation, particularly on the skin and eyes.

Gas Plasma

A gas plasma is a highly ionised body of gas produced through the action of either very high temperatures or strong electric or magnetic fields. It is composed of positive ions and electrons together with ionised neutral molecules. Plasmas produced by arcs or plasma jets are described as high-temperature plasmas with temperatures in excess of $4500°$ and are of little use in sterilisation. Low-temperature plasmas including glow discharges and corona discharges show greater potential as sterilants.

Low-temperature plasmas are generated in an enclosed chamber under vacuum using radiofrequency or microwave energy to excite the contained gas molecules. The level of vacuum in the chamber is important since greater energy and reactivity of the plasma is attained under very low vacuum. A vacuum in the range 10 Pa to 100 Pa is usually required for applications in sterilisation. The precursor gas used in the system can be inert (for example, argon, helium or nitrogen) or reactive (for example, air, oxygen, hydrogen, nitrous oxide, or hydrogen peroxide vapour). In general, more reactive plasmas are generated from reactive precursors. It is also desirable to select those precursors whose chemical residues or by-products are non-toxic. The mechanisms by which gas plasmas induce microbial death have not been established but free radicals and reactive species, micro-incineration, and ultraviolet radiation emitted by the plasma have all been implicated.

Low-temperature plasmas have average electron energies in the range 1 to 10 eV. They therefore have low penetrative powers and are only applicable to sterilisation of surfaces. Since they are generated at low pressure they cannot be used for sterilisation of liquids. Plasmas initiated in air by a Q-switched ruby laser and coupled with a microwave field have been used to sterilise glass vials. Sterilising conditions have also been produced using hydrogen peroxide vapour, at a concentration of 0.2 mg/litre, as the precursor in either a microwave discharge system or an inductive radio-frequency discharge system. The temperature of the gas plasma is around $40°$. Furthermore, if sufficient time is allowed for the precursor gas to diffuse through the packaging, the gas plasma can be generated inside the package thereby facilitating the sterilisation of packaged materials such as surgical instruments. Gas plasmas are routinely used to remove thin proteinaceous films and other contaminants from surfaces and surface modification of some materials, for example stainless steel, may occur during sterilisation.

Gaseous Sterilisation

Chemical vapours can be used to sterilise articles that cannot withstand the temperatures employed in moist heat and dry heat sterilisation or the high radiation doses used in radiation sterilisation. Of the many compounds available only a limited number have been found to be generally suitable and then only when the critical conditions of concentration, temperature, relative humidity, and exposure time are carefully controlled. As it is not always practicable to monitor all of the factors operating during gaseous sterilisation by physical or chemical means, it is necessary to include biological indicators in every load. In view of the critical nature of gaseous sterilisation procedures it is inadvisable to use them if more reliable methods are available.

Ethylene Oxide

At atmospheric pressure and ambient temperature ethylene oxide is a colourless gas which liquefies at $10.8°$ and freezes at $-111.3°$. Pure ethylene oxide gas is inflammable and explosive in mixtures of concentration greater than 3.6% in air and efficient air removal is required if it is used as a sterilant. The explosion hazard can be reduced by admixture with an inert carrier such as carbon dioxide, nitrogen, or chlorofluorocarbons. A 10% mixture with carbon dioxide has a high vapour pressure and is often preferred for use in large industrial sterilisers. A 12% mixture with dichlorofluoromethane is used in smaller sterilisers. The use of chlorofluorocarbons is being phased out because of their adverse effect on the earth's protective ozone layer and the use of alternative diluent gases including hydrochlorofluorocarbons is being investigated. Admixture of ethylene oxide with diluent gases also minimises polymerisation which can occur in the liquid phase.

Ethylene oxide is a direct-acting mutagen and a suspected human carcinogen. The symptoms of acute toxicity resulting from inhalation include headache, nausea, vomiting, and respiratory and conjunctival irritation. Dermal contact causes skin burns and sensitisation. Chronic exposure may be associated with neurological, ocular, and haematological effects. The use of ethylene oxide is therefore controlled to protect the environment and the health and safety of workers and patients. In the UK the maximum exposure level as a time weighted average (TWA) over eight hours is 5 ppm.

Ethylene oxide is a potent alkylating agent and its antimicrobial activity is attributed to alkylation of sulphydryl, hydroxyl, carboxyl, and amino groups on proteins, and amino groups on nucleic acids. It is active against all micro-organisms and, under the controlled conditions used in sterilisation, produces log-linear survivor curves. Microbial lethality of ethylene oxide is a function of the water content of the organisms, the gas concentration, the temperature, and the exposure time. It is generally considered that the relative humidity range 33% to 60% is critical for the action of ethylene oxide and must be maintained throughout the sterilisation process. At relative humidities above 60% ethylene oxide may be hydrolysed to less active ethylene glycol. Dehydrated organisms are resistant to ethylene oxide and, as they rehydrate slowly, they must be equilibrated to the required relative humidity before exposure to ethylene oxide. Organisms on hygroscopic materials, occluded in crystals or protected by organic matter or gas-impermeable deposits are resistant to inactivation by ethylene oxide. Controlled pre-humidification of materials before sterilisation is therefore essential and packaging must be permeable to air, water vapour, and ethylene oxide. Ethylene oxide at a concentration of 50 mg/litre is sporicidal but higher concentrations are used for sterilisation to reduce the exposure time.

Antimicrobial activity of ethylene oxide increases with increasing temperature and to reduce exposure times it is desirable to use as high a temperature as possible. Since ethylene oxide sterilisation is designed as a low temperature process the temperature range usually used is 40° to 60°. Over this temperature range, and at the gas concentrations usually employed, the Q_{10} for microbial lethality is 2 to 3.

Because of the complex interrelationships between the factors that affect the activity of ethylene oxide there is no standard cycle for ethylene oxide sterilisation. Cycles in use employ a range of conditions which include gas concentrations 250 mg/litre to 1500 mg/litre, relative humidity 30% to 90%, temperature 30° to 65°, and exposure times 1 hour to 30 hours. The characteristics of a particular product also influence the conditions that can be used and thus the sterilisation cycle must be specifically designed for that product and validated microbiologically using reference organisms.

An ethylene oxide steriliser comprises a gas-tight jacketed stainless steel chamber capable of withstanding high pressure and vacuum. To increase the efficacy of the process and reduce the cycle time the relative humidity of the load is usually controlled by preconditioning before sterilisation. The load is placed in the steriliser chamber in a defined configuration and a vacuum drawn to around 2 kPa to ensure air removal and ethylene oxide penetration. Pulses of subatmospheric steam are admitted to the chamber to humidify the load and replace moisture lost during the evacuation stage, and to condition the load to the sterilisation temperature. Ethylene oxide gas is then admitted via a heated vaporiser. Forced gas circulation using fans or external recirculation loops is used to ensure homogeneity within the chamber. Gas concentration is controlled by the pressure within the chamber and monitored independently, either by chemical analysis, or more usually by weight loss from the supply cylinder. At the end of the exposure period the gas is exhausted and either subjected to acid hydrolysis, or catalytic oxidation, or recycled. Vacuum/sterile air purges are introduced to disperse residual traces of the gas. Sterilisers may operate either subatmospheric cycles using pure ethylene oxide or supra-atmospheric cycles using ethylene oxide gas mixtures and should be automatically controlled. A European Standard specification for ethylene oxide sterilisers is in preparation.

Ethylene oxide is highly penetrant and residues, including the toxic reaction products ethylene chlorohydrin and ethylene glycol, must be removed from the sterilised products. Post-sterilisation quarantine under controlled temperature and airflow conditions, often for 7 to 10 days, is required to allow residues to degas from the load. The *European Pharmacopoeia* specifies maximum ethylene oxide residues of 10 ppm, as determined by a specific method, for sterile single-use plastic syringes and sets for transfusion of blood and blood products. International and European Standards for limits and test methods for ethylene oxide residues in medical products are in preparation. In spite of its high reactivity, few materials are damaged by ethylene oxide. The major use of ethylene oxide is in the terminal sterilisation of medical devices including dressings, catheters and tubing, intravenous infusion sets, syringes and needles, prostheses, intraocular lenses, fibre-optic endoscopes, pacemakers, and dialysers. Ethylene oxide has also been used to sterilise plastic containers and some thermolabile powders.

Low-temperature Steam and Formaldehyde

Formaldehyde gas is colourless with a characteristic odour and is non-explosive and non-flammable in air. It has low penetrative power, a high affinity for water, and polymerises readily on surfaces at temperatures below 80°. Formaldehyde gas is toxic to humans but, in contrast to ethylene oxide, can be detected by smell at concentrations well below toxic levels. Symptoms of acute toxicity are respiratory and conjunctival irritation. Formaldehyde gas, unlike aqueous solutions of formaldehyde, does not induce type IV, T-cell mediated delayed hypersensitivity and is not a potent skin sensitiser. Formaldehyde is a direct-acting mutagen and a possible human carcinogen. In the UK the maximum exposure level as an eight-hour TWA is 2 ppm.

Formaldehyde is an alkylating agent which is active against all types of micro-organisms including bacterial spores. Its activity is influenced by the water content of the organisms and relative humidity levels between 75% and 100% are required for optimal activity. Activity is also influenced by temperature, gas concentration, and exposure time and is markedly reduced in the presence of organic matter.

The addition of dry saturated steam at subatmospheric pressure enhances the sporicidal activity of formaldehyde and produces sterilising conditions. Low temperature steam and formaldehyde (LTS/F) cycles have used formaldehyde concentrations 3 mg/litre to 100 mg/litre, temperatures 60° to 80° and exposure times one hour to six hours. In the UK the recommended LTS/F cycle uses 14 mg/litre formaldehyde in combination with dry saturated steam at 73° ± 2° (35 ± 3 kPa).

The LTS/F steriliser is similar in design and construction to a porous load steriliser. Automatic sterilisation cycles employing formaldehyde and steam pulses are preferred to ones having a single formaldehyde injection and hold period. A vacuum is first drawn to remove air from the load and assist gas penetration. An initial steam flush is provided to heat the load. Formaldehyde, generated by vaporisation of formalin in a steam jacketed vaporiser, is admitted to the chamber and allowed to diffuse through the load for about two minutes. This is followed by an injection of steam to the operating temperature and re-evacuation of the chamber. Up to twenty formaldehyde and steam pulses are introduced during the sterilisation period. Formaldehyde is removed from the chamber by steam flushing and the load is dried and aerated by a series of vacuum/sterile air pulses. British Standard 3970:Part 6:1993 details the specifications for LTS/F sterilisers.

Prehumidification of the load is not a requirement for LTS/F sterilisation. Load configuration is critical to ensure a homogeneous distribution of sterilant within the steriliser chamber. Since formaldehyde gas has high affinity for water, care is taken to ensure the absence of free water. A biological indicator in a Line-Pickerill helix (see Biological Methods below) is used to test for efficient gas penetration. Although absorption of formaldehyde onto materials does occur, residual levels are much lower than with ethylene oxide and the post-sterilisation degassing period is therefore reduced.

LTS/F has been used to sterilise a range of medical devices including nephrostomy tubes, laparoscopes, fibre-optic devices, and electrodes, and is used as an alternative to ethylene oxide in hospitals in the UK.

Vapour Phase Hydrogen Peroxide

Aqueous hydrogen peroxide has been recognised for many years as an effective disinfectant for inert surfaces and has been used in aseptic packaging technology. Although active against a range of micro-organisms it is only sporicidal at high concentrations with long contact times and this has precluded its use as a sterilant. Recently a sterilisation process has been developed that uses vapour phase hydrogen peroxide (VHP) generated by micro-flash vaporisation of a 30% solution of hydrogen peroxide. The process operates at low temperatures (4° to 80°) and with low concentrations of hydrogen peroxide vapour (0.5 mg/litre to 5 mg/litre) that are claimed to be non-corrosive. Sterilisation cycle times of less than 90 minutes have been achieved.

Vapour phase hydrogen peroxide has been used in a single injection and hold period cycle for surface sterilisation of enclosures (for example, transfer isolators and biological safety cabinets) or in multiple pulse cycles for sterilisation of equipment (for example, freeze driers). In each case the relative humidity is reduced to approximately 10% before admission of the sterilant. At the end of the sterilisation cycle the hydrogen peroxide vapour is removed by aeration and/or catalytically decomposed. The process is 'environmentally friendly' as the decomposition products of hydrogen peroxide are non-toxic water and oxygen. The occupational exposure standard as an eight-hour TWA for hydrogen peroxide is 1 ppm in the UK. Vapour phase hydrogen peroxide cannot be used to sterilise liquids and is incompatible with highly porous cellulosic materials and nylon.

Ozone

Ozone is an allotropic form of oxygen which is used commercially for disinfection of water. It is produced by the action of ultraviolet radiation or electrical discharge on air or oxygen and owes its potent antimicrobial activity to its powerful oxidising properties. Ozone is also active against endotoxins. Acute exposure to ozone causes respiratory, conjunctival, and mucous membrane irritation. The occupational exposure standard as an eight-hour TWA for ozone is 0.1 ppm in the UK. Ozone decomposes rapidly to oxygen when exposed to air or water and must therefore be generated at the point of use.

A sterilisation process has recently been developed that uses ozone gas humidified to 75% to 90% relative humidity. The sterilant gas flows continuously through the steriliser chamber during the sterilisation cycle. The process operates at low temperatures (25°) and low ozone concentration (2 mg/litre to 5 mg/litre). The high relative humidity and oxidising properties of the sterilant gas cause corrosion of metals other than high grade stainless steel and degradation of rubber and many plastics and this is a major limitation to its use.

Chlorine Dioxide

Chlorine dioxide has been extensively used in the treatment of water but has only recently been promoted as a gaseous sterilant. It causes mucosal irritation on acute exposure but is claimed to be non-carcinogenic and of low general toxicity. The occupational exposure standard as an eight-hour TWA for chlorine dioxide is 0.1 ppm in the UK.

Chlorine dioxide is generated at the point of use by reacting sodium chloride with dilute chlorine gas. The sterilisation process requires prehumidification to high relative humidity (greater than 80%) but operates at low temperatures (25° to 30°) with concentrations of chlorine dioxide of less than 25 mg/litre. Chemical neutralisation of the chlorine dioxide is required at the end of the sterilisation cycle. Chlorine dioxide is corrosive and degrades silk, unbleached paper, and uncoated aluminium foil but is compatible with many plastics, cellulosics, silicone rubber, and stainless steel.

Liquid Chemical Sterilisation

With the exception of the chemicals discussed under Gaseous Sterilisation most antimicrobial agents are unsuitable for sterilisation purposes. They tend to be selective in their action towards micro-organisms, are often toxic and reactive with the materials treated, and cannot be easily eliminated after treatment. In addition, many organisms, for example *Mycobacterium tuberculosis*, and most bacterial spores are highly resistant to them, requiring prolonged exposure to high concentrations under controlled conditions of pH and temperature for inactivation. Generally, liquid chemicals are only suitable for the sterilisation of clean, hard, impenetrable surfaces. Most liquid sterilants are affected by the presence of organic material so that all surfaces must be thoroughly cleaned before sterilisation. After treatment aseptic washing and handling of items is needed to remove residual chemical and prevent recontamination. Liquid chemicals are used only in extreme circumstances to sterilise materials that are incapable of sterilisation by any other means, for example heart valves and vascular prostheses prepared from animal material. Liquid chemical sterilisation is also used in hospitals to process fibre-optic endoscopes and bronchoscopes.

Glutaraldehyde

Glutaraldehyde is a saturated five-carbon dialdehyde which is highly reactive particularly with sulphydryl, carboxyl, and amino groups of proteins. A concentration of 2% in aqueous solution has a broad spectrum of activity against micro-organisms and a rapid rate of kill. The sporicidal activity of glutaraldehyde is greater at alkaline pH than at acid pH and therefore 0.3% sodium bicarbonate is added to 'activate' the solution to pH 7.5 to 8.5. Total immersion at 20° for three hours is recommended. Glutaraldehyde is more stable at acid pH. Alkaline solutions polymerise and are only stable at 20° for about two weeks. Glutaraldehyde retains a considerable degree of activity in the presence of organic matter and is non-corrosive to metals or rubber; however, rubber and some plastics may absorb significant amounts. It is irritant to the skin, eyes, and mucous membranes and cases of skin sensitisation have been reported. The occupational exposure standard (10 minute exposure) for glutaraldehyde is 0.2 ppm in the UK.

Formaldehyde

Immersion in aqueous solutions of formaldehyde at a concentration of 6% to 8% at temperatures of 40° or more can be used for sterilisation. Antimicrobial activity can be enhanced by combining the formaldehyde with 65% to 70% isopropanol. This process is only sporicidal if the concentration is maintained and the exposure prolonged for up to 18 hours or longer. The temperature must be maintained to prevent polymerisation. The characteristics, toxicity, and exposure limits for formaldehyde are given under Low-temperature Steam and Formaldehyde sterilisation above.

Peracetic Acid

Peracetic acid is a colourless liquid which may in certain situations be corrosive and at high concentrations, in the absence of stabilisers, can be explosive. It is a powerful oxidising agent and produces irreversible oxidation damage to cellular components. Peracetic acid has a broad spectrum of activity against micro-organisms and is an effective sporicide. It is more active than hydrogen peroxide and its activity is not unduly affected by the presence of organic matter. The decomposition products of peracetic acid are non-toxic water, oxygen, and acetic acid and residues are not a major problem. Peracetic acid aerosols at a concentration of 0.1% to 0.5% have been used to sterilise isolators and surgical instruments. A liquid immersion process using 0.2% peracetic acid has recently been developed for sterile processing of fibre-optic endoscopes.

Filtration Sterilisation

Aqueous solutions may be sterilised by filtration through a suitable bacteria-proof filter. The method is rapid, can be conducted at any temperature, and is particularly suitable for solutions containing thermolabile ingredients that cannot be heat sterilised, even using short time-high temperature protocols. Oils, viscous fluids, and organic solvents can be sterilised by filtration and the process can also be applied to air and other gases.

A **filter** is a porous solid that retains particles when a particle-laden fluid is passed through it and therefore in filtration sterilisation, in contrast to other sterilisation processes, suspended micro-organisms are physically removed rather than inactivated. A filter cannot distinguish between viable micro-organisms and non-viable micro-organisms or particles and will remove all types of particle with dimensions larger than the stated pore size.

Micro-organisms are removed from suspension by sieving out particles larger than the stated pore size, adsorption, deposition in the filter bed, and retention in capillary films. Membrane filters are often described as screen filters and are considered to act primarily by sieving effects although other mechanisms may be operating to lesser extents. Other types of filter, which are described as depth filters, appear to function by a combination of all four mechanisms. Filters have either a nominal or an absolute pore size rating and for filtration sterilisation of pharmaceuticals should have a nominal pore size rating of 0.22 micrometre or less. The filter, its holder, and any downstream distribution equipment must be capable of being sterilised, preferably by moist heat.

The pores in a filter consist of a range of sizes characterised by its pore size distribution. There is a very small but finite probability that a viable micro-organism will pass through a pore at the large pore size extreme of the size distribution. The other mechanisms involved in filtration are also probability functions and hence the process of filtration sterilisation is itself a probability function and must not be regarded as absolute. Filtration sterilisation is not a terminal sterilisation process since it must be followed by aseptic transference of the sterilised solution to final sterile containers which are then sealed. Since recontamination can occur during these stages filtration sterilisation is a highly skilled operation demanding good aseptic technique and sterility tests are required on the final product.

Filters for Fluid Sterilisation

Regulatory authorities require that filters used with pharmaceutical products should not shed fibres or leach undesirable material into the solution being filtered. This has restricted the types of filters that can be used for filtration sterilisation to those made of sintered glass or metal, or polymeric materials.

Sintered Glass/Metal Filters. The bacteriological grade of sintered glass filter was originally described as No.5 and is defined in British Standard 1752:1989 as P1.6 with a maximum pore size of 1.6 micrometres. Since this grade is fragile, it is usually superimposed on a coarser grade, the two being fused into a suitable holder. Sintered glass filters have low solute adsorption properties and are easily cleaned by soaking in nitric/sulphuric acid followed by thorough back flushing with water. The filters can be re-sterilised although repeated heat sterilisation can cause loss of adhesion of the component glass particles in the filter bed with consequent enlargement of the pore size. They should therefore be tested before use to ensure that their efficiency has not become impaired. Sintered glass filters act as depth filters and consequently can exhibit problems of microbial 'grow through' and fluid retention. They are no longer in widespread use in filtration sterilisation and are mainly employed in the sterilisation of viscous preparations, organic solvents, and corrosive fluids.

Similar filters of sintered metal, for example stainless steel or silver, have been manufactured that have good mechanical strength but these may be susceptible to corrosion by sodium chloride and citrates.

Membrane Filters. These are generally composed of cellulose esters (acetate or nitrate) but can be obtained in polyvinyl chloride, polypropylene, polycarbonate, nylon, and other polymers. Membranes have also been developed for specific applications, for example hydrophobic membranes for removal of viruses and pyrogens. Cast polymeric membranes are prepared by mixing the components with a suitable solvent, allowing the mixture to gel, and then casting it onto a smooth belt to provide a uniform thin film. The resultant membranes have good strength and flexibility and have a high filtration rate, because of their high pore density. They have low fluid retention and low solute adsorption but some types are affected by certain organic solvents which cause swelling and solution of the membranes.

Polyester and polycarbonate membranes have been prepared by irradiation-etching in which a thin film of polymer is exposed to charged particles in a nuclear reactor. The resultant fission tracks through the film are etched into round cylindrical pores. These membranes are thin, strong, and flexible, possess greater uniformity than cast polymeric membranes, and have a lower porosity. These membranes are true screen filters, acting almost entirely by sieving.

Membrane filters can be sterilised by moist heat or ethylene oxide. They are intended for single use and should not be cleaned and re-sterilised. The filters are available as discs in a range of diameters to handle liquid volumes up to 20 litres. Multiple plate filtration systems and pleated membrane cartridges are available for industrial scale filtration sterilisation. A problem associated with membrane filters is clogging, arising from their low 'dirt' handling capacity. This may be overcome by the inclusion of a pre-filter upstream of the membrane filter.

Filtration sterilisation can be carried out under negative or positive pressure, but in order to minimise foaming, it is usually carried out under positive pressure using air or nitrogen gas pressure. One situation in which negative pressure filtration is used is in sterility testing where solutions are filtered through a sterile membrane to trap any contained micro-organisms and the membrane, after washing, is transferred to suitable culture medium and incubated to encourage growth.

Testing of Filters for Fluid Sterilisation. Filtration sterilisation is not amenable to reliable in-process validation and, therefore, confidence in this method is reliant upon stringent testing of filter efficiency. Challenge testing of filters uses a procedure that is sufficiently sensitive to detect the passage of particles of interest. For sterilisation filters a typical challenge test assesses the biological capacity of a filter using *Pseudomonas diminuta* (ATCC 19146), minimum dimension approximately 0.3 micrometre, as the test micro-organism at a minimum challenge of $10^7/cm^2$. A volume of culture medium containing the requisite concentration of organisms is passed through the filter under defined pressure and then incubated. The filter passes the challenge test if no growth is observed.

An important aspect of filtration sterilisation is the requirement to be able to test filter integrity before and after each filtration. Challenge testing is destructive and cannot be used for this purpose. Non-destructive tests have therefore been developed based on applying air pressure to a wetted filter and observing the flow of air. Non-destructive integrity tests should be carried out on the complete filtration system and not the filter in isolation. The values recorded in these tests will be influenced by the characteristics of the wetting fluid. The most widely used of these tests is the **bubble point test**. At zero air pressure there is no passage of gas through the wetted filter as the pores are filled with liquid. If the air pressure is gradually increased the pressure at which a gas bubble is first observed is the bubble point. The bubble point is therefore a measure of the largest pore size of the filter. If the air pressure is gradually increased further until there is a general eruption of bubbles over the entire surface of the filter, this second end point pressure can be used to calculate the mean pore size.

When applied to large filter areas the bubble point test can be insensitive and inaccurate and this has led to the development of diffusion or forward flow tests, particularly for testing cartridge filters. These tests are based on the theory that, at differential pressures below the bubble point, air flows through water-filled pores in a filter by a diffusion process. Pressure is applied to the wetted filter at approximately 80% of the established bubble point pressure and the volume of air displaced is measured. Pressure-hold tests have also been developed in which pressure loss per unit time is measured. These methods can be used to assess pore size distribution.

In order for a filtration sterilisation process to give a sterility assurance level of 1×10^{-6}, the biological capacity of the filter should be 10^6 times the total microbial challenge of the process. It is therefore essential that the microbial contamination (bioburden) of the solution being processed is maintained at as low a level as possible.

Filters for Air Sterilisation

Sterile filtration of small volumes of air, for example for venting sterilisers, or medical gases, can be achieved using hydrophobic membrane filters. For the provision of large volumes of air with low particulate levels, for instance in aseptic production areas, the following filters are used:

Fibrous Filters. These are composed of glass wool, slag wool, or long-staple cotton wool. When loosely packed they may be used for pre-filtration, removing approximately 99.9% of particles down to 5 micrometres with very low resistance to airflow. Oil-wetted disposable glass-fibre filters can also be used for this purpose. The usual use of fibrous filters is as a prefilter to terminal HEPA filters.

HEPA Filters. HEPA (high efficiency particulate air) filters consist of water-repellent micro-glass material, having individual fibre diameters of around 0.1 micrometre, bonded with resin or acrylic binders. They are pleated to provide the maximum filtration area, each pleat being spaced by separators that provide support and ensure even packing. The filter and separators are bonded into rigid panels. Modern HEPA filters achieve greater volume flow capacity by using bonded glass threads or ribbons instead of separators. HEPA filters are most efficient when the velocity of air passing through them is in the range 0.025 to 0.050 m/s. Filters that are 99.9997% efficient against 0.3 micrometre particles are suitable for pharmaceutical applications. HEPA filters must

be installed with prefilters to minimise clogging and prolong their life since they are single-use units that cannot be cleaned.

Filtration of gases is achieved by a combination of four different mechanisms; sieving and inertial impaction of particles greater than 1 micrometre, electrostatic retention of particles between 0.5 micrometre and 1 micrometre, and diffusion retention of particles smaller than 0.5 micrometre.

Testing of Filters for Air Sterilisation. The efficiency of filters for air sterilisation is tested by generating particles of defined size into the airflow upstream of the filter and detecting their appearance downstream of the filter. In the **DOP smoke test**, dioctylphthalate (DOP) is thermally vaporised to generate an aerosol of particles of approximately 0.3 micrometre which can be detected by a suitable photoelectric device. British Standard 3928:1969 describes a sodium flame test in which rapid evaporation of an aerosol, produced from a sodium chloride solution, produces sodium chloride particles of defined size that can be detected by flame photometry.

VALIDATION AND ROUTINE MONITORING OF STERILISATION PROCESSES

Sterilisation is a process that cannot be verified by subsequent inspection and testing of the finished product. For statistical reasons a practical sterility test that can give absolute assurance of sterility has not yet been devised. Sterility assurance is therefore achieved only by careful product design and process development and by subsequent validation of the sterilisation process before use. This fundamental principle is summarised in the *British Pharmacopoeia 1993* which states 'The effect of the chosen sterilisation process on the product (including its final container or package) should be investigated and the procedure validated before being applied in practice. Failure to follow meticulously a validated process involves the risk of a non-sterile product or of a deteriorated product'.

Validation

Validation is defined as a documented procedure for obtaining, recording, and interpreting data required to show that a process will consistently comply with pre-determined specifications; it is discussed in detail in the Validation chapter. In the validation of sterilisation processes two distinct types of data are required. Commissioning data give evidence that the process equipment has been provided and installed in accordance with its specifications and that it is safe to use and functions within pre-determined limits when operated in accordance with documented operating instructions. The data will include certificates of calibration for instruments used to control, monitor, or record the parameters of the process. Performance qualification data provide evidence that the commissioned process equipment will produce a product with an acceptable assurance of sterility when operated in accordance with the operating instructions. Performance qualification can be further subdivided into physical qualification and biological qualification.

Physical performance qualification provides evidence that the specified sterilising conditions are attained within every part of the product in its final packaging and are maintained throughout the sterilisation cycle. Data must be obtained from the product at the location within the sterilisers that is least accessible to the sterilant. The measurements performed will depend upon the process being validated and may include temperature, pressure, relative humidity, chemical concentration, irradiation dose, and filter integrity. Physical performance qualification also demonstrates that the process has no deleterious effects on the product or its packaging. The data required may include assay of formulation components and their degradation products, assessment of product function and determination of packaging integrity.

Biological performance qualification provides evidence that the specified sterilising conditions deliver the required microbial lethality to the product. This is usually achieved by measuring the inactivation of reference micro-organisms with known resistance to the sterilant either presented on carriers or inoculated directly on or in the product. Microbial inactivation data are not normally required when accepted sterilisation conditions are used, where the microbial inactivation kinetics of the process are already known and documented, and where the required physical performance qualification is attained. However, if a process is used for which accepted sterilisation conditions have not been defined (for example, gaseous and liquid chemical processes) or if the process is non-standard or novel, microbial inactivation data would be required.

Performance qualification relates to a defined product, product packaging, and loading pattern; if changes are introduced in any of these, performance requalification is required. Performance requalification is also carried out routinely, typically annually, and may be required after any modification and recommissioning of the sterilisers. International and European Standards for the validation of sterilisation processes (ISO 11134, 11135, and 11137, and EN 550, 552, and 554) are in press.

Routine Monitoring

Sterility assurance also requires that the performance of a sterilising process is monitored routinely. This is emphasised in the statement in the *British Pharmacopoeia 1993* that 'having established a process, knowledge of its performance in routine use should, whenever possible, be gained by monitoring and suitably recording the physical and, where relevant, chemical conditions achieved within the load in the chamber throughout each sterilising cycle'. Physical, chemical, and biological methods are available for routine monitoring of sterilisation processes.

Physical Methods

Measurement of **heat** distribution within the steriliser chamber or load is usually undertaken using thermocouples. These are usually copper/constantan (Type T) selected and certified, and connected to electronic recording instruments. Resistance temperature detectors (RTDs) are sensitive but are not generally sufficiently corrosion-resistant or robust for use in sterilisers and are more commonly used for calibration studies. A Process Master Record (PMR) is prepared during validation and this is then used as a reference for the Batch Process Record (BPR) obtained from a thermocouple placed in each load.

Pressure measurement is by means of bourdon type pressure gauges or through pressure transducers connected to electronic recording instruments.

Physical measurement of **relative humidity** in sterilisers is difficult since dew point hygrometers are incapable of withstanding the pressures and temperatures of sterilisation cycles and techniques such as direct calorimetry are too slow to be of use. For all physical measurements separate sensors must be used for the control of the sterilisation cycle and for the recording equipment. Physical measurements are only reliable if the instruments are correctly maintained and regularly calibrated. Microprocessor-controlled sterilisers utilise multichannel recording systems that are able to handle large amounts of data from physical instruments and give a more detailed control and monitoring of the sterilisation cycle. Physical methods for testing the integrity of filters used for fluid sterilisation and for testing filters for air sterilisation are discussed above.

Chemical Methods

Chemical monitoring is based on the ability of the sterilisation process to produce sufficient change in the physical and/or chemical characteristics of chemical substances to be detected visually or by physical instrumentation. In general, chemical indicators (CIs) undergo melting and/or colour changes. In an ideal indicator, the change should only occur after completion of a satisfactory sterilisation cycle. In practice, this ideal is not always achieved and consequently chemical indicators are classified into a number of categories.

Process Indicators. These are intended for use with individual packs of sterilised product to distinguish between those that have been exposed to the sterilisation process and those that are unprocessed. They have a defined end-point and may be designed to react to one or more of the critical process variables. These indicators do not confirm that the pack has been exposed to a satisfactory sterilisation process since the end-point reaction may occur after exposure to sub-optimal levels of the process variable. Process indicators may be printed directly onto packaging materials or be in the form of self-adhesive labels or tapes (for example, autoclave tape).

Single Variable Indicators. These are designed to respond to the attainment of the required value of one critical variable in the sterilisation process and may have a graduated response or defined end-point reaction. An example of this type of indicator consists of a chemical having a specific melting point with a characteristic colour change on melting, sealed into a glass tube (for example, Temptubes™).

Multi-variable Indicators. These are designed to respond to the attainment of the required value of two or more critical variables in the sterilisation process. Examples of this type of indicator are Browne's tubes which contain a reaction mixture that requires exposure to specific time-at-temperature to complete the reaction and produce a colour change.

Integrating Indicators. These are designed to respond to a defined combination of the critical variables in the sterilisation process at a level normally associated with a satisfactory sterilisation process and are therefore quantitative indicators. Examples are the liquid and solid dosimeters used in radiation sterilisation. The liquid dosimeters are acidified solutions of ferric ammonium sul-

phate or ceric sulphate which respond to radiation by dose-related changes in their ultraviolet spectra. Solid dosimeters comprise strips of polymethacrylate (Perspex™) which when irradiated, show a dose-related change from colourless to red that can be determined photometrically.

A further category of chemical indicator includes those defined for use in specific tests. An example is the indicator used in the **Bowie Dick Test**. The Bowie Dick Test is the standard test for rapid and even steam penetration. It is performed on porous load sterilisers on each day of operation. A small standardised test pack containing a chemical indicator in its centre to detect the presence of steam is exposed to the sterilisation cycle. The indicator is examined at the end of the cycle and will show a uniform colour change if the cycle is satisfactory. The presence of air within the pack will result in inadequate steam penetration and an uneven colour change in the indicator. The test as originally described used a pack of 'Huckaback' towels and a diagonal cross of autoclave tape. European Standards in preparation describe tests that use cotton sheets and other materials, in combination with chemical indicator sheets.

The performance of chemical indicators may be affected by conditions of storage before and after use, and the method of use. They should only be used for the sterilisation process for which they are intended. International and European Standards for Non-Biological Systems for use in Sterilisers (chemical indicators) are in preparation.

Biological Methods

A biological indicator (BI) consists of a defined number of viable micro-organisms, usually bacterial spores, of known resistance to the specific sterilisation process, inoculated onto a suitable carrier. The inoculated carrier is placed within a primary pack which provides protection from contamination and damage without preventing penetration of the sterilant. After exposure to the sterilisation cycle, the inoculated carrier is aseptically removed from the primary pack, transferred to a suitable culture medium, and incubated to determine the presence or absence of survivors.

In the self-contained biological indicator, the recovery medium is an integral part of the unit thus eliminating the need for aseptic manipulation of the inoculated carrier after use of the indicator. Two types are available. The first type consists of a glass ampoule containing spores suspended in culture medium. The second type consists of an inoculated carrier and a sealed ampoule of culture medium contained in a vial that is permeable to the sterilant. After use the culture medium ampoule is broken to allow its contents to come into contact with the inoculated carrier. Self-contained biological indicators usually have pH indicators added to the culture medium to aid detection of growth.

In some industrial applications suspensions of bacterial spores are used to directly inoculate the product to be sterilised.

Bacterial spores that are used in biological indicators for specific sterilisation processes are:

Moist heat: *Bacillus stearothermophilus* (NCTC 10003, ATCC 7953, and ATCC 12980), *Clostridium sporogenes* (NCTC 8594)

Dry heat: *Bacillus subtilis* var. *niger* (NCIMB 8058)

Ionising radiation: *Bacillus pumilus* (NCTC 8241)

Ethylene oxide: *Bacillus subtilis* var. *niger* (NCTC 10073 and ATCC 9372)

Low temperature steam and formaldehyde: *Bacillus stearothermophilus* (NCTC 10003 and NCIMB 8224).

Biological indicators for routine monitoring should contain not less than 10^6 viable spores. Other concentrations may be required for biological indicators used in validation. The perceived advantage of biological indicators is that they measure sterilisation directly and are able to integrate all of the parameters of a sterilisation process. In order to provide reliable and reproducible data the methods of production, use, and recovery of the biological indicators must be carefully standardised. This involves the provision of pure cultures, grown under defined sporulation conditions and harvested to ensure freedom from any medium residues that may affect spore resistance to the sterilant. The resistance of the spores in the biological indicator must be specified and the conditions and methodology for resistance determination must be defined. Directions for storage and use and details of conditions for recovery and culturing of the spores after exposure to the sterilisation process must also be specified. International and European Standards for biological systems for testing sterilisers are in preparation.

Biological indicators should only be used for the sterilisation process for which they are intended and only in accordance with the manufacturers directions. They should be placed at the location which is least accessible to the sterilant. They may be presented in a process challenge device, that is, an object that simulates worst case conditions. An example is the Line-Pickerell helix in which the biological indicator is contained in a capsule at the end of a helical, stainless steel tube. The length:bore ratio (1500:1) provides a rigorous test for gas penetration in low temperature steam and formaldehyde sterilisation. Biological indicators are less reliable for monitoring than physical methods and are only recommended for routine use in gaseous sterilisation.

Biological indicators and chemical indicators should always be used in combination with physical monitoring or dosimetry. If the latter indicate that a process variable is outside its specified limits, the sterilisation cycle must be considered unsatisfactory, irrespective of the results attained with biological indicators or chemical indicators. With moist heat, dry heat, and radiation sterilisation products can be released on the basis of physical process data rather than on the basis of product testing or biological indicator data. This is defined as **parametric release**. With gaseous sterilisation, the relevant process parameters are not always clearly understood and, as a consequence, parametric release is usually not feasible and product release is reliant on biological indicator data.

Guidance on the installation, commissioning, and maintenance of sterilisers is given in the Health and Technical Memorandum (HTM) No.10(1980) which is currently under revision.

Tests for Sterility

Tests for sterility are procedures that attempt to prove that materials and products purported to be sterile are in fact free from living organisms. They have regulatory and legal implications and detailed procedures for conducting the tests are given in the official compendia. There are a number of problems associated with tests for sterility and these can be summarised as microbiological limitations and statistical limitations.

Microbiological Limitations

In microbiological terms, routine tests for sterility are limited in their scope. As normally conducted, they will not detect the presence of viruses, protozoa, exacting parasitic bacteria, or the majority of thermophilic and psychrophilic bacteria. In addition, organisms that have been stressed or damaged by sublethal exposure to a sterilant may have specialised recovery requirements in terms of nutrients and incubation temperature and the routine test may not be able to provide these. Damaged spores may have long germination periods and may not grow within the period of testing. It is therefore apparent that since the status and identity of all potential contaminants in the product being tested are not known, their detection in a test for sterility cannot be guaranteed.

Two types of culture media are commonly used in tests for sterility. Fluid Mercaptoacetate Medium (Fluid Thioglycollate Medium) incubated at 30° to 35° is used for the detection of anaerobic bacteria and will detect some aerobic bacteria. Soya Bean Casein Digest Medium is used for the detection of aerobic bacteria when incubated at 30° to 35° and for the detection of fungi when incubated at 20° to 25°.

Statistical Limitations

Testing an item for the presence of viable organisms involves adding the item to a suitable culture medium which is then incubated and examined for growth. The test procedure breaches the sterility of the item and is therefore a destructive test which cannot be used to examine the whole of a product batch. It is therefore necessary to examine random samples from the batch and make inferences regarding the sterility of the remaining items in the batch on the basis of the sterility or otherwise of the samples. The statistical aspects of random sampling is one of the most critical considerations in sterility testing. The reliability with which the state of a batch can be inferred from sampling depends upon the number of items sampled (n) and the probability of contamination (P) in the batch and is independent of the batch size. The probability of obtaining n non-contaminated items in a sample of n items, that is, of accepting a contaminated batch, is $(1 - P)^n$. Compendial tests for sterility give recommendations on the number of items to be tested in a batch in relation to the batch size and product type. Table 3 shows the probability of accepting different size batches with different levels of contamination based on the sample sizes recommended in the *British Pharmacopoeia 1993*, for parenteral solutions.

Table 3
Probability of accepting batches of different percent contamination (a) in a single British Pharmacopoeia test for sterility and (b) after a single retest

Batch size	Sample size		0.1	1	10	20	50
			\multicolumn{5}{c}{% Contaminated items in the batch}				
40	4	(a)	0.996	0.961	0.656	0.410	0.063
100–500	10	(a)	0.990	0.904	0.349	0.107	0.001
>500	20	(a)	0.980	0.818	0.122	0.012	<0.0001
		(b)	>0.999	0.967	0.229	0.024	<0.0001

The probability of accepting a contaminated batch decreases with increasing sample size. It also decreases with increasing levels of contamination and is only acceptable at high contamination levels. At very low contamination levels (those to be expected in terminally sterilised products) the probability of accepting a batch is extremely high. Furthermore, if the total amount of each item in the sample cannot be examined and an aliquot of each is tested, this proportionate sampling results in a dramatic increase in the probability of accepting contaminated batches.

Since the test for sterility breaches the sterility of the item, it creates the risk of accidental contamination and allowance is made for this by permitting the test to be repeated. In statistical terms a retest procedure using the same sample size does not in fact improve the chances of making the correct decision since the probability of accepting a contaminated batch is increased from $(1 - P)^n$ to $(1 - P)^n [2 - (1 - P^n)]$ (see Table 3). It must also be noted that these statistical calculations assume an ideal situation and take no account of the microbiological limitations on detecting contamination outlined above.

Test Methods

Membrane Filtration Method. Fluid samples are passed through a sterile membrane of nominal pore size not greater than 0.45 micrometre and any contaminating organisms are collected on its surface. The latter are then freed of any residual product by washing with a suitable diluent, for example 0.1% peptone solution. The washed membrane is then aseptically divided into the required number of portions and each portion transferred to an appropriate culture medium. Media are usually incubated for a minimum of seven days.

Membrane filtration is the method of choice since it can be used with a wide range of test materials including aqueous products, water-soluble or oil-soluble powders and preparations, and ointments. The latter may be dispersed in low viscosity non-toxic esters such as isopropyl myristate or in aqueous solutions of suitable dispersing agents. The method is also applicable to products containing inhibitory constituents such as antibiotics, preservatives, and antoxidants. Furthermore, since large volumes may be sampled with a single membrane, the method eliminates the need for proportionate sampling.

Direct Inoculation Method. In this method, the test samples are introduced directly into the appropriate culture medium and incubated, usually for a minimum of 14 days. The method can be used with solid materials, aqueous solutions and suspensions, and ointments and creams diluted in a suitable sterile diluent. If a suitable emulsifying agent is added to the culture medium, the method is also applicable to oily liquids. In all cases, a maximum feasible ratio of medium volume to inoculum volume is recommended to avoid reducing the nutritive properties of the medium and this may result in the need to use proportionate sampling. For large volume samples, the culture medium may be added to the sample in its original container such that the resultant mixture is equivalent to single-strength culture medium. In all cases measures must be taken to neutralise any inhibitory constituents in the product.

Controls. The culture media must be shown to be capable of initiating and maintaining the vigorous growth of small numbers of viable micro-organisms, both in the presence and absence of the product being tested. The *British Pharmacopoeia 1993* uses *Staphylococcus aureus, Bacillus subtilis, Clostridium sporogenes,* and *Candida albicans* as representative examples. Controls must also be conducted to demonstrate the sterility of the culture media and to confirm that the method used to inactivate inhibitory constituents in the product has been successful.

Interpretation of Results. All controls must be satisfactory, with vigorous growth in all media inoculated with organisms, before the test can be considered valid. If any control is unsatisfactory, the whole test must be repeated. If there is no growth in any of the test series and growth in the inactivation controls the batch passes the test for sterility. If growth occurs in any of the test series, the requisite retest procedures must be carried out. It is clear from microbiological and statistical considerations that the test for sterility cannot, by itself, give assurance that an adequate sterility assurance level has been achieved for a batch of product. It will, however, detect gross contamination and total process failure and for this reason is mandatory for products sterilised by filtration or manufactured under aseptic conditions where adequate in-process monitoring is not possible. Tests for sterility are exacting and should be carried out under aseptic conditions by trained and experienced personnel. The continued requirement for sterility testing has encouraged the application of new technologies. The use of computer controlled robotic systems and isolator technology have been reported to significantly reduce the occurrence of false-positive sterility tests and the need to retest products.

FURTHER INFORMATION

Akers MJ, editor. Parenteral quality control. New York: Marcel Dekker, 1985.

Association for the Advancement of Medical Instrumentation (AAMI). Guideline for gamma radiation sterilisation (ANSI/AAMI ST32-1991). Arlington, VA: The Association, 1992.

Block SS, editor. Disinfection, sterilization and preservation. 3rd ed. Philadelphia: Lea and Febiger, 1983.

British pharmacopoeia 1993. London: HMSO, 1993.

British Standards Institution. British Standard 1752:1983(1989). Specification for laboratory sintered or fitted filters including porosity grading. London: The Institution, 1983.

British Standards Institution. British Standard 3928:1969. Method for sodium flame test for air filters (other than for air supply to IC engines and compressors). London: The Institution, 1969.

British Standards Institution. British Standard 3970:1990. Sterilising and disinfecting equipment for medical products. Part 1. Specification for steam sterilisers for aqueous fluids in sealed rigid containers. London: The Institution, 1990.

British Standards Institution. British Standard 3970:1991. Sterilising and disinfecting equipment for medical products. Part 2. Specification for general requirements. London: The Institution, 1991.

British Standards Institution. British Standard 3970:1990. Sterilising and disinfecting equipment for medical products. Part 3. Specification for steam sterilisers for wrapped goods and porous loads. London: The Institution, 1990.

British Standards Institution. British Standard 3970:1990. Sterilising and disinfecting equipment for medical products. Part 4. Specification for transportable steam sterilisers for unwrapped instruments and utensils. London: The Institution, 1990.

British Standards Institution. British Standard 3970:1993. Sterilising and disinfecting equipment for medical products. Part 6. Specification for sterilisers using low temperature steam with formaldehyde. London: The Institution, 1993.

Carleton FJ, Agalloco JP, editors. Validation of aseptic pharmaceutical processes. New York: Marcel Dekker, 1986.

Council of Europe. The European pharmacopoeia. 2nd ed. Saint Ruffine: Maisonneuve.

Denyer SP, Baird RM, editors. Guide to microbiological control in pharmaceuticals. London: Ellis Horwood, 1990.

Department of Health and Social Security. Health Equipment Information 185. Evaluation of portable steam sterilisers. London: HMSO, 1988.

Department of Health and Social Security. Health Equipment Information 196. Evaluation of transportable steam sterilisers. London: HMSO, 1990.

Department of Health and Social Security. Health Technical Memorandum No.10, Sterilisers. London: HMSO, 1980 (under revision).

Health and Safety Executive; Guidance Note EH40/93. Occupational exposure limits. London: HMSO, 1993.

Health Industry Manufacturers Association (HIMA). Proceedings of Sterilisation in the 1990s Conference. Washington, DC: The Association, 1989.

Pflug IJ, editor. Selected papers on the microbiology and engineering of sterilisation processes. 5th ed. Minneapolis, MN: Environmental Sterilisation Laboratory, 1988.

Russell AD, Hugo WB, Ayliffe GAJ, editors. Principles and practice of disinfection, sterilisation and preservation. 2nd ed. Oxford: Blackwell, 1992.

Stumbo CR, editor. Thermobacteriology in food processing. 2nd ed. New York: Academic Press, 1973.

United States pharmacopeia XXII. National formulary XVII. Rockville: United States Pharmacopeial Convention Inc, 1990.

Documents and guidelines on aspects of the sterilisation of medical products are issued by the following:

UK Department of Health (DoH)

United States Food and Drug Administration (FDA)

Association for the Advancement of Medical Instrumentation (AAMI)

Health Industry Manufacturers' Association (HIMA)

European Confederation of Medical Suppliers Associations (EUCOMED)

The Parenteral Drug Association, Inc. (PDA)

The Parenteral Society

Aseptic Processing

Injections, eye drops, eye lotions, eye ointments, and implants are required to be sterile. The ideal method of manufacture is to place and seal them in final containers that are impervious to micro-organisms and terminally sterilise them, thus providing immediate protection from further contamination. Unfortunately, a number of products would be chemically or physically degraded by terminal sterilisation; they must therefore be sterilised by an alternative method (usually bacteria-proof filtration) and filled into previously sterilised containers with the avoidance of recontamination. Such a transfer and sealing operation constitutes aseptic processing as it is usually carried out in the pharmaceutical industry.

Aseptic processing is undertaken in hospital pharmacies when specialised formulations are prepared from sterile components for administration to a particular patient. This is often necessary for parenteral nutrition formulations and individually calculated doses of cytotoxic and radiopharmaceutical injections. To reduce the chance of contamination during aseptic transfer, aseptic dispensing makes maximum use of syringes and needles. Although this may result in final containers having rubber stoppers that are pierced, they provide a bacteria-tight receptacle for the relatively short time before administration.

Aseptic processing of any kind will rarely provide the same level of sterility assurance as terminal sterilisation and is therefore regarded as a method that should be avoided where possible. Cleanroom technology is invariably required to ensure an acceptably low level of contamination.

OPERATING AND ENTRY PROCEDURES

The room environment for aseptic processing is provided by standard cleanroom technology as described in the Cleanrooms for Pharmaceutical Production chapter. It is very unusual to find pharmaceutical cleanrooms that have a horizontal or vertical unidirectional airflow of the type provided by banks of filters covering a wall or ceiling. Ventilation is usually provided by ceiling diffusers and the air is extracted for recycling at a number of points positioned low on the walls; this results in conventional or non-unidirectional airflow. Within the room, one or more 'critical areas' are then established where unidirectional airflow can be supplied to allow the filling or transfer of products to take place. This may be provided by vertical unidirectional airflow from a filter bank fitted above a filling machine and surrounded by some kind of material that allows partial containment, often a curtain of heavy gauge polyethylene strips. Alternatively, it may be a cabinet that provides a vertical or horizontal flow of filtered air. These critical areas can achieve a significantly lower bacterial concentration than the rest of the room due to the unidirectional sweeping action of the clean air and the exclusion of all but the hands and arms of the personnel involved.

Operating procedures for aseptic processing should be devised to conform with the concept that the perimeter of an aseptic processing area is a boundary where everything entering should be sterilised (Fig. 1); failing this, the microbial count must be reduced as much as possible. Ventilation air, filtered free from bacteria as it passes through the high efficiency filters in the ceiling, conforms to the concept. For containers, closures, tools, and miscellaneous materials, the best method of sterilisation is moist heat and therefore a pass-through autoclave is the entry of choice. A pass-through oven or ethylene oxide steriliser is an alternative in appropriate cases. Liquids that cannot be heated, probably the chief reason for employing an aseptic process in the first place, may be sterilised by bacteria-proof filtration as they pass through the boundary of the aseptic area. When none of these measures is appropriate, entry of materials must be through a cabinet-type hatch or air-lock, but at that point, some process of disinfection by immersion or wiping must be employed. This method gives much less assurance than a sterilising process and therefore care must be taken to make it as effective as possible. Entry of items sterilised outside the facility may be simplified by having them double-wrapped or triple-wrapped. The outermost wrappers can then be left behind in stages during entry.

The remaining entry point in the perimeter is the changing room. It should not be used for the entry of anything except personnel. The only way that personnel can respond to the principle of disinfection at the aseptic room boundary is to wash

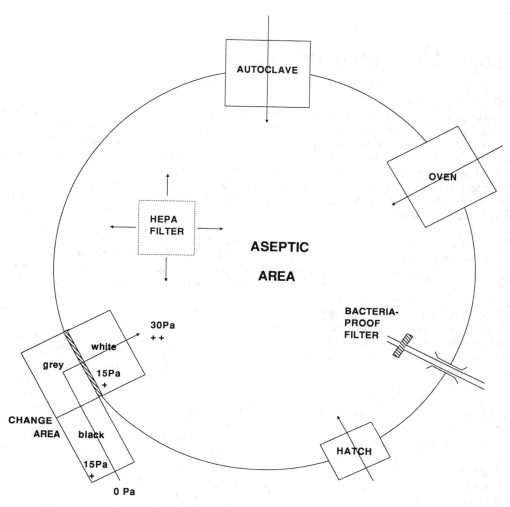

Fig. 1
Asepsis boundary concept.

adequately and don cleanroom clothing and gloves. The changing room is most conveniently arranged to provide three separate areas (commonly called black, grey, and white) for successive stages in the entry process. The black area is used to remove and store outer clothing and jewellery and to change into shoes suitable for wearing inside cleanroom clothing. Personnel then enter the grey area, stepping on to a sticky mat to remove loose soiling from their shoes. The grey area is used for a preliminary hand wash which is typically a one-minute wash and rinse, using a detergent-based skin disinfectant such as chlorhexidine solution, drying with a non-shedding sterile wipe. Use of a sterile soft nailbrush and nail pick

aids the process. The grey area is separated from the white area by a low threshold-bench that provides a distinct floor boundary beyond which only cleanroom clothing may be worn. The threshold-bench also provides sitting space to facilitate the donning of the cleanroom suit. The legs should be swung over the bench one at a time as the boots are put on. The one-piece suit is put on over the boots, taking care that the suit does not touch the floor. The legs of the suit are then tucked into the boots which are tied just below the knee. The hood is put on next and its skirted base is tucked into the neck of the suit which is then firmly fastened. A small quantity of a final hand treatment, such as chlorhexidine and an emollient dissolved in isopropyl alcohol, is then rubbed into the hands until dry. Finally, sterile gloves, usually of latex rubber and with a low particle count, are put on in such a way that working surfaces of the gloves are not touched by the ungloved hands. Gloves should have gauntlets long enough to provide an adequate seal over the cuffs of the suit.

CONTAMINATION: SOURCES AND CONTROL

The major source of microbial contamination in any aseptic process is the operator, who sheds skin scales continuously in large numbers at a rate that is directly related to his or her level of physical activity. These scales are unacceptable both as particles and because approximately a tenth of them carry bacteria. It is the job of cleanroom clothing to minimise their escape into the aerial environment. Bacteria unassociated with skin scales form a negligible proportion of the aerial microbial contamination.

The main effort to minimise microbial contamination will centre on keeping the number of operating staff low, on the quality of the cleanroom clothing, and on the discipline involved in wearing it properly. Cleanroom clothing able to provide a complete barrier to the airborne dispersion of the bacteria-carrying skin particles would also be a barrier to the exchange of air and water vapour and would subject the wearer to an intolerable level of discomfort unless piped ventilation were provided to the suit. Therefore, it has to be accepted that cleanroom clothing, as used in pharmacy, is a compromise between the opposing requirements of containment and comfort. The compromise at present is typically a fabric of man-made monofilament polyester yarn, close woven and made up into a one-piece coverall with hood and boots of the same material. The fabric, when submitted to a bubble-point test, will have a pore diameter in the range 20 to 40 micrometres. The bacteria shed from a person can be reduced by about 95% by such a suit, but bacteria will still remain as a feature of the cleanroom air. It is therefore necessary to remove as many of these airborne bacteria as possible by ventilation.

A secondary source of contamination occurs mainly on the horizontal surfaces of the cleanroom due to the sedimentation of the bacteria shed by the personnel. These bacteria are not normally spore-formers and have a limited life under cleanroom conditions. An equilibrium is established between the settling rate and the death rate. Organisms that have settled on bench surfaces constitute a hazard to aseptic processing by the contact route, for instance transferring them to open containers by the gloved hand of an operator. Effective aseptic technique requires that nothing is touched unnecessarily and that gloves are frequently disinfected with an isopropanol wipe. Organisms that have settled on the floor are not resuspended into the air in large numbers by walking over them. The best way to deal with contamination on benches and floors is by thorough washing with an efficient detergent. The use of a disinfectant will provide an additional kill. In a similar way, mops and receptacles used for cleaning are themselves best cleaned by being thoroughly washed and stored dry. Again, the use of a disinfectant provides an additional kill. Cleaning utensils should be returned to the aseptic area through the autoclave.

A further source of contamination may occur because of 'tracking' of organisms on the footwear of the staff into the cleanroom by way of the changing room floor. This type of contamination may contain a significant proportion of spores (which are more frequently found in the outside environment) and are, therefore, relatively more resistant to the action of disinfectants. The entire changing room floor area should be thoroughly cleaned by washing supplemented by the use of a disinfectant. The changing procedure must ensure that the threshold-bench does in fact provide an effective break of foot contact between the floors of the grey and white areas. The floor contamination of the grey area can be reduced substantially by providing a sticky mat at the entrance; the mat is best used by placing the feet upon it three successive times.

The development of pharmaceutical cleanroom technology aims at the separation of people from products. This, in the short term, means highlighting the importance of cleanroom clothing and, in the longer term, adopting isolation technology that involves separation by a physical barrier. On the industrial scale, the large throughput of containers suggests that a semi-isolation technology, with protected entry and exit, may be more appropriate, backed up by more automation.

VERIFICATION

Verification is the process of checking that the procedures, components, equipment, and room used for the production of sterile pharmaceuticals can yield a product of the required quality. To achieve this in the aseptic processing context, levels of microbiological contamination must be determined in the components delivered to the cleanroom; the use of the equipment involved must have been authorised as a result of satisfactory commissioning procedures; and the cleanroom must comply with the microbial and particle standards stipulated by the regulatory authorities for the type of work planned for it. Compliance levels for particles and micro-organisms are considered in the chapter on Cleanrooms for Pharmaceutical Production. An alternative strategy is to begin with a specified standard of chance of contamination for the pharmaceutical dosage form and work backwards through the production process, establishing the conditions necessary to achieve the specified standard.

Component Sterilisation

The components that are brought together to be assembled into the final, sealed, sterile product are sterilised by methods that must be validated. Containers, closures, apparatus used to fill containers, and apparatus used to bring about sterilisation by filtration all require to be sterilised by appropriate methods. There are well known 'overkill' methods, established by the *British Pharmacopoeia* for instance, such as steam at 121° for 15 minutes and dry heat at 170° for one hour. In these cases, validation would not involve verifying that such a treatment would kill any reasonable number of bacteria present, but would take the form of thermocouple tests of the autoclave or oven to establish that all parts of the proposed loads would be maintained at these temperatures for the times stated. Ethylene oxide sterilisation is a less dependable process requiring optimal humidity levels; validation is required on every cycle by means of biological indicators included in the load.

Bacteria-proof filtration, the process that is applied to what is usually the most important component of all (the liquid in the dosage container), has little in common with the methods of sterilisation that kill bacteria. The physical characteristics of the liquid to be filtered influence the bacteria-retention properties of a filter and validation should be carried out to confirm that *Pseudomonas diminuta* added to samples of the liquid to be filtered can be removed satisfactorily. This service is now provided by the customer support laboratory of at least one membrane filter manufacturer.

While much of the work involved in sterilising components will be carried out in-house, consideration should always be given to the possibility of buying ready-made sterile components. This is of particular relevance to hospital aseptic dispensing. In such cases, validation should take the form of obtaining satisfactory certification from the supplier that the product conforms to requirements. Documentation is an important part of the validation process and should not be neglected.

Standard of Asepsis

Simulation Method

It is desirable to be able to quantify the risk of contamination in any aseptic fill or transfer. What appears at first sight to be the most direct way to do this is to simulate the aseptic transfer by substituting a microbial growth medium for the product. After incubation, the containers showing turbidity (from bacterial growth) in this 'broth fill' will be those contaminated by an organism that can multiply in the medium and at the temperature selected. However, the better the result expected, the greater will be the number of transfers that have to be carried out to demonstrate it.

In large-scale repetitive filling, it is usual to express the target contamination rate as a vulgar fraction with a numerator of 1 and then fill a number of containers equal to three times the denominator. For example, to prove that a contamination rate is no worse than 1 in 3000 containers, 9000 are filled and this should give an expected number of contaminations of three. Statistically, if the target rate is true, there will in fact be a 0.95 probability that at least one contaminated container will be found. New procedures or equipment should be validated by carrying out three separate broth fills which will show more accurately what the true rate is. Broth filling may be carried out using Soybean-Casein Digest medium. An occasional substitution of Fluid Thioglycollate medium may detect micro-aerophilic organisms and is a useful opportunity to test the aseptic functioning of any nitrogen flushing and filling apparatus.

Small-scale dispensing can be validated in a similar way by having personnel perform aseptic transfers of broth between containers to simulate the typical operations undertaken. Such exercises are useful during training but any realistic number of these transfers will detect, in the short term, only major faults.

In 1973, the World Health Organization was of the opinion that 0.3% was a reasonable maximum for the contamination rate of aseptically-filled dosage forms. In 1980, this was improved to 0.1% by the United States Parenteral Drug Association. As standards continue to improve, validation by the broth fill method has practical restrictions because of the limit on the number of containers that can be filled. Theoretical means of calculating the chance of contamination are therefore desirable.

Calculation Methods

Volumetric. A first step in the theoretical calculation of the chance of contamination of an aseptic process is to establish the microbial concentration in the air surrounding the operation. This can be done using instruments such as a slit-sampler or a centrifugal sampler, although these are intrusive and may modify the airflows in which they operate. Having established the bacterial concentration, an equation can be applied that governs the number of particles (N) falling into a container under the influence of gravity in unit time:

$$N = v_g cAt$$

where v_g is the velocity of the particle under gravity, c is the concentration of particles in the air, A is the area of the neck of the container, and t is the time for which the container is exposed. Because bacteria occur in the air almost exclusively on skin scales with an average equivalent diameter of 12 micrometres, a settling velocity of 0.46 cm per second can be substituted for v_g. If, in addition, c is expressed as bacteria per m^3, A in cm^2, and t in hours, the equation can be customised for pharmaceutical asepsis as:

$$N = cAt/602$$

For example, using 'closed' ampoules with a neck area of 0.3 cm^2 which are melted open and sealed within five seconds at a point of fill conforming to the European Community Guide requirement of not more than one organism per cubic metre will result in a maximum of $(1 \times 0.3 \times 0.0014)/602 = 7 \times 10^{-7}$ organisms per ampoule, that is a chance of contamination from the air not exceeding one in 1.4 million.

Proportional. Settle plates provide a less obtrusive method of measuring chance of contamination and have the advantage of detecting bacteria by the same mechanism as that which results in product contamination. Thus a settle plate can be looked upon as a wide diameter, shallow vial containing nutrient agar. The chance of contamination can be estimated by directly comparing the two diameters.

For example, a 140-mm settle plate, with an area of 154 cm^2, would have given a result of 0.26 colony forming units per hour in an environment containing one organism per cubic metre and the calculation would be $0.26 \times (0.3/154) \times (0.0014/1) = 7 \times 10^{-7}$ organisms per ampoule as before.

Conditions Needed for a Specified Standard of Asepsis

The reduction of the chance of contaminating containers exposed in an aseptic environment depends upon minimising the chance of organisms gaining access both by the contact route and the aerial route. The contact route is the less important and can be controlled by paying attention to disinfection of work surfaces and gloves at frequent intervals using disinfectant wipes. The aerial route is the more important route in determining the chance of contamination and is the aspect considered in the remainder of this section.

It will be seen from the formula $N = cAt/602$ that the chance of contamination is directly proportional to, and therefore markedly affected by, the area of the open neck of the containers being filled and also by the time for which the containers are exposed during filling. For example, when filling ampoules, there is distinct advantage to be gained from the use of the reduced vacuum (so-called 'closed') type. Conversely, any procedure that involves leaving containers open for a long time, for instance in a hopper, will result in an average time of exposure for a container equal to half the time taken to fill and seal the whole content of the hopper. For example, vials with a neck area of 0.8 cm^2 exposed in a filling machine hopper in lots of 1000 and stoppered immediately after filling in an operation that takes 10 minutes, amid an environmental bacterial concentration of one organism per cubic metre, would result in a maximum of $(1 \times 0.8 \times 0.083)/602 = 1.1 \times 10^{-4}$ organisms per vial, that is a chance of contamination not exceeding 1 in 9091.

The environmental standards used in a cleanroom will not define the area of the neck of the containers to be filled nor will it define the time for which the containers are to be exposed, although it is obvious that these two parameters have a directly proportional effect on the chance of contamination of the product. Preparing sterile products aseptically in a cleanroom validated to regulatory guideline standards will not guarantee an acceptably small chance of contamination of the product. However, as the calculations on chance of contamination show, it is possible to stipulate a contamination standard for the product and to work backwards to derive the cleanroom standard that could achieve it. That standard might be higher or lower than present regulatory guidelines which could in turn result in either greater expenditure or possible economies. While regulatory cleanroom standards remain fixed, such calculations can nevertheless be used to obtain the best possible results for the product.

MONITORING

Monitoring of an aseptic operation involves routine checks to obtain continued assurance that the standards that have been validated continue to be maintained. Monitoring procedures can be divided into parts that apply to the sterile components that are brought together in the aseptic environment, the aseptic environment itself, and the personnel involved.

Sterility of Components

Effective monitoring includes the checking and retention of signed temperature-time charts from autoclaves and ovens; these verify their correct functioning during the sterilisation cycles. This operation should be supplemented by a system of applying the appropriate type of indicator tape to packages to show that they have been through the sterilisation process.

In the case of liquid filtration, a bubble point or air diffusion test should be carried out before and after filtration to check on filter integrity. A viable count of the bacterial bioburden of the solution immediately before filtration should also be obtained. Solutions prepared in a Grade C environment from solid ingredients that are in a normal state of bacterial cleanliness will be able to meet a bioburden standard of a few organisms per millilitre. For hospital aseptic dispensing, similar principles will apply to components produced in-house. Certification of sterile components purchased from outside suppliers should be obtained from their manufacturers.

Environment

Monitoring of the aseptic environment may be carried out using such instruments as slit-samplers or centrifugal samplers but these are both labour-intensive operations and would be difficult to use for continuous monitoring. It is also possible that they may disturb and alter the aerial quality of the location being measured. For reasons stated earlier, settle plates can be used to solve these problems provided that they are of adequate surface area and are exposed for a sufficiently long period

of time. Plates of 140 mm diameter containing 150 mL of media can be exposed in a unidirectional airflow for 6 hours without excessive loss of moisture, or in a room with conventional airflow for 24 hours. Thus, they are ideally suited to the provision of economical continuous monitoring and can be deployed, for instance, on the basis of one settle plate per half working day at the point of fill and one per working day in a conventionally ventilated room.

Settle plates made in-house should be carefully prepared in an aseptic environment under conditions that make an assiduous attempt to eliminate incidental contamination. This will require that the cardboard (spore-bearing) outer containers of Petri dishes are irradiated before delivery so that external disinfection of the polythene bags of dishes within can be simplified at the point of entry to the aseptic area. Plates should be poured and dried aseptically, heat-sealed in individual sterile polythene bags, and pre-incubated at 37° to check sterility. A nutrient agar containing 0.5% polysorbate 80 should be used to encourage the growth of the lipophilic skin bacteria.

The equation $N = cAt/602$ given earlier can be used to provide a bacterial concentration value at the point of exposure and, therefore, provides a monitoring function. For example, the number of organisms falling into the plate per hour at a point where compliance with a limit of one organism per cubic metre is being monitored, should not exceed $(1 \times 154 \times 1)/602 = 0.26$ colony forming units per hour.

The United States Food and Drug Administration has stated clearly that they would not accept for monitoring purposes, settle plate counts uncorroborated by measurements made by other methods. It is not clear why this should be so since the mechanism of entry of bacteria to settle plates seems to be self-evidently the same as the entry of bacteria to product containers.

Personnel

Because personnel are the prime source of bacteria in the aseptic processing environment, monitoring of their microbiological condition and of their actions are of the greatest importance. A basic expectation is that staff who work in the controlled area will maintain a high level of personal hygiene and that they will declare any relevant clinical condition.

It is also important to be able to detect personnel who, although not showing clinical symptoms, may pose a threat to the product being aseptically filled because they shed an excessive number of organisms or because the organisms are of a type that are capable of multiplying in the product (for example, Gram-negative bacteria in aqueous injections). Monitoring is best done by periodic testing, during which the subject does a simple exercise routine in a dispersion box fitted with microbiological monitoring equipment. If such a box is not available, sampling of the surface of cleanroom clothing immediately before discard may reveal excessive or unusual shedders.

Monitoring within the aseptic area is carried out by 'finger dab' spot checks; this involves the subject pressing the pad of each gloved finger in turn on to the surface of a nutrient agar plate which is then incubated. Such spot checks have to be followed by regloving to eliminate the possibility of contamination from nutrient residues on the gloves.

OFFICIAL GUIDELINES AND REGULATORY ASPECTS

Volume IV of the *Rules Governing Medicinal Products in the European Community* (the 'European Guide') includes a table of the particulate and microbial standards that are specified for the environment in which sterile products should be manufactured (see Table 3 in Cleanrooms for Pharmaceutical Production chapter). Aseptic processing demands the highest grade of standards in the table, acknowledging the fact that live microorganisms introduced during a transfer have an altogether greater significance for aseptically assembled pharmaceutical products than for those that are terminally sterilised.

The European Guide complies with the concept of critical areas in the cleanroom by requiring aseptic processes to be carried out in a Grade A environment within a Grade B room. A microbiological standard of less than one organism per cubic metre is set for Grade A and five organisms per cubic metre for Grade B. The standard for inanimate particles for Grade A equates to United States Federal Standard 209E, Class M3.5 and for Grade B, it is, surprisingly, the same. However, the European Guide directs that the measurement of particle concentrations should be carried out in the unmanned condition (which is not relevant to the manufacturing process). In practice, the room in the manned condition will conform to a standard of not more than 50 organisms per cubic metre and to the European Guide particle standard for Grade C.

Now that it is possible, and necessary, for the micro-electronics industry to have ever better cleanrooms, the divergence of pharmaceutical requirements from those of micro-electronics is apparent. Injections need to be as free as possible only from particles greater than 5 micrometres in size and as free as possible from live bacteria; the standards for the cleanroom environment for the manufacture of micro-electronics are much more demanding, involving particles down to 0.02 micrometres in size in some cases.

SPECIAL HAZARDS OF CYTOTOXIC PREPARATIONS AND OF RADIOPHARMACEUTICALS

The handling of cytotoxic preparations and radiopharmaceuticals can pose particular problems (see Cytotoxic Drugs: Handling Precautions, and Radiopharmaceuticals chapters).

Under normal circumstances, aseptic processing and dispensing are carried out in a critical area that is copiously supplied with a unidirectional flow of bacteria-free air directed out of the critical area towards the operator. As the operator presents the greatest microbial threat to the success of the aseptic operation, this cycle of air movement ensures that the product is protected from the operator. However, when the process material is hazardous, the operator also requires to be protected from the product. The simultaneous protection of each from the other is usually effected by the use of a microbiological safety cabinet conforming to Class II, British Standard 5726 (Fig. 2). This type of workstation allows the product to be surrounded by sterile air that descends from the ceiling of the cabinet; the overspill is drawn through a grille that is situated along the front edge of the

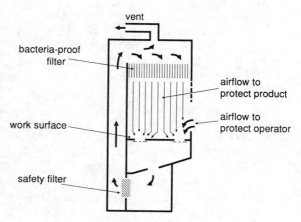

Fig. 2
Dual protection cabinet.

work surface. Operator protection is provided by taking air from around the operator and drawing it down through the same grille. The rate of air admission to the cabinet will add to the recirculating air in the cabinet and will require a compensating loss. This air exhaust must be carefully filtered and, if the hazardous material is not particulate, led to the outside of the building to a position where it will not be a hazard to the general public.

Spillage, both of cytotoxic and radioactive fluids, is a possibility that must be anticipated. The work surface can be modified by fitting what amounts to a large, very shallow rectangular tray. This can be lined with a commercially available disposable material that is absorbent on the top surface and impervious underneath. The safety and the aseptic aspects are both enhanced if transfers are made with syringes between 'closed' containers, that is, vials with rubber stoppers.

Radiopharmaceuticals and radionuclide generators pose additional problems due to radiation. In such cases lead shielding must be placed at the front of the workstation in such a way that the proper airflow configuration (checked by smoke)

is maintained. The primary method to contain radiation is, of course, at source. Radionuclide generators come fitted with lead shielding. Vials for the dispensed doses should be provided with lead pots suitably painted to prevent metal shedding.

FURTHER INFORMATION

Bell NDS. Design criteria in relation to protection of the product. In: Kristensen K, Norbygaard E, editors. Safety and efficacy of radiopharmaceuticals. Boston: Martinus Nijhoff, 1984:311–25.

Carleton FJ, Agalloco JP, editors. Validation of aseptic pharmaceutical processes. New York: Marcel Dekker, 1986.

Commission of the European Communities. The rules governing medicinal products in the European Community, Volume IV: Good manufacturing practice for medicinal products. Luxembourg: The Commission, 1992.

Institute of Environmental Sciences. RP003, Recommended practice for garments required in cleanrooms and controlled environmental areas. Mount Prospect (IL): The Institute.

Olson WP, Groves MJ, editors. Aseptic pharmaceutical manufacturing. Prairie View (IL): Interpharm Press, 1987.

Parenteral Drug Association, Inc. Technical monograph No. 2. Validation of aseptic filling for solution drug products. Philadelphia (PA): The Association, 1980.

Whyte W. Sterility assurance and models for assessing airborne bacterial contamination. J Parenter Sci Technol 1986;40(5):188–97.

Cleanrooms for Pharmaceutical Production

Pharmaceuticals are manufactured in cleanrooms to minimise the entry of bacteria and inert particles into the product. This chapter describes the design of cleanrooms, how they operate, the standards of cleanliness required for different pharmaceutical processes, and how cleanrooms are tested to ensure that they achieve and maintain the correct standards of cleanliness.

CLEANROOM DESIGN

Types of Cleanroom

There are two basic types of cleanroom; these are identified by the method of ventilation, namely, the **non-unidirectional** type (sometimes called conventional turbulent) and the more effective **unidirectional** type (sometimes called laminar flow). The unidirectional type can be divided into **crossflow** and **downflow**. Non-unidirectional cleanrooms (Fig. 1) have a ventilation supply system similar to that found in offices and shops where ceiling diffusers supply filtered, conditioned air which mixes and dilutes the contaminated room air. Cleanroom ventilation differs because:

- the air filters are of a high efficiency and installed in a terminal position in the supply ducts
- the air supply to the room is much greater than that needed for comfort
- the cleanroom is at a higher pressure than adjacent areas to ensure that contamination does not move from a less clean area to a cleaner one.

Unidirectional cleanrooms (Fig. 2) are ventilated through a complete ceiling or wall of high efficiency filters. The velocity is usually about 0.30 m/s in downflow rooms and 0.45 m/s in crossflow. Contamination is thus swept in a unidirectional manner to the exhaust system ensuring that the particle and bacterial contamination is usually between 10 and 100 times better than that found in conventionally ventilated rooms. Unidirectional cleanrooms use substantially more conditioned air than conventionally ventilated rooms and are, therefore, more expensive to build and run. They are only used where products, such as microelectronic components (which are extremely

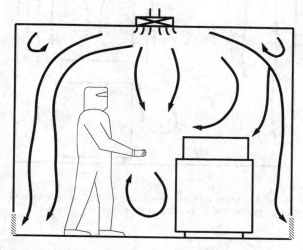

Fig. 1
Non-unidirectional airflow cleanroom.

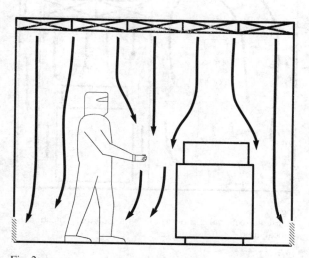

Fig. 2
Vertical unidirectional airflow cleanroom.

sensitive to very low concentrations of small particles) are manufactured.

Mixed flow systems (Fig. 3) are used in most pharmaceutical applications. The ventilation of the background room area is non-unidirectional whereas in the critical area, where the product is open to contamination, airflow is unidirectional. There has, however, been a trend towards protecting

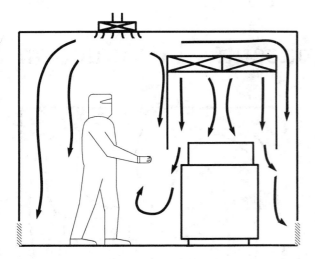

Fig. 3
Mixed flow room with non-unidirectional airflow in room and unidirectional airflow protection for critical area.

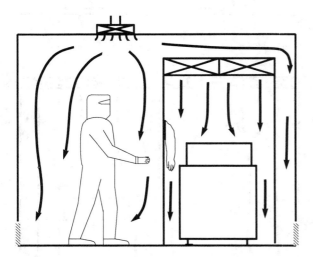

Fig. 4
Non-unidirectional airflow room with isolator protection for critical area.

the critical area with **isolators**. Isolators (Fig. 4) give almost complete protection from room contamination as they are positively pressurised with air supplied through high efficiency air filters. The operator works outside the system using glove ports to make contact with the containers and the filling and sealing machinery.

High Efficiency Filters

High efficiency particulate air (HEPA) filters are essential to the correct performance of a clean-

room. They use glass fibre paper as a filter medium, which has a much higher pressure drop across it than the more open fibrous material used in ordinary air filters. To ensure that sufficient air can pass through, the filter medium must be pleated. Aluminium foil is used to form spacers in the traditional type of HEPA filter shown in Fig. 5, but in the more modern 'mini pleat' type of construction spacers are not necessary, resulting in a more compact form of filter.

Filters may be damaged during delivery or installation and the seal between the filter and its housing may also be faulty. Therefore, all filters should be checked using the methods described later in this chapter. Problems can be minimised by using housings built either to the German DIN 1948 standard, where the seal can be checked by a pressure testing method, or by the use of housings with jelly-like fluid seals which prevent contamination leaking through the interface between the filter and its housing.

Cleanroom Suites

Pharmaceutical manufacturing is not carried out in one cleanroom but in a suite of cleanrooms. The highest quality of cleanroom is used for the container filling and sealing part of the operation when the risk of product contamination is particularly high. Cleanrooms with less stringent specifications can be used for other functions, for example changing into and out of cleanroom clothing or the preparation of solutions that are sterilised by

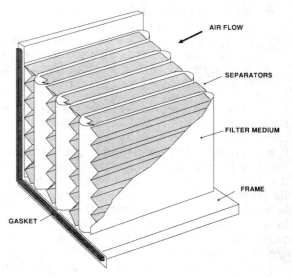

Fig. 5
Section through a high efficiency filter showing its construction.

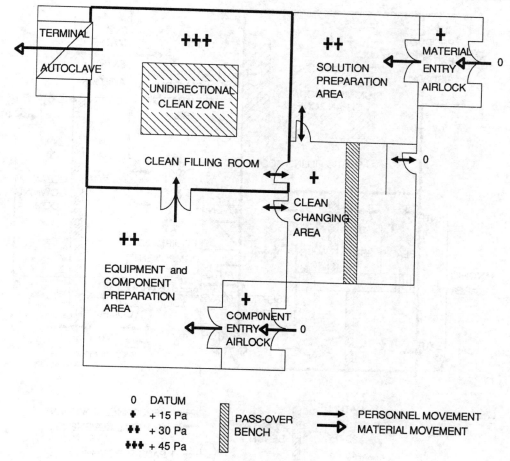

TERMINAL AUTOCLAVE

+++

UNIDIRECTIONAL CLEAN ZONE

CLEAN FILLING ROOM

++

SOLUTION PREPARATION AREA

+

MATERIAL ENTRY AIRLOCK

0

0

+

CLEAN CHANGING AREA

++

EQUIPMENT and COMPONENT PREPARATION AREA

+

COMPONENT ENTRY AIRLOCK

0

0	DATUM
+	+ 15 Pa
++	+ 30 Pa
+++	+ 45 Pa

PASS-OVER BENCH

PERSONNEL MOVEMENT
MATERIAL MOVEMENT

Fig. 6
Typical suite of rooms for terminally sterilised injectables.

filtration. Further information on cleanroom clothing and entry procedures (for personnel) are discussed in the Aseptic Processing chapter.

Two common pharmaceutical manufacturing tasks are the filling of products that will be terminally sterilised and the aseptic filling of non-terminally sterilised products; the latter is clearly the more exacting process. The different requirements of these two processes are reflected in the difference in design between the typical cleanroom suites shown in Figs. 6 and 7. These show the pressure differentials established between rooms to prevent airborne contamination moving from a less clean room to a cleaner room. It is generally accepted that a pressure differential of 10 to 15 Pascals (Pa) is satisfactory for this purpose.

Also shown in Figs. 6 and 7 are the flow patterns of personnel, who must pass in and out through a changing area, and goods which must pass

through air locks, hatches, or sterilisers. To minimise the transfer of contamination, doors in changing areas, air locks, or pass-through hatches have interlocks to prevent both ends being open at the same time.

STANDARDS AND REGULATIONS

The most widely known cleanroom standard used to define the quality of a cleanroom is Federal Standard 209. It was first published in the USA in 1963 and the present version is 209E. The Standard defines the quality of the air of a cleanroom by reference to the log number of airborne particles, of size 0.5 micrometres or greater, per cubic metre. Thus the limit for a Class 2M room is 100 particles per cubic metre and the limit for a Class 3M room is 1000 particles. Other sizes of particles can also be used to define these limits as shown in Table 1. Details of British Standard 5295:1989, the UK

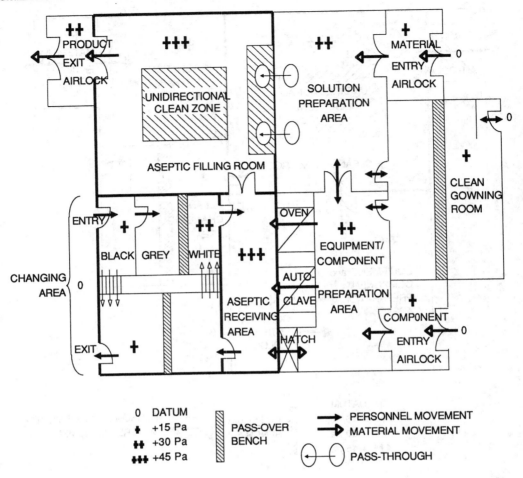

Fig. 7
Typical suite of rooms for aseptic production.

Table 1
Federal Standard 209E airborne particulate cleanliness classes

Class name		≥0.1 μm volume units		≥0.2 μm volume units		≥0.3 μm volume units		≥0.5 μm volume units		≥5.0 μm volume units	
SI	English	(m³)	(ft³)	(m³)	(ft³)	(m³)	(ft³)	(m³)	(ft³)	(m³)	(ft³)
M 1		350	9.91	75.7	2.14	30.9	0.875	10.0	0.283	—	—
M 1.5	1	1240	35.0	265	7.50	106	3.00	35.5	1.00	—	—
M 2		3500	99.1	757	21.4	309	8.75	100	2.83	—	—
M 2.5	10	12 400	350	2650	75.0	1060	30.0	353	10.0	—	—
M 3		35 000	991	7570	214	3090	87.5	1000	28.3	—	—
M 3.5	100	—	—	26 500	750	10 600	300	3530	100	—	—
M 4		—	—	75 700	2140	30 900	875	10 000	283	—	—
M 4.5	1000	—	—	—	—	—	—	35 300	1000	247	7.00
M 5		—	—	—	—	—	—	100 000	2830	618	17.5
M 5.5	10 000	—	—	—	—	—	—	353 300	10 000	2470	70.0
M 6		—	—	—	—	—	—	1 000 000	28 300	6180	175
M 6.5	100 000	—	—	—	—	—	—	3 530 000	100 000	24 700	700
M 7		—	—	—	—	—	—	10 000 000	283 000	61 800	1750

equivalent to the Federal Standard, are given in Table 2.

Both of these standards are routinely applied to cleanrooms of all kinds. However, the European Community guide to good manufacturing practice is a more important document to Pharmacy as it contains the regulatory framework and standards to which pharmaceutical cleanrooms should be built. Details of the specifications of the European document for different grades of air quality are shown in Table 3. The classes of cleanroom required for various pharmaceutical manufacturing processes are shown in Tables 4 and 5.

VERIFICATION AND MONITORING

When a cleanroom is built and 'handed over' to the purchaser, it must be verified to ensure that it is working correctly. During its operational lifetime it must be monitored at regular intervals to ensure that it continues to perform satisfactorily. The tests used to verify and monitor a cleanroom are similar,

Table 2
Summary of British Standard 5295 requirements

| Class of environmental cleanliness | Maximum permitted number of particles per m^3 (equal to, or greater than, stated size) | | | | | Maximum floor area per sampling position for cleanrooms (m^2) | Minimum pressure difference* | |
	0.3 μm	0.5 μm	5 μm	10 μm	25 μm		Between classified areas and unclassified areas (Pa)	Between classified areas and adjacent areas of lower classification (Pa)
C	100	35	0	NS	NS	10	15	10
D	1000	350	0	NS	NS	10	15	10
E	10 000	3500	0	NS	NS	10	15	10
F	NS	3500	0	NS	NS	25	15	10
G	100 000	35 000	200	0	NS	25	15	10
H	NS	35 000	200	0	NS	25	15	10
J	NS	350 000	2000	450	0	25	15	10
K	NS	3500 000	20 000	4500	500	50	15	10
L	NS	NS	200 000	45 000	5000	50	10	10
M	NS	NS	NS	450 000	50 000	50	10	NA

* This applies only to cleanrooms and totally enclosed devices
NS = No specified limit
NA = Not applicable as no limit specified

Table 3
Air classifications given in the European Community Guide to Good Manufacturing Practice

| Grade | Maximum permitted number of particles per m^3 equal to or above: | | Maximum permitted number of viable micro-organisms per m^3 |
	0.5 μm	5 μm	
A Laminar air flow work station	3500	none	less than 1*
B	3500	none	5*
C	350 000	2000	100
D	3 500 000	20 000	500

* low values are only reliable when a large number of air samples are taken

Notes.
- Laminar air flow systems should provide a homogeneous air speed of 0.30 m/s for vertical flow and 0.45 m/s for horizontal flow.
- In order to reach the B, C, and D air grades, the number of air changes should generally be higher than 20 per hour in a room with a good air flow pattern and appropriate HEPA filters.
- The guidance given for the maximum permitted number of particles corresponds approximately to the US Federal Standard 209C as follows: Class 100 (Grades A and B), Class 10 000 (Grade C) and Class 100 000 (Grade D).
- It is accepted that it may not always be possible to demonstrate conformity with particulate standards at the point of fill when filling is in progress, due to generation of particles or droplets from the product itself.

Table 4
Conditions for terminally-sterilised products

Operation	Cleanliness requirement
Preparation of solutions for filtration and sterilisation	Grade C. Grade D permissible if additional steps are taken to minimise contamination, for example, closed vessels
Filling large and small volume parenterals	Grade A with Grade C background conditions
Preparation and filling of ointments, creams, suspensions, and emulsions	Grade C before terminal sterilisation

Table 5
Conditions for aseptic preparations

Operation	Cleanliness requirement
Handling of starting materials and preparation of solutions	Grade A with Grade B background but Grade C if sterilisation by filtration follows later in the process
Handling of filling of prepared products including large and small volume parenterals	Grade with Grade B background
The preparation and filling of ointments, creams, suspensions, and emulsions, if preparation occurs in open containers and without filtration	Grade A with Grade B background

although verification is more thorough. Useful sources of information on the verification and monitoring of cleanrooms are given in the 'Further Information' list at the end of this chapter. The monitoring frequencies that ensure compliance with British Standard 5295 are summarised in Table 6.

To ensure that a suite of pharmaceutical cleanrooms is working correctly, it is necessary to establish the following:

- correct air supply rates
- air supplies of the correct quality
- minimal movement of contamination from a less clean to a cleaner room
- ventilation is sufficient to all parts of the cleanroom
- the concentration of airborne contaminants

  within the rooms is not greater than that specified.

These variables can be checked at verification and during monitoring as follows:

Air Supply

The rate of air supplied to the non-critical part of the cleanroom should be checked when a cleanroom is commissioned and at regular intervals during its use. The frequency of air supply monitoring is not specified in standards but the time intervals given for the installation leak test in Table 6 are reasonable and could be used.

The velocity of air at a number of points in the unidirectional flow within the critical area of the cleanroom should be checked at validation and at regular intervals. Sampling protocols that give the number of sampling points and their positions are given in the Institute of Environmental Sciences Recommended Practice RP002.

Air Quality

The air supply must not contribute to the contamination in a cleanroom. Filters must, therefore, be

Table 6
Summary of minimum monitoring frequencies (British Standard 5295)

Parameter	Action	Minimum monitoring frequency			
		Classes C and D	Classes E and F	Classes G to J	Classes K to M
Air pressure difference	Indication	|————————————————— Continuous —————————————————|			
	Check	|——————————————————— Hourly ———————————————————|			
	Record	Every 8 hr of operational use or hourly during periods of non-compliance			
Installation leak test	Test and record	6 monthly	6 monthly	12 monthly	On revalidation
Induction leak test	Test and record	|————————————————— On revalidation ————————————————|			
Particulate contamination	Test and record	Daily	Weekly	Monthly	Quarterly

checked to verify that they are not damaged and the filter frame-to-housing interfaces should be checked to ensure that they are not leaking. A test smoke is introduced upstream of the frame and filter and the surface immediately downstream is then scanned for smoke penetration; not more than 0.01% of the original upstream concentration should be detected by a photometer. Various oils can be used to produce a test smoke and as long as they are not toxic they can be used. Optical particle counters can be used as an alternative to a photometer but care must be taken to ensure that the optical system is not coated with oil caused by too great a concentration of smoke upstream of the filter. An optical particle counter is more sensitive than a photometer, so smaller quantities of smoke can be used. If an optical particle counter is available which measures particles of 0.3 micrometre, or smaller, it may be found that the naturally occurring particles may be a sufficient challenge.

Air Movement Between Rooms

Air should move within the cleanrooms suite from clean to less clean rooms. The correct movement of air when the doors are shut will be ensured if the appropriate pressure differentials are achieved. These should be checked by a fixed or portable manometer.

Air Movement Within Rooms

To ensure that there are no poorly ventilated areas within the cleanroom, air movement checks are carried out. In non-critical parts of the room this is done by release of smoke and observation of its speed of removal. Any poor air movement can be quantified by seeding that area with smoke particles and measuring their decay rate by means of a particle counter. This decay rate can be used to calculate the air change rate which can then be compared with the expected values.

It is often suggested in cleanroom guides that unidirectional airflow be checked to ensure that its flow lines are parallel. However, this will only be found where there are no obstructions. It is more useful to concentrate on ensuring that the clean area within a unidirectional work station or cabinet is not being contaminated with dirty air drawn from its outside environment. This can be done by releasing smoke outside the workstation and measuring, by means of a particle counter, the amount of smoke which penetrates the clean area.

Checking for good air movement should generally only be necessary when verifying a new cleanroom. If the air movement within the room is found at verification to be satisfactory it is likely that as long as no changes are made to the cleanroom and the correct air supply rate is maintained no problems should occur over the time the room is in use.

Airborne Contamination

Particles

Airborne contamination of the cleanroom can be measured under three sets of conditions:

- when it is empty
- when it has production machinery installed and running but in the absence of personnel
- during production.

The empty room is normally validated at 'handover' so that the contractor can be paid. This is not altogether satisfactory but measurement of the rate and quality of air supply, air movement, and the overpressures between cleanrooms ought to indicate that the cleanroom will function correctly when production begins. Particle counts must be made during production to ensure that the products are indeed being subjected to the correct conditions.

Airborne particles are normally sized and counted by optical particle counters although the time-consuming microscopic examination of membranes through which air has been drawn is recommended if an accurate measurement of particles greater than 5 micrometres is required.

The location of sampling positions and the number of samples to be taken at each position are determined by the size and class of the room. The larger the room or the higher its standard, the greater is the amount of sampling required. Sampling protocols are given in British Standard 5295:1989 and Federal Standard 209E.

Microbial Contamination

Possible sources of microbial contamination in a cleanroom environment are from the air supply, adjacent rooms, and people working in the room. Most come from personnel within the room. The air supply is effectively checked by a particle challenge (smoke test) to the filters and no microbial checks of the air supply should, therefore, be necessary. Contamination from adjacent areas is checked by differential pressure testing or by observation of smoke movement through doorways. Sampling for microbial contamination is therefore only necessary when people are in the room, that is, during production. To ensure that the ventilation system and the use of cleanroom clothing are achieving the required environmental standards, microbial contamination should be routinely monitored.

Air sampling is either by volumetric sampling, where the bacteria are thrown out of the air on to an agar surface, or by the use of settle plates, where bacteria-carrying particles are deposited by gravity. A problem with air sampling in a cleanroom is the lack of sensitivity of sampling methods that were devised in an era of lower air standards. A typical air sampling rate of a bacterial sampler is in the region of 40 litre/minute. To check the aerial contamination limit appropriate to the filling of aseptic products would require a 25-minute sample to collect one bacterium. Air sampling must, therefore, be for a suitable period of time. Care must also be taken that bacteria are not inadvertently introduced during preparation or handling of nutrient agar plates, which should be pre-incubated to check sterility. Settle plates have similar problems of reduced sensitivity but larger plates (140 mm) and extended sampling times of more than four hours will achieve reasonable accuracy.

Although airborne contamination has been shown to be a major source of contamination of pharmaceuticals, contact contamination from surfaces in the cleanroom is also a potential problem. Cleanroom surfaces should be checked for microbial contamination. This is normally carried out by the use of contact plates which allow an agar surface to be pressed on to a cleanroom surface. Microbes thus removed are revealed by incubation. Further information on microbial sampling is given in the chapter on Aseptic Processing.

FURTHER INFORMATION

British Standards Institution. British Standard 5295:1989. Environmental cleanliness in enclosed spaces. Parts 0, 1, 2, 3, 4. London: The Institution, 1989.

Commission of the European Communities. The rules governing medicinal products in the European Community, Volume IV: Good manufacturing practice for medicinal products. Luxembourg: The Commission, 1992.

Institute of Environmental Sciences. Federal Standard 209. Clean room and work station requirements, controlled environment. Illinois: The Institute.

Institute of Environmental Sciences. Recommended Practice-006, Testing cleanrooms. Illinois: The Institute.

Institute of Environmental Sciences. Recommended Practice-002, Laminar flow clean air devices. Illinois: The Institute.

The Parenteral Society. Technical monograph No.2 (1989). Environmental contamination control practice. Swindon: The Society, 1989.

Whyte W, editor. Cleanroom design. Chichester: John Wiley & Sons, 1991.

Acknowledgement—Figures 6 and 7 are reprinted by permission of John Wiley & Sons, Ltd from the book *Cleanroom Design* edited by W. Whyte. Tables 2 and 6 are reproduced by permission of the British Standards Institution.

Disinfectants and Antiseptics

The following definitions are in accordance with the Glossary of terms relating to disinfectants, British Standard 5283:1986(1991). **Disinfection** is defined as the destruction of micro-organisms, but not usually bacterial spores; it does not necessarily kill all micro-organisms but reduces them to a level that is acceptable for a defined purpose, for example, a level which is harmful neither to health nor to the quality of perishable goods. A **disinfectant** is a chemical agent that under defined conditions is capable of disinfection.

The term **sterile** is defined as 'free from all living micro-organisms' and **sterilisation** is a process that renders an item sterile. Therefore, the term 'chemical sterilising agent' should not be used as a synonym for disinfectant.

Antisepsis is the destruction or inhibition of micro-organisms on living tissues having the effect of limiting or preventing the harmful results of infection. It is not a synonym for disinfection. An **antiseptic** is a chemical agent used in antisepsis. The original meaning of the term was a substance that opposes sepsis, putrefaction, or decay.

A **bactericide** is a chemical agent that, under defined conditions, is capable of killing bacteria but not necessarily bacterial spores. A **bacteriostat** is a chemical agent that, under defined conditions, induces **bacteriostasis**, which is a state of bacterial population in which multiplication is inhibited. A **fungicide** is a chemical agent that, under defined conditions, is capable of killing fungi, including their spores. A **fungistat** is a chemical agent that, under defined conditions, induces **fungistasis**, which is a state of fungal population the development of which is inhibited. A **sporicide** is a chemical agent that, under defined conditions, is capable of killing bacterial spores, and a **virucide** is a chemical agent that, under defined conditions, is capable of killing or inactivating viruses.

A **biocide** is a chemical agent capable of killing or inactivating micro-organisms. It embraces the more specific terms algicide, bactericide, fungicide, sporicide, and virucide.

The term **germicide** is vague and should be avoided. It refers to an agent that, under defined conditions, is capable of killing germs.

Sanitisation is a term used mainly in the food and catering industry to describe a process of both cleaning and disinfecting utensils, equipment, and surfaces. A **sanitiser** is a chemical agent used for sanitisation.

TYPES OF DISINFECTANTS

Disinfectants and antiseptics are a heterogeneous group of compounds that vary greatly with respect to chemical structure, mode of action, range of activity, and method of use. Disinfectants belonging to a particular chemical group often possess antimicrobial properties characteristic of the group as a whole. Within a group, modification of chemical structure can produce changes in activity. However, the disinfectant action of a compound cannot be completely characterised by its chemical and physical properties. The activity of a disinfectant is dependent on many factors including temperature, concentration, and pH. Other substances present in the disinfectant preparation may enhance activity, and material at the site of usage (for example, blood or organic matter) may reduce activity by physical processes or chemical reaction.

The groups of disinfectants discussed in this chapter are arranged alphabetically and include alcohols, aldehydes, cationic surfactants, chlorhexidine, dyes, gaseous disinfectants, halogens, oxidising agents, and phenols.

Alcohols

The aliphatic alcohols are bactericidal and fungicidal. They are active against mycobacteria but have little effect on spores. Activity against viruses is variable. Alcohol precipitates the protein in tissues or body fluids associated with viruses and this protects the viruses from the inhibitory action of the alcohol. The antimicrobial activity of aliphatic alcohols increases, at first, with chain length and molecular weight. Chain structure as well as length influences activity and a straight-chain primary alcohol is more active than its isomers.

Alcohol (ethanol) 70% and **isopropanol** 60% to 70% are effective and rapidly acting disinfectants and antiseptics with the advantage that they leave the surfaces dry. However, they have poor penetrative powers and should only be used on clean surfaces. Ethanol at concentrations between 60%

and 95% is rapidly bactericidal against most vegetative cells. A concentration of 70%, often as methylated spirits, is optimal for killing organisms *in vitro*. Lower concentrations are bactericidal if the contact time is increased. At concentrations above 95% the activity is markedly reduced. Ethanol affects cell membrane permeability causing a release of cellular material. This effect has been shown to be maximal at concentrations of 50% to 60% for some organisms. The action of alcohols is reduced in the presence of organic material. Ethanol is used for skin disinfection before injection, venepuncture, or surgical procedures. It is also used to disinfect hands and clean surfaces. Ethanol is not recommended for the disinfection of equipment such as syringes because it is not sporicidal and is inactivated by organic material; it may be used to disinfect clean thermometers. Ethanol is also used as a solvent and preservative in pharmaceutical preparations. Isopropanol at concentrations above 70% is slightly more active than ethanol against vegetative cells and the undiluted form also has antimicrobial properties. It is used for pre-operative skin cleansing and is an ingredient in preparations for disinfection of hands and surfaces.

Benzyl alcohol, which has bacteriostatic and weak local anaesthetic and antipruritic properties, and **phenethyl alcohol**, which is primarily active against Gram-negative bacteria, are used as preservatives. Some chlorinated alcohols have also been used as antibacterial agents.

Aldehydes

Formaldehyde and glutaraldehyde are used as solutions and vapours for disinfection and sterilisation. Other compounds that are thought to act by releasing formaldehyde include noxythiolin and polynoxylin (see below), and the antimicrobial drugs hexamine and taurolidine.

Formaldehyde solution is active against bacteria, fungi, and many viruses, with a slow action against bacterial spores. Formaldehyde does not penetrate well and readily polymerises to paraformaldehyde, which condenses on surfaces. Formaldehyde solution is sometimes known as formalin or just formaldehyde, which has caused confusion in interpreting the strength and the form actually used. Formaldehyde is available as Formaldehyde Solution BP, which contains 34% to 38% of CH_2O, with methanol as a stabilising agent to delay polymerisation of the formaldehyde. Formaldehyde Solution is diluted before use, the percentage strength often being expressed in terms of Formaldehyde Solution rather than formaldehyde (CH_2O).

The antimicrobial action of formaldehyde results from its ability to inactivate proteins by condensing with free amino groups on proteins to form azomethines and other compounds. Formaldehyde can also cause cell wall lysis and micro-organisms may be inhibited by concentrations that do not have any observable effect on cell proteins. The action of formaldehyde increases with rising temperature. Its activity is reduced in the presence of organic material such as protein. Formaldehyde gas has little penetrating power and readily polymerises and condenses on surfaces. Its effectiveness depends on it dissolving in a film of moisture before acting on micro-organisms: a relative humidity of 80% to 90% is necessary. Formaldehyde has been used in the disinfection of blankets, bedding, and membranes in dialysis equipment. Although formaldehyde is required in some instances for fumigation and may sterilise if used with sub-atmospheric steam, solutions of formaldehyde are too irritant for use as general disinfectants.

Glutaraldehyde is active against Gram-positive and Gram-negative bacteria. It is also active against *Mycobacterium tuberculosis*, some fungi, and viruses, including hepatitis B virus and human immunodeficiency virus (HIV), and is slowly effective against bacterial spores. Glutaraldehyde may be irritant to the eyes, skin, and respiratory mucosa. Glutaraldehyde has two active carbonyl groups, which can react with amino acid groups on proteins. It also combines with other groups including the thiol (—SH) groups of essential membrane enzymes and cytoplasmic constituents. High concentrations of glutaraldehyde coagulate cell cytoplasm. The lethal action of glutaraldehyde is probably due to the cumulative effects of several inhibitory actions. It does not penetrate organic material but its action is reported to be unaffected by up to 20% serum.

Aqueous solutions of glutaraldehyde show optimum activity when buffered to pH 7.5 to 8.5 with sodium bicarbonate, but these have a limited shelf-life of about two weeks. In alkaline conditions, glutaraldehyde is polymerised and this reaction is rapid at pH values above 9. A 2% aqueous solution buffered to a pH of about 8 (activated glutaraldehyde; alkaline glutaraldehyde) is used for the sterilisation of endoscopic and dental instruments, rubber or plastic equipment, and for other equipment that cannot be sterilised by heat. Glutaraldehyde is non-corrosive towards most materials. Complete immersion in the solution for 15 to 20 minutes is sufficient for rapid disinfection of thoroughly cleansed instruments, but exposure for 10 hours is necessary for sterilisation.

Both formaldehyde and glutaraldehyde are controlled under the 1988 Control of Substances Hazardous to Health (COSHH) regulations due to their irritant properties and limits are set for exposure to them in the working environment.

Paraformaldehyde is a solid used as a source of formaldehyde vapour for the disinfection of rooms. Paraformaldehyde tablets used for this purpose should be coloured by the addition of a suitable blue dye. **Noxythiolin** may act by slowly releasing formaldehyde. It is used as an aqueous solution for bladder irrigation. **Polynoxylin** is a condensation product of formaldehyde and urea which may act by releasing formaldehyde. It has been used in topical preparations to treat skin infections, and in lozenges to treat mouth infections.

Cationic Surfactants

The cationic surfactants are quaternary ammonium compounds or pyridinium compounds with activity against a wide range of Gram-positive bacteria, some Gram-negative bacteria, lipophilic viruses, and fungi. Resistant Gram-negative organisms include *Pseudomonas* species. Cationic surfactants are ineffective against bacterial spores and acid-fast bacteria, and are inactivated by soaps, anionic surfactants, and organic matter, and by adsorption onto some plastics and fabrics.

Cationic surfactants are bacteriostatic at concentrations far lower than those which are bactericidal. They are adsorbed onto the negatively-charged cell surface and this results in changes in cell membrane permeability and leakage of low molecular weight cytoplasmic contents; at bacteriostatic concentrations the membrane damage may be reversible. Cationic surfactants dissociate in aqueous solution to provide a relatively large and complex cation, which is responsible for the surface activity, and a smaller anion. Their activity is pH dependent although they remain ionised at all pH values. They are almost completely inactive at pH values below 3.5; activity increases with pH to a maximum at neutral or slightly alkaline pH. The action of cationic surfactants against Gram-negative bacilli may be improved by the addition of a chelating agent.

Solutions of **benzalkonium chloride** are used for cleansing skin, mucous membranes, and wounds, and as a vaginal douche. Aqueous solutions have also been used for irrigation of the bladder and urethra, and retention lavage of the bladder. It is also used as a preservative in eye drops. **Benzethonium chloride** is used as a skin disinfectant and has also been used in the food and dairy industry for cleaning utensils, and for the control of algal growth in swimming pools. **Cetylpyridinium chloride** and **domiphen bromide** are used in preparations applied to the mouth and throat. **Cetrimide** consists chiefly of trimethyltetradecylammonium bromide together with smaller amounts of dodecyl- and hexadecyl-trimethylammonium bromides. It has greater bactericidal activity against Gram-positive bacteria than Gram-negative bacteria. It is ineffective against bacterial spores, has variable antifungal activity, and is effective against some viruses. Cetrimide has been used for cleansing skin, wounds, and burns. However, a mixture of cetrimide with chlorhexidine (see below) has often been preferred to cetrimide alone. **Methylbenzethonium chloride** has been used in the prevention and treatment of ammoniacal dermatitis, and skin irritation due to contact with urine, faeces, or perspiration.

Chlorhexidine and Other Diguanides

Chlorhexidine is active against both Gram-positive and Gram-negative bacteria, although it is less effective against some species of *Pseudomonas* and *Proteus*. It inhibits mycobacteria and some viruses, and is active against some fungi. It is inactive against bacterial spores at room temperature. Chlorhexidine is most commonly used as the gluconate, although the acetate and hydrochloride are also utilised.

Cationic or nonionic surfactants are sometimes added to aqueous solutions of chlorhexidine to improve wetting and detergent properties. They also solubilise less soluble salts and improve the compatibility of chlorhexidine with hard water. However, an excess of nonionic surfactant may cause a decrease in antibacterial activity. Chlorhexidine is incompatible with soaps and other anionic materials including bicarbonates, borates, carbonates, chlorides, citrates, nitrates, phosphates, and sulphates, forming salts of low solubility.

Chlorhexidine, because of its cationic nature, is most active at pH 8; the activity decreases with a lowering of pH, and at pH 5.2 there is little or no antibacterial activity. Chlorhexidine is a membrane active antibacterial agent. It is adsorbed by bacterial cells and it reacts with negatively-charged groups on the cell surface. The effect produced depends on chlorhexidine concentration and the number and species of bacteria. It damages bacterial cell membranes causing changes in membrane permeability. With low concentrations of chlorhexidine this results in leakage of low molecular weight cytoplasmic contents. High concentrations of chlorhexidine cause coagulation of the cytoplasm and there is less leakage of cell contents. Chlorhexidine may also arrest anaerobic cellular functions by inhibition of the membrane enzyme, adenosine triphosphatase.

Detergent solutions containing chlorhexidine gluconate 4% are available, which are effective for the disinfection of surgeons' hands and have a good persistent effect due to a residue on the skin after rinsing and drying. A preparation containing chlorhexidine and cetrimide is available for cleansing dirty wounds. Cetrimide is a good cleansing agent and enhances the antimicrobial activity of chlorhexidine. Chlorhexidine is also available combined with isopropanol or ethanol.

Chlorhexidine gluconate 4% detergent solution or chlorhexidine acetate or gluconate 0.5% in ethanol (70%) are used in pre-operative skin disinfection and hand disinfection. Chlorhexidine in the form of a solution, tulle dressing, or cream is effective for disinfection of wounds, burns, or other skin damage. Chlorhexidine gluconate has been used as a dental gel and mouthwash for the prevention of plaque and the prevention and treatment of gingivitis, and as an aqueous solution and as a cream in obstetrics. The cream is also used as a barrier against bacterial hand infection. Chlorhexidine hydrochloride is also available, with neomycin, as a cream for the management of nasal staphylococcal infections.

An alcoholic solution of chlorhexidine acetate or gluconate may be used for the disinfection of clean instruments, and an aqueous solution has been used for the storage and disinfection of clean instruments.

Picloxydine has been used as the gluconate with benzalkonium chloride and octoxinol as an equipment and surface disinfectant in hospitals. The hydrochloride salt has also been used in eye drops for the management of conjunctivitis and chlamydial infections. **Alexidine** has also been used. It is a bisbiguanide disinfectant with similar properties to chlorhexidine.

Dyes

The main classes of antibacterial dyes are the acridine derivatives and the triphenylmethane derivatives (pararosanilines).

The **acridine derivatives**, proflavine, acriflavine, aminacrine, ethacridine, and euflavine, are slow-acting disinfectants. They are bacteriostatic against many Gram-positive bacteria, but less active against Gram-negative bacteria. They are ineffective against spores. Their activity is increased in alkaline conditions and is not reduced by tissue fluids. The acridine derivatives have been used for the treatment of infected wounds or burns and for skin disinfection. They have also been used for the treatment of local infections of the ear, nose, and throat. Bacteria may develop resistance to the acridines.

Triphenylmethane dyes are bacteriostatic and more active against Gram-positive than Gram-negative bacteria. They are also fungistatic but they are ineffective against acid-fast bacteria and spores. The triphenylmethane dyes are cationic compounds and antibacterial activity increases with increased ionisation. Antibacterial activity is decreased in the presence of organic material. **Brilliant green** has been used in a gel with lactic acid for the treatment of skin ulcers. A solution containing brilliant green 0.5% and crystal violet 0.5% has been used as a skin disinfectant, but concern at possible animal carcinogenicity with crystal violet has led to its decline in use. However, a solution of brilliant green and crystal violet (Bonney's Blue) may be used for skin marking before surgery. **Crystal violet** has been applied topically for the treatment of bacterial and fungal infections, but its use is now restricted to unbroken skin because of concern about animal carcinogenicity.

Malachite green, magenta, and acid fuchsine have all formerly been used.

Gaseous Disinfectants

Ethylene oxide is a bactericidal, fungicidal, and sporicidal gaseous disinfectant, effective against most micro-organisms including viruses. Its principal disadvantage is that it forms explosive mixtures with air, but this may be overcome by using mixtures containing halogenated hydrocarbons or carbon dioxide, or removing at least 95% of the air from the apparatus. Ethylene oxide is used for the gaseous sterilisation of heat-labile pharmaceutical and surgical materials.

Formaldehyde and **glutaraldehyde** are aldehydes used as liquids or gases for disinfection (see above) and sterilisation.

Propiolactone vapour is an irritant, mutagenic, and possibly carcinogenic disinfectant that is effective against most micro-organisms including viruses. It is less active against spores. It has been used for the sterilisation of pharmaceutical and surgical materials, and for disinfecting large enclosed areas.

Halogens

The disinfectant properties of the halogens are mainly due to their oxidising properties. Chlorine and iodine preparations have been used extensively as disinfectants although for many purposes they have been replaced by newer preparations. Bromine has not been widely used because it is very irritant. Brominated salicylanilides (bromsalans) have antibacterial and antifungal properties and have been used in medicated soaps.

Inorganic Chlorine Compounds

Chlorine and **hypochlorites** are rapidly bactericidal and fungicidal; they are also active against most viruses, yeasts, protozoa, and algae, but they are less active against spores. The potency of chlorine and chlorine compounds is expressed as the 'available' chlorine, which is based on the concept of chlorine gas as the reference substance. Two atoms of chlorine ($2 \times Cl$) yield in water only one molecule of hypochlorous acid (on which activity is based), whereas hypochlorites and chloramines yield one molecule of hypochlorous acid for each atom of chlorine as shown in the following equations:

$$Cl_2 + H_2O = HOCl + H^+ + Cl^-$$

$$NaOCl + H_2O = HOCl + NaOH$$

Thus, the assayed chlorine in such compounds has to be multiplied by 2 to produce 'available chlorine'. In the presence of water these compounds produce hypochlorous acid (HOCl) and hypochlorite ion (OCl^-) and it is generally considered that the lethal action on organisms is due to chlorination of cell protein or enzyme systems by unionised hypochlorous acid, although the hypochlorite ion may also contribute. The activity of these compounds decreases with increase in pH, the activity of solutions of pH 4 to 7 being greater than those of higher pH values. However, stability is usually greater at an alkaline pH.

Chlorine compounds are useful for the disinfection of relatively clean impervious surfaces, such as babies' feeding bottles, baths, and food and dairy equipment because they have relatively low residual toxicity. Solutions containing 10 000 ppm 'available chlorine' are used to disinfect surfaces contaminated with spilled blood or body fluids; this strength is effective against hepatitis B virus and HIV. Solutions of chlorine-releasing compounds are also used in wound desloughing and disinfection.

Chlorinated Soda Solution (Dakin's Solution) is prepared from **chlorinated lime** and has been used to cleanse and disinfect wounds, although there have been reports of wound cell toxicity and delayed healing. Eusol (Edinburgh University Solution of Lime; Chlorinated Lime and Boric Acid Solution BP) is a solution of calcium hypochlorite containing not less than 0.25% w/v of 'available chlorine', buffered with boric acid to a pH of 7.5 to 8.5. Milton™ solution is a commercially available solution containing sodium hypochlorite 1% and sodium chloride 16.5%. It is used in a 1 in 80 dilution to sterilise babies' feeding utensils. For wound management purposes, a 1 in 4 dilution is generally used, which contains 0.25% 'available chlorine'. The use of diluted hypochlorite solutions to cleanse and disinfect wounds has declined since it was shown that their toxicity to wound cells could delay healing.

For use in small swimming pools, sodium or calcium hypochlorite may be added daily to maintain a free residual 'available chlorine' concentration of 1 to 3 ppm. Chloramine, chlorinated lime, and the isocyanurates may also be used.

On a large scale, chlorine gas is used to disinfect public water supplies. On a smaller scale, the use of chlorine compounds is more convenient and sodium hypochlorite, chlorinated lime, chlorine dioxide, and the organic compounds chloramine and halazone are used. After satisfying the chlorine demand (the amount of chlorine needed to react with organic matter and other substances), a free residual content of 0.2 to 0.4 ppm 'available chlorine' should be maintained, although more is required for alkaline waters with a pH of 9 or more. For the disinfection of potentially contaminated water, a concentration of 1 ppm is recommended. Excessive residual chlorine may be removed by the addition of smaller amounts of sodium thiosulphate or citric acid.

Organic Chlorine Compounds

Several organic chlorine compounds are used as disinfectants. Their spectrum of activity and mode of action are similar to chlorine and the hypochlorites, but they are more stable. The organic chlorine compounds are less irritant and toxic than chlorine or hypochlorites.

Chloramine has been used as a wound disinfectant and general surgical antiseptic. It is also used to disinfect water for drinking purposes and in swimming pools. Chloramine B has been used similarly.

Chloroazodin has been used as a wet dressing and for irrigating infected wounds. **Dichlordimethylhydantoin** is used for sterilising food and dairy equipment and disinfecting babies' feeding bottles. **Sodium dichloroisocyanurate** has been used similarly, as well as for the treatment of swimming pool water, for soft contact lens care, and in commercial scouring powders and bleach detergents. **Halazone** is used to disinfect contaminated drinking water and **oxychlorosene** is used as a 0.4% solution for cleansing wounds, and in urological and ophthalmological disinfection.

Inorganic Iodine Compounds

Iodine is a non-selective bactericide and sporicide that acts rapidly at the concentrations usually employed; it is also effective against fungi, protozoa, and viruses. The presence of iodides in aqueous solutions of iodine results in periodide or tri-iodide formation and loss of activity; this reaction only becomes significant if there is a large excess of iodide to complex with free iodine. In alkaline solutions, iodine is converted to hypoiodous acid; at pH 8.5 the ratio of iodine to hypoiodous acid is 1:1 and bactericidal and sporicidal activity is markedly reduced.

The activity is thought to be due to the oxidising properties of free molecular iodine and may also be due to the combination of free iodine with cell proteins. Chemically-combined iodine does not possess bactericidal or sporicidal properties. The activity of iodine is reduced in the presence of organic material.

Solutions such as Alcoholic Iodine Solution BP are used for the treatment of minor wounds and abrasions. It has been used as a pre-operative disinfectant for unbroken skin, and as a throat paint as a 2% solution in glycerol. Iodine has also been used to disinfect water.

Iodophores

Iodophores are complexes of iodine with surfactants, which are not volatile. Bactericidal activity increases with temperature up to about 43°; at higher temperatures they decompose liberating iodine.

Nonionic surfactants form the most stable iodophores but only nonionic surfactants that are iodine carriers and sufficiently water soluble can be used. Iodophores may solubilise up to 25% by weight of iodine; some iodine is chemically combined but usually 70% to 80% may be released as available iodine. Iodophores provide a means of formulating aqueous iodine preparations without the use of iodides and the loss of iodine as tri-iodide.

Solutions of iodophores that release iodine on contact with skin or mucous membranes are used in pre-operative skin disinfection. **Povidone-iodine** is a complex of iodine with povidone containing 9% to 12% of available iodine calculated on the dried basis. It is used as a disinfectant mainly for the treatment of contaminated wounds and pre-operative preparation of the skin and mucous membranes. Preparations containing 1% of povidone-iodine are available as a mouthwash or gargle and as 10% solution, gel, or pessaries for vaginal infections or cleansing. Iodine may be absorbed and affect thyroid function.

Oxidising Agents

Oxidising agents (chiefly, peroxides and permanganates) are used as disinfectants, antiseptics, and deodorants. Magnesium peroxide, urea, hydrogen peroxide, zinc peroxide, and zinc permanganate have also been used. Sodium perborate and sodium percarbonate have been used similarly to hydrogen peroxide.

Hydrogen peroxide solution (20 volumes) contains 5% to 7% of H_2O_2. Hydrogen peroxide is an unstable compound with a relatively weak germicidal action of short duration. In contact with tissues hydrogen peroxide decomposes rapidly to form water and oxygen; the antimicrobial action is due to oxidation of cell materials. Hydrogen peroxide will oxidise thiol and other oxidisable groups within bacterial cells; in the presence of heavy metal ions a self-propagating chain reaction can occur. Hydrogen peroxide has been found to affect ribosomes but this is not thought to be a primary action. The antimicrobial action of peroxides is reduced in the presence of other oxidisable material such as protein.

Hydrogen peroxide solution is used for cleansing wounds and ulcers. The disinfectant and deodorant action occurs during the release of oxygen. The solution does not penetrate well but the effervescence provides a mechanical means for detachment of dead tissue and bacteria from inaccessible parts of wounds. It should not be used in closed body cavities.

Hydrogen peroxide solutions are used for the disinfection of soft contact lenses, tonometers, and ventilators. Diluted solutions are used as gargles and mouthwashes. Nebulised solutions have been used to disinfect ventilators, and aerosols have been used to disinfect rooms. Hydrogen peroxide ear drops have been used to remove wax. Hydrogen peroxide is used in industry as a bleach and oxidising agent.

Potassium permanganate is an oxidising agent with disinfectant, deodorising, and astringent properties. The antimicrobial action of permanganates is reduced in the presence of other oxidisable material. A concentration of 0.01% is usually bactericidal within an hour. Concentrations of 0.025% to 0.1% are used similarly to peroxides for cleansing wounds and as mouthwashes and gargles; more dilute solutions have been used as vaginal and bladder irrigations. Solutions are also used as wet dressings and in baths in various skin conditions where there is secondary infection. A 1% solution has been used to treat mycotic infections. It is liable to stain the skin. A 0.02% solution in water was formerly used as a stomach washout in the treatment of morphine, opium, and strychnine poisoning.

Phenol and its Derivatives

Phenol has been used as a disinfectant since the nineteenth century but its usefulness is limited by its corrosive properties. The spectrum of activity and toxicity of phenol have been modified by the introduction of substituents into the phenol molecule. The alkyl and halogenated derivatives are less corrosive than phenol, but as their substituents are lipophilic their activity is more markedly reduced by organic material. Some of the halogenated derivatives are also diphenyl derivatives. Nitration of phenol alters the mode of action.

Alkyl Derivatives

Phenol and its alkyl derivatives are active against Gram-positive and Gram-negative bacteria. The action is bacteriostatic or bactericidal depending on concentration and bacterial species; the antibacterial activity is greater with increases in temperature. They are also active against fungi and viruses but have little activity against acid-fast bacteria and spores.

The alkyl derivatives of phenol are compatible with anionic surfactants and their bactericidal and sporicidal activity may be enhanced by the addition of soap. This is associated with the formation of mixed micelles of the soap and phenol, and depends on the properties and proportions of the soap and phenol in the system.

The alkyl derivatives of phenol are more active than phenol. The activity is greater with increasing alkyl-chain length up to *n*-amyl. This is paralleled by increases in lipid solubility and ability to associate with cell membrane lipids. The decrease in activity associated with substituents of longer chain length is due to very low water solubility. The position of the alkyl group in relation to the hydroxy group does not seem to be an important factor in antimicrobial activity as *o*-, *m*-, and *p*-isomers of alkyl-substituted phenols have been shown to possess similar activities. Primary alkyl-phenols are more active than secondary or tertiary isomers. Phenol and its derivatives are more active in acid than in alkaline conditions. The activity of phenol depends on the presence of undissociated molecules. This may also be linked to lipid solubility as undissociated phenol molecules are more lipid soluble than phenolate ions. The pK_a of phenol is 10.0, therefore, in acidic conditions it is mainly in the undissociated form. Phenols being lipophilic have high oil/water partition coefficients and solutions in oils, glycerol, and organic solvents have reduced antimicrobial activities and are also less corrosive. Similarly the reduction of activity in the presence of organic material is caused by partition of the phenol into lipid material.

Phenol and its derivatives damage bacterial cell walls thus causing changes in membrane permeability and loss of certain essential cell constituents. High concentrations coagulate cell proteins.

Phenol (carbolic acid) in concentrations up to 1% is bacteriostatic; higher concentrations are bactericidal. Solutions containing up to 2% have been used to treat minor wounds and higher concentrations (5%) have been used to disinfect excreta. Preparations of phenol in glycerol have been used as a gargle or mouthwash. Phenol in glycerol is used by intrathecal injection to alleviate chronic low-back pain or spasticity.

Cresol is a mixture of cresols and other phenols obtained from coal tar. Concentrations of 0.3% to 0.6% cresol will kill vegetative cells including mycobacteria in about 10 minutes. Cresol is used as a preservative for some injections. Cresol and Soap Solution (Lysol) has been used to disinfect contaminated hospital equipment and as a general domestic disinfectant, but has largely been superseded by other less irritant phenolic disinfectants.

Amylmetacresol is a phenolic disinfectant used in the treatment of minor infections of the mouth and throat.

Tar acids are obtained by the distillation of coal tar or petroleum fractions. The lowest boiling fraction (distilled at 188° to 205°) consists of mixed cresol isomers. The middle fraction (distilled at 205° to 230°) consists of cresols and xylenols, and the high-boiling tar acids (distilled at 230° to 290°) consist mainly of alkyl homologues of phenol, with naphthalenes and other hydrocarbons. Tar acids are used to prepare 'Black Fluids' and 'White Fluids' which are used as household and general disinfectants. The activity depends on the tar acid fraction used, the 'lowest boiling fraction' being least active and the 'high-boiling tar acids' most active. The 'high-boiling tar acids' have a more selective action than the other fractions and their activity is substantially reduced by organic material.

Black fluids are solutions of coal tar acids or similar acids derived from petroleum or mixtures of these with or without hydrocarbons and with an emulsifying agent; they form stable emulsions when diluted with water and they are preferred when the undiluted fluid is required to be stable for prolonged periods near freezing point.

White fluids are finely dispersed emulsions of coal tar acids or similar acids derived from petroleum or a mixture of these with or without hydrocarbons. They are diluted with water and mix readily with hard water or sodium chloride solutions. White fluids are more stable after dilution than black fluids.

Modified black fluids and modified white fluids contain additional ingredients and may be less corrosive.

Thymol is a phenolic disinfectant with bactericidal and antifungal activity. Its use is limited by its low water solubility; it is also inactivated by organic material. It is used as a deodorant in mouthwashes and has been used in dusting powders to treat fungal infections of the skin.

Halogenated Derivatives

The halogenated derivatives of phenol are active against Gram-positive bacteria; their activity is bacteriostatic or bactericidal depending on concentration and bacterial species. They are almost inactive against spores and some Gram-negative bacteria including *Pseudomonas aeruginosa*, *Proteus vulgaris*, and some *Salmonella* species. Some halogenated derivatives are used for their antifungal properties.

The activity of phenol is increased by halogenation. The halogenated phenolic disinfectants are mainly chlorinated compounds. Dichloro- and trichlorophenols are more active than the monochloroderivatives but further halogenation does not increase activity. Halogenation of alkyl-phenols enhances activity and this is most marked when the alkyl group is ortho to the hydroxy group and the halogen para to the hydroxy group. The activity of the halogenated derivatives, like that of the alkyl derivatives of phenol, depends on lipid solubility and pH.

Some halogenated phenols are also diphenyl derivatives. These compounds are derivatives of phenylphenol in which the two rings are either linked directly or separated by an alkyl group, a nitrogen-containing group, or by sulphur or oxygen atoms. The activity of compounds in which the rings are separated by an alkyl group increases with increased alkyl-chain length up to butyl; longer alkyl chains are associated with reduced activity against Gram-negative organisms. In general, alkylation of diphenyl derivatives does not result in enhancement of activity produced by corresponding alkylation of phenol.

Chlorocresol is used as a skin and wound disinfectant. It has bactericidal activity against Gram-positive and Gram-negative bacteria and is effective against fungi, but has little activity against bacterial spores. Chlorocresol is used as a preservative in creams, and in aqueous injections supplied in multidose containers. Injections prepared with chlorocresol should not be injected into the cerebrospinal fluid, the heart, or the eye.

Chloroxylenol is used as a skin and wound disinfectant. It is bactericidal against most Gram-positive bacteria but is less active against staphylococci and Gram-negative bacteria, and is often inactive against *Pseudomonas* species. A mixture of chloroxylenol and disodium edetate has been shown to be active against *Pseudomonas aeruginosa*. It is thought that edetate chelates the cations that form cross-links between the phosphate groups of the lipopolysaccharides in the outer membrane of Gram-negative cells; chloroxylenol then enters the cell through the damaged outer membrane and exerts its bactericidal effect. It is inactive against bacterial spores. Dichloroxylenol is similarly used. **Orthophenylphenol** has similar properties to chloroxylenol and is used for skin and hard surface disinfection. It is also used with **amylphenol** in a lubricant gel and sterile dressing. **Chlorophene** was formerly used as a disinfectant in solutions and soaps. **Chlorothymol** is a chlorinated phenolic derivative that has been used for skin disinfection and for topical treatment of fungal infections. **Fentichlor** is a derivative of phenol active against some bacteria, *Candida albicans*, *Microsporum*, and *Trichophyton* species. It is used to treat skin infections. Fentichlor has caused photosensitivity reactions and cross-sensitivity with bithionol has been reported.

Hexachlorophane is a chlorinated bisphenol derivative active against Gram-positive bacteria. Hexachlorophane has little activity against Gram-negative cells and preparations are sometimes contaminated with *Pseudomonas* and *Salmonella* species. Its activity is reduced in the presence of blood. Soaps and creams containing hexachlorophane 0.23% to 3% are used as skin disinfectants in hospitals to prevent staphylococcal cross-infection. Single applications are not effective; repeated applications over several days are required to accumulate an effective concentration in the skin. Hexachlorophane was formerly widely used for the skin care of infants. However, its use was restricted following reports of brain damage, sometimes fatal, due to absorption of excessive amounts through intact and broken skin. If used with adequate precautions it is still of value in the control of staphylococcal infection.

Parachlorophenol is a potent chlorinated phenolic antiseptic, but it is more toxic and irritant than phenol. Parachlorophenol solution 0.25% in sodium chloride 0.9% has been used for the irrigation of sinus tracts. **Triclosan** is active against Gram-positive and most Gram-negative bacteria; it is poorly active against *Pseudomonas* species. Triclosan is used in soaps, creams, and solutions as a skin disinfectant.

Nitrophenols

Trinitrophenol has antibacterial properties. Nitration increases the antibacterial activity of phenol; it also increases the systemic toxicity. Nitrophenols are most active in acidic conditions and most of the activity is due to undissociated molecules. In contrast to phenol, the ionic form of dinitrophenol has been shown to contribute to the activity in less acidic conditions. Nitrophenols act by uncoupling oxidation from phosphorylation in bacterial and fungal cells. This action prevents energy from being stored as ATP (adenosine triphosphate). Trinitrophenol 1% aqueous solution was formerly used to treat burns. Other nitrophenols are used as fungicides, insecticides, and herbicides.

Miscellaneous Disinfectants

Acids

For many years acids have been used to prevent food spoilage. In addition, the antimicrobial action of some other antimicrobial agents is enhanced under acidic conditions. The resistance of spores to heat is also reduced under acidic conditions.

The antimicrobial action of inorganic acids is mainly due to the presence of hydrogen ions, whereas organic acids owe their antimicrobial activity to the undissociated molecule. Inorganic acids are too corrosive for general use, but a number of organic acids (for example, acetic acid) are used as antimicrobial agents. Benzoic acid and *p*-hydroxybenzoate esters are used as preservatives.

Acetic acid 5% solution is bactericidal or fungicidal to a number of micro-organisms including *Pseudomonas aeruginosa* and some *Trichomonas*, *Candida*, and *Haemophilus* species, while lower concentrations are bacteriostatic or fungistatic. It has been used for its antifungal and antiprotozoal properties in vaginal gels and douches, and to disinfect dialysers and inhalation therapy equipment. Potential uses as a spermicide, astringent lotion, surgical dressing, and as a treatment for jellyfish stings have been investigated.

Boric acid and **borax** (sodium borate) are weak bacteriostatic and antifungal agents, which have been used in topical preparations such as eye lotions, mouthwashes, and gargles. Boric acid has been used to treat napkin rash. Solutions of boric acid were formerly used to wash out body cavities and as applications to wounds and ulcers, but their use for these purposes is inadvisable owing to the possibility of absorption. Boron toxicity, sometimes fatal, resulting from the use of boric acid and borax preparations has led to the use of more effective and less toxic compounds.

Peracetic acid is a strong oxidising agent that has been used as a 0.2% solution, to disinfect surgeons' hands and as a spray to disinfect air. It is corrosive to the skin.

Amidines

The amidines were initially used to treat protozoal infections. Pentamidine is used as a trypanocide, but dibromopropamidine and propamidine are used as disinfectants. The amidines are structurally related to another group of disinfectants, the diguanides (see above).

Dibromopropamidine isethionate is bactericidal against Gram-positive bacteria, but is less active against Gram-negative bacteria and spore-forming organisms. It also has antifungal properties. Dibromopropamidine has been used as a cream for the treatment of skin infections and minor burns, and as eye ointment or eye drops for the treatment of eye infections.

Propamidine isethionate is active against Gram-positive bacteria, but is less active against Gram-negative bacteria and spore-forming organisms. It also has antifungal properties. An ophthalmic solution has been used for the treatment of blepharitis and conjunctivitis.

Ampholytic Surfactants

The ampholytic (or amphoteric) surfactants are derivatives of long-chain N-substituted amino acids having the general formula $RNHCH_2COOH$, where R is an alkyl radical, an acyl radical, or one containing an aminoethyl substituent of aminoacetic acid. These compounds can be anionic, nonionic, or cationic depending on the pH; they are anionic at pH values above their isoelectric point and cationic at pH values below it. They have the detergent properties of the anionic surfactants and the disinfectant properties of the cationic surfactants. They are bactericidal and fungicidal and their activity is not reduced in the presence of organic matter.

Dodicin is mainly used for surface and instrument disinfection in hospitals. The hydrochloride is also used. Dodicin has also been used for skin disinfection. Ampholytic disinfectants are also used in the food and dairy industries.

Metals

Most heavy metal ions possess some antibacterial properties, and inorganic salts or organic compounds of copper, mercury, and silver have been used as disinfectants.

Copper sulphate and other cupric salts are bacteriostatic and to some extent bactericidal; they are effective against fungi and algae and have weak virucidal activity. The inhibitory action of cupric salts is due to the ability of the cupric ion to combine with essential thiol groups of the bacterial cell. Higher concentrations may precipitate protein.

Copper sulphate has been used to prevent algal growth in swimming pools and reservoirs, as an antifungal spray for fruit trees, and as a molluscicide.

Silver nitrate is used for its astringent, caustic, and antibacterial properties. The inhibitory action of silver compounds is due to the ability of the silver ion to combine with essential thiol groups of the bacterial cell. The silver ion also combines with carboxyl, phosphate, amino, and other groups within the bacterial cell. The action of the silver ion is not restricted to bacterial cells; bactericidal concentrations are also toxic to tissues. High concentrations will precipitate proteins. Silver nitrate is bactericidal at a concentration of 1 in 1000 and it is bacteriostatic at lower concentrations. It is more active against Gram-negative than Gram-positive bacteria. Ophthalmic solutions containing silver nitrate 1% have been used for the prophylaxis of ophthalmia neonatorum. Silver nitrate compresses have been applied to severe burns to prevent infection. **Silver sulphadiazine** has broad antimicrobial activity against Gram-positive and Gram-negative organisms and yeasts and is used for the prevention of infection, particularly by *Pseudomonas aeruginosa*, in severe burns. Silver protein, mild silver protein, methargen, and silver acetate have also been used as antibacterial agents. **Mercury** and its inorganic salts and organic compounds have bacteriostatic properties due to the presence of mercuric ions (Hg^{2+}) which combine with the thiol (—SH) groups of essential membrane enzymes and cytoplasmic constituents. Inorganic mercury salts such as mercuric chloride are seldom used now because more efficient and less toxic preparations are available. Organic compounds of mercury used as antibacterial agents include **hydrargaphen**, **nitromersol**, and **thiomersal**. Hydrargaphen was formerly used as a solution or tincture for treating wounds, as pessaries for the treatment of vaginal candidiasis, and as a cream. Nitromersol and thiomersal have been used as alcoholic solutions for skin disinfection. **Mercurochrome** has also been used for skin disinfection, and for bladder and urethral irrigation. Phenylmercuric acetate, borate, and nitrate, and thiomersal are used as preservatives.

Quinoline Derivatives

Hydroxyquinoline (oxine) was formerly used as an antimicrobial agent and several halogenated derivatives are still in use. Dequalinium chloride and other 4-aminoquinaldinium derivatives are also used as antiseptics. Hydroxyquinoline and its derivatives are active against fungi and Gram-positive bacteria but possess little activity against Gram-negative bacteria; some have anti-amoebic properties. Hydroxyquinoline and its derivatives are chelating agents. They are active in the presence of divalent iron or copper ions; in the absence of these ions, hydroxyquinoline can enter bacterial or fungal cells but it will not be inhibitory. The active antimicrobial agent is a complex of hydroxyquinoline or its derivative and iron or copper.

Hydroxyquinoline sulphate is applied topically in the treatment of skin infections and a concentration of 0.001% has been used as a preservative and antoxidant.

Potassium hydroxyquinoline sulphate is an equimolecular mixture of potassium sulphate and hydroxyquinoline sulphate. It is used in topical preparations to treat fungal infections and minor bacterial skin infections.

Chlorquinaldol has been used in the treatment of skin conditions and vaginal infections.

Dequalinium chloride is a 4-aminoquinaldinium derivative and a cationic surfactant. It is more active against Gram-positive than Gram-negative bacteria and it is also active against *Borrelia vincentii*, *Candida albicans*, and some *Trichophyton* species. Dequalinium chloride lozenges are used for the treatment of mouth and throat infections. **Bisdequalinium diacetate** has similar properties to dequalinium chloride and is used for the treatment of minor skin infections.

Laurolinium acetate is a 4-aminoquinaldinium derivative and a cationic surfactant, which has been used for skin disinfection.

USES OF DISINFECTANTS

Disinfectants are used to reduce the number of micro-organisms to levels that are unlikely to be harmful to health. Disinfection can be carried out using heat or chemical disinfectants and in many instances thorough cleaning can replace disinfection.

Effective chemical disinfection depends on the correct use of suitable disinfectants. The efficiency of disinfectants also depends on the design of the premises or objects to be treated; for example, inaccessible areas or rough surfaces are difficult to clean and disinfect.

Use in Hospitals

The presence of virulent micro-organisms is a potential hazard in hospital environments where patients are living in a relatively small area; body fluids and discharges and objects contaminated with them are also a potential source of infection. Both staff and patients are at risk. Staff may acquire infections by contact with contaminated materials from patients. Patients may have increased susceptibility to infection because of lowered resistance resulting from disease or drug therapy. There is also the danger of infection in patients with burns and wounds and during surgery when susceptible tissue may be exposed to infection.

Infection in hospitals may be due to self-infection, which is caused by the transfer of micro-organisms from the skin or mucous membranes to a lesion or to the mouth. Cross-infection may result from contact with hands, clothes, equipment, food, and even disinfectants contaminated with virulent micro-organisms; it may also result from airborne organisms in dust and particles and in droplets shed by personnel and from dressings. Hospital-acquired infection often necessitates a prolonged stay in hospital, and in patients with a very low resistance it may cause death. It is therefore important that adequate measures should be taken to minimise the risk of hospital-acquired infection. Staff should be aware of the sources and routes of infection and should be trained to use procedures which minimise the risk of cross-infection. 'No-touch' dressing techniques should be employed. The risk of cross-infection may be reduced by isolating infected patients from uninfected patients; high risk patients may be barrier nursed. Patients' resistance to infection may be enhanced by good surgical procedures and, where necessary, by prophylactic antibiotic therapy.

The main area of control considered in this section is the inactivation and removal of virulent micro-organisms. The method used depends upon the source of infection and the likelihood of infection being transmitted to patients and staff.

Heat treatment has many advantages over chemical treatment; it can be used for disinfection and because it is lethal to all micro-organisms including spores it can be used to sterilise materials. Other physical methods of treatment include irradiation and filtration. In the absence of spores, chemical disinfectants can produce sterile conditions but as a rule they cannot be regarded as sterilising agents. Many disinfectants have a narrow spectrum of activity; they may be inactivated by organic matter or other materials and may have limited stability in solution. It is, therefore, important to use freshly prepared solutions because inactivated and unstable solutions may support the growth of micro-organisms and be a source of infection.

Hospital Disinfectant Policies

Hospital disinfectant policies have been devised to rationalise the use of chemical disinfectants in hospitals. In many hospitals a confusing number of different disinfectants and dilutions have been used, often inappropriately, and at considerable expense. The aim of all disinfectant policies should be the effective control of infection by the most efficient and economical methods possible.

Hospital disinfectant policies require consultation between the microbiologist, infection control doctor, infection control nurse, pharmacist, supplies officer, and representatives of medical, nursing, and domestic staff. All requests for disinfectants should be approved by the hospital pharmacist who can check whether they are in agreement with the hospital policy.

A hospital disinfectant policy should consider the following principles:

- identify the purposes for which disinfectants are required
- establish when heat sterilisation could be used, when sterilisation is required, when thorough cleaning is adequate, or where disposable products could economically be used
- select the smallest practicable number of disinfectants for the remaining uses, including alternatives for situations where patients or staff are sensitive to the routine disinfectant, instruments may be damaged, or the disinfectant is inappropriate for a given purpose
- distribute disinfectants at the correct use-dilution or provide equipment for appropriate dilution
- all disinfectant users should receive information on the appropriate disinfectant and concentration to be used for each task, and should be aware of the shelf-life of solutions, suitable containers for use, the frequency at which solutions should be changed, materials that react with the disinfectant, and measures required for the protection of personnel
- the policy should be monitored and changes implemented where necessary.

Chemical disinfection is used for the disinfection of skin and mucous membranes; pre-operative skin disinfection and surgical scrubbing are not usually within the scope of disinfection policies. Chemical disinfectants are used in food hygiene and to clean surfaces from which there is little risk of infection. They are also used to make contaminated objects and equipment safe to handle and to disinfect equipment that would be damaged by heat.

The disinfectants selected should be used at dilutions that are known to be effective; the use of a wide range of disinfectants should be avoided but those used should be suitable for their intended use. Solutions should be prepared with freshly distilled or freshly boiled and cooled water and transferred to thoroughly cleansed containers; cork liners or closures should not be used. Disinfectants should be distributed at the correct use-dilution and frequently renewed; the contents should not be used later than one week after opening the container. Containers should be thoroughly cleaned and dried before they are refilled; bottles containing partly used solutions should not be topped up. All staff using disinfectants should be instructed on their correct use with particular emphasis being placed on correct dilution and the problems of incompatibility and inactivation. The action of chemical disinfectants should be examined routinely by use-dilution and in-use tests.

Other factors that influence the choice of disinfectants are toxicity, corrosiveness, detergency, cost, and acceptability on aesthetic grounds.

Disinfection of the Skin and Mucous Membranes

The microbial population of the skin can be divided into resident and transient organisms. The resident organisms, with the exception of *Staphylococcus aureus*, are usually harmless. These organisms are situated in the crevices and lower layers of the skin and mainly persist after washing with soap and water. Persistent organisms may also be acquired by contact of the skin with contaminated material such as faeces. The mucous membranes of the mouth, nose, and vagina contain large numbers of resident bacteria. Transient bacteria are deposited on the surface of the skin. They do not multiply on the skin and are usually removed by washing with soap and water.

Disinfection of Hands. It is essential that the hands and arms of surgeons and staff involved in wound dressing be efficiently disinfected because gowns cannot adequately prevent the transfer of bacteria from the arms, and surgical gloves may become punctured. Preparations of chlorhexidine and povidone-iodine are widely used for this purpose because the soap and water scrub-up is time consuming and is not an efficient method for removing resident organisms. Soap inactivates cationic agents such as chlorhexidine.

A significant reduction in bacterial counts on the hands may be achieved by hand washing with chlorhexidine gluconate 4% in a detergent solution, instead of soap. Bacterial counts on the hands may also be reduced effectively by the application, with rubbing, of chlorhexidine gluconate 0.5% in water or ethanol (70%). The ethanol also exerts an antibacterial effect; because of its volatile nature ethanol leaves the skin dry but its action is of short duration.

Povidone-iodine solutions, containing 0.75% to 1% of available iodine, and other iodophores are also used as surgical hand scrubs. Povidone-iodine solutions do not produce such an immediate reduction in bacterial numbers on the hands as some chlorhexidine preparations, but when used for successive hand washes over two days their antibacterial activities appear similar.

Triclosan 0.5% in isopropanol 70% is also used for the disinfection of physically clean hands. It is applied to the palm of the hand, and then the hands, wrists, and forearms are rubbed until dry. Triclosan is compatible with soap.

Pre-operative Skin Disinfection. A rapidly acting disinfectant is required for pre-operative disinfection of the skin. Solutions of chlorhexidine 0.5%, iodine 1% in ethanol 70%, or alcoholic povidone-iodine applied with friction for at least two minutes are generally used to reduce resident skin flora at operation sites. Alcoholic solutions are preferred to aqueous solutions as they are more rapidly effective.

A benzalkonium chloride solution (0.01% to 0.1%) is also used for pre-operative skin disinfection.

Disinfection of Mucous Membranes. An aqueous solution of iodine (for example, Lugol's iodine or povidone-iodine) or an aqueous chlorhexidine solution is used for the disinfection of mucous membranes.

Elimination of organisms such as staphylococci from the nasal vestibule can be achieved by the use of a cream containing chlorhexidine hydrochloride 0.1% and neomycin 0.5%. A nasal ointment containing mupirocin is also available, but should probably be reserved for resistant cases.

The instillation of a chlorhexidine gluconate solution 0.01% to 0.02% is used for disinfection of the bladder after gynaecological surgery. A povidone-iodine vaginal douche, followed by povidone-iodine vaginal gel or pessaries, may be used for disinfection of vaginal mucosa.

Hexachlorophane should not be applied to mucous membranes.

Wound and Burn Toilet. Disinfectants are used to prevent and treat infected wounds and burns. The use of disinfectant solutions such as chlorhexidine gluconate with cetrimide is effective for cleaning dirty wounds. Hypochlorite solutions such as Chlorinated Lime and Boric Acid Solution BP (Eusol) and Surgical Chlorinated Soda Solution BPC (Dakin's Solution) are often used as debriding agents. These preparations have been used undiluted for wound and ulcer cleansing, but are no longer recommended as they are considered too irritant. Chlorhexidine is less toxic to cells and has been shown to reduce the emergence of infection in minor burns. Silver sulphadiazine is commonly used, particularly for Gram-negative infections such as pseudomonal infections in second- and third-degree burns, infected leg ulcers, and pressure sores. There is some evidence that the wound exudate may contain an antibacterial substance and complete removal of all wound exudate may be undesirable.

Disinfection of Clean Surfaces

Floors, Walls, and Furniture. Cleaning with soap or detergent and water is usually sufficient to reduce microbial contamination on floors, walls, and furniture to acceptable levels. Walls and other vertical surfaces are not readily contaminated and, if dry, do not support the growth of many microorganisms. Except in operating theatres, microorganisms deposited on walls are not an important source of infection as they are held by electrostatic forces and are not easily removed by air currents; they are more readily removed by contact. Floors and other horizontal surfaces are quickly recontaminated after cleaning. Cleaning is as efficient as combined cleaning and disinfection in most circumstances and the use of disinfectants does not decrease the rate of recontamination to any extent. Locker tops and ward furniture should be washed daily with soap or detergent and water; furniture may also be damp-dusted.

Disinfection is not required unless contamination is known to have occurred. Surface disinfection is necessary where there is soilage or in infectious disease units and high risk areas such as operating theatres, intensive care units, and nurseries; clear soluble phenolic disinfectants, at the recommended dilutions, are suitable in most instances. In areas where surfaces are heavily contaminated with blood, a hypochlorite solution should be used. Terminal disinfection of wards or rooms and their contents is used only in special circumstances. The rooms are usually disinfected by fumigation with formaldehyde. Terminal disinfection may also be carried out by fogging. The disinfectant fog is produced by a special spray and the disinfectant is deposited on the surfaces. This method cannot be used instead of cleaning as repeated fogging leads to a build-up of layers of old disinfectant. Terminal disinfection may be considered after an outbreak of infection by a specific resistant pathogen. Cleaning equipment, such as mops, brushes, and buckets, is a potential source of infection. This equipment should be cleaned, disinfected by heat if possible, and then dried; preliminary cleaning of this equipment is particularly important if chemical disinfection is used. Chemical disinfection is only effective if there is adequate penetration and no inactivation by mop head materials.

Ward Bathrooms and Lavatories. Baths, sinks, and wash-basins should be cleaned with detergent, daily and after use. Non-abrasive powders containing hypochlorite are suitable for the disinfection of relatively clean surfaces. Hypochlorite-detergent solutions are also suitable. Lavatory seats should be washed at least daily with detergent. During outbreaks of infection, disinfection with hypochlorite or phenolic solutions, followed by rinsing, may be necessary.

Disposable paper towels should be used for cleaning baths, sinks, and wash-basins. Where disposable equipment is not available, quick-drying nylon brushes may be used. Non-disposable cloths should be washed and dried after use. Toilet brushes should be rinsed in the flushing water of the lavatory pan and stored dry.

Ward Kitchen Equipment. Work surfaces are cleaned and then disinfected with suitable dilutions of hypochlorite or cationic surfactants. Crockery and cutlery are washed in a dish-washing machine that gives a final rinse temperature of 80°; the temperature should be high enough to ensure spontaneous drying. Where dish-washing machines are not available, for most purposes, crockery and cutlery may be washed in hot water with detergent. Disinfection should only be used on advice from the microbiologist. Disinfectants suitable for kitchen use are hypochlorite solutions, giving 120 to 250 ppm of available chlorine, or where hypochlorites might cause erosion, cationic surfactants. Phenolic disinfectants should not be used in kitchens as they may taint food even at low concentrations.

Disinfection of Equipment

Non-medical Equipment. Patients should have their own plastic wash-bowls which should be washed after use with soap or detergent and hot water, dried, and stored inverted. The bowls should be disinfected by heat, with a hypochlorite solution, or with a clear soluble phenolic compound before being issued to another patient. Nail-brushes and soap dishes are not usually necessary. Nail-brushes are often contaminated with Gram-negative bacteria even when stored in disinfectant; sterile nail-brushes should be used when required for aseptic procedures.

Razors and shaving brushes for pre-operative use should be sterile; disposable sterile razors and brushless shaving cream are often used. Communal razors and shaving brushes used by the hospital barber should be immersed in ethanol 70% or isopropanol 70% for five minutes after each shave; electric razor heads should also be immersed in ethanol 70% for five minutes.

Bed frames, bed-cradles, and plastic covers on pillows and mattresses should be washed with soap or detergent and water. Bed-linen cannot readily be disinfected if it becomes contaminated; it should be enclosed within a waterproof cover, which can be wiped with a detergent solution for decontamination. Clear soluble phenolic disinfectants can make covers permeable and should be avoided if possible. If disinfection is necessary, a hypochlorite solution, providing 1000 ppm available chlorine, should be used before rinsing well.

Medical and Surgical Equipment. In this section the use of disinfectants to make objects safe to handle and the disinfection of equipment which cannot be heat treated is discussed.

Trolley tops are disinfected with ethanol 70%, isopropanol 70%, or recommended dilutions of clear soluble phenolic disinfectants. Instruments should be supplied packed and sterilised. Instruments can be disinfected, but not sterilised, in boiling water for 5 to 10 minutes. Immersion of clean instruments in ethanol 70%, or glutaraldehyde 2%, for 10 minutes will disinfect, but is not as reliably effective as hot water or steam. Instruments immersed in glutaraldehyde should be thoroughly rinsed in water to remove irritant residues before use. Sterile water should be used for invasive items. The use of glutaraldehyde in wards and clinics should be avoided if possible. Wiping with ethanol 70% is a rapid and useful method for disinfecting surfaces, but is less appropriate for instruments such as scissors. Cheatle's forceps should be autoclaved or boiled daily and may be stored in solutions of clear soluble phenolic disinfectants. Soiled instruments are immersed in solutions containing a phenolic disinfectant and a compatible detergent.

The necks of ampoules should be swabbed with sterile cotton wool and ethanol 70% or isopropanol 70%.

Oral thermometers should be stored dry because those stored in disinfectant solutions are often contaminated with Gram-negative bacteria. If used for an individual patient, the thermometer may be cleaned with an alcoholic wipe. Terminal disinfection of thermometers is achieved by their immersion for at least 10 minutes in ethanol 70%, isopropanol 70%, or a clear phenolic solution. Disposable thermometers for application to the skin are now commonly used.

Contamination of rectal thermometers is reduced by the use of disposable plastic sleeves; for terminal disinfection, rectal thermometers may be treated as for oral thermometers

Re-usable bedpans should be disinfected by heat after sluicing and washing. If facilities for heat disinfection are not available, bedpans may be disinfected by placing in boiling water for 5 to 10 minutes. In emergency situations, or in countries with limited facilities, chemical disinfection may be used. The entire surface of the cleaned bedpan should be wiped with a clear phenolic disinfectant or hypochlorite solution, before rinsing and drying. Hypochlorite solutions may damage stainless steel bedpans. Immersion tanks should be avoided as they encourage the growth of resistant strains of Gram-negative bacteria. Disposable bedpans and urine bottles are available and in common use in most hospitals. Staff should always wash their hands after handling bedpans and urinals, and staff carrying out disinfection procedures should wear gloves and plastic gowns.

A clear soluble phenolic disinfectant or a hypochlorite solution is used in laboratory discard jars. Hypochlorite is inactivated by organic material and its activity should be checked routinely; if it is found to be unsatisfactory, it should be replaced by a suitable dilution of a phenolic disinfectant. Dilute solutions should be accurately and regularly prepared and the jars should be washed before refilling.

Many of the new operative endoscopes are flexible and damaged by heat. They should be cleaned thoroughly and, if possible, sterilised with ethylene oxide or low temperature steam and formaldehyde. Immersion in glutaraldehyde 2% for three hours is a suitable alternative, but this method is less reliable due to the possible presence of air bubbles and recontamination on subsequent rinsing. Shorter immersion times of 10 to 20 minutes are usually used, and provided that the endoscope is well cleaned before disinfection the risk of infection is small, although there is a risk of infection due to spore-forming organisms.

Pasteurisation of cystoscopes in a water bath at 70° to 80° for 10 minutes is an alternative to chemical disinfection, but the manufacturer should be consulted about heat tolerance. Another alternative is ethanol 70% for five minutes, but this may damage the instrument if immersion is prolonged beyond that recommended by the manufacturer.

Flexible gastro-intestinal endoscopes may be disinfected using activated glutaraldehyde 2%. The British Society of Gastroenterology has recommended thorough cleaning of all channels and external surfaces followed by immersion in glutaraldehyde 2% for four minutes after each patient. The period of immersion should be extended to one hour for patients with known, or suspected, pulmonary tuberculosis. For immunocompromised patients, the endoscope should be disinfected for one hour before and after the procedure. An alternative method involves cleaning the endoscope with a detergent followed by ethanol 70%. It is a less effective method and immersion in alcohol for longer than five minutes may damage epoxy lens cements.

Presterilised disposable catheters, cystoscopes, and endoscopes are available.

Disinfection of ventilators after use by each patient is advised, but may not be necessary with ventilators that are protected by bacteria-impermeable filters. Ventilators can usually be disinfected with nebulised hydrogen peroxide or formaldehyde gas. Smaller ventilators and humidifiers can be decontaminated with low temperature steam or glutaraldehyde 2%. Chlorhexidine 0.1% may be used to prevent bacterial growth in the evaporator type of humidifier in infant incubators, but not in the nebuliser type.

Viruses

The virus causing Creutzfeldt-Jakob disease is resistant to several disinfection procedures. Immersion in sodium hydroxide 1M for one hour at room temperature provides full inactivation and is the treatment of choice. Decontamination has been carried out by autoclaving, or disinfection with sodium hypochlorite 0.5% or povidone-iodine.

Hepatitis B virus can be inactivated by boiling for one minute, autoclaving, ethylene oxide gas sterilisation, glutaraldehyde 2%, formaldehyde 8%, or sodium hypochlorite 0.5%. Phenolic disinfectants, hexachlorophane, and cationic surfactants are not effective.

Heat is the most effective method of eliminating the human immunodeficiency virus (HIV). Chemical disinfectants should only be used if other methods are not available and must not be used for needles or syringes. Cleaned instruments may be disinfected by immersion in glutaraldehyde 2% or hydrogen peroxide 6% for 30 minutes followed by thorough rinsing. Spillages of blood and body fluids should be managed with absorbent materials and chlorine-releasing disinfectants (see below).

Spillages of Blood and Body Fluids

Spillages of blood and body fluids should be absorbed into disposable towels and treated with a chlorine-releasing compound (giving 10 000 ppm available chlorine) such as hypochlorite solution, chlorinated lime, sodium dichloroisocyanurate, or chloramine. After ten minutes the whole spill is wiped up with fresh absorbent material and placed in a container for contaminated waste. An alternative is to use a granular form of chlorine, which helps to contain the spillage. The surface should then be disinfected. Gloves should be worn throughout the procedure.

Alcohols are not suitable for spillages as they rapidly evaporate and also coagulate, and do not penetrate, organic material.

Use in the Home

The correct use of disinfectants in the home is governed by the same principles that apply to their use in hospitals. In most circumstances there is little risk of transmitting infection in the home and the serious consequences that can arise from the transmission of infection in hospital are unlikely to occur. General disinfectants used in the home should have a wide range of activity and the activity should not be markedly reduced by organic matter or mop-head materials.

Baths, wash-basins, and sinks can be adequately cleaned with an abrasive powder containing sodium hypochlorite. Lavatories may be cleaned and disinfected with hypochlorite solutions. Many commercially available preparations used as household disinfectants are clear soluble phenolic disinfectants. These preparations are relatively cheap and retain much of their activity in the presence of organic matter and mop-head materials. Preparations containing pine oil or other aromatic oils are relatively ineffective as disinfectants but they are often used routinely for the 'clean' smell they impart regardless of whether disinfection is necessary. Products containing white or black fluids are strong smelling but are inexpensive and have a wide range of antibacterial activity. They are used for lavatories and drains although their activity may be significantly reduced by dilution and the presence of plastics and other mop-head materials. Generally, however, except in the presence of contaminated or infective material, thorough cleansing alone is adequate.

Cationic surfactants, diguanides, and chlorinated phenols are available in over-the-counter preparations for use in the first-aid treatment of minor cuts, wounds, and burns. Acridine derivatives are also available for the treatment of minor burns. Amylmetacresol, dequalinium chloride, and chlorinated phenols are used in mouthwashes, gargles, and throat lozenges.

Use on Farms

Disinfectants are used on farms to control disease of animals and to cleanse and decontaminate dairy equipment.

Diseases of Animals. In Great Britain approved disinfectants and their maximum rates of dilution for general use during outbreaks of foot-and-mouth disease, swine vesicular disease, fowl pest, tuberculosis, and other diseases are listed in schedules of the Diseases of Animals (Approved Disinfectants) Order 1978 (SI 1978:No 32), the Diseases of Animals (Approved Disinfectants) (Amendment) Order 1992, and the Diseases of Animals (Approved Disinfectants) (Amendment) (No 2) Order 1992.

Disinfection of Air

In many occupied buildings the airborne micro-organisms are mainly Gram-positive cocci but in hospitals many other pathogens may be present. The micro-organisms may be dry and associated with dust particles or with shed hair and skin particles; they may also be expelled from the respiratory tract and enclosed in droplets which on drying are enclosed in a protective layer of dried mucus. Air conditioning systems may become contaminated with Gram-negative, aerobic non-sporing bacilli of the genus *Legionella*. Acute infections of the respiratory tract may be caused by *Legionella pneumophila* (Legionnaires' disease). Air outside buildings is usually less contaminated and the organisms present are mainly bacterial spores with some mould spores. The particles are usually smaller than those found in enclosed air as they are not associated with dust or other particles.

Chemical Disinfection. The use of chemical disinfectants for the disinfection of rooms is limited by their irritant nature. Air filtration techniques are now more widely used (see below).

Formaldehyde solution is used to fumigate rooms. The gas may be generated by the addition of 170 g of potassium permanganate to 500 mL of Formaldehyde Solution; this results in rapid boiling and the generation of moist formaldehyde gas. Rooms are sealed during fumigation and the temperature and relative humidity should be controlled to remain above 18° and 60%, respectively. It has been suggested that water should, if necessary, be sprayed into the air to maintain adequate humidity. After initiating the fumigation, the room should be kept sealed for 48 hours.

Sulphur dioxide has formerly been employed as a fumigant. The gas may be generated by burning sulphur.

Filtration. This method is used to sterilise large volumes of air in the fermentation stage of antibiotic production and it is also used on a smaller scale to produce an environment of sterile air in which to perform aseptic procedures (see Cleanrooms for Pharmaceutical Production chapter).

Ultraviolet Irradiation. This technique has been used in hospitals to reduce the bacterial contamination of the air but it is not a very efficient method. Spores and those vegetative cells protected by a layer of organic material are resistant to ultraviolet irradiation. It is only active against bacterial cells if the contact time is long and the cells are close to the source of radiation.

Disinfection of Water

Water may be disinfected by physical means such as ultraviolet irradiation or filtration, or by chemicals. The physical methods are more expensive; ultraviolet irradiation has many disadvantages and filters require constant maintenance and may not prevent the passage of micro-organisms. Public water supplies, small volumes of drinking water, and water in swimming pools are usually subjected to chemical disinfection.

Drinking Water. The main reasons for disinfecting drinking water are to eradicate pathogens, maintain a protective barrier against pathogens entering the distribution system, and suppress bacterial regrowth in the pipe environment.

A European Community (EC) directive on drinking water specifies that no faecal coliforms or streptococci should be present in water at the point of human consumption and the World Health Organization (WHO) recommends similar standards for water entering the distribution systems. It also specifies that water may be considered of a suitable virological quality when a turbidity of 1NTU (nephelometric turbidity unit) is achieved with at least 500 micrograms/litre of free residual chlorine after a contact period of at least 30 minutes.

The use of chlorine, chlorine dioxide, or ozone is preferable, although for chlorine the pH should be less than 8.0. Because chloramines are only slowly biocidal, their use as primary disinfecting agents for water treatment purposes is not recommended, although they may be used for the maintenance of residuals in distribution systems where the contact time is longer.

Maintenance and monitoring of a chlorine residual offers two benefits. A chlorine residual will suppress the growth of organisms within the system and may afford some protection against contamination entering through cross-connection or leakage. The sudden disappearance of the residual provides an immediate indication of the entry of oxidisable matter into the system or of a malfunction of the treatment process. If chlorine is employed, it is desirable that a free chlorine residual of 0.2 to 0.5 mg/litre be maintained and monitored daily throughout the entire system.

Any organic particulate matter present in potable water during distribution exerts a chlorine demand which reduces the available free chlorine residual, especially in dead-end sections of a system. Regular flushing of mains is desirable to avoid such accumulations.

Swimming Pools. Sodium hypochlorite, generated by the electrolysis of a dilute brine solution external to the swimming pool, may be used as a means of disinfection. The Department of the Environment National Water Council have recommended that the free chlorine residual concentration is maintained in the range 1 to 3 mg/litre; ideally, between 1.5 and 2.0 mg/litre. Pool operators should maintain the pH in the range 7.2 to 7.8; ideally, in the range 7.4 to 7.6.

At the time of installation, consideration should be given to the incorporation of pH control, normally by acid addition, using either automatic or manually controlled dosage pumps. Other disinfectant systems that have been used for swimming pools include calcium hypochlorite, sodium dichloroisocyanurate, trichloroisocyanuric acid, ozone with residual free chlorine, elemental liquid bromine, and bromochlorodimethylhydantoin.

Air Conditioning Plants and Water Storage Tanks. Static water may be contaminated with indigenous micro-organisms which will readily multiply at ambient temperatures. Mild and acute infections may arise from such contaminated water (for example, Legionnaires' disease). Regular cleansing and disinfection of cooling towers and water storage tanks is essential to prevent the build-up of micro-organisms.

FACTORS AFFECTING THE EFFICIENCY OF DISINFECTANTS

The process of disinfection is influenced by several factors and to obtain reproducible results in some tests certain conditions are standardised. The influence of changes in these factors on the efficiency of disinfectants in the non-standard conditions met in practice should be noted.

Temperature

The rate of disinfection increases with rises in temperature and the increase varies with the type of disinfectant used. The temperature coefficient, which is characteristic for a particular disinfectant under standard conditions, is a measure of the change in velocity of disinfection per degree (or per 10°) rise in temperature. It cannot be estimated but must be assessed by direct measurement over the desired temperature range and is given by:

temperature coefficient (per 10° rise)

$$= \frac{\text{time to kill at x}°}{\text{time to kill at (x + 10)}°}$$

The coefficient is an exponential factor and as the temperature increases arithmetically the rate of disinfection increases geometrically. The action of a disinfectant with a high temperature coefficient is more influenced by temperature changes than that of a disinfectant with a low temperature coefficient.

The influence of temperature changes on disinfectant action is also associated with the temperature-dependent rates of microbial growth. The temperature coefficient will depend on the test organisms. In methods for testing disinfectants it is important that the recovery incubation temperature is optimal for growth of the test organism.

Concentration

The rate of disinfection is directly proportional to disinfectant concentration. For a particular disinfectant, the dilution coefficient is the slope of the line obtained when the logarithm of the time to kill an inoculum is plotted against the logarithm of concentration. It can be expressed by the equation:

$$n \log c + \log t = k$$

where c is the concentration, t is the time to kill, n is the dilution coefficient, and k is a constant.

The action of a disinfectant that has a high dilution coefficient is markedly reduced by dilution (for example, phenolic agents, $n = 4$ to 10). Disinfectants with a low dilution coefficient retain a signifi-

cant amount of activity on dilution (for example, cationic surfactants, $n = 0.8$ to 2.5). In practice, it is obviously important to know the effect of dilution on disinfectant action. Additionally, in disinfectant tests the effect of dilution influences the type of inactivation required.

Contact Time

The time during which a disinfectant must remain in contact with the inoculum to exert its effect will be influenced by many factors such as temperature and concentration, which affect the rate of disinfection.

pH

The influence of pH on the activity of disinfectants is complex. Microbial growth is influenced by pH as well as by temperature; the optimum pH for the growth of many species of bacteria is in the range 6 to 8. The ability of a disinfectant to interact with a bacterial cell depends on the charge on the cell surface which in turn depends on the pH of the environment. The rate of reaction between disinfectant and target groups within the cell may also be pH dependent.

The activity of some disinfectants is due to undissociated molecules, and changes in pH which promote ion formation will reduce the activity. Conversely, disinfectants that are only active in the ionised form will be less active when pH changes favour formation of the unionised form. Thus the activity of cationic disinfectants is increased with increases in pH. The stability of some disinfectants is altered by changes in pH and compounds may not be most active at the pH of greatest stability.

Types of Micro-organisms and Extent of Contamination

The purposes for which a particular disinfectant can be used effectively are limited by its spectrum of activity. The efficiency of chlorhexidine and other disinfectants that are adsorbed in significant amounts onto cells is markedly reduced where there is gross contamination. This effect may be countered to some extent by the use of higher concentrations of disinfectant and longer contact times. In evaluations of the activity of this type of disinfectant it is essential to know the inoculum size.

Organic Material

The presence of organic material such as food, body fluids, faeces, fabrics, and plastic is known to reduce the efficiency of many disinfectants. The disinfectant may be inactivated by chemical reaction or adsorbed onto, or dissolved in, the organic material. The organic material may form a protective layer round the micro-organisms. Methods for evaluating disinfectants should, therefore, take into account the influence of these materials on activity.

Formulation

The activity of lipid-soluble disinfectants, such as phenols, may be reduced by the use of organic solvents. The amount of available disinfectant is in effect reduced by partition into the organic phase. The activity of some cationic disinfectants is greater in alcoholic than in aqueous solution and the addition of acid to some disinfectants renders them sporicidal.

Soaps and other surfactants are used to solubilise relatively insoluble disinfectants. The antibacterial effect may be enhanced by reduced surface tension and increased permeability of microbial cell membranes. The activity of cationic compounds is antagonised by anionic surfactants and, in some instances, by nonionic surfactants.

METHODS FOR TESTING DISINFECTANTS

No single test can be used to evaluate all antimicrobial activity. Tests must be modified to measure antibacterial and antifungal activity, and different methods must be applied to determine lethal and inhibitory activities. Although these tests provide an indication of the relative activities of disinfectants, the tests are devised to be reproducible under laboratory conditions and the results must not be used in isolation to draw conclusions about the in-use situation. Methods for testing disinfectants have been devised which take account of the in-use conditions and the use of these tests with the long-established laboratory tests can give useful information on disinfectant action.

Organisations that have published details of test methods include the British Standards Institution (BSI); the Association Francaise de Normalisation (AFNOR); the Association of Official Analytical Chemists (AOAC); and the Deutsche Gesellschaft fur Hygiene und Mikrobiologie (DGHM).

Bacteriostatic Tests

Bacteriostatic tests demonstrate the ability of the disinfectant to inhibit the growth and reproduction of the test organism. The tests may be either quantitative (for example, serial dilution tests) or qualitative (for example, agar diffusion tests).

Serial Dilution Tests

Serial dilutions of disinfectant solutions are prepared by transferring solution from one tube to a second tube containing diluent; further similar transferences are then carried out to produce a series of dilute solutions. These solutions are then added to nutrient media and inoculated with test organisms. An agar plate can be inoculated with several test organisms but a sample in a liquid medium must be inoculated with a single test organism. Following a suitable incubation period the samples are observed. The point at which no growth occurs is taken as the bacteriostatic concentration or minimum inhibitory concentration (MIC). It is possible to examine the samples spectrophotometrically to determine the MIC. The end-point varies with the inoculum size which should therefore always be defined. The use of these tests in the evaluation of disinfectants is limited because disinfectants are required to have bactericidal rather than bacteriostatic activity.

Agar Diffusion Tests

These tests, when applied to disinfectants, are usually qualitative rather than quantitative. They depend on the ability of the disinfectant to diffuse through agar and are used to show the activity of an antibacterial agent which has to be released from a solid or semi-solid preparation before it exerts its effect.

Agar Cup Tests. Suitable solutions or disinfectant formulations are placed in cups cut out of the agar in an inoculated agar plate. After incubation the widths of the zones of inhibition on the plate are recorded and used as a measure of activity.

Surface Contact Tests. Filter-paper disks impregnated with the test disinfectant or small sterile fish-spine insulator beads touched with the test solution are placed on the surface of inoculated agar plates. Solid samples which do not change in consistency at 37° can be placed directly on the agar plate. After incubation the zones of inhibition are measured to determine activity.

Ditch Plate Test. The test solution is placed in a ditch cut in an agar plate. The test organisms are streaked over the plate at right-angles to the ditch. The plates are incubated under suitable conditions for 24 hours and the plates are then examined for zones of inhibition.

Gradient Plate Method. The agar plate is prepared by pouring agar containing the disinfectant into a plate held at an angle so that the agar sets as a wedge. Agar is then poured onto the plate held horizontally. The test organisms are streaked across the plate so that each streak covers the range of disinfectant concentrations. The plate is incubated and the point on the streak at which inhibition occurs is noted. This test is only of value if the disinfectant can diffuse through the agar to produce a concentration gradient.

Tests for Combined Action. Two test solutions are applied on paper strips at right-angles to each other on an inoculated agar plate. After incubation the plates are examined and the synergistic or antagonistic effects of the disinfectants can be determined from the size and shape of the zones of inhibition.

Bactericidal Tests

Bactericidal tests measure the ability of the disinfectant to kill the test organism. The effects of the disinfectant must therefore be neutralised before incubation in order to prevent bacteriostatic effects.

Phenol Coefficient Tests

Phenol coefficient tests are used to determine bactericidal activity. The activity of a disinfectant against *Salmonella typhi* is compared with that of phenol under test conditions and expressed as a ratio. In Great Britain, the Rideal-Walker and Chick-Martin tests have been standardised by the British Standards Institution (see below). The standard tests are used to compare phenols and the phenol coefficients obtained are accepted parameters in the specifications of phenolic disinfectants.

The activities of non-phenolic disinfectants of similar structure can be compared by measuring their phenol coefficients. However, these tests are not designed to give a useful comparison of disinfectants with totally different modes of action.

The Rideal-Walker Test. Details of the original Rideal-Walker test were published in 1903 and this test was one of the first designed to quantify disinfectant activity. Over the years the test has been modified and the standard test is described in British Standard 541:1985(1991), the method for determination of the Rideal-Walker coefficient of disinfectants. The method applies only to disinfectants based on coal tar derivatives and/or substituted phenols. The test compares disinfectants in aqueous solutions, and the apparatus, reagents

(including test organism), test conditions, and technique are all standardised. The effects of five suitable dilutions of the disinfectant under test are compared with those of five standard dilutions of phenol against *Salmonella typhi* (NCTC 786) during specified contact periods of up to 10 minutes. The Rideal-Walker coefficient is calculated by dividing the dilution of the test disinfectant which contains viable bacteria at $2\frac{1}{2}$ and 5 minutes but not at $7\frac{1}{2}$ and 10 minutes by the dilution of phenol which is similarly bactericidal at $7\frac{1}{2}$ and 10 minutes, but not at $2\frac{1}{2}$ and 5 minutes.

In British Standard 5197:1976(1991), the specification for aromatic disinfectant fluids, the antimicrobial values of the disinfectant are designated PA, PB, PC, and PD and represent Rideal-Walker coefficients of 3.0 to 5.0, 5.1 to 7.0, 7.1 to 10.0, and above 10.0, respectively. The Standard applies to light-duty aromatic disinfectant fluids containing substituted phenols. To comply with this specification, manufacturers must give the minimum value for the Rideal-Walker coefficient claimed for a particular disinfectant fluid. The use-dilution recommended for disinfectant fluids should not exceed one part in twenty times the claimed Rideal-Walker coefficient.

The Rideal-Walker coefficient gives an indication of the activity of a disinfectant under the specified conditions of the test and provides a quantitative comparison of one disinfectant with another under those test conditions.

The Chick-Martin Test. This test was designed by Chick and Martin in 1908 to determine disinfectant activity in the presence of organic material. As disinfectants are frequently used in the presence of organic material this test modification went some way to simulate the conditions met in practice. In the original test 3% dried human faeces was included but later dried yeast was used as a suitable organic alternative. Chick and Martin also extended the contact time of 10 minutes used in the Rideal-Walker test up to 30 minutes. The modified Chick-Martin test is described in British Standard 808:1986(1991), the method for assessing the efficacy of disinfectants by the modified Chick-Martin test. The apparatus, reagents (including test organism), and test conditions and techniques are all controlled by the Standard.

The phenol coefficient is the quotient of the mean of the highest concentration of phenol permitting growth in a challenge medium and the lowest concentration not permitting such growth to the corresponding mean concentration of the disinfectant under test. The phenol coefficient may show whether the action of a disinfectant is reduced in the presence of organic material but the results cannot be assumed to be exactly those that would be observed with organic material other than yeast.

The Crown Agents' Test. This test is intended to be used for testing of white disinfectant fluids only; these are finely dispersed emulsions of coal tar acids, or similar acids derived from petroleum, or any mixture of these, with or without hydrocarbons and containing a colloidal protectant. It is a phenol coefficient test. The Crown Agents' test is a modified version of the tests described above in which the test disinfectant is diluted in sterile artificial sea water; gelatin and rice starch are included as organic material. The test is described in British Standard 2462:1986(1991), the specification for black and white disinfectant fluids.

AOAC Phenol Coefficient Test. This is a modification of the Rideal-Walker test specified by the AOAC (Association of Official Analytical Chemists). In this test there is a choice of three subculture media to eliminate the carry-over of bacteriostatic effects and it specifies three test organisms, *Salmonella typhi*, *Pseudomonas aeruginosa*, and *Staphylococcus aureus*.

Limitations of Phenol Coefficients. *Salmonella typhi* was chosen as a suitable test organism when typhoid fever was a relatively common disease. Other pathogenic organisms, often more resistant than *Salmonella typhi* to the action of disinfectants, are routinely encountered in hospitals. The use of *Salmonella typhi* as test organism has led to the use of a correction factor to obtain information on the action of disinfectants against more resistant organisms; the use of correction factors means that the results are further removed from those found in practice because they do not take into account the effect of concentration changes on the activity of various disinfectants. It has been suggested that *Escherichia coli* or *Pseudomonas aeruginosa* would be suitable alternative test organisms (for example, AOAC test). The day-to-day maintenance of the test organism under standard conditions is essential for reproducible results but even under carefully controlled conditions variations in sensitivity to phenol can occur. Phenol was originally chosen as the standard because at the time it was regarded as an important disinfectant. It is water soluble and although many of the disinfectants used today are phenols,

they are often insoluble and formulated as emulsions or in a solubilised form.

Variability in results can also be attributed to a total kill end-point; towards the end-point it becomes a matter of statistical chance whether the loopful withdrawn contains viable cells. Variation in inoculum size from a 4 mm loop is a further source of error; larger volumes cannot be used because they could cause bacteriostasis in the small volumes of nutrient broth used in the recovery incubation period.

The incubation temperature of 37° has been criticised as not being the optimum for the recovery of damaged cells because it is now known that damaged cells recover better at temperatures below their normal optimum. In addition, the variation in disinfectant activity with temperature depends on the type of disinfectant. The ratio of activities of the test disinfectant and phenol may be very different at 37° from that at room temperature.

In the Rideal-Walker test the contact time of 10 minutes is too short. It is possible that the rate of kill at the times of sampling is high and this will cause wide variations in the end-point result. The 30-minute contact time used in the Chick-Martin test is more reliable. Changes in composition of the nutrient medium will obviously affect results but some changes in ingredients have become necessary because of the unavailability of the original test materials.

Finally, major limitations of these tests are, as previously stated, that they can only be used to compare compounds with similar modes of action and that the results obtained give an indication of disinfectant activity under test conditions that are unlikely to be those found in practice.

Viable Counts

The bactericidal activity of disinfectants may be estimated from viable cell counts obtained after various contact times. The proportion of viable cells observed after a specific contact time is also used to characterise bactericidal activity.

Disinfectant-bacteria mixtures are prepared and after the required period of time 0.5- to 1.0-mL dilutions of the mixture are added to molten agar at about 46°; the inoculated agar is poured onto a plate and incubated at a suitable temperature for 48 to 72 hours. The cell colonies, each of which is assumed to be produced from a single cell, are counted and the number of viable cells in the original sample is calculated. These techniques are also known as quantitative suspension tests.

In viable count techniques the disinfectant activity in a sample must be neutralised as soon as the sample is removed from the test mixture. Inactivation of phenols and alcohols is achieved by dilution but with other disinfectants a specific inactivating compound must be added to the sample. Chlorhexidine and quaternary ammonium compounds are inactivated by a nonionic surfactant (Lubrol™ W) and egg lecithin, mercurials by thioglycollic acid, halogens by sodium thiosulphate, acridine dyes by nucleic acid, hexachlorophane by polysorbate 80 (Tween™ 80), and formaldehyde by ammonium ions.

Bacterial cells that have been damaged by the action of a disinfectant may suffer more damage by contact with hot agar; this additional damage may prevent cell recovery and lead to an inaccurate estimation of bactericidal activity. This problem may be overcome by using surface inoculation of agar plates.

The assumption that each colony is produced from a single cell may be misleading. If cell clumping occurs on the plate the number of viable cells may be underestimated. Ionic disinfectants which affect the cell surface charge on bacteria often cause cell clumping and this effect can be minimised by the addition of certain nonionic surfactants.

The Kelsey-Sykes Test

Over the years attempts have been made to devise methods for testing disinfectants which both simulate conditions met in practice and overcome the limitations inherent in phenol coefficient tests. Several capacity use-dilution tests have been devised and the Kelsey-Sykes test for hospital disinfectants was developed from a test specified in British Standard 3286:1960(1991), method for laboratory evaluation of disinfectant activity of quaternary ammonium compounds by suspension test procedure.

The test allows variations in several parameters including test organism, contact time, and presence of organic material. The test organisms are *Pseudomonas aeruginosa* (NCTC 6749), *Staphylococcus aureus* (NCTC 4163), and *Proteus vulgaris* (NCTC 4635); they were chosen because they cause major problems in hospitals and because they are highly resistant to disinfectants.

An 'improved Kelsey-Sykes test' that is a modified version of the original test was developed. The test organisms are grown in a chemically defined medium in an attempt to improve reproducibility. Organisms used for the test under 'clean' conditions are in a watery suspension and the organic material added to represent 'dirty' conditions is yeast; horse serum is not allowed as an alternative; the recovery medium contains 3% Tween™ 80. This test was originally considered suitable for evaluating all types of disinfectants used in hospitals. More recent data suggest that the improved Kelsey-Sykes test is only suitable for certain phenolic disinfectants. The modified Kelsey-Sykes test is described in British Standard 6905:1987, method for estimation of concentration of disinfectants used in 'dirty' conditions in hospitals by the modified Kelsey-Sykes test.

An In-use Test for Hospital Disinfectants

Routine testing to check the performance of disinfectants is recommended in most hospital disinfectant policies. Samples are collected from disinfectant dilutions following their use in disinfectant procedures and from dilutions in closed containers awaiting use. One mL of sample is diluted to 10 mL with a suitable diluent; phenols and alcohols may be diluted with quarter-strength compound sodium chloride solution, hypochlorites and iodophores with nutrient broth containing 0.5% of sodium thiosulphate, and diguanides with nutrient broth containing 3% of polysorbate 80. Ten drops are placed separately on each of two agar plates. The plates are incubated for up to 72 hours, one at room temperature and the other at 37°. Growth from more than 5 of 10 drops on either plate indicates inadequate disinfectant activity.

Evaluation of Skin Disinfectants

Skin disinfectants may be tested under conditions approaching those found in practice. The tests used are either skin infection tests or skin disinfection tests.

Skin infection tests are used to evaluate preparations for use in the treatment of wounds. In these tests, wounds or the abraded skin of experimental *animals* are inoculated with a virulent or non-virulent strain of bacteria and then treated with the test disinfectant. The efficacy of the disinfectant is measured as a function of either the survival of the test *animals* or the reduction of the lesions.

Skin disinfection tests are of three main types: hand-washing tests; direct swabbing; and the replica method.

Hand-washing Tests. These tests were devised to test antiseptic soaps but have been adopted for other skin disinfectants. In the basic method, the hands and arms are scrubbed with an ordinary soap for 1 minute and rinsed for several 15-second periods with water. The bacterial count of each rinse is estimated by viable counts. The procedure is then repeated using the test preparation and disinfectant activity is evaluated by comparison of the number of bacteria at each rinsing.

The split-use procedure is a modified version in which one hand is covered by a rubber glove while the other is washed with soap and rinsed. The glove is then removed, the washed hand is gloved, and the unwashed hand treated with the test preparations and rinsed. Again the activity of the disinfectant is evaluated by viable count techniques.

The glove test is also a modified version of the basic hand-washing test. In this, rubber gloves are put on after washing the hands. After two hours, the gloves are removed and the insides rinsed with water. One-mL samples of the water are plated. The procedure is repeated using the test preparation. If the test disinfectant is effective it should produce a significant reduction in the counts.

Direct Swabbing. This method can be used to test the retention of activity of skin disinfectants other than soaps. Two loopfuls of each of a number of dilutions of the test disinfectant are spread over half-inch squares of the basal internodes of the backs of the fingers. After two hours a loopful of a diluted culture of *Staphylococcus aureus* is spread over each area. Ten minutes later the area is thoroughly swabbed; the swab is mixed with nutrient broth and samples of this are plated.

Replica Method. This technique involves taking contact impressions from areas of skin such as the fingertips onto an agar plate. It has been used to measure the ability of disinfectants to reduce skin flora.

Surface Disinfectant Tests

Surfaces should be cleansed before they are disinfected because in situations such as those found in the food and dairy industry, bacteria may be dried on surfaces and protected by contact with organic material or by the uneven or porous nature of some surfaces. The activity of a disinfectant against organisms in suspension may be very different from that against bacteria on surfaces because of differences in access.

Lisboa Tube Test. In the dairy industry the disinfectant action of compounds may be tested using milk churns soiled with poor quality milk (Hoy can test). The Lisboa tube test is a less cumbersome method.

A steel tube (33 cm × 3.25 cm internal diameter) is soiled with raw milk and then closed at both ends with rubber caps and incubated at 30° for 4 hours. Fifty mL of disinfectant is added and the tube is rolled horizontally. After one minute the tube is quickly drained and 25 mL of neutralising solution is added; the residual milk film is removed and the solution obtained is plated for surviving organisms.

Test for Spray Disinfectants. Glass slides are inoculated with the test organism, allowed to dry in air, and then sprayed with disinfectant. After a contact time of 10 minutes, the slides are cultured in suitable media containing, if necessary, an inactivator of the disinfectant. The AOAC specifies a method suitable for determining the effectiveness of sprays and pressurised spray products as spot disinfectants for contaminated surfaces. Test organisms used are *Trichophyton mentagrophytes*, *Salmonella choleraesuis*, *Staphylococcus aureus*, and *Pseudomonas aeruginosa*.

Tuberculocidal Test

The AOAC specifies two tests suitable for assessing the tuberculocidal activity of disinfectants used on inanimate objects. The first is a presumptive screening test *in vitro* using *Mycobacterium smegmatis* and the second is a confirmative test *in vitro* for determining tuberculocidal activity using *Mycobacterium bovis* var. *BCG*. From these tests the maximum safe use-dilution for practical tuberculocidal disinfection can be calculated.

Tests for Agricultural Disinfectants

Disinfectants intended for agricultural use are subject to the MAFF disinfectant approval test, which is published as the Diseases of Animals (Approved Disinfectants) Order 1978 (SI 1978:No 32), the Diseases of Animals (Approved Disinfectants) (Amendment) Order 1992, and the Diseases of Animals (Approved Disinfectants) (Amendment) (No 2) Order 1992. Disinfectants intended for agricultural use were formerly evaluated by the Chick-Martin test.

Sporicidal Tests

Methods for assessing sporicidal activity are specified by the AOAC. The method is suitable for determining the sporicidal activity of liquid and gaseous disinfectants. It is a surface disinfection test using silk sutures and porcelain cylinders as carriers. It allows the use of any *Clostridium* or *Bacillus* species as the test organism but suggests

Clostridium sporogenes ATCC No. 3584 and *Bacillus subtilis* ATCC No. 19659 for routine evaluation.

Sporicidal activity may also be determined by viable counts.

Antifungal Tests

Some of the methods used to determine bacteriostatic and bactericidal activity may be used, with suitable modifications, to test for fungistatic and fungicidal activity.

Fungal spore suspensions and yeast cultures are used as test organisms and Sabouraud's glucose agar, Sabouraud's glucose broth, and tryptone soy agar are suitable nutrients. Incubation temperatures are usually lower and incubation periods longer than those used in tests for antibacterial activity.

Rapid Evaluation of Disinfectants and Antiseptics

The development of rapid evaluation techniques in microbiology allows early detection of the action of antimicrobial agents. Thus, the inhibition of impedance changes, light production (bioluminescence), or heat generation, all of which may be early indicators of cell multiplication, will provide a measure of antimicrobial activity in a much shorter time than conventional methods. These techniques have considerable potential for screening compounds for antimicrobial activity before applying the established testing procedures.

FURTHER INFORMATION

Ayliffe GAJ, Coates D, Hoffman PN. Chemical disinfection in hospitals. London: Public Health Laboratory Service, 1984.

Ayliffe GAJ, Lowbury EJL, Geddes AM, Williams JD, editors. Control of hospital infection: a practical handbook. 3rd ed. London: Chapman and Hall, 1992.

Block SS, editor. Disinfection, sterilization, and preservation. 3rd ed. Philadelphia: Lea and Febiger, 1983.

British Medical Association. A code of practice for sterilisation of instruments and control of cross-infection. London: The Association, 1989.

Department of Health and Social Security. Code of practice for the prevention of infection in clinical laboratories and post-mortem rooms. London: HMSO, 1978.

Department of the Environment. Swimming pool disinfection systems using sodium hypochlorite and calcium hypochlorite: a survey of the efficacy of disinfection. London: HMSO, 1981.

Department of the Environment. Swimming pool disinfection systems using electrolytically generated sodium hypochlorite: monitoring the efficacy of disinfection. London: HMSO, 1983.

Department of the Environment. The treatment and quality of swimming pool water. London: HMSO, 1984.

Gardner JF, Peel MM, editors. Introduction to sterilization and disinfection. London: Churchill Livingstone, 1986.

Harvey SC. Antiseptics, disinfectants and spermaticides. In: Gennaro AR, editor. Remington's pharmaceutical sciences. 18th ed. Easton: Mack, 1990:1163-73.

Leaper DJ, Simpson RA. The effect of antiseptics and topical antimicrobials on wound healing. J Antimicrob Chemother 1986;2:135-7.

Linton AH, Hugo WB, Russell AD, editors. Disinfection in veterinary and farm animal practice. Oxford: Blackwell, 1987.

Maurer IM. Hospital hygiene. 3rd ed. London: Edward Arnold, 1985.

Russell AD, Hugo WB, Ayliffe GAJ, editors. Principles and practice of disinfection, preservation and sterilization. 2nd ed. London: Blackwell, 1992.

World Health Organization. Guidelines for drinking-water quality; vol 2. Health criteria and other supporting information. Geneva: WHO, 1984.

World Health Organization. Guidelines for drinking-water quality; vol 3. Drinking-water quality control in small-community supplies. Geneva: WHO, 1985.

World Health Organization. Guidelines on sterilization and disinfection methods effective against human immunodeficiency virus (HIV). WHO AIDS series 2. 2nd ed. Geneva: WHO, 1989.

Section 5 Electrolyte Replacement, Nutrition Fluids, and Dialysis Solutions

Electrolyte Powders and Oral Rehydration Fluids

In acute diarrhoea, loss of water and electrolytes can, if sufficiently severe, lead to significant dehydration and metabolic imbalance. Without appropriate treatment, this may have fatal consequences, particularly in infants. In all but mild cases, attempts to correct dehydration by oral administration of water alone is likely to lead to increased loss of electrolyte, as is oral dosing with a simple solution of glucose.[1] Isotonic sodium chloride 0.9% solution given orally in an attempt to replace lost electrolyte results only in increased loss of water due to the osmotic effect exerted by the salt in the intestine.[2] If, however, a solution containing appropriate concentrations of both glucose and sodium chloride 0.9% solution is administered orally, absorption of both sodium and water is greatly enhanced. This effect is due to the action of glucose as a carrier molecule in the transport of one ion of sodium, together with water, from the intestinal lumen; a mechanism of absorption which is largely unaffected by acute diarrhoea. Sucrose and starches exert a similar effect as they release glucose in the intestine. Coupled absorption of sodium also occurs with amino acids and dipeptides via a mechanism that is independent of glucose-promoted absorption.[3]

The oral administration of fluid that contains a suitable combination of carbohydrate and electrolytes is known as **oral rehydration therapy (ORT)**; since its introduction in developing nations, a significant reduction in mortality due to diarrhoea has been reported.[2] It has been shown that ORT is a highly effective means of treating or preventing dehydration and electrolyte imbalance associated with acute watery diarrhoea. Only in the most severe cases of dehydration (or where shock or unconsciousness exist) should intravenous treatment with electrolyte solutions be necessary. Even in the presence of vomiting, oral rehydration solutions can still be administered successfully by mouth or by nasogastric tube.[4]

The composition of carbohydrate-electrolyte mixtures used in ORT varies, principally in sodium content, according to whether they are intended for initial rehydration or for the subsequent maintenance of hydration whilst diarrhoea continues.

Preparations intended for maintenance have lower sodium contents than those used for rehydration. Mixtures with lower sodium contents have also been recommended[3,5,6] for the treatment of dehydration in temperate climates where the types of diarrhoea encountered are less likely to cause excessive sodium depletion than the secretory diarrhoeas which are common in tropical regions. The simplest preparation used in ORT is an aqueous solution of sugar and salt which can be prepared in the home. However this preparation is only considered suitable for mild cases of diarrhoeal dehydration or for first aid use.[2,3,7,8] Of the more complete, balanced formulations available, the most widely used is the **oral rehydration salts (ORS) solution** which is recommended by both the World Health Organization (WHO) and the United Nations International Children's Emergency Fund (UNICEF).

The major disadvantage of all the currently available standard formulations for use in ORT is that they do not affect the volume, frequency, or duration of diarrhoea. In addition, they offer little nutritional value and may be unpalatable. Their use in developing countries may be limited by cost and availability and also by lack of education. For all these reasons, research into the formulation of the ideal carbohydrate-electrolyte combination continues.

FORMULATION AND PRESENTATION

In most instances, generic formulations are presented as powders which are premixed or prepared extemporaneously and are intended for solution in water immediately before use. The most common generic formulations are shown in Table 1. Various proprietary preparations are also available; these may be presented as powders, solution tablets, concentrates, or ready-made solutions.

The individual components of oral rehydration preparations are considered below:

Sodium

In general, solutions intended for initial rehydration contain between 60 and 90 mmol/litre of sodium. The latter concentration was chosen for

Table 1
Common generic formulations of oral rehydration preparations

	BP 1988 ORS (Formula A)	WHO/UNICEF/ BP 1988 ORS–bicarbonate (Formula B)	WHO/UNICEF/ BP 1988 ORS–citrate (Formula C)[‡]	'First aid'
Sodium chloride	1.0 g	3.5 g	3.5 g	1 × 5 mL spoonful (level)
Potassium chloride	1.5 g	1.5 g	1.5 g	–
Sodium bicarbonate	1.5 g	2.5 g	–	–
Sodium citrate dihydrate	–	–	2.9 g	–
Glucose, anhydrous	36.4 g or	20.0 g[†] or	20.0 g[†]	–
Glucose, monohydrate	40.0 g	22.0 g[*]	–	–
Sucrose	–	–	–	8 × 5 mL spoonfuls (level)

All the above preparations are intended for solution in 1 litre of water.
[*]In the BP 1988 Formula B, glucose monohydrate may be used when the sodium bicarbonate is packaged separately.
[†]In the WHO/UNICEF formulae, glucose monohydrate (22 g) or sucrose (40 g) may be used as alternatives but only where the preparation is intended for immediate use.[9]
[‡]The BP 1993 includes only Formula C, as recommended by the WHO.

the WHO-UNICEF ORS formulations to replace the high losses of sodium which occur in patients with cholera. For maintenance of hydration, the WHO-UNICEF ORS solutions should be given with additional water; one volume of water for every two volumes of ORS solution is recommended for infants.[7]

In temperate climates, where the prevalent types of diarrhoea result in less drastic losses of sodium, concern about the risk of hypernatraemia have led to the use of solutions that contain sodium levels below 60 mmol/litre for maintenance of hydration and even for initial rehydration therapy.[3,6]

Chloride

According to Walters and Robinson,[6] chloride is required for maintenance of a normally expanded plasma compartment and is an essential constituent of ORS preparations for replacement of faecal losses. Booth and Smith[10] have also drawn attention to the chloride deficit which exists in diarrhoeal dehydration and they questioned the marketing in the United Kingdom of a proprietary effervescent tablet intended for the preparation of a chloride-free oral rehydration solution. Short-term use of such a preparation in patients (other than infants or those where large chloride losses have already occurred or are expected) is defended by Leiper and Maughan[11] who point out that large chloride reserves are normally present in adults.

Potassium

Significant losses of potassium can occur in children with diarrhoeal illness and there is little difference in the amount lost between the various types of diarrhoea.[3] Therefore, to prevent the development of hypokalaemia, rehydration solutions should provide adequate amounts of potassium. Most oral rehydration solutions contain between 20 to 25 mmol/litre although solutions containing up to 35 mmol/litre of potassium have been tolerated without adverse effects.[5]

Base

The inclusion of a base in oral rehydration solutions is required to correct or prevent the acidosis which often accompanies dehydration. Acidosis can result not only from faecal loss of bicarbonate but also from decreased renal excretion of acid.[3] The original WHO-UNICEF ORS formulation contained bicarbonate as the base but the alternative formulation containing citrate was subsequently introduced because of stability considerations. Studies have shown citrate and bicarbonate to be equally effective in preventing or correcting acidosis. Mazumder and co-workers[12] also found that both the stool volume during the first 24 hours of rehydration and the oral fluid requirements were less in patients with acute diarrhoea who received citrate than in those who received bicarbonate-containing rehydration solutions. These findings may have been related to enhanced absorption of the citrate solution and/or to its lower osmolality. Bases other than citrate and bicarbonate, such as lactate, are used in some proprietary rehydration preparations. Citrate and lactate are metabolised to bicarbonate.

Carbohydrate

Sugars

Although glucose is used as the carbohydrate in almost all currently available oral rehydration preparations, various studies have shown that sucrose, which is cheaper and more readily available, is equally or only marginally less effective in promoting the absorption of sodium and water. Black and co-workers,[13] in a study of the treatment of children suffering from rotavirus-associated diarrhoea, found that sucrose could be substituted for glucose in oral rehydration solutions with only minimal loss of efficacy. The slightly higher failure rate with the sucrose-containing solution was largely attributed (particularly in non-dehydrated to mildly dehydrated patients) to the higher rates of vomiting found with this solution. Vomiting may have been related to the increased rate of intake of the sucrose-containing solution, possibly due to its greater palatability.

The concentration of glucose included in oral rehydration fluids should be appropriate to maximise the coupled absorption of water with sodium. Optimal solutions should be isotonic (that is, 310 mosmol/kg) with a molar ratio of glucose to sodium close to 1:1.[5] If the concentration of glucose is too high, the resultant fluid will be hypertonic; this will result in osmotic diarrhoea due to unabsorbed carbohydrate, with no further enhancement of sodium absorption.[3] The dangers associated with the administration of an inappropriate hypertonic fluid for the treatment of gastro-enteritis have been highlighted by Bucens and Catto-Smith.[14] Although the official ORS preparations are approximately isotonic, hypotonic solutions with lower sugar contents may be effective in the treatment of the mild to moderate dehydration usually encountered in European countries.[15, 16]

Optimal ranges of concentrations of glucose in oral rehydration preparations have been reported as 56 to 140 mmol/litre,[6] 80 to 120 mmol/litre,[5] and 2.0% to 2.5%.[3]

Glucose polymers such as maltodextrin have also been examined as possible replacements for glucose in the WHO ORS solution. In one study[17] the results suggested that a maltodextrin-containing solution provided no advantage over the standard glucose-containing solution in the treatment of mild to moderate dehydration in children with acute diarrhoea.

Cereals and Other Starches

Much of the research aimed at developing an oral carbohydrate-electrolyte preparation which would not only be effective for rehydration and maintenance of hydration but would also reduce the frequency, volume and duration of diarrhoea has centred around replacement of glucose or sucrose by various cereals or other starches used as food. Starches are digested intraluminally and slowly release glucose for absorption with sodium, and because of their low osmolality, starches result in less osmotic backflow of water into the intestine.[2] Amino acids are also released during digestion, improving the potential for further increasing sodium absorption. It has been argued that such food-based products would also be cheaper and more readily available in developing countries.[3]

Rice-based products containing either rice water (the supernatant obtained after boiling rice) or more commonly, rice powder have been the subject of much research. Home-made solutions of rice water and salt[18] and rice powder and salt[19] have been reported to be well-accepted methods of preventing and treating dehydration. Mehta and Subramaniam[20] found that in infants under 6 months with acute gastro-enteritis, rice water and a rice-electrolyte solution were superior to the WHO-UNICEF ORS solution in reducing the frequency and volume of stool output and in promoting weight gain. In a study of patients with acute diarrhoea due to *Vibrio cholerae* or *Escherichia coli*, Molla and co-workers[21] also demonstrated that a rice powder-electrolyte solution was as effective as a sucrose-electrolyte solution in correcting dehydration and maintaining hydration although significant differences in stool output were not detected. In later studies, however, Molla and co-workers[22, 23] did show significant reduction in stool output when a rice flour-electrolyte solution was compared to the standard WHO-UNICEF ORS solution.

Studies to date do indicate that rice-based solutions are not only as effective as glucose-based solutions in rehydration and maintenance of hydration but also offer the advantage of reduced duration and volume of diarrhoea.[24] From a meta-analysis of 13 clinical trials, Gore and co-workers[25] concluded that the benefits produced by rice-ORS solution were sufficiently great to justify its use in cholera patients. In patients with non-cholera diarrhoea, benefits were less pronounced.

Nevertheless, some resistance to the use of home-made rice-based solution as an alternative to sugar-salt solution has been detected.[26] Prepackaged rice-based oral rehydration salts have also been reported[27] to be more expensive than the corresponding WHO-UNICEF ORS packets.

Other cereals and starches which have been shown to be effective for rehydration and for reduction of stool output and duration of diarrhoea include sorghum[22, 23, 28] and maize, millet, wheat and potato.[22, 23] A note of caution, however, has been introduced by Behrens and Tomkins[29] with reference to the possible sensitisation of intestinal mucosal cells by cereal-based ORS preparations, particularly those containing millet, sorghum, or wheat.

Amino Acids and Peptides

As amino acids and dipeptides stimulate absorption of sodium and water by a mechanism which is independent of the glucose-facilitated transport system, their addition to oral rehydration formulations might be expected to enhance effectiveness.

In adults and older children who were suffering from severe diarrhoea associated with *Vibrio cholerae* or enterotoxigenic *Escherichia coli*, Patra and co-workers[30] reported that an oral rehydration solution containing alanine together with glucose showed improved efficacy over the standard WHO ORS solution. However, in patients with less severe dehydration resulting from infection with rotavirus or enterotoxigenic *Escherichia coli*, the improvement shown by the alanine-containing solutions was much less pronounced.[31] Bhan and co-workers[32] demonstrated that there was no significant therapeutic advantage in using a glycine, glycyl-glycine and maltodextrin-based oral rehydration solution, rather than the standard WHO ORS solution, in the treatment of moderate dehydration caused mainly by rotavirus, although other reported studies had indicated improved efficacy of glycine-containing oral rehydration solutions in cholera.

Flavour and Colour

Although flavour and colour are included in many proprietary oral rehydration preparations, the use of such additives in the WHO formulations has until the present time been resisted, principally because of theoretical concerns with regard to possible over-consumption leading to hypernatraemia. It is widely recognised that the solution prepared from the WHO-UNICEF ORS formulation is unpalatable but this does not appear to be a problem in the treatment of dehydrated babies.[9] The *British Pharmacopoeia*, however, permits the inclusion of suitable flavourings in its formulae and the WHO is reported[33] to be sponsoring an investigative study on the inclusion of flavouring and colouring agents to improve acceptability of the standard ORS formulation.

STABILITY CONSIDERATIONS

Chemical and Physical Stability

On storage, particularly under conditions of high temperature and humidity, powder mixtures of oral rehydration salts are hygroscopic and those containing bicarbonate are especially prone to discoloration due to decomposition of glucose. The stability of ORS has been examined by Izgü and Baykara[34] and by Siewert and Gnekow.[35] A method for determination of 5-hydroxymethyl-2-furfuraldehyde (the major decomposition product of glucose) has been proposed by Santoro and co-workers.[36]

The choice of packaging for mixtures intended to be stored is, therefore, of critical importance; laminated aluminium foil sachets are preferred. These are generally presented in unit or daily doses to avoid problems associated with segregation in bulk powder mixtures. When sealed and stored properly, a shelf-life of at least three years can be expected for a citrate-containing ORS powder.[2] However, the necessity to use sachets significantly increases the cost of treatment, which is a major consideration in poorer nations.

As a means of reducing the problem of hygroscopicity and the need for specialised packaging, Ombaka, Alkan and Groves[37] examined the possibility of presenting ORS mixtures in tablet form. They found that a solution tablet was feasible provided that the electrolytes were separated from the glucose either by film coating the electrolyte granules with a resin or by compression coating precompressed electrolyte granules with glucose.

Microbiological Considerations

Due to the risk of microbial contamination, it is recommended that solutions prepared from ORS powders should either be used within 24 hours or discarded. However, Santosham and co-workers[38] found that solutions prepared from bicarbonate-containing ORS did not support the growth of 1000 colonies of *Escherichia coli* when stored in a refrigerator for 24 hours. Furthermore, the concentration of bicarbonate, which it was thought might decrease in the presence of bacterial contamination, remained unchanged even after a week at 26°. In a further study,[39] solutions contaminated with 1000 organisms of one of three different strains of *Escherichia coli* or *Salmonella* or *Shigella* did not support growth after 24 or 48 hours at refrigerator temperatures. At room temperature (26°), growth of all organisms, except *Shigella*, was supported. Solutions containing acetate or citrate in place of bicarbonate offered no advantage in this respect. Acra and co-workers[40] reported that exposure to sunlight destroyed bacteria in a bicarbonate-containing ORS solution prepared with water that had been contaminated with sewage. Solar irradiation did not affect the bicarbonate concentration or the pH of the solution.

PRODUCTION

Electrolyte powders and oral rehydration fluids can be produced domestically, or on a small-scale (for example, in hospital pharmacies or field clinics), or commercially. Activities which can be undertaken in the home include mixing simple salt and carbohydrate solutions, addition of carbohydrate to and dilution of concentrated solutions, and reconstitution of pre-prepared ORS powders; the use of freshly boiled and cooled water is recommended, particularly during the preparation of solutions intended for administration to infants. Several studies have, however, identified wide variation in the composition and osmolality of home-made preparations. Dibley and co-workers[5] reported marked variability in the contents of sodium and glucose in salt and sugar mixtures and reconstituted glucose and electrolyte solutions prepared both by mothers in the home and by medical workers in a hospital kitchen; the osmolality levels of the solutions varied from 90 to 478 mosmol/kg. In a similar investigation by Fontana and co-workers,[41] wide ranges were again found in the sodium contents and osmolality of domestic preparations, in particular in salt and sugar mixtures. The contents of sodium ranged from 23 to 134 mmol/litre and osmolalities from 147 to 623 mosmol/kg; the corresponding expected values were 50 mmol/litre and 210 mosmol/kg. It has been found that variation in osmolality is particularly pronounced in solutions that contain glucose rather than sucrose and in some instances, the osmolality values recorded were dangerously high. Harland and co-workers[42] determined a mean osmolality value of 1216 mosmol/litre (range 212 to 3000 mosmol/litre) for glucose/water solutions prepared by Jamaican mothers whereas the corresponding value for sucrose/water solutions was 809 mosmol/litre (range 401 to 2397 mosmol/litre). In a study carried out in the United Kingdom,[43] mothers were provided with a concentrated electrolyte mixture which required dilution and addition of either glucose or sucrose. Analysis of the resultant solutions showed osmolalities of from 192 to 600 mosmol/kg for the glucose-containing solutions and from 145 to 360 mosmol/kg for those containing sucrose; the correct values were 315 mosmol/kg and 216 mosmol/kg, respectively.

For the preparation of simple sodium chloride and sucrose mixtures, special double-ended spoons are available[7, 8, 44] and these have been shown to improve the accuracy of solutions made domestically.[42]

Special spoons are also available for use by health workers for the preparation of the WHO-UNICEF ORS powder.[45]

USAGE

The amount of carbohydrate-electrolyte solution required to treat dehydration is dependent on the age and bodyweight of the patient and the severity of diarrhoea. For children with severe dehydration, Cutting[7] suggests 100 mL of ORS fluid for every kilogram of bodyweight administered over a period of three to four hours. The fluid should be given in small amounts to reduce vomiting. For maintenance purposes, the quantity of fluid administered should be related to the number of watery stools passed. As a simple approximation, 50 mL per stool should be given to a small infant, ranging to 400 mL per stool for an adult. During the maintenance phase other low-solute fluids should also be given.[3]

Many authors stress the importance of not starving infants during treatment of diarrhoea.[2, 3, 7, 46, 47] Breast feeding may be continued throughout the course of mild diarrhoea and may be resumed after initial rehydration in severe cases.[3] In bottle-fed infants, milk is usually withheld during the rehydration phase and re-introduced initially at half strength.[3] Feeding of solids may be resumed after the acute rehydration phase.[7]

REFERENCES

1. Nalin DR. Br Med J 1985;290:473.
2. Merson MH. Int Pharm J 1987;1:52.
3. Casteel HB, Fiedorek SC. Pediatr Clin North Am 1990;37:295.
4. Mackenzie A, Barnes G. Br Med J 1991;303:393.
5. Dibley M, Phillips F, Mahoney TJ, Berry RJ. Med J Aust 1984;140:341.
6. Walters EG, Robinson GC. Pharm J 1989;243:237.
7. Cutting WAM. Pharm J 1982;228:725.
8. Cutting WAM, Elliott KM. Br Med J 1983;287:1141.
9. D'Arcy PF. Int Pharm J 1987;1:26.
10. Booth IW, Smith DE. Lancet 1988;1:540.
11. Leiper JB, Maughan RJ. Lancet 1988;1:945.
12. Mazumder RN, Nath SK, Ashraf H, Patra FC, Alam AN. Br Med J 1991;302:88.
13. Black RE, Merson MH, Taylor PR et al. Pediatrics 1981;67:79.

14. Bucens IK, Catto-Smith AG. Med J Aust 1991;155:128.
15. Elliott EJ, Walker-Smith JA, Farthing MJ, Hunt J, Cameron D. Clin Ther 1990;12(Suppl A):86.
16. Mallet E, Guillot M, Le Luyer B, Morin C, Pollet F, De Meynard C. Clin Ther 1990;12(Suppl A):104.
17. Akbar MS, Baker KM, Aziz MA, Khan WA, Salim AF. J Diarrhoeal Dis Res 1991;9:33.
18. Roesel C, Schaffter T. Lancet 1989;1:620.
19. Rahman ASMM, Bari A, Molla AM, Greenough WB. Lancet 1985;2:539.
20. Mehta MN, Subramaniam S. Lancet 1986;1:843.
21. Molla AM, Sarker SA, Hossain M, Molla A, Greenough WB. Lancet 1982;1:1317.
22. Molla AM, Molla A, Nath SK, Khatun M. Lancet 1989;2:429.
23. Molla AM, Molla A, Bari A. Clin Ther 1990;12:113.
24. Lebenthal E. J Pediatr Gastoenterol Nutr 1990;11:293.
25. Gore SM, Fontaine O, Pierce NF. Br Med J 1992;304:287.
26. Chowdhury AM, Karim F, Rohde JE, Ahmed J, Abed FH. Bull WHO 1991;69:229.
27. Rahman AM, Bari A. J Diarrhoeal Dis Res 1990;8:18.
28. Lepage P, Hitimana D-G, Goethem CV, Ntahorutaba M, Nsengumuremyi F. Lancet 1989;2:868.
29. Behrens RH, Tomkins AM. Lancet 1989;2:868.
30. Patra PC, Sack DA, Islam A, Alam AN, Mazumder RN. Br Med J 1989;298:1353.
31. Sazawal S, Bhatnagar S, Bhan MK et al. J Pediatr Gastroenterol Nutr 1991;12:461.
32. Bhan MK, Sazawal S, Bhatnagar S, Bhandari N, Guha DK, Aggarwal SK. Acta Paediatr Scand 1990;79:518.
33. Int Pharm J 1988;2:197.
34. Izgü E, Baykara T. J Clin Hosp Pharm 1981;6:135.
35. Siewert M, Gnekow H. Pharm Ztg 1983;128:1169.
36. Santoro MIRM, Hackmann ERM, Magalhaes JF, Vernengo MJ. Rev Farm Bioquim Univ Sao Paulo 1986;22:77.
37. Ombaka EMA, Alkan MH, Groves MJ. J Pharm Pharmacol 1989;41:737.
38. Santosham M, Sack RB, Lochlear E, Foster S, Garret S, Rousey D et al. Lancet 1982;1:797.
39. Santosham M, Benson L, Foster S, Roncone R. Lancet 1982;2:724.
40. Acra A, Karahagopian Y, Raffoul Z, Dajani R. Lancet 1980;2:1257.
41. Fontana M, Zuin G, Paccagnini S, Palmieri M, Beretta P, Principi N. Acta Paediatr Scand 1991;80:720.
42. Harland PSEG, Cox DL, Lyew M, Lindo F. Lancet 1981;1:600.
43. Hutchins P, Lawrie B, Matthews THJ, Manly J, Walker-Smith JA. Lancet 1978;1:1211.
44. Lancet 1979;1:939.
45. Morley D, King M. Lancet 1978;1:53.
46. Easton HG. Br Med J 1984;289:1541.
47. Edwards C, Waterston AJR. Pharm J 1990;246:599.

FURTHER INFORMATION

Banwell JG. Worldwide impact of oral rehydration therapy. Clin Ther 1990;12:29.

da Cunha Ferreira RM, Cash RA. History of the development of oral rehydration therapy. Clin Ther 1990;12:2.

Guandalini S. Current controversies in oral rehydration solution formulation. Clin Ther 1990;12:38.

Sack DA. Use of oral rehydration therapy in acute watery diarrhoea. A practical guide. Drugs 1991;41:566.

Schedl HP. Scientific rationale for oral rehydration therapy. Clin Ther 1990;12:14.

Parenteral and Enteral Nutrition Fluids

Parenteral nutrition fluids are complex pharmaceuticals, which, when given in appropriate combinations, provide all the nutrients that would otherwise be absorbed via the gastro-intestinal tract from a normal diet. Parenteral nutrition may be the sole source of nutrition (**total parenteral nutrition**, TPN) or it may supplement oral or tube-feeding. Parenteral nutrition is indicated when adequate nutrition cannot be provided via the alimentary tract. This situation arises after major surgery, trauma, or burns; during prolonged or severe disorders of the gastro-intestinal tract; and when the patient is unconscious. Parenteral nutrition is also used occasionally when preparing malnourished patients for surgery, chemotherapy or radiation therapy, and in patients with renal or hepatic failure. Long-term parenteral nutrition, administered in the patient's home, (**home parenteral nutrition**, HPN) is indicated for patients suffering from 'gut failure'. These patients have insufficient gastro-intestinal tissue for adequate digestion and absorption of nutrients, as a result of surgery or disease. Some patients in this category have been nourished by HPN for periods of ten years or more.

A parenteral nutrition regimen must contain amino acids, an energy source (carbohydrate and, usually, fat), vitamins, electrolytes, trace elements, and water. Individual nutritional products are commonly compounded to make complex TPN mixtures, which are variously described as 'three-in-one' or 'all-in-one' mixtures, or total nutrient admixtures. There are many advantages associated with this approach, including decreased risk of contamination due to frequent manipulations, improved nutrient utilisation, and cost-savings at all stages. The compounding process should be carried out under pharmaceutical supervision to ensure the chemical and microbiological integrity of the final product.

The pharmacist contributes both technical and clinical expertise to the management of parenteral nutrition. Successful compounding of parenteral nutrition fluids requires a sound knowledge of the factors that influence the physical, chemical, and microbiological stability of the final product. Effective management of parenteral nutrition in both acute and chronic settings, should be achieved through a multi-disciplinary nutrition team. The team pharmacist is responsible for providing pharmaceutical advice at ward and clinic level, educating patients, and liaising with colleagues in the community and with home-care agencies.

Enteral nutrition is usually managed by a dietitian, but when used to treat specific conditions, certain food products have the status of drugs. The products that fall into this category are described as 'borderline substances' and are listed as an Appendix in the *British National Formulary*.

This chapter reviews the products that are used to prepare compounded parenteral nutrition mixtures and the factors that influence the design and preparation of these complex pharmaceuticals. Enteral nutrition products are also reviewed.

PARENTERAL NUTRITION

The fluids used in parenteral nutrition include large-volume products, which provide water and the major nutrients, and a range of small-volume solutions, which provide minerals, trace elements, and vitamins. Some are single-ingredient items (for example, glucose 20%, magnesium sulphate 50%), but many are complex mixtures (for example, amino acid and electrolyte mixtures, vitamin mixtures, trace element mixtures). In the UK, almost all parenteral nutrition fluids are manufactured by large pharmaceutical companies and compounded in hospital pharmacies. A useful comparison of the large-volume fluids is given in the *British National Formulary* chapter, Drugs affecting Nutrition and Blood.

Constituents of Parenteral Nutrition Products

Amino Acid Solutions

Amino acid solutions are mixtures of essential and non-essential synthetic L-amino acids. The proportions of individual amino acids vary but the clinical significance of this is not known in most situations. In renal and hepatic failure, and in neonatal TPN, the amino acid profile is important and specifically designed products are available.

The total concentration of amino acids ranges from 4% to 14% w/v, but the content is usually expressed in terms of grams of nitrogen per litre. This figure is easier to use in the clinical situation as nitrogen losses are described in the same way. The content may also be described in terms of grams of protein per litre. One gram of amino-acid nitrogen is approximately equivalent to 6.25 grams of protein.

Most amino acid solutions contain some electrolytes and a few also contain small amounts of glucose. All amino acid solutions are hypertonic, with osmolarities ranging from approximately 400 to 1300 mosmol/L; this contributes significantly to the final osmolarity of the compounded product. The pH of amino acid solutions generally lies between 5 and 6.

Energy Sources

Energy sources may be carbohydrate or fat. Clinical and pharmaceutical considerations govern the choice of proportions of each (see Compounding of Parenteral Nutrition Products below).

Carbohydrate. Glucose is the most commonly used carbohydrate although small amounts of fructose, sorbitol, and alcohol are present in some products. Glucose and other sugars provide 4.0 kcal/g (16.7 kJ/g) whilst alcohol provides 7.0 kcal/g (29.3 kJ/g). The glucose solutions that are used for parenteral nutrition range from 10% to 50% w/v and are all hypertonic; together with the amino acid mixtures, these exert the greatest effect on the osmolarity of the compounded product. The pH of glucose may fall as low as 3 during autoclaving, owing to the formation of the acidic decomposition products, formic and laevulinic acids.

Fat. Fat is given intravenously as oil-in-water emulsions of soya oil, usually in concentrations of 10% or 20% w/v. Most products contain exclusively long-chain triglycerides (LCTs); however, one product containing both medium-chain triglycerides (MCTs) and LCTs is now also available (Lipofundin MCT/LCT™, Braun). It should be noted that linoleic and α-linolenic acids, which are essential nutrients, are long-chain fatty acids and are therefore absent from MCTs.

The fat is emulsified with egg-yolk lecithin, which is mainly phosphatidylcholine with small amounts of acidic lipids. The emulsifier forms a negatively charged film at the surface of the lipid droplets. The size of the droplets is comparable to that of the chylomicra which are formed in the blood after a fatty meal (average diameter 200 to 400 nm).

Fat provides 9 kcal/g (37.6 kJ/g). Both the 10% and 20% emulsions are effectively isotonic with plasma and have a neutral pH. Fat emulsions can be mixed with other parenteral nutrition fluids, subject to compatibility considerations, or may be given separately, either concurrently or sequentially. In some patients they are used only as a source of essential fatty acids (linoleic and α-linolenic acids) and not as an energy source. Fat emulsion is also a useful vehicle for administration of lipid-soluble vitamins.

Electrolytes and Trace Elements

The essential electrolytes (those that are routinely measured in clinical practice) comprise: sodium, potassium, magnesium, calcium, chloride, phosphate, and bicarbonate. These are required in relatively large amounts, whereas the doses of the trace elements can generally be measured in micromoles. A wide range of electrolyte injections is available (see Table 1) and this gives a degree of flexibility to the formulation design process.

It should be noted that chloride is the most commonly used anion. If it becomes necessary to limit chloride input, acetate salts can sometimes be substituted. The anions acetate and phosphate are usually delivered as the sodium or potassium salts

Table 1
Electrolyte content of electrolyte injections

Electrolyte injection	Content of electrolyte (mmol/L)						
	Na^+	K^+	Ca^{2+}	Mg^{2+}	Phosphate	Cl^-	Acetate
Addiphos™ (Kabi Pharmacia)	1500	1500	—	—	2000	—	—
Calcium chloride 15%	—	—	1000	—	—	2000	—
Calcium gluconate 10%	—	—	223	—	—	—	—
Magnesium sulphate 50%	—	—	—	2040	—	—	—
Potassium acetate 19.6%	—	2000	—	—	—	—	2000
Potassium acid phosphate 13.6%	—	1000	—	—	1000	—	—
Potassium chloride 15%	—	2000	—	—	—	2000	—
Potassium phosphate 17.42%	—	2000	—	—	1000	—	—
Sodium acetate 54.4%	4000	—	—	—	—	—	4000
Sodium chloride 0.9%	150	—	—	—	—	150	—
Sodium chloride 1.8%	300	—	—	—	—	300	—
Sodium chloride 30%	5100	—	—	—	—	5100	—

Table 2
Content of trace element sources

Product	Volume	Content of trace elements										
		Ca^{2+} mmol	Mg^{2+} mmol	Fe^{3+} μmol	Zn^{2+} μmol	Mn^{2+} μmol	Cu^{2+} μmol	Cr^{3+} μmol	Se^{4+} μmol	Mo^{6+} μmol	F^- μmol	I^- μmol
Addamel™ (Kabi Pharmacia)	10 mL	5	1.5	50	20	40	5	—	—	—	50	1
Additrace™ (Kabi Pharmacia)	10 mL	—	—	20	100	5	20	0.2	0.4	0.2	50	1
Nutracel™ 400 (Clintec)	500 mL	7.5	9	—	40	40	—	—	—	—	—	—
Nutracel™ 800 (Clintec)	1000 mL	7.5	9	—	40	40	—	—	—	—	—	—
Ped-El™ (Kabi Pharmacia)	20 mL	3	0.5	10	3	5	1.5	—	—	—	15	0.2

and this must be taken into account when calculating the final total electrolyte input. Most amino acid mixtures also contain a quantity of electrolytes.

Trace elements can be divided into the macro-trace elements, comprising zinc, iron, iodine, and fluorine, and the micro-trace elements, comprising copper, manganese, selenium, cobalt, molybdenum, and chromium. There are several products available that provide trace element supplements for adults and infants (see Table 2). Single-ingredient products are also available to supplement zinc, copper, selenium, chromium, and iron. Cobalt is not supplemented as it is provided as hydroxocobalamin (vitamin B_{12}).

Vitamins

A number of vitamin mixtures are manufactured for addition to individual parenteral nutrition fluids or compounded mixtures, namely, Solivito N^{TM}, which contains water-soluble vitamins, and Vitlipid N^{TM} (infant and adult), which is an emulsion of fat-soluble vitamins. The mixtures are designed to provide the reference nutrient intake for each component. In practice, they all exceed these values.

Multibionta™ (Merck) contains both fat-soluble and water-soluble vitamins and is used in parenteral nutrition, although it is not specifically designed for this purpose. Vitamin B_{12}, folic acid, and biotin are absent from Multibionta™ and need to be added separately.

An American product, MVI-12™ (Lyphomed, USA), is used in some hospitals in the UK. It contains a balanced mixture of fat-soluble and water-soluble vitamins.

Combination Products

Most parenteral nutrition products require compounding before use, but there are some terminally sterilised products that can be used with little or no further manipulation. One type is the pre-mixed amino acid, glucose, and electrolyte mixture. The second is the type that provides a 'kit' of terminally sterilised products, either as two-compartment bags or in separate bottles. The individual components are mixed by a simple manoeuvre immediately before use. These products are generally suitable only for short-term or emergency use as they are nutritionally incomplete.

Contaminants

Some TPN products have been found to contain traces of aluminium, cadmium, and lead. The amounts detected are unlikely to cause harm, although neonates and patients with renal failure are potentially at risk, as these metals undergo renal excretion. No official limits exist for metal contaminants in parenteral nutrition products.

Compounding of Parenteral Nutrition Products

The design of a parenteral nutrition product must take into account both clinical and pharmaceutical factors. Regardless of the details of individual regimens, any compounded parenteral nutrition fluid will have the following features: it will be hypertonic, with an osmolarity up to 2000 mosmol/L; it will deliver a large acid load (pH 5 to 6); and for adult patients, it will occupy a volume of approximately three litres.

Clinical Factors

Protein (nitrogen). Nitrogen input has to be sufficient to meet the requirements for both tissue repair and growth. Additional nitrogen will be required for patients whose losses are unusually large as a result of protein-losing enteropathies or hypercatabolic states (such as trauma or sepsis). For most patients, an input of 1.5 to 1.75 g/kg/day of protein is adequate, as greater protein inputs do not achieve additional benefits; this is equivalent to 75 to 87.5 g of protein per day (approximately 12 to 14 g nitrogen) for a 50 kg patient. Modified inputs are required for patients with renal failure and liver failure: Nephramine™

(Kendall), which provides essential amino acids only, and Hepanutrin™ (Geistlich), which provides mainly branched-chain amino acids, have been designed with these situations in mind.

Energy. Energy expenditure may be measured by means of indirect calorimetry or estimated using established formulae such as the Harris-Benedict equation for the calculation of basal metabolic rate (BMR).
For males:

$$BEE = 66.7 + 13.8\,w + 5.0\,h - 6.8\,a$$

where BEE is the basal energy expenditure in kcal, w is the weight in kg, h is the height in cm, and a represents age in years.
For females:

$$BEE = 665 + 9.5\,w + 1.8\,h - 4.7\,a$$

The calculated BEE is then adjusted to take account of activity, injury, and thermal factors. This method tends to overestimate calorific requirements and, in practice, a total calorie intake of 25 to 35 kcal/kg/day is found to be effective. Alternatively, multiplication of the BEE by 1.2 to 1.5 also gives a good approximation.
If insufficient energy is given, glucose will be derived from amino acids and growth and tissue repair delayed or prevented. The energy content of a nutritional regimen is always calculated as 'non-protein calories' (those derived from fat and carbohydrate only).
The normal diet provides energy as both carbohydrate and fat, ideally with 30% of energy coming from fat. This is also the ideal situation for parenteral nutrition; in practice, clinical problems may dictate otherwise. Occasionally, patients experience adverse reactions to fat emulsions, such as fever and shivering or nausea, and are given mainly or exclusively glucose calories. This may, itself, give rise to problems: administration of excess glucose confers no nutritional benefit, but in addition to hyperglycaemia and osmotic diuresis it also causes increased lipogenesis and carbon dioxide production. Clinically, this leads to fatty infiltration of the liver and increased respiratory effort. In order to achieve the best balance, it is recommended that glucose be given at the optimal rate for its utilisation, 4 to 5 mg/kg/min, and the remainder of calories as fat.
Fat is the preferred energy substrate in septic patients, and this group may require a greater proportion of fat-derived calories in order to avoid respiratory problems.

Fluids and Electrolytes. Most patients require a minimum fluid input of 1.5 L per day, along with 120 to 150 mmol sodium and 60 to 80 mmol potassium. Total parenteral nutrition regimens should also provide calcium, magnesium, and phosphorus but the exact quantities will depend on metabolic status and renal function.
Losses of fluid and electrolytes from fistulae or burns can be several litres per day; these will need to be matched, for fluid and electrolyte content, by additional parenteral nutrition fluids.

Pharmaceutical Factors

Stability of Fat Emulsions. The lipid droplets in fat emulsions for parenteral nutrition have a size distribution similar to that of naturally occurring chylomicra, that is, average diameters of 200 to 400 nm. However, when fat emulsions are mixed with electrolyte and amino acid mixtures, the physical stability characteristics of the emulsion are altered and the lipid droplets can increase in size. This is undesirable clinically, as the intravenous infusion of particles greater than 600 nm is known to be associated with adverse reactions. Changes in the characteristics of the emulsion may even result in 'creaming', as aggregates of droplets form a visible layer on top of the mixture; this is readily dispersed by gentle agitation. If the emulsion is more seriously disturbed, the lipid droplets may flocculate and form a dense 'cream' layer which cannot be redispersed. Finally, the emulsion may 'crack' and free oil droplets will be visible on the surface of the mixture.
The major determinants of fat emulsion stability are the electrolyte composition and the pH of the final mixture. Cations interact with emulsified droplets both electrically (non-specifically) and chemically (specifically).[1]
Non-specific adsorption (Fig. 1) occurs when cations are bound by electrostatic forces to the negatively charged surface of an emulsified droplet. As the electrolyte concentration increases, more ions are adsorbed and the zeta potential (surface charge) approaches zero. Eventually, the point is reached at which the repulsive electrostatic force becomes equal to the attractive Van der Waals force. This is the point at which flocculation begins and it is known as the **critical flocculation concentration** (CFC).
Specific adsorption (Fig. 2) occurs when, in addition to electrostatic attraction, an ion is bound to the droplet surface by chemical binding or complexation. In this way, a droplet adsorbs more of an ion than is necessary to neutralise its charge.

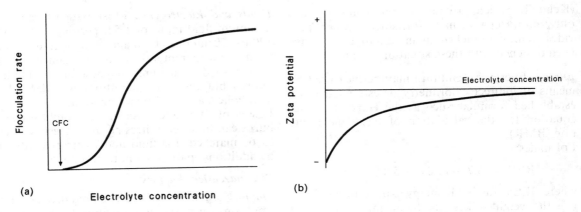

Fig. 1
Non-specific adsorption. The relationship between (a) zeta potential and electrolyte concentration and (b) flocculation rate and electrolyte concentration.

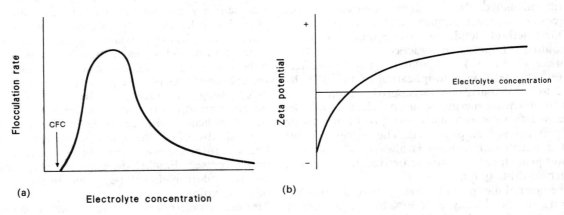

Fig. 2
Specific adsorption. The relationship between (a) zeta potential and electrolyte concentration and (b) flocculation rate and electrolyte concentration.

As a result, the zeta potential may pass through zero and become positive; this phenomenon is known as charge-reversal. It follows that there is a maximum rate of flocculation at intermediate concentrations, when the zeta potential is close to zero.

There have been attempts to predict the stability of emulsions in relation to the concentration of cations in the aqueous phase by manipulation of the Schultze-Hardy rule; however, the issue is not straightforward. According to the Schultze-Hardy rule, the CFC depends inversely on the sixth power of the ion charge, thus, for monovalent, divalent, and trivalent cations, the CFCs should be in the ratio 1:1/64:1/729:1. However, the contributions of the individual ions cannot be added together because they function competitively, rather than additively, at droplet surfaces. Furthermore, the rule applies only to electrolytes that are non-specifically adsorbed, but parenteral nutrition fat emulsions adsorb monovalent ions, such as sodium and potassium, non-specifically and adsorb divalent ions, such as calcium and magnesium, specifically. In practice it is most useful to limit the quantity of divalent cations. Guidelines are provided in the stability matrices produced by manufacturers.

The **pH** of the final mixture influences the surface charge on lipid droplets through the specific adsorption of protons and the consequent alteration of the ionisation status of the phospholipid. At a pH of approximately 3.0, the surface charge is neutralised.

Glucose solutions may significantly reduce the pH of the final TPN fluid and would be expected to increase the rate of flocculation of lipid droplets; however, high concentrations of glucose have also been shown to reduce flocculation suggesting that other processes are involved.[2]

Amino acids stabilise lipid emulsions against the flocculating effects of electrolytes. This was thought to be due to their buffering action but recent work suggests that the effects may be more complex, and involve features such as increasing the mechanical strength of the surfactant barrier and ligand formation with metal ions, resulting in a reduction in the number of free cations.

The addition of **heparin** causes extensive and rapid flocculation of lipid droplets, when calcium is also present. This effect is only seen when the droplet charge is positive, which suggests that the negatively charged heparin acts as a bridging flocculant in this situation.[3] The evidence suggests that heparin should be avoided in TPN mixtures that contain fat emulsions. Low-molecular-weight heparins may offer an alternative solution.[4]

Vitamins. The stability of vitamins in TPN mixtures depends on a number of factors including pH, amino acid profile, concentration, temperature, light, and the presence of trace elements, sodium metabisulphite, or dissolved oxygen. Most vitamins are relatively stable in TPN mixtures but vitamin A, folic acid, thiamine, riboflavine, and ascorbic acid (vitamin C) represent the major exceptions.

Ascorbic acid is the least stable vitamin. It is rapidly oxidised and the reaction is catalysed by copper ions; degradation can be prevented by excluding oxygen from the container. Riboflavine is also oxidised, but less readily than ascorbic acid. Losses of thiamine are accelerated by reducing agents such as sodium metabisulphite, which is included in some amino acid solutions. Folic acid may be lost by adsorption on to plastics, such as polyvinyl chloride; however, it is very poorly soluble in acidic solutions and precipitation is a more likely cause of losses observed during storage. Vitamin A is very sensitive to ultraviolet light and should be protected from daylight.

In general, vitamins should be added to TPN fluids shortly before use. Other measures that enhance the stability of added vitamins include the prevention of aeration during compounding, prevention of oxygen ingress during storage, and protection from light. Compounded mixtures containing fat emulsions afford some protection from light by virtue of their opacity. In some hospitals, vitamins and trace elements are given on alternate days in order to minimise vitamin losses catalysed by metal ions.

Calcium Phosphate Precipitation. The concentrations of calcium and phosphate in a parenteral nutrition mixture are critical. If the solubility product for a particular calcium phosphate salt is exceeded then a precipitate will form. The maximum permissible concentrations are given in the stability matrices provided by the manufacturers of parenteral nutrition fluids.

Amino Acid Stability. Most of the amino acids are stable in solution; however, degradation of cysteine has been observed and this process is accelerated by the presence of dissolved oxygen. It is possible that some interactions may occur between trace elements and amino acids. Zinc, copper, and iron are known to bind to a variety of amino acids but the significance of this in practice is uncertain.

Stability Matrices. Each of the manufacturers of parenteral nutrition fluids produces a table which shows the proportions of each product that may be combined to form a stable mixture. The tables also show the maximum amounts of electrolytes that may be added without compromising the stability of the final product. All tables of this type refer to specific products and it cannot be assumed that, for example, an alternative lipid emulsion or amino acid solution can be used. The reader is referred to product literature for further information.

Addition of Drugs

Drugs are occasionally added to TPN mixtures or administered through the same intravenous line using a Y-connector. Although this is undesirable as a rule, it may be useful in specific situations. Neonates and infants may have only one intravenous line, and so TPN may have to be interrupted several times during the day to give antibiotics and other medications; frequent manipulation of the line increases the potential for sepsis and the loss of calories may be considerable. In adults, the loss of infusion time may be less important, but the addition of drugs to the TPN mixture may still be beneficial in the critically ill: some drugs are more effective when given by continuous infusion and the volume burden in fluid-restricted patients can be minimised.

Drugs should only be added to a TPN mixture if the following criteria are satisfied:

- the dosage regimen is stable over 24 hours
- the drug kinetics are appropriate for continuous infusion
- the drug is physically compatible with the components of the TPN mixture, including other possible drugs
- the drug/TPN mixture is chemically stable over 24 hours
- the TPN infusion rate is constant.

Drugs that have been added to compounded parenteral nutrition mixtures have been reviewed.[5, 6] It is advisable to research the stability of any proposed combination carefully before making the addition.

Compounding Techniques

Equipment. Compounding of TPN solutions must be carried out under aseptic conditions (Class 1, European Guidelines[7]). The process may be manual or semi-automatic. The filling time for TPN bags may be reduced by the use of a vacuum chamber, which draws fluid into the bag instead of relying on gravity alone; however, this can lead to excessive aeration of the mixture. Microcomputer-controlled programmable compounding machines are available. In practice, these are most useful for paediatric compounding where the volumes required are small and the reservoir containers can be used to compound a number of mixtures.

Procedure. The sequence of compounding is important in preserving the integrity of the lipid emulsion. The most critical aspect is to ensure that the electrolytes are fully diluted before they are mixed with the lipid emulsion; in practice, this means that the electrolytes are first added to the amino acids and glucose, and the fat emulsion is added last. Small-volume additives are added to bulk fluids to avoid the risk of their being left in the dead space of the compounding equipment. The compounding procedure must be carefully controlled so as to minimise the opportunity for microbial contamination. The environment should conform to Class 1 (European Guidelines[7]) standards and the operators should be fully trained. Ideally, they should perform regular 'broth tests' to ensure that the standard of their technique is maintained. Readers are referred to the manufacturers' guidelines for exact instructions.

Vacuum chambers and other pumping devices all accelerate the flow of the component solutions and, inevitably, this increases the degree of aeration of the fluid. As it is desirable to minimise the amount of dissolved oxygen in the final product, the filling technique must be carefully controlled to ensure steady flow rates with minimal turbulence. Attempts to drain the last few drops from containers should be avoided as this can introduce significant amounts of air. Finally, as much air as possible should be squeezed out of the bag before it is sealed.

Particulate contamination may be minimised by passing all additives through a suitable filter. Fat emulsions cannot pass through a 0.2 micrometre filter but a 5.0 micrometre filter is suitable and effective. Modern TPN bags are made with an integral 15.0 micrometre filter in the filling line, so that all components are filtered as the product is made. Other measures to minimise particulate contamination include the use of rounded-bevel needles to reduce rubber fragmentation ('coring') and measures to reduce glass splintering. Contamination with glass spicules can be minimised by the adoption of careful techniques for opening ampoules and by drawing up ampoule contents from the upper corner of the ampoule, rather than from the lower corner where glass particles collect.

Microbiological Factors. Compounding under correct aseptic conditions minimises the risk of microbial contamination during preparation; contamination during use is more likely. Compounded TPN solutions support the growth of *Escherichia coli*, *Staphylococcus epidermidis*, and *Candida* species. They also support the growth of some common pathogens although these are unlikely to survive beyond 72 hours.[8]

Packaging

Compounded TPN fluids are filled directly into empty, sterile intravenous bags of appropriate size. Bags with pre-mounted filling sets are preferred as they minimise the risks of bacterial contamination during compounding.

In the past, polyvinyl chloride (PVC) bags were used, but they were unsatisfactory for mixtures containing fat as the plasticiser was leached out into the product. Bags for parenteral nutrition fluids are now made of other plastics, such as ethyl vinyl acetate (EVA), which contains no plasticiser and are suitable for use with lipids. EVA bags are, however, relatively permeable to oxygen and, if extended storage is planned, 'multilayer' bags are preferred: these are made of plastic materials in five or seven layers, with an inert EVA inner layer, a polyethylene outer layer, and a polyvinylidene chloride layer sandwiched in the middle. Oxygen permeability of the multilayer bags is only 1% of that of EVA bags and they have been shown to enhance the stability of cysteine and ascorbic acid. It is important to exclude light, if vitamins are included in the parenteral nutrition fluid, but it is also necessary to examine the mixture periodically. Most manufacturers provide opaque overwrappers suitable for the purpose of excluding light. Any opaque material is acceptable but, in practice, heavy-duty polyethylene or aluminium foil are the most useful; heavy-duty polyethylene is less likely to tear in use than aluminium foil.

If compounded TPN bags have to be transported any distance they should be sealed in an over-wrapper and packed in a rigid container. They should also be kept cool, at between 2° and 8°. In this way the ports will be protected from bacterial contamination and the bag protected from puncture damage.

Storage

Compounded TPN fluids should be cooled to 4° if they are not to be used immediately. This reduces the rate of chemical degradation and minimises the opportunity for multiplication of any microbial contaminant. They should also be protected from light. Under these conditions it is possible to store some fat-free compounded TPN mixtures for up to 90 days, without evidence of significant degradation. Certain fat-containing compounded TPN mixtures can be stored for up to 30 days. Readers are referred to manufacturers' stability matrices for further details.

Freezing

Parenteral nutrition solutions containing final concentrations of amino acids 4.25% and glucose 35% have been packed in polyvinyl chloride bags and stored frozen at −20° for 60 days. Both microwave and room-temperature thawing techniques were used. Analysis of the contents showed that the amino acids, electrolytes, and glucose were unchanged after 60 days frozen storage and subsequent thawing by either method.[9] Compounded mixtures containing fat emulsions cannot be frozen. In practice, mixtures without fat are not frozen either, because they can be stored satisfactorily at refrigerator temperatures (0° to 4°) for long periods, providing vitamins, trace elements, and heparin have not been added.

Special Considerations for Neonatal and Paediatric TPN

The nutritional requirements of neonates and infants are qualitatively and quantitatively different from those of adults and this is reflected in the formulation of compounded TPN products for these groups.

Fluid

The fluid requirements of neonates may be proportionately larger, because they have significant insensible fluid losses owing to their thin skin and large surface area:body mass ratio. Renal regulation of fluid and electrolyte excretion is less effective in pre-term babies than in full-term infants. Many babies who require TPN will also be receiving other intravenous drug treatment and this should be taken into account in the calculation of the total fluid input.

Protein

Babies have immature hepatic enzyme systems and are unable to synthesise the otherwise non-essential amino acids (histidine, taurine, cysteine, and tyrosine); they are at risk of accumulating high, neurotoxic concentrations of phenylalanine. Amino acid mixtures for infants are designed with these factors in mind.

Energy

The energy requirement of a parenterally fed (pre-term) infant has been estimated to be 85 to 130 kcal/kg/day (355 to 543 kJ/kg/day). The optimum energy:nitrogen ratio is 630 to 1050 kJ (non-protein) per gram of nitrogen. Glucose is the only suitable carbohydrate for neonates. Glucose 10% provides 167 kJ/100 mL and is given to provide up to 10 mg/kg/minute. Very low birthweight infants may have difficulty handling this amount of glucose and may develop glycosuria.

Pre-term babies have a lower capacity to utilise fats. In order to avoid lipid overload, the fat should be started at 0.5 g/kg/day for pre-term babies and 1 g/kg/day for full-term babies; this may be increased to a maximum of 3 g/kg/day. This is usually given over 20 hours with a four-hour break to allow for blood sampling. Lipid overload is associated with emboli in the pulmonary circulation, thrombocytopenia, anaemia, and neurological abnormalities. Furthermore, free fatty acids may displace bilirubin from albumin and increase the risk of kernicterus.

Electrolytes

Calcium and phosphorus are taken up in large amounts by the foetus in the last trimester of pregnancy (calcium 3.2 mmol/day and phosphorus 2.45 mmol/day) and it is difficult to match these amounts in stable TPN mixtures for premature babies. Alternate-day administration of calcium and phosphate is an established technique, but a different approach is to use α-D-glucose-1-phosphate (G-1-P) as the phosphorus source. Unlike inorganic phosphates this does not interact with calcium in solution, but it is readily hydrolysed *in vivo*.[10] Using this compound it is possible to make stable neonatal TPN mixtures containing G-1-P 13.6 mmol/L and calcium 9.5 mmol/L.

Vitamins and Trace Elements

Premature babies are born with minimal vitamin stores, and so supplements must be provided immediately to prevent the development of deficiencies. Similarly, pre-term babies should receive supplementary trace elements, but full-term babies will only need them if parenteral feeding continues for two weeks or longer.

Recent evidence suggests that supplementation with inositol significantly improves respiratory function in premature babies with respiratory distress syndrome.[11]

Administration

All-in-one TPN mixtures are not generally used for neonates and infants; instead, the fluids are given through two lines, joined by a Y-connector near the patient. The amino acids, glucose, and electrolytes are compounded together (with vitamin and trace element additives) for one line and the lipid emulsion (containing added fat-soluble vitamins) is given using the other line. In this way, the lipid can easily be withdrawn, if problems develop, without removing all other nutrition and fluid.

Administration Equipment

Mixtures for TPN are usually administered via a central venous catheter, although some types of peripheral venous catheters are also suitable. For short-term parenteral nutrition a conventional polyvinyl chloride catheter usually sited in the subclavian vein is used; but for long-term feeding a Silastic catheter, anchored in a skin tunnel, is preferred. Implantable subcutaneous infusion ports are cosmetically more attractive, but are rarely used. When TPN is administered by this means, a large needle is required to pierce the skin and penetrate the catheter hub; if TPN is given daily the skin overlying the hub soon becomes badly macerated. Good catheter-care protocols are essential to avoid bacterial contamination. If the catheter tip becomes colonised by bacteria, then it is almost impossible to eradicate the infection without removing the catheter. Careless handling of the catheter and connections may lead to contamination of the compounded TPN mixture. In use, the mixture is not protected by a low temperature and some mixtures will support growth of potential pathogens.

In order to maximise the life of a parenteral nutrition catheter, it is usual to avoid using it for any other purpose, for example, blood sampling or drug administration. In situations where venous access sites are limited (for example, in bone marrow transplant patients), a triple lumen catheter is used and one channel is reserved for TPN administration.

Compounded TPN mixtures should be administered using a volumetric pump. Because of the volumes involved, gravity feed alone is not satisfactory; the flow rates cannot be controlled accurately and there is always the risk of accidental overadministration if the clamp on the administration set slips. Most modern pumps are programmable in such a way that the patient can be 'weaned' on and off the TPN mixture. This is important to avoid problems with glucose handling. A 'keep vein open' feature is also useful. This means that the pump switches to an administration rate of 5 mL/hour when the last 100 mL of fluid is reached. In this way, the risk of a clot forming in or on the TPN catheter is avoided.

Parenteral nutrition may be given through an in-line filter (depending on local protocols). A minimum pore size of 15 micrometres is required and, in practice, a 25 micrometre filter is most commonly used.

Home Parenteral Nutrition

Home parenteral nutrition (HPN) programmes have developed considerably over the past ten years. As a result, patients with 'gut failure' are able to lead relatively normal lives, in spite of their inability to absorb much, if anything, from the gastro-intestinal tract. Gut failure may be a temporary or permanent phenomenon. Some patients require supplementary HPN for 12 to 18 months, while their gastro-intestinal function recovers or adapts; others require total parenteral feeding for life. HPN patients often return to work and several women have conceived and borne healthy babies whilst receiving HPN.

Successful HPN depends on a scheme that translates all the processes that take place in a specialist ward into something that patients can undertake, unaided, in their own home. Most patients can be trained for HPN, provided that they have the necessary motivation and manual dexterity. Patients are taught an aseptic technique, so that they can correctly handle their catheter and TPN bags. They are trained to carry out all the necessary manipulations, including dressing changes, addition of vitamins to TPN bags, connection and disconnection of the pump, and 'heparin-locking' (the procedure for filling the catheter with a dilute heparin solution when it is not in use). Finally, they are trained to monitor themselves for signs of infection or other problems. Often, adaptations have to be made in the home to provide storage space and an area in which to carry out the manipulations.

A suitable TPN formulation has to be designed for home use. In many instances, in the UK, it will be prescribed by the general practitioner and delivered by a home-care agency. The compounded product has to be stable for a minimum of three weeks to allow for bulk deliveries. Vitamins and trace elements are usually omitted from HPN formulations and added by the patient immediately before administration.

Pharmacists are involved in training patients for HPN, providing information to the GPs involved, and monitoring patients in the HPN clinic.

Future Developments

Future developments in the field of parenteral nutrition will include more 'ready-to-use' products, and new protein and calorie sources.

Oligopeptides can safely be given by the intravenous route and their use may offer several advantages: firstly, the less stable amino acids are more stable in the form of short-chain peptides; secondly, peptides are, weight for weight, less osmotically active than amino acids; and thirdly, oligopeptides represent a means of delivering larger quantities of poorly soluble amino acids.

As the metabolic roles of specific amino acids become better understood, it is likely that formulations of amino acid solutions will be modified accordingly. Ornithine appears to be important in preserving normal functions, and branched chain amino acids may have a sparing effect on muscle protein in some situations; glutamine has to be provided for critically ill patients in order to balance losses. The provision of glutamine and growth hormone together has been shown to promote anabolic activity without requiring a large additional energy input.

The use of glucose polymers as energy substrates with lower osmotic activity has been considered, but has been no more than moderately successful. Conventional fat emulsions are based on long-chain triglycerides, but energy can be derived more efficiently from medium-chain triglycerides; however, medium-chain fatty acids are relatively toxic and so efforts are currently directed towards finding the best balance for safe intravenous delivery. Other products under investigation include nucleosides, triacetin, insulin-like growth factor (IGF_1), glutathione monoester, and taurine.

ENTERAL NUTRITION

Enteral nutrition products are used to supplement or replace the normal diet. Most of these products may be prescribed under the National Health Service for patients who are unable to eat, swallow, or absorb sufficient conventional food. A complete list of the products available in the UK and the conditions for which they may be prescribed is given in the *British National Formulary* (Borderline substances).

Enteral nutrition products comprise 'complete' feeds that provide all the elements of a balanced diet and 'supplements' that provide specific components only. There are also some products designed for particular clinical situations, such as renal failure.

All enteral nutrition products are given as liquids. They are unlike puréed food in several respects: they have a high nutrient density, a relatively low viscosity, and often contain pre-digested components. Some can be taken orally as 'sip' feeds, but all can be given by nasogastric or gastrostomy feeding tubes.

Constituents of Enteral Nutrition Products

Complete enteral feeds contain protein and energy sources together with essential fatty acids, minerals, and vitamins. Some also provide non-starch polysaccharide (fibre). The form in which the nutrients are provided influences clinical choice.

Protein

Protein may be present as whole protein or as short-chain peptides (usually di- and tri-peptides); elemental diets contain individual amino acids but these have a strong, disagreeable smell and taste. Elemental diets are always free of milk protein, whereas most of the whole protein feeds contain milk protein. Enteral nutrition products are almost always gluten free.

Energy

Complete enteral nutrition products provide approximately one-third of energy as fat and the remainder as carbohydrate. Some products provide at least a proportion of the fat as medium-chain triglycerides, which do not require digestion before absorption. All complete enteral nutrition products satisfy the current recommendations for essential fatty acids (linoleic and α-linolenic acids). Carbohydrates are provided as a combination of sugars, such as glucose and sucrose, and carbohydrate polymers, such as glucose polymer and hydrolysed maize starch. Carbohydrate polymers provide large amounts of energy without unacceptable osmotic effects.

Vitamins and Minerals

Complete products contain sufficient vitamins and minerals to meet the Estimated Average Requirement (EAR) when taken in the full daily 'dose' of 1500 to 2000 mL.

Non-starch Polysaccharide (Fibre)

Several products containing non-starch polysaccharide (NSP) are available; this is valuable for long-term enteral nutrition patients, who often become constipated as a result of the low residue diet. The NSP in enteral feeds does not form a sediment and the products are suitable for administration by tube.

Special Application Feeds

Specific formulations are available that are enriched with essential amino acids and branched-chain amino acids, for renal and hepatic failure, respectively. There is also a product with a high fat:carbohydrate ratio, which is designed for patients with a low respiratory reserve, and there are low-sodium products. These specifically designed products are all complete feeds.

Flavouring

Complete feeds are available in a range of sweet and savoury flavours. Even though the products are often given through a tube, patients usually become aware of their taste, and flavouring is an important factor in enhancing the acceptability of the treatment.

Osmolarity

Many enteral feeds are hypertonic. This presents no problem if the feed is taken orally or via a gastrostomy tube; however, for patients with a feeding jejunostomy, ingestion of the product may cause symptoms similar to 'dumping syndrome' (weakness, dizziness, palpitations, sweating, diarrhoea, and nausea after meals). Although the aetiology of this condition is not fully understood, it is primarily related to the 'dumping' of hypertonic carbohydrates into the small intestine. It can be minimised by feeding slowly.

Microbial Contamination

Enteral feeds are excellent media for the growth of micro-organisms. Most products do not require reconstitution and are presented as sterile products in cans or bottles; they should be handled with the same attention to hygiene as for any other food product. Outbreaks of food-poisoning have been traced to enteral nutrition products and this has usually been because of poor practice. Sensible precautions include aseptic handling, the use of closed systems, and limitation of the hang-time and giving-set life to 24 hours.

Drug Interactions

Many patients who are receiving enteral nutrition are unable to take solid food and so their medication must also be presented in liquid form. Crushed tablets should be avoided at all costs, as they may easily block the fine-bore feeding tube. Liquid medications should not, as far as possible, be mixed with the feed as they may cause it to flocculate or separate. Many administration systems incorporate a separate port for the administration of drugs; however, the line should be flushed with water both before and after medications are given in order to minimise the possibility of blockage. Clearly, drugs that should not be given with food, such as tetracyclines or colloidal bismuth, should not be given with enteral nutrition, for the same reasons. Enteral nutrition products contain relatively high levels of vitamin K, and this may be a problem for patients who are already stabilised on warfarin.

Administration Systems

Enteral nutrition is given using a fine-bore feeding catheter or via a gastrostomy or jejunostomy tube. An electronic pump is usually used to ensure a constant rate of administration. The pumps are designed for enteral nutrition and are not interchangeable with intravenous pumps. Similarly, the connections on enteral nutrition hardware are incompatible with those on intravenous hardware. Feeding tubes are male-ended, whereas central venous catheters are female-ended. Unfortunately the system is not totally foolproof and conversion kits are available.

REFERENCES

1. Washington C. Int J Pharmaceutics 1990;66:1–21.
2. Washington C, Athersuch A, Kynoch D. Int J Pharmaceutics 1990;64:217–22.
3. Johnson OL, Washington C, Davis SS, Schaupp K. Int J Pharmaceutics 1989;53:237–40.
4. Durand M-C, Barnett MI. Brit J Intensive Care 1992;2:10–20.
5. Manning RJ, Washington C. Int J Pharmaceutics 1992;81:1–20.
6. Driscoll DF, Baptista RJ, Mitrano FP, Mascioli EA, Blackburn GL, Bistrian BR. DICP Ann Pharmacother 1991;25:276–83.
7. Commission of the European Communities. The rules governing medicinal products in the European Community, Volume IV: Good manufacturing practice for medicinal products. Luxembourg: The Commission, 1992.
8. Lawrence J, Turner M, Gilbert P. J Clin Pharm Ther 1988;13:151–7.
9. Ausman RK, Kerkhof K, Holmes CJ et al. Drug Intell Clin Pharm 1981;15:440–3.
10. Hardy G, Jiminez-Torres NV [letter]. Pharm J 1987;239:641–2.
11. Hallman M, Bry K, Hoppu K, Lappi M, Pohjavourin P. New Engl J Med 1992;326:1233–9.

FURTHER INFORMATION

Allwood MC. The stability of vitamins in total parenteral nutrition mixtures. Clinical Nutrition, 1992 Sept.

Ball PA, Booth IW, Puntis JWL. Paediatric parenteral nutrition. KabiVitrum, 1988.

Baptista RJ, Dumas GJ, Bistrian BR, Condella F, Blackburn GL [letter]. Compatibility of total nutrient admixtures and secondary cardiovascular medications. Am J Hosp Pharm 1985;42:777–8.

Barnett MI, Corslett AG, Duffield JR, Evans DA, Hall SB, Williams DR. Parenteral nutrition: pharmaceutical problems of compatibility and stability. Drug Safety 1990;5(Suppl 1):101–6.

Brown R, Quercia RA, Sigman R. Total nutrient admixture—a review. J Parenter Enteral Nut 1986;10:650–7.

Department of Health. Dietary reference values: a guide. London: HMSO, 1991.

Driscoll DF, Blackburn GL. Total Parenteral Nutrition 1990. A review of its current status in hospitalised patients and the need for patient-specific feeding. Drugs 1990;40(3):346–63.

Grimble GK, Payne-James JJ, Rees RGP, Solk DBA. Novel nitrogen substrates. In: Nutrition support, theory and practice. London: Medical Tribune UK, 1990:118–34.

Grimble GK, Payne-James JJ, Rees RGP, Solk DBA. Novel energy substrates. In: Nutrition support, theory and practice. London: Medical Tribune UK, 1990:136–52.

Home parenteral nutrition. In: Harman RJ. Patient care in the community practice. London: Pharmaceutical Press, 1989:187–201.

Johnson OL, Washington C, Davis SS, Schaupp K. The destabilization of parenteral feeding emulsions by heparin. Int J Pharmaceutics 1989;53:237–40.

Menon G. Parenteral nutrition for the neonate; composition and administration of P.N. Brit J Intensive Care 1992;5:185–92.

Payne-James JJ. Enteral nutrition and the critically ill:infection risk minimisation. Brit J Intensive Care 1991;12:135–41.

Trissel LA, editor. Handbook on injectable drugs. 7th ed. Bethesda: American Society of Hospital Pharmacists, 1992.

Washington C. The stability of intravenous fat emulsions in total parenteral nutrition mixtures. Int J Pharmaceutics 1990;66:1–21.

Peritoneal Dialysis and Haemodialysis Preparations

This chapter presents an overview of the principles of dialysis that are of relevance to the pharmacist. Topics examined are the clinical indications for dialysis; the circulation techniques and equipment employed; the formulation and processing methods for dialysis fluids; and practice-related considerations.

Impairment of renal function results in physiological and biochemical changes as the homoeostatic balance of water and electrolytes (sodium, potassium, calcium, magnesium, chloride, phosphate) is disturbed and the excretion of metabolic products is decreased; the result is an elevation of the toxic end-products of nitrogen metabolism (principally creatinine and urea) in the blood together with fluid overload.

During the last 30 years, the prognosis for the patient with end-stage renal failure (ESRF) has improved considerably. The development of dialysis procedures, improvements in bioengineering technology for both dialysis and monitoring, and the overall advance in biochemical knowledge have been of major benefit to patients with varying degrees of renal failure.

Dialysis and filtration procedures are now widely employed as artificial means to correct electrolyte imbalance, eliminate fluid overload, and remove metabolites in acute and chronic renal failure (ARF, CRF). Dialysis may be employed as a temporary measure pending spontaneous recovery or until a kidney transplant is available. However, some patients are not suitable for transplantation and dialysis may be used for prolonged periods. In addition, there is a selective but useful role for dialysis in the removal of other endogenous poisons, drugs, and exogenous poisons in addition to its value in the treatment of renal disease or injury.

DIALYSIS

Dialysis processes depend on the use of a semipermeable membrane to separate a flowing stream of blood and a dialysis solution. The membrane is permeable to water and small ions, and molecules that can diffuse in either direction; the membrane is not permeable to blood cells, lipids, or plasma proteins. Control of the properties and flow of the dialysis solution allows removal of water and waste products from the blood and the restoration of homoeostatic balance; blood pressure and bodyweight should be monitored.

Transport across the membrane may be by the following mechanisms:

- convective transport
- diffusion–movement along a concentration gradient
- hydrostatic ultrafiltration–movement along a pressure gradient
- osmotic ultrafiltration–movement of water along an osmotic pressure gradient.

Peritoneal Dialysis

In peritoneal dialysis the peritoneum acts as the dialysis membrane for exchange between the blood and dialysis solution. A dialysis solution is introduced into the peritoneal cavity through a temporary or permanent indwelling catheter and dialysis occurs. The fluid is then drained and the cycle repeated.

An ultrafiltration pressure gradient is derived from the osmotic effect of high glucose concentrations in the dialysis fluid. The concentration of glucose in the solution determines the amount of fluid that is withdrawn from the patient.

Peritoneal dialysis procedures impose minimal restrictions on the dietary and fluid intake of the patient. Once corrected, fluid and electrolyte levels remain fairly constant and there is no significant blood loss or anaemia. Some protein is lost through the peritoneum in dialysis and the losses are increased in the presence of peritonitis. Dialysis solutions must be sterile and apyrogenic; patients must be competent in the exchange of bags using strict aseptic techniques. Peritoneal infection can be a recurrent problem (see below).

Different techniques have been adopted to control the delivery and the frequency of changes of peritoneal dialysis fluids.

Continuous Ambulatory Peritoneal Dialysis (CAPD)

Most patients are now trained to use this relatively simple and inexpensive procedure that allows patient mobility and requires no specialised apparatus. The dialysis solution is warmed to body temperature before introduction into the peritoneal cavity. About two litres of dialysis solution is drained by gravity from a 3-litre capacity bag into the peritoneal cavity. The empty bag is then rolled-up and stored in a pouch or pocket until the fluid is ready to be drained off. Dialysis proceeds over about 4 to 6 hours (dwell time) and the fluid is then siphoned from the abdomen into the original bag. The cycle is repeated continuously with replacement bags of fresh dialysis solution. The number of daily exchanges is usually 3 or 4, with the longest dwell time being 8 to 10 hours overnight. The patient is weighed daily.[1]

Sometimes a Y-connection and second bag is incorporated in the system. This enables fresh dialysis solution to be introduced without risking contamination from the effluent and significantly reducing the risk of infection.

The CAPD solution exchange is fully illustrated in *Patient Care in Community Practice* (Harman, Pharmaceutical Press).

Intermittent Peritoneal Dialysis (IPD)

This technique is employed in acute uraemia when there is a need for rapid and frequent exchange. It is used much less frequently than CAPD or haemodialysis, but it is an established technique. In IPD, the fluid remains in the peritoneum for 15 to 20 minutes, although inflow and outflow times add about 20 minutes to the complete cycle. The dialysis solution can be pumped into and out of the peritoneum with a peritoneal dialysis cycler and the total time the patient must be connected to the machine is about 12 hours. The process is usually carried out overnight and is repeated 2 to 4 times a week.

Continuous Cycle Peritoneal Dialysis (CCPD)

This technique was developed from CAPD and IPD. A machine provides pump-assisted delivery of fluid, bag heating, and controls the volume and cycling sequence. Patients are able to dialyse themselves overnight for 8 to 10 hours, rather than perform CAPD or spend long periods on IPD. In CCPD, 2 litres of dialysis solution is pumped into the peritoneal cavity. After a dialysis period of about 2½ hours, the fluid is drained out, the volume checked, and a further 2 litres run in. CCPD is less frequently used than CAPD.

Haemodialysis and Haemofiltration

In haemodialysis, blood is removed from the body, combined with an anticoagulant (usually heparin), and passed over a semi-permeable membrane across which solutes are transferred to and from the dialysis solution before the blood is returned to the body. To increase the surface area and to achieve counter-circulation of blood and dialysis fluid, three designs of semi-permeable membrane, commonly made from cellulose or cellulose acetate, have evolved. In the **flat-plate type**, stacks of membranes are separated by ridged plates of polypropylene. An advantage of the flat-plate type is that pressure can be applied to the blood to induce ultrafiltration and the removal of excess water. The efficient **coil dialyser** is based on a flattened tubular membrane coiled round a central core. The **hollow-fibre type** is compact and compresses bundles of hollow capillaries through which the blood flows, while the tubes are surrounded by rinsing fluid flowing in the opposite direction. Membrane materials may be cellulose based or synthetic (for example, polyacrylonitrile, polysulphone, polycarbonate). Disposable units reduce problems of cleaning and infection. The patient is connected via the extracorporeal access to the machine, which has the dialysis cycles pre-programmed.

Haemodialysis is used in chronic renal failure and in poisoning by certain agents such as salicylates, phenobarbitone, methanol, ethylene glycol, and lithium. Haemodialysis is more efficient than peritoneal dialysis in the removal of metabolic products.

Many procedures related to haemodialysis have been developed.

Continuous Arteriovenous Haemofiltration (CAVH)

Blood pressure drives heparinised blood through a conventional hollow-fibre dialyser with a highly permeable membrane. Ultrafiltration occurs together with convection and there is good urea clearance. Unlike haemodialysis, blood is not pumped through a dialyser.

Continuous Arteriovenous Haemodialysis (CAVHD) or Haemodiafiltration

The procedure is similar to CAVH except that dialysis fluid flows through the dialyser under gravity. Convection and diffusion effects are combined with osmosis-enhanced ultrafiltration.

Continuous Venovenous Haemofiltration (CVVH) and Continuous Venovenous Haemodialysis (CVVHD)

The major difference between these techniques and CAVH and CAVHD is that pumps are required to compensate for the absence of arteriovenous pressure. Output of filtrate is larger than with CAVH and CAVHD but the apparatus is more complex.

Haemoperfusion

In haemoperfusion, toxins are adsorbed on activated charcoal or ion exchange resins. This technique may be useful for reducing the blood concentration of lipid soluble or protein-bound drugs, such as medium- and short-acting barbiturates and theophylline, in the treatment of poisoning.

Formulation

Solutions for either peritoneal dialysis or haemodialysis are formulated in accord with the same principles, that is, they are solutions of electrolytes in concentrations similar to those of normal extracellular body fluid. Glucose is usually a constituent and either lactate or acetate is used as the source of bicarbonate ions.

The composition of solutions varies slightly between sources and is influenced by factors such as the source of the bicarbonate ions, the osmolality required, and the need for potassium ions to be present. Table 1 shows the concentration of ions at 'in-use' dilution.

Table 1
Concentration ranges of ions (mmol per litre) in dialysis solutions

	Peritoneal dialysis solutions (mmol/L)	Haemodialysis solutions (mmol/L)
Sodium	130–140	130–140
Potassium	–	0–3
Calcium	1.5–2.0	1–2
Magnesium	0.5–0.75	0.25–1.0
Bicarbonate equivalent (as acetate or lactate)	35–45	32–40
Chloride	90–102	95–110

Dialysis solutions contain sodium ions, calcium ions, and magnesium ions, in association with chloride ions and bicarbonate ions. Either lactate or acetate is used as the source of bicarbonate ions. Glucose is the main determinant of osmolality. Potassium is incorporated in haemodialysis solutions, but is added to peritoneal dialysis solutions only when clinically indicated; alternatively, it may be administered separately.

Examples of typical formulations:

PERITONEAL DIALYSIS SOLUTION

Sodium chloride	5.60 g
Calcium chloride	0.26 g
Magnesium chloride	0.15 g
Sodium lactate*	5.00 g
Anhydrous glucose	13.60 g
Water for injections	to 1000 mL

*Sodium lactate is prepared from lactic acid, sodium hydroxide, and dilute hydrochloric acid in accord with the method of the *British Pharmacopoeia 1980* for sodium lactate injection. Due allowance must be made for the sodium chloride that is a product of the reaction.

A formulation closely resembling the above appeared in the *British Pharmaceutical Codex 1973*; the only difference was that sodium metabisulphite 0.005% was also present in the *BPC* formulation.

This solution has an osmolality of 346 mosmol/kg and usually contains no antimicrobial agents or buffers.

CONCENTRATED HAEMODIALYSIS SOLUTION
(35× concentrate)

Sodium chloride	204.75 g
Potassium chloride	3.92 g
Calcium chloride	9.00 g
Magnesium chloride	5.32 g
Sodium acetate	166.60 g
Purified water	to 1000 mL

Glucose may be added to give a concentration of 0.1% to 0.2% when diluted.

Haemodialysis solutions are produced as concentrates for convenience of handling. Unless clinical reasons direct that the solution should be sterile and apyrogenic, the above preparation would be diluted immediately before use with 34 parts of purified water, potable water, or with distilled water subject to certain provisos (see Water Quality below). Accurate dilution is essential and this is achieved by proportion either in tanks or in the dialyser and mixing pumps. The concentrate must be stored at a suitably elevated temperature to prevent crystallisation.

Buffer Selection

Originally, sodium bicarbonate was used as the buffer substrate to counter uraemic acidosis; the pH was raised by bubbling carbon dioxide through the solution to prevent precipitation of calcium and magnesium. An acetic acid/electrolyte haemodialysis concentrate, to which bicarbonate is added before use, has also been utilised. Both acetate and lactate are metabolised *in vivo* to bicarbonate and each has served as a source of bicarbonate ions. Sodium acetate has certain advantages over lactate; it is less susceptible to bacterial growth and causes less caramelisation of glucose on autoclaving. Disadvantages are that acetate intolerance has been reported but this has been challenged;[2] acetate may also be a cause of peritoneal sclerosis.[1] Lactate is currently preferred as the bicarbonate source for peritoneal dialysis solutions.

The pH of dialysis solutions is in the range 5.0 to 5.5, but when in use, solutions equilibrate rapidly to pH 7.2 to 7.4.

Osmotic Effects

Glucose increases osmotic pressure and thereby determines the rate of fluid transfer and facilitates ultrafiltration in peritoneal dialysis. Solutions that contain concentrations of 1.36%, 2.27%, 3.86%, and 6.36% anhydrous glucose are produced for clinical use. The osmolality of a glucose 1.36% solution is similar to that of plasma and more rapid fluid removal is facilitated by solutions with higher concentrations of glucose. However, these higher concentrations can lead to protein loss, hyperlipidaemia, and excessive dehydration.

Sterilisation

During autoclaving of peritoneal dialysis solutions, the possibility of caramelisation of glucose increases due to the presence of minerals and to the pH of the fluid being greater than 5. The length of time required for heating-up and cooling during the autoclave cycle, particularly of large volume solutions, is an additional indicator of the need for efficient and rapid cooling autoclaves.

Bisulphite has been included as an antoxidant but this may cause toxic effects and is now omitted. Sorbitol has been tried as a replacement for glucose; although it eliminates the caramelisation problem and enhances water removal, it is slowly metabolised and may lead to dehydration.[1,3,4]

Water Quality

For the dilution of haemodialysis concentrates, large volumes of water are required. Water should preferably be freshly distilled and collected in conditions designed to minimise the risk of contamination. Purified water that meets the microbiological standards of potable water may be used provided that due regard is paid to the possible presence of water treatment residues and trace elements. In the absence of freshly distilled water or purified

water of low microbial content, potable water may be used provided that it has been subjected to chemical analysis, so that adjustments can be made to the ionic content of the concentrate. It should meet the same limits as purified water for acidity/alkalinity and content of nitrates, nitrites, ammonium, heavy metals, and oxidisable substances. Mains water varies in quality depending on the source; its principal contaminants are:

- aluminium from aluminium sulphate used in water treatment as a flocculent
- calcium and magnesium extracted in hard water areas
- chloramines added as antimicrobials
- copper leached from piping systems
- fluoride added for dental reasons
- nitrates leached in agricultural areas
- other trace metals – mercury, tin, zinc, heavy metals
- nitrites, phosphates, sulphates, free chlorine, ozone
- pyrogens arising from bacterial contamination
- particulate matter that blocks membranes.

If high amounts of these contaminating elements are present in mains water it must be treated by sequential combinations of reverse osmosis, ion exchange, or activated carbon filtration. Subsequently, the water should be de-gassed to control pH and to minimise bubbling.

Aluminium in the dilution water is a particularly serious problem. The kidney is the major route for aluminium excretion so that, as renal function fails, aluminium concentrations rise with the consequent risk of encephalopathy. A 'safe' upper limit of $1.0 \, \mu mol/L$ has been suggested for aluminium in water used for dialysis.[5] The problem is exacerbated by the concurrent oral administration of a phosphate binder if it contains aluminium; the use of calcium carbonate as a phosphate binder is gaining in popularity .

Conservation of the water supply can be achieved by re-use of dialysis fluid using the REDY™ sorbent cartridge system. The fluid is subjected to enzymatic decomposition of urea, cation exchange through zirconium phosphate, anion exchange through zirconium oxide, and absorption of creatinine, uric acid, and phenols by activated carbon.

Microbial Contamination

Peritoneal dialysis solutions are prepared under the same stringent conditions as intravenous fluids, packed in plastic bags and autoclaved in accordance with pharmacopoeial requirements. The major problem with peritoneal dialysis is the incidence of peritonitis and it has been established[6] that problems of infection usually arise as a consequence of failure in aseptic technique during catheter connection, leakage of fluid, or to microbial proliferation at the exit site. Any additions made to a container should be under aseptic conditions. The preparation, storage, dilution, and use of haemodialysis solutions should all be under conditions designed to minimise microbial contamination. The solutions should be used immediately after dilution.

For clinical reasons, sterile apyrogenic haemodialysis solutions are sometimes required. These and peritoneal dialysis solutions should comply with tests for pyrogens and sterility.

Disinfection has an important role in prevention of solution contamination and peritonitis. Dialysis equipment requires careful and regular disinfection with agents such as formaldehyde, hypochlorite, peracetic acid, ethylene oxide, and subsequent rinsing with water at 90° to 95°. Skin at entry sites should be swabbed regularly with povidone-iodine. In-line 0.22-micrometre filters have been used in an attempt to reduce infection but this increases the amount of manipulation required and seems to be counter-productive.

Production and Technology

Peritoneal dialysis solutions are dilute and ready for use. Plastic containers should meet pharmacopoeial standards and CAPD bags should have the capacity to accommodate increased volume after dialysis.

Haemodialysis solutions are prepared as 35× or 40× concentrates under suitable hygienic conditions (see Microbial Contamination). Order of dissolution is important: calcium, magnesium, and potassium salts first, then sodium chloride, sodium acetate, and finally glucose. Solubilisation can be hastened by use of an ultrasonic machine.[8] Suitable filtration equipment is also required to prevent crystallisation that may be initiated by particulate matter on storage.

The formulation may require modification in accordance with the composition of the diluting water (see Water Quality). The calcium and magnesium ions required in the diluted haemodialysis solution may be obtained in some areas simply by using the unsoftened mains water to dilute the concentrate. Concentrates are corrosive and produc-

tion equipment should be made of stainless steel and thoroughly cleaned after use.

The quality control of peritoneal dialysis and haemodialysis solutions is essential. Their electrolyte concentrations are analysed by atomic absorption spectroscopy.[9]

Labelling

Pharmacopoeial labelling requirements include, as appropriate:

- name of the solution
- formula in g/L or percentage
- ionic formula of solution or diluted solution in mmol/L
- volume in the container
- whether the solution is sterile, apyrogenic, or both
- storage conditions
- 'do not use if solid particles are present, if solution is cloudy, or if container is damaged'
- dilute immediately before use with water of suitable quality
- instructions for dilution
- 'not for intravenous use' or 'for intraperitoneal use only'
- 'discard any unused portion'
- check compatibility with additives
- expiry date
- batch number.

Packaging

Solutions should be packaged in airtight, tamper-evident containers of plastic, glass or other suitable material which does not release toxic or particulate matter into the solution (see Pharmaceutical Packaging chapter).

Catheter Access

Peritoneal Dialysis

A semi-rigid catheter with multiple side holes may be inserted into the pouch of Douglas in the peritoneal cavity but this requires frequent manipulation and change. More usually a soft Silastic Tenckhoff catheter with two Dacron cuffs is used. One cuff is sited in the peritoneum, the other in the abdominal wall. Scar tissue seals the site, preventing leakage and immobilising the catheter. Daily visual checks are made for any sign of infection and the site is disinfected with povidone-iodine.

Peritoneal dialysis solutions are packed in volumes ranging from 300 mL (for children) to 2 litres and haemodialysis solutions in 5- or 10-litre containers.

Haemodialysis

Extracorporeal dialysis may be carried out by introducing a catheter (for example, Teflon, polyurethane, or silicone rubber) into the subclavian or femoral vein. The catheter may be cuffed for anchorage at the site of entry and may have a single or double lumen. Permanent vascular access is through an arteriovenous (AV) fistula or, very occasionally now, a shunt in the wrist or ankle. In a Cimino AV fistula, the simplest and most satisfactory junction is created surgically in the non-dominant arm by anastomosing the radial artery and cephalic vein. After about three months, the vein above the shunt is dilated sufficiently to allow repeated needle insertion. Alternatively, an AV Scribner shunt can be created by forming a Teflon-Silastic loop between the radial artery and cephalic vein.

Potential Contaminants

In addition to the water and microbial contaminants already discussed, there is a slight risk from the equipment in use. Problems arising from silicone particles[7] and anaphylactoid reactions from ethylene oxide[10] have been recorded.

Warming of Solutions

Hot solutions should never be used for dialysis. Dialysis solutions should be used at body temperature attained by use of a thermostatically controlled purpose-designed heater; this improves exchange and causes the patient less discomfort. Wet heat should not be used due to the risk of contamination should there be a leak in the container (a common cause of *Pseudomonas aeruginosa* infections). Suitably controlled microwave ovens have been designed to give rapid and accurate warming,[11] but domestic ovens may cause caramelisation of the glucose, deterioration in the structure and possibly rupture of the plastic bag.

Drug Administration

The possibility of adsorption of drugs on polyvinyl chloride (PVC) bags and tubing should be considered when calculating dosage. The stability of drugs in PVC bags should also be monitored.[6, 12] In renal disease there are changes in absorption, metabolism, and clearance of drugs that affect the pharmacokinetics of dosage and dialysis.[13-15] Certain drugs, particularly insulin, antibiotics, and some cytotoxic drugs, can be administered intra-peritoneally.

Drug Overdosage

Drug overdosage or poisoning may be treated by peritoneal dialysis or more effectively by haemodialysis, particularly if the drug is of low molecular weight, has a low protein binding capacity, a volume of distribution of less than one litre/kg, high water solubility, and a high degree of renal clearance. Dialysis has been tried in many cases of drug overdosage with varying success.[3]

Complications

Peritonitis is a major problem in peritoneal dialysis. The most common causative organisms are *Staphylococcus epidermidis* and *Staphylococcus aureus* from skin. It has been shown that mishandling during connection is the main source of the problem. Dialysis-associated peritonitis is managed with vancomycin or teicoplanin with gentamicin added to the dialysis fluid. Gentamicin or vancomycin can be discontinued when the sensitivity of the infecting organisms are known. Treatment should be for 5 to 10 days.

Adhesions or obstruction may necessitate transference to haemodialysis.

Nutrition

Dietary management is less of a problem during peritoneal dialysis than in haemodialysis. Anaemia is a common side-effect from multifactorial causes requiring prophylactic treatment; failure of the kidney to produce erythropoietin may necessitate replacement therapy. Protein loss in dialysis necessitates a high protein diet. Vitamin supplements are also required. Intake of sodium, refined carbohydrates, and fluid may need to be restricted.

Mechanical Problems

Leakage at catheter sites and mechanical obstruction can cause problems. The latter can be minimised in haemodialysis by administration of an anticoagulant such as heparin.

REFERENCES

1. Coles GA. Manual of peritoneal dialysis. Dordrecht: Kluwer Academic Publishers, 1990.
2. Mansell MA, Wing AJ. Br Med J 1983;287:308–9.
3. Mattocks AM, El-Bassiouni EA. J Pharm Sci 1971;60:1767–82.
4. Maher JF. Replacement of renal function by dialysis. 3rd ed. Dordrecht: Kluwer Academic Publishers, 1989.
5. Platts MM, Owen G, Smith S. Br Med J 1984;288:969–72.
6. Chard CAM. Pharm J 1981;227:323–5.
7. Leong AS-Y, Disney APS, Gove DW. Lancet 1981;2:210.
8. Myers JA. Chemist Drugg 1967;188:138–9.
9. Calder G, Neil JM, Barnett JW. Pharm J 1969;202:339–40.

10. Nicholls AJ, Platts MM. Br Med J 1982;285:1607–9.
11. Hudson S, Stewart WK. Br Med J 1985;290:1989.
12. Maine JE. Br J Pharm Pract 1987;9:298–304.
13. Bunn TJ, Smith S. Pharm J 1990;244:413–14.
14. Maine JE. Br J Pharm Pract 1987;9:178–9.
15. Maine JE. Br J Pharm Pract 1987;9:240–9.

FURTHER INFORMATION

Bunn RJ, Smith S. Drug dosing during renal replacement therapies. Pharm J 1990;244:413–14.

Coles GA. Manual of peritoneal dialysis. Dordrecht: Kluwer Academic Publishers, 1990.

Gokal R. Peritoneal dialysis. In: Cameron S, Davidson AM, Grunfeld J-P, Kerr D, Ritz E, editors. Oxford textbook of clinical nephrology. Oxford: Oxford University Press, 1992:147–505.

Gokal R, Mallick N. Continuous ambulatory peritoneal dialysis. Prescribers' J 1992;32(6):251–6.

Harman RJ, editor. Patient care in community practice. A handbook of non-medicinal health-care. London: Pharmaceutical Press, 1989.

Marriott JF, Gibson SP. Dialysis in the renal patient. Pharm J 1990;244:390–3.

Michael J. Chronic renal failure–end-stage management. Med Inter 1991;86:3569–75.

Section 6 Nomenclature and Miscellaneous Data

Nomenclature of Organic Compounds

The principal source of modern chemical nomenclature is the body of rules issued by the Commission on the Nomenclature of Organic Chemistry of the International Union of Pure and Applied Chemistry (IUPAC). Rules for compounds such as amino acids, carbohydrates, and steroids are issued jointly by the IUPAC Commission on the Nomenclature of Organic Chemistry and the IUPAC/International Union of Biochemistry Commission on Biochemical Nomenclature. These organisations publish Tentative Rules for discussion and eventually Definitive Rules or Recommendations. A list of the relevant publications is given at the end of this chapter.

Although the IUPAC rules are internationally accepted as the source of chemical nomenclature, problems of interpretation still arise. IUPAC nomenclature is a codification of existing practice and where acceptable alternatives exist the rules do not always indicate which is preferred. This and the complexity of some drug molecules mean that the literature may contain several chemical names for the same compound.

The rules contain clauses designed to cover every possible type of compound. In this chapter only the main rules are discussed but these, together with the tables of prefixes, radicals, principal groups, and parent structures, constitute a reference system which should enable most chemical names to be interpreted. The appropriate rules should be consulted for more detailed information. The chapter is organised along the following lines: the section up to and including Conventions deals with general principles and definition of terms. Pharmaceutical examples are included at an early stage to illustrate particular points. This is followed by sections on naming particular kinds of structures: chain structures, ring structures, compounds with characteristic groups, special classes of compounds of pharmaceutical importance, and stereochemistry. The chapter is concluded with sections on approved names and recommended names for radicals and groups.

CHEMICAL NAMES

Chemical names should represent three-dimensional structures in linear form, without the loss of any essential information. To achieve this the elements of the name have to be arranged in a very precise way. The rules of nomenclature provide a system of priorities enabling every part to be assigned to its correct place.

In general, the progress of nomenclature has been in the direction of reducing the number of trivial names for relatively complex structures and replacing them with names built from single groups.

It should be noted that there is also an opposing tendency in modern nomenclature: where a recognisable class of compounds exists, derivable from a relatively complex parent structure, a trivial name for that parent structure is often used as a basis for naming such compounds, for example penicillanic acid, tetracycline. Such names are also used in discussing derivatives and metabolites, where the repetition of the full name would be tedious.

Increasing use has been made of the Sequence Rule method of denoting the configuration of geometrical and optical isomers (see under Stereochemistry).

Definition of Terms

Systematic Name. A name composed entirely of specially coined or selected syllables, each denoting a structural feature, for example pentane, in which the ending -ane denotes the homologous series of alkanes (paraffins) and pent- denotes that member of the series which contains five carbon atoms.

Trivial Name. A name of which no part is used in a systematic sense. It is an arbitrary label which bears no logical relationship to the structure of the compound, for example valeric acid for the five-carbon carboxylic acid systematically named pentanoic acid. A trivial name can be assigned to a compound of unknown structure.

Semi-systematic or Semi-trivial Name. A name in which only a part is used in a systematic sense. Many of the chemical names encountered in pharmacy belong to this class.

EXAMPLE

5-ethyl-5-phenyl barbituric acid

systematic   trivial

(Phenobarbitone)

The reason for the use of semi-systematic rather than fully systematic names in such cases is that the full name is cumbersome and obscures the relationship between related compounds. Since all the barbiturates contain the barbituric acid nucleus, it is convenient to name only the substituents systematically.

Approved Name. The official title by which drugs are known. British Approved Names (BAN) are coined by the British Pharmacopoeia Commission. In this chapter approved names or, occasionally, accepted trivial names are given where appropriate. Approved names are also known as adopted names in the USA (USAN) and those proposed or recommended by the World Health Organization are known as international nonproprietary names (pINN or rINN respectively). A section on Approved Names is included towards the end of this chapter.

Parent. That part of a name from which the particular name is derived by a prescribed variation. Thus alcohols, ketones, and acids are formally derived from the 'parent' alkane by attachment of the appropriate suffix, for example hexanol, hexanone, and hexanoic acid from hexane. For the purpose of nomenclature one compound is regarded as the parent of another in a formal sense only; chemical parentage is not implied.

Chain. A linear assembly of atoms which may be branched but may not be linked to form a ring.

Ring. A cyclic assembly of atoms.

Group or Radical. A combination of atoms common to a number of compounds. They may be simple, for example —OH, —COOH, or complex (see List of Common Radicals). The term 'radical' as used in nomenclature should not be confused with the term 'free radical'.

Characteristic Group. An atom or group that is incorporated into a parent compound other than by a direct carbon-carbon linkage, but including groups —CN and —C(=X)— where X is O, S, Se, Te, NH, or substituted NH (see Compounds with Characteristic Groups).

Principal Group. That characteristic group which is expressed as the suffix in substitutive nomenclature. The principal group is selected according to a list of priorities. Citation as the principal group does not necessarily imply that the fundamental activity of the compound is defined by that group.

Functional Class Name. The name for a class of compounds containing the same principal group, which is used in the formation of radicofunctional names, for example ethyl *alcohol*, diethyl *ether*, dimethyl *ketone*, etc.

Substituent. Strictly, any atom or group replacing hydrogen in a parent compound. In this chapter its use is restricted to those groups not cited as principal groups.

Locant. A symbol which denotes the position of an atom or group or structural feature within a molecule. It may be a numeral or a Greek or Roman letter.

Hetero-atom. An atom other than carbon or hydrogen incorporated in an organic structure.

GRAPHIC FORMULAE

There are many ways in which chemical structures may be illustrated graphically. In general, acyclic structures are drawn with the bonds represented by straight lines or points and the atoms represented by atomic symbols. Repeating subunits may be placed in square brackets. Bonds linking substituent hydrogen to the main atom in a group are not drawn unless stereochemistry is to be shown; similarly with other atoms in commonly encountered groups such as —CHO, —OH, etc.

EXAMPLE

$$CH_3CH_2CH_2CH_2CH_3$$

or $CH_3 \cdot CH_2 \cdot CH_2 \cdot CH_2 \cdot CH_3$

or $CH_3[CH_2]_3CH_3$

Cyclic structures are drawn as lines (bonds) and the carbon atoms in these structures are represented by the angular junctions of two bonds whilst hetero-atoms are represented by the appropriate atomic symbols. Substituent hydrogen is not usually drawn unless stereochemistry is to be shown or unless the hydrogen is attached to a hetero-atom.

EXAMPLE

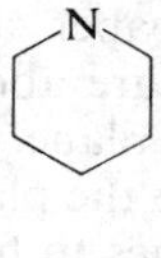

is equivalent to

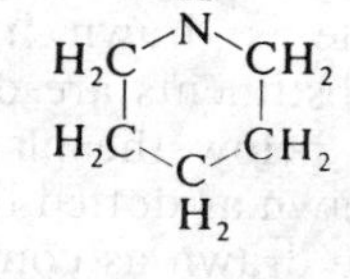

Multiple bonds are represented by the appropriate number of lines or points, and benzene rings are represented either as a conjugated ring system (a) or as a delocalised electron cloud system (b):

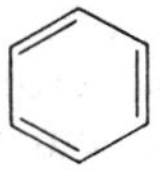

(a)

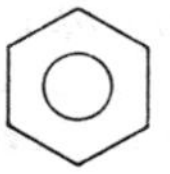

(b)

These two representations are also used to indicate other rings with delocalised electrons:

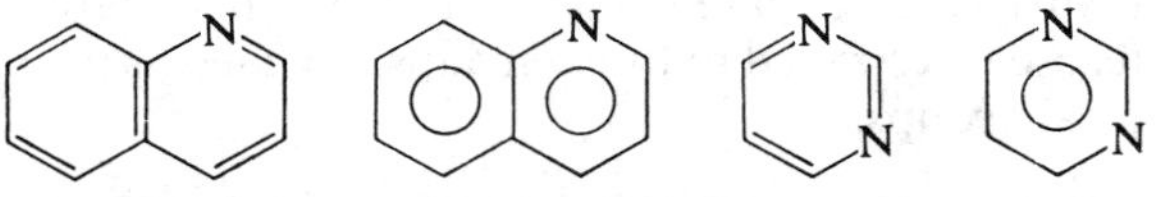

The conjugated ring system is increasingly preferred. Additional symbols have been introduced which can replace the atomic-symbol representation for certain common groups. These symbols, which are not a part of IUPAC nomenclature, are Ac(acetyl), Bu^n (butyl), Bu^i (isobutyl), Bu^s (*sec*-butyl), Bu^t (*tert*-butyl), Et (ethyl), Me (methyl), Ph (phenyl), Pr^n (propyl), Pr^i (isopropyl).

EXAMPLE

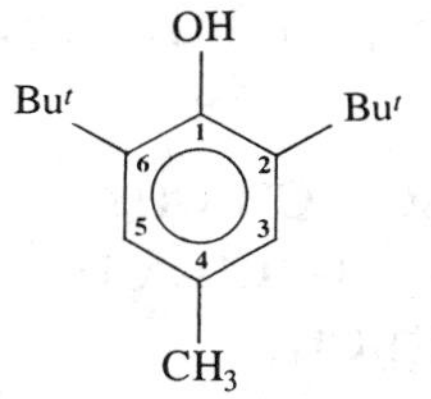

2,6-di-*tert*-butyl-*p*-cresol
(Butylated hydroxytoluene)

Many graphic formulae are drawn without any indication of stereochemistry but it is now common practice to indicate configuration where possible and there are a number of conventions that may be used to achieve a representation of stereochemistry on paper. In general, the main plane of a molecule is drawn in the plane of the paper and substituents are drawn as though they are above or below the plane. Bonds below the plane are drawn as dotted lines while bonds above the plane are drawn as continuous lines (sometimes in **bold** type). In the example (hydrocortisone) substituents at positions 9, 14, and 17 are below the plane and those at 8, 10, 11, 13, and 17 are above the plane of the paper.

EXAMPLE

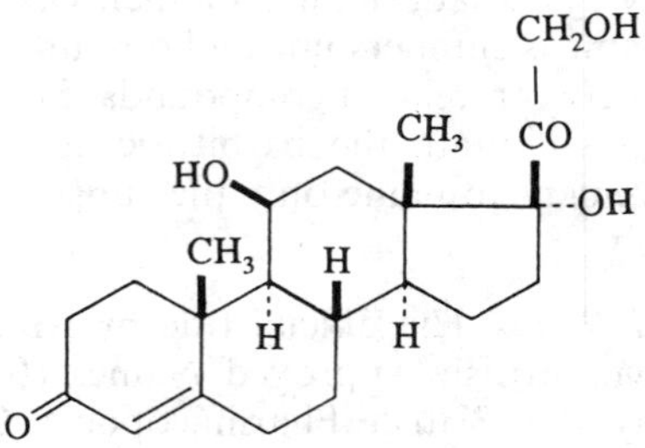

11β,17α,21-trihydroxypregn-4-ene-3,20-dione
(Hydrocortisone)

Alternatively, the main ring structure in a molecule may be drawn as a projection in a plane perpendicular to the plane of the paper with the substituents in the plane of the paper, as in the Haworth representation of carbohydrates.

Other specialised conventions (such as Fischer and Newman projections) are described under Stereochemistry.

NAMING A COMPOUND

Nomenclature Systems

Substitutive Nomenclature

In this system, names are derived by the substitution of an atom or group into a parent structure, one hydrogen atom being lost in the process. One group, the principal group, is denoted by a suffix to the parent name and the other substituents are arranged in alphabetical order before the parent.

EXAMPLE

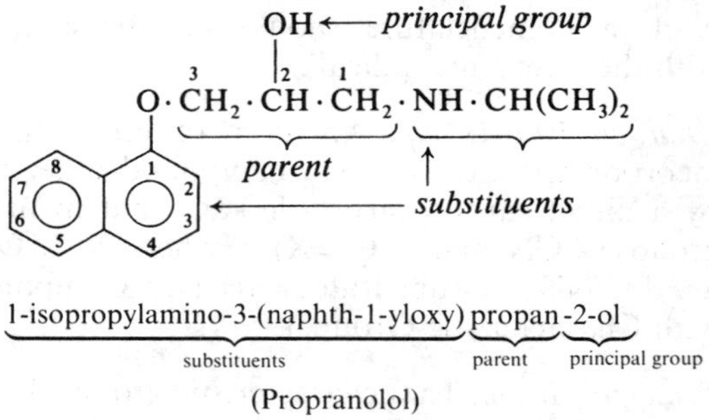

1-isopropylamino-3-(naphth-1-yloxy) propan -2-ol

substituents   parent   principal group

(Propranolol)

This is the most widely used method of nomenclature and the principles involved in selecting the principal group, parent, and substituents are explained in detail under Principles, below.

Radicofunctional Nomenclature

Whereas substitutive names generally consist of one often very lengthy word, radicofunctional names are binomial, comprising a functional class name preceded by a radical name, for example ethyl alcohol, diethyl ether, dimethyl ketone.

Conjunctive Nomenclature

This type of nomenclature can be used in cases where a chain carrying characteristic groups is attached to a ring structure. The process can be considered formally as the combination of two parent structures, two hydrogen atoms being lost in the process. In substitutive nomenclature such compounds are named by placing the name of the radical derived from the ring before the name of the chain structure.

EXAMPLE

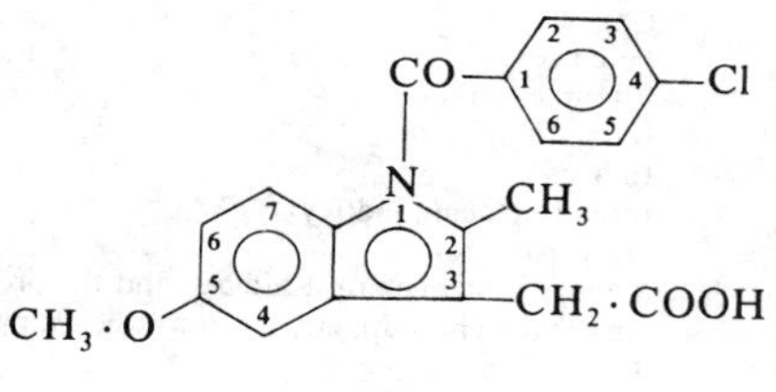

Conjunctive: 1-(4-chlorobenzoyl)-5-methoxy-2-methyl*indole-3-acetic acid*
Substitutive: 1-(4-chlorobenzoyl)-5-methoxy-2-methylindol-3-yl*acetic acid*
(Indomethacin)

This seems at first sight to be a trivial difference but it can have important consequences. For classification, chemical names are usually placed in alphabetical order of the parent names. In the substitutive system indomethacin would be indexed under acetic acid together with many other only tenuously related compounds. The conjunctive name, however, would be indexed under indoleacetic acid, thus bringing together more closely related compounds. This method is used extensively in the USA but British practice has favoured substitutive nomenclature.

Additive Nomenclature

Additive nomenclature relates to the chemical process of addition, which differs from substitution in that no atoms are lost in the process. It may be used to denote addition across double bonds, especially the use of hydro-prefixes to denote addition of hydrogen to unsaturated polycyclic compounds.

It may also be used when an element in a compound increases its valency, as in the case of oxides.

EXAMPLE

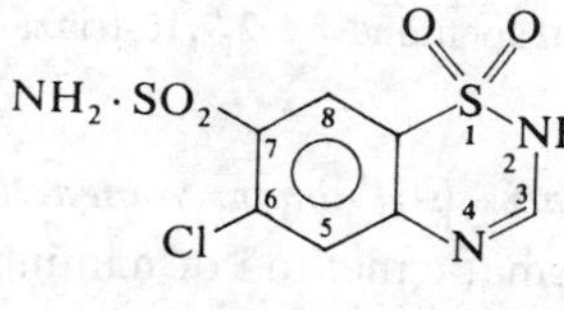

6-chloro-7-sulphamoyl-2*H*-benzo-1,2,4-thiadiazine 1,1-dioxide
(Chlorothiazide)

Subtractive Nomenclature

Certain compounds can be named as derivatives of a parent compound by subtraction of atoms or groups. Thus the endings -ene and -yne to denote alkenes and alkynes represent the loss of hydrogen atoms from alkanes. The prefix de- followed by the name of an atom or group denotes its replacement by hydrogen. This procedure is useful with complex alkaloids which are difficult to name systematically, for example deserpidine, which is methyl 11-demethoxy-18-*O*-(3,4,5-trimethoxybenzoyl) reserpate. Dehydro (strictly didehydro) is sometimes used to denote the loss of hydrogen atoms from structures with trivial names.

Deoxy, which denotes the replacement of hydroxyl by hydrogen, is mainly used in the naming of carbohydrates. Nor-, which denotes loss of a —CH_2— group from a chain or contraction of a ring by one —CH_2— group, is used in steroid nomenclature and in naming natural products. The prefix anhydro-, denoting the loss of the elements of water from a molecule, is used mainly in carbohydrate nomenclature.

Replacement Nomenclature

Some compounds containing a hetero-atom as an integral part of a chain or ring can be named by adding prefixes denoting the hetero-atom to the corresponding hydrocarbon name. In this method, also known as 'a' nomenclature, the hetero-atom is considered formally to have replaced a carbon atom. Prefixes commonly employed, in order of citation, are:

oxa-	oxygen	phospha-	phosphorus
thia-	sulphur	arsa-	arsenic
selena-	selenium	sila-	silicon
aza-	nitrogen	mercura-	mercury

EXAMPLES

$$CH_3 \cdot \overset{5}{N}H \cdot \overset{4}{C}H_2 \cdot \overset{3}{O} \cdot \overset{2}{C}H_3 \quad \overset{1}{C}H_3$$

2-oxa-4-azapentane   2,7,10-triaza-anthracene

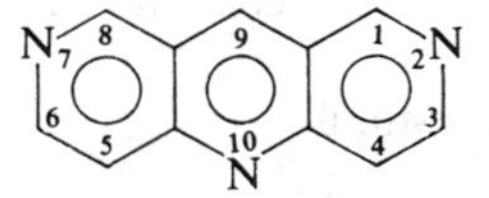

Extended Hantzsch-Widman Nomenclature

This is a systematic method of naming monocyclic compounds containing hetero-atoms. It is described under Heterocyclic Compounds.

Fusion Nomenclature

Polycyclic structures can be named as simple ring structures fused together. This method is described for hydrocarbons and for heterocycles later in this chapter.

Principles

Choice of Nomenclature System

Substitutive nomenclature is the preferred system and the other systems should only be used where this proves inadequate. Some of the situations in which alternative systems can be used are outlined in the section on Nomenclature Systems above.

Choice of Principal Group

It might be supposed that in approaching a new structure the first step would be to identify the largest familiar component, probably a ring system. In fact the choice of a parent structure depends on which of the characteristic groups is considered to be the principal group. The principal group is that characteristic group which has highest priority in the following list; it is always expressed by a suffix.

1. 'Onium and similar cations
2. Acids (in the order COOH, C(=O)OOH, then successively their S and Se derivatives, followed by sulphonic, sulphinic acids, etc.
3. Derivatives of acids: in the order anhydrides, esters, acyl halides, amides, hydrazides, imides, amidines, etc.
4. Nitriles (cyanides), then isocyanides
5. Aldehydes, then successively their S and Se analogues; then their derivatives
6. Ketones, then their analogues and derivatives, in the same order as for aldehydes

7. Alcohols, then phenols; then S and Se analogues of alcohols; then esters of alcohols with inorganic acids (except esters of hydrogen halides, which are named by means of prefixes); then similar derivatives of phenols in the same order
8. Hydroperoxides
9. Amines; then imines, hydrazines, etc.
10. Ethers; then successively their S and Se analogues
11. Peroxides

The following characteristic groups are always expressed by a prefix.

Characteristic group	Prefix
—Br	Bromo
—Cl	Chloro
—ClO	Chlorosyl
—ClO₂	Chloryl
—ClO₃	Perchloryl
—F	Fluoro
—I	Iodo
—IO	Iodosyl
—IO₂	Iodyl (replacing iodoxy)
—I(OH)₂	Dihydroxyiodo
—IX₂	X may be halogen or a radical, and the prefix names are dihalogenoiodo, etc., or, for radicals, patterned on diacetoxyiodo
=N₂	Diazo
—N₃	Azido
—NO	Nitroso
—NO₂	Nitro
—OR	R-oxy
—SR	R-thio

EXAMPLE

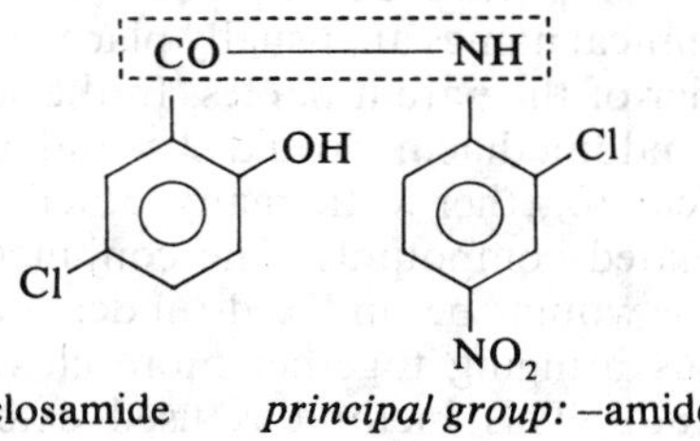

Niclosamide   *principal group:* –amide

In the above example, of the characteristic groups present, chloro- and nitro- are compulsory prefixes and the amide group has higher priority than hydroxy-; the suffix will thus be -amide. The fact that the amide group is substituted on the nitrogen atom does not alter its status as principal group. Should there be no characteristic group from the first list present, there will be no suffix and the name will end with the parent name.

Choice of Parent Structure

The parent structure is that chain or ring which carries the principal group. It is not necessarily the largest ring or the longest chain.

EXAMPLE

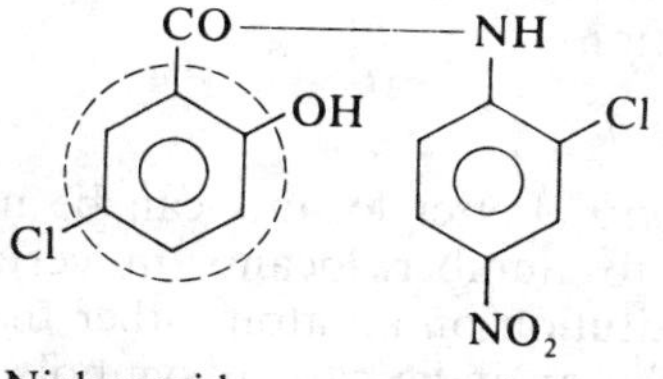

Niclosamide   *parent:* benzene

Niclosamide comprises two benzene rings. That which carries the amide group is the parent; the other is a substituent of the amide group.

Naming Substituents

The groups which remain after selection of the principal group are the substituent groups. Unlike the principal group, these are not ranged in any order of priority but are placed in alphabetical order before the parent. The substituents themselves are often substituted, that is, they are complex substituents. Complex substituents are named by a similar procedure to that described above, substituents being placed in alphabetical order before a parent radical name.

EXAMPLE

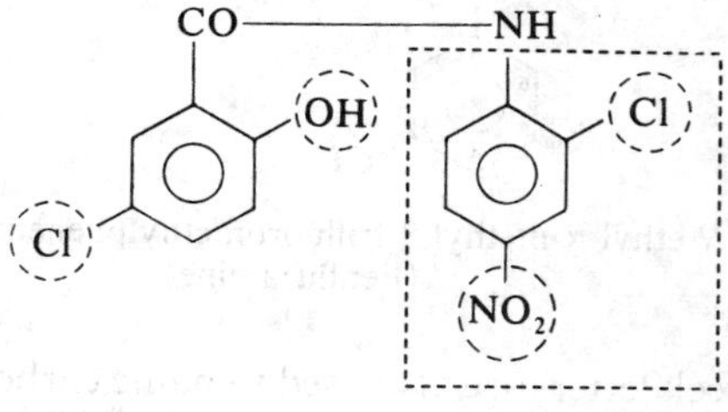

Niclosamide   *simple substituents:*   chloro–,
                                        hydroxy–.
             complex substituent: phenyl–,
                                        chloro–.
                                        nitro–,

Numbering

The numbering of parent structures and radicals is described under Chain Structures and Ring Structures. The presence of a principal group can mod-

ify the parent numbering in some cases. Where there is a choice, the numbering system should give the lowest locant to the principal group. In complex radicals the free valency takes priority over substituents for assignment of the lowest locant.

EXAMPLE

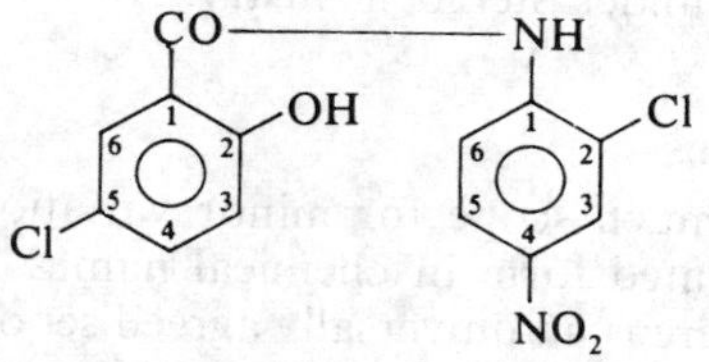

Niclosamide

In niclosamide, position 1 of the parent ring is assigned to the carbon carrying the principal group. The ring is then numbered in the direction that gives the lowest locants for the substituents, at the first point of difference: in this case, clockwise (locants of 2 and 5 compared to 3 and 6 when numbered in an anti-clockwise direction). The substituent benzene ring (named phenyl) is numbered so that the point of attachment to the principal group has the locant 1 and the substituents have the lowest locants (2, 4 lower than 4, 6). The position of attachment of the complex substituent is given by the letter locant *N*, which indicates its attachment to the nitrogen atom of the amide group. The complex substituent is enclosed in parentheses. The parts of the name can now be listed with their locants.

EXAMPLE
Parent and   benzamide (contraction of
principal group: benzeneamide)

Substituents: 5-chloro-
                    N-(2-chloro-4-nitrophenyl)-
                    2-hydroxy-

Assembly

The components are assembled in the order: substituents, parent, principal group. The substituents are placed in alphabetical order.

EXAMPLE
Niclosamide: 5-chloro-*N*-(2-chloro-4-nitrophenyl)-2-hydroxybenzamide

Multiplying prefixes, di-, tri-, etc., are ignored for simple substituents, for example dimethyl is alphabetised under 'm'. However, complex substituents beginning with a multiplying prefix, for example dimethylamino-, are alphabetised under the first letter. In compounds where alternative three-dimensional configurations are possible, stereochemical prefixes are added to the completed name. The procedure for selecting these prefixes is described under Stereochemistry.

Conventions

There is much scope for minor variations in the actual printed form of chemical names. Unfortunately, there is no universally agreed set of conventions even within the English-speaking world.
The IUPAC rules follow the conventions of *Chemical Abstracts* with regard to spelling and punctuation and in recent years British practice has moved closer to the American, whilst retaining certain distinctive features. In this chapter British spelling has been used for chemical names; it is a matter of editorial discretion whether 'f' should be substituted for 'ph' in sulph- and 'e' for 'oe' in oestr-, etc.

Brackets. Complex substituents are enclosed in brackets to avoid ambiguity. Where more than one set of brackets is necessary they are arranged in the order {[()]}. The brace is not a part of IUPAC nomenclature but it is widely used.

Detachable and Non-detachable Prefixes. Non-detachable prefixes are those relating to alterations to the parent structure, for example bicyclo-, nor-, *H*- (indicated hydrogen). They always immediately precede the parent name. Detachable prefixes are those denoting substitution and are arranged in alphabetical order before the parent name. The prefix hydro- is detachable despite the fact that it represents a fundamental alteration to the parent structure.

Elision of Vowels. The terminal -e of a parent structure is omitted before a suffix beginning with a vowel, for example ethanol from ethane and -ol. In fusion names 'o' is omitted before a vowel, for example benzindole from benzoindole. In certain names 'y' is omitted before a vowel, for example carboxamide from carboxyamide. In some cases, whole syllables are elided on the grounds of euphony, for example benzamide from benz(ene)amide.

Italic Prefixes. Italic prefixes are ignored for the purpose of arranging prefixes in alphabetical order. The prefixes *sec-* and *tert-* for secondary and tertiary radicals are thus ignored but iso- and neo- are not italic and are alphabetised. In British practice s- and t- have often been used in place of *sec-* and *tert-* and these are taken into account in alphabetisation.

Letter Locants. Letter locants can be used as an alternative to number locants in certain situations. Substitution on an atom other than carbon is denoted by an italic capital symbol of the element concerned.

EXAMPLE

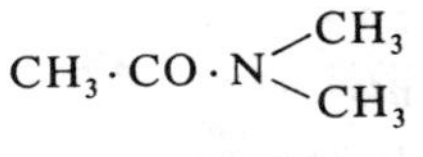

$$CH_3 \cdot CO \cdot N \diagdown_{CH_3}^{CH_3}$$

NN-dimethylacetamide

Greek letters, α, β, γ, etc., are used with trivial names of radicals in which a chain is attached to a benzene ring, for example benzyl, phenethyl, styryl. The α-position is assigned to the atom carrying the free valency.

EXAMPLE

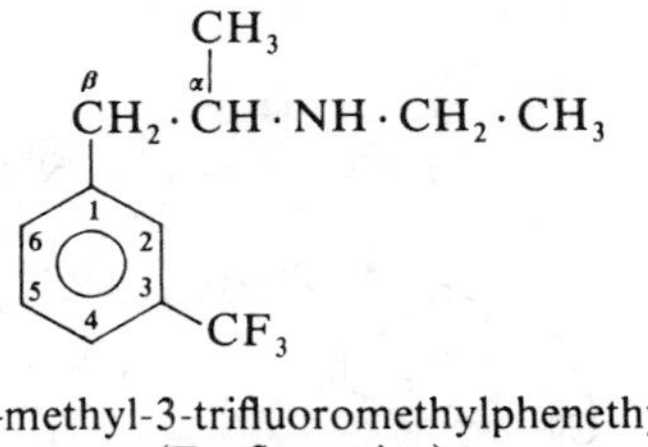

N-ethyl-α-methyl-3-trifluoromethylphenethylamine
(Fenfluramine)

Greek letters are also used to name carboxylic acids and their derivatives, in which the α-position is equivalent to the atom adjacent to the carboxyl group (see Carboxylic Acids).
Other common letter locants are *o*, *m*, and *p*, which are used for 1,2-, 1,3-, and 1,4-disubstituted benzene derivatives. Number locants can be used as an alternative to these but the letter locants enable the minimum use to be made of brackets, for example hydroxyephedrine which may be named as 1-*p*-hydroxyphenyl-2-methylaminopropanol or 1-(4-hydroxyphenyl)-2-methylaminopropanol.

Multiplying Prefixes. The following multiplying prefixes are used for simple, unsubstituted groups:

1	mono or hen*	23	tricosa
2	di or do*	30	triaconta
3	tri	31	hentriaconta
4	tetra	32	dotriaconta
5	penta	40	tetraconta
6	hexa	100	hecta
7	hepta	121	heneicosahecta†
8	octa	200	dicta
9	nona	300	tricta
10	deca	400	tetracta
11	undeca	500	pentacta
12	dodeca	1000	kilia
13	trideca	2000	dilia
20	eicosa†	3000	trilia
21	heneicosa†	4000	tetralia
22	docosa	5000	pentalia

*The terms hen- and do- are used when the numbers 1 and 2 are combined with other numerical terms; the exception is the number 11 which is represented by undeca.

†icosa is also used.

EXAMPLE
    542   dotetracontapentacta

The prefixes bis, tris, tetrakis etc., are used for identically substituted complex groups, for example bis(2-chloroethyl)-, bisdimethylamino-. The Latin prefixes bi-, ter-, quater-, quinque-, sexi-, septi-, octi-, novi-, deci-, are used for assemblies of two or more rings (see Ring Assemblies).

Number Locants. Locants are attached to the groups they qualify by hyphens. Locants denoting two or more identical groups are separated by commas, for example 1,2-dimethyl. Practice differs concerning the position of locants within a name. In Britain, locants for endings are generally placed immediately before the ending. This has the effect of splitting names into short syllables rather than words, and in American practice locants are placed as far to the left as possible to avoid this. In France, locants are placed after the ending.

EXAMPLE
French	propanediol-1,2
British	propane-1,2-diol
American	1,2-propanediol

Where mixtures of number and letter locants occur they are placed in the order: number, Roman letter, Greek letter, for example 2,N,α-trimethyl-. Multiple letter locants are sometimes written without commas, for example $NN\alpha$-trimethyl-. This is merely a typographical convention and has no structural significance.

Primed Locants. Primed locants (a prime is ′) may be used in several different situations. When a compound contains substituents attached to two or more identical rings, primes are used to indicate to which ring the substituents are attached. The ring which contains the lowest numbered substituent is assigned the unprimed locants.

EXAMPLE

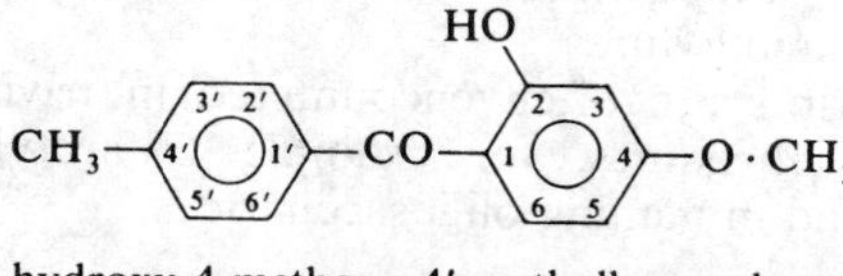

2-hydroxy-4-methoxy-4′-methylbenzophenone
(Mexenone)

When a compound contains substituents attached to two or more hetero-atoms, primes can be used to differentiate them. This is an alternative to the use of superscript numbers. In general, number locants are now preferred.

EXAMPLE

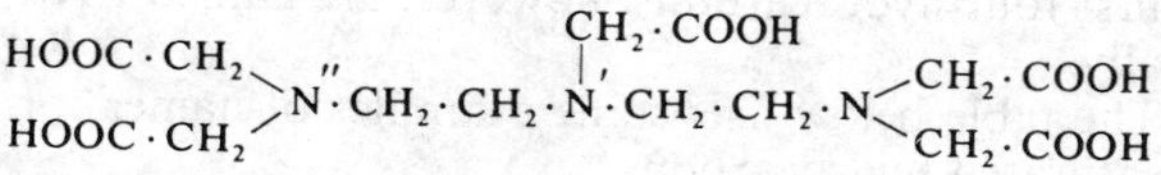

diethylenetriamine-$NNN'N''N''$-penta-acetic acid
(Pentetic Acid)

In pentetic acid (above) the three nitrogen atoms are denoted by N, N', and N''. The terminal nitrogen atoms both have two acetic acid groups attached to them; their locants are thus N,N and N'',N''. The locant for attachment of acetic acid to the central nitrogen atom is N'.

Primes may sometimes be used as an alternative to brackets. In compounds containing complex substituents, the parent structure is assigned unprimed locants and the substituents primed locants.

EXAMPLE

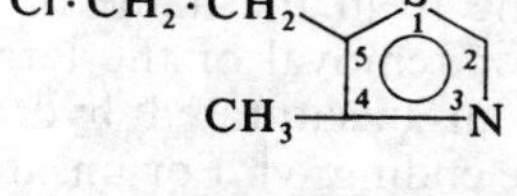

5-2′-chloroethyl-4-methylthiazole
or 5-(2-chloroethyl)-4-methyl-1,3-thiazole
(Chlormethiazole)

Superscript Numbers. Superscript numbers have often been used attached to letter locants in compounds containing two or more hetero-atoms. Primed locants fulfil the same purpose in such cases but number locants are now generally preferred.

EXAMPLE

$$\overset{3}{CH_3} \cdot \overset{2}{NH} \cdot \overset{1}{CO} \cdot \overset{}{NH} \cdot CH_3$$

$N^1 N^2$-dimethylurea, NN'-dimethylurea, *or* 1,3-dimethylurea

Superscripts are often encountered in trivial or semi-trivial names, for example O^6-acetylmorphine, and in naming oligosaccharides.

CHAIN STRUCTURES

Hydrocarbon chains are named by taking the appropriate numerical term, generally derived from the Greek, to indicate the number of atoms in the chain, followed by the endings -ane for **alkanes** (saturated hydrocarbons), -ene for **alkenes** (hydrocarbons with double bonds), and -yne for **alkynes** (hydrocarbons with triple bonds). The first four hydrocarbons, however, are named trivially.

The table below lists some examples of names for saturated hydrocarbons.

Number of carbon atoms	Name of saturated hydrocarbon	
1	methane	(CH_4)
2	ethane	(C_2H_6)
3	propane	(C_3H_8)
4	butane	(C_4H_{10})
5	pentane	(C_5H_{12})
6	hexane	(C_6H_{14})
7	heptane	(C_7H_{16})
8	octane	(C_8H_{18})
9	nonane	(C_9H_{20})
10	decane	$(C_{10}H_{22})$
11	undecane	$(C_{11}H_{24})$
12	dodecane	$(C_{12}H_{26})$
20	eicosane	$(C_{20}H_{42})$
21	heneicosane	$(C_{21}H_{44})$
30	triacontane	$(C_{30}H_{62})$
31	hentriacontane	$(C_{31}H_{64})$

Univalent radicals are derived by the removal of the ending -ane from the name of the saturated hydrocarbon or removal of the terminal -e from the name of an unsaturated hydrocarbon, and addition of the ending -yl. For unsaturated hydrocarbons with double bonds the endings become -ene and -enyl respectively, and -yne and -ynyl for hydrocarbons with triple bonds.

Branched chains are named by prefixing the radical name of the side-chain to the name of the longest chain. In numbering saturated hydrocarbons, one of the terminal methyl groups is assigned locant 1, substituent groups being assigned the lowest possible locants.

EXAMPLES

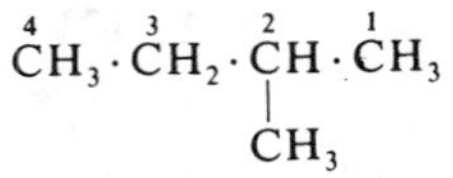

$$\overset{4}{CH_3} \cdot \overset{3}{CH_2} \cdot \overset{2}{CH} \cdot \overset{1}{CH_3}$$
$$| \atop CH_3$$

2-methylbutane

$$\overset{4}{CH_3} \cdot \overset{3}{CH} \cdot \overset{2}{CH_2} \cdot \overset{1}{CH_2} \cdot \overset{}{CH_3}$$
$$\overset{5}{CH_2} \cdot \overset{6}{CH_2} \cdot \overset{7}{CH_3}$$

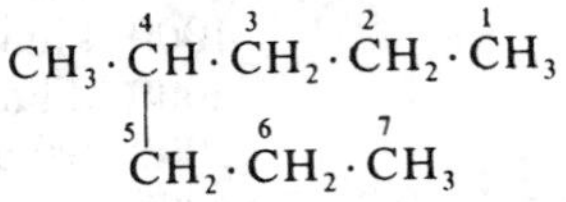

4-methylheptane (*not* 2-propylpentane)

In numbering hydrocarbon chain radicals, the locant 1 is assigned to the carbon atom with the free valency. The locant 1 is usually omitted from the name of an unsubstituted radical.

EXAMPLES

$$\overset{3}{CH_3} \cdot \overset{2}{CH_2} \cdot \overset{1}{CH_2} -$$

propyl (for prop-1-yl)

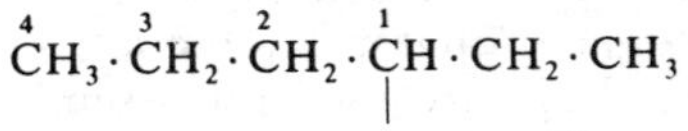

$$\overset{4}{CH_3} \cdot \overset{3}{CH_2} \cdot \overset{2}{CH_2} \cdot \overset{1}{CH} \cdot CH_2 \cdot CH_3$$
$$|$$

1-ethylbutyl *not* hex-3-yl

The numbering in unsaturated hydrocarbons is dictated by the positions of the unsaturated bonds, which are assigned the lowest possible locants but one of the terminal atoms is still assigned the locant 1.

EXAMPLES

$$\overset{5}{CH_3} \cdot \overset{4}{CH_2} \cdot \overset{3}{CH} : \overset{2}{CH} \cdot \overset{1}{CH_3}$$

pent-2-ene

$$\overset{5}{CH_3} \cdot \overset{4}{CH} : \overset{3}{CH} \cdot \overset{2}{CH_2} \cdot \overset{1}{CH_2} -$$

pent-3-enyl

In branched chains, the locant of the side-chain is given the lowest possible locant but when the branched chain is unsaturated the double or triple bonds take priority for assignment of the lowest locants.

EXAMPLES

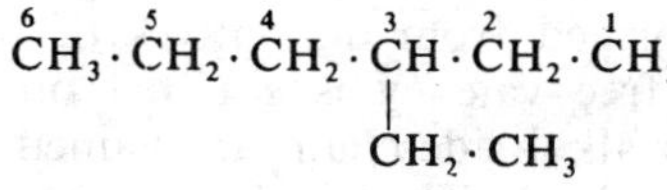

$$\overset{6}{C}H_3 \cdot \overset{5}{C}H_2 \cdot \overset{4}{C}H_2 \cdot \overset{3}{C}H \cdot \overset{2}{C}H_2 \cdot \overset{1}{C}H_3$$
$$CH_2 \cdot CH_3$$

3-ethylhexane

$$\overset{6}{C}H_3 \cdot \overset{5}{C}H_2 \cdot \overset{4}{C}H \cdot \overset{3}{C}H : \overset{2}{C}H \cdot \overset{1}{C}H_3$$
$$CH_2 \cdot CH_3$$

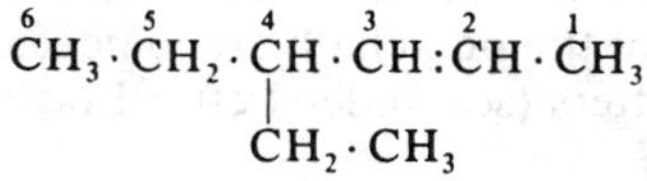

4-ethylhex-2-ene

When the branched chain contains two or more side-chains, they are cited in alphabetical order and when they are in equivalent positions, the side-chain that is cited first is given the lowest locant.

If more than one unsaturated bond is present in a chain then multiple terms or composite endings are used such as -atriene, -adiene, -enyne, -adienyne, etc.

EXAMPLE

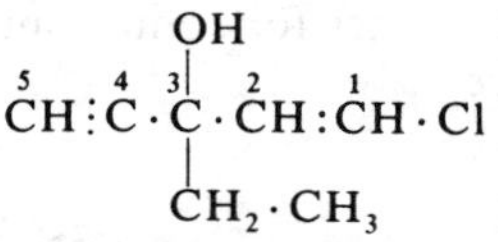

$$OH$$
$$\overset{5}{C}H : \overset{4}{C} \cdot \overset{3}{C} \cdot \overset{2}{C}H : \overset{1}{C}H \cdot Cl$$
$$CH_2 \cdot CH_3$$

1-chloro-3-ethylpent-1-en-4-yn-3-ol
(Ethchlorvynol)

A bivalent or multivalent radical of a hydrocarbon chain is named by the addition of the terms -idene or -idyne to the radical name of the hydrocarbon when the bi- or multivalent radical results from the removal of hydrogen from the free valency carbon atom.

EXAMPLE

$$\overset{3}{C}H_3 \cdot \overset{2}{C}H_2 \cdot \overset{1}{C}H=$$

propylidene

When hydrogen atoms are removed from each of the two terminal carbon atoms of a chain the radicals are named methylene, ethylene, trimethylene, etc.

EXAMPLE

$$-CH_2 \cdot CH_2 \cdot CH_2-$$

trimethylene

The name methylene is also retained for $CH_2=$ and propylene is retained for

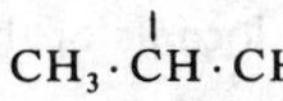

$$CH_3 \cdot CH \cdot CH_2-.$$

When more than one hydrogen atom is removed from each of the two terminals of the chain, endings such as -diylidene or -diylidyne are added to the name of the saturated hydrocarbon.

EXAMPLE

$$=CH \cdot CH_2 \cdot CH=$$

propanediylidene

Multivalent radicals in which there are three or more free valency carbon atoms are named by the use of the endings -triyl, -tetryl, -diylylidene, etc. which are added to the hydrocarbon name.

There are several names for branched-chain hydrocarbons which are not systematic but which are retained. These are:

isobutane	(2-methylpropane)
isohexane	(2-methylpentane)
isopentane	(2-methylbutane)
neopentane	(2,2-dimethylpropane)

The use of iso- and neo- in naming other branched-chain hydrocarbons has been discontinued. In addition, there are a number of branched-chain radicals which retain similar non-systematic (semi-trivial) names. These are:

isopropyl	(1-methylethyl)
isobutyl	(2-methylpropyl)
sec-butyl*	(1-methylpropyl)
tert-butyl*	(1,1-dimethylethyl)
isopentyl	(3-methylbutyl)
tert-pentyl*	(1,1-dimethylpropyl)
neopentyl	(2,2-dimethylpropyl)
isohexyl	(4-methylpentyl)

*sec- and *tert*- are sometimes abbreviated to s- and t-.

All these non-systematic names have been retained for use with unsubstituted hydrocarbons or radicals only. Trivial names have been retained for some unsaturated hydrocarbons and radicals. These are:

acetylene	(ethyne)
allyl	(prop-2-enyl)
isopropenyl	(1-methylethenyl)
vinyl	(ethenyl)

The name isoprene is retained for the unsubstituted form of 2-methylbuta-1,3-diene.

Chains containing hetero-atoms are named by the same procedures as those described above with the additional use of replacement nomenclature to indicate the types and locants of the hetero-atoms.

RING STRUCTURES

Cyclic Hydrocarbons

Saturated Monocyclic Hydrocarbons

These hydrocarbons are named by the introduction of the prefix cyclo- into the name of the acyclic hydrocarbon containing the same number of carbon atoms. Such compounds are referred to as **cycloalkanes**, and individual members of this series are cyclopropane, cyclobutane, cyclopentane, etc.

Unsaturated Monocyclic Hydrocarbons

These are named in a similar way by employing the characteristic unsaturated endings -ene and -yne. The ring is so numbered that the multiple bonds are given the lowest possible locants and the numbering proceeds in a clockwise direction. Radicals are numbered beginning with the free valency and giving the lowest possible locant to the multiple bonds.

EXAMPLES

cyclohepta-1,3-diene   cyclohex-3-enyl

The name **benzene** is retained to describe the parent aromatic hydrocarbon C_6H_6:

All the positions are equivalent in the unsubstituted benzene; the numbering of substituted benzenes is usually decided by the presence of a principal group which has the locant 1. The letter locants o- (ortho), m- (meta), and p- (para) are retained as alternatives to number locants for 1,2-, 1,3-, and 1,4-disubstituted benzenes.

Trivial names still acceptable for use in naming derivatives of benzene include toluene for methylbenzene, o-, m-, and p-xylene for the three isomeric dimethylbenzenes, and styrene for vinylbenzene.

Univalent and bivalent aromatic radicals are named **aryl** and **arylene** respectively. The univalent radical derived from benzene is named phenyl.

Univalent radicals derived from toluene and xylene are named tolyl and xylyl respectively.

Radicals formed from derivatives of benzene in which the free valency is situated on a carbon atom of an alkyl side-chain are named as substituted alkyl radicals. The trivial names benzyl, cinnamyl, phenethyl, styryl, and trityl are retained (for formulae, see List of Common Radicals). The carbon atoms of the side-chain are indicated by means of Greek letters (see under Letter Locants).

Unsaturated Polycyclic Hydrocarbons

Polycyclic systems in which two rings have two atoms in common are said to be ortho-fused; those in which one ring contains two atoms in common with each of two or more rings of a contiguous series of rings are ortho- and peri-fused.

Fused polycyclic hydrocarbons with the maximum number of alternate double bonds are generally named by means of trivial names. They all have the ending -ene. Systematic names are given to linear arrangements of more than four benzene rings: the suffix -acene is added to a prefix denoting the number of rings, giving pentacene, hexacene, etc.

Accepted trivial names for some common polycyclic structures are:

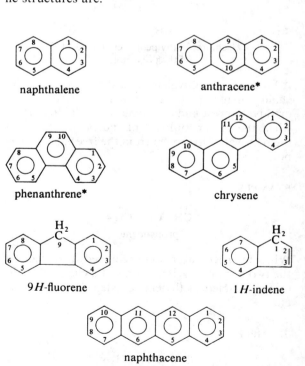

naphthalene   anthracene*

phenanthrene*   chrysene

9H-fluorene   1H-indene

naphthacene

*This numbering is an exception to the usual systematic numbering.

Univalent radicals are named by replacing the ending -ene by -enyl. The radicals derived from naphthalene, anthracene, and phenanthrene are named naphthyl, anthryl, and phenanthryl.

Orientation and Numbering. For the purpose of numbering, a polycyclic system is oriented so that (a) the greatest number of rings are in a horizontal row and (b) the maximum number of rings are above and to the right of the horizontal row, that is, in the upper right quadrant. When two or more orientations fulfil these requirements, the one is chosen which has as few rings as possible in the lower left quadrant.

EXAMPLE

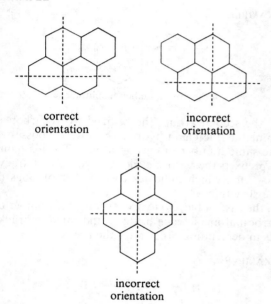

correct orientation   incorrect orientation

incorrect orientation

The system thus oriented is numbered in a clockwise direction beginning with the carbon atom not engaged in ring-fusion of the uppermost ring farthest to the right, and omitting the atoms common to two or more rings.

EXAMPLE

It is important to appreciate that formulae are always oriented for numbering this way and that this system involves complete renumbering of

many systems named by adding prefixes to trivial names (see the Fusion Principle below).

The atoms common to two or more rings are designated by the addition of the letters a, b, c, etc. to the number of the atom immediately preceding. Interior atoms follow the highest number, a clockwise sequence being taken whenever there is a choice.

EXAMPLES

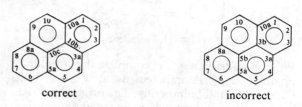

correct   incorrect

Indicated Hydrogen. Where possible, when a name applies equally to two or more isomeric fused ring systems with the maximum number of alternate double bonds, that name is made specific by indicating the position of one or more hydrogen atoms in the structure. This is accomplished by preceding the name with the locant(s) of the position(s) bearing the hydrogen atom(s) and designating each number by the italic capital *H*. These atoms are known as 'indicated hydrogen'. The same principle is applied to radicals and compounds derived from these systems and to heterocyclic systems where necessary.

EXAMPLES

1*H*-indene   2*H*-indene

The Fusion Principle. Non-linear polycyclic hydrocarbons that do not possess a trivial name are regarded as two or more simple ring systems fused together. Such structures are named by adding a prefix of the form benzo-, naphtho-, anthra-, etc. to the trivial name of the larger ring system. Prefixes are generally derived by replacement of the terminal -e of the hydrocarbon by 'o' (sometimes with contraction).

The position of fusion in the main component is indicated by the use of italicised letters which are assigned to the peripheral sides of this component; *a* being given to the side formed by carbon atoms C-1 and C-2; *b* to the side formed by C-2 and C-3; and so on around the cyclic system.

Numerals are employed to denote the position of attachment in the second component if this is necessary to distinguish between isomers, and these are placed, together with the appropriate italicised letters, in brackets after the prefix.

EXAMPLE

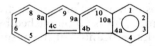

indeno[1,2-a]indene

When the fusion name is complete the structure is oriented and renumbered as described under Orientation and Numbering. The original numbering is only retained when one component is a stereoparent, in which case the name connotes a particular numbering system.

EXAMPLE

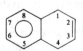

indeno[1,2-a]indene

Hydrogenated Polycyclic Hydrocarbons

Compounds containing less than the maximum number of alternate double bonds are named as hydrogenated derivatives of the fully unsaturated systems by the use of the appropriate prefix, dihydro-, tetrahydro-, etc. The lowest possible numbers are assigned to the carbon atoms bearing the additional hydrogen atoms. Fully hydrogenated systems are named by means of the prefix perhydro-.

EXAMPLES

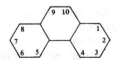

1,4-dihydronaphthalene   perhydrophenanthrene

The name indan is retained for the structure:

Bridged Hydrocarbons

Bridged hydrocarbons are molecules possessing two or more carbon atoms which are common to

more than one ring. They fall into two categories: (a) those which are *ortho*-fused or *ortho*- and *peri*-fused; (b) those polycyclic hydrocarbons which do not conform to (a). In the first category, additional hydrocarbon bridges may occur which are not part of the fused system. These bridges are named as prefixes to the fused ring system by taking the name of the hydrocarbon with the same number of carbon atoms as the bridge and replacing the ending -ane or -ene by -ano or -eno. These prefixes are non-detachable and their locants of attachment to the parent compound should be as low as possible. The atoms of the bridge are numbered so as to give the lowest locant to the atom adjacent to the highest numbered bridgehead.

EXAMPLE

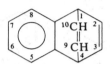

1,4-dihydro-1,4-ethenonaphthalene

In the second group, the bridged hydrocarbon is named as the chain hydrocarbon which possesses the same number of carbon atoms. To this name is prefixed the term bicyclo-, tricyclo-, or tetracyclo-, etc., which indicates the number of rings in the structure.

In the case of bicyclo hydrocarbons, the number of carbon atoms in each bridge is indicated in brackets in descending order after the prefix.

EXAMPLE

$$H_2C_8 \text{---} CH_1 \text{---} CH_2{}^2$$
$$^9CH_2 \qquad ^3CH_2$$
$$^4CH_2$$
$$H_2C^7 \text{---} CH_6 \text{---} CH_2{}^5$$

bicyclo[4.2.1]nonane

The structure in the above example is composed of three bridges which link two tertiary carbon atoms (1 and 6). The tertiary carbon atoms are referred to as bridgeheads. It can be seen that the bridges possess four, two, and one carbon atoms respectively. The bridgeheads are not included in counting the number of atoms in a bridge. The numbering of these structures starts from one bridgehead and follows the path of the longest bridge to the second bridgehead, then along the next longest bridge and so on until all the carbons are numbered.

Naming structures with three or more rings follows a similar procedure but the brackets contain, in decreasing order, the number of carbon atoms in the two branches of the main ring, the number in the main bridge, and finally the numbers in the secondary bridges.

EXAMPLES

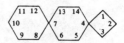

tricyclo[4.2.2.0^{2,5}]decane
(a)

tricyclo[3.3.1.1^{3,7}]decane (adamantane)
(b)

In example (a) above, the bridge between carbons 2 and 5 is a secondary bridge.

If this is temporarily disregarded, the main structure can be named according to the system described for bicyclic structures and the secondary bridge can then be described by the last entry in the brackets, which shows the number of atoms in the bridge, and the locants of the secondary bridgeheads, which are shown by superscripts.

Spiro-hydrocarbons

Spiro-hydrocarbons contain a single carbon atom common to two rings and are generally named by placing the prefix spiro- before the name of the hydrocarbon containing the same total number of carbon atoms as the bicyclic spiro-system. The number of carbon atoms in each ring, excluding the spiro-atom itself, is indicated in brackets in ascending order after the prefix spiro-.

EXAMPLE

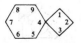

spiro[3.5]nonane

The system is numbered beginning with the carbon atom in the smaller ring adjacent to the spiro-atom as shown above for spiro[3.5]nonane.

Molecules containing more than one spiro-junction are named by the appropriate prefixes dispiro-, trispiro-, etc. The number of carbon atoms in each bridge that links the spiro-atoms is indicated in brackets and they are arranged in the same order as the numbering proceeds around the ring.

EXAMPLE

dispiro[3.2.5.2]tetradecane

There is an alternative system for structures in which one ring of the spiro compound is larger than the other(s). In this case the name of the larger component is followed by the word spiro- and the name of the smaller component. Between the word spiro- and the names of the components are inserted the positions of the spiro- atoms in each ring.

EXAMPLE

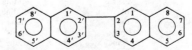

cyclohexanespirocyclobutane
(alternative to spiro[3.5]nonane, above)

Ring Assemblies

Ring assemblies are structures in which two or more ring systems are linked by single bonds to form a chain.

Identical Ring Assemblies. These structures are indicated by the numerical prefixes bi- (2), ter- (3), quater- (4), quinque- (5), sexi- (6), septi- (7), octi- (8), novi- (9), and deci- (10). These prefixes are placed before the hydrocarbon name or corresponding radical. Points of attachment are indicated by the appropriate locant and the use of primes to identify the ring components.

EXAMPLE

2,2′-binaphthalene *or* 2,2′-binaphthyl

Assemblies of benzene rings are named using the appropriate prefix and the term phenyl.

EXAMPLE

biphenyl

Non-identical Ring Assemblies. These structures are named by taking the parent ring structure and naming other rings as substituents.

EXAMPLE

2-cyclopentyl-1*H*-indene

Heterocyclic Compounds

Monocyclic Systems

Monocyclic compounds containing three to ten ring atoms and incorporating one or more hetero-atoms are named systematically by the use of a prefix or prefixes to indicate the nature of the hetero-atom(s), attached to a suffix denoting the number of atoms in the ring and the degree of saturation. The terminal -a of the prefix is elided where necessary. This is known as the **extended Hantzsch-Widman system**. Prefixes most commonly employed are:

oxa-	oxygen	sila-	silicon
thia-	sulphur	bora-	boron
selena-	selenium	mercura-	mercury
aza-	nitrogen	phospha-	phosphorus
arsa-	arsenic		

The suffixes used for **nitrogen-containing systems** are:

Number of atoms in ring	Unsaturated systems*	Saturated systems
3	-irine	-iridine
4	-ete	-etidine
5	-ole	-olidine
6	-ine	-inane
7	-epine	-epane
8	-ocine	-ocane
9	-onine	-onane
10	-ecine	-ecane

*Unsaturated systems are those containing the maximum number of alternate double bonds.

For heterocyclic systems that do not contain nitrogen, the following suffixes are employed:

Number of atoms in ring	Unsaturated systems	Saturated systems
3	-irene	-irane
4	-ete	-etane
5	-ole	-olane
6	-ine*	-ane†
7	-epine	-epane
8	-ocine	-ocane
9	-onine	-onane
10	-ecine	-ecane

*The stem -inine is used for systems containing the heteroatoms, As, B, and P.
†The stem -inane is used for systems containing the heteroatoms, As, B, P, and Si.

EXAMPLES

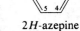

oxetane   2*H*-azepine

The presence of two or more identical hetero-atoms is indicated by the use of the multiplying prefixes di-, tri-, tetra-, etc. When hetero-atoms of different types are present, the appropriate prefixes are used, and these are cited in the name in descending order of group number in the Periodic Table, as in the list above, oxa- for example, taking precedence over aza-. If both hetero-atoms lie within the same group of the Periodic Table, then the order in the name is determined by increasing atomic number, with oxa- preceding thia- which in turn precedes selena-. The appropriate suffix is determined by the least preferred heteroatom.

Numbering. Systematic numbering of heterocyclic systems begins on a hetero-atom, preference being given to the hetero-atom cited first in the order of priority, oxygen, sulphur, selenium, nitrogen, phosphorus, arsenic, silicon, boron, and mercury. The ring is then numbered so as to give the lowest possible number preferentially to any other hetero-atoms and then to any substituent.

EXAMPLES

1,3-diazetidine   1,2,4-oxadiazole   1,3,5-triazine

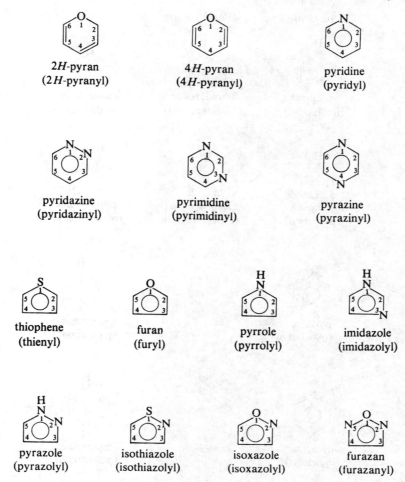

2H-pyran
(2H-pyranyl)

4H-pyran
(4H-pyranyl)

pyridine
(pyridyl)

pyridazine
(pyridazinyl)

pyrimidine
(pyrimidinyl)

pyrazine
(pyrazinyl)

thiophene
(thienyl)

furan
(furyl)

pyrrole
(pyrrolyl)

imidazole
(imidazolyl)

pyrazole
(pyrazolyl)

isothiazole
(isothiazolyl)

isoxazole
(isoxazolyl)

furazan
(furazanyl)

Univalent radicals derived from heterocycles by removal of a hydrogen atom from the ring are named by adding -yl to the name of the parent compound, with elision of the terminal -e if present. The numbering system of the parent compound is retained. There are a few exceptions to this method of naming radicals, some of which are indicated in the next paragraph.

Accepted Trivial Names. Many monocyclic hetero-systems are still known by trivial names; the more important of these (with their radical names in parentheses) are shown above.

Saturated and partially saturated derivatives can be named by use of the appropriate prefix, dihydro- or tetrahydro-. Saturated and partially saturated derivatives of pyrrole, imidazole, pyrazole, pyridine, and pyrazine have the following trivial names:

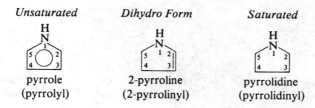

Unsaturated	*Dihydro Form*	*Saturated*
pyrrole	2-pyrroline	pyrrolidine
(pyrrolyl)	(2-pyrrolinyl)	(pyrrolidinyl)

Unsaturated	*Dihydro Form*	*Saturated*
imidazole (imidazolyl)	2-imidazoline (2-imidazolinyl)	imidazolidine (imidazolidinyl)
pyrazole (pyrazolyl)	2-pyrazoline (2-pyrazolinyl)	pyrazolidine (pyrazolidinyl)
pyridine (pyridyl)	—	piperidine (piperidino*)
pyrazine (pyrazinyl)	—	piperazine (piperazinyl)

*Piperidino is the preferred name for piperid-1-yl-. Radicals in which the free valency is at any position other than 1 must be named systematically.

Morpholine (rather than the systematic name perhydro-1,4-oxazine) is used to describe the saturated system shown opposite.
The radical derived from morpholine with the free valency on the nitrogen atom is called morpholino- rather than morpholin-4-yl-.

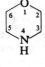

Polycyclic Systems
Trivial names are widely employed for bi- and tricyclic systems, and include:

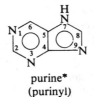

purine* (purinyl)

1*H*-indazole (1*H*-indazolyl)

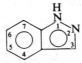

indolizine† (indolizinyl)

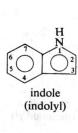

indole
(indolyl)

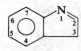

3H-indole
(3H-indolyl)

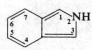

isoindole
(isoindolyl)

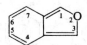

isobenzofuran
(isobenzofuranyl)

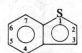

benzo[b]thiophene
(benzo[b]thienyl)
[replacing thianaphthene]

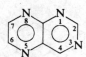

pteridine
(pteridinyl)

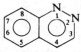

cinnoline
(cinnolinyl)

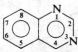

quinazoline
(quinazolinyl)

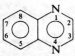

quinoxaline
(quinoxalinyl)

phthalazine
(phthalazinyl)

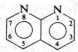

naphthyridine
(naphthyridinyl)

4H-quinolizine†
(4H-quinolizinyl)

quinoline
(quinolyl)

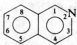

isoquinoline
(isoquinolyl)

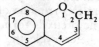

2H-chromene
(2H-chromenyl)

β-carboline
(β-carbolinyl)

carbazole*
(carbazolyl)

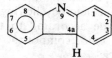

4aH-carbazole*
(4aH-carbazolyl)

naphtho[2,3-b]thiophene
(naphtho[2,3-b]thienyl)
[replacing thiophanthrene]

phenarsazine
(phenarsazinyl)

phenoxazine
(phenoxazinyl)

phenothiazine
(phenothiazinyl)

phenazine
(phenazinyl)

perimidine
(perimidinyl)

acridine*
(acridinyl)

phenanthridine
(phenanthridinyl)

xanthene
(xanthenyl)

phenoxathiin
(phenoxathiinyl)

thianthrene
(thianthrenyl)

phenanthroline
(phenanthrolinyl)
[1,7– shown]

* This is an exception to the usual numbering system.
† Note that when a hetero-atom occupies a position of ring-fusion it is included in the peripheral numbering scheme.

The Fusion Principle. Polycyclic systems not possessing a trivial name are named by an extension of the fusion principle, described for unsaturated polycyclic hydrocarbons. The basic method involves the attachment of a prefix denoting one ring or ring system to the name of the senior ring or ring system. The prefix is formed by adding to the name of the heterocycle the ending -o, with prior elision of -e if necessary, for example pyrano- from pyran, indolo- from indole. The following prefixes are irregular: furo-, imidazo-, isoquino-, pyrido-, quino- , and thieno-.
The selection of one heterocyclic ring as the senior component is made according to the following priority list. The senior component should be, in order of preference:

1. a nitrogen-containing component
2. a component containing a hetero-atom (other than nitrogen), in the order O, S, Se, P, As, Si, B, Hg
3. a component containing the greatest number of rings
4. a component containing the largest possible individual ring
5. a component containing the greatest number of hetero-atoms of any kind

6. a component containing the greatest variety of hetero-atoms
7. a component containing the greatest number of hetero-atoms having priority in the order O, S, Se, N, P, As, Si, B, Hg
8. a component containing the lowest locants before fusion for the hetero-atoms.

The position of fusion is indicated by the method used for unsaturated polycyclic hydrocarbons.

EXAMPLES

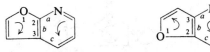

furo[2,3-*b*]pyridine   furo[3,2-*b*]pyridine

In the above example, the direction of numbering of the two rings is reflected in the order of the locants; 2,3 when the rotation is synchronised; 3,2 when it is counter.
When the locants of fusion have been determined the new ring skeleton is renumbered. The principle of numbering is essentially that described under Orientation and Numbering, but there is one important difference: when a hetero-atom occupies

a position of fusion it is included in the peripheral numbering scheme.

EXAMPLE

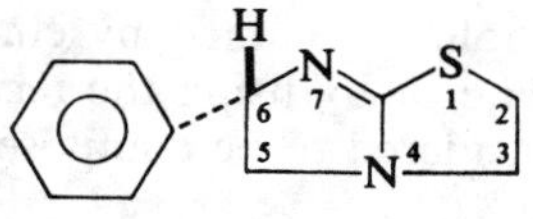

(−)-(*S*)-2,3,5,6-tetrahydro-6-phenylimidazo[2,1-*b*]thiazole
(Levamisole)

Two-ring structures containing benzene are named by a modification of this system. The locants of the hetero-atoms are given by numbers prefixing benzo- in the fusion name.

EXAMPLE

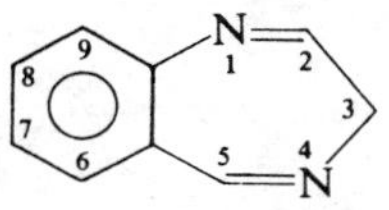

3*H*-1,4-benzodiazepine

For the purposes of fusion nomenclature the rings are considered to possess the maximum possible number of alternate double bonds. Hydrogenated derivatives are named by adding hydro- prefixes to the fusion names.
An alternative method of naming complex heterocyclic systems is Replacement Nomenclature.

Bridged Systems

In the *ortho*-fused and *ortho*- and *peri*-fused systems containing additional hetero-atom bridges, the bridges are named by the appropriate heteroatom prefix, such as epoxy (—O—), epimino or imino (—NH—), epithio (—S—), etc., along with the locants of bridge attachment.

EXAMPLE

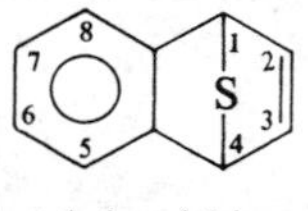

1,4-dihydro-1,4-epithionaphthalene

In other heterocyclic systems the nomenclature used is similar to that used in naming bridged hydrocarbon systems with the exception that the hetero-atoms are indicated by replacement nomenclature.

EXAMPLE

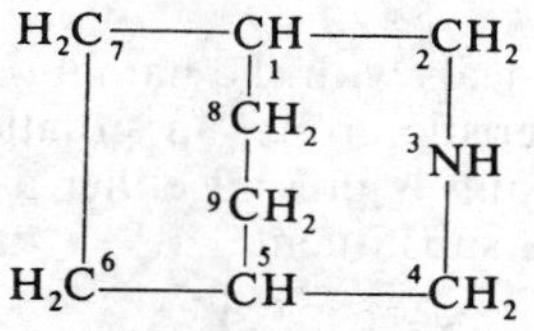

3-azabicyclo[3.2.2]nonane

The trivial name quinuclidine is retained for 1-azabicyclo[2.2.2]octane and tropane, although not a part of IUPAC nomenclature, is often used for 8-methyl-8-azabicyclo[3.2.1]octane. Additional prefixes to indicate hetero-atom bridges may be found in the List of Common Radicals.

Spiro-systems

Heterocyclic spiro-systems are named in a similar manner to hydrocarbon spiro-systems with the exception that the hetero-atoms are indicated by replacement nomenclature or, in the case of *ortho*-fused or *ortho*- and *peri*-fused heterocyclic components, by the use of trivial names.

EXAMPLE

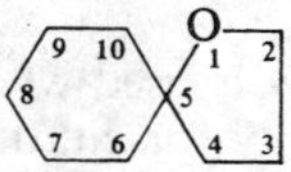

1-oxaspiro[4.5]decane
or cyclohexanespiro-2'-tetrahydrofuran

If trivial or semi-trivial names are used, then a heterocyclic component takes priority over a carbocyclic component of the same size.
An example of a drug which possesses a spiro-structure is fluspirilene which has the following structure:

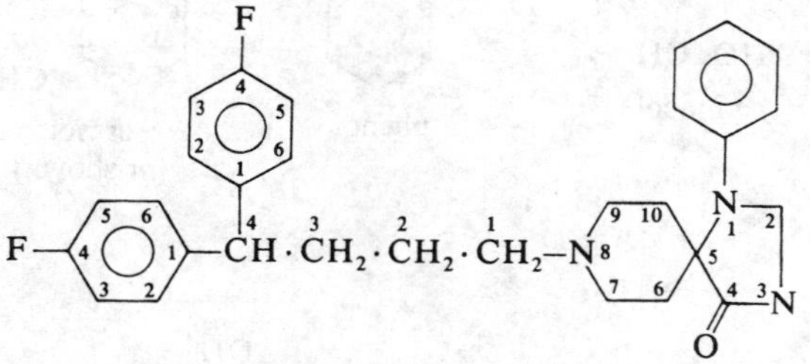

8-[4,4-bis(4-fluorophenyl)butyl]-1-phenyl-1,3,8-triazaspiro[4.5]decan-2-one

Ring Assemblies

Heterocyclic ring assemblies are named in a similar manner to hydrocarbon ring assemblies.

COMPOUNDS WITH CHARACTERISTIC GROUPS

This section deals with the naming of compounds with characteristic groups in situations where the particular group is present either as the principal group or as a substituent.

Alcohols and Phenols

Alcohols and phenols (ROH) are named by elision of the terminal -e from the name of the parent structure, followed by addition of the suffix -ol as in pyridin-2-ol and butan-2-ol.

Simple alcohols may also be named by radicofunctional nomenclature in which the radical derived from the parent hydrocarbon is placed before the word alcohol.

EXAMPLE

$$CH_3OH$$
methanol *or* methyl alcohol

The prefix hydroxy- is used when there is another group taking priority for citation as the principal group.

A number of trivial names are retained which consist of radicofunctional names based on trivial names for the radical R, for example benzyl alcohol, or which describe the entire molecule, such as the following examples.

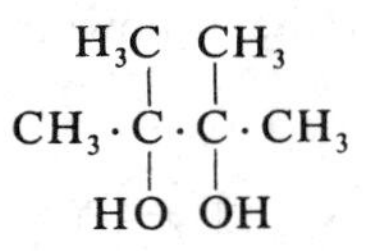

pinacol

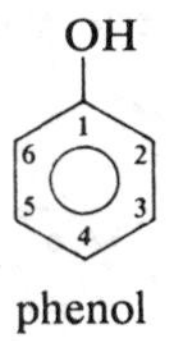

phenol

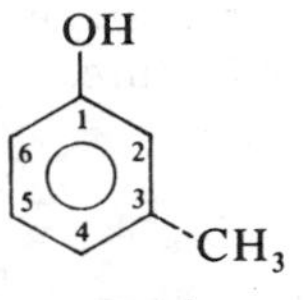

cresol
(*m*-shown)

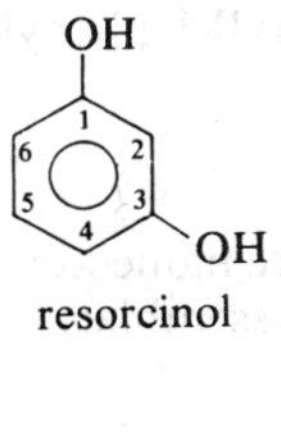

resorcinol

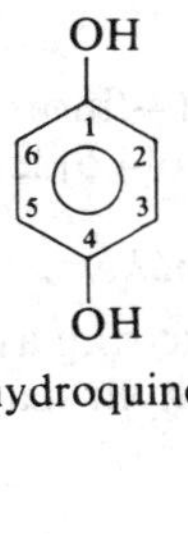

hydroquinone

The radical RO— is named by adding the term -oxy to the name of the radical R. For hydrocarbon radicals, up to and including the butyl isomers, and for phenyl, the -yl is elided forming such names as methoxy, phenoxy, propoxy etc.

Salts of alcohols are named by changing the -ol ending to -olate or by using the term oxide when the salt is considered to be composed of an anion and a cation.

EXAMPLES

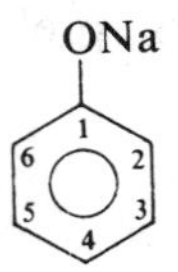

sodium phenolate

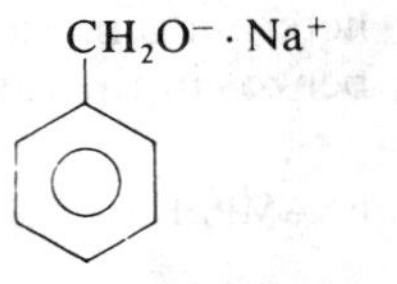

sodium benzyl oxide

Aldehydes

Aldehydes (RCHO) are named by the attachment of the characteristic suffix -al to the name of the hydrocarbon with the same number of carbon atoms, with elision of the terminal -e. Dialdehydes are denoted by the suffix -dial.

EXAMPLE

$$\overset{4}{C}H_3 \cdot \overset{3}{C}H_2 \cdot \overset{2}{C}H_2 \cdot \overset{1}{C}HO$$
butanal

When another group has priority for citation as the principal group, the prefix formyl- is employed. Cyclic compounds in which an aldehyde group is directly attached to a ring system are named by adding the suffix -carbaldehyde to the name of the ring system (conjunctive nomenclature).

EXAMPLE

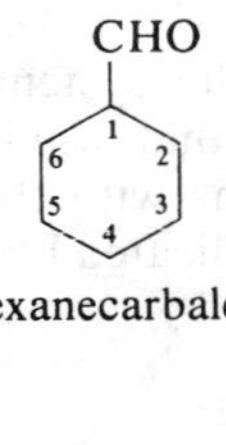

cyclohexanecarbaldehyde

Trivial names are also in common use. Many of these are derived from the trivial name of the corresponding carboxylic acid by replacement of the ending -oic acid or -ic acid by -aldehyde; for example formaldehyde from formic acid, acetaldehyde from acetic acid, benzaldehyde from benzoic acid, and nicotinaldehyde from nicotinic acid.

Carboxylic Acids and their Derivatives

Many carboxylic acids (RCOOH) retain trivial or semi-trivial names such as formic acid (HCOOH), acetic acid (CH_3COOH), and valeric acid ($CH_3[CH_2]_3COOH$). It is not possible to list all of these here but their radicals (RCO—) are shown in the List of Common Radicals. The names caproic, caprylic, and capric acid (for hexanoic, octanoic, and decanoic acid) have been abandoned by IUPAC but may still sometimes appear in the pharmaceutical literature.

Systematic names are based either upon replacement of a hydrogen atom by a carboxyl group (—COOH), in which case the ending -carboxylic acid is added to the name of the chain or ring to which it is attached, or upon replacement of a —CH_3 group by —COOH, in which case the terminal -e of the parent hydrocarbon is replaced by the ending -oic acid. When the ending -carboxylic acid is used, it is assigned the lowest possible locant of attachment; when a trivial name or the ending -oic acid is used, numbering begins with the carboxyl group.

EXAMPLE

$$\overset{5}{C}H_3 \cdot \overset{4}{C}H_2 \cdot \overset{3}{C}H_2 \cdot \overset{2}{C}H_2 \cdot \overset{1}{C}H_2 \cdot COOH$$

$$\overset{6}{C}H_3 \cdot \overset{5}{C}H_2 \cdot \overset{4}{C}H_2 \cdot \overset{3}{C}H_2 \cdot \overset{2}{C}H_2 \cdot \overset{1}{C}OOH$$

pentane-1-carboxylic acid or hexanoic acid

When acids are named trivially or as -oic acids Greek letters may be used, in which case locants 2, 3, 4, and 5 may be alternatively expressed as α, β, γ, and δ.

EXAMPLE

$$\overset{\delta}{C}H_3 \cdot \overset{\gamma}{C}H_2 \cdot \overset{\beta}{C}H_2 \cdot \overset{\alpha}{C}H_2 \cdot COOH$$

pentanoic acid

Carboxylic acid groups attached directly to ring structures are named by the addition of -carboxylic acid to the ring name as in cyclopentanecarboxylic acid. Trivial names, such as benzoic

acid (C_6H_5COOH), are retained for some structures. Dicarboxylic acids can be named systematically by use of the ending -dioic acid but many trivial names are retained.

When a carboxyl group is linked to a chain at the other end of which is a ring structure, the name may be derived from the name of the hydrocarbon chain by using the ending -oic acid. The ring is named either as a substituent by using the appropriate radical name or by conjunctive nomenclature, in which case the name of the cyclic component prefixes the name of the acid.

EXAMPLE

$$\overset{7}{C}H_2 \cdot \overset{6}{C}H : \overset{5}{C}H \cdot \overset{4}{C}H_2 \cdot \overset{3}{C}H_2 \cdot \overset{2}{C}H_2 \cdot \overset{1}{C}OOH$$

7-cyclopentylhept-5-enoic acid or
7-cyclopentanehept-5-enoic acid

When there is a group possessing higher priority in the molecule, the carboxyl group is denoted by the prefix carboxy-.

Radicals formed by removal of the hydroxyl group are named by replacing the ending -oic acid by -oyl or by replacing the words carboxylic acid by the ending -carbonyl. Radical names derived from trivial names are formed by replacing the ending -ic acid by -yl. The use of these radicals is described under Ketones.

Where components of a carboxyl group have been replaced by =NH, —NHOH, —NH_2, =N·NH_2, or —NHC_6H_5 the acid endings -oic acid or -carboxylic acid are replaced by the endings in the table below.

Acid type	Acid ending	Radical ending
$NH_2CORCOOH$	-amic acid* (used with trivial names of dicarboxylic acids)	-amoyl
$C_6H_5NHCORCOOH$	-anilic acid (used for N-phenyl derivatives of amic acids)	-aniloyl
$RC(=NH)OH$	-imidic acid -carboximidic acid	-imidoyl
$RC(NNH_2)OH$	-hydrazonic acid -carbohydrazonic acid	-hydrazonoyl
$RC(=NOH)OH$	-hydroximic acid -carbohydroximic acid	-hydroximoyl
$RCONHOH$	-hydroxamic acid -carbohydroxamic acid	-hydroxamoyl

*Carbamic acid and oxamic acid are retained for NH_2COOH and $NH_2COCOOH$ respectively.
The letters 'e' and 'o' are sometimes inserted between these endings and a preceding consonant.

EXAMPLE

$$CH_3\cdot CH_2\cdot C{\overset{\displaystyle \nearrow N\cdot NH_2}{\underset{\displaystyle \searrow OH}{}}}$$

propanehydrazonic acid

α-Amino acids [$RCH(NH_2)COOH$] are described separately.

Acid Anhydrides

Symmetrical anhydrides [$(RCO)_2O$] are named by replacing the word acid by anhydride.

EXAMPLE

$$(CH_3\cdot CO)_2O$$

acetic anhydride

Mixed anhydrides (RCOOCOR′) are named by citing, in alphabetical order, the first parts of the two acid names followed by the word anhydride.

EXAMPLE

$$CH_3\cdot CO\cdot O\cdot CO\cdot CH_2\cdot CH_2\cdot CH_3$$

acetic butyric anhydride

Cyclic anhydrides are named as acid anhydrides despite their heterocyclic structure.

EXAMPLE

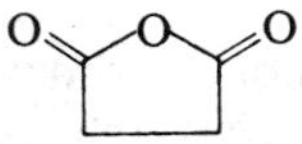

succinic anhydride

Esters and Salts

Esters (RCOOR′) are named by taking the name of the radical R′, derived from the alcohol R′OH, followed by the name of the acid, the acid endings -ic or -oic acid being replaced by -ate or -oate.

EXAMPLE

$$CH_3\cdot CO\cdot O\cdot CH_2\cdot CH_3$$

ethyl acetate

Esters of dicarboxylic acids may be formed by esterification at one or both acid groups. When both are esterified, either the same or different alcohols may be involved. Monosubstitution is indicated by insertion of the word hydrogen between the radical and the acid name.

EXAMPLES

$$\begin{array}{l} CH_2\cdot CO\cdot O\cdot CH_3 \\ | \\ CH_2\cdot CO\cdot O\cdot C_2H_5 \end{array}$$

ethyl methyl succinate

$$\begin{array}{l} CH_2\cdot CO\cdot O\cdot C_2H_5 \\ | \\ CH_2\cdot COOH \end{array}$$

ethyl hydrogen succinate

Where a group with higher priority is present, the ester group linkage is named by the prefixes ...carbonyloxy- (RCOO—) or ...oxycarbonyl- (ROCO—). Acetoxy is retained for CH_3COO—. Salts are named in the same way. For example, CH_3COONa is named sodium acetate. When a salt group is cited as a prefix the ending -ate is changed to -ato.

Lactones

Lactones are cyclic esters formed by intramolecular loss of water from a hydroxy acid. They may be named as heterocyclic compounds such as tetrahydrofuran-2-one or as lactones by substituting -olactone for -ic or -oic acid in cases where the hydroxy acid has a trivial name. Butyrolactone and valerolactone are permitted names for lactones derived from the non-hydroxylated acids butyric acid and valeric acid.

EXAMPLE

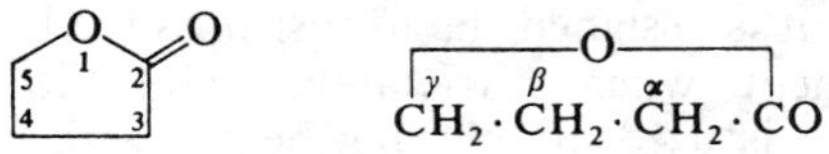

tetrahydrofuran-2-one *or* γ-butyrolactone

Alternatively, when the lactone is formed from an aliphatic acid it is named by adding the ending -olide to the name of the parent hydrocarbon with the same number of carbon atoms, with elision of the terminal -e.

EXAMPLE

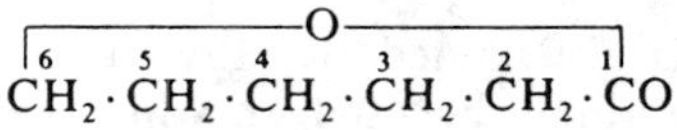

6-hexanolide (the locant indicates the position of ring closure) *or* oxepan-2-one

The trivial name coumarin is retained for the following lactone:

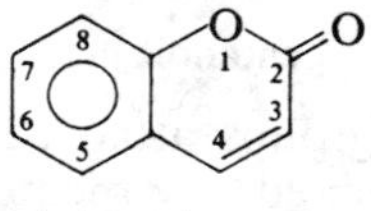

Compounds containing the groups —CONH— or —C(OH):N— which form cyclic structures in the

same manner as lactones may be named as -lactam or -lactim respectively in place of -olide or they may be named as heterocyclic compounds.

EXAMPLE

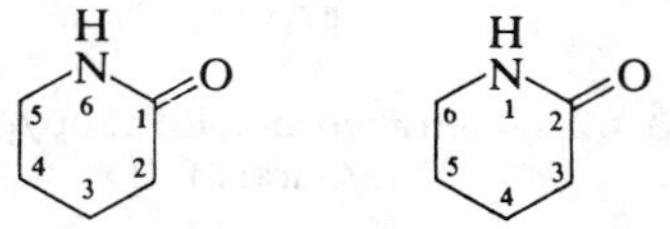

5-pentanelactam *or* piperidin-2-one

Ethers

Ethers (ROR′) may be named by either substitutive or radicofunctional nomenclature.

With substitutive nomenclature, the radical name for RO— is cited as a prefix to the hydrocarbon name corresponding to R′. The radical names for RO— are formed in a similar way to the method described for alcohols and phenols.

With radicofunctional nomenclature, the radicals R and R′ are cited before the generic term ether.

EXAMPLE

$$\overset{3}{C}H_3 \cdot \overset{2}{C}H_2 \cdot \overset{1}{C}H_2 \cdot O \cdot CH_3$$

1-methoxypropane *or* methyl propyl ether

When two identical groups that have a higher priority than the ether group are linked by oxygen, the prefix oxy- (—O—) may be used.

EXAMPLE

$$HOOC \cdot \overset{2}{C}H_2 \cdot O \cdot \overset{2'}{C}H_2 \cdot \overset{1'}{C}OOH$$

2,2′-oxydiacetic acid

If the oxygen atom links members of a chain or ring, it is termed epoxy. In linear polymers where several ether linkages occur, the molecules may be named as a single chain by replacement nomenclature.

Ketones

Ketones contain the carbonyl group —C(=O)— as the principal group and are named by using the suffix -one. Where another group has priority for citation as principal group the prefix oxo- is employed. For acyclic ketones the suffix is attached to the name of the parent hydrocarbon containing the same number of carbon atoms, that is, the group —C(=O)— is considered to have replaced —CH₂—.

EXAMPLES

$$\overset{4}{C}H_3 \cdot \overset{3}{C}H_2 \cdot \overset{2}{C}O \cdot \overset{1}{C}H_3 \qquad \overset{6}{C}H_3 \cdot \overset{5}{C}H_2 \cdot \overset{4}{C}O \cdot \overset{3}{C}H_2 \cdot \overset{2}{C}O \cdot \overset{1}{C}H_3$$

butan-2-one   hexane-2,4-dione

Radicals derived from ketones in which the free valency is on the carbonyl carbon are named by changing the ending of the corresponding acid from -oic acid or -carboxylic acid to -oyl or -carbonyl.

EXAMPLES

$$\overset{6}{C}H_3 \cdot \overset{5}{C}H_2 \cdot \overset{4}{C}H_2 \cdot \overset{3}{C}H_2 \cdot \overset{2}{C}H_2 \cdot \overset{1}{C}O-$$

hexanoyl

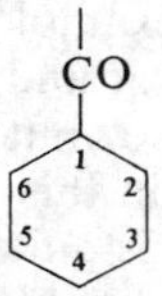

cyclohexanecarbonyl *or* cyclohexylcarbonyl

Many such radicals have trivial names which are preferred to the systematic names. These may be found in the List of Common Radicals. The name cyclohexylcarbonyl in the foregoing example can be regarded as a compound radical.

Many drugs are **cyclic ketones**, that is, the carbonyl group is part of a ring structure. Well-known classes include the hydantoins, barbiturates, benzodiazepines, and the pyrazole analgesics. These compounds are difficult to name systematically and there has been some disagreement. The problem concerns the degree of hydrogenation of the ring containing the carbonyl group.

Two principal alternative methods have been used:

Method 1. The carbonyl group is expressed by the suffix -one and the position of saturated ring atoms is denoted by added hydrogen, the locant and an italic *H* being placed immediately behind the locant for the principal group.

EXAMPLE

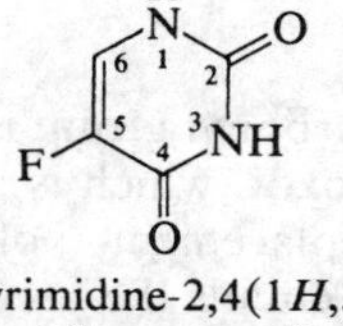

5-fluoropyrimidine-2,4(1*H*,3*H*)-dione
(Fluorouracil)

The added hydrogen may be omitted when the degree of hydrogenation follows unambiguously from the position of the carbonyl groups.

EXAMPLE

pyrimidine-2,4,6-trione
(Barbituric Acid)

Strictly, in the above example, hydrogen should be added at positions 1, 3, and 5 giving pyrimidine-2,4,6(1H,3H,5H)-trione but because the compound can only exist in this degree of hydrogenation the shorter name is quite clear.

This added hydrogen should be distinguished from indicated hydrogen. Indicated hydrogen is a property of the parent ring system, added hydrogen belongs to the ketone structure. Ketones derived from parent structures with indicated hydrogen normally retain indicated hydrogen in the ketone name, although this may be omitted without ambiguity in some cases.

EXAMPLE

4H-pyran-4-one or pyran-4-one

In this case there is only one possible structure containing the maximum number of double bonds; indicated hydrogen is thus redundant.

Contracted names are sometimes used for heterocyclic ketones, for example 4-pyrone for the example given above.

Method 2. The carbonyl group is expressed by the use of the prefix oxo-, which is used rigorously to denote the replacement of —CH$_2$— by —C(=O)—. This entails the use of hydro- prefixes to obtain the correct degree of hydrogenation.

EXAMPLE

5-fluoro-1,2,3,4-tetrahydro-2,4-dioxopyrimidine
(Fluorouracil)

Ketones in which the carbonyl group is attached to an acyl chain and either a benzene or naphthalene ring are named by changing the endings -ic acid or -oic acid to -ophenone or -onaphthone.

EXAMPLES

acetophenone

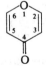

γ-[4-p-chlorophenyl-4-hydroxypiperidino]-p-fluorobutyrophenone
(Haloperidol)

The trivial name propiophenone is retained for the structure:

In cases where the carbonyl group is attached to two complex structures substitutive nomenclature is unsatisfactory. Radicofunctional nomenclature is then used. At its simplest this produces names exemplified by ethyl methyl ketone. The principle is the same for more complex compounds: the two structures attached to the carbonyl group are named as radicals and placed before the generic name 'ketone'.

EXAMPLE

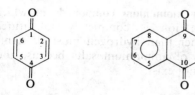

p-fluorophenyl 4-*p*-fluorophenyl-4-hydroxy-1-methylpiperid-3-yl ketone
(Flazalone)

Quinones. Quinones are di- and tetra-ketones, derived from aromatic compounds, in which the carbonyl groups are conjugated with the ring structure. They are named by adding the suffix -quinone to the parent name (sometimes with contractions).

EXAMPLES

p-benzoquinone   anthraquinone

Nitrogen-containing Compounds

Amides

Amides ($RCONH_2$) are named by changing the ending of the corresponding acid from -oic acid, -ic acid, or carboxylic acid to -amide or -carboxamide. When another group has priority for citation as the principal group the prefix carbamoyl- ($NH_2CO—$) is used. Radicals $RCONH—$ derived from amides by loss of hydrogen from the nitrogen are named by changing the ending to -amido-.
N-Substituted amides are frequently encountered. These are named by means of the letter locant *N*-, thus preserving amide as the principal group.

EXAMPLE

2,2-dichloro-*N*-[($\alpha R,\beta R$)-β-hydroxy-α-hydroxymethyl-4-nitrophenethyl]acetamide
(Chloramphenicol)

Amides in which the nitrogen is substituted by a phenyl group may be named by means of the suffix -anilide.

EXAMPLES

acetanilide (*or N*-phenylacetamide)

benzanilide (*or N*-phenylbenzamide)

Amines

Amines (RNH_2) are named by adding the suffix -amine either to the radical derived from a parent name (for simple compounds) or to the parent name itself. The use of the radical name rather than the parent is justified mainly on grounds of euphony.

EXAMPLES

cyclohexylamine   benzofuran-2-amine

When another group has priority for citation as the principal group the prefix amino- is used. Radicals derived from amines in which the free valency is on the nitrogen atom are named as substituted amino-groups.

EXAMPLES

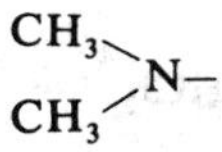

dimethylamino

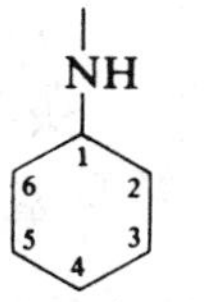

cyclohexylamino

The following trivial names are retained: aniline, anisidine, phenetidine, toluidine, xylidine (for formulae, see List of Common Radicals).

Heterocyclic bases containing nitrogen are sometimes regarded as amines but the endings -ine and -ole are not considered to be suffixes. Amines derived from such bases are thus named in the same manner as simple amines.

EXAMPLE

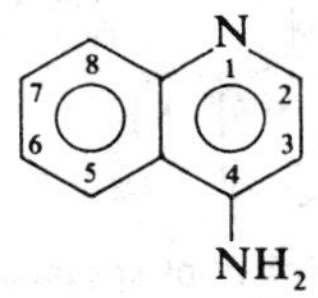

quinol-4-ylamine *or* quinolin-4-amine

Secondary and tertiary amines are named in a variety of ways depending on their complexity. Secondary and tertiary amines possessing identical alkyl groups are named by adding the prefix di- or tri- to the name of the corresponding primary amine.

EXAMPLES

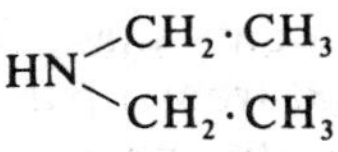

diethylamine

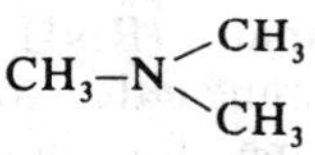

trimethylamine

Secondary and tertiary amines possessing non-identical groups are named (a) by means of primes, (b) by treating them as *N*-substituted primary amines, or (c) by enclosing the radicals in brackets before the suffix -amine.

EXAMPLE

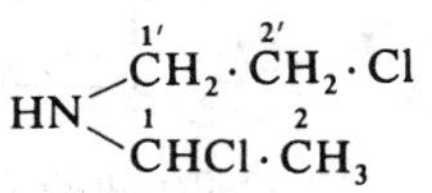

a) 1,2'-dichlorodiethylamine
b) 1-chloro-*N*-(2-chloroethyl)ethylamine
c) (1-chloroethyl)(2-chloroethyl)amine

Complex linear polyamines are named most simply by means of replacement nomenclature.

Ammonium Compounds and other Cations

When a nitrogenous base forms a salt the nitrogen becomes protonated and can be formally considered to be a derivative of the ammonium ion NH_4^+. Such compounds can be named as substituted ammonium salts. When the nitrogen is part of a ring structure the ion is named by adding the suffix -ium to the heterocycle name, with elision of the terminal -e. Cations have the highest priority for citation as the principal group so that salt formation can completely alter the appearance of the name of the base. To preserve the integrity of the base name a non-systematic method is often used for naming salts: the name of the anion is added to the unchanged name of the base (for salts of halo-acids the anion is represented by hydrogen halide).

EXAMPLE

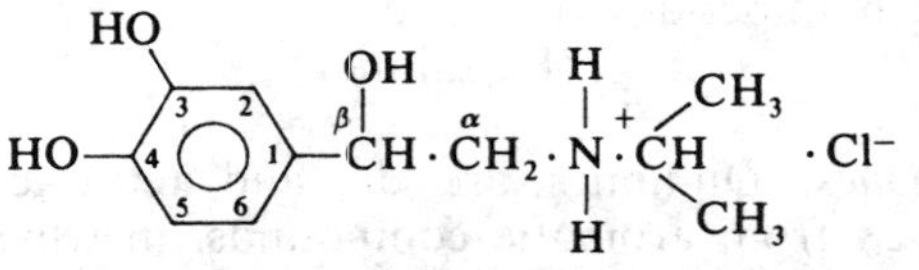

isopropyl(β,3,4-trihydroxyphenethyl)ammonium chloride
or 1-(3,4-dihydroxyphenyl)-2-isopropylaminoethanol hydrochloride
(Isoprenaline Hydrochloride)

Quaternary ammonium compounds in which the ammonium ion is completely substituted by groups other than hydrogen must be named as derivatives of ammonium salts because the free base does not exist.

EXAMPLE

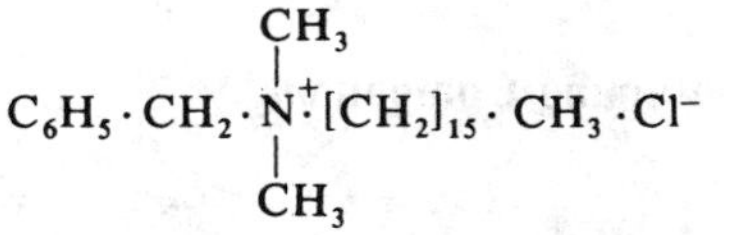

$$C_6H_5 \cdot CH_2 \cdot \overset{CH_3}{\underset{CH_3}{\overset{|}{N^+}}}[CH_2]_{15} \cdot CH_3 \cdot Cl^-$$

benzylhexadecyldimethylammonium chloride
(Cetalkonium Chloride)

Peroxides

Peroxides (R·O·OH) are named as hydroperoxides or, if there is a group present with higher priority, as hydroperoxy-derivatives. When the hydrogen atom is replaced by a radical R' to form compounds of the type RO·OR', they are named as peroxides.

EXAMPLES

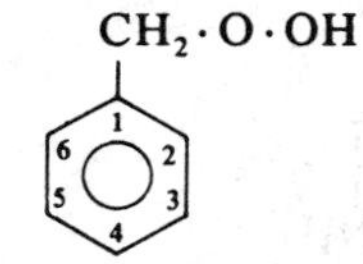

$$CH_2 \cdot O \cdot OH$$

benzyl hydroperoxide

$$CO{-}O \cdot O{-}CO$$

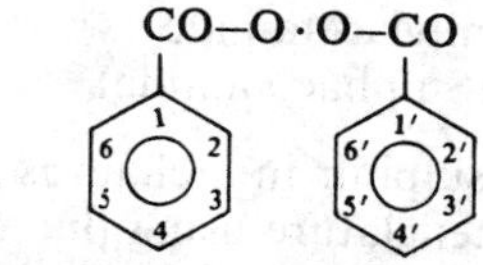

dibenzoyl peroxide (benzoyl peroxide)

When the —O·O— group links two components in which there is a group with higher priority, then it is referred to as dioxy-.

EXAMPLE

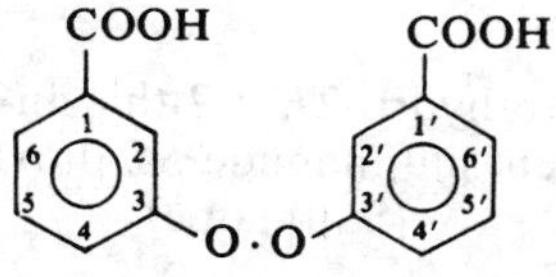

3,3'-dioxydibenzoic acid

If the —O·O— group links two members of a ring or chain, then it is referred to as epidioxy-.

Sulphur-containing Compounds

Sulphur compounds are named by the use of the term thio- which indicates the replacement of oxygen in a group by sulphur, by the use of the stem sulpho- to indicate the presence of sulphur in a group, or by a combination of both methods.

In general, suffixes denoting a sulphur group are used with the full name of the chain or ring to which it is attached, for example benzenesulfonamide, ethanesulfonic acid, and purine-6(1H)-thione.

The term thio- is placed in front of the name of the oxygen-containing group in which an oxygen atom has been replaced or, if the molecule in question is simple, in front of the trivial or semi-trivial name of the molecule.

EXAMPLES

$$\overset{3}{C}H_3 \cdot \overset{2}{C}H_2 \cdot \overset{1}{C}H_2 \cdot CS \cdot NH_2$$

propanethioamide

$$\overset{3}{N}H_2 \cdot \overset{2}{C}S \cdot \overset{1}{N}H_2$$

thiourea

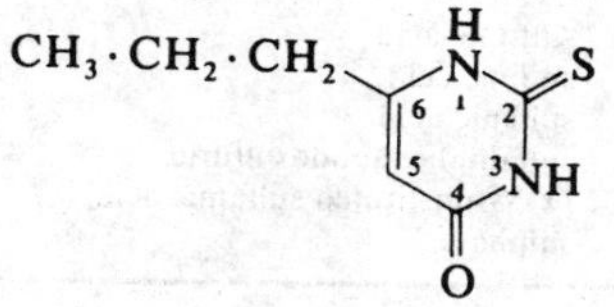

2,3-dihydro-6-propyl-2-thioxopyrimidin-4(1H)-one

(Propylthiouracil)

The following tables show examples of the use of thio in naming commonly encountered groups in which oxygen is replaced by sulphur.

Oxygen-containing group

Type	Suffix
—OH	-ol
—COOH	-carboxylic acid
	-oic acid
=O	-one
—CHO	-aldehyde
	-al
—CONH$_2$	-amide
	-carboxamide
—O—	ether

Sulfur-containing group

Type	Suffix	Prefix
—SH	-thiol	mercapto-
—CS·OH	-carbothioic acid	thiocarboxy-
or		[or hydroxy-
—CO·SH	-thioic acid	(thiocarbonyl)- for HO·SC— and mercaptocarbonyl- for HS·CO—]
—CS·SH	-carbodithioic acid	dithiocarboxy-
	-dithioic acid	
=S	-thione	thioxo-
—CHS	-thialdehyde	thioformyl-
	-thial	
—CSNH$_2$	-thioamide	thiocarbamoyl-
	-carbothioamide	
—S—	sulfide*	thio-

*The term thioether is not used; note also that these compounds can be named by radicofunctional nomenclature or by substitutive nomenclature.

Esters of thioic acids may be substituted on either the oxygen or sulphur atoms of the acid group. When known, the type of ester linkage is indicated by the use of O- or S-.

Sulphur-containing acid groups in which carbon atoms are absent are named as follows:

Type	Acid name	Prefix
RSO₃H	sulfonic acid	sulfo-
RSO₂H	sulfinic acid	sulfino-
RSOH	sulfenic acid	sulfeno-
RNHSO₃H	sulfamidic, amidosulfuric, or N-substituted sulfamic acid	sulfoamino-
ROSO₂OR′	sulphate	sulfonyldioxy-

EXAMPLE

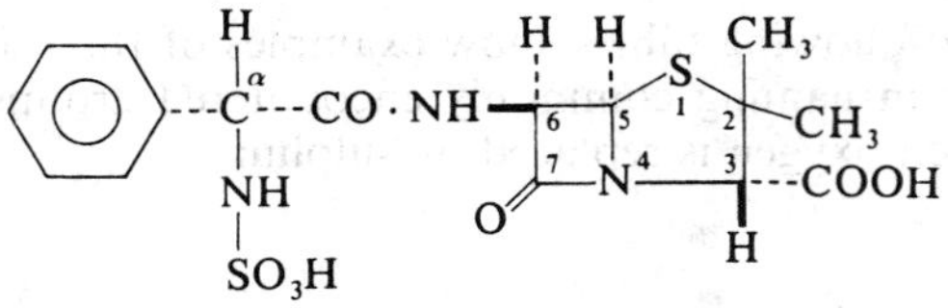

(6R)-6-(α-phenyl-α-D-sulfoaminoacetamido)
penicillanic acid
(Suncillin)

Examples of derivatives whose names are based on the above acid parents are shown in the table below:

Group	Suffix	Prefix(es)
RSOR′	-sulfoxide	sulfinyl-
RSO₂R′	-sulfone	sulfonyl-
RSNH₂	-sulfenamide	sulfenamoyl- (sulfenamido for RSNH—)
RSONH₂	-sulfinamide	sulfinamoyl- (sulfinamido for RSONH—)
RSO₂NH₂	-sulfonamide	sulfamoyl- (sulfonamido- or sulfonylamino- for RSO₂NH—)*
RSO₂NHC₆H₅	-sulfonanilide	phenylsulfamoyl-
RNHSO₂NHR′	-sulfamide	

*Note benzenesulfonamido- but phenylsulfonylamino-.

EXAMPLES

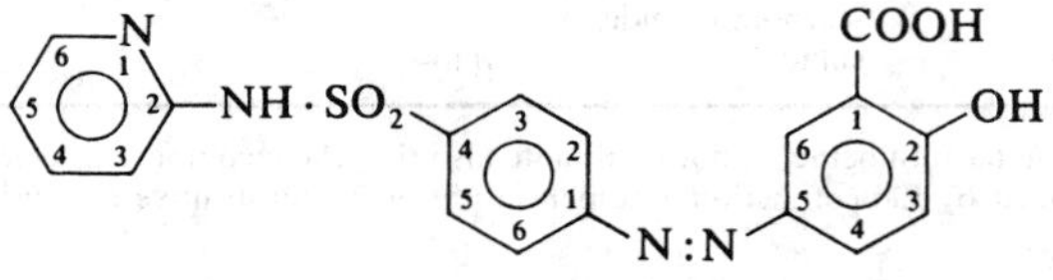

2-hydroxy-5-[4-(pyrid-2-ylaminosulfonyl)
phenylazo]benzoic acid or 5-(4-pyrid-2-
ylsulfamoylphenylazo)salicylic acid
(Sulphasalazine)

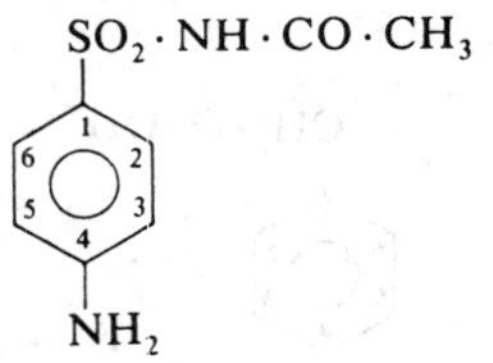

N-(4-aminophenylsulfonyl)acetamide
or N-sulfanilylacetamide
(Sulphacetamide)

The presence of sulphur in a chain is indicated by replacement nomenclature using the term thia-.
The presence of sulphur in a ring structure is indicated by replacement nomenclature, by use of the term thia- in the extended Hantzsch-Widman method, or by use of trivial or semi-trivial names as described in the section on heterocycles.

EXAMPLES

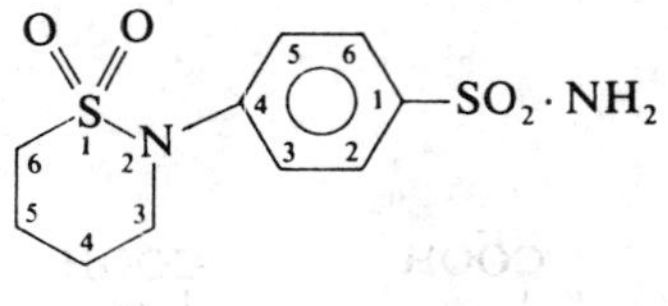

4-(tetrahydro-2H-1,2-thiazin-2-yl)
benzenesulfonamide SS-dioxide
(Sulthiame)

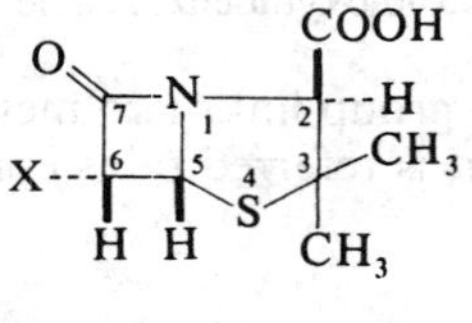

(2S,5R)-3,3-dimethyl-7-oxo-4-thia-1-azabicyclo
[3.2.0]heptane-2-carboxylic acid
(Penicillanic acid)

SPECIAL CLASSES OF COMPOUND

Amino Acids and Peptides

The nomenclature of α-amino acids and peptides is described in Nomenclature and symbolism for amino acids and peptides (IUPAC-IUB Joint Commission on Biochemical Nomenclature, Recommendations 1983) Eur J Biochem 1984;138:9–37.
Amino acids contain the group —CH(NH₂)COOH. Although they can be named systematically, trivial names are preferred. For the purpose of naming peptides (up to about 50 amino acids) the trivial names of amino acids are often contracted to 3-letter symbols. One-letter symbols, however, are used

for long chain peptides (proteins). Names, symbols, and structures for the most common amino acids are:

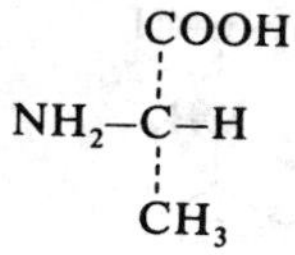

$$\begin{array}{c} COOH \\ | \\ NH_2-C-H \\ | \\ CH_3 \end{array}$$

Alanine (Ala)

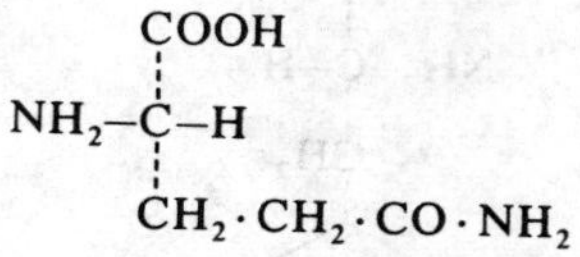

$$\begin{array}{c} COOH \\ | \\ NH_2-C-H \\ | \\ CH_2 \cdot CH_2 \cdot CO \cdot NH_2 \end{array}$$

Glutamine (Gln)

$$\begin{array}{c} COOH \\ | \\ NH_2-C-H \\ | \\ CH_2 \cdot [CH_2]_2 \cdot NH \cdot \underset{\underset{NH}{\|}}{C} \cdot NH_2 \end{array}$$

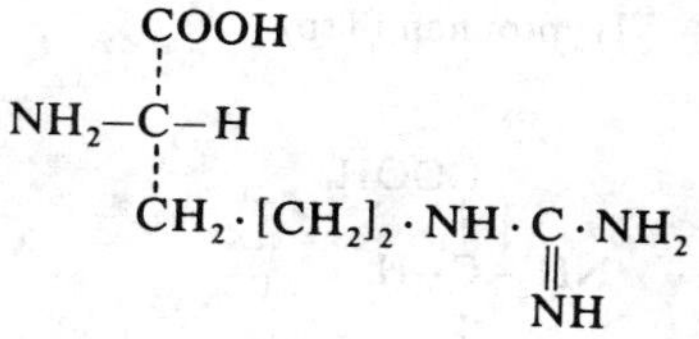

Arginine (Arg)

$$NH_2 \cdot CH_2 \cdot COOH$$

Glycine (Gly)

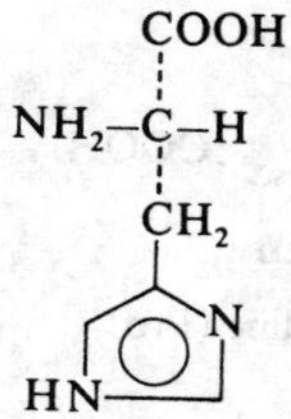

$$\begin{array}{c} COOH \\ | \\ NH_2-C-H \\ | \\ CH_2 \cdot CO \cdot NH_2 \end{array}$$

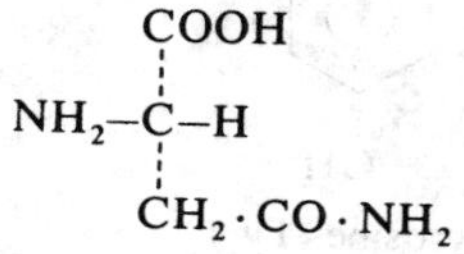

Asparagine (Asn)

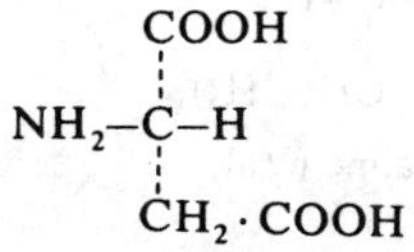

$$\begin{array}{c} COOH \\ | \\ NH_2-C-H \\ | \\ CH_2 \end{array}$$

Histidine (His)

$$\begin{array}{c} COOH \\ | \\ NH_2-C-H \\ | \\ CH_2 \cdot COOH \end{array}$$

Aspartic Acid (Asp)

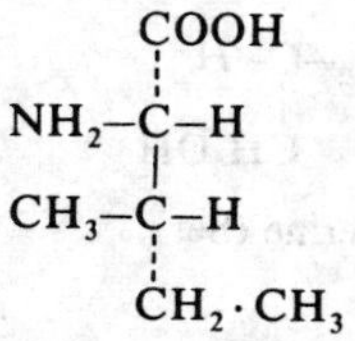

$$\begin{array}{c} COOH \\ | \\ NH_2-C-H \\ | \\ CH_3-C-H \\ | \\ CH_2 \cdot CH_3 \end{array}$$

Isoleucine (Ile)

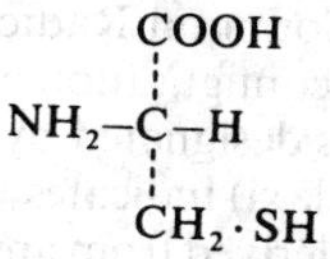

$$\begin{array}{c} COOH \\ | \\ NH_2-C-H \\ | \\ CH_2 \cdot SH \end{array}$$

Cysteine (Cys)

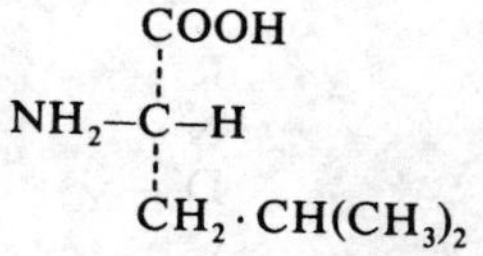

$$\begin{array}{c} COOH \\ | \\ NH_2-C-H \\ | \\ CH_2 \cdot CH(CH_3)_2 \end{array}$$

Leucine (Leu)

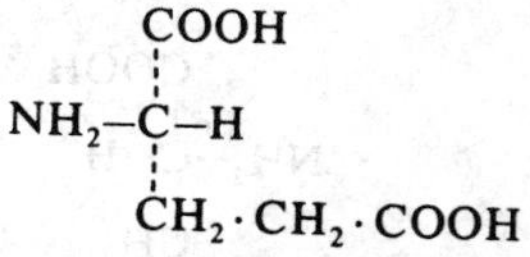

$$\begin{array}{c} COOH \\ | \\ NH_2-C-H \\ | \\ CH_2 \cdot CH_2 \cdot COOH \end{array}$$

Glutamic Acid (Glu)

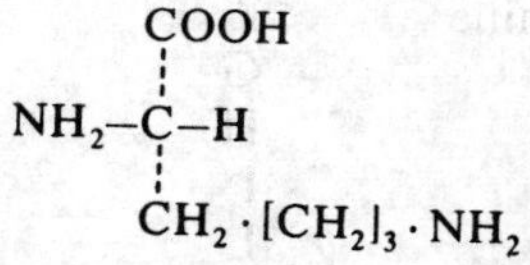

$$\begin{array}{c} COOH \\ | \\ NH_2-C-H \\ | \\ CH_2 \cdot [CH_2]_3 \cdot NH_2 \end{array}$$

Lysine (Lys)

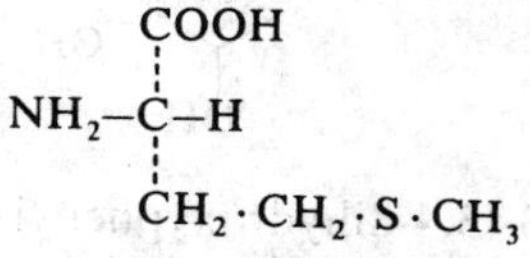

$$\begin{array}{c} COOH \\ | \\ NH_2-C-H \\ | \\ CH_2 \cdot CH_2 \cdot S \cdot CH_3 \end{array}$$

Methionine (Met)

$$\begin{array}{c} COOH \\ | \\ NH_2-C-H \\ | \\ H-C-OH \\ | \\ CH_3 \end{array}$$

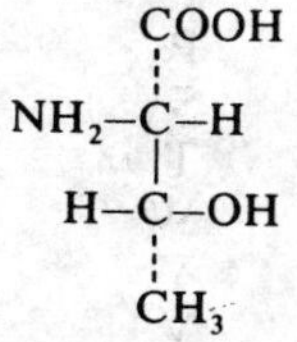

Threonine (Thr)

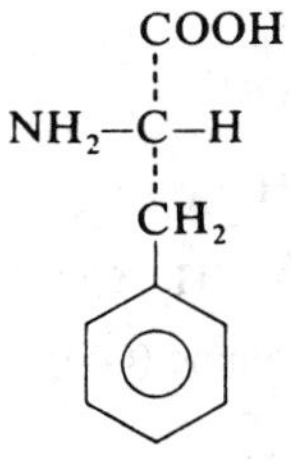

Phenylalanine (Phe)

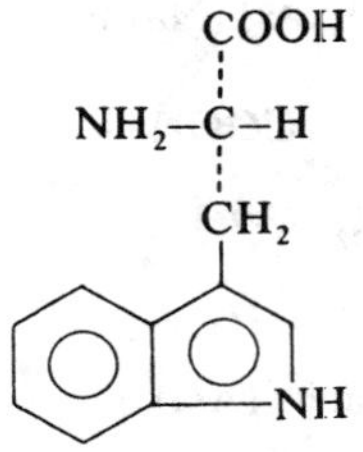

Tryptophan (Trp)

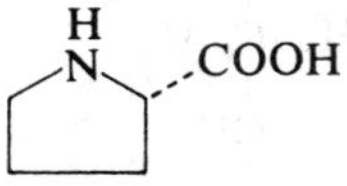

Proline (Pro)

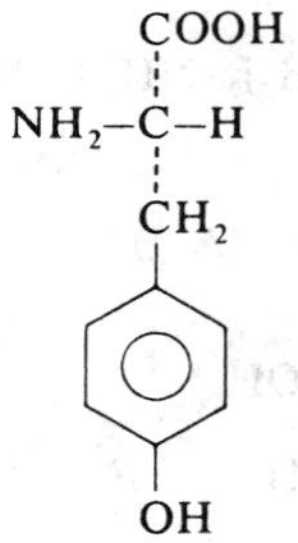

Tyrosine (Tyr)

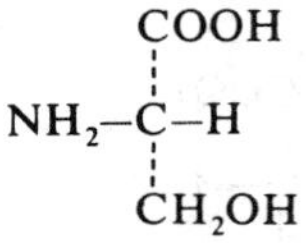

Serine (Ser)

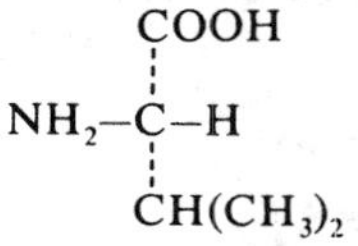

Valine (Val)

The following one-letter abbreviations are used for amino acids in proteins:

Alanine	A
Arginine	R
Asparagine	N
Aspartic Acid	D
Cysteine	C
Glutamic Acid	E
Glutamine	Q
Glutaminic Acid or Glutamine	Z
Glycine	G
Histidine	H
Isoleucine	I
Leucine	L
Lysine	K
Methionine	M
Phenylalanine	F
Proline	P
Serine	S
Threonine	T
Tryptophan	W
Tyrosine	Y
Valine	V
Unknown or 'other' amino acid	X

Radicals derived by removal of the hydroxyl group are named by replacing the endings -ine, etc., by -yl (see List of Common Radicals).

The absolute configuration at the α-carbon of the α-amino acids is designated by D- and L-notation. The prefix ξ (Greek xi) indicates unknown configuration. Compounds derived from amino acids may be named either as amino-acid derivatives or systematically.

EXAMPLE

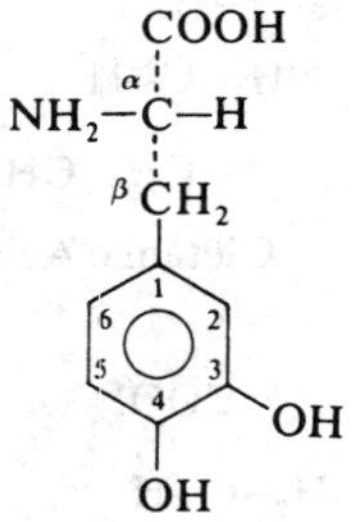

(−)-3-(3,4-dihydroxyphenyl)-L-alanine
or (−)-(S)-2-amino-3-(3,4-
dihydroxyphenyl)propionic acid
(Levodopa)

Peptides are named by joining together the name of the amino-acid radicals involved. Where this would result in a name of unwieldy length the 3-letter or 1-letter symbols are used. The first radical to be cited is that which contains the free carboxyl group. Peptides are generally considered to contain up to 50 amino-acid residues. Proteins contain more than 50 residues and the 1-letter symbols are commonly used to show their structure.

EXAMPLES

N-tert-butyloxycarbonyl-β-alanyl-L-tryptophyl-L-methionyl-L-aspartyl-L-phenylalanine amide
(Pentagastrin)

Ser-Tyr-Ser-Met-Glu-His-Phe-Arg-Trp-Gly-Lys-Pro-Val-Gly-Lys-Lys-Arg-Arg-Pro-Val-Lys-Val-Tyr-Pro

(Tetracosactrin)

MTPLGPASSL PQSFLLKCLE QVRKIQGDGA ALQEKLCATY KLCHPEELVL

LGHSLGIPWA PLSSCPSQAL QLAGCLSQLH SGLFLYQGLL QALEGISPEL

GPTLDTLQLD VADFATTIWQ QMEELGMAPA LQPTQGAMPA FASAFQRRAG

GVLVASHLQS FLEVSYRVLR HLAQP
(Filgrastim)

Many peptides can be named by reference to a natural peptide having a trivial name.

EXAMPLE

Cys-Tyr-Ile-Gln-Asn-Cys-Pro-Leu-Gly-NH$_2$
3-isoleucine-8-leucine-vasopressin (Oxytocin)

Carbohydrates

The nomenclature of carbohydrates (IUPAC-IUB Joint Commission on Biochemical Nomenclature) is described, as a series of papers, in Biochemical nomenclature and related documents. 2nd ed. London: Portland Press, 1992.

Carbohydrates have the general formula $C_x(H_2O)_y$ and are classified as monosaccharides, oligosaccharides, and polysaccharides. Many drugs, especially antibiotics, have structures related to carbohydrates and are named by means of carbohydrate nomenclature.

Monosaccharides

Reducing sugars contain an aldehydic group and are known as aldoses. They may exist in either a chain or a ring form. Trivial names exist for many aldoses—see below under Configuration. Systematic names for aldoses consist of a configurational prefix derived from the corresponding trivial name, a prefix denoting the number of carbon atoms, and the suffix -ose. In the cyclic form of aldoses the carbonyl group condenses with a hydroxyl to produce a heterocyclic ring. Six-membered rings are called pyranoses and five-membered rings furanoses. The carbonyl carbon is numbered 1; in the cyclic form this carbon is known as the anomeric, glycosidic, or potential carbonyl carbon.

Ketoses contain a keto rather than an aldehydic group and are non-reducing. They are named by means of a prefix denoting the number of carbon atoms and the ending -ulose. The position of the carbonyl group is indicated by a number locant. The most common position for the carbonyl group is position 2 and this locant is often omitted. Certain ketoses have trivial names of which fructose is the most important.

Configuration. The structures of monosaccharides may be represented either by Fischer projection formulae or by Haworth representations. The Fischer form usually denotes acyclic structures but can represent the cyclic forms; the Haworth form can only be used for cyclic structures.

In the Fischer projection the structure is written as a vertical chain with the anomeric carbon, numbered 1, at the top. The configurational prefix D- or L- is assigned on the basis of the configuration at the highest numbered asymmetric carbon (the reference carbon). If the hydroxyl group at this position is to the right, the configuration is D (by relation to D-glyceraldehyde, which has only one asymmetric centre and the hydroxyl group on the right). If the hydroxyl at the reference carbon is to the left of the chain the configuration is L. In the cyclic forms there are further configurational possibilities at the anomeric carbon. Considering the Fischer projection, if the orientation at the anomeric carbon is the same as that at the reference carbon (*cis*) the prefix α- is used, if the orientations are opposed (*trans*) the prefix is β-.

To convert a Fischer projection to a Haworth representation, the ring is drawn with carbon 1 to the right and should be imagined to be perpendicular to the plane of the paper with the oxygen bridge behind the paper. Substituent groups to the right in the Fischer formula then appear below the ring in Haworth. In the pyranose form of D-aldohexoses the terminal —CH$_2$OH group (C-6) always lies above the ring; in the furanose form C-5 and C-6 will lie above the ring if the oxygen atom at C-4 is on the right and below the ring if this oxygen is on the left.

EXAMPLES

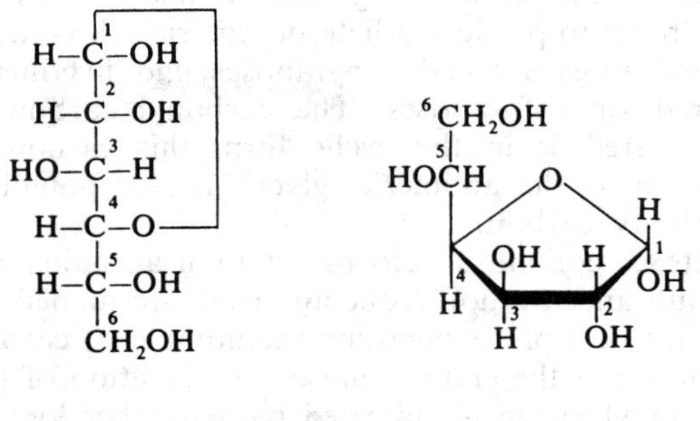

```
     1
 H—C—OH
     |2
 H—C—OH
     |3
HO—C—H
     |4
 H—C—O——
     |5
 H—C—OH
     |6
   CH₂OH
```

```
    6 CH₂OH
   5
HOCH      O
        OH  H   H
      4         1
     H        OH
        3   2
       H   OH
```

α-D-glucofuranose
(Fischer)   (Haworth)

```
     1
 H—C—OH
     |2
 H—C—OH
     |3
HO—C—H
     |4
 H—C—OH
     |5
 H—C—O——
     |6
   CH₂OH
```

```
      6 CH₂OH
     5
  H  H      O
 4              H
    OH    H   1
HO            OH
    3    2
   H    OH
```

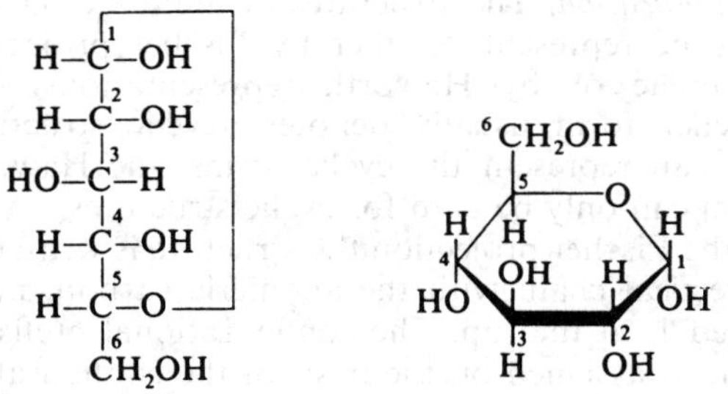

α-D-glucopyranose
(Fischer)   (Haworth)

The trivial names for the acyclic aldoses are retained and are used as the basis for systematic names. The aldoses are:

triose	glyceraldehyde
tetroses	erythrose, threose
pentoses	arabinose, lyxose, ribose, xylose
hexoses	allose, altrose, galactose, glucose, gulose, idose, mannose, talose

The prefix D- or L- refers only to the configuration at one centre–the asymmetric carbon atom with the highest locant. The configuration of consecutive and contiguous asymmetric centres is denoted by an italic prefix derived from the trivial names of aldohexoses. The configurations are:

one $>$CHOH group:

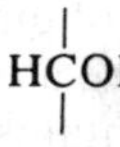

```
   |
 HCOH
   |
```

D-*glycero*–

two $>$CHOH groups:

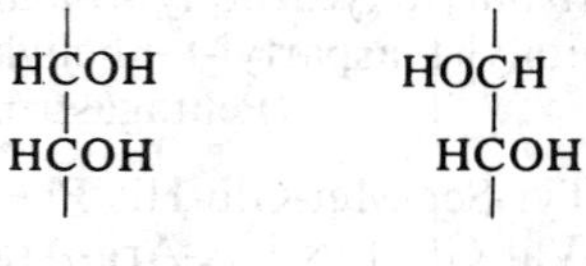

```
   |           |
 HCOH        HOCH
 HCOH        HCOH
   |           |
```

D-*erythro*–   D-*threo*–

three $>$CHOH groups:

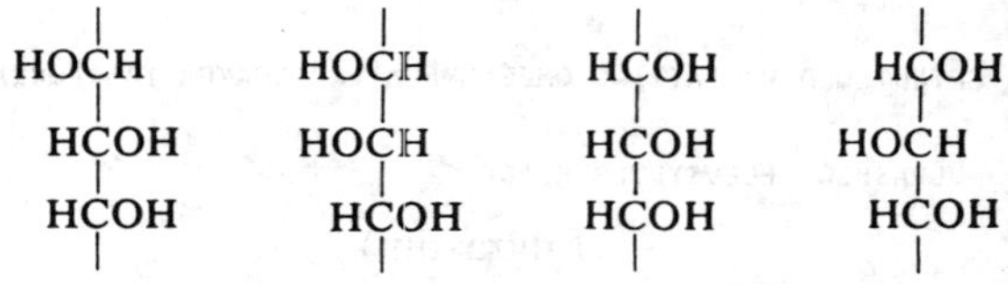

```
   |         |         |         |
 HOCH      HOCH      HCOH      HCOH
 HCOH      HOCH      HCOH      HOCH
 HCOH      HCOH      HCOH      HCOH
   |         |         |         |
```

D-*arabino*– D-*lyxo*– D-*ribo*– D-*xylo*–

four $>$CHOH groups:

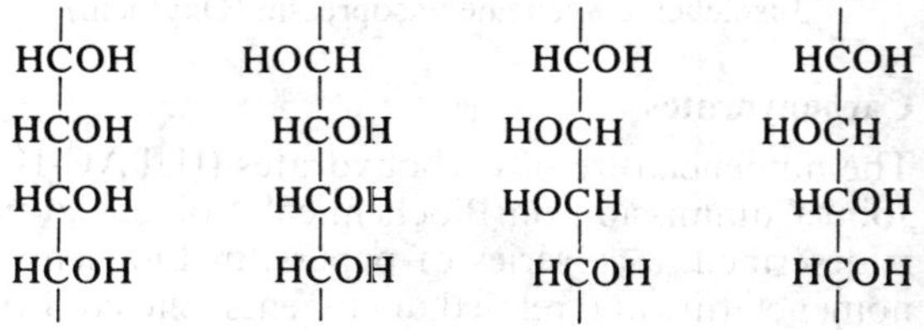

```
   |         |         |         |
 HCOH      HOCH      HCOH      HCOH
 HCOH      HCOH      HOCH      HOCH
 HCOH      HCOH      HOCH      HCOH
 HCOH      HCOH      HCOH      HCOH
   |         |         |         |
```

D-*allo*– D-*altro*– D-*galacto*– D-*gluco*–

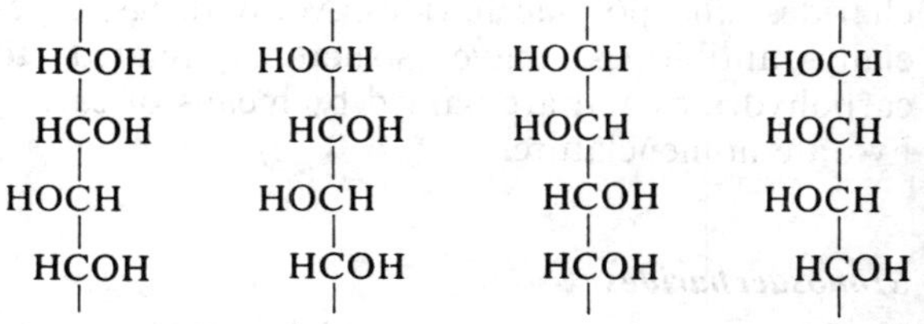

```
   |         |         |         |
 HCOH      HOCH      HOCH      HOCH
 HCOH      HCOH      HOCH      HOCH
 HOCH      HOCH      HCOH      HCOH
 HCOH      HCOH      HCOH      HCOH
   |         |         |         |
```

D-*gulo*– D-*ido*– D-*manno*– D-*talo*–

In the L-series all the asymmetric centres have the reversed configuration.

In the UK and the USA these prefixes have been used to denote consecutive but not necessarily contiguous asymmetric groups.

Systematic names for cyclic aldoses are formed by adding the configurational prefix to the name denoting the number of carbon atoms and the size of the ring. Thus glucose is named D-*gluco*-hexopyranose, although the shorter form, D-gluco-pyranose, is usually preferred.

Monosaccharides containing more than four contiguous asymmetric carbon atoms are named systematically by adding two or more configurational prefixes, one prefix denoting the first four asymmetric carbons. The prefix referring to the highest numbered carbon atom is cited first in the name. The anomeric prefix α- or β- is assigned by comparing the configurations at the anomeric carbon and the reference carbon, the reference carbon being the highest numbered asymmetric carbon in the whole structure. The prefix α- or β- is placed before that part of the name which contains the reference carbon.

Derivatives. The replacement of a hydroxyl- group by hydrogen is denoted by the prefix deoxy-. Replacement of hydroxyl by a group other than hydrogen is denoted by a deoxy- prefix and the name of the substituent. Substitution on carbon is denoted by the letter locant C. Replacement of a hydroxyl hydrogen is denoted by the letter locant O. All the substituents also have number locants denoting their position in the ring. All prefixes denoting substitution are arranged in alphabetical order.

EXAMPLE

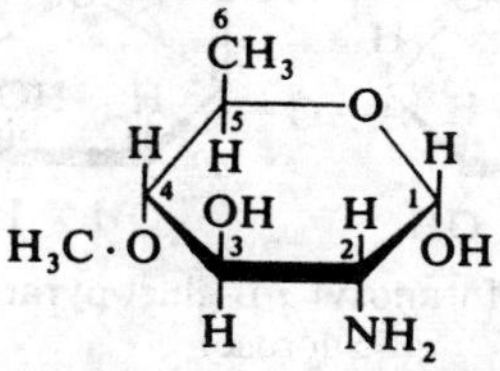

2-amino-2,6-dideoxy-4-O-methyl-α-D-glucopyranose

Glycosides are derivatives in which the hydroxyl group attached to the anomeric carbon (position 1) of cyclic monosaccharides is replaced by a group of the form —OR, where R may be an alkyl or aryl group or, in the case of oligosaccharides, another monosaccharide. Glycosides are named by replacing the terminal -e of the monosaccharide name by the ending -ide, the substituent being denoted by the appropriate radical name. The non-sugar component of a glycoside is termed the aglycone.

EXAMPLE

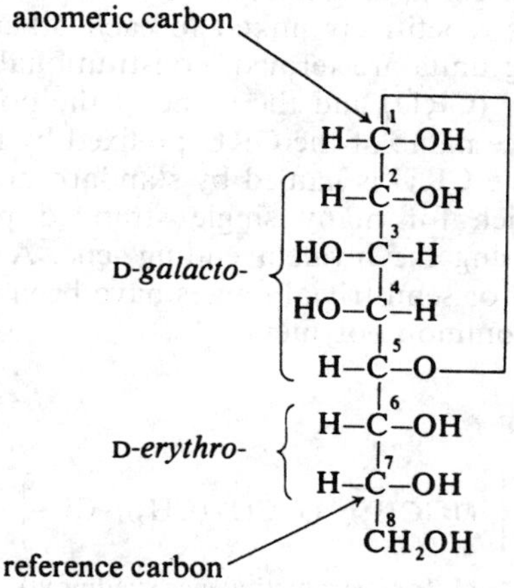

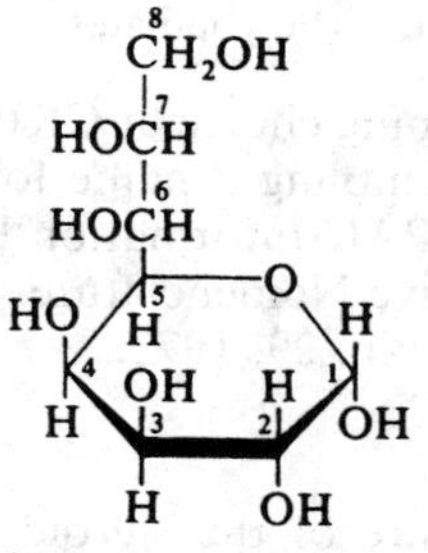

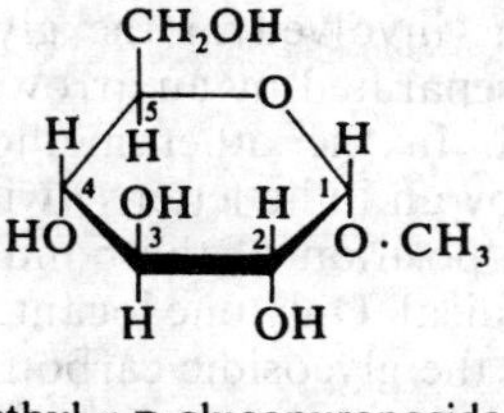

α-D-*erythro*-D-*galacto*-octopyranose

EXAMPLE

methyl α-D-glucopyranoside

Oligosaccharides. Oligosaccharides are glycosides containing from two to ten monosaccharide units. The most common oligosaccharides are the disaccharides, many of which, like cellobiose, lactose, maltose, and sucrose, are best known by trivial names. The link between monosaccharides is glycosidic and the compounds are named differently depending on whether they are reducing or non-reducing sugars. Non-reducing sugars are named as glycosyl glycosides, the monosaccharides being placed in alphabetical order.

EXAMPLE

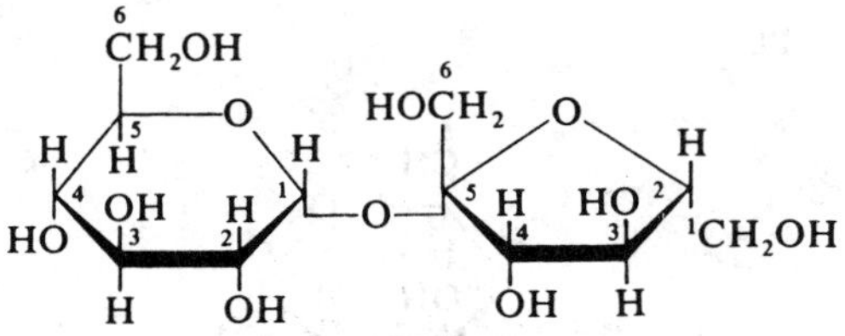

β-D-fructofuranosyl α-D-glucopyranoside
(Sucrose)

Reducing sugars are named as glycosylglycoses, the monosaccharides again being placed in alphabetical order.

EXAMPLE

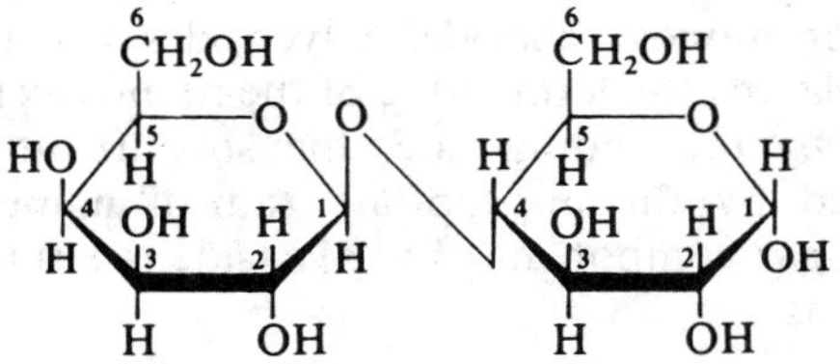

4-*O*-β-D-galactopyranosyl-α-D-glucopyranose
(α-Lactose)

Trisaccharides and higher oligosaccharides are named in a similar manner but two alternative methods of representing the glycosidic linkage are commonly used. In one method the locants of the carbon atoms involved in the glycosidic linkage are written, separated by an arrow, after each glycosyl radical. In the other method the bond is represented by an italic letter *O* with a superscript denoting the position of the bond. This is placed before the radical. Only one locant is strictly necessary because the glycosidic carbon is always numbered 1.

EXAMPLE

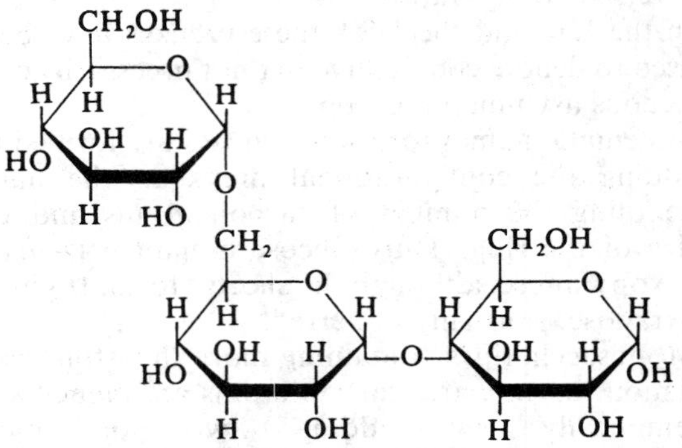

O-α-D-glucopyranosyl-(1 → 6)-*O*-α-D-glucopyranosyl-(1 → 4)-α-D-glucopyranose *or* O^4-(O^6-α-D-glucopyranosyl-α-D-glucopyranosyl)-α-D-glucopyranose

Polysaccharides. These are polymeric carbohydrates of high molecular weight. They are usually named trivially, for example, cellulose, glycogen, and amylose.

Polymers

Polymers are defined as substances composed of molecules containing many of one or more species of atoms repetitively linked to each other. These repeating units are termed 'constitutional repeating units' (CRU) and the name of the polymer is simply the name of the CRU prefixed by the term poly-. The CRU is named by standard nomenclature which for many single stranded polymers means using the bivalent ending -ene. A number of trivial or semi-trivial names have been retained for the common polymers.

EXAMPLE

poly(oxytetramethyleneoxyadipoyl)
(Polybutilate)

The rules governing choice of CRU and the details involved in assembling a name for a polymer are discussed in IUPAC Information Bulletin, Appendices on Tentative Nomenclature, Symbols, Units, and Standards, No. 29, 1972.

Steroids

The nomenclature of the steroids is described in detail in The nomenclature of steroids (IUPAC-

IUB Joint Commission on Biochemical Nomenclature, Recommendations 1989) Eur J Biochem 1989;186:429–58.

The numbering of the steroidal skeleton and the labelling of its constituent rings are as follows:

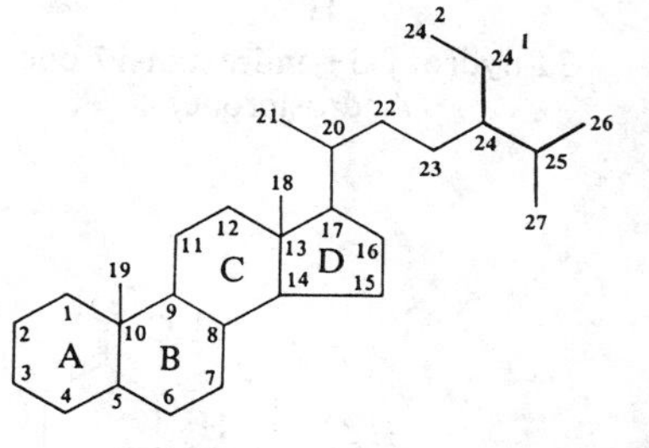

If one of the methyl groups at C-25 is substituted it becomes C-26. If both are substituted, that with the substituent cited first alphabetically is C-26. C-24[1] and C-24[2] were formerly numbered C-28 and C-29. There are a number of parent steroid structures each having different alkyl substituents and each possessing a specific stereochemical configuration. The common parent structures are listed below.

If there are two carbon chains at C-17, one of which appears in the above table, and the steroid possesses methyl groups at C-18 and C-19, the steroid is named as a 17-alkyl derivative of the corresponding parent steroid. If neither of the carbon chains at C-17 is in the table then the steroid is named as a dialkylandrostane.

The ring structures in the steroid nucleus may exist in a number of configurations. However, only two configurations are commonly encountered and they differ only in the stereochemistry of the ring-A/ring-B junction, which may be cis or trans. The other ring junctions are usually trans (the cardiac glycosides and fusidic acid are exceptions).

By convention, substituents projecting above the general plane of the steroid nucleus are designated β and those projecting below the plane are designated α. The substituents at C-10 and C-13 project above the plane. When the ring-A/ring-B junction is cis the hydrogen atom at C-5 will also project above the plane (designated β) and when the ring-A/ring-B junction is trans the C-5 hydrogen will be below the plane (designated α). The perspective formulae below depict the two configurations.

Parent	R_1	R_2	R_3
gonane	H	H	H
estrane	H	CH_3	H
androstane	CH_3	CH_3	H
pregnane	CH_3	CH_3	CH_2CH_3
cholane	CH_3	CH_3	$CH(CH_3)CH_2CH_2CH_3$
cholestane	CH_3	CH_3	$CH(CH_3)CH_2CH_2CH_2CH(CH_3)_2$
ergostane	CH_3	CH_3	$CH(CH_3)CH_2CH_2CH(CH_3)CH(CH_3)_2$
stigmastane	CH_3	CH_3	$CH(CH_3)CH_2CH_2CH(CH_2CH_3)CH(CH_3)_2$

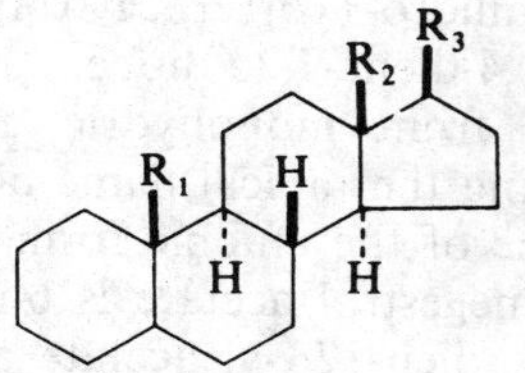

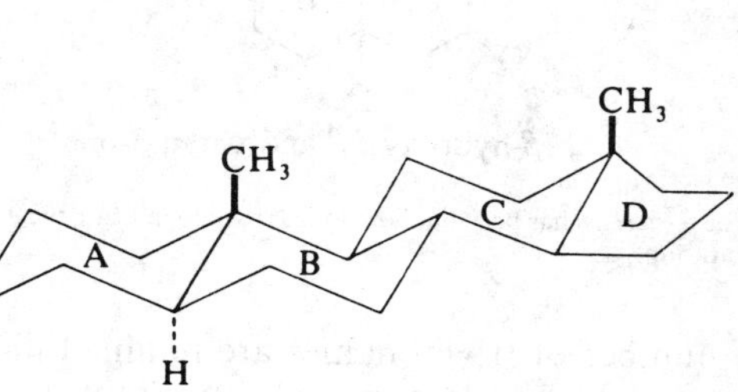

A/B trans: 5α-androstane

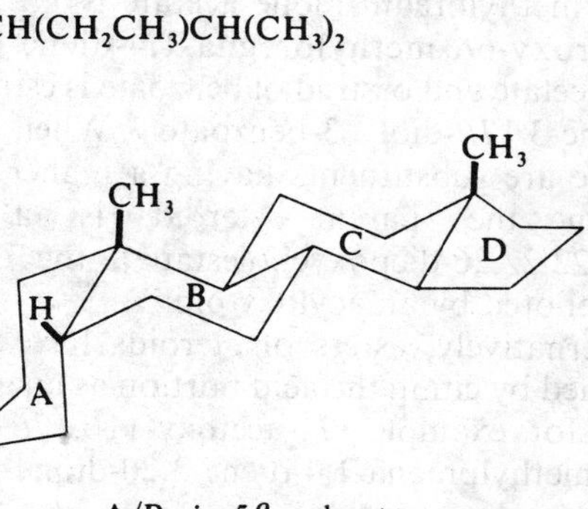

A/B cis: 5β-androstane

Thus the assignment of α or β to the C-5 hydrogen atom will unambiguously define the stereochemistry of the parent steroid structures. If the configuration is unknown then the symbol ξ (Greek xi) is used. The terms allo and normal have been but are no longer used to indicate 5α- or 5β-steroids respectively.

Stereochemistry about carbon atoms on side chains is denoted by the R- and S-system.

Configurations at C-20 were formerly denoted by an α/β notation, based on a Fischer projection, but the use of the R/S is now recommended. Substituents to the right of C-20 used to be termed α whilst those to the left were termed β.

Complete stereochemical inversions are denoted by *ent* (short for enantio) whilst partial inversions are denoted by the use of the α/β or R- and S-notations. Racemic mixtures are denoted by *rac*.

Examples of androstane derivatives are shown opposite.

Derivatives of steroidal hydrocarbons are named by substitutive nomenclature using standard prefixes and suffixes. Rules for describing unsaturation are the same as those relating to unsaturated hydrocarbons generally. For example, fluoxymesterone is 9α-fluoro-11β,17β-dihydroxy-17α-methylandrost-4-en-3-one, oestriol is estra-1,3,5(10)-triene-3,16α,17β-triol, and dexamethasone is 9α-fluoro-11β,17α,21-trihydroxy-16α-methylpregna-1,4-diene-3,20-dione.

Esters derived from monohydric alcohols are named by placing the radical name of the steroid before the name of the anionic form of the acid. For example, megestrol acetate is 6-methyl-3,20-dioxopregna-4,6-dien-17α-yl acetate and nandrolone phenylpropionate is 3-oxo-estr-4-en-17β-yl 3-phenylpropionate.

Esters derived from polyhydric alcohols are named by placing the full name of the steroid polyol before the name of the anionic form of the acid. For example, methylprednisolone acetate is 11β,17α,21-trihydroxy-6α-methylpregna-1,4-diene-3,20-dione 21-acetate and oestradiol benzoate is estra-1,3,5(10)-triene-3,17β-diol 3-benzoate. When, however, there are substituents having a higher priority or when the parent steroid is a spirostan (16,22:22,26-diepoxycholestane), the ester group is denoted by an acyloxy prefix.

Alternatively, esters of steroids have often been named by citing the acid portion as an acyloxy prefix, for example, 21-acetoxy-11β,17α-dihydroxy-6α-methylpregna-1,4-diene-3,20-dione (methylprednisolone acetate).

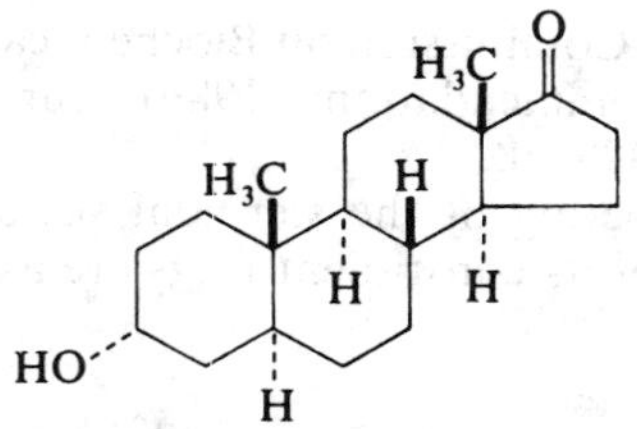

3α-hydroxy-5α-androstan-17-one
(Androsterone)

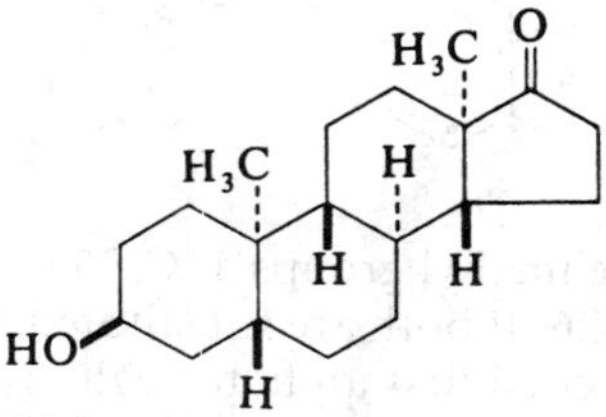

ent-3α-hydroxy-5α-androstan-17-one
(*ent*-Androsterone)

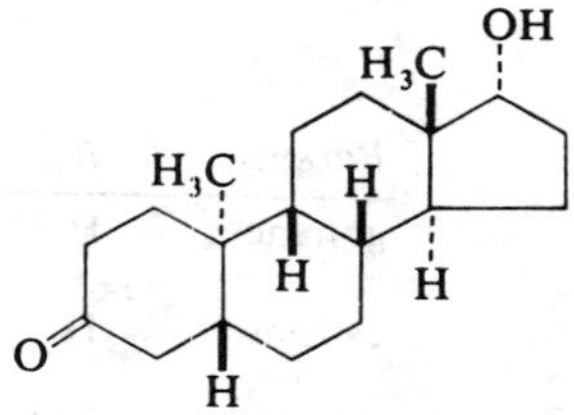

17α-hydroxy-5β,9β,10α-androstan-3-one*

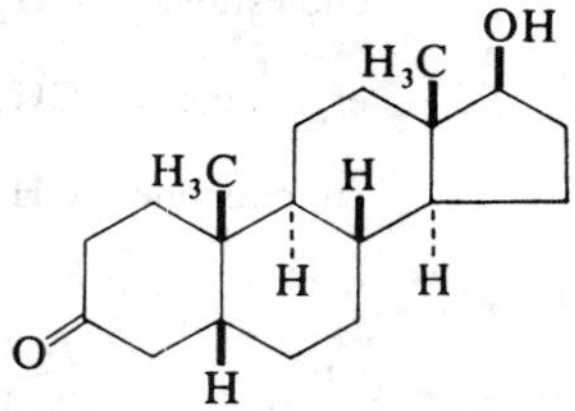

17β-hydroxy-5β-androstan-3-one

*The term *retro* has been but is no longer used to indicate the 9β,10α-configuration.

A number of trivial names are retained in current usage which relate mainly to natural steroids. These are:

aldosterone
androsterone
cholecalciferol
cholesterol
cholic acid
corticosterone
cortisol (acetate)
cortisone (acetate)
deoxycorticosterone
ergocalciferol

ergosterol
lanosterol
lithocholic acid
oestradiol-17α (and -17β)
(estradiol-17α and -17β)
oestriol (estriol)
oestrone (estrone)
progesterone
testosterone

Testane and coprostane have been used in the past as alternatives to 5β-androstane and 5β-cholestane respectively but these are no longer used.

Another trivial name which appears in the literature is etianic acid which is androstane-17-carboxylic acid. This name may still be used but the systematic name is preferred.

Extra rings formed by direct linkage between two carbon atoms of the steroid nucleus are indicated by the term cyclo-.

EXAMPLE

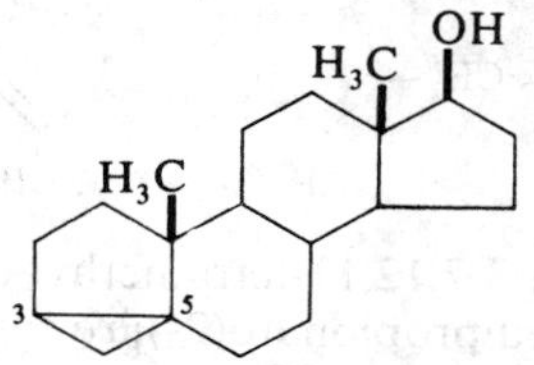

3β,5-cyclo-5β-androstan-17β-ol

Cyclic modifications of the side chains at C-17 are indicated by the use of trivial names such as cardanolide, bufanolide, spirostan, and furostan. Each trivial name represents a specific type of cyclisation and a particular stereochemical configuration. When hetero-atoms are present in the steroid nucleus they are denoted by replacement nomenclature. If however the molecule has changed to such an extent that it may have lost its 'steroidal' character then the systematic fusion name should be used.

Loss of methyl groups or methylene groups (ring contraction) is denoted by the term nor-.

EXAMPLES

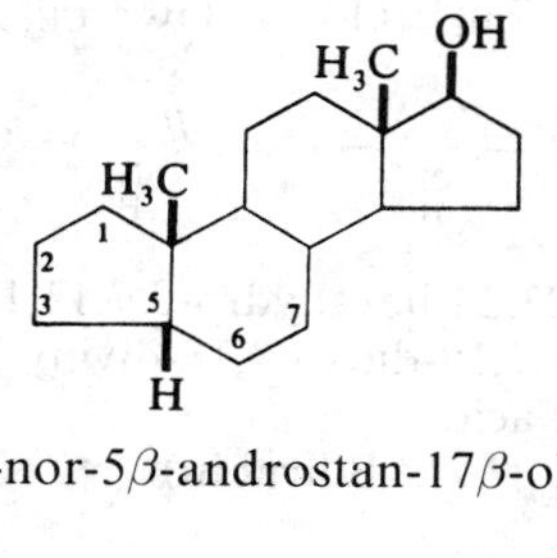

4-nor-5β-androstan-17β-ol*

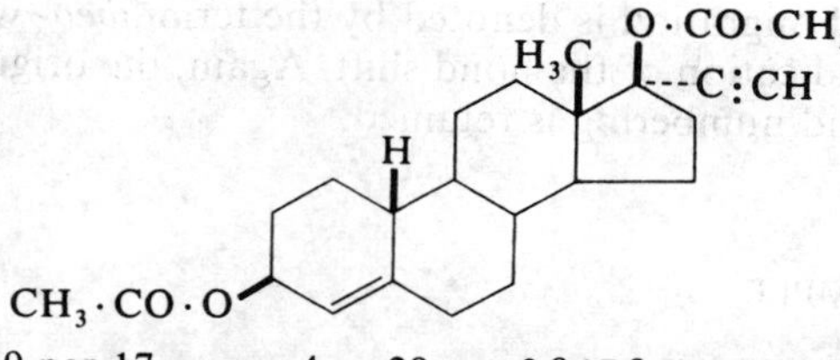

19-nor-17α-pregn-4-en-20-yne-3β,17β-diol diacetate
(Ethynodiol Diacetate)

*The original numbering is retained and the highest number of the contracted ring, excluding ring junctions, is deleted.

If a two-carbon chain (for example, ethynyl) is present at C-17 and one or both of the C-18 and C-19 methyl groups are missing then the preferred name appears to be norpregnane or dinorpregnane.

Ring enlargement by one methylene is denoted by the term homo- and enlargement by two methylenes by dihomo- , preceded in each case by the locant(s) of the carbon atom(s) inserted. If the methylene group is not inserted between directly linked bridgeheads or between C-13 and C-17 with a side chain, the letter a, b, etc. is added to the locant of the highest numbered atom of the ring that is not a bridgehead.

EXAMPLE

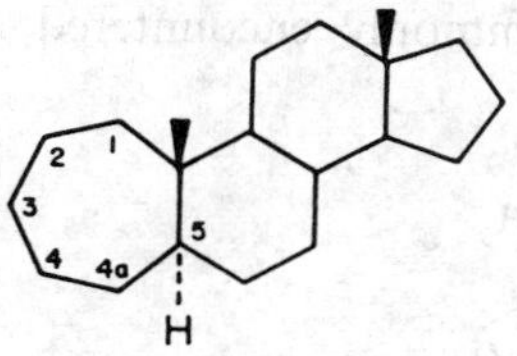

4a-homo-5α-androstane

Bond fission in the ring systems of a steroid is indicated by the term seco-. The original steroid numbering is retained.

EXAMPLE

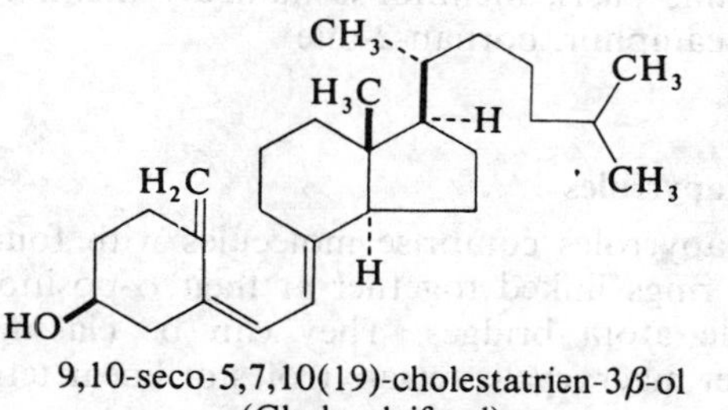

9,10-seco-5,7,10(19)-cholestatrien-3β-ol
(Cholecalciferol)

Bond migration is denoted by the term *abeo-* with an indication of the bond shift. Again, the original steroid numbering is retained.

EXAMPLE

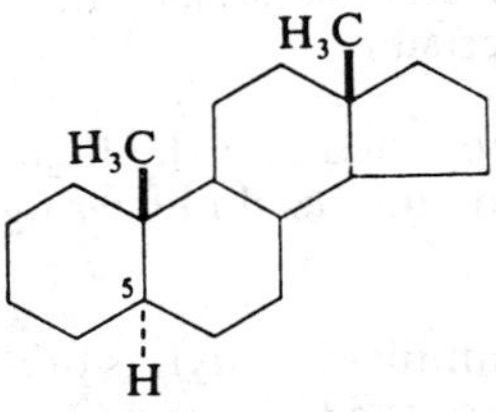

5α-androstane 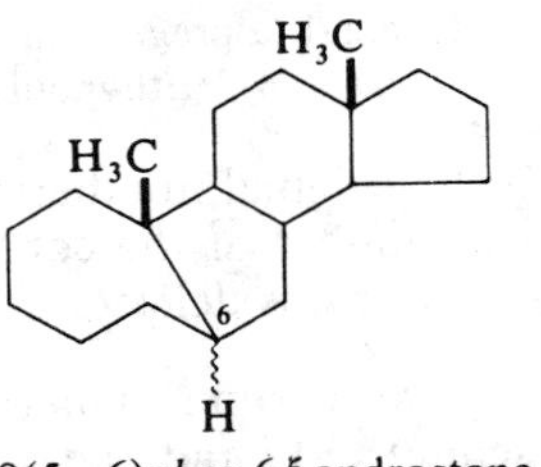   10(5→6)abeo-6ξ-androstane

Thus cholecalciferol is (5Z,7E)-(3S)-9,10-secocholesta-5,7,10(19)-trien-3-ol. The systematic and trivial names for vitamin D compounds are given in the 1989 Recommendations on steroids.

Terpenes

Although terpenes are easily named by systematic methods the older terpene nomenclature is still in use. Acyclic terpenes are named systematically but cyclic terpenes are named on the basis of trivial names for fundamental structural types. Two structures commonly encountered are menthane and bornane:

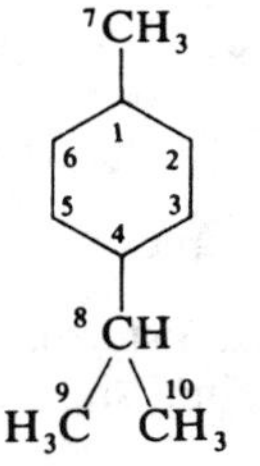

p-menthane 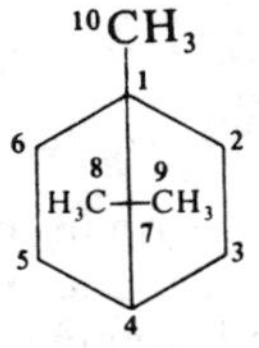   bornane

On this basis, menthol is named *p*-menthan-3-ol and camphor, bornan-2-one.

Tetrapyrroles

Tetrapyrroles comprise molecules with four pyrrole rings linked together at their α-positions by single atom bridges. They can be classified as either macrocyclic tetrapyrroles or linear tetrapyrroles.

Macrocyclic Tetrapyrroles. The fundamental structure is named porphyrin, the numbering system of which is shown below:

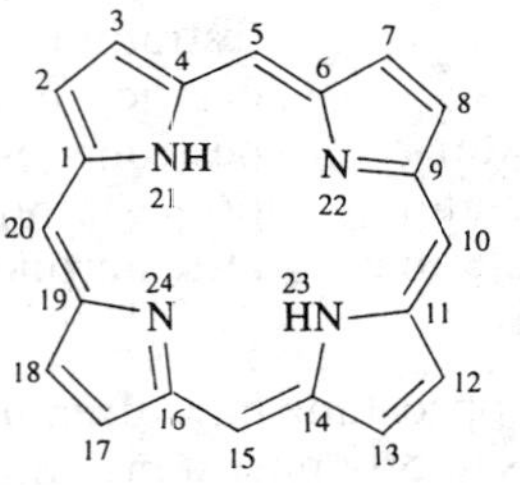

(Porphyrin)

A typical example of a macrocyclic tetrapyrrole is haem:

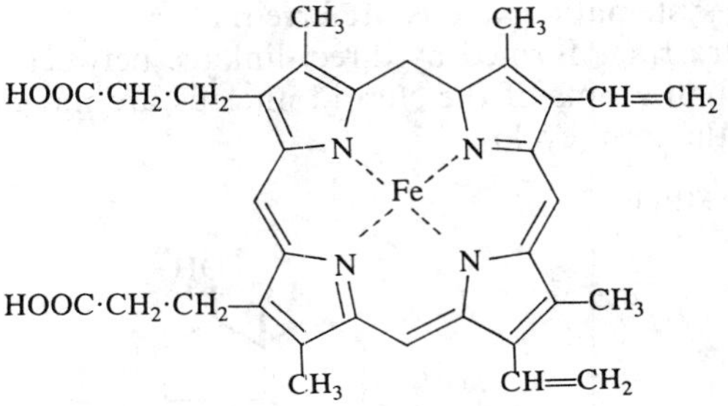

[dihydrogen 3,7,12,17-tetramethyl-8,13-divinyl-2, 18-porphinedipropionato(2-)]iron
(Haem)

Linear Tetrapyrroles. The fundamental structure is named bilane, the numbering system of which is shown below (omitting C-20):

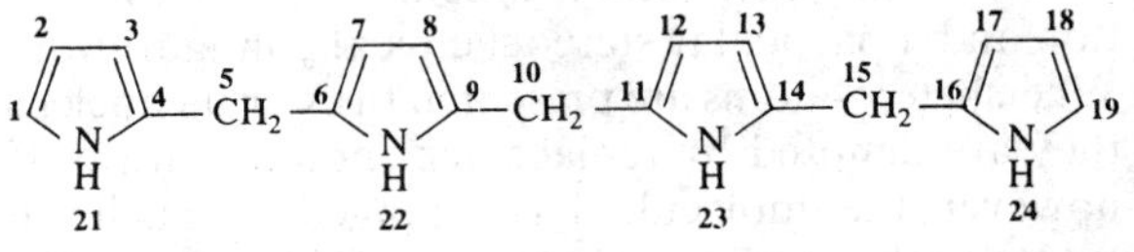

A typical example of a linear tetrapyrrole is bilirubin:

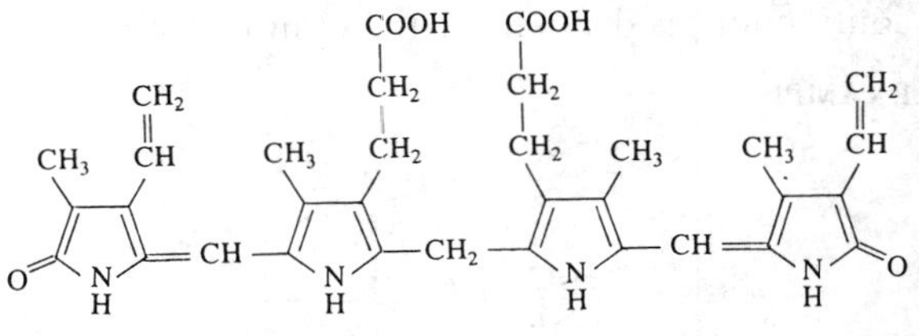

1,10,19,22,23,24-hexahydro-2,7,13,17-tetramethyl-1,19-dioxo-3,18-divinylbiline-8,12-dipropionic acid
(Bilirubin)

SOME OTHER CLASSES OF PHARMACOLOGICALLY ACTIVE COMPOUNDS

There are a number of drug classes whose names are based upon a trivial name derived from the parent compound of the class. Many of these trivial names do not form a part of IUPAC nomenclature. In some cases the parent name implicitly denotes a precise stereochemical configuration. This type of parent is sometimes referred to as a stereoparent. Chemical Abstracts Service uses a large number of these stereoparents and their use is gaining increasing acceptance, especially in names for natural compounds. Other classes may be named by one or more alternative methods and systematic names may, at first sight, appear to be too complicated for ready interpretation. The sections that follow briefly indicate some of these nomenclature difficulties.

Aminoglycosides

The aminoglycosides, for example, gentamicin, kanamycin, neomycin, paromomycin, and streptomycin, all contain the cyclitol structure, streptamine, to which is attached, by a glycosidic linkage, one or more amino-sugar moieties. They are named by glycoside nomenclature. A typical example is kanamycin; its structure and alternative chemical names are shown below:

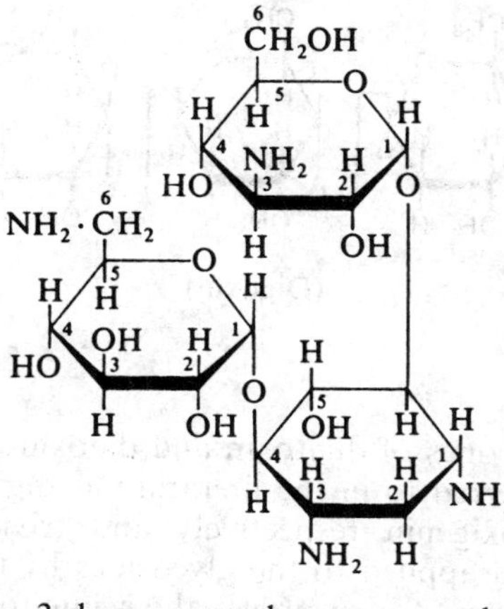

O-3-amino-3-deoxy-α-D-glucopyranosyl-(1 → 6)-
O-[6-amino-6-deoxy-α-D-glucopyranosyl-(1 → 4)]-
2-deoxy-D-streptamine
or 6-O-(3-amino-3-deoxy-α-D-glucopyranosyl)-4-
O-(6-amino-6-deoxy-α-D-glucopyranosyl)-2-deoxy-
streptamine
or O^6-(3-amino-3-deoxy-α-D-glucopyranosyl)-O^4-
(6-amino-6-deoxy-α-D-glucopyranosyl)-2-deoxy-
streptamine

Barbiturates

Names for the barbiturate group of drugs are based on the parent compound, pyrimidine-2,4,6-trione, for which the trivial name barbituric acid is retained. All active barbiturates are disubstituted at the 5-position. The numbering of a typical barbiturate is shown below:

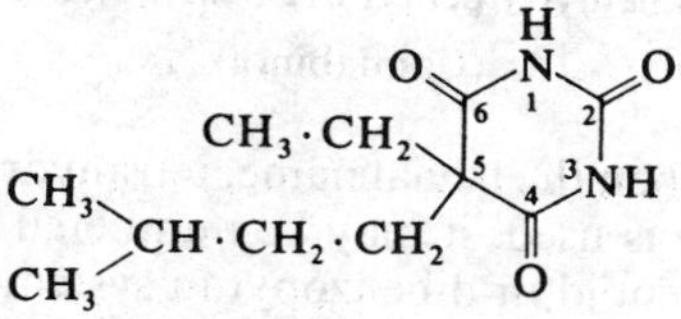

5-ethyl-5-isopentylbarbituric acid
or 5-ethyl-5-(3-methylbutyl)pyrimidine-
2,4,6(1H,3H,5H)-trione
(Amylobarbitone)

Cannabinoids

The four most important cannabinoids are cannabidiol, cannabinol, and the two isomers of tetrahydrocannabinol. Each may be named according to different nomenclature systems each with its own numbering system. Cannabidiol, for example, may be named and numbered as a terpene derivative or, by systematic nomenclature, as a benzenediol derivative (terpene numbering shown).

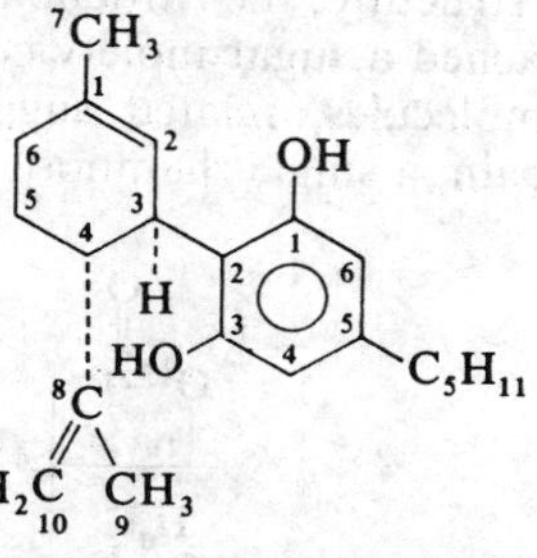

(3R,4R)-2-p-mentha-1,8-dien-3-yl-5-pentylresorcinol
or (1R,6R)-2-[3-methyl-6-(1-methylethenyl)cyclohex-2-
en-1-yl]-5-pentylbenzene-1,3-diol
(Cannabidiol)

The other three cannabinoids mentioned above may be named as dibenzopyrans or as benzochromenes (dibenzopyran numbering shown).

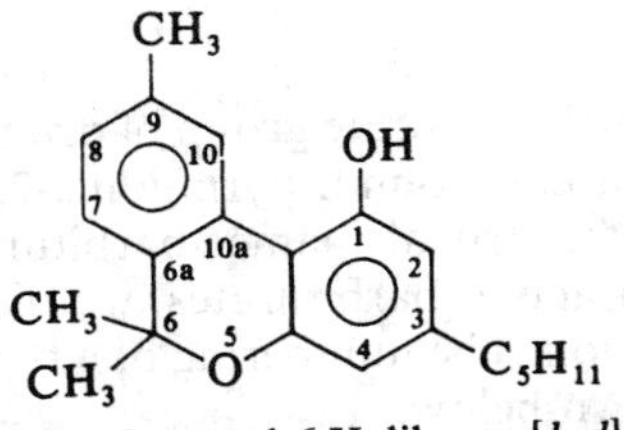

6,6,9-trimethyl-3-pentyl-6*H*-dibenzo[*b,d*]pyran-1-ol
or 6,6,9-trimethyl-3-pentyl-6*H*-benzo[*c*]chromen-1-ol

(Cannabinol)

Further, when the trivial name, tetrahydrocannabinol (THC) is used, it may be numbered according to the terpenoid or dibenzopyran systems resulting in the names Δ^1-THC and Δ^9-THC for one form and the names Δ^{1-6}-THC and Δ^8-THC for the other. The superscripts attached to Δ indicate the position of the double bond in the left-hand ring.

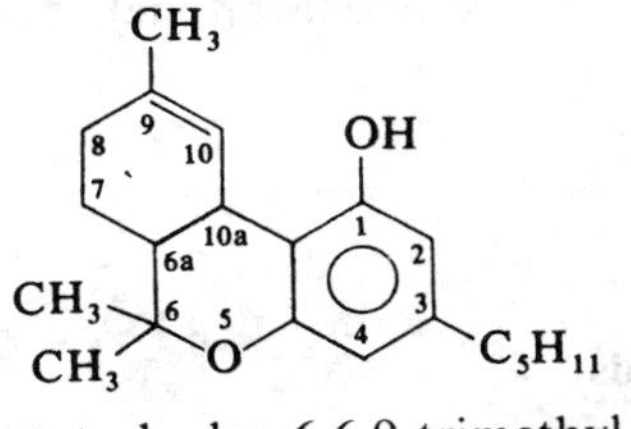

6a,7,8,10a-tetrahydro-6,6,9-trimethyl-3-pentyl-
6*H*-dibenzo[*b,d*]pyran-1-ol
(Δ^1- *or* Δ^9-Tetrahydrocannabinol)

The dibenzopyran names for cannabinol and the tetrahydrocannabinols are preferred.

Cardiac Glycosides

The cardiac glycosides all possess a steroidal aglycone parent structure, the cardenolide skeleton, to which is attached a sugar moiety containing three digitoxose molecules, related sugars, or, in the case of ouabain, a single rhamnose molecule.

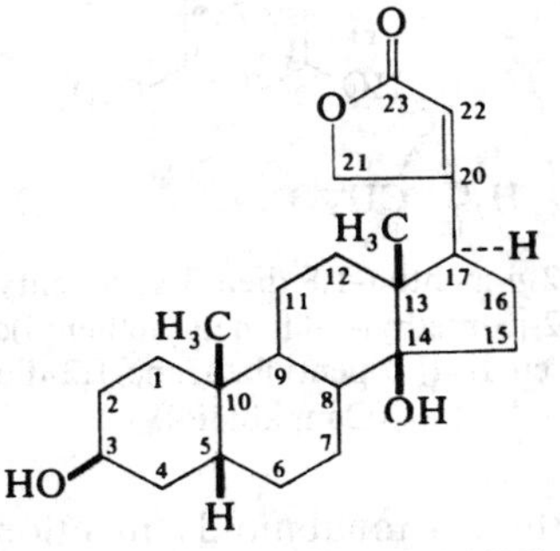

3β,14-dihydroxy-5β,14β-card-20(22)-enolide
(Digitoxigenin)

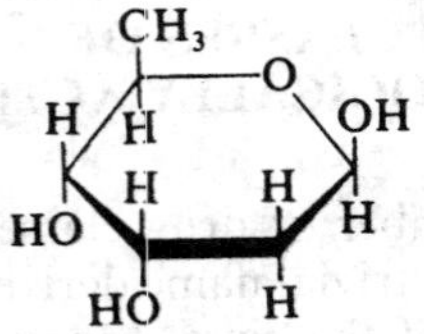

2,6-dideoxy-*ribo*-hexopyranose
(Digitoxose)

The cardenolide structure differs in stereochemistry from the usual steroidal ring nucleus since the ring-C and ring-D fusion is *cis* and not *trans*.

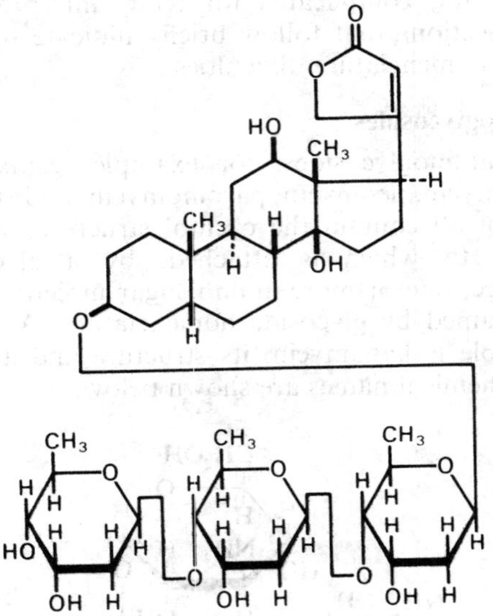

(Digoxin)

The aglycones of digitoxin and digoxin are sometimes referred to in the literature as digitoxigenin and digoxigenin respectively and trivial names have been applied to the glycosides by the use of these names, for example, the tridigitoxoside of digitoxigenin (digitoxin). The full chemical name for digitoxin is: 3-[*O*-2,6-dideoxy-β-D-*ribo*- hexopyranosyl-(1 → 4)-*O*-2,6-dideoxy-β-D-*ribo*-hexopyranosyl-(1 → 4)-*O*-2,6-dideoxy-β-D-*ribo*-hexopyranosyloxy]-14-hydroxy-3β,5β,14β-card-20(22)-enolide.

The main cardiac glycosides differ only in the substituents on the aglycone moiety.

Cephalosporins

The cephalosporins may be named by reference to the trivial names cephem or cephalosporanic acid, or by means of systematic bicyclo-nomenclature. The systematic and trivial names employ different numbering systems.

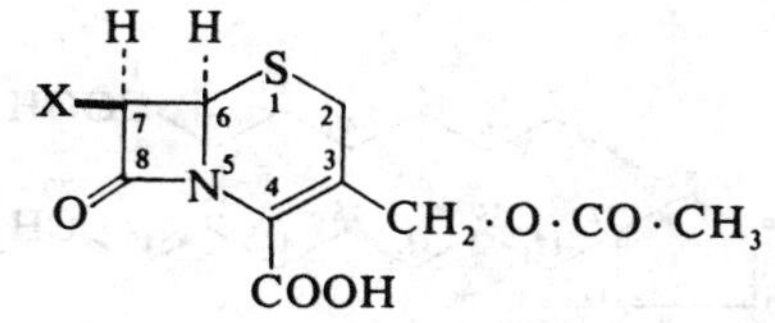

cephalosporanic acid

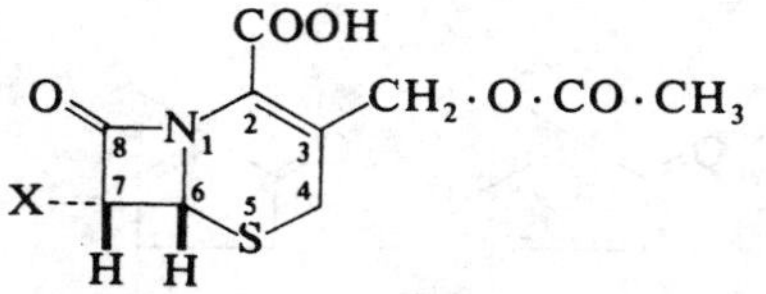

(6R)-3-acetoxymethyl-8-oxo-5-thia-1-azabicyclo[4.2.0]oct-2-ene-2-carboxylic acid

Cephem is (6R)-8-oxo-5-thia-1-azabicyclo[4.2.0] oct-2-ene. The numbering system is identical to that of cephalosporanic acid. All the cephalosporins have an acylamino side-chain at position 7 (in both numbering systems) and this always has the configuration R.

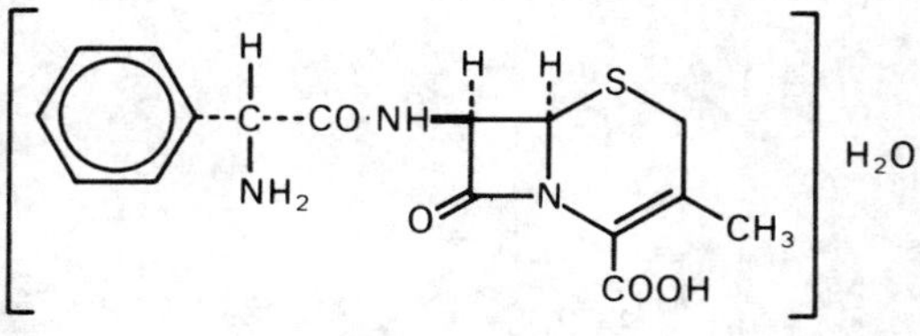

Cephalexin

Macrolides

The macrolides are large cyclic lactone structures which possess a number of substituents, including some sugar moieties. They have been named in the literature as lactones, glycosides, or ketones. The structure and alternative chemical names for erythromycin, an important member of this class, are shown below:

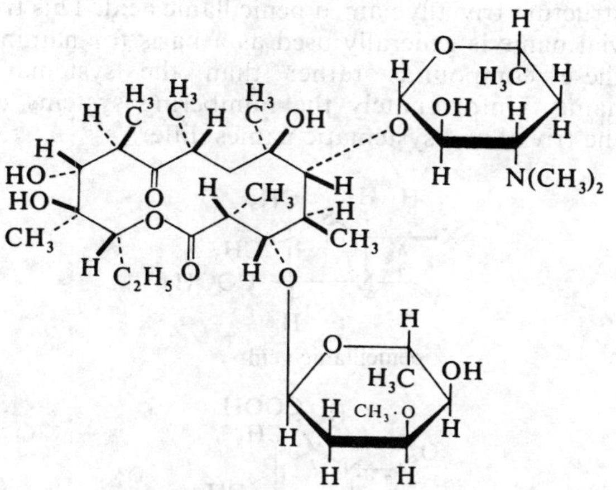

14-ethyl-7,12,13-trihydroxy-3,5,7,9,11,13-hexamethyl-2,10-dioxo-6-[3,4,6-trideoxy-3-(dimethylamino)-β-L-*xylo*-hexopyranosyloxy] oxacyclotetradec-4-yl 2,6-dideoxy-3-*C*-methyl-3-*O*-methyl-α-L-*ribo*-hexopyranoside

or (2R,3S,4S,5R,6R,8R,10R,11R,12S,13R)-5-(3-amino-3,4,6-trideoxy-*NN*-dimethyl-β-D-*xylo*-hexopyranosyloxy)-3-(2,6-dideoxy-3*C*,3*O*-dimethyl-α-L-*ribo*-hexopyranosyloxy)-13-ethyl-6,11,12-trihydroxy-2,4,6,8,10,12-hexamethyl-9-oxotridecan-13-olide

(Erythromycin)

It can be seen that not only does the choice of parent compound and characteristic group differ between these names but also the numbering since the locant 1 is assigned in the one case to the hetero-atom in the ring structure and in the other to the carbon atom in the lactone group.

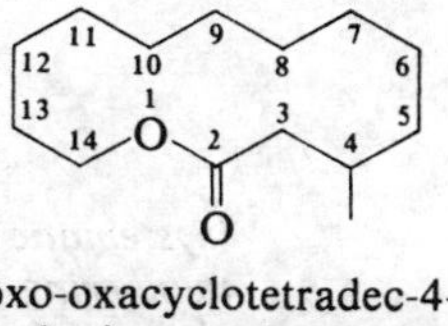

2-oxo-oxacyclotetradec-4-yl
(numbering as a heterocycle;
named by replacement nomenclature)

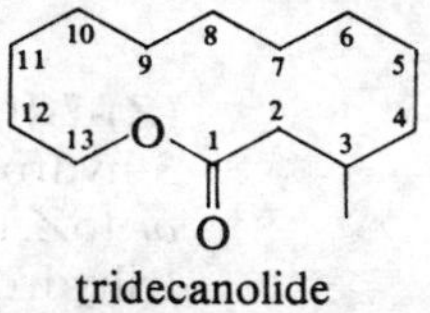

tridecanolide
(name and numbering as a lactone)

Penicillins

The penicillins are all derivatives of a β-lactam ring structure trivially named penicillanic acid. This trivial name is generally used as a basis for naming these compounds rather than the systematic name. Unfortunately the numbering systems of the trivial and systematic names differ:

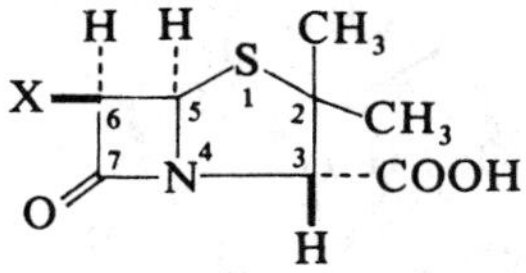

penicillanic acid

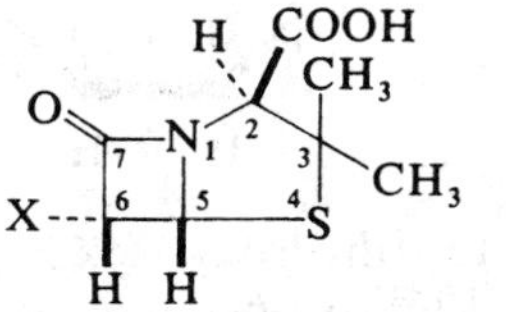

(2S,5R)-3,3-dimethyl-7-oxo-4-thia-1-aza-bicyclo[3.2.0]heptane-2-carboxylic acid

All the penicillins have an acylamino side-chain at position 6 (in both numbering systems) and this always has the configuration R.

EXAMPLE

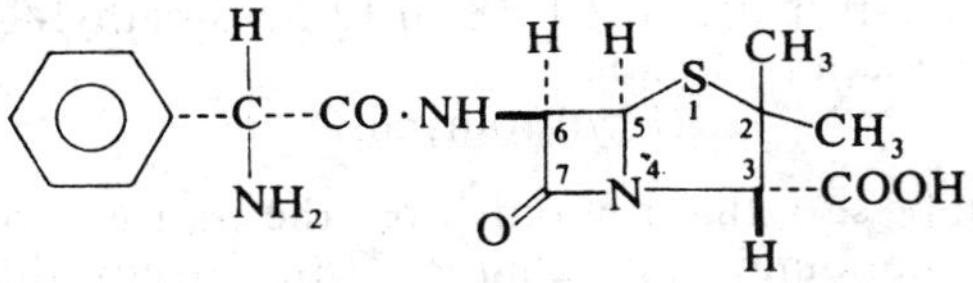

(6R)-6-(α-D-phenylglycylamino)penicillanic acid
(Ampicillin)

Prostaglandins

Prostaglandins are structures comprising a cyclopentane ring, two aliphatic side chains, and a terminal carboxyl group. Trivial names are based on the hypothetical parent, prostanoic acid. They are categorised into four series, E, F, A, and B. These categories are based upon the presence of different groups on the cyclopentane ring.

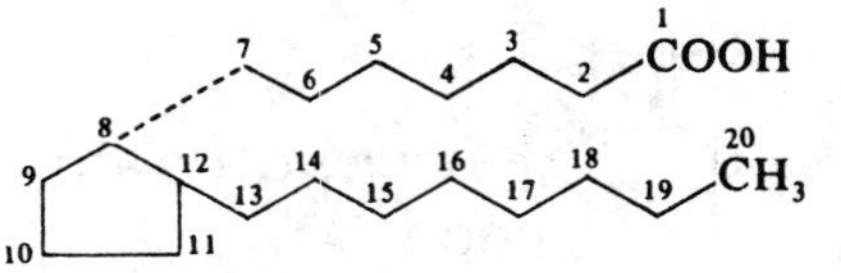

Prostanoic acid

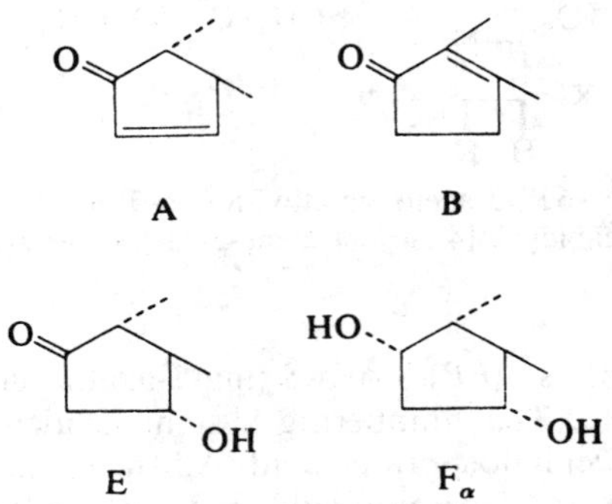

A   B

E F_α

Prostaglandin series

Systematically they are named as octenylcyclopentylheptenoic acids or variants thereof.

EXAMPLE

(systematic numbering shown)

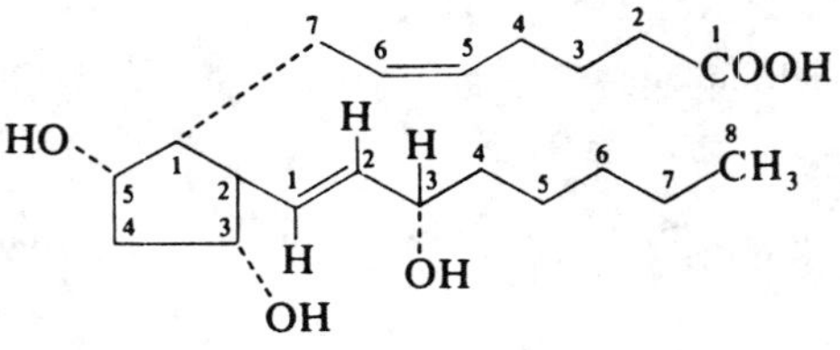

(Z)-7-{(1R,2R,3R,5S)-3,5-dihydroxy-2-[(E)-(3S)-3-hydroxyoct-1-enyl]cyclopentyl}hept-5-enoic acid
or (5Z,13E)-(9S,11R,15S)-9,11,15-trihydroxyprosta-5,13-dienoic acid
(Dinoprost; Prostaglandin $F_{2\alpha}$)

Tetracyclines

Tetracycline itself possesses the following structure and chemical name:

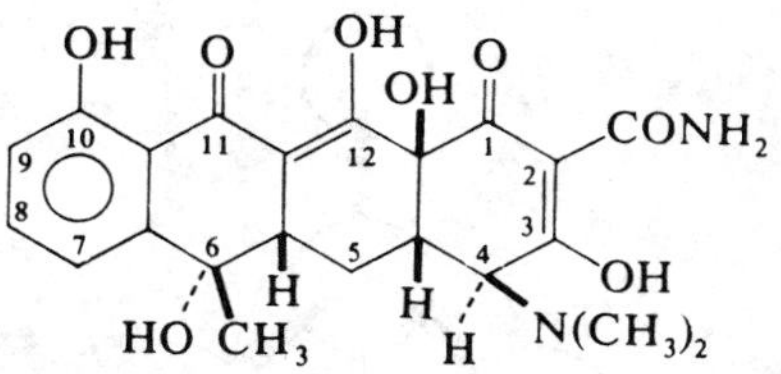

(4S,4aS,5aS,6S,12aS)-4-dimethylamino-1,4,
4a,5,5a,6,11,12a-octahydro-3,6,10,12,12a-
pentahydroxy- 6-methyl-1,11-
dioxonaphthacene-2-carboxamide

For other tetracyclines, derivative names are commonly used. The name tetracycline implies, as shown above, a particular stereochemistry and only additional steric relations need be added to the derived name.

EXAMPLE

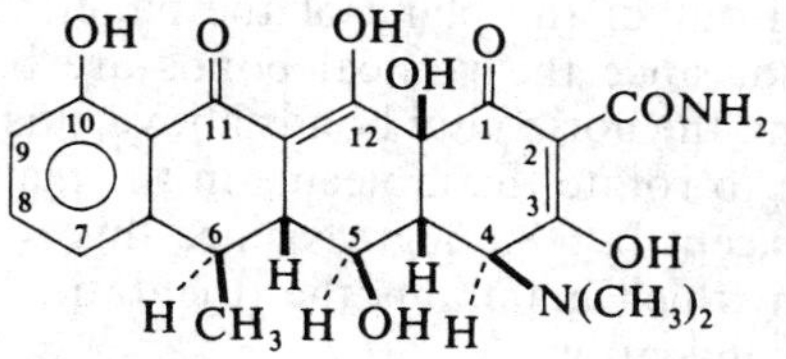

6-deoxy-5β-hydroxytetracycline
(Doxycycline)

EXAMPLES

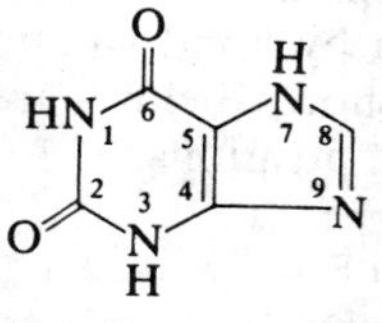

xanthine (2,6-dioxopurine)

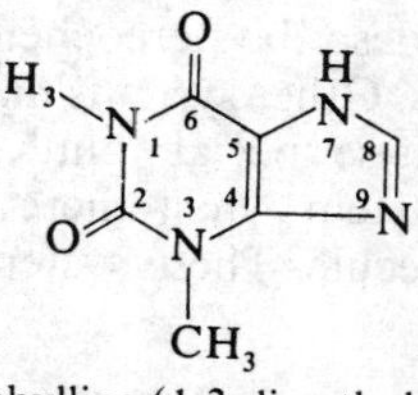

theophylline (1,3-dimethylxanthine)

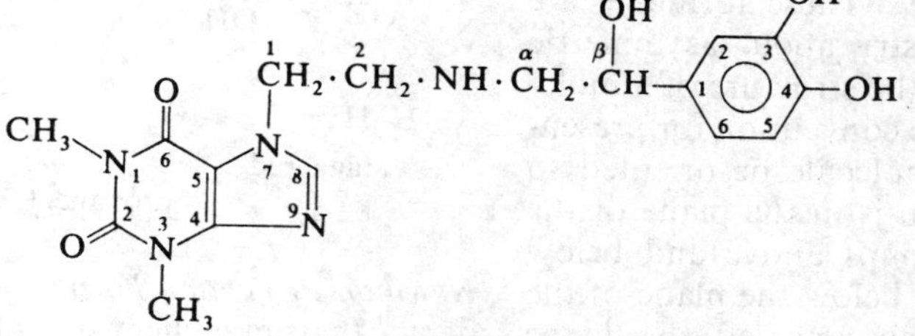

7-[2-(3,4,β-trihydroxyphenethylamino)-
ethyl]theophylline
(Theodrenaline)

Tropane Alkaloids

The tropane alkaloids include atropine, hyoscine, and their derivatives. They all contain the bicyclic structure tropane, which is systematically named (8s)-N-methyl-8-azabicyclo[3.2.1]octane, and are esters of an acid trivially named tropic acid.

EXAMPLE

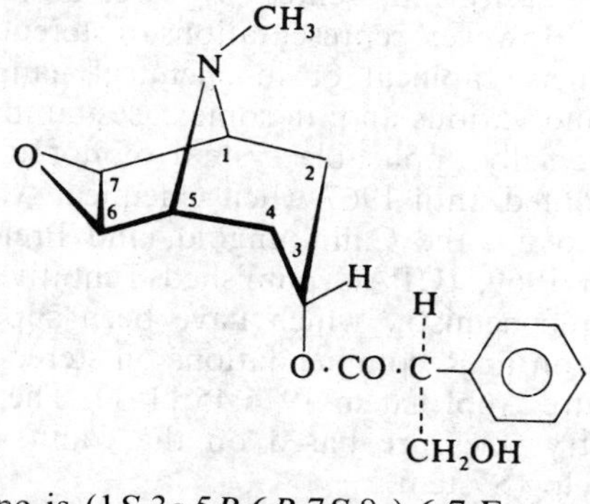

Hyoscine is (1S,3s,5R,6R,7S,8s)-6,7-Epoxy-3-[(S)-tropoyloxy]tropane.

Xanthines

Xanthines are derivatives of purine and include caffeine, theobromine, and theophylline. They may be named as purines, xanthines, or, in the case of 1,3-dimethylxanthines, as theophyllines. Examples are shown below.

It should be noted that all the parent names use the purine numbering system, which is not typical.

STEREOCHEMISTRY

Stereochemical configuration, the spatial arrangements of atoms or groups of atoms within molecules, is easily represented by three-dimensional models. However, representations of stereochemistry, either graphical or in chemical names, are many and various and, in some cases, ambiguous. A universally applicable system of notation was not adopted until 1967 when Chemical Abstracts began to use the Cahn, Ingold, and Prelog system. In 1969, IUPAC published Tentative Rules on Stereochemistry which have been superseded by Section E: Recommendations on stereochemistry—Pure Appl Chem 1976;45:11-30. The stereochemistry rules are based on the Cahn, Ingold, and Prelog System.

The following brief description introduces aspects of stereochemical nomenclature recommended by IUPAC and also indicates some of the other systems still in use.

Graphic Representations of Stereochemistry

A number of specialised graphic systems have been used to project 3-dimensional structures on to paper. The system described under Graphic Formulae at the beginning of this chapter is generally applicable and may be used to describe stereochemistry under most circumstances. Other systems may be necessary in order to emphasise special points or to supplement the general system when there is more than one plane in a molecule. These systems are briefly described below.

Fischer Projection Formulae. These formulae are used to show stereochemistry about asymmetric carbon atoms, and project the structure of a molecule in two dimensions. The convention for presentation demands that the molecule be oriented so that the asymmetric carbon is in the plane of the paper. The substituent groups above and below the central atom should be below the plane of the paper and those to the right and left should be above the plane of the paper. The principal chain must be on the vertical axis with the lowest numbered member of the chain at the top. The derivation of a Fischer projection for L-lactic acid is shown below:

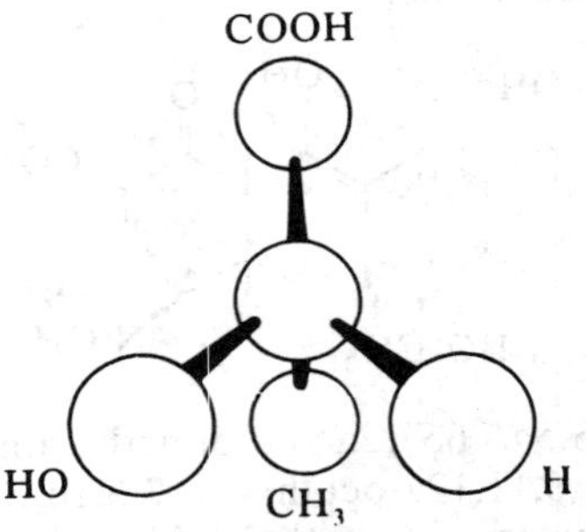

stereochemical model

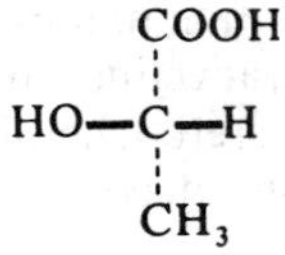

general convention 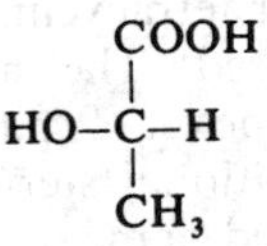   Fischer projection

When manipulating these formulae, they must not be lifted out of the plane of the paper or turned over and, since the vertical bonds are below the plane and the horizontal bonds above, it is not permissible to rotate the molecule in the plane of the paper except by 180 degrees since this is the only rotation which maintains the orientation dictated by the convention.

Sawhorse Projections. These projections are three-dimensional representations of the steric relations of groups about a single bond and how they are affected by bond rotation. The two extreme positions, shown below, are called the staggered and eclipsed positions.

EXAMPLE

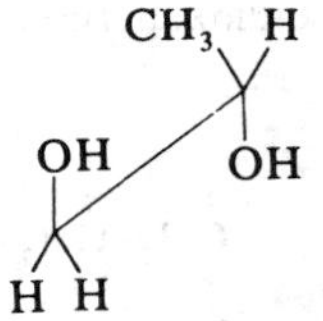

staggered 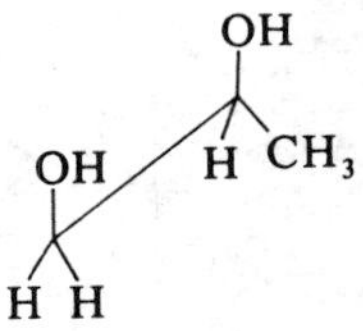   eclipsed

propane-1,2-diol

Newman Projection Formulae. These formulae also depict the stereochemistry of a molecule with two carbon atoms linked by a single bond. The molecule is viewed along the bond linking the two atoms. The nearer atom is drawn as a circle and in such a position that it eclipses the second atom. Bonds linking substituents to the nearer atom are drawn to the centre of the circle whilst bonds linking groups to the second atom are drawn to the circumference of the circle.

EXAMPLE

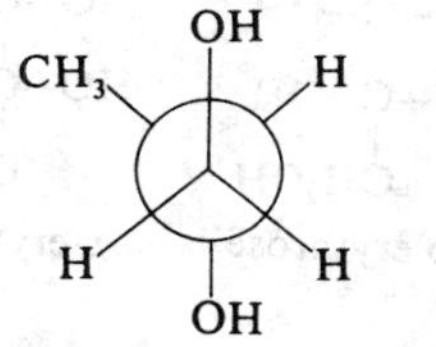

propane-1,2-diol (staggered form)

Flying-wedge Formulae. These formulae have been used instead of, but are now used to supplement, the general system already described under Graphic Formulae. The major plane of a molecule is drawn in the plane of the paper and substituents are drawn above or below the plane. This is indicated by the use of a wedge, the thick end representing the nearer part of a bond and the thin end the most distant part of the bond.

EXAMPLE

flying wedge   general convention

L-lactic acid

This system is used to depict the stereochemistry of chains attached to larger structures.

EXAMPLE

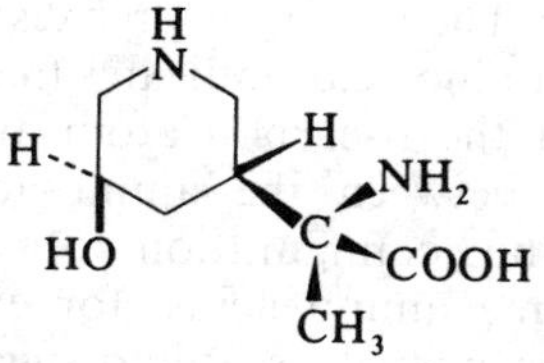

Stereochemical Notation in Chemical Names

Stereochemical isomerism falls into two categories, geometrical isomerism and optical isomerism. The term geometrical isomerism is now restricted to mean isomerism that does not depend upon asymmetry of the molecule. Optical isomerism results from the presence of an asymmetric structure in the molecule. Since optical activity is only a consequence of the asymmetry in a molecule, the term optical isomerism has been replaced by the term **chirality**. An object is said to possess the property of chirality when the object and its mirror image are not superimposable. All asymmetric molecules (molecules without any elements of symmetry) are chiral. However not all chiral molecules are asymmetric since they may possess axes of symmetry (axes of rotation). All chiral molecules are optically active, which means they can rotate the plane of polarised light.

The most basic chiral structure in an organic molecule is a carbon atom to which four other atoms or groups, each different from the others, are attached. Lactic acid, shown below, is a typical example. It exists in two forms, one being the non-superimposable mirror image of the other:

L-(+)-lactic acid   D-(−)-lactic acid
(a)   (b)

Stereochemistry within a chemical name has been specified by the use of a number of specialised systems each designed to describe the stereochemistry of particular classes of compounds. A universally applicable system, based upon the *R*- and *S*-system devised by Cahn, Ingold, and Prelog, has now gained international acceptance. Many of the specialised systems have been retained such as D and L for carbohydrates, amino acids, cyclitols, and, sometimes, for penicillins; α and β for steroids, alkaloids, certain antibiotics, and other compounds; (+) and (−) for optical isomerism where absolute configuration is unknown; and *cis* and *trans* or *Z* and *E* for geometrical isomerism about planes and double bonds. *Endo* and *exo* are retained for use with bridges and bicyclo-systems.

Optical Activity

The two forms of lactic acid (described above) being chiral are optically active and they rotate the plane of polarised light in different directions. The optical isomer in formula (a) is dextrorotatory (rotates the plane to the right) and the isomer in formula (b) is laevorotatory (rotates the plane to the left). The terms dextro- and laevo-rotatory are abbreviated to (+) and (−) respectively or, in the older literature, to *d* and *l* respectively. The

(+)- and (−)-forms of lactic acid constitute an optically active pair. Such optically active pairs are called **enantiomers**.

It must be emphasised that optical activity is related to chirality and not to asymmetric carbon atoms. For example, tartaric acid, shown below, possesses asymmetric carbon atoms but may exist in chiral or achiral forms:

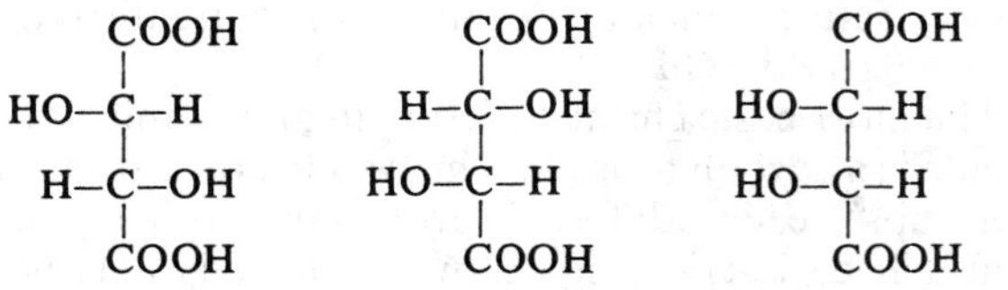

```
       COOH              COOH              COOH
        |                 |                 |
  HO—C—H            H—C—OH            HO—C—H
        |                 |                 |
   H—C—OH            HO—C—H            HO—C—H
        |                 |                 |
       COOH              COOH              COOH

(−)-tartaric acid   (+)-tartaric acid   meso-tartaric acid
```

The achiral form, *meso*-tartaric acid, can be divided into two parts, one part being the mirror image of the other. The optical activity of one half is counteracted or compensated by the activity of the other. The term *meso-* is used to indicate this form of internal compensation.

A mixture of equal parts of enantiomers will also be inactive since the optical activity of one enantiomer will be compensated by the other. This type of mixture is referred to as a racemate (denoted by the prefixes (±)- or *rac-*).

Diastereoisomerism

Compounds containing two or more unequal asymmetric carbon atoms have more than two possible stereoisomeric arrangements. In general, the number of stereoisomers for a compound with n asymmetric atoms is 2^n. Consider the tetroses, erythrose and threose shown opposite.

The two erythroses are members of an enantiomeric pair as are the two threoses but erythrose is not an enantiomer of threose. Erythrose and threose are referred to as diastereoisomers which means that they are stereoisomers but not mirror images of each other.

It is convenient to represent molecules of this type by Fischer projections. The configuration of these molecules is represented by the use of the prefixes D- or L- which indicate the configuration of the asymmetric atom bearing the highest numbered locant, whilst the relative positions of the atoms

or groups attached to the other asymmetric atom or atoms are denoted by a second prefix such as *erythro* or *threo*. These prefixes are used mainly in the naming of carbohydrates.

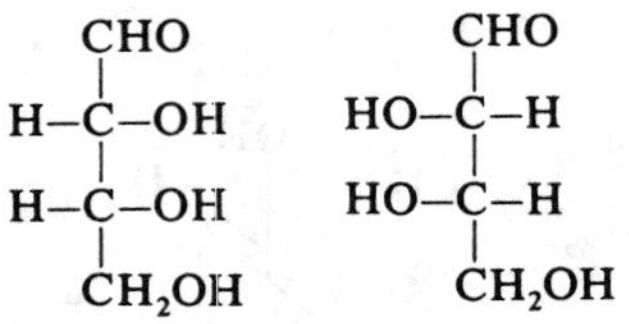

```
    CHO               CHO
     |                 |
 H—C—OH           HO—C—H
     |                 |
 H—C—OH           HO—C—H
     |                 |
   CH2OH             CH2OH

 D-erythrose       L-erythrose
```

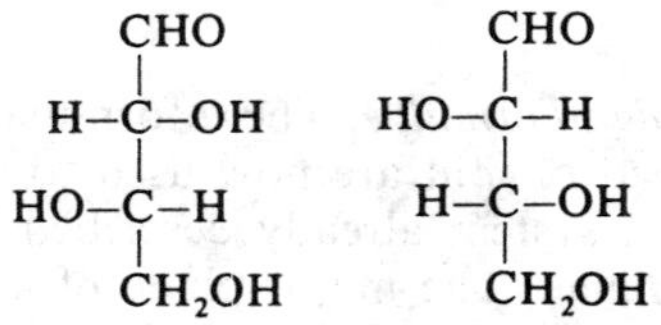

```
    CHO               CHO
     |                 |
 H—C—OH           HO—C—H
     |                 |
 HO—C—H            H—C—OH
     |                 |
   CH2OH             CH2OH

  L-threose         D-threose
```

D- *and* L-*Notation*

This notation is used to denote relative or absolute configuration of compounds with respect to their classes and is used as an alternative to the *R*- and *S*- system. Amino acids, carbohydrates, cyclitols, and their derivatives are all described by this system. It should be emphasised that D and L bear no relationship to the sign of optical rotation.

Amino Acids. The use of the prefixes D- or L- in the names of α-amino acids indicates the absolute configuration at the α-carbon atom and indicates a relationship between the amino-acid configuration and the configuration of either D- or L-serine. Some amino acids, for example threonine, may be named as amino-sugar derivatives, in which case the prefixes D- or L- indicate the absolute configuration at the highest numbered asymmetric carbon atom and demonstrate a relationship between the amino-acid configuration and the configuration of either D- or L-glyceraldehyde. To avoid confusion the two systems are identified by the subscripts s (for serine) and g (for glyceraldehyde).

EXAMPLES

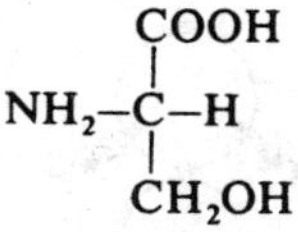

L-serine 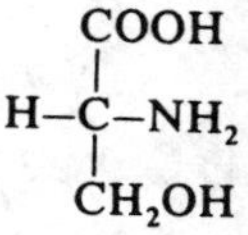 D-serine 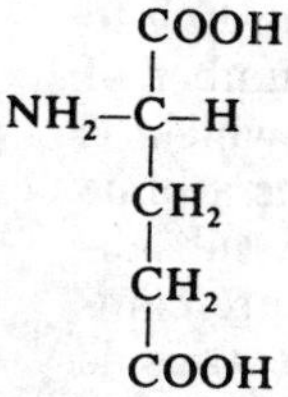 L-glutamic acid Lₛ-threonine or 2-amino-2,4-dideoxy-Dₛ threonic acid

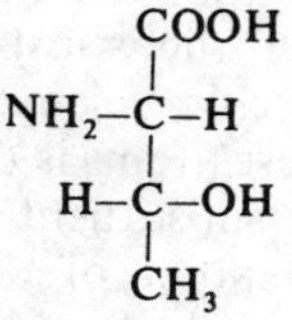

Carbohydrates. The use of the prefixes D- and L- denotes a relationship between glyceraldehyde and the highest numbered asymmetric carbon atom in the carbohydrate molecule. This system is based upon the early work of Fischer and Rosanoff who suggested that glyceraldehyde should be a reference point for establishing the configuration of other compounds. The prefix D- was arbitrarily assigned to the glyceraldehyde configuration that was dextrorotatory and then other substances with the same configuration were designated as the D-series. Similarly with the use of L- for laevorotatory glyceraldehyde and its related series. About sixty years later the absolute configuration of D-glyceraldehyde was determined and was shown to possess the configuration shown below in which the hydroxyl group is on the right hand side of the asymmetric carbon atom. The configurations of a large number of compounds have subsequently been determined and the stereochemical relationship between them and D- or L-glyceraldehyde established.

α- and β-Notation

These symbols are used to indicate the relative stereochemistry about atoms in ring structures such as steroids, certain alkaloids, and related compounds, and have also been adapted for use in other classes such as the tetracyclines. This notation is applicable to molecules which possess a ring system which may be represented as a structure falling within a single plane.

Graphically, these structures are represented as being in the plane of the paper and substituents are drawn either above or below the plane. In the case of steroids, those above the plane, indicated by the use of bold bonds, are denoted by the symbol β and those below the plane, indicated by the use of dotted bonds, are denoted by the symbol α. In steroids the reference methyl groups at C-10 and C-13 are always above the plane and are therefore β, unless there is some specialised stereochemical inversion.

EXAMPLE

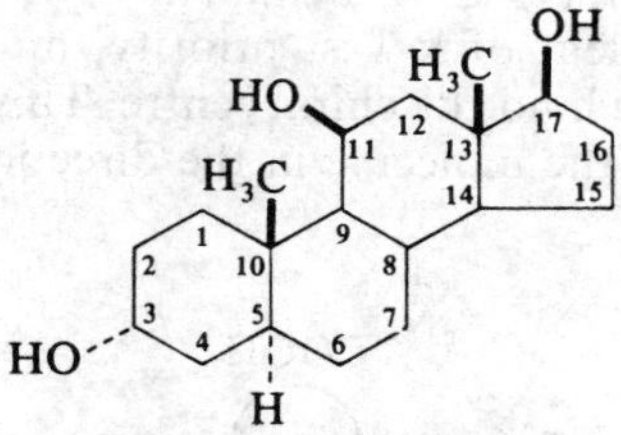

5α-androstane-3α,11β,17β-triol

EXAMPLES

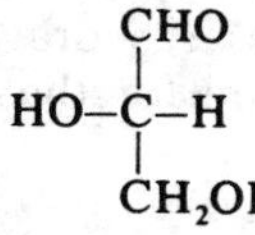

L-(−)-glyceraldehyde D-(+)-glyceraldehyde

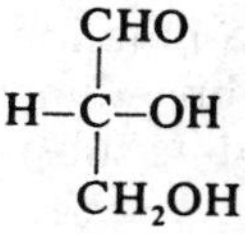

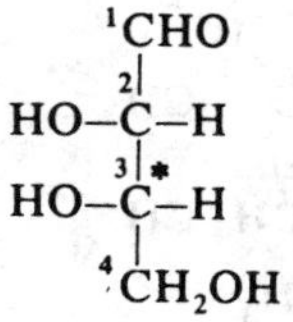

L-(+)-erythrose D-(−)-lactic acid

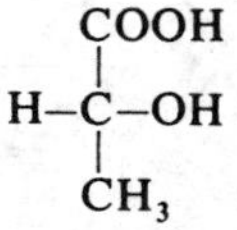

*Highest numbered asymmetric carbon atom.

R- and S-Notation

The D- and L-notation described above is derived from projections of three-dimensional structures. The R- and S-notation, sometimes referred to as the Sequence Rule, enables configuration to be assigned directly from the three-dimensional structure. In order to assign configuration, the substituent atoms or groups about a chiral centre, plane, or axis are placed in sequence according to a priority rule based upon the atomic number of the atom in each of the substituents which is directly linked to the chiral element. If the atomic number of each of these atoms is the same, subsidiary atoms within the substituent groups are compared until the first point of difference (this is described in detail under the Sequence Rule). Atoms with a higher atomic number have a higher priority. Having established the priority sequence, the molecule is oriented so that the molecule can be viewed with the substituent atom or group of lowest priority at the back of the chiral centre. Consider, for example, L-lactic acid which has the following Fischer projection:

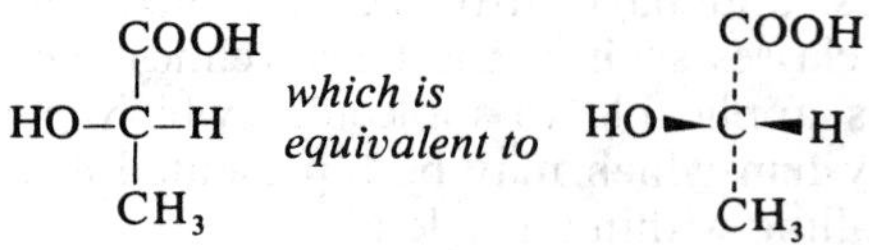

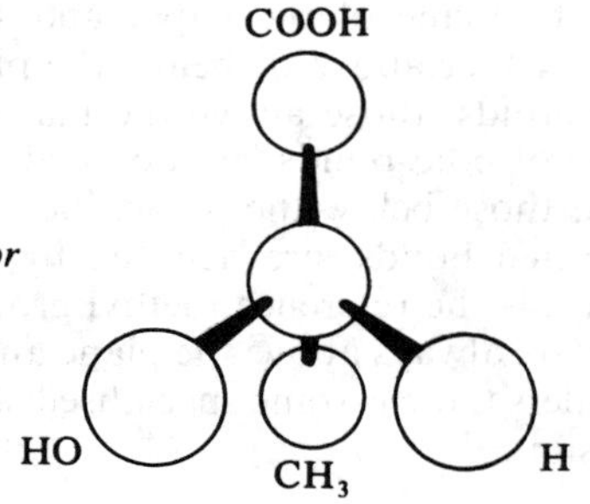

The priorities of the four substituents are: OH > COOH > CH$_3$ > H. The hydrogen atom, the substituent of lowest priority, must therefore be placed behind the chiral centre. This is achieved by viewing the molecule in the direction shown in (a) below.

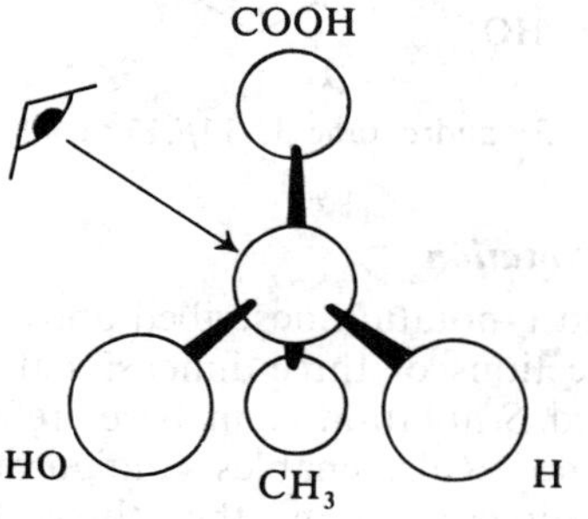

(a)

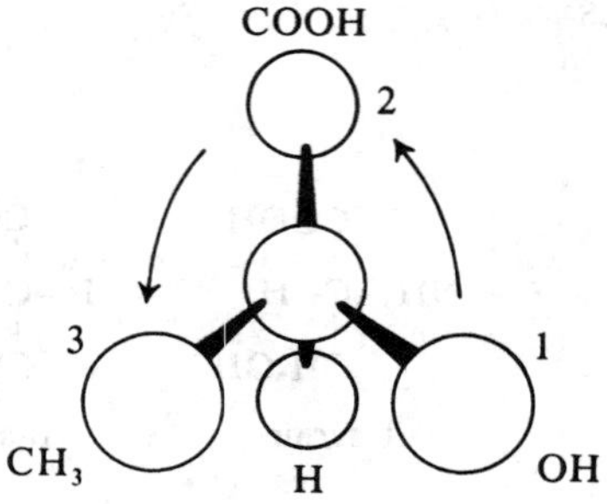

(b)

The priorities of the three remaining groups (OH, COOH, CH$_3$) are compared and the direction of decreasing priority discerned. If the direction is clockwise the configuration is R (rectus) and if the direction is anticlockwise the configuration is S (sinister). In the case of L-lactic acid the direction is anticlockwise and the molecule has the S-configuration as shown in (b) above.

As a more complex example, consider the structure of griseofulvin shown below:

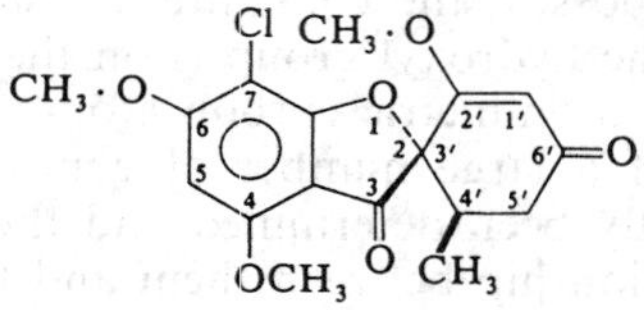

The chiral atoms are at positions 2 and 4'. By selecting the appropriate position from which to view the molecule, it is possible to determine the R- and S-notation without necessarily drawing a further three-dimensional structure for the chiral atom and its substituents.

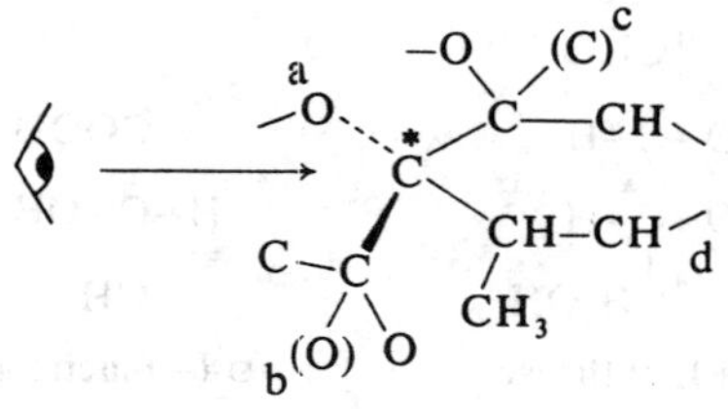

priority order a > b > c > d

By viewing the chiral atom at position 2 (asterisked above) from the direction indicated, the substituent with the lowest priority will be behind the chiral atom and the following view will be obtained:

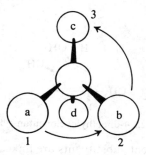

The order of decreasing priority is in an anticlockwise direction which indicates the S-configuration. The 4'-position (asterisked below), if viewed from the direction indicated, will give the view shown in formula (b) which shows the configuration at the 4'-position to be R.

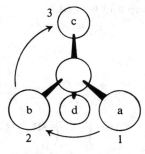

priority order a > b > c > d
(a)

R-configuration
(b)

R- and S-notation is cited as a prefix, to which the appropriate locant has been added, to the full chemical name and is placed in brackets. The full name for griseofulvin is therefore: $(2S,4'R)$-7-chloro-2',4,6-trimethoxy-4'-methylspiro[benzofuran-2-(3H),3'-cyclohexene]-3,6'-dione.

Manipulation of graphic formulae in order to obtain the correct orientation for the determination of R and S may take some time to grasp. The use of a model of the tetrahedral arrangement of substituents about a central carbon atom will do much to alleviate any problems.

When only the relative configurations of chiral centres are known the prefixes R^*- and S^*- are used. These terms are assigned as before but the chiral centre with the lowest locant is arbitrarily assigned the R^*-configuration. The term *rel-* may be used as an alternative to R^* and S^* in complex cases.

An atom which is bonded to one pair of substituent groups which are stereoisomers (enantiomeric pair or geometrical isomeric pair) and to two different substituents is termed pseudoasymmetric. Pseudoasymmetry is denoted by the symbols r and s which are determined in the same way as R and S. However, since two substituents differ only in their steric relations the rule for deciding priority is that R precedes S and *cis* precedes *trans*.

Geometrical Isomerism

This is a form of stereoisomerism caused by different arrangements of groups or atoms around ethylenic double bonds or cyclic compounds.

Stereoisomerism around double bonds is not normally associated with optical activity since the double bond possesses a plane of symmetry but stereoisomerism around cyclic structures may produce chirality and optical activity.

The configurations of compounds containing ethylenic double bonds were indicated by *cis*- and *trans*-notation. These terms have been replaced for such compounds by a system utilising the Sequence Rule and incorporating the symbols Z and E. This system removes some of the ambiguities inherent in the *cis*- and *trans*-system when applied to ethylenic double bonds. Both R- and S- and *cis*- and *trans*-notations are retained for cyclic structures.

cis- and *trans*-Notation. Consider the following structures:

$$\underset{b}{\overset{a}{>}}C=C\underset{c}{\overset{a}{<}}$$

cis-isomer
(1)

$$\underset{c}{\overset{a}{>}}C=C\underset{a}{\overset{b}{<}}$$

trans-isomer
(2)

The letters a, b, and c denote different substituents about the double bonds in each of the structures. In formula (1) it can be seen that the 'a' groups are on the same side of the double bond and in formula (2) they are on opposite sides of the double bond. These two relative positions are designated *cis* and *trans* respectively. In deciding which atoms or groups are to be compared it is usual to choose those which are similar, or, in the case where all four substituents are different, those which are most alike.

EXAMPLE

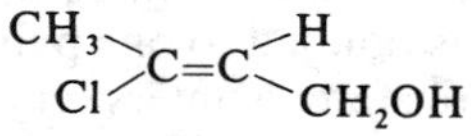

$$CH_3 \diagdown \diagup H$$
$$Cl \diagup C=C \diagdown CH_2OH$$

trans when comparing the methyl– and hydroxymethyl– groups

Alternatively, the choice may be made according to the context in which the chemical names are used, in which case those substituents which are most important to the discussion are compared.
Configuration in dienes or polyenes must be defined with reference to all double bonds.

EXAMPLES

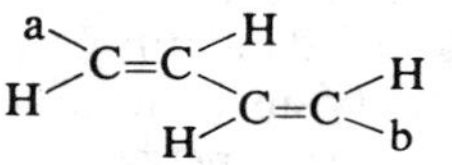

$$a \diagdown C=C \diagup H$$
$$H \diagup \qquad \diagdown C=C \diagdown H$$
$$H \diagup \qquad \diagup b$$

trans-trans-isomer

$$H \diagdown C=C \diagup b$$
$$a \diagdown C=C \diagup \diagdown H$$
$$H \diagup \diagdown H$$

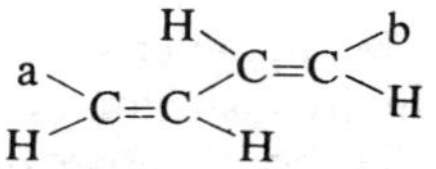

cis-trans-isomer

When the *cis-* and *trans-* prefixes are applied to substituents in ring systems they refer to the positions of the groups relative to each other and to the plane of the ring. The absolute configuration of such structures is given by *R-* and *S-*notation.
When one hydrogen atom and one substituent are each attached to two members of a ring, the two substituents are compared.

EXAMPLE

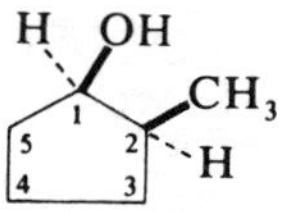

$$H \quad OH$$
$$CH_3$$
$$H$$

*cis-*2-methylcyclopentanol

When one hydrogen atom and one substituent are each attached to more than two members of a ring, steric relations are denoted by comparison of substituents to a reference substituent, indicated by *r*,

and the terms *cis* and *trans* are abbreviated to *c* and *t*. The reference substituent is chosen as the one with the lowest-numbered locant.

EXAMPLE

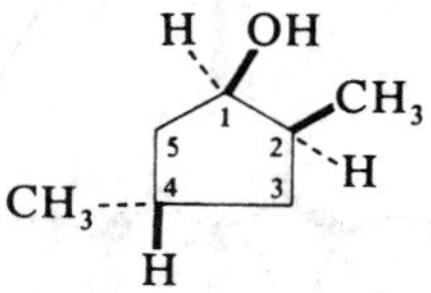

$$H \quad OH$$
$$CH_3$$
$$CH_3$$
$$H$$

c-2,*t*-4-dimethylcyclopentan-*r*-1-ol

When different substituents are linked to the same ring member their steric relations are indicated by *c* or *t* with reference to the lowest numbered group cited as suffix.

EXAMPLE

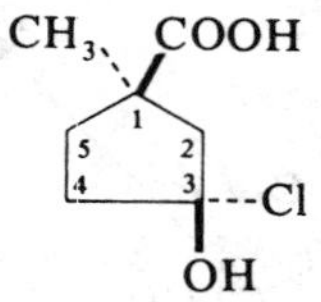

$$CH_3 \quad COOH$$
$$Cl$$
$$OH$$

t-3-chloro-3-hydroxy-1-methylcyclopentane-*r*-1-carboxylic acid

If there are no groups cited as suffix, then from the lowest numbered pair of substituents, that substituent preferred by the sequence rule is selected as reference group and termed *r*.

EXAMPLE

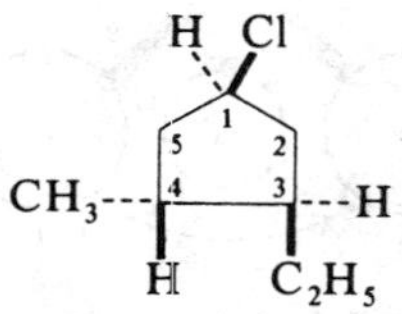

$$H \quad Cl$$
$$CH_3$$
$$H$$
$$H \quad C_2H_5$$

r-1-chloro-*c*-3-ethyl-*t*-4-methylcyclopentane

Steric relations in fused ring structures may again be indicated by *cis* or *trans*. Steric relations at saturated bridgeheads, for example, are indicated by the relative positions of the exocyclic atoms or groups at the bridgehead and are termed *cis-* or *trans-*fused. *cis-* or *trans-*fused systems may, for certain classes of compound, be indicated by the use of α or β to show the positions, relative to the plane of the ring system, of the atoms or groups attached to the bridgeheads, for example, steroids.

EXAMPLE

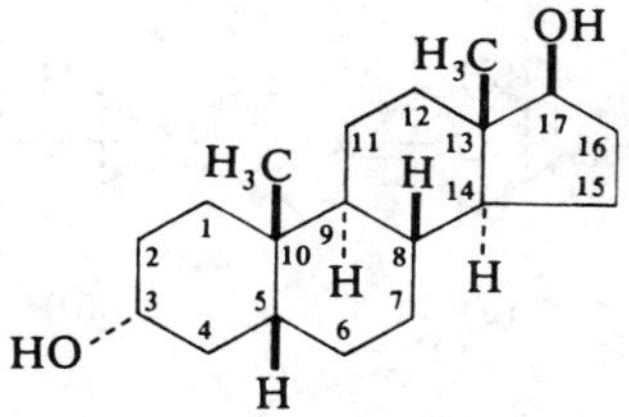

5β-androstane-3α,17β-diol

When more than one pair of saturated bridgeheads are present their relations to each other may be indicated by the terms *cisoid* or *transoid*. The nearest atoms from each bridgehead are compared but when there is a choice the nearest atom-pair which includes the lowest numbered atom is used. Thus in the above steroid example, the bridge at carbons 5 and 10 is *cis*, that at 8 and 9 is *trans*, and that at 13 and 14 is *trans*. The relationships between the bridges are *transoid* between bridges at 5(10) and 8(9) (comparison of bridgehead substituents at 9 and 10) and *transoid* between the bridges at 8(9) and 13(14) (comparison of bridgehead substituents at 8 and 14). The steric relations of the rings in this example may therefore be written as: *cis-transoid*-9,10-*trans-transoid*-8,14-*trans*-androstane. Formerly the terms *syn* and *anti* were used as alternatives to *cisoid* and *transoid* but these are no longer recommended.

Z- and E-Notation. In order to overcome the inherent ambiguities in the *cis-* and *trans*-notation it has been recommended by IUPAC that choice of atoms for comparison when defining steric relations across double bonds should be made by the Sequence Rule and the symbols *Z* (*zusammen*; together) and *E* (*entgegen*; opposite) should be used. In many cases *Z-* and *E*-notation will coincide with the *cis-* and *trans*-notation but this is not necessarily the case.

When adding the *Z-* and *E*-terms to a chemical name, they are cited as prefixes along with the lower locants of the bonds concerned and are placed in brackets. When these prefixes relate to a substituent then they are placed in front of the substituent name.

EXAMPLES

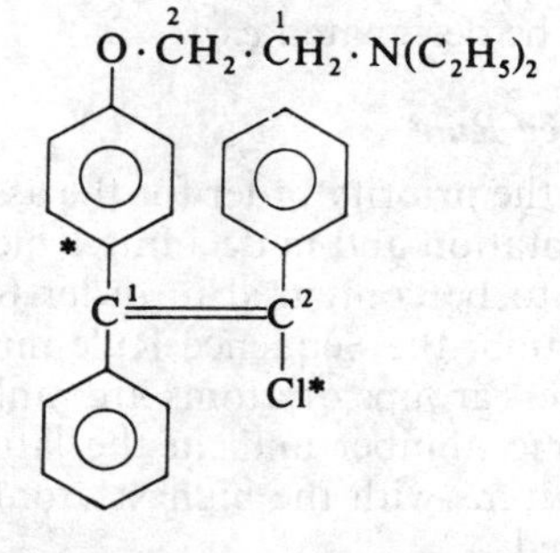

(*E*)-2-[4-(2-chloro-1,2-diphenylvinyl) phenoxy]triethylamine
(Enclomiphene)

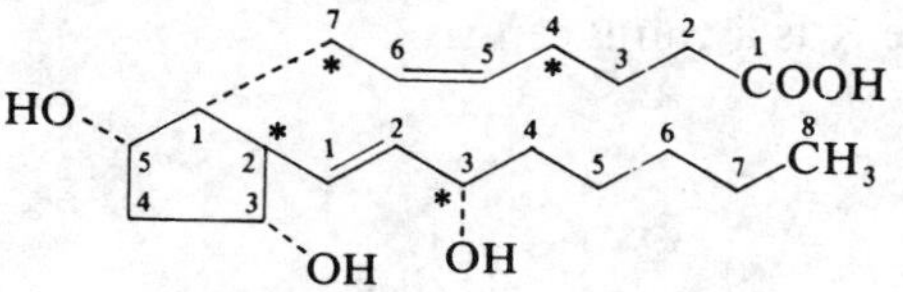

(1*R*,2*R*,3*R*,5*S*)-7-{3,5-dihydroxy-2-[(3*S*-3-hydroxyoct-1-(*E*)-enyl]cyclopentyl}hept-5-(*Z*)-enoic acid

(Dinoprost)

The groups for comparison, determined by the Sequence Rule, are indicated by asterisks in the two examples above. Enclomiphene is the *E*-isomer of clomiphene.

endo- and exo-Notation. These terms are used to indicate steric relations in bridged systems. Etorphine, for example, is (6*R*,7*R*,14*R*)-7,8-dihydro-7-[(1*R*)-1-hydroxy-1-methylbutyl]-6-*O*-methyl-6,14-*endo*-ethenomorphine.

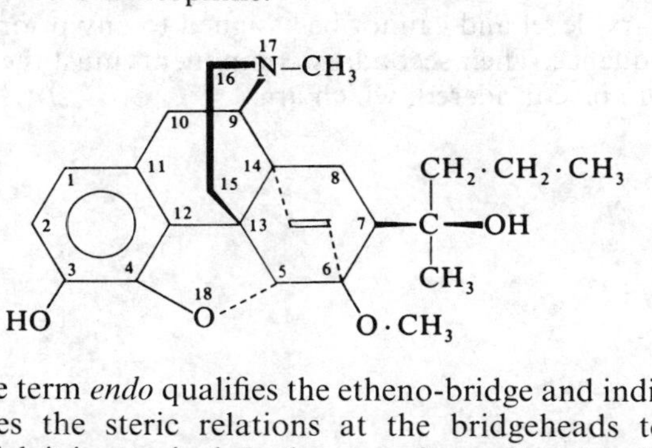

The term *endo* qualifies the etheno-bridge and indicates the steric relations at the bridgeheads to which it is attached. In the case of etorphine it indicates that the *etheno*-bridge is on the opposite side of the phenanthrene ring structure compared to the iminoethano-bridge. If the two bridges were on the same side of the phenanthrene ring structure then they would be designated *exo*.

The Sequence Rule

In deciding the priority order for the assignment of *R*- and *S*-notation and in deciding which atoms or groups are to be compared in order to assign *Z*- and *E*-notation, the Sequence Rule must be used. In the former, groups or atoms are ranked according to atomic number and, in the latter, the two groups or atoms with the highest atomic numbers are compared.

When only atoms are to be compared there is no difficulty but when groups are to be compared, deciding which group has priority is more complex. Consider, for example, the following groups where X is a chiral centre.

$$d-X-b$$

with a above X and c below X.

$$a = -\overset{\text{H}}{\underset{\text{OH}}{\text{C}}}-CH_2OH \qquad b = -\overset{\text{H}}{\underset{\text{OH}}{\text{C}}}-CH_3$$

$$c = -\overset{\text{H}}{\underset{\text{H}}{\text{C}}}-OH \qquad d = -\overset{\text{H}}{\underset{\text{H}}{\text{C}}}-CH_2OH$$

All four groups are linked to the chiral centre by a carbon atom. They are therefore similar at 'primary' level and cannot be assigned to any priority sequence. Their secondary components must therefore be considered, which are:

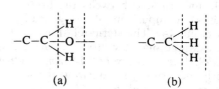

(a)   (b)

(c)   (d)

By taking the first points of difference it can be seen that the group (d) has the lowest priority since the atom with highest atomic number is carbon (6) whilst all the other groups possess an oxygen (8). However group (c) possesses one O-atom and two H-atoms whilst groups (a) and (b) each possess one O-atom, one C-atom, and one H-atom. Group (c) therefore has a lower priority than (a) or (b). To decide which of groups (a) and (b) has the highest priority, tertiary linked components must be considered.

(a)   (b)

Here it can be seen that (a) must have the higher priority since it possesses an O-atom at tertiary level, whilst (b) possesses only H-atoms. The priority sequence of these four groups is therefore a > b > c > d.

Examples of the priority rule order are shown in the following list in which the order is that of decreasing priority.

I—	R_3COCO—
Br—	ROCO—
Cl—	HOOC—
RSO_3—	NH_2OC—
RSO_2—	RCO—
RSO—	HCO—
RS—	o-substituted C_6H_5—
HS—	m-substituted C_6H_5—
F—	p-substituted C_6H_5—
RSO_2O—	C_6H_5—
RSOO—	CH:C—
RCOO—	CH_2:$C(CH_3)$—
HCOO—	$(CH_3)_3C$—
RO—	CH_3CH:CH—
HO—	C_6H_{11}—(cyclohexyl)
O_2N—	$RCH_2CH(CH_3)$—
ON—	CH_2:CH_2—
RN:N—	$(CH_3)_2CH$—
R_3N^+—	C_6H_5CH—
R_2N—	CH:CCH_2—
ROCONH—	$(CH_3)_3CCH_2$—
RCONH	CH_2:$CHCH_2$—
RNH—	$(CH_3)_2CHCH_2$—
H_3N^+—	$(CH_3)_2CHCH_2CH_2$—
H_2N—	—RCH_2—
Cl_3C—	CH_3—
ClOC—	H—

APPROVED NAMES

In the UK, names for new chemical entities are proposed by manufacturers or licence holders to the British Pharmacopoeia Commission, whose Nomenclature Committee examines the proposed names for conformity with guiding principles and modifies them as necessary. Names chosen should be suitable as potential titles for a monograph in the *British Pharmacopoeia*. Names are generally proposed around the time the new drug is undergoing clinical trials.

After consultation with other national nomenclature authorities through the World Health Organization in Geneva a final name is taken as the British Approved Name (BAN) and published by the Health Ministers on the recommendation of the Medicines Commission. In the USA a similar process is used for the United States Adopted Name (USAN).

When necessary, names are also approved for salts, esters, or radicals as well as for carrier substances used with radionuclides or other diagnostic media.

The guiding principles followed in the selection of approved names are that the names should:

- be distinctive in spelling and sound
- not be inconveniently long
- not be liable to confusion with names in common use
- be free from conflict with trade marks
- indicate, where appropriate, the relationship for substances within a pharmacological group or therapeutic class
- avoid conveying explicitly to a patient an anatomical, physiological, pathological, or therapeutic suggestion.

In general, the use of isolated letters or numbers or hyphens in names is avoided. Examples are, however, to be found among biotechnology products and polymers. The co- prefix is used in names for substance-combinations.

Proposed names from various countries are published by the World Health Organization in their journal, WHO Drug Information, about twice a year as Proposed International Nonproprietary Names (pINN). If no objections are lodged the name is republished as a Recommended International Nonproprietary Name (RecINN or rINN). This lengthy worldwide consultation process helps to ensure that an approved name can be used safely throughout the world. There are numerous examples from before the early 1960s, when international nomenclature became established, of different names being used in different countries. Most of the differences occurred between Europe and the USA but some differences remain between Europe and the UK. Many of these names were in existence before the 1960s. WHO and national nomenclature authorities discourage the incorporation in proprietary trade marks of syllables used in established approved names since this may interfere with the creation of appropriate new names for closely related drugs.

Some letters or letter combinations are difficult or pronounced differently in certain languages and should be avoided. For this reason *f* should normally be used instead of *ph*, *t* instead of *th* and *i* instead of *y* in new names. Examples include sulfadoxine, tioconazole, and ciclacillin. The letters h and k are now avoided in new names.

Preferential consideration for a British Approved Name is given to existing International Nonproprietary Names, official names in other countries, or names proposed by the originator of the drug, provided the name is in accordance with the guiding principles.

Common Stems

Common stems should be used in approved names to indicate group relationships, for example the -olol suffix common to the beta-adrenoceptor antagonists such as atenolol. Examples of the stems used in approved names are listed below. Such stems are constantly evolving as new pharmacological and therapeutic groups and subgroups are discovered.

-ac	anti-inflammatory agents of the ibufenac group
-actide	synthetic polypeptides with a corticotrophin-like action
-adol	analgesics
andr	steroids, androgens
-ast	anti-asthmatics, anti-allergics when not acting primarily as antihistamines
-astine	antihistamines, not otherwise classifiable
-azepam	substances of the diazepam group
-bactam	beta-lactamase inhibitors
bol	steroids, anabolic
-buzone	anti-inflammatory analgesics of the phenylbutazone group
-cain-	antifibrillants with local anaesthetic activity
-caine	local anaesthetics
cef-	antibiotics, derivatives of cephalosporanic acid
-cillin	antibiotics, derivatives of 6-aminopenicillanic acid
-conazole	systemic antifungals of the miconazole group
cort	corticosteroids, except those of the prednisolone group
-cycline	antibiotics of the tetracycline group
-dipine	calcium ion channel blockers of the nifedipine group
estr	oestrogenic substances
-fibrate	substances of the clofibrate group
gest	steroids, progestogens
gli	sulphonamide hypoglycaemics
io-	iodine-containing contrast media
-ium	quaternary ammonium compounds
-metacin	anti-inflammatory substances of the indomethacin group
-mycin	antibiotics produced by *Streptomyces* strains
-nidazole	antiprotozoal substances of the metronidazole group
-olol	beta-adrenoceptor antagonists
-orex	anorectic agents, phenethylamine derivatives
-oxacin	antibacterial agents of the cinoxacin group
-pramine	substances of the imipramine group
-pride	substances of the sulpiride group
-pril	inhibitors of angiotensin-converting enzyme
-prilat	inhibitors of angiotensin-converting enzyme
-profen	anti-inflammatory substances of the ibuprofen group
prost	prostaglandins
-racetam	substances of the piracetam group
-relin	hypophyseal hormone release-stimulating peptides
-stat	enzyme inhibitors
-steine	substances of the acetylcysteine group
-sulpha-	sulphonamides, anti-infective
-terol	bronchodilators, phenethylamine derivatives
-tidine	H_2-receptor antagonists of the cimetidine group
-verine	spasmolytics with a papaverine-like action
vin	vinca-type alkaloids

A more extensive list of stems with examples is included in the USAN and the USP Dictionary of Drug Names.

Co- Names

The BP Commission has adopted names for a series of substance-combinations commonly prescribed in the UK where the generic name of preparations would otherwise be unwieldy. The distinguishing prefix *co*- is used to signal the presence of two substances in the names, for example co-trimoxazole for the antibacterials trimethoprim and sulphamethoxazole in the proportions, by weight, of 1 part to 5 parts respectively.

In a few cases the proportions of the two drugs differ in different dosage forms, in which case the nominal amounts of the two ingredients per unit dose are expressed in the form x/y, where x and y are the respective amounts in milligrams of the two components in the order implied in the name. For oral liquids the unit dose is taken as 5 mL. For parenteral preparations x and y are the nominal amounts in milligrams of the components in the single-dose container.

In the USA, such names have been issued by the United States Pharmacopeial Convention as Pharmacy Equivalent Names (PEN). The USPC intends the names to be informative and to discourage the use of trivial names and undefined abbreviations.

Substance-Combination Names

Co-amilofruse
Amiloride hydrochloride and frusemide in the proportions, by weight, 1 part to 8 parts respectively

Co-amilozide
Amiloride hydrochloride and hydrochlorothiazide in the proportions, by weight, 1 part to 10 parts respectively

Co-amoxiclav
Amoxycillin (as the trihydrate or as the sodium salt) and clavulanic acid (as potassium clavulanate); the proportions are expressed in the form x/y, where x and y are the strengths in milligrams of amoxycillin and clavulanic acid respectively

Co-beneldopa
Benserazide (as the hydrochloride) and levodopa in the proportions, by weight, 1 part to 4 parts respectively

Co-careldopa
Carbidopa and levodopa; the proportions are expressed in the form x/y, where x and y are the strengths in milligrams of carbidopa and levodopa respectively

Co-codamol
Codeine phosphate and paracetamol; the proportions are expressed in the form x/y, where x and y are the strengths in milligrams of codeine phosphate and paracetamol respectively

Co-codaprin
Codeine phosphate and aspirin in the proportions, by weight, 1 part to 50 parts respectively

Co-danthramer*
Danthron and poloxamer 188; the proportions are expressed in the form x/y, where x and y are the strengths in milligrams of danthron and poloxamer respectively

Co-danthrusate
Danthron and docusate sodium in the proportions, by weight, 5 parts to 6 parts respectively

Co-dydramol
Dihydrocodeine tartrate and paracetamol in the proportions, by weight, 1 part to 50 parts respectively

*The definition of co-danthramer has been modified to include combinations of danthron and poloxamer 188 in the proportions 3 parts to 40 parts respectively, a combination previously known as *Strong Co-danthramer*.

Co-fluampicil
Flucloxacillin and ampicillin in equal proportions by weight

Co-flumactone
Hydroflumethiazide and spironolactone in equal proportions by weight

Co-magaldrox
Magnesium hydroxide and aluminium hydroxide; the proportions are expressed in the form x/y where x and y are the strengths in milligrams per unit dose of magnesium hydroxide and aluminium hydroxide respectively

Co-phenotrope
Diphenoxylate hydrochloride and atropine sulphate in the proportions, by weight, 100 parts to 1 part respectively

Co-prenozide
Oxprenolol hydrochloride and cyclopenthiazide in the proportions, by weight, 640 parts to 1 part respectively

Co-proxamol
Dextroproxyphene hydrochloride and paracetamol in the proportions, by weight, 1 part to 10 parts respectively

Co-simalcite
Activated dimethicone and hydrotalcite; the proportions are expressed in the form x/y where x and y are the strengths in milligrams of activated dimethicone and hydrotalcite respectively

Co-tenidone
Atenolol and chlorthalidone in the proportions, by weight, 4 parts to 1 part respectively

Co-tetroxazine
Tetroxoprim and sulphadiazine in the proportions, by weight, 2 parts to 5 parts respectively

Co-triamterzide
Triamterene and hydrochlorothiazide in the proportions, by weight, 2 parts to 1 part respectively

Co-trifamole
Trimethoprim and sulphamoxole in the proportions, by weight, 1 part to 5 parts respectively

Co-trimazine
Trimethoprim and sulphadiazine in the proportions, by weight, 1 part to 5 parts respectively

Co-trimoxazole
Trimethoprim and sulphamethoxazole in the proportions, by weight, 1 part to 5 parts respectively

LIST OF COMMON RADICALS

Radical name and formula

Acetamido $CH_3 \cdot CO \cdot NH—$
Acetimidoyl $CH_3 \cdot C(:NH)—$
Acetoacetyl $CH_3 \cdot CO \cdot CH_2 \cdot CO—$
Acetohydrazonoyl $CH_3 \cdot C(:N \cdot NH_2)—$
Acetohydroximoyl $CH_3 \cdot C(:N \cdot OH)—$
Acetonyl $CH_3 \cdot CO \cdot CH_2—$
Acetonylidene $CH_3 \cdot CO \cdot CH=$
Acetoxy $CH_3 \cdot CO \cdot O—$
Acetyl $CH_3 \cdot CO—$
Acryloyl $CH_2 \colon CH \cdot CO—$
Adipoyl $—CO \cdot [CH_2]_4 \cdot CO—$
Alanyl $CH_3 \cdot CH(NH_2) \cdot CO—$
β-Alanyl $H_2N \cdot CH_2 \cdot CH_2 \cdot CO—$
Allyl $CH_2 \colon CH \cdot CH_2—$
Allylidene $CH_2 \colon CH \cdot CH=$
Allyloxy $CH_3 \cdot CH(NH_2) \cdot CO—$
Amidino $H_2N \cdot C(:NH)—$
Amino $NH_2—$
Aminomethyleneamino $H_2N \cdot CH \colon N—$
Ammonio $^+H_3N—$
Amyl, *see* Pentyl
Anilino $C_6H_5 \cdot NH—$
Anisidino (*o-, m-,* or *p-*) $CH_3 \cdot O \cdot C_6H_4 \cdot NH—$
Anisoyl (*o-, m-,* or *p-*) $CH_3 \cdot O \cdot C_6H_4 \cdot CO—$
Anisyl $CH_3 \cdot O \cdot C_6H_4 \cdot CH_2—$
Arginyl $NH_2 \cdot C(:NH) \cdot NH \cdot [CH_2]_3 \cdot CH(NH_2) \cdot CO—$
Asparaginyl $NH_2 \cdot CO \cdot CH_2 \cdot CH(NH_2) \cdot CO—$
Aspartoyl $—CO \cdot CH_2 \cdot CH(NH_2) \cdot CO—$
α-Aspartyl $HO_2C \cdot CH_2 \cdot CH(NH_2) \cdot CO—$
β-Aspartyl $HO_2C \cdot CH(NH_2) \cdot CH_2 \cdot CO—$
Atropoyl $C_6H_5 \cdot C(:CH_2) \cdot CO—$
Azelaoyl (*unsubstituted only*) $—CO \cdot [CH_2]_7 \cdot CO—$
Azido $N_3—$
Azino $=N \cdot N=$
Azo $—N \colon N—$
Azoxy $—N(O) \cdot N—$

Benzamido $C_6H_5 \cdot CO \cdot NH—$
Benzenesulfonamido $C_6H_5 \cdot SO_2 \cdot NH—$
Benzenetriyl $C_6H_3\!\!<$
Benzhydryl (*alternative to Diphenylmethyl*) $(C_6H_5)_2CH—$
Benzhydrylidene (*alternative to Diphenylmethylene*) $(C_6H_5)_2C=$
Benzidino $p\text{-}NH_2 \cdot C_6H_4 \cdot C_6H_4 \cdot NH—$
Benziloyl $(C_6H_5)_2C(OH) \cdot CO—$
Benzimidoyl $C_6H_5 \cdot C(:NH)—$
Benzoyl $C_6H_5 \cdot CO—$
Benzoyloxy $C_6H_5 \cdot CO \cdot O—$
Benzyl $C_6H_5 \cdot CH_2—$
Benzylidene $C_6H_5 \cdot CH=$
Benzylidyne $C_6H_5 \cdot C\equiv$
Bromo $Br—$
Butanoyl, *see* Butyryl
Butenoyl, *see* Crotonoyl *and* Isocrotonoyl
2-Butenyl $CH_3 \cdot CH \colon CH \cdot CH_2—$
Butoxy $CH_3 \cdot [CH_2]_2 \cdot CH_2 \cdot O—$
*sec-*Butoxy (*unsubstituted only*) $C_2H_5 \cdot CH(CH_3) \cdot O—$
*tert-*Butoxy (*unsubstituted only*) $(CH_3)_3C \cdot O—$
Butyl $CH_3 \cdot [CH_2]_2 \cdot CH_2—$
*sec-*Butyl (*unsubstituted only*) $C_2H_5 \cdot CH(CH_3)—$
*tert-*Butyl (*unsubstituted only*) $(CH_3)_3C—$
Butyryl $CH_3 \cdot CH_2 \cdot CH_2 \cdot CO—$

Radical name and formula

Caproyl, *see* Hexanoyl
Carbamoyl $NH_2 \cdot CO—$
Carbazido, *see* Carbonohydrazido
Carbazono $HN \colon N \cdot CO \cdot NH \cdot NH—$
Carbazoyl $NH_2 \cdot NH \cdot CO—$
Carbodiazono $HN \colon N \cdot CO \cdot N \colon N—$
Carbonimidoyl $—C(:NH)—$
Carbonohydrazido $H_2N \cdot NH \cdot CO \cdot NH \cdot NH—$
Carbonyl $—C—$
Carbonyldioxy $—O \cdot CO \cdot O—$
Carboxamido $—CO \cdot NH—$
Carboxy $HO_2C—$
Carboxylato $—OOC—$
Chloro $Cl—$
Cinnamoyl $C_6H_5 \cdot CH \colon CH \cdot CO—$
Cinnamyl $C_6H_5 \cdot CH \colon CH \cdot CH_2—$
Cinnamylidene $C_6H_5 \cdot CH \colon CH \cdot CH=$
Crotonoyl $CH_3 \cdot CH \colon CH \cdot CO—$ (*trans*)
Cumenyl (*o-, m-,* or *p-*) $(CH_3)_2CH \cdot C_6H_4—$
Cyanato $NCO—$
Cyano $NC—$
Cysteinyl $HS \cdot CH_2 \cdot CH(NH_2) \cdot CO—$
Cystyl $—CO \cdot CH(NH_2) \cdot CH_2 \cdot S \cdot S \cdot CH_2 \cdot CH(NH_2) \cdot CO—$

Diazo $N_2=$
Diazoamino $—N \colon N \cdot NH—$
Dimethylamino $(CH_3)_2N—$
Dioxy $—O \cdot O—$
Diphenylmethyl (*alternative to Benzhydryl*) $(C_6H_5)_2CH—$
Diphenylmethylene (*alternative to Benzhydrylidene*) $(C_6H_5)_2C=$
Dithio $—S \cdot S—$
Dithiocarboxy $HS \cdot SC—$
Dithiosulfo $HOS_3—$

Elaidoyl $CH_3 \cdot [CH_2]_7 \cdot CH \colon CH \cdot [CH_2]_7 \cdot CO—$ (*trans*)
Epidioxy (*as bridge*) $—O \cdot O—$
Epidithio (*as bridge*) $—S \cdot S—$
Epimino (*as bridge*) $—NH—$
Epithio (*as bridge*) $—S—$
Epoxy (*as bridge*) $—O—$
Ethanediylidene $=CH \cdot CH=$
Ethoxy $C_2H_5 \cdot O—$
Ethyl $CH_3 \cdot CH_2—$
Ethynyl $HC \colon C—$

Fluoro $F—$
Formamido $OCH \cdot NH—$
Formimidoyl $CH(:NH)—$
Formyl $OHC—$
Formyloxy $H \cdot CO \cdot O—$
Fumaroyl $—CO \cdot CH \colon CH \cdot CO—$ (*trans*)
Furancarbonyl, *see* Furoyl

$$CH_2—$$
Furfuryl (2- *only*) $\overline{CH \colon CH \cdot O \cdot C} \colon CH$
Furoyl (3- *shown*) $\overline{CH \colon CH \cdot O \cdot CH \colon C} \cdot CO—$
3-Furylmethyl $\overline{CH \colon CH \cdot O \cdot CH \colon C} \cdot CH_2—$

Galloyl $3,4,5\text{-}(HO)_3C_6H_2 \cdot CO—$
Glutaminyl $NH_2 \cdot CO \cdot CH_2 \cdot CH_2 \cdot CH(NH_2) \cdot CO—$
Glutamoyl $—CO \cdot CH_2 \cdot CH_2 \cdot CH(NH_2) \cdot CO—$
α-Glutamyl $HOOC \cdot [CH_2]_2 \cdot CH(NH_2) \cdot CO—$

Radical name and formula	*Radical name and formula*

γ-Glutamyl $HOOC \cdot CH(NH_2) \cdot [CH_2]_2 \cdot CO—$
Glutaryl $—CO \cdot [CH_2]_3 \cdot CO—$
Glyceroyl $HO \cdot CH_2 \cdot CH(OH) \cdot CO—$
Glycoloyl $HO \cdot CH_2 \cdot CO—$
Glycyl $NH_2 \cdot CH_2 \cdot CO—$
Glyoxyloyl $OHC \cdot CO—$
Guanidino $NH_2 \cdot C(:NH) \cdot NH—$

Hexanoyl (*replacing Caproyl*) $CH_2 \cdot [CH_2]_4 \cdot CO—$
Hippuroyl $C_6H_5 \cdot CO \cdot NH \cdot CH_2 \cdot CO—$
Histidyl $N_2C_3H_3 \cdot CH_2 \cdot CH(NH_2) \cdot CO—$
Homocysteinyl $HS \cdot CH_2 \cdot CH_2 \cdot CH(NH_2) \cdot CO—$
Homoseryl $HO \cdot CH_2 \cdot CH_2 \cdot CH(NH_2) \cdot CO—$
Hydantoyl $NH_2 \cdot CO \cdot NH \cdot CH_2 \cdot CO—$
Hydratropoyl $C_6H_5 \cdot CH(CH_3) \cdot CO—$
Hydrazino $NH_2 \cdot NH—$
Hydrazono $NH_2 \cdot N=$
Hydroperoxy $HO \cdot O—$
Hydroseleno $HSe—$
Hydroxy $HO—$
Hydroxyamino $HO \cdot NH—$
Hydroxyimino $HO \cdot N=$

Imino $—HN—$ *or* $HN=$
Iminomethylamino $HN:CH—NH—$
Iodo $I—$
Isobutyl (*unsubstituted only*) $(CH_3)_2CH \cdot CH_2—$
Isobutyryl (*unsubstituted only*) $(CH_3)_2CH \cdot CO—$
Isocrotonoyl $CH_3 \cdot CH:CH \cdot CO—$ (*cis*)
Isocyanato $OCN—$
Isocyano $CN—$
Isohexyl (*unsubstituted only*) $(CH_3)_2CH \cdot [CH_2]_2 \cdot CH_2—$
Isoleucyl $C_2H_5 \cdot CH(CH_3) \cdot CH(NH_2) \cdot CO—$
Isonicotinoyl $NC_5H_4 \cdot CO—$
Isopentyl (*unsubstituted only*) $(CH_3)_2CH \cdot CH_2 \cdot CH_2—$
Isophthaloyl $—CO \cdot C_6H_4 \cdot CO—$ (*m-*)
Isopropenyl (*unsubstituted only*) $CH_2:C(CH_3)—$
Isopropoxy (*unsubstituted only*) $(CH_3)_2CH \cdot O—$
Isopropyl (*unsubstituted only*) $(CH_3)_2CH—$
Isosemicarbazido $H_2N \cdot NH \cdot C(OH):N—$ (and tautomers)
Isothiocyanato $SCN—$
Isothioureido $HN:C(SH) \cdot NH—$ *or* $H_2N \cdot C(SH):N—$
Isoureido $HN:C(OH) \cdot NH—$ *or* $H_2N \cdot C(OH):N—$
Isovaleryl (*unsubstituted only*) $(CH_3)_2CH \cdot CH_2 \cdot CO—$

Lactoyl $CH_3 \cdot CH(OH) \cdot CO—$
Lanthionyl $—CO \cdot CH(NH_2) \cdot CH_2 \cdot S \cdot CH_2 \cdot CH(NH_2) \cdot CO—$
Lauroyl (*unsubstituted only*) $CH_3 \cdot [CH_2]_{10} \cdot CO—$
Leucyl $(CH_3)_2CH \cdot CH_2 \cdot CH(NH_2) \cdot CO—$
Lysyl $NH_2 \cdot [CH_2]_4 \cdot CH(NH_2) \cdot CO—$

Maleoyl $—CO \cdot CH:CH \cdot CO—$ (*cis*)
Malonyl $—CO \cdot CH_2 \cdot CO—$
Maloyl $—CO \cdot CH(OH) \cdot CH_2 \cdot CO—$
Mercapto $HS—$
Mesityl $2,4,6-(CH_3)_3C_6H_2—$
Mesoxalo $HOOC \cdot CO \cdot CO—$
Mesoxalyl $—CO \cdot CO \cdot CO—$
Mesyl $CH_3 \cdot SO_2—$
Methacryloyl $CH_2:C(CH_3) \cdot CO—$
Methanesulfonyl, *see* Mesyl
Methionyl $CH_3 \cdot S \cdot CH_2 \cdot CH_2 \cdot CH(NH_2) \cdot CO—$
Methoxalyl $CH_3OOC \cdot CO—$

Methoxy $CH_3O—$
Methyl $CH_3—$
Methylene $—CH_2—$ *or* CH_2
Methylenedioxy $—O \cdot CH_2 \cdot O—$
Methylsulfonyl, *see* Mesyl
Morpholino (*4-position only*) $\overline{CH_2 \cdot CH_2 \cdot O \cdot CH_2 \cdot CH_2 \cdot N}—$
Myristoyl (*unsubstituted only*) $CH_3 \cdot [CH_2]_{12} \cdot CO—$

Naphthoyl $C_{10}H_7 \cdot CO—$
Naphthyloxy $C_{10}H_7 \cdot O—$
Neopentyl (*unsubstituted only*) $(CH_3)_3C \cdot CH_2—$
Nicotinoyl (*3-pyridinecarbonyl only*) $NC_5H_4 \cdot CO—$
Nitrilo $N≡$
Nitro $O_2N—$
aci-Nitro $HO(O:)N=$
Nitroso $ON—$
Norleucyl $CH_3 \cdot [CH_2]_3 \cdot CH(NH_2) \cdot CO—$
Norvalyl $CH_3 \cdot CH_2 \cdot CH_2 \cdot CH(NH_2) \cdot CO—$

9-Octadecenoyl, *see* Elaidoyl *and* Oleoyl
Octyl $CH_3 \cdot [CH_2]_6 \cdot CH_2—$
Oleoyl $CH_3 \cdot [CH_2]_7 \cdot CH:CH \cdot [CH_2]_7 \cdot CO—$ (*cis*)
Ornithyl $NH_2 \cdot [CH_2]_3 \cdot CH(NH_2) \cdot CO—$
Oxalacetyl $—CO \cdot CH_2 \cdot CO \cdot CO—$
Oxalo $HOOC \cdot CO—$
Oxalyl $—CO \cdot CO—$
Oxamoyl $NH_2 \cdot CO \cdot CO—$
Oxido $^-O—$
Oxo $O=$
Oxonio $^+H_2O—$
Oxy $—O—$

Palmitoyl (*unsubstituted only*) $CH_3 \cdot [CH_2]_{14} \cdot CO—$
Pentanoyl, *see* Valeryl
Pentyl (*replacing Amyl*) $CH_3 \cdot [CH_2]_3 \cdot CH_2—$
tert-Pentyl (*unsubstituted only*) $C_2H_5 \cdot C(CH_3)_2—$
Phenacyl $C_6H_5 \cdot CO \cdot CH_2—$
Phenethyl $C_6H_5 \cdot CH_2 \cdot CH_2—$
Phenetidino (*o-, m-,* or *p-*) $C_2H_5O \cdot C_6H_4 \cdot NH—$
Phenoxy $C_6H_5 \cdot O—$
Phenyl $C_6H_5—$
Phenylacetyl $C_6H_5 \cdot CH_2 \cdot CO—$
Phthalamoyl $NH_2 \cdot CO \cdot C_6H_4 \cdot CO—$ (*o-*)
Phthalazinyl $N_2C_8H_5—$
Phthalidyl $\overline{C_6H_4 \cdot CO \cdot O \cdot CH}—$
Phthalimido $\overline{CO \cdot C_6H_4 \cdot CO \cdot N}—$
Phthaloyl $—CO \cdot C_6H_4 \cdot CO—$ (*o-*)
Picryl $2,4,6-(NO_2)_3C_6H_2—$
Pimeloyl (*unsubstituted only*) $—CO \cdot [CH_2]_5 \cdot CO—$
Piperidino (*1 only*) $C_5H_{10}N—$
Piperidyl $NC_5H_{10}—$
Piperonyl $3,4-CH_2O_2:C_6H_3 \cdot CH_2—$
Pivaloyl (*unsubstituted only*) $(CH_3)_3C \cdot CO—$

Prolyl $\overline{NH \cdot CH_2 \cdot CH_2 \cdot CH_2 \cdot CH} \cdot CO—$
Propanoyl, *see* Propionyl
2-Propenyl, *see* Allyl
Propioloyl $CH:C \cdot CO—$
Propionamido $CH_3 \cdot CH_2 \cdot CO \cdot NH—$
Propionyl $CH_3 \cdot CH_2 \cdot CO—$

Radical name and formula

Propoxy $CH_3 \cdot CH_2 \cdot CH_2 \cdot O$—
Propyl $CH_3 \cdot CH_2 \cdot CH_2$—
Protocatechuoyl $3,4\text{-}(HO)_2C_6H_3 \cdot CO$—
Pyridinio $^+NC_5H_5$—
Pyruvoyl $CH_3 \cdot CO \cdot CO$—

Salicyl $o\text{-}HO \cdot C_6H_4 \cdot CH_2$—
Salicylidene $o\text{-}HO \cdot C_6H_4 \cdot CH=$
Salicyloyl $o\text{-}HO \cdot C_6H_4 \cdot CO$—
Sarcosyl $CH_3 \cdot NH \cdot CH_2 \cdot CO$—
Sebacoyl (*unsubstituted only*) $—CO \cdot [CH_2]_8 \cdot CO$—
Semicarbazido $H_2N \cdot CO \cdot NH \cdot NH$—
Semicarbazono $H_2N \cdot CO \cdot NH \cdot N=$
Seryl $HO \cdot CH_2 \cdot CH(NH_2) \cdot CO$—
Stearoyl (*unsubstituted only*) $CH_3 \cdot [CH_2]_{16} \cdot CO$—
Styryl $C_6H_5 \cdot CH{:}CH$—
Suberoyl (*unsubstituted only*) $—CO \cdot [CH_2]_6 \cdot CO$—
Succinamoyl $NH_2 \cdot CO \cdot CH_2 \cdot CH_2 \cdot CO$—

Succinimido $\overline{CO \cdot CH_2 \cdot CH_2 \cdot CO \cdot N}$—
Succinimidoyl $—C({:}NH) \cdot CH_2 \cdot CH_2 \cdot C({:}NH)$—
Succinyl $—CO \cdot CH_2 \cdot CH_2 \cdot CO$—
Sulfamoyl $NH_2 \cdot SO_2$—
Sulfanilamido $p\text{-}NH_2 \cdot C_6H_4 \cdot SO_2 \cdot NH$—
Sulfanilyl $p\text{-}NH_2 \cdot C_6H_4 \cdot SO_2$—
Sulfenamoyl $NH_2 \cdot S$—
Sulfeno $HO \cdot S$—
Sulfido ^-S—
Sulfinamoyl $NH_2 \cdot SO$—
Sulfino HO_2S—
Sulfinyl $—SO$—
Sulfo $HO \cdot SO_2$—
Sulfoamino $HO_3S \cdot NH$—
Sulfonato ^-O_3S—
Sulfonio ^+H_2S—
Sulfonyl $—SO_2$—
Sulfonyldioxy $—O \cdot SO_2 \cdot O$—

Tartaroyl $—CO \cdot CH(OH) \cdot CH(OH) \cdot CO$—
Tartronoyl $—CO \cdot CH(OH) \cdot CO$—
Tauryl $H_2N \cdot CH_2 \cdot CH_2 \cdot SO_2$—
Terephthaloyl $—CO \cdot C_6H_4 \cdot CO$— (*p-*)
Thenoyl (*2 shown*) $S \cdot CH{:}CH \cdot CH{:}C \cdot CO$—

Thenyl $SC_4H_3 \cdot CH_2$—
Thio $—S$—
Thioacetyl $CH_3 \cdot CS$—

Radical name and formula

Thiobenzoyl $C_6H_5 \cdot CS$—
Thiocarbamoyl $H_2N \cdot CS$—
Thiocarbazono $HN{:}N \cdot CS \cdot NH \cdot NH$— (and tautomers)
Thiocarbodiazono $HN{:}N \cdot CS \cdot N{:}N$— (and tautomers)
Thiocarbonohydrazido $H_2N \cdot NH \cdot CS \cdot NH \cdot NH$—
Thiocarbonyl $—CS$—
Thiocarboxamido $—CS \cdot NH$—
Thiocarboxy $HSOC$—
Thiocyanato NCS—
Thioformyl SCH—
Thiosemicarbazido $H_2N \cdot CS \cdot NH \cdot NH$—
Thiosulfino HOS_2—
Thiosulfo HO_2S_2—
Thioureido $H_2N \cdot CS \cdot NH$—
Thioxo $S=$
Threonyl $CH_3 \cdot CH(OH) \cdot CH(NH_2) \cdot CO$—
Thyronyl $p\text{-}(p\text{-}HO \cdot C_6H_4 \cdot O) \cdot C_6H_4 \cdot CH_2 \cdot CH(NH_2) \cdot CO$—
Toluidino (*o-, m-,* and *p-*) $CH_3 \cdot C_6H_4 \cdot NH$—
Toluoyl (*o-, m-,* and *p-*) $CH_3 \cdot C_6H_4 \cdot CO$—
Tolyl (*o-, m-,* and *p*) $CH_3 \cdot C_6H_4$—
Tosyl $p\text{-}CH_3 \cdot C_6H_4 \cdot SO_2$—
Triazano $H_2N \cdot NH \cdot NH$—
Triphenylmethyl (*alternative to Trityl*) $(C_6H_5)_3C$—
Trithiosulfo $HS \cdot S_3$—
Trityl (*alternative to Triphenylmethyl*) $(C_6H_5)_3C$—
Tropoyl $C_6H_5 \cdot CH(CH_2 \cdot OH) \cdot CO$—
Tryptophyl $NC_8H_6 \cdot CH_2 \cdot CH(NH_2) \cdot CO$—
Tyrosyl $p\text{-}HO \cdot C_6H_4 \cdot CH_2 \cdot CH(NH_2) \cdot CO$—

Ureido $NH_2 \cdot CO \cdot NH$—
Ureylene $—NH \cdot CO \cdot NH$—

Valeryl $CH_3 \cdot [CH_2]_3 \cdot CO$—
Valyl $(CH_3)_2CH \cdot CH(NH_2) \cdot CO$—
Vanilloyl $3,4\text{-}CH_3O \cdot (HO)C_6H_3 \cdot CO$—
Vanillyl $3,4\text{-}CH_3O \cdot (HO)C_6H_3 \cdot CH_2$—
Vanillylidene $3,4\text{-}CH_3O(HO)C_6H_3 \cdot CH=$
Veratroyl $3,4\text{-}(CH_3O)_2C_6H_3 \cdot CO$—
Veratryl $3,4\text{-}(CH_3O)_2C_6H_3 \cdot CH_2$—
Vinyl $CH_2{:}CH$—
Vinylene $—CH{:}CH$—
Vinylidene $CH_2{:}C=$

Xylidino $(CH_3)_2C_6H_3 \cdot NH$—
Xylyl $(CH_3)_2C_6H_3$—

The spelling *f* and *ph* are interchangeable in many radicals (for example, sul*f*o- and sul*ph*o-).

RECOMMENDED NAMES FOR RADICALS AND GROUPS

Some substances for which a nonproprietary name has been established may be of complex composition and it is then inconvenient to refer to them in systematic chemical nomenclature. The following contractions are used by the indicated organisations for the radicals and groups shown.

Contraction	Chemical name
acetonide (BAN)	isopropylidene ether of a dihydric alcohol
aceturate (BAN, USAN, INN)	N-acetylglycinate
acistrate (USAN, INN)	2′-acetate (ester) and octadecanoate (salt)
acoxil (INN)	acetoxymethyl
amsonate (BAN, INN)	4,4′-diaminostilbene-2,2′-disulphonate
axetil (BAN, USAN, INN)	1-acetoxyethyl
besilate (INN), besylate (BAN, USAN)	benzenesulphonate
bezomil (INN)	(benzoyloxy)methyl
buciclate (INN)	trans-4-butylcyclohexanecarboxylate
bunapsilate (INN)	3,7-di-tert-butylnaphthalene-1,5-disulphonate
buteprate (USAN, INN)	butyrate propionate
camsilate (INN), camsylate (BAN, USAN)	camphor-10-sulphonate
caproate (USAN)	hexanoate
carbesilate (INN)	4-carboxybenzenesulphonate
ciclotate (INN), cyclotate (USAN)	4-methylbicyclo[2.2.2]oct-2-ene-1-carboxylate
cipionate (INN), cypionate (BAN, USAN)	β-cyclopentylpropionate
closilate (INN), closylate (BAN, USAN)	4-chlorobenzenesulphonate
crobefate (INN)	(±)-(E)-6-hydroxy-4′-methoxy-3-(p-methoxybenzylidene) flavanone, phosphate, ion (2-)
cromacate (INN)	[(6-hydroxy-4-methyl-2-oxo-2H-1-benzopyran-7-yl)oxy]acetate
cromesilate (BAN, INN)	6,7-dihydroxycoumarin-4-methanesulphonate
cyclotate (USAN)	see ciclotate (INN)
cypionate (BAN, USAN)	see cipionate (INN)
deanil (INN)	2-dimethylaminoethyl
decil (INN)	decyl
dibudinate (INN)	2,6-di-tert-butylnaphthalene-1,5-disulphonate
dibunate (INN)	2,6-di-tert-butylnaphthalenesulphonate
digolil (INN)	2-(2-hydroxyethoxy)ethyl
diolamine (USAN, INN)	diethanolamine
docosil (INN)	docosyl
dofosfate (INN)	octadecyl hydrogen phosphate
edetate (USAN)	ethylenediamine-N,N,N′,N′-tetra-acetate
edisilate (INN), edisylate (BAN, USAN)	ethane-1,2-disulphonate
embonate (BAN, INN), pamoate (USAN)	4,4′-methylenebis(3-hydroxy-2-naphthoate)
enantate (INN), enanthate (BAN, USAN)	heptanoate
erbumine (BAN, USAN, INN)	tert-butylamine
esilate (INN), esylate (BAN, USAN)	ethanesulphonate
estolate (USAN, INN)	propionate dodecyl sulphate
esylate (BAN, USAN)	see esilate (INN)
etabonate (USAN, INN)	(ethoxycarbonyl)oxy
farnesil (INN)	(2E,6E)-3,7,11-trimethyl-2,6,10-dodecatrienyl
fendizoate (INN)	2-[(2′-hydroxybiphenyl-4-yl)carbonyl]benzoate
gluceptate (BAN, USAN, INN)	glucoheptonate
hibenzate (INN), hybenzate (USAN)	2-(4-hydroxybenzoyl)benzoate
hyclate (USAN, INN)	monohydrochloride hemiethanolate hemihydrate
isethionate (BAN, USAN), isetionate (INN)	2-hydroxyethanesulphonate
lauril (INN)	dodecyl
laurilsulfate (INN)	dodecylsulphate
megallate (BAN, INN)	3,4,5-trimethoxybenzoate
meglumine (USAN)	1-methylamino-1-deoxy-D-glucitol
mesilate (INN), mesylate (BAN, USAN)	methanesulphonate
metembonate (INN)	4,4′-methylenebis(3-methoxy-2-naphthoate)
metilsulfate (INN)	methylsulphate
mofetil (USAN, INN)	2-(4-morpholinyl)ethyl
napadisilate (INN), napadisylate (BAN)	naphthalene-1,5-disulphonate
napsilate (INN), napsylate (BAN, USAN)	naphthalene-2-sulphonate

Contraction	Chemical name
octil (INN)	octyl
olamine (USAN, INN)	ethanolamine
oxoglurate (INN)	2-oxopentanedioate
pamoate (USAN)	see embonate (BAN, INN)
pendetide (INN)	N^6-{N-[2-({2-[bis(carboxymethyl)amino]ethyl} (carboxymethyl)amino)ethyl]-N-(carboxymethyl)glycyl}-N^2-(N-glycyl-L-tyrosyl)-L-lysine
phenpropionate (USAN)	3-phenylpropionate
pivalate (BAN, USAN, INN)	trimethylacetate
pivetil (INN)	1-hydroxyethyl pivalate (ester)
pivoxetil (BAN, USAN, INN)	1-(2-methoxy-2-methylpropionyloxy)ethyl
pivoxil (USAN, INN)	(2,2-dimethyl-1-oxopropoxy)methyl; (pivaloyloxy)methyl
proxetil (BAN, USAN, INN)	1-[(isopropoxycarbonyl)oxy]ethyl
steaglate (INN)	octadecanoyloxyacetate
suleptanate (BAN)	sodium 7-[methyl(2-sulphonatoethyl)-carbamoyl]heptanoyl
tebutate (USAN, INN)	tertiary butyl acetate
tenoate (INN)	thiophene-2-carboxylate
teoclate (INN), theoclate (BAN)	8-chlorotheophyllinate
teprosilate (INN)	1,2,3,6-tetrahydro-1,3-dimethyl-2,6-dioxopurine-7-propanesulphonate
theoclate (BAN)	see teoclate (INN)
tofesilate (INN)	1,2,3,6-tetrahydro-1,3-dimethyl-2,6-dioxopurine-7-ethanesulphonate
tosilate (INN), tosylate (BAN, USAN)	toluene-4-sulphonate
triclofenate (INN)	2,4,5-trichlorophenolate
triflutate (USAN, INN)	trifluoroacetate
trolamine (USAN, INN)	triethanolamine
troxundate (BAN, INN)	3,6,9-trioxaundecanoate
xinafoate (BAN, USAN, INN)	1-hydroxy-2-naphthoate

FURTHER INFORMATION

Biochemical Nomenclature and Related Documents. 2nd ed. London: Portland Press, 1992. A compendium of recommendations published previously in one or more of the biochemical journals represented by the Committee of Editors of Biochemical Journals (CEBJ).

British Approved Names are published by the British Pharmacopoeia Commission on the recommendation of the Medicines Commission in British Approved Names 1990. London: HMSO. Supplements are published about twice a year.

International Union of Pure and Applied Chemistry (IUPAC). Nomenclature of organic chemistry. Oxford: Pergamon Press 1979 (The Blue Book).

Section A: Hydrocarbons
Section B: Fundamental Heterocyclic Systems
Section C: Characteristic Groups containing Carbon, Hydrogen, Oxygen, Nitrogen, Halogen, Sulphur, Selenium, and/or Tellurium
Section D: Organic Compounds containing elements which are not exclusively Carbon, Hydrogen, Oxygen, Nitrogen, Halogen, Sulphur, Selenium, and Tellurium
Section E: Stereochemistry
Section F: Natural Products and Related Compounds
Section H: Isotopically Modified Compounds

Lees R, Smith AF, editors. Chemical nomenclature usage. Chichester: Ellis Horwood, 1983.

New rules of the IUPAC Commission on the Nomenclature of Organic Chemistry and the IUPAC/IUB Commission on Biochemical Nomenclature are published in the IUPAC Information Bulletin, Pure Appl Chem, and journals such as the Journal of Biological Chemistry and the European Journal of Biochemistry. These sources should be consulted as they appear in order to obtain information on new rules.

Proposed and Recommended International Nonproprietary Names are published about twice a year in WHO Drug Information. Published names are collected in International Nonproprietary Names (INN) for Pharmaceutical Substances: Lists 1-65 of Proposed INN and Lists 1-31 of Recommended INN Cumulative List No. 8. Geneva: World Health Organization. 1992.

Treatment of variable valence in organic nomenclature (IUPAC Commission on Nomenclature of Organic Chemistry, Recommendations 1983). Pure Appl Chem 1984;56:769–78.

United States Adopted Names (USAN) are published annually in USAN and the USP Dictionary of Drug Names. Rockville, MD: United States Pharmacopeial Convention Inc. New and proposed names are generated by the USAN Council published in USP DI Update and Pharmacopeial Forum by USP Convention Inc.

Amino Acids. Nomenclature and symbolism for amino acids and peptides (IUPAC-IUB Joint Commission on Biochemical Nomenclature, Recommendations 1983). J Biol Chem 1985;260:14–42.

Carbohydrates. Abbreviated terminology of oligosaccharide chains (IUPAC-IUB Joint Commission on Biochemical Nomenclature, Recommendations 1980). J Biol Chem 1982;257:3347–51 and Eur J Biochem 1982; 126:433–7.

Conformational nomenclature for five- and six-membered ring forms of monosaccharides and their derivatives (IUPAC-IUB Joint Commission on Biochemical Nomenclature, Recommendations 1980). Eur J Biochem 1980;111:295–8.

Nomenclature of branched-chain monosaccharides (IUPAC-IUB Joint Commission on Biochemical Nomenclature, Recommendations 1980). Eur J Biochem 1981;119:5–8.

Nomenclature of unsaturated monosaccharides (IUPAC-IUB Joint Commission on Biochemical Nomenclature, Recommendations 1980). Eur J Biochem 1981;119:1–3.

Polysaccharide nomenclature (IUPAC-IUB Joint Commission on Biochemical Nomenclature, Recommendations 1980). J Biol Chem 1982;257:3352-4 and Eur J Biochem 1982;126: 439–41.

Symbols for specifying the conformation of polysaccharide chains (IUPAC-IUB Joint Commission on Biochemical Nomenclature, Recommendations 1981). Eur J Biochem 1983;131: 5–7.

Folates. Nomenclature and symbols for folic acid and related compounds. (IUPAC-IUB Joint Commission on Biochemical Nomenclature, Recommendations 1986). Eur J Biochem 1987;168:251–3.

Pesticides. Recommended common names for pesticides. BS 1831:1969.

Retinoids. Nomenclature of retinoids. (IUPAC-IUB Joint

Commission on Biochemical Nomenclature, Recommendations 1981). Eur J Biochem 1982;129:1–5.

Steroids. The nomenclature of steroids: recommendations 1989. IUPAC-IUB Joint Commission on Biochemical Nomenclature. Eur J Biochem 1989;186:429–58.

Tetrapyrroles. Nomenclature of tetrapyrroles (IUPAC-IUB Joint Commission on Biochemical Nomenclature, Recommendations 1986). Eur J Biochem 1988;178:277–328.

Tocopherols. Nomenclature of tocopherols and related compounds (IUPAC-IUB Joint Commission on Biochemical Nomenclature, Recommendations 1981). Eur J Biochem 1982;123:473-5.

Vitamin D. Nomenclature of vitamin D. (IUPAC-IUB Joint Commission on Biochemical Nomenclature, Recommendations 1981). Eur J Biochem 1982;124:223–7.

Miscellaneous Data

Atomic Weights of the Elements $^{12}C=12$

Atomic Number	Name	Symbol	Atomic Weight	Atomic Number	Name	Symbol	Atomic Weight
89	Actinium	Ac	227.0278	57	Lanthanum	La	138.9055
13	Aluminium	Al	26.98154	103	Lawrencium	Lr	(260)
95	Americium	Am	(243)	82	Lead	Pb	207.2
51	Antimony	Sb	121.75	3	Lithium	Li	6.941
18	Argon	Ar	39.948	71	Lutetium	Lu	174.967
33	Arsenic	As	74.9216	12	Magnesium	Mg	24.305
85	Astatine	At	(210)	25	Manganese	Mn	54.9380
56	Barium	Ba	137.33	101	Mendelevium	Md	(258)
97	Berkelium	Bk	(247)	80	Mercury	Hg	200.59
4	Beryllium	Be	9.01218	42	Molybdenum	Mo	95.94
83	Bismuth	Bi	208.9804	60	Neodymium	Nd	144.24
5	Boron	B	10.811	10	Neon	Ne	20.179
35	Bromine	Br	79.904	93	*Neptunium	Np	237.0482
48	Cadmium	Cd	112.41	28	Nickel	Ni	58.69
55	Caesium	Cs	132.9054	41	Niobium	Nb	92.9064
20	Calcium	Ca	40.078	7	Nitrogen	N	14.0067
98	Californium	Cf	(251)	102	Nobelium	No	(259)
6	Carbon	C	12.011	76	Osmium	Os	190.2
58	Cerium	Ce	140.12	8	Oxygen	O	15.9994
17	Chlorine	Cl	35.453	46	Palladium	Pd	106.42
24	Chromium	Cr	51.9961	15	Phosphorus	P	30.97376
27	Cobalt	Co	58.9332	78	Platinum	Pt	195.08
29	Copper	Cu	63.546	94	Plutonium	Pu	(244)
96	Curium	Cm	(247)	84	Polonium	Po	(209)
66	Dysprosium	Dy	162.50	19	Potassium	K	39.0983
99	Einsteinium	Es	(252)	59	Praseodymium	Pr	140.9077
68	Erbium	Er	167.26	61	Promethium	Pm	(145)
63	Europium	Eu	151.96	91	*Protactinium	Pa	231.0359
100	Fermium	Fm	(257)	88	*Radium	Ra	226.0254
9	Fluorine	F	18.998403	86	Radon	Rn	(222)
87	Francium	Fr	(223)	75	Rhenium	Re	186.207
64	Gadolinium	Gd	157.25	45	Rhodium	Rh	102.9055
31	Gallium	Ga	69.723	37	Rubidium	Rb	85.4678
32	Germanium	Ge	72.59	44	Ruthenium	Ru	101.07
79	Gold	Au	196.9665	62	Samarium	Sm	150.36
73	Hafnium	Hf	178.49	21	Scandium	Sc	44.95591
2	Helium	He	4.002602	34	Selenium	Se	78.96
67	Holmium	Ho	164.9304	14	Silicon	Si	28.0855
1	Hydrogen	H	1.00794	47	Silver	Ag	107.8682
49	Indium	In	114.82	11	Sodium	Na	22.98977
53	Iodine	I	126.9045	38	Strontium	Sr	87.62
77	Iridium	Ir	192.22	16	Sulphur	S	32.066
26	Iron	Fe	55.847	73	Tantalum	Ta	180.9479
36	Krypton	Kr	83.80	43	Technetium	Tc	(98)

Atomic Number	Name	Symbol	Atomic Weight
52	Tellurium	Te	127.60
65	Terbium	Tb	158.9254
81	Thallium	Tl	204.383
90	Thorium	Th	232.0381
69	Thulium	Tm	168.9342
50	Tin	Sn	118.710
22	Titanium	Ti	47.88
74	Tungsten	W	183.85
106	Unnilhexium	Unh	(263)
105	Unnilpentium	Unp	(262)
104	Unnilquadium	Unq	(261)
92	Uranium	U	238.0289
23	Vanadium	V	50.9415
54	Xenon	Xe	131.29
70	Ytterbium	Yb	173.04
39	Yttrium	Y	88.9059
30	Zinc	Zn	65.39
40	Zirconium	Zr	91.224

Values in parentheses are used for certain radioactive elements whose atomic weights cannot be quoted precisely without knowledge of origin; the value given is the atomic mass number of the most stable known isotope of that element. The atomic weight of elements marked (*) is that of the best known isotope.

Mensuration Formulae

Area of a circle $= \pi r^2$, where r is the radius.
Area of a cone (curved surface) $= \pi r \sqrt{r^2 + h^2}$, where h is the height and r the radius of the base.
Area of a cylinder (curved surface) $= 2\pi rh$, where h is the height and r the radius of the base.
Area of an ellipse $= \pi ab$, where a and b are the semi-axes.
Area of a parallelogram $=$ base $\times$ height.
Area of a rectangle $=$ base $\times$ height.
Area of a rhombus $= \dfrac{\text{diagonal } a \times \text{diagonal } b}{2}$
Area of surface of a sphere $= 4\pi r^2$, where r is the radius.
Area of a trapezoid $= \frac{1}{2}(a + b)h$, where a and b are the parallel sides and h the height.
Area of a triangle $= \frac{1}{2}(\text{base} \times \text{height})$.
Circumference of a circle $= 2\pi r$, where r is the radius.
Circumference of an ellipse $= \pi\sqrt{(2a^2 + 2b^2)}$, where a and b are the semi-axes.

Volume of a cone $= \dfrac{\pi r^2 h}{3}$ where h is the height and r the radius of the base.
Volume of a cylinder $= \pi r^2 h$ where h is the height and r the radius of the base.
Volume of a pyramid
$$= \frac{\text{area of base} \times \text{perpendicular height}}{3}$$
Volume of a sphere $= \frac{4}{3}\pi r^3$ where r is the radius.

Mathematical Notation

$ab, a \cdot b, a \times b$	a multiplied by b
$a/b, \dfrac{a}{b}, ab^{-1}$	a divided by b
a^n	a raised to power n
$a^{\frac{1}{2}}, \sqrt{a}$	square root of a
$a^{\frac{1}{n}}, a^{1/n}, \sqrt[n]{a}$	nth root of a
$\langle a \rangle, \bar{a}$	mean value of a
$f(x), \mathrm{f}(x)$	function of x

Mathematical Signs and Symbols

$+$	plus
$-$	minus
$\pm$	plus or minus; more or less
$\times$	multiplied by
$\div$	divided by
$=$	equal to
$\mathrm{d} \stackrel{e}{=} \mathrm{f}$	is equal by definition to
$\neq$	not equal to
$\equiv$	identically equal to
$\approx$	approximately equal to
$\simeq$	asymptotically equal to
$\hat{=}$ or $\wedge$	corresponds to
$\propto$	proportional to, varies directly as
∞	infinity
$>$	greater than
$<$	less than
$\geq$	equal to or greater than
$\leq$	equal to or less than
$\gg$	much greater than
$\ll$	much less than
$\rightarrow$	approaches
$\parallel$	parallel to
$\perp$	perpendicular to
$\sum$	sum of
$\int$	indefinite integral
$\prod$	product of
$\sqrt{}$	square root of
$()$	parentheses
$[]$	brackets
$\{\}$	braces

'brackets'

Weights and Measures

A. The International System of Units (SI)

The International System of Units has been generally accepted in the United Kingdom and certain other countries for use in medical sciences and pharmacy. The base units of SI are:

metre (m) (length)
kilogram (kg) (mass)
second (s) (time)
ampere (A) (electric current)
kelvin (K) (thermodynamic temperature)
mole (mol) (amount of substance)
candela (cd) (luminous intensity)

The following units, derived from the base units, have special names.

hertz	$Hz = s^{-1}$	frequency
newton	$N = m\,kg\,s^{-2}$	force
pascal	$Pa = m^{-1}\,kg\,s^{-2}$	pressure
joule	$J = m^2\,kg\,s^{-2}$	energy
watt	$W = m^2\,kg\,s^{-3}$	power
coulomb	$C = s\,A$	electric charge
volt	$V = m^2\,kg\,s^{-3}\,A^{-1}$	electric potential difference
ohm	$\Omega = m^2\,kg\,s^{-3}\,A^{-2}$	electric resistance
siemens	$S = m^{-2}\,kg^{-1}\,s^3\,A^2$	electric conductance
farad	$F = m^{-2}\,kg^{-1}\,s^4\,A^2$	electric capacitance
becquerel	$Bq = s^{-1}$	activity of a radioactive source
gray	$Gy = J\,kg^{-1}$	absorbed dose of ionising radiation

Certain other units are not part of SI but will continue to be used in appropriate circumstances for the foreseeable future. They include:

minute	min	
hour	h	time
day	d	
litre	l	volume
degree Celsius	°C	temperature
electronvolt	eV	energy

The following units are in common use for various purposes and are expected to continue in use for a limited time.

ångström	Å	length
dyne	dyn	force
erg	erg	energy
stokes	St	kinematic viscosity
poise	P	dynamic viscosity
inch	in	length
pound (avoirdupois)	lb	mass
calorie	cal	energy
millimetre of mercury	mmHg	pressure
degree Fahrenheit	°F	temperature
curie	Ci	activity of a radioactive source
rad	rad	absorbed dose of ionising radiation
röntgen	R	exposure to ionising radiation

Decimal multiples and submultiples of units are denoted by the following prefixes. In practice, it is preferable to use only the thousandfold multiples, e.g. gram, milligram, microgram, nanogram.

Prefix	Symbol	Multiple or Submultiple	
exa	E	10^{18}	= 1 000 000 000 000 000 000
peta	P	10^{15}	= 1 000 000 000 000 000
tera	T	10^{12}	= 1 000 000 000 000
giga	G	10^9	= 1 000 000 000
mega	M	10^6	= 1 000 000
kilo	k	10^3	= 1 000
hecta	h	10^2	= 100
deca	da	10^1	= 10
deci	d	10^{-1}	= 0.1
centi	c	10^{-2}	= 0.01
milli	m	10^{-3}	= 0.001
micro	μ	10^{-6}	= 0.000 001
nano	n	10^{-9}	= 0.000 000 001
pico	p	10^{-12}	= 0.000 000 000 001
femto	f	10^{-15}	= 0.000 000 000 000 001
atto	a	10^{-18}	= 0.000 000 000 000 000 001

Mass (Weights)

1 kilogram (kg) is the mass of the International Prototype Kilogram

1 gram (g)	=	the 1000th part of 1 kilogram
1 milligram (mg)	=	the 1000th part of 1 gram
1 microgram (μg)	=	the 1000th part of 1 milligram
1 nanogram (ng)	=	the 1000th part of 1 microgram

Capacity (Volumes)

The litre (L) is now defined in the United Kingdom by the Units of Measurement Regulations 1986 (S.I. 1986: No. 1082) as 1 cubic decimetre.
The litre is the accepted term for general use but should not be used for measurements of high precision.

1 litre (L or l)	=	$1000\,cm^3$
1 millilitre (mL or ml)	=	the 1000th part of 1 litre
1 microlitre (μL or μl)	=	the 1000th part of 1 millilitre

Length

1 metre (m) is the Metre as defined in the Weights and Measures (International Definitions) Order 1963

1 decimetre (dm)	=	the 10th part of 1 metre
1 centimetre (cm)	=	the 100th part of 1 metre
1 millimetre (mm)	=	the 1000th part of 1 metre
1 micrometre (μm)	=	the 1000th part of 1 millimetre
1 nanometre (nm)	=	the 1000th part of 1 micrometre

Radioactivity

The curie (Ci) has been replaced as the unit of activity of radionuclides by the becquerel (Bq).

1 curie (Ci)	=	3.7×10^{10} disintegrations per second
	=	3.7×10^{10} becquerels
1 millicurie (mCi)	=	3.7×10^7 becquerels
1 microcurie (μCi)	=	3.7×10^4 becquerels

For further information on these units see the Radiopharmaceuticals chapter.

B. Imperial System of Weights and Measures

The Imperial System is no longer used in medicine and pharmacy in the United Kingdom, but is still used for domestic and general trade purposes.

Mass (Weights)

1 pound (avoirdupois) (lb) is the Imperial Pound as defined in the UK Weights and Measures Act, 1963, Schedule 1

1 ounce (avoirdupois) (oz)	= the 16th part of 1 pound
	= 437.5 grains
1 grain (gr)	= the 7000th part of 1 pound

Capacity (Volumes)

1 gallon (gal) is now defined in the United Kingdom under the Units of Measurement Regulations 1986 (S.I. 1986: No. 1082) as 4.546 09 cubic decimetres.

1 pint (pt)	= the 8th part of 1 gallon
	= 20 fluid ounces
1 fluid ounce (fl oz)	= the 20th part of 1 pint
	= 8 fluid drachms
1 fluid drachm (fl dr)	= the 8th part of 1 fluid ounce
	= 60 minims
1 minim (min)	= the 60th part of 1 fluid drachm

Relation of Capacity to Weight

The following equivalents are stated to five significant figures:

1 minim	= the volume at 16.7° (62°F) of 0.911 46 grain of water
1 fluid drachm	= the volume at 16.7° (62°F) of 54.688 grains of water
1 fluid ounce	= the volume at 16.7° (62°F) of 1 ounce (avoirdupois) or 437.5 grains of water
109.71 minims*	= the volume at 16.7° (62°F) of 100 grains of water

*Usually taken as 110 minims

Length

1 yard (yd) is the Imperial Yard as defined in the Weights and Measures Act, 1963, Schedule 1

| 1 foot (ft) | = the 3rd part of 1 yard |
| 1 inch (in.) | = the 12th part of 1 foot |

C. SI Unit Equivalents of other Metric Units

Length

1 ångström (Å) $= 10^{-10}$ metre $= 10^{-1}$ nanometre (nm)
1 micron (μ) $= 10^{-6}$ metre = 1 micrometre (μm)

Volume

1 millilitre (mL or ml) = 1 cubic centimetre (cm^3)
1 litre (L or l) = 1 cubic decimetre (dm^3)

Energy

1 kilocalorie (kcal) $= 4.186\ 8 \times 10^3$ joules
1 erg (erg) $= 10^{-7}$ joule
1 electronvolt (eV) $= 1.602\ 2 \times 10^{-19}$ joule

Pressure

1 millimetre of mercury (mmHg) = 133.322 pascals
1 bar (bar) $= 10^5$ pascals

Viscosity, Dynamic

1 poise (P) $= 10^{-1}$ pascal second (Pa s)
1 centipoise (cP) $= 10^{-3}$ pascal second
$= 10^{-3}$ newton second per square metre (N s m^{-2})

Viscosity, Kinematic

1 stokes (St) $= 10^{-4}$ square metre per second (m^2 s^{-1})
1 centistokes (cSt) $= 10^{-6}$ square metre per second

Temperature

1 degree Celsius (°C) = 1 kelvin (K)
1 degree Fahrenheit (°F) $= \frac{5}{9}$ kelvin

D. Imperial Equivalents of Metric and SI Units
Weights or Measures of Mass

1 picogram (pg)	$= 15.432 \times 10^{-12}$ grain
1 nanogram (ng)	$= 15.432 \times 10^{-9}$ grain
1 microgram (μg)	$= 15.432 \times 10^{-6}$ grain
1 milligram (mg)	= 0.015 432 grain
1 gram (g)	= 15.432 grains
	= 0.032 15 ounce (apothecaries')
	= 0.035 27 ounce (avoirdupois)
1 kilogram (kg)	= 2.204 6 pounds

Measures of Capacity

1 millilitre (mL or ml)	= 16.894 minims
1 litre (L or l)	= 0.219 97 gallon
	= 1.759 75 pints
	= 35.195 1 fluid ounces

Measures of Length

1 ångström (Å)	$= 3.9370 \times 10^{-9}$ inch
1 nanometre (nm)	$= 3.9370 \times 10^{-8}$ inch
1 micrometre (μm)	$= 3.9370 \times 10^{-5}$ inch
1 millimetre (mm)	= 0.039 370 inch
1 centimetre (cm)	= 0.393 70 inch
1 decimetre (dm)	= 3.937 0 inches
1 metre (m)	= 39.370 inches
1 kilometre (km)	= 0.621 37 mile

Pressure

1 bar (bar) = 14.50 pounds force per square inch (lbf/in^2)

E. SI and Metric Equivalents of Imperial Weights and Measures
Weights or Measures of Mass

1 grain (gr)	= 0.064 799 gram
1 ounce (avoirdupois) (437.5 gr) (oz)	= 28.350 grams
1 ounce (apothecaries') (480 gr)	= 31.104 grams
1 pound (lb)	= 453.592 grams

Measures of Capacity

1 minim (min)	= 0.059 194 millilitre
1 fluid drachm (fl dr)	= 3.551 6 millilitres
1 fluid ounce (fl oz)	= 28.413 millilitres
	= 0.028 413 litre
1 pint (pt)	= 568.261 millilitres
	= 0.568 261 litre
1 gallon (gal)	= 4.546 09 litres
1 gallon (US)	= 3.785 41 litres
	= 0.832 674 gallon (UK)

Measures of Length

1 inch (in.)	= 25.400×10^7 ångströms
	= 25.400×10^6 nanometres
	= 25.400×10^3 micrometres
	= 25.400 millimetres
1 foot (ft)	= 304.80 millimetres
1 yard (yd)	= 914.40 millimetres
1 mile	= 1.609 3 kilometres

Pressure

1 pound force per square inch (lbf/in^2) = 0.068 97 bar

Dilution of Ethanol

Dilute ethanol of various strengths may be prepared by diluting ethanol (95 per cent) with distilled water in the proportions given in the following table. Before the mixture is finally adjusted to volume it is cooled to the same temperature, about 20°, as that at which the ethanol (95 per cent) is measured.

Strength of ethanol required (v/v)	Volume of ethanol (95 per cent)	Final volume of mixture
90 per cent	947 ml	1000 ml
80 per cent	842 ml	1000 ml
70 per cent	737 ml	1000 ml
60 per cent	632 ml	1000 ml
50 per cent	526 ml	1000 ml
45 per cent	474 ml	1000 ml
25 per cent	263 ml	1000 ml
20 per cent	210 ml	1000 ml

If strengths other than those above are required, the following equation may be used:

Volume of ethanol to be used

$$= \frac{\text{volume required} \times \% \text{ required}}{\% \text{ used}}$$

EXAMPLES

(i) If 95% ethanol is available and 1000 mL of 65% ethanol is required:

$$\text{Volume to be used} = \frac{1000 \times 65}{95}$$
$$= 684\,\text{mL}$$

that is, 684 mL of 95% ethanol diluted to 1000 mL with water, gives 1000 mL of 65% ethanol.

(ii) If 71% ethanol is available and 1000 mL of 45% ethanol is required:

$$\text{Volume to be used} = \frac{1000 \times 45}{71}$$
$$= 634\,\text{mL}$$

that is, 634 mL of 71% ethanol diluted to 1000 mL with water, gives 1000 mL of 45% ethanol.

If the strength of the ethanol available is unknown, it may be determined from the specific gravity and then appropriately adjusted to the strength required. The specific gravity is determined at 20° by means of a hydrometer and the corresponding percentage of alcohol is read off from the table below. If, for example, the specific gravity at 20° is found to be 0.883, the strength of the alcohol is 71.6 per cent v/v.

Specific Gravity and Percentage by Volume of Ethanol/Water Mixtures

Specific gravity 20°/20°	Percentage of ethanol v/v	Specific gravity 20°/20°	Percentage of ethanol v/v	Specific gravity 20°/20°	Percentage of ethanol v/v	Specific gravity 20°/20°	Percentage of ethanol v/v
1.000	0						
0.999	0.67	0.939	46.22	0.879	73.17	0.819	93.34
8	1.34	8	46.76	8	73.56	8	93.61
7	2.02	7	47.30	7	73.94	7	93.88
6	2.72	6	47.83	6	74.33	6	94.15
5	3.43	5	48.36	5	74.71	5	94.41
4	4.15	4	48.88	4	75.09	4	94.67
3	4.88	3	49.40	3	74.46	3	94.93
2	5.62	2	49.92	2	75.84	2	95.18
1	6.38	1	50.43	1	76.22	1	95.44
0	7.16	0	50.94	0	76.59	0	95.69
989	7.94	929	51.44	869	76.96	809	95.93
8	8.75	8	51.93	8	77.33	8	96.17
7	9.57	7	52.42	7	77.71	7	96.41
6	10.40	6	52.90	6	78.08	6	96.65
5	11.25	5	53.39	5	78.44	5	96.89
4	12.11	4	53.87	4	78.81	4	97.12
3	12.98	3	54.35	3	79.19	3	97.35
2	13.87	2	54.82	2	79.53	2	97.58
1	14.77	1	55.30	1	79.89	1	97.80
0	15.68	0	55.77	0	80.25	0	98.02
979	16.59	919	56.24	859	80.61	799	98.24
8	17.53	8	56.70	8	80.96	8	98.46
7	18.46	7	57.16	7	81.32	7	98.67
6	19.38	6	57.62	6	81.67	6	98.88
5	20.31	5	58.08	5	82.02	5	99.09
4	21.24	4	58.54	4	82.37	4	99.29
3	22.16	3	58.99	3	82.72	3	99.49
2	23.08	2	59.44	2	83.07	2	99.69
1	23.98	1	59.88	1	83.41	1	99.89
0	24.88	0	60.33	0	83.75	0.7904	100.0
969	25.77	909	60.77	849	84.09		
8	26.65	8	61.20	8	84.43		
7	27.51	7	61.64	7	84.77		
6	28.36	6	62.07	6	85.10		
5	29.19	5	62.51	5	85.44		
4	30.01	4	62.95	4	85.77		
3	30.80	3	63.38	3	86.10		
2	31.58	2	63.81	2	86.42		
1	32.34	1	64.23	1	86.75		
0	33.09	0	64.66	0	87.07		
959	33.82	899	65.08	839	87.39		
8	34.54	8	65.50	8	87.71		
7	35.23	7	65.92	7	88.03		
6	35.92	6	66.34	6	88.34		
5	36.61	5	66.76	5	88.65		
4	37.28	4	67.17	4	88.96		
3	37.94	3	67.58	3	89.27		
2	38.59	2	67.99	2	89.58		
1	39.23	1	68.40	1	89.88		
0	39.85	0	68.80	0	90.18		
949	40.46	889	69.21	829	90.48		
8	41.07	8	69.61	8	90.78		
7	41.67	7	70.01	7	91.07		
6	42.26	6	70.41	6	91.36		
5	42.84	5	70.81	5	91.65		
4	43.42	4	71.21	4	91.94		
3	43.99	3	71.60	3	92.23		
2	44.56	2	72.00	2	92.51		
1	45.12	1	72.39	1	92.79		
0	45.68	0	72.78	0	93.06		

Temperatures of Various Freezing Mixtures

Components	Proportions by weight	Temperature (°C) at commencement	Temperature (°C) attained by the mixture
Sodium acetate (cryst.) / Water	17 / 20	10	−5
Sodium thiosulphate / Water	11 / 10	10	−8
Calcium chloride ($CaCl_2$, $6H_2O$) / Snow, or powdered ice	100 / 246	0	−9
Ammonium chloride / Snow, or powdered ice	1 / 4	0	−15
Sodium nitrate / Snow, or powdered ice	1 / 2	0	−18
Sodium chloride / Snow, or powdered ice	1 / 2	0	−18
Sodium chloride / Snow, or powdered ice	3 / 10	0	−21
Sulphuric acid, 66.1% / Snow, or powdered ice	100 / 432	0	−25
Sulphuric acid, 66.1% / Snow, or powdered ice	100 / 252	0	−30
Sulphuric acid, 66.1% / Snow, or powdered ice	10 / 11	0	−37
Calcium chloride ($CaCl_2$, $6H_2O$) / Snow, or powdered ice	100 / 81	0	−40
Calcium chloride ($CaCl_2$, $6H_2O$) / Snow, or powdered ice	4 / 3	0	−48
Calcium chloride ($CaCl_2$, $6H_2O$) / Snow, or powdered ice	10 / 7	0	−55
Alcohol at 4° / Solid carbon dioxide	— / —	below 0	−72
Chloroform / Solid carbon dioxide	— / —	below 0	−77
Ether / Solid carbon dioxide	— / —	below 0	−77

Constant Humidity Solutions

In an enclosed space a constant humidity can be maintained at a given temperature by the presence of a saturated aqueous solution in contact with an excess of solute.

The table shows the percentage relative humidity above saturated solutions at various temperatures.

Saturated salt solution	Temperature °C										
	0	5	10	15	20	25	30	35	40	50	60
Potassium Sulphate, K_2SO_4	99	98	98	97	97	97	96	96	96	96	96
Lead Nitrate, $Pb(NO_3)_2$	—	—	—	—	98	—	—	—	—	—	—
Sodium Phosphate, Na_2HPO_4, $12H_2O$	—	—	—	—	95	—	—	—	—	—	—
Potassium Nitrate, KNO_3	97	96	95	94	93	92	91	89	88	85	82
Ammonium Dihydrogen Orthophosphate, $NH_4H_2PO_4$	—	—	—	—	93	93	—	—	—	—	—
Zinc Sulphate, $ZnSO_4$, $7H_2O$	—	—	—	—	90	—	—	—	—	—	—
Potassium Chromate, K_2CrO_4	—	—	—	—	88	—	—	—	—	—	—
Potassium Chloride, KCl	89	88	88	87	86	85	84	83	82	81	80
Potassium Bisulphate, $KHSO_4$	—	—	—	—	86	—	—	—	—	—	—
Potassium Bromide, KBr	—	—	—	—	84	—	—	—	—	—	—
Ammonium Sulphate, $(NH_4)_2SO_4$	83	82	82	81	81	80	80	80	79	79	78
Ammonium Chloride, NH_4Cl	—	—	—	—	79	79	—	—	—	—	—
Sodium Chloride, NaCl	76	76	76	76	76	75	75	75	75	75	75
Sodium Acetate, $NaC_2H_3O_2$, $3H_2O$	—	—	—	—	76	—	—	—	—	—	—
Sodium Chlorate, $NaClO_3$	—	—	—	—	75	—	—	—	—	—	—
Sodium Nitrite, $NaNO_2$	—	—	—	—	66	65	63	62	62	59	59
Ammonium Nitrate, NH_4NO_3	77	74	72	69	65	62	59	55	53	47	42
Sodium Bromide, $NaBr$, $2H_2O$	—	—	—	—	58	—	—	—	—	—	—
Magnesium Nitrate, $Mg(NO_3)_2$, $6H_2O$	60	58	57	56	55	53	52	50	49	46	43
Sodium Dichromate, $Na_2Cr_2O_7$, $2H_2O$	60	59	58	56	55	54	52	51	50	47	—
Potassium Thiocyanate, KSCN	—	—	—	—	47	—	—	—	—	—	—
Potassium Carbonate, K_2CO_3	—	—	47	44	44	43	43	43	42	—	—
Zinc Nitrate, $Zn(NO_3)_2$, $6H_2O$	—	—	—	—	42	—	—	—	—	—	—
Chromium Trioxide, CrO_3	—	—	—	—	35	—	—	—	—	—	—
Magnesium Chloride, $MgCl_2$, $6H_2O$	35	34	34	34	33	33	33	32	32	31	30
Calcium Chloride, $CaCl_2$, $6H_2O$	—	—	—	—	—	*31	—	—	—	—	—
Potassium Acetate, $KC_2H_3O_2$	25	24	24	23	23	22	22	21	20	—	—
Lithium Chloride, $LiCl$, H_2O	15	14	13	13	12	12	12	12	11	11	11
Potassium Hydroxide, KOH	—	14	13	10	9	8	7	6	6	6	5

*at 24.5°.

Concentrations of Some Acids

Acid R = reagent	Molecular weight	Percent w/w	Wt per mL (g)	Grams per litre	Moles per litre
Acetic acid (CH_3CO_2H)	60.05				
Acetic acid, anhydrous R EurP, R BP		99.6	1.052[†]	1048.8	17.5
Acetic acid, glacial BP, R EurP		98.0	1.052[†]	1031.5	17.2
Acetic acid R EurP		30.0*	—	300.0	5.00
Acetic acid BP		33.0	1.041	343.5	5.72
Acetic acid, dilute R EurP		12.0*	—	120.0	2.00
Acetic acid (6%) BP		6.0	1.005	60.3	1.00
Formic acid (HCO_2H)	46.03				
Formic acid, anhydrous R EurP, R BP		98.0	1.22[†]	1195.6	26.0
Formic acid R BP		90.0	1.2	1080.0	23.5
Formic acid, dilute		25.0	1.05	262.5	5.70
Hydriodic acid (HI)	127.9				
Hydriodic acid R BP (constant boiling)		55.0	1.7	935.0	7.31
Hydriodic acid, dilute		10.0	1.1	110.0	0.86
Hydrobromic acid (HBr)	80.92				
Hydrobromic acid R BP		47.0	1.47	—	—
Hydrobromic acid, dilute		10.0	1.073	107.3	1.33
Hydrochloric acid (HCl)	36.46				
Hydrochloric acid, concentrated EurP (Hydrochloric acid BP)		36	1.18	430.7	11.8
Hydrochloric acid, dilute EurP, BP		10.0	1.046	104.6	2.87
Hydrocyanic acid (HCN)	27.03				
Stronger hydrocyanic acid		4	0.99	39.6	1.47
Dilute hydrocyanic acid		2	0.997	19.94	0.74
Hydrocyanic acid solution R BP		0.3	—	3.0	0.11
Hydrofluoric acid (HF)	20.01				
Hydrofluoric acid R EurP, R BP		40.0	1.13	452.0	22.6
Hydrofluorosilicic acid (H_2SIF_6)	144.1	30.0	1.27	381.0	2.64
Hypophosphorus acid (H_3PO_2)	66.99				
Hypophosphorus acid		31.0	1.14	353.4	5.35
Hypophosphorus acid, dilute R EurP, R BP		10.0	1.04	103.8	1.57
Lactic acid ($CH_3 \cdot CHOH \cdot CO_2H$)	90.08				
Lactic acid EurP, BP		90.0	1.2[†]	1080.0	12.0
Nitric acid (HNO_3)	63.10				
Nitric acid, fuming R EurP, R BP		95.0	1.5	1425	22.5
Nitric acid R EurP, R BP		70.0	1.42	990.5	16
Nitric acid, dilute R EurP		12.6*	—	126	2.00
Perchloric acid ($HClO_4$)	100.46				
Perchloric acid R EurP, R BP		72.0	1.7[†]	1224	12
Perchloric acid R BP		60.0	1.54	—	—
Perchloric acid, dilute BP		2.5*	—	25	0.25
Phosphoric acid (H_3PO_4)	98.00				
Phosphoric acid, concentrated EurP (Phosphoric acid BP)		87.5	1.7[†]	1488	15.2
Phosphoric acid, dilute EurP		10.0	1.054	105.4	1.08
Sulphuric acid (H_2SO_4)	98.08				
Sulphuric acid EurP, BP		98.0	1.84	1785	18.0
Sulphuric acid, dilute EurP, BP		10.0	1.067	106.7	1.09
Sulphurous acid (H_2SO_3)	82.08				
Sulphurous acid BP		5.0	1.03	66.63	0.81

*Percent w/v

[†] Relative density ≡ specific gravity

Drying Agents

Agent	Formula
Aluminium (III) oxide	Al_2O_3
Barium (II) oxide	BaO
Barium (II) perchlorate	$Ba(ClO_4)_2$
Calcium (II) bromide	$CaBr_2$
Calcium (II) chloride, fused or granular	$CaCl_2$
Calcium (II) oxide	CaO
Calcium (II) sulphate, anhydrous	$CaSO_4$
Copper (II) sulphate, anhydrous	$CuSO_4$
Magnesium (II) oxide	MgO
Magnesium (II) perchlorate, anhydrous	$Mg(ClO_4)_2$
Phosphorus (V) oxide	P_2O_5
Potassium (I) hydroxide, fused or sticks	KOH
Silica gel	$(SiO_2)_x$
Sodium (I) hydroxide, fused or sticks	NaOH
Sulphuric acid, concentrated	H_2SO_4
Zinc (II) bromide	$ZnBr_2$
Zinc (II) chloride, fused	$ZnCl_2$

Standard Wire Gauge

SWG Number	Diameter mm	SWG Number	Diameter mm
11	2.946	26	0.4572
12	2.642	27	0.4166
13	2.337	28	0.3759
14	2.032	29	0.3454
15	1.829	30	0.3150
16	1.6256	31	0.2946
17	1.4224	32	0.2743
18	1.2192	33	0.2540
19	1.0160	34	0.2337
20	0.9411	35	0.2134
21	0.8128	36	0.1930
22	0.7112	37	0.1727
23	0.6096	38	0.1524
24	0.5588	39	0.1321
25	0.5080	40	0.1219

Metric standards for metallic materials are given in British Standard 6722:1986

Roman Numerals

I	1	XX	20	CC	200
II	2	XXX	30	CCC	300
III	3	XL	40	CD	400
IV	4	L	50	D	500
V	5	LX	60	DC	600
VI	6	LXX	70	DCC	700
VII	7	LXXX	80	DCCC	800
VIII	8	XC	90	CM	900
IX	9	C	100	M	1000
X	10				

Greek Alphabet

Greek letter	Greek name	English equivalent	Greek letter	Greek name	English equivalent
A α	Alpha	a	N ν	Nu	n
B β	Beta	b	Ξ ξ	Xi	x
Γ γ	Gamma	g	O ο	Omicron	ŏ
Δ δ	Delta	d	Π π	Pi	p
E ε	Epsilon	ĕ	P ρ	Rho	r
Z ζ	Zeta	z	Σ σ	Sigma	s
H η	Eta	ē	T τ	Tau	t
Θ θ	Theta	th	Y υ	Upsilon	u
I ι	Iota	i	Φ φ	Phi	ph
K κ	Kappa	k	X χ	Chi	ch
Λ λ	Lambda	l	Ψ ψ	Psi	ps
M μ	Mu	m	Ω ω	Omega	ō

Abbreviations used in Prescriptions

While the use of Latin abbreviations in writing prescriptions has greatly declined in Great Britain, the practice is still current in many countries and the Latin abbreviations in the following lists are still occasionally encountered in prescriptions originating from abroad.

a.c.   ante cibum, *before food*
a.h.   alternis horis, *every other hour*
a.j.   ante jentaculum, *before breakfast*
a.m.   ante meridiem, *before noon*
a.p.   ante prandium, *before dinner*
aa.   ana, *of each*
ad   { 2 vic.   ad duas vices, *for two times* (twice)
       3 vic.   ad tres vices, *for three times* (thrice)
ad lib.   ad libitum, *at pleasure, to any extent*
ad neutral.   ad neutralisandum, *to neutralisation*
ad part. dolent.   ad partes dolentes, *to the painful parts*
ad sat.   ad saturandum, *to saturation*
add.   adde, *add* (imperative)
Add.   Addendum, a
addend.   { addendus, a, um, *to be added*
             addendo, *by adding* (gerund with accusative)
admov.   { admove, *apply* (imperative);
             admoveatur, *let it be applied*
             admoveantur, *let them be applied*
adv.   adversus *or* adversum (with accusative), *against*
aeg.   aeger, aegra, *the patient*
alt.   altera (pars), *the remainder;* alternus, a, um, *alternate*
altern. d.   alterno die,
altern. dieb.   alternis diebus, } *every other day*
amp.   amplus, a, um, *full, large; also* ampulla, *ampoule*
ante, *before*   { coen.   coenam, *supper* (often *dinner*)
                    jentac.   jentaculum, *breakfast*
                    prand.   prandium, *dinner*
aper.   aperiens, *an aperient*
applic.   { applicandus, a, um, *to be applied*
            applicatio, *an application*
            applicetur, applicentur, *let it, let them, be applied*
aq.   aqua, *water*
Aq. ad—   Aquam ad— (governed by Recipe), *water up to*—
aq. bull.   aqua bulliens, entis, *boiling water*
aq. calid.   aqua calida, *warm or hot water*

aq. comm.   aqua communis, *common or plain water*
aq. dest.   aqua destillata, *distilled water*
aq. ferv.   aqua fervens, entis, *boiling water*
aq. gel.   aqua gelida, *cold water*
aq. pur.   aqua pura, *pure water*
Aquae ad—(quantum sufficiat, *or* quantitatem sufficientem *understood*), *water up to*—
arg.   argentum, *silver*
aug.   augeatur, *let it be increased*
aur.   aurum, *gold;* auris, *the ear*
aur. dextr. (laev.)   auri dextrae (laevae), *to right (left) ear*
   ad aur.   ad aurem, *to the ear*
   p. aur.   pone aurem, *behind the ear*
aurist, auristillae, *ear-drops*

b.   bis, *twice*
B.N.F.   *British National Formulary*
B.P.   *British Pharmacopoeia*
B.P.C.   *British Pharmaceutical Codex*
B.P.(Vet.)   *British Pharmacopoeia (Veterinary)*
B. Vet. C.   *British Veterinary Codex*
baln.   balneum, *bath*
bals.   balsamum, *balsam*
bib.   bibe, *drink* (imperative)
bid.   biduum, *two days*
bis   { d.   bis die
        d.d.   bis de die } *or* bis in d.: bis in die, *twice a day*
brach.   brachium, *the arm*
brev.   brevis, e, *short*
buginar.   buginarium, *a bougie*
bull.   bulliens, *boiling;* bulliat, *let it boil*

C.   congius, *a gallon;* C. centum, *100;* c. cum, *with*
c.c.   *cubic centimetre*
c.l.q.s.   cuilibet quantum sufficiat, *as you please, a sufficient quantity*
c.m.   cras mane, *tomorrow morning;* c.m.s.: cras mane sumendus, a, um, *to be taken tomorrow morning*
c.n.   cras nocte, *tomorrow night*
c.v.   cras vespere, *tomorrow evening*
c. vin.   cyathus vinosus *or* vinarius, *a wine-glass*
calid.   calidus, a, um, *warm or hot*
cap.   { capiat, *let him take*
         capiatur, *let it be taken*
         capiantur, *let them be taken*
         capsula, *a capsule*
cataplasm,   cataplasma, *a poultice*
cib.   cibus, *food*

circ.   circa, *around; or* circiter, *about*

co.   compositus, a, um, *compound*

cochleat.   cochleatim, *by spoonfuls*

collut.   collutorium, *a mouth-wash*

collyr.   collyrium, *an eye lotion*

comp.   compositus, a, um, *compound*

conc.   concentratus, a, um, *concentrated; or* concisus, a, um, *sliced*

conf.   confectio, *a confection*

cong.   congius, *a gallon*

conserv.   conserva, ae, *a conserve;* conserva, *keep* (imperative)

conspers.   conspersus, *a dusting-powder*

cont.   contusus, a, um, *bruised*

contrit.   contritus, a, um, *pounded*

coq.   coque, *boil* (imperative)

corp.   corpori, *to the body*

cort.   cortex, corticis, *bark*

crast.   crastinus, a, um, *of tomorrow; tomorrow's*

crem.   cremor, *a cream*

cryst.   crystallus, *a crystal;* crystallisatus, a, um, *crystallised*

cuj.   cujus, *of which*

cujusl.   cujuslibet, *of any*

cyath.   cyathus, *glass*

cyath. vinos.   cyathus vinosus, *wine-glass*

d.   dosis, *dose; or* dies, *a day*

d.d.   de die, *daily*

d. in dup.   detur in duplo, *let twice as much be given*

d. in p. aeq.   divide in partes aequales, *divide into equal parts*

d.p.   directione propria, *with proper direction*

d.p.c.   dosi pedetentim crescente, *the dose gradually increasing*

D.P.F.   *Dental Practitioners' Formulary*

d.s.   { da, signa, *give and label*
       { detur, signetur, *let it be given and labelled*

d. secund., tert., etc.   diebus secundis, tertiis, etc., *every second, third day,* etc.

d. seq.   die sequente, *on the following day*

D.T.   *Drug Tariff*

d. t. d.   dentur tales doses, *let such doses be given*

D.T.F.   *Drug Tariff Formulary*

dand.   dandus, a, um, *to be given*

de d. in d.   de die in diem, } *daily, or*

de d.   de die, } *from day to day*

dec.   decoctum, *a decoction*

decub.   decubitus, *lying down*

deglut.   deglutiatur, *let it be swallowed*

dent. ad scat.   dentur ad scatulam, *let them be put in a box*

dest.   destillatus, a, um, *distilled*

det.   detur, *let it be given*

dext. lat.   dextro lateri, *to the right side*

dieb. altern.   diebus alternis, *every other day*

dil.   dilutus, a, um, *diluted*

dim.   dimidium (subs.), *the half;* dimidius, a, um, *half*

div.   divide, *divide* (imperative)

dol. urg.   dolore urgente, *when the pain is severe*

dolent. part.   dolenti parti, *to the afflicted part*

donec dol. exulav.   donec dolor exulaverit [*also* exsulaverit], *until the pain is relieved*

dos.   dosis, *a dose*

dr.   drachma, *a drachm*

dulc.   dulcis, e, *sweet*

dup. }
dx. } duplex, *double*

dur.   durus, a, um, *hard*

dur. dol.   durante dolore, *while the pain lasts*

e.m.p.   ex modo praescripto, *in the manner prescribed*

e paul. aq.   e paulo aquae, *in a little water*

e quol. vehic. idon.   e quolibet vehiculo idoneo, *in any suitable vehicle*

ead.   eadem, *the same*

ejusd.   ejusdem, *of the same*

elect.   electuarium, *an electuary*

elect. [*commercial*] electus, a, um, *picked, select, choice*

emet.   emeticum, *an emetic*

emp.   emplastrum, *a plaster*

enem.   enema, *an enema*

esur.   esuriens, *fasting,* i.e. *before food*

ex aq.   ex aqua, *in water*

ex. aq. coch. ampl.   ex aquae cochleari amplo, *in a tablespoonful of water*

ex. aq. cyath. vinos.   ex aquae cyatho vinoso, *in a wine-glass of water*

ex paul.   ex paulo (e paulo), *in a little*

exprim. exprime, *express, squeeze out* (imperative)

ex.   extractum, *an extract*

extempl.   extemplo, *immediately*

extend.   extende, *spread* (imperative)

f., ft.   fiat (fiant), *let it (them) be made*

f. m. *or* ft. mist.   fiat mistura, *let a mixture be made*

filtr.   filtra, *filter;* filtrum, *a filter*

fl.   fluidus, *liquid*

flav.   flavus, a, um, *yellow*

fol.   folium, *a leaf*

fort.   fortis, e, *strong*

freq.   frequenter, *frequently*

frigid. frigidus, a, um, *cold*

frust. frustillum, *a small portion;* frustillatim, *in small pieces*

ft. haust. fiat haustus, *let a draught be made*

ft. pil. fiat pilula, *or* fiant pilulae, *let a pill,* or *pills, be made*

ft. pulv. fiat pulvis, *let a powder be made*

fusc. fuscus, a, um, *brown*

G., g., gm., grm. gramma, *a gram*

gall. gallicus, *French*

garg. gargarisma, *a gargle*

gr. granum, *a grain*

grad. gradatim, *by degrees*

gtt. guttae, *drops;* guttat.: guttatim, *drop by drop*

guttur. appl. gutturi applicandus, a, um, *to be applied to the throat*

h. hora [ablative], *at the hour of*

h. d. hora decubitus, *at bedtime*

h. s. hora somni, *at bedtime*

hab. habeat, *let him have* (or *take*); habeantur, *let them be taken*

hac noct. hac nocte, *tonight*

haust. haustus, *a draught*

i.c. inter cibos, *between meals*

id. idem, *the same*

impet. efferv. impetu effervescentiae, *during effervescence*

imprans. impransus, a, um, *fasting*

in d. in dies, *from day to day*

in loc. frig. in loco frigido, *in a cool place*

in p. aeq. in partes aequales, *in* (i.e. *into*) *equal parts*

incis. incisus, a, um, *cut, sliced*

inf. infusum, *an infusion*

infric. { infricetur, *let it be rubbed in* / infricandus, a, um, *to be rubbed in*

infund. infunde, *pour in* (imperative)

infus. infusa, *infuse* (imperative)

inj. injectio, *an injection*

inj. enem. injiciatur enema, *let an enema be administered*

insip. insipidus, a, um, *tasteless*

insp. inspissare, *to thicken*

insuff. insufflatio, *an insufflation*

int. inter, *between*

intim. intime, *intimately*

involv. involvere, *to roll in*

irrig. irrigatio, *an irrigation*

jentac. jentaculum, *breakfast*

jusc. jusculum, *broth*

l. lac, *milk;* litra, atis, *or* litrum, *litre*

laev. laevus, a, um, *left, on the left side*

lat. dol. lateri dolenti, *to the affected side*

lb., lib. libra, *a pound*

lig. lignum, *wood*

liq. liquor, *a solution*

lot. lotio, *a lotion*

luc. p. luce prima, *early in the morning (at the first light)*

m. mane, *in the morning*

m. minimum, *a minim*

m. misce, *mix* (bene), *well;* (intime), *thoroughly* (s.a. secundum artem), *pharmaceutically*

m. d. more dicto, *as directed*

M. D. S. misce, da, signa, *mix, give, and label*

m. d. u. more dicto utendus, a, um, *to be used as directed*

m. et v. mane et vespere, *morning and evening*

m. ft. mist. misce, fiat mistura, *mix, and let a mixture be made*

m. p. mane primo, *early in the morning;* or massa pilularum, *a pill mass*

m. q. dx. mitte quantitatem duplicem, *send double quantity*

m. s. more solito, *in the usual manner*

m. seq. mane sequenti, *on the following morning*

mass. massa, *a pill mass*

min. minimum, *a minim*

mist. mistura, *a mixture*

mitt. mitte, *send;* mittatur, *let it be sent;* mittantur, *let them be sent*

mitt. in phial. mittantur in phialam, *let them be put into a phial*

mod. *or* { dict.   modo *or* { dicto,
mor.   { praes. }   more   { praescripto, }
  as prescribed

moll. mollis, e, *soft*

n. nocte, *at night*

n. a. non altera, *no alternative*

n. et m. *or* n. mque. nocte maneque, *night and morning*

N.F. *National Formulary*

n.p. nomen proprium, *the proper name;* or nomine proprio, *with (by) the proper name*

N.W.F. *National War Formulary*

narist. naristillae, *nasal drops*

neb. nebula, *a spray*

nig.   niger, ra, rum, *black*

nim.   nimis, *too much*

no.   numero, *in number*

noct.   nocte, *at night*

non rep.   non repetatur, *do not repeat it*

nov.   novus, a, um, *new*

O.   octarius, *a pint*

o. alt. hor.   omnibus alternis horis, *every other hour*

o. h.   omni hora, *every hour*

o. m.   omni mane, *every morning*

o.n.   omni nocte, *every night*

ocul.   oculo, *to (for) the eye*

oculent.   oculentum, *an eye ointment*

ol.   oleum, *oil*

omn. bid.   omni biduo, *every two days*

op.   ope, *by means of*

opt.   optimus, a, um, *best*

ov.   ovum, *an egg*

oz.   uncia, *an ounce (avoidupois)*

P.   pondere, *by weight*

p. a. a.   parti affectae applicandus, a, um, *to be applied to the affected part*

p. aeq.   partes aequales, *equal parts*

p. c.   per centum, *per cent;* or post cibum, *after food*

p. d.   pro dosi, *for a dose*

p. m.   post meridiem, *afternoon;* primo mane, *early in the morning*

p. r. n.   pro re nata, *occasionally, when required*

part. affect.   parti affectae, *to the affected part*

part. dolent.   parti dolenti, *to the painful part*

part. vic.   partitis vicibus, *in divided doses*

parv.   parvus, a, um, *small*

past.   pasta, *a paste;* pastillus, *a pastille*

ped.   pedetentim, *gradually*

per bid., trid.   per biduum, triduum, *for a period of two,* or *three, days*

pess.   pessus, *a pessary*

Ph. Eur.   Pharmacopoeia Europaea, *European Pharmacopoeia*

Ph.I.   Pharmacopoea Internationalis, *International Pharmacopoeia*

phial.   phiala, *a phial*

pig.   pigmentum, *a paint*

poc.   poculum, *a cup*

pond.   ponderosus, a, um, *heavy*

post jentac.   post jentaculum, *after breakfast*

post prand.   post prandium, *after dinner*

ppt.   praecipitatus, a, um, *precipitated*

praep.   praeparatus, a, um, *prepared*

pro pot. s.   pro potu sumendus, a, um, *to be taken as a drink*

pro rat. aet.   pro ratione aetatis, *according to age*

prox. luc.   proxima luce, *on the next day*

pulv.   { pulverisatus, a, um, *powdered* / pulvis, *a powder* }

pv.   parvus, a, um, *small*

q. d.   quater die, *four times a day*

q. dx.   quantitas duplex, *a double quantity*

q. l.   quantum libet, / q. p.   quantum placet, } *as much as you please*

q. s.   quantum sufficiat, quantitas sufficiens, *or* quantum satis, *sufficient*

q. v.   quantum volueris, *as much as you please*

q. v.   quod vide, *which see*

qq.   quaque, *every*

q. q. h., 4ta qq. hor.   quarta quaque hora, *every fourth hour*

quart.   quartus, a, um, *the fourth*

quat.   quater, *four times*

-que,   *and* (enclitic)

quol. man.   quolibet mane, *any morning*

quot.   quotidie, *daily*

R.   recipe, *take*

r. in pulv.   redactus in pulverem, *reduced to powder*

rad.   radix, *a root*

rect.   rectificatus, a, um, *rectified*

redig. in pulv.   redigatur in pulverem, *let it be reduced to powder*

reg.   regioni, *to the region*

reg.   { cor. / epigast. / hepat. / umbilic. } regioni { cordis, *of the heart* / epigastricae, *pit of the stomach* / hepatis, *of the liver* / umbilici, *of the navel* }

rep.   { repetat, *let him repeat* / repetatur, *let it be repeated* / repetantur, *let them be repeated* }

s.   { sumat, *let him take* / sumatur, *let it be taken* / sumantur, *let them be taken* / sumendus, a, um, *to be taken* }

s.g. or sp. gr.   *specific gravity*

s.o.s.   si opus sit, *if there is need, if occasion requires, if necessary*

s.s.s.   stratum super stratum, *layer upon layer*

S.V.M.   spiritus vini methylatus, *methylated spirit*

S.V.R.   spiritus vini rectificatus, *rectified spirit*
S.V.T.   spiritus vini tenuior, *proof spirit*
scat.   scatula, *a box*
sem. in die   semel in die, *once a day*
semih.   semihora, *half an hour*
seq. luc.   sequenti luce, *the following day*
serv.   serva, *keep* (imperative)
sesquih.   sesquihora, *an hour and a half*
sesunc.   sesuncia, *an ounce and a half*
sig.   signa, signetur, signentur, *label, let it (them) be labelled*
sing.   singulorum, *of each*
sing. auror.   singulis auroris, *every morning*
sing. hor. quad.   singulis horae quadrantibus, *every quarter of an hour*
sinist.   sinister, *left, on the left*
solv.   solve, *dissolve; also* solvellae, *solution-tablets*
sp.   spiritus, *spirit*
ss.   semisse (ablative), *from* semis, semissis (genitive), *the half*
st.   stet, stent, *let it (them) stand*
stat.   statim, *immediately*
stat. eff.   statu effervescentiae, *whilst effervescing*
succ.   succus, *juice*
suff.   sufficiens, *sufficient*
sug.   sugatur, *let it be sucked*
sugend.   sugendus, a, um, *to be sucked*
sum.   { sumat, *let him take*
sumatur, *let it be taken*
sumantur, *let them be taken*
sumendus, a, um, *to be taken.*
sum. tal.   sumat talem, tales, *let the patient take one (or more) such*

sumend.   sumendus, a, um, *to be taken*
supp.   suppositorium, *a suppository*
syr.   syrupus, *syrup*

t.   ter, *thrice*
t. d. d.   ter de die, *thrice a day*
t. d. s.   ter die sumendus, a, um, *to be taken three times a day*
t. i. d.   ter in die, *three times a day*
tab.   tabletta, *or* tabella, *a tablet*
tinct.   tinctura, *a tincture*
tr.   tinctura, *a tincture*
trit.   tritura, *triturate* (imperative)
troch.   trochiscus, *a lozenge*
tuss.   tussis, *a cough*
tuss. urg.   tussi urgente, *when the cough is troublesome*

u.   utendus, a, um, *to be used*
ult. praescrip.   ultimo praescriptus, a, um, etc., *the last ordered*
ung.   unguentum, *an ointment*
U.S.P.   *Pharmacopeia of the United States of America*
ut ant.   ut ante, *as before*
ut dict.   ut dictum, *as directed*
ut direct.   ut directum, *as directed*
ut supr.   ut supra, *as above*
utend.   utendus, a, um, *to be used*

v.   vespere, *in the evening*
vap.   vapor, *an inhalation*
vitrell.   vitrella, *a crushable glass ampoule*

Displacement Values of Powder Injections

Reconstitution and dosage guidelines for powder injections
(compiled by Mr Peter Mulholland, Southern General Hospital, Glasgow)

Drug	Displacement volume	Reconstitute with	Final volume	Dosage guide
Cardiovascular system				
Alteplase 50 mg (Actilyse, Boehringer)	Zero	50 mL water	50 mL	1 mg in 1 mL
Anistreplase 30 units (Eminase, SB)	0.1 mL/30 units	4.9 mL water	5 mL	6 units in 1 mL
Epoprostenol 500 µg (Flolan, Wellcome)	Negligible	50 mL diluent	50 mL	10 µg in 1 mL
Hydralazine 20 mg (Apresoline, Ciba)	0.14 mL/ 20 mg	0.86 mL water	1 mL	20 mg in 1 mL
Sodium Nitroprusside 50 mg (Nipride, Roche)	Negligible	2 mL diluent	2 mL	25 mg in 1 mL
Streptokinase 1,500,000 units (Streptase, Hoechst)	Zero	50 mL sodium chloride	50 mL	30,000 units in 1 mL
Urokinase 5,000 units (Leo)	Zero	2 mL water	2 mL	2,500 units in 1 mL
Central nervous system				
Amylobarbitone Sodium 500 mg	0.33 mL/ 500 mg	49.67 mL water	50 mL	For a 1% solution
(Sodium Amytal, Lilly)		4.67 mL water	5 mL	For a 10% solution
Botulinum Toxin 500 units (Dysport, Porton)	Zero	2.5 mL water	2.5 mL	200 units in 1 mL
Diamorphine 5 mg (Napp)	0.06 mL/ 5 mg	0.94 mL water	1 mL	5 mg in 1 mL
Sodium Valproate 400 mg (Epilim I/V, Sanofi)	0.35 mL/ 400 mg	3.65 mL diluent	4 mL	100 mg in 1 mL
Infections				
Acyclovir 250 mg (Zovirax, Wellcome)	Negligible	10 mL water	10 mL	25 mg in 1 mL
Amoxycillin 250 mg (Amoxil, Bencard)	0.2 mL/ 250 mg	1.8 mL water	2 mL	125 mg in 1 mL
Amphotericin 50 mg (Fungizone, Squibb)	Negligible	10 mL water	10 mL	5 mg in 1 mL
Amphotericin Liposomal 50 mg (AmBisome, Vestar)	0.5 mL/50 mg	12 mL water	12.5 mL	4 mg in 1 mL
Ampicillin 250 mg (Penbritin, Beecham)	0.2 mL/ 250 mg	1.8 mL water	2 mL	125 mg in 1 mL
Ampiclox (Beecham)	0.4 mL/ 500 mg	1.6 mL water	2 mL	250 mg in 1 mL
Azlocillin 500 mg (Securopen, Bayer)	0.37 mL/ 500 mg	4.63 mL water	5 mL	100 mg in 1 mL
Aztreonam 500 mg (Azactam, Squibb)	0.4 mL/ 500 mg	3.6 mL water	4 mL	125 mg in 1 mL

Drug	Displacement volume	Reconstitute with	Final volume	Dosage guide
Benzylpenicillin 600 mg (Crystapen, Brittania)	0.4 mL/ 600 mg	1.6 mL water	2 mL	300 mg in 1 mL
Capreomycin 1 g (Capastat, Dista)	0.7 mL/ gram	2.3 mL water	3 mL	300 mg in 0.9 mL
Carbenicillin 1 g (Pyopen, Goldshield)	0.75 mL/ gram	3.25 mL water	4 mL	250 mg in 1 mL
Cefodizime 1 g (Timecef, Roussel)	0.56 mL/ gram	3.44 mL water	4 mL	250 mg in 1 mL
Cefotaxime 500 mg (Claforan, Roussel)	0.2 mL/ 500 mg	1.8 mL water	2 mL	250 mg in 1 mL
Cefoxitin 1 g (Mefoxin, MSD)	0.5 mL/ gram	2 mL water	2.5 mL	400 mg in 1 mL
Cefsulodin 1 g (Monaspor, Ciba)	0.65 mL/ gram	3.35 mL water	4 mL	250 mg in 1 mL
Ceftazidime 500 mg (Fortum, Glaxo)	0.45 mL/ 500 mg	1.55 mL water	2 mL	250 mg in 1 mL
Ceftizoxime 500 mg (Cefizox, Wellcome)	0.3 mL/ 500 mg	2.2 mL water	2.5 mL	200 mg in 1 mL
Ceftriaxone 250 mg (Rocephin, Roche)	0.19 mL/ 250 mg	4.81 mL water	5 mL	50 mg in 1 mL
Cefuroxime 250 mg (Zinacef, Glaxo)	0.18 mL/ 250 mg	1.82 mL water	2 mL	125 mg in 1 mL
Cephamandole 500 mg (Kefadol, Dista)	0.35 mL/ 500 mg	1.15 mL water	1.5 mL	250 mg in 0.75 mL
Cephazolin 500 mg (Kefzol, Dista)	0.3 mL/ 500 mg	2.2 mL water	2.5 mL	200 mg in 1 mL
Cephradine 500 mg (Velosef, Squibb)	0.4 mL/ 500 mg	2.1 mL water	2.5 mL	200 mg in 1 mL
Chloramphenicol 300 mg (Chloromycetin, Parke Davis)	0.25 mL/ 300 mg	11.75 mL water	12 mL	25 mg in 1 mL
Chloramphenicol 1 g (Kemicetine, Farmitalia)	0.8 mL/ gram	9.2 mL water	10 mL	100 mg in 1 mL
Chloramphenicol 1.2 g (Chloromycetin, Parke Davis)	1 mL/1.2 g	11 mL water	12 mL	100 mg in 1 mL
Cloxacillin 250 mg (Orbenin, Beecham)	0.2 mL/ 250 mg	1.8 mL water	2 mL	125 mg in 1 mL
Co-Amoxiclav 600 mg (Augmentin, Beecham)	0.5 mL/ 600 mg	9.5 mL water	10 mL	60 mg in 1 mL
Co-Fluampicil 500 mg (Magnapen, Beecham)	0.4 mL/ 500 mg	1.6 mL water	2 mL	250 mg in 1 mL
Colistin 1 megaunit (Colomycin, Pharmax)	0.02 mL/ million units	1.98 mL water	2 mL	500,000 units in 1 mL

Drug	Displacement volume	Reconstitute with	Final volume	Dosage guide
Erythromycin 1 g (Abbott)	Allowed for	20 mL water	22 mL	Contains 1 g in 20 mL 50 mg in 1 mL
Flucloxacillin 250 mg (Floxapen, Beecham)	0.2 mL/ 250 mg	1.8 mL water	2 mL	125 mg in 1 mL
Fusidate Sodium 500 mg (Fucidin, Leo)	Negligible	10 mL buffer	10 mL	50 mg in 1 mL
Ganciclovir 500 mg (Cymevene, Syntex)	0.29 mL/ 500 mg	9.71 mL water	10 mL	50 mg in 1 mL
Imipenem/Cilastatin 250 mg (Primaxin, MSD)	Negligible	50 mL water	50 mL	5 mg in 1 mL
Kanamycin 1 g (Kannasyn, Sanofi Winthrop)	0.8 mL/g	4.2 mL water	5 mL	200 mg in 1 mL
Mecillinam 400 mg (Selexidin, Leo)	0.1 mL/ 400 mg	1.9 mL water	2 mL	200 mg in 1 mL
Methicillin 1 g (Celbenin, Goldshield)	0.7 mL/g	1.8 mL water	2.5 mL	400 mg in 1 mL
Pentamidine 300 mg (Pentacarinat, RPR)	0.15 mL/ 300 mg	3.85 mL water	4 mL	75 mg in 1 mL
Piperacillin 1 g (Pipril, Lederle)	0.73 mL/g	3.27 mL water	4 mL	250 mg in 1 mL
Polymyxin B Sulphate 500,000 units (Aerosporin, Wellcome)	Zero	1 mL water	1 mL	500,000 units in 1 mL
Procaine Penicillin 3 megaunits (Bicillin, Brocades)	1.4 mL/vial	4.6 mL water	6 mL	500,000 units in 1 mL
Rifampicin 300 mg (Rifadin, Merrell; Rimactane, Ciba)	0.24 mL/ 300 mg	4.76 mL solvent	5 mL	60 mg in 1 mL
Spectinomycin 2 g (Trobicin, Upjohn)	1.8 mL/2 g	3.2 mL diluent	5 mL	400 mg in 1 mL
Streptomycin 1 g (Evans)	0.75 mL/g	1.25 mL water	2 mL	500 mg in 1 mL
Tazocin 2.25 g (Lederle)	0.7 mL/g	13.4 mL water	15 mL	150 mg in 1 mL
Teicoplanin 200 mg (Targocid, Merrell)	Allowed for	3 mL diluent	3 mL	50 mg in 0.75 mL
Temocillin 500 mg (Temopen, Bencard)	0.35 mL/ 500 mg	1.65 mL water	2 mL	250 mg in 1 mL
Tetracycline 100 mg (Achromycin, Lederle)	0.3 mL/ 100 mg	2.2 mL water	2.5 mL	40 mg in 1 mL
Tetracycline 250 mg (Achromycin I/V, Lederle)	0.15 mL/ 250 mg	4.85 mL water	5 mL	50 mg in 1 mL
Ticarcillin 1 g (Ticar, Goldshield)	0.7 mL/g	3.3 mL water	4 mL	250 mg in 1 mL
Timentin 800 mg (Beecham)	0.55 mL/ 800 mg	4.45 mL water	5 mL	160 mg in 1 mL
Vancomycin 500 mg (Vancocin, Lilly)	0.3 mL/ 500 mg	9.7 mL water	10 mL	50 mg in 1 mL

Drug	Displacement volume	Reconstitute with	Final volume	Dosage guide
Endocrine system				
Calcitonin 160 units (Calcitare, RPR)	Negligible	1 mL diluent	1 mL	160 units in 1 mL
Glucagon 1 unit (Lilly)	0.04 mL	0.96 mL diluent	1 mL	1 unit in 1 mL
Hydrocortisone Sodium Succinate 100 mg (Solu-Cortef, Upjohn)	0.05 mL/ 100 mg	1.95 mL water	2 mL	50 mg in 1 mL
Liothyronine 20 μg (Triiodothyronine, Evans)	Zero	1 mL water	1 mL	20 μg in 1 mL
Methylprednisolone 40 mg (Solu-Medrone, Upjohn)	Zero	1 mL diluent	1 mL	40 mg in 1 mL
Obstetrics and gynaecology				
Indomethacin 1 mg (Indocid PDA, Morson)	Zero	2 mL water	2 mL	500 μg in 1 mL
Malignant disease and immunosuppression				
Aclarubicin 20 mg (Aclacin, Lundbeck)	Zero	10 mL water	10 mL	2 mg in 1 mL
Actinomycin D 500 μg (Cosmegen Lyovac, MSD)	Allowed for	1.1 mL water		500 μg in 1 mL
Azathioprine 50 mg (Imuran, Wellcome)	0.05 mL/ 50 mg	4.95 mL water	5 mL	10 mg in 1 mL
Bleomycin 15 units (Lundbeck)	Weight varies as preparation has been purified. Ampoules contain 7 to 8 mg of powder			
Carmustine 100 mg (BiCNU, Bristol Myers)	Negligible	3 mL diluent then 27 mL water	30 mL	100 mg in 30 mL
Corynebacterium Parvum 7 mg (Coparavax, Wellcome)	Negligible	1 mL sodium chloride 0.9%	1 mL	7 mg in 1 mL
Cristantaspase 10,000 units (Erwinase, Porton)	Zero	1 mL water	1 mL	10,000 units in 1 mL
Cyclophosphamide 100 mg (Farmitalia)	0.1 mL/ 100 mg	4.9 mL water	5 mL	20 mg in 1 mL
Cytarabine 100 mg (Cytosar, Upjohn)	0.06 mL/ 100 mg	4.94 mL water	5 mL	20 mg in 1 mL
Dacarbazine 100 mg (DTIC Dome, Bayer)	0.1 mL/ 100 mg	9.9 mL water	10 mL	10 mg in 1 mL
Doxorubicin 10 mg (Doxorubicin RD, Farmitalia)	0.03 mL/ 10 mg	4.97 mL water	5 mL	2 mg in 1 mL
Epirubicin 10 mg (Pharmorubicin RD, Farmitalia)	0.03 mL/ 10 mg	4.97 mL water	5 mL	2 mg in 1 mL
Idarubicin 5 mg (Zavedos, Farmitalia)	Negligible	5 mL water	5 mL	1 mg in 1 mL

Drug	Displacement volume	Reconstitute with	Final volume	Dosage guide
Ifosfamide 500 mg (Mitoxana, ASTA)	Final volume of solution = $\dfrac{(\text{Conc ifosfamide (\%)} \times \text{mL water added} \times 0.7)}{100}$ +ml water added eg, Add 6.25 mL water to 500 mg vial to give 8% solution then final volume $= \dfrac{(8 \times 6.25 \times 0.7)}{100} + 6.25$ $= 6.6\,\text{mL}$ (100 mg in 1.32 mL)			
Interferon 3 megaunits (Intron A, Schering Plough)	Zero	1 mL water	1 mL	3 megaunits in 1 mL
Interferon 3 megaunits (Roferon A, Roche)	0.1 mL	0.9 mL water	1 mL	3 megaunits in 1 mL
Melphalan 100 mg (Alkeran, Wellcome)	Negligible	1.8 mL Wellcome Acid-Alcohol solvent followed by 9 mL Wellcome diluent	100 mg in in 10.8 mL	
Mitomycin 2 mg (Mitomycin C Kyowa, Martindale)	Negligible	5 mL water	5 mL	400 μg in 1 mL
Mustine 10 mg (Boots)	Negligible	10 mL water	10 mL	1 mg in 1 mL
Plicamycin 2.5 mg (Mithracin, Pfizer)	0.1 mL/ 2.5 mg	4.9 mL water	5 mL	500 μg in 1 mL
Polyestradiol Phosphate 40 mg (Estradurin, Kabi Pharmacia)	0.05 to 0.25 mL	2 mL water	2.05 to 2.25 mL	

Drug	Displacement volume	Reconstitute with	Final volume	Dosage guide
Thiotepa 15 mg (Lederle)	0.1 mL	1.4 mL water	1.5 mL	10 mg in 1 mL
Treosulphan 250 mg (Medac)	2.5 mL/5 g	97.5 mL water	100 mL	2.5 mg in 1 mL
Vinblastine 10 mg (Velbe, Lilly)	Negligible	10 mL diluent	10 mL	1 mg in 1 mL
Vindesine 5 mg (Eldisine, Lilly)	Negligible	5 mL diluent	5 mL	1 mg in 1 mL
Nutrition and blood				
Desferrioxamine 500 mg (Desferal, Ciba)	0.4 mL/ 500 mg	4.6 mL water	5 mL	100 mg in 1 mL
Erythropoietin 2,000 units (Recormon, Boehringer Mannheim)	Zero	2 mL water	2 mL	1,000 units in 1 mL
Solivito N (Kabi Pharmacia)	0.3 mL	9.7 mL water	10 mL	
Musculoskeletal and joint diseases				
Hyaluronidase 1,500 units (Hyalase, CP)	Zero	1 mL water	1 mL	1,500 units in 1 mL
Anaesthesia				
Methohexitone 100 mg (Brietal, Sodium, Lilly	0.07 mL/ 100 mg	9.93 mL water	10 mL	For a 1% solution
Thiopentone 2.5 g (Intraval, RPR)	1.5 mL/ 2.5 g	98.5 mL water	100 mL	For a 2.5% solution

Part II Monographs on Drug Substances

Acetazolamide (BAN, rINN)

Carbonic anhydrase inhibitor

Acetazolam
N-(5-Sulphamoyl-1,3,4-thiadiazol-2-yl)acetamide;   *N*-[5-(amino-sulphonyl)-1,3,4-thiadiazol-2-yl]-acetamide
$C_4H_6N_4O_3S_2 = 222.2$

Acetazolamide Sodium (BANM, rINNM)

$C_4H_5N_4O_3S_2$, Na = 244.2
CAS—59-66-5 (acetazolamide); 1424-27-7 (acetazolamide sodium)

Pharmacopoeial status

BP, USP (acetazolamide)

Preparations

Compendial
Acetazolamide Tablets BP.
Tablets containing, in each, 250 mg are usually available.
Acetazolamide Tablets USP.
Sterile Acetazolamide Sodium USP. A freshly prepared solution (1 in 10) has a pH of 9.0 to 10.0.

Non-compendial
Diamox (Lederle). *Capsules* (Diamox SR), sustained release, acetazolamide 250 mg.
Tablets, acetazolamide 250 mg.
Injection (Sodium Parenteral), powder for reconstitution, acetazolamide (as sodium salt) 500 mg, with sodium hydroxide to adjust pH to approximately 9.2. To be reconstituted with at least 5 mL of water for injections before use. Reconstituted solutions contain no preservative and should be used immediately or within 24 hours if stored in a refrigerator (2° to 8°).

Containers and storage

Solid state
Acetazolamide USP should be preserved in well-closed containers.

Dosage forms
Acetazolamide Tablets USP should be preserved in well-closed containers.
Sterile Acetazolamide Sodium USP should be preserved in containers for sterile solids, preferably of Type III glass.
Diamox tablets and Diamox Sodium Parenteral should be stored at controlled room temperature (15° to 25°) in their original packs or in containers that protect from moisture.
Diamox SR capsules should be stored at controlled room temperature (15° to 30°) in the original pack or in well-closed dispensing containers which prevent access of light and moisture.

PHYSICAL PROPERTIES

Acetazolamide is a fine, white to yellowish-white, odourless, crystalline powder.

Melting point

Acetazolamide melts at about 260°, with decomposition.

Dissociation constants

pK_a 7.2, 9.0 (25°)

Solubility

Acetazolamide is soluble 1 in 1400 of water, 1 in 400 of ethanol, and 1 in 100 of acetone; practically insoluble in carbon tetrachloride, in chloroform, and in ether; soluble in solutions of alkali hydroxides.

Effect of cosolvents
Ibrahim and Shawky[1] investigated the effect of glycerol, propylene glycol, various macrogols, dimethyl sulphoxide, and dimethylacetamide on the solubility of acetazolamide. Solubility was enhanced by each of the solvents tested. The effect was greatest with dimethyl sulphoxide and dimethylacetamide and least with glycerol. Solubility was also determined in mixtures of dioxan with methanol, ethanol, or water.

Dissolution

The USP specifies that for Acetazolamide Tablets USP not less than 80% of the labelled amount of $C_4H_6N_4O_3S_2$ is dissolved in 60 minutes. Dissolution medium: 900 mL of 0.1N hydrochloric acid; Apparatus 1 at 100 rpm.

STABILITY

Hydrolysis of acetazolamide in sodium hydroxide (0.1N) follows first-order kinetics; the principal degradation products are acetic acid and 5-amino-1,3,4-thiadiazole-2 sulphonamide. In a solution (0.25 mg/mL) at approximately pH 12, the rate constant[2] was found to be 0.0495/day at 25°.
In an earlier study,[3] degradation rate constants for acetazolamide in alkaline solutions (pH 14) were reported to be 2.9×10^{-3}/min, 4.8×10^{-3}/min, and 1.0×10^{-2}/min at 60°, 70°, and 80°, respectively.
In preformulation studies of an oral liquid dosage form of acetazolamide,[4] the optimum pH of stability appeared to be pH 4. Less than 5% of the initial concentration of acetazolamide was lost when solutions at pH 4 (phosphate buffer) were stored for up to 310 days at 25° in amber glass bottles. Changes in buffer concentration or in ionic strength did not affect degradation constants. From results of stability tests at 37° to 80° the activation energy at pH 4 was determined to be about 69.4 kJ/mol.
In stored solutions of acetazolamide sodium[5] in infusion fluids (glucose 5% or sodium chloride 0.9%) mean potency losses were less than 7.1% after 5 days at 25°, less than 5.4% after 44 days at 5°, and less than 2.9% after 44 days at −10°.

FURTHER INFORMATION. A stability-indicating first-derivative spectrophotometric assay of acetazolamide and its use in dissolution and kinetic studies—Khamis EF, Abdel-Hamid M, Hassan EM, Eshra A, Elsayed MA. J Clin Pharm Ther 1993;18:97–101.

INCOMPATIBILITY/COMPATIBILITY

The physical compatibility of acetazolamide sodium with infusion solutions in common use was demonstrated by Kirkland et al.[6]

Sorption to infusion bags, administration sets, and syringes

Kowaluk and her colleagues[7,8] observed no significant sorption of acetazolamide to various plastic materials from solutions (19 mg/L) in sodium chloride 0.9% infusion when kept under the following conditions:

Container	Storage conditions
Polyvinyl chloride infusion bags	1 week in the dark at room temperature (15° to 20°)
Infusion bottle: glass, sealed with a rubber closure.	
Administration set: cellulose propionate burette chamber plus 170-cm polyvinyl chloride tubing	7-hour infusion
Syringe pump system: 20-cm polyethylene tubing or 50-cm Silastic tubing plus glass syringe	at least 1-hour infusion
Syringe: polypropylene barrel with polyethylene plunger	25 mL sample, 24 hours at room temperature in the dark

FORMULATION

Excipients

Excipients that have been used in presentations of acetazolamide include:

Sustained-release capsules: beeswax; ethylcellulose; gelatin; glycerol; liquid paraffin; magnesium stearate; methyl and propyl hydroxybenzoates; monoglycerides and diglycerides; propylene glycol; silica; starch; sucrose; Sumatra benzoin; talc; vanillin.
Tablets: calcium carbonate; calcium hydrogen phosphate; gelatin; magnesium stearate; povidone; sodium starch glycollate; wheat starch.
Suspensions (of crushed acetazolamide tablets): benzoic acid; chloroform water; orange syrup; tragacanth.
Creams: hydrous wool fat; liquid paraffin; methyl and propyl hydroxybenzoates; propylene glycol; self-emulsifying wax.

Modified-release preparations

Development data obtained *in vitro* and *in vivo* have been presented for sustained-release dosage forms in which 125 mg or 250 mg of the anhydrous acetazolamide are delivered at rates of 15 mg or 20 mg per hour, respectively, by an osmotic pump.[9]

Bioavailability

A comparison of the bioavailability of two oral dosage forms of acetazolamide has been performed by Ledger-Scott and Hurst.[10] In a crossover study, acetazolamide concentrations in plasma were measured over 24 hours in five healthy subjects following administration of a 250 mg tablet, or a 500 mg sustained-release capsule. In all subjects, peak plasma concentrations were significantly higher from the tablet than from the capsule formulation; the extent of absorption from the 500 mg capsule was less than half of that from the 250 mg tablet. Ocular pressure response (by applanation tonometry) was similar for both dosage forms but unrelated to plasma concentrations. It was suggested that the higher incidence of adverse reactions observed with a regimen of four tablets of 250 mg daily compared with two capsules of 500 mg daily, could be the result of the higher steady-state concentrations achieved with the tablet regimen.

When discussing the results of the study[10] described above, Kelly[11] commented that in evaluating the bioavailability of sus-

tained-release presentations of acetazolamide, consideration must be given to the non-linear relationship between plasma and blood concentrations. He also concluded that acetazolamide pharmacokinetics cannot be derived from plasma concentrations alone, following single oral dosage, as the drug preferentially partitions into erythrocytes.

In a randomised, crossover study using 18 healthy males, Schoenwald *et al*[12] compared the bioavailability of two sustained-release preparations of acetazolamide 500 mg (Diamox Sequels, Lederle, USA, and a test presentation) and an immediate-release dosage form (a capsule containing acetazolamide 250 mg). The sustained-release preparations were each administered as a single dose whereas the immediate-release form was given in divided doses, four hours apart. The capsule contents were dispersed in water before administration. Concentrations of acetazolamide in plasma were measured during the 36 hours after dosing, using an enzymatic method. The areas under the plasma concentration versus time curves were significantly higher for the immediate-release preparation than for each of the sustained-release forms, indicating the reduced bioavailability of the latter. The authors suggested that a 40% reduction in acetazolamide dosage could be achieved by using rapid-release presentations.

Bioinequivalence

Yakatan *et al*[13] determined acetazolamide concentrations in plasma following the administration of a 250 mg tablet to 20 healthy subjects. Five separate batches of tablets from the same manufacturer were studied and the results obtained suggested bioinequivalence between batches with respect to peak plasma concentration. Tablet disintegration times were measured *in vitro* and dissolution behaviour was studied using both the *USP XIX* dissolution apparatus and rotating-filter, stationary-basket apparatus. Data obtained from the rotating-filter, stationary-basket apparatus correlated better with observed results *in vivo*, but the authors suggested that refinement of *in-vitro* test procedures is necessary before *in-vivo* bioinequivalence of acetazolamide tablets can be predicted with certainty from *in-vitro* results.

Oral liquids

Further to previous preformulation studies,[4] two 'reasonably stable' oral liquid dosage forms of acetazolamide (pH 4.0; with potential for paediatric use) were formulated.[14] Inactive ingredients included in the formulations were macrogol 400, propylene glycol, sorbitol solution (70% w/w), syrup, saccharin sodium, aspartame, sodium benzoate, brilliant blue FCF (133), allura red AC (E129), raspberry flavour, menthol, ethanol, and buffer (phosphate or citrate). Final preparations were stable (less than 10% loss of acetazolamide content) for 179 days at 37° and a tentative shelf-life of 2 years at 25° was assigned.

Alexander *et al*[15] prepared an extemporaneous suspension of acetazolamide 25 mg/mL; powdered tablets of acetazolamide (Lederle, USA) were levigated with 70% sorbitol solution and mixed with a suspension vehicle of aluminium magnesium silicate, carmellose sodium, and water. Other excipients were Syrup USP, glycerol, methyl and propyl hydroxybenzoates, propylene glycol, allura red AC (E129), and strawberry flavour; the pH was adjusted to 5 with hydrochloric acid. Less than 6% of the initial concentration of acetazolamide was lost after storage, in amber glass bottles, at 5°, 22°, or 30° for 79 days. However, more than 10% was lost after similar storage at 40° and 50° for 79 days and 32 days, respectively. Throughout the study suspensions remained homogeneous, showed no evidence of caking, and had good redispersibility.

Capsule excipients

When acetazolamide was mixed in a 1:1 ratio with each of various excipients, dissolution from capsules was affected by the pH of the medium.[16] At pH 1.12, capsules containing aluminium magnesium silicate, colloidal silica, magnesium carbonate, or microcrystalline cellulose showed greater dissolution than those with lactose, mannitol, calcium hydrogen phosphate, or aluminium hydroxide. At pH 7.4, calcium hydrogen phosphate, magnesium carbonate, or aluminium hydroxide retarded dissolution.

FURTHER INFORMATION. Equivalence of conventional and sustained release oral dosage formulations of acetazolamide in primary open angle glaucoma—Joyce PW, Mills KB, Richardson T, Mawer GE. Br J Clin Pharmacol 1989;27:597–606.

REFERENCES

1. Ibrahim SA, Shawky S. Pharm Ind 1984;46:412–16.
2. Das Gupta V, Parasrampuria J. Drug Dev Ind Pharm 1987;13:147–57.
3. Yamana T, Mizukami Y, Niikawa Y, Murakami Y, Yamamoto Y, Setokawa K [Japanese]. Yakuzaigaku 1963;23:72–3.
4. Parasrampuria J, Das Gupta V. J Pharm Sci 1989;78(10):855–7.
5. Parasrampuria J, Das Gupta V, Stewart KR. Am J Hosp Pharm 1987; 44:358–60.
6. Kirkland WD, Jones RW, Ellis JR, Schultz CG. Am J Hosp Pharm 1961;18:694–9.
7. Kowaluk EA, Roberts MS, Blackburn HD, Polack AE. Am J Hosp Pharm 1981;38:1308–14.
8. Kowaluk EA, Roberts MS, Polack AE. Am J Hosp Pharm 1982;39:460–7.
9. Urquhart J, editor. Controlled-release pharmaceuticals. Washington: American Pharmaceutical Association Academy of Pharmaceutical Sciences, 1981:81.
10. Ledger-Scott M, Hurst J. Pharm J 1985;235:451.
11. Kelly RG [letter]. J Pharm Pharmacol 1986;38:863–4.
12. Schoenwald RD, Garabedian ME, Yakatan GJ. Drug Dev Ind Pharm 1978; 4:599–609.
13. Yakatan GJ, Frome EL, Leonard RG, Shah AC, Doluisio JT. J Pharm Sci 1978;67:252–6.
14. Parasrampuria J, Das Gupta V. J Pharm Sci 1990;79(9):835–6.
15. Alexander KS, Haribhakti RP, Parker GA. Am J Hosp Pharm 1991;48:1241–4.
16. Hashim F, El-Din EZ. Acta Pharm Fenn 1989;98:197–204.

Acetylcysteine (BAN, USAN, rINN)

Mucolytic; Paracetamol antidote

N-Acetylcysteine
N-Acetyl-L-cysteine
$C_5H_9NO_3S = 163.2$
CAS—616-91-1

```
              NH·CO·CH3
               |
  SH·CH2---C---COOH
               |
               H
```

Pharmacopoeial status

BP, USP

Preparations

Compendial
Acetylcysteine Solution USP.

Non-compendial
Fabrol (Zyma). *Granules*, acetylcysteine 200 mg/sachet. To be dissolved in water before administration. Other drugs should not be added to the Fabrol solution.
Ilube (Cusi). *Eye drops*, acetylcysteine 5%, hypromellose 0.35%, preserved with benzalkonium chloride 0.01%.
Parvolex (Evans). *Injection*, acetylcysteine 200 mg/mL, adjusted to pH 7 with sodium hydroxide. *Diluent*: glucose 5% injection. Incompatible with rubber and metals, particularly, iron, copper, and nickel. Silicone rubber and plastic can be used with Parvolex.

Containers and storage

Solid state
Acetylcysteine BP should be kept in a well-closed container, protected from light, and stored at a temperature not exceeding 15°. Acetylcysteine USP should be preserved in tight containers.

Dosage forms
Acetylcysteine Solution USP should be preserved in single-unit or in multiple-unit tight containers that effectively exclude oxygen. Ilube eye drops should be stored below 25° and protected from light.
Parvolex injection should be stored below 25°.

PHYSICAL PROPERTIES

Acetylcysteine is a white crystalline deliquescent powder with a slight acetic odour.
Aqueous solutions of acetylcysteine, as the sodium salt, are colourless and have the characteristic odour and taste of hydrogen sulphide.[1]

Melting point

Acetylcysteine melts at about 108° (BP) or between 104° and 110° (USP).

pH

A 1% w/v solution of *acetylcysteine* has a pH of 2.0 to 2.8.

Dissociation constant

pK_a 9.5 (30°)

Solubility

Acetylcysteine is soluble 1 in 8 of water and 1 in 2 of ethanol; it is practically insoluble in chloroform and in ether.

STABILITY

In solution, the major route of degradation of acetylcysteine is reported to be oxidation to *N,N'*-diacetylcysteine; a minor degradation product is hydrogen sulphide. The reaction is catalysed by metal ions. Solutions of acetylcysteine may become discoloured and liberate hydrogen sulphide when subjected to autoclaving, although the presence of a light purple colour in a solution does not necessarily indicate a significant change in the potency of the product.[1–3]

Stabilisation

The protection afforded by disodium edetate (0.05%) to aqueous solutions of acetylcysteine adjusted to pH 7 was demonstrated by Hamlow and Peck;[2] oxidation, catalysed by metal ions, was 'effectively controlled' during nebulisation into oxygen. A solution containing acetylcysteine (as the sodium salt), disodium edetate, sodium hydroxide, and purified water has been commercially available in the USA for administration by inhalation from a nebuliser, or by direct tracheal instillation. When packaged in ampoules under nitrogen such a solution was stated to be stable 'indefinitely'.[4]

Acetylcysteine injection (neutralised with sodium bicarbonate and containing 0.05% disodium edetate) in ampoules in the absence of oxygen stored at elevated temperatures (100° and 120°) showed very slow decomposition which followed first-order kinetics.[5]

INCOMPATIBILITY/COMPATIBILITY

There is a possibility of physical or chemical incompatibility between acetylcysteine and the following: amphotericin, ampicillin sodium, chlortetracycline hydrochloride, chymotrypsin, erythromycin lactobionate, most metals (in particular copper, iron, nickel), oxygen and oxidising substances, oxytetracycline hydrochloride, rubber, tetracycline hydrochloride, trypsin.

Some antibiotics may be inactivated if nebulised with acetylcysteine.

FURTHER INFORMATION. Compatibility study between acetylcysteine and some commonly used tablet excipients—Kerc J, Srcic S, Urleb U, Kanalec A, Kofler B, Smid-Korbar J. J Pharm Pharmacol 1992;44:515–18.

FORMULATION

Excipients

Excipients that have been used in presentations of acetylcysteine include:

Tablets: aspartame; colloidal silica; lactose; magnesium stearate; microcrystalline cellulose.

Granules and powder (for oral solution): acacia; β-carotene (E160a); colloidal silica; dextrin; glycine; maltodextrin; saccharin; sodium ascorbate; sodium citrate; sodium methyl hydroxybenzoate; sucrose; sunset yellow FCF (E110); DL-α-tocopherol; xylitol.

Solutions (for nebulisation or local instillation): disodium edetate; sodium hydroxide.

Eye drops: benzalkonium chloride; disodium edetate; hypromellose; sodium hydroxide.

Injections: disodium edetate; sodium hydroxide.

Packaging

A primary package developed by Hamlow *et al*[4] for an acetylcysteine solution (that contained acetylcysteine, disodium edetate, sodium hydroxide to pH 7, and water) comprised a polyethylene plug closure with a rubber diaphragm below an aluminium seal fitted to a glass vial and was suitable for aseptic packaging of a sterile solution. Solutions lost less than 5% of their acetylcysteine content after 2 years at room temperature.

REFERENCES

1. Lintner CJ. In: Cooper MS, editor. Quality control in the pharmaceutical industry; vol 2. London: Academic Press, 1973:181.
2. Hamlow EE, Peck GE. Anesthesiology 1967;28:934–5.
3. Talley JR, Magarian RA, Sommers EB. Am J Hosp Pharm 1973;30:526–30.
4. Hamlow EE, Blankenship DR, Bryan HD. Bull Parent Drug Ass 1968;22:122–6.
5. Van Loenen AC, De Jong A, Van der Meer YG, Schwietert HR [German]. Pharm Weekbl 1985;120:313–17.

Acyclovir (BAN, USAN)   *Antiviral*

Aciclovir (rINN); acycloguanosine
9-(2-Hydroxyethoxymethyl)guanine;   2-amino-1,9-dihydro-9-[(2-hydroxyethoxy)methyl]-6*H*-purin-6-one
$C_8H_{11}N_5O_3 = 225.2$

Acyclovir Sodium (BANM, USAN)

Aciclovir Sodium (rINNM)
$C_8H_{10}N_5NaO_3 = 247.2$
CAS—59277-89-3 (acyclovir); 69657-51-8 (acyclovir sodium)

Pharmacopoeial status

BP, USP (acyclovir)

Preparations

Non-compendial

Zovirax (Wellcome). *Tablets*, acyclovir 200 mg, 400 mg, and 800 mg (Shingles Treatment Pack).

Suspension, sugar free, acyclovir 200 mg/5 mL. *Diluent*: equal volume of syrup or sorbitol solution (70%), non-crystallising grade. Life of diluted suspension 28 days at 25°, but it is recommended that dilutions are freshly prepared.

Cream, acyclovir 5% w/w in an aqueous cream basis. Should not be diluted or used as a basis for the incorporation of other medicaments.

Ophthalmic ointment, acyclovir 3% w/w in a white soft paraffin basis.

Intravenous infusion (Zovirax I.V.), powder for reconstitution. Vials containing the equivalent of 250 mg and 500 mg of sterile acyclovir (as sodium salt), for reconstitution with water for injections or sodium chloride 0.9% injection to provide a solution of acyclovir 25 mg/mL. When reconstituted, pH is about 11. For further dilution, Zovirax I.V. is compatible with: sodium chloride 0.9% injection; sodium chloride 0.45% injection; sodium chloride 0.18% and glucose 4% injection; sodium chloride 0.45% and glucose 2.5% injection; or compound sodium lactate injection. Reconstitution and dilution should be performed immediately before use and under full aseptic conditions (product contains no antimicrobial preservative). The infusion is stable for up to 12 hours at 20° when reconstituted and diluted as recommended; solutions should not be refrigerated.

Containers and storage

Solid state

Acyclovir BP should be kept in a well-closed container.
Acyclovir USP should be preserved in tight containers.

Dosage forms

Zovirax tablets, suspension, cream, ophthalmic ointment, and Zovirax I.V. should be stored below 25°; the cream, and the reconstituted and diluted infusion should not be refrigerated. The 200 mg tablets and Shingles Treatment Pack should be kept dry.

PHYSICAL PROPERTIES

Acyclovir is a white or almost white, crystalline powder.

Melting point

Acyclovir is stated to melt at about 230°, with decomposition (BP) or at temperatures higher than 250°, with decomposition (USP).

Dissociation constants

pK_a 2.27, 9.25[1]

From determinations of partition coefficients Kristl *et al*[2] calculated the ionisation constants for acyclovir (by two linear regression methods) to be: pK_{a1} 2.41 ± 0.27 or 2.39 and pK_{a2} 9.06 ± 0.88 or 9.31, at room temperature.

Partition coefficient

Kristl *et al*[2] calculated values for apparent partition coefficients of acyclovir between water and *n*-octanol over a range of pH values at room temperature. Values for the 'real partition coefficient' (*P*) calculated, using two sets of results, by two linear regression methods were 0.024 and 0.022.

Solubility

Acyclovir is slightly soluble in water; insoluble in ethanol; practically insoluble in most organic solvents; soluble in dilute aqueous solutions of alkali hydroxides and mineral acids.

Acyclovir sodium is soluble 1 in 10 of water.

The manufacturers of Zovirax (Burroughs Wellcome, USA) state that the maximum solubility of free acyclovir in water at 37° is 2.5 mg/mL. Kenley *et al*[3] report an intrinsic solubility of 1 mg/mL.

The same workers[3] attempted to enhance the water solubility of acyclovir at neutral pH by the formation of complexes with ligands such as nicotinamide and caffeine. Formation constants (K_1) were determined from a series of phase-solubility experiments and correlation was demonstrated between the formation constant and hydrophobicity of the ligand. The low K_1 values obtained for acyclovir complexes dictate that a high concentration of ligand is necessary to achieve solubilities at therapeutically active levels (acyclovir-caffeine $K_1 = 12.4$ M^{-1}, acyclovir-nicotinamide = 3.34 M^{-1}). To achieve solubility enhancement, the calculated amount of caffeine and nicotinamide required to be tolerated per dose (500 mg acyclovir) is 4.4 g and 9.4 g, respectively. The authors concluded that caffeine and nicotinamide were of limited value as solubility enhancers in parenteral formulations of acyclovir.

Dissolution

Automated dissolution testing with flow-injection analysis, dissolution profiles for the antiviral drugs, DHPG and acyclovir, in capsule formulations — Kenley RA, Jackson SE, Visor GC, Winterle JS. Drug Dev Ind Pharm 1987;13:39–56.

STABILITY

Refrigeration of reconstituted solutions of acyclovir sodium can result in the formation of a precipitate. The precipitate redissolves at room temperature.

Acyclovir exhibited greater stability in an alkaline solution than in an acidic solution during the development of a stability-indicating HPLC method for quantitation of acyclovir in capsules, ointments, and injections.[4] When acyclovir was boiled for 10 minutes in 1N sulphuric acid and in 1N sodium hydroxide, loss of 'potency' was about 12% and 5%, respectively. Similarly, Das Gupta *et al*[5] measured a 27% and 13% loss of acyclovir when it was boiled for 30 minutes in suphuric acid and in sodium hydroxide, respectively.

Negligible decomposition of acyclovir sodium was detected (by HPLC) when solutions of acyclovir sodium (Burroughs Wellcome) 5 mg/mL in sodium chloride 0.9% injection or in glucose 5% injection were stored in Viaflex plastic bags at 5° and 25° for 37 days.[5] However, at 5°, precipitation of acyclovir was evident although the precipitate redissolved when the temperature was increased to 25°.

INCOMPATIBILITY/COMPATIBILITY

Acyclovir sodium sterile powder (Zovirax, Burroughs Wellcome, USA) is incompatible with hydroxybenzoates; precipitation may occur if it is reconstituted with bacteriostatic water for injection which contains hydroxybenzoates. Further dilution of reconstituted acyclovir solution with blood products or colloidal proteins is not recommended.

On admixture (in glucose 5% injection) of acyclovir sodium 5 mg/mL (Burroughs Wellcome) with dopamine hydrochloride 1.6 mg/mL (Abbott) or dobutamine hydrochloride 1 mg/mL (Lilly), brown discoloration was apparent after 2 hours and 1 hour, respectively.[6] Das Gupta *et al*[5] attributed such discoloration to oxidation of dopamine or dobutamine; no loss of acyclovir was detected after 2 hours at 25° in admixtures of acyclovir sodium (5 mg/mL) in a 1:1 ratio with dopamine (Solopak, USA) 1.6 mg/mL or dobutamine (Lilly, USA) 1 mg/mL. Solutions were prepared in glucose 5% injection.

Acyclovir sodium was determined to be visually compatible with 50 commonly used intravenous drugs (under conditions simulating Y-site injection) during a 4-hour study period at 25° under fluorescent light.[6]

FORMULATION

Excipients

Excipients that have been used in presentations of acyclovir include:

Capsules: lactose; magnesium stearate; maize starch; sodium lauryl sulphate.

Tablets: lactose; magnesium stearate; microcrystalline cellulose; povidone; sodium starch glycollate.

Creams: aqueous cream; cetostearyl alcohol; liquid paraffin; poloxamer 407; propylene glycol; sodium lauryl sulphate.

Ointments: macrogols.

Ophthalmic ointments: white soft paraffin.

Topical preparations

Penetration of acyclovir through excised human skin was slow from a macrogol ointment; 8-fold and 60-fold increases in the flux of acyclovir were shown, respectively, from a modified aqueous cream vehicle and a dimethyl sulphoxide vehicle, compared to the macrogol vehicle. Formulations contained acyclovir 5%.[7]

In *guinea pigs* and *mice*, acyclovir 5% presented in an aqueous cream (which contained 40% propylene glycol to increase the aqueous solubility of acyclovir) was found to be more effective than acyclovir 5% in a macrogol ointment basis in the treatment of experimental herpes simplex infections.[8]

In a detailed study,[9] Okamoto *et al* investigated and discussed the effects of four vehicles (propylene glycol, ethanol, isopropanol, and isopropyl myristate) and four penetration enhancers (1-alkyl- and 1- alkenyl-azacycloalkanone derivatives) on the penetration of acyclovir through excised hairless *mouse* and *rat* skin. A combination of a relatively hydrophilic vehicle and a hydrophobic enhancer produced a good enhancing effect.

Bioavailability

In an evaluation of oral acyclovir therapy, Fletcher and Bean reported that oral absorption of acyclovir is slow and variable and that oral bioavailability is in the range 15% to 30%.[10]

FURTHER INFORMATION. Estimation of a concentration profile of acyclovir in the skin after topical administration—Yamashita F, Koyama Y, Sezaki H, Hashida M. Int J Pharmaceutics 1993;89:199–206. Controlled (trans)dermal delivery [dermal patches] of an antiviral agent (acyclovir). I: an *in vivo* animal model for efficacy evaluation in cutaneous HSV-1 infections—Gonsho A, Imanidis G, Vogt P, Kern ER, Tsuge H, Su M-H *et al.* Int J Pharmaceutics 1990;65:183–94. Water-soluble, solution-stable, and biolabile *N*-substituted (aminomethyl)benzoate ester prodrugs of acyclovir—Bundgaard H, Jensen E, Falch E. Pharm Res 1991;8:1087–93.

REFERENCES

1. American Society of Hospital Pharmacists. Drug information 86. Acyclovir. Bethesda: The Society, 1986:324.
2. Kristl A, Mrhar A, Kozjek F, Kobe J. Int J Pharmaceutics 1989;57:229–34.
3. Kenley RA, Jackson SE, Winterle JS, Shunko Y, Visor GC. J Pharm Sci 1986;75:648–53.
4. Pramar Y, Das Gupta V, Zerai T. Drug Dev Ind Pharm 1990;16(10):1687–95.
5. Das Gupta V, Pramar Y, Bethea C. J Clin Pharm Ther 1989;14:451–6.
6. Forman JK, Lachs JR, Souney PF. Am J Hosp Pharm 1987;44:1408–9.
7. Freeman DJ, Sheth NV, Spruance SL. Antimicrob Agents Chemother 1986;29:730–2.
8. Collins P, Oliver NM. Am J Med 1982;73:96–9.
9. Okamoto H, Muta K, Hashida M, Sezaki H. Pharm Res 1990;7:64–8.
10. Fletcher C, Bean B. Drug Intell Clin Pharm 1985;19:518–24.

Adrenaline (BAN)

Sympathomimetic agent; Beta-adrenoceptor agonist
Epinephrine (rINN); epirenamine; levorenin; suprarenin
(*R*)-1-(3,4-Dihydroxyphenyl)-2-methylaminoethanol; (*R*)-4-[1-hydroxy-2-(methylamino)ethyl]-1,2-benzenediol; (−)-3,4-dihydroxy-A- [(methylamino)methyl]benzyl alcohol
$C_9H_{13}NO_3 = 183.2$

Adrenaline Acid Tartrate (BANM)

Epinephrine Bitartrate (rINNM)
$C_9H_{13}NO_3, C_4H_6O_6 = 333.3$

Adrenaline Hydrochloride

$C_9H_{13}NO_3, HCl = 219.7$
CAS—51-43-4 (adrenaline); 51-42-3 (adrenaline acid tartrate); 55-31-2 (adrenaline hydrochloride)

Pharmacopoeial status

BP (adrenaline, adrenaline acid tartrate); USP (epinephrine, epinephrine bitartrate)

Preparations

Compendial
Adrenaline Solution BP (Adrenaline Tartrate Solution). An isotonic solution containing adrenaline acid tartrate 0.18% w/v with a suitable combination of an antoxidant and an antimicrobial preservative in purified water. pH 2.7 to 3.6.
Adrenaline Eye Drops BP (Neutral Adrenaline Eye Drops). A sterile solution of adrenaline in purified water. pH 5.5 to 7.6. Eye drops containing 0.5% w/v and 1% w/v are usually available.
Adrenaline Injection BP (Adrenaline Tartrate Injection). A sterile isotonic solution containing adrenaline acid tartrate 0.18% w/v in water for injections. pH 2.8 to 3.6.
Bupivacaine and Adrenaline Injection BP. A sterile solution of bupivacaine hydrochloride and adrenaline acid tartrate in water for injections. pH 3.0 to 5.5.
Lignocaine and Adrenaline Injection BP. A sterile solution of lignocaine hydrochloride and adrenaline acid tartrate in water for injections. pH 3.0 to 4.5.
Epinephrine Inhalation Aerosol USP.
Epinephrine Bitartrate Inhalation Aerosol USP.
Epinephrine Inhalation Solution USP.
Epinephrine Nasal Solution USP.
Epinephrine Ophthalmic Solution USP. pH 2.2 to 4.5.
Epinephrine Bitartrate Ophthalmic Solution USP. pH 3.0 to 3.8.
Epinephrine Bitartrate for Ophthalmic Solution USP.
Epinephryl Borate Ophthalmic Solution USP. pH 5.5 to 7.6.
Epinephrine Injection USP. pH 2.2 to 5.0.
Sterile Epinephrine Oil Suspension USP.

Non-compendial
Epifrin (Allergan). *Eye drops*, adrenaline (as hydrochloride) 1%.
Eppy (S&N Pharm). *Eye drops*, adrenaline 1% in an isotonic buffered ophthalmic solution. Eppy should not be diluted and should not be used if the solution has darkened. It should only be dispensed from the original container.
Medihaler-epi (3M). *Aerosol inhalation*, adrenaline acid tartrate 14 mg/mL (containing 280 micrograms/metered inhalation) in aerosol propellant.
Min-I-Jet Adrenaline (IMS). *Injection*, adrenaline (as hydrochloride) 1 in 1000 (1 mg/mL).
Injection, adrenaline (as acid tartrate) 1 in 10 000 (100 micrograms/mL).
Simplene (S&N Pharm). *Eye drops*, adrenaline 0.5% or 1% in a viscous, buffered solution. It should not be diluted and should not be used if the solution has darkened. It should only be dispensed from the original container.
Adrenaline injections of various salts and strengths are also available from Boots, Evans, Hillcross, Martindale, Penn.

Containers and storage

Solid state
Adrenaline BP should be kept in a well-closed container, which is preferably filled with nitrogen, and protected from light.

Adrenaline Acid Tartrate BP should be kept in airtight containers, or preferably in sealed tubes under vacuum or under inert gas, and protected from light.
Epinephrine USP and Epinephrine Bitartrate USP should be preserved in tight, light-resistant containers.

Dosage forms
Adrenaline Solution BP should be kept in well-filled, well-closed containers, and protected from light.
Adrenaline Eye Drops BP, Adrenaline Injection BP, Bupivacaine and Adrenaline Injection BP, and Lignocaine and Adrenaline Injection BP should be protected from light.
Epinephrine Inhalation Aerosol USP and Epinephrine Bitartrate Inhalation Aerosol USP should be preserved in small, non-reactive, light-resistant containers equipped with metered-dose valves and provided with oral inhalation actuators.
Epinephrine Inhalation Solution USP, Epinephrine Nasal Solution USP, Epinephrine Bitartrate Ophthalmic Solution USP, and Epinephryl Borate Ophthalmic Solution USP should be preserved in small, well-filled, tight, light-resistant containers.
Epinephrine Ophthalmic Solution USP should be preserved in tight, light-resistant containers.
Epinephrine Bitartrate for Ophthalmic Solution USP should be preserved in containers suitable for sterile solids.
Epinephrine Injection USP should be preserved in single-dose or multiple-dose, light-resistant containers, preferably of Type I glass.
Sterile Epinephrine Oil Suspension USP should be preserved in single-dose, light-resistant containers, preferably of Type I or Type III glass.
Eppy and Simplene ophthalmic solutions should be stored, in their cartons, in a cool place (Simplene at 8° to 15°), away from strong sunlight. Simplene plastic dropper bottles are over-wrapped by a nitrogen-filled pouch to ensure a long shelf-life.
Medihaler-epi should be stored in a cool place, protected from frost and sunlight. The vial is pressurised and should not be punctured or disposed of by burning.

PHYSICAL PROPERTIES

Adrenaline exists as white or creamy-white, odourless, sphaero-crystalline powder or granules. It darkens on exposure to air and light.
Adrenaline acid tartrate is a white to greyish-white or light-brownish grey, odourless, crystalline powder. It slowly darkens on exposure to air and light.

Melting point

Adrenaline melts at about 212°, with decomposition, the rate of rise of temperature being 10° per minute.
Adrenaline acid tartrate melts in the range 147° to 152°, with decomposition.

pH

Solutions of *adrenaline* are alkaline to litmus.
Solutions of *adrenaline acid tartrate* are acidic, with a pH of about 3.5.

Dissociation constants

pK_a 8.7, 10.2, 12.0 (20°)

Solubility

Adrenaline is sparingly soluble in water; practically insoluble in ethanol, in chloroform, in ether, in fixed and volatile oils, and in petroleum spirit. It dissolves in solutions of mineral acids, of

sodium hydroxide, and of potassium hydroxide, but not in solutions of ammonia or of the alkali carbonates.
Adrenaline acid tartrate is soluble 1 in 3 of water; slightly soluble in ethanol; practically insoluble in chloroform and in ether.

Effect of pH
The solubility of adrenaline in water is pH-dependent, with minimum solubility at pH 9.4. Its solubility increases as the pH moves away from 9.4 owing to the formation of water-soluble species bearing net positive or negative charges.[1]

STABILITY

Solutions of adrenaline and its salts gradually turn pink, red, and finally brown on exposure to air and light owing to oxidation. Degradation is also promoted by heat. In the solid state, adrenaline is also susceptible to decomposition. The initial stage in the oxidation of adrenaline is believed to involve the formation of adrenaline-*o*-quinone with further changes resulting in the formation of indole derivatives and other compounds. It is the formation of adrenochrome and other coloured products that produces the reddish discoloration. Oxidative discoloration of adrenaline solution occurs more rapidly as pH increases. Adrenaline solutions are most stable at pH 3.2 to 3.6.
Solutions of adrenaline also lose potency due to racemisation, which follows first-order kinetics, is accelerated by light, and is believed to be acid catalysed.
Thoma and Struve[2] reported on the considerable influence of temperature, pH, and daylight and xenon irradiation on the rate of degradation of adrenaline in solution. Solutions (that had not been treated with nitrogen) had $t_{10\%}$ values of 31 days and 4 days at 40° and 60°, respectively. After storage for 200 days at 30°, an increase in the pH of similar solutions from 2.5 to 4.5 resulted in a two-fold increase in degradation (from 5% to 10%). Exposure to daylight and xenon irradiation resulted in rapid oxidation of adrenaline.
Adrenaline reacts with salts of sulphurous acid to form a derivative of sulphonic acid, 1-(3,4-dihydroxyphenyl)-2-methyl-aminoethane sulphonic acid, which is biologically inactive.[1,3] This interaction may be important when the oxygen content is low and the molar ratio of sodium metabisulphite to adrenaline in a formulation approaches unity. In medicines in which an excess of adrenaline is present, interaction with sodium metabisulphite reduces the biological activity only slightly.
Results from a study by Milano *et al*[4] of solutions containing lignocaine hydrochloride and adrenaline indicated that aluminium (often present in chlorobutyl rubber closures) catalysed the adrenaline-bisulphite addition reaction. In a later study by Milano and Williams[5] it was demonstrated that at pH 4, aluminium chelated adrenaline through its catechol structure in a 1:1 ratio.
Allwood[6] assessed the stability of adrenaline 16 mg/L in glucose 5% injection during storage in Viaflex minibags at 5°, protected from light for 30 days; based on $t_{5\%}$ values, the solution was assigned a shelf-life of 20 days at 5°.
Lignocaine and adrenaline were stable in pH-adjusted (with alkali to pH 6.5 or 7.05) parenteral solutions for at least 6 hours.[7]

Stabilisation

The oxidation of adrenaline may be retarded by antioxidants and by traces of mineral acids. Synergists such as chelating agents can enhance the antioxidant effect.
Solutions containing adrenaline with sodium metabisulphite as an antioxidant can be stabilised by the addition of boric acid provided that the oxygen content is low; stabilisation is due to

chelation of adrenaline by the boric acid and the degree of chelation is enhanced by an increase in pH.

FURTHER INFORMATION. Chelating agents as colour stabilisers for epinephrine [adrenaline] hydrochloride solutions—Roscoe CW, Hall NA. J Am Pharm Assoc Sci Ed 1956;45:464–70. A kinetic study of acid-catalysed racemisation of epinephrine [adrenaline]—Schroeter LC, Higuchi T. J Am Pharm Assoc Sci Ed 1958;47:426–30. Degradation of epinephrine [adrenaline] induced by bisulphite—Schroeter LC, Higuchi T, Schuler EE. J Am Pharm Assoc Sci Ed 1958;47:723–8. Stabilisation of epinephrine [adrenaline] against sulphite attack—Riegelman S, Fischer EZ. J Pharm Sci 1962;51:206–10. Kinetics of sulphite-induced anaerobic degradation of epinephrine [adrenaline]—Hajratwala BR. J Pharm Sci 1975;64:45–8. Sulphite-induced anaerobic degradation of epinephrine [adrenaline] in lidocaine [lignocaine] hydrochloride injection—Hajratwala BR. Drug Dev Ind Pharm 1977;3:65–72. Inhibition of epinephrine [adrenaline] oxidation in weak alkaline solutions—Bonevski R, Momirovic-Culjat J, Balint L. J Pharm Sci 1978;67:1474–6. Thermal stability of various epinephrine [adrenaline] formulations—Lee IP, Burton H. Drug Dev Ind Pharm 1981;7:397–403. Stability of Adrenaline Injection BP following resterilisation—Patterson MJ, Tjokrosetio R, Ilett KF. Aust J Hosp Pharm 1981;11:21–2. Stability of adrenaline ophthalmic solutions on sterilisation and storage—Sixsmith DG, Watkins WM, Kokwaro GO. J Clin Hosp Pharm 1982;7:205–7. Effect of sodium metabisulphite and anaerobic processing conditions on the oxidative degradation of adrenaline injection BP—Taylor JB, Sharma SC, Simpkins DE. Pharm J 1984;232:646–8. The effect of anaerobic conditions on epinephrine stability in solutions containing lignocaine and sodium metabisulphite, with or without citric acid—Fyhr P, Brodin A. Acta Pharm Suec 1987;24(3):89–96. Stabilisation of epinephrine [adrenaline] in a local anaesthetic injectable solution using reduced levels of sodium metabisulfite and EDTA—Grubstein B, Milano E. Drug Dev Ind Pharm 1992;18(14):1549–66.

INCOMPATIBILITY/COMPATIBILITY

Adrenaline and its salts are rapidly destroyed in solution with oxidising agents, alkalis, copper, iron, silver, zinc, and other metals, gums, and tannin. Incompatibility has also been reported with aminophylline, cephapirin sodium, hyaluronidase, iodine and other halogens, mephentermine sulphate, and warfarin sodium.
Adrenaline has been reported to deteriorate rapidly when stored in certain types of amber glass because of the leaching of iron from the glass.
The interaction of adrenaline with sulphites and with aluminium is discussed under Stability, above.

FORMULATION

ADRENALINE SOLUTION BP
The following formula was given in the *British Pharmacopoeia 1980*:

Adrenaline acid tartrate	1.8 g
Chlorbutol	4 g
Chlorocresol	1 g
Sodium metabisulphite	1 g
Sodium chloride	8 g
Purified water	to 1000 mL

Contains the equivalent of adrenaline 0.1% w/v.

ADRENALINE INJECTION BP
The following formula was given in the *British Pharmacopoeia 1980*:

Adrenaline acid tartrate	0.18 g
Sodium metabisulphite	0.1 g
Sodium chloride	0.8 g
Water for injections	to 100 mL

Contains the equivalent of adrenaline 0.1% w/v.

The sodium metabisulphite should be dissolved in 10 mL of water for injections and the adrenaline acid tartrate added; the sodium chloride should then be dissolved in 75 mL of water for injections. The two solutions should be mixed and sufficient water for injections added to produce 100 mL. Sterilised by heating in an autoclave.

Excipients

Excipients that have been used in presentations of adrenaline (as the acid tartrate or hydrochloride in some instances) include:
Aerosol inhalations: ascorbic acid; benzoic acid; ethanol; fluorocarbons; hydrochloric acid; potassium chloride; propellants 11, 12, and 114; sodium bisulphite; sodium chloride; sodium sulphite; sorbitan trioleate.
Eye drops: ascorbic acid; benzalkonium chloride; borax; boric acid; chlorhexidine acetate; disodium edetate; glycerol; hydroxyquinoline sulphate; hypromellose; isoascorbic acid; phenylmercuric acetate; phenylmercuric nitrate; polyoxyl 40 stearate; povidone; sodium ascorbate; sodium hydroxide; sodium metabisulphite; thiomersal.
Injections: ascorbic acid; chlorbutol; disodium edetate; glycerol; hydrochloric acid; phenol; sodium bisulphite; sodium chloride; sodium metabisulphite; sodium hydroxide; sodium thioglycollate.

Aerosols

Results from studies by Sciarra *et al*[8] indicated that the formulation of adrenaline salts (acid tartrate, fumarate, malate, and maleate) as an aerosol dosage form should involve the use of a cosolvent or a dispersion system. The solubility of all four salts was greater in difluoroethane than in the other fluorocarbon propellants studied. Adrenaline maleate and fumarate exhibited the greatest solubility. Preliminary studies showed adrenaline maleate and acid tartrate to have greater stability than the malate or fumarate.

FURTHER INFORMATION. Faster and more reliable absorption of adrenaline by aerosol inhalation than by subcutaneous injection—Mellem H, Lande K, Kjeldsen SE, Westheim A, Eide I, Ekholt PF *et al*. Br J Clin Pharmacol 1991;31:677–81.

PROCESSING

Sterilisation

Adrenaline injection, a solution containing adrenaline acid tartrate, can be sterilised by heating in an autoclave.

REFERENCES

1. Szulczewski DH, Hong W-h. In: Florey K, editor. Analytical profiles of drug substances; vol 7. London: Academic Press, 1978:193–229.
2. Thoma K, Struve M [German]. Pharm Acta Helv 1986;61(1):2–9.
3. Higuchi T, Schroeter LC. J Am Chem Soc 1960;82:1904–7.

4. Milano EA, Waraszkiewicz SM, Dirubio R. J Parenter Sci Technol 1982;36:232–6.
5. Milano EA, Williams DA. J Parenter Sci Technol 1983;37:165–9.
6. Allwood MC. J Clin Pharm Ther 1991;16:337–40.
7. Bonhomme L, Postaire E, Touratier S, Benhamou D, Marte-Sauvageon H, Preaux N. J Clin Pharm Ther 1988;13:257–61.
8. Sciarra JJ, Patel JM, Kapoor AL. J Pharm Sci 1972;61:219–23.

Allopurinol (BAN, USAN, rINN)

Xanthine-oxidase inhibitor

HPP; isopurinol
1*H*-Pyrazolo[3,4-*d*]pyrimidin-4-ol; 1,5-dihydro-4*H*-pyrazolo[3,4-*d*]pyrimidin-4-one
$C_5H_4N_4O = 136.1$
CAS—315-30-0 (allopurinol); 17795-21-0 (allopurinol sodium)

Pharmacopoeial status

BP, USP

Preparations

Compendial
Allopurinol Tablets BP. Tablets containing, in each, 100 mg and 300 mg are usually available.
Allopurinol Tablets USP.

Non-compendial
Caplenal (Berk). *Tablets*, allopurinol 100 mg and 300 mg.
Hamarin (Nicholas). *Tablets*, allopurinol 100 mg and 300 mg.
Zyloric (Wellcome). *Tablets*, allopurinol 100 mg and 300 mg (Zyloric-300).
Allopurinol tablets are also available in various strengths from APS, Ashbourne (Xanthomax), Cox, CP, DDSA (Cosuric), Evans, Kerfoot, Rima (Rimapurinol).

Containers and storage

Solid state
Allopurinol USP should be preserved in well-closed containers.

Dosage forms
Hamarin tablets should be stored in a cool, dry place.
Zyloric and Zyloric-300 tablets should be stored below 25° and kept dry.

PHYSICAL PROPERTIES

Allopurinol is a white or almost white powder.

Melting point

Allopurinol has no characteristic melting point but above 300° it darkens, becomes charred, and ultimately decomposes.

Dissociation constant

pK_a 9.4
Benezra and Bennett[1] determined a pK_a value of 10.2 using a spectrophotometric method.

Partition coefficients

Log *P* (octanol/water), pH 1.2, 25°, −0.62[1]; pH 6.0, 25°, −0.48[1]; 22°, −0.55.[2]

Solubility

Allopurinol is very slightly soluble in water and in ethanol; practically insoluble in chloroform and in ether; soluble in dimethylformamide and in dilute solutions of alkali hydroxides.

Solubility enhancement
To increase the aqueous solubility of allopurinol, *N*-hydroxymethyl,[3] *N*-acyl and *N*-acyloxymethyl,[2] and *N*-substituted (aminomethyl)benzyloxymethyl[4] derivatives have been prepared. Some derivatives were sufficiently water soluble and lipophilic to allow the formulation of rectal and parenteral preparations.[2,4] After administration via either of these routes to *rabbits*, the prodrugs were rapidly hydrolysed in plasma, resulting in the regeneration of allopurinol.

FURTHER INFORMATION. Influence of certain hydrotropic and complexing agents [sodium salicylate, sodium benzoate, and nicotinamide] on solubilisation of allopurinol—Hamza YE, Kata M. Pharm Ind 1989;51(10):1159–62. Influence of certain non-ionic surfactants [Tween 80, Tween 20, Myrj 59, Myrj 53, Brij 58, Brij 35, Pluronic F 127, Pluronic F 68] on solubilisation and *in vitro* availability of allopurinol—Hamza YE, Kata M. Pharm Ind 1989;51(12):1441–4.

Dissolution

The USP specifies that for Allopurinol Tablets USP not less than 75% of the labelled amount of $C_5H_4N_4O$ is dissolved in 45 minutes. Dissolution medium: 900 mL of 0.1N hydrochloric acid; Apparatus 2 at 75 rpm.

STABILITY

The main decomposition product of allopurinol is 3-aminopyrazole-4-carboxamide, which forms in both acidic and basic media. Further decomposition to 3-aminopyrazole-4-carboxylic acid and 3-aminopyrazole can occur in basic solutions; 3-aminopyrazole-4-carboxylic acid is not formed in acidic media.[1]
Gressel and Gallelli[5] studied the decomposition of allopurinol using ion-exchange chromatographic separation and spectrophotometric analysis. Degradation of allopurinol in alkaline media approximated to first-order kinetics and rate constants were calculated. The activation energy for the decomposition of an allopurinol solution (5 mg/mL) in an unbuffered medium (pH 10.8) was calculated to be 106.7 kJ/mol. Values of $t_{10\%}$ for allopurinol solutions (5 mg/mL) in alkaline media at 25° were determined to be 28.5 days at pH 10.7 (buffered) and 150 days at pH 10.8 (unbuffered).
A suspension comprising crushed allopurinol tablets (Burroughs Wellcome, USA) in Cologel, syrup, and cherry syrup lost less than 3% of the initial allopurinol concentration (20 mg/mL) after storage, in amber glass bottles, for 56 days at 5° and at ambient room temperature.[6]
Allopurinol sodium 300 mg in 5 to 10 mL of sodium chloride 0.9% or glucose 5% is reported to be stable for 7 days at 4° to 8°. At 105°, allopurinol solutions exhibit maximum stability in the pH range 3.1 to 3.4; decomposition is rapid at high pH values.[1]

INCOMPATIBILITY/COMPATIBILITY

Solutions of allopurinol sodium in sodium chloride 0.9% and glucose 5% are incompatible with prednisolone sodium succinate and acidic materials. In glucose 5% injection, allopurinol sodium is physically incompatible with mercaptopurine sodium and methotrexate sodium.

FORMULATION

Excipients

Excipients that have been used in presentations of allopurinol include:

Capsules: arachis oil; polysorbate 80; soya lecithin; soya oil, hydrogenated; vegetable oil, partially hydrogenated; yellow beeswax.

Tablets: lactose; magnesium stearate; povidone; starch (maize, potato); sunset yellow FCF (E110), lake.

Suspensions: carmellose sodium; ethanol; glycerol; methylcellulose; methyl hydroxybenzoate; saccharin sodium; syrup; vanilla flavour; wild cherry syrup.

Suppositories

Allopurinol 300 mg suppositories have been compounded extemporaneously from tablets (Zyloprim, USA) using either a theobroma oil basis or a macrogol basis (comprising 96% macrogol 1000 and 4% macrogol 4000). Although such suppositories appeared to be effective in the prophylaxis of hyperuricaemia in patients receiving cytotoxic drugs, Appelbaum et al[7] found that in six healthy adults, allopurinol was not absorbed from rectal suppositories prepared using these bases. These findings were corroborated by Chang et al,[8] although trace amounts of a metabolite of allopurinol (oxipurinol) were detected in the plasma of volunteers after administration of the theobroma oil suppositories.

Prodrugs

The formation of water-soluble prodrug derivatives of allopurinol led to the formulation of suppositories that were found to have superior bioavailability in comparison to allupurinol alone when tested in *rabbits*.[2,4] See Solubility, above.

Mouthwashes

An extemporaneously formulated mouthwash of allopurinol (one crushed allopurinol 300 mg tablet; Cologel 100 mL; syrup:cherry syrup [2:1] to 300 mL) was found (by HPLC) to be stable during storage at room or refrigerated temperatures for at least eight months in amber containers.[9] No evidence of systemic allopurinol absorption was detected in ten healthy volunteers following use of multiple small doses of allopurinol as a mouthwash.

Bioequivalence

There were no significant differences in any of the pharmacokinetic parameters examined when two US commercial brands of allopurinol tablets were compared in 32 healthy subjects in a randomised, crossover study.[10]

FURTHER INFORMATION. A comparative study of the bioavailability and the pharmacodynamic effects of 5 allopurinol preparations [tablets and slow-release tablets]—Jaeger H, Russmann D, Rasper J, Blome J [German]. Arzneimittelforschung 1982;32:438–43.

REFERENCES

1. Benezra SA, Bennett TR. In: Florey K, editor. Analytical profiles of drug substances; vol 7. London: Academic Press, 1978:1–17.

2. Bundgaard H, Falch E, Pedersen SB, Nielsen GH. Int J Pharmaceutics 1985;27:71–80.

3. Bansal PC, Pitman IH, Higuchi T. J Pharm Sci 1981;70:855–7.

4. Bundgaard H, Jensen E, Falch E, Pedersen SB. Int J Pharmaceutics 1990;64:75–87.

5. Gressel PD, Gallelli JF. J Pharm Sci 1968;57:335–8.

6. Dressman JB, Poust RI. Am J Hosp Pharm 1983;40:616–18.

7. Appelbaum SJ, Mayersohn M, Perrier D, Dorr RT [letter]. Drug Intell Clin Pharm 1980;14:789.

8. Chang S-L, Kramer WG, Feldman S, Ballentine R, Frankel LS. Am J Hosp Pharm 1981;38:365–8.

9. Loprinzi CL, Burnham NL, O'Connell MJ, Svingen PA, Peterson DA. Hosp Pharm 1989;24:353–4,373.

10. Marcus M, Tse FLS, Kleinberg SI. Int J Clin Pharmacol Ther Toxicol 1982;20:302–5.

Amethocaine (BAN)   *Local anaesthetic*

Tetracaine (rINN)
2-Dimethylaminoethyl 4-butylaminobenzoate; 2-(dimethylamino)ethyl ester of 4-(butylamino)-benzoic acid
$C_{15}H_{24}N_2O_2 = 264.4$

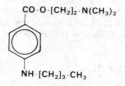

Amethocaine Hydrochloride (BANM)

Dicainum; Tetracaine Hydrochloride (rINNM)
$C_{15}H_{24}N_2O_2, HCl = 300.8$
CAS—94-24-6 (amethocaine); 136-47-0 (amethocaine hydrochloride)

Pharmacopoeial status

BP (amethocaine hydrochloride); USP (tetracaine, tetracaine hydrochloride)

Preparations

Compendial

Amethocaine Eye Drops BP. A sterile solution of amethocaine hydrochloride in purified water. Eye drops containing 0.5% w/v and 1.0% w/v are usually available.
Tetracaine Ointment USP.
Tetracaine Ophthalmic Ointment USP.
Tetracaine Hydrochloride Cream USP.
Tetracaine Hydrochloride Ophthalmic Solution USP. pH 3.7 to 6.0.
Tetracaine Hydrochloride Topical Solution USP.
Tetracaine Hydrochloride Injection USP. pH 3.2 to 6.0.
Tetracaine Hydrochloride in Dextrose Injection. pH 3.5 to 6.0.
Sterile Tetracaine Hydrochloride USP. Tetracaine hydrochloride suitable for parenteral use. A 1% solution has a pH of 5.0 to 6.0.

Non-compendial

Minims Amethocaine Hydrochloride (S&N Pharm). *Eye drops*, amethocaine hydrochloride 0.5% and 1%, in single-use units.

Containers and storage

Solid state
Amethocaine Hydrochloride BP should be kept in a well-closed container, protected from light.
Tetracaine USP should be preserved in tight, light-resistant containers.
Tetracaine Hydrochloride USP should be preserved in tight, light-resistant containers.

Dosage forms
Amethocaine Eye Drops BP should be protected from light.
Tetracaine Ointment USP should be preserved in collapsible ointment tubes.
Tetracaine Ophthalmic Ointment USP should be preserved in collapsible ophthalmic ointment tubes.
Tetracaine Hydrochloride Cream USP should be preserved in collapsible tubes, of lined metal.
Tetracaine Hydrochloride Ophthalmic Solution USP should be preserved in tight, light-resistant containers.
Tetracaine Hydrochloride Topical Solution USP should be preserved in tight, light-resistant containers.
Tetracaine Hydrochloride Injection USP and Tetracaine Hydrochloride in Dextrose Injection USP should be preserved in single-dose or in multiple-dose containers, preferably of Type I glass, under refrigeration, protected from light.
Sterile Tetracaine Hydrochloride USP should be preserved in containers suitable for sterile solids, preferably of Type I glass.
Minims Amethocaine Hydrochloride should be stored in a cool place (8° to 15°), and should not be exposed to strong light.

PHYSICAL PROPERTIES

Amethocaine is a white or light yellow, waxy solid.
Amethocaine hydrochloride is a white, odourless, crystalline, slightly hygroscopic powder.

Melting point

Amethocaine melts in the range 41° to 46°.
Amethocaine hydrochloride melts at about 148°; two polymorphic forms melt at about 134° and 139°, respectively; mixtures of the forms melt in the range 134° to 147°. Amethocaine hydrochloride, recrystallised from ethanol and absolute ether, has been reported to have a melting point[1] of 151° to 152°.

pH

A 1% w/v solution of *amethocaine hydrochloride* in water has a pH of 4.5 to 5.5.

Dissociation constant

pK_a 8.5 (20°)

Solubility

Amethocaine is very slightly soluble in water; soluble 1 in 5 of ethanol, 1 in 2 of chloroform, and 1 in 2 of ether; soluble in benzene.
Amethocaine hydrochloride is soluble 1 in 7.5 of water, 1 in 40 of ethanol, 1 in 30 of chloroform; soluble in glycerol; practically insoluble in acetone, in ether, and in benzene.

Critical micelle concentration

The critical micelle concentration of amethocaine hydrochloride in glucose-free, citrate-buffered medium (pH 6.5) was deduced to be 5 mg/mL.[2]

Crystal and molecular structure

Polymorphs
Thermodynamic data (transition temperature, heat of transition, and melting points) for the transition between the three forms of amethocaine hydrochloride have been presented by Burger and Ramberger.[3]

STABILITY

In aqueous solution, amethocaine hydrochloride degrades by hydrolysis to *n*-butylaminobenzoic acid and 2-dimethylaminoethanol; both compounds are colourless. The *n*-butylaminobenzoic acid formed can become decarboxylated to form butylaniline, which can be further oxidised to various purple-coloured products. The hydrolysis of amethocaine is both acid-catalysed and base-catalysed. At 25°, solutions are most stable at about pH 3.5.
The low aqueous solubility of the decomposition product, *n*-butylaminobenzoic acid, may result in its deposition in amethocaine hydrochloride injection solutions during long-term storage. In solutions degraded at 85°, crystal deposits formed when the content of *n*-butylaminobenzoic acid exceeded 0.6 mg/mL at pH 3.15 to 5.15. An HPLC method has been developed to simultaneously determine amethocaine and *n*-butylaminobenzoic acid.[4]
The time required for 10% decomposition ($t_{10\%}$) of amethocaine in solutions at pH values of 5 and 6.8 has been determined.[5] At pH 5, the $t_{10\%}$ at 25° was calculated to be 3 years and at 120° to be 5.5 hours. The equivalent values at pH 6.8 were 2 weeks at 25° and 2 minutes at 120°.
Göber *et al*[6] estimated that an amethocaine hydrochloride solution buffered at pH 3.1 would degrade to 90% of the label claim (owing to hydrolysis) over a period of 14.7 years.
Chalardsunthornvatee and Thomas[7] found that decomposition of amethocaine hydrochloride was greater with increasing amounts of sodium chloride up to a limiting concentration of about 4%. Decomposition was also accelerated by heat and by hydroxide ions.

Sterilisation

Following an investigation to determine the effects of autoclaving a series of amethocaine hydrochloride 2% solutions with different pH values (3.2 to 6.0), Vervloet *et al*[8] concluded that the solutions should be sterilised for 30 minutes at 100° and then stored at room temperature.
Zöllner[9] reported that heat sterilisation at 120° for 30 minutes resulted in 0.5% decomposition of amethocaine in solution (pH 4 to 6). Further sterilisation for a total of 5 hours resulted in 3.5% degradation.
Workers in Hungary formulated a 1% amethocaine aqueous solution for spinal anaesthesia which was reported to be stable to heat sterilisation.[10]
According to Chalardsunthornvatee and Thomas,[7] aqueous solutions of amethocaine hydrochloride may be sterilised by heating with a bactericide at 98° to 100° for 30 minutes and ampoules may be sterilised in an autoclave without serious decomposition. Repeated and prolonged autoclaving is undesirable. Injections of amethocaine hydrochloride containing electrolytes should be prepared aseptically.
However, Whittet[11] recommended that amethocaine solutions should not be sterilised by autoclaving. An amethocaine solution (0.1% in sodium chloride solution 0.3%, pH 5.4) lost more than 10% of its initial activity during autoclaving at 115° for 1 hour and the pH reduced to 4.80. A solution of

amethocaine hydrochloride (1% in glucose 6.3% solution, pH 4.8) lost about 4% and the pH reduced to 4.7.

Norton[12] reported that during autoclaving at 115° for 30 minutes, a 1% solution of amethocaine hydrochloride, at pH 5.6, hydrolysed by 3.5%. In a similar solution that had been initially adjusted to pH 4 the extent of hydrolysis was less than 1%.

Stabilisation

The addition of caffeine to solutions of amethocaine hydrochloride has been reported to result in a reduction in the rate of hydrolysis.[1]

The stability of amethocaine in aqueous solutions has been reported to be unaffected by the addition of glucose.[13]

INCOMPATIBILITY/COMPATIBILITY

Addition of alkali hydroxides or carbonates to solutions of amethocaine hydrochloride results in precipitation of the free base as an oily liquid.

Amethocaine hydrochloride is incompatible with iodides, bromides, inorganic silver and mercury salts, copper ions, and with polysorbate 80.[14]

In a study of the use of preservatives in amethocaine eye drops, amethocaine was found to be compatible with phenylmercuric nitrate, thiomersal, and benzalkonium chloride but incompatible with chlorhexidine.

Neels[15] reported that hydromorphone hydrochloride (Knoll, USA), final concentration 4.38 mg/mL, and amethocaine hydrochloride (Winthrop, USA), final concentration 1.25 mg/mL, were visually compatible in sodium chloride 0.9% injection following storage in a disposable plastic syringe at 25° for 30 days. Microbiological cultures were also found to be free of any signs of growth after incubation for 30 days.

FORMULATION

Excipients

Excipients that have been used in presentations of amethocaine include:

Lollipops: lemon flavour; potassium acid tartrate; sucrose.
Lozenges: lactose; magnesium stearate; starch; sucrose.
Topical solutions: benzalkonium chloride; cetyldimethylethylammonium bromide; hydrochloric acid; methyl and propyl hydroxybenzoates.
Topical sprays: chlorhexidine gluconate; poloxamer.
Eye drops: acetic acid/sodium acetate; benzalkonium chloride; boric acid; chlorbutol; disodium edetate; phenylmercuric acetate; phenylmercuric nitrate; sodium metabisulphite; sulphur dioxide.
Isobaric solutions (for spinal anaesthesia): sodium chloride.

Effects of excipients

Povidone and methylcellulose form complexes with amethocaine which contribute to the delayed release of the local anaesthetic.[16] Povidone has also been found to prolong the duration of action of a 0.5% amethocaine solution in a sodium chloride isotonic solvent *in vitro*.[17] The prolongation was directly proportional to the molecular weight of the povidone added.

The use of benzalkonium chloride as a preservative in amethocaine eye drop formulations is not recommended as there is a danger that combinations of topical anaesthetics and benzalkonium may reduce or abolish the blink reflex. In addition, the detergent action of benzalkonium removes the protective oily layer of the pre-corneal water film; this results in a greater risk of the surface of the eye drying out.

FURTHER INFORMATION. Percutaneous penetration characteristics of amethocaine [gels] through porcine and human skin— Woolfson AD, McCafferty DF, McGowan KE. Int J Pharmaceutics 1992;78:209–16.

REFERENCES

1. Lachman L, Higuchi T. J Am Pharm Assoc (Sci) 1957;46:32–6.
2. Salt WG, Traynor JR. J Pharm Pharmacol 1979;31:41–2.
3. Burger A, Ramberger R. Mikrochim Acta 1979;ii:273–316.
4. Menon GN, Norris BJ. J Pharm Sci 1981;70:569–70.
5. Dolder R. In: Mainz V, editor. Ophthalmica; band 1. Stuttgart: Wissenschaftliche Verlagsgesellschaft mbH, 1975:82–99.
6. Göber B, Timm U, Pfeifer S [German]. Pharmazie 1979;34:161–4.
7. Chalardsunthornvatee P, Thomas RE. Australas J Pharm 1961;42:800–2.
8. Vervloet E, Ariens E, Lammers J, Witte GJ. Pharm Weekbl (Sci) 1986;8:318.
9. Zöllner EI [Hungarian]. Acta Pharm Hung 1964;34:145–51.
10. Mezey G, Lazar-Mozga E, Szigeti J, Boros M, Kalovics M [Hungarian]. Acta Pharm Hung 1979;49:201–6.
11. Whittet TD. Anaesthesia 1954;9:271–80.
12. Norton DA. J Hosp Pharm 1967;48:328–38.
13. Harb N. J Hosp Pharm 1969;26:44–5.
14. Dolder R, Skinner FS. In: Mainz V, editor. Ophthalmica; band II. Stuttgart: Wissenschaftliche Verlagsgesellschaft mbH, 1978:565–9.
15. Neels JT [letter]. Am J Hosp Pharm 1991;48:1682–3.
16. Thoma K, Ullman E, Mohrschulz P [German]. Arch Pharm 1978;311:205–13.
17. Tsvykh LA [Russian]. Farmatsiya (Moscow) 1979;28:24–6.

Amikacin (BAN, rINN) *Antibacterial aminoglycoside*

6-*O*-(3-Amino-3-deoxy-α-D-glucopyranosyl)-4-*O*-(6-amino-6-deoxy-α-D-glucopyranosyl)-N^1-[(2S)-4-amino-2-hydroxybutyryl]-2-deoxystreptamine; (S)-*O*-3-amino-3-deoxy-α-D-glucopyranosyl-(1 → 6)-*O*-[6-amino-6-deoxy-α-D-glucopyranosyl-(1 → 4)]-N^1-(4-amino-2-hydroxy-1-oxobutyl)-2-deoxy-D-streptamine
$C_{22}H_{43}N_5O_{13} = 585.6$

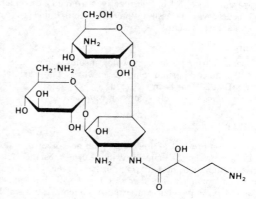

Amikacin Sulphate (BANM, rINNM)
Amikacin Sulfate (USAN)
$C_{22}H_{43}N_5O_{13}, 2H_2SO_4 = 781.8$

CAS—37517-28-5 (amikacin); 39831-55-5 (amikacin sulphate 1:2); 56086-43-2 (amikacin sulphate 1:1); 75282-58-5 (amikacin carbonate 1:1)

Pharmacopoeial status

USP (amikacin)

Preparations

Compendial
Amikacin Sulfate Injection USP. pH 3.5 to 5.5.

Non-compendial
Amikin (Bristol-Myers). *Injection*, amikacin 250 mg (as sulphate)/mL.
Paediatric injection, amikacin 50 mg (as sulphate)/mL. For intravenous use, may be diluted with sodium chloride 0.9%, glucose 5%, compound sodium lactate injection, or compound sodium lactate injection with glucose 5%. Once diluted the solution should be used as soon as possible and not stored.
Amikin should not be physically mixed with other antibacterial agents in syringes, infusion bottles, or any other equipment.

Containers and storage

Solid state
Amikacin USP should be preserved in tight containers.

Dosage forms
Amikacin Sulfate Injection USP should be preserved in single-dose or multiple-dose containers, preferably of Type I or Type III glass.

PHYSICAL PROPERTIES

Amikacin is a white crystalline powder.

Melting point

Amikacin melts in the range 201° to 204°, with decomposition.
Amikacin sulphate, amorphous form, melts in the range 220° to 230°, with decomposition.

pH

A 1% aqueous solution of *amikacin* has a pH of 9.5 to 11.5.

Dissociation constant

An apparent pK_a of 8.1 has been derived from an electrometric titration curve with the assumption that all four amine groups in amikacin are equivalent.[1]

Solubility

Amikacin is sparingly soluble in water; insoluble in ethanol.
At pH 10.4, an equilibrium solubility in water of approximately 185 mg/mL at 25° has been recorded.[2]
Amikacin sulphate is freely soluble in water.

STABILITY

A degradation product of amikacin, 4-amino-2-hydroxybutyric acid, may be present as an impurity in the drug substance. Other materials that may be present as impurities are the synthetic precursors and kanamycin together with isomers of amikacin.
Amikacin base in powder form, exposed to temperatures of 56° and 45° for 4 months, showed a loss of activity not greater than 14.3% and 3.9%, respectively; at 37° the greatest loss after 6 months was 11.2%. At 25° the average loss of activity after 2 years was 3.9%.[2]

Aqueous solutions of amikacin are subject to air oxidation which causes colour darkening. This colour change does not affect potency but can be prevented by the inclusion of an antoxidant.
An aqueous solution of amikacin base (18.5% w/v) autoclaved at 120° for 30 minutes changed in colour from white to light yellow or amber, but no loss of potency was detected.[2]
Undiluted solutions of amikacin sulphate for injection (Amikin) are reported by the manufacturer to be stable at 25°. Darkening of such solutions from colourless to pale yellow may occur, but does not indicate a loss of potency.
Kaplan *et al*[2] studied the stability of aqueous solutions of amikacin sulphate for parenteral use. The solutions contained preservatives, antoxidants, and buffers, and had a pH of 4.5 to 6.8. The average loss of activity was not greater than 10% after storage at 56° and 45° for 4 months, at 37° for 12 months, and at 25° for up to 36 months. Stability was not affected by the presence or absence of methyl and propyl hydroxybenzoates or by pH differences. In similar solutions (pH 4.5, 6.0, and 6.8), autoclaved for one hour at 120° in glass vials stoppered with butyl rubber, losses of activity were less than 10% and no physical changes were evident.
The effects of freeze-thaw treatment on amikacin sulphate (2% w/v) in glucose 5% infusion in polyvinyl chloride minibags have been assessed.[3] After storage for 30 days at −20° and subsequent thawing by microwave radiation or exposure to ambient temperatures, mean antibiotic activity was not less than 90% of the original value. Solutions kept for a further 24 hours at room temperature after freeze-thaw treatment showed negligible change in activity.

INCOMPATIBILITY/COMPATIBILITY

It is recommended that solutions of amikacin sulphate for injection should not be physically mixed with other antibacterial agents but should be administered separately.
The mixing of amikacin with β-lactam antibiotics may lead to significant mutual inactivation although amikacin is reported to be less affected than other aminoglycosides.[4,5]
Amikacin sulphate is reported to be incompatible with the following antimicrobial agents: amphotericin, benzylpenicillin potassium, erythromycin gluceptate, chlortetracycline hydrochloride, oxytetracycline hydrochloride, tetracycline hydrochloride, and with the sodium salts of ampicillin, carbenicillin, cephazolin, cephalothin, cephapirin, methicillin, oxacillin, nitrofurantoin sodium, novobiocin, and sulphadiazine.
Incompatibility has also been reported with aminophylline, chlorothiazide sodium, dexamethasone sodium phosphate, heparin sodium, phenytoin sodium, potassium chloride, thiopentone sodium, vitamin B complex with vitamin C, and warfarin sodium.
Roberts *et al*[6] studied the chemical stability of a combination of amikacin and azlocillin in continuous ambulatory peritoneal dialysis fluid (Dianeal 1.36% adjusted to approximately pH 7.2), during storage for 8 hours at 37°. Approximately 30% degradation of amikacin (initial concentration 20 mg/L) was observed. Azlocillin, 500 mg/L, showed no appreciable loss of activity.
The compatibility and stability of amikacin sulphate injection in 30 commonly used infusion solutions has been studied by Nunning and Granatek.[7] After 24 hours at room temperature all simple admixtures (with an amikacin activity equivalent to 0.25 or 5.0 mg/mL) exhibited satisfactory physical and chemical compatibility.
The results of a study by Zbrozek *et al*[8] showed that clindamycin phosphate (87.6 mg/mL, Upjohn, USA) and amikacin

sulphate (29.04 micrograms/mL, Bristol, USA) were chemically and physically stable in admixture in sodium chloride 0.9% injection for 48 hours in polypropylene syringes at constant room temperature under fluorescent light.

FORMULATION

Excipients

Excipients that have been used in presentations of amikacin sulphate include:

Injections: sodium bisulphite; sodium citrate; sodium metabisulphite; sulphuric acid.

FURTHER INFORMATION. Amikacin liposomes: characterization, aerosolization, and *in-vitro* activity against *Mycobacterium avium-intracellulare* in alveolar macrophages—Wichert BV, Gonzalez-Rothi RJ, Straub LE, Wichert BM, Schreier H. Int J Pharmaceutics 1992;78:227–35. Improvement of ocular penetration of amikacin sulphate by association to poly(butylcyanoacrylate) nanoparticles—Losa C, Calvo P, Castro E, Vila-Jato JL, Alonso MJ. J Pharm Pharmacol 1991;43:548–52.

REFERENCES

1. Monteleone PM, Muhammad N, Brown RD, McGrory JP, Hanna SA. In: Florey K, editor. Analytical profiles of drug substances; vol 12. London: Academic Press, 1983:41.
2. Kaplan MA, Coppola WP, Nunning BC, Granatek AP. Curr Ther Res 1976;20:352–8.
3. Holmes CJ, Ausman RK, Kundsin RB, Walter CW. Am J Hosp Pharm 1982;39:104–8.
4. Farchione LA. J Antimicrob Chemother 1981;8 (Suppl A):27–36.
5. Tindula RJ, Ambrose PJ, Harralson AF. Drug Intell Clin Pharm 1983;17:906–8.
6. Roberts DE, Cross MD, Thomas PH, Walters TH. Br J Pharm Pract 1987;9:98–9.
7. Nunning BC, Granatek AP. Curr Ther Res 1976;20:359–68.
8. Zbrozek AS, Marble DA, Bosso JA, Bair JN, Townsend RJ. Drug Intell Clin Pharm 1987;21:806–10.

Aminophylline (BAN, pINN)

Xanthine bronchodilator

Euphyllinum; metaphyllin; theophyllaminum; theophylline and ethylenediamine

Theophylline compound with ethylenediamine (2:1); 3,7-dihydro-1,3-dimethyl-1*H*-purine-2,6-dione compound with 1,2-ethanediamine (2:1)

Aminophylline is a stable mixture or combination of theophylline and ethylenediamine. Theophylline is the subject of a separate monograph.

$(C_7H_8N_4O_2)_2, C_2H_8N_2 = 420.4$

Aminophylline Hydrate (BANM, pINNM)

$(C_7H_8N_4O_2)_2, C_2H_8N_2, 2H_2O = 456.5$
CAS—317-34-0 (aminophylline); 5877-66-5 (aminophylline hydrate)

Pharmacopoeial status

BP (aminophylline, aminophylline hydrate); USP (aminophylline)

Preparations

Compendial

Aminophylline Tablets BP. Tablets containing, in each, 100 mg of aminophylline are usually available.

Aminophylline Injection BP. A sterile solution of aminophylline or aminophylline hydrate in water for injections free from carbon dioxide, pH 8.8 to 10. It may be prepared by dissolving theophylline or theophylline hydrate in a solution of ethylenediamine hydrate in water for injections free from carbon dioxide. Ethylenediamine hydrate additional to that necessary for the formation of aminophylline may be added but the total amount of ethylenediamine should not exceed 0.295 g for each gram of anhydrous theophylline present. The solution should not be allowed to come into contact with metal. Injections containing 250 mg aminophylline in 10 mL and 500 mg of aminophylline in 2 mL are usually available.

Aminophylline Tablets USP.
Aminophylline Oral Solution USP.
Aminophylline Enema USP.
Aminophylline Suppositories USP.
Aminophylline Injection USP. pH 8.6 to 9.0.

Non-compendial

Pecram (Zyma). *Tablets*, slow release, aminophylline hydrate 225 mg.
Phyllocontin Continus (Napp). *Tablets*, controlled release, aminophylline hydrate 225 mg.
Forte tablets, controlled release, aminophylline hydrate 350 mg.
Paediatric tablets, controlled release, aminophylline hydrate 100 mg.
Modified-release tablets containing aminophylline 225 mg and 350 mg are also available from Ashbourne (Amnivent).
Aminophylline injection containing aminophylline 25 mg/mL is available from Evans, IMS (Min-I-Jet).

Containers and storage

Solid state

Aminophylline BP and Aminophylline Hydrate BP should be kept in well-filled, airtight containers and protected from light. Aminophylline USP should be preserved in tight containers.

Dosage forms

Aminophylline Tablets BP should be kept in an airtight container and protected from light.
Aminophylline Tablets USP and Aminophylline Oral Solution USP should be preserved in tight containers.
Aminophylline Enema USP should be preserved in single-dose or multiple-dose containers.
Aminophylline Suppositories USP should be preserved in well-closed containers, in a cold place.
Aminophylline Injection USP should be preserved in single-dose containers of Type I glass, from which carbon dioxide should be excluded. It should be protected from light.
Pecram tablets should be stored in a cool dry place, protected from light.
Phyllocontin preparations should be stored at room temperature in a dry place, protected from light.

PHYSICAL PROPERTIES

Aminophylline and *aminophylline hydrate* are white or slightly yellowish powders or granular powders; odourless or with a slight ammoniacal odour.

Solubility

Both *aminophylline* and *aminophylline hydrate* are soluble 1 in 5 of water (the solutions may become cloudy in the presence of carbon dioxide). The addition of ethylenediamine or ammonia solution may be necessary to produce complete solution. *Aminophylline* and *aminophylline hydrate* are practically insoluble in absolute ethanol and in ether.

Dissolution

The USP specifies that for Aminophylline Tablets (uncoated or plain coated) USP not less than 75% of the labelled amount of $C_7H_8N_4O_2$ (anhydrous theophylline) is dissolved in 45 minutes. Dissolution medium: 900 mL of water; Apparatus 2 at 50 rpm.

STABILITY

Aminophylline can absorb carbon dioxide from the air resulting in liberation of theophylline. Aqueous solutions absorb carbon dioxide from the air resulting in precipitation of theophylline. In solutions exposed to sunlight and oxygen, aminophylline has been found to degrade to 1,3-dimethylallantoin, *N,N*-dimethyloxamide, and ammonia.[1]

Tablets

Aminophylline tablets repackaged into single-unit containers were found to discolour after 21 weeks when stored at 24° and 35% to 75% relative humidity. Water absorption was observed, with 1% absorbed over the 21-week period.[2] An amber colour imparted to unit-dose packaging containing uncoated aminophylline tablets and observed within 3 months when stored at room temperature was found to be caused by the release of ethylenediamine.[3] The quantity of ethylenediamine required to discolour packaging material is very small and tablets stored in the packaging under test still met the USP requirements for ethylenediamine content after 13 months.

Suppositories

Brower et al[4] determined that during storage of aminophylline suppositories at room temperature for one month, a reduction in ethylenediamine content and an increase in melting point of the suppositories had occurred. An accelerated decomposition study, which involved storage at 40° for 3 months, resulted in complete loss of ethylenediamine. Diamide products were found to have formed in the suppositories stored both at room temperature and at the elevated temperature. These diamides were thought to form through a reaction of ethylenediamine with fatty acids present in coconut and palm kernel oils.

Similarly, diamide decomposition products were reported[5] to form in aminophylline suppositories (stored, for example, at 32° for 12 weeks) due to reaction between ethylenediamine and the triglyceride suppository basis.

Solutions and injections

In the presence of lactose and other sugars, aminophylline solutions develop a yellow or brown colour on standing.

Parker[6] measured the aminophylline content of solutions in glucose 5% during storage for 48 hours at pH values of 3.5, 4.9, 6.0, 7.0, and 8.6; aminophylline breakdown during the study period was negligible. Boddapati et al,[7] prompted by reports of yellow discoloration in mixtures of glucose and aminophylline injections, characterised the physicochemical properties of these mixtures. It was found that on storage for 48 hours, 24 hours, and 6 hours at 25°, 35°, and 55°, respectively, a yellow colour developed; discoloration was possibly due to the formation of hydroxymethylfurfural. A solution stored in a refrigerator remained colourless over the seven days of the study. Control solutions of glucose 5% remained clear and colourless when stored at 25° for 48 hours. On the basis of HPLC analyses it was concluded that the yellow coloration does not alter the physicochemical properties or the concentration of the active ingredient. The admixture was visually and chemically stable for at least 48 hours when stored at 25° and at 5°.

Adams et al[8] reported that when aminophylline injection was added to sodium chloride 0.9% injection (aminophylline concentration of 250 mg/260 mL) no discoloration was apparent, whereas when it was added to glucose 5% injection, or glucose 4% and sodium chloride 0.18% injection a yellow colour developed on standing. The intensity of discoloration was dependent upon the content of ethylenediamine. The content of theophylline was found to be significantly lowered only when the solution was very discoloured.

Aminophylline injection 250 mg/10 mL and 500 mg/20 mL diluted in 50 mL of glucose 5% injection was stable when stored in glass intravenous containers for 96 hours in a refrigerator. There was little change in pH or in concentration of active ingredient and the solutions remained clear and colourless when brought to room temperature.[9]

Aminophylline stability in glucose solutions has been the subject of many studies, prompted by concern over the pH of glucose 5% solution, which could be too low to maintain aminophylline stability. Hadgraft,[10] however, found that when the appropriate concentration of aminophylline is added to glucose 5% injection, the resultant pH is about 8.5. Similar findings in aminophylline admixtures with glucose and glucose/sodium chloride solutions were reported by Edward[11] who determined pH values between 8.35 and 8.6.

The stability of aminophylline in glucose 5%, 10%, and 20% injections and in neonatal parenteral nutrition solutions over a 24-hour period was examined by Kirk and Sprake.[12] At a concentration of 250 micrograms/mL aminophylline was stable in all the glucose solutions when stored in a polypropylene syringe or glass flask at room temperature over a 24-hour period. A yellow discoloration was observed after 2 hours. The aminophylline concentration of 4.4 mg/150 mL in a standard total parenteral nutrition (TPN) solution did not change appreciably. The solutions were stored in polyvinyl chloride minibags, glass containers, and polypropylene burettes. The stability of the other constituents of the TPN solution was not assessed.

The stability of aminophylline in three parenteral nutrition solutions containing glucose was the subject of an investigation by Niemiec et al.[13] Aminophylline was added to 100 mL portions of prepared nutrition solutions to produce final concentrations of 0.25, 0.50, 1.00, and 1.50 mg/mL. Assessment of visual compatibility and measurement of pH and theophylline concentrations were undertaken at 1 hour, 24 hours, and 48 hours from the time of preparation. It was concluded that in the parenteral nutrition solutions studied, aminophylline injection was stable for 24 hours at 25° at concentrations up to 1.5 mg/mL. Swerling[14] examined the stability of dilute oral and intravenous aminophylline preparations. The intravenous solution was prepared by dilution of Aminophylline Injection USP 25 mg/mL to a concentration of 4 mg/mL using sterile water for injections. The oral solution was prepared using Somophylline (Fisons, USA) 105 mg/5 mL which was diluted with sterile water for injections to a concentration of 5 mg/mL and stored in amber bottles. Although both solutions showed acceptable stability over the 86 days of the test, a shelf-life of one month was assigned because of microbiological considerations.

When aminophylline was added to total parenteral nutrition mixtures containing lipids in ethyl vinyl acetate bags,[15] the concentration of theophylline remained stable over a 24-hour study period at 25°.

FURTHER INFORMATION. Aminophylline suppository decomposition: an investigation using differential scanning calorimetry—Pryce-Jones RH, Eccleston GM, Abu-Bakar BB. Int J Pharmaceutics 1992;86:231–7. Polymorphism of fatty acid diamides of ethylenediamine and their detection in aged aminophylline suppositories—Pryce-Jones RH, Grant KM, Eccleston GM. J Pharm Pharmacol 1989;41:106P. Aminophylline suppository decomposition: GC mass spectrometry and GC-mass spectrometry of the decomposition products—Pryce-Jones RH, Johnson DG, Watson DG, Eccleston GM. J Pharm Pharmacol 1990;42:111P. Direct observation using high-field ^{1}H NMR of reactions occurring in aminophylline suppositories—Eccleston GM, Gray AI, Pryce-Jones RH, Waigh RD. J Pharm Pharmacol 1992;44(Suppl):1079. Stability of aminophylline in bacteriostatic water for injection stored in plastic syringes at two temperatures—Nahata MC, Morosco RS, Hipple TF. Am J Hosp Pharm 1992;49:2962–3.

INCOMPATIBILITY/COMPATIBILITY

Incompatibility has been reported between aminophylline or aminophylline hydrate and bleomycin sulphate, chlorpromazine hydrochloride, clindamycin phosphate, corticotrophin, dimenhydrinate, doxorubicin, erythromycin gluceptate, hydralazine hydrochloride, hydroxyzine hydrochloride, opioid analgesics, oxytetracycline hydrochloride, phenytoin sodium, procaine hydrochloride, prochlorperazine salts, promazine hydrochloride, promethazine hydrochloride, sulphafurazole diethanolamine, and vancomycin hydrochloride.

Aminophylline is incompatible with acids. In the presence of lactose and other sugars, a yellow or brown colour develops on standing; in the presence of copper, solutions develop a blue colour.

Hartauer and Guillory[16] used Fourier-transform infrared spectroscopy to demonstrate that brown discoloration such as that which appeared when aminophylline:lactose (1:5 w/w) mixtures were stored for three weeks at 60° was due to a chemical reaction between ethylenediamine and lactose.

Aminophylline injection should not be mixed with alkali-labile drugs.

The visual compatibility of dobutamine hydrochloride (Dobutrex, Eli Lilly, USA) 1 mg/mL with aminophylline (Elkins-Sinn, USA) was investigated by Hasegawa and Eder.[17] At an aminophylline concentration of 2.5 mg/mL in glucose 5% injection or sodium chloride 0.9% injection, a white precipitate was evident after 12 hours. The solutions were stored in glass vials. Kirschenbaum et al[18] prepared admixtures of dobutamine hydrochloride (Eli Lilly, USA) 1 mg/mL and aminophylline (Searle, USA) 1 mg/mL in either glucose 5% injection or sodium chloride 0.9% injection. After six hours the solutions became cloudy.

Admixtures of bretylium tosylate (Bretylol, American Critical Care, USA) 1 mg/mL with aminophylline (Elkins-Sinn, USA) 1 mg/mL in sodium chloride 0.9% injection or glucose 5% injection were found to be visually compatible when observed over a 48-hour period.[19]

Lignocaine 2 mg/mL is reported to be visually compatible for 24 hours with aminophylline in sodium chloride 0.9% injection, glucose 5% injection, or compound sodium lactate injection.[20] Jhunjhunwala and Bhalla[21] investigated the compatibility of mephentermine sulphate (equivalent to 300 mg mephentermine) with aminophylline (250 mg) in glucose 5% injection (400 mL). They suggested that the admixture was stable for at least 24 hours under the test conditions. The solutions were stored in USP Type I glass containers at temperatures of 3°, 30°, and 45°.

A transient precipitate was evident when aminophylline injection (Searle, USA) was added to verapamil hydrochloride (Knoll, USA) in glucose 5% injection or sodium chloride 0.9% injection.[22] It was postulated that precipitation resulted from a change in pH at the point of mixing.

Verapamil hydrochloride injection at final concentrations of 0.1 or 0.4 mg/mL was incompatible with aminophylline 1.0 mg/mL in glucose 5% injection as manifested by a decrease in the concentration of verapamil hydrochloride and turbidity or microscopic precipitation.[23] Precipitation of verapamil was attributed to the pH of the admixtures, which exceeded pH 8.

An apparent decrease in glyceryl trinitrate (American Critical Care, USA) concentration over a period of 48 hours at 23° was noted in admixture with aminophylline (manufacturer Invenex) in glucose 5% injection and in sodium chloride 0.9% injection. However, the decrease (about 5%) was not statistically significant. Aminophylline concentration was not monitored.[24]

Neil[25] reported that a precipitate was formed immediately when gentamicin sulphate 80 mg/2 mL was added to aminophylline 250 mg in glucose injection (500 mL) via the drip-tubing. Additional compatibility information was given for various aminophylline/intravenous fluid admixtures. It was recommended that aminophylline should only be added to glucose 5%, glucose/sodium chloride, compound sodium lactate, or sodium chloride 0.9% injections.

Aminophylline 500 mg and cimetidine hydrochloride 1200 mg were visually and chemically compatible for 48 hours at room temperature in one litre of glucose 5% injection.[26]

When aminophylline injection was administered as a manual retrograde injection through a system delivering neonatal total parenteral nutrition solutions, precipitation occurred in most solutions; this was attributed to precipitation of calcium and phosphate (as calcium phosphate).[27] In solutions with high concentrations of amino acids, low pH, and low concentrations of calcium and phosphate, precipitation was thought to be less likely to occur.

Sorption to plastics

The percentage loss of aminophylline to four brands of plastic 2-mL syringe was declared as being less than 5% after storage for 18 hours at room temperature.[28] Three brands of syringe had a polypropylene barrel and one had a polypropylene/polystyrene barrel.

FURTHER INFORMATION. Compatibility of ceftazidime and aminophylline admixtures for different methods of intravenous infusion—Pleasants RA, Vaughan LM, Williams DM, Fox JL. Ann Pharmacother 1992;26:1221–6. Stability and compatibility of fluconazole and aminophylline in intravenous admixtures—Johnson CE, Jacobson PA, Pillen HA, Woycik CL. Am J Hosp Pharm 1993;50:703–6.

FORMULATION

Excipients

Excipients that have been used in presentations of aminophylline include:

Tablets: acacia; maize starch; magnesium stearate; potassium phosphate; sodium sulphate; sodium sulphite; talc.
Tablets (sustained-release): cetostearyl alcohol; hydroxyethylcellulose; magnesium stearate; povidone; talc.
Oral liquids: acid fuchsine D; saccharin sodium.
Suppositories: theobroma oil.

Bioavailability

Although seven aminophylline suppositories commercially available in the Netherlands met Dutch Pharmacopoeial requirements, only three products had relative bioavailabilities greater than 80% when compared with that of an oral hydro-alcoholic solution of aminophylline in twelve healthy volunteers (four-way Latin square study).[42] Results of in-vitro dissolution tests could not be used to predict in-vivo bioavailability. The authors concluded that the products tested were bioinequivalent and were not interchangeable.

In a non-randomised, multidose, crossover study[43] a liquid preparation of aminophylline, intermittently administered via a nasogastric tube or a gastrostomy tube to critically ill, mechanically ventilated patients, was bioequivalent with continuous intravenous infusion of a similar liquid.

Tablets

Hammouda et al[29] prepared tablets by mixing aminophylline with sodium chloride, as a directly compressible filler, in the ratios 20:80, 40:60, 60:40, and 80:20; magnesium stearate 1% was also included in the formulation. The degree of compressibility was found to decrease as the proportion of aminophylline was increased. Tablets could not be obtained using pure aminophylline. The inclusion of sodium chloride with aminophylline at a ratio of 60:40 produced tablets with the most desirable properties.

Suppositories

The melting behaviour of aminophylline suppositories prepared using eight different bases and stored at 4°, 22°, and 30° for periods of up to 15 months was investigated by de Blaey and Rutten-Kingma.[30] Considerable changes in melting behaviour were detected in vitro but the significance of these changes to in-vivo release was not determined. The same authors examined (in vitro) the effect of method of preparation and storage conditions on the release rate of ageing aminophylline suppositories.[31] As a result of in-vitro dissolution studies, Nissen and Juul[32] concluded that after storage for one year at room temperature there should be no reduction in the extent of absorption of aminophylline from suppositories manufactured using macrogols 100 and 3000 (65:35). However, Taylor and Simpkins[33] demonstrated that the in-vitro dissolution rate of theophylline from aminophylline suppositories prepared using fatty bases is decreased on storage. Shelf-lives could be less than 12 months and storage at temperatures not exceeding 15° is recommended. Aminophylline suppositories were withdrawn from the UK market in 1990 because of reports of bioavailability problems with erratic absorption and unpredictable response.[34] Ethylenediamine was thought to react with the fatty basis of the suppository to produce fatty acid amides; this reaction caused an increase in the melting point of the suppository and a corresponding decrease in theophylline release.

Controlled release

Although in-vivo studies[35-37] have claimed that various controlled-release tablets of aminophylline (two in each study) may be bioequivalent, it is generally accepted that controlled-release preparations of aminophylline are not interchangeable.[38-40]

Smart et al[41] demonstrated that when the dissolution properties of two controlled-release aminophylline tablets (Phyllocontin Continus, Napp UK, and Pecram, Zyma UK) were compared in vitro, release profiles in water were similar but when the dissolution medium was acid at pH 2 for one hour and then buffer at pH 6 for 23 hours, a reduction was observed in the rate of release of Phyllocontin Continus tablets; the results suggested that release from the two products may differ in vivo.

FURTHER INFORMATION. Aminophylline enema for paediatric patients [stability and bioavailability]—Vinuales A, Alfaro J, Napal V, Irvin A [Spanish]. Farm Clin 1986;3:389–98. Physical stability of aminophylline suppositories—Kassem AA, El-Din IN, El-Shamy AHA. Bull Fac Pharm Cairo Univ 1969;8:193–202. Formulation and stability of aminophylline suppositories—Kassem AA, El-Shamy AHA. J Drug Res Egypt 1972;4:53–9. Prolonged storage of aminophylline suppositories. The impact on physical parameters and bioavailability—Tukker JJ, de Blaey CJ. Pharm Weekbl (Sci) 1984;6:96–8. The gastrointestinal transit investigation of a controlled release aminophylline formulation [tablet]—Davis SS, Parr GD, Feely L, Leslie ST, Malkowska S, Lockwood GF. Int J Pharmaceutics 1989;49:183–8. Design and evaluation of a sustained-release aminophylline tablet [in vitro and in vivo]—Boles MG, Deasy PB, Donnellan MF. Drug Dev Ind Pharm 1993;19(3):349–70.

PROCESSING

Sterilisation

Aminophylline injection can be sterilised by heating in an autoclave.

REFERENCES

1. Ishiguro Y, Sawada M, Tanaka Y, Kawabe K [Japanese]. Yakugaku Zasshi 1980;100:1048–53.
2. Das Gupta V, Stewart KR, Gupta A [letter]. Am J Hosp Pharm 1980;37:165–9.
3. Estabrook DR, Stennett DJ, Ayres JW [letter]. Am J Hosp Pharm 1980;37:1046.
4. Brower JF, Juenge EC, Page DP, Dow ML. J Pharm Sci 1980;69:942–5.
5. Pryce-Jones RH, Eccleston GM, Abu-Baka B, Das Gupta AH. J Pharm Pharmacol 1987;39:50P.
6. Parker EA. Am J Hosp Pharm 1970;27:67–9.
7. Boddapati S, Yang K, Murty R. Am J Hosp Pharm 1982;39:108–12.
8. Adams PS, Haines-Nutt RF, Ross ID. Proceedings of the Guild 1988;25:41–4.
9. Zatz L, Sethia P, Sherman NE. Hosp Pharm 1981;16:548.
10. Hadgraft JW [letter]. Lancet 1970;2:1254.
11. Edward M. Am J Hosp Pharm 1967;24:440–9.
12. Kirk B, Sprake JM. Br J Intravenous Ther 1982;3:4,6,8.
13. Niemiec PW, Vanderveen TW, Hohenwarter MW, Gadsden RH. Am J Hosp Pharm 1983;40:428–32.
14. Swerling R. Am J Hosp Pharm 1981;38:1359–60.
15. Andreu A, Cardona D, Pastor C, Bonal J [letter]. Ann Pharmacother 1992;26:127–8.
16. Hartauer KJ, Guillory JK. Drug Dev Ind Pharm 1991;17(4):617–30.
17. Hasegawa GR, Eder JF. Am J Hosp Pharm 1984;41:949–51.
18. Kirschenbaum HL, Aronoff W, Piltz GW, Perentesis GP, Cutie AJ. Am J Hosp Pharm 1983;40:1690–1.
19. Perentesis GP, Piltz GW, Kirschenbaum HL, Navalakha P, Aronoff W, Cutie AJ. Am J Hosp Pharm 1983;40:1010-12.
20. Kirschenbaum HL, Aronoff W, Perentesis GP, Piltz GW, Cutie AJ. Am J Hosp Pharm 1982;39:1013–15.
21. Jhunjhunwala VP, Bhalla HL. Am J Hosp Pharm 1981;38:1922–4.
22. Cutie MR. Am J Hosp Pharm 1981;38:231.
23. Johnson CE, Lloyd CW, Mesaros JL, Rubley GJ. Am J Hosp Pharm 1989;46:97–100.

24. Klamerus KJ, Veda CT, Newton DW. Am J Hosp Pharm 1984;41:303–5.
25. Neil JM. The prescribing and administration of IV additives to infusion fluids. Thetford: Travenol, 1976:2/3, 3/3.
26. Baptista RJ, Mitrano FP. Drug Intell Clin Pharm 1988;22:592–3.
27. Kirkpatrick AE, Holcombe BJ, Sawyer WT. Am J Hosp Pharm 1989;46:2496–500.
28. Simmons A, Allwood MC. J Clin Hosp Pharm 1981;6:71–3.
29. Hammouda Y, Eshra AG, El-Banna HM. Pharm Ind 1978;40:987–92.
30. de Blaey CJ, Rutten-Kingma JJ. Pharm Acta Helv 1976;51:186–92.
31. de Blaey CJ, Rutten-Kingma JJ. Pharm Acta Helv 1977;52:11–14.
32. Nissen P, Juul G [Danish]. Arch Pharm Chemi 1979;136:117–25.
33. Taylor JB, Simpkins DE. Pharm J 1981;227:601–3.
34. Pharm J 1990;244:764.
35. Lin S-Y, Chang H-N, Yang J-C, Kao Y-H, Cheng L-F. Curr Ther Res 1988;44(4):585–92.
36. Crawford FE, Guy GW, Tilson RM. Pharm J 1989;243:221–4.
37. Lin S-Y, Kao Y-H, Chang H-N. J Pharm Sci 1990;79(4):326–30.
38. Caldwell J [letter]. Pharm J 1989;243:204.
39. Caldwell J, Teeman M [letters]. Pharm J 1989;243:263–4.
40. Tucker GT [letter]. Pharm J 1989;243:362.
41. Smart JD, Barnes MS, Norris MJ. J Pharm Pharmacol 1992;44:623–5.
42. Tukker JJ, Crombeen JP, Breimer DD, de Blaey CJ. Pharm Weekbl (Sci) 1981;3:221–31.
43. Shalansky KF, Vaughan LM, Ustad C, Tweeddale MG, Sahn SA. Am J Hosp Pharm 1992;49:1556, 1559.

Amitriptyline (BAN, rINN)   *Tricyclic antidepressant*

3-(10,11-Dihydro-5*H*-dibenzo[*a,d*]cyclohepten-5-ylidene)-propyldimethylamine; 3-(10,11-dihydro-5*H*-dibenzo[*a,d*]cyclohepten-5-ylidene)-*N*,*N*-dimethyl-1-propanamine
$C_{20}H_{23}N = 277.4$

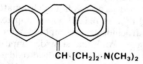

CH·[CH₂]₂·N(CH₃)₂

Amitriptyline Embonate (BANM, rINNM)
$(C_{20}H_{23}N)_2, C_{23}H_{16}O_6 = 943.2$

Amitriptyline Hydrochloride (BANM, rINNM)
$C_{20}H_{23}N, HCl = 313.9$
CAS—50-48-6 (amitriptyline); 17086-03-2 (amitriptyline embonate); 549-18-8 (amitriptyline hydrochloride)

Pharmacopoeial status

BP (amitriptyline embonate, amitriptyline hydrochloride); USP (amitriptyline hydrochloride)

Preparations

Compendial

Amitriptyline Tablets BP. Tablets containing, in each, 10 mg, 25 mg, and 50 mg of amitriptyline hydrochloride are usually available.

Amitriptyline Oral Suspension BP (Amitriptyline Embonate Mixture, Amitriptyline Syrup). A suspension of amitriptyline embonate in a suitable flavoured vehicle. An oral suspension containing the equivalent of 10 mg of amitriptyline in 5 mL is usually available. pH 5.0 to 7.0.

Amitriptyline Hydrochloride Tablets USP.

Amitriptyline Hydrochloride Injection USP. pH between 4.0 and 6.0.

Non-compendial

Domical (Berk). *Tablets*, amitriptyline hydrochloride 10 mg, 25 mg, and 50 mg.

Lentizol (P–D). *Capsules*, sustained release, amitriptyline hydrochloride 25 mg and 50 mg.

Tryptizol (Morson). *Capsules*, slow release, amitriptyline hydrochloride 75 mg in a pelleted formulation.

Tablets, amitriptyline hydrochloride 10 mg, 25 mg, and 50 mg.

Syrup, sugar-free suspension, amitriptyline 10 mg (as embonate)/5 mL. Diluent: syrup, life of diluted syrup 14 days.

Injection, amitriptyline hydrochloride 10 mg/mL.

Amitriptyline tablets are also available from APS, Cox, DDSA (Elavil), Evans, Kerfoot.

Containers and storage

Solid state

Amitriptyline Embonate BP should be protected from light.

Amitriptyline Hydrochloride BP and Amitriptyline Hydrochloride USP should be stored in well-closed containers.

Dosage forms

Amitriptyline Tablets USP should be preserved in well-closed containers.

Amitriptyline Hydrochloride Injection USP should be preserved in single-dose or multiple-dose containers, preferably of Type I glass.

Lentizol capsules should be stored in a dry place at a temperature not exceeding 25°

Tryptizol preparations should be kept in well-closed containers and stored below 25°, protected from light; protect the injection and syrup from freezing.

PHYSICAL PROPERTIES

Amitriptyline is a colourless oil that turns yellow on standing.

Amitriptyline embonate is a pale yellow to brownish-yellow powder; odourless or almost odourless.

Amitriptyline hydrochloride appears as a white or practically white, crystalline powder or as small crystals; odourless or practically odourless.

Melting point

Amitriptyline embonate melts at about 140°.

Amitriptyline hydrochloride melts in the range 195° to 199°.

pH

A 1% aqueous solution of *amitriptyline hydrochloride* has a pH of 5.0 to 6.0.

Dissociation constant

pK_a 9.4 (24° ± 1°);[1] pK_a 9.31 (37°);[2] pK_a 9.5[3]

Partition coefficients

Log *P* (octanol/pH 7.4), 3.0

Log *P* values for amitriptyline hydrochloride[2] in an octanol/aqueous (Sørensen's) buffer system at 37°:

pH	Log P
2.10	1.30
3.00	1.34
4.00	1.46
5.80	1.73
5.97	1.84
6.19	2.06
6.80	2.59

Solubility

Amitriptyline is practically insoluble in water; solubility[1] in 0.01 M sodium hydroxide at 24° ± 1° is 1 in 100 000.

Amitriptyline embonate is practically insoluble in water; soluble 1 in 120 of ethanol; soluble 1 in 6 of acetone and 1 in 8 of chloroform.

Amitriptyline hydrochloride is soluble 1 in 1 of water, 1 in 5 of ethanol, 1 in 1 of methanol, 1 in 2 of chloroform, 1 in 56 of acetone; practically insoluble in ether.

Blessel *et al*[4] have reported the solubility of *amitriptyline hydrochloride* in ether to be 1 in 2000.

Critical micelle concentration

As determined by tensiometry,[5] the critical micelle concentration (cmc) of amitriptyline hydrochloride in acetate buffer pH 5.0 was 1.56×10^{-2} mol/L, and in sodium chloride 0.9% the cmc was 1.27×10^{-2} mol/L.

Dissolution

The USP specifies that for Amitriptyline Hydrochloride Tablets USP not less than 75% of the labelled amount of $C_{20}H_{23}N, HCl$ is dissolved in 45 minutes. Dissolution medium: 900 mL of 0.1 N hydrochloric acid; Apparatus 1 at 100 rpm.

Dissolution properties

Amitriptyline hydrochloride tablets were subjected to dissolution tests before and after storage for between 9 and 46 days in automatic tablet counter containers. The average daily temperature of the containers ranged from 22.2° to 26.1°. The data indicated that the dissolution properties of the tablets were not affected by the environmental conditions of the tablet counter containers.[6]

Statistically significant differences in dissolution rates were demonstrated by formulations of amitriptyline supplied by different manufacturers; ion-selective electrodes were used as sensors in an air-segmented continuous flow analyser.[7] Dissolution curves illustrated that a dependence on the pH of the medium was shown by only two products.

STABILITY

Enever *et al*[8] proposed that the initial step in the decomposition of aqueous solutions of amitriptyline hydrochloride, buffered at pH 6.8 and autoclaved at 115° to 116° for periods of up to 6 hours, involves the formation of 3-(propa-1,3-dienyl)-1,2:4,5-dibenzocyclohepta-1,4-diene; this is subsequently oxidised to dibenzosuberone and 3-(2-oxoethylidene)-1,2:4,5-dibenzocyclohepta-1,4-diene.

Henwood[9] noted the instability of amitriptyline as the free base and that the colourless oil made from a tablet for reference purposes turned yellow on standing; this was attributed to oxidation to form a ketonic product, 10,11-dihydro-5*H*-dibenzo[*a,d*]cycloheptene-5-one (dibenzosuberone).

Bouche[10] implicated anthraquinone as a possible product of the decomposition of amitriptyline at room temperature. Anthraquinone is formed by boiling amitriptyline in an alkaline permanganate solution or when dibenzosuberone is heated to 200° in the presence of oxygen.

At room temperature and in daylight, Buckles and Walters[11] found the principal product of decomposition of amitriptyline hydrochloride to be dibenzosuberone. Solutions of the drug in purified water (1% w/v) were stable during storage for at least 8 weeks either at room temperature or in a refrigerator, protected from light.

Stability of a commercial parenteral product

Although the buffered solutions examined by Enever *et al*[12] showed losses of between 5% and 90% after storage at 80° for 30 days, Roman *et al*[13] found no detectable degradation of amitriptyline hydrochloride in an unbuffered (pH between 4 and 6) commercial parenteral preparation (Elavil, MSD, USA) stored at 80° for up to 90 days. The enhanced stability was attributed to the low ratio of head space to liquid (1:6) in the multidose vial which was considerably less than that (4:1) for the solutions studied by Enever *et al*.[12] In intact vials from three batches stored at room temperature for 5 years, no decomposition products could be detected by HPLC.[11]

Effect of temperature

The effects of elevated temperature and exposure to light on the stability of amitriptyline hydrochloride in the solid state have been studied. Amitriptyline hydrochloride was found to be stable for more than 2 months at room temperature and at 45°, but some decomposition was measured after 2 months at 100°; a brownish discoloration was observed when the bulk powder was exposed to light. Aqueous solutions (1% w/v) were found to be stable at 0°, room temperature, and at 45°, as well as for a period of 60 hours at 100°.[4]

Effect of additives

Solutions of amitriptyline hydrochloride (0.2% w/v) in buffer (pH 3.0 or pH 5.0) were filled into 10 mL clear or amber glass ampoules and stored in the dark at 80°.[12] Rates of decomposition were determined using gas liquid chromatography (GLC). It was calculated that, in pH 3.0 buffer, approximately 68% of amitriptyline hydrochloride decomposed after 20 days in the clear glass ampoules. An initial slow decomposition rate which then accelerated indicated a free-radical oxidation mechanism. This theory was confirmed by the absence of decomposition when the ampoules were sealed under nitrogen and also by the observed acceleration of decomposition following the addition of cupric acetate or ferric chloride $(2 \times 10^{-4}$ M). Inclusion of the chelating agent disodium edetate (0.1% w/v) significantly reduced the decomposition rate and further confirmed that metal ion contaminants are a major cause of degradation. The authors postulated that amber glass containers are potential sources of iron contaminants which are leached as metal ions into solutions. This phenomenon is used to explain the greater decomposition rates observed for solutions stored in amber ampoules than for those stored in clear glass.

The antioxidants propyl gallate (0.05% w/v) and, to a lesser extent, hydroquinone (0.01% w/v) were found to slow the rate of degradation of amitriptyline hydrochloride in aqueous solution whereas sodium metabisulphite, although initially observed to have no effect, subsequently resulted in an acceleration of the decomposition rate.[12]

INCOMPATIBILITY/COMPATIBILITY

Admixtures of methadone hydrochloride 10 mg (Eli Lilly, USA) and amitriptyline hydrochloride 25 mg (Hoffmann-La Roche, USA) in cherry syrup (15 mL) showed no visual change or appreciable variation in pH over two weeks.[14]

Amitriptyline Oral Suspension BP is incompatible with alkaline preparations such as aluminium hydroxide gel, and with vehicles that may raise the pH of the preparation and give rise to the formation of amitriptyline base.

The decomposition of amitriptyline hydrochloride in solution is accelerated by sodium metabisulphite and by cupric and ferric ions.

In suspensions, amitriptyline has been stated to be physically incompatible with xanthan gum (Keltrol, Kelco International) used as a suspending agent.[15]

FORMULATION

Excipients

Excipients that have been used in presentations of amitriptyline include:

Capsules, amitriptyline hydrochloride: sucrose.
Tablets, amitriptyline hydrochloride: acacia; allura red AC (E129); brilliant blue FCF (133); calcium hydrogen phosphate; cellulose; colloidal anhydrous silica; diethyl phthalate; ethylcellulose; hydroxypropylcellulose; hypromellose; indigo carmine (E132); iron oxide; lactose; macrogol 3350; magnesium stearate; methylcellulose; microcrystalline cellulose; povidone; propylene glycol; quinoline yellow (E104); starch; stearic acid; sucrose; sunset yellow FCF (E110); talc; tartrazine (E102); titanium dioxide (E171).
Oral liquids, amitriptyline embonate: methyl and propyl hydroxybenzoates; sorbitol; tragacanth.
Oral drops, amitriptyline: ethanol; glycerol.
Injections, amitriptyline hydrochloride: glucose; methyl and propyl hydroxybenzoates; sodium chloride.

Suspensions

The preparation of an amitriptyline suspension (50 mg/5 mL) from crushed tablets of amitriptyline hydrochloride resulted in a product that was not only very bitter but also anaesthetised the tongue. The problem was overcome by the replacement of the hydrochloride salt by amitriptyline embonate in the formulation.[16]

Bioavailability

The pharmacokinetic parameters of a sustained-release form of amitriptyline (Lentizol) were compared with those of ordinary tablets (Saroten, Warner, UK) by Burch and Hullin.[17] In a crossover study, single doses were administered to six depressed patients. At identical amitriptyline doses, Lentizol produced marginally higher plasma concentrations 24 hours after administration, but the difference was of doubtful significance.

In a review of controlled-release preparations, Garcia *et al*[18] drew attention to reports of the bioequivalence of a daily regimen of amitriptyline 50 mg administered as a single dose in a controlled-release formulation (Lentizol) and a 75 mg daily dose of the drug given in three divided doses as conventional tablets.

Administration of a pelleted presentation of amitriptyline (Tryptacap, Merck, USA) in single daily doses of 75 mg over one week to 12 healthy volunteers appeared to produce an equivalent effect to that produced by an 8-hourly regimen of standard amitriptyline 25 mg tablets[19].

REFERENCES

1. Green AL. J Pharm Pharmacol 1967;19:10–16.
2. Irwin WJ, Li Wan Po A. Int J Pharmaceutics 1979;4:47–56.
3. Thoma K, Albert K [German]. Arch Pharm 1981;314:1053–5.
4. Blessel KW, Rudy BC, Senkowski BZ. In: Florey K, editor. Analytical profiles of drug substances; vol 3. London: Academic Press, 1974:127–48.
5. Thoma K, Albert K [German]. Pharm Acta Helv 1979;54(11):330–6.
6. Knapp GG, Page DP. Am J Hosp Pharm 1983;40:623–5.
7. Mitsana-Papazoglou A, Christopoulos TK, Diamandis EP, Koupparis MA. J Pharm Sci 1987;76(9):724–30.
8. Enever RP, Li Wan Po A, Millard BJ, Shotton E. J Pharm Sci 1975;64:1497–9.
9. Henwood CR. Nature 1967;216:1039–40.
10. Bouche R [letter]. J Pharm Sci 1972;61:986–7.
11. Buckles J, Walters V. J Clin Pharm 1976;1:107–12.
12. Enever RP, Li Wan Po A, Shotton E. J Pharm Sci 1977;66:1087–9.
13. Roman R, Cohen GM, Christy ME, Hagerman WB. J Pharm Sci 1979;68:1329–30.
14. Little TL, Tielke VM, Carlson RK. Am J Hosp Pharm 1982;39:646–7.
15. UKCPA Symposium. Pharm J 1986;237:665.
16. Anderson S. Proc Guild Hosp Pharm 1977;3:68–82.
17. Burch JE, Hullin RP. J Pharm Pharmacol 1982;34:260–1.
18. Garcia CR, Siqueiros A, Benet LZ. Pharm Acta Helv 1978;53:99–109.
19. Hucker HB, Stauffer SC, Clayton FG, Nakra BRS, Gaind R. J Clin Pharmacol 1975;15:168–72.

Ammonium Chloride   *Urine acidifier; Expectorant*

$NH_4Cl = 53.5$
CAS—12125-02-9

Pharmacopoeial status

BP, USP

Preparations

Compendial

Ammonium Chloride Mixture BP (Ammonium Chloride Oral Solution). Contains 10% w/v ammonium chloride in a suitable vehicle containing aromatic ammonia solution and liquorice liquid extract. It should be recently prepared. See Formulation below.

Ammonium Chloride and Morphine Mixture BP (Ammonium Chloride and Morphine Oral Solution). Contains 3% w/v ammonium chloride, 2% w/v ammonium bicarbonate, and 3% v/v chloroform and morphine tincture in a suitable vehicle containing liquorice liquid extract. It should be recently prepared. See Formulation below.

Ammonium Chloride Delayed-release Tablets USP.

Ammonium Chloride Injection USP. pH between 4.0 and 6.0.

Containers and storage

Solid state

Ammonium Chloride USP should be preserved in tight containers.

Dosage forms

Ammonium Chloride Tablets USP should be preserved in tight containers.

Ammonium Chloride Injection USP should be preserved in single-dose or in multiple-dose containers preferably of Type I or Type II glass.

PHYSICAL PROPERTIES

Ammonium chloride exists as odourless, colourless crystals or as a white crystalline powder; hygroscopic.

Melting point

Ammonium chloride sublimes without melting.

pH

A 0.5% solution of *ammonium chloride* in water has a pH of 4.6 to 6.0. At 25°, aqueous solutions of ammonium chloride 1%, 3%, and 10% are reported to have pH values of 5.5, 5.0, and 5.1, respectively.

Solubility

Ammonium chloride is soluble in 2.7 parts of water, in 100 parts of ethanol, and in 8 parts of glycerol; soluble in methanol; almost insoluble in acetone, in ether, and in ethyl acetate.

Effect of temperature
Approximate solubilities in water: 1 in 4.4 (0°); 1 in 3.8 (15°); 1 in 3.5 (25°); 1 in 2.5 (80°).
It has also been reported that ammonium chloride is soluble in 1.4 parts of boiling water.

STABILITY

In the solid state, ammonium chloride has a high vapour pressure. It tends to lose ammonia and therefore becomes more acid on storage. The vapour resulting from the sublimation of ammonium chloride does not consist of molecular ammonium chloride but mainly of equal volumes of ammonia and hydrogen chloride.
Exposure of highly concentrated solutions of ammonium chloride to low temperatures may result in crystallisation. This phenomenon can be reversed by warming the affected solutions to room temperature in a water bath.

Stabilisation

Solutions of ammonium chloride for parenteral use have been stabilised with disodium edetate 2 mg/mL.

INCOMPATIBILITY/COMPATIBILITY

Ammonium chloride 400 mEq/L (2.14% w/v) was reported to be physically compatible with 60 parenteral solutions (Abbott, USA). These included: dextran 6% in glucose 5%; dextran 6% in sodium chloride 0.9%; glucose-sodium choride 0.9% combinations; glucose 2.5%, 5%, and 10%; sodium lactate injection; compound sodium lactate injection; sodium chloride 0.45%; sodium chloride 0.9%; sodium lactate 0.167M.[1]
Ammonium chloride is incompatible with alkalis, carbonates of alkaline earths, and lead and silver salts.
There was loss of clarity when intravenous solutions of ammonium chloride were mixed with dimenhydrinate, codeine phosphate, anileridine hydrochloride, levorphanol tartrate, methadone hydrochloride, and with sulphafurazole diethanolamine.[2]

FORMULATION

AMMONIUM CHLORIDE MIXTURE BP

Ammonium chloride	100	g
Aromatic ammonia solution	50	mL
Liquorice liquid extract	100	mL
Water to	1000	mL

AMMONIUM CHLORIDE AND MORPHINE MIXTURE BP

Ammonium chloride	30	g
Ammonium bicarbonate	20	g
Chloroform and morphine tincture	30	mL
Liquorice liquid extract	50	mL
Water to	1000	mL

Excipients

Excipients that have been used in presentations of ammonium chloride include:
Tablets: acacia; castor oil; cellacephate; gelatin; magnesium stearate; sucrose; talc; white beeswax.
Oral liquids: aromatic ammonia solution; concentrated chloroform water; ipecacuanha tincture; liquorice liquid extract; methyl hydroxybenzoate.
Injections (additive solution for addition to sodium chloride 0.9%): disodium edetate; hydrochloric acid.
Cowley[3] reported that the taste of ammonium chloride could be masked by citric acid and by liquorice and raspberry syrups.

FURTHER INFORMATION. Conductivity and hardness changes in aged compacts—Bhatia RP, Lordi NG. J Pharm Sci 1979; 68:896–9; Use of sorption isotherms to study the effect of moisture on the hardness of aged compacts—Lordi N, Shiromani P. Drug Dev Ind Pharm 1983;9:1399–416; Mechanism of hardness of aged compacts—Lordi N, Shiromani P. Drug Dev Ind Pharm 1984;10:729–52.

PROCESSING

Sterilisation

Solutions of ammonium chloride have been sterilised by heating in an autoclave or by filtration.

REFERENCES

1. Kirkland WD, Jones RW, Ellis JR, Schultz CG. Am J Hosp Pharm 1961;18:694–9.
2. Patel JA, Phillips GL. Am J Hosp Pharm 1966;23:409–11.
3. Cowley E. J Hosp Pharm 1967;24:299–302.

Amoxycillin (BAN)   *Antibacterial*

Amoxicillin (rINN)
(6*R*)-6-(α-D-*p*-Hydroxyphenylglycylamino)penicillanic acid
$C_{16}H_{19}N_3O_5S = 365.4$

Amoxycillin Sodium (BANM)
Amoxicillin Sodium (rINNM)
$C_{16}H_{18}N_3NaO_5S = 387.4$

Amoxycillin Trihydrate (BANM)

Amoxicillin (USAN); Amoxicillin Trihydrate (rINNM)
$C_{16}H_{19}N_3O_5S$, $3H_2O = 419.4$
CAS—26787-78-0 (amoxycillin); 34642-77-8 (amoxycillin sodium); 61336-70-7 (amoxycillin trihydrate)

Pharmacopoeial status

BP (amoxycillin sodium, amoxycillin trihydrate); USP (amoxicillin)

Preparations

Compendial
Amoxicillin Capsules BP. Contain amoxycillin trihydrate. Capsules containing, in each, the equivalent of 250 mg and 500 mg of amoxycillin are usually available.
Amoxicillin Oral Suspension BP (Amoxycillin Mixture; Amoxycillin Syrup). A suspension of amoxycillin trihydrate in a suitable flavoured vehicle. It is prepared by dispersing the dry ingredients in the specified volume of water just before issue for use. pH 4.0 to 7.0. If the oral suspension is diluted, the diluted oral suspension should be freshly prepared.
Amoxicillin Injection BP (Amoxycillin Sodium for Injection). A sterile solution of amoxycillin sodium in water for injections, prepared by dissolving amoxycillin sodium for injection in the requisite amount of water for injections immediately before use.
Amoxicillin Capsules USP.
Amoxicillin Tablets USP.
Amoxicillin Oral Suspension USP.
Amoxicillin for Oral Suspension USP.

Non-compendial
Almodan (Berk). *Injection*, powder for reconstitution, amoxycillin (as sodium salt), 250-mg vial and 500-mg vial.
Amoxil (Bencard). *Capsules*, amoxycillin (as trihydrate) 250 mg and 500 mg.
Dispersible tablets, sugar free, amoxycillin (as trihydrate) 500 mg.
Fiztab (chewable tablets), sugar free, amoxycillin (as trihydrate) 125 mg, 250 mg, and 500 mg.
Syrup SF, sugar free, amoxycillin (as trihydrate) for reconstitution with water, 125 mg/5 mL and 250 mg/5 mL. *Diluent:* water.
Paediatric suspension, amoxycillin 125 mg (as trihydrate) per 1.25 mL when reconstituted with water. It may be diluted with water or syrup.
Sachets SF, powder, sugar free, amoxycillin 750 mg (as trihydrate)/sachet, for reconstitution in water.
Injection, powder for reconstitution, amoxycillin (as sodium salt) 250-mg vial, 500-mg vial, and 1-g vial. Amoxil should not be mixed with blood products, other proteinaceous fluids such as protein hydrolysates or with intravenous lipid emulsions. If Amoxil is prescribed concurrently with an aminoglycoside, the antibiotics should not be mixed in the syringe, intravenous fluid container, or giving set because loss of activity of the aminoglycoside can occur under these conditions.
Flemoxin Solutab (Brocades). *Dispersible tablets*, sugar free, amoxycillin (as trihydrate) 375 mg and 750 mg.
Amoxicillin capsules and oral suspensions are also available in various strengths from APS, Ashbourne (Amix), Berk (Almodan), BHR (Amrit), Cox, CP, Eastern (Amoram), Evans, Galen (Galenamox), Kerfoot, Lagap, Norton, Rima (Rimoxallin).

Compound preparations
Co-amoxiclav is the British Approved Name for compounded preparations of amoxycillin (as the trihydrate or as the sodium salt) and clavulanic acid (as potassium clavulanate); the proportions are expressed in the form x/y where x and y are the strengths in milligrams of amoxycillin and clavulanic acid, respectively. Preparation: Augmentin (Beecham).

Containers and storage

Solid state
Amoxicillin Trihydrate BP should be kept in an airtight container and stored at a temperature not exceeding 30°.
Amoxicillin USP should be preserved in tight containers, at controlled room temperature.

Dosage forms
Amoxicillin Oral Suspension BP. The dry ingredients should be stored at a temperature not exceeding 25°.
Amoxicillin Capsules USP, Amoxicillin Tablets USP, and Amoxicillin for Oral Suspension USP should be preserved in tight containers, at controlled room temperature.
Amoxicillin Oral Suspension USP should be preserved in multiple-dose containers equipped with a suitable dosing pump.
Almodan injection should be administered immediately after reconstitution.
Amoxil oral presentations should be stored in a dry place. Amoxil sachets SF and Fiztab tablets should be stored in a dry place below 25°. Amoxil injections should be stored in a cool, dry place. Once dispensed, Amoxil syrups SF and Amoxil paediatric suspension should be used within the period stated on the label and any remainder discarded. Amoxil injection (for intramuscular or direct intravenous use) should be administered immediately after reconstitution. The package leaflet gives recommended stability times (dependent upon concentration and temperature) in various infusion fluids.

PHYSICAL PROPERTIES

Amoxycillin trihydrate is a white or almost white, almost odourless microcrystalline powder.
Amoxycillin sodium is a white powder.

pH

The pH of a 10% solution of *amoxycillin sodium* is in the range 8.0 to 10.0. The pH of a 0.2% w/v aqueous solution of *amoxycillin trihydrate* is in the range 3.5 to 5.5 (BP), or 3.5 to 6.0 (USP).

Dissociation constants

pK_a 2.4 (carboxyl), 7.4 (aromatic hydroxyl), 9.6 (α-ammonium)
Values of pK_a of 2.63, 7.16, and 9.55 were determined at 35° by Tsuji *et al.*[1]

Partition coefficient

Log *P* (octanol), 0.87

Solubility

Amoxycillin trihydrate is soluble 1 in 400 of water, 1 in 1000 of ethanol, and 1 in 200 of methanol; practically insoluble in chloroform and in ether; dissolves in dilute solutions of acids and alkali hydroxides.
Amoxycillin sodium is soluble 1 in less than 1 of water.

Effect of pH
The pH-solubility profile of amoxycillin trihydrate was determined, at 37° and ionic strength 0.5, to be a U-shaped curve with minimum solubility at pH close to the isoelectric point[1]. Van't Hoff plots indicated a linear relationship between the equilibrium solubilities of amoxycillin to temperature in the range 20° to 50°.

Dissolution

The USP specifies that for Amoxicillin Capsules USP, not less than 80% of the labelled amount of $C_{16}H_{19}N_3O_5S$, $3H_2O$ is dissolved in 90 minutes. Dissolution medium: 900 mL of water; Apparatus 1 at 100 rpm.

STABILITY

Amoxycillin is subject, in common with all penicillins, to hydrolytic degradation of the β-lactam ring to produce, under alkaline conditions, the penicilloic acid which subsequently decomposes to the penilloic acid by decarboxylation. The reaction rate is first-order. Under acidic conditions, amoxycillin hydrolyses to form penicillenic acid. At the same time, base-catalysed self-aminolysis (dimerisation) occurs, by nucleophilic attack of the β-lactam carbonyl moiety of one molecule by the free side-chain amino group of a neighbouring molecule. Concentrations of amoxycillin and the pH of the solution determine the corresponding input of hydrolysis and aminolysis to the overall degradation reaction.

Tsuji et al[1] measured the degradation rate of amoxycillin trihydrate (0.005M) over the pH range 0.3 to 10.5 at 35°. At constant pH with excess buffer degradation followed first-order kinetics. Beta-lactam cleavage of amoxycillin was subject to general acid-base catalysis.

Solid state

In a study of the rate of decomposition of amoxycillin in the solid state, Méndez and co-workers[2] demonstrated that amoxycillin trihydrate (zwitterion form) was more stable than amoxycillin sodium (anionic form). Thermal degradation of both salts at 37°, 80°, 90°, 100°, and 110° was examined. Calculated activation enthalpies of amoxycillin trihydrate and amoxycillin sodium were 90.75 kJ/mol and 99.5 kJ/mol, respectively. The $t_{10\%}$ values of amoxycillin trihydrate and amoxycillin sodium were 3.2 years and 1.25 years, respectively at 20°.

Solutions

Unbuffered solutions of amoxycillin sodium are most stable at pH 5.8 and solutions in citrate buffer solution are most stable at pH 6.5.

Intravenous infusion fluids

Amoxycillin sodium 5% w/v was less stable than either the 1% or 2% solutions at 25° in water and in ten intravenous infusion fluids. Stability in the different vehicles decreased in the following order: water = sodium chloride 0.9% = sodium chloride 0.9% with potassium chloride 0.3% > compound sodium lactate = sodium lactate 0.167M > sodium bicarbonate 8.4% > glucose 5% = dextran 40 10% in sodium chloride 0.9% > dextran 40 10% in glucose 5% > sorbitol 30%.[3]

Effect of temperature

Values for $t_{10\%}$ (hours) for amoxycillin sodium 1% w/v in two infusion fluids:[4]

Infusion fluid	Storage temperature (°C)								
	−26.0	−19.2	−15.0	−13.7	−8.9	−6.5	0.0	10.0	25.0
Sodium chloride 0.9% w/v	55.0	14.0	11.0	10.0	8.5	8.0	252.0	91.2	24.0
Glucose 5% w/v	25.5	8.4	4.5	4.0	2.1	2.5	12.5	5.2	1.8

Concannon et al[5] found that the $t_{10\%}$ of amoxycillin sodium (10 mg/mL in water) increased from 1.2 days to 2 days as temperature decreased in the range 19.5° to 0°. Between 0° and −7° the $t_{10\%}$ of solutions that appeared to be frozen decreased from 2 days to 1.08 hours. Below −7° the rate of degradation decreased and the solution was completely frozen at −30°; at this temperature the $t_{10\%}$ increased to 13 days. The authors recommended storage at temperatures below −30° if admixtures of amoxycillin sodium are to be stored frozen.

Reconstitution and repackaging

Repackaging of oral liquids of antibiotics has become more commonplace and may be expected to affect the subsequent stability of the preparation. Sylvestri et al[6] did not detect any significant difference between the potency of a commercially available reconstituted oral suspension of amoxycillin trihydrate repackaged in clear polypropylene unit-dose oral syringes and stored at 25°, 40°, 60°, and 80° for up to 90 days, 35 days, 27 hours, and 6 hours, respectively, and the potency of the same suspensions stored in the original containers under identical conditions. The $t_{10\%}$ for repackaged solutions at 25° was approximately 78 days. Accelerated stability studies at 40°, 60°, and 80° indicated $t_{10\%}$ values of 240, 7, and 1.5 hours, respectively. The authors stated that the manufacturer's recommended expiry date of 7 days for reconstituted suspensions stored in original containers at room temperature would be suitable for the repackaged suspensions.

FURTHER INFORMATION. Polymerisation of penicillins. II. Kinetics and mechanism of dimerisation and self-catalysed hydrolysis of amoxycillin in aqueous solution—Bundgaard H. Acta Pharm Suec 1977;14:47–66.

INCOMPATIBILITY/COMPATIBILITY

Workers in Egypt[7] determined that amoxycillin trihydrate was adsorbed from solution by attapulgite and aluminium magnesium silicate (Veegum) but not by magnesium trisilicate or kaolin in the pH range 2.1 to 3.2. Methylcellulose 0.5% and polysorbate 80 0.05% suppressed adsorption of amoxycillin onto Veegum by 33% and 43.3%, respectively.

FORMULATION

Excipients

Excipients that have been used in presentations of amoxycillin include:
Capsules, amoxycillin: colloidal silica; lactose; magnesium stearate; titanium dioxide (E171).
Amoxycillin trihydrate: magnesium stearate; sodium lauryl sulphate.
Tablets, amoxycillin trihydrate: lactose; sorbitol.
Oral suspensions/syrups, powder for reconstitution, amoxycillin: β-carotene; carmellose sodium; citric acid; colloidal silica; erythrosine (E127); fruit flavours; sodium benzoate; sodium citrate; sorbitol; sucrose; sunset yellow FCF (E110).
Amoxycillin trihydrate: ammoniated liquorice; citric acid; disodium edetate; fruit flavours; Hercules casting colour 27–75; microcrystalline cellulose; silica; sodium benzoate; sodium citrate; sodium edetate; sodium propionate; sorbitol; sucrose.
Injections, amoxycillin sodium: benzyl alcohol.

Effect of excipients

The ability of sorbitol (instant and crystalline) to adsorb amoxycillin trihydrate (and other antibiotics) was examined by Nikolakakis and Newton[8] using an air-sieving technique. The adsorption capacity and binding strength of instant sorbitol was greater than that of the crystalline form in dry powder blends.

Bioavailability

Dutch workers[9] reported that the relative bioavailabilities of a new tablet formulation of amoxycillin (when swallowed or dispersed) and an oral suspension (Flemoxin solutab and Flemoxin forte suspension, Gist-Brocades) were higher than that of a commercially available capsule when tested in twelve healthy volunteers. Results indicated that the method of ingestion of the new tablet, which can also be sucked or chewed, would not influence bioavailability.

FURTHER INFORMATION. *In vitro* and *in vivo* evaluation of an oral sustained-release floating dosage form of amoxycillin trihydrate—Hilton AK, Deasy PB. Int J Pharmaceutics 1992;86:79–88.

REFERENCES

1. Tsuji A, Nakashima E, Hamano S, Yamana T. J Pharm Sci 1978;67(8):1059–66.
2. Méndez R, Alemany MT, Jurado C, Martin J. Drug Dev Ind Pharm 1989;15(8):1263–74.
3. Cook B, Hill SA, Lynn B. J Clin Hosp Pharm 1982;7:245-50.
4. McDonald C, Sunderland VB, Lau H, Shija R. J Clin Pharm Ther 1989;14:45–52.
5. Concannon J, Lovitt H, Ramage M, Tai LH, McDonald C, Sunderland VB. Am J Hosp Pharm 1986;43:3027–30.
6. Sylvestri MF, Makoid MC, Frost GL. Drug Dev Ind Pharm 1988;14(6):819–30.
7. Khalil SAH, Mortada LM, El-Khawas M. Int J Pharmaceutics 1984;18:157–67.
8. Nikolakakis I, Newton JM. J Pharm Pharmacol 1989;41:145–8.
9. Cortvriendt WRE, Verschoor JSC, Hespe W. Arzneimittelforschung 1987;37(II) Nr 8:977–9.

Amphotericin (BAN)   *Antifungal*

Amphotericin B (rINN)

Amphotericin is a mixture of antifungal polyenes produced by the growth of certain strains of *Streptomyces nodosus* or by any other means. It consists largely of amphotericin B which is (3R,5R,8R,9R,11S,13R,15S, 16R,17S,19R,34S,35R,36R,37S)-19-(3-amino-3,6-dideoxy-β-D-mannopyranosyloxy)-16-carboxy-3, 5,8,9,11,13,15,35-octahydroxy-34,36- dimethyl-13,17-epoxyoctatriaconta-20,22,24,26,28,30,32-heptaen-37-olide.

$C_{47}H_{73}NO_{17} = 924.1$

CAS—1397-89-3

Pharmacopoeial status

BP, USP

Preparations

Compendial

Amphotericin Lozenges BP. Contain amphotericin. Lozenges containing, in each, the equivalent of 10 mg of amphotericin are usually available. Prepared by compression.

Amphotericin B Cream USP.

Amphotericin B Lotion USP.

Amphotericin B Ointment USP.

Amphotericin B for Injection USP. An aqueous solution containing amphotericin 1%, pH 7.2 to 8.0.

Non-compendial

AmBisome (Vestar). *Intravenous infusion*, powder for reconstitution with cold (2° to 8°) sterile water for injections without a bacteriostatic agent, amphotericin 50 mg encapsulated in liposomes. *Diluent*: glucose 5% injection; infusion of AmBisome should commence within 6 hours of dilution. AmBisome powder/cake and reconstituted solution should not be mixed with sodium chloride 0.9% solution or with other drugs or electrolytes. The manufacturer provides detailed instructions for the reconstitution, dilution, and administration of the product. Aseptic technique must be employed in all handling.

Fungilin (Squibb). *Tablets*, amphotericin 100 mg.

Lozenges, amphotericin 10 mg.

Suspension, sugar free, amphotericin 100 mg/mL. Should not be diluted. Discard any unused suspension 4 days after opening.

Fungizone (Squibb). *Intravenous infusion*, powder for reconstitution with sterile water for injections without a bacteriostatic agent, amphotericin (as sodium deoxycholate complex) 50 mg. The reconstituted solution containing 5 mg/mL should be diluted with glucose 5% injection. If the pH of the glucose is below 4.2, 1 or 2 mL of sterile buffer with the following composition should be added: anhydrous sodium phosphate 1.59 g, anhydrous sodium acid phosphate 0.96 g, water for injections to 100 mL. Sodium chloride 0.9% solution should not be used for reconstitution. Precipitation of amphotericin may occur if diluents other than those recommended, or which contain a bacteriostatic agent, are used. Other injection preparations should not be mixed with Fungizone Intravenous solution or administered concurrently via the same cannula. Aseptic technique must be employed in all handling.

Containers and storage

Solid state

Amphotericin BP should be kept in well-closed containers, protected from light, and stored at 2° to 8°.

Amphotericin B USP should be preserved in tight, light-resistant containers, in a cold place.

Dosage forms

Amphotericin Lozenges BP should be protected from light.

Amphotericin B Cream USP and Amphotericin B Ointment USP should be preserved in collapsible tubes or in other well-closed containers.

Amphotericin B Lotion USP should be preserved in well-closed containers.

Amphotericin B for Injection USP should be preserved in containers suitable for sterile solids, in a refrigerator and protected from light.

Unopened vials of lyophilised AmBisome should be stored under refrigeration at 2° to 8°. Following reconstitution, the concentrate may be stored for up to 24 hours at 2° to 8°. Unopened vials, the concentrate, and diluted solutions should be protected against exposure to light and should not be frozen. Partially-used vials should not be stored for future use.

Fungilin tablets and lozenges should be stored at room temperature.

Fungilin suspension should be stored in a cool place, protected from direct sunlight.

Fungizone powder for reconstitution should be stored in a refrigerator. The concentrate (after reconstitution with sterile water for injections) should be stored, protected from light, for not more than 8 hours at room temperature or 24 hours in a refrigerator. Solutions for intravenous infusion should be protected from light during administration and should be used promptly after preparation.

PHYSICAL PROPERTIES

Amphotericin is a yellow to orange powder.

Melting point

Amphotericin decomposes gradually above 170°.

pH

A 3% aqueous suspension of *amphotericin* has a pH of 6.0 to 8.0.

Dissociation constants

pK_a 5.5, 10.0

Solubility

Amphotericin is practically insoluble in water, in ethanol, in chloroform, in ether, in benzene, and in toluene; soluble in dimethyl sulphoxide and in propylene glycol; slightly soluble in dimethyl formamide and in methanol.

The solubility of amphotericin in water can be increased by the addition of sodium lauryl sulphate or sodium deoxycholate.

From a study[1] of 18 solvent systems (suitable for intravenous use) only two systems yielded amphotericin solubility greater than 1.0 mg/mL at 25°. These were macrogol 400:propylene glycol (50:50 v/v) and dimethylacetamide. The solubility of amphotericin in the latter solvent was markedly increased (from 7.6 to 152.4 mg/mL) with the addition of 6% sodium deoxycholate; data suggested the underlying mechanism for this increased solubility was not micellar but involved ion pair formation.

STABILITY

Amphotericin in the solid state appears to be stable for long periods of time when stored at moderate temperature and protected from light and air.

The major route of degradation of amphotericin, in aqueous solution, is thought to be epoxidation and *trans-cis* isomerism, although degradation products have not been identified. Dilute solutions are light-sensitive. Amphotericin is inactivated at low pH values.

In aqueous solution at pH 4 to 8, degradation has been shown to follow first-order kinetics. The activation energy for the degradation of amphotericin at pH 7.0 in McIlvaine's buffer was reported[2] to be 69 kJ/mol; the half-life of amphotericin in aqueous solution was calculated to be 34 days at 4°. Maximum stability of amphotericin in the presence of phosphate-citrate buffer at 37° was observed at pH 5 to 7.

The activity of amphotericin in aqueous colloidal dispersions is reported to be retained if frozen, but colloidal coagulation may be accelerated.[3]

Washington *et al*[4] reported amphotericin (1 mg/mL and 2 mg/mL) to be stable over 7 months in 20% fat emulsions (stabilised with parenteral egg lecithin) at 20°.

FURTHER INFORMATION. A stability study of amphotericin B in aqueous media using factorial design [effects of temperature, pH, ionic strength, surfactant concentration, oxygen, and light]—Hung CT, Lam FC, Perrier DG, Souter A. Int J Pharmaceutics 1988;44:117-23. A study of the chemical stability of amphotericin in *N,N*-dimethylacetamide—Dicken CM, Rossi TM, Rajagopalan N, Ravin LJ, Sternson LA. Int J Pharmaceutics 1988;46:223-9.

INCOMPATIBILITY/COMPATIBILITY

Many drugs have been reported to be incompatible with amphotericin including the following antimicrobial agents: amikacin sulphate, ampicillin, benzylpenicillin potassium, benzylpenicillin sodium, carbenicillin sodium, chlortetracycline hydrochloride, gentamicin sulphate, kanamycin sulphate, nitrofurantoin sodium, oxytetracycline hydrochloride, polymyxin B sulphate, streptomycin sulphate, tetracycline hydrochloride, and viomycin sulphate. Amphotericin has also been reported to be incompatible with calcium chloride, calcium gluconate, chlorpromazine hydrochloride, cimetidine hydrochloride, diphenhydramine hydrochloride, dopamine hydrochloride, lignocaine hydrochloride, metaraminol tartrate, methyldopate hydrochloride, potassium chloride, procaine hydrochloride, prochlorperazine mesylate, ranitidine hydrochloride, sodium calciumedetate, sodium chloride, verapamil hydrochloride, vitamins, and solutions for total parenteral administration.

There have been conflicting reports on the compatibility of amphotericin with heparin and with certain corticosteroids; amphotericin appears to be compatible with limited amounts of heparin sodium, hydrocortisone sodium succinate, and methylprednisolone sodium succinate.

Within three hours of admixture of amphotericin injection 40 or 80 micrograms/mL (Fungizone, Squibb, USA) with magnesium sulphate injection (International Medication Systems, USA) in glucose 5% injection there was a reduction in visible clarity and a decrease in amphotericin concentration.[5] However, the same mixture was physically compatible and amphotericin was chemically stable over a period of six hours when infused as separate solutions mixed at the Y-site of an intravenous administration set.

The use of any diluent for infusion other than the recommended glucose 5%, for example sodium chloride 0.9%, glucose 5% in sodium chloride 0.9%, compound sodium lactate injection, glucose 5% in compound sodium lactate injection,[6] or a solution containing amino acids 4.25% and glucose 25%[7] may lead to precipitation. The presence of an antimicrobial preservative such as benzyl alcohol in the diluent may also lead to precipitation. The same effect may occur if pH has been adjusted using hydrochloric acid or sodium hydroxide.

Recent studies have shown amphotericin (Fungizone, Squibb, USA) to be chemically stable and physically compatible in glucose 5% injection at concentrations of 0.47, 0.66, and 0.75 mg/mL in polyolefin containers when stored at 25° for up to 24 hours.[8] Previous work by the same authors had demonstrated that stability was maintained at concentrations of 0.92, 1.20, and 1.40 mg/mL during storage at 6° and 25° for up to 36 hours.[9]

Wiest *et al*[10] demonstrated the stability of amphotericin (Fungizone Intravenous, Squibb, USA) 100 micrograms/mL in glucose 5%, 10%, 15%, and 20% injections during storage for up to 24 hours at 15° to 25° in polyvinyl chloride bags, protected from light.

Moore and Tindula[11] reported on the development of visible precipitation when admixtures of amphotericin (Squibb) and glucose 5% injection were prepared in evacuated intravenous containers. This apparent incompatibility was thought to be due either to small amounts of buffer remaining in the container (Abbott) or to the remnants of sodium chloride 0.9% injection present for sterilisation of the containers (Travenol), before admixture preparation. Admixtures prepared in evacuated containers which contained only small amounts of sterile water (McGaw) remained clear.

FORMULATION

Excipients

Excipients that have been used in presentations of amphotericin include:

Capsules: acacia; lactose; magnesium stearate; maize starch; povidone.

Tablets: ethylcellulose; lactose; maize starch; magnesium stearate; saccharin sodium; talc.

Lozenges: acacia powder; D-mannitol; magnesium stearate; polyvinyl alcohol; talc.

Suspensions: carmellose sodium; citric acid; erythrosine (E127); ethanol; flavours; glycerol; methyl and propyl hydroxybenzoates; potassium chloride; saccharin sodium; sodium benzoate; sodium phosphate; sodium acid phosphate, anhydrous; sunset yellow FCF (E110).

Creams: activated dimethicone; benzyl alcohol; cetostearyl alcohol; glyceryl monostearate; macrogol monostearate; methyl and propyl hydroxybenzoates; propylene glycol; sorbic acid; sorbitol; thiomersal; titanium dioxide (E171); white soft paraffin.

Lotions: activated dimethicone; cetyl alcohol; glyceryl monostearate; guar gum; macrogol monostearate; methyl and propyl hydroxybenzoates; polysorbate 20; propylene glycol; sodium citrate; sorbic acid; sorbitan monopalmitate; stearyl alcohol; thiomersal; titanium dioxide (E171).

Ointments: liquid paraffin; Plastibase; titanium dioxide (E171).

Intravenous infusions (powder for reconstitution): deoxycholic acid; phosphoric acid; sodium hydroxide; sodium phosphate; sodium acid phosphate.

Intravenous infusions (liposomal, powder for reconstitution): cholesterol; disodium succinate hexahydrate; distearoylphosphatidylglycerol; hydrogenated soy phosphatidylcholine; sucrose; α-tocopherol.

FURTHER INFORMATION. Practical guidelines for preparing and administering amphotericin B [injections]—Kintzel PE, Smith GH. Am J Hosp Pharm 1992;49:1156–64. Formulation and toxicity studies in *mice* using amphotericin liposomes derived from proliposomes—Payne NI, Cosgrove RF, Green AP, Liu L. J Pharm Pharmacol 1987;39:24–8. The influence of Myrj 59 [macrogol (100) stearate, Codibel] on the solubility, toxicity and activity of amphotericin B—Tasset C, Preat V, Roland M. J Pharm Pharmacol 1991;43:297–302. Effect of polyoxyethyleneglycol [macrogol] (24) cholesterol on the solubility, toxicity and activity of amphotericin B—Tasset C, Goethals F, Preat V, Roland M. Int J Pharmaceutics 1990;58:41–8. Novel antifungal drug delivery: stable amphotericin B-cholesterol sulfate discs—Guo LSS, Fielding RM, Lasic DD, Hamilton RL, Mufson D. Int J Pharmaceutics 1991;75:45–54.

REFERENCES

1. Rajagopalan N, Dicken CM, Ravin LJ, Sternson LA. J Parenter Sci Technol 1988;42:97–102.
2. Hamilton-Miller JMT. J Pharm Pharmacol 1973;25:401–7.
3. Kirschenbaum BE, Latiolais CJ. Am J Hosp Pharm 1976;33:767–91.
4. Washington C, Lutz O, Davis SS. J Pharm Pharmacol 1991;43 Suppl:93P.
5. Raymond GG, Davis RL. DICP Ann Pharmacother 1991;25:123–6.
6. Jurgens RW, DeLuca PP, Papadimitrion D. Am J Hosp Pharm 1981;38:377–8.
7. Athanikar N, Boyer B, Deamer R, Harbison H, Henry RS, Jurgens R et al. Am J Hosp Pharm 1979;36:511–13.
8. Kintzel PE, Kennedy PE [letter]. Am J Hosp Pharm 1991;48:1681.
9. Kintzel PE, Kennedy PE. Am J Hosp Pharm 1991;48:283–5.
10. Wiest DB, Maish WA, Garner SS, El-Chaar GM. Am J Hosp Pharm 1991;48:2430–3.
11. Moore BR, Tindula R [letter]. Am J Hosp Pharm 1987;44:1312.

Ampicillin (BAN, USAN, rINN)   *Antibacterial*

Aminobenzylpenicillin; anhydrous ampicillin
(6*R*)-6-(α-D-phenylglycylamino)penicillanic acid; 6-[(aminophenylacetyl)amino]-3,3-dimethyl-7-oxo-4-thia-1-azabicyclo[3.2.0]heptane-2-carboxylic acid
$C_{16}H_{19}N_3O_4S = 349.4$

Ampicillin Sodium (BANM, USAN, rINNM)
$C_{16}H_{18}N_3NaO_4S = 371.4$

Ampicillin Trihydrate (BANM, rINNM)
$C_{16}H_{19}N_3O_4S, 3H_2O = 403.5$
CAS — 69-53-4 (ampicillin); 69-52-3 (ampicillin sodium); 7177-48-2 (ampicillin trihydrate)

Pharmacopoeial status

BP (ampicillin, ampicillin sodium, ampicillin trihydrate); USP (ampicillin–permits anhydrous or trihydrate)

Preparations

Compendial

Ampicillin Capsules BP. Capsules containing in each, 250 mg and 500 mg of ampicillin or an equivalent amount of ampicillin trihydrate are usually available.

Ampicillin Oral Suspension BP (Ampicillin Mixture; Ampicillin Syrup). A suspension of ampicillin or ampicillin trihydrate in a suitable flavoured vehicle, prepared by dispersion of the dry ingredients in the specified volume of water immediately before issue for use; pH 4.0 to 7.0.

Ampicillin Injection BP (Ampicillin Sodium for Injection). A sterile solution of ampicillin sodium in water for injections, prepared by dissolving ampicillin sodium for injection in the requisite amount of water for injections immediately before use. pH of a 10% w/v solution 8.0 to 10.0.

Ampicillin Capsules USP. Contain ampicillin or ampicillin trihydrate.

Ampicillin Tablets USP. Chewable tablets containing ampicillin (anhydrous or as trihydrate).

Ampicillin for Oral Suspension USP. Contains ampicillin (anhydrous or as trihydrate).

Sterile Ampicillin for Suspension USP. Contains sterile ampicillin trihydrate.
Sterile Ampicillin USP. Contains ampicillin trihydrate for parenteral use.
Sterile Ampicillin Sodium USP.

Non-compendial

Amfipen (Brocades). *Capsules*, ampicillin 250 mg and 500 mg.
Syrup, ampicillin 125 mg/5 mL when reconstituted with purified water. *Syrup forte*, ampicillin 250 mg/5 mL when reconstituted with purified water.
A shelf-life of 7 days is recommended for the reconstituted syrups if stored in a cool place. It is recommended that the bottles be well shaken before reconstitution of the syrups in order to ensure a homogeneous suspension.
Penbritin (Beecham). *Capsules*, ampicillin (as trihydrate) 250 mg and 500 mg.
Syrup, ampicillin (as trihydrate) 125 mg/5 mL when reconstituted with water.
Syrup forte, ampicillin (as trihydrate) 250 mg/5 mL when reconstituted with water. Syrup is recommended as a suitable diluent of reconstituted syrups.
Paediatric Suspension, ampicillin (as trihydrate) 125 mg/1.25 mL when reconstituted with water.
Once dispensed the oral liquids remain stable for 7 days if kept in a cool place.
Injection, powder for reconstitution, ampicillin (as sodium salt), 250-mg and 500-mg vials. Penbritin solutions for injection should be used immediately. Penbritin may be added to most intravenous fluids, such as water for injections, sodium chloride 0.9%, glucose 5%, and sodium chloride 0.18% with glucose 4%. In intravenous solutions containing glucose or other carbohydrate it should be infused within one hour of preparation. In water for injections or sodium chloride 0.9% it should be infused within 24 hours of preparation. If these extended storage times are required, the infusion must be prepared under the appropriate aseptic conditions. Penbritin should not be mixed with blood products or other proteinaceous fluids or with intravenous lipid emulsions. It should not be mixed with aminoglycosides in the syringe, intravenous fluid container or giving set.
Vidopen (Berk). *Injection*, powder for reconstitution, ampicillin (as sodium salt) 250-mg and 500-mg vials.
Ampicillin capsules and oral suspensions are also available in various strengths from APS, Berk, Cox, Evans, Kerfoot, Lagap, Norton, Rima (Rimacillin). Ampicillin capsules are also available from CP.

Compound preparations

Co-fluampicil is the British Approved Name for a mixture of equal parts by weight of flucloxacillin and ampicillin. Preparations: Magnapen (Beecham). Co-fluampicil capsules are also available from Generics (Flu-Amp) and Norton.

Containers and storage

Solid state

Ampicillin BP, Ampicillin Sodium BP, and Ampicillin Trihydrate BP should be stored in airtight containers at temperatures not exceeding 30°.
Ampicillin Sodium BP, if sterile, should be kept in a tamper-evident, sealed, sterile container so as to exclude micro-organisms. Ampicillin USP should be preserved in tight containers.

Dosage forms

Ampicillin Oral Suspension BP. The dry ingredients should be stored at a temperature not exceeding 25°. The oral suspension

and diluted oral suspension should be stored at the temperature, and used within the period, stated on the label.
Ampicillin Injection BP. The sealed container should be stored at temperatures not exceeding 25°. Ampicillin injection should be used immediately after preparation.
All Ampicillin USP preparations should be preserved in tight containers.
Sterile Ampicillin USP (trihydrate) should be preserved in a container suitable for sterile solids. Sterile Ampicillin Sodium USP should be preserved in a container suitable for sterile solids and the constituted solutions should be protected from freezing.
Amfipen and Penbritin preparations should be stored in a cool, dry place.

PHYSICAL PROPERTIES

Ampicillin (anhydrous) is a white, crystalline powder.
Ampicillin sodium is a white to off-white, crystalline or amorphous, hygroscopic powder; odourless or almost odourless.
Ampicillin trihydrate is a white, crystalline powder; odourless. Both *ampicillin* and *ampicillin trihydrate* absorb insignificant amounts of moisture at 25° and relative humidities up to 80%, but absorb significant amounts at higher humidities.

Melting point

Ampicillin melts in the range 199° to 203°, with decomposition. *Ampicillin sodium* melts at about 205°, with decomposition.

pH

pH of a 0.25% w/v solution (BP) of *ampicillin* is 3.5 to 5.5.
pH of a 10 mg/mL solution (USP) of *ampicillin* is 3.5 to 6.0.
A 10% w/v solution (BP) of *ampicillin sodium* and a solution (USP) of *sterile ampicillin sodium* containing 10 mg ampicillin per mL have a pH of 8.0 to 10.0.
The pH of a 0.25% w/v solution (BP) of *ampicillin trihydrate* is 3.5 to 5.5.

Dissociation constants

pK_a 2.5 (—COOH), 7.3 (—NH$_2$) at 25°

Solubility

Ampicillin is sparingly soluble in water; practically insoluble in ethanol, in acetone, in chloroform, in ether, and in fixed oils. It dissolves in dilute solutions of acids and alkali hydroxides.
Ampicillin sodium is soluble 1 in 2 of water; soluble 1 in 50 of acetone; slightly soluble in chloroform; practically insoluble in ether, in liquid paraffin and in fixed oils. A colloidal dispersion which gels on standing is formed with ethanol.
Ampicillin trihydrate is soluble 1 in 150 of water; practically insoluble in ethanol, in chloroform, in ether, and in fixed oils. It dissolves in dilute solutions of acids and of alkali hydroxides.

Effect of pH

Hou and Poole[1] demonstrated a minimum solubility of ampicillin (3.98×10^{-2} M) at ionic strength 0.5 and 25° at pH 4.9, where ampicillin exists as the zwitterion; however at lower or higher pH, solubility was greater.

Effect of cosolvents

The solubility of ampicillin at 25° in mixtures of 80% of water and 20% of organic solvent (methanol, ethanol, *n*-propanol, isopropanol, acetone, dimethyl sulphoxide, *p*-dioxan, or tetrahydrofuran) in the presence of potassium chloride was lower than that in water alone, but increased with increased salt concentration, especially in the presence of *p*-dioxan and tetrahydrofuran.[1]

Dissolution

The USP specifies that for Ampicillin Capsules USP and Ampicillin Tablets USP not less than 75% of the labelled amount of $C_{16}H_{19}N_3O_4S$ is dissolved in 45 minutes. Dissolution medium: 900 mL of water; Apparatus 1 at 100 rpm.

Dissolution properties

The intrinsic dissolution rates, in micrograms/cm^2/s, of anhydrous ampicillin and ampicillin trihydrate, measured at 37° by a flow-cell method, were 3.94 and 3.85, respectively in water, and 35.0 and 32.6, respectively in 0.053 N hydrochloric acid.[2] The rates of dissolution from loose-filled gelatin capsules in the acid were similar for both forms. In-vivo studies revealed a similar oral bioavailability for both compounds.

Greek workers[3] investigated factors affecting the rate of dissolution of ampicillin trihydrate from capsules, including the length of time of mixing before encapsulation of the materials, ampicillin particle size, lubricant content (magnesium stearate), and the relative humidity maintained during storage. Results indicated that the particle size of ampicillin was the most important factor controlling drug release.

Crystal and molecular structure

Polymorphs

Three solvent-crystallised polymorphic modifications of ampicillin sodium and an amorphous form produced by lyophilisation or spray-drying were analysed by Chinese workers.[4] All crystalline forms were more stable than the amorphous form when subjected to a moisture-absorption test (relative humidity 52%) and a thermal stability test.

STABILITY

Kinetics

Ampicillin is amphoteric and, in solution, can exist as the anion, cation, or zwitterion. At 35°, degradation of ampicillin in buffered solution (ionic strength 0.5) at pH values between 0.8 and 10.0 followed pseudo-first-order kinetics.[5] The rate of degradation was significantly influenced by general acid and general base catalysis. Reaction rates in acidic solution (0.08 M hydrochloric acid, pH 1.2) increased owing to a positive salt effect but were retarded by the addition of ethanol. Activation energy values at pH 1.35, 4.93, and 9.78 were 68.6, 76.5, and 38.5 kJ/mol, respectively. In buffered solution at 35°, maximum stability was achieved at pH 4.85 (the isoelectric point) whereas in solution in the absence of buffers the pH of maximum stability was about 5.8. This finding has been attributed to the greater stability of ampicillin as the zwitterion.

Rates of degradation of ampicillin sodium are known to be accelerated in neutral and weakly alkaline solutions of carbohydrates (glucose, fructose, dextrans, and sucrose) and polyhydric alcohols (sorbitol).[6,7]

Mechanism of degradation and degradation products

Hydrolytic cleavage of the β-lactam ring has been cited[5] as the initial reaction of the degradation of ampicillin in solution. The decomposition products, α-aminobenzylpenicilloic acid and α-aminobenzylpenilloic acid were identified in alkaline solutions, whereas α-aminobenzylpenicillinic acid and α-aminobenzylpenillic acid were among the probable products in acidic solutions. The greater stability of ampicillin in acid appeared to be influenced by the amino group of the side chain. Other degradation products of ampicillin[8] formed within a few days in aqueous solution (initial concentration 20% ampicillin) at pH 8.5 and room temperature (23° ± 2°) were polymeric substances formed by an aminolytic chain reaction. Structures of a dimer, tetramer, and hexamer have been confirmed and subsequently the three forms were quantitatively determined.[9]

In a further investigation of degradation mechanisms in aqueous solution at pH 6.3 to 7.4 and 37°, Bundgaard and Hansen[10] examined the catalytic effect of phosphate buffers. Evidence was presented to support a nucleophilic mechanism, with the formation of penicilloyl phosphate as an intermediate. Major degradation products of ampicillin were a stable piperazine-2,5-dione derivative and α-aminobenzylpenicilloic acid. The major products of the nucleophilic reaction between ampicillin and carbohydrates or alcohols in mild alkaline solution[7] were penicilloyl esters which then yielded a piperazine-2,5-dione derivative by intramolecular aminolysis and α-aminobenzylpenicilloic acid by hydrolysis.

Tablets

Ampicillin tablets stored at either 22° or 37° and 60% relative humidity[11] showed no change in physical properties or dissolution profiles over 24 months and 7 months, respectively. Calculated $t_{10\%}$ values under these conditions were 57 months and 48 months, respectively, and a shelf-life of 4 years was predicted.

Capsules

The physical and chemical stability of ampicillin trihydrate capsules over a period of 42 months under ambient conditions was demonstrated by workers in France.[12] Although dissolution rates first decreased and finally increased over the period, comparative bioavailability studies (in six healthy volunteers) of a recent batch and 42-month-old capsules indicated bioequivalence.

There was no significant degradation of ampicillin trihydrate in capsules (equivalent to 250 mg ampicillin) during transit (by road and sea) from Sweden to Port Sudan.[13] After dispersal to centres within Sudan, the extent of the hydrolytic degradation that occurred was attributed to the water in the ampicillin trihydrate molecule. It was suggested that anhydrous ampicillin might be less liable to hydrolytic degradation.

Oral liquids

Differences in stability among reconstituted oral suspensions of ampicillin from five commercial sources in the USA (SK-Ampicillin, Polycillin, Principen, Penbritin, Omnipen) were noted[14] after storage at 5°, 25°, and 35°; the differences were most apparent at 25°. The trihydrate form was generally more stable than the anhydrous form. Potency was maintained at over 90% of the original ampicillin concentration for at least 7 days at room temperature in all products tested.

Evidence of segregation of the granulated constituents of a commercial product and the effects of different diluents (water and water/syrup) on the stability of ampicillin oral suspensions (when reconstituted by non-approved procedures) led Hempenstall et al[15] to affirm that reconstitution and dilution should always be undertaken in accordance with the manufacturer's recommendations. During storage at 25° degradation exceeded 10% within 7 days in dilutions of one product which contained anhydrous ampicillin.

When workers in Egypt[16] examined the effect of temperature (5°, 25°, 40°) on the stability and bioavailability of four locally available brands of ampicillin oral suspension (in original containers), they found that immediately after reconstitution, none of the suspensions met the USP potency requirement. Only one brand met the label claim for stability after storage under the recommended refrigeration and room temperature conditions. At 25°, suspensions of the trihydrate form showed greater stability than those of the anhydrous form. Bioavailability studies involving five healthy volunteers revealed statistically significant inter-brand variations.

At least 90% of the initial concentration of ampicillin trihydrate in suspension (Principen '125' for oral suspension, Squibb, USA), repackaged in amber, plastic (polypropylene) oral syringes, was maintained during storage at $-20°$, $4°$, and $25°$ for at least 30 days. Stability was decreased significantly at $60°$ and $80°$ ($t_{10\%}$ less than 2 hours).[17] These data concurred with the manufacturer's recommended shelf-lives (following reconstitution and in the original containers) of 7 days at room temperature and 14 days if refrigerated.

Intravenous infusions

Shelf-life and stability data for solutions of ampicillin sodium in various intravenous infusions appear in the literature but are rarely amenable to precise comparison. Findings tend to vary with the method of analysis. However, there is agreement on certain aspects which can be broadly summarised as follows:

- as the ampicillin concentration increases, the rate of degradation increases[18-20]
- degradation rate increases with temperature above $4°$ and is also enhanced under some freezing conditions[18, 21]
- as ampicillin concentration increases, pH values tend to rise, owing to alkalinity of the sodium salt; subsequent decreases in pH are due to the formation of degradation products; hydrolysis rates are directly dependent on pH at concentrations between 2% and 10%[20]
- stability on dilution with intravenous infusions varies; it is similar in sodium chloride 0.9% and in water but is reduced by more than half in glucose 5% injection; in glucose solutions, pH ranged between 8 and 9 and the anion was the predominant species.[19, 20, 22]

A summary of shelf-life and stability data for solutions of ampicillin sodium is presented in Table 1.

Effect of freezing and thawing by microwave

The instability of ampicillin sodium when diluted with glucose 5% injection and stored at $-20°$ for 30 days is well established. Holmes et al[21] found the degree of degradation to be greater than 10% in similar dilutions that had been stored for 30 days at $-30°$. Stability was maintained in glucose 5% injection after storage at $-70°$ (for 30 days) and microwave-thawing, but potency was reduced to 70.5% when the solutions were kept at room temperature for 8 hours after thawing. Dilutions in sodium chloride 0.9% also lost more than 10% potency after 30 days at $-20°$ but less than 10% of their initial concentration was lost during storage at $-30°$ and $-70°$ for the same time period. During further storage at ambient temperature after thawing, the concentration of ampicillin fell to 70.5% and 51.9% of the original after 8 and 24 hours, respectively.

Suppositories

Suppositories of ampicillin (anhydrous and the sodium salt), formulated with Witepsol H15, Witepsol H15 plus 0.1% polysorbate 80, Novata BD, or macrogol bases showed little change in disintegration time and no discoloration or crystal growth after storage at $4°$ for 240 days.[26]

Stabilisation

The maintenance of aqueous solutions of ampicillin sodium and sucrose at pH 6.0 to 6.5 is recommended to minimise the formation of sucrose penicilloate.[6]

FURTHER INFORMATION. Stabilization of ampicillin analogs in aqueous solution. II. Kinetic analysis of the mechanism of degradation of ampicillin with benzaldehyde in aqueous solution—Fujiwara H, Kawashima S, Ohhashi M. Chem Pharm Bull 1982;30(6):2181–8. Potential improvement in the shelf-life of parenterals using the prodrug approach: bacampicillin and talampicillin hydrolysis kinetics and utilisation time—Ngoyen NA, Mortaoa LM, Notari RE. Pharm Res 1988;5:288–96. Stability testing of pharmaceuticals by isothermal heat conduction calorimetry: Ampicillin in aqueous solution—Oliyai R, Lindenbaum S. Int J Pharmaceutics 1991;73:33–6. Penicillins and cephalosporins—Physicochemical properties and analysis in pharmaceutical and biological matrices [review article]—Van Krimpen PC, Van Bennekom WP, Bult A. Pharm Weekbl (Sci) 1987;9:1–23.

INCOMPATIBILITY/COMPATIBILITY

Ampicillin sodium has been reported to be incompatible with adrenaline, amikacin sulphate, aminoglycosides, atropine sulphate, calcium chloride, calcium gluconate, chloramphenicol sodium succinate, chlorpromazine hydrochloride, chlortetracycline, clindamycin phosphate, dopamine hydrochloride, erythromycin ethylsuccinate, erythromycin lactobionate, gentamicin sulphate, heparin sodium, hydralazine hydrochloride, hydrocortisone sodium succinate, kanamycin sulphate, lincomycin hydrochloride, metoclopramide, metaraminol tartrate, metronidazole, noradrenaline, novobiocin, oxytetracycline hydrochloride, pentobarbitone, phenobarbitone, polymyxin B sulphate, prochlorperazine edisylate, prochlorperazine mesylate, sodium bicarbonate, suxamethonium, tetracycline hydrochloride, thiopentone sodium.

Ampicillin sodium may be added to most intravenous fluids but should not be mixed with blood products or other proteinaceous fluids. In intravenous injections of sodium chloride 0.9% containing 1% of ampicillin sodium, 90% of the potency may be expected to be retained for 24 hours at $25°$. In glucose 5% infusion ampicillin is much less stable; the solution should be infused within one hour of preparation or the drug may be administered by bolus injection into the infusion tubing.

FORMULATION

Excipients

Excipients that have been used in presentations of ampicillin include:

Capsules, ampicillin: lactose; magnesium stearate.
Ampicillin trihydrate: colloidal silica; lactose; magnesium stearate; microcrystalline cellulose; talc.
Syrups and suspensions (powder for reconstitution), ampicillin trihydrate: acacia, powdered; amaranth (E123); ammoniated liquorice; carmellose sodium; carmoisine (E122); β-carotene (E160a); fruit flavours; lactose; microcrystalline cellulose; pectin; polysorbate 40; quinoline yellow (E104); saccharin sodium; silica; sodium benzoate; sodium chloride; sodium citrate (anhydrous); sodium propionate; sucrose; sunset yellow FCF (E110); trisodium citrate; vanilla.
Ampicillin free acid: amaranth (E123); cetomacrogol 1000; compound orange spirit; compound tartrazine solution; ethanol; methyl and propyl hydroxybenzoates; sodium benzoate; sodium citrate; sucrose; sunset yellow FCF (E110).

Bioavailability

In comparison with intravenous administration, the absolute bioavailabilities of ampicillin 500 mg as an intramuscular injection solution, capsules, or syrups (from two manufacturers;

Table 1
A summary of shelf-life and stability data for solutions of ampicillin sodium

Vehicle	Concentration of ampicillin	Initial pH	Temp	Storage time	Extent of degradation	Reference
Sodium chloride 0.9%	2%	8.8	4°	4 days	>10%	18
			24°	4 days	>30%	
			−7°	4 days	>30%	
Water	20%	9.7	24°	1 day	>61%	
	0.01 M	9.1	24°	1 day	5.8%	
Glucose 5%	0.2%, 0.4%, 1%	8.5 to 8.9	20° to 25°	1 to 24 hours	5% to 12% in 2 hours	19
Sodium chloride 0.9%	0.2%, 0.4%, 1%	8.6 to 8.9	20° to 25°	1 to 24 hours	up to 10% in 24 hours	
Glucose 5%	2%, 5%, 10%	8.0 to 9.3	26° ± 1°	2.12 to 6.9 hours	10%	20
Sodium chloride 0.9%	2%, 5%, 10%	8.0 to 9.2	26° ± 1°	3.86 to 17 hours	10%	
Water, sterile	2%, 5%, 10%	8.0 to 9.15	26° ± 1°	2.7 to 26 hours	10%	
Glucose 5.5%	2, 5, or 15 g/L	8.5 to 9.0	25°	2 to 3.5 hours	10%	22
Glucose/fructose	2, 5, or 10 g/L	7.8 to 8.6	25°	1 to 3 hours	10%	
Invert sugar (10%)	2, 5, or 10 g/L	7.8 to 8.7	25°	1.5 to 5.6 hours	10%	
Sodium chloride, 0.9%	2, 5, or 15 g/L	8.5 to 8.95	25°	33 to >48 hours	10%	
Glucose			30°	1 day	10%	23
Glucose/sodium chloride			30°	1 day	10%	
			−10°	1.4 days	10%	
Sodium chloride 0.9%			30°	1 day	10%	
			−10°	2.2 days	10%	
Water, double-distilled			30°	1.2 days	10%	
			−10°	2.8 days	10%	
Glucose 5%			25°	1 hour ('stability period')		24
Sodium chloride 0.9%	<1.5% w/v		0° to 5°	168 hours		
	1.5 to 2.0%		0° to 5°	72 hours		
			25°	24 hours		
Glucose 5%	20 mg/mL	8.50	25°	2 days	62.4%	25
	10 mg/mL	8.20	25°	2 days	66.4%	
	20 mg/mL	8.6	4°	7 days	59.3%	
	10 mg/mL	7.95	4°	7 days	54.7%	
Sodium chloride 0.9%	20 mg/mL	8.60	25°	2 days	12.4%	
	10 mg/mL	8.20	25°	2 days	17.6%	
	20 mg/mL	8.83	4°	7 days	18.5%	
	10 mg/mL	8.28	4°	7 days	18.4%	

Beecham and Pliva) were determined to be 84%/83%, 33%/37%, and 33%/32%, respectively.[27] A marked absorption window effect (a limited section of the gastro-intestinal tract involved in absorption) was apparent with the capsules and syrups. The Beecham and Pliva ampicillin 500 mg forms were found to be bioequivalent.

Bioequivalence

A comparison of two brands of ampicillin 250 mg capsules (Omnipen, Wyeth, USA [anhydrous form] and Penbritin, Beecham, UK [trihydrate form]) in ten healthy volunteers[28] indicated significantly greater bioavailability of ampicillin from Omnipen. However, when each capsule was compared with its respective 'pure drug' form, Omnipen had a lower bioavailability than the pure anhydrous form, whereas Penbritin had better bioavailability than the pure trihydrate form. The authors concluded that these differences were due to both the state of hydration and the formulation of the drug.

The comparative bioavailability of ampicillin capsules 500 mg as trihydrate from eight different manufacturers was determined in five healthy volunteers, by Ali[29] using Omnipen (Wyeth, USA; anhydrous ampicillin) as a reference product. No inter-brand bioequivalence could be demonstrated. In addition, bioequivalence could not be demonstrated between two brands of ampicillin capsules, commercially available in Sudan, when urine samples from five healthy volunteers were assayed by chemical and microbiological means.[30]

Workers in the USA[31] found no difference in bioavailability between 17 commercially available ampicillin capsules given to 14 healthy volunteers in a single-dose study.

Suspensions

Egyptian workers[32] examined the ability of kaolin in the presence of other additives (glycerol, sorbitol, macrogol, propylene glycol, povidone, acacia, tragacanth, syrup, Gifford's buffer) to adsorb anhydrous ampicillin in suspension. The physical properties of suspensions were improved by all additives except acacia. Sorbitol 70% was the most effective additive in respect of sedimentation volume and redispersibility. Kaolin was shown to adsorb ampicillin from suspension but when other excipients (except propylene glycol or Gifford's buffer, pH 8.6) were present, adsorption was reduced.

Modified-release preparations

Dissolution rate studies by Lauwo et al[33] at 30° in distilled water compared three different tablets of ampicillin (100 mg, 150 mg, or 200 mg) as trihydrate. The ampicillin 150 mg tablet contained Eudragit-RS in a 2:1 co-precipitate and the 200 mg tablet contained Eudragit-RS in a 1:1 co-precipitate. Dissolution rates of the co-precipitate tablets were considerably lower than that of the 100mg tablet prepared using the drug powder.

Rectal absorption

The addition of 0.16 M sodium decanoate (an absorption promoter) to an aqueous solution (pH 7.4) of ampicillin sodium (15 mg/mL) enhanced the rectal bioavailability of ampicillin (from 8% ± 7% to 79% ± 30%) when delivered in a rate-controlled manner to rats.[34]

Powders for reconstitution

The densities and displacement values of sucrose solutions (10% to 60% w/v) were calculated by Gibbins and James[35] at 23°. The displacement values of the dispersible powders ampicillin trihydrate, phenoxymethylpenicillin potassium, compound tragacanth powder, lactose, and glucose were also derived from their respective measured densities. The volume of water required for reconstitution of a given weight of powder ('dry syrup') into an oral suspension ('wet syrup') could then be calculated. This value is often an inconvenient volume (not easily measured in the dispensary) for which the authors provide an equation to transform it into a more convenient volume. Problems associated with sedimentation due to the relative insolubility of ampicillin trihydrate were overcome by the incorporation of a suspending agent (compound tragacanth powder) into the formulation. Displacement values of the suspending agent, buffer solutions, and any other excipients in high enough concentration would have to be considered and determined in any formulation.

Adsorption to sorbitol

The ability of sorbitol (instant and crystalline) to adsorb ampicillin trihydrate (and other antibiotics) was examined by Nikolakakis and Newton[36] using an air-sieving technique. The adsorption capacity and binding strength of instant sorbitol was greater than that of the crystalline form in dry powder blends.

FURTHER INFORMATION. The uptake of ampicillin and amoxycillin by some adsorbents [in vitro, by attapulgite, magnesium trisilicate, Veegum, and three types of kaolin, under simulated in vivo conditions with respect to pH changes]—Khalil SAH, Mortada LM, EL-Khawas M. Int J Pharmaceutics 1984;18:157–67. Enhancement of the rectal absorption of sodium ampicillin by N-acylamino acids in rats—Wu WM, Murakami T, Higashi Y, Yata N. J Pharm Sci 1987;76(7):508–12. Calcium ion sequestration by N-acylamino acids within the rectal membrane and the enhancement of the rectal absorption of sodium ampicillin in rats—Wu WM, Murakami T, Yamajo R, Higashi Y, Yata N. J Pharm Sci 1989;78(6):499–503.

REFERENCES

1. Hou JP, Poole JW. J Pharm Sci 1969;58(12):1510–15.
2. Hill SA, Jones KH, Seager H, Taskis CB. J Pharm Pharmacol 1975;27:594–8.
3. Georgarakis M, Hatzipantou P, Kountourliss JE. Drug Dev Ind Pharm 1988;14(7):915–23.
4. Ni W-H, Gu Y-L, Deng Z-M [Chinese]. Acta Pharmaceutica Sinica 1987;22(2):130–5.
5. Hou JP, Poole JW. J Pharm Sci 1969;58(4):447–54.
6. Bundgaard H, Larsen C. Int J Pharmaceutics 1978;1:95–104.
7. Bundgaard H, Larsen C. Int J Pharmaceutics 1979;3:1–11.
8. Bundgaard H, Larsen C. Int J Pharmaceutics 1977;132(1):51–9.
9. Larsen C, Bundgaard H. J Chromatogr 1978;147:143–50.
10. Bundgaard H, Hansen J. Int J Pharmaceutics 1981;9:273–83.
11. Acartürk F. J Fac Pharm Gazi 1988;5:139–46.
12. Mohamad H, Renoux R, Aiache S, Aiache J-M, Sirot J, Kantelip J-P [French]. STP Pharma 1986;2(20/21):912–17.
13. Abu-Reid IO, El-Samani SA, Hag Omer AI, Khalil NY, Mahgoub KM, Everitt G et al. Int Pharm J 1990;4(1):6–10.
14. Jaffe JM, Certo NM, Pirakitikulr P, Colaizzi JL. Am J Hosp Pharm 1976;33:1005–10.
15. Hempenstall JM, Irwin WJ, Li Wan Po A, Andrews AH. Int J Pharmaceutics 1985;23:131–46.
16. Boraie NA, El-Fattah SA, Hassan HM. Drug Dev Ind Pharm 1988;14(6):831–54.
17. Sylvestri MF, Makoid MC. Am J Hosp Pharm 1986;43:1496–8.

18. Gupta VD, Shah KA, De La Torre M. Can J Pharm Sci 1981;16(1):61–5.
19. Ashwin J, Lynn B. Pharm J 1975;214:487–9.
20. Stratton M, Sandmann BJ. Bull Parenter Drug Assoc 1975;29(6):286–95.
21. Holmes CJ, Ausman RK, Kundsin RB, Walter CW. Am J Hosp Pharm 1982;39:104–7.
22. Stjernström G, Olson OT, Nyqvist H, Lundgren P. Acta Pharm Suec 1978;15:33–50.
23. Sánchez-Morcillo J, Sellés E, Marin MT [Spanish]. Boll Chim Farm 1980;119:221–8.
24. Fletcher NR, Fletcher P, Yates RJ. Br J Pharm Prac 1988;10(10):442,444,448,453.
25. James MJ, Riley CM. Am J Hosp Pharm 1985;42:1095–100.
26. Hosny EA, Kassem AA, El-Shattawy HH. Drug Dev Ind Pharm 1990;16(9):1585–9.
27. Plavsic F, Wolf-Coporda A, Vrhovac B. Acta Pharm Jugosl 1989;39:53–61.
28. Ali AA, Farouk A. Int J Pharmaceutics 1981;9:239–43.
29. Ali HM. Int J Pharmaceutics 1981;7(4):301–6.
30. Ali HM, Farouk A, Khalil SAH, El-Nakeeb MA. Int J Pharmaceutics 1981;9:233–8.
31. Whyatt PL, Slywka GWA, Melikian AP, Meyer MC. J Pharm Sci 1976;65(5):652–5.
32. Hosny EA, Kassem A, El-Shattawy HH. Drug Dev Ind Pharm 1988;14(6):779–89.
33. Lauwo JAK, Agrawal DK, Emenike IV. Drug Dev Ind Pharm 1990;16(8):1375–89.
34. Van Hoogdalem EJ, De Boer AG, Breimer DD. Pharm Weekbl (Sci) 1988;10:76–9.
35. Gibbins LB, James KC. Int J Pharmaceutics 1980;4:353–5.
36. Nikolakakis I, Newton JM. J Pharm Pharmacol 1989;41:145–8.

Apomorphine (BAN)

Emetic

(R)-10,11-Dihydroxy-6a-aporphine; 6aβ-aporphine-10,11-diol; (R)-5,6,6a,7-tetrahydro-6-methyl-4H-dibenzo[de,g]quinoline-10,11-diol
$C_{17}H_{17}NO_2 = 267.3$

Apomorphine Hydrochloride (BANM)
Apomorphine hydrochloride hemihydrate
$C_{17}H_{17}NO_2, HCl, \frac{1}{2}H_2O = 312.8$
CAS—58-00-4 (apomorphine); 314-19-2 (apomorphine hydrochloride, anhydrous); 41372-20-7 (apomorphine hydrochloride, hemihydrate)

Pharmacopoeial status

BP, USP (apomorphine hydrochloride)

Preparations

Compendial
Apomorphine Hydrochloride Tablets USP.

Containers and storage

Solid state
Apomorphine Hydrochloride BP should be stored in an airtight container, protected from light.
Apomorphine Hydrochloride USP should be preserved in small, tight, light-resistant containers. Containers from which the powder is to be recovered for immediate dispensing should contain not more than 350 mg.

Dosage forms
Apomorphine Hydrochloride Tablets USP should be preserved in tight, light-resistant containers.

PHYSICAL PROPERTIES

Apomorphine hydrochloride exists as white to grey-white glistening crystals or as a white to grey-white microcrystalline powder; odourless. Samples become green on exposure to air and light.

Melting point

Apomorphine melts at about 195°, with decomposition.
Apomorphine hydrochloride melts between 225° and 236°, with decomposition.

pH

A 1% w/v solution of *apomorphine hydrochloride*, prepared without heating, has a pH of 4.0 to 5.0.

Dissociation constants

pK_a 7.2, 8.9 (15°)

Solubility

At about 25°, *apomorphine* is soluble in ethanol, in acetone, and in chloroform; slightly soluble in water, in benzene, in ether, and in petroleum spirit.
Apomorphine hydrochloride is soluble 1 in 50 of water and 1 in 50 of ethanol; practically insoluble in chloroform; very slightly soluble in ether.

Effect of temperature
The solubility of apomorphine hydrochloride increases with increasing temperature; in water, it is soluble 1 in 50 at 20°, and 1 in 20 at 80°.

STABILITY

Apomorphine hydrochloride undergoes oxidation on exposure to light and air. In aqueous solution apomorphine degrades to various quinolinedione derivatives which impart an emerald-green colour to the medium. Unfortunately, the depth of colour is not a reliable indicator of the extent of oxidation. In a discussion of the degradation of apomorphine, Burkman[1] stated that a deeply pigmented solution could still contain 98% of the original substance.
The decomposition of apomorphine hydrochloride is influenced by the concentration of atmospheric or dissolved oxygen and by pH. The oxidation products are devoid of any emetic properties. Using spectrophotometric and biological assay procedures, Burkman[2] investigated the autoxidation of 0.05% w/v apomorphine hydrochloride solutions in buffered (initial pH 6.0) and unbuffered (initial pH 5.5) sodium chloride 0.9%. The solutions were kept at 30° for 61 days, in the presence of excess oxygen. The buffered solutions became biologically inert, as evidenced by a gradual diminution in the intensity of the pecking syndrome of *pigeons*, after 16 days, whereas the unbuffered solutions

retained approximately 75% of their activity after 61 days; the unbuffered solutions had, however, turned dark green with a black precipitate. There appeared to be a correlation between the loss of biological activity and the disappearance of unoxidised apomorphine (spectrophotometrically). A reduction in pH was observed in all degraded solutions.

In a further study, Burkman[1] determined, by spectrophotometry, the rates of degradation of 0.05% w/v apomorphine hydrochloride at different temperatures and pH values. At 30°, the decomposition rate increased considerably as the pH rose from 5.2 to 5.8; the increase was less marked in the pH range 5.8 to 6.8. At a fixed pH of 6.0, solutions stored at 40° degraded 1.9 times faster than solutions stored at 30°. Lundgren and Landersjö[3] observed that copper (II) and, to a lesser extent, iron (II) ions catalyse the autoxidation process.

Effect of sterilisation

Powdered samples (30 mg) of Apomorphine Hydrochloride Tablets USP (6 mg) in sealed vials were autoclaved at 120° for 20 minutes.[4] It was found that this process, followed by 62 days storage in darkness at room temperature, caused a 13% potency loss and the production of a slight green tint when samples were brought into solution. In sealed vials, apomorphine hydrochloride 0.3% w/v solutions, stabilised with 1% w/v ascorbic acid and autoclaved at 120° for 20 minutes, turned amber then dark brown upon ageing in the dark. When the air in the vials was replaced by nitrogen before sterilisation, the shelf-life of 0.6% w/v solutions was extended, although this did not prevent the eventual appearance of a precipitate. When 0.3% apomorphine solutions containing 1% w/v ascorbic acid were sterilised by filtration (0.22 micrometre Millipore filter) and sealed under nitrogen, no measurable loss of potency or water clarity was evident after storage for 371 days at 5° in the dark. Maloney[5] recommended that solutions of apomorphine hydrochloride for subcutaneous injection should be sterilised by aseptic filtration rather than by autoclaving. It was claimed that the injection solution (sterilised by filtration) was stable for one year if stored below 8° and protected from light.

Various injection formulations of apomorphine hydrochloride were prepared, each containing one or a combination of the following antioxidants: sodium metabisulphite, disodium edetate, and ascorbic acid.[6] After sterilisation by autoclaving, decomposition was not greater than 4.3% in any of the solutions, although only the solution that contained disodium edetate and ascorbic acid remained clear, colourless, and acceptable in terms of apomorphine concentration and presence of the quinone oxidation product.

Lundgren and Landersjö[3] studied the effect of heat sterilisation on five injection formulations of 0.5% apomorphine hydrochloride. The effect of inclusion of 0.01% disodium edetate, 0.1% sodium metabisulphite, or both, and the removal of dissolved air by carbon dioxide were examined. It was concluded that only the complete removal of air would result in a colourless preparation after heat treatment. It was also noted that a slow reaction occurred between sodium metabisulphite and apomorphine.

Stabilisation

The rate of oxidation of apomorphine hydrochloride in solution can be retarded by the addition of dilute hydrochloric acid, to adjust the pH to between 3 and 4, and sodium metabisulphite; the solution should be free of dissolved oxygen.

Several studies have been undertaken to evaluate the role of various excipients in stabilising apomorphine hydrochloride in aqueous solution. Lundgren and Landersjö[3] investigated its stability in oral solutions and flavoured mixtures that contained 0.05% w/v apomorphine hydrochloride with different combinations of 0.1% w/v sodium metabisulphite, 0.01% w/v disodium edetate, 0.3% w/v hydrochloric acid (0.1 M), and distilled water. Samples were stored unopened at 25° and between 2° and 8°, and at 25° with frequent opening of the containers. After 205 days not more than 10% apomorphine degradation had occurred in any preparation. The degradation was found to be less in the apomorphine mixtures than in the solutions. This was explained by the organic acid content of the blackcurrant syrup which was included in the mixture formulations and which lowered their effective pH. Disodium edetate did not appear to have any stabilising effect in these formulations and frequent opening of the bottle did not lead to accelerated degradation. Sodium metabisulphite, however, was observed to protect the apomorphine.

Wilcox et al,[7] using HPLC and bioassay techniques, demonstrated that ascorbic acid 10% w/v or sodium bisulphite 0.052% w/v and 2% w/v limited degradation to less than 10% when 0.02% w/v aqueous solutions of apomorphine hydrochloride were stored at room temperature (22° to 25°) for 3 days. Control solutions prepared without the inclusion of antioxidants contained only 82.3% of their initial drug content after a similar period of time. Refrigeration at 5° was found to be an effective means of stabilising apomorphine solutions for periods of up to 7 days.[4]

Pandolfo et al[8] investigated the stability of solutions of apomorphine hydrochloride 1% w/v designed for parenteral use that contained sodium metabisulphite 0.2% and edetic acid 0.01% as possible stabilising agents. Solutions were sterilised by filtration, sealed in ampoules under nitrogen, and then stored at room temperature. After 4 years, the solutions were colourless and still contained ±10% of their initial drug content. The same workers also observed that lyophilisation did not result in a significant improvement in stability, and that the stability of the solution was not affected by steam sterilisation at 100° for 30 minutes.

INCOMPATIBILITY/COMPATIBILITY

Apomorphine hydrochloride is incompatible with oxidising agents, iron salts, tannins, alkalis, and iodides. A green colour is formed in the presence of iodine and a purple colour in the presence of nitric acid.

FORMULATION

Excipients

Excipients that have been used in presentations of apomorphine hydrochloride include:

Oral liquids: ascorbic acid; disodium edetate; ethanol; hydrochloric acid; sodium metabisulphite; blackcurrant, cherry, liquorice, and simple syrups.

Suppositories

In-vitro studies[9] of the release of apomorphine from suppositories prepared with either Witepsol, macrogol, or gelatin, indicated that the gelatin basis had the most desirable release properties under 'physiological' conditions in sodium chloride 0.9% at 36°.

FURTHER INFORMATION. Apomorphine hydrochloride stabilisation and oral liquid formulations—Engelhardt RJ, Schell FM, Lichtin JL. J Am Pharm Assoc 1968;NS8:198–9.

REFERENCES

1. Burkman AM. J Pharm Sci 1965;54:325–6.
2. Burkman AM. J Pharm Pharmacol 1963;15:461–5.
3. Lundgren P, Landersjö L. Acta Pharm Suec 1970;7:133–48.
4. Decker WJ, Corby DG, Combs HF. Clin Toxicol 1981;18:763–72.
5. Maloney TJ. Aust J Hosp Pharm 1985;15:34.
6. Brookes RW, McLaughlin JP, Moore AC, Simpson C. Pharm J 1991;247 (Pharm Pract Res Suppl 6657):R11.
7. Wilcox RE, Humphrey DW, Riffee WH, Smith RV. J Pharm Sci 1980;69:974–6.
8. Pandolfo V, Tanini R, Polidori G, Santoni G [Italian]. Boll Chim Farm 1984;123:449–52.
9. Neef C, Troost S, van Laar T, Essink G, Jansen E. Pharm Weekbl(Sci) 1991;13(6) Suppl L:L4.

Aspirin (BAN) *Analgesic; Anti-inflammatory; Antipyretic*

Acetylsalicylic acid; salicylic acid acetate

NOTE. The use of the name Aspirin is limited; in some countries it is a trademark.

O-Acetylsalicylic acid; 2-(acetyloxy)benzoic acid
$C_9H_8O_4 = 180.2$
CAS—50-78-2

Pharmacopoeial status

BP, USP

Preparations

Co-codaprin is the British Approved Name for compounded preparations of codeine phosphate and aspirin in the proportions, by weight, of 1 part to 50 parts, respectively.

Compendial
Aspirin Tablets BP (Acetylsalicylic Acid Tablets). Tablets containing, in each, 75 mg, 150 mg, 300 mg, 450 mg, and 500 mg are usually available.
Dispersible Aspirin Tablets BP. Tablets containing, in each, 75 mg, 300 mg, and 500 mg are usually available.
Effervescent Soluble Aspirin Tablets BP (Effervescent Aspirin Tablets). Tablets containing, in each, 75 mg, 100 mg, 300 mg, and 500 mg are usually available.
Aspirin and Caffeine Tablets BP.
Co-codaprin Tablets BP. Tablets containing, in each, 400 mg of aspirin and 8 mg of codeine phosphate are usually available.
Dispersible Co-codaprin Tablets BP. Tablets containing, in each, 400 mg of aspirin and 8 mg of codeine phosphate are usually available.

NOTE. When Soluble Aspirin Tablets are prescribed, Dispersible Aspirin Tablets shall be dispensed.
Aspirin Capsules USP.
Aspirin Delayed-release Capsules USP.
Aspirin Tablets USP.
Buffered Aspirin Tablets USP.
Aspirin Delayed-release Tablets USP.
Aspirin Extended-release Tablets USP.
Aspirin Effervescent Tablets for Oral Solution USP.
Aspirin Suppositories USP.

Non-compendial
Angettes 75 (Bristol-Myers). *Tablets*, aspirin 75 mg.
Caprin (Monmouth). *Tablets*, enteric coated, aspirin 324 mg.
Nu-seals Aspirin (Lilly). *Tablets*, enteric coated, aspirin 300 mg.
Platet (Nicholas). *Tablets*, effervescent, aspirin 100 mg and 300 mg.
Aspirin tablets (300 mg) are also available from APS, Evans, Kerfoot.
Aspirin dispersible tablets of various strengths are also available from APS, Cox, Evans, Kerfoot, R&C (Solprin 75).

Compound preparations
Co-codaprin tablets and co-codaprin dispersible tablets are available from Cox.

Containers and storage

Solid state
Aspirin BP should be kept in airtight containers.
Aspirin USP should be preserved in tight containers.

Dosage forms
Dispersible Aspirin Tablets BP and Effervescent Soluble Aspirin Tablets BP should be kept in well-closed containers and stored at a temperature not exceeding 25°.
Co-codaprin Tablets BP and Dispersible Co-codaprin Tablets BP should be protected from light.
All USP Capsule and Tablet preparations of aspirin should be preserved in tight containers. Flavoured or sweetened Aspirin Tablets USP of 81-mg size or smaller should be preserved in containers holding not more than 36 tablets each.
Aspirin Suppositories USP should be preserved in well-closed containers, in a cool place.
Angettes 75 tablets should be stored at room temperature.
Caprin tablets should be stored in a cool, dry place.
Containers for Nu-seals Aspirin should be kept tightly closed.
Platet tablets should be stored in a dry place, at room temperature.

PHYSICAL PROPERTIES

Aspirin exists as colourless or white crystals or as a white crystalline powder; odourless or with a faint odour of acetic acid.

Melting point
Aspirin melts at about 143°.

Dissociation constant
pK_a 3.5 (25°)

Partition coefficients
Log *P* (octanol/pH 7.4), −1.1
Log *P* (octanol/pH 1.05),[1] 1.2

Solubility
Aspirin is soluble 1 in 300 of water, 1 in 7 of ethanol, 1 in 17 of chloroform, and 1 in 20 of ether; sparingly soluble in absolute ether; soluble, with decomposition, in solutions of acetates and citrates and in solutions of alkali hydroxides and carbonates.

Effect of temperature
The aqueous solubilities of aspirin at different temperatures are as follows:

Temperature	Solubility
25°	1 in 300
37°	1 in 100
100°	1 in 33

Dissolution

The USP specifies that for Aspirin Tablets USP not less than 80% of the labelled amount of $C_9H_8O_4$ is dissolved in 30 minutes. Dissolution medium: 500 mL of 0.05 M acetate buffer, prepared by mixing 2.99 g of sodium acetate trihydrate and 1.66 mL of glacial acetic acid with water to obtain a 1000 mL solution having a pH of 4.50 ± 0.05; Apparatus 1 at 50 rpm.

Aspirin Capsules USP. The dissolution test procedure and limits are identical to those described for Aspirin Tablets USP except that the test is conducted at 100 rpm.

Buffered Aspirin Tablets USP. The dissolution test procedure and limits are identical to those described for Aspirin Tablets USP except that the test is conducted using Apparatus 2 at 75 rpm.

Dissolution properties

It has been reported that the intrinsic dissolution rate of aspirin is dependent upon crystal habit.[2–4]

The rate of absorption of aspirin from the gastro-intestinal tract is markedly influenced by its solubility.[5] Therefore, a great deal of effort has been channelled into designing *in-vitro* dissolution tests that correlate with *in-vivo* absorption.[6–8]

Crystal and molecular structure

Polymorphs

In a study of the dissolution rates of single crystals, Tawashi[9] characterised two polymorphic forms of aspirin, each with different melting points. Subsequently, Summers *et al*[10] claimed to have identified several more polymorphs. However, the existence of different polymorphic forms of aspirin has been questioned.[11–13]

Mitchell and Saville[14] demonstrated that polymorphic forms of aspirin can be distinguished by their intrinsic dissolution rates. Samples containing different mixtures of polymorphs may appear identical using techniques such as infrared and X-ray diffraction.

STABILITY

Aspirin is stable in dry air but in contact with moisture or in aqueous solution, it undergoes hydrolysis to yield acetic and salicylic acids. The stability of aspirin has been reviewed by Kelly.[15]

The rate of decomposition is both acid and base catalysed and is accelerated by heat. Maximum stability is observed at pH values between 2 and 3. The kinetics involved in the hydrolysis of aspirin have been described by Edwards.[16] Reepmeyer[17] reported that linear salicylate oligomers and various other compounds may also be products of the thermal decomposition of aspirin.

Solid state and tablets

The decomposition of aspirin has been studied in the solid state.[18,19] The extent of the decomposition is mainly dependent on water vapour pressure and on temperature.[19] Samples of aspirin stored at 35°, 45°, 60°, 80°, 100°, and 110° in the absence of moisture showed negligible decomposition after 50 days. A possible mechanism for the solid state decomposition of aspirin was suggested to involve initial sorption of moisture by each particle to form a water layer, diffusion of aspirin into solution, and subsequent decomposition by acid-catalysed hydrolysis. Yang and Brooke[20] established a rate equation for the sorbed-moisture model for the degradation of aspirin in the solid state. Decomposition of aspirin in the solid state was later shown to be dependent on the amount of moisture present; in a closed system in the presence of limited amounts of moisture,

at[21] 62.5° and at five other temperatures (40° to 65°),[22] the decomposition kinetics proposed by Leeson and Mattocks[19] were not followed. Other models were investigated.

Significant changes in the disintegration behaviour of enteric-coated tablets of aspirin were noted after 4 weeks storage at 30° in cyclic and isothermal heating conditions and under cyclic and constant humidity control (moderate stress conditions).[23] Similarly,[24] significant increases in the dissolution rates of enteric-coated aspirin tablets (with a shellac-type coating) were measured following storage at 22° and 60% relative humidity, or 33° and 60% relative humidity, for 42 days.

In studies where the concentration of salicylic acid was used to follow the extent of aspirin hydrolysis, Gore *et al*,[25] warned that sublimation and subsequent loss of salicylic acid may lead to erroneous results and an overestimation of aspirin stability.

Effects of additives and stabilisation

Neri *et al*[26] reported that a water-soluble salt of aspirin, lysine acetylsalicylate, was stable for two years at 25°.

Blaug and Wesolowski[27] investigated the effect of temperature, concentration, and the influence of certain additives on the stability of aqueous aspirin suspensions. Unbuffered suspensions (pH 2.5) were found to have longer half-lives than buffered suspensions (pH 3.0). The increased stability was attributed to the lower pH of 2.5 which coincides with the pH of maximum aspirin stability. As was expected for zero-order reactions, more concentrated suspensions exhibited longer half-lives. Of the additives studied, crystalline sorbitol 50% w/v was the most effective stabilising agent.

Munson *et al*[28] demonstrated that sodium bisulphite had a marked catalytic effect on the hydrolysis of aspirin at 40° in the pH range of 6.5 to 7.5. Folkers *et al*[29] reported that the hydrolysis of aspirin is catalysed by thiols.

The addition of between 1% and 3% of the polymer, poly(methylvinyl ether/maleic anhydride), to various dosage forms of aspirin, was found to exert a stabilising effect.[30]

In tablet formulations containing aspirin and constant concentrations of starch, silica exhibited a maximum stabilising effect against aspirin hydrolysis at a concentration of 3%.[31] This was explained by the fact that tablets prepared with silica 3% usually had a smaller pore size and were therefore less accessible to the entry of water vapour. Ager *et al*[32] reported that aspirin degraded to some extent in both 1:1 and in 1:10 aspirin:silica solid-state admixtures in the absence of moisture; however, no decomposition was detected in 15:4 mixtures. Alumina gave almost identical results indicating that aspirin degradation can be catalysed in the solid state by both acids and bases, as is the case for aspirin solutions. The addition of potato starch in identical proportions had no significant effect on decomposition rates. Rates of decomposition were measured in both solid admixtures and in tablets. Gore and Banker[33] studied the possible use of colloidal silica to stabilise aspirin in solid matrices.

The accelerated decomposition of aspirin in capsule formulations containing an alkali stearate can be inhibited by the inclusion of 20% by weight of malic, hexamic, or maleic acids.[34] Maulding *et al*[35] reported that a powder mix of aspirin containing hexamic acid 10% showed relatively little degradation. In the same study, a calcium stearate 5% preparation showed less aspirin decomposition than a mix containing magnesium stearate 5%. Aluminium hydroxide 10% had a stabilising effect on an aspirin powder mixture. This was ascribed to the relative insolubility of the aluminium acetylsalicylate salt and the adsorbent properties of aluminium hydroxide.

The effects of temperature (40° or 60°), excipient (microcrystalline cellulose [Avicel PH 101], dicalcium phosphate dihydrate

[Emcompress], or lactose), and mechanical treatment (ball milling) on the stability of aspirin in suspension were investigated in a factorially designed study.[36] The degradation rate of aspirin was significantly increased by an increase in temperature or the inclusion of Emcompress in the formulation. Milling produced an insignificant increase in degradation rate, although the effect may have been concealed by effects of temperature. In a similar factorially designed study,[37] significant increases in the degradation of aspirin in the solid state were attributed to several factors (relative humidity, temperature, and the presence of Avicel or Emcompress) and 'interactions' between factors were demonstrated.

When aspirin was incorporated in physical mixtures or co-precipitates with either urea or povidone, it exhibited enhanced decomposition rates under accelerated storage conditions. El-Banna et al[38] suggested that the acceleration may be due to the polar and perhaps the hygroscopic nature of the two excipients. Two amino acids, methionine and histidine, adversely affected the stability of aspirin in propylene glycol.[39]

Chang and Whitworth[40] reported a linear relationship between water content and the degradation rate constants of aspirin in mixed polar solvents. The surfactant, polysorbate 20, was observed to accelerate decomposition, possibly by a transesterification mechanism. A similar mechanism was implicated in polyglycerol ester suspensions of aspirin where the greatest stability was evident in those vehicles with low hydroxyl values and high viscosities.[41] Vehicles with low hydroxyl values have few hydroxyl groups that can be acetylated by aspirin. They therefore help prevent the formation of salicylic acid.

First-order rate constants observed for the acid-catalysed hydrolysis of aspirin were reduced[42] by the presence of polyoxyl stearates (Myrj 52, Myrj 53, and Myrj 59), at $37°$ over the pH range 1 to 2. Rate constants decreased as the concentration of polyoxyl stearate increased (1% to 10%).

A two-fold to three-fold reduction in the apparent first-order rate constants for the hydrolysis of aspirin was demonstrated in the presence of aqueous solutions and gels of poloxamines (Tetronic 1508) in the pH range 1 to 10 at $50°$, although at pH 5 to 8 no such reduction was apparent.[43] The observed rate constant decreased with an increase in the concentration of polymer (0% w/w to 25% w/w), except in the pH range 5 to 8. These effects were not as large as predicted; viscosity characteristics were considered as an explanation.

Asker and Whitworth[44] found that 0.3 g of aspirin suspended in 9.7 g of dimethylpolysiloxane fluids was stable for eight weeks at $4°$ and at $26°$.

Jun et al[45] reported that when aspirin 10% was incorporated into macrogol bases, rapid decomposition to salicylic acid and to acetylated macrogol by transesterification occurred at $45°$ and $60°$, even in the absence of moisture. Blocking of the free hydroxide groups of the macrogols should increase stability by inhibiting a transesterification reaction. With this in mind, Whitworth et al[46] studied monosubstituted methoxymacrogol 550 and macrogol 400 acetate as suitable liquid and semi-solid bases for aspirin. The results of this[46] and similar studies[47, 48] supported the theory that enhanced stability would be achieved in systems where aspirin is suspended in substituted macrogols. Whitworth and Pongpaibul[49] studied the effects of five nonionic surfactants (sorbitan monopalmitate, sorbitan monostearate, polysorbate 60, Tween 61, and polysorbate 65) on the stability of aspirin when added at concentrations of 5% and 20% to an oleaginous suppository preparation. All surfactants decreased aspirin stability, possibly by a transesterification reaction. Schneider and Stanislaus[50] reported that decreasing the hydroxyl number of suppository bases increased aspirin stability.

FURTHER INFORMATION. Influence of temperature and hydrophobic group-associated icebergs on the activation energy of drug decomposition [hydrolysis of aspirin] and its implication in drug shelf-life prediction—Kishore AK, Nagwekar JB. Pharm Res 1990;7(7):730–5. Decomposition of aspirin in the solid state in the presence of limited amounts of moisture. II. Kinetics and salting-in of aspirin in aqueous acetic acid solutions—Carstensen JT, Attarchi F. J Pharm Sci 1988;77(4):314–17. The effect of selected direct compression excipients [dibasic calcium phosphate dihydrate, lactose, microcrystalline cellulose, pregelatinised starch] on the stability of aspirin as a model hydrolysable drug—Patel NK, Patel IJ, Cutie AJ, Wadke DA, Monkhouse DC, Reier GE. Drug Dev Ind Pharm 1988;14(1):77–98. The stability of aspirin in a moisture containing direct compression tablet formulation—Snavely MJ, Price JC, Jun HW. Drug Dev Ind Pharm 1993;19(6):729–38. Influencing the stability of acetylsalicylic acid adsorbates with silicon dioxide [silica] auxiliary substances. Part 1. Comparison of different [silica] products—Rupprecht H, Kerstiens B [German]. Pharm Ztg 1986;131:421–5. ibid. Part 2. Influence of storage conditions on the stability of the adsorbates—Kerstiens B, Rupprecht H [German]. Pharm Ztg 1986;131:1154–9. Stability of aspirin in propoxyphene compound dosage forms—Goldberg R, Nightingale CH. Am J Hosp Pharm 1977;34:267–9.

INCOMPATIBILITY/COMPATIBILITY

A sticky mass is produced when aspirin is triturated with acetanilide, amidopyrine, phenacetin, phenazone, hexamine, phenol, salol, potassium acetate, or sodium phosphate. Aspirin is incompatible with free acids, iron salts, phenobarbitone sodium, quinine salts, potassium and sodium iodides, and with alkali hydroxides, carbonates, and stearates.

Hydrolysis of aspirin occurs in admixture with salts containing water of crystallisation. Solutions of alkali acetates and citrates, as well as alkalis, dissolve aspirin but the resulting solution rapidly hydrolyses to form salicylic acid and acetic acid.

In solid admixture, aspirin has been reported to acetylate other drugs such as paracetamol, homatropine, ephedrine, phenylpropanolamine, and codeine phosphate. Aspirin has also been reported to be incompatible with antihistamines.

FORMULATION

Excipients

Excipients that have been used in presentations of aspirin include:

Capsules: benzyl alcohol; cellacephate; cetyl alcohol; cetylpyridinium chloride; colloidal silica; erythrosine (E127); gelatin; glyceryl monostearate; purified talc; sodium lauryl sulphate; sunset yellow FCF (E110); wheat starch.

Tablets: aluminium glycinate; calcium carbonate; cellulose; colloidal silica; ethylcellulose; hypromellose; lactose; magnesium carbonate; maize starch; maize starch, pregelatinised; saccharin sodium; sodium lauryl sulphate; triacetin.

Effervescent tablets: citric acid; docusate; lemon flavouring; malic acid; mannitol; povidone; saccharin sodium; sodium bicarbonate; sodium carbonate.

Enteric-coated and coated tablets: acacia; activated dimethicone emulsion; aluminium glycinate; candelilla wax; carnauba wax; cellacephate; colloidal silica; diethyl phthalate; gelatin; hypromellose; liquid paraffin; macrogol 3350; magnesium carbonate; maize starch; maize starch, pregelatinised; methyl and propyl hydroxybenzoates; microcrystalline cellulose; polysorbate 20; povidone; propylene glycol; quinoline yellow (E104); sodium starch glycollate; sorbitan monolaurate; stearic acid; sucrose; sunset yellow FCF (E110); talc; titanium dioxide (E171); vanillin; white beeswax; zinc stearate.

Suspensions: chloroform; compound tragacanth powder.

Suppositories: macrogol 1500; macrogol 6000.

Effects of additives

Mital studied the use of methylcellulose in non-aqueous solvents as a granulating agent for aspirin.[51] The study was prompted by the fact that aspirin hydrolysis is greatest in tablets prepared using water. Jaminet and Louis[52] found that glyceryl monostearates were more suitable tablet lubricants than either magnesium stearate or macrogol 6000. The glyceryl esters provided better protection for aspirin against the deleterious effects of moisture. In a study of tablet disintegrants, calcium sulphate was found to be the most suitable.[53] Maulding et al[54] reported that stearic acid increased the rate of decomposition of aspirin when included in tablet and powder formulations. See also under Stability above.

Javaid and Cadwallader[55] studied eleven different buffering agents to determine their effects on the dissolution of aspirin from tablets. In general, buffering agents such as sodium bicarbonate, magnesium carbonate, and calcium carbonate resulted in more rapid dissolution. However,[56] dissolution rates of aspirin in McIlvaine's buffer, pH 6.8 at 37°, were decreased by the addition of 5% or 10% of taurine, glycine or sorbitol (alone or in various combinations); this was attributed to an increase in viscosity of the dissolution medium by the additives. Blaug and Wesolowski[27] found that both macrogol 6000 and povidone stabilised aspirin suspensions. Unfortunately, the use of such agents was found to result in precipitation. The influence of suspending agents on the release of aspirin from suspensions *in vitro* has been studied by Barzegar-Jalali and Richards.[57] A rank order relationship was observed between the first-order rate constant for the release of aspirin and the viscosity of the medium. See also Absorption and Bioavailability below.

Suppositories

Displacement values: theobroma oil and other fatty bases, 1.1; Witepsol H15, 1.56.

Several studies have been concerned with the influence of various suppository bases on the *in-vitro* release[58, 59] and on the *in-vivo* absorption[59-61] of aspirin from rectal dosage forms. Macrogol bases showed the best *in-vitro* release results for aspirin in a study carried out by Trivdi and Patel.[58] Lowenthal et al[61] reported that commercial aspirin suppositories, comprising a water-soluble basis, produced lower peak-plasma concentrations and bioavailability compared to extemporaneously prepared suppositories of aspirin comprising theobroma oil, macrogols, or a synthetic fatty basis, when administered to *dogs*. However, the commercial suppositories produced peak-plasma concentrations more quickly than the extemporaneous preparations. Parrott[59] demonstrated that the rectal absorption of aspirin from suppositories prepared using theobroma oil was influenced by particle size. In a 12-hour period the total salicylate excretion was 1.5-times greater for a suppository containing powdered aspirin (163 micrometres particle size) than for a suppository prepared using aspirin discs (3175 micrometres in diameter). No correlation between dissolution *in vitro* and bioavailability was shown.

Crospovidone has been used by Palmieri et al[62] as a disintegrant to increase the dissolution rate of aspirin from suppositories prepared with a macrogol basis. In a subsequent study, Palmieri[63] investigated the effects of ageing on these suppositories. Whit-worth et al[64] found that the addition of vegetable fats (at a concentration of 10%) had little effect on the stability of aspirin suppositories prepared using a macrogol basis; the most effective means of preventing decomposition was by refrigeration. Both citric acid (5% and 10%) and tartaric acid (10%) were found to inhibit decomposition of aspirin in macrogol basis[65] at 4°, 26°, and 45°.

Bioavailability

The rate of absorption of aspirin was shown to be dependent on the solubility of the oral preparation.[5] In healthy subjects, rates of aspirin absorption from commercially available buffered or effervescent preparations were greater than from a 'plain' aspirin preparation. A solution of the sodium salt of aspirin was also rapidly absorbed.

In healthy subjects, the bioavailabilities of four types of aspirin tablets available in Egypt (compared to the bioavailability of an aqueous solution) were as follows: effervescent aspirin (Effervescent Aspo-Cid, Chemical Industries Development), 100%; aluminium derivative of aspirin (Alexoprine forte, Alexandria), 88.9%; soluble aspirin (Dispirin, Reckitt and Colman), 83.27%; buffered aspirin (Alkaspirin, Kahira), 69.36%. However, absorption rate constants of the aspirin preparations were in the order: effervescent > soluble > buffered > aluminium derivative.[66]

Anslow et al[67] found that enteric-coated aspirin granules (Encaprin, Proctor and Gamble) led to more rapid and reliable absorption in the small intestine than a conventional enteric-coated tablet preparation (Ecotrin, SKF).

In a study in twelve healthy subjects, Orton et al[68] found no difference between the absorption profiles of effervescent and soluble aspirin preparations.

Absorption of aspirin was determined to be rapid and complete (total dose absorbed) from two buffered preparations (Ascriptin and Ascriptin A/D, Rorer) and complete from a compressed tablet (Aspro, Bauty) following a randomised crossover study involving six healthy subjects; results were calculated using urinary excretion data.[69] Absorption was slower from an enteric-coated tablet (Cemirit, Bayer) with about 90% of the total dose absorbed.

An absolute bioavailability of 95% was calculated for aspirin from a German sustained-release preparation (Contrheuma retard, that contained 300 mg aspirin as an initial dose and 350 mg aspirin in a 'retard' formulation) compared to an intravenous solution in a crossover study with six healthy subjects.[70] Statistically significant differences in plasma concentrations of the metabolite, salicylic acid, were detected.

During the first six-hour period after dosing, urinary salicylate concentrations were found to be almost identical for 680.4 mg of aspirin given in the form of a chewing gum and 648 mg of aspirin administered in the form of tablets.[71] However, in a study of the recovery of total salicylates from urine after administration of aspirin gum, only 63.5% of the administered dose was recovered; this compared with 91.2% for aspirin tablets.

Parrott[72] compared the fractions of a 600-mg dose of aspirin recovered as urinary salicylate over 24 hours following administration of capsules (oral) or macrogol suppositories (rectal) to healthy volunteers; the fraction of the rectal dose recovered was 0.9 compared to the oral dose. However, in a study of commercial suppositories, when retention time in the bowel was limited to two hours, Gibaldi and Grundhofer[73] found that at best only about 40% of the dose was absorbed in healthy subjects. The absorption rate was slow for all the commercial products with complete absorption in most instances only occurring after retention of the suppositories for periods in excess of ten hours.

Moolenaar *et al*[74] found that concentrations of aspirin in plasma after administration of a rectal micro-enema (20 mL, pH 4.0) may approach the plasma concentrations found after oral administration of a solution. The low pH of the enema suspension resulted in higher plasma concentrations of aspirin than enemas prepared at pH 7.0. Suppositories containing aspirin with an optimised particle size, produced much lower concentrations of aspirin in plasma than an oral preparation at an equivalent dose.

Further to investigations *in vitro*,[57] *in-vivo* studies using *rabbits*[75] indicated that the amounts of aspirin absorbed from 4% suspensions varied significantly when different macromolecular suspending agents were used (sodium alginate 1.15% w/v, methylcellulose 1.5% w/v, carmellose sodium 1% w/v, povidone 7% [mol. wt. 700 000], xanthan gum 1% w/v, tragacanth powder 1% w/v, or compound tragacanth powder 4% w/v). However, rates of absorption did not differ significantly. Compared to the suspension in distilled water, the extents of aspirin absorption from all other suspensions over a nine-hour period were greater; most absorption was apparent from the 1% w/v xanthan gum suspension. Differences were attributed to effects of viscosity on gastric emptying rates.

Modified-release preparations

Slower release of aspirin was demonstrated[76] from tablets prepared with aspirin 74% and either polymethylmethacrylate (Eudragit RSPM), polyvinyl chloride (Pevicon PE 737P), or carbomer (Carbopol 934P) at each of three concentrations (10%, 15%, or 20%), compared to conventional aspirin tablets, in 0.05 M acetate buffer, pH 4.5, at 37°. Rates of release decreased as the concentration of polymer was increased. The bioavailability of the preparation containing carbomer 15% was evaluated using urinary salicylate excretion data from six healthy volunteers.

Novel dosage forms

During the development of 'microdispersed' enteric tablets of aspirin, Dechesne[77] demonstrated that when aspirin crystals were coated with an aqueous acrylic latex (Eudragit L30D), inclusion of the plasticiser propylene glycol (at 30% w/w compared to the Eudragit) conferred good gastric resistance properties on compressed tablets of the formulation; gastric resistance studies were performed in 0.1 M hydrochloric acid for three hours in USP dissolution apparatus 2.

Watanabe *et al*[78] developed and demonstrated the pH-independent, controlled-release nature of 'enteric' granules of aspirin (as a model drug) prepared by coating aspirin crystals with Poemu S100V, Riken Vitamin Japan (a commercially available glyceryl monostearate) or by coating an aspirin/Poemu S100V 'mass' with glyceryl trilaurate. Poemu S100V and glyceryl trilaurate are broken down by lipase and bile salts in intestinal juice. Studies of dissolution *in vitro* and absorption in volunteers were performed.

FURTHER INFORMATION. Analgesics and antipyretics: Aspirin formulations—Colbert JC, editor. Controlled action drug forms. New Jersey: Noyes Data Corporation, 1974:245–54. Kinetics of dissolution and disintegration using a modified starch [STA-Rx-1500]—Joachim J, Joachim G, Acquier R, Maillols H, Delonca H [French]. Labo Pharma Probl Tech 1984;32:592–7. Influence of *in vitro* test conditions on release of aspirin from commercial tablets—Nikolic L, Djuric Z, Jovanovic M. J Pharm Sci 1992;81(4):386-91. Effect of thermal constraints on the *in vitro* release of the drug from the suppository form [Witepsol H15]: study of [aspirin]—Lasserre Y, Peneva B, Jacob M, Puech A [French]. J Pharm Belg 1986;41:12–16.

Aspirin, bioavailability monograph—Mayersohn M. J Am Pharm Assoc 1977;NS17:107–12. A pharmacokinetic approach to the establishment of biopharmaceutic characteristics of different [aspirin] formulations [conventional, buccal, effervescent, buffered, soluble, and enteric-coated tablets] in man—Raghoebar M, Vrancx F, Van Ginneken CAM. Biopharm Drug Dispos 1986;7:183–95. Kinetics and mechanism of hydrolysis of 1-(2′-acetoxybenzoyl)-2-deoxy-α-D-glucopyranose, a novel aspirin prodrug—Hussain A, Truelove J, Kostenbauder H. J Pharm Sci 1979;68:299–301. Enteric-coated and sustained-release [aspirin] dosage forms. Comparative bioavailability and effect of food on salicylate levels in serum—Kahela P, Anttila M. Acta Pharm Fenn 1983;92:249–57. Influence of type and concentration of carboxymethyl starches on bioavailability of aspirin in tablets—Tape LG, Robert H, Guyot-Hermann AM [French]. Farmaco Ed Prat 1982;37:128–38. Study of the compressibility of rosin-coated aspirin microcapsules—Pathak YV, Dorle AK. East Pharm 1989;32:121–3. Bioinequivalence of four 100 mg oral aspirin formulations in healthy volunteers—Bochner F, Somogyi AA, Wilson KM. Clin Pharmacokinet 1991;21:394–9.

PROCESSING

Waltersson and Lundgren[79] warned that processes such as milling or spray-drying may cause chemical degradation of drugs susceptible to hydrolytic degradation, such as aspirin, through a mechanical activation mechanism.

Aspirin tablets prepared by direct compression or by wet granulation showed greater stability at high humidity than those prepared by microencapsulation.[80] In later work on the three types of tablet,[81] the directly-compressed tablets were found to have the fastest dissolution rate. Correlation between *in-vitro* and *in-vivo* data (in five healthy subjects) was demonstrated.

The material tensile strength of convex-faced tablets of aspirin crystals, compacted under controlled conditions at pressures of 40 MPa and 320 MPa, was investigated by Pitt *et al*.[82] For a given tablet shape, compaction at 320 MPa produced tablets that had a two- to four-fold greater strength than those compacted at 40 MPa. The influence of tablet thickness on material tensile strength was also studied.

FURTHER INFORMATION. Determination of precompression and compression force levels to minimise tablet friability using simplex—Masilungan FC, Kraus KF. Drug Dev Ind Pharm 1989;15(11):1771–8.

REFERENCES

1. Thompkins L, Lee KH. Can J Pharm Sci 1968;3:10–13.
2. Mitchell AG, Saville DJ. J Pharm Pharmacol 1967;19:729–34.
3. Bauer K, Voege H [German]. Pharm Ind 1972;34(12):960–3.
4. Watanabe A, Yamaoka Y, Takada K. Chem Pharm Bull (Tokyo) 1982;30:2958–63.
5. Leonards JR. Clin Pharmacol Ther 1963;4:476–9.
6. Doelker E, Schwyter H, Mordier D [French]. Pharm Acta Helv 1975;50:24–7.
7. Johansen H. Arch Pharm Chemi Sci 1979;7:33–40.
8. Needham TE, Shah K, Kotzan J, Zia H. J Pharm Sci 1978;67(8):1070–3.
9. Tawashi R. Science 1968;160:76.
10. Summers MP, Carless JE, Enever RP [letter]. J Pharm Pharmacol 1970;22:615–16.
11. Mulley BA, Rye RM, Shaw P [letter]. J Pharm Pharmacol 1971;23:902–4.

12. Pfeiffer RR [letter]. J Pharm Pharmacol 1971;23:75–6.
13. Schwartzman G [letter]. J Pharm Pharmacol 1972;24:169–70.
14. Mitchell AG, Saville DJ. J Pharm Pharmacol 1969;21:28–34.
15. Kelly CA. J Pharm Sci 1970;59(8):1053–79.
16. Edwards LJ. Trans Faraday Soc 1950;46:723–35.
17. Reepmeyer JC [letter]. J Pharm Sci 1983;72(3):322–3.
18. Hasegawa J, Hanano M, Awazu S. Chem Pharm Bull 1975;23:86–97.
19. Leeson LJ, Mattocks AM. J Am Pharm Assoc (Sci) 1958;47:329–33.
20. Yang W-H, Brooke D. Int J Pharmaceutics 1982;11:271–6.
21. Carstensen JT, Attarchi F, Hou X-P. J Pharm Sci 1985;74(7):741–5.
22. Carstensen JT, Attarchi F. J Pharm Sci 1988;77(4):318–21.
23. Ondari CO, Prasad VK, Shan VP, Rhodes CT. Pharm Acta Helv 1984;59:149–53.
24. Hoblitzell JR, Thakker KD, Rhodes CT. Pharm Acta Helv 1985;60(1):28–32.
25. Gore AY, Naik KB, Kildsig DO, Peck GE, Smolen VF, Banker GS. J Pharm Sci 1968;57(11):1850–4.
26. Neri G, Cambieri M, Bruzzese T [Italian]. Boll Chim Farm 1976;115:845–57.
27. Blaug SM, Wesolowski JW. J Am Pharm Assoc (Sci) 1959;48:691–4.
28. Munson JW, Hussain A, Bilous R. J Pharm Sci 1977;66(12):1775–6.
29. Folkers G, Chang DW, Roth HJ [German]. Arch Pharm (Weinheim) 1984;317:962–4.
30. Chalhoub E, El-Shibini HAM, Daabis NA. Sci Pharm 1980;48:24–33.
31. Gucluyildiz H, Banker GS, Peck GE. J Pharm Sci 1977;66(3):407–14.
32. Ager DJ, Alexander KS, Bhatti AS, Blackburn JS, Dollimore D, Koogan TS. J Pharm Sci 1986;75(1):97–101.
33. Gore AY, Banker GS. J Pharm Sci 1979;68(2):197–202.
34. Zoglio MA, Maulding HV, Haller RM, Briggen S. J Pharm Sci 1968;57(11):1877–80.
35. Maulding HV, Zoglio MA, Pigois FE, Wagner M. J Pharm Sci 1969;58(11):1359–62.
36. Waltersson J-O. Acta Pharm Suec 1986;23:129–38.
37. Ahlneck C, Waltersson J-O. Acta Pharm Suec 1986;23:139–50.
38. El-Banna HM, Daabis NA, Abd El-Fattah S. J Pharm Sci 1978;67(11):1631–3.
39. Narang PK, Lim JK. J Pharm Sci 1979;68(5):645–8.
40. Chang R-K, Whitworth CW. Drug Dev Ind Pharm 1984;10(3):515–26.
41. Whitworth CW, Asker AF. J Pharm Sci 1975;64(12):2018–20.
42. Ismail S, Mohamed AA, Abd-El-Mohsen MG. Bull Pharm Sci Assiut Univ 1989;12(1):52–67.
43. Spancake CW, Mitra AK, Kildsig DO. Int J Pharmaceutics 1991;75:231–9.
44. Asker AF, Whitworth CW. J Pharm Sci 1974;63(10):1630–1.
45. Jun HW, Whitworth CW, Luzzi LA. J Pharm Sci 1972;61(7):1160–2.
46. Whitworth CW, Jun HW, Luzzi LA. J Pharm Sci 1973;62(7):1184–5.
47. Whitworth CW, Asker AF. J Pharm Sci 1974;63(11):1790–2.
48. Jun HW, Whitworth CW, Luzzi LA. J Pharm Sci 1974;63(1):133–5.
49. Whitworth CW, Pongpaibul Y. Can J Pharm Sci 1979;14:36–8.
50. Schneider GF, Stanislaus F [German]. Acta Pharm Technol 1981;27:159–67.
51. Mital HC. Pharm Acta Helv 1968;43:91–4.
52. Jaminet F, Louis G. Pharm Acta Helv 1968;43:153–7.
53. Delonca H, Puech A, Segura G, Youakim Y. J Pharm Belg 1969;24:243–52.
54. Maulding HV, Zoglio MA, Johnston EJ. J Pharm Sci 1968;57(11):1873–6.
55. Javaid KA, Cadwallader DE. J Pharm Sci 1972;61(9):1370–3.
56. Mahmud A, Li Wan Po A. Drug Dev Ind Pharm 1991;17(5):709–24.
57. Barzegar-Jalali M, Richards JH. Int J Pharmaceutics 1979;2:195–201.
58. Trivdi BM, Patel LD. Indian J Hosp Pharm 1982;19:218–23.
59. Parrott EL. J Pharm Sci 1975;64(5):878–80.
60. Samelius U, Åström A. Acta Pharmacol Toxicol 1958;14:240–50.
61. Lowenthal W, Borzelleca JF, Corder CD. J Pharm Sci 1970;59(9):1353–5.
62. Palmieri A, Dummer C, Groben W, Jukka R. Drug Dev Ind Pharm 1984;10:137–56.
63. Palmieri A. Drug Dev Ind Pharm 1986;12:1477–502.
64. Whitworth CW, Luzzi LA, Thompson BB, Jun HW. J Pharm Sci 1973;62(8):1372–4.
65. Whitworth CW, Jun HW, Luzzi LA. J Pharm Sci 1973;62(10):1721–2.
66. Gadalla MAF, Ismail AA, Abd El-Hameed MH. Drug Dev Ind Pharm 1989;15(3):447–72.
67. Anslow JA, Greene DS, Hooper JW, Wagner GS. Curr Ther Res 1984;36:811–18.
68. Orton D, Treharne Jones R, Kaspi T, Richardson R [letter]. Br J Clin Pharmacol 1979;7:410–12.
69. Latini R, Cerletti C, de Gaetano G, Dejana E, Galletti F, Urso R et al. Int J Clin Pharmacol Ther Toxicol 1986;24(6):313–18.
70. Lücker PW, Swoboda M, Wetzelsberger N [German]. Arzneimittelforschung 1989;39(I)Nr 3:391–4.
71. Woodford DW, Lesko LJ. J Pharm Sci 1981;70(12):1341–3.
72. Parrott EL. J Pharm Sci 1971;60(6):867–72.
73. Gibaldi M, Grundhofer B. J Pharm Sci 1975;64(6):1064–6.
74. Moolenaar F, Oldenhof NJJ, Groenewoud W, Huizinga T. Pharm Weekbl(Sci) 1979;114(1):243–53.
75. Barzegar-Jalali M, Richards JH. Int J Pharmaceutics 1979;3:133–41.
76. Capan Y, Senel S, Calis S, Takka S, Hincal AA. Pharm Ind 1989;51(4):443–8.
77. Dechesne J-P. Int J Pharmaceutics 1987;37:203–9.
78. Watanabe Y, Kogoshi T, Amagai Y, Matsumoto M. Int J Pharmaceutics 1990;64:147–54.
79. Waltersson J-O, Lundgren P. Acta Pharm Suec 1985;22:291–300.
80. Nouh AT, El-Sabbagh HM, Abd El-Gawad AH, El-Shaboury M. Bull Pharm Sci Assiut Univ 1985;8(2):25–46.
81. El-Sabbagh HM, Nouh AT, El-Saboury MH. Pharm Ind 1986;48(6):666–9.
82. Pitt KG, Newton JM, Richardson R, Stanley P. J Pharm Pharmacol 1989;41:289–92.

Atenolol (BAN, USAN, pINN)

Beta-adrenoceptor antagonist

4-(2-Hydroxy-3-isopropylaminopropoxy)phenylacetamide
$C_{14}H_{22}N_2O_3 = 266.3$
CAS—29122-68-7

Pharmacopoeial status

BP

Preparations

Compendial
Atenolol Tablets BP. Tablets containing, in each, 25 mg, 50 mg, and 100 mg are usually available.

Non-compendial
Antipressan (Berk). *Tablets*, atenolol 50 mg and 100 mg.
Tenormin (Stuart). '25' *Tablets*, atenolol 25 mg.
LS Tablets, atenolol 50 mg.
Tablets, atenolol 100 mg.
Syrup, sugar free, atenolol 0.5% w/v (equivalent to 25 mg/5 mL).
Injection, atenolol 500 micrograms/mL. *Diluents*: glucose 5% injection, sodium chloride 0.9% injection, or sodium chloride and glucose injection.
Totamol (CP). *Tablets*, atenolol 25 mg, 50 mg, and 100 mg.
Atenolol tablets of various strengths are also available from APS, Ashbourne (Atenix), Cox, Evans, Kerfoot, Norton, Shire (Vasaten).

Compound preparations
Co-tenidone is the British Approved Name for compounded preparations of atenolol and chlorthalidone in the proportions, by weight, 4 parts to 1 part respectively. Preparations: Tenoret 50 (Stuart), Tenoretic (Stuart). Co-tenidone tablets are also available from Ashbourne (Atenix Co), Cox, Kerfoot.

Containers and storage

Dosage forms
Antipressan tablets should be protected from light and moisture. Tenormin, Tenormin 25, and Tenormin LS tablets should be stored at room temperature and protected from light and moisture.
Tenormin syrup and injection should be stored at room temperature and protected from light.
Totamol tablets should be stored below 25°.

PHYSICAL PROPERTIES

Atenolol is a white or almost white powder; odourless or almost odourless.

Melting point

Atenolol has been reported to melt in the ranges 146° to 148°, 150° to 152°, and 152° to 155°.

Dissociation constant

pK_a 9.6 (24°)

Partition coefficient

Log *P* (octanol), 0.23
A value of log *P* (octanol) of 0.16 at 25° was reported by Burgot et al[1] for atenolol.

Solubility

Atenolol is sparingly soluble in water; soluble in absolute ethanol and in methanol; practically insoluble in ether.

Crystal and molecular structure

Liquid chromatographic analysis of atenolol enantiomers in human plasma and urine—Mehvar R. J Pharm Sci 1989;78(12):1035–9.

STABILITY

Atenolol as powder and in tablets was reported to remain stable and unchanged in appearance after storage at 50% to 60% relative humidity and 45° to 50° for seven days.[2]

FORMULATION

Excipients

Excipients that have been used in presentations of atenolol include:
Tablets: carnauba wax; colloidal silica (Aerosil 200); diethyl phthalate; ethylcellulose; gelatin; glycerol; hypromellose; lactose; macrogol 400; heavy magnesium carbonate; magnesium stearate; maize starch; microcrystalline cellulose; povidone; quinoline yellow (E104); sodium lauryl sulphate; sodium starch glycollate; starch; stearic acid; sunset yellow FCF (E110); sunset yellow FCF (E110) lake; talc; titanium dioxide (E171).
Oral liquids: citric acid; ethanol 95%; lemon and lime flavour; methyl and propyl hydroxybenzoates; orange syrup; saccharin sodium; sodium citrate; sorbitol; xanthan gum.
Injections: citric acid; citric acid/sodium citrate; sodium chloride; sodium hydroxide.

Compatibility with excipients

Under the conditions (30° to 250°) of differential scanning calorimetry atenolol was found to be compatible in 1:1 physical mixtures with starch, directly compressible starch (Sta-Rx 1500), sodium starch glycollate (Primojel), microcrystalline cellulose (Avicel PH 101), a cross-linked form of carmellose sodium (Ac-Di-Sol), cross-linked povidone, magnesium stearate, calcium sulphate dihydrate, dicalcium phosphate, and icing sugar.[3] Changes in endotherms that were attributed to interactions were observed for mixtures of atenolol with povidone, lactose, and stearic acid.

Eye drops

Eye drops of atenolol (1%, 2%, and 4%) in an aqueous vehicle adjusted to pH 6 and preserved with benzalkonium chloride 0.02% v/v were evaluated in 16 patients with intraocular pressures of 22 mg Hg or higher.[4] A fall in intra-ocular pressure began within one hour and reached a maximum (6.3 mm Hg) after two to three hours; the intra-ocular pressure regained its original value after seven hours.

Bioavailability

Atenolol is poorly absorbed and bioavailability values by the oral route range between 50% and 65%; by injection, bioavailability is reported to be from 85% to 100%.

Bioequivalence

Concern has been expressed about the bioequivalence of atenolol from non-branded (generic) sources when substituted for Tenormin.[5] However, Weller[6] found no major differences in the *in-vitro* dissolution characteristics of atenolol 100 mg tablets from three generic sources and from the proprietary manufacturer.

FURTHER INFORMATION. Reduced bioavailability of atenolol in man: the role of bile acids—Barnwell SG, Laudanski T, Dwyer M, Story MJ, Guard P, Cole S *et al.* Int J Pharmaceutics 1993;89:245–50.

REFERENCES

1. Burgot G, Serrand P, Burgot J-L. Int J Pharmaceutics 1990;63:73–6.
2. Caplar V, Mikotic-Mihun Z, Hofman H, Kuftinec J, Kajfez F, Nagl A, Blazevic N. In: Florey K, editor. Analytical profiles of drug substances; vol 13. London: Academic Press, 1984;1:25.
3. Botha SA, Lötter AP. Drug Dev Ind Pharm 1990;16(12):1945–54.
4. Wettrell K, Pandolfi M. Br J Ophthal 1977;61:334–8.
5. Pharm J 1987;239:472.
6. Weller PJ. Br J Pharm Pract 1990;12:388–90.

Atropine (BAN)   *Antimuscarinic*

(±)-Hyoscyamine
(1*R*,3*r*,5*S*)-Tropan-3-yl (±)-tropate; (1*R*,3*r*,5*S*,8*r*)-tropan-3-yl (*RS*)-tropate; α-(hydroxymethyl)-8-methyl-8-azabicyclo[3.2.1] oct-3-yl ester endo-(±)-benzeneacetic acid
$C_{17}H_{23}NO_3$ = 289.4

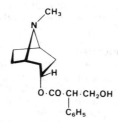

Atropine Methobromide (BANM)
$C_{18}H_{26}BrNO_3$ = 384.3

Atropine Methonitrate (BANM, rINN)
Methylatropine Nitrate (USAN)
$C_{18}H_{26}N_2O_6$ = 366.4

Atropine Sulphate (BANM)
Atropine Sulfate
$(C_{17}H_{23}NO_3)_2, H_2SO_4, H_2O$ = 694.8
CAS—51-55-8 (atropine); 2870-71-5 (atropine methobromide); 52-88-0 (atropine methonitrate); 55-48-1 (atropine sulphate, anhydrous); 5908-99-6 (atropine sulphate, monohydrate)

Pharmacopoeial status

BP (atropine methobromide, atropine methonitrate, atropine sulphate); USP (atropine, atropine sulfate)

Preparations

Compendial

Atropine Tablets BP. Tablets containing, in each, 600 micrograms of atropine sulphate are usually available.
Atropine Eye Drops BP. Eye drops containing 1% w/v atropine sulphate in purified water are usually available.
Atropine Eye Ointment BP. An eye ointment containing 1% w/w atropine sulphate in a suitable basis is usually available.
Atropine Injection BP (Atropine Sulphate Injection). Injections containing 400 micrograms, 600 micrograms, 800 micrograms, 1 mg, and 1.25 mg of atropine sulphate in 1 mL of water for injections; and 600 micrograms of atropine sulphate in 0.5 mL of water for injections are usually available. pH 2.8 to 4.5.
Morphine and Atropine Injection BP.
Atropine Sulfate Tablets USP.
Atropine Sulfate Ophthalmic Ointment USP.
Atropine Sulfate Ophthalmic Solution USP. pH 3.5 to 6.0.
Atropine Sulfate Injection USP. pH 3.0 to 6.5.

Non-compendial

Isopto Atropine (Alcon). *Eye drops*, atropine sulphate 1%, hypromellose 0.5%.
Minims Atropine Sulphate (S&N Pharm). *Eye drops* (single use), atropine sulphate 1%.
Min-I-Jet Atropine Sulphate (IMS). *Injection*, atropine sulphate 100 micrograms/mL.

Containers and storage

Solid state

Atropine Methobromide BP, Atropine Methonitrate BP, and Atropine Sulphate BP should be kept in well-closed containers and protected from light.
Atropine USP should be preserved in tight, light-resistant containers.
Atropine Sulfate USP should be preserved in tight containers.

Dosage forms

Atropine Sulfate Tablets USP should be preserved in well-closed containers.
Atropine Sulfate Ophthalmic Ointment USP should be preserved in collapsible ophthalmic ointment tubes.
Atropine Sulfate Ophthalmic Solution USP should be preserved in tight containers.
Atropine Sulfate Injection USP should be preserved in single-dose or in multiple-dose containers, preferably of Type I glass.
Isopto Atropine should be stored in a cool place away from direct sunlight. The container should be kept tightly closed.
Minims Atropine Sulphate should be stored in a cool place (8° to 15°) and should not be exposed to strong light.

PHYSICAL PROPERTIES

Atropine exists as colourless crystals or as a white crystalline powder; odourless or almost odourless.
Atropine methobromide and *atropine methonitrate* exist as colourless crystals or as white crystalline powders.
Atropine sulphate exists as colourless crystals or as a white crystalline powder; odourless. It effloresces in dry air.

Melting point

Atropine melts in the range 114° to 118°.
Atropine methobromide melts at about 219°, with decomposition.
Atropine methonitrate melts at about 167°.
Atropine sulphate melts at about 190°, with decomposition, after drying at 135° for 15 minutes.

pH

A 2% w/v aqueous solution of *atropine sulphate* has a pH of 4.5 to 6.2.

Dissociation constant

pK_a 9.9 (20°)

Partition coefficient

Log P (octanol), 1.8

Solubility

Atropine is soluble 1 in 400 of water, 1 in 3 of ethanol, 1 in 1 of chloroform, 1 in 60 of ether, and 1 in 30 of glycerol; soluble in dilute acids.

Atropine methobromide is soluble 1 in 1 of water and 1 in 20 of ethanol; very slightly soluble in absolute ethanol; practically insoluble in chloroform and in ether.

Atropine methonitrate is soluble 1 in less than 1 of water and 1 in 13 of ethanol; practically insoluble in chloroform and in ether.

Atropine sulphate is soluble 1 in less than 1 of water and 1 in 4 of ethanol; practically insoluble in chloroform and in ether.

Effect of temperature

The aqueous solubility of *atropine* increases with increasing temperature; it is soluble 1 in 90 of water at 80° and 1 in 50 of boiling water.

Atropine sulphate is soluble 1 in 0.5 of water at 25° and 1 in 2.5 of boiling water. It is soluble 1 in 5 of ethanol at 25°; its solubility is increased in boiling ethanol.

Crystal and molecular structure

Enantiomers

Atropine is optically inactive but it usually contains a small proportion of laevorotatory hyoscyamine.

STABILITY

In aqueous solution, atropine hydrolyses to tropine and tropic acid; decomposition at room temperature occurs very slowly. Hydrolysis of atropine is catalysed by hydrogen ions and hydroxide ions. At 25°, the rate of hydrolysis is at a minimum at pH 3.8. Dehydration of atropine to apoatropine may also occur. The rate of dehydration contributes significantly to the decomposition rate in the pH range 2 to 4.[1] Apoatropine hydrolyses to tropine and atropic acid.

Both the hydrolysis and dehydration of atropine were taken into account in the construction of the table below. Half-lives ($t_{50\%}$ years) of atropine as determined by Lund and Waaler;[1] under various conditions of pH and temperature were as follows:

Temperature (°C)	pH 2.0	pH 3.0	pH 4.0
20	74.8	1710	728
50	3.76	33.4	17.0
80	0.31	1.27	0.76
90	0.15	0.48	0.30
100	0.07	0.19	0.13

In an evaluation of ^{1}H NMR as a method for the determination of hydrolysis rates, aqueous solutions of atropine sulphate 1% were studied[2] at pH 8 over the range 60° to 88°. First-order rate constants for the hydrolysis reaction were about 2.95×10^{-3}/min (60°), 9.66×10^{-3}/min (70°), 2.02×10^{-2}/min (80°), and 4.95×10^{-2}/min (88°); an activation energy of about 47.6 kJ/mol for the hydrolysis of atropine was calculated.

Fahmy *et al*[3] subjected atropine sulphate solutions in Pyrex containers to continuous boiling for 15 minutes. The solutions contained 100 micrograms of atropine and were adjusted to cover the pH range 1 to 5. At pH 1.2, 3% of the atropine had decomposed; at about pH 5.6, the level of degradation was 21%.

Aqueous solutions of atropine methonitrate are reported to be unstable; stability is enhanced in acid solutions of pH below 6. However, a study has concluded that dilute aqueous solutions of atropine methonitrate are stable and may be sterilised by heating without loss of activity. The methods studied included autoclaving, steaming at 98° to 100° for 30 minutes. No decomposition products were detected in a solution prepared from atropine methonitrate that had been subjected to dry heat at 150° for 1 hour.[4]

Alcoholic solutions of atropine methonitrate are stable for 12 months but such solutions should be kept in airtight containers to prevent concentration of the solution by partial evaporation of the solvent.

Effect of light

Atropine sulphate is slowly affected by light. Fahmy *et al*[3] exposed 10 mL aliquots of atropine sulphate solution at pH 6.5, containing 200 micrograms of atropine, to ultraviolet radiation. About 50% decomposition occurred within 30 minutes and more than 95% after 3 hours.

Microbiological stability

In addition to deterioration caused by chemical and physical factors, instability of atropine solutions has also been attributed to bacterial and fungal contamination.

Kedzia *et al*[5] determined that of 744 strains of micro-organisms, 54 had the ability to break down atropine; of these, 38 belonged to the genus *Pseudomonas*.

FURTHER INFORMATION. The effect of autoclaving on stability of solutions of certain thermolabile substances—Murphy JT, Stoklosa MJ. Bull Am Soc Hosp Pharmsts 1952;9:94–7. The kinetics of the hydrolysis of atropine—Zvirblis P, Socholitsky I, Kondritzer AA. J Am Pharm Assoc (Sci) 1956;45:450–4. [Stability of atropine]—Wagner G, Luthardt K [German]. Pharmazie 1956;11:129–33. Stability of atropine in aqueous solution—Kondritzer AA, Zvirblis P. J Am Pharm Assoc (Sci) 1957;46:531–5. Stability of atropine solutions: biological and chemical assays—Lu FC, Hummel BCW. J Pharm Pharmacol 1960;12:698–702. On the analytics and stability of atropine sulphate and scopolamine hydrobromide. Part I. Quantitative detection of alkaloids in the presence of their decomposition products—Jira T, Pohloudek-Fabini R [German]. Pharmazie 1982;37:645–9; Part 3. [Use of plastic containers for liquid pharmaceuticals]—Jira T, Pohloudek-Fabini R [German]. Pharmazie 1983;38:520–3. Stability of tropane alkaloids (hyoscyamine, atropine) in syrups—Kahn-Borenstein C [French]. J Pharm Belg 1986;41:5–11. Bioassay of stored atropine solutions—Huycke EJ. JAMA 1957;46:160–3. Decomposition of an atropine sulphate solution irradiated with gamma rays—Cospito M, Contarini M, Gangemi G [Italian]. Boll Chim Farm 1966;105:109–14. Effects of radiosterilisation on atropine ophthalmic preparations—Trigger DJ, Caldwell ADS. J Hosp Pharm 1968;25:259–65. Identification of barium sulphate crystals in [atropine sulphate] parenteral solutions—Boddapati S, Butler LD, Im S, DeLuca PP [letter]. J Pharm Sci 1980;69(5):608–10.

INCOMPATIBILITY/COMPATIBILITY

Atropine and its salts are reported to be incompatible with bromides, iodides, iodine, alkalis, tannic acid, quinine, and mercury salts. Atropine methobromide is also incompatible with silver salts.

In intravenous admixture, atropine sulphate has been reported to be incompatible with pentobarbitone sodium. Atropine sulphate was incompatible with cimetidine and pentobarbitone sodium when the three drugs were combined in a syringe.[6]

Compatibility of eye drop preservatives

From the results of compatibility studies it was concluded that phenylmercuric nitrate 0.001% and 0.002%, thiomersal 0.01%, and benzalkonium chloride 0.01% were compatible with both atropine methonitrate 1% and atropine sulphate 1%. Chlorhexidine acetate 0.01% was compatible with atropine methonitrate but was deemed incompatible with atropine sulphate.[7]

Packaging

Atropine sulphate 1% eye drops (pH 6.4 to 6.8), packed in amber soda glass bottles, have been reported to become cloudy after autoclaving at 115° for 30 minutes or after steaming at 98° to 100° for 30 minutes. The turbidity was explained by leached alkali from the soda glass causing hydrolysis of the atropine and the subsequent precipitation of insoluble decomposition products. It was, therefore, considered important to use neutral or surface-treated glass containers when atropine solutions were to be sterilised. The pH of atropine sulphate 1% eye drops in neutral glass ampoules and surface-treated glass bottles was 4.8 and 4.5, respectively. Surface-treated eye drop bottles should not be autoclaved more than once.[8]

Sorption onto plastics

Gotz[9] studied the sorption characteristics of aqueous atropine sulphate solutions (at normal therapeutic concentrations) onto polyethylene and polyvinyl chloride plastics. Sorption was not apparent during prolonged storage, or under conditions of elevated temperature at different concentrations and pH values.

FURTHER INFORMATION. A comparative study of some of the effects of filter media on atropine sulphate and vitamin B_{12} solutions—Hernandez L, Mody DS, Avis KE. Bull Parent Drug Ass 1961;15:16–23. The adsorption of atropine from aqueous solution by kaolin—Ridout CW. Pharm Acta Helv 1968;43:42–9. The effect of pH on the adsorption of atropine from aqueous solutions by kaolin—Ridout CW. Pharm Acta Helv 1968;43:177–81. The adsorption of atropine sulphate and hyoscyamine hydrobromide by various antacids—Singh A, Mital HC. Acta Pharm Technol 1979;25:217–24. Investigations of adsorption of atropine sulphate on some pharmaceutical adjuvants—Hincal AA. Eczacilik Bul 1979;21:20–3.

FORMULATION

Excipients

Excipients that have been used in presentations of atropine include:
Oral liquids, atropine sulphate: raspberry syrup.
Eye drops, atropine: boric acid; chlorhexidine acetate.
Atropine methonitrate: chlorocresol; sodium chloride.
Atropine sulphate: benzalkonium chloride; boric acid; chlorocresol; disodium edetate; glycine; hypromellose; phenylmercuric acetate; phenylmercuric borate; phenylmercuric nitrate; sodium borate; sodium chloride.
Oily solutions, atropine: benzyl alcohol; Miglyol 812.

Eye ointments, atropine sulphate: liquid paraffin; wool fat; yellow soft paraffin.
Injections, atropine sulphate: dilute sulphuric acid; sodium chloride.

Ointment bases

Whitworth and Stephenson[10] examined the diffusion of atropine 5% from four ointment bases. Each basis contained one of three liquid additives at a concentration of 1%, 2%, or 5%. The bases studied were a water-in-oil basis, an oil-in-water basis, a hydrogenated cottonseed oil basis, and a macrogol basis; the additives were dimethyl sulphoxide, ethanol, and water. Apart from 'three instances at 1% concentrations', all the additives increased atropine diffusion. Without the inclusion of an additive the macrogol basis permitted the greatest release. Both water and ethanol increased atropine diffusion from the macrogol basis. In this respect both solvents were more effective than dimethyl sulphoxide. This observation was reversed in both the water-in-oil and oil-in-water bases where dimethyl sulphoxide produced the greatest increase in atropine release.

FURTHER INFORMATION. Preparation of atropine sulphate ampoules for high-dose therapy—Berman JM, Bertoldi IM [letter]. Am J Hosp Pharm 1985;42:1046. Leaching of zinc from rubber stoppers into the contents of automatic atropine injector—Ellin RI, Kaminskis A, Zvirblis P, Sultan WE, Shutz MB, Matthews R. J Pharm Sci 1985;74:788–90.

PROCESSING

Sterilisation

Atropine injection can be sterilised by heating in an autoclave. See Stability, above.

Lyophilisation

Korey and Schwarz[11] established that after lyophilisation of an aqueous solution of atropine sulphate 10% w/v, the atropine sulphate was present in the amorphous form as compared to the 100% crystalline state exhibited before lyophilisation. However, results indicated that some excipients, at certain concentrations, induced crystallisation of atropine sulphate during the lyophilisation process; these include glycine, alanine, serine, methionine, urea, or nicotinamide.

FURTHER INFORMATION. An examination of the sterilisation of atropine eye drops using ultraviolet light—Box JA, Sugden JK, Younis NMT. J Parenter Sci Technol 1984;38:115–21.

REFERENCES

1. Lund W, Waaler T. Acta Chem Scand 1968;22:3085–97.
2. Ferdous AJ, Dickinson NA, Waigh RD. J Pharm Pharmacol 1991;43:860–2.
3. Fahmy IR, Ahmed ZF, Karawia S, Eid SA. J Chem Un Arab Repub 1961;3:209–28.
4. *PSGB Lab Report P807* 1961.
5. Kedzia W, Lewon J, Wisniewski T. J Pharm Pharmacol 1961;13:614–16.
6. Yuhas EM, Lofton FT, Baldinus JG. Am J Hosp Pharm 1981;38:1173–4.
7. *PSGB Lab Report P/65/5* 1965.
8. Lund W, John EG. Pharm J 1969;203:217–18.
9. Gotz M [Hungarian]. Gyogyszereszet 1980;24:209–14.
10. Whitworth CW, Stephenson RE. J Pharm Sci 1971;60:48–51.
11. Korey DJ, Schwarz JB. J Parenter Sci Technol 1989;43(2):80–3.

Azathioprine (BAN, USAN, rINN)

Immunosuppressant

6-(1-Methyl-4-nitroimidazol-5-ylthio)purine;   6-[(1-methyl-4-nitro-1*H*-imidazol-5-yl)thio]-1*H*-purine

$C_9H_7N_7O_2S = 277.3$

CAS—446-86-6

Pharmacopoeial status

BP, USP

Preparations

Compendial

Azathioprine Tablets BP. Tablets containing, in each, 25 mg or 50 mg of azathioprine are usually available.

Azathioprine Tablets USP.

Azathioprine Sodium for Injection USP. pH 9.8 to 11.0.

Non-compendial

Berkaprine (Berk). *Tablets*, azathioprine 50 mg.

Imuran (Wellcome). *Tablets*, azathioprine 25 mg and 50 mg. *Injection*, powder for reconstitution with water for injections, azathioprine 50 mg (as the sodium salt) per vial. The solution should be preferably prepared immediately before use, and any remainder discarded. *Diluents*: sodium chloride injection (0.9% and 0.45%) or sodium chloride 0.18% and glucose 4% injection. The solution must be discarded if visible turbidity or crystallisation appears in the reconstituted or diluted preparation. Addition of reconstituted Imuran injection to any other infusion solution or intravenous admixture is not recommended. Azathioprine tablets are also available from APS, Ashbourne (Immunoprin), Cox, CP, Evans, Kerfoot, Penn (Azamune).

Containers and storage

Solid state

Azathioprine BP should be stored in well-closed containers and protected from light.

Azathioprine USP should be stored in tight, light-resistant containers.

Dosage forms

Azathioprine Tablets BP and Azathioprine Tablets USP should be protected from light.

Azathioprine Sodium for Injection USP should be preserved in containers suitable for sterile solids, at controlled room temperature.

Berkaprine tablets, Imuran tablets, and Imuran injection should be stored below 25°, protected from light. Berkaprine tablets and Imuran powder for reconstitution should be kept dry.

PHYSICAL PROPERTIES

Azathioprine is a pale yellow, odourless powder.

Melting point

Azathioprine melts at about 238°, with decomposition.

Dissociation constant

pK_a 8.2 (25°)

By spectrophotometric and solubility methods,[1] thermodynamic pK_a values of 7.87 and 7.99, respectively, were measured for azathioprine at 25°.

Partition coefficients

Log *P* (octanol/0.01N acetic acid pH 3.6), 1.25 (25°)[1]

Log *P* (octanol/0.04M phosphate buffer pH 7.4), 1.04 (37°)[1]

Solubility

Azathioprine is practically insoluble in water, in ethanol, and in chloroform; soluble in dimethyl sulphoxide and in macrogol 400; sparingly soluble in dilute mineral acids. It is soluble in dilute solutions of alkali hydroxides, but decomposes in stronger solutions.

Effect of pH

The solubility of azathioprine in water at 25° was determined to be 0.13 mg/mL, whereas in 0.02N acetate buffer at pH 4.08, the intrinsic solubility was found to be 0.124 mg/mL.[1]

Azathioprine is practically insoluble in water but it is soluble in 0.02M sodium hydroxide.[2]

Dissolution

The USP specifies that for Azathioprine Tablets USP not less than 65% of the labelled amount of $C_9H_7N_7O_2S$ is dissolved in 45 minutes. Dissolution medium: 900 mL of water; Apparatus 2 at 50 rpm.

STABILITY

In most instances the initial reaction in the decomposition of azathioprine is cleavage of the sulphide bond between the imidazole and purine rings. Although 6-mercaptopurine is the main degradation product, 1-methyl-4-nitro-5-thioimidazole and 1-methyl-4-nitro-5-hydroxyimidazole may also be found.[2]

In the solid state and when stored in well-closed light-resistant containers, azathioprine is reported to be stable for at least 2 years when kept between 5° and 37°, but for only 1 year at 50°.[3] Azathioprine is stable in neutral and acidic solutions.[3,4] Under alkaline conditions azathioprine is subject to decomposition, the rate of degradation increasing with increasing alkali concentration.[4]

Mitra and Narurkar[5] determined the kinetics of azathioprine degradation to 6-mercaptopurine and 1-methyl-4-nitro-5-hydroxyimidazole in buffered aqueous solution at 73° over the pH range 1 to 13 at an ionic strength of 0.5. Maximum stability was achieved at pH 5.5 to 6.5. When the rate of degradation of azathioprine was determined at 55°, 65°, 73°, and 85° at pH 1.2 and ionic strength 0.5, the calculated activation energy was 80.48 kJ/mol.

Using HPLC, Singh and Gupta[6] demonstrated the degradation of azathioprine by different reaction pathways in two pH regions (acidic and alkaline).

Azathioprine sodium injection 10 mg/mL (Imuran, Burroughs Wellcome, USA) when reconstituted with water has a pH of approximately 9.6; it is claimed to be stable for 24 hours at 15° to 30°.

In developing a stability-indicating HPLC assay for azathioprine, Fell *et al*[2] investigated the degradation of azathioprine in sodium chloride 0.9% injection when subjected to ultraviolet radiation or elevated temperatures. Two vials of the lyophilised sodium salt (Imuran injection, Wellcome) were added to the contents of 100-mL bags of sodium chloride 0.9% injection to give an initial concentration of about 1 mg/mL. Some bags were stored in diffuse light in water baths at room temperature or at 85°; others were subjected to ultraviolet radiation from a mercury lamp at room temperature. In the sample stored at 85° the concentration of azathioprine had fallen by 6.8% after 5 hours. At room temperature, exposure to ultraviolet radiation had a similar effect over 5 hours, the concentration falling by 4.4%. In diffuse light at room temperature, the concentration fell by only 0.4% in 5 hours. The principal products of thermal and photolytic degradation were identified and their distribution determined.

INCOMPATIBILITY/COMPATIBILITY

The compatibility and stability of azathioprine sodium with several intravenous fluids were investigated by Johnson and Porter.[7] Containers used in the study included the manufacturer's vial, plastic syringes, and plastic minibags. Azathioprine sodium was apparently chemically stable and physically compatible in all the containers with glucose 5% injection after 8 days at 4° in the dark and at 23° under constant illumination; however, a precipitate formed in the glucose solution after 16 days. Azathioprine sodium was physically compatible and chemically stable in sodium chloride 0.45% and 0.9% injections for 16 days at 4° and 23°. Reconstituted azathioprine sodium stored in either the manufacturer's vial or plastic syringe at 4° formed a precipitate after 4 days. The precipitate redissolved on heating to 70° but by day 16 the precipitate could not be dispersed by this treatment.

In solution, azathioprine is converted to 6-mercaptopurine in the presence of sulphydryl compounds such as cysteine, glutathione, and hydrogen sulphide.

FURTHER INFORMATION. Dielectric constant effects on degradation of azathioprine in solution—Singh S, Gupta RL. Int J Pharmaceutics 1988;46:267–70. Complexation behaviour of azathioprine with metal ions—Singh S, Gulati M, Gupta RL. Int J Pharmaceutics 1991;68:105–10.

FORMULATION

Excipients

Excipients that have been used in presentations of azathioprine include:
Tablets: lactose; magnesium stearate; povidone; starch (maize and potato); stearic acid.
Suspensions: carmellose sodium; Cologel; glycerol; methylcellulose; methyl hydroxybenzoate; syrup; vanillin; wild cherry syrup.
Injections: sodium hydroxide.
Dressman and Poust[8] investigated the stability of an extemporaneously prepared suspension of crushed azathioprine tablets in Cologel (Lilly) and simple syrup:wild cherry syrup (2:1). Greater than 90% of the initial concentration of azathioprine (measured by ultraviolet absorption) was retained when the suspension was stored at room temperature for 56 days and at 5° for 84 days. Although no reference was made to the physical or microbiological quality of the product, the authors concluded that the azathioprine suspension was stable for at least 14 days at room temperature.

PROCESSING

Azathioprine is cytotoxic; general guidelines on handling and disposal are given in the chapter entitled Cytotoxic Drugs: Handling Precautions.

REFERENCES

1. Newton DW, Ratanamaneichatara S, Murray WJ. Int J Pharmaceutics 1982;11:209–13.
2. Fell AF, Plag SM, Neil JM. J Chromatogr 1979;186:691–704.
3. Wilson WP, Benezra SA. In: Florey K, editor. Analytical profiles of drug substances; vol 10. London: Academic Press, 1981:39.
4. Elion GB, Callahan S, Bieber S, Hitchings GH, Rundles RW. Cancer Chemother Rep 1961;14:93–8.
5. Mitra AK, Narurkar MM. Int J Pharmaceutics 1986;35:165–71.
6. Singh S, Gupta RL. Int J Pharmaceutics 1988;42:263–6.
7. Johnson CA, Porter WA. Am J Hosp Pharm 1981;38:871–5.
8. Dressman JB, Poust RI. Am J Hosp Pharm 1983;40:616–18.

Bacitracin (BAN, rINN)   *Antibacterial*

Bacitracin consists of one or more of the antimicrobial polypeptides produced by certain strains of *Bacillus licheniformis* and by *B. subtilis* var. *Tracy*.
Bacitracin yields on hydrolysis the amino acids L-cysteine, D-glutamic acid, L-histidine, L-isoleucine, L-leucine, L-lysine, D-ornithine, D-phenylalanine, and DL-aspartic acid.

Bacitracin Zinc (BANM, rINNM)
A zinc complex of bacitracin.
CAS—1405-87-4 (bacitracin); 1405-89-6 (bacitracin zinc)

Pharmacopoeial status

BP, USP (bacitracin, bacitracin zinc)

Preparations

Compendial
Bacitracin Ointment USP.
Bacitracin Ophthalmic Ointment USP.
Sterile Bacitracin USP.
Bacitracin Zinc Ointment USP.
Sterile Bacitracin Zinc USP.

Containers and storage

Solid state
Bacitracin BP should be kept in an airtight container and stored at a temperature of 8° to 15°. If it is intended for the preparation of eye drops, the container should be sterile, tamper-evident and sealed so as to exclude micro-organisms.
Bacitracin Zinc BP should be kept in an airtight container. If it is intended for administration by spraying into internal body cavities, the container should be sterile, tamper-evident and sealed so as to exclude micro-organisms.
Bacitracin USP and Bacitracin Zinc USP should be preserved in tight containers and stored in a cool place.

Dosage forms
Sterile Bacitracin USP and Sterile Bacitracin Zinc USP should be preserved in containers suitable for sterile solids and stored in a cool place.
Ophthalmic ointments containing Bacitracin USP or Bacitracin Zinc USP should be preserved in collapsible ophthalmic ointment tubes.
Bacitracin Ointment USP and Bacitracin Zinc Ointment USP should be preserved in well-closed containers containing not more than 60 g, unless labelled solely for hospital use, preferably at controlled room temperature.

PHYSICAL PROPERTIES

Bacitracin is a white or almost white, hygroscopic powder; odourless or with a slight odour.
Bacitracin zinc is a white or pale yellowish-grey or pale tan, hygroscopic powder; odourless or with a slight odour.

pH

The pH of a 1% w/v solution of *bacitracin* lies between 6.0 and 7.0.
The pH of a solution containing 10 000 *bacitracin* units/mL lies between 5.5 and 7.5.
The pH of a saturated solution of *bacitracin zinc* (approximately 10% w/v) lies between 6.0 and 7.5.

Solubility

Bacitracin is freely soluble in water and in ethanol; soluble in methanol and in glacial acetic acid; and practically insoluble in chloroform and in ether. *Bacitracin zinc* is soluble 1 in 900 of water and 1 in 500 of ethanol; very slightly soluble in ether; and practically insoluble in chloroform.

STABILITY

Bacitracin powder is reported to be relatively thermostable. Gross[1] found no significant differences in stability between bacitracin of high potency (63 to 71 units/mg) and of low potency (45 to 59 units/mg).
In an extensive review of bacitracin biosynthesis, its chemical and physical properties, manufacturing procedures, therapeutic and other applications, Hickey[2] reported that bacitracin is precipitated from aqueous solutions by many heavy metal ions. However, the stability of bacitracin is enhanced by its conversion to bacitracin zinc, a high potency product with greater stability during storage and a less bitter taste.

Ointments

Bacitracin was found to retain 'most of its potency' for up to six months when mixed with the following ointment bases: Jelene (a combination of mineral oils and heavy hydrocarbon waxes), white soft paraffin, liquid paraffin, white beeswax, hydroquinone, ascorbyl palmitate, cetyl alcohol, calamine, zinc oxide, and ethyl aminobenzoate.[3] However, bacitracin was inactivated slowly in ointments with Carbowax bases (Carbowax 4000 with propylene glycol), sodium lauryl sulphate, some Spans, cholesterol, stearyl alcohol, and some Tweens, and was rapidly inactivated in ointments with water, macrogol 400, ichthammol, glycerol, tannic acid, phenol, and propylene glycol.

Solutions

Bacitracin is unstable in water at room temperature. Maximum stability of bacitracin in aqueous solution[2] is shown in the pH range 4.0 to 5.0. It is rapidly inactivated in aqueous solutions of pH below 4.0 or above 9.0. Prolonged exposure of bacitracin solutions to light also results in inactivation.
Souney *et al*[4] demonstrated that aqueous solutions of bacitracin (5000 units/mL) could be stored at −15° for up to 20 weeks in glass vials or plastic syringes without any loss of activity.
In each of three commercial brands of hypromellose 0.5% artificial tear solutions (Lacril, Tearisol and Isoptotears) in plastic squeeze bottles,[5] bacitracin (reconstituted from sterile powder according to the manufacturers' directions) was found to retain a relative potency of at least 83%, compared to control solutions, over a period of seven days at −10° or 25°.

FORMULATION

NEOMYCIN AND BACITRACIN OINTMENT
The following formula was given in the *British Pharmaceutical Codex 1973*:

Neomycin sulphate	5 g
Bacitracin zinc	500 000 units
Liquid paraffin	100 g
White soft paraffin	to 1000 g

Melt the white soft paraffin, incorporate the liquid paraffin, and stir until cold. Triturate the neomycin sulphate and the bacitracin zinc with a portion of the basis and gradually incorporate the remainder of the basis. The ointment may be expected to retain its potency for two years provided the moisture content of the ointment does not exceed 0.2%. When materials complying with BPC 1973 requirements are used, the moisture content may be expected to be below this figure.

Excipients

Excipients that have been used in presentations of bacitracin include:
Ointments: liquid paraffin; white soft paraffin.

FURTHER INFORMATION. Brewer GA. In: Florey K, editor. Analytical profiles of drug substances; vol 9. London: Academic Press, 1980:2–45.

REFERENCES

1. Gross HM. J Am Pharm Assoc (Sci) 1955;44(11):704–5.
2. Hickey RJ. Bacitracin, its manufacture and uses. In: Hockenhull DJD, editor. Progress in industrial microbiology; vol V. London: Temple Press Books, 1964:93–150.
3. Plaxco JM, Husa WJ. J Am Pharm Assoc (Sci) 1956;45(3):141–5.
4. Souney PF, Braun L, Steele L, Fanikos J. Am J Hosp Pharm 1987;44:1125–6.
5. Osborn E, Baum JL, Ernst C, Koch P. Am J Ophthalmol 1976;82(5):775–80.

Baclofen (BAN, USAN, rINN)

Skeletal muscle relaxant
Aminomethyl chlorohydrocinnamic acid
4-Amino-3-(4-chlorophenyl)butyric acid; β-(aminomethyl)-4-chlorobenzenepropanoic acid
$C_{10}H_{12}ClNO_2 = 213.7$
CAS—1134-47-0

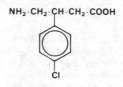

Pharmacopoeial status

BP, USP

Preparations

Compendial
Baclofen Tablets BP. Tablets containing, in each, 10 mg are usually available.
Baclofen Tablets USP.

Non-compendial
Lioresal (Geigy). *Tablets*, baclofen 10 mg.
Liquid, sugar free, baclofen 5 mg/5 mL. *Diluent*: purified water, freshly boiled and cooled; life of diluted liquid 14 days at room temperature. Bioequivalence is claimed for the tablet and liquid formulations.
Baclofen tablets are also available from APS, Ashbourne (Baclospas), Cox, Evans, Kerfoot, Norton.

Containers and storage

Solid state
Baclofen USP should be preserved in tight containers.

Dosage forms
Baclofen Tablets USP should be preserved in well-closed containers.
Lioresal tablets should be protected from heat. Lioresal liquid should be protected from heat and light and should not be refrigerated.

PHYSICAL PROPERTIES

Baclofen is a white or creamy-white crystalline powder; odourless or practically odourless.
The water absorption isotherm of baclofen at 40° has been determined[1] using the Karl Fischer method. During 14 days, at relative humidities of between 30% and 90% equilibrium moisture contents remained at about 0.4% to 0.6% whereas at relative humidities of 90% to 100% they increased to values of about 1.2%.

Melting point

Baclofen melts at about 207°.
The melting range of baclofen is variable owing to the rapid formation of lactam as heating proceeds, especially above 160°. The range has also been reported[1] as being from 192° to 193° and as 189° to 191°. See Stability, below.

Dissociation constants

pK_a 3.9, 9.6 (20°)

Partition coefficient

Log P (octanol/pH 7.4, aqueous phosphate buffer), −0.96 (23°)[1]

Solubility

Baclofen is slightly soluble in water (4.3 mg/mL); practically insoluble in most organic solvents; very slightly soluble in methanol. It dissolves in dilute mineral acids and alkali hydroxides; in phosphate buffer (pH 7.4) solubility is 5 mg/mL at ambient temperature.[1]

Dissolution

The USP specifies that for Baclofen Tablets USP not less than 75% of the labelled amount of $C_{10}H_{12}ClNO_2$ is dissolved in 30 minutes. Dissolution medium: 0.1N hydrochloric acid, 500 mL for tablets containing 10 mg or less of baclofen, 1000 mL for tablets containing more than 10 mg of baclofen; Apparatus 2 at 50 rpm.

Crystal and molecular structure

Baclofen crystals are reported to be orthorhombic.[1]

Enantiomers
The findings of a study of biological activity in *cats*, *mice*, and *rats* in which Olpe *et al*[2] compared the two enantiomers, and the racemate, of baclofen indicated that the therapeutic potency of the racemate was attributable to the laevorotatory enantiomer.

STABILITY

In the solid state, baclofen is relatively stable at ambient temperatures and humidity. At temperatures above 160°, it undergoes cyclisation with the release of one molecule of water to form its corresponding γ-lactam, 4-(4-chlorophenyl)-2-pyrrolidone.[1,3] The melting point of the γ-lactam is 117° to 118°, compared to the 207° value for baclofen itself. The rate of decomposition of baclofen[3] accelerates with increasing temperature above 160°. Compendial specifications limit the content of lactam in baclofen tablets and in baclofen powder (USP only). The principal degradation product of baclofen when the drug is in solution is also 4-(4-chlorophenyl)-2-pyrrolidone. Lactam formation in aqueous solutions of baclofen at 70°, 80°, and 90° appears to be most rapid at pH 9 to 10; solutions show greatest stability at pH 7.
Predictions from studies of aqueous solutions at elevated temperatures indicate that at 25° and at pH values of 7, 9, and 10 it would take 11.2, 2.0, and 2.0 years, respectively, for 10% decomposition to occur.[1]

FURTHER INFORMATION. Quantitation of baclofen in tablets using high-performance liquid chromatography [little decomposition noted during heating with dilute sulphuric acid or sodium hydroxide]—Das Gupta V. J Liq Chromatogr 1987;10(4):749–55. Quantitation of 4-(4-chlorophenyl)-2-pyrrolidinone in baclofen powder and tablets [by HPLC]—Das Gupta V, Parasrampuria J. Drug Dev Ind Pharm 1988;14(11):1623–8.

FORMULATION

Excipients

Excipients that have been used in presentations of baclofen include:
Tablets: magnesium stearate; microcrystalline cellulose; povidone; maize starch and wheat starch.
Oral liquids: Cologel; glycerol; methyl and propyl hydroxybenzoates; syrup.

Intrathecal injections

Intrathecal injections which contain baclofen at concentrations of 50 micrograms per mL (in 1 mL and 4 mL ampoules) and of 250 or 1000 micrograms per mL (in 12 mL vials for domestic use with implantable medication reservoirs) are manufactured in Belfast hospitals. The injection is prepared in sodium chloride 0.9% injection and adjusted to pH 6 for optimum stability. It is sterilised by filtration. Incomplete stability trials indicate stability for up to nine months.[4]

FURTHER INFORMATION. Production and testing of baclofen solutions [sterile solutions for intrathecal injection; stable for one year when stored below 25°]—Baum S, Schuster F [German]. Pharm Ztg 1988 April;133:28–32. Epidural baclofen for intractable spasticity—Jones RF, Anthony M, Torda TA, Poulos C [letter]. Lancet 1988;1:527.

REFERENCES

1. Ahuja S. In: Florey K, editor. Analytical profiles of drug substances; vol 14. London: Academic Press, 1985:527–48.
2. Olpe H-R, Demiéville H, Baltzer V, Bencze WL, Koella WP, Wolf P *et al*. Eur J Pharmacol 1978;52:133–6.
3. Borka L. Acta Pharm Suec 1979;16:345–8.
4. Millership SM, Crowe DE [letter]. Pharm J 1987;238:186.

Barium Sulphate

Radio-opaque substance (contrast medium)

Barium Sulfate (USAN)
Sulphuric acid, barium salt (1:1)
$BaSO_4 = 233.4$
CAS—7727-43-7

Pharmacopoeial status

BP (barium sulphate); USP (barium sulfate)

Preparations

Compendial
Barium Sulphate for Suspension BP. A dry mixture of barium sulphate, containing not less than 85.0% w/w $BaSO_4$, with suitable flavours, antimicrobial preservatives, and a suitable dispersing agent.
Barium Sulphate Oral Suspension BP (Barium Sulphate Suspension). A suspension of Barium Sulphate for Suspension in a suitable aqueous vehicle. Contains not less than 75.0% w/v $BaSO_4$. pH, 4.5 to 7.0.
Barium Sulfate for Suspension USP.

Non-compendial
Baritop 100 (Bioglan). *Suspension*, barium sulphate 100% w/v, with carbon dioxide as an effervescent agent.
Baritop Plus (Bioglan). *Granules*, for suspension in water, barium sulphate.
Micropaque (Nicholas). *Powder for suspension* (Micropaque HD), barium sulphate 96% w/w. To be reconstituted with water.
Suspension (Micropaque Standard), barium sulphate 100% w/v. A brown supernatant layer may form; this is normal and will disappear on shaking the bottle. The suspension may be diluted with water.
A suspension of barium in a prefilled enema bag is also available from S&N Pharm (EPI-C Barium Dispersion).

Containers and storage

Solid state
Barium Sulfate USP should be preserved in well-closed containers.

Dosage forms
Barium Sulfate for Suspension USP should be preserved in well-closed containers.
Baritop 100 should be stored in a warm place. Baritop Plus should be stored in a dry place.
Micropaque HD should be stored at room temperature in a dry place. Reconstituted suspensions should be used as soon as possible, in any event within 2 hours of adding water. Micropaque Standard should be stored at room temperature and should not be frozen. Shake before use.

PHYSICAL PROPERTIES

Barium sulphate is a fine, heavy, white, odourless powder; free from grittiness.

pH

A 5% aqueous suspension of *barium sulphate* is neutral to litmus.

Solubility

Barium sulphate is practically insoluble in water and in organic solvents; very slightly soluble in acids and in alkali hydroxides.

STABILITY

Barium sulphate decomposes above 1600°.
Suspensions of barium sulphate are liable to be affected on storage by sulphate-splitting micro-organisms, especially in the presence of small amounts of ethanol and saccharin.

FORMULATION

Excipients

Excipients that have been used in presentations of barium sulphate include:
Powders (for oral suspensions): activated dimethicone; caramel, cherry, strawberry, and vanilla flavours; carbon dioxide; carrageenan; cocoa powder; erythrosine (E127); macrogol mono-oleate; saccharin sodium; sodium citrate; sorbitol; sucrose.
Powders (for rectal suspensions): bentonite; carmellose sodium; sodium citrate; titanium dioxide (E171).
Oral pastes: butterscotch, caramel, and vanilla flavours; chloroform; disodium edetate; ethanol; glycerol; potassium sorbate; saccharin sodium; sodium benzoate; sodium methyl hydroxybenzoate; sodium propyl hydroxybenzoate; sorbitol; sulphuric acid; xanthan gum.
Oral suspensions: carmellose sodium; citric acid; dimethicone emulsion; disodium edetate; formaldehyde; glycine; potassium sorbate; saccharin sodium; silicones; sodium ascorbate; sodium benzoate; sodium citrate; sodium methyl hydroxybenzoate; sorbitol; sucrose; xanthan gum.

Pharmaceutical requirements

The formulation of barium sulphate preparations is influenced by the need to create a uniform layer on the gastro-intestinal mucosa, which is free from flocculation, bubbles and lumps, and is not too thick. Barium sulphate preparations must have high density to ensure good contrast, low viscosity to enable adequate coverage of the area under investigation, and is resistant to flocculation by the gastric contents. A simple barium sulphate/water mixture fails to satisfy many of these criteria, and is unpalatable. The quality of barium sulphate radiographs is highly dependent on particle size, with 0.5 micrometre particles giving the best results.[1]

Powders

Two basic processes are used in the manufacture of barium sulphate powders. Wet manufacturing involves the formulation of a suspension having the predetermined properties of the finished product when reconstituted with water. The water is then removed by a drying process such as drum drying, spray drying, or vacuum drying. Wet manufacturing results in products which are easily reconstituted and are without grittiness. Dry blending is a simple weighing, milling, and blending process that requires precise formulation, since adjustments cannot be made once the process has started. Products that have been dry-blended do not reconstitute as readily as those prepared by wet formulation and they may be slightly gritty.[2]

Suspensions

The high specific gravity (4.5) of barium sulphate necessitates a viscous suspending medium to maintain the suspension and to provide a satisfactory shelf-life for the product. Suspending agents such as carmellose sodium, aluminium magnesium silicate, and pectin have been used for this purpose. High-shear mixing and milling should also be employed to ensure adequate mixing of the ingredients.[2]

Flocculation of barium sulphate suspensions can occur on administration because of the action of human gastric juice. This problem can be partly overcome by including defloccu- lants, such as tragacanth, kaolin, gelatin, and aluminium hydro- xide gel. Certain physiologically inert salts can also be used as deflocculants for example, the salts of an alkali metal and the ammonium salt of a poly acid monomer; these agents act by increasing the negative charge on the surface of barium sul- phate particles.[2]

Barium sulphate formulations may also contain humectants (such as sorbitol), antifoaming agents (such as activated dimethicone), and various flavours.

Cellulose derivatives have been examined as barium sulphate suspension stabilisers. On the small scale it was found that 0.5% of carmellose sodium (50 centipoises viscosity) produced an acceptable preparation. The concentration of carmellose sodium required depends on the particle size of the barium sul- phate employed, the scale of manufacture, and the apparatus being used for dispersion. Methylcellulose and hypromellose were found to induce froth when products were shaken.

Embring and Mattsson[3] found that suspensions prepared with carmellose sodium and methylcellulose were not suitable for mucosal relief studies as they were too viscous; however, the pre- sentations were stable. Dextrans in the molecular weight range 15 000 to 200 000, povidone, and Sephadex were also consid- ered but again poor relief rendering was obtained. Mixing these materials with wetting agents such as polysorbates, sodium lauryl sulphate, and saponins improved mucus miscibility, but foaming prevented a critical evaluation of mucosal detail. The same workers noted that a high degree of stability was obtained when various salts of multibasic organic acids were included in such formulations. Results indicated that sodium citrate pro- duced the most stable suspensions, and that the effect was sub- stantially intensified by sorbitol.

Flavouring

Although most proprietary presentations of barium sulphate are flavoured, the need to flavour extemporaneous preparations may occasionally arise. The unpalatable chalk-like taste of bar- ium sulphate/water mixtures can be improved by choosing a good suspending agent and an appropriate flavour. Flavours for barium sulphate suspensions should also be capable of mask- ing the tastes of other adjuvants such as preservatives. Liquid flavours can be sprayed onto powdered barium sulphate in small amounts and then thoroughly mixed, thus giving a dry product that is convenient for storing and packing. Powdered flavours can be mixed directly with barium sulphate, but the resulting flavour is influenced by particle size. Fine powdered materials will adhere to coarser particles, and if two powdered flavours are included it will be the flavour of the finer materials that will be experienced first. The use of more than one flavour- ing agent is recommended to ensure that no particular taste, sweetness, or texture predominates.[4]

Ultra-fine milling and the addition of flavouring agents that do not cause over-secretion of gastric juices are suggested as means by which the chalky taste of barium sulphate/water mixtures can be improved.[1]

FURTHER INFORMATION. Radiopaques—a review—Chenoy NC. Pharm J 1965;194:663–9. A new deflocculant and protective col- loid for barium sulphate [degraded carrageenan with ghatti gum]—Anderson W [letter]. J Pharm Pharmacol 1961;13:64. A study of barium sulphate preparations used as X-ray opaque media—particle size and particle charge—James AM, Goddard GH. Pharm Acta Helv 1971;46:708–20. Barium meals: a physi- cal chemical study of the adsorption of hydrocolloids by bar-

ium sulphate—James AM, Goddard GH. Pharm Acta Helv 1972;47:244–56. Behaviour of enteric-coated granules [of bar- ium sulphate] administered in controlled-release matrices to the stomach of a fed dog—Heinamaki J. Acta Pharm Fenn 1991;100:27–34.

REFERENCES

1. Bentley A [review]. Pharm J 1987;238:138–9.
2. McKee MW, Jurgens RW [review]. Am J Hosp Pharm 1986;43:145–8.
3. Embring G, Mattsson O. Acta Radiol 1968;7:245–56.
4. Miller RE [overview]. Am J Roentgenol 1966;96:484–7.

Benzocaine (BAN, rINN)   *Local anaesthetic*

Anesthamine; éthoforme
Ethyl 4-aminobenzoate; ethyl *p*-aminobenzoate
$C_9H_{11}NO_2 = 165.2$
CAS—94-09-7

Pharmacopoeial status

BP, USP

Preparations

Compendial
Benzocaine Topical Aerosol USP. Benzocaine Cream USP. Ben- zocaine Ointment USP. Benzocaine Topical Solution USP. Ben- zocaine Otic Solution USP.

Containers and storage

Solid state
Benzocaine BP should be protected from light.
Benzocaine USP should be preserved in well-closed containers.

Dosage forms
Benzocaine Topical Aerosol USP should be preserved in pres- surised containers, avoiding exposure to excessive heat.
Benzocaine Cream USP, Benzocaine Ointment USP, and Ben- zocaine Topical Solution USP should be preserved in tight con- tainers, protected from light. Prolonged exposure to temperatures greater than 30° should be avoided.
Benzocaine Otic Solution USP should be preserved in tight, light- resistant containers.

PHYSICAL PROPERTIES

Benzocaine appears as colourless crystals or a white crystalline powder; almost odourless.

Melting point

Benzocaine melts between 89° and 92° (BP). The USP states that *benzocaine* melts between 88° and 92°, but the range between the beginning and end of melting should not exceed 2°.

Dissociation constant

pK_a 2.8 (25°)

Solubility

Benzocaine is soluble 1 in 2500 of water, 1 in 8 of ethanol, 1 in 2 of chloroform, 1 in 4 of ether, and 1 in 50 of fixed oils; it is soluble in dilute mineral acids and in liquid paraffin.

Effect of cosolvents

Rubino and Yalkowsky[1] measured the solubility of benzocaine in various cosolvent-water mixtures. Cosolvents that were studied included propylene glycol, 1,3-butanediol, glycerol, sorbitol, macrogol 200 or 400, ethanol, and methanol. A logarithmic increase in solubility with increasing volume fraction of the cosolvent was generally noted; the magnitude of the increase was in agreement with the order of polarity of the cosolvent. In the case of 1,3-butanediol, a decrease in solubility was noted with increasing concentration of the cosolvent.

Dissolution

Saleh and York[2] demonstrated that the dissolution rate of benzocaine in water at 37° was increased by the presence of sodium salicylate and by macrogol 300. It was suggested that the surface-tension-lowering properties of these two agents may have resulted in more efficient wetting of the benzocaine particles. A synergistic effect on the dissolution rate was observed when sodium salicylate and macrogol 300 were combined with benzocaine.

Solid dispersions

The dissolution rate of benzocaine from solid dispersions has been examined by Sirenius et al.[3] Dissolution rates from xylitol dispersions were greater than that observed from tablets made from the simple drug; the increase was greatest when the drug content of the dispersions was lowest. When the benzocaine content of the dispersions exceeded about 20% w/v to 30% w/v, the dissolution rate per unit area was almost constant.

Suppositories

Roseman et al[4] developed a continuous flow bead-bed apparatus to investigate the release of benzocaine from two suppository formulations. The apparatus consisted of a bed of glass beads surrounding the suppository, through which there was a continuous flow of water at a constant rate. Two suppository bases were selected representing low melting (Witepsol H-15) and high melting (Witepsol E-76) types. Initial benzocaine release rates were similar for both bases, but at later times faster release was exhibited by the lower melting basis. Temperature of the dissolution medium had a marked effect on benzocaine release from the high melting basis. There was an increase in release from 33° to 37°, a decrease at 39° and 40° where the release was equivalent to that at 33°, and an increase to a maximum value at 45°. At 39° and 40°, the glass beads were observed to penetrate the suppository basis thus reducing the available surface area for drug release.

A comparative study between the continuous flow bead-bed apparatus of Roseman et al[4] and a rotating basket technique was undertaken by McElnay and Nicol.[5] The dosage units employed were suppositories of benzocaine (0.481% w/v) in Witepsol E-75. During the 2-hour test period, 29.9% of the initial benzocaine content had dissolved using the rotating basket apparatus. This compared favourably with the 27% benzocaine release measured using the flow-through bead-bed apparatus. A temperature-dependent release profile similar to that noted by Roseman et al was observed when using the continuous flow bead-bed device. However, with the rotating basket technique, there was no inflection at 39° and dissolution simply increased with increasing temperature.

STABILITY

Benzocaine is stable in air.

Benzocaine undergoes specific acid-catalysed and base-catalysed hydrolysis to yield ethanol and *p*-aminobenzoic acid. The reaction is temperature dependent. The rate constant at pH 9 and 30° is 6.31×10^{-8}/s; this corresponds to a half-life of about 127 days. The first-order rate constant for the hydrolysis of benzocaine in 0.5M perchloric acid (pH 0.3) at 97.3° was determined by Marcus and Baron[6] to be 140/s; the activation energy under these conditions was calculated to be 77.8 kJ/mol. Hamid and Parrott[7] calculated the activation energy for the alkaline hydrolysis of benzocaine (pH 8) to be in the range 50.2 to 62.8 kJ/mol. Benzocaine stability studies have been undertaken at various conditions of temperature (25°, 40°, 60°, and 70°) and pH (2, 7, and 11) by Narang et al.[8] At 25°, degradation was greatest at pH 11, intermediate at pH 2, and slowest at pH 7. In the presence of phosphate buffer (0.1M), benzocaine was found to be 8.0, 7.3, and 1.3 times more stable at pH 11, pH 2, and pH 7 respectively, than in non-buffered solutions at equivalent pH values.

Stabilisation

The stability of benzocaine is improved by reducing contact with water, bases, and acids. The small quantities of water present in most benzocaine formulations, such as lozenges, suppositories, and ointments, ensure that hydrolysis is minimal.

Benzocaine stability can be improved by protecting the molecule from water contact using complexation and micellar solubilisation techniques.

Complexation

Complexation with large molecules has been examined as a means of increasing the apparent water solubility and stability of benzocaine. Complexing molecules may inhibit hydrolysis by sterically hindering the approach of catalytic species to the ester linkage. Alternatively, electronic effects induced by the complexing agent may alter the affinity of the carbonyl group for the catalyst. This latter effect may result in an increase or a decrease in the rate of hydrolysis.

Caffeine[9] and a homologue of caffeine, 1-ethyltheobromine,[10] have been studied as suitable complexing agents for the stabilisation of benzocaine in solution. Caffeine interacted more readily with benzocaine than 1-ethyltheobromine and whereas caffeine formed 1:1 complexes with benzocaine, 1-ethyltheobromine formed at least two complex species. Of the two additives, caffeine was observed to be the better stabilising agent. On inclusion of either caffeine 2.5% w/v or 1-ethyltheobromine 2.5% w/v, the half-life of benzocaine in 0.04N barium hydroxide (at 30°) increased by a factor of 5.5 or 4.6, respectively. However, 1-ethyltheobromine, being more soluble than caffeine, may prove the more useful stabilising agent as it can be used at higher concentrations.

The use of cyclodextrins to form inclusion complexes with benzocaine has been studied by Chin et al.[11] Both α-cyclodextrin and β-cyclodextrin produced an increase in the half-life of benzocaine under alkaline conditions. The most effective of the two stabilisers was β-cyclodextrin. A 1:1 complex was noted between benzocaine and β-cyclodextrin with total inclusion of the drug within the β-cyclodextrin molecule. This inclusion provided protection from nucleophilic attack by the alkoxide ions of the β-cyclodextrin molecule itself and by hydroxyl ions from the solution. Hydrolysis was stated to be due only to the free ester in solution, formed from the dissociation of the inclusion complex. Lach and Pauli[12] considered the suitability of the following agents for the complexation of benzocaine, and the subsequent stabilisation of aqueous solutions of the drug: povidone, *N*-methyl-2-pyrrolidone, *N,N*-dimethylacetamide, dimethyl urea, macrogol 4000, urea, thiourea, deoxycholic acid, and cholic acid. All the compounds tested increased the stability of benzocaine in barium hydroxide solution (0.04N) at 30°, but none achieved a stabilising effect greater than that produced by caffeine. Results obtained using cholic acid and deoxycholic acid, however, indicated their potential value for the stabilisation of benzocaine.

Micellar solubilisation

Surfactants have been examined as a means of increasing the apparent solubility of benzocaine, and its stability against alkaline hydrolysis. When included at levels greater than their critical micelle concentrations, anionic, cationic and nonionic surfactants have been found to increase the stability of benzocaine. The stabilising properties of surfactants are due to the affinity of benzocaine for the hydrophobic medium within the micelles. Differences in solubilisation and stabilisation effects between surfactants, are a function of the chemical structure of the surfactant, especially its charge and the chain length of the monomers.

In a study of the effects of surfactants on the hydroxide-ion catalysed hydrolysis of benzocaine, Riegelman[13] reported that an anionic surfactant, sodium lauryl sulphate, extended the half-life up to eighteen-fold; this stabilising effect was attributed to the polar head group which shielded solubilised benzocaine in the deeper parts of the micelle from the approach of hydroxide ions. A similar effect was observed with the cationic surfactant, cetyltrimethylammonium bromide, but only where its concentration was much greater than the critical micelle concentration. However, for a surfactant concentration only just above the critical micelle concentration, benzocaine was hydrolysed slightly faster than was a simple solution of the drug; it was suggested that at very low concentrations of surfactant the micelles were loosely arranged and permitted the penetration of hydroxide ions, which were attracted to the cationic polar heads. The nonionic surfactants, cetyl alcohol polyoxyethylene ethers, gave less protection against the hydrolysis of benzocaine than did sodium lauryl sulphate; the half-life was enhanced less than four-fold. It was postulated that benzocaine was solubilised in the hydrated polyoxyethylene palisade layer of the nonionic micelles, where hydroxide ions could readily attack the drug.

Hamid and Parrott[7] considered the effectiveness of polyoxyethylene lauryl ether and polysorbate 80 in retarding the hydrolysis of benzocaine, in a 0.04N hydroxide ion concentration at several temperatures. At 30°, the half-life of benzocaine solubilised with 15% w/v polyoxyethylene lauryl ether was increased 1825 times; and when solubilised with 15% w/v polysorbate 80 the half-life was increased 180 times.

Meakin *et al*[14] studied the effect of the cationic surfactant, cetyltrimethylammonium bromide, on the rate of base-catalysed hydrolysis of benzocaine. Inclusion of the surfactant at a concentration of 0.02M resulted in a 2.8-fold reduction in the observed hydrolytic rate constant (at pH 10.39 in Sørensen's glycine buffer at 50°).

An examination of the effects of the surfactant cetyltrimethylammonium bromide on the radiation sensitivity of benzocaine in aqueous solution has been reported by Chingpaisal *et al*.[15] Aqueous solutions of benzocaine 1.2×10^{-4}M containing various concentrations of the surfactant were irradiated using a ^{60}Co source, and the degrading effects of two of the radiolytic products of water were studied spectrophotometrically. Although the results suggested that cetyltrimethylammonium bromide increased benzocaine breakdown by the hydrated electron, it protected the drug from the hydroxyl radical, especially above its critical micelle concentration.

Sheth[16] demonstrated that at concentrations below the critical micelle concentration (cmc), four nonionic surfactants had no significant effect on the half-life of benzocaine in a solution with a 0.04N hydroxide ion concentration at 30°. At concentrations above the cmc, however, an increase in half-life was observed. The stabilising properties of the surfactants followed the order: Brij 35 (Atlas, USA) = Triton WR-1339 (Winthrop, USA) > Tetronic 908 (Wyandotte, USA) > Pluronic F68 (Wyandotte, USA).

INCOMPATIBILITY/COMPATIBILITY

An acidic solution of benzocaine gives a precipitate with iodine and is incompatible with oxidising agents. Benzocaine forms coloured mixtures with bismuth subnitrate. In admixture with camphor, menthol, and resorcinol, benzocaine forms a liquid or semi-liquid. Benzocaine is reported to be incompatible with cetomacrogol, citric acid, liquid glucose, and natural cherry flavour.

Sorption

Bray and Meakin[17] have studied the permeability and sorption characteristics associated with the interaction between benzocaine and polyvinyl chloride. It was demonstrated that an increase in benzocaine permeability accompanied an increase in the concentration of the plasticisers, di-2-ethylhexylphthalate and acetyl tri-*n*-butyl citrate; benzocaine permeability also rose with temperature. Sorption increased with plasticiser concentration but decreased with temperature. Overall, the effects of acetyl tri-*n*-butyl citrate on the sorption and permeability characteristics of benzocaine were greater than those of di-2-ethylhexylphthalate.

Interaction between benzocaine and polyvinyl acetate phthalate in propylene glycol or in a mixture of propylene glycol and ethanol (stored in glass bottles at room temperature) was manifest as a yellow discoloration, with formation of a crystalline product in the solutions;[18] 4-phthalimidobenzoic acid ethyl ester was isolated and characterised. The authors commented that the primary amine group of benzocaine makes it susceptible to interaction with compounds that contain a carbonyl group.

FURTHER INFORMATION. Fractional factorial experimental design study of the incompatibility of benzocaine in throat lozenges—Kabasakalian P, Cannon G, Pinchuk G. J Pharm Sci 1969;58:45–7. Incompatibility of nonionic surfactants with oxidisable drugs—Azaz E, Donbrow M, Hamburger R. Pharm J 1973;211:15. Influence of sunscreening agents [such as benzocaine as protective agent] on colour stability of tablets coated with certified dyes III: [sunset yellow FCF (E110)]—Hajratwala BR, Hennig AJ. J Pharm Sci 1977;66:107–9.

FORMULATION

COMPOUND BENZOCAINE LOZENGES
The following formula was given in the *British Pharmaceutical Codex 1973*:

For each lozenge:

Benzocaine	100 mg
Menthol	3 mg

Prepared by compression, with the addition of menthol dissolved in a little ethanol to the dried granules. Each lozenge weighs about 1 g.

COMPOUND BENZOCAINE OINTMENT

The following formula was given in the *British Pharmaceutical Codex 1973*:

Benzocaine	100 g
Hamamelis ointment	450 g
Zinc ointment	450 g

The benzocaine should be triturated with a portion of the hamamelis ointment until smooth and gradually incorporated into the remainder of the hamamelis ointment and the zinc ointment.

Excipients

Excipients that have been used in presentations of benzocaine include:

Lozenges: brilliant blue FCF (133); maize syrup; FD&C Red No.4; glycerol; liquid glucose; sucrose.

Dental gels: acid fuchsine D; carbomer 934P; clove oil; disodium edetate; glycerol; macrogols; saccharin; tragacanth powder.

Ointments: liquid paraffin; yellow soft paraffin.

Lotions: aloe vera gel; carbomer 934P; glycerol; glyceryl monostearate; lanolin alcohols, fractionated; menthol; methyl and propyl hydroxybenzoates; simethicone; triethanolamine.

Aerosol sprays: aloe vera oil; macrogol 400 monolaurate; menthol; methyl hydroxybenzoate; polysorbate 85.

Topical liquids: brilliant blue FCF (133); D&C Green No. 5; isopropanol; macrogol; menthol; quinoline yellow (E104).

Suspensions

The effect of nonionic surfactants (polyoxyethylene nonylphenols) and added salts on the flocculation of benzocaine suspensions has been studied using measurements of apparent viscosity, sedimentation behaviour, and refiltration. Flocculation was found to be influenced by surfactant concentration, polyoxyethylene chain length, and benzocaine particle size. The results of the three techniques correlated well except in the case of surfactants with less than or equal to 9 polyoxyethylene units per molecule.[19] Addition of various salts to suspensions stabilised with polyoxyethylene nonylphenols initially produced a decrease in flocculation, and then, at a critical salt concentration, a rapid increase in flocculation occurred. The flocculating properties of the salts decreased in the order: sodium sulphate > magnesium sulphate > sodium chloride > calcium chloride.[20]

Topical preparations

A cellulose membrane dialysis technique has been used to study benzocaine release from oleaginous, absorption, emulsion (water-in-oil and oil-in-water), and water-soluble ointment bases. A comparison of the release from some commercial products (available in the United States) with that from experimental formulations has also been undertaken.[21] Wide variations in the amount of benzocaine dialysed were noted, with benzocaine release from the bases following the order: water-soluble macrogol basis > oil-in-water emulsion > water-in-oil emulsion > abtion basis > white soft paraffin. An increase in benzocaine concentration in the vehicle generally led to a rise in the quantity of dialysed drug, except with the macrogol basis. This was attributed to a marked decrease in benzocaine solubility (at concentrations greater than 5%) in water-macrogol solutions and its subsequent precipitation due to a diffusion of water through the membrane to the donor compartment.

Nannipieri *et al*[22] investigated the influence of formulation, manufacturing variables and temperature, on the *in-vitro* release of benzocaine from gel-type oily vehicles, that contained differing proportions of isopropyl myristate, white soft paraffin, and hard paraffin. Drug release was inversely related to the hard paraffin content of the basis, and directly related to the temperature. The rate of benzocaine release from the hard paraffin:white soft paraffin:isopropyl myristate (10:60:30% w/w) basis was also observed to be influenced by the method of manufacture. Rates of release were higher for bases prepared by slow cooling than those manufactured by a rapid cooling procedure.

An investigation of benzocaine-vehicle interactions in anhydrous macrogol ointment bases indicated a high affinity of benzocaine for low molecular weight macrogols. The observed interactive phenomena were ascribed to hydrogen bonding effects.[23]

Belmonte and Tsai[24] considered the diffusion, penetration, and surface effects of benzocaine in macrogol ointment bases on human stratum corneum. In this *in-vitro* study, a decrease in drug diffusion was observed in the presence of relatively high amounts of the lower molecular weight macrogols. Scanning electron microscopy was used to show that both the bases (combinations of macrogol 4000 and macrogol 600) and benzocaine altered the surface structure of the stratum corneum. The basis effect appeared to be principally a function of the content of macrogol 600.

An evaluation of benzocaine-containing ophthalmic vehicles was made by Bottari *et al*[25] using *rabbits*. Micronised benzocaine in yellow soft paraffin exhibited a significantly faster onset of anaesthetic action than 'macrosize' benzocaine in the same vehicle. A carboxyvinyl aqueous gel which contained micronised benzocaine produced a greater peak anaesthetic action and a longer duration of effect than either of the two yellow soft paraffin preparations.

Rectal absorption

The rectal absorption in *rats* of ^{3}H-benzocaine in five different ointment bases has been measured by Ayers *et al*.[26] The five ointment bases studied were white soft paraffin, an absorption vehicle, an oil-in-water emulsion, a water-in-oil emulsion, and a water-soluble macrogol vehicle. Levels of radioactivity measured in blood samples were used to measure absorption rates. No benzocaine could be detected *in vivo* and all the radioactivity was attributed to metabolised drug. Over five hours, the levels of benzocaine absorbed from the bases followed the order: macrogol > oil-in-water emulsion > water-in-oil emulsion > absorption basis = white soft paraffin. These results compare favourably with a previous *in-vitro* study by Ayres and Laskar,[21] in which benzocaine diffusion from the same five ointment bases was examined using a cellulose membrane dialysis technique.

A study in *rats* to compare the effect of suppository vehicles, drug concentrations, and the inclusion of nonionic hydrophilic or lipophilic surfactants, on the *in-vitro* release of benzocaine and the *in-vivo* absorption of ^{3}H-benzocaine was carried out by Ayres *et al*.[27] Both *in vitro* and *in vivo*, drug release was greater from a water-soluble basis (75% w/w macrogol 1000 and 25% w/w macrogol 4000) than from an oleaginous basis (theobroma oil). When the concentration of ^{3}H-benzocaine in both the water-soluble and the oleaginous basis was increased, a higher total count of radioactivity was measured in blood samples. Although an increase in the benzocaine concentration from 3% w/v to 10% w/v in a single vehicle led to the release of a larger quantity of drug *in vitro*, the amount released represented a smaller percentage of the initial drug concentration. The effects of added surfactants were variable. Inclusion of a hydrophilic or lipophilic surfactant had statistically insignificant effects on ^{3}H-benzocaine release from macrogol suppositories. Addition of either type of surfactant to the theobroma oil basis produced an increased drug release *in vitro*, but a similar result was not observed under *in-vivo* conditions.

FURTHER INFORMATION. [Release data of benzocaine from hydrophilic gels]—Bottari F, Carelli V, Di Colo G, Saettone MF, Serafini MF. Int J Pharmaceutics 1979;2:63–79. Vehicle effects in percutaneous absorption: *in vitro* study of influence of solvent power and microscopic viscosity of vehicle on benzocaine release from suspension hydrogels—Di Colo G, Carelli V, Giannaccini B, Serafini MF, Bottari F. J Pharm Sci 1980;69:387–91. Effect of nonionic surfactants on penetration of dissolved benzocaine through hairless *mouse* skin—Dalvi UG, Zatz JL. J Soc Cosmet Chem 1981;32:87–94. Effect of skin binding on percutaneous transport of benzocaine from aqueous suspensions and solutions—Dalvi UG, Zatz JL. J Pharm Sci 1982;71:824–6. Influence of drug-surfactant and skin-surfactant interactions on percutaneous absorption of two model compounds [including benzocaine] from ointment bases *in vitro*—Di Colo G, Giannessi C, Nannipieri E, Serafini MF, Vitale D. Int J Pharmaceutics 1989;50:27–34. Release of benzocaine, procaine, 2-aminothiazole and 4-amino-4H-1,2,4-triazole from polymer carriers—Kolli M, Montheard JP, Vergnaud JM. Int J Pharmaceutics 1992;81:103–10. Solvent interaction with polydimethylsiloxane membranes and its effects on benzocaine solubility and diffusion—Gelotte KM, Lostritto RT. Pharm Res 1990;7:523–9.

REFERENCES

1. Rubino JT, Yalkowsky SH. J Parenter Sci Technol 1985;39:106–11.
2. Saleh AM, York P. Pharm Ind 1978;40:1076–80.
3. Sirenius I, Krogerus VE, Leppänen T. J Pharm Sci 1979;68:791–2.
4. Roseman TJ, Derr GR, Nelson KG, Lieberman BL, Butler SS. J Pharm Sci 1981;70:646–51.
5. McElnay JC, Nicol AC. Int J Pharmaceutics 1984;19:89–96.
6. Marcus AD, Baron S. J Am Pharm Assoc 1959;48:85–90.
7. Hamid IA, Parrott EL. J Pharm Sci 1971;60:901–6.
8. Narang PK, Bird G, Crouthamel WG. J Pharm Sci 1980;69:1384–7.
9. Higuchi T, Lachman L. J Am Pharm Assoc 1955;44:521–6.
10. Lachman L, Guttman D, Higuchi T. J Am Pharm Assoc 1957;46:36–8.
11. Chin T-F, Chung P-H, Lach JL. J Pharm Sci 1968;57:44–8.
12. Lach JL, Pauli WA. Drug Stand 1959;27:104–8.
13. Riegelman S. J Am Pharm Assoc 1960;49:339–43.
14. Meakin BJ, Winterborn IK, Davies DJG. J Pharm Pharmacol 1971;23(Suppl):25S–32S.
15. Chingpaisal P, Fletcher G, Davies DJG. J Pharm Pharmacol 1977;29(Suppl):47P.
16. Sheth PB [abstract]. Diss Abstr 1967;28:974B–5B.
17. Bray CS, Meakin BJ. J Pharm Pharmacol 1977;29(Suppl):49P.
18. Kumar V, Banker GS. Int J Pharmaceutics 1992;79:61–5.
19. Liao W-C, Zatz JL. J Soc Cosmet Chem 1980;31:107–21.
20. Liao W-C, Zatz JL. J Soc Cosmet Chem 1980;31:123–31.
21. Ayres JW, Laskar PA. J Pharm Sci 1974;63:1402–6.
22. Nannipieri E, Di Colo G, Saettone MF, Serafini MF, Vitale D. Farmaco(Prat) 1981;36:235–48.
23. Di Colo G, Carelli V, Lofiego G, Nannipieri E. Farmaco(Prat) 1983;38:323–33.
24. Belmonte AA, Tsai W. J Pharm Sci 1978;67:517–20.
25. Bottari F, Giannaccini B, Peverini D, Saettone MF, Tellini N. Can J Pharm Sci 1979;14:39–43.
26. Ayres JW, Lorskulsint D, Lock A. J Pharm Sci 1975;64:1958–61.
27. Ayres JW, Lorskulsint D, Lock A, Kuhl L, Laskar PA. J Pharm Sci 1976;65:832–8.

Benzylpenicillin (BAN, rINN)   *Antibacterial*

Crystalline penicillin G; penicillin; penicillin G
(6R)-6-(2-Phenylacetamido)penicillanic acid
$C_{16}H_{18}N_2O_4S = 334.4$

Benethamine Penicillin (BAN, rINN)
The N-benzylphenethylamine salt of benzylpenicillin
$C_{15}H_{17}N, C_{16}H_{18}N_2O_4S = 545.7$

Benzathine Penicillin (BAN)
Benzathine Benzylpenicillin (rINN); penicillin G benzathine.
The N,N'-dibenzylethylenediamine salt of benzylpenicillin
$C_{16}H_{20}N_2, (C_{16}H_{18}N_2O_4S)_2 = 909.1$

Benzylpenicillin Potassium (BANM, rINNM)
Benzylpenicillin; crystalline penicillin G; penicillin G; penicillin G potassium
$C_{16}H_{17}KN_2O_4S = 372.5$

Benzylpenicillin Sodium (BANM, rINNM)
Benzylpenicillin; crystalline penicillin G; penicillin G; penicillin G sodium
$C_{16}H_{17}N_2NaO_4S = 356.4$

Procaine Penicillin (BAN)
Benzylpenicillin novocaine; penicillin G procaine; procaine benzylpenicillin
$C_{13}H_{20}N_2O_2, C_{16}H_{18}N_2O_4S, H_2O = 588.7$
CAS—751-84-8 (benethamine penicillin); 1538-09-6 (benzathine penicillin, anhydrous); 5928-83-6 (benzathine penicillin, monohydrate); 41372-02-5 (benzathine penicillin, tetrahydrate); 61-33-6 (benzylpenicillin); 113-98-4 (benzylpenicillin potassium); 69-57-8 (benzylpenicillin sodium); 54-35-3 (procaine penicillin, anhydrous); 6130-64-9 (procaine penicillin, monohydrate)

Pharmacopoeial status

BP (benethamine penicillin, benzathine penicillin, benzylpenicillin potassium, benzylpenicillin sodium, procaine penicillin); USP (penicillin G benzathine, penicillin G potassium)

Preparations

Compendial
Benzylpenicillin Injection BP (Benzylpenicillin for Injection). A sterile solution of benzylpenicillin potassium or benzylpenicillin sodium in water for injections. It is prepared by dissolving benzylpenicillin for injection in the requisite amount of water for injections. Sealed containers each containing the equivalent of 600 mg of benzylpenicillin are usually available. pH of a 10% w/v solution, 5.5 to 7.5.
Fortified Benethamine Penicillin Injection BP (Fortified Benethamine Penicillin for Injection). A sterile suspension of benethamine penicillin and procaine penicillin in water for injections containing benzylpenicillin sodium in solution. It is prepared by dissolving fortified benethamine penicillin for injection in the requisite amount of water for injections. Sealed containers each containing 475 mg of benethamine penicillin, 300 mg of benzylpenicillin sodium and 250 mg of procaine penicillin are usually available.

Fortified Procaine Penicillin Injection BP (Fortified Procaine Penicillin for Injection). A sterile suspension of procaine penicillin in water for injections containing benzylpenicillin potassium or benzylpenicillin sodium. It is prepared by adding the requisite amount of water for injections to fortified procaine penicillin for injection (which contains a mixture of five parts of procaine penicillin and one part of benzylpenicillin potassium or benzyl-penicillin sodium) immediately before use. Sealed containers each containing 3 g of procaine penicillin and 600 mg of benzyl-penicillin sodium are usually available.

Procaine Penicillin Injection BP (Procaine Penicillin for Injection). A sterile suspension of procaine penicillin in water for injections. It is either issued as a suspension or prepared by suspending procaine penicillin for injection in water for injections. An injection containing 3 g in 10 mL and sealed containers each containing 3 g are usually available.

Penicillin G Benzathine Tablets USP.

Penicillin G Benzathine Oral Suspension USP.

Sterile Penicillin G Benzathine USP.

Sterile Penicillin G Benzathine Suspension USP. pH between 5.0 and 7.5.

Penicillin G Potassium Capsules USP.

Penicillin G Potassium Tablets USP.

Penicillin G Potassium for Oral Solution USP.

Penicillin G Potassium Tablets for Oral Solution USP.

Penicillin G Potassium for Injection USP. pH between 6.0 and 8.5, in a solution containing 6% w/v or where packaged for dispensing, in the solution constituted as directed in the labelling.

Sterile Penicillin G Potassium USP.

Sterile Penicillin G Procaine USP. pH between 5.0 and 7.5, in a (saturated) solution containing about 30% w/v.

Sterile Penicillin G Procaine Suspension USP. pH between 5.0 and 7.5.

Sterile Penicillin G Procaine for Suspension USP. pH between 5.0 and 7.5, when constituted as directed in the labelling.

Penicillin G Sodium for Injection USP. pH between 6.0 and 7.5, in a solution containing 6% w/v.

Sterile Penicillin G Sodium USP. pH between 5.0 and 7.5, in a solution containing 6% w/v.

Sterile Penicillin G Benzathine and Penicillin G Procaine Suspension USP. pH between 5.0 and 7.5.

Non-compendial

Bicillin (Brocades). *Injection* (intramuscular), powder for reconstitution with water for injections, procaine penicillin 1.8 g, ben-zylpenicillin sodium 0.36 g in each 6-mL multidose vial.

Crystapen (Britannia). *Injection*, powder for reconstitution, ben-zylpenicillin sodium (unbuffered) 600 mg.

Containers and storage

Solid state

Benethamine Penicillin BP and Benzathine Penicillin BP should be kept in an airtight container and stored at a temperature not exceeding 30°. Benzylpenicillin Potassium BP, Benzylpenicillin Sodium BP, and Procaine Penicillin BP should be kept in an air-tight container, protected from moisture and stored at a temperature not exceeding 30°. For all these BP solid state compounds, if the contents are intended for use in the manufacture of a parenteral dosage form, the container should be sterile, tamper-evident, and sealed so as to exclude micro-organisms. Penicillin G Benzathine USP and Penicillin G Potassium USP should be preserved in tight containers.

Dosage forms

The sealed containers of Benzylpenicillin Injection BP and of Fortified Benethamine Penicillin Injection BP should be stored at a temperature not exceeding 30°, and the sealed container of Fortified Procaine Penicillin Injection BP at a temperature not exceeding 15°.

Procaine Penicillin Injection BP should be protected from light and stored at a temperature of 8° to 15°.

Benzylpenicillin Injection BP, Fortified Benethamine Penicillin Injection BP, Fortified Procaine Penicillin Injection BP, and Procaine Penicillin Injection BP (prepared by dissolving the contents of a sealed container in water for injections) should be used immediately after preparation but, in any case, within the period recommended by the manufacturer when prepared and stored strictly in accordance with the manufacturer's instructions.

Penicillin G Benzathine Tablets USP, Penicillin G Potassium Capsules USP, Penicillin G Potassium Tablets USP, Penicillin G Potassium Tablets for Oral Solution USP, and Penicillin G Potassium for Oral Solution USP should all be preserved in tight containers.

Sterile Penicillin G Benzathine USP, Penicillin G Potassium for Injection USP, Sterile Penicillin G Potassium USP, Sterile Penicillin G Procaine USP, Penicillin G Sodium for Injection USP, and Sterile Penicillin G Sodium USP should all be preserved in containers suitable for sterile solids.

Sterile Penicillin G Benzathine Suspension USP should be preserved in single-dose or in multiple-dose containers, preferably of Type I or Type II glass, in a refrigerator.

Sterile Penicillin G Procaine Suspension USP should be preserved in single-dose or in multiple-dose containers, preferably of Type I or Type III glass, in a refrigerator.

Sterile Penicillin G Procaine for Suspension USP and Sterile Penicillin G Benzathine and Penicillin G Procaine Suspension USP should be preserved in single-dose or in multiple-dose containers, preferably of Type I or Type III glass.

Bicillin should be stored in a cool place. When reconstituted the preparation is for single-dose use only; it may be kept at 2° to 8° for up to 24 hours after constitution but must be discarded after the first usage or after the first 24 hours after constitution.

PHYSICAL PROPERTIES

Benethamine penicillin, *benzathine penicillin*, and *procaine penicillin* exist as white crystalline powders.

Benzylpenicillin potassium and *benzylpenicillin sodium* exist as white or almost white crystalline powders.

Melting point

Benzathine penicillin melts at about 131°, with decomposition.

Benzylpenicillin potassium melts in the range 214° to 217°, with decomposition.

pH

The pH values of 10% w/v solutions of *benzylpenicillin potassium* and of *benzylpenicillin sodium* are in the range 5.5 to 7.5. The pH of a 6% w/v solution of *benzylpenicillin potassium* is in the range 5.0 to 7.5.

Benzathine penicillin has a pH between 4.0 and 6.5, in a solution prepared by dissolving 50 mg in 50 mL of dehydrated alcohol, adding 50 mL of water, and mixing.

Dissociation constant

pK_a 2.8 (benzylpenicillin), 25°

FURTHER INFORMATION. Ionisation constants of some penicillins and of their alkaline and penicillinase hydrolysis products—Rapson HDC, Bird AE. J Pharm Pharmacol 1963;15:222T–231T.

Partition coefficient

Log P (octanol/water) at 37° for unionised benzylpenicillin,[1] 1.7

Solubility

Benethamine penicillin is very slightly soluble in water; slightly soluble in ethanol; sparingly soluble in acetone and in chloroform.

Benzathine penicillin is very slightly soluble in water and in chloroform; slightly soluble in ethanol; soluble 1 in 7 of dimethylformamide and 1 in 10 of formamide; practically insoluble in ether.

Benzylpenicillin potassium and *benzylpenicillin sodium* are very soluble in water; practically insoluble in chloroform, in ether, in fixed oils, and in liquid paraffin.

Procaine penicillin is slightly soluble in water; sparingly soluble in ethanol.

Dissolution

The USP specifies that for Penicillin G Potassium Tablets USP not less than 70% of the labelled amount of Penicillin G Units is dissolved in 60 minutes. Dissolution medium: 900 mL of pH 6.0 phosphate buffer; Apparatus 2 at 75 rpm.

The USP specifies that for Penicillin G Potassium Capsules USP not less than 75% of the labelled amount of Penicillin G Units is dissolved in 45 minutes. Dissolution medium: 900 mL of 1% phosphate buffer, pH 6.0; Apparatus 1 at 100 rpm.

STABILITY

Solid state

The stability of benzylpenicillin depends mainly on its moisture content; provided that it contains less than 0.5% water, it can be stored at room temperature for 2 to 3 years without significant loss of potency. Benzylpenicillin is not affected by air or light. When stored protected from moisture at room temperature, dry benzathine penicillin retains its potency for up to 5 years.

Solutions

Benzylpenicillin and its soluble salts are unstable in aqueous solution. Benzylpenicillin sodium or potassium undergoes hydrolysis of the β-lactam ring in aqueous solution; hydrolysis is accelerated by increased temperature or under alkaline conditions. Degradation in acidic conditions also occurs. The pH of maximum stability is pH 6 to 7. The overall hydrolysis exhibits first-order kinetics at constant temperature and pH.

The relatively water-insoluble salts procaine penicillin and benzathine penicillin exhibit improved stability in suspension. In aqueous suspensions degradation follows pseudo-zero-order kinetics as only material in solution degrades.

Degradation routes and kinetics

In solution, several decomposition products of benzylpenicillin sodium or potassium form depending on the reaction conditions.[2] In neutral and alkaline conditions, initial cleavage of the β-lactam ring yields benzylpenicilloic acid which may further decompose. In acidic conditions, initial cleavage of the β-lactam ring yields benzylpenicillenic acid, benzylpenillic acid, and benzylpenicilloic acid, all of which can further decompose to benzylpenilloic acid. Benzylpenamaldic acid may be formed during degradation under various conditions.

Formation of acidic degradation products lowers the pH and causes a progressive increase in the rate of decomposition. Activation energies of approximately 73.6 kJ/mol, 87.9 kJ/mol, and 95.0 kJ/mol at pH 1.2, 4.54, and 9.57, respectively, have been reported.

Jemal *et al*[3] demonstrated, by differential pulse polarography, that in neutral media penicillamine was a product of benzylpenicillenic acid degradation. Bird *et al*[4] showed that in unbuffered 2% aqueous solutions of benzylpenicillin that had been stored for 4 days at 37° the extent of formation of N-formylpenicillamine was 15%. Storage of four major degradation products of benzylpenicillin at pH 5 for up to 6 hours indicated that the penicilloic, penilloic, and penillic acids of benzylpenicillin produced a small amount of penicillamine but no N-formylpenicillamine; benzylpenicillenic acid, however, rapidly produced N-formylpenicillamine but no penicillamine.

Results of an investigation of the kinetics of degradation of benzylpenicillin potassium in solution at pH 2.7 at 37° indicated that benzylpenicillin degraded to benzylpenicillenic acid, with subsequent formation of benzylpenamaldic acid and benzylpenillic acid.[5] The final products detected were penicillamine (from benzylpenamaldic acid) and benzylpenilloic acid (from benzylpenamaldic acid via benzylpenicilloic acid and from benzylpenillic acid).

Effects of vehicles, buffers, and metal ions

The stability of benzylpenicillin potassium or sodium in vehicles for intravenous administration is dependent upon the pH of the final admixture (that is, within the pH range for acceptable stability of benzylpenicillin, pH 5.5 to 8.0). Discrepancies between published results for the stability of benzylpenicillin potassium or sodium may depend on the use of buffered or unbuffered material.

In a study of the kinetics and mechanisms of degradation of benzylpenicillin sodium at 35°, pH greater than 6, in aqueous solutions containing various carbohydrates[6,7] or polyhydric alcohols,[6] a linear relationship was apparent between the degradation rate of benzylpenicillin and the concentration (up to 10%) of glucose, fructose, sucrose, dextran, sorbitol, mannitol, or glycerol. The rate-accelerating effect of these compounds was directly proportional to the hydroxide ion concentration up to about pH 10.5. The reaction proceeded through a nucleophilic pathway with penicilloyl esters formed as intermediates (for example, penicilloyl sucrose esters[7]). Formation of these esters (which may contribute to allergic reactions to penicillins) was reduced or prevented[6] by adjusting the pH to between 6 and 6.5.

Hem *et al*[8] determined that benzylpenicillin potassium formed a 1:1 molar complex with sucrose in solution. The rate of degradation of complexed benzylpenicillin in solution at pH 7.0 and 45° with 0.06M citrate buffer was five to six times the rate of uncomplexed benzylpenicillin, although the degradation pathway was unchanged.

The stability of benzylpenicillin potassium 0.01M in solution was not affected by ionic strength up to 0.5 unless one of the ions that contributed to the ionic strength was catalytic.[9] In solutions buffered with 0.06M citrate buffer to pH less than 6.5, monohydrogen citrate and dihydrogen citrate ions were found to be catalytic. Addition of sodium chloride (to increase the ionic strength) to citrate-buffered solutions caused an increase in the degradation rate when the pH was less than 6.5 but not at pH 7.

In aqueous solutions of benzylpenicillin sodium at 60°, dihydrogen citrate ions, monohydrogen phosphate ions, and borate ions were found to have catalytic effects on the degradation of the benzylpenicillinate ion, whereas acetic acid catalysed the degradation of benzylpenicillinic acid.[10]

Bicarbonate ions (at pH 8.1) and phosphate buffer (at pH 6.5 but to a lesser extent at pH 5.4) were found to exert a significant positive catalytic effect on the degradation of benzylpenicillin sodium 0.12% solutions at 25°.[11] Lactate ions caused rapid degradation of benzylpenicillin at pH 6.4, although this effect was reduced in the presence of citrate buffer.

When iron(II), copper(II), chromium(III), or manganese(II) ions, each at 0.2×10^{-3} mg/mL, were added to a solution of benzylpenicillin sodium 3.3×10^{-3}M at pH 6.4 and 25°, there was a 'moderate increase' in the degradation rate of benzylpenicillin.[12] The effect of zinc(II) ions at the same concentrations was greater. In the presence of sodium lactate at 0.1M, however, the effects of these metal ions were greatly enhanced. When a chelating agent (disodium edetate at 0.3 mM) was added, lactate did not affect the decomposition of benzylpenicillin within the pH range 5 to 10. Sodium citrate (10 mM) also had a stabilising effect.

Eye drops

Deeks et al[13] investigated (by HPLC) the stability of benzylpenicillin in various buffer solutions at 2° to 8° and in an eye drop formulation. Degradation half-lives were 1.9 days in phosphate buffer (pH 4.0), 23.1 days in acetate buffer (pH 5.5), 95.7 days in phosphate buffer (pH 7.0), 198 days in citrate buffer (pH 7.2), and 50.6 days in phosphate buffer (pH 8.0). The eye drops contained benzylpenicillin sodium 300 mg or 150 mg, sodium chloride 800 mg, sodium citrate 500 mg, phenylmercuric acetate 2 mg, and water to 100 mL. When stored at 2° to 8°, a shelf-life of 30 days was predicted and, for unopened bottles, a shelf-life of 6 weeks was suggested.

Benzylpenicillin sodium eye drops (prepared using vials of the injectable drug mixed in isotonic citrate buffer at pH 5, 6, 6.5, 7, and 8) were stored at 2° to 4° and at 25° (room temperature).[14] At all pH values studied, the degradation rate was lower at 2° to 4°; in this temperature range, benzylpenicillin stability was greatest at pH 6.5 whereas at 25°, stability was greatest in the pH range 6.5 to 7.0. Studies in vitro of the uptake of benzyl[^{14}C]penicillin into the cornea and aqueous humour of sheep eyes indicated greatest uptake from the eye drops at pH 6.5.

Freezing and thawing

Benzylpenicillin potassium 2×10^6 units in 50 mL of sodium chloride 0.9% injection or glucose 5% injection was stable (microbiological agar gel diffusion assay) when stored in polyvinyl chloride minibags frozen at −20° for 30 days and thawed for 3 hours at 21° to 23°.[15]

Stiles et al[16] examined the stability of benzylpenicillin sodium (reconstituted in sterile water for injections) in prefilled drug reservoirs and in glass vials (as controls) that were stored at −20° for 30 days, thawed at 5° for four days, and then placed on portable infusion pumps for a one-day pumping cycle at 37°. No colour changes or precipitation were observed. Although stability was maintained until after the thawing process at 5°, only $83.9\% \pm 0.6\%$ and $87.9\% \pm 0.9\%$ of the initial concentration of benzylpenicillin sodium remained in the drug reservoir and the glass vials, respectively, after the one-day pumping cycle (day 35). It was recommended that after such a freeze-thaw procedure, benzylpenicillin sodium infusions should not be administered for more than 12 hours.

Benzylpenicillin was found to be stable when an injection of benzylpenicillin sodium (reconstituted in sterile water) was added to 50-mL polyvinyl chloride minibags that contained glucose 5% injection and stored at −20° for up to 39 days.[17] During subsequent refrigeration at 5° there was a progressive loss in benzylpenicillin concentration (HPLC analysis); after 31 days approximately 90% of the initial concentration remained in one batch (of three bags) and 94% to 99% of initial concentration remained in a second batch (of three bags).

Irradiation

When benzylpenicillin was subjected to Cobalt-60 irradiation, benzylpenaldic acid and benzylpenilloaldehyde were detected as hydrolytic degradation products.[18,19] The rate of degradation was 0.6 %/Mrad.[19]

Stabilisation

Aqueous solutions of benzylpenicillin (sodium or potassium) are stabilised by buffering to pH 6 to 7 with buffers that do not catalyse the degradation at this pH (see Stability, above). Similarly, powders for reconstitution usually contain buffering agents to maintain the pH within the optimum range.

FURTHER INFORMATION. Kirschbaum J. In: Florey K, editor. Analytical profiles of drug substances [penicillin G potassium]; vol 15. London: Academic Press, 1986:427–507. Penicillins and cephalosporins: physicochemical properties [stability], and analysis in pharmaceutical and biological matrices [review]—Van Krimpen PC, Van Bennekom WP, Bult A. Pharm Weekbl (Sci) 1987;9:1–23. Pharmaceutics of penicillin [review of stability]—Schwartz MA, Buckwalter FH. J Pharm Sci 1962;51(12):1119–28. Kinetics and mechanism of the rearrangement of penicillin to penicillenic acid in acidic aqueous solution—Bundgaard H. Arch Pharm Chemi (Sci) 1980;8:161–80. Thermal decomposition of amorphous β-lactam antibacterials [effect of water]—Pikal MJ, Lukes AL, Lang JE. J Pharm Sci 1977;66(9):1312–16. Nucleophilic phosphate-catalysed degradation of penicillins [benzylpenicillin and ampicillin]: demonstration of a penicilloyl phosphate intermediate and transformation of ampicillin to a piperazinedione—Bundgaard H, Hansen J. Int J Pharmaceutics 1981;9:273–83. The effect of buffering on the stability of reconstituted benzylpenicillin injection—Allwood MC, Brown PW. Int J Pharm Pract 1992 Aug;1:242–4. The stability of benzylpenicillin injections [unbuffered and buffered]—Allwood MC. Pharm J 1991;247:R12. Comparative stability of antibiotic admixtures in minibags and minibottles [benzylpenicillin potassium]—Dinel BA, Ayotte DL, Behme RJ, Black BL, Whitby JL. Drug Intell Clin Pharm 1977;11:226–39. [A comprehensive review of the stability of benzylpenicillin preparations under frozen conditions]—Trissel LA, editor. Handbook on injectable drugs. 7th ed. Bethesda: American Society of Hospital Pharmacists, 1992:701–23.

INCOMPATIBILITY/COMPATIBILITY

In this section benzylpenicillin means either the sodium or potassium salt.

Benzylpenicillin is incompatible with acids and alkalis. It is inactivated by penicillinase.

Benzylpenicillin is also reported to be incompatible with traces of heavy metal ions (such as copper, lead, mercury, and zinc), and some rubbers (because of compounds leached from vulcanised rubber). Its stability is affected by ionic and nonionic surfactants, oxidising and reducing agents, alcohols, glycerol, glycols, macrogols and other hydroxy compounds, cetostearyl alcohol, wool alcohols (with a high peroxide content), some paraffins, organic peroxides, oxidised cellulose, zinc oxide, some preservatives (such as chlorocresol and thiomersal), carbohydrate solutions at alkaline pH, fat emulsions, blood and blood products, and viscosity modifiers.

Incompatibility or loss of activity has also been recorded between benzylpenicillin and aminacrine hydrochloride, aminophylline, amphotericin, ascorbic acid, cephaloridine, cephalothin sodium, chlorpromazine hydrochloride, cysteine, ephedrine, erythromycin ethyl succinate, heparin sodium, hydroxyzine hydrochloride, iodine/iodides, lincomycin hydrochloride, metaraminol tartrate, metoclopramide hydrochloride, noradrenaline acid tartrate, oxytetracycline hydrochloride, phenytoin sodium, pentobarbitone sodium, procaine hydrochloride, prochlorperazine salts, promazine hydrochloride, promethazine hydrochloride, resorcinol, sodium bicarbonate, streptomycin sulphate, tetracycline hydrochloride, thiamine hydrochloride, thiopentone sodium, trometamol, and vancomycin hydrochloride. Incompatibility with gentamicin sulphate or tobramycin sulphate in human serum has also been reported.

Although high concentrations of ethanol should be avoided, rigorous exclusion of ethanol from preparations is unnecessary and it can be used to wipe caps of bottles containing either the dry powder or solutions for injection.

Low concentrations of glycerol (for example 10%) have little effect on the deterioration of aqueous solutions of benzylpenicillin, but high concentrations increase the loss of activity; impurities present in glycerol may be responsible for some of the inactivation. Similar effects occur with propylene glycol.

At pH 5.4, no effects on the degradation of benzylpenicillin sodium were produced by the addition of glucose (5% and 10%), fructose (5% and 15%), invert sugar (4% and 8%), ethanol (up to 20%), or macrogol 400 (1% to 5%).[11]

Das Gupta and Stewart[20] concluded that benzylpenicillin potassium injection (as powder, 20 million units, Pfizer) was stable (less than 10% of the initial concentration was lost) when mixed with metronidazole injection 5 mg/mL (Searle) and stored for 3 days at 25° or for 12 days at 5°. A slight fall in pH, from 5.95 to 5.4, during the study periods was not considered to influence stability. In contrast,[21] when benzylpenicillin potassium injection (1.2 million units, Ayerst, Canada; pH 7.3) was mixed with metronidazole injection 5 mg/mL (Flagyl, Rhône-Poulenc Pharma) the pH fell to 5.35. During 3 days storage at 23° the admixture pH fell further to 4.6. Such decreases in pH were thought to indicate that benzylpenicillin potassium injection should not be mixed with metronidazole.

Degradation of benzylpenicillin potassium in aqueous solution (distilled water[22] or glucose 5% injection[23]) with magnesium sulphate was attributed to a fall in pH of the solutions during storage at 25°. For example,[23] although no change in clarity of the solutions was noted over a period of 20 hours, about 12% of the initial concentration of benzylpenicillin potassium (5 mg/mL) was lost during the same time period in the presence of magnesium sulphate (10 mg/mL). However, the effect of magnesium sulphate on the stability of benzylpenicillin potassium was negligible[22] if the pH of the solutions was maintained by, for example, using 0.1M acetate buffer or by adding extra amounts of citrate buffer to increase the buffer capacity of commercial benzylpenicillin potassium powder.

Koshiro and Fujita[24] investigated the interaction of penicillins (including benzylpenicillin potassium) with high molecular weight components of plasma expanders such as dextran, 6-hydroxyethylstarch, and polygeline. Following incubation at 20° for 24 hours the formation of penicilloyl polysaccharides and smaller amounts of penicilloyl polygeline was demonstrated by ultrafiltration and gel filtration.

FURTHER INFORMATION. Compatibility [visual] of narcotic analgesic solutions with various antibiotics [including benzylpenicillin potassium] during simulated Y-site injection—Nieves-Cordero AL, Luciw HM, Souney PF. Am J Hosp Pharm 1985;42:1108–9.

FORMULATION

Excipients

Excipients that have been used in presentations of benzylpenicillin include:

Tablets, benzylpenicillin potassium: brilliant blue FCF (133); calcium carbonate; lactose; magnesium stearate; maize starch; povidone; sodium benzoate; talc; tartrazine (E102).

Oral suspensions (powder for reconstitution), benzylpenicillin potassium: saccharin sodium; sodium phosphate; sucrose; sunset yellow FCF (E110); tartrazine (E102).

Injections (aqueous suspensions), benzathine penicillin: carmellose; lecithin; methyl and propyl hydroxybenzoates; polyoxyethylene sorbitan monopalmitate; povidone; sodium citrate; sorbitan monopalmitate.

Procaine penicillin: carmellose; carmellose sodium; lecithin; methyl and propyl hydroxybenzoates; povidone; sodium citrate; sorbitol solution.

Benzathine penicillin with procaine penicillin: carmellose; lecithin; methyl and propyl hydroxybenzoates; polyoxyethylene sorbitan monopalmitate; povidone; sodium citrate; sorbitan monopalmitate.

Injections (powder for reconstitution), benzathine penicillin: carmellose; povidone; sodium citrate.

Benzylpenicillin potassium: citric acid; sodium citrate.

Benzylpenicillin sodium: citric acid; sodium citrate.

Benethamine penicillin with benzylpenicillin sodium: dimethicone; hexamine; macrogol oleate; sodium citrate, anhydrous.

Procaine penicillin with benzylpenicillin sodium: carmellose sodium; lecithin; sodium citrate, dried.

Bioavailability

When benzylpenicillin (600 000 units in 5 mL of sodium chloride 0.9%) was administered to nine healthy volunteers by either the intraduodenal or intramuscular routes,[25] similar peak concentrations in serum were detected. However, high plasma concentrations were sustained for longer and areas under the serum concentration versus time curves were greater following intramuscular administration.

FURTHER INFORMATION. Fatty peptides. VI. Penicillin and cephalosporin esters with increased lipophilic character—Toth I, Hughes RA, Ward P, McColm AM, Cox DM, Anderson GI et al. Int J Pharmaceutics 1991;77:13–20. Solubilization and stabilization of a benzylpenicillin chemical delivery system by 2-hydroxypropyl-β-cyclodextrin—Pop E, Loftsson T, Bodor N. Pharm Res 1991;8:1044–9.

REFERENCES

1. Tsuji A, Kubo O, Miyamoto E, Yamana T. J Pharm Sci 1977;66(12):1675–9.
2. Van Krimpen PC, Van Bennekom WP, Bult A [review]. Pharm Weekbl (Sci) 1987;9:1–23.
3. Jemal M, Hem SL, Knevel AM. J Pharm Sci 1978;67(3):302–5.
4. Bird AE, Jennings KR, Marshall AC. J Pharm Pharmacol 1986;38:913–17.
5. Blaha JM, Knevel AM, Kessler DP, Mincy JW, Hem SL. J Pharm Sci 1976;65(8):1165–70.
6. Bundgaard H, Larsen C. Arch Pharm Chemi (Sci) 1978;6:184–200.
7. Bundgaard H, Larsen C. Int J Pharmaceutics 1978;1:95–104.
8. Hem SL, Russo EJ, Bahal SM, Levi RS. J Pharm Sci 1973;62(2):267–70.
9. Lindsay RE, Hem SL. J Pharm Sci 1972;61(2):202–6.
10. Finholt P, Jürgensen G, Kristiansen H. J Pharm Sci 1965;54(3):387–93.
11. Lundgren P, Landersjö L. Acta Pharm Suec 1970;7:509–26.
12. Landersjö L, Stjernström G, Lundgren P. Acta Pharm Suec 1978;15:161–8.

13. Deeks T, Nash S, Sihre G. Pharm J '984;233:233–4, 254.
14. Zinyemba E, Morton DJ. J Clin Pharm Ther 1991;16:477–81.
15. Dinel BA, Ayotte DL, Behme RJ, Black BL, Whitby JL. Drug Intell Clin Pharm 1977;11:542–8.
16. Stiles ML, Tu Y-H, Allen LV. Am J Hosp Pharm 1989;46:1408–12.
17. Rayani S, Jamali F. Can J Pharm Sci 1985;38(6):162–3.
18. Tsuji K, Goetz JF, Vanmeter W. J Pharm Sci 1979;68(9):1075–80.
19. Tsuji K, Rahn PD, Steindler KA. J Pharm Sci 1983;72(1):23–6.
20. Das Gupta V, Stewart KR. J Parenter Sci Technol 1985;39(3):145–9.
21. Bisaillon S, Sarrazin R. J Parenter Sci Technol 1983;37(4):129–32.
22. Das Gupta V, Stewart KR. Am J Hosp Pharm 1985;42:598–602.
23. Das Gupta V, Stewart KR. J Clin Hosp Pharm 1985;10:67–72.
24. Koshiro A, Fujita T. Drug Intell Clin Pharm 1983;17:351–6.
25. Gonciarz Z, Checinska J, Cholewka A, Staszalek K, Garstka E. Int J Clin Pharmacol Ther Toxicol 1986;24(11):622–4.

Betamethasone (BAN, USAN, rINN)

Corticosteroid

Flubenisolone; 9α-fluoro-16β-methylprednisolone

9α-Fluoro-11β,17α,21-trihydroxy-16β-methylpregna-1,4-diene-3,20-dione; (11β,16β)-9-fluoro-11,17,21-trihydroxy-16-methylpregna-1,4-diene-3,20-dione; 9-fluoro-11β,17,21-trihydroxy-16β-methylpregna-1,4-diene-3,20-dione

$C_{22}H_{29}FO_5 = 392.5$

Betamethasone Acetate (BANM, rINNM)

Betamethasone 21-acetate
$C_{24}H_{31}FO_6 = 434.5$

Betamethasone Benzoate (BANM, USAN, rINNM)

Betamethasone 17α-benzoate
$C_{29}H_{33}FO_6 = 496.6$

Betamethasone Dipropionate (BANM, USAN, rINNM)

Betamethasone 17α,21-dipropionate
$C_{28}H_{37}FO_7 = 504.6$

Betamethasone Sodium Phosphate (BANM, rINNM)

Betamethasone 21-(disodium phosphate)
$C_{22}H_{28}FNa_2O_8P = 516.4$

Betamethasone Valerate (BANM, USAN, rINNM)

Betamethasone 17α-valerate
$C_{27}H_{37}FO_6 = 476.6$
CAS—378-44-9 (betamethasone); 987-24-6 (betamethasone acetate); 22298-29-9 (betamethasone benzoate); 5593-20-4 (betamethasone dipropionate); 151-73-5 (betamethasone sodium phosphate); 2152-44-5 (betamethasone valerate)

Pharmacopoeial status

BP (betamethasone, betamethasone sodium phosphate, betamethasone valerate); USP (betamethasone, betamethasone acetate, betamethasone benzoate, betamethasone dipropionate, betamethasone sodium phosphate, betamethasone valerate)

Preparations

Compendial

Betamethasone Tablets BP. Tablets containing, in each, 250 micrograms and 500 micrograms are usually available.

Betamethasone Sodium Phosphate Tablets BP. Tablets containing, in each, the equivalent of 500 micrograms of betamethasone are usually available.

Betamethasone Valerate Scalp Application BP. An application containing the equivalent of 0.1% w/v of betamethasone, in a suitable liquid basis, is usually available.

Betamethasone Valerate Cream BP. Creams containing the equivalent of 0.025% w/w and 0.1% w/w of betamethasone, in a suitable basis, are usually available.

Betamethasone Valerate Lotion BP. A lotion containing the equivalent of 0.1% w/v of betamethasone, in a suitable vehicle, is usually available.

Betamethasone Valerate Ointment BP. Ointments containing the equivalent of 0.025% w/w and 0.1% w/w of betamethasone, in a suitable basis, are usually available.

Betamethasone Eye Drops BP. A sterile solution of betamethasone sodium phosphate in purified water. pH 7.0 to 8.5. Eye drops containing 0.1% w/v of betamethasone sodium phosphate are usually available.

Betamethasone Injection BP (Betamethasone Sodium Phosphate Injection). A sterile solution of betamethasone sodium phosphate in water for injections. An injection containing the equivalent of 4 mg of betamethasone in 1 mL is usually available. pH 8.0 to 9.0.

Betamethasone Tablets USP.

Betamethasone Syrup USP.

Betamethasone Cream USP.

Betamethasone Benzoate Gel USP.

Betamethasone Dipropionate Ointment USP.

Sterile Betamethasone Sodium Phosphate and Betamethasone Acetate Suspension USP.

Betamethasone Valerate Cream USP.

Betamethasone Valerate Lotion USP.

Betamethasone Valerate Ointment USP.

Non-compendial

Betnelan (Evans). *Tablets*, betamethasone 500 micrograms.

Betnesol (Evans). *Tablets*, soluble, betamethasone 500 micrograms (as sodium phosphate).

Drops (for ear, eye, or nose), betamethasone sodium phosphate 0.1%.

Eye ointment, betamethasone sodium phosphate 0.1%.

Injection, betamethasone 4 mg (as sodium phosphate)/mL.

Betnovate (Glaxo). *Cream*, betamethasone 0.1% (as valerate) in a water-miscible basis.

Cream (Betnovate-RD), betamethasone 0.025% (as valerate) in a water-miscible basis (1 in 4 dilution of Betnovate cream).

Ointment, betamethasone 0.1% (as valerate) in an anhydrous paraffin basis.

Ointment (Betnovate-RD), betamethasone 0.025% (as valerate) in an anhydrous paraffin basis (1 in 4 dilution of Betnovate ointment).

Lotion, betamethasone 0.1% (as valerate).

Scalp application, betamethasone 0.1% (as valerate) in a thickened alcoholic basis.

Diprosone (Schering-Plough). *Cream*, betamethasone 0.05% (as dipropionate) in a water-miscible basis.
Ointment, betamethasone 0.05% (as dipropionate).
Lotion, betamethasone 0.05% (as dipropionate) in a thickened alcoholic basis.
Vista-Methasone (Daniel). *Drops* (for ear, eye, or nose), betamethasone sodium phosphate 0.1%.

Containers and storage

Solid state
Betamethasone BP and Betamethasone Sodium Phosphate BP should be stored in well-closed containers, protected from light.
Betamethasone Valerate BP should be protected from light.
Betamethasone USP and Betamethasone Dipropionate USP should be preserved in well-closed containers.
Betamethasone Acetate USP, Betamethasone Benzoate USP, Betamethasone Sodium Phosphate USP, and Betamethasone Valerate USP should be preserved in tight containers.

Dosage forms
Betamethasone Tablets BP, Betamethasone Sodium Phosphate Tablets BP, Betamethasone Valerate Scalp Application BP, Betamethasone Valerate Cream BP, Betamethasone Valerate Lotion BP, and Betamethasone Valerate Ointment BP should be protected from light.
Betamethasone Injection BP should be stored at a temperature not exceeding 30° and protected from light.
Betamethasone Eye Drops BP should be protected from light and stored at a temperature not exceeding 25°.
Betamethasone Tablets USP and Betamethasone Syrup USP should be preserved in well-closed containers.
Betamethasone Cream USP, Betamethasone Benzoate Gel USP, and Betamethasone Valerate Cream USP should be preserved in collapsible tubes or in tight containers.
Betamethasone Dipropionate Ointment USP should be preserved in collapsible tubes or in well-closed containers.
Sterile Betamethasone Sodium Phosphate and Betamethasone Acetate Suspension USP should be preserved in multiple-dose containers, preferably of Type I glass.
Betamethasone Valerate Lotion USP should be preserved in tight, light-resistant containers, at controlled room temperature.
Betamethasone Valerate Ointment USP should be preserved in collapsible tubes or in tight containers, avoiding exposure to excessive heat.
Betnelan tablets and Betnesol injection should be protected from light.
Betnesol eye, ear and nose preparations should be used within four weeks of the container being opened.
Diprosone preparations should be stored in a cool place.

PHYSICAL PROPERTIES

Betamethasone is a white to almost white crystalline powder.
Betamethasone acetate is a white to creamy-white powder.
Betamethasone benzoate is a white powder.
Betamethasone dipropionate is a white or creamy-white powder.
Betamethasone sodium phosphate is a white or almost white powder; odourless or almost odourless; hygroscopic.
Betamethasone valerate is a white to creamy-white powder.

Melting point

Betamethasone melts at around 240°, with decomposition.
Betamethasone acetate melts at about 165°, and with decomposition at 200° to 220°.
Betamethasone benzoate melts at about 220°, with decomposition.

Betamethasone dipropionate melts at 170° to 179°, with decomposition.
Betamethasone valerate melts at about 190°, with decomposition.

pH

A 0.5% w/v solution of Betamethasone Sodium Phosphate BP has a pH of 7.5 to 9.0.

Partition coefficients

Log P (octanol/pH 7), 2.01 (betamethasone)[1]
Log P (octanol/pH 7), 3.60 (betamethasone valerate)[1]

Solubility

Betamethasone is practically insoluble in water; soluble 1 in 75 of ethanol and 1 in 15 of warm ethanol; sparingly soluble in acetone, in dioxan, and in methanol; very slightly soluble in chloroform and in ether.
Betamethasone acetate is practically insoluble in water; soluble 1 in 9 of ethanol and 1 in 16 of chloroform; freely soluble in acetone.
Betamethasone benzoate is practically insoluble in water; soluble in ethanol, in chloroform, and in methanol.
Betamethasone dipropionate is practically insoluble in water; sparingly soluble in ethanol; freely soluble in acetone and in chloroform.
Betamethasone sodium phosphate is soluble 1 in 2 of water; slightly soluble in absolute ethanol; freely soluble in methanol; practically insoluble in acetone, in chloroform, and in ether.
Betamethasone valerate is practically insoluble in water and in petroleum spirit; soluble 1 in 12 of ethanol, 1 in 2 of chloroform, and 1 in 50 of isopropanol; freely soluble in acetone; slightly soluble in ether.

Dissolution

The USP specifies that for Betamethasone Tablets USP not less than 75% of the labelled amount of $C_{22}H_{29}FO_5$ is dissolved in 45 minutes. Dissolution medium: 900 mL of water; Apparatus 2 at 50 rpm.

Crystal and molecular structure

Polymorphs
Perrier *et al*[2] suggest that *betamethasone acetate* exists in two polymorphic forms, and that *betamethasone dipropionate* does not exhibit polymorphism.

FURTHER INFORMATION. Operational possibilities of betamethasone acetate modifications in aqueous suspensions [German]— Seiller VE, Nürnberg E. Pharm Ind 1990;52(1):104–7.

STABILITY

Betamethasone

Dekker and Beijnen[3] postulated that, under anaerobic alkaline (pH 8.3) conditions, the decomposition products of betamethasone are the 17-deoxy-17-carboxylic acid and the 17-deoxy-20-hydroxy-21-acid derivatives.

Betamethasone dipropionate

Betamethasone dipropionate is highly stable in aqueous suspensions because of its low water solubility and diester structure. Any hydrolysis results in the formation of betamethasone alcohol. Maximum stability is achieved at pH 4.
No evidence of degradation is observed when betamethasone dipropionate is heated at 75° for 6 months in the presence of air; minor decomposition is reported after prolonged exposure to fluorescent light.

Betamethasone sodium phosphate

Aqueous solutions of betamethasone sodium phosphate with a pH of about 8 are stable if protected from light. Particular care must be taken to prevent microbial contamination as hydrolysis of the ester by phosphatase enzymes, which are a common product of microbial metabolism, can occur.

Betamethasone valerate

In the presence of acid or base, 17-α monoesters of corticosteroids are unstable and undergo a rearrangement to the corresponding 21-monoester; betamethasone 17-valerate is no exception. Bundgaard and Hansen[4] found that, in addition to a water-catalysed or spontaneous reaction, the degradation of betamethasone valerate, at 60°, is subject to both specific acid and base catalysis. First-order reaction kinetics were followed for more than four half-lives when measured at constant pH and temperature. The rate constants at various pH values are shown in the table below. The minimum degradation rate was found to occur at pH 3.5. The effect of temperature was determined over the range 30° to 60°, in a 0.1M phosphate buffer solution at pH 7.5 (ionic strength 0.5); the activation energy was found to be 32.8 kJ/mol. Observed pseudo-first-order rate constants (K_{obs}) for the overall degradation of betamethasone valerate in solutions of different pH (ionic strength 0.5, 60°) were as follows:

pH	$K_{obs} \times 10^2$ (per hour)
1.15	1.5
3.39	0.21
5.48	1.8
6.47	12
7.98	394

The degradation of betamethasone 17-valerate in propylene glycol solution, catalysed by ethanolamine, was studied by Li Wan Po et al.[5] The following reaction sequence was elucidated: betamethasone 17-valerate first rearranges to betamethasone 21-valerate which subsequently undergoes hydrolysis to betamethasone. Betamethasone itself may undergo a condensation reaction to a 21-hydroxy-ethylimine derivative. Rate constants were determined for each of the reaction mechanisms.

Stability of diluted betamethasone valerate creams and ointments Yip and Li Wan Po[6] determined the decomposition rates of diluted betamethasone valerate ointment preparations. The diluents tested were Plastibase, white soft paraffin, and emulsifying ointment. Observed rate constants (h^{-1}) for the decomposition of diluted betamethasone 17-valerate ointment preparations were:

Betamethasone ointment:Plastibase (3:1)	3×10^{-3}	(25°)
Betamethasone ointment:Plastibase (1:1)	4.74×10^{-1}	(22.5°)
Betamethasone ointment:white soft paraffin (1:1)	6.13×10^{-5}	(22.5°)
Betamethasone ointment:emulsifying ointment (3:1)	2.21×10^{-1}	(22.5°)
Betamethasone ointment:emulsifying ointment (3:1) + phosphoric acid 0.005%	3.85×10^{-3}	(22.5°)

Dilution with white soft paraffin formed the most stable product, with a $t_{10\%}$ value of 71.6 days. The $t_{10\%}$ for the betamethasone ointment:Plastibase (1:1) combination was 0.22 hours.

Stabilisation of the emulsifying ointment dilution was attempted by acidifying the preparation with phosphoric acid 0.005%; the rationale being that the decomposition is base-catalysed. Although the pH of the system was virtually unaltered by the addition, stability was improved.

The stability at room temperature of dilutions (1 in 4) of betamethasone valerate ointment (Betnovate, Glaxo) in emulsifying ointment was studied over a period of one month by Mehta and Calvert.[7] The half-lives for the conversion of the 17-valerate ester to the 21-valerate derivative in 5 batches ranged from 4 to 5 hours. The subsequent hydrolysis of betamethasone 21-valerate to betamethasone proceeded more slowly ($t_{50\%} = 8$ days).

The chemical stability and clinical efficacy of betamethasone 17-valerate ointment preparations (Betnovate, Glaxo) diluted with Unguentum Merck (1:4, 1:16, and 1:32) were assessed by Ryatt et al.[8] Analysis by HPLC showed no loss of the steroid from any of the dilutions after 2 months and no loss from a 5-month-old 1 in 4 dilution. Clinical efficacy was satisfactory and it was concluded that Unguentum Merck is a suitable diluent for Betnovate ointment.

Beeler's basis (sodium lauryl sulphate 2 g, cetyl alcohol 15 g, white beeswax 1 g, propylene glycol 10 g, water 72 g) and a commercial cold cream preparation were used as diluents for betamethasone 17-valerate cream. The steroid was stable in the diluted creams for at least 30 days at room temperature. Increasing the temperature to 40° resulted in degradation in some of the preparations. It was found that preparations diluted with Beeler's basis, and which had a higher pH, were more stable. A reduction in potency, as determined by the skin blanching test, was not achieved by any of the dilutions prepared using Beeler's basis.[9]

FURTHER INFORMATION. Photostability testing of betamethasone [valerate solution] with different methods of exposure [German]—Thoma VK, Kerker R, Weissbach C. Pharm Ind 1987;49(9):961–3. Stability of betamethasone sodium phosphate, hydrocortisone sodium phosphate, and prednisolone sodium phosphate injections submitted by US hospitals—Kreienbaum MA. Am J Hosp Pharm 1986;43:1747–50. The influence of cyclodextrin complexation on the stability of betamethasone 17-valerate—Andersen FM, Bundgaard H. Int J Pharmaceutics 1984;20:155–62.

INCOMPATIBILITY/COMPATIBILITY

Betamethasone valerate is incompatible with alkalis, heavy metals, and metabisulphites. It is inactivated by coal tar, salicylic acid, and many other substances.

In a study conducted in the Pharmaceutics Laboratory of the Royal Pharmaceutical Society, the physical compatibility of betamethasone valerate cream 0.1% with two formulations of cetomacrogol cream was assessed. The creams were Cetomacrogol Cream BP 1988—Formula A and a modified form where some of the water is replaced by propylene glycol. Formulae of diluents for betamethasone valerate creams were as follows:

	Cetomacrogol Cream BP 1988— Formula A	Modified Cetomacrogal Cream BP 1988
Cetomacrogol emulsifying ointment	30 g	30 g
Chlorocresol	0.1 g	0.15 g
Propylene glycol	—	20 g
Purified water, freshly boiled and cooled	69.9 g	49.85 g

A 1 in 10 and a 1 in 2 dilution of the betamethasone cream were prepared. Over a 14-day period in the dark at 25°, no physical incompatibility was detected.

FORMULATION

Excipients

Excipients that have been used in presentations of betamethasone or the betamethasone esters include:

Tablets, betamethasone: lactose; magnesium stearate; maize starch; patent blue V (E131).

Buccal tablets, betamethasone valerate: acacia; lactose; magnesium stearate.

Soluble tablets, betamethasone sodium phosphate: erythrosine (E127); povidone; saccharin sodium; sodium acid citrate; sodium bicarbonate; sodium benzoate.

Delayed-release tablets, betamethasone: acacia; beeswax; calcium carbonate; carnauba wax; cetyl alcohol; gelatin; lactose; magnesium stearate; maize starch; methyl hydroxybenzoate; patent blue V (E131); shellac; sucrose; talc.

Oral drops, betamethasone: citric acid; disodium edetate; propylene glycol; sodium benzoate; sodium phosphate; sorbitol; sucrose.

Topical aerosols, betamethasone dipropionate: caprylic/capric triglyceride; liquid paraffin; isopropanol; propellants: isobutane and propane.

Creams, betamethasone benzoate: cetyl alcohol; citric acid; glyceryl stearate; light liquid paraffin; propylene glycol.

Betamethasone dipropionate: carbomer 940; cetomacrogol 1000; cetostearyl alcohol; chlorocresol; cyclomethicone; liquid paraffin; phosphoric acid; propylene glycol; sodium acid phosphate; sodium hydroxide; sorbitol; titanium dioxide (E171); white beeswax; white soft paraffin.

Betamethasone valerate: cetomacrogol 1000; cetostearyl alcohol; cetyl alcohol; chlorocresol; liquid paraffin; methyl hydroxybenzoate; sodium acid phosphate; phosphoric acid; propylene glycol; sodium hydroxide; stearyl alcohol; white soft paraffin.

Gels, betamethasone benzoate: carbomer; diisopropanolamine; disodium edetate; ethanol; propylene glycol.

Lotions, betamethasone benzoate: cetyl alcohol; methyl, propyl, and butyl hydroxybenzoates; propylene glycol; sodium lauryl sulphate; stearyl alcohol.

Betamethasone dipropionate: carbomer; isopropanol; phosphoric acid; sodium hydroxide.

Betamethasone valerate: carbomer; cetomacrogol 1000; cetostearyl alcohol; cetyl alcohol; citric acid; diethylene glycol monostearate; glycerol; isopropanol; liquid paraffin; methyl hydroxybenzoate; phosphoric acid; sodium citrate; sodium hydroxide; stearyl alcohol.

Ointments, betamethasone benzoate: glyceryl stearate; light liquid paraffin; modified food starch.

Betamethasone dipropionate: liquid paraffin; propylene glycol; propylene glycol monostearate; white beeswax; white soft paraffin.

Betamethasone valerate: hydrogenated wool fat; liquid paraffin; white soft paraffin.

Rectal solutions, betamethasone sodium phosphate: disodium edetate; methyl and propyl hydroxybenzoates; sodium citrate; sodium hydroxide.

Eye, ear, and nose drops, betamethasone sodium phosphate: benzalkonium chloride.

Solutions for injection, betamethasone sodium phosphate: disodium edetate; phenol; sodium bisulphite; sodium chloride; sodium hydroxide; sodium metabisulphite; sodium phosphate.

Suspensions for injection, betamethasone acetate and betamethasone sodium phosphate: benzalkonium chloride; disodium edetate; sodium acid phosphate; sodium phosphate.

Betamethasone dipropionate and betamethasone sodium phosphate: benzyl alcohol; carmellose sodium; disodium edetate; macrogol 4000; methyl and propyl hydroxybenzoates; polysorbate 80; sodium chloride; sodium phosphate.

Betamethasone and betamethasone sodium phosphate: benzyl alcohol; disodium edetate; hydroxyethylcellulose; sodium chloride; sodium citrate; sodium hydroxide; sodium metabisulphite.

Preparation of solid dosage forms

Betamethasone should be used in the form of an ultrafine powder in order to achieve a satisfactory rate of dissolution.

Topical preparations

Lippold and Schneemann[10] discussed the bioavailability (in 23 healthy subjects) of betamethasone benzoate in various ointment bases. The penetration rate across the skin barrier achieved by suspension-type ointment bases was found to be independent of the solubility of the drug. However, with solution-type ointment bases, the skin penetration rate was found to increase with increasing drug concentrations and to be at a maximum when it contained a concentration equal to the solubility of the drug in the vehicle.

Seven ointment bases were used by Pepler *et al*[11] to prepare betamethasone benzoate 0.025% ointment. The ointments were applied, in turn, to both forearms of 18 subjects. Betamethasone benzoate in white soft paraffin:propylene glycol (95:5) and in white soft paraffin:isopropyl myristate (95:5) produced vasoconstriction which was significantly greater than that observed with any of the other ointments studied.

The use of penetration enhancers to increase the percutaneous absorption of betamethasone benzoate was investigated by Barry *et al*.[12] The only agent which significantly increased the bioavailability of the steroid was *N*-methyl-2-pyrrolidone.

Betamethasone valerate was found to be released more rapidly (at 37° *in vitro*) from creams than from ointments.[13] The release rate was increased following dilution of one of the test creams with cold cream (w/o emulsion) but was not markedly different following dilution with the creams (o/w emulsions), Filovit (Filoderm) and Nutraderm (Alcon Laboratories).

Barnes *et al*[14] reported inadequate stability of betamethasone dipropionate (0.05% w/w as Diprosone ointment, Kirby-Warwick, UK) and betamethasone valerate (0.1% w/w ointment, Harris, UK) when each were diluted 1:10 in Compound Zinc Paste BP, and concluded that extemporaneous dilution on this basis could not be recommended. Betamethasone dipropionate exhibited first-order degradation at 25° and at 32° with $t_{10\%}$ values of about 11 days and 4.4 days, respectively.

FURTHER INFORMATION. The behaviour of bioadhesive betamethasone tablets [betamethasone valerate with high viscosity carmellose sodium] in the mouth—Tucker IG, Szylkarski HAM, Romaniuk K. J Clin Pharm Ther 1989;14:153–8. Bioequivalence (bioavailability) of generic topical corticosteroids [betamethasone valerate 0.1% creams were not all equivalent; quantitative modification of the vasoconstrictor assay]—Jackson DB, Thompson C, McCormack JR, Guin JD. J Am Acad Dermatol 1989;20:791–6.

PROCESSING

Sterilisation

Betamethasone injection, an aqueous solution containing betamethasone sodium phosphate, can be sterilised by filtration.

REFERENCES

1. Caron JC, Shroot B. J Pharm Sci 1984;73:1703–6.
2. Perrier R, Chauvet A, Masse J [French]. Thermochim Acta 1981;44:189–201.
3. Dekker D, Beijnen JH. Acta Pharm Suec 1981;18:185–92.
4. Bundgaard H, Hansen J. Int J Pharmaceutics 1981;7:197–203.
5. Li Wan Po A, Irwin WJ, Yip YW. J Chromatogr 1979;176:399–405.
6. Yip YW, Li Wan Po A. J Pharm Pharmacol 1979;31:400–2.
7. Mehta AC, Calvert RT. Br J Pharm Pract 1982;4:10–13.
8. Ryatt KS, Cotterill JA, Mehta A. J Clin Hosp Pharm 1983;8:143–5.
9. Boonsaner P, Remon JP, De Rudder D. J Clin Hosp Pharm 1986;11:101–6.
10. Lippold BC, Schneemann H. Int J Pharmaceutics 1984;22:31–43.
11. Pepler AF, Woodford R, Morrison JC. Br J Derm 1971;85:171–6.
12. Barry BW, Southwell D, Woodford R. J Invest Dermatol 1984;82:49–52.
13. Rekkas DM, Dallas PP, Hatzis J, Choulis NH. Drug Dev Ind Pharm 1989;15(11):1881–8.
14. Barnes AR, Nash S, Watkiss SB. J Clin Pharm Ther 1991;16:103–9.

Bretylium Tosylate (BAN, USAN)

Anti-arrhythmic

Bretylium Tosilate (rINN)
2-Bromobenzyl-*N*-ethyldimethylammonium toluene-4-sulphonate
$C_{11}H_{17}BrN,C_7H_7O_3S = 414.4$
CAS—59-41-6 (bretylium); 61-75-6 (bretylium tosylate)

Preparations

Non-compendial

Bretylate (Wellcome). *Injection*, bretylium tosylate 50 mg/mL. Should be diluted to not more than 10 mg/mL with glucose 5% injection or sodium chloride 0.9% injection. When diluted, the injection is stable for up to 24 hours.
Min-I-Jet Bretylium Tosylate (IMS). *Injection*, bretylium tosylate 50 mg/mL.

Containers and storage

Bretylate injection should be stored at a temperature below 25° and protected from light. It should not be frozen.

PHYSICAL PROPERTIES

Bretylium tosylate is a white, odourless, crystalline powder with a very bitter taste.
In the solid state, *bretylium tosylate* is hygroscopic.

Melting point

Bretylium tosylate melts at about 98°.

Solubility

Bretylium tosylate is soluble 1 in 1 of water and 1 in less than 1 of ethanol; freely soluble in methanol; practically insoluble in ether, in ethyl acetate, and in hexane.

STABILITY

In solution, bretylium tosylate is stable[1] in the pH range 2 to 12. Bretylol, an injectable preparation of bretylium tosylate available in the USA (American Critical Care), is adjusted to a pH of 5 to 7 with either hydrochloric acid or sodium hydroxide and has a shelf-life of 3 years.[1]
No decomposition was observed when solutions of bretylium tosylate 50 mg/mL, prepared in either 1M hydrochloric acid, 1M sodium hydroxide, or 10% hydrogen peroxide, were heated at 90° for one hour.[2]

INCOMPATIBILITY/COMPATIBILITY

Bretylium tosylate (Bretylol, American Critical Care) was found to be stable in admixtures (10 mg/mL) with eleven of the common large-volume parenteral solutions (glucose 5% in sodium chloride 0.45%; sodium chloride 0.9%; glucose 5%; glucose 5% in compound sodium lactate; sodium lactate; compound sodium lactate; glucose 5% in sodium chloride 0.9%; sodium bicarbonate 5%; mannitol 20%; calcium chloride 54.4 mEq/L in glucose 5%; potassium chloride 40 mEq/L in glucose 5%).[3] The test conditions to which these admixtures were subjected included exposure to intense light (1.50×10^4 to 2.15×10^4 lx), ambient room temperature with normal light, storage at 40°, and refrigeration at 4°. Analyses of bretylium content (by HPLC) after 1, 2, and in some instances 7 days, showed no significant change in potency. Mannitol (but not bretylium tosylate) precipitated from mannitol admixtures stored at 4°.
Perentesis *et al*[4] demonstrated that bretylium tosylate (Bretylol, American Critical Care) at a concentration of 1 mg/mL was stable at 25° in glucose 5% injection, in sodium chloride 0.9% injection, and in compound sodium lactate injection over a 4-week study period under normal fluorescent light. There were no apparent differences between the stability of the admixtures when stored in containers of either glass or polyvinyl chloride.
In the study reported above,[4] admixtures of bretylium tosylate were prepared in glucose 5% injection and in sodium chloride 0.9% injection with each of the following: aminophylline, calcium gluconate, digoxin, insulin, lignocaine hydrochloride, phenytoin sodium, procainamide hydrochloride, and quinidine gluconate. All the solutions were visually compatible for 48 hours except for the admixture with phenytoin sodium which immediately formed a precipitate of translucent, needle-like crystals.
Lee *et al*[5] found that bretylium tosylate (10 mg/mL) was stable and compatible in parenteral admixture with each of four cardiovascular drugs (dopamine hydrochloride, lignocaine hydrochloride, procainamide hydrochloride, and glyceryl trinitrate) for at least 24 hours. The solutions were subjected to four storage conditions: intense light (1.50×10^4 to 2.15×10^4 lx) at 25°, normal light at room temperature, and temperatures of 40° and 4°. The drugs were added at their maximum recommended dosage levels to glass and Viaflex (Travenol) plastic containers containing either glucose 5% injection or sodium chloride 0.9% injection.

FORMULATION

Excipients

Excipients that have been used in presentations of bretylium tosylate include:
Injections: hydrochloric acid; sodium hydroxide.

REFERENCES

1. Bryan CK, Darby MH. Am J Hosp Pharm 1979;36:1189–92.
2. Carter JE, Amann AH, Baaske DM. In: Florey K, editor. Analytical profiles of drug substances; vol 9. London: Academic Press, 1980:11–86.
3. Lee Y-C, Baaske DM, Amann AH, Carter JE, Mooers MA, Wagenknecht DM, *et al.* Am J Hosp Pharm 1980;37:803–8.
4. Perentesis GP, Piltz GW, Kirschenbaum HL, Navalakha P, Aronoff W, Cutie AJ. Am J Hosp Pharm 1983;40:1010–12.
5. Lee Y-C, Malick AW, Amann AH, Baaske DM, Shah JJ, Wagenknecht DM, *et al.* Am J Hosp Pharm 1981;38:183–7.

Buprenorphine (BAN, rINN)   *Opioid analgesic*

(2S)-2-[(−)-(5R,6R,7R,14S)-9a-Cyclopropylmethyl-4,5-epoxy-3-hydroxy-6-methoxy-6,14-ethanomorphinan-7-yl]-3,3-dimethyl-butan-2-ol;   [5α,7α   (S)]-17-(cyclopropylmethyl)-α-(1,1-dimethylethyl)-4,5-epoxy-18,19-dihydro-3-hydroxy-6-methoxy-α-methyl-6,14-ethenomorphinan-7-methanol
$C_{29}H_{41}NO_4 = 467.6$

Buprenorphine Hydrochloride (BANM, USAN, rINNM)
$C_{29}H_{41}NO_4, HCl = 504.1$
CAS—52485-79-7 (buprenorphine); 53152-21-9 (buprenorphine hydrochloride)

Preparations

Non-compendial
Temgesic (R&C). *Tablets (sublingual)*, buprenorphine (as hydrochloride) 200 micrograms and 400 micrograms.
Injection, buprenorphine (as hydrochloride) 300 micrograms/mL, in a glucose 5% solution, adjusted to pH range 3.5 to 5.5 with hydrochloric acid. It may be diluted with glucose 5% injection or sodium chloride 0.9% injection.

Containers and storage

Dosage forms
Temgesic sublingual tablets should be stored in a cool place. Temgesic injection should be kept cool and protected from light.

PHYSICAL PROPERTIES

Buprenorphine hydrochloride is a white crystalline powder.

Melting point

Buprenorphine melts at 209°.

Dissociation constants

pK_a 8.5 (ammonium group), 10.0 (phenol group)

Solubility

Buprenorphine is very slightly soluble in water at pH 7.
Buprenorphine hydrochloride is slightly soluble in water.

Effect of pH
Approximate solubilities of buprenorphine in buffer solutions:[1]

pH	Solubility (µg/mL)
6	1401
7	236
7.6	66
10	18

STABILITY

Cone *et al*[2] isolated an acid-catalysed and heat-catalysed rearrangement product of buprenorphine in aqueous solutions (5 to 10 micrograms/mL) at pH values up to 1. The rearrangement product was not detected in any sample above pH 3 when a range of solutions (pH up to 12) were kept for 24 hours at the following temperatures: 0° to 4°, 26° to 28°, and 36° to 38°. Significant degradation (83%) was evident in samples buffered at pH 7.4 that were autoclaved (112° and 75.8 kN/m²) for 30 minutes. The degradation occurred via other hydrolytic pathways, rather than by rearrangement, to form products of unknown composition. Only trace amounts of the rearrangement product were detected in samples at pH 5 stored for 10 weeks at 26° to 28°.
Studies by Garrett and Chandran[1] indicated that at fixed hydrogen and hydroxide ion concentrations, the degradation of buprenorphine apparently followed first-order kinetics. Half-lives at 25° were calculated to be 12.5 years at pH 2 and 125 years at pH 3. The authors claimed that complete stability of buprenorphine can be assumed at neutral pH even at elevated temperatures. The degradation of buprenorphine was neither enhanced nor inhibited by bubbling oxygen through acidic solutions.

INCOMPATIBILITY/COMPATIBILITY

Buprenorphine injection 0.3 mg/mL has been reported to be physically and chemically compatible with the following solutions for at least 7 hours: sodium chloride 0.9%, compound sodium lactate, glucose 5% in sodium chloride 0.9%, and glucose 5%. It is reported to be compatible with hyoscine hydrobromide, haloperidol, glycopyrronium bromide, droperidol, and hydroxyzine hydrochloride and to be incompatible with diazepam and lorazepam.[3]

FORMULATION

Excipients

Excipients that have been used in presentations of buprenorphine hydrochloride include:
Tablets, sublingual: lactose.
Injections: glucose; hydrochloric acid.

Bioavailability

Bullingham *et al*[4] observed a delay of between 15 and 45 minutes in the onset of analgesia following sublingual administration of buprenorphine. By comparing the blood concentrations achieved after sublingual and intravenous administration of equivalent doses, the systemic availability of sublingual buprenorphine was estimated to be 31% after 3 hours. Although the resulting blood concentrations were low, sublingual administration resulted in an unexpectedly strong analgesic effect.

A mean bioavailability of 48.2 ± 8.3%, compared to that after intravenous administration, was reported following single-dose administration of 0.3 mg of buprenorphine by nasal spray in a crossover study with nine healthy volunteers.[5] The buprenorphine spray solution contained buprenorphine hydrochloride 2 mg/mL in glucose 5%; the solution was adjusted to pH 5.

FURTHER INFORMATION. Sublingual versus subcutaneous buprenorphine in opiate abusers—Jasinski DR, Fudala PJ, Johnson RE. Clin Pharmacol Ther 1989;45:513–19.

REFERENCES

1. Garrett ER, Chandran VR. J Pharm Sci 1985;74:515–24.
2. Cone EJ, Gorodetzky CW, Darwin WD, Buchwald WF. J Pharm Sci 1984;73:243–6.
3. Smith C [letter]. Hosp Pharm 1986;21:362–3.
4. Bullingham RES, McQuay HJ, Dwyer D, Allen MC, Moore RA. Br J Clin Pharmacol 1981;12:117–22.
5. Eriksen J, Jensen N-H, Kamp-Jensen M, Bjarnø H, Friis P, Brewster D. J Pharm Pharmacol 1989;41:803–5.

Caffeine (BAN)   *Central nervous stimulant*

Anhydrous caffeine; guaranine; methyltheobromine; 7-methyltheophylline

1,3,7-Trimethylpurine-2,6(3H,1H)-dione; 3,7-dihydro-1,3,7-trimethyl-1H-purine-2,6-dione

$C_8H_{10}N_4O_2 = 194.2$

Caffeine Citrate (BANM)

$C_8H_{10}N_4O_2, C_6H_8O_7 = 386.3$

Caffeine Hydrate (BANM)

$C_8H_{10}N_4O_2, H_2O = 212.2$

CAS—58-08-2 (caffeine); 69-22-7 (caffeine citrate); 5743-12-4 (caffeine hydrate)

Pharmacopoeial status

BP (caffeine, caffeine hydrate); USP (caffeine, anhydrous or monohydrate)

Preparations

Compendial
Aspirin and Caffeine Tablets BP.
Caffeine and Sodium Benzoate Injection USP. pH 6.5 to 8.5.

Containers and storage

Solid state
Caffeine BP and Caffeine Hydrate BP should be kept in well-closed containers.
Caffeine (anhydrous) USP should be kept in well-closed containers.
Caffeine (hydrous) USP should be preserved in tight containers.

PHYSICAL PROPERTIES

Both *caffeine* and *caffeine hydrate* exist as silky white crystals, usually matted together, or as a white crystalline powder; sublimation occurs readily in both substances; they are odourless with a bitter taste.

Melting point

Caffeine melts in the range 234° to 239°.

Dissociation constant

pK_a 14.0 (25°)

Partition coefficient

Log P (octanol/pH 7.4),0.0

Solubility

Caffeine is soluble 1 in 60 of water, 1 in 130 of ethanol, and 1 in 7 of chloroform; slightly soluble in ether.
Caffeine hydrate is soluble 1 in 60 of water and 1 in 110 of ethanol; soluble with separation of water in chloroform.

Effect of temperature
Caffeine is soluble 1 in 1.5 of boiling water.

Effect of cosolvents
In a study of the solubility of methylxanthines in mixed solvents, the solubility graphs of caffeine in various binary solvent systems were determined. The solvent systems were: dioxan/formamide, water/macrogol 400, and glycerol/propylene glycol.[1]

Effect of additives
Caffeine citrate is a mixture of caffeine and citric acid containing between 47% and 50% anhydrous caffeine. The presence of citric acid increases the solubility of caffeine. This mixture is soluble in approximately four parts of warm water, but adding more water causes some of the caffeine to separate out. This caffeine can be redissolved by further dilution. An increase in the pH of caffeine-citric acid solutions (as can occur when buffer salts are present) may however cause a substantial reduction in the solubility of caffeine.

The solubility of caffeine in citric acid solution at various pH values was investigated by Anderson and Pitman.[2] When the pH of such solutions is raised above 5.0, the solubility of caffeine is reduced.

The aqueous solubility of caffeine is increased by the inclusion of either sodium benzoate, sodium iodide, or sodium salicylate in the solution.

The mechanism by which sodium benzoate enhances the solubility of caffeine seems to be complex formation. It has been found[3] that at temperatures between 37° and 90° no molecular combination or definite double salt can exist between caffeine and sodium benzoate; only mixtures of the two substances are obtained. Below 37°, the enhancement of solubility of caffeine by benzoate appears to be due to the formation of several complexes. Complex formation has also been reported by Higuchi and Zuck[4] and by Rohdewald and Baumeister.[5]

Crystal and molecular structure

Polymorphs
Sabon et al[6] have identified two stable polymorphic forms of caffeine. Form I melts at 235° and Form II is transformed into Form I at 162°. The two forms show slight differences in solubility over a range of temperatures. Form I exhibits more rapid dissolution than Form II.

STABILITY

Caffeine is a weak base and is decomposed by strong solutions of caustic alkalis. Salts of caffeine are hydrolysed by water.

Caffeine hydrate effloresces on exposure to dry air. It loses its water of crystallisation when heated, becoming anhydrous at 100°.

The stability of caffeine citrate solutions for injection and enteral use was examined by Eisenberg and Kang.[7] The injection was prepared in sterile water and autoclaved at 121° for fifteen minutes. The enteral solution was prepared by dissolving caffeine citrate powder in sterile water and adding syrup and cherry syrup (2:1 ratio) as flavouring. It was found that these preparations were stable for at least three months.

An injectable form of caffeine (10 mg/mL) was prepared by Nahata et al[8] in sterile water for injections with benzyl alcohol as preservative. It was found to be stable for 24 hours at room temperature when diluted to yield caffeine 5 mg/mL in several admixtures (glucose 5% injection; glucose 5% with sodium chloride 0.2% injection; glucose 5% with sodium chloride 0.2% and 20 mEq/L of potassium chloride injection; glucose 10% injection; and glucose 10% with sodium chloride 0.2% and 5 mEq/L of potassium chloride injection) and in parenteral nutrition solutions (1.1%, 2.2%, or 4.25% amino acids with electrolytes, prepared in glucose 10% injection). In a further study, the same authors[9] demonstrated the stability of the caffeine 10 mg/mL injection in both plastic and in glass syringes during storage for 2 months at room temperature or at 4°.

INCOMPATIBILITY/COMPATIBILITY

Caffeine is incompatible with silver salts and with strong solutions of caustic alkalis. In the presence of hydrochloric acid and iodine, caffeine forms a red-brown precipitate. Tannic acid causes caffeine to precipitate but when tannic acid is in excess, caffeine is dissolved.

FORMULATION

Excipients

Excipients that have been used in presentations of caffeine include:
Gels: Carbopol; ethanol; triethanolamine.
Injections: sodium benzoate.

Tablets

The effect of hardness on the dissolution rate and the disintegration of caffeine tablets (uncoated) was studied by Kitazawa *et al.*[10] The tablets consisted of caffeine 5% w/w, talc 0.6% w/w, magnesium stearate 1.4% w/w, potato starch 3% w/w, and lactose (containing 3% hydroxypropylcellulose) 90% w/w. Eight compression pressures were used and the tablet weights were 0.3 g. It was found that an increase in hardness prolonged the disintegration time and, in general, reduced the dissolution rate. Theories about the dissolution pattern were presented.

In a study by Chan and Doelker,[11] the relationship between compression pressure and polymorphic transformation of caffeine during tableting was examined. Tablets were made using the two polymorphic forms of caffeine. Transformation of Form A (transition temperature 141°) to Form B (m.p. 236°) was not uniform throughout the tablet. The upper surface transformed rapidly with increasing pressure reaching a 25% maximum transformation. The maximum transformation in the middle region was 18%. Transformation on the lower surface was slower but still attained a maximum of 18%. Although a

maximum transformation of 23% was reached at the side of the tablets, this process was slow at low pressures but increased from 250 MPa onwards. Form B was found to be stable on compression. Both polymorphic forms were stable during storage at room temperature.

PROCESSING

Sterilisation

Solutions of caffeine and sodium benzoate are sterilised by autoclaving or by filtration, as are solutions of caffeine and sodium salicylate.

REFERENCES

1. Martin A, Paruta AN, Adjei A. J Pharm Sci 1981;70:1115–20.
2. Anderson JR, Pitman IH. Aust J Pharm Sci 1979;8:117–22.
3. Osol A, Farrar GE, editors. United States Dispensatory. 25th ed. Philadelphia: Lippincott, 1955:208.
4. Higuchi T, Zuck DA. J Am Pharm Assoc (Sci) 1953;42:132–8.
5. Rohdewald P, Baumeister M [letter]. J Pharm Pharmacol 1969;21:867–9.
6. Sabon F, Alberola S, Terol A, Jeanjean B [French]. Trav Soc Pharm Montpellier 1979;39:19–24.
7. Eisenberg MG, Kang N. Am J Hosp Pharm 1984;41:2405–6.
8. Nahata MC, Zingarelli JR, Durrell DE. DICP Ann Pharmacother 1989;23:466–7.
9. Nahata MC, Zingarelli JR, Durrell DE [letter]. DICP Ann Pharmacother 1989;23:1035.
10. Kitazawa W, Johno I, Ito Y, Teramura S, Okado J. J Pharm Pharmacol 1975;27:765–70.
11. Chan HK, Doelker E. Drug Dev Ind Pharm 1985;11:315–32.

Captopril (BAN, USAN, rINN)   *Antihypertensive*

1-[(2S)-3-Mercapto-2-methylpropionyl]-L-proline; (S)-1-(3-mercapto-2-methyl-l-oxopropyl)-L-proline; 1-[(2S)-3-mercapto-2-methyl-1-oxopropyl]-L-proline
$C_9H_{15}NO_3S = 217.3$
CAS—62571-86-2

Pharmacopoeial status

USP

Preparations

Compendial
Captopril Tablets USP.

Non-compendial
Acepril (Squibb). *Tablets,* captopril 12.5 mg, 25 mg, and 50 mg.
Capoten (Squibb). *Tablets,* captopril 12.5 mg, 25 mg, and 50 mg.

Containers and storage

Solid state
Captopril USP should be preserved in tight containers.

Dosage forms
Captopril Tablets USP should be preserved in tight containers. Acepril and Capoten tablets should be stored at room temperature.

PHYSICAL PROPERTIES

Captopril is a white to off-white crystalline powder. It may have a characteristic sulphide-like odour.

Melting point

Captopril melts in the range 104° to 110°. See also Crystal and molecular structure, below.

Dissociation constants

pK_a 3.7, 9.8

Partition coefficients

During preparation of sustained-release dosage forms of captopril,[1] partition coefficients between octanol and water at 37° were calculated as 0.19, 0.17, 0.03, and 0.01 at pH values of 2.0, 3.0, 4.0, and 7.4, respectively.

Solubility

Captopril is freely soluble in water, in ethanol, in chloroform, and in methanol.

Dissolution

The USP specifies that for Captopril Tablets USP not less than 80% of the labelled amount of $C_9H_{15}NO_3S$ is dissolved in 20 minutes. Dissolution medium: 900 mL of 0.1N hydrochloric acid; Apparatus 1 at 50 rpm.

Crystal and molecular structure

Polymorphs
Two polymorphic forms of captopril have been identified, an unstable and a stable form, which melt at 88° and 106°, respectively.

STABILITY

Although captopril demonstrates excellent stability in the solid state, it readily oxidises when mixed with certain excipients which release moisture. The rate of excipient-mediated degradation in the solid state depends upon factors such as moisture content, temperature, and oxygen pressure. Pure captopril is not hygroscopic under normal conditions.
Captopril undergoes a free-radical oxidation reaction in aqueous solution to yield captopril disulphide. The reaction is oxygen facilitated and occurs via the thiol group. An alternative degradation pathway via hydrolysis of the amide function is of minimal importance; such a reaction requires acidic conditions and elevated temperatures.
The stability of captopril in aqueous solution is influenced by factors such as concentration, pH, oxygen tension, and the presence of metal ions. Timmins et al[2] identified the oxidative and hydrolytic degradation products of captopril and studied the effects of temperature, pH, and additives on the decomposition rates. In McIlvaine buffers (pH range 2.1 to 5.6) of constant ionic strength (at 50°), captopril solutions (5 mg/mL) demonstrated maximum oxidative stability at pH values below 4.0.

The degradation rate of captopril in aqueous solution (5 mg/mL) in a citric acid/sodium citrate buffered medium (pH 4.0) increased in the presence of 5 ppm of either copper or iron ions.[2] Similarly, the addition of either 0.05% w/v propyl gallate, an antoxidant that breaks free-radical chain reactions, or 0.1% w/v sodium metabisulphite 5 mg/mL, a reducing agent, decreased the stability of 5 mg/mL solutions buffered at pH 4.0 and stored at 50°.
When captopril 25 mg tablets (Capoten, Squibb, USA) were crushed and added to tap water (final concentration of captopril 1 mg/mL), $t_{10\%}$ values of 28 days, 11.8 ± 1.2 days, 3.6 ± 0.4 days, and 2.0 ± 0.1 days after storage at 5°, 25°, 50°, and 75°, respectively, were calculated.[3]

Containers

Captopril 12.5 mg tablets (Capoten, Squibb, USA) were powdered and triturated with lactose to a final concentration of captopril 2 mg in 100 mg of powder.[4] When powder papers were prepared and stored in either 'class A prescription vials', plastic zip-lock bags, or in moisture-proof barrier bags (Baxa, USA), all at room temperature and protected from light, captopril was physically and chemically stable for at least 12 weeks.

Stabilisation

Increased stability of captopril in aqueous solution is achieved by adjusting the pH to a value below 4, by using sodium edetate as a chelating agent to remove metal ions, and by employing a nitrogen purge to eliminate oxygen. In addition, the oxidation rate can be further reduced by increasing the concentration of captopril in solution and by using a non-aqueous solvent such as methanol. In the solid state, contact with moisture-releasing excipients must be avoided and control of humidity and temperature during storage is essential.
Jarrott et al[5] found that standard solutions of captopril (0.001M), prepared by dissolving the pure drug in aqueous solutions of sodium edetate (0.001M) which had previously been purged with nitrogen, were stable for at least seven days when stored at 4°.

FURTHER INFORMATION. Stability of captopril in some aqueous systems—Pramar Y, Das Gupta V, Bethea C. J Clin Pharm Ther 1992;17:185–9.

FORMULATION

Excipients

Excipients that have been used in presentations of captopril include:
Tablets: lactose; maize starch; microcrystalline cellulose; stearic acid.
Powders: lactose.

Modified-release preparations

Seven 'prolonged-action' dosage forms of captopril were designed and prepared by Seta et al;[1] detailed formulations were presented for coated slow-release granules, four modified-release tablets, enteric coated granules, and an oily semi-solid suspension (comprising soybean oil and glyceryl monostearate) filled into capsules. Oral administration to *dogs* (under non-fasting conditions) revealed a greater area under the plasma concentration versus time curve (AUC) and a more sustained plasma-captopril concentration from the oily semi-solid preparation than from the coated slow-release granules. However, the AUC for the oily semi-solid preparation was only about 50% of that for conventional tablets. Further developments of the oily semi-solid matrix dosage form of captopril were investigated *in vitro* and *in vivo*, in *dogs*[6] and in eight human subjects.[7] In the latter study, the inclusion of ascorbic acid in an amount more than five times that of captopril by weight produced a dosage form suitable for sustained-release pharmacokinetics; in a single-dose, crossover study AUC values were 'almost equal' following oral administration of the oily semi-solid matrix preparation containing ascorbic acid and conventional tablets.

FURTHER INFORMATION. Novel drug delivery system for capto-pril—Matharu RS, Sanghavi NM. Drug Dev Ind Pharm 1992;18:1567–74.

REFERENCES

1. Seta Y, Higuchi F, Kawahara Y, Nishimura K, Okada R. Int J Pharmaceutics 1988;41:245–54.
2. Timmins P, Jackson IM, Wang Y-J. Int J Pharmaceutics 1982;11:329–36.
3. Pereira CM, Tam YK. Am J Hosp Pharm 1992;49:612–15.
4. Taketomo CK, Chu SA, Cheng MH, Corpuz RP. Am J Hosp Pharm 1990;47:1799–801.
5. Jarrott B, Anderson A, Hooper R, Louis WJ. J Pharm Sci 1981;70(6):665–7.
6. Seta Y, Higuchi F, Otsuka T, Kawahara Y, Nishimura K, Okada R *et al*. Int J Pharmaceutics 1988;41:255–62.
7. Seta Y, Otsuka T, Tokiwa H, Naganuma H, Kawahara Y, Nishimura K *et al*. Int J Pharmaceutics 1988;41:263–9.

Carbamazepine (BAN, USAN, rINN)

Anticonvulsant

5*H*-Dibenz[*b*, *f*]azepine-5-carboxamide
$C_{15}H_{12}N_2O = 236.3$
CAS—298-46-4

Pharmacopoeial status

BP, USP

Preparations

Compendial
Carbamazepine Tablets BP. Tablets containing in each, 100 mg, 200 mg, and 400 mg are usually available.
Carbamazepine Tablets USP.
Carbamazepine Oral Suspension USP.

Non-compendial
Tegretol (Geigy). *Tablets*, carbamazepine 100 mg, 200 mg, and 400 mg.
Chewtabs, carbamazepine 100 mg and 200 mg.
Liquid, sugar free, carbamazepine 100 mg/5 mL. *Diluent*: traga-canth mucilage for 1:1 dilution, life of diluted liquid 14 days.
Tegretol Retard (Geigy). *Tablets*, modified release, carbamaze-pine 200 mg and 400 mg.

Containers and storage

Solid state
Carbamazepine BP should be kept in an airtight container.
Carbamazepine USP should be preserved in tight containers.

Dosage forms
Carbamazepine Tablets USP should be preserved in tight con-tainers preferably of glass. Dispense in a container labelled 'Store in a dry place. Protect from moisture.'
Carbamazepine Oral Suspension USP should be preserved in tight, light-resistant containers, protected from freezing and from excessive heat.
Tegretol chewtabs should be protected from heat and moisture.
Tegretol liquid should be kept in a tightly closed container, pro-tected from heat.
Tegretol Retard tablets should be stored below 25° and pro-tected from moisture.

PHYSICAL PROPERTIES

Carbamazepine is a white to yellowish-white crystalline powder.

Melting point

Carbamazepine melts in the range 189° to 193°.

Solubility

Carbamazepine is practically insoluble in water and in ether; sparingly soluble in ethanol and in acetone; soluble 1 in 10 of chloroform; soluble in propylene glycol.

Enhancement of solubility
The solubility of carbamazepine was increased in aqueous solu-tions of eight nonionic surfactants (Tweens 20, 40, 60 and 80; Myrjs 51 and 52; and Brijs 35 and 98)[1] over a concentration range of surfactant up to 0.09M at 37°. Solubilisation was also demonstrated to increase with increased concentration of the bile salt sodium deoxycholate.
Significant enhancement of the solubility of carbamazepine was achieved by complexation with dimethyl-*β*-cyclodextrin, hydr-oxypropyl-*β*-cyclodextrin, 2-hydroxyethyl-*β*-cyclodextrin, *γ*-cyclodextrin, or hydroxypropyl-*γ*-cyclodextrin.[2] In the concen-tration range 1% to 10% w/v, the *β*-cyclodextrin derivatives were superior to the *γ*-cyclodextrin derivatives in the enhance-ment of drug solubility.

Dissolution

The USP specifies that for Carbamazepine Tablets USP not less than 75% of the labelled amount of $C_{15}H_{12}N_2O$ is dissolved in 60 minutes. Dissolution medium: 900 mL of water containing 1% sodium lauryl sulphate; Apparatus 2 at 75 rpm.

Dissolution properties
Carbamazepine can exist in an anhydrous form and as the dihy-drate. Kahela *et al*[3] demonstrated that the dihydrate exhibited faster dissolution than the anhydrous form in a medium of hydrochloric acid (0.01M). The experiment was extended to include a wetting agent, polysorbate 80 (0.01%), in the med-ium. In this instance, the initial dissolution rate of the anhy-drous form was greater than that of the dihydrate. However, after one hour, the pattern was reversed and the dissolution rate of the dihydrate was again greater. In studies *in vivo*, it was found that anhydrous carbamazepine was absorbed more slowly than the dihydrate. Crystal transformation and crystal growth may have contributed to the differences in the dissolu-tion and absorption behaviour of the two forms.

Crystal and molecular structure

Polymorphs
Carbamazepine has been reported to exist in several different polymorphic forms. Pöhlmann *et al*[4] identified six crystalline forms. Lefebvre *et al*[5,6] reviewed and studied the polymorph-

ism of carbamazepine. Commercial carbamazepine is usually the β-form (ground crystals); however, a small quantity of the α-form (narrow needles) can also be present. In aqueous suspensions carbamazepine exists as the dihydrate (needles). Alpha-carbamazepine can be prepared by heating the β-form at 170° for two hours; the dihydrate can be prepared by dispersion of the α-form in water. See also Processing, below.

Several authors[3,7] have discussed the properties of the dihydrate of carbamazepine.

FURTHER INFORMATION. On the crystallographic behaviour of carbamazepine under compression pressure—Kala H, Haack U, Wenzel U, Zessin G, Pollandt P [German]. Pharmazie 1987;42:524-7. Physicochemical properties and X-ray structural studies of the trigonal [α] polymorph of carbamazepine [comparison with monoclinic (β) polymorph]—Lowes MMJ, Caira MR, Lötter AP, Van der Watt JG. J Pharm Sci 1987;76(9):744-52. Relations between several polymorphic forms and the dihydrate of carbamazepine—Krahn FU, Mielck JB. Pharm Acta Helv 1987;62(9):247-54. [Speed of dissolution and polymorphism of carbamazepine: study of different preparations]—Lefebvre C, Guyot-Hermann AM, Draguet-Brughmans M, Bouché R [French]. Pharm Acta Helv 1987;62(12):341-7. Kinetics of transition of anhydrous carbamazepine to carbamazepine dihydrate in aqueous suspensions—Young WWL, Suryanarayanan R. J Pharm Sci 1991;80(5):496-500. Kinetics of the thermal transition of carbamazepine polymorphic forms in the solid state—Umeda T, Ohnishi N, Yokoyama T, Kuroda K, Kuroda T, Tatsumi E [Japanese]. Yakugaku Zasshi 1984;104:786-92. Heat of fusion measurement of a low melting polymorph of carbamazepine that undergoes multiple-phase changes during differential scanning calorimetry analysis—Behme RJ, Brooke D. J Pharm Sci 1991;80(10):986-90.

STABILITY

Solid state

Carbamazepine is relatively stable at room temperature.

The physical and chemical stability of three crystalline phases of carbamazepine prepared by Krahn and Mielck[8] were investigated after mixing with colloidal silica 40% w/w and storage under 'climatic stress' at 56° to 72° and 41% to 71% relative humidities for 200 days. The three phases were needle-shaped (tempered) crystals of Form 1, beam-shaped (anhydrous) crystals of Form 1 and prismatic Form 3. The anhydrous Form 1 transformed under all conditions to Form 3 whereas other phases were physically stable. Carbamazepine degraded chemically to iminostilbene by hydrolysis; about 10% of carbamazepine had degraded at the highest stress (72°) after 200 days. The influence of relative humidity could not be detected. Other degradation products identified by TLC and HPLC were 9-methylacridine, acridine-9-carboxylic acid, acridine, and acridone.

Tablets

Crystal growth was demonstrated on the surface of carbamazepine tablets containing stearic acid following storage at 50° and 80° for six weeks and five days, respectively, but was not apparent on tablets stored for six weeks at 35° or on tablets that did not contain stearic acid.[9] Results showed that carbamazepine was soluble in molten stearic acid and crystal growth was only noted in tablets stored above the melting point of stearic acid. The US Food and Drug Administration reported[10] that carbamazepine could lose one third of its efficacy if stored in humid conditions; tablets hardened and subsequently showed poor dis-

solution in test liquids. Lowes[11] suggested that these phenomena could be attributed to the formation of dihydrate crystals.

Suspensions

Carbamazepine suspension 20 mg/mL (Tegretol, Ciba-Geigy, USA), repackaged in amber glass vials, polypropylene vials, amber polypropylene syringes, and amber glass oral syringes, was stable for at least eight weeks when stored at room temperature under continuous fluorescent light. Although no physical changes or changes in pH were noted after twelve weeks, there were significant decreases in carbamazepine concentration.[12]

INCOMPATIBILITY/COMPATIBILITY

Significant loss of carbamazepine was reported when carbamazepine suspension 100 mg/5 mL (Tegretol, Ciba-Geigy, USA) was administered, undiluted, by various methods, through polyvinyl chloride nasogastric feeding tubes;[13] carbamazepine in undiluted suspensions was thought to 'adhere' to the tube. No significant losses were noted from diluted suspensions (50% with sterile water, sodium chloride 0.9%, or glucose 5% solutions). The presence of diluent was thought to decrease the extent of adhesion of carbamazepine.

FORMULATION

Excipients

Excipients that have been used in presentations of carbamazepine include:

Tablets: Aerosil; allura red AC (E129); carmellose sodium; colloidal silica; gelatin; glycerol; magnesium stearate; microcrystalline cellulose; polyethoxylated castor oils; starch; stearic acid.

Chewable tablets: colloidal silica; erythrosine (E127); gelatin; glycerol; magnesium stearate; sodium starch glycollate; sorbitol; starch; stearic acid; sucrose.

Oral liquids: caramel flavour; cherry syrup; Cologel; dispersible cellulose; hydroxyethylcellulose; methyl and propyl hydroxybenzoates; polyoxyl 8 stearate; polyethoxylated castor oils; propylene glycol; saccharin sodium; sorbic acid; sorbitol solution (70%); syrup.

Bioavailability

A controlled-release form of carbamazepine (Tegretol CR Divitabs, Ciba-Geigy) showed apparent bioavailability comparable with that of conventional carbamazepine tablets (Tegretol, Ciba-Geigy) when tested in eight healthy subjects in single-dose and multiple-dose studies of double-blind, crossover design.[14]

In a comparative bioavailability study of carbamazepine,[15] six healthy subjects received the drug either as three 200 mg tablets (Ciba-Geigy, Australia) or as 30 mL of a 100 mg/5 mL syrup formulation (Ciba-Geigy, Australia). The two regimens were found to be equally bioavailable although the syrup was absorbed faster and produced higher peak plasma concentrations.

Maas et al[16] found no significant difference in bioavailability (although significant differences in maximum concentrations of carbamazepine in plasma were noted) between a conventional carbamazepine tablet and a chewable tablet formulation (both Ciba-Geigy) in a single-dose, randomised, crossover study involving ten healthy volunteers. Marked inter-subject and intra-subject variation was noted in pharmacokinetic parameters.

The absorption of carbamazepine from a mixture of carbamazepine 20 mg/mL, sorbitol 300 mg/mL, and water (Macrepan, Huhtamäki, Finland) administered to eight healthy volunteers was slower via the rectal route than the oral route.[17] However, bioavailability was similar.

In a randomised, crossover study with twelve healthy volunteers, the bioavailability of carbamazepine from an unflavoured extemporaneously prepared 20 mg/mL suspension (carbamazepine 200 mg tablets, Tegretol, Ciba-Geigy, in a vehicle of syrup, methylcellulose gel, and sodium benzoate) was 94.5% ± 20.4% relative to the bioavailability of the tablets.[18] However, earlier and higher peak concentrations of carbamazepine were produced by the suspension.

Bioequivalence

A study conducted at steady-state in epileptic patients showed that a generic carbamazepine tablet (Ethical Generics, UK) had a similar extent and rate of absorption and equivalent pharmacokinetics to those of the proprietary brand (Tegretol, Ciba-Geigy), although the initial dissolution rate of carbamazepine (in 0.1M hydrochloric acid at 37°) was greater from the generic tablet.[19]

Suspensions

Burckart et al[20] investigated the stability of suspensions of carbamazepine in sorbitol solution (70%), in syrup, and in two hospital suspending vehicles (HUP and HUP-A). The formulae for HUP (modified Hospital of the University of Pennsylvania Suspending Vehicle) and HUP-A (dilute HUP) are as follows:

	HUP	HUP-A
Sucrose	125.0 g	95.0 g
Sorbitol solution (70%)	50.0 mL	40.0 mL
Glycerol	12.5 mL	8.5 mL
Saccharin sodium	250.0 mg	170.0 mg
Methyl hydroxybenzoate	500.0 mg	340.0 mg
Methylcellulose 400	6.9 g	4.7 g
Methylcellulose 4000	3.1 g	2.1 g
FD&C yellow	750.0 mg	510.0 mg
Lemon/lime flavour	1.5 mL	1.0 mL
Purified water to	500.0 mL	500.0 mL

The suspensions (200 mg/5 mL) were made using crushed carbamazepine tablets (Tegretol 200 mg, Ciba-Geigy, USA). Each suspension was packed in amber glass bottles and in unit-dose syringes. The bottles were stored at 4°, 25°, and 37°, and the syringes at 4°; samples prepared using dilute HUP were stored at 4° only. Both chemical and physical stability were assessed. Suspensions prepared using sorbitol solution (70%), syrup, and HUP-A retained at least 90% of their potency over the 90-day test period at all the temperatures studied. Carbamazepine in sorbitol solution (70%) froze when refrigerated but resuspended with vigorous shaking after thawing. The product prepared using syrup separated over 90 days but also resuspended on vigorous shaking. Carbamazepine in HUP was difficult to pour but the product formulated with HUP-A was less viscous and easy to pour; both products were homogeneous. It was concluded that pharmaceutically acceptable suspensions can be obtained using sorbitol solution (70%), syrup, or the HUP-A vehicle. Sorbitol solution (70%), however, is stated to be clinically unacceptable as a vehicle because of its gastro-intestinal side-effects.

Injections

Jain et al[21] formulated an aqueous injection of carbamazepine (3.6 mg/mL) in sodium salicylate 50% w/v. The injection was sterilised by filtration. Results of accelerated stability studies suggested that the injection should be stored at 8° (under refrigeration), although 97.5% of undecomposed carbamazepine remained after 7 weeks at room temperature (23°). At higher temperatures (50° and above) rapid decomposition was observed, manifested by a change of colour to deep yellow.

Further to studies of enhancement of solubility by modified cyclodextrins, Brewster et al[2] developed aqueous parenteral formulations of carbamazepine 10.3 mg/mL, 27.3 mg/mL, and 39.5 mg/mL in 20% w/v, 40% w/v, and 60% w/v hydroxypropyl-β-cyclodextrin, respectively. No significant decomposition of carbamazepine was detected when solutions in glass ampoules were stored at room temperature for 2 months or were autoclaved at 123° for 35 minutes and stored at 4°, room temperature, or 60° for 2 months. Pharmacological and toxicological properties of such solutions were examined following intravenous administration to rats.

Suppositories

The in-vitro dissolution rate (in ethanol at 37°) of carbamazepine from suppositories formulated in a Witepsol H15 basis was enhanced by the addition of each of four surfactants (polyoxyethylene 23-lauryl ether, polyoxyethylene 50-stearate, polysorbate 20, or polysorbate 80) at 0.5%, 2%, or 5%; the dissolution increased from 54% released at 30 minutes (without surfactant) to 100% released at 30 minutes (with 2% polysorbate 80).[22]

Modified-release preparations

Slow release of carbamazepine from granules, prepared by Giunchedi et al,[23] was demonstrated in in-vitro dissolution tests in gastric fluid pH 1.2, and rapid release was demonstrated in intestinal fluid, pH 7.5. The granules contained croscarmellose sodium (Ac-Di-Sol) and one of the following three enteric polymers at 20% or 25% w/w: cellulose acetate trimellitate; cellacephate; or methacrylic acid/methacrylic acid methyl ester copolymer (Eudragit S100). In-vitro release from sustained-release tablets prepared using these granules and tableted with hypromellose was variable, and depended on the type and amount of enteric polymer constituting the granules and the amount of hypromellose present. The same workers had previously demonstrated[24] an enhancement in dissolution rate of carbamazepine in water from carbamazepine:croscarmellose sodium (1:4) systems prepared by physical mixing, solvent evaporation, or a spraying method.

FURTHER INFORMATION. Relationship between systemic drug absorption and gastrointestinal transit after the simultaneous oral administration of carbamazepine as a controlled-release system [Oros osmotic pump] and as a suspension of ^{15}N-labelled drug to healthy volunteers—Wilding IR, Davis SS, Hardy JG, Robertson CS, John VA, Powell ML et al. Br J Clin Pharmacol 1991;32:573–9. Improvement of oral bioavailability of carbamazepine by inclusion in 2-hydroxypropyl-β-cyclodextrin—Choudhury S, Nelson KF. Int J Pharmaceutics 1992;85:175–80. pH dependent zero order release from glassy hydrogels: penetration vs. diffusion control—Shah SS, Kulkarni MG, Mashelkar RA. J Controlled Release 1991;15:121–32.

PROCESSING

Problems may be encountered with carbamazepine tablets prepared by wet granulation if the granules are not thoroughly dried before processing. If any dihydrate is retained in the prepared tablets, it may act as a nucleus for further rehydration when the humidity rises or the tablets come into contact with moisture. This can result in the recrystallisation of the drug throughout the tablet which may affect disintegration properties and possibly absorption. Manufacturing and storage conditions must be well controlled to prevent dihydrate build-up.[25]

Lefebvre *et al*[5] have shown that polymorphic changes can be induced by certain pharmaceutical processes. They investigated the behaviour of the α-form, β-form, and dihydrate form of carbamazepine subjected to compression and grinding conditions. The dihydrate was found to be the most compressible form of carbamazepine. However, X-ray diffraction patterns of the dihydrate indicated that about half of the total concentration was converted to the β-form on compression. The α-form had good compression characteristics although some stickiness was observed. The β-form could not be compressed into tablets. Grinding had little effect on the α-form. The β-form exhibited differences in its differential scanning calorimetry (DSC) curve after grinding, as did the dihydrate. The particular DSC curve obtained with the dihydrate depended on the duration of grinding; water was apparently lost during the grinding process. Loss of water was noted to begin below 30°. See also Crystal and molecular structure, above.

REFERENCES

1. Samaha MW, Gadalla MAF. Drug Dev Ind Pharm 1987;13(1):93–112.
2. Brewster ME, Anderson WR, Estes KS, Bodor N. J Pharm Sci 1991;80(4):380–3.
3. Kahela P, Aaltonen R, Lewing E, Anttila M, Kristoffersson E. Int J Pharmaceutics 1983;14:103–12.
4. Pöhlmann H, Gulde C, Jahn R, Pfeifer S [German]. Pharmazie 1975;30:709–11.
5. Lefebvre C, Guyot-Hermann AM, Draguet-Brughmans M, Bouché R, Guyot JC. Drug Dev Ind Pharm 1986;12:1913–27.
6. Lefebvre C, Guyot-Hermann AM, Draguet-Brughmans M, Bouché R, Guyot JC. In: Rubinstein MH, editor. Pharmaceutical technology: tabletting technology; vol I. Chichester: Ellis Horwood, 1987:166–77.
7. Laine E, Tuominen V, Ilvessalo P, Kahela P. Int J Pharmaceutics 1984;20:307–14.
8. Krahn FU, Mielck JB. Int J Pharmaceutics 1989;53:25–34.
9. Matthews GP, Lowther N, Shott MJ. Int J Pharmaceutics 1989;50:111–15.
10. Am J Hosp Pharm 1990;47:958.
11. Lowes MMJ [letter]. Am J Hosp Pharm 1991;48:2130–1.
12. Lowe DR, Fuller SH, Pesko LJ, Garnett WR, Karnes HT. Am J Hosp Pharm 1989;46:982–4.
13. Clark-Schmidt AL, Garnett WR, Lowe DR, Karnes HT. Am J Hosp Pharm 1990;47:2034–7.
14. Larkin GJA, McLellan A, Munday A, Sutherland M, Butler E, Brodie MJ. Br J Clin Pharmacol 1989;27:313–22.
15. Hooper WD, King AR, Patterson M, Dickinson RG, Eadie MJ. Ther Drug Monit 1985;7:36–40.
16. Maas B, Garnett WR, Pellock JM, Comstock TJ. Ther Drug Monit 1987;9:28–33.
17. Neuvonen PJ, Tokola O. Br J Clin Pharmacol 1987;24:839–41.
18. Bloomer D, Dupuis LL, MacGregor D, Soldin SJ. Clin Pharm 1987;6:646–9.
19. Hartley R, Aleksandrowicz J, Bowmer CJ, Cawood A, Forsythe WI. J Pharm Pharmacol 1991;43:117–19.
20. Burckart GJ, Hammond RW, Akers MJ. Am J Hosp Pharm 1981;38:1929–31.
21. Jain NK, Agrawal RK, Singhai AK. Pharmazie 1990;45:221–2.
22. Fontan JE, Arnaud P, Chaumeil JC. Int J Pharmaceutics 1991;73:17–21.
23. Giunchedi P, Conte U, La Manna A. Drug Dev Ind Pharm 1991;17(13):1753–64.
24. Giunchedi P, Conte U, La Manna A. Boll Chim Farm 1990;129(1):17–20.
25. Stahl PH. In: Breimer DD, editor. Towards better safety of drugs and pharmaceutical products. Amsterdam: Elsevier/North Holland Biomedical Press, 1980:271–4.

Cefotaxime (BAN, rINN)   *Antibacterial*

(*Z*)-7-[2-(2-Amino-1,3-thiazol-4-yl)-2-methoxyiminoacetamido]-cephalosporanic acid; [6*R*-[6α,7β(*Z*)]]-3-[(acetyloxy)methyl]-7-[[(2-amino-4-thiazolyl)(methoxyimino)acetyl]amino]-8-oxo-5-thia-1-azabicyclo[4.2.0]oct-2-ene-2-carboxylic acid
$C_{16}H_{17}N_5O_7S_2 = 455.5$

Cefotaxime Sodium (BANM, USAN, rINNM)
$C_{16}H_{16}N_5NaO_7S_2 = 477.44$
CAS—60846-21-1, 63527-52-6 (cefotaxime); 64485-93-4 (cefotaxime sodium)

Pharmacopoeial status

USP (cefotaxime sodium)

Preparations

Compendial
Cefotaxime Sodium Injection USP. pH 5.0 to 7.5.
Sterile Cefotaxime Sodium USP.

Non-compendial
Claforan (Roussel). *Injection*, powder for reconstitution, cefotaxime (as sodium salt). Vials contain 0.5 g, 1 g, and 2 g. Reconstitute with water for injections to form a straw-coloured solution. Freshly prepared solutions may vary in intensity of colour. When stored under refrigeration, Claforan retains its potency for up to 24 hours when mixed with the following intravenous infusion fluids: water for injections; sodium chloride injection; glucose 5% injection; glucose and sodium chloride injection; or compound sodium lactate injection. Freshly prepared solutions are also compatible with lignocaine 1%.

Containers and storage

Solid state
Cefotaxime Sodium USP should be preserved in tight containers.

Dosage forms
Cefotaxime Sodium Injection USP should be preserved in single-dose containers and maintained in the frozen state.
Sterile Cefotaxime Sodium USP should be preserved in containers suitable for sterile solids.
Claforan (as dry powder) should be protected from light and stored away from heat.

PHYSICAL PROPERTIES

Cefotaxime sodium is a white to slightly cream-coloured, odourless powder.

Melting point

Cefotaxime sodium melts, with decomposition, in the range 162° to 163°.

pH

A 10% solution of *cefotaxime sodium* has a pH value in the range 4.5 to 6.5.

Dissociation constants

The following approximate pK_a values were determined by potentiometric titration of an aqueous solution of cefotaxime sodium (2.8×10^{-3}M) at 20°: pK_{a1}, 2.1 (carboxylic group); pK_{a2}, 3.4 (terminal amino group of side chain at position 7); pK_{a3}, 10.9 (amino group in the α-carbonyl position of side chain at position 7).[1]

Solubility

Cefotaxime sodium is freely soluble in water; slightly soluble in ethanol (95%); insoluble in chloroform.

STABILITY

Solutions

In aqueous solution, cefotaxime sodium decomposes via two parallel reactions that follow pseudo-first-order kinetics: hydrolysis of the acetoxy ester group at the C-3 position and cleavage of the β-lactam ring occur simultaneously. The initial degradation product of hydrolysis is desacetylcefotaxime; under acidic conditions (pH < 4) an internal ring closure within this product results in the formation of desacetylcefotaxime lactone. The β-lactam ring of desacetylcefotaxime is also susceptible to cleavage.[1,2]

Berge *et al*[2] reported the activation energies for the degradation reaction in buffer solutions (35°, ionic strength 0.5) at pH 2.23, 5.52, and 8.94 to be 88.3 kJ/mol, 103.3 kJ/mol, and 39.3 kJ/mol respectively.

The rate constant-pH profile for the degradation of cefotaxime sodium in solution has a characteristic 'U'-shape. Hydrogen ion catalysis occurs in the pH range 1.6 to 3.0 and at pH values greater than 7.0 the reaction is catalysed by hydroxide ions; no pH dependency is apparent within the pH range 3.0 to 7.0.[1] Das Gupta[3] reported that the stability of cefotaxime sodium (1.0 mg/mL) in aqueous solution was optimum in the pH range 4.3 to 6.2 (phosphate buffer).

Inclusion of carbonate (pH 8.5) or borate (pH 9.5 and 10.0) buffer significantly increased the rate of degradation of cefotaxime sodium whereas citrate (pH 2.2 and 3.0) and phosphate (pH 6.0 and 7.5) buffers had no influence on the rate of reaction.[1]

Solutions for peritoneal dialysis

Cefotaxime sodium was stable in peritoneal dialysis solutions that contained either glucose 1.5% or glucose 4.25% during storage at 25° and 37° for 24 hours and 6 hours, respectively.[4]

Intravenous admixtures

Admixtures of cefotaxime sodium 1 g/100 mL (Claforan, Hoechst-Roussel) in either glucose 5% or sodium chloride 0.9% injections stored in plastic bags at 24° and 4° were stable for 24 hours and 22 days, respectively; similar solutions stored at −10° were stable for at least 63 days.[5] A subsequent study by Das Gupta[3] found that the admixtures were stable for at least 112 days at −10° and only 5% degradation was observed after storage for 224 days at that temperature.

Photodegradation

The susceptibility of cefotaxime sodium in aqueous solution to ultraviolet radiation (at 254 nm) was demonstrated by Lerner *et al*;[6] during exposure for 45 minutes and 4 hours, the respective extents of degradation were 50% and about 95%. Two competitive processes were involved in the decomposition reaction. Initially, photo-isomerisation of the methoxy-imino linkage resulted in the formation of the less active anti-isomer of cefotaxime sodium as the main decomposition product. Following exposure for approximately one hour, photolysis of the Δ3-cephem ring was the major decomposition reaction; a corresponding intense yellow coloration of the solution was observed.

FURTHER INFORMATION. Automated liquid chromatography for non-isothermal kinetic studies—Kipp JE, Jensen MM, Kronholm K, McHalsky M. Int J Pharmaceutics 1986;34:1–8.

INCOMPATIBILITY/COMPATIBILITY

Cefotaxime sodium has been reported to be incompatible with alkaline solutions such as those containing sodium bicarbonate. It should be administered separately from aminoglycosides.

Cefotaxime sodium (2 g, Claforan, Hoechst-Roussel) was shown to be compatible with clindamycin phosphate (900 mg, Cleocin, Upjohn) following aseptic transfer into either glass bottles or polyvinyl chloride bags that contained 100 mL of either sodium chloride 0.9% injection or glucose 5% injection, and storage at 24° ± 2° for 24 hours.[7]

Rivers *et al*[8] demonstrated that admixtures of cefotaxime sodium (Claforan, Hoechst-Roussel, USA) and metronidazole (ready-to-use injection, Abbott, USA) at final concentrations of 10 mg/mL and 5 mg/mL, respectively, were stable in glass bottles at 8° for 72 hours.

FORMULATION

Excipients

Excipients that have been used in presentations of cefotaxime sodium include:

Injections: glucose; hydrochloric acid; sodium citrate, hydrated; sodium hydroxide.

REFERENCES

1. Fabre H, Hussam Eddine N, Berge G. J Pharm Sci 1984;73(5):611–18.
2. Berge SM, Henderson NL, Frank MJ. J Pharm Sci 1983;72(1):59–63.
3. Das Gupta V. J Pharm Sci 1984;73(4):565–7.
4. Paap CM, Nahata MC. Am J Hosp Pharm 1990;47:147–50.
5. Das Gupta V, Stewart KR, Gunter JM. Am J IV Ther Clin Nutr 1983;10:20–9.
6. Lerner DA, Bonnefond G, Fabre H, Mandrou B, Simeon de Buochberg M. J Pharm Sci 1988;77(8):699–703.
7. Foley PT, Bosso JA, Bair JN, Townsend RJ. Am J Hosp Pharm 1985;42:839–43.
8. Rivers TE, McBride HA, Trang JM. Am J Hosp Pharm 1991;48:2638–40.

Cefuroxime (BAN, USAN, rINN)   *Antibacterial*

(Z)-3-Carbamoyloxymethyl-7-[2-(2-furyl)-2-methoxyimino-acetamidol]-3-cephem-4-carboxylic acid
$C_{16}H_{16}N_4O_8S = 424.4$

Cefuroxime Axetil (BANM, USAN, rINNM)
$C_{20}H_{22}N_4O_{10}S = 510.5$

Cefuroxime Pivoxetil (BANM, USAN, rINNM)
$C_{23}H_{28}N_4O_{11}S = 568.6$

Cefuroxime Sodium (BANM, rINNM)
$C_{16}H_{15}N_4NaO_8S = 446.4$
CAS—55268-75-2 (cefuroxime); 64544-07-6 (cefuroxime axetil); 100680-33-9 (cefuroxime pivoxetil); 56238-63-2 (cefuroxime sodium)

Pharmacopoeial status

USP (cefuroxime sodium)

Preparations

Compendial
Sterile Cefuroxime Sodium USP. Cefuroxime sodium suitable for parenteral use.
Cefuroxime Sodium Injection USP. pH 5.0 to 7.5.

Non-compendial
Zinacef (Glaxo). *Injection*, powder for reconstitution with water for injections, cefuroxime (as sodium salt). *Diluents*: sodium chloride 0.9% injection, glucose 5% injection, sodium chloride 0.18% plus glucose 4% injection, compound sodium lactate injection, 5% xylitol injection. Should not be mixed in the syringe with aminoglycoside antibiotics or diluted with 2.74% w/v sodium bicarbonate injection.
Zinnat (Glaxo). *Tablets*, cefuroxime (as cefuroxime axetil) 125 mg and 250 mg. The manufacturer states that Zinnat tablets should not be crushed.
Suspension, cefuroxime (as cefuroxime axetil) 125 mg/5 mL when reconstituted with water.
Sachets, cefuroxime (as cefuroxime axetil) 125 mg/sachet. The constituted suspension should be used immediately.

Containers and storage

Solid state
Cefuroxime Sodium USP should be preserved in tight containers.

Dosage forms
Sterile Cefuroxime Sodium USP should be preserved in containers suitable for sterile solids.
Cefuroxime Sodium Injection USP should be preserved in containers suitable for injections and should be maintained in the frozen state.
Zinacef injection should be protected from light. It is preferable to use freshly prepared solutions or suspensions but diluted solutions or suspensions may be stored in a refrigerator (2° to 8°) for up to 24 hours.
Zinnat tablets should be stored below 30°.

Zinnat suspension granules (in multidose bottles) should be stored below 25°, preferably in a refrigerator. The constituted suspension (in multidose bottles) for up to 10 days when stored below 25°.

PHYSICAL PROPERTIES

Cefuroxime is a white, crystalline solid.
Cefuroxime sodium is a white to faintly yellow powder.

pH

The pH of a 10% solution of *cefuroxime sodium* in water is in the range 6.0 to 8.5.

Dissociation constant

pK_a about 2.5

Solubility

Sterile *cefuroxime sodium* is soluble in water; sparingly soluble in ethanol; insoluble in chloroform, in toluene, in ether, in ethyl acetate, and in acetone.

STABILITY

Unbuffered aqueous solutions of cefuroxime sodium are stable for about 12 hours at room temperature, but about 15% decomposition occurs after 24 hours. Liquids may darken or become yellowish on storage.
Maximum stability of cefuroxime sodium in aqueous solution was observed[2] in the pH range 4.5 to 7.3. Both unbuffered and buffered solutions followed first-order decomposition in clear glass containers; the rate of decomposition was unaffected by ionic strength. In glucose 5% injection and sodium chloride 0.9% injection, cefuroxime sodium (0.5% and 1% w/v) was stable in Viaflex bags and in clear glass bottles for one day at 25° and for at least 30 days at 5°. At −10° there was negligible decomposition after 30 days. Thawing the frozen solutions in a microwave oven caused the development of an orange colour in the solutions and a considerable reduction in potency.
Reconstituted cefuroxime sodium injection (750 mg and 1.5 g) was added to 50-mL polyvinyl chloride minibags of sodium chloride 0.9% injection and glucose 5% injection, and stored protected from light.[3] For both concentrations $t_{10\%}$ was 20 days and 24 hours at 4° and 25°, respectively, in both infusion solutions.
Cefuroxime axetil suspensions (10 mg/mL, from crushed tablets) in three vehicles containing sucrose were stable for at least 28 days at 5° in amber bottles. There was no change in either pH or physical appearance.[1] However, it should be noted that the manufacturer of Zinnat tablets (Glaxo) recommends that tablets should not be crushed.
During storage for 24 hours, maximum losses of cefuroxime (0.5% w/v as the sodium salt) of 10% at 25° and 2% at 4° were demonstrated (no physical deterioration) in seven commonly used parenteral fluids: sodium chloride 0.9% injection; glucose 5% injection; sodium chloride 0.18% and glucose 4% injection; compound sodium lactate injection; dextran 40; dextran 70; intraperitoneal dialysis fluid (lactate).[6] A reduction in potency of approximately 15% and significant yellowing of the solution were observed when cefuroxime sodium was admixed with 2.74% w/v sodium bicarbonate injection.

FURTHER INFORMATION. Penicillins and cephalosporins. Physicochemical properties and analysis in pharmaceutical and biological matrices [review of stability, degradation routes and analysis]—Van Krimpen PC, Van Bennekom WP, Bult A. Pharm Weekbl (Sci) 1987;9:1–23. Particulate matter content of

11 cephalosporin injections: conformance with USP limits—Parkins DA, Taylor AJ. Am J Hosp Pharm 1987;44:1111–18. Relationship of diastereomer hydrolysis kinetics to shelf-life predictions for cefuroxime axetil—Nguyen NA. Pharm Res 1991;8:893–8. Stability of ceftazidime (with arginine) and of cefuroxime sodium in infusion-pump reservoirs—Stiles ML, Allen LV, Fox JL. Am J Hosp Pharm 1992;49:2761–4.

INCOMPATIBILITY/COMPATIBILITY

Cefuroxime sodium injection should not be mixed with sodium bicarbonate injection or aminoglycosides.

At 25°, cefuroxime sodium 750 mg in 10 mL of water for injection (Zinacef injection, Glaxo) in metronidazole injection (500 mg in 100-mL polyvinyl chloride infusion bags) degraded by first-order kinetics (rate constant 7.04×10^{-2} per day) but at 4° the kinetics approximated to zero-order over the 20-day study period. The physical appearance of the admixture changed only at 25° with intensification throughout the study period of a yellow discoloration of the solution. The $t_{10\%}$ values at 25° and 4° were 36 hours and 20 days, respectively. At 4°, the admixture was given a 7-day shelf-life.

Cefuroxime sodium 1.5 g reconstituted with 15 mL of water for injections was reported to be stable in admixture with azlocillin (1 g/15 mL) during a period of 24 hours in a refrigerator, azlocillin (5 g/50 mL) during a period of 6 hours below 25°, and metronidazole (500 mg/100 mL) during 24 hours below 25°.[5] Compatibility with lignocaine 1% was also reported.

FORMULATION

Excipients

Excipients that have been used in presentations of cefuroxime include:

Tablets, cefuroxime axetil: colloidal silica; croscarmellose sodium; hydrogenated vegetable oil; hypromellose; methyl and propyl hydroxybenzoates; microcrystalline cellulose; propylene glycol; sodium lauryl sulphate.

Bioavailability

When 24 healthy volunteers were given single oral doses of cefuroxime axetil 1 g in a comparison of its bioavailability with that of intravenous cefuroxime (as the sodium salt), mean absolute bioavailability in male and female subjects (in the fasting state) was 0.35 and 0.32, respectively, and (in the non-fasting state) 0.45 and 0.41, respectively.[7]

Eye drops

The stability of several formulations of cefuroxime eye drops, prepared using cefuroxime sodium powder for injection (Zinacef, Glaxo) was investigated by HPLC.[8] A simple aqueous solution (pH about 7.5, without preservative) containing the equivalent of 5% cefuroxime, in low density polyethylene bottles, remained stable for 21 days in a refrigerator at 2°, but for only 24 hours at room temperature. Degradation was shown by a darkening of the solution. Buffering of the solution within the pH range 6.0 to 7.3 had little effect on stability. Storage at −30° for 12 months resulted in a negligible loss of potency; solutions thawed at room temperature were stable for a further 21 days at 2° and for 14 days at 8°. Cefuroxime eye drops were less stable in low density polyethylene bottles than in amber glass bottles.

FURTHER INFORMATION. Review of the new second-generation cephalosporins: cefonicid, ceforanide, and cefuroxime—Tartaglione TA, Polk RE. Drug Intell Clin Pharm 1985;19(3):188–98.

REFERENCES

1. Pramar Y, Das Gupta V, Bethea C, Zerai T. J Clin Pharm Ther 1991;16:341–4.
2. Das Gupta V, Stewart KR. J Clin Pharm Ther 1986;11:47–54.
3. Small D. Pharm J 1992;248:HS40.
4. Barnes AR. J Clin Pharm Ther 1990;15:187–96.
5. Fletcher NR, Fletcher P, Yates RJ. Br J Pharm Pract 1988;10:442, 444, 448, 453.
6. Hartley MJ, Coomber PA, Andrews GD, Wallis T. Pharm J 1978;221:288–90.
7. Williams PEO, Harding SM. J Antimicrob Chemother 1984;13:191–6.
8. Oldham GB. Int J Pharm Pract 1991;1:19–22.

Cephalexin (BAN, USAN)   *Antibacterial*

Cefalexin (pINN)
7-α-D-Phenylglycylamino-3-methyl-3-cephem-4-carboxylic acid monohydrate;   (7R)-3-methyl-7-(α-D-phenylglycylamino)-3-cephem-4-carboxylic acid monohydrate
$C_{16}H_{17}N_3O_4S, H_2O = 365.4$ (monohydrate)
$C_{16}H_{17}N_3O_4S = 347.4$ (anhydrous)

Cephalexin Hydrochloride (BANM, USAN)
Cefalexin Hydrochloride (pINNM)
$C_{16}H_{17}N_3O_4S, HCl, H_2O = 401.9$
CAS—23325-78-2 (cephalexin, monohydrate); 15686-71-2 (cephalexin, anhydrous); 105879-42-3 (cephalexin hydrochloride)

Pharmacopoeial status

BP (cephalexin); USP (cephalexin, cephalexin hydrochloride)

Preparations

Compendial
Cephalexin Capsules BP. Capsules containing, in each, the equivalent of 250 mg and 500 mg of anhydrous cephalexin are usually available.
Cephalexin Tablets BP. Tablets containing, in each, the equivalent of 250 mg and 500 mg of anhydrous cephalexin are usually available.
Cephalexin Oral Suspension BP (Cephalexin Mixture). A suspension of cephalexin in a suitable flavoured vehicle. It is prepared by dispersion of the dry ingredients in the specified volume of water just before issue for use. If the oral suspension is diluted, it should be freshly prepared.
Cephalexin Capsules USP.
Cephalexin Tablets USP. Contain cephalexin or cephalexin hydrochloride.
Cephalexin for Oral Suspension USP.

Non-compendial
Ceporex (Glaxo). *Capsules*, cephalexin 250 mg and 500 mg.
Tablets, cephalexin 250 mg, 500 mg, and 1 g.
Syrup, prepared by reconstitution of cephalexin granules with water, giving a suspension containing 125 mg, 250 mg, or

500 mg in each 5 mL. *Diluent:* water, life of diluted syrup 7 days.
Paediatric drops, reconstituted with water to give 10 mL suspension containing 125 mg cephalexin in 1.25 mL.
Suspension, ready-prepared, suspension in vegetable oil, containing 125 mg or 250 mg cephalexin in 5 mL. The suspension must not be diluted with water or syrup.
Keflex (Lilly). *Capsules,* cephalexin 250 mg and 500 mg.
Tablets, cephalexin 250 mg and 500 mg.
Suspension, granules for reconstitution with water, cephalexin 125 mg/5 mL or 250 mg/5 mL. Where dilution is unavoidable, syrup should be used after the suspension has been prepared according to the manufacturer's instructions.

Containers and storage

Solid state

Cephalexin BP should be kept in a well-closed container, protected from light and stored at a temperature not exceeding 30°.
Cephalexin USP and Cephalexin Hydrochloride USP should be preserved in tight containers.

Dosage forms

All BP Cephalexin preparations should be stored at a temperature not exceeding 30°.
The dry ingredients of Cephalexin Oral Suspension BP should be kept in a well-closed container and protected from light.
All USP Cephalexin preparations should be preserved in tight containers.
Ceporex tablets and capsules should be protected from light. Ceporex suspension should not be refrigerated. Reconstituted Ceporex syrups retain their potency for 10 days when kept in a cool place, preferably a refrigerator.
Keflex tablets and capsules should be kept in tightly closed containers. After mixing, Keflex suspensions should be stored in a cool place (6° to 15°) or in a refrigerator (2° to 8°) and be used within 10 days.

PHYSICAL PROPERTIES

Cephalexin is a white to almost white, slightly hygroscopic crystalline powder.
Cephalexin hydrochloride is a white to almost white crystalline powder.

pH

The BP states that the pH of a 0.5% w/v aqueous solution of *cephalexin* is in the range 4.0 to 5.5.
The USP states that the pH of a 5% aqueous suspension of *cephalexin* lies between 3.0 and 5.5, and that the pH of a 1% solution of *cephalexin hydrochloride* lies between 1.5 and 3.0.

Dissociation constants

In 66% dimethylformamide, pK_a values of 5.2 (carboxyl group) and 7.3 (amine group) have been recorded.
Tsuji *et al*[1] reported pK_a values for cephalexin monohydrate, at 37° and ionic strength 0.5 in aqueous solution, of 2.67 (4-carboxylic acid) and 6.96 (7/α ammonium chain).
Yamana and Tsuji[2] determined pK_a values of 2.56 and 6.88 in aqueous solution at 35° and ionic strength 0.5.

FURTHER INFORMATION. Ionisation constants of cephalosporin zwitterionic compounds—Streng WH, Huber HE, De Young JL, Zoglio MA. J Pharm Sci 1976;65:1034–8.

Partition coefficients

Log P (octanol), 0.65, −0.85

FURTHER INFORMATION. l-Octanol-water partition coefficients of the anionic and zwitterionic species of diprotic zwitterionic cephalosporin antibiotics [effect of pH].—Irwin VP, Quigley JM, Timoney RF. Int J Pharmaceutics 1988;43:187–8.

Solubility

Cephalexin is slightly soluble in water (1 in 100) and practically insoluble in ethanol, in chloroform, and in ether; it is soluble in 30 parts of dilute hydrochloric acid (0.2% w/v).
Cephalexin hydrochloride is soluble to the extent of 1% w/v in water, in ethanol, in acetone, in dimethylformamide, and in methanol; practically insoluble in chloroform, in ether, in ethyl acetate, and in isopropanol.
Workers in Japan[1] determined the solubilities of several aminocephalosporins in aqueous solution as a function of pH at 37° and ionic strength 0.5. The intrinsic solubility of cephalexin monohydrate was 17.2 mg/mL at isoelectric pH.

Effect of pH

The solubility-pH profile of cephalexin in water at 37° is a U-shaped curve with values ranging from 120 mg/mL at pH 2.3, 12 mg/mL at pH 5.0, and 100 mg/mL at pH 8.2.

FURTHER INFORMATION. Solubility of cephalexin crystals—Otsuka M, Kaneniwa N [Japanese]. Yakugaku Zasshi 1982;102(10):967–71.

Dissolution

The USP specifies that for Cephalexin Capsules USP and Cephalexin Tablets USP not less than 75% of the labelled amount of $C_{16}H_{17}N_3O_4S$ is dissolved in 45 minutes. Dissolution medium: 900 mL of water; Apparatus 1 at 100 rpm (for the Capsules and where the Tablets contain cephalexin) or Apparatus 1 at 150 rpm (where the Tablets contain cephalexin hydrochloride).

Crystal and molecular structure

Enantiomers

The D-isomer of cephalexin exhibits more biological activity than the L-isomer.

Crystal forms

Cephalexin occurs in a wide range of solvated crystal forms as discussed by Pfeiffer *et al*;[3] using solubility versus solvent composition diagrams. Other factors that influence the extent of crystal formation and stability are relative humidity and vapour pressure. At room temperature, cephalexin crystallises from aqueous solutions as the dihydrate but converts to the monohydrate when relative humidity is below 70%.

FURTHER INFORMATION. Stereospecific absorption and degradation of cephalexin [in *rat* intestine]—Tamai I, Ling H-Y, Timbul S-M, Nishikido J, Tsuji A. J Pharm Pharmacol 1988;40:320–4.

STABILITY

Aqueous solutions and suspensions of cephalexin degrade rapidly in neutral or alkaline systems; under acidic conditions they are stable for several days if refrigerated. Stability is optimal at pH 4.5.
In aqueous solution degradation of cephalexin occurs by simultaneous hydroxide ion-catalysed β-lactam hydrolysis and intramolecular aminolysis by the C-7 side chain amino group on the β-lactam moieties.[4] The ratio of these reactions is affected by pH. The primary degradation product at 35° is a piperazine-2,5-dione. The reaction is both specific base and general acid-base catalysed.

Further decomposition of the primary degradation product in neutral aqueous solution results in formation of 3-aminomethylene-6-phenyl-piperazine-2,5-dione and 3-hydroxy-4-methyl-2(5H) thiophenone. Degradation kinetics were also studied.[5] Cephalexin is degraded by strong acids and alkalis, ultraviolet light, and β-lactamase (cephalosporinase) produced by some bacteria.

Effect of pH

At 25°, no loss of cephalexin activity occurred over 72 hours in the pH range 3.0 to 5.0, but at pH 6.0 and 7.0 the rate of degradation was 3% and 18% per day, respectively. Under refrigeration no appreciable loss had occurred after 72 hours over the pH range 3.0 to 7.0.

At 37° in USP hydrochloric acid buffer (pH 1.2) and in phosphate buffer (pH 6.5) cephalexin lost 5% and 45% of its initial activity, respectively, in 24 hours.

In a study of the comparative stability of six cephalosporins by Yamana and Tsuji[2] the rate-pH profile of cephalexin was determined at 35°, ionic strength 0.5. Rate constants for cephalexin were pH-independent below pH 5.0.

Effect of additives

An analysis of the effect of several additives on the stability of cephalexin at pH 6.5, 37° and ionic strength 0.25 led Yasuhara et al[6] to conclude that degradation was 'protected' in the presence of anionic surfactants (such as sodium lauryl sulphate) and enhanced by cationic surfactants (such as hexadecyltrimethylammonium bromide [CTAB] or benzalkonium chloride) above their critical micelle concentration. The pseudo-first-order rate constant for cephalexin degradation was 0.045/h in the absence of surfactant, 0.6482/h in the presence of cationic CTAB (20 mM), and 0.0317/h in the presence of anionic sodium lauryl sulphate (20 mM). Calculated activation energies in the presence and absence of CTAB were 75 kJ/mol and 79 kJ/mol, respectively. The effect of CTAB was reduced when the ionic strength was increased.

Effect of temperature and repackaging

The chemical stability of reconstituted cephalexin monohydrate suspension (either stored in original containers or repackaged into polypropylene syringes) was examined by American workers[7] over the temperature range −20° to 80°. Significant first-order degradation was observed at 40°, 60°, and 80° after 3 days, 4 hours, and 1 hour, respectively; less than 10% degradation occurred at −20°, 4°, and 25° in either container over the 90-day study period. Cephalexin monohydrate suspension was chemically stable in both original and polypropylene containers under ambient, refrigerated, and frozen storage conditions.

Photochemical effects

Samples of cephalexin monohydrate suspension (2.5% in liquid paraffin) were packaged in amber bottles and kept in artificial light (60.3 to 62.4 kilolux) at room temperature (19° to 21°) for 30 days.[8] Photochemical degradation followed first-order kinetics with predicted $t_{50\%}$ of 259 days and 305 days, identified by microbiological and spectrophotometric methods, respectively.

FURTHER INFORMATION. Penicillins and cephalosporins—Physicochemical properties and analysis in pharmaceutical and biological matrices [comprehensive review]—Van Krimpen PC, Van Bennekom WP, Bult A. Pharm Weekbl(Sci)1987;9:1–23. A comparison of the stability of commercial cephradine and cephalexin capsules—Conine JW, Johnson DW, Coleman DL. Curr Ther Res 1978;24(8):967–79.

FORMULATION

Excipients

Excipients that have been used in presentations of cephalexin monohydrate include:

Capsules: brilliant blue (133); erythrosine (E127); FD&C Yellow 10; gelatin; iron oxide—black (E172); magnesium stearate; microcrystalline cellulose; quinoline yellow (E104); silica; sodium lauryl sulphate; starch; sunset yellow FCF (E110); talc; titanium dioxide (E171).

Tablets: allura red AC (E129); brilliant blue FCF (133); hypromellose; magnesium stearate; maize starch; microcrystalline cellulose; povidone; quinoline yellow (E104); sodium benzoate; stearic acid; sunset yellow FCF (E110); titanium dioxide (E171).

Suspensions: allura red AC (E129); methylcellulose; silicone; sodium lauryl sulphate; sucrose; sunset yellow FCF (E110).

Granules (for reconstitution): citric acid, anhydrous; erythrosine (E127); sodium citrate; sucrose; sunset yellow FCF (E110); vanillin.

Bioavailability

A crossover study by Finkelstein et al[9] involving nine healthy volunteers who received cephalexin tablets (1 g) and capsules (500 mg) in 5 oral doses over 24 hours indicated that the pharmacokinetics of the two products were equivalent.

Oral liquids

Formation of 'ordered mixtures' between several antibiotics (including cephalexin monohydrate) and sorbitol (instant or crystalline) was assessed in a study preliminary to the formulation of a sucrose-free dry powder for reconstitution.[10] The adsorption capacity and binding strength of instant sorbitol were greater than those of crystalline sorbitol. Adsorption of cephalexin monohydrate was assumed to occur at sites on the surface of sorbitol particles.

Modified-release preparations

Studies undertaken by Spanish workers[11] who compared 3 different 'punch pressures' during production of cephalexin tablets containing 10% Eudragit RS indicated that drug release was controlled by diffusion through matrix pores. Total porosity, identified as the chief variable governing cephalexin release from the matrices studied, was inversely related to punch pressure during tablet production. A comparison of the bioavailability of the tablet formulations with each other and with that of a capsule was reported to show that the proportion of the dose absorbed decreased with increasing punch pressure.

FURTHER INFORMATION. A bioequivalence study of six brands of cephalexin ['bioequivalence' of tablets and capsules]—Suleiman MS, Najib NM, El-Sayed YM, Abdulhameed ME. J Clin Pharm Ther 1988;13:65–72. Bioavailability of cephalexine dosage forms [no significant differences in extent of absorption of tablets, capsules, and suspension when compared to that of a solution]—Jung H, Perez R, Hernandez L, Fuentes I, Rodriguez JM. Drug Dev Ind Pharm 1991;17(16):2173–83. Percutaneous diffusion of cephalexin, sulfamethoxazole and diphenhydramine from ointments [through *mouse* skin]—Ezzedeen FW, Shihab FA, Husain EJ. Pharmazie 1990;45:512–14.

REFERENCES

1. Tsuji A, Nakashima E, Yamana T. J Pharm Sci 1979;68(3):308–11.
2. Yamana T, Tsuji A. J Pharm Sci 1976;65(11):1563–74.

3. Pfeiffer RR, Yang KS, Tucker MA. J Pharm Sci 1970;59(12):1809–15.
4. Bundgaard H. Arch Pharm Chemi Sci 1976(4):25–43.
5. Bundgaard H. Arch Pharm Chemi Sci 1977(5):149–55.
6. Yasuhara M, Sato F, Kimura T, Muranishi S, Sezaki H. J Pharm Pharmacol 1977;29:638–40.
7. Sylvestri MF, Makoid MC, Cox BE. Am J Hosp Pharm 1988;45:1353–6.
8. de Oliveira AG, Petrovick PR [Portuguese]. Rev Cienc Farm 1984;6:63–6.
9. Finkelstein F, Quintiliani R, Lee R, Bracci A, Nightingale CH. J Pharm Sci 1978;67(10):1447–50.
10. Nikolakakis I, Newton JM. J Pharm Pharmacol 1989;41:145–8.
11. Martinez-Pacheco R, Vila-Jato JL, Conchiero A, Souto C, Losa CM, Ramos T. Int J Pharmaceutics 1988;47:37–42.

Chloral Hydrate (BAN)

Hypnotic

Chloral
2,2,2-Trichloroethane-1,1-diol
$C_2H_3Cl_3O_2 = 165.4$
CAS—302-17-0

Pharmacopoeial status

BP, USP

Preparations

Compendial
Chloral Mixture BP (Chloral Oral Solution; Chloral Hydrate Mixture). A solution containing 10% w/v of chloral hydrate in a suitable vehicle. For extemporaneous preparation see Formulation, below.
Paediatric Chloral Elixir BP (Paediatric Chloral Oral Solution). A solution containing 4% w/v of chloral hydrate in a suitable vehicle with a blackcurrant flavour. For extemporaneous preparation see Formulation, below.
Chloral Hydrate Capsules USP.
Chloral Hydrate Syrup USP.

Non-compendial
Noctec (Squibb). *Capsules*, chloral hydrate 500 mg in solution.
Welldorm (S&N Pharm). *Tablets*, chloral betaine 707 mg (equivalent to chloral hydrate 414 mg).
Elixir, chloral hydrate 143 mg/5 mL. *Diluent*: syrup.

Containers and storage

Solid state
Chloral Hydrate BP should be stored in airtight containers.
Chloral Hydrate USP should be preserved in tight containers.

Dosage forms
Chloral Hydrate Capsules USP should be preserved in tight containers, preferably at controlled room temperature.
Chloral Hydrate Syrup USP should be preserved in tight, light-resistant containers.
Noctec capsules should be stored in a cool place; avoid freezing.
Welldorm tablets should be stored in a dry place below 25°.
Welldorm elixir should be stored in a well-stoppered bottle away from direct sunlight.

PHYSICAL PROPERTIES

Chloral hydrate exists as colourless, transparent or white crystals with an aromatic pungent odour and a bitter caustic taste.

Melting point

Chloral hydrate melts at about 55°.

pH

pH of a 10% solution of *chloral hydrate* in carbon dioxide-free water, 3.5 to 5.5.

Dissociation constant

pK_a 10.0

Partition coefficient

Log P (octanol), 0.6

Solubility

At 20° (BP), *chloral hydrate* is soluble 1 in 0.3 of water, 1 in 0.2 of ethanol, 1 in 3 of chloroform; freely soluble in ether.
At 25° (USP), *chloral hydrate* is soluble 1 in 0.25 of water, 1 in 1.3 of ethanol, 1 in 2 of chloroform, 1 in 1.5 of ether; very soluble in olive oil.
Ethanolic solutions may deposit crystals of chloral ethanolate.
Chloral hydrate is soluble in fixed and volatile oils.

Effect of temperature
The solubility of chloral hydrate in water has been reported to increase from 2.4 g/mL at 0°, to 8.3 g/mL at 25°, and to 14.3 g/mL at 40°.

Crystal and molecular structure

Polymorphs
Biedenkapp and Weiss[1] reported the existence of two crystal modifications of chloral hydrate, only one of which is stable at room temperature. Using differential thermal analysis, Ogawa[2] found that the crystal structure of chloral hydrate transformed on heating to a form that melts between 55.0° and 64.5°.

STABILITY

Chloral hydrate volatilises slowly in air as chloral ('anhydrous chloral') and water which, on condensation, revert to chloral hydrate. In an airtight container volatilisation ceases as soon as the vapour pressure has reached equilibrium.
After melting at about 55°, chloral hydrate boils at 98° with dissociation into water and trichloroacetaldehyde.
In the presence of excess free oxygen, and after a considerable lag-phase, chloral hydrate degrades to form phosgene, carbon dioxide, and hydrochloric acid. A solid polymer, thought to be metachloral, is also formed. In the absence of oxygen, chloral hydrate does not degrade significantly in the presence of sunlight.
'Anhydrous chloral' undergoes autoxidation in air to trichloroacetic acid, dichloroacetaldehyde, carbon dioxide, and hydrochloric acid; light appears to be necessary to initiate the reaction.
At pH 7, chloral hydrate in solution degrades by an oxidation-reduction process to form dichloroacetaldehyde, trichloroacetic acid, and hydrochloric acid. Under normal storage conditions, decomposition is slow but the rate is greatly accelerated by exposure to ultraviolet light.[3] The application of heat to neutral or slightly acid solutions also results in decomposition by the same process.
Strong sulphuric acid polymerises chloral to α-parachloral and β-parachloral whereas in more dilute acid, amorphous metachloral is produced. Chloral hydrate decomposes in alkaline solution to yield chloroform and formate ions. It may also be degraded by the action of micro-organisms, by high energy ultrasound, and by exposure to irradiation with X-rays, γ-rays or β-rays.

Aqueous solutions of chloral hydrate are susceptible to the development of mould growth.

INCOMPATIBILITY/COMPATIBILITY

Chloral hydrate forms molecular complexes or adducts with acetone, alcohols, caffeine, diazepam, ether, glucose, oxytetracycline, phenacetin, tetracyline, and urea. Because of its acidity in aqueous solution, it is incompatible with most bases and substances that bear hydroxyl groups.

Other incompatible compounds include: alkali carbonates, arachis oil, soluble barbiturates, borax, calcium phosphate, castor oil, cetomacrogol 1000, glucose, soluble iodides, lactose, macrogols, maize oil, mannitol, olive oil, permanganates, peroxides, piperidine, sesame oil, sodium phosphate, stearic acid, sucrose, tannin, hydrous wool fat.

A liquid or soft mass forms when chloral hydrate is triturated with a number of compounds; for example, camphor, menthol, phenol, thymol, quinine salts, theobromine, sodium salicylate, salol, phenazone, urea, and urethane.

FORMULATION

CHLORAL MIXTURE BP

Chloral hydrate	100 g
Syrup	200 mL
Water sufficient to produce	1000 mL

The mixture should be recently prepared.

Antimicrobial activity
In the above mixture the pH is relatively low (3.45) and the concentration of dissolved solids (approximately 27%) is high; a low potential for microbial proliferation could therefore be expected. However, the growth of moulds cannot be precluded. When samples of this BP mixture were submitted to microbial challenge tests similar to the test protocol of the USP XIX they were found to be rapidly bactericidal and sporicidal.[4] There was no marked difference between unpreserved samples and samples which contained benzoic acid 0.1% (as the BPC solution).

Compatibility with preservatives
From studies of samples of chloral mixture with each of three preservative systems (mixtures of methyl and propyl hydroxybenzoate 8:2, 0.2%; benzoic acid 0.1%, as the BPC solution; and sorbic acid 0.2%, as the potassium salt 0.268%) it was concluded that the most suitable, on the grounds of physical and chemical stability, was benzoic acid 0.1%.[5]

Stability
In a comparison of the stability of Chloral Mixture BPC (1973) with that of a similar mixture containing benzoic acid 0.1% over 48 weeks at 25° in the dark there were negligible losses of chloral hydrate in both mixtures although the pH fell from the initial values.[6]

PAEDIATRIC CHLORAL MIXTURE BP

Chloral hydrate	40 g
Water	20 mL
Blackcurrant syrup	200 mL
Syrup sufficient to produce	1000 mL

It should be recently prepared as follows: dissolve the chloral hydrate in the water, add the blackcurrant syrup and add sufficient syrup to produce 1000 mL and mix.

Excipients

Excipients that have been used in presentations of chloral hydrate include:
Capsules: erythrosine (E127); macrogol; methyl and propyl hydroxybenzoates; quinoline yellow (E104).
Oral liquids: anise water, concentrated; chloroform spirit; chloroform water, concentrated; citric acid monohydrate; glycerol; methyl and propyl hydroxybenzoates; propylene glycol; saccharin sodium; theobroma oil; syrups (blackcurrant, orange, raspberry).
Suppositories: theobroma oil.

Flavouring

Flavours that have been used to mask the taste of chloral hydrate in liquid medicines include peppermint, liquorice, blackcurrant, orange, and raspberry.

Bioavailability

Simpson and Parrott[7] studied the oral and rectal bioavailability of a 1:1 complex of chloral hydrate and betaine; the complex was demonstrated in a previous study to reduce the bitter taste and gastric irritation of the hypnotic. After oral administration to 9 healthy subjects no significant difference in absorption was observed between chloral hydrate and chloral betaine complex; similarly, no difference in absorption of these compounds was observed after rectal administration.[7] However, a significant difference in absorption was observed between oral and rectal administration of chloral hydrate and between oral and rectal administration of chloral betaine complex.

Suppositories

Chloral hydrate displacement value = 1.5 (fatty basis)
The formulation of chloral hydrate suppositories poses many problems, several of which were discussed by Schumacher.[8] Chloral hydrate liquefies many hydrophilic bases and softens certain fatty bases such as theobroma oil. Suppositories that have been toughened with a high melting point ingredient, however, often have a brittle consistency and they frequently crack and crumble. Several formulae for suppository production based on self-emulsifying glyceryl monostearate and propylene glycol monostearate are reported.
It has been stated that an unsatisfactory product is produced when theobroma oil is used as the sole basis.[9]
Del Pozo and Cemeli[10] found that 20% chloral hydrate incorporated in Witepsol H15 had only a slight effect on the melting and solidification temperatures of the basis.

FURTHER INFORMATION. [Disintegration *in vitro* of capsules containing chloral hydrate and dissolution rate of chloral hydrate]—Cox HLM, Breimer DD, Freeke G [Dutch]. Pharm Weekbl 1974;109:1018–26.

REFERENCES

1. Biedenkapp D, Weiss A. Z Naturforsch 1967;22a:1124–6.
2. Ogawa K. Bull Chem Soc Jpn 1963;36:610–16.
3. Danckwortt PW [German]. Arch Pharm 1942;280:197–212.
4. *PSGB Lab Report DPS P/78/3* 1978.
5. *PSGB Lab Report DPS P/77/14* 1977.
6. *PSGB Lab Report DPS P/78/6* 1978.
7. Simpson M, Parrott EL. J Pharm Sci 1980;69:227–8.
8. Schumacher GE. Am J Hosp Pharm 1966;23:110.
9. The Pharmaceutical Society of Australia. Australian pharmaceutical formulary and handbook. 14th ed. Deakin: The Society, 1988:433.
10. Del Pozo A, Cemeli J. J Galenica Acta 1954;7:137–55.

Chlorambucil (BAN, rINN)   *Cytotoxic*

4-[4-Bis(2-chloroethyl)aminophenyl]butyric acid; 4-[bis(2-chloroethyl)amino]-benzenebutanoic acid; 4-[*p*-[bis(2-chloroethyl)-amino]phenyl]butyric acid
$C_{14}H_{19}Cl_2NO_2 = 304.2$
CAS—305-03-3

Pharmacopoeial status

BP, USP

Preparations

Compendial
Chlorambucil Tablets BP. Tablets containing, in each, 2 mg and 5 mg are usually available. They are coated.
Chlorambucil Tablets USP.

Non-compendial
Leukeran (Wellcome). *Tablets*, chlorambucil 2 mg and 5 mg.

Containers and storage

Solid state
Chlorambucil BP should be kept in well-closed containers and protected from light.
Chlorambucil USP should be preserved in tight, light-resistant containers.

Dosage forms
Chlorambucil Tablets USP should be preserved in well-closed containers; uncoated tablets should be preserved in light-resistant containers.
Leukeran tablets should be stored at 2° to 8° in a dry place.

PHYSICAL PROPERTIES

Chlorambucil is a white crystalline powder or an off-white, slightly granular powder.

Melting point

Chlorambucil melts in the range 64° to 69°.

Dissociation constants

In aqueous solution in the pH range 1.5 to 10, the amino and carboxylic acid groups of chlorambucil are ionised to varying degrees; the compound also exists in the undissociated state and as a zwitterion.

Basic (nitrogen mustard) group
Between pH 5 and pH 10, the amino group is unionised. Below pH 5 protonation of the amino group occurs; pK_a values of about 2.5 have been reported.[1,2]

Acid groups
Ionisation of the carboxylic group at about pH 5 was postulated by Chatterji *et al*;[3] proposed pK_a values[2-4] were 4.46, 4.9 and about 5.8. In solutions of low concentration zwitterion formation was negligible.[2]

Partition coefficient

Log *P* (octanol/pH 7.4), 1.7

Solubility

Chlorambucil is practically insoluble in water; it is soluble in 1.5 parts of ethanol, in 2 parts of acetone, and in 2.5 parts of chloroform; it dissolves in ether.

Effect of pH
Chlorambucil is readily soluble in water at alkaline pH values; below pH 7, solubility decreases, but increases again at about pH 2.5.

Effect of cosolvents
To obtain chlorambucil solutions of the concentration necessary for parenteral administration cosolvent mixtures have been used. Stewart and Owen[5] examined decomposition rates of chlorambucil in absolute ethanol and in ethanol/water and propylene glycol/water mixtures (see Stability below).

Dissolution

The effect of 2-hydroxypropyl-β-cyclodextrin on the simultaneous dissolution and degradation of chlorambucil [improved dissolution characteristics in aqueous media]—Loftsson T, Olafsdóttir BJ. Int J Pharmaceutics 1990;66:289–92.

STABILITY

Chlorambucil rapidly decomposes in aqueous systems by a hydrolytic reaction that involves a unimolecular nucleophilic substitution at the amino group; in the step-wise reaction unstable cyclic ethyleneimmonium intermediates form. Ehrsson *et al*[2] identified the degradation product as 4-[*p*-(2-chloroethyl-2-hydroxyethylamino)phenyl]butyric acid. The reaction follows first-order kinetics and the rate depends on the degree of protonation of the amino (nitrogen mustard) group. The carboxylic group appears to make only a small contribution to the reactivity of chlorambucil.

Effect of temperature

Hydrolysis is markedly influenced by temperature. Arrhenius plots derived by Stewart and Owen[5] for aqueous and cosolvent systems demonstrate the limited stability of such formulations at elevated temperatures and the unsuitability of heating as a method of sterilisation. Ehrsson *et al*[2] calculated the activation energy at pH 7 to be 102 kJ/mol.

Effect of pH

When chlorambucil is in the free base (unprotonated) form, rates of hydrolysis are rapid and essentially independent of hydrogen ion and hydroxide ion concentration in the pH range 5 to 10. Below pH 5, as the amine group becomes protonated, the reaction rate is retarded; maximum stability is at about pH 2. Hydrolysis rates are independent of buffer species and drug concentration. In aqueous solution at 75°, $t_{5\%}$ values at pH 4.5 and pH 1.5 were 9.1 and 99.7 minutes, respectively.[5]

Effect of added salts

Chatterji *et al*[3] found that an excess of chloride (common) ions has a stabilising effect in buffered chlorambucil solutions. As chloride ion concentration increased (at a particular pH and buffer concentration) there was a linear decrease in the rate of hydrolysis. The chloride ion is thought to reverse the formation of the cyclic ethyleneimmonium intermediates.
Acetate, borate, and nitrate ions (non-common) had negligible effect on reaction rates.[1]

As ionic strength (in borate buffer, adjusted with potassium nitrate) increased from 0.025 to 0.1 there was a small increase in the rate of hydrolysis.[1]

Effect of solvents

In mixtures of ethanol (up to 40%) or propylene glycol (up to 45%) with water, rates of hydrolysis decreased with solvent polarity but were not linearly related to the dielectric constant.[1,5]

Stability of preparations

Crushed tablets of chlorambucil (equivalent to 2 mg/mL) suspended with Cologel in a mixture of simple and wild cherry syrups decomposed rapidly; there was 10% reduction in potency,[6] after one day at room temperature, and after 7 days at 5°.

Stabilisation

In a perfusion fluid with a vehicle of propylene glycol 45% in phosphate buffer pH 9, the shelf-life ($t_{5\%}$) of chlorambucil was found to be only 45 minutes at 25°.[5] A convenient means of storing chlorambucil in readiness for the preparation of the perfusion fluid is as a concentrate in absolute (anhydrous) ethanol under refrigeration or freezing conditions. Shelf-lives were calculated as 6.3 days (4°) and 31.1 days (−10°).[5] For maximum stability chlorambucil should be kept in the solid state.

FORMULATION

Excipients

Excipients that have been used in presentations of chlorambucil include:
Tablets: black PN; sucrose.

Parenteral presentation

For details of the vehicle used in a perfusion fluid of chlorambucil and in a concentrate used to prepare perfusion fluids see Stability (stabilisation) above. The concentrate should be anhydrous and carefully protected from moisture during storage.

PROCESSING

Sterilisation

In propylene glycol/water systems high rates of hydrolysis at 100° and 115° preclude the adoption of heat sterilisation techniques.[5]

Safety and handling precautions

CAUTION. Chlorambucil is irritant; avoid inhalation of particles and contact with skin and mucous membranes.
Chlorambucil is cytotoxic; general guidelines on handling and disposal are given in the chapter entitled Cytotoxic Drugs: Handling Precautions.

REFERENCES

1. Owen WR, Stewart PJ. J Pharm Sci 1979;68:992–6.
2. Ehrsson H, Eksborg S, Wallin I, Nilsson S-O. J Pharm Sci 1980;69:1091–4.
3. Chatterji DC, Yeager RL, Gallelli JF. J Pharm Sci 1982;71:50–4.
4. Linford JH. Biochem Pharmacol 1963;12:317–24.
5. Stewart PJ, Owen WR. Aust J Pharm Sci 1980;9:15–18.
6. Dressman JB, Poust RI. Am J Hosp Pharm 1983;40:616–18.

Chloramphenicol (BAN, rINN)   *Antibacterial*

Chloranfenicol; cloranfenicol
2,2-Dichloro-*N*-[($\alpha R,\beta R$)-β-hydroxy-α-hydroxymethyl-4-nitro-phenethyl]-acetamide
$C_{11}H_{12}Cl_2N_2O_5 = 323.1$

Chloramphenicol Cinnamate (BANM, rINNM)
$C_{20}H_{18}Cl_2N_2O_6 = 453.3$

Chloramphenicol Palmitate (BANM, rINNM)
Chloramphenicol α-palmitate
$C_{27}H_{42}Cl_2N_2O_6 = 561.5$

Chloramphenicol Sodium Succinate (BANM, rINNM)
Chloramphenicol α-sodium succinate
$C_{15}H_{15}Cl_2N_2NaO_8 = 445.2$
CAS—56-75-7 (chloramphenicol); 14399-14-5 (chloramphenicol cinnamate); 530-43-8 (chloramphenicol palmitate); 982-57-0 (chloramphenicol sodium succinate)

Pharmacopoeial status

BP (chloramphenicol, chloramphenicol palmitate, chloramphenicol sodium succinate); USP (chloramphenicol, chloramphenicol palmitate)

Preparations

Compendial
Chloramphenicol Capsules BP. Capsules containing, in each, 250 mg are usually available.
Chloramphenicol Ear Drops BP. A solution of chloramphenicol in a suitable vehicle. Ear drops containing 5% w/v and 10% w/v are usually available.
Chloramphenicol Eye Drops BP. A sterile solution of chloramphenicol in purified water. Eye drops containing 0.5% w/v are usually available. pH 7.0 to 7.5.
Chloramphenicol Eye Ointment BP is a sterile preparation containing chloramphenicol in a suitable basis. An eye ointment containing 1% w/w is usually available.
Chloramphenicol Oral Suspension BP (Chloramphenicol Palmitate Mixture; Chloramphenicol Suspension) is a suspension of chloramphenicol palmitate in a suitable flavoured vehicle. The method of manufacture must be such that the content of the biologically inactive chloramphenicol palmitate polymorph A is within the prescribed limit in the final product. If the oral suspension is diluted, the diluted oral suspension should be freshly prepared. An oral suspension containing the equivalent of 125 mg of chloramphenicol in 5 mL is usually available.
Chloramphenicol Sodium Succinate Injection BP (Chloramphenicol Sodium Succinate for Injection). A sterile solution of chloramphenicol sodium succinate in water for injections. It is prepared by dissolving chloramphenicol sodium succinate for injection in the requisite amount of water for injections. Sealed containers each containing the equivalent of 300 mg, 1000 mg,

and 1200 mg of chloramphenicol are usually available. The pH of a 25% w/v solution is 6.0 to 7.0.
Chloramphenicol Capsules USP.
Chloramphenicol Tablets USP.
Chloramphenicol Oral Solution USP.
Chloramphenicol Cream USP.
Chloramphenicol Otic Solution USP.
Chloramphenicol Ophthalmic Ointment USP.
Chloramphenicol Ophthalmic Solution USP.
Chloramphenicol for Ophthalmic Solution USP.
Sterile Chloramphenicol USP is chloramphenicol suitable for parenteral use.
Chloramphenicol Injection USP. pH of 1:1 dilution in water, 5.0 to 8.0.
Chloramphenicol Palmitate Oral Suspension USP.
Sterile Chloramphenicol Sodium Succinate USP.

Non-compendial
Chloromycetin (P–D). *Capsules*, chloramphenicol 250 mg. *Suspension*, chloramphenicol 125 mg (as palmitate)/5 mL. *Diluent*: syrup, life of diluted suspenion 14 days.
Injection, powder for reconstitution, chloramphenicol (as sodium succinate) 300-mg and 1.2-g vials.
Ophthalmic ointment, chloramphenicol 1%.
Redidrops (eye drops), chloramphenicol 0.5%.
Kemicetine (Farmitalia Carlo Erba). *Injection*, powder for reconstitution, chloramphenicol (as sodium succinate) 1 g per vial. The injection should be reconstituted with water for injections, sodium chloride 0.9% injection, or glucose 5% injection.
Sno Phenicol (S&N Pharm). *Eye drops*, chloramphenicol 0.5% in a viscous vehicle.
Minims Chloramphenicol (S&N Pharm). *Eye drops*, single-use, chloramphenicol 0.5%.
Chloramphenicol ear drops 5% and 10% as chloramphenicol in a propylene glycol vehicle are usually available.

Containers and storage

Solid state
Chloramphenicol BP should be protected from light. If the material is intended for use in the manufacture of a parenteral dosage form without further appropriate procedure of sterilisation, the container should be sterile, tamper-evident, and sealed so as to exclude micro-organisms.
Chloramphenicol Palmitate BP should be protected from light. Chloramphenicol Sodium Succinate BP should be kept in an airtight container and protected from light. If the substance is sterile, it should be kept in a sterile, tamper-evident container and sealed so as to exclude micro-organisms.
Chloramphenicol USP and Chloramphenicol Palmitate USP should be preserved in tight containers.

Dosage forms
Chloramphenicol Ear Drops BP, Chloramphenicol Eye Drops BP, Chloramphenicol Oral Suspension BP, and the sealed container of Chloramphenicol Sodium Succinate Injection BP should all be protected from light. In addition, the injection should be used immediately after preparation, but in any case, within the period recommended by the manufacturer when prepared according to the instructions.
Chloramphenicol Capsules USP, Chloramphenicol for Ophthalmic Solution USP, Chloramphenicol Otic Solution USP, Chloramphenicol Oral Solution USP, and Chloramphenicol Tablets USP should be preserved in tight containers.
Chloramphenicol Cream USP should be preserved in collapsible tubes or in tight containers.

Chloramphenicol Ophthalmic Ointment USP should be preserved in collapsible ophthalmic ointment tubes.
Chloramphenicol Ophthalmic Solution USP should be preserved in tight containers and stored in a refrigerator until dispensed. The containers or individual cartons are sealed and tamper-proof so that sterility is assured at time of first use.
Chloramphenicol Palmitate Oral Suspension USP should be preserved in tight, light-resistant containers.
Chloramphenicol Injection USP should be preserved in single-dose or in multiple-dose containers.
Sterile Chloramphenicol Sodium Succinate USP should be preserved in containers suitable for sterile solids.
Chloromycetin capsules and suspension should be stored at temperatures not exceeding 30° and protected from light. Chloromycetin redidrops should be stored between 2° and 8° and protected from light. Chloromycetin ophthalmic ointment should be stored at temperatures not exceeding 30°. Chloromycetin injection should be stored at temperatures not exceeding 30° and protected from light; the reconstituted solution should be used once only, immediately after preparation.
Minims Chloramphenicol eye drops should be stored between 2° and 8°, it should not be frozen.
Sno Phenicol should be stored between 2° and 8°, it should not be frozen; do not dilute; dispense from original container.

PHYSICAL PROPERTIES

Chloramphenicol exists as a white to greyish-white or yellowish-white, fine crystalline powder or fine crystals, needles, or elongated plates.
Chloramphenicol cinnamate is a white or yellowish-white crystalline powder.
Chloramphenicol palmitate is a fine, white or almost white unctuous crystalline powder, with a faint odour.
Chloramphenicol sodium succinate is a white or yellowish-white hygroscopic powder.

Melting point

Chloramphenicol melts in the range 149° to 153°.
Chloramphenicol cinnamate melts at about 119°.
Chloramphenicol palmitate melts in the range 87° to 95°.

pH

A 2.5% w/v aqueous suspension of *chloramphenicol* has a pH between 4.5 and 7.5.
A solution of sterile *chloramphenicol sodium succinate*, containing the equivalent of chloramphenicol 25% w/v, has a pH between 6.4 and 7.0.

Dissociation constant

pK_a 5.5

Partition coefficient

Log P (octanol), 1.1

Solubility

Chloramphenicol is slightly soluble in water (1 in 400), in chloroform and in ether; freely soluble in ethanol (1 in 2.5), in propylene glycol (1 in 7), in acetone, and in ethyl acetate.
Chloramphenicol cinnamate is very slightly soluble in water; soluble 1 in 25 of ethanol, 1 in 50 of chloroform, and 1 in 500 of ether.
Chloramphenicol palmitate is practically insoluble in water; sparingly soluble in ethanol (1 in 45); freely soluble in chloroform (1 in 6) and in acetone; soluble in ether (1 in 14) and in ethyl acetate; very slightly soluble in hexane.

Chloramphenicol sodium succinate is soluble 1 in less than 1 of water and 1 in 1 of ethanol; practically insoluble in chloroform and in ether.

Dissolution

The USP specifies that for Chloramphenicol Capsules USP not less than 85% of the labelled amount of $C_{11}H_{12}Cl_2N_2O_5$ is dissolved in 30 minutes. Dissolution medium: 900 mL of 0.1N hydrochloric acid; Apparatus 1 at 100 rpm.

Crystal and molecular structure

Polymorphs

Chloramphenicol palmitate occurs in three crystalline forms and in one amorphous form. Only one polymorph (known as B) is active. Any polymorph may be used to make preparations that contain chloramphenicol palmitate in the solid form, but the manufacturing process must be of a design that will ensure that the final product contains the desired polymorph B.

Polymorph B (the α-form) of chloramphenicol palmitate is the biologically active form and was found to be stable at room and at elevated temperatures. Borka[1] isolated a third form which he called the C-form. It was less stable, converting into the biologically inactive polymorph A (β-form) at elevated temperatures. Polymorph B was stable in aqueous suspension but in saturated solutions in organic solvents, rapid transformation from polymorph B to polymorph A, and from C-form to polymorph A was observed.

When polymorphs A and B of chloramphenicol palmitate were ground in the presence or absence of different quantities of Avicel PH 102 as diluent, a stable form (Form A*) with low crystallinity was obtained.[2] This stable form had all the characteristics of inactive Form A; however, it had an *in-vitro* hydrolysis rate constant four times greater than that of Form B from commercially available chloramphenicol palmitate.

Workers in South Africa[3] heated the B polymorph of chloramphenicol palmitate at 82° for 26.67 hours and found that it changed completely to the less soluble and less bioavailable polymorph A. When the most soluble polymorph C was ground for a prolonged period it changed, via polymorph B, to polymorph A. A sample of polymorph C stored at 50° and 75° changed to polymorph B, but, after 53.33 hours, only the sample kept at 75° changed into polymorph A.

FURTHER INFORMATION. Solid state transitions and CAP [chloramphenicol] availability in surface solid dispersions of chloramphenicol stearate polymorphs—Forni F, Coppi G, Iannuccelli V, Vandelli MA, Bernabei MT. Drug Dev Ind Pharm 1988;14(5):633–47. Surface area and crystallinity of Form A of chloramphenicol palmitic and stearic esters: which one is the limiting factor in the enzymatic hydrolysis?—Forni F, Iannuccelli V, Cameroni R. J Pharm Pharmacol 1987;39:1041–3. Effect of seed crystals on solid-state transformation of polymorphs of chloramphenicol palmitate during grinding—Otsuka M, Kaneniwa N. J Pharm Sci 1986;75(5):506–11. The influence of crystal structure on drug formulation [review]—Pearson JT, Varney G. Mfg Chem 1973;44(12):35–8.

STABILITY

Chloramphenicol in the solid state can remain stable over a prolonged period of time provided that recommended storage conditions are adhered to.

Solutions

In aqueous solution, chloramphenicol degrades mainly by amide hydrolysis, at pH below 7, with the formation of 1-*p*-nitrophe-nylpropan-1,3-diol-2-amine and dichloroacetic acid. Dichloroacetic acid hydrolyses further, with release of chloride ions. Hydrolysis of the covalent chlorine of the dichloroacetamide moiety occurs at pH values above 6. Chloramphenicol may also degrade by a photolytic reaction to *p*-nitrobenzaldehyde and other products. Hydrolysis is independent of pH in the range 2 to 7, but is catalysed by monohydrogen phosphate ions, monohydrogen and dihydrogen citrate ions, and undissociated acetic acid.

Maximum stability is reported at pH 6.0.

Shih[4] demonstrated that aqueous solutions of chloramphenicol were liable to photodegradation by sunlight, ultraviolet light, and light from a tungsten lamp. The major degradation products were: hydrochloric acid; *p*-nitrobenzaldehyde; *p*-nitrobenzoic acid; *p*-aminophenyl-2-acetamido-1,3,propanediol; and 4,4′ azoxybenzoic acid. Aqueous solutions of chloramphenicol in the presence of light underwent oxidation, reduction, and condensation reactions.[4]

Over a period of 24 days at room temperature, aqueous solutions of chloramphenicol (pH 1 to 14) degraded with the formation of *p*-nitrobenzaldehyde (oxidation product) and the arylamine (reduction product).[5] The products of decomposition were also found in some dosage forms (creams and capsules) but not in water-free ophthalmic ointments stored under 'normal conditions'.

Mubarak et al[6] proposed a reaction pathway for the photolytic degradation of chloramphenicol (0.25% w/v) and investigated the rate of the reaction in Clark Lubs borate buffer (pH 7.8). Yellow discoloration, which darkened with time, was observed. The same workers also examined the photochemical reactions of chloramphenicol in aqueous solution (0.86% w/v) containing 1,3-butandiol (19.6% w/v) under nitrogen and atmospheric conditions, and identified the degradation product 2-(4-nitrophenyl)-4-methyl-1,3-dioxane in both environments.[7]

Eye drops

Boer and Pijnenburg[8] used a reversed-phase HPLC method to monitor the degradation of two chloramphenicol eye drop solutions (0.25%, pH 4.7 and 0.5%, pH 7.2) containing boric acid, borax, or both, stored at 4° or 21°; or heated at 100° or 120° (for 30 minutes or 20 minutes, respectively). Degradation occurred in both solutions stored at 4° and 21°; the number of moles of 1-(4′-nitrophenyl)-2-amino-1,3-propanediol corresponded with the decrease in the number of moles of chloramphenicol. After 53 weeks at 4° and 21°, the losses of chloramphenicol due to amide hydrolysis were 1% and 15%, respectively, for the solution at pH 7.2 and 11% and 44% for the solution at pH 4.7. Reaction rates at 100° and 120° were higher in the solution at pH 7.2 (chloramphenicol level reduced to 95% and 77%) than in the solution at pH 4.7 (chloramphenicol level reduced to 97% and 91%). Exposure to daylight for several hours caused the development of a yellow to yellow-brown discoloration with photodegradation products present (mainly 4-nitrobenzaldehyde) only in the chloramphenicol 0.5% (pH 7.2) solution.

Exposure of chloramphenicol (eye drops, 10 mg/L, buffered to pH 7.0 with phosphate buffer) to sunlight caused 80% degradation within 45 minutes;[9] 30% was converted into *p*-nitrobenzaldehyde. The products *p*-nitrobenzoic acid and *p*-nitrosobenzoic acid were also identified. The authors warn of the dangers of conversion of chloramphenicol to nitroso compounds either in the eye or on the skin on exposure to sunlight. Accelerated stability studies[10] generated $t_{10\%}$ values for Chloramphenicol Eye Drops BPC of 29 minutes at 115°, 85 minutes at 100°, 4 months at 20°, and 31 months at 4°.

Chloramphenicol ointment and eye ointment were stable for 2 years at 20° to 25°. Chloramphenicol ear drops and eye drops (BPC) and chloramphenicol cream (DTF) retained more than 90% of their potencies after 2 years, 3 to 4 months, and 5 months, respectively. After heating the eye drops at 115° to 116° for 30 minutes, 15% hydrolysis occurred, and after heating with a bactericide at 100° for 30 minutes, 3% to 4% hydrolysis occurred.[11]

Eye ointments

The uniformity of chloramphenicol distribution in an eye ointment was measured by Powell[12] using a specially developed HPLC method that could detect variations in chloramphenicol content that remained undetected by the BP method. A clear oil (identified as liquid paraffin) separated from the ointment mass; chloramphenicol was concentrated in the remaining ointment.

The stability of chloramphenicol 1% in some ophthalmic ointment bases (absorption bases, and oil-in-water and water-in-oil emulsions) at 25° and 35° was studied.[13] Ingredients in the formulations included white soft paraffin, benzalkonium chloride, and some of the following: cetyl alcohol, wool fat, propylene glycol, liquid paraffin, sodium metabisulphite, disodium edetate, polysorbate 40 (Tween 40), sorbitan monopalmitate (Span 40), and distilled water. Chloramphenicol was more stable during the 12-month storage period in the absorption basis containing wool fat than in that containing cetyl alcohol. Stability was improved during storage at 35° by the addition of sodium metabisulphite and disodium edetate. In general, stability at 25° over 12 months decreased in the order: absorption bases > oil-in-water emulsion > water-in-oil emulsion, all containing sodium metabisulphite and disodium edetate.

Suspensions

Chloramphenicol palmitate suspension pH 6.7 (in a syrup basis with chloroform spirit, methyl and propyl hydroxybenzoates, sorbic acid, Tween 80, colloidal aluminium magnesium silicate (Veegum), and carmellose) curdled and discoloured after two years storage in rigid, transparent, amber polyvinyl chloride bottles.[14] Suspensions stored in amber glass bottles kept well during the same study period.

Stabilisation

Since hydrolysis of chloramphenicol is catalysed by both phosphate and citrate buffers, borax/boric acid solution has been recommended as a buffer for chloramphenicol solutions. Photodegradation can be avoided by protecting the solutions from light.

FURTHER INFORMATION. Stability of chloramphenicol in pharmaceutical preparations—Kister G, Esteve G, Catterini A, Chonal J, Fromental L, Personne JC [French]. Trav Soc Pharm Montpellier 1977;37(3):173–82. Nonisothermal kinetics applied to drugs in pharmaceutical suspensions—Waltersson J-O, Lundgren P. Acta Pharm Suec 1983;20:145–54. Effect of additives on the photostability of chloramphenicol in Clark Lubs borate buffer at pH 7.8—Mubarak SIM, Stanford JB, Sugden JK. Pharm Acta Helv 1985;60(7):187–92. Some aspects of the antimicrobial and chemical properties of phenyl boronate esters of chloramphenicol [faster photodegradation in simulated sunlight than the parent drug]—Mubarak SIM, Stanford JB, Sugden JK. Drug Dev Ind Pharm 1984;10(7):1131–60.

INCOMPATIBILITY/COMPATIBILITY

Chloramphenicol sodium succinate is reported to be incompatible with the following compounds: aminophylline, ampicillin, ascorbic acid, calcium chloride, carbenicillin sodium, chlorpromazine hydrochloride, erythromycin salts, gentamicin sulphate, hydrocortisone sodium succinate, hydroxyzine hydrochloride, methicillin sodium, methylprednisolone sodium succinate, nitrofurantoin sodium, novobiocin sodium, oxytetracycline hydrochloride, phenytoin sodium, polymyxin B sulphate, prochlorperazine salts, promazine hydrochloride, promethazine hydrochloride, sulphafurazole diethanolamine, tetracycline hydrochloride, tripelennamine hydrochloride, vancomycin hydrochloride, vitamin B complex.

FORMULATION

Excipients

Excipients that have been used in presentations of chloramphenicol include:

Capsules, chloramphenicol: lactose.

Tablets, chloramphenicol: acacia; gelatin; maize starch, pregelatinised; magnesium stearate; quinoline yellow (E104); rice starch; spermaceti; sucrose; talc; wheat flour; white shellac; white beeswax.

Oral liquids, chloramphenicol: wild cherry syrup.

Chloramphenicol palmitate: carmellose sodium; citric acid; custard powder, imitation; ethanol; glycerol; povidone; propylene glycol; sodium benzoate; sorbitan monolaurate; sucrose; Veegum.

Ophthalmic drops, chloramphenicol: borax; boric acid; chlorhexidine acetate; dextran; macrogol 1540; methyl and propyl hydroxybenzoates; phenylmercuric acetate; phenylmercuric nitrate; polysorbate; sodium chloride; sodium hydroxide; thiomersal sodium.

Ophthalmic ointments, chloramphenicol: cholesterol; liquid paraffin; polyethylene; yellow soft paraffin.

Ear drops, chloramphenicol: propylene glycol.

Creams, chloramphenicol: cetyl alcohol; liquid paraffin; propyl hydroxybenzoate; sodium lauryl sulphate; sodium phosphate.

Injections, chloramphenicol sodium succinate: sodium hydroxide.

Bioavailability

Chloramphenicol has a low solubility in water and thus the method of formulation may have a considerable effect on its rate of absorption. Studies of bioavailability show significant variations in both the peak concentrations in blood and the times at which these occur. These variations may be related to disintegration or dissolution rates or to particle sizes. Chloramphenicol palmitate has several polymorphic forms each having different absorption characteristics.

Topical preparations

Safwat et al[15] investigated the use of cellulose acetate butyrate films as a topical drug delivery system for chloramphenicol. The incorporation of plasticisers (5% to 20%) was found to increase chloramphenicol release from films; their effects reduced in the order: dimethyl phthalate > diethyl phthalate > propylene glycol > castor oil > unplasticised films. A kinetic study showed that release data followed a diffusion-controlled release model.

Twenty-four emulsion bases were prepared by adding aqueous or lipid phase to six different ambiphilic bases (lipid phase 47%, aqueous phase 46%, emulsifiers 7%). The lipid content of the 24 bases ranged from 22% to 75%. Release of chloramphenicol through a semi-permeable haemodialysis membrane into an aqueous medium was greater from the o/w bases than from the w/o or mixed bases.[16]

Ophthalmic ointments

Further to previous stability studies,[13] the extent of chloramphenicol release at 35° from an absorption basis containing wool fat was shown to be higher than from that containing cetyl alcohol.[17] The addition of sodium metabisulphite and disodium edetate improved the release of chloramphenicol from the ointments. Rheological data revealed that 'plastic viscosity' played a major role in drug release from ointment bases. Release of chloramphenicol (which was first order in all instances) from ointment bases decreased in the order: water-in-oil emulsion > oil-in-water emulsion > absorption basis.

Ford and co-workers[18] measured the rheology, particle size distribution, and drug release of five commercially available Chloramphenicol Eye Ointments BP by dissolution and agar diffusion techniques. All ointments showed structural decomposition during continuous shear rheology. Differences in release and particle size distribution were detected between the preparations studied, depending on the experimental method used.

Four different formulations containing chloramphenicol 1% and chlortetracycline hydrochloride 0.5% were prepared by Attia and co-workers in Egypt.[19] All bases contained benzalkonium chloride 0.01% w/w, sodium metabisulphite 0.5% w/w, and disodium edetate 0.3% w/w. The two absorption bases contained white soft paraffin, liquid paraffin, and either wool fat or cetyl alcohol. The two emulsion bases both contained white soft paraffin, cetyl alcohol, and distilled water, either liquid paraffin or propylene glycol, and either Span 40 or Tween 40. The availability of chloramphenicol to the different tissues of the eye (of *rabbits*) depended mainly on the composition of the ointment basis and whether the drug was concentrated in the aqueous or the oily phase of the basis.

Suppositories

The release *in vitro* of L-chloramphenicol from various suppository bases containing 5% of the drug (50 mg/suppository) at 38° was examined by Kassem *et al*.[20] Release from hard fat bases was lower than from water-soluble bases. Witepsol H15 showed best release rates of the hard fat bases tested. Release from bases containing surfactants decreased in rank order: Brij > Myrj > Tweens > Arlacels. Release was dependent on drug solubility in the basis, solubility of the basis in the test medium, and the composition and melting point of the basis.

FURTHER INFORMATION. Interactions between macromolecular adjuvants and drugs. Part 28: The influence of starch derivatives on dissolution characteristics of chloramphenicol—Keipert SG, Hildebrandt S [German]. Pharmazie 1990;45:111–16. The release rate of chloramphenicol in EVA [ethylene vinyl acetate] film [laminated, semilaminated and unlaminated]—Honyun L, Fengwen L, Zhongkai S [Japanese]. Nanjing Yaoxueyan Xuebao 1984;15(1):57–60. Accuracy of delivery of cefazolin, chloramphenicol, and vancomycin by a controlled-release membrane infusion device [MICROS]—Nahata MC, Durrell DE, Miller MA. Am J Hosp Pharm 1988;45:2358–60. Influence of vehicle on antimicrobial efficiency of topical dosage forms of chloramphenicol—Cajkovak M, Kupinic M. Pharmazie 1987;42:327–9. Aminomethylbenzoate esters of chloramphenicol as a novel prodrug type for parenteral administration—Jensen E, Bundgaard H. Int J Pharmaceutics 1991;70:137–46. Studies of cyclodextrin inclusions: 1. Inclusion between α- and β-cyclodextrins and chloramphenicol in aqueous solution—Aboutaleb A-E, Abdel-Rahman A-A, Ismail S. STP Pharma 1986;2(13):116–21. *In vitro* comparative release studies on suppository bases—Trivdi BM, Patel LD. Ind J Hosp Pharm 1982;19:218–23. The effect of storage on the dissolution rate of some drug-polyethylene glycol 6000 [macrogol 6000] solid dispersions—Dubois JL, Chaumeil JC, Ford JL. STP Pharma 1985;1(8):711–14.

PROCESSING

Sterilisation

Solutions of chloramphenicol in propylene glycol are sterilised by filtration.

Buffered aqueous solutions for use as eye drops are sterilised by filtration.

REFERENCES

1. Borka L. Acta Pharm Suec 1971;8:365–72.
2. Cameroni R, Coppi G, Forni F, Bernabei MT [Italian]. Il Farmaco (Prat) 1984;39:76–86.
3. De Villiers MM, van der Watt JG, Lötter AP. Drug Dev Ind Pharm 1991;17(10):1295–1303.
4. Shih IK. J Pharm Sci 1971;60(12):1889–90.
5. Shih IK. J Pharm Sci 1971;60(5):786–7.
6. Mubarak SIM, Stanford JB, Sugden JK. Pharm Acta Helv 1982;57(8):226–30.
7. Mubarak SIM, Stanford JB, Sugden K. Pharm Acta Helv 1983;58(12):343–7.
8. Boer Y, Pijnenburg A. Pharm Weekbl (Sci) 1983;5:95–101.
9. de Vries H, Beijers Bergen van Henegouwen GMJ, Huf FA. Int J Pharmaceutics 1984;20:265–71.
10. Heward M, Norton DA, Rivers SM. Pharm J 1970;204:386–7.
11. James KC, Leach RH. J Pharm Pharmacol 1970;22:607–11.
12. Powell EGP. J Pharm Pharmacol 1985;37:124P.
13. Attia MA, El-Sourady HA, El-Shanawany SM. Pharmazie 1985;40:629–31.
14. Shah RC, Raman PV, Shah BM. Pharm J 1978;221:58–9.
15. Safwat SM, Hafez E, El-Monem HA, Ibrahim EA. Bull Pharm Sci Assiut Univ 1989;12:152–72.
16. Cajkovac M. Acta Pharm Technol 1984;30(3):248–52.
17. Attia MA, El-Sourady HA, El-Shanawany SM. Pharm Ind 1986;48(10):1196–9.
18. Ford JL, Rubinstein MH, Duffy TD, Ireland DS. Drug Dev Ind Pharm 1983;9(1 and 2):21–33.
19. Attia MA, El-Sourady HA, El-Shanawany SM. Acta Pharm Technol 1985;31(2):85–9.
20. Kassem AA, Nour El-Dine, Abd El-Bary A, Faddel HM. Pharmazie 1975;30(H7):472–5.

Chlordiazepoxide (BAN, rINN)   *Anxiolytic*

Methaminodiazepoxide
7-Chloro-2-methylamino-5-phenyl-3H-1,4-benzodiazepine 4-oxide
$C_{16}H_{14}ClN_3O = 299.8$

Chlordiazepoxide Hydrochloride (BANM, USAN, rINNM)

$C_{16}H_{14}ClN_3O, HCl = 336.2$
CAS—58-25-3 (chlordiazepoxide); 438-41-5 (chlordiazepoxide hydrochloride)

Pharmacopoeial status

BP, USP (chlordiazepoxide, chlordiazepoxide hydrochloride)

Preparations

Compendial

Chlordiazepoxide Capsules BP. Contain chlordiazepoxide hydrochloride. Capsules containing, in each, 5 mg and 10 mg are usually available.

Chlordiazepoxide Tablets BP. Contain chlordiazepoxide. Tablets containing, in each, 5 mg, 10 mg, and 25 mg are usually available.

Chlordiazepoxide Hydrochloride Tablets BP. Tablets containing, in each, the equivalent of 5 mg, 10 mg, and 25 mg of chlordiazepoxide are usually available.

Chlordiazepoxide Hydrochloride Capsules USP.

Chlordiazepoxide Tablets USP.

Sterile Chlordiazepoxide Hydrochloride USP. Suitable for parenteral use.

Non-compendial

Librium (Roche). *Capsules*, chlordiazepoxide hydrochloride 5 mg and 10 mg.

Tablets, chlordiazepoxide 5 mg, 10 mg, and 25 mg.

Chlordiazepoxide capsules are also available from APS, Cox, DDSA (Tropium), Kerfoot, Norton.

Containers and storage

Solid state

Chlordiazepoxide BP and Chlordiazepoxide Hydrochloride BP should be kept in well-closed containers and protected from light.

Chlordiazepoxide USP and Chlordiazepoxide Hydrochloride USP should be preserved in tight, light-resistant containers.

Dosage forms

Chlordiazepoxide Capsules BP should be protected from light.

Chlordiazepoxide Tablets BP and Chlordiazepoxide Hydrochloride Tablets BP should be stored at a temperature not exceeding 25°.

Chlordiazepoxide Hydrochloride Capsules USP and Chlordiazepoxide Tablets USP should be preserved in tight, light-resistant containers.

Sterile Chlordiazepoxide Hydrochloride USP should be preserved in containers suitable for sterile solids, and protected from light.

Librium capsules and Librium tablets should be stored at a maximum temperature of 30° and 25°, respectively.

PHYSICAL PROPERTIES

Chlordiazepoxide is an almost white or light yellow crystalline powder; sensitive to sunlight.

Chlordiazepoxide hydrochloride is a white or slightly yellow crystalline powder; affected by sunlight.

Melting point

Chlordiazepoxide melts in the range 240° to 244°.

Chlordiazepoxide hydrochloride melts between 212° and 218°, with decomposition.

pH

A 10% solution of *chlordiazepoxide hydrochloride* has a pH of 2 to 3.

Dissociation constant

pK_a 4.6 (20°)

Partition coefficient

Log P (octanol/pH 7.4), 2.5

Solubility

Chlordiazepoxide is practically insoluble in water; soluble 1 in 50 of ethanol, and 1 in 130 of ether; slightly soluble in chloroform.

Chlordiazepoxide hydrochloride is soluble 1 in 10 of water, and 1 in 40 of ethanol; practically insoluble in chloroform and in ether.

Dissolution

The USP specifies that for Chlordiazepoxide Hydrochloride Capsules USP not less than 85% of the labelled amount of $C_{16}H_{14}ClN_3O,HCl$ is dissolved in 30 minutes. Dissolution medium: 900 mL of water; Apparatus 1 at 100 rpm.

The USP specifies that for Chlordiazepoxide Tablets USP not less than 85% of the labelled amount of $C_{16}H_{14}ClN_3O$ is dissolved in 30 minutes. Dissolution medium: 900 mL of simulated gastric fluid TS prepared without pepsin; Apparatus 1 at 100 rpm.

Crystal and molecular structure

Polymorphs

Crystalline modification of chlordiazepoxide—Singh D, York P, Shields L, Marshall PV. J Pharm Pharmacol 1992;44(Suppl):1050.

STABILITY

Chlordiazepoxide undergoes hydrolysis to demoxepam by loss of the methylamino group.[1] Demoxepam undergoes further degradation by two parallel consecutive reactions: the major route involves rupture of the 4,5-azomethine linkage to form an intermediate compound which is subsequently converted to 2-amino-5-chlorobenzophenone; in the parallel reaction, demoxepam forms a second intermediate, by hydrolysis of the 1,2-amide bond, which subsequently yields glycine N-oxide. The hydrolysis of chlordiazepoxide to demoxepam may proceed uncatalysed or may be catalysed by specific acids and bases. Reaction rates were determined at various temperatures.

Photodegradation

Chlordiazepoxide undergoes a heat-reversible isomerisation under sunlight to form an oxaziridine.

When a solution of chlordiazepoxide (10^{-3}M) was irradiated with ultraviolet light (at 350 nm) the intermediate decomposition product, oxaziridine, was produced which on further irradiation yielded a mixture of two photoisomers: the quinoxaline derivative (1-benzoyl-7-chloro- 1,3,dihydro-3-methylaminoquinoxaline) and the benzoxadiazocine derivative (9-chloro-5-methylamino-2-phenyl-4H-benzo[g]-1,3,6-oxidiazo-cine.[2] Further decomposition products were described.

Subsequent studies[3] confirmed that the wavelength of light used to irradiate chlordiazepoxide (254, 300, or 350 nm) determined only the concentrations of the decomposition products formed, not their character. On irradiation of ^{14}C-labelled chlordiazepoxide, dissolved in methanol or methanol-water (pH 7.4), an oxaziridine was formed, which was subsequently converted into a quinoxaline and a benzoxadiazocine derivative. However, by irradiation in the presence of glutathione, the rate of decomposition was increased and the reduced form of chlordiazepoxide (deoxygenated) and an unidentified conjugate were formed. It was established that the oxaziridine reacted spontaneously with glutathione at room temperature in the absence of light.

Effect of surfactants

Studies of the solubilisation of chlordiazepoxide in aqueous micellar solutions of the cationic surfactant hexadecyltrimethylammonium bromide (CTAB) or the nonionic surfactant polyoxyethylene(23)dodecanol (Brij 35), revealed that micellar effects on the hydrolytic degradation of chlordiazepoxide were strongly pH-dependent; catalysis occurred in the pH range below the pK_a of chlordiazepoxide and inhibition occurred at higher pH. Thermodynamic parameters were calculated for chlordiazepoxide solutions containing 5% w/w surfactant.

FURTHER INFORMATION. Practical kinetics III: Benzodiazepine hydrolysis—Maulding HV, Nazareno JP, Pearson JE, Michaelis AF. J Pharm Sci 1975;64(2):278–84. High performance liquid chromatographic determination of chlordiazepoxide and major related impurities in pharmaceuticals—Butterfield AG, Matsui FF, Smith SJ, Sears RW. J Pharm Sci 1977;66(5):684–7. High performance liquid chromatographic separation and determination of chlordiazepoxide hydrochloride and two of its decomposition products—Ali SL. Int J Pharmaceutics 1980;5:85–90. Correlations between phototoxicity of some 7-chloro-1,4-benzodiazepines and their (photo)chemical properties—De Vries H, Beijersbergen van Henegouwen GMJ, Wouters PJHH. Pharm Weekbl (Sci) 1983;5:302–7. Simultaneous high performance liquid chromatographic determination of chlordiazepoxide and amitryptyline hydrochloride in two-component tablet formulations—Burke D, Sokoloff H. J Pharm Sci 1980;69(2):138–40.

INCOMPATIBILITY/COMPATIBILITY

Sorption to plastic

The compatibility of chlordiazepoxide hydrochloride (1 mg/mL or 2 mg/mL) was demonstrated with glucose 5% in water, sodium chloride 0.9%, and compound sodium chloride injection in glass containers stored at room temperature for 4 hours.[5] Acceptable potency was also maintained for 4 hours in glucose 5% in water and in compound sodium chloride injection in Viaflex plastic bags. However, in the solutions of concentration 1 mg/mL or 2 mg/mL in sodium chloride 0.9% in Viaflex plastic bags, potency was maintained for only 2 hours or 30 minutes, respectively. Some sorption of chlordiazepoxide to the plastic bag was assumed, the extent of which was dependent on time and the type of vehicle used.

FORMULATION

Excipients

Excipients that have been used in presentations of chlordiazepoxide include:
Capsules, chlordiazepoxide and *chlordiazepoxide hydrochloride*: lactose; maize starch; talc.
Tablets, chlordiazepoxide: brilliant blue FCF (133); ethylcellulose; hypromellose; indigo carmine (E132); lactose; magnesium stearate; microcrystalline cellulose; quinoline yellow (E104); saccharin; starch; sunset yellow FCF (E110); talc; triacetin.
Injections, chlordiazepoxide hydrochloride: benzyl alcohol; maleic acid.

Solid matrices

The stability of chlordiazepoxide in various solid matrices was greatest when microcrystalline cellulose, calcium phosphate, or maltose-glucose granules were excipients in the formulations. The tablet matrices were obtained by direct compression.[6]

PROCESSING

Sterilisation

Sterility of powder ampoules containing chlordiazepoxide hydrochloride was achieved by radiosterilisation with ^{60}Co at a dose of 4.5 Mrad (ascertained by bacteriological assay).[7]

REFERENCES

1. Han WW, Yakatan GJ, Maness DD. J Pharm Sci 1976;65(8):1198–1204.
2. Cornelissen PJG, Beijersbergen van Henegouwen GMJ, Gerritsma KW. Int J Pharmaceutics 1979;3:205–20.
3. Cornelissen PJG, Beijersbergen van Henegouwen GMJ. Pharm Weekbl (Sci) 1980;115:547–56.
4. Buur A, Gravsholt S. Arch Pharm Chemi (Sci Ed) 1982;10:1–16.
5. Morris ME, Parker WA. Can J Pharm Sci 1981;16(1):43–5.
6. Valls LM [Spanish]. Cienc Ind Farm 1978;10:31–40.
7. Jacob VBP, Leupin K [German]. Pharm Acta Helv 1974;49:1–11.

Chlormethiazole (BAN)

Hypnotic; Sedative; Anticonvulsant

Clomethiazole (rINN)
5-(2-Chloroethyl)-4-methylthiazole
$C_6H_8ClNS = 161.6$

Chlormethiazole Edisylate (BANM)

Clomethiazole Edisilate (rINNM)
$(C_6H_8ClNS)_2, C_2H_6O_6S_2 = 513.5$
CAS—533-45-9 (chlormethiazole); 1867-58-9 (chlormethiazole edisylate)

Pharmacopoeial status

BP (chlormethiazole, chlormethiazole edisylate)

Preparations

Compendial
Chlormethiazole Capsules BP. Contain a solution of chlormethiazole in a suitable fixed oil. Capsules containing, in each, 192 mg are usually available.

Non-compendial
Heminevrin (Astra). *Capsules*, chlormethiazole base 192 mg in an oily basis.
Syrup, sugar-free aqueous solution of chlormethiazole edisylate 50 mg/mL.
Intravenous infusion 0.8%, chlormethiazole edisylate 8 mg/mL.

Containers and storage

Solid state
Chlormethiazole BP and Chlormethiazole Edisylate BP should be kept in well-closed containers. Chlormethiazole BP should be stored at a temperature of 2° to 8°.

Dosage forms
Heminevrin syrup should be stored in a cool place.
Heminevrin infusion should be stored at a temperature of 5° to 8°.

PHYSICAL PROPERTIES

Chlormethiazole is a colourless to slightly yellowish-brown oily viscous liquid with a characteristic odour.
Chlormethiazole edisylate is a white crystalline powder with a characteristic odour which becomes more distinct and unpleasant when the substance is heated.

Melting point

Chlormethiazole edisylate melts at about 128°.

pH

The pH of a 0.5% w/v solution of *chlormethiazole* is 5.5 to 7.0.

Dissociation constant

pK_a 3.2
Gustavii and Ekstrand-Asker[1] determined the acid dissociation constant for chlormethiazole (at ionic strength 0.2) to be 2.96 at 25°.

Partition coefficient

The apparent octanol-water (pH 7.4) partition coefficient of chlormethiazole edisylate has been reported[2] to be 132 (log *P*, 2.12).

Solubility

Chlormethiazole is soluble 1 in 100 of water. It is miscible in ethanol, in ether, and in chloroform.
Chlormethiazole edisylate is freely soluble in water; soluble in ethanol; practically insoluble in ether.

STABILITY

Gustavii and Ekstrand-Asker[1] studied the stability of buffered aqueous solutions of chlormethiazole edisylate. Degradation was by hydrolysis and followed pseudo-first-order kinetics. For solutions (0.001M and ionic strength 0.2) in phosphate buffer the apparent first-order rate constant at 120° and pH 7.0 was 8.1/day while at 35° and pH 6.87 it was 9.1×10^{-4}/day. Two main degradation products were identified together with a quaternary dimer. At pH less than 9, the major product was 4-methyl-5-(2-hydroxyethyl)-thiazole and the reaction was catalysed by water. The dominant degradation product at pH greater than 9 was 4-methyl-5-vinylthiazole; hydroxide ions acted as the catalyst. Both degradation products were formed directly from chlormethiazole edisylate.

Shelf-life

Infusion and injection solutions (8 mg/mL) stored at 5° for 36 to 38 months showed degradation of 1.0% to 3.1%; a 20% solution stored at 20° for 36 months degraded by 5%. Infusion solutions heated to 120° for 20 minutes or at 105° for 80 minutes degraded by 10.3% and 9.0%, respectively.[1]

INCOMPATIBILITY/COMPATIBILITY

Sorption to plastics

Kowaluk *et al*[3] investigated the interaction between chlormethiazole edisylate in aqueous solutions and polyvinyl chloride infusion bags (and tubing) and cellulose propionate burette chambers. After storage for 200 hours at 20°, solutions (0.2% to 0.8%) in infusion bags and in burette chambers lost from 30% to 50% and 20% to 30% chlormethiazole edisylate, respectively. Losses were concentration dependent. There were marked losses from solutions infused through polyvinyl chloride tubing, but control samples in glass containers showed negligible loss. Sorption appeared to be the main mechanism for the losses found after storage in bags and burettes and infusion through tubing. Both permeation and evaporation appeared to contribute to the remaining loss through polyvinyl chloride components but these processes were not associated with migration to cellulose propionate burettes. The polyvinyl chloride was found to soften on storage as the concentration of chlormethiazole edisylate increased, confirming results of earlier studies.[2]
Lee[4] reported about 40% to 50% loss of potency from chlormethiazole edisylate 0.8% infusion due to sorption to polyvinyl chloride administration sets; 10% to 15% sorption occurred onto adjoining cellulose propionate burettes. There was also a reduction of 7% to 13% in potency with polybutadiene administration sets, but sorption did not occur onto accompanying methacrylate butadiene styrene burettes.
Roberts *et al*[5] were unable to detect any loss of chlormethiazole from an aqueous solution after storage for 24 hours in an all-plastic syringe (polypropylene barrel and polyethylene plunger) or in glass containers. Plastic syringes of other types with rubber plunger seals were excluded from the study because of leaching of a benzothiazole from the seal.
Sorption of chlormethiazole (Heminevrin, Astra) infusion to plastic syringes (Becton Dickinson) was also investigated by Allwood.[6] After 24 hours at ambient temperature, under simulated clinical conditions, about 8.5% of the original concentration of chlormethiazole had been sorbed into the barrel and rubber plunger of the syringe. Up to 85% chlormethiazole was sorbed to polyvinyl chloride extension tubing at slow flow rates. In comparison, only about 20% of the initial concentration was sorbed to polyethylene tubing. As flow rate was increased, sorption decreased slightly whereas an increase in the length of the line resulted in a non-proportional increase in sorption. No evidence of softening of the tubing was observed.

FORMULATION

Excipients

Excipients that have been used in presentations of chlormethiazole include:
Capsules, chlormethiazole: Miglyol 812.
Tablets, chlormethiazole edisylate: acacia; beeswax; carmellose sodium; carnauba wax; castor oil; colloidal anhydrous silica; gelatin; lactose; light calcium carbonate; light magnesium oxide; magnesium stearate; maize starch; rice starch; shellac; sucrose; talc.
Syrups, chlormethiazole edisylate: cineole; ethanol; methanol; sodium hydroxide; sorbitol.
Intravenous infusions, chlormethiazole edisylate: arginine; ethanol; glucose, anhydrous; sodium hydroxide.

REFERENCES

1. Gustavii K, Ekstrand-Asker K. Acta Pharm Suec 1986;23:21–30.
2. Kowaluk EA, Roberts MS, Blackburn HD, Polack AE. Am J Hosp Pharm 1981;38:1308–14.
3. Kowaluk EA, Roberts MS, Polack AE. J Pharm Sci 1984;73:43–7.
4. Lee MG. Am J Hosp Pharm 1986;43:1945–50.
5. Roberts MS, Cossum PA, Kowaluk EA, Polack AE, Flukes WK [letter]. Med J Aust 1981;2:580–1.
6. Allwood MC. Proceedings of the Guild 1988;25:61-5.

Chloroquine (BAN, rINN)

Antimalarial; Anti-amoebic; Antirheumatic

Cloroquina
4-(7-Chloro-4-quinolylamino)pentyldiethylamine;   7-chloro-4-
(4-diethylamino-1-methylbutylamino)quinoline
$C_{18}H_{26}ClN_3 = 319.9$

Chloroquine Hydrochloride (BANM, rINNM)
$C_{18}H_{26}ClN_3, 2HCl = 392.8$

Chloroquine Phosphate (BANM, rINNM)
Chingaminum; chloroquine diphosphate; quingamine
$C_{18}H_{26}ClN_3, 2H_3PO_4 = 515.9$

Chloroquine Sulphate (BANM, rINNM)
$C_{18}H_{26}ClN_3, H_2SO_4, H_2O = 436.0$
CAS—54-05-7 (chloroquine); 3545-67-3 (chloroquine hydrochloride); 50-63-5 (chloroquine phosphate); 132-73-0 (chloroquine sulphate, anhydrous)

Pharmacopoeial status

BP (chloroquine phosphate, chloroquine sulphate); USP
(chloroquine, chloroquine phosphate)

Preparations

Compendial
Chloroquine Phosphate Tablets BP. Tablets containing, in each,
250 mg are usually available (250 mg of chloroquine phosphate
is approximately equivalent to 155 mg of chloroquine base).
They are coated.
Chloroquine Sulphate Tablets BP. Tablets containing, in each,
200 mg are usually available (200 mg of chloroquine sulphate
is approximately equivalent to 146 mg of chloroquine base).
They are coated.
Chloroquine Phosphate Injection BP. A sterile solution of chloroquine phosphate in water for injections. pH 3.5 to 4.5. An injection containing the equivalent of 200 mg of chloroquine base in
5 mL is usually available (40 mg of chloroquine base is approximately equivalent to 64.5 mg of chloroquine phosphate).
Chloroquine Sulphate Injection BP. A sterile solution of chloroquine sulphate in water for injections. pH 4.0 to 5.5. Injections
containing 80 mg of chloroquine base in 2 mL and 200 mg of
chloroquine base in 5 mL are usually available (40 mg of chloroquine base is approximately equivalent to 55 mg of chloroquine sulphate).
Chloroquine Phosphate Tablets USP.
Chloroquine Hydrochloride Injection USP. pH 5.5 to 6.5.

Non-compendial
Avloclor (ICI). *Tablets*, chloroquine phosphate 250 mg.
Nivaquine (Rhône-Poulenc Rorer). *Tablets*, chloroquine sul-
phate 200 mg.
Syrup, chloroquine sulphate 68 mg/5mL.
Injection, chloroquine sulphate 54.5 mg/mL. During administra-
tion by slow intravenous infusion it is mixed with sodium chlor-
ide 0.9% injection.

Containers and storage

Solid state
Chloroquine Phosphate BP and Chloroquine Sulphate BP
should be kept in airtight containers and protected from light.
Chloroquine USP and Chloroquine Phosphate USP should be
preserved in well-closed containers.

Dosage forms
Chloroquine Phosphate Tablets USP should be preserved in
well-closed containers.
Chloroquine Hydrochloride Injection USP should be preserved
in single-dose containers, preferably of Type I glass.
Avloclor tablets should be stored at room temperature. When in
plastic containers they should be protected from light and moisture.
Nivaquine tablets and injection should be protected from light.
Nivaquine syrup should be stored below 25° and protected from
light.

PHYSICAL PROPERTIES

Chloroquine base is a white or slightly yellow, odourless, crystalline powder with a bitter taste.
Chloroquine phosphate is a white or almost white, odourless,
crystalline powder with a bitter taste. It is hygroscopic.
Chloroquine sulphate is a white or almost white, odourless, crystalline powder.

Melting point

Chloroquine base melts in the range 87° to 92°.
Chloroquine phosphate exists in two polymorphic forms; one
form melts in the range 193° to 195° and the other melts in the
range 210° to 218°.
Chloroquine sulphate melts in the range 205° to 210°.

pH

A 10% w/v solution of *chloroquine phosphate* has a pH of 3.8 to
4.3. A 1% w/v solution has a pH of about 4.5.
An 8% w/v solution of *chloroquine sulphate* has a pH of 4.0 to
5.0.

Dissociation constants

Chloroquine, pK_a 8.4, 10.8
Chloroquine phosphate, pK_a 8.1 (base) and 9.94 (base)
Chloroquine base has two sites of ionisation and can exist in
either the diprotonated, monoprotonated, or neutral state. Ferrari and Cutler[1] investigated the temperature dependence of
ionisation, using nonlinear regression analysis to calculate pK_a
values. As the temperature was increased in the range 0° to
37°, pK_a values decreased. At 20°, values of 8.5 and 10.87
were determined for chloroquine in the ground state. The
most common tautomeric form of chloroquine is protonated
at the alkylamino nitrogen and the other is protonated at the
quinoline ring nitrogen.

Solubility

Chloroquine is very slightly soluble in water; soluble in chloroform, in ether, and in dilute acids.
Chloroquine phosphate is freely soluble (1 in 4) in water, although
solubility is reduced at neutral or alkaline pH. It is practically
insoluble in ethanol and in benzene; very slightly soluble in
chloroform, in ether, and in methanol.
Chloroquine sulphate is soluble 1 in 3 of water and very slightly
soluble in ethanol; freely soluble in methanol; practically insoluble in acetone, in chloroform, and in ether.

Dissolution

The USP specifies that for Chloroquine Phosphate Tablets USP not less than 75% of the labelled amount of $C_{18}H_{26}ClN_3, 2H_3PO_4$ is dissolved in 45 minutes. Dissolution medium: 900 mL of water; Apparatus 2 at 100 rpm.

Crystal and molecular structure

Polymorphs

Van Aerde et al[2] identified the polymorphic type of two batches of chloroquine phosphate (CDP1, Rhône-Poulenc and CDP2, Sigma). Differential thermal analysis (DTA) produced a trace with one endothermic peak at 196° for CDP2, whereas the trace representative of CDP1 had peaks at 196° and 216° indicating that two polymorphic modifications were present in that batch. A heating microscope was used to examine the melting behaviour of the powders; CDP2 was completely melted at 200°, however the formation of small, regular crystals was observed between 200° and 210° in the sample CDP1. These crystals melted at 216°, corresponding with the second peak on the DTA thermogram.

FURTHER INFORMATION. Separation of chloroquine enantiomers by high performance liquid chromatography—Ibrahim KE, Fell AF. J Pharm Biomed Anal 1990;8:449–52.

STABILITY

Chloroquine phosphate absorbs insignificant amounts of moisture at relative humidities up to about 80% at temperatures up to 37°.

Solutions of chloroquine phosphate of pH 4 to 6 are stable when heated but sensitive to light.

Following ultraviolet irradiation of chloroquine phosphate at pH 8 using a 254 nm lamp, a spectral shift was observed.[3] When chloroquine phosphate in phosphate buffer solution (pH 8) was irradiated with a 366 nm ultraviolet lamp, the spectral changes that occurred were accompanied by the appearance of a pink coloration. Further investigations indicated that ultraviolet irradiation led to the production of at least four decomposition products; chloroquine (as the phosphate in phosphate buffer) formed fluorescent compounds which further decomposed, with production of a pink coloration and quenching of fluorescence.

Nord et al[4] investigated the photodegradation of chloroquine in oxygen-containing solutions. Following irradiation of solutions of chloroquine in isopropanol at 240 nm to 600 nm and in phosphate buffer (pH 7.4) at 320 nm to 600 nm, the main degradation products were 4-amino-7-chloroquinoline and desethylchloroquine. Further analysis of solutions in isopropanol revealed other compounds (seven of which were isolated and identified) some of these compounds were attributed to a reaction between isopropanol and chloroquine fragments. The observed half-life of chloroquine in isopropanol (3.2 mg/mL) under continuous light at 240 nm to 600 nm was 3.5 hours.

INCOMPATIBILITY/COMPATIBILITY

Sorption

The rate and extent of binding of chloroquine (phosphate) to different grades of glass was examined by Yahya et al.[5] Binding to soda glass wool was dependent upon pH and concentration; in general, an increase in the drug concentration resulted in a reduction in the percentage of chloroquine phosphate bound. Binding was greatest at concentrations below 0.25 micrograms/mL and at physiological pH. Binding to soda glass test-tubes also decreased with increasing drug concentration; pH studies demonstrated that the amount of drug bound was greatest at pH 7.4 and least at pH values of 4 and 9.5. Binding to borosilicate glass test-tubes was negligible.

The above workers undertook a further study to examine the binding of chloroquine (phosphate) to various plastic materials with different physicochemical characteristics.[6] Minimal binding to polystyrene Petri dishes was evident. However, the other plastics tested all demonstrated sorption of chloroquine (phosphate); the degree of drug bound decreased in the order: cellulose propionate > methacrylate butadiene styrene > polypropylene > polyvinyl chloride > ethyl vinyl acetate > polyethylene. It was suggested that the drug molecules were bound by an absorption and diffusion mechanism. Sorption was greatest at pH 9.5 and least at pH 4. As the chloroquine phosphate concentration of the test solutions was increased, the amount of drug bound also increased. Following exposure to polyvinyl chloride for 12 hours, an equilibrium state was attained. Immediate and extensive binding (pH-dependent) to cellulose acetate membrane filters was demonstrated.

In an in-vitro study to examine the effects of filtration on the activities of some standard antimalarial agents against Plasmodium falciparum, Baird and Lambros[7] tested four commercially available membrane filters of different composition. Binding of chloroquine phosphate was greatest with a fluorocarbon filter unit. At high drug concentration (2 g/L) no reduction in drug activity was evident after filtration; however, an appreciable reduction in activity was observed when solutions of low concentration (10 mg/L) were filtered. Detergents or other components of the filters may also have been present in the filtrate. It was recommended that antimalarial drug solutions be filtered at high concentration, followed by aseptic serial dilution of the filtrate. An alternative method of preparing sterile solutions was suggested which involved the initial dissolution of the drug in ethanol with subsequent serial dilutions performed aseptically.

FURTHER INFORMATION. Adsorption of paracetamol and chloroquine phosphate by some antacids—Iwuagwu MA, Aloko KS. J Pharm Pharmacol 1992;44:655–8. An in vitro chemical interaction between promethazine and chloroquine phosphate—Abubakar AA, Mustapha A, Wambebe OC. Int Pharm J 1993;7:14–18.

FORMULATION

Excipients

Excipients that have been used in presentations of chloroquine include:

Tablets, chloroquine phosphate: acacia; calcium hydrogen phosphate; carnauba wax; erythrosine (E127); gelatin; glucose; kaolin; magnesium stearate; maize starch; sucrose; talc; yellow beeswax.

Chloroquine sulphate: gelatin; glucose; magnesium stearate; silica (hydrated); starch; sugar.

Syrups, chloroquine phosphate: glycerol; cherry syrup; syrup.

Chloroquine sulphate: amaranth (E123); caramel; citric acid; coffee extract; methyl and propyl hydroxybenzoates; monosodium glutamate; saccharin sodium; sugars; tartrazine (E102).

Injections, chloroquine sulphate: potassium sulphite (anhydrous); sodium sulphite.

Bioavailability

Workers in Egypt[8] prepared chloroquine phosphate suppositories with Witepsol H15 as basis, and compared their in-vitro release and in-vivo bioavailability with those of commercial tablets containing the same dose of drug (250 mg). The partition coefficient of the drug in the suppositories was markedly affected by pH and this was linked to the higher potential of the drug to be absorbed at rectal pH than at the pH of the stomach. Drug release from both the suppositories and the tablets appeared to follow first-order kinetics. After 60 minutes, the amount of drug released (in vitro) from the tablets and suppositories were 90% and 70%, respectively. In-vivo tests showed that urinary excretion levels peaked after 2 hours following administration of the suppositories and after 3 hours following tablet administration and drug release from the two preparations was 60% and 48%, respectively. It was concluded that the suppository formulation tested could be considered as a suitable dosage form for chloroquine phosphate administration.

However, a relative bioavailability of 10% to 53% was calculated for chloroquine from suppositories (chloroquine phosphate in Witepsol H15) compared to that of oral tablets (Resochin, Bayer, Germany) in a study involving ten healthy volunteers.[9]

Chloroquine was rapidly absorbed (peak plasma concentration reached within 15 minutes) following administration by the intramuscular and intravenous routes to healthy Nigerian volunteers.[10] All patients who received intramuscular chloroquine had side-effects. Controversy surrounds the intramuscular administration of this drug and the results of this study supported the view that this route is not advisable where the drug could be administered orally. Slow intravenous infusion of 5 mg/kg over 2 to 4 hours was considered the preferable alternative to oral administration.

Tablets

Megwa et al[11] compared cassava starch with the commercial product Sta Rx 1500 (directly compressible starch) as direct compression excipients for chloroquine phosphate tablets. The inclusion of starch produced tablets with short disintegration times. Cassava starch formulations were less compressible and release of chloroquine phosphate from these preparations was faster than from tablets prepared with Sta Rx 1500. Disintegration and dissolution from the tablets investigated was a function of the hardness of the formulation.

Dissolution of chloroquine phosphate (as a model drug) from matrix tablets obeyed first-order kinetics.[12] The tablets contained polyvinyl alcohol (Mowiol 20-98), ethylcellulose, talc, magnesium stearate and, in one formulation, calcium sulphate. About 55% of chloroquine phosphate was released in 60 minutes with the remainder released more slowly by 4 to 6 hours.

Oral liquids

The use of cellulose derivatives as viscosity-imparting agents in formulations of chloroquine phosphate syrup was assessed by Odusote and Nasipuri.[13] A degree of interaction appeared to take place between the drug and carmellose sodium although no complexation was evident between chloroquine phosphate and methylcellulose. A syrup was prepared using methylcellulose (1.12%) as the basis and 0.05% w/v Talin (Tate & Lyle) as a sweetening agent. The stability of this preparation was compared with that of a preparation containing 85% w/v sucrose syrup as basis and sweetener with the same viscosity or flow rate. Following storage at 5°, room temperature, or 40° for 12 weeks, no change in concentration of chloroquine phosphate was observed. When stored in colourless plain bottles and stored under diffused light in a chamber fitted with a fluorescent lamp, the degradation rates of both the sucrose syrup and methylcellulose solution were similar. Degradation in amber-coloured bottles was minimal.

The antimicrobial activity of a number of preservatives (methyl and propyl hydroxybenzoates and sorbic acid), individually and in combination, in chloroquine phosphate syrup was assessed.[14] The preservatives were tested for their efficacy against Staphylococcus aureus, Escherichia coli, Candida albicans, Aspergillus niger, and Debaromyces hansenu. A. niger demonstrated greatest resistance against the preservatives tested. It was concluded that sorbic acid, in combination with citric acid to adjust the pH to a value of about 4, was the most suitable preservative. A formulation, based on these findings, was suggested.

Suppositories

A suppository basis consisting of a mixture of macrogols 1000 and 6000 (7:3) and the absorption promoter polysorbate 80 (0.5% w/w) was used to prepare suppositories containing chloroquine phosphate 200 mg or 300 mg (displacement value 1.18).[15] After administration to children of average age 21 months, rectal absorption and elimination parameters were studied and compared with literature values reported after administration of a single oral dose. The results suggested that the suppositories may be a useful alternative to oral formulations of chloroquine phosphate, subject to further investigation.

The physicochemical characteristics of chloroquine phosphate suppositories in four different bases were evaluated by Ifudu and Odimgbe.[16] The bases studied were theobroma oil (displacement value 1.47 ± 0.25) and three macrogol mixtures composed of various combinations of macrogols 400, 1000, 1500, 4000, 6000 (displacement values 1.22 ± 0.14, 1.24 ± 0.19, 1.19 ± 0.2, respectively). At 37°, theobroma oil suppositories melted at a much greater rate than the macrogol-based preparations. At low concentrations of chloroquine phosphate (5% or less) drug release (in vitro) from the macrogol-based (water-soluble) suppositories was higher than from the theobroma oil (water-insoluble) ones. However, this pattern was reversed when the drug concentration was increased to 10%.

The above workers undertook a further study to investigate the rectal absorption of chloroquine phosphate from the bases examined in their initial study and to identify any correlation between in-vitro and in-vivo results.[17] Theobroma oil melted at body temperature, releasing the drug, with rapid partitioning into the rectal fluid. Dissolution of the vehicle in the rectal fluid appeared to be the rate limiting step of absorption from macrogol formulations. Ten hours after administration, there was no significant difference in the cumulative amounts of drug and its metabolites excreted from the different bases. Higher drug concentrations were produced from the theobroma oil basis and one of the macrogol mixtures, and these two bases were used in a study comparing oral and rectal administration of chloroquine phosphate which indicated that the two routes compared favourably. Rectal administration reduced the type and number of side-effects and produced a more steady urinary excretion profile compared with that of the oral route. See also Bioavailability, above.

Emulsions

Multiple water-in-oil-in-water emulsions were prepared that consisted of an aqueous phase of chloroquine phosphate (10 mg/mL) with 2% w/v of either acacia, gelatin, or povidone, an oil phase of soybean oil with 10% w/v sorbitan monooleate (Span 80), and a secondary emulsifier phase of water with 1% Tween 80.[18] Release of chloroquine phosphate in vitro was slower from emulsions than from an aqueous solution; the emulsions prepared with acacia prolonged release most effectively. Following storage of the emulsions at room temperature for two weeks, reduced release rates were observed.

FURTHER INFORMATION. Liquid dosage form of chloroquine—Closson RG [letter]. Drug Intell Clin Pharm 1988;22:347. Comment: liquid dosage form of chloroquine—Dupuis L, Rappaport P; Lee H; Williams FE; Closson RG [letters]. Drug Intell Clin Pharm 1988;22:828–9. Comparative bioavailability of rectal and oral formulations of chloroquine—Tjoeng MM, Hogeman PHG, Kapelle H, De Ridder MLJ, Verhaar H. Pharm Weekbl (Sci) 1991;13(4):176–8. The disposition of chloroquine in healthy Nigerians after single intravenous and oral doses—Walker O, Salako LA, Alvan G, Ericsson O, Sjoqvist F. Br J Clin Pharmacol 1987;23:295–301. The parenteral controlled release of liposomal encapsulated chloroquine in *mice*—Titulaer HAC, Eling WMC, Crommelin DJA, Peeters PAM, Zuidema J. J Pharm Pharmacol 1990;42:529–32. Effect of chloroquine on the globule structure of certain water-in-oil-in-water multiple emulsions—Okor RS. Pharm World 1988;5:312–16. Some properties of chloroquine phosphate and quinine hydrochloride microcapsules—Chukwu A, Adikwu MU. STP Pharma Sci 1991;1:117–20.

PROCESSING

Sterilisation

Chloroquine phosphate injection and chloroquine sulphate injection can be sterilised by heating in an autoclave. Solutions for injection have also been sterilised by filtration (see Incompatibility, above).

REFERENCES

1. Ferrari V, Cutler DJ. J Pharm Sci 1987;76(7):554–6.
2. Van Aerde P, Remon JP, De Rudder D, Van Severen R, Braeckman P. J Pharm Pharmacol 1984;36:190–1.
3. Owoyale JA. Int J Pharmaceutics 1989;52:179–81.
4. Nord K, Karlsen J, Tønnesen HH. Int J Pharmaceutics 1991;72:11–18.
5. Yahya AM, McElnay JC, D'Arcy PF. Int J Pharmaceutics 1985;25:217–23.
6. Yahya AM, McElnay JC, D'Arcy PF. Int J Pharmaceutics 1986;34:137–43.
7. Baird JK, Lambros C. Bull Wld Hlth Org 1984;62(3):439–44.
8. Abdel-Gawad AGH, Zein El-Din E.E-S. Drug Dev Ind Pharm 1989;15:2681–93.
9. Tjoeng M, Hogeman PHG, Kapelle H, De Ridder MLJ, Verhaar H. Pharm Weekbl (Sci) 1991;13(4):176–8.
10. Fadeke Aderounmu A, Salako LA, Lindstrom B, Walker O, Ekman L. Br J Clin Pharmacol 1986;22:559–64.
11. Megwa SA, Obiakor CO, Aly SAS. STP Pharma 1988;4:392-6.
12. Gaizer SN, Pintye-Hodi K, Selmeczi B. Pharm Ind 1989;51:1444–6.
13. Odusote MO, Nasipuri RN. Pharm Ind 1988;50(3):367–9.
14. Van Doorne H, Wieringa NF, Bosch EH, De Meijer R. Pharm Weekbl (Sci) 1988;10:170–2.
15. Okor RS, Nwankwo MU. J Clin Pharm Ther 1988;13:219–23.
16. Ifudu ND, Odimgbe JO. Arch Pharm Chemi (Sci) 1987;15:1–7.
17. Ifudu ND, Odimgbe JO. Arch Pharm Chemi (Sci) 1987;15:8–14.
18. Omotosho JA. Int J Pharmaceutics 1990;62:81–4.

Chlorpheniramine (BAN)

Histamine H_1-receptor antagonist

Chlorphenamine (rINN); chlorprophenpyridamine

3-(4-Chlorophenyl)-3-(2-pyridyl)propyldimethylamine; (±)-3-(4-chlorophenyl)-*N*-*N*-dimethyl-3-(2-pyridyl)propylamine

$C_{16}H_{19}ClN_2 = 274.8$

Chlorpheniramine Maleate (BANM)

Chlorphenamine Maleate (rINNM)

$C_{16}H_{19}ClN_2, C_4H_4O_4 = 390.9$

CAS—132-22-9 (chlorpheniramine); 42882-96-2 (chlorpheniramine, ±); 113-92-8 (chlorpheniramine maleate)

Pharmacopoeial status

BP, USP (chlorpheniramine maleate)

Preparations

Compendial

Chlorpheniramine Tablets BP. Contain chlorpheniramine maleate. Tablets containing, in each, 4 mg are usually available.

Chlorpheniramine Oral Solution BP (Chlorpheniramine Elixir). A solution of chlorpheniramine maleate in a suitable flavoured vehicle. If diluted, the oral solution should be freshly prepared. An oral solution containing 2 mg in 5 mL is usually available.

Chlorpheniramine Injection BP. A colourless, sterile solution of chlorpheniramine maleate in water for injections free from dissolved air. pH 4.0 to 5.2. An injection containing 10 mg in 1 mL is usually available.

Chlorpheniramine Maleate Extended-release Capsules USP.

Chlorpheniramine Maleate Tablets USP.

Chlorpheniramine Maleate Syrup USP.

Chlorpheniramine Maleate Injection USP. pH between 4.0 and 5.2.

Non-compendial

Piriton (A&H). *Tablets*, chlorpheniramine maleate 4 mg.

Syrup, chlorpheniramine maleate 2 mg/5 mL.

Injection, chlorpheniramine maleate 10 mg/mL.

Chlorpheniramine tablets are also available from Cox.

Containers and storage

Solid state

Chlorpheniramine Maleate BP should be kept in a well-closed container and protected from light.

Chlorpheniramine Maleate USP should be preserved in tight, light-resistant containers.

Dosage forms

Chlorpheniramine Oral Solution BP should be protected from light and stored at a temperature not exceeding 25°.

Chlorpheniramine Injection BP should be protected from light.

Chlorpheniramine Maleate Tablets USP and Extended-release Capsules USP should be preserved in tight containers and Chlorpheniramine Maleate Syrup USP should be kept in tight, light-resistant containers.

Chlorpheniramine Maleate Injection USP should be preserved in single-dose or in multiple-dose containers, preferably of Type I glass, protected from light.

Piriton tablets should be stored below 30°. Piriton injection should be stored below 25° and protected from light.

PHYSICAL PROPERTIES

Chlorpheniramine is an oily liquid.
Chlorpheniramine maleate is a white crystalline powder; odourless with a bitter taste.

Melting point

Chlorpheniramine maleate melts in the range 130° to 135°.

pH

pH of a 1% solution of *chlorpheniramine maleate*, 4.0 to 5.0.

Dissociation constant

pK_a 9.1 (25°)

Solubility

Chlorpheniramine maleate is freely soluble in water (1 in 4); soluble in ethanol (1 in 10) and in chloroform (1 in 10); slightly soluble in ether and in benzene.

Dissolution

The USP specifies that for Chlorpheniramine Maleate Tablets USP not less than 75% of the labelled amount of $C_{16}H_{19}ClN_2, C_4H_4O_4$ is dissolved in 45 minutes. Dissolution medium: 500 mL of water; Apparatus 2 at 50 rpm.

FURTHER INFORMATION. Chlorpheniramine dissolution and relative urinary excretion from [sustained-release and immediate-release] commercial products [six combination preparations and one single-entity preparation]—Hsu H-Y, Ayres JW. J Pharm Sci 1989;78(10):844–7.

STABILITY

No degradation of chlorpheniramine maleate was reported when aqueous solutions containing 15 mg/5 mL, (buffered to pH 2, 4, 6, and 8), in sealed glass ampoules, were stored under fluorescent light or in the dark for 3 months at 25°.[1]

INCOMPATIBILITY/COMPATIBILITY

Physical incompatibilities have been reported between intravenous solutions of chlorpheniramine maleate and calcium chloride, noradrenaline acid tartrate, or pentobarbitone sodium.[2]

Chlorpheniramine maleate injection has also been reported to be incompatible with kanamycin sulphate and iodipamide meglumine.

Sanchez Camazano *et al*[3] investigated the adsorption of chlorpheniramine maleate by sodium montmorillonite using X-ray diffraction and infrared spectroscopy. In aqueous solution, chlorphenirammonium ions penetrated and were adsorbed into the interlayer space of montmorillonite to form a complex by a cation-exchange mechanism. Further work[4] demonstrated that the amount of chlorpheniramine adsorbed increased as the pH of aqueous suspensions (50 mL) of chlorpheniramine maleate 0.2 mEq with 100 mg sodium montmorillonite was increased. A Langmuir plot of adsorption data followed a straight line.

FORMULATION

Excipients

Excipients that have been used in presentations of chlorpheniramine maleate include:

Capsules (timed-release): acid fuchsine D; allura red AC (E129); benzyl alcohol; cetylpyridinium chloride; erythrosine (E127); ethylcellulose; fast green FCF; gelatin; hydrogenated castor oil; silica; sodium lauryl sulphate; starch; sucrose; sunset yellow FCF (E110).

Tablets: lactose.

Ointments and transdermal devices

The rate of release of chlorpheniramine maleate from several semi-solid ointment bases decreased in the order: water-in-oil emulsion > oil-in-water emulsion > anhydrous ointments.[5] Formulations were presented, and experiments were performed using a Sartorius Absorption Simulator (buffer at pH 7.2). The addition of a Tween 80-Span 80 mixture to the oil-in-water emulsion ointment increased the release rate, whereas the addition of propylene glycol or glycerol had no effect. An increase in chlorpheniramine maleate concentration (from 3% to 5%) produced increased release rates from oil-in-water and water-in-oil emulsion ointments.

Studies of devices for transdermal delivery of chlorpheniramine across hairless *mouse* skin *in vitro* have been published. Two novel devices were examined: hydrogel patches that contained poly(hydroxyethyl methacrylate) with other excipients;[6] and a hydrogel system that contained a copolymer of N-morpholinoethyl methacrylate, 2-hydroxyethyl acrylate, and glycerol or triacetin.[7]

Correlation was observed between flux *in vitro* and plasma concentrations (in humans) of chlorpheniramine produced from transdermal patch formulations.[8]

Studies of the release of chlorpheniramine maleate from a polymeric gel basis, a modified hydrophilic basis, and a modified hydrophilic petrolatum basis indicated that greatest release was from the gel basis.[9] Tests were performed *in vitro* through a cellulose membrane and across hairless *mouse* skin. The effect of additives (urea, ethanol, and dimethyl sulphoxide) on release was investigated.

Modified-release preparations

Sprockel *et al*[10] examined a sustained-release oral liquid preparation of chlorpheniramine maleate. Particles of a complex of chlorpheniramine maleate and carboxylic acid cation-exchange resin were coated with cellulose acetate butyrate, and the resulting microcapsules were suspended in an aqueous solution of methylcellulose 1500. Release of chlorpheniramine was more rapid from smaller microcapsules, and faster in simulated gastric fluid (pH 1.2) than in simulated intestinal fluid (pH 7.5). In a crossover study with four *dogs*, absolute bioavailabilities of an oral solution of chlorpheniramine maleate and the microcapsule suspension were 92.1% and 83.3%, respectively.

The dissolution rate *in vitro* of chlorpheniramine maleate from gelatin micropellets, which were 'rigidised' with formaldehyde vapour for 90 hours, compared favourably with that from a commercial sustained-release product (Zeet SR, Alembic, India).[11]

In a single-dose, crossover study,[12] 15 healthy volunteers received the following preparations: chlorpheniramine maleate as conventional-release tablets (Chlortrimeton, Schering, USA); a syrup (Chlortrimeton Syrup, Schering, USA); coated, slow-release bead capsules (Teldrin Spansules, SKF, USA) and 'repeat-action' tablets (Chlortrimeton Repetabs, Schering,

USA). From the area under plasma concentration versus time curves, bioavailability of the controlled-release products was shown to be lower than that of the immediate-release products. However, large intra-subject and inter-subject variations were noted.

Coated beads

Bodmeier and Paeratakul[13] prepared aqueous ethyl cellulose pseudolatexes (by a microfluidisation-solvent evaporation method, with dibutyl sebacate as a plasticiser) that were used to coat chlorpheniramine maleate-loaded beads. The release of chlorpheniramine maleate from coated preparations and from beads coated with a commercial ethyl cellulose pseudolatex (Aquacoat) was studied in 0.1M hydrochloric acid and pH 7.4 buffer solutions; the effects of the curing and coating temperatures and of the composition of pseudolatexes were investigated. When sodium lauryl sulphate was present in the pseudolatex, release was greatest at pH 7.4. Increasing the concentration of cetyl alcohol (a cosurfactant) in the pseudolatex decreased the amount of drug released.

FURTHER INFORMATION. Skin permeation [*in vitro*] of chlorpheniramine maleate and detection of demethylated metabolites by high-performance liquid chromatography [metabolism in skin]—Zbaida S, Touitou E [letter]. J Pharm Sci 1988;77(2):188–90. Evaluation of sustained-action chlorpheniramine-pseudoephedrine dosage form in humans [bioavailability study]—Yacobi A, Stoll RG, Chao GC, Carter JE, Baaske DM, Kamath BL, Amann AH, Lai C-M. J Pharm Sci 1980;69(9):1077–81. Release of chlorpheniramine maleate from fatty acid ester matrix disks prepared by melt-extrusion—Prapaitrakul W, Sprockel OL, Shivanand P. J Pharm Pharmacol 1991;43:377–81. Dissolution profiles of resin-based oral suspensions [chlorpheniramine polistirex]—Ogger KE, Noory C, Gabay J, Shah VP, Skelly JP. Pharmaceut Technol 1991 Sept;15:84, 86, 88, 90–1.

PROCESSING

Sterilisation

Chlorpheniramine injection can be sterilised by heating in an autoclave.

REFERENCES

1. Eckhart CG, McCorkle T. In: Florey K, editor. Analytical profiles of drug substances; vol 7. London: Academic Press, 1978:43–80.
2. Patel JA, Phillips GL. Am J Hosp Pharm 1966;23:409–11.
3. Sanchez Camazano M, Sanchez MJ, Vicente MT, Dominguez-Gil A. J Pharm Sci 1980;69(10):1142–4.
4. Sanchez Camazano M, Sanchez MJ, Vicente MT, Dominguez-Gil A. Int J Pharmaceutics 1980;6:243–51.
5. Velissaratou AS, Papaioannou G. Int J Pharmaceutics 1989;52:83–6.
6. Song SZ, Rashidbaigi ZA, Mehta SC, Nesbitt RU, Fawzi MB. J Pharm Sci 1987;76(11):C07-Z-38,S56.
7. Song SZ, Rashidbaigi ZA, Mehta SC, Nesbitt RU, Fawzi MB. J Pharm Sci 1987;76(11):C07-Z-39,S57.
8. Smith D, Dey M, Enever R, Leonard T, Mulvana D, Thone G. J Pharm Sci 1987;76(11):D06-W-30,S68.
9. Babar A, Bhandari RD, Plakogiannis FM. Drug Dev Ind Pharm 1991;17(16):2145–56.
10. Sprockel OL, Price JC, Jennings R, Tackett RL, Hemingway S, Clark B et al. Drug Dev Ind Pharm 1989;15(9):1393–1404.
11. Sista SM, Das SK, Gupta BK. Indian J Pharm Sci 1987;49:62–4.
12. Kotzan JA, Vallner JJ, Stewart JT, Brown WJ, Viswanathan CT, Needham TE et al. J Pharm Sci 1982;71(8):919–23.
13. Bodmeier R, Paeratakul O. Int J Pharmaceutics 1991;70:59–68.

Chlorpromazine (BAN, rINN)

Antipsychotic; Anti-emetic
3-(2-Chlorophenothiazin-10-yl)propyldimethylamine; 2-chloro-*N,N*-dimethyl-10*H*-phenothiazine-10-propanamine
$C_{17}H_{19}ClN_2S = 318.9$

Chlorpromazine Embonate (BANM, rINNM)
$(C_{17}H_{19}ClN_2S)_2, C_{23}H_{16}O_6 = 1026.1$

Chlorpromazine Hydrochloride (BANM, rINNM)
$C_{17}H_{19}ClN_2S, HCl = 355.3$
CAS—50-53-3 (chlorpromazine); 69-09-0 (chlorpromazine hydrochloride)

Pharmacopoeial status

BP, USP (chlorpromazine, chlorpromazine hydrochloride)

Preparations

Compendial
Chlorpromazine Tablets BP. Tablets containing, in each, chlorpromazine hydrochloride 10 mg, 25 mg, 50 mg, and 100 mg are usually available.
Chlorpromazine Oral Solution BP (Chlorpromazine Elixir). Contains chlorpromazine hydrochloride in a flavoured vehicle. An oral solution containing 25 mg in 5 mL is usually available. If dilution is required, the solution should be freshly prepared.
Chlorpromazine Suppositories BP. Contain chlorpromazine in a suitable suppository basis. Suppositories containing, in each, 100 mg are usually available.
Chlorpromazine Injection BP. A sterile solution containing chlorpromazine hydrochloride in water for injections free from dissolved air. Injections containing 25 mg in 1 mL and 50 mg in 2 mL are usually available. pH 5.0 to 6.5.
Chlorpromazine Hydrochloride Tablets USP.
Chlorpromazine Hydrochloride Oral Concentrate USP.
Chlorpromazine Hydrochloride Syrup USP.
Chlorpromazine Suppositories USP.
Chlorpromazine Hydrochloride Injection USP. pH 3.4 to 5.4.

Non-compendial
Largactil (Rhône-Poulenc Rorer). *Tablets*, chlorpromazine hydrochloride 10 mg, 25 mg, 50 mg, and 100 mg.
Syrup, chlorpromazine hydrochloride 25 mg/5 mL. *Diluent*: syrup (without preservative), life of diluted syrup 14 days.
Suspension forte, sugar free, chlorpromazine embonate 145 mg/5 mL (equivalent to chlorpromazine hydrochloride 100 mg/5 mL). *Diluent*: syrup (without preservative), life of diluted suspension 7 days.

Injection, chlorpromazine hydrochloride 25 mg/mL. pH 5.0 to 6.5. If pink or yellow discoloration develops, as may occur on exposure to light, the solution should be discarded. Injection solutions are incompatible with benzylpenicillin potassium, pentobarbitone sodium, and phenobarbitone sodium.
Chlorpromazine hydrochloride tablets of various strengths are also available from APS, DDSA (Chloractil), Norton.
Chlorpromazine suppositories are available from Penn.

Containers and storage

Solid state

Chlorpromazine BP should be stored in well-closed containers, protected from light.
Chlorpromazine Hydrochloride BP should be stored in airtight containers, protected from light.
Chlorpromazine USP and Chlorpromazine Hydrochloride USP should be preserved in tight, light-resistant containers.

Dosage forms

Chlorpromazine Oral Solution BP, Chlorpromazine Suppositories BP, and Chlorpromazine Injection BP should be protected from light.
Chlorpromazine Hydrochloride Tablets USP and Chlorpromazine Suppositories USP should be preserved in well-closed, light-resistant containers at controlled room temperature.
Chlorpromazine Hydrochloride Oral Concentrate USP and Chlorpromazine Hydrochloride Syrup USP should be preserved in tight, light-resistant containers.
Chlorpromazine Hydrochloride Injection USP should be preserved in single-dose or multiple-dose containers, preferably of Type I glass, protected from light.
Largactil tablets should not be crushed and solutions should be handled carefully as there is a risk of contact dermatitis.
Largactil preparations should be protected from light. Largactil tablets should be stored below 30° and other Largactil products below 25°.

PHYSICAL PROPERTIES

Chlorpromazine is a white or creamy-white powder or waxy solid; odourless or with an amine-like odour; darkens on prolonged exposure to light.
Chlorpromazine embonate is a pale yellow powder.
Chlorpromazine hydrochloride is a white or almost white crystalline powder; odourless; decomposes on exposure to air and light becoming yellow, pink, then violet.

Melting point

Chlorpromazine melts in the range 56° to 60°.
Chlorpromazine hydrochloride melts in the range 195° to 198°.

pH

A solution of *chlorpromazine hydrochloride* 10% w/v in water, freshly prepared, has a pH of 3.5 to 4.5.

Dissociation constant

pK_a 9.3 (20°)

Partition coefficients

Log P (octanol/pH 7.4), 3.4
Whelpton[1] determined the log P (octanol/water) for chlorpromazine to be 5.3.
Cheng *et al*[2] developed a mathematical model and evaluated thermodynamic parameters for the partitioning of chlorpromazine hydrochloride between octanol and aqueous acetate buffers, over ranges of pH, buffer concentration, and temperature.

Solubility

Chlorpromazine is practically insoluble in water; it is soluble 1 in 2 of ethanol, 1 in less than 1 of chloroform, and 1 in 1 of ether; it is practically insoluble in dilute alkali hydroxides but freely soluble in dilute mineral acids.
Chlorpromazine embonate is very slightly soluble in water and soluble in acetone.
Chlorpromazine hydrochloride is soluble 1 in 0.4 of water, 1 in 1.3 of ethanol, and 1 in 1 of chloroform; it is practically insoluble in ether and soluble in methanol.

Critical micelle concentration

Measurements of the critical micelle concentrations of mixtures of chlorpromazine hydrochloride and polysorbate 80, by pH titration, suggested that in mixtures with less than 0.8 mole fraction of chlorpromazine some interaction between the two components occurred in the premicellar concentration range; in mixtures with more than 0.8 mole fraction of chlorpromazine the micellisation process was suggested to occur in two or more steps.[3]

Dissolution

The USP specifies that for Chlorpromazine Hydrochloride Tablets USP not less than 80% of the labelled amount of $C_{17}H_{19}ClN_2S$, HCl is dissolved in 30 minutes. Dissolution medium: 900 mL of 0.1N hydrochloric acid; Apparatus 1 at 50 rpm.
Changes in disintegration and dissolution behaviour of compressed chlorpromazine tablets subjected to moderate temperature (room temperature to 30°) and humidity (up to 90% relative humidity) under cyclic conditions for one to four weeks were investigated by Ondari *et al*.[4] Film-coated and sugar-coated chlorpromazine tablets (50 mg, from commercial sources) in amber safety-lock bottles were compared with a prednisone 10 mg calibrator tablet. Dissolution profiles (USP paddle) and disintegration test (USP) results indicated acceptable stability for film-coated tablets but changes in the properties of sugar-coated tablets were significant. The authors suggested that ageing effects were more likely to be associated with the sugar-coating than with the tablet core.
When El-Fattah and Khalil[5] examined three commercial brands of sugar-coated chlorpromazine tablets (10 mg, 25 mg, and 100 mg); all samples from 14 batches passed the USP test for disintegration time and content uniformity but none complied with the specification for dissolution. There were also significant differences between batches in the rate and extent of dissolution. Poor dissolution was attributed to the slow break-up of the sugar coating.
Marked differences in the dissolution rates of chlorpromazine, determined in a continuous flow analyser with drug ion-selective electrodes, were observed between formulations from different manufacturers.[6] Dissolution rates were faster at pH 1 than at pH 6.5.

STABILITY

Chlorpromazine, in powder form or in aqueous solution, degrades by photochemical oxidation to form chlorpromazine sulphoxide (chlorpromazine-5-oxide) and various phenolic compounds; the sulphoxide may undergo further oxidation to form a sulphone. Degradation occurs rapidly in alkaline solution. Degraded solutions become discoloured and solutions of chlorpromazine hydrochloride for injection that are yellow or pink should not be used.
Storage of chlorpromazine hydrochloride syrup for 18 months in filled 125-mL amber bottles resulted in about 0.5% degradation

with the formation of chlorpromazine sulphoxide, determined by difference spectrophotometry. Storage for 18 months in bottles that were only one-fifth full resulted in about 28% degradation.[7] Dugas[8] studied the effects of various storage conditions on the stability, after repackaging, of chlorpromazine hydrochloride solutions (50, 200, and 500 mg/15 mL) made by dilution of an oral concentrate 100 mg/mL (Thorazine, SK&F, USA). When stored for up to 20 weeks at 27° either under fluorescent light or in darkness, the maximum loss of chlorpromazine was 40% from clear glass vials and 13% from unit dose containers of amber glass. Bottles of undiluted oral concentrate that were either opened frequently under simulated use conditions or kept improperly closed, increased in concentration (to 115% or 124%, respectively, after 33 days at 27°). Evaporation of the vehicle may have obscured chlorpromazine degradation.

A diluted and repackaged solution of chlorpromazine hydrochloride solution (1 mg/mL in sodium chloride 0.9%) kept in 5-mL vials for 30 days in the dark at 18° to 23° exhibited negligible potency loss.[9]

FURTHER INFORMATION. The determination of chlorpromazine, related impurities and degradation products in pharmaceutical dosage forms [review of literature]—Chagonda LFS, Millership JS. J Pharm Biomed Anal 1989;7:271–8.

INCOMPATIBILITY/COMPATIBILITY

Chlorpromazine hydrochloride is reported to be incompatible with aminophylline, amphotericin, benzylpenicillin potassium, chloramphenicol sodium succinate, cimetidine hydrochloride, cyanocobalamin, dexamethasone, dimenhydrinate, ethamivan, kanamycin, paraldehyde, sodium bicarbonate, thioridazine, vitamin B complex with vitamin C, and with the sodium salts of ampicillin, benzylpenicillin, cephalothin, chlorothiazide, cloxacillin, heparin, methicillin, methohexitone, pentobarbitone, phenobarbitone, secobarbitone, sulphadiazine, and thiopentone.

Precipitation occurred when chlorpromazine and morphine were mixed in a syringe; the precipitate formed as a result of an interaction between chlorpromazine and chlorocresol, the preservative present in the morphine preparation.[10]

Yellow discoloration developed after two weeks storage protected from light in an extemporaneous mixture comprising chlorpromazine hydrochloride injection (Elkins-Sinn), promethazine hydrochloride injection (Elkins-Sinn), and pethidine hydrochloride injection preserved with *m*-cresol (Winthrop).[11] This discoloration was attributed to an interaction between chlorpromazine hydrochloride and *m*-cresol; mixtures prepared with preservative-free pethidine hydrochloride injection (Wyeth) remained colourless after storage for three months protected from light.

Sorption to plastics

Kowaluk *et al*[12,13] reported a loss of 41%, due to sorption, of chlorpromazine hydrochloride from solution following infusion at a rate of 1 mL/minute for 7 hours via an infusion set consisting of a cellulose propionate burette chamber and polyvinyl chloride tubing, and a loss of 79% following infusion at a rate of 0.08 mL/minute for one hour from a glass syringe infused through Silastic tubing. Negligible loss was reported from solutions in glass syringes with polyethylene tubing.

FORMULATION

Excipients

Excipients that have been used in presentations of chlorpromazine include:

Tablets, chlorpromazine hydrochloride: benzoic acid; croscarmellose sodium; erythrosine (E127); gelatin; hydrated silica; hypromellose; indigo carmine (E132); lactose; macrogol; magnesium stearate; methyl and propyl hydroxybenzoates; quinoline yellow (E104); starch; sucrose; sunset yellow FCF (E110); talc; titanium dioxide (E171).

Capsules, sustained release, chlorpromazine hydrochloride: benzyl alcohol; calcium sulphate; cetylpyridinium chloride; gelatin; glyceryl distearate; glyceryl monostearate; iron oxide; povidone; silica; sodium lauryl sulphate; starch; sucrose; sunset yellow FCF (E110); titanium dioxide (E171); wax.

Oral liquid concentrates, chlorpromazine hydrochloride: citric acid; hypromellose; propylene glycol; saccharin sodium; sodium benzoate; sodium calcium edetate.

Suspensions, chlorpromazine embonate: ethanol; methyl and propyl hydroxybenzoates; sodium benzoate; sorbitol; sunset yellow FCF (E110).

Syrups, chlorpromazine hydrochloride: citric acid; sodium benzoate; sodium metabisulphite; sodium sulphite; sugars.

Suppositories, chlorpromazine: glycerol; glyceryl monopalmitate; glyceryl monostearate; hydrogenated coconut oil fatty acids; hydrogenated palm kernel oil fatty acids; Witepsol H15.

Injections, chlorpromazine hydrochloride: anhydrous potassium sulphite; anhydrous sodium sulphite; ascorbic acid; benzyl alcohol; cysteine hydrochloride; potassium metabisulphite; sodium acetate; sodium bisulphite; sodium chloride; sodium citrate; sodium metabisulphite.

Bioequivalence

Two analytical methods were used to compare the bioavailability of film-coated tablets of chlorpromazine hydrochloride (Thorazine 25 mg, SK&F, USA) and sugar-coated tablets (Thorazine 25 mg, SK&F, USA) in a single-dose, two-way crossover study involving 36 healthy subjects. Bioequivalence of the two formulations was demonstrated.[14]

Syrups

From an evaluation of formulations of chlorpromazine hydrochloride syrup (0.2%) under accelerated storage conditions (at 62° under a 100 W lamp for 14 days), Gadalla and Ismail[15] predicted that the most stable vehicle formulation would contain: sucrose (66% w/w); sodium metabisulphite (0.1% w/v); methyl hydroxybenzoate (0.12% w/v) and propyl hydroxybenzoate (0.02% w/v); and propylene glycol (10% v/v). Inclusion of amaranth and citrus flavours was recommended.

Suppositories

The stability of chlorpromazine hydrochloride in various suppository bases was claimed to be dependent on light, whereas physicochemical properties (melting point, deformation time and hardness) and release characteristics depended on the basis and on the nature and concentration of surfactant.[16] Among the bases studied were Witepsols H-15, W-35, and E-75, alone or in combination with polysorbates (Tweens 20, 40, 60, or 80), and macrogols.

Modified-release preparations

Chlorpromazine base was used as the model drug (because of its low aqueous solubility) in a study of the control of drug release from microspheres composed of mixtures of the polymers polycaprolactone and cellulose propionate.[17] Drug release was mainly by permeation followed by diffusion. Pure polycaprolactone was more rapidly permeable to chlorpromazine than cellulose propionate; as the polycaprolactone content in the microsphere was increased, release of the drug was enhanced.

Vyas and Dixit[18] developed 'controlled-release osmo-regulated' coated granules of chlorpromazine hydrochloride ('osmo-sino-sules'); granules of chlorpromazine hydrochloride with sucrose and soluble lactose were coated with a polybutylmethacry-late:polyvinylacetate (80:20) semipermeable film. A water-in-oil emulsion of the coating solution was developed in order to ensure uniform distribution of macrogol 4000 (a channelling agent). Release of chlorpromazine hydrochloride *in vitro* followed zero-order kinetics. Concentrations of chlorpromazine in plasma, following administration of the 'sinosules' to *dogs*, were maintained at peak levels over about eight hours.

FURTHER INFORMATION. Controlled release chlorpromazine hydrochloride system based on polymer grafted starch—Vyas SP, Jain CP, Dixit VK. Pharmazie 1991;46:224–5. Physicochemical characterization of a phase change produced during the wet granulation of chlorpromazine hydrochloride and its effects on tableting—Wong MWY, Mitchell AG. Int J Pharmaceutics 1992;88:261–73. Effect of interpolymer complex formation of chitosan with pectin or acacia on the release behaviour of chlorpromazine HCl—Meshali MM, Gabr KE. Int J Pharmaceutics 1993;89:177–81.

PROCESSING

Sterilisation

Chlorpromazine injection can be sterilised by heating in an autoclave.

REFERENCES

1. Whelpton R. J Pharm Pharmacol 1989;41:856–8.
2. Cheng SW, Shanker R, Lindenbaum S. Pharm Res 1990;7:856–62.
3. Paiment J. J Pharm Pharmacol 1984;36:614–15.
4. Ondari CO, Prasad VK, Shah VP, Rhodes CT. Pharm Acta Helv 1984;59:149.
5. El-Fattah SA, Khalil SAH. Int J Pharmaceutics 1984;18:225–34.
6. Mitsana-Papazoglou A, Christopoulos TK, Diamandis EP, Koupparis MA. J Pharm Sci 1987;76:724–30.
7. Davidson AG. J Pharm Pharmacol 1977;29(Suppl):13P.
8. Dugas JE [letter]. Am J Hosp Pharm 1981;38:1276.
9. DeVane CL, Wailand LA, Jusko WJ [letter]. Can J Hosp Pharm 1984;37:9.
10. Crapper JB [letter]. Br Med J 1975;1:33.
11. McSherry TJ [letter]. Am J Hosp Pharm 1987;44:1574.
12. Kowaluk EA, Roberts MS, Polack AE. Am J Hosp Pharm 1982;39:460–7.
13. Kowaluk EA, Roberts MS, Polack AE. Am J Hosp Pharm 1983;40:118–19.
14. Midha KK, McKay G, Chakraborty BS, Young M, Hawes EM, Hubbard JW *et al.* J Pharm Sci 1990;79(3):196–201.
15. Gadalla MAF, Ismail AA. Pharm Ind 1983;45:814–16.
16. Meshali M, Helmy A, Gabr K. J Drug Res Egypt 1987;17:1–8.
17. Chang R-K, Price JC, Whitworth CW. Pharm Tech 1986;10:24, 26, 29, 32–3.
18. Vyas SP, Dixit VK. Drug Dev Ind Pharm 1990;16(15):2325–38.

Chlorthalidone (BAN, USAN)

Diuretic; Antihypertensive

Chlortalidone (rINN)

2-Chloro-5-(1-hydroxy-3-oxoisoindolin-1-yl) benzene-sulphonamide; 2-chloro-5-(2,3-dihydro-1-hydroxy-3-oxo-1*H*-isoindol-1-yl)benzenesulphonamide

$C_{14}H_{11}ClN_2O_4S = 338.8$

CAS—77-36-1

Pharmacopoeial status

BP, USP

Preparations

Compendial

Chlorthalidone Tablets BP. Tablets containing, in each, 50 mg and 100 mg are usually available.

Chlorthalidone Tablets USP.

Non-compendial

Hygroton (Geigy). *Tablets*, chlorthalidone 50 mg.

Compound preparations

Co-tenidone is the British Approved Name for compounded preparations of atenolol and chlorthalidone in the proportions, by weight, 4 parts to 1 part respectively. Preparations: Tenoret 50, Tenoretic (Stuart).

Co-tenidone tablets are also available from Ashbourne (Atenix Co), Cox, Kerfoot.

Containers and storage

Solid state

Chlorthalidone USP should be preserved in well-closed containers.

Dosage forms

Chlorthalidone Tablets USP should be preserved in well-closed containers.

PHYSICAL PROPERTIES

Chlorthalidone is a white or yellowish white crystalline powder; odourless or almost odourless.

Melting point

Chlorthalidone melts at about 220°, with decomposition.

A melting point range of 215° to 222°, with decomposition above this range, has been reported.[1]

Dissociation constant

pK_a 9.4

A thermodynamic dissociation constant for chlorthalidone was calculated by Fleuren *et al*[2] to be 9.35 at 25°; the mean of four determinations (by potentiometric titration) of the apparent dissociation constant of the first chlorthalidone acid group was 9.24 ± 0.02 (mean ± SEM).

Solubility

Chlorthalidone is practically insoluble in water; soluble 1 in 150 of ethanol; practically insoluble in chloroform and in ether; soluble 1 in 25 of methanol; soluble in acetone and in dilute solutions of alkali hydroxides.

Solubilities of chlorthalidone in macrogol 400:water mixtures, 20:80% v/v, 80:20% v/v, and 100:0% v/v were reported as 0.98 mg/mL, 67.8 mg/mL, and 141.5 mg/mL respectively, after shaking for 65 hours at room temperature.[1]

Effect of pH

As the pH of aqueous solutions of chlorthalidone was increased, solubility was observed to increase;[1] the effect was especially marked above pH 10. Reported solubility values at room temperature were: 0.167 mg/mL (pH 4.9), 0.180 mg/mL (pH 7.0), 0.597 mg/mL (pH 9.6), and 9.911 mg/mL (pH 10.9).

Effect of temperature

Solubility values in water of 12 mg/100 mL at 20° and 27 mg/100 mL at 37° have been reported.[1]

Effect of cosolvents

Each of the following cosolvents enhanced the solubility of chlorthalidone in mixed aqueous solvent systems:[3] glycerol, 1,2-propylene glycol, macrogol 300, macrogol 400, polypropylene glycol 420, dimethylacetamide, and dimethyl sulphoxide. Glycerol had the lowest solubility enhancing effect and dimethyl sulphoxide had the greatest effect. Optimum dielectric constants of cosolvent mixtures and mechanisms of solubility enhancement were discussed.

Dissolution

The USP specifies that for Chlorthalidone Tablets USP not less than 50% of the labelled amount of $C_{14}H_{11}ClN_2O_4S$ is dissolved in 60 minutes. Dissolution medium: 900 mL of water; Apparatus 2 at 100 rpm.

STABILITY

Stability-indicating assay for chlorthalidone formulation: Evaluation of the USP analysis and the high-performance liquid chromatographic analysis [decomposition during assay of the preparation]—Bauer J, Quick J, Krogh S, Shada D. J Pharm Sci 1983;72(8):924–8.

FORMULATION

Excipients

Excipients that have been used in presentations of chlorthalidone include:
Tablets: brilliant blue FCF (133); colloidal silica; gelatin; glycerol; methyl and propyl hydroxybenzoates; lactose; magnesium stearate; maize starch; microcrystalline cellulose; povidone; sodium starch glycollate; sunset yellow FCF (E110); sunset yellow FCF (E110), aluminium lake; talc.

Bioavailability

In a single-dose, crossover study of 4×4 Latin square design, twelve healthy volunteers received chlorthalidone 50 mg as: two 25 mg tablets from two manufacturers (USV Laboratories and Mylan Pharmaceuticals); a 10% water-macrogol 4000 solution of chlorthalidone 50 mg/100 mL; and an aqueous solution/suspension of chlorthalidone (50 mg/100 mL).[4] Ten other subjects received only tablets (Mylan Pharmaceuticals) and the solution in water-macrogol. The results demonstrated that the bioavailability of chlorthalidone from the water-macrogol solution was significantly lower than from the tablets (Mylan) and suggested that it was also lower than from the other commercial tablet (USV) or from the aqueous solution/suspension.

PROCESSING

Narurkar *et al*[5] evaluated three methods for the reduction of the particle size of chlorthalidone; they also studied the dissolution characteristics (USP XX paddle apparatus at 75 rpm in 900 mL of purified water) of chlorthalidone from prepared tablets containing chlorthalidone 25 mg and propranolol hydrochloride 80 mg. An air jet mill (fluid energy milling) and an Alpine Mill, but not a Fitzpatrick Mill, produced the desired particle size of chlorthalidone. However, decomposition of chlorthalidone (to chlorthalidone carboxylic acid) occurred in the Alpine Mill, whereas no degradation was noted following fluid energy milling. Dissolution studies indicated that to achieve the maximum dissolution rate from the tablets, a minimum effective specific surface area of chlorthalidone of 3.5 m²/g was required.

REFERENCES

1. Singer JM, O'Hare MJ, Rehm CR, Zarembo JE. In: Florey K, editor. Analytical profiles of drug substances; vol 14. London: Academic Press, 1985:1–35.
2. Fleuren HLJ, van Ginneken CAM, van Rossum JM. J Pharm Sci 1979;68(8):1056–8.
3. Ibrahim SA, Shawky S. Pharm Ind 1984;46(4):412–16.
4. Williams RL, Blume CD, Lin ET, Holford NHG, Benet LZ. J Pharm Sci 1982;71(5):533–5.
5. Narurkar A, Sheen PC, Hurwitz EL, Augustine MA. Drug Dev Ind Pharm 1987;13(2):319–28.

Cimetidine (BAN, USAN, rINN)

Histamine H₂-receptor antagonist
2-Cyano-1-methyl-3-[2-(5-methylimidazol-4-yl-methylthio)-ethyl]-guanidine; N-cyano-N'-methyl-N''-[2-[[(5-methyl-1H-imidazol-4-yl)methyl]thio]ethyl]-guanidine;
$C_{10}H_{16}N_6S = 252.3$
CAS—51481-61-9

Pharmacopoeial status

BP, USP

Preparations

Compendial
Cimetidine Tablets USP.

Non-compendial
Dyspamet (SK&F). *Chewable tablets*, sugar free, cimetidine 200 mg.
Suspension, sugar free, cimetidine 200 mg/5 mL. Dilution of the suspension is not recommended.
Tagamet (SK&F). *Tablets*, cimetidine 200 mg, 400 mg, and 800 mg.
Effervescent tablets, sugar free, cimetidine 400 mg.
Syrup, cimetidine 200 mg/5 mL.
Injection, cimetidine 100 mg/mL.

Intravenous infusion, flexible plastic containers, cimetidine 4 mg/mL in sodium chloride 0.9%. The manufacturer states compatibility with 'electrolyte and glucose solutions commonly used for intravenous infusion'.

Cimetidine tablets of various strengths are also available from APS, Ashbourne (Peptimax), Cox, CP, Evans, Galen (Galenamet), Kerfoot, Norton.

Containers and storage

Solid state

Cimetidine BP should be kept in an airtight container, protected from light.

Cimetidine USP should be preserved in tight, light-resistant containers at controlled room temperature.

Dosage forms

Cimetidine Tablets USP should be preserved in tight, light-resistant containers at controlled room temperature.

Dyspamet tablets should be stored in a dry place. Dyspamet suspension should be stored at a temperature not exceeding 25°.

Tagamet effervescent tablets should be stored in a dry place and the cap replaced after use. Tagamet syrup should be kept below 25° and Tagamet ampoules below 30°. Both should be protected from light. Tagamet infusion bags should be stored below 25° and protected from light except during use.

PHYSICAL PROPERTIES

Cimetidine is a white or almost white crystalline powder with an unpleasant odour.

Melting point

Cimetidine melts in the range 139° to 144°.

Dissociation constant

pK_a 6.8

pK_a 7.09 (25°), in 0.1M sodium chloride[1]

Partition coefficient

Apparent chloroform/water partition coefficient,[2] 0.061

Solubility

Cimetidine is soluble 1 in 200 of water, 1 in 18 of ethanol, 1 in 1000 of chloroform; insoluble in ether. It is practically insoluble in dichloromethane and in ether. It dissolves in dilute mineral acids.

Effect of pH

The solubility of cimetidine in water is increased by the addition of dilute hydrochloric acid.

Effect of temperature

At 37° cimetidine is soluble 1 in 88 of water.

Dissolution

The USP specifies that for Cimetidine Tablets USP not less than 75% of the labelled amount of $C_{10}H_{16}N_6S$ is dissolved in 15 minutes. Dissolution medium: 900 mL of water. Apparatus 1 at 100 rpm. See also Bioavailability, below.

Crystal and molecular structure

Polymorphs

Shibata *et al*[3] have characterised four crystalline forms of cimetidine. Three of these are anhydrous (A,B,D) and the fourth is a monohydrate (C). Form A is the most stable form and Form C exhibits more rapid dissolution than the other forms. On dehydration, Form C is converted into Form A.

FURTHER INFORMATION. Polymorphism of cimetidine [4 anhydrous and 3 monohydrate modifications]—Hegedus B, Gorog S. J Pharm Biomed Anal 1985;3:303–13. Bioavailability and inhibitory effect for stress ulcer of cimetidine polymorphs in *rats*—Kokubo H, Morimoto K, Ishida T, Inoue M, Morisaka K. Int J Pharmaceutics 1987;35:181–3.

STABILITY

An oral liquid preparation of cimetidine hydrochloride was stable for up to 180 days at 4° and 25° when repackaged into either polypropylene oral syringes or glass vials.[4] At 4° and 25° no significant difference was found between the cimetidine concentration of solutions packed in polypropylene syringes and glass vials. At higher temperatures (44° to 76°) degradation was greater in polypropylene syringes. The predicted shelf-life ($t_{10\%}$) at 25° was 317 days in polypropylene syringes and 332 days in glass vials. Storage at temperatures greater than 25° adversely affects the stability of oral liquid.[4]

Kac and Uvodic[5] subjected cimetidine parenteral solution (100 mg/mL) to elevated temperatures (50°, 60°, 70°, and 80°) for periods of 7 to 180 days. The activation energy for thermal degradation was determined as 81.1 kJ/mol. At room temperature (20°), the first-order rate constant was predicted to be 5×10^{-6}/day. The shelf-life ($t_{10\%}$) was calculated as 2.1×10^4 days. A long-term room temperature study confirmed the predicted shelf-life.

Cimetidine (300 mg, as the hydrochloride) prepared in either glucose 5% injection or sodium chloride 0.9% injection, in 50-mL and 100-mL polyvinyl chloride bags, respectively, was investigated for stability to freezing, at −10°, and microwave thawing. After freezing for 28 days some of the bags were thawed at room temperature and some in a microwave oven. It was concluded that microwave thawing did not adversely affect cimetidine stability.[6]

INCOMPATIBILITY/COMPATIBILITY

Cimetidine hydrochloride was found to be visually and chemically stable for at least one week at ambient room temperature in each of 22 commonly used intravenous fluids.[7] A similar study assessed that cimetidine hydrochloride was compatible with and stable in a further 19 intravenous fluids for at least one week.[8]

Cimetidine hydrochloride (SK&F) was shown to be chemically stable and physically compatible in glucose 5% injection when in admixture with aminophylline (Invenex, USA) for 48 hours at room temperature,[9] with cefoperazone sodium (Pfizer, USA) for 48 hours at 4° and 25°,[10] and with methylprednisolone sodium succinate (Solu-Medrol, Upjohn) for 24 hours at 24°.[11]

Over a period of 24 hours no visible or chemical incompatibility was observed between cimetidine hydrochloride injection (30 mg/100 mL) and four types of total parenteral nutrition solution. The solutions were stored in 100-mL polyvinyl chloride bags at 4° or at room temperature.[12]

Cimetidine hydrochloride at concentrations of 600 mg, 1200 mg, and 1800 mg per 1500 mL was added to a total parenteral nutrition (TPN) solution consisting of 5% amino acid injection, 20% glucose injection, and 3% intravenous fat emulsion in 2-litre ethylene vinyl acetate bags. Cimetidine concentration did not alter significantly over 48 hours and pH was also maintained. There were no visible signs of incompatibility. The particle size distribution of the samples was compared with that of a control TPN solution, without cimetidine, after 24 and 48 hours storage. There was no significant change in particle size distribution in any of the samples after 24 hours, however, after 48 hours an increase in particle size was observed in the admixture containing 600 mg cimetidine hydrochloride. It was concluded that cimetidine hydrochloride at concentrations up to 1800 mg/1500 mL could be mixed with the TPN solution studied and stored for up to 24 hours at room temperature without a loss of stability or change in the fat emulsion.[13]

El-Mallakh[14] reported on the incompatibilities of cimetidine with cefamandole nafate and cefazolin sodium. A precipitate was formed immediately upon addition of cimetidine (300 mg/2 mL, as the hydrochloride) to either of the two drugs, presented at a concentration of 1 g/5 mL. A precipitate was also formed after 36 to 48 hours when cimetidine hydrochloride was added to cephalothin sodium (1 g/5 mL), penicillin sodium (1 million units/5 mL), or sodium chloride (12 mEq/5 mL); cimetidine was stable in 0.9% sodium chloride for at least 48 hours.

Yuhas et al[15] investigated the stability of cimetidine hydrochloride in admixture with 37 intravenous additives. Incompatibility was observed with amphotericin B, cefamandole nafate, cefazolin sodium, and cephalothin sodium. It is possible that these incompatibilities may be a function of concentration.

Souney et al[16] investigated the compatibility of 21 common preoperative injectable preparations with cimetidine hydrochloride. Chlorpromazine hydrochloride and quinalbarbitone sodium were incompatible with cimetidine hydrochloride, producing a haze and precipitate respectively, immediately on mixing. The difference in pH between cimetidine hydrochloride (pH 4.4) and quinalbarbitone sodium (pH 9.5) can explain the incompatibility, but the interaction with chlorpromazine hydrochloride (pH 4.0) was unexpected.

Interactions with containers

Only a minimal loss of cimetidine was observed when an aqueous solution was stored in a polyvinyl chloride bag in the dark at room temperature (15° to 20°) for up to three months.[17] The loss of cimetidine from a sodium chloride 0.9% solution during simulated infusion was found to be negligible.[18] The study was conducted by simulating infusion through plastic infusion sets, through syringe-pump systems, and by storage in plastic syringes. Variants in the study were drug concentration, pH, flow rate, infusion times, and tubing length and radius.

FORMULATION

Excipients

Excipients that have been used in presentations of cimetidine include:

Tablets, cimetidine: aspartame; carmellose sodium; cellulose; ferric oxides (black and yellow); hydroxypropylcellulose; hypromellose; indigo carmine (E132); lactose; magnesium stearate; maize starch; microcrystalline cellulose; povidone; propylene glycol; quinoline yellow (E104); sodium lauryl sulphate; sodium starch glycollate; sorbitol; starch; titanium dioxide (E171).

Effervescent tablets, cimetidine: aspartame; dimethicone; saccharin sodium; sodium benzoate; sodium bicarbonate; sodium dihydrogen citrate.

Cimetidine hydrochloride: aspartame; saccharin sodium; silicone oil; sodium benzoate.

Oral liquids, cimetidine: ethanol; butyl, methyl, and propyl hydroxybenzoates; sorbitol; sucrose; sunset yellow FCF (E110).

Cimetidine hydrochloride: ethanol; methyl and propyl hydroxybenzoates; propylene glycol; saccharin sodium; sodium chloride; sodium phosphate; sorbitol.

Injections, cimetidine: hydrochloric acid.

Cimetidine hydrochloride: phenol.

Infusions, cimetidine: hydrochloric acid; sodium chloride; sodium hydroxide.

Bioavailability

The oral bioavailability of cimetidine as Tagamet (SK&F) or Histodil (RG, Hungary) tablets was shown to be 73% to 74% of that of Histodil injection in a crossover study involving six healthy volunteers.[19]

Britton et al[20] demonstrated equivalent bioavailability of cimetidine administered separately as cimetidine tablets (Tagamet) with alginate liquid or tablets (Gaviscon), and as fixed-dose alginate-cimetidine combination tablets (Algitec), in a single-dose crossover study with twelve healthy subjects.

Bioequivalence

In-vitro studies of seven commercially available cimetidine tablets showed vast differences in dissolution rate, disintegration time, tablet hardness, polymorphic form, and drug content. The authors suggested that without standardisation of formulation the bioavailability of these products is unlikely to be comparable.[21]

Complete bioequivalence of an oral 800 mg cimetidine tablet and a single dose of two 400 mg tablets (commercially available in the USA) was demonstrated in a randomised crossover study involving 23 healthy subjects.[22]

Modified-release preparations

Modified release of cimetidine from ethylcellulose micropellets was demonstrated by Chattaraj and Das.[23] *In-vitro/in-vivo* correlation (in *rabbits*) revealed that the dissolution process was the rate determining step in drug absorption. Cimetidine micropellets prepared with a higher concentration of ethylcellulose exhibited better modified-release properties.

REFERENCES

1. Vochten R, Remant G, Huybrechts W. J Pharm Pharmacol 1980;32:863–6.
2. El-Ridy MS, Mayer PR, Peck GE, Kildsig DO. Drug Dev Ind Pharm 1983;9:453–8.
3. Shibata M, Kokubo H, Morimoto K, Morisaka K, Ishida T, Inoue M. J Pharm Sci 1983;72:1436–42.
4. Christensen JM, Lee R-Y, Parrott KA. Am J Hosp Pharm 1983;40:612–15.
5. Kac M, Uvodic F. Acta Pharm Jugosl 1981;31:171–5.
6. Elliott GT, McKenzie MW, Curry SH, Pieper JA, Quinn SL. Am J Hosp Pharm 1983;40:1002–6.
7. Rosenberg HA, Dougherty JT, Mayron D, Baldinus JG. Am J Hosp Pharm 1980;37:390–2.
8. Yuhas EM, Lofton FT, Mayron D, Baldinus JG, Rosenberg HA. Am J Hosp Pharm 1981;38:879–81.
9. Baptista RJ, Mitrano FP. Drug Intell Clin Pharm 1988;22:592–3.
10. Lee DKT, Wang D-P, Lee A. Am J Hosp Pharm 1991;48:111–13.
11. Strom IG, Miller SW. Am J Hosp Pharm 1991;48:1237–41.
12. Tsallas G, Allen LC. Am J Hosp Pharm 1982;39:484–5.
13. Baptista RJ, Palombo JD, Tahan SR, Valicenti AJ, Bistrian BR, Arkin CF, Blackburn GL. Am J Hosp Pharm 1985;42:2208–10.
14. El-Mallakh R [letter]. Am J Hosp Pharm 1979;36:1024.
15. Yuhas EM, Lofton FT, Rosenberg HA, Mayron D, Baldinus JG. Am J Hosp Pharm 1981;38:1919–22.
16. Souney PF, Solomon MA, Stancher D. Am J Hosp Pharm 1984;41:1840–1.

17. Kowaluk EA, Roberts MS, Blackburn HD, Polack AE. Am J Hosp Pharm 1981;38:1308–14.
18. Kowaluk EA, Roberts MS, Polack AE. Am J Hosp Pharm 1982;39:460–7.
19. Vereczkey L, Kozma M, Kerpel-Fronius S. Acta Pharm Hung 1985;55:217–20.
20. Britton AM, Nichols JD, Draper PR. J Pharm Pharmacol 1991;43:122–3.
21. Choulis NH. Drug Dev Ind Pharm 1985;11:2099–107.
22. Randolph WC, Peace KE, Seaman JJ, Frank WO, Putterman K. Curr Ther Res 1986;39:767–72.
23. Chattaraj SC, Das SK. Drug Dev Ind Pharm 1990;16(2):283–93.

Cisplatin (BAN, USAN, rINN)   *Cytotoxic*

cis-DDP; *cis*-platinum II; Peyrone's Salt
cis-Diamminedichloroplatinum (II)
$H_6Cl_2N_2Pt = 300.0$
CAS—15663-27-1

Pharmacopoeial status
BP, USP

Preparations

Compendial
Cisplatin for Injection USP. pH 3.5 to 6.2. A sterile, lyophilised mixture of cisplatin, mannitol, and sodium chloride.

Non-compendial
Cisplatin (Farmitalia Carlo Erba). *Powder for injection*, cisplatin 50 mg. For reconstitution with water for injections; reconstituted solution contains cisplatin 1 mg/mL. Cisplatin reconstituted solution should be diluted in two litres of sodium chloride 0.9% or a glucose/sodium chloride solution (to which 37.5 g of mannitol may be added). The manufacturer warns that cisplatin degrades when in contact with aluminium.
Cisplatin (Lederle). *Injection*, cisplatin 10 mg, 25 mg, or 50 mg in each vial at a concentration of 1 mg/mL. *Diluents*: sodium chloride 0.9% injection or sodium chloride 0.9% and glucose 5% injection. Cisplatin injection should be added directly into the infusion fluid before administration.
Powder for injection, cisplatin 10 mg or 50 mg; the lyophilised powder should be reconstituted with 10 mL or 50 mL of water for injections, respectively, before addition to the infusion fluid. Cisplatin interacts with aluminium, therefore administration sets, cannulae, and syringes containing aluminium must not be used with this product. Mannitol 37.5 g may be added to infusion solutions.

Containers and storage

Solid state
Cisplatin BP should be kept in an airtight container and protected from light.
Cisplatin USP should be preserved in tight containers, protected from light.

Dosage forms
Cisplatin for Injection USP should be preserved in containers suitable for sterile solids and protected from light.
Unopened vials of Cisplatin (Farmitalia Carlo Erba) freeze-dried powder should be stored at room temperature, protected from light. Solutions of cisplatin should be stored at room temperature protected from light and used within 20 hours. If cooled or refrigerated, precipitation may occur. It is recommended that, during administration, diluted infusion solutions of cisplatin should be protected from light.
Cisplatin Injection and Cisplatin Powder (Lederle) should be stored at controlled room temperature (15° to 30°) and protected from light. Refrigeration of the injection or the reconstituted solution will result in precipitation. The reconstituted solution is stable for 24 hours at controlled room temperature. For details of handling of cisplatin see Processing below.

PHYSICAL PROPERTIES

Cisplatin exists as a yellow powder or as yellow or orange–yellow crystals.

Melting point
Cisplatin melts at about 270°, with decomposition and blackening.

pH
The pH of a 0.1% w/v solution of *cisplatin* in sodium chloride 0.9% w/v prepared with carbon dioxide-free water is 4.5 to 6.0.

Solubility
Cisplatin is slightly soluble in water; practically insoluble in ethanol; sparingly soluble in dimethylformamide.

Crystal and molecular structure
Enantiomers
Diamminedichloroplatinum exists in two isomeric forms, *cis* and *trans*. The *cis* isomer is the therapeutically active form.

STABILITY

Cisplatin, in the solid state, is reported to be stable to light and air at room temperature, but decomposes to platinum metal at 270°.

Solutions
In aqueous solution, degradation occurs via nucleophilic displacement involving one or both chloride ligands, resulting in the formation of mono-aquo and di-aquo species.
Cheung *et al*[1] demonstrated the stability of cisplatin 0.3 mg/mL for 24 hours in solutions containing sodium chloride (contributed by drug and infusion solution) at concentrations of 0.3% or greater.
Kristjanssen and co-workers[2] failed to demonstrate the presence of the oligomers di-μ-hydroxo-bis(*cis*-diammineplatinum II) and tri-μ-hydroxy-tris(*cis*-diammineplatinum II) as degradation products of cisplatin in solutions of cisplatin (1 mg/mL) in sodium chloride 0.9% with mannitol 10 g/L that had been stored in glass vials at 5° or 40° for 10 months followed by one year in a refrigerator at 5°. At the end of the storage period a 15% loss of cisplatin was observed in the solution stored at 40°, a 4% loss was recorded in the samples stored at 5°; the degradation route was not identified.
Solutions of cisplatin 1 mg/mL reconstituted with double distilled water from sterile powder for injection (which also contained sodium chloride and mannitol) were stored either protected from light or exposed for 24 hours to intense fluorescent light or normal room fluorescent light.[3] Differences in absorption spectra, measured by ultraviolet spectroscopy, were found in all solutions, but to a lesser extent in those exposed to normal fluorescent light. In aqueous solution, decomposition was found to be primarily due to the reversible formation of

cis-diammineaquochloroplatinum and one chloride ion per molecule, and was dependent on the drug concentration and the amount of chloride in solution. Maximum cisplatin stability was achieved in sodium chloride 0.9% when 3% decomposition occurred (equilibrium established between cisplatin and chloride ions) in the first hour and the drug remained stable thereafter for 24 hours at room temperature. However, when stored at refrigerated temperatures (2° to 6°), cisplatin (in sodium chloride 0.9% injection) precipitated in a manner that was dependent on time and concentration. The authors recommended that infusion solutions should have a concentration of less then 0.6 mg/mL to allow storage under refrigeration. At this concentration precipitation was observed after 48 hours, whereas at a concentration of 1 mg/mL precipitation was observed within one hour.

Reconstituted solutions of cisplatin (1 mg/mL in sterile water) which also contained sodium chloride 0.9% and mannitol (10 mg/mL) were stored in polyvinyl chloride containers, clear and amber glass flasks, and plastic syringes at 22° to 25° either in the dark or exposed to measured amounts of light for 96 days.[4] Decomposition was shown to be pH-dependent with trichloroammineplatinate II (TCAP, identified by HPLC) as the major degradation product in all solutions. At pH 4.3 and 6.3, in solutions kept in the dark, there was approximately 0.04% and 0.21% cisplatin degradation to TCAP per week. Storage in amber glass flasks protected the solutions from ambient light-induced degradation whereas solutions in clear glass containers underwent significant decomposition with an accompanying rise in pH. Cisplatin was more sensitive to short-wavelength light (350 to 490 nm) than to longer wavelength light (above 580 nm). The addition of ethylene oxide (which may be used to sterilise polyvinyl chloride containers and giving sets) to the solutions also effected a rise in pH and subsequent acceleration of cisplatin degradation. Isomerisation of cisplatin to transplatin was not observed.

Hincal *et al*[5] used HPLC to study the stability of cisplatin 50 and 500 micrograms/mL in aqueous parenteral vehicles. At 25°, in water, an initial rapid loss of cisplatin occurred but equilibrium was reached within 48 hours, with 9% and 30% cisplatin remaining in the 50 and 500 micrograms/mL solutions, respectively. The rate of loss of cisplatin was demonstrated to be concentration-dependent; the more concentrated solutions degraded more rapidly. Neither light nor the presence of glucose or mannitol in solution had any significant effect on cisplatin stability. Sodium chloride exerted a stabilising effect at concentrations of 0.1% up to 0.9%, while sodium bicarbonate had a deleterious effect with precipitation in some instances.

LaFollette *et al*[6] reported that solutions (in polyvinyl chloride bags) of cisplatin (50 or 200 micrograms/mL) in admixture with glucose 5% and sodium chloride 0.45% solution containing mannitol (18.75 mg/mL) and magnesium sulphate (1 or 2 mg/mL) were stable for up to 48 hours at 25°; for up to 4 days at 4° followed by 2 days at 25°; and for up to 30 days at −15° with an additional 2 days at 25°.

Holmes *et al*[7] reported that cisplatin injection (1 mg/mL) in sodium chloride 0.9% injection stored in polyvinyl chloride minibags at 25° for 28 days did not support rapid growth of the micro-organisms *Aspergillus niger*, *Candida albicans*, *Escherichia coli*, *Pseudomonas cepacia*, or *Staphylococcus aureus*. However, Parti and Wolf[8] suggested that storage of cisplatin injection at room temperature for 28 days would probably result in hydrolysis of the drug to mono-aquo and di-aquo species which are toxic and therapeutically inactive. One manufacturer states that the reconstituted solution is stable for 20 hours at room temperature (27°).

Stabilisation

The stability of cisplatin in aqueous solution is increased by the addition of chloride ions.

FURTHER INFORMATION. Extent of cisplatin formation in carboplatin admixtures—Perrone RK, Kaplan MA, Bogardus JB [letter]. Am J Hosp Pharm 1989;46:258–9. Stability of cisplatin in sodium chloride 0.9% intravenous solution related to the container's material (glass, PE, PP, PVC)—Cubells MP, Aixela JP, Brumos VG, Pou SD, Flaque MV. Pharm World Sci 1993;15(1):34–6.

INCOMPATIBILITY/COMPATIBILITY

A reaction between cisplatin (10^{-4}M in pH 4.2, 0.5M acetate buffer) and sodium bisulphite (0.005M to 0.2M solutions), which resulted in enhanced ultraviolet absorbance at 280 nm, was reported by Hussain *et al*.[9]

Intravenous admixtures

Cisplatin (200 micrograms/mL, Platinol, Bristol, USA) was found to be compatible with etoposide (200 or 400 micrograms/mL, VePesid Injection, Bristol, USA) in admixture in sodium chloride 0.9%, or in glucose 5% and sodium chloride 0.45%, during storage in polyvinyl chloride bags or glass bottles at room temperature, with or without fluorescent light, for 24 hours.[10] However, when mannitol and potassium chloride were added to the admixture (in sodium chloride 0.9%) an unidentified precipitate was formed. An increased loss of cisplatin concentration was observed from solutions stored in light.

A similar study with admixtures of cisplatin and fluorouracil (200 microgams/mL and 1000 micrograms/mL respectively, or 500 micrograms/mL and 10 000 micrograms/mL respectively)[11] in sodium chloride 0.9% injection in polyvinyl chloride bags, at 24° to 26°, indicated that $t_{10\%}$ values for cisplatin were 1.5 hours and 1.2 hours at the lower and higher concentrations, respectively. Less than 75% of the initial cisplatin concentrations remained after 4 hours and 3 hours, respectively. Neither light nor initial concentrations of either drug had any effect on the rate of decline of cisplatin concentration following preparation of the admixture.

The incompatibility of cisplatin with Reglan Injectable (AH Robins, containing metoclopramide, sodium metabisulphite, and sodium chloride) was established by Garren and Repta[12] following attempts to mix both drugs in a single parenteral fluid. Cisplatin was stable in solution with metoclopramide alone but degraded rapidly with sodium metabisulphite. At concentrations similar to those used in a clinical setting (cisplatin 0.2 mg/mL, sodium metabisulphite 0.148 mg/mL, metoclopramide 0.5 mg/mL) there was a total loss of cisplatin in 30 minutes at room temperature.

Aluminium

Cisplatin interacts with aluminium. Cisplatin (Platinol, Bristol, 1 mg/mL) was noted to react rapidly with the aluminium in a chemotherapy dispensing pin[13] resulting in the formation of a black precipitate and gas. The avoidance of any aluminium-containing device during reconstitution or administration of cisplatin is recommended.

FURTHER INFORMATION. Compatibility of cisplatine, carboplatine and dacarbazine with PVC infusion bags—Benaji B, Dine T, Goudaliez F, Luyckx M, Brunet C, Cazin JC et al. Pharm Weekbl (Sci) 1992;14(5)Suppl F:F49.

FORMULATION

Excipients

Excipients that have been used in presentations of cisplatin include:

Injections, solutions and powders for reconstitution: hydrochloric acid; mannitol; sodium chloride.

Microencapsulation

Cisplatin microcapsules with a relatively slow release rate (80% to 100% in 24 hours) were prepared with ethylcellulose (viscosity 45 mPa for a 5% w/w solution) by a coacervation process in the presence of low-density polyethylene.[14] No alteration of the cisplatin chemical structure could be detected (by HPLC) after microencapsulation.

FURTHER INFORMATION. Formation and characterisation of cisplatin loaded poly(*d,l*-lactide) microspheres for chemoembolisation—Spenlehauer G, Veillard M, Benoît J-P. J Pharm Sci 1986;75(8):750–5. Preparation and characterisation of cisplatin-loaded polymethyl methacrylate microspheres—Mestiri M, Puisieux F, Benoit JP. Int J Pharmaceutics 1993;89:229–34. Soluble polymers [and other macromolecular carriers] as carriers of cis-platinum [DNA, proteins, hyaluronic acid, synthetic copolymer divinyl ether-maleic anhydride, poly(D-glutamic acid), poly(L-aspartic acid), carboxymethyl dextran]—Schechter B, Neumann A, Wilchek M, Arnon R. J Controlled Release 1989;10:75–87.

PROCESSING

Handling precautions

CAUTION. Cisplatin is potentially cytotoxic. Great care should be taken to avoid exposure to skin and to prevent inhalation of particles.

Cisplatin injection should be reconstituted in a designated area and the work surface should be covered with disposable, plastic-backed, absorbent paper. It has been recommended that personnel handling cisplatin, during reconstitution or administration, should wear two pairs of gloves; a latex pair beneath a polyvinyl chloride pair. Any contamination of the skin or eyes should be immediately washed with water. Any spillage, waste, or other contaminated materials may be disposed of by incineration at 800°. Cisplatin is reduced to elemental platinum by zinc powder under acidic conditions. General guidelines on the handling and disposal of cytotoxic drugs are given in the chapter entitled Cytotoxic Drugs: Handling Precautions.

REFERENCES

1. Cheung Y-W, Cradock JC, Vishnuvajjala BR, Flora KP. Am J Hosp Pharm 1987;44:124–30.
2. Kristjanssen F, Sternson LA, Lindenbaum S. Int J Pharmaceutics 1988;41:67–74.
3. Greene RF, Chatterji DC, Hiranaka PK, Gallelli JF. Am J Hosp Pharm 1979;36:38–43.
4. Zeiske PA, Koberda M, Hines JL, Knight CC, Sriram R, Raaghavan NV *et al.* Am J Hosp Pharm 1991;48:1500–6.
5. Hincal AA, Long DF, Repta AJ. J Parenter Drug Assoc 1979;33(3):107–16.
6. LaFollette JM, Arbus MH, Lauper RD [letter]. Am J Hosp Pharm 1985;42:2652.
7. Holmes CJ, Kubey WY, Love DI. Am J Hosp Pharm 1988;45:1089–91.
8. Parti R, Wolf W [letter]. Am J Hosp Pharm 1989;46:259.
9. Hussain AA, Haddadin M, Iga K [letter]. J Pharm Sci 1980;69(3):364–5.
10. Stewart CF, Hampton EM. Am J Hosp Pharm 1989;46:1400–4.
11. Stewart CF, Fleming RA. Am J Hosp Pharm 1990;47:1373–7.
12. Garren KW, Repta AJ. Int J Pharmaceutics 1985;24:91–9.
13. Ogawa GS, Young R, Munar M [letter]. Am J Hosp Pharm 1985;42:1044–5.
14. Hecquet B, Fournier C, Depadt G, Cappelaere P. J Pharm Pharmacol 1984;36:803–7.

Clindamycin (BAN, USAN, rINN)   *Antibacterial*

NOTE. The name clinimycin was formerly used for clindamycin.
Chlorodeoxylincomycin
Methyl 6-amino-7-chloro-6,7,8-trideoxy-*N*-[(2*S*,4*R*)-1-methyl-4-propylprolyl]-1-thio-β-L-*threo*-D-*galacto*-octopyranoside; (7*S*)-chloro-7-deoxylincomycin
$C_{18}H_{33}ClN_2O_5S = 425.0$

Clindamycin Hydrochloride (BANM, rINNM)
$C_{18}H_{33}ClN_2O_5S, HCl = 461.4$

Clindamycin Palmitate Hydrochloride (BANM, USAN, rINNM)
$C_{34}H_{63}ClN_2O_6S, HCl = 699.9$

Clindamycin Phosphate (BANM, USAN, rINNM)
$C_{18}H_{34}ClN_2O_8PS = 505.0$
CAS—18323-44-9 (clindamycin); 21462-39-5 (clindamycin hydrochloride,anhydrous); 58207-19-5 (clindamycin hydrochloride, monohydrate); 36688-78-5 (clindamycin palmitate); 25507-04-4 (clindamycin palmitate hydrochloride); 24729-96-2 (clindamycin phosphate)

Pharmacopoeial status

BP (clindamycin hydrochloride, clindamycin phosphate); USP (clindamycin hydrochloride, clindamycin palmitate hydrochloride, clindamycin phosphate)

Preparations

Compendial
Clindamycin Capsules BP. Contain clindamycin hydrochloride. Capsules containing, in each, the equivalent of 75 mg and 150 mg of clindamycin are usually available.
Clindamycin Injection BP. A sterile solution of clindamycin phosphate in water for injections. pH 5.5 to 7.0.
Clindamycin Hydrochloride Capsules USP.
Clindamycin Palmitate Hydrochloride for Oral Solution USP.
Clindamycin Phosphate Topical Solution USP.
Clindamycin Phosphate Injection USP. pH 5.5 to 7.0.
Sterile Clindamycin Phosphate USP.

Non-compendial

Dalacin C (Upjohn). *Capsules*, clindamycin (as hydrochloride) 75 mg and 150 mg.

Paediatric suspension, sucrose-based granules, clindamycin (as palmitate hydrochloride) 75 mg/5 mL when reconstituted with purified water (freshly boiled and cooled). *Diluent*: purified water (freshly boiled and cooled).

Dalacin C Phosphate Sterile Solution (Upjohn). *Injection*, the equivalent of 150 mg clindamycin base (as clindamycin phosphate) per mL. It is physically incompatible with ampicillin, phenytoin, barbiturates, aminophylline, calcium gluconate, and magnesium sulphate.

Dalacin T (Upjohn). *Topical solution*, clindamycin (as phosphate) 1% in an aqueous alcoholic basis.

Lotion, emulsion containing clindamycin (as phosphate) 1% in an aqueous basis.

Containers and storage

Solid state

Clindamycin Hydrochloride BP should be kept in an airtight container and stored at a temperature not exceeding 30°.

Clindamycin Phosphate BP should be kept in a well-closed container and stored at a temperature of 2° to 8°. If the substance is sterile, the container should be sterile, tamper-evident and sealed so as to exclude micro-organisms.

Clindamycin Hydrochloride USP, Clindamycin Palmitate Hydrochloride USP and Clindamycin Phosphate USP should all be preserved in tight containers.

Sterile Clindamycin Phosphate USP should be preserved in containers suitable for sterile solids.

Dosage forms

Clindamycin Injection BP should be stored at a temperature of 8° to 30°.

Clindamycin Hydrochloride Capsules USP, Clindamycin Palmitate Hydrochloride for Oral Solution USP and Clindamycin Phosphate Topical Solution USP should be preserved in tight containers.

Clindamycin Phosphate Injection USP should be preserved in single-dose or in multiple-dose containers, preferably of Type I glass, or in suitable plastic containers.

Dalacin C paediatric granules should be stored within the temperature range 18° to 25°; under these conditions the shelf-life will be at least 24 months. Following reconstitution, the paediatric suspension is stable for up to 2 weeks at room temperature.

Dalacin C Phosphate sterile solution should be stored at room temperature. Avoid refrigeration.

Dalacin T topical solution and lotion should be stored at room temperature. The topical solution is inflammable.

PHYSICAL PROPERTIES

Clindamycin is a yellow, amorphous solid.

Clindamycin hydrochloride is a white or almost white, crystalline powder; odourless or with a slight mercaptan-like odour, and a bitter taste.

Clindamycin palmitate hydrochloride is a white to off-white amorphous powder with a characteristic odour.

Clindamycin phosphate is a white or almost white, hygroscopic crystalline powder; odourless or practically odourless with a bitter taste.

Melting point

Clindamycin hydrochloride melts in the range 141° to 143°.

pH

The pH of a 10% w/v solution of *clindamycin hydrochloride* in water lies in the range 3.0 to 5.5.

The pH of a 1% solution of *clindamycin phosphate* in water is 3.5 to 4.5.

The pH of a 1% solution of *clindamycin palmitate hydrochloride* is 2.8 to 3.8.

Dissociation constant

pK_a 7.7 (25°)

FURTHER INFORMATION. Determination of phosphate functional group acid dissociation constants of clindamycin 2-phosphate using ^{31}P Fourier transform NMR spectrometry—Kipp JE, Smith WJ, Myrdal PB. Int J Pharmaceutics 1991;74:215–20.

Solubility

Clindamycin hydrochloride is freely soluble in water, in methanol, and in dimethylformamide; slightly soluble in ethanol; very slightly soluble in chloroform; practically insoluble in acetone.

Clindamycin palmitate hydrochloride is freely soluble in water, in ethanol, in chloroform, and in ether; very soluble in dimethylformamide.

Clindamycin phosphate is soluble 1 in 2.5 of water; slightly soluble in dehydrated ethanol; practically insoluble in chloroform and in ether; very slightly soluble in acetone.

Effect of pH

Rowe[1] demonstrated that the solubility of clindamycin palmitate hydrochloride, at 25°, decreased with an increase in pH in the range 3.7 to 7.4. At pH 7.4 the observed solubility was below the detection limit of the assay. Monomeric solubility of the protonated drug, below pH 4.0, was over 1000 times greater than the base solubility.

Critical micelle concentration

Clindamycin-2-palmitate hydrochloride has an amphiphilic structure conducive to surface activity and micellar aggregation. The high solubility of the compound, at 25°, is due to micelle formation. The critical micelle concentration, observed experimentally, was[1] 3.4×10^{-4} mol/L at 25°.

Dissolution

The USP specifies that for Clindamycin Hydrochloride Capsules USP not less than 80% of the labelled amount of $C_{18}H_{33}ClN_2O_5S$ is dissolved in 30 minutes. Dissolution medium: 900 mL of water; Apparatus 1 at 100 rpm.

STABILITY

Clindamycin is a semi-synthetic chlorinated derivative of lincomycin. Oesterling[2] investigated the mechanisms and kinetics of degradation of clindamycin hydrochloride in buffered aqueous solution in the pH range 0.4 to 12.0. Maximum stability was observed between pH 3 and 5. Below pH 4.0, degradation occurred mainly via thioglycoside hydrolysis. The major decomposition products were *1*-dethiomethyl-*1*-hydroxy clindamycin and methyl mercaptan. The rate of degradation increased as the pH decreased in the range 4.0 to 0.4. Between pH 5.0 and 9.0, conversion of clindamycin to lincomycin occurred; the extent of this reaction was dependent on the degree of protonation of the *N*-methyl-4-propylpyrrolidine moiety. The rate of conversion to lincomycin increased as pH increased up to 9.0 and then became constant. Amide hydrolysis was thought to occur throughout the entire pH range. The degradation of clindamycin followed apparent first-order kinetics. The activation energies for clindamycin degradation in 0.1M hydrochloric acid and at pH 5.0 were about 159.0 kJ/mol and 121.8 kJ/mol, respectively. It was predicted that during storage for 2 years at 25° the degree of degradation of clindamycin in pharmaceutical formulations adjusted to between pH 1 and 6.5 should not exceed 10%.

Clindamycin-2-phosphate in aqueous solution between pH 6.0 and 9.0 was shown[3] to degrade by three major routes at 90°. Below pH 6.0, apparent first-order hydrolyses of the thioglycoside and phosphate ester predominated. Above pH 6.0, 'scission' of the 7(S)—Cl to form the 7(R)—OH analogue was reported to take precedence. The rate of hydrolysis was found to increase as pH decreased. The activation energy for clindamycin-2-phosphate hydrolysis was 137.6 kJ/mol at pH 7.5. Clindamycin phosphate was predicted to be most stable in solution in the pH range 3.5 to 6.5.

Topical formulations

The degradation of topical solutions of clindamycin hydrochloride and clindamycin phosphate, formulated in three different mixed solvent systems, was followed at 25°, 40°, and 50° in glass and in polypropylene bottles, and compared with that of a standard clindamycin topical solution.[4] All formulations were more stable in glass containers than in plastic containers. The formulation (for both clindamycin hydrochloride and clindamycin phosphate) that had greatest stability at 25° contained (as the solvent) ethanol 40%, acetone, polysorbate 20, fragrance, and water; the pH was 5.0. At pH values below 4.0, the stability of all formulations decreased. Rate constants for decomposition of clindamycin hydrochloride and clindamycin phosphate in this solvent (at room temperature) pH 5.0 were 6.67×10^{-3}/month and 8.64×10^{-3}/month, respectively, in glass bottles, and 6.9×10^{-3}/month and 9.21×10^{-3}/month, respectively, in plastic bottles.

An assessment of the stability of two clindamycin topical formulations, containing clindamycin hydrochloride or clindamycin phosphate, (see Formulation—Topical preparations, below) revealed no significant decomposition in either solution after storage at room temperature for three months.[5]

Intravenous admixtures

An intravenous solution of clindamycin phosphate 300 mg in glucose 5% injection in polyvinyl chloride bags retained over 90% of its initial concentration when microwave-thawed after storage at −20° for 30 days, and after subsequent storage at room temperature for 24 hours.[6]

Stability of clindamycin phosphate (6, 9, or 12 mg clindamycin/mL) was maintained in both glass bottles and polyvinyl chloride minibags containing sodium chloride 0.9% injection, glucose 5% injection, or compound sodium lactate injection for 8 weeks at −10°, 32 days at 4°, and 16 days at 25°.[7]

Bosso[8] determined the stability of clindamycin phosphate injection at two dosage levels (300 mg and 900 mg) when diluted in 20 mL of glucose 10%, and stored in glass containers under refrigerated conditions. Stability was maintained for at least 30 days at 10°.

Das Gupta et al[9] demonstrated that a generic clindamycin phosphate injection, 600 mg/4 mL (Quad Pharm) was stable when diluted to 6 mg/mL and 12 mg/mL in glucose 5% injection and in sodium chloride 0.9% injection in Viaflex plastic bags, and stored at 25°, 5°, and −10° for at least 22 days, 54 days, and 68 days, respectively.

Similarly, clindamycin phosphate (Cleocin Phosphate, Upjohn, USA) was stable in admixture with glucose 5% injection when stored frozen at −20° in polyolefin containers for 30 days and then refrigerated at 4° (after thawing at 25°) for 14 days.[10]

INCOMPATIBILITY/COMPATIBILITY

The stability of clindamycin phosphate in admixture with β-lactam antibiotics,[11–13] cephalosporins,[13–15] and aminoglycosides[14,16–18] has been extensively investigated by various workers under a variety of conditions of storage and temperature. Vehicles most commonly used were sodium chloride 0.9% injection and glucose 5% injection. Tobramycin sulphate (Dista, USA) was not stable in admixture with clindamycin phosphate (Upjohn, USA); a cloudy, white precipitate formed at room temperature in sodium chloride 0.9% and when frozen at −20° in glucose 5%.[17,18] Cefazolin sodium (SK&F, USA), in admixture with clindamycin phosphate (Upjohn, USA) and gentamicin sulphate (Elkins-Sinn, USA) was unstable after 4 hours in glucose 5% and after 12 hours in sodium chloride 0.9% at room temperature.[19] Gentamicin sulphate retained over 90% of its initial concentration for 48 hours.

No sorption to polyvinyl chloride, polypropylene or glass containers was demonstrated in any of the studies.

FURTHER INFORMATION. Mechanism of adsorption of clindamycin and tetracycline by montmorillonite—Porubcan LS, Serna CJ, White JL, Hem SL. J Pharm Sci 1978;67(8):1081–7. Incompatibility of undiluted clindamycin and gentamicin sulfate [precipitation of a zinc-clindamycin complex]—Baker RP [letter]. Am J Hosp Pharm 1992;49:2144.

FORMULATION

Excipients

Excipients that have been used in presentations of clindamycin include:

Capsules, clindamycin hydrochloride: brilliant blue FCF (133); erythrosine sodium; gelatin; indigo carmine (E132); lactose; magnesium stearate; maize starch; talc; tartrazine (E102); titanium dioxide (E171).

Granules for oral solution, clindamycin palmitate hydrochloride: cherry flavour; dextrin; ethyl hydroxybenzoate; poloxamer (Pluronic F68); polymethylsiloxane; saccharin; sucrose.

Topical solutions, clindamycin phosphate: isopropanol; propylene glycol.

Topical gels, clindamycin phosphate: allantoin; carbomer 934P; methyl hydroxybenzoate; macrogol 400; propylene glycol; sodium hydroxide.

Injection solutions, clindamycin phosphate: benzyl alcohol; disodium edetate.

Topical preparations

American workers[20] developed extemporaneous preparations of topical clindamycin lotion from clindamycin hydrochloride capsules (a method for extraction is given). Clindamycin hydrochloride was not sufficiently soluble in alcoholic systems to form a stable solution unless sufficient water was added to the cosolvent system. The following solvent mixture was recommended: isopropanol or ethanol 70% v/v, propylene glycol 10% v/v, water 20% v/v. The preparation was given a shelf-life of 6 to 8 weeks.

Lee and Richards[21] recommend the following formulations for topical use:

1. Clindamycin hydrochloride 1 g, isopropanol 70 mL, propylene glycol 10 mL, water to 100 mL. The pH of the solution is 4.0 and it is stable for 6 months at room temperature.

2. Clindamycin injection (150 mg/mL) 6.6 mL, propylene glycol 10 mL, ethanol (70%) to 100 mL. The pH of this solution is 6.5 to 7.0.

The same formulations are given by Richards *et al*[5] for topical preparations of clindamycin hydrochloride and clindamycin phosphate.

Drug absorption

Concomitant administration of clindamycin hydrochloride (150 mg) capsules (Cleocin hydrochloride, Upjohn, USA) and kaolin-pectin suspension in 16 healthy volunteers resulted in a dramatic reduction in the rate of absorption of clindamycin but had no effect on the extent of absorption.[22]

FURTHER INFORMATION. Topical clindamycin for acne. Part 1: Current prescribing practices—Lacina NC, Orr RJ, Peters LS, Flynn GL. Am Pharm 1978 Oct;NS18:30–3. Liposomes with clindamycin hydrochloride in the therapy of acne vulgaris—Skalko N, Cajkovac M, Jalsenjak I. Int J Pharmaceutics 1992;85:97–101.

REFERENCES

1. Rowe EL. J Pharm Sci 1979;68(10):1292–6.
2. Oesterling TO. J Pharm Sci 1970;59(1):63–7.
3. Oesterling TO, Rowe EL. J Pharm Sci 1970;59(2):175–9.
4. Migton JM, Kennon L, Sideman M, Plakogiannis FM. Drug Dev Ind Pharm 1984;10(4):563–73.
5. Richards S, Lee MG, Parry P. Proc Guild Hosp Pharm 1985;20:31–6.
6. Holmes CJ, Ausman RK, Kundsin RB, Walter CW. Am J Hosp Pharm 1982;39:104–8.
7. Porter WR, Johnston CA, Cohon MS, Gillespie W. Am J Hosp Pharm 1983;40:91–4.
8. Bosso JA [letter]. DICP Ann Pharmacother 1990;24:1008–9.
9. Das Gupta V, Parasrampuria J, Bethea C, Wright W. Can J Hosp Pharm 1989;42(3):109–12.
10. Sarkar MA, Rogers E, Reinhard M, Wells B, Karnes HT. Am J Hosp Pharm 1991;48:2184–6.
11. James MJ, Riley CM. Am J Hosp Pharm 1985;42:1984–6.
12. Marble DA, Bosso JA, Townsend RJ. Am J Hosp Pharm 1986;43:1732–6.
13. Marble DA, Bosso JA, Townsend RJ. Drug Intell Clin Pharm 1988;22:54–7.
14. Foley PT, Bosso JA, Bair JN, Townsend RJ. Am J Hosp Pharm 1985;42:839–43.
15. Bosso JA, Townsend RJ. Am J Hosp Pharm 1985;42:2211–14.
16. Mansur JM, Abramowitz PW, Lerner SA, Smith RB, Townsend RJ. Am J Hosp Pharm 1985;42:332–5.
17. Marble DA, Bosso JA, Townsend RJ. Drug Intell Clin Pharm 1986;20:960–3.
18. Zbrozek AS, Marble DA, Bosso JA, Bair JN, Townsend RJ. Drug Intell Clin Pharm 1987;21:806–10.
19. Zbrozek AS, Marble DA, Bosso JA. Drug Intell Clin Pharm 1988;22:873–5.
20. Orr RJ, Lacina NC, Peters LS, Flynn GL. Am Pharm 1978 Nov;NS18,(12):23–6.
21. Lee MG, Richards S [letter]. Pharm J 1983;230:448.
22. Albert KS, DeSante KA, Welch RD, DiSanto AR. J Pharm Sci 1978;67(11):1579–82.

Cloxacillin (BAN, rINN)   *Antibacterial*

(6R)-6-(3-o-Chlorophenyl-5-methyl-1,2-oxazole-4-carboxamido)-penicillanic acid; (6R)-6[3-(2-chlorophenyl)-5-methyl-isoxazole-4-carboxamido]-penicillanic acid
$C_{19}H_{18}ClN_3O_5S = 435.9$

Cloxacillin Sodium (BANM, USAN, rINNM)
$C_{19}H_{17}ClN_3NaO_5S, H_2O = 475.9$
CAS—61-72-3 (cloxacillin); 642-78-4 (cloxacillin sodium, anhydrous); 7081-44-91 (cloxacillin sodium, monohydrate)

Pharmacopoeial status

BP, USP (cloxacillin sodium)

Preparations

Compendial

Cloxacillin Capsules BP. Capsules containing cloxacillin sodium. Capsules containing, in each, the equivalent of 250 mg and 500 mg of cloxacillin are usually available.
Cloxacillin Oral Solution BP (Cloxacillin Elixir, Cloxacillin Syrup). A solution of cloxacillin sodium in a suitable flavoured vehicle. It is prepared by dissolving the dry ingredients in the specified volume of water just before issue for use. If the oral solution is diluted, the diluted oral solution should be freshly prepared. pH 4.0 to 7.0.
Cloxacillin Injection BP (Cloxacillin Sodium for Injection). A sterile solution of cloxacillin sodium in water for injections, prepared by dissolving cloxacillin sodium for injection in the requisite amount of water for injections. pH of a 10% w/v solution, 5.0 to 7.0. Sealed containers each containing the equivalent of 250 mg, 500 mg, and 1 g of cloxacillin are usually available.
Cloxacillin Sodium Capsules USP.
Cloxacillin Sodium for Oral Solution USP.

Non-compendial

Orbenin (Beecham). *Capsules,* cloxacillin (as sodium salt) 250 mg and 500 mg.
Injection, powder for reconstitution. Vials containing 250 mg and 500 mg cloxacillin (as sodium salt). Orbenin injection may be added to most intravenous fluids such as water for injections, sodium chloride 0.9% injection, glucose 5% injection, sodium chloride 0.18% with glucose 4% injection. See also under Incompatibility, below. A solution for nebulisation can be prepared by dissolving 125 mg to 250 mg of the injection vial powder contents in 3 mL of sterile water.

Containers and storage

Solid state

Cloxacillin Sodium BP should be kept in an airtight container and stored at a temperature not exceeding 25°. If the substance is sterile the container should be sterile, tamper-evident and sealed so as to exclude micro-organisms.
Cloxacillin Sodium USP should be preserved in tight containers, at a temperature not exceeding 25°.

Dosage forms

Cloxacillin Oral Solution BP. The dry ingredients should be kept in a well-closed container and stored at a temperature not exceeding 25°. The oral solution and the diluted oral solution should be stored at the temperature and used within the period stated on the label.

Cloxacillin Injection BP. The sealed container should be kept at a temperature not exceeding 25°. The injection should be stored in accordance with the manufacturer's instructions. It should be used immediately after preparation but, in any case, within the period recommended by the manufacturer.

Orbenin capsules and vials for injection should be stored in a cool, dry place. Solutions of Orbenin injection for intramuscular or direct intravenous injection should usually be administered within 30 minutes of preparation. Aqueous solutions of Orbenin injection, however, retain their activity for up to 24 hours at room temperature (25°) and up to 72 hours in a refrigerator (5°). Intravenous solutions for infusion, stored up to 25°, should be used within 24 hours. If these extended storage times are required, reconstitution and preparation must be carried out under appropriate aseptic conditions.

PHYSICAL PROPERTIES

Cloxacillin sodium is a white or almost white, odourless, crystalline powder; it is hygroscopic and has a bitter taste.

Melting point

Cloxacillin (free acid) melts at 126° to 127°, with decomposition. *Cloxacillin sodium* melts at 170°, with decomposition.

pH

A 10% w/v solution of *cloxacillin sodium* has a pH of 5.0 to 7.0. A 1% w/v solution of *cloxacillin sodium* has a pH of 4.5 to 7.5.

Dissociation constant

The pK_a of the carboxyl group of *cloxacillin* has been determined under various conditions:
pK_a 2.70 ± 0.03 and 2.73 ± 0.04 (25°; 0.0025M in water)[1]
pK_a 2.68 ± 0.05 (35°; 0.0025M)[2]
An apparent pK_a value for cloxacillin of 2.78 at 37° was determined by potentiometric titration in ethanol-water mixtures and extrapolation of the results to a solution in water.[3]

Partition coefficient

Using values of apparent partition coefficients for cloxacillin measured over a range of pH, Tsuji *et al*[3] calculated an intrinsic partition coefficient for unionised cloxacillin: log P (octanol/water), 2.43 (37°).
Log P (octanol/water), 2.44; measurements at pH 3 and pH 4.[4]

Solubility

Cloxacillin sodium is soluble 1 in 2.5 of water, 1 in 30 of ethanol, and 1 in 500 of chloroform; freely soluble in methanol.

Critical micelle concentration

Using light scattering methods, Attwood and Agarwal[5] studied micelle formation by cloxacillin sodium in aqueous solutions. At 30°, the critical micelle concentration for cloxacillin sodium was determined to be 0.135 mol/kg in water and 0.075 mol/kg in 0.15M sodium chloride. The aggregation number was 5 in both instances.

Dissolution

The USP states that for Cloxacillin Sodium Capsules USP not less than 75% of the labelled amount of cloxacillin ($C_{19}H_{18}ClN_3O_5S$) is dissolved in 45 minutes. Dissolution medium: 900 mL of water; Apparatus 1 at 100 rpm.

STABILITY

Cloxacillin is susceptible to hydrolysis of the β-lactam ring by hydroxide ions or other nucleophiles to form the corresponding penicilloic acid or penicilloyl derivative.[6] It is resistant to most penicillinase enzymes (β-lactamases) which can catalyse this reaction.

Solid state

In the dry solid state cloxacillin sodium is stable for at least 3 years at room temperature, but moisture content is an important factor in influencing this stability. In a review of the pharmaceutical aspects of semi-synthetic penicillins, Lynn[7] reported that when exposed to dry heat of 110° cloxacillin sodium was stable for one hour and was decomposed by 2% to 3% after 3 hours; it was unstable at 150°.

Solutions

In solution, hydrolysis of cloxacillin sodium is catalysed by hydrogen ions and hydroxide ions and is accelerated by lactate ions. Unbuffered solutions containing cloxacillin sodium 2.5% to 20% may lose about 5% of their initial activity during storage for 7 days at 5°. After storage for 4 days at 25° losses of up to 15% may occur.

Bundgaard and Ilver[2] investigated the effect of pH, buffer species, ionic strength, and temperature on the degradation of aqueous solutions of cloxacillin sodium. Hydrolysis followed pseudo-first-order kinetics with respect to cloxacillin sodium. Of the buffers studied, only citrate buffer (0.02M) did not significantly catalyse hydrolysis; an activation energy of 79.6 kJ/mol was determined in this buffer at pH 6.3, the pH of maximum stability. Predicted $t_{10\%}$ values (pH 6.3) at 4° and 25° were 140 days and 13 days, respectively. It was suggested that reconstituted preparations of cloxacillin sodium should be buffered to pH 6.0 to 6.5 as hydrolysis is accelerated outside this range. A precipitate (suggested to be cloxacillinic acid) may form in solutions of low pH.

Effects of freezing

Reconstituted intravenous solutions of cloxacillin sodium (1 g in 5 mL sterile water) were added to sodium chloride 0.9% or glucose 5% solutions in 50-mL polyvinyl chloride minibags and stored frozen[8] at −27°. All solutions in minibags removed after 1, 2, 3, 6, and 9 months, and thawed in a microwave oven for 2.5 minutes, retained at least 95% of their initial cloxacillin potency. After storage of the thawed solutions for 24 hours at 4°, at least 92% of the initial cloxacillin concentration was still retained. A yellow discoloration (attributed to reactions of the isoxazolyl group) was apparent in the solutions in glucose 5% stored for 6 and 9 months. The authors warn that these discoloured solutions would not be suitable for administration to patients.

Less than 2% degradation of cloxacillin was reported when reconstituted intravenous solutions of cloxacillin (Beecham), added aseptically to sodium chloride 0.9% injection solutions in minibags, were stored at −20° for up to 100 days.[9]

FURTHER INFORMATION. Studies on the stability and compatibility of drugs in infusion fluids. III. Factors affecting the stability of cloxacillin [effect of pH, electrolytes, buffers (acetate, bicarbonate, citrate, lactate and phosphate), carbohydrates (glucose and fructose) and temperature]—Landersjö L, Källstrand G, Lundgren P. Acta Pharm Suec 1974;11:563–80. β-lactam antibiotics: their physicochemical properties and biological activities in relation to structure [review article]—Hou JP, Poole JW. J Pharm Sci 1971;60(4):503–27.

INCOMPATIBILITY/COMPATIBILITY

In a review of work on parenteral penicillins,[10] it was reported that solutions of cloxacillin sodium (Orbenin, Beecham), equivalent to cloxacillin 1% w/v, retained 99% activity for 24 hours when added to three solutions (sodium chloride 0.9%, glucose 5%, and glucose-sodium chloride injections) containing 0.02% w/v hydrocortisone sodium succinate. The mixtures were also visually compatible.

Intramuscular solutions of cloxacillin sodium (Orbenin, Beecham) have been reported to be visually compatible with lignocaine hydrochloride and procaine hydrochloride.[10]

Cloxacillin sodium should not be mixed with blood products or other proteinaceous fluids such as protein hydrolysates or with intravenous lipid emulsions.

Aminoglycosides should not be mixed with cloxacillin sodium in the same syringe, intravenous fluid container, or giving set. In studies of gentamicin sulphate (Cidomycin, Roussel) compatibility,[11] a visible precipitate formed with cloxacillin sodium injection (Orbenin, Beecham) in intravenous infusion fluids.

Visual incompatibilities have also been observed between cloxacillin sodium (Orbenin, Beecham) and tetracycline hydrochloride, oxytetracycline hydrochloride, erythromycin ethylsuccinate, or polymyxin B sulphate.

Intravenous infusion fluids

In a review by Lynn[7] cloxacillin sodium (Orbenin, Beecham) was reported to be stable at 23° for up to 24 hours in sodium chloride 0.9%, glucose 5%, and glucose-sodium chloride injections and for up to 6 hours in 0.167M sodium lactate injection.

Plasma expanders

The formation of macromolecular penicilloates such as penicilloyl polysaccharides and penicilloyl polygeline was detected by ultrafiltration when cloxacillin sodium was incubated with plasma expanders[12] for 24 hours at 20°. Such products were attributed to an interaction between cloxacillin and high molecular weight components of plasma expanders such as dextran, 6-hetastarch, and polygeline. Formation of penicilloyl esters with glucose or lactic acid was also detected.

FORMULATION

Excipients

Excipients that have been used in presentations of cloxacillin sodium include:

Capsules: black PN (E151); colloidal silica; erythrosine (E127); gelatin; iron oxide, yellow (E172); lactose; magnesium stearate; sunset yellow FCF (E110); titanium dioxide (E171).

Syrups, (powder for reconstitution): disodium edetate; erythrosine (E127); fruit flavours; lactose; monosodium glutamate; sodium benzoate; sodium chloride; sodium citrate, dried; sucrose; sunset yellow FCF (E110).

Suspensions: anise oil; chloroform water; saccharin solution.

Dosage form development

Formation of 'ordered mixtures' between several antibiotics (including cloxacillin sodium) and sorbitol was assessed in a study preliminary to the formulation of a sucrose-free dry powder for reconstitution.[13] Instant sorbitol and crystalline sorbitol were compared. Adsorption of cloxacillin sodium, assumed to occur at sites on the surface of sorbitol particles, was influenced by the nature and size of the antibiotic particles. The adsorption capacity and binding strength of instant sorbitol were greater than those of crystalline sorbitol. Studies with 'moisturised

spray-dried' sorbitol[14] demonstrated that the number of adsorption sites for cloxacillin sodium on sorbitol increased in the presence of water.

REFERENCES

1. Rapson HDC, Bird AE. J Pharm Pharmacol 1963;15(Suppl):222T–31T.
2. Bundgaard H, Ilver K. Dansk Tidsskr Farm 1970;44:365–80.
3. Tsuji A, Kubo O, Miyamoto E, Yamana T. J Pharm Sci 1977;66(12):1675–9.
4. Bird AE, Marshall AC. J Chromatogr 1971;63:313–19.
5. Attwood D, Agarwal SP. J Pharm Pharmacol 1984;36:563–4.
6. Van Krimpen PC, Van Bennekom WP, Bult A. Pharm Weekbl (Sci) 1987;9:1–23.
7. Lynn B. J Hosp Pharm 1970;28:71–86.
8. Sanburg AL, Lyndon RC, Sunderland B. Aust J Hosp Pharm 1987;17(1):31–4.
9. Brown AF, Harvey DJ, Hoddinott DJ, Britton KJ. Br J Parent Ther 1986;7:42–4.
10. Lynn B. J Hosp Pharm 1971;29:183–95.
11. Noone P, Pattison JR. Lancet 1971;2:575–8.
12. Koshiro A, Fujita T. Drug Intell Clin Pharm 1983;17:351–6.
13. Nikolakakis I, Newton JM. J Pharm Pharmacol 1989;41:145–8.
14. Nikolakakis I, Newton JM. J Pharm Pharmacol 1988;40:67P.

Codeine (BAN)   *Opioid analgesic; Antitussive; Antidiarrhoeal*

Morphine methyl ether
(5R,6S)-7,8-Didehydro-4,5-epoxy-3-methoxy-N-methylmorphinan-6-ol monohydrate; 7,8-didehydro-4,5-epoxy-3-methoxy-17-methyl-(5α,6α)-morphinan-6-ol monohydrate
$C_{18}H_{21}NO_3, H_2O = 317.4$

Codeine Hydrochloride (BANM)
$C_{18}H_{21}NO_3, HCl, 2H_2O = 371.9$

Codeine Phosphate (BANM)
Codeine phosphate hemihydrate
$C_{18}H_{21}NO_3, H_3PO_4, \frac{1}{2}H_2O = 406.4$

Codeine Phosphate Sesquihydrate (BANM)
$C_{18}H_{21}NO_3, H_3PO_4, 1\frac{1}{2}H_2O = 424.4$

Codeine Sulphate (BANM)
Codeine sulfate
$(C_{18}H_{21}NO_3)_2, H_2SO_4, 3H_2O = 750.9$
CAS—76-57-3 (codeine, anhydrous); 6059-47-8 (codeine, monohydrate); 1422-07-7 (codeine hydrochloride, anhydrous); 52-28-8 (codeine phosphate, anhydrous); 41444-62-6 (codeine phosphate,

hemihydrate); 5913-76-8 (codeine phosphate, sesquihydrate); 1420-53-7 (codeine sulphate, anhydrous); 6854-40-6 (codeine sulphate, trihydrate)

Pharmacopoeial status

BP (codeine, codeine hydrochloride, codeine phosphate, codeine phosphate sesquihydrate); USP (codeine, codeine phosphate, codeine sulfate)

Preparations

Compendial
Codeine Phosphate Tablets BP. Contain codeine phosphate or codeine phosphate sesquihydrate. Tablets containing, in each, 15 mg, 30 mg, and 60 mg of codeine phosphate are usually available.
Codeine Linctus BP is a solution containing 0.3% w/v of codeine phosphate or an equivalent concentration of codeine phosphate sesquihydrate in a suitable flavoured vehicle. The title 'Diabetic Codeine Linctus' may be used for a preparation that complies with the requirements of the monograph for Codeine Linctus but which is formulated with a vehicle appropriate for administration to diabetics.
Paediatric Codeine Linctus BP is a solution containing 0.06% w/v of codeine phosphate or an equivalent concentration of codeine phosphate sesquihydrate in a suitable flavoured vehicle. It may be prepared extemporaneously by diluting Codeine Linctus with a suitable vehicle according to the manufacturer's instructions.
Codeine Phosphate Oral Solution BP (Codeine Phosphate Syrup) is a solution containing 0.5% w/v of codeine phosphate or an equivalent concentration of codeine phosphate sesquihydrate in a suitable flavoured vehicle. For extemporaneous preparation, see under Formulation.
Co-codamol is the British Approved Name for compounded preparations of codeine phosphate 2 parts and paracetamol 125 parts. Preparation: Co-codamol Tablets BP (Codeine Phosphate and Paracetamol Tablets). Tablets containing, in each, 8 mg of codeine phosphate and 500 mg of paracetamol are usually available.
Co-codaprin is the British Approved Name for compounded preparations of codeine phosphate 1 part and aspirin 50 parts. Preparations: Co-codaprin Tablets BP (Aspirin and Codeine Tablets). Tablets containing, in each, 400 mg of aspirin and 8 mg of codeine phosphate are usually available.
Dispersible Co-codaprin Tablets BP (Dispersible Aspirin and Codeine Tablets). Tablets containing, in each, 400 mg of aspirin and 8 mg of codeine phosphate are usually available.
Codeine Phosphate Tablets USP.
Codeine Sulfate Tablets USP.
Codeine Phosphate Injection USP. pH 3.0 to 6.0.

Non-compendial
Galcodine (Galen). *Linctus*, sugar free, codeine phosphate 15 mg/5 mL.
Paediatric linctus, sugar free, codeine phosphate 3 mg/5 mL.
Codeine linctus (codeine phosphate 15 mg/5 mL) is available from APS, Evans, Kerfoot.
Codeine linctus paediatric (codeine phosphate 3 mg/mL) is available from Evans.

Compound preparations
Co-codamol tablets are available from APS, Cox, Evans, Galen (Parake), Kerfoot, Norton, Sterling Health (Panadeine).
Dispersible or effervescent co-codamol tablets are available from Fisons (Paracodol), Sterwin. Capsules are available from Fisons (Paracodol).

Co-codaprin tablets and dispersible tablets are available from Cox.

Containers and storage

Solid state
Codeine BP, Codeine Hydrochloride BP, Codeine Phosphate BP, and Codeine Phosphate Sesquihydrate BP should be kept in well-closed containers, protected from light.
Codeine USP, Codeine Phosphate USP, and Codeine Sulfate USP should be preserved in tight, light-resistant containers.

Dosage forms
Codeine Phosphate Tablets BP, Codeine Linctus BP, Paediatric Codeine Linctus BP, Codeine Phosphate Oral Solution BP, Co-codaprin Tablets BP, and Dispersible Co-codaprin Tablets BP should be protected from light.
Codeine Phosphate Tablets USP should be preserved in well-closed, light-resistant containers.
Codeine Sulfate Tablets USP should be preserved in well-closed containers.
Codeine Phosphate Injection USP should be preserved in single-dose or in multiple-dose containers, preferably of Type I glass, protected from light.

PHYSICAL PROPERTIES

Codeine exists as an odourless, white crystalline powder or as colourless crystals.
Codeine hydrochloride exists as a white crystalline powder or small, colourless crystals.
Codeine phosphate exists as a white crystalline powder or small, colourless crystals.
Codeine phosphate sesquihydrate exists as a white crystalline powder or small, colourless crystals.
Codeine sulphate exists as white crystals, or as a white crystalline powder.

Melting point

Codeine melts in the range 155° to 159°.
Codeine hydrochloride melts at about 280°, with some decomposition.

pH

A 0.5% w/v solution of *codeine* has a pH greater than 9. A saturated aqueous solution of *codeine* has a pH of 9.8.

Dissociation constant

pK_a 8.2 (20°); pK_a 6.05 (15°)

Partition coefficient

Log P (octanol/pH 7.4), 0.6

Solubility

Solubility of codeine and codeine salts in various solvents:

	Water	Ethanol	Chloroform	Ether
Codeine	1 in 120	1 in 2	1 in 0.5	1 in 50
Codeine hydrochloride	1 in 20	1 in 100	practically insoluble	practically insoluble
Codeine phosphate	1 in 4	slightly soluble	practically insoluble	practically insoluble
Codeine sulphate	1 in 30	1 in 1300	practically insoluble	practically insoluble

At 25°, codeine is soluble in 13 parts of benzene. Codeine is freely soluble in methanol, in pentanol, and in dilute acids; almost insoluble in petroleum ether or in solutions of alkali hydroxides.

Effect of temperature

Effect of temperature on the solubility of codeine and codeine salts in water and ethanol:

	Water (20°)	Water (80°)	Water (100°)	Ethanol (20°)	Ethanol (hot)	Ethanol (boiling)
Codeine	1 in 120	1 in 60	1 in 15	1 in 2	1 in 1.2	—
Codeine hydrochloride	1 in 20	—	1 in 1	—	—	—
Codeine phosphate	—	—	—	slightly soluble	—	1 in 125
Codeine sulphate	1 in 30	1 in 6.5	—	—	—	—

Dissolution

The USP specifies that for Codeine Phosphate Tablets USP not less than 75% of the labelled amount of $C_{18}H_{21}NO_3, H_3PO_4, \frac{1}{2}H_2O$ is dissolved in 45 minutes. Dissolution medium: 900 mL of water; Apparatus 2 at 50 rpm.
The USP specifies that for Codeine Sulfate Tablets USP not less than 75% of the labelled amount of $(C_{18}H_{21}NO_3)_2, H_2SO_4, 3H_2O$ is dissolved in 45 minutes. Dissolution medium: 500 mL of water; Apparatus 1 at 100 rpm.

Dissolution properties

Dissolution studies on the various polymorphic forms of codeine have shown differences in solubility and in dissolution rate.[1] Both Form II and Form III exhibited a faster dissolution rate than Form I (stable form). Form III was at least ten times more soluble than Form I.
A further study by the same authors[2] investigated the factors affecting the dissolution rate of Form III. Particle size affected the dissolution rate slightly. Addition of povidone to the dissolution medium resulted in an increase in dissolution rate, possibly caused by the increased viscosity of the medium and retardation of the transition of Form III to Form I. It was also found that when the dissolution rates of tablets of either Form I or Form III, prepared by wet granulation, were compared there was little difference. However, when the tablets were prepared by direct compression, Form III dissolved approximately three times faster than Form I. See also under Crystal and molecular structure, below.

Crystal and molecular structure

According to Ebian and El-Gindy,[1] codeine exists in three polymorphic forms. Form I and Form II are the hydrous and anhydrous forms respectively, and Form III is a solvate. Form I is transformed to Form II on heating which is consistent with loss of water of hydration. When all forms were suspended in water the resulting form was Form I. Transformation took longer for Form III than for Form II. Polymorphs I and III were converted to Form II on dry grinding.
In a further study, El-Gindy and Ebian[2] investigated the thermodynamic parameters of the polymorphs of codeine. Differences in the heats of solution and the free energy change between forms were found. See also Dissolution, above.

STABILITY

Codeine is affected by light. On exposure to air, codeine phosphate loses water of hydration. Its stability is affected by light. Codeine sulphate effloresces in dry air, as does codeine.

A study of the stability of liquid dosage forms of codeine demonstrated that at room temperature (22°), 40°, and 50° the main degradation product was codeine N-oxide.[3]
According to Gundermann and Pohloudek-Fabini,[4] the degradation of codeine phosphate in aqueous solution followed first-order kinetics. Degradation was dependent on temperature, light, and pH. Codeine phosphate solutions appeared to be relatively stable at a pH of 3.5. In another study by Polish workers,[5] however, a gradual increase in degradation rate from pH 1.6 to pH 10.5 was observed for codeine and codeine phosphate solutions.
Powell[6] presented pH-rate profiles for codeine sulphate degradation at 60°, 80°, and 100°. Again, first-order degradation was observed. Phosphate buffers accelerated the rate of codeine degradation, one of the primary degradation products being norcodeine; higher rate constants were recorded when greater amounts of buffer were used.
On dissolution, codeine phosphate produces phosphate ions which will act as a catalyst for codeine degradation. This is borne out when the rate constant for codeine phosphate degradation at 25° (3.0×10^{-9}/s) is compared[6] with the rate constant for codeine sulphate degradation at 25° (7.6×10^{-11}/s).
Galante et al[7] reported on the formation of acetylcodeine phosphate as a result of a solid-state interaction between aspirin and codeine phosphate. It was concluded that this reaction could occur in solid dosage forms containing aspirin and codeine phosphate even when moisture levels are low. The physiological activity of acetylcodeine is thought to be about the same as codeine.

Stabilisation

The stability of a codeine liquid preparation that also contained ipecacuanha extract, ephedrine hydrochloride, anise oil, fennel oil, ethanol 95%, and purified water was investigated.[3] Iron (III), zinc (II), and copper (II) ions (in the ipecacuanha extract), as well as light, were found to have most influence on the rate of oxidation of codeine. Butylated hydroxyanisole and tartaric acid (both 0.01%) were found to have a stabilising effect which was independent of pH.
It has been found that citric acid and thiourea reduce the rate of degradation of codeine phosphate solutions. Low-density polyethylene containers are suitable for the storage of such solutions.[4]
Reports of discoloration of codeine phosphate aqueous solutions on autoclaving prompted a study of this effect.[8] Simple aqueous solutions of codeine phosphate (50 mg/mL) were prepared with and without sodium metabisulphite (0.1%). The solutions were filtered and packed in neutral glass ampoules either under nitrogen or without further treatment. All the ampoules except some retained as controls were autoclaved at 115° for 30 minutes and then examined for signs of deterioration. Half the autoclaved ampoules were subjected to another autoclave cycle. All the autoclaved solutions that did not contain metabisulphite showed a faint yellow discoloration which was not apparent in those with added metabisulphite. The discoloration was even more marked after a second autoclave cycle. Sealing under nitrogen did not appear to affect the results.
Although earlier studies have shown citric acid and tartaric acid to have a stabilising effect on codeine in liquid dosage forms, they may contribute to the degradation of codeine phosphate in effervescent tablet formulations. In a paracetamol-codeine effervescent preparation, codeine phosphate was found to react with citric acid to form citrate esters of codeine at room temperature and at 37°. The esterification was confirmed by a solid-state reaction at a higher temperature. Tartaric acid was also found to form an ester with codeine phosphate.[9]

INCOMPATIBILITY/COMPATIBILITY

Codeine and codeine salts are incompatible with bromides, iodides, alkalis, the majority of alkaloidal precipitants, ammonium chloride, valerates, and salts of copper, iron, or lead. Tannins may also cause precipitation. Many metal oxides or hydroxides are precipitated from solutions of metal salts by the action of a saturated solution of codeine (pH 9.8). Iodides will only form a precipitate with codeine salts at specified concentrations. At a codeine concentration of 1% and a potassium iodide concentration of 3% to 5% or a hydroiodic acid concentration of 2.5% to 3%, insoluble codeine iodide is formed. At lower concentrations, clear solutions are formed. Ethanol at a concentration of 10% to 20% can prevent or retard precipitation in more concentrated solutions.

FORMULATION

CODEINE LINCTUS
The following formula was given in the *British Pharmacopoeia 1980*:

Codeine phosphate	3 g
Water	20 mL
Compound tartrazine solution	10 mL
Benzoic acid solution	20 mL
Chloroform spirit	20 mL
Lemon syrup	200 mL
Syrup	to 1000 mL

Dissolve the codeine phosphate in water, add 500 mL of syrup, and mix; the remaining ingredients should then be added. Make up to volume with syrup. Protect from light. Diluent, syrup. Shelf-life of diluted linctus 14 days.

DIABETIC CODEINE LINCTUS
The following formula was given in the *British Pharmaceutical Codex 1973*:

Codeine phosphate	3 g
Citric acid	5 g
Lemon spirit	1 mL
Compound tartrazine solution	10 mL
Benzoic acid solution	20 mL
Chloroform spirit	20 mL
Water	20 mL
Sorbitol solution, non-crystallising grade	to 1000 mL

Dissolve the codeine phosphate and the citric acid in the water, add 750 mL of the sorbitol solution, and mix. The remaining ingredients should then be added. Make up to volume with the sorbitol solution.

CODEINE PHOSPHATE ORAL SOLUTION BP

Codeine phosphate	5 g
Water	15 mL
Chloroform spirit	25 mL
Syrup	to 1000 mL

Dissolve the codeine phosphate in the water, add 750 mL of the syrup and mix. Add the chloroform spirit and sufficient of the syrup to produce 1000 mL and mix. The oral solution should be recently prepared.

Excipients

Excipients that have been used in presentations of codeine include:
Oral liquids, codeine phosphate: chloroform spirit; concentrated chloroform water; eucalyptol; glycerol; menthol; methyl hydroxybenzoate; syrup.

Pastilles, codeine phosphate: caramel; eucalyptus oil; glucose; honey; menthol; sucrose; thymol.
Injections, codeine phosphate: chlorbutol; sodium acetate buffer; sodium bisulphite; sodium metabisulphite.

Suppositories

Codeine phosphate has the following displacement values in the bases listed:
Witepsol 1.25
Imitation theobroma oil 1.2
Theobroma oil 1.1

Novel presentations

The release of codeine base from poly(alkyl)cyanoacrylate films was investigated by El Egakey and Speiser.[10] It was found that poly(methyl)cyanoacrylate and poly(ethyl)cyanoacrylate produced the most satisfactory release characteristics. The quantity of drug released was approximately proportional to the initial drug content and was independent of pH change from 1.2 to 7.2.

PROCESSING

Sterilisation

Solutions of codeine and codeine salts can be sterilised by heating in an autoclave or by filtration.
A Russian research team investigated the possibility of sterilising alkaloidal pharmaceuticals by radiation.[11] Injectable solutions and codeine phosphate powder were exposed at low temperatures to radiation doses of 266 ± 3 rad/s (total dose 2.3997 Mrad). Decomposition was detected and changes in biological activity and increased toxicity were also apparent. It was concluded that sterilisation by radiation is not suitable for codeine phosphate.

REFERENCES

1. Ebian AR, El-Gindy NA. Sci Pharm 1978;46:1–7.
2. El-Gindy NA, Ebian AR. Sci Pharm 1978;46:8–16.
3. Nägler H-J, Graf E [German]. Acta Pharm Technol 1982;28:66–72.
4. Gundermann P, Pohloudek-Fabini R [German]. Pharmazie 1983;38:92–4.
5. Pawelczyk E, Wachowiek R [Polish]. Herba Pol 1974;20:253–63.
6. Powell MF. J Pharm Sci 1986;75:901–3.
7. Galante RN, Visalli AJ, Patel DM. J Pharm Sci 1979;68:1494–8.
8. *PSGB Lab Report P/76/8* 1976.
9. Silver B, Sundholm EG. J Pharm Sci 1987;76:53–5.
10. El Egakey MA, Speiser PP. Acta Pharm Technol 1982;28:103–9.
11. Grachev SA, Chakchir BA, Ryabykh LD [Russian]. Khim Farm Zh 1973;7:47–50.

Cortisone (BAN, rINN)   *Corticosteroid*

Compound E; 11-dehydro-17-hydroxycorticosterone
17α,21-Dihydroxypregn-4-ene-3,11,20-trione
$C_{21}H_{28}O_5 = 360.4$

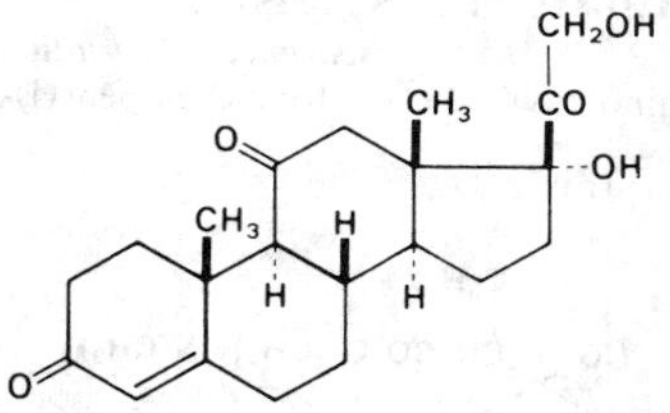

Cortisone Acetate (BANM, rINNM)

$C_{23}H_{30}O_6 = 402.5$
CAS—53-06-5 (cortisone); 53-04-4 (cortisone acetate)

Pharmacopoeial status

BP, USP (cortisone acetate)

Preparations

Compendial
Cortisone Tablets BP. Tablets containing, in each, cortisone
acetate (as fine powder) 5 mg and 25 mg, are usually available.
Cortisone Acetate Tablets USP.
Sterile Cortisone Acetate Suspension USP. pH between 5.0 and
7.0.

Non-compendial
Cortistab (Boots). *Tablets*, cortisone acetate 5 mg and 25 mg.
Cortisyl (Roussel). *Tablets*, cortisone acetate 25 mg.

Containers and storage

Solid state
Cortisone Acetate BP should be protected from light and stored
in a well-closed container.
Cortisone Acetate USP should be preserved in well-closed containers.

Dosage forms
Cortisone Tablets BP should be protected from light.
Cortisone Acetate Tablets USP should be preserved in well-
closed containers.
Sterile Cortisone Acetate Suspension USP should be preserved
in single-dose or multiple-dose containers, preferably of Type I
glass.
Cortistab tablets should be stored in a cool dry place and protected from light.

PHYSICAL PROPERTIES

Cortisone exists as crystals (rhombohedral platelets).
Cortisone acetate is a white or almost white, odourless crystalline powder.

Melting point

Cortisone melts in the range 217° to 224°, with some decomposition.
Cortisone acetate melts at about 240°, with some decomposition.

Partition coefficients

A mean value of log $P = 1.40$ (ether/water, at 23° ± 1°) was
determined for cortisone by Flynn[1] from experimental values
of 1.35 and 1.44.

Caron and Shroot[2] determined the partition coefficients of cortisone and cortisone acetate by HPLC using a persilylated octa-
decylisilane phase saturated with 1-octanol and eluted with 1-
octanol-saturated phosphate buffer (pH 7): log $P = 1.5$ for cortisone and log $P = 2.45$ for cortisone acetate.
Data obtained by Ponec et al[3] also produced a value for log P of
1.5 for cortisone (1-octanol and pH 7.4 aqueous buffer).

Solubility

Cortisone is very slightly soluble in water; soluble in ethanol; and
sparingly soluble in chloroform and in ether.
Cortisone acetate is practically insoluble in water; slightly soluble in ethanol, in methanol, and in ether; freely soluble in chloroform (1 in 4); soluble in 1,4-dioxan; sparingly soluble in acetone.

Dissolution

The USP specifies that for Cortisone Acetate Tablets USP not
less than 60% of the labelled amount of $C_{23}H_{30}O_6$ is dissolved
in 30 minutes. Dissolution medium: 900 mL of a mixture containing 3 volumes of isopropyl alcohol and 7 volumes of dilute
hydrochloric acid (1 in 100); Apparatus 1 at 100 rpm.

Dissolution properties
The dissolution rates of several corticosteroids prepared as solid
dispersions with glucose, galactose, or sucrose were significantly
increased when compared to the dissolution rates of the corticosteroid powders alone.[4] Glass dispersions prepared with glucose and sucrose displayed faster release times than those
made with galactose. The times for 50% and 100% dissolution
for cortisone acetate in glucose carrier were less than 2 minutes
and 20 minutes, respectively.

Crystal and molecular structure

Polymorphs
Cortisone acetate exists in several polymorphic forms. Early
attempts to suspend crystalline cortisone acetate in an aqueous
medium resulted, after a few hours, in caking and sedimentation of the less soluble polymorph (Form V). Florence and Attwood[5] postulate the existence of more than seven forms of
cortisone acetate and observe that 'authentic' Cortisone Acetate BP is Form II whereas Form III is recommended as 'authentic' by the USP and WHO.
Spectroscopic and calorimetric evidence for three anhydrous
(Forms I, II, and III) and two hydrated (Forms IV and V) crystalline modifications of cortisone acetate was presented by Carless et al.[6] Methods for the preparation of the different forms are
strongly dependent upon solvent composition, as shown below:

Polymorphic form	Solvent
I	(obtained by heating any other form to 200°)
II	chloroform; benzene
III	30% v/v water in acetone; water at 100°
IV	95% aqueous ethanol
V	carbon tetrachloride: anhydrous methanol (3:1 v/v)

During storage for two weeks at room temperature, the polymorphic form in aqueous suspensions of cortisone acetate
(initially present in any polymorphic form) changed to Form
IV. Form III was produced when all forms (except IV) were continuously ground under water in an agate mortar for 45 minutes.
In a later study, the same workers[7] showed that crystal growth,
initiated mainly by polymorphic transformation from Form II

to Form III, was controlled by the lattice energy, the heat of wetting, and the heat of solution of different crystal forms. Further work examined the effects of crystal form, saturation with cortisone alcohol, and agitation, on crystal growth of cortisone acetate in aqueous suspensions.[8]

FURTHER INFORMATION. The kinetics of thermal dehydration and transformation of solid cortisone acetate—Carless JE, Moustafa MA, Rapson HDC. J Pharm Pharmacol 1972;24:130P. Pharmaceutical applications of polymorphism [review article]—Haleblian J, McCrone W. J Pharm Sci 1969;58(8):911–29.

STABILITY

Cortisone acetate rapidly decomposes in alkaline media and in strong acids. Hansen and Bundgaard[9] reported that the degradation of cortisone in acidic aqueous solution at 70° followed first-order kinetics and was dependent upon the concentrations of both the steroid and hydrogen ions in the test solution (within the range 0.5M to 2.0M hydrochloric acid). Specific acid-catalysed degradation of cortisone in aqueous solution at 70° produced a molar yield of the main product of decomposition (the 17-deoxy glyoxal derivative) of 80% to 97%.

In an examination of the feasibility of sterilisation by irradiation Kane and Tsuji[10] measured the radiolytic degradation of a number of corticosteroids, including cortisone and cortisone acetate. The two main routes of decomposition were: loss of the C-17 side chain to produce the C-17 ketone and oxidation of the C-11 alcohol (if present) to the C-11 ketone. Most of the corticosteroids in the solid state were stable to irradiation by cobalt-60 at dose levels between 0.5 and 6 Mrads.

Stabilisation

When aqueous suspensions of cortisone acetate are prepared, all particles should be converted to the most stable of the polymorphic forms in order to avoid crystal growth.

FORMULATION

Excipients

Excipients that have been used in presentations of cortisone acetate include:

Tablets: gelatin; lactose; magnesium stearate; starch; sucrose; talc.

Suspensions (for intramuscular injection only): benzyl alcohol; carmellose sodium; citric acid; methylcellulose; methyl hydroxybenzoate; polysorbate 80; sodium benzoate; sodium chloride; syrup.

REFERENCES

1. Flynn GL. J Pharm Sci 1971;60:345–53.
2. Caron JC, Shroot B. J Pharm Sci 1984;73(12):1703–6.
3. Ponec M, Kempenaar J, Shroot B, Caron JC. J Pharm Sci 1986;75(10):973–5.
4. Allen LV, Yanchick VA, Maness DD. J Pharm Sci 1977;66:494–6.
5. Florence AT, Attwood D. Physicochemical principles of pharmacy. 2nd ed. London: McMillan, 1986:30.
6. Carless JE, Moustafa MA, Rapson HDC. J Pharm Pharmacol 1966;18:190S-197S.
7. Carless JE, Moustafa MA, Rapson HDC. J Pharm Pharmacol 1968;20:630–8.
8. Carless JE, Moustafa MA, Rapson HDC. J Pharm Pharmacol 1968;20:639–45.
9. Hansen J, Bundgaard H. Arch Pharm Chemi (Sci) 1980;8:5–14.
10. Kane MP, Tsuji K. J Pharm Sci 1983;72:30–5.

Cyclopentolate (BAN, rINN)

Antimuscarinic; Mydriatic (ophthalmic)

2-Dimethylaminoethyl 2-(1-hydroxycyclopentyl)-2-phenylacetate

$C_{17}H_{25}NO_3 = 291.4$

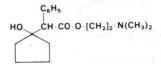

Cyclopentolate Hydrochloride (BANM, rINNM)

$C_{17}H_{25}NO_3, HCl = 327.9$

CAS—512-15-2 (cyclopentolate); 5870-29-1 (cyclopentolate hydrochloride)

Pharmacopoeial status

BP, USP (cyclopentolate hydrochloride)

Preparations

Compendial

Cyclopentolate Eye Drops BP. A sterile solution of cyclopentolate hydrochloride in purified water. Eye drops containing 0.5% w/v and 1% w/v are usually available. pH 3.0 to 5.5.

Cyclopentolate Hydrochloride Ophthalmic Solution USP. pH 3.0 to 5.5.

Non-compendial

Alnide (Cusi). *Eye drops*, cyclopentolate hydrochloride 0.5% and 1%, buffered to pH 5.0.

Minims Cyclopentolate (S&N Pharm). *Eye drops*, single use, cyclopentolate hydrochloride 0.5% and 1%.

Mydrilate (Boehringer Ingelheim). *Eye drops*, cyclopentolate hydrochloride 0.5% and 1.0%, buffered to pH 5.0.

Containers and storage

Solid state

Cyclopentolate Hydrochloride USP should be preserved in tight containers and stored in a cold place.

Dosage forms

Cyclopentolate Hydrochloride Ophthalmic Solution USP should be preserved in tight containers and stored at controlled room temperature.

Minims cyclopentolate hydrochloride should be stored in a cool place (8° to 15°) and should not be exposed to strong light.

Alnide and Mydrilate should be stored below 15° and protected from light. They should not be diluted, or dispensed from any container other than the original bottle and should be discarded one month after opening.

PHYSICAL PROPERTIES

Cyclopentolate hydrochloride is a white crystalline powder; odourless or with an odour of phenylacetic acid.

Melting point

The melting point of *cyclopentolate hydrochloride* is in the range 135° to 138°.

pH

The pH of a 1% solution of *cyclopentolate hydrochloride* is between 4.5 and 5.5.

Dissociation constant

pK_a 7.9

Solubility

Cyclopentolate hydrochloride is soluble 1 in less than 1 of water and 1 in 5 of ethanol; insoluble in ether.

STABILITY

Cyclopentolate hydrochloride (as Mydrilate eye drops) has been reported[1] to become chemically unstable above pH 6.0.

FORMULATION

Excipients

Excipients that have been used in presentations of cyclopentolate hydrochloride include:
Eye drops and eye solutions: benzalkonium chloride; boric acid; dibasic potassium phosphate; disodium edetate; hydrochloric acid; monobasic potassium phosphate; phenylmercuric nitrate; potassium chloride; sodium carbonate; sodium chloride.

Eye drops

Wang and Hammarlund[2] reported that eye drops comprising phenylephrine 1% plus cyclopentolate hydrochloride 0.1%, buffered with isotonic sterile sodium borate 2.6% solution, exerted a mydriatic effect similar to that of unbuffered solutions that were ten times more concentrated.

FURTHER INFORMATION. Plasma concentrations and ocular effects of cyclopentolate after ocular application of three formulations—Lahdes K, Huupponen R, Kaila T, Monti D, Saettone MF, Salminen L. Br J Clin Pharmacol 1993;35:479–83.

REFERENCES

1. Granger CD. Ophthalmic Optician 1964;4:1161–2.
2. Wang ESN, Hammarlund ER. J Pharm Sci 1970;59(11):1559–62.

Cyclophosphamide (BAN, rINN)   *Cytotoxic*

2-[Bis(2-chloroethyl)amino]perhydro-1,3,2-oxazaphosphorinane 2-oxide monohydrate; *N,N*-bis(2-chloroethyl)tetrahydro-2*H*-1,3,2-oxazaphosphorin-2-amine 2-oxide monohydrate
$C_7H_{15}Cl_2N_2O_2P, H_2O = 279.1$
CAS—6055-19-2 (monohydrate); 50-18-0 (anhydrous)

Pharmacopoeial status

BP, USP

Preparations

Compendial
Cyclophosphamide Tablets BP. Coated tablets containing, in each, 10 mg, 50 mg, and 53.5 mg are usually available.

Cyclophosphamide Injection BP (Cyclophosphamide for Injection). A sterile isotonic solution of cyclophosphamide in water for injections. It is prepared by dissolving cyclophosphamide for injection in the requisite amount of water for injections immediately before use; pH of a freshly prepared 2% w/v solution, 4.0 to 6.0. Sealed containers each containing the equivalent of 100, 200, 500, and 1000 mg of anhydrous cyclophosphamide (107, 214, 535, and 1070 mg of cyclophosphamide) are usually available.
Cyclophosphamide Tablets USP.
Cyclophosphamide for Injection USP.

Non-compendial
Cyclophosphamide (Farmitalia Carlo Erba). *Tablets*, cyclophosphamide 53.5 mg (equivalent to 50 mg of anhydrous cyclophosphamide).
Injection, powder for reconstitution in clear glass vials containing 107, 214, 535, and 1070 mg of cyclophosphamide (equivalent to 100, 200, 500, and 1000 mg of anhydrous cyclophosphamide, respectively). For reconstitution with water for injections.
Endoxana (ASTA Medica). *Tablets*, cyclophosphamide 50 mg.
Injection, powder for reconstitution in vials containing 107, 214, 535, and 1069 mg of cyclophosphamide (equivalent to 100, 200, 500, and 1000 mg of anhydrous cyclophosphamide, respectively). For reconstitution with water for injections. The injection is compatible with glucose/sodium chloride injections and when mixed, such solutions are chemically stable for 24 hours at room temperature or for 6 days under refrigeration. However, such solutions should be used within 8 hours unless prepared under aseptic conditions. An oral elixir may be prepared by dissolving the dry powder contents of the vials in Aromatic Elixir USP shortly before administration.

Containers and storage

Solid state
Cyclophosphamide USP should be preserved in tight containers, at a temperature between 2° and 30°.

Dosage forms
Cyclophosphamide Injection BP deteriorates on storage and should be used immediately after preparation.
Cyclophosphamide Tablets USP should be preserved in tight containers. Storage at a temperature not exceeding 25° is recommended; although tablets will withstand brief exposure to temperatures up to 30°, they should be protected from temperatures above 30°.
Cyclophosphamide for Injection USP should be preserved in containers suitable for sterile solids. Storage at a temperature not exceeding 25° is recommended; although it will withstand brief exposure to temperatures up to 30°, it should be protected from temperatures above 30°.
Cyclophosphamide (Farmitalia Carlo Erba) tablets should be stored in a cool dry place, protected from light; the injection should be stored in a cool place protected from light. It is recommended that the products are not stored in places where heat build-up may occur because, if heated above 32°, cyclophosphamide may decompose to a 'damp-looking gel'. After reconstitution, the injection will remain stable for 2 to 3 hours at room temperature.
Endoxana tablets and injection should be stored below 25°, protected from light.

PHYSICAL PROPERTIES

Cyclophosphamide exists as a fine, white crystalline powder, which discolours on exposure to light; odourless or almost odourless. It liquefies on loss of its water of crystallisation.

Melting point

Cyclophosphamide melts at 49.5° to 53°.
Anhydrous cyclophosphamide melts at 53.5°.[1]

pH

The USP states that, 30 minutes after its preparation, a 1% solution of *cyclophosphamide* has a pH between 3.9 and 7.1.

Solubility

Cyclophosphamide is soluble 1 in 25 of water and 1 in 1 of ethanol; slightly soluble in ether.

Crystal and molecular structure

Cyclophosphamide is a monohydrate but the anhydrous form of cyclophosphamide has been shown to be stable; the monohydrate converted to the anhydrate if the relative humidity fell below 70% and the temperature was above 30°.[1] Transition between the forms was reversible.

STABILITY

Degradation pathways and kinetics

In aqueous solution, degradation of cyclophosphamide occurs primarily by hydrolysis, particularly at temperatures greater than 30°; the products and reaction pathways are reported to be pH-dependent. The rate of reaction is independent of pH in the range 2 to 10, although specific acid and specific base catalysis occur outside this pH range.[2] A slight fall in pH generally accompanies decomposition of cyclophosphamide but this is not thought to influence the kinetics of degradation significantly.[2,3] Under acidic conditions the final degradation products have been reported to be phosphoric acid, propanolamine, and nor-nitrogen mustard, although the initial hydrolysis may follow one of three pathways.[2] At pH 1 or less, degradation of cyclophosphamide yields bis(2-chloroethyl)amine and 3-aminopropan-1-ol. Under neutral or basic conditions the main degradation product, formed from an initial intramolecular *N*-alkylation with the liberation of chloride ions and subsequent reactions, is *N*-(2-hydroxyethyl)-*N'*-(3-hydroxypropyl)ethylenediamine.[2,4]

An activation energy of approximately 112 kJ/mol was calculated from rate constants for the hydrolysis of cyclophosphamide in solution at pH 7 (phosphate buffer) measured at 40°, 50°, 60°, and 80°.[5]

When solutions of cyclophosphamide (21 mg/mL) were heated to 50° or 60° for 15 minutes, negligible loss of concentration of cyclophosphamide, compared to an unheated solution, occurred (analysis by vapour phase chromatography).[3] However, when heated to 70° and 80° for 15 minutes, losses of about 9.8% and 22.5%, respectively, were measured.

Vehicles and containers

Gallelli[6] noted that when solutions of cyclophosphamide 4 mg/mL in sodium chloride 0.9% injection were stored at 25°, unprotected from light, about 3.5% and 12% decomposition occurred after 24 hours and 7 days, respectively. However, negligible decomposition was apparent during storage of similar solutions protected from light at 5° for the same time periods. In a comprehensive study Brooke *et al*[7] prepared solutions of cyclophosphamide in various aqueous parenteral vehicles using a cyclophosphamide/sodium chloride blend equivalent to Cytoxan for Injection (Mead Johnson). At room temperature (24° to 27°), first-order rate constants for the decomposition of cyclophosphamide monohydrate (initial concentrations 0.1 mg/mL and 3.1 mg/mL) were 0.0167/day and 0.027/day, respec-

tively, in glucose 5% injection, and 0.0229/day and 0.0216/day, respectively, in glucose 5%/sodium chloride 0.9% injection. Similarly, at room temperature, first-order rate constants (initial concentration of cyclophosphamide monohydrate of 21 mg/mL) were 0.0263/ day, 0.028/day, and 0.0405/day in bacteriostatic water for injections preserved with hydroxybenzoates, in sterile water for injections, and in bacteriostatic water for injections preserved with benzyl alcohol, respectively. It was suggested that benzyl alcohol may catalyse the decomposition of cyclophosphamide. When stored at 5° (under refrigeration), rate constants in all solutions were lower than those at room temperature.

Similarly, the first-order decomposition of cyclophosphamide monohydrate 2 mg/mL in Aromatic Elixir USP was studied during storage in clear glass bottles at 30° to 45° (in an oven), at 24° to 26° (room temperature), or at 4° to 8° (in a refrigerator).[8] An activation energy of approximately 117.9 kJ/mol was calculated and it was concluded that the vehicle was suitable for solutions stored for short periods in a refrigerator; it was estimated that a maximum loss of 1.5% of cyclophosphamide would occur during storage for 14 days at 4° to 8°.

More than 90% of the initial concentration of cyclophosphamide remained after 24 hours when an injection of cyclophosphamide (Mead Johnson), reconstituted with sterile water, was added to glucose 5% injection and stored in polyvinyl chloride bags or partly filled glass bottles, unprotected from light, at room temperature.[9]

The stability of cyclophosphamide injection (Carlo Erba, UK), reconstituted under aseptic conditions with water for injections to a concentration of 20 mg/mL, was examined (by HPLC) under various storage conditions.[10] In sealed glass ampoules at room temperature (20° to 23°), 4°, and −20.5° (thawed in a microwave) approximately 36%, 0.5%, and 2.8%, respectively, of the initial concentration of cyclophosphamide was lost after 4 weeks. After one week at room temperature 13% had degraded. In sealed polypropylene syringes at 4°, losses of about 2.4% after 4 weeks and 10% after 11 to 14 weeks were detected. When stored in similar syringes at −20.5° for 19 weeks (then microwave thawed) the concentration loss was about 4%. At cyclophosphamide concentrations greater than 8 mg/mL precipitation of cyclophosphamide occurred during microwave thawing; the precipitate redissolved after vigorous shaking for five minutes. In addition, storage at −20° in polypropylene syringes was not recommended as a transient contraction of the syringe plunger was observed on cooling. When the injection was further diluted to 4 mg/mL with sodium chloride 0.9% injection and stored in polyvinyl chloride bags, there was no appreciable degradation after 4 weeks but about 8% degradation occurred after 19 weeks at either 4° or −20.5° (with microwave thawing).

FURTHER INFORMATION. Chemical stability of two sterile, parenteral formulations of cyclophosphamide (Endoxan) after reconstitution and dilution in commonly used infusion fluids— Beijnen JH, van Gijn R, Challa EE, Kaijser GP, Underberg WJM. J Parenter Sci Technol 1992;46(4):111–16.

FORMULATION

Excipients

Excipients that have been used in presentations of cyclophosphamide include:

Tablets: acacia; brilliant blue FCF (133); lactose; magnesium stearate; quinoline yellow (E104); aluminium lake; saccharin; sodium benzoate; sodium ethyl hydroxybenzoate; sodium propyl hydroxybenzoate; starch; stearic acid; talc; titanium dioxide (E171).

Oral liquids: Aromatic Elixir USP.

Injections (powder for reconstitution): mannitol; sodium chloride.

Lozenges: acacia; gelatin; lactose; magnesium carbonate; magnesium stearate; shellac; starch; sucrose; talc.

Lyophilised products

Kovalcik and Guillory prepared lyophilised products that contained cyclophosphamide with mannitol, lactose, sodium bicarbonate,[11] urea, povidone 40, or dextran.[12] All produced 'well-formed cakes'. A lyophilised product containing cyclophosphamide and sorbitol formed a 'collapsed mass'.[11] At room temperature, cyclophosphamide in the solid state was shown to degrade rapidly; $t_{10\%}$ values were about 15 days in the cakes with mannitol, lactose, or sodium bicarbonate and were less than 30 days for those with urea, povidone 40, or dextran. For products exposed to moisture, analysis by powder X-ray diffraction and differential scanning calorimetry revealed that in cakes containing mannitol, sodium bicarbonate, or urea, cyclophosphamide was converted from the amorphous form to the monohydrate and stability was improved. However, in cakes containing lactose or dextran, cyclophosphamide was not converted to the monohydrate and stability was not improved. Cakes with povidone 40 formed a clear, semi-solid with poor stability on exposure to moisture.

FURTHER INFORMATION. Synthesis and evaluation of 3-halocyclophosphamides and analogous compounds as novel anticancer 'pro-drugs'—Zon G, Ludeman SM, Özkan G, Chandrasegaran S, Hammer CF, Dickerson R *et al. J Pharm Sci* 1983;72(6):687–91.

PROCESSING

Handling and disposal

CAUTION. Cyclophosphamide should be handled with great care as it is a potent cytotoxic agent.

The manufacturer of Endoxana recommends that if contamination of the eyes or skin occurs the area should be washed thoroughly with copious water. Non-mucous membranes should then be washed with soap and water.

The manufacturer of Endoxana also recommends that protective clothing, goggles, masks, and disposable polyvinyl chloride or latex gloves should be worn when handling cyclophosphamide injection. Reconstitution should be performed in a designated area, preferably under a laminar-airflow system, and the work surface should be protected by a disposable, plastic-backed, absorbent paper.

Unopened vials of cyclophosphamide may be destroyed by incineration at 900°.[13]

General guidelines on the handling and disposal of cytotoxic drugs are given in the chapter entitled Cytotoxic Drugs: Handling Precautions.

FURTHER INFORMATION. IARC Scientific Publications No 73, Laboratory decontamination and destruction of carcinogens in laboratory wastes: some antineoplastic agents [a method for the destruction of cyclophosphamide using alkaline hydrolysis in the presence of dimethylformamide]—Castegnaro M, Adams J, Armour MA *et al*, editors. London: International Agency for Research on Cancer, 1985:57.

REFERENCES

1. Laine E, Tuominen V, Jalonen H, Kahela P. Acta Pharm Fenn 1983;92:243–8.

2. Connors KA, Amidon GL, Stella VJ, editors. Chemical stability of pharmaceuticals: a handbook for pharmacists. 2nd ed. New York: John Wiley & Sons, 1986:385–93.

3. Brooke D, Scott JA, Bequette RJ. Am J Hosp Pharm 1975;32:44–5.

4. Friedman OM, Bien S, Chakrabarti JK. J Am Chem Soc 1965;87:4978–9.

5. Kensler TT, Behme RJ, Brooke D. J Pharm Sci 1979;68(2):172–4.

6. Gallelli JF. Am J Hosp Pharm 1967;24:425–33.

7. Brooke D, Bequette RJ, Davis RE. Am J Hosp Pharm 1973;30:134–7.

8. Brooke D, Davis RE, Bequette RJ. Am J Hosp Pharm 1973;30:618–20.

9. Benvenuto JA, Anderson RW, Kerkof K, Smith RG, Loo TL. Am J Hosp Pharm 1981;38:1914–18.

10. Kirk B, Melia CD, Wilson JV, Sprake JM. Br J Parenter Ther 1984;5:90–7.

11. Kovalcik TR, Guillory JK. J Parenter Sci Technol 1988;42:29–37.

12. Kovalcik TR, Guillory JK. J Parenter Sci Technol 1988;42:165–73.

13. Garner S, Ross M, Wilson J. Pharm J 1988;241(Hosp Suppl):H532.

Cyclosporin (BAN)   *Immunosuppressant*

Ciclosporin (rINN); Cyclosporine (USAN); cyclosporin A
Cyclo[-[4-(*E*)-but-2-enyl-*N*,4-dimethyl-L-threonyl]-L-homoalanyl-(*N*-methylglycyl)-(*N*-methyl-L-leucyl)-L-valyl-(*N*-methyl-L-leucyl)-L-alanyl-D-alanyl-(*N*-methyl-L-leucyl)-(*N*-methyl-L-leucyl)-(*N*-methyl-L-valyl)-]
$C_{62}H_{111}N_{11}O_{12} = 1202.6$
CAS—59865-13-3

Pharmacopoeial status

USP

Preparations

Compendial
Cyclosporine Capsules USP.
Cyclosporine Oral Solution USP.
Cyclosporine Concentrate for Injection USP.

Non-compendial
Sandimmun (Sandoz). *Capsules*, cyclosporin 25 mg, 50 mg, and 100 mg.
Oral solution, oily, sugar free, cyclosporin 100 mg/mL. If the taste of the oral solution needs to be masked, the solution may be diluted with milk, chocolate drink, or fruit juice immediately before being taken.
Concentrate for intravenous infusion, oily, cyclosporin 50 mg/mL. To be diluted 1:20 to 1:100 with sodium chloride 0.9% or glucose 5% before use.

Containers and storage

Solid state
Cyclosporine USP should be preserved in tight, light-resistant containers.

Dosage forms
Cyclosporine Capsules USP and Cyclosporine Oral Solution USP should be preserved in tight containers.
Cyclosporine Concentrate for Injection USP should be preserved in single-dose or in multiple-dose containers.

All dosage forms of Sandimmun may be stored at room temperature not exceeding 30°. Sandimmun capsules should be kept in their blister-pack until required for use.

Sandimmun oral solution should not be refrigerated as precipitation may occur. It should be used within two months of opening the bottle.

Once an ampoule of Sandimmun concentrate is opened the contents should be used immediately. Polyethoxylated castor oil contained in the concentrate can cause phthalate leaching from polyvinyl chloride.

PHYSICAL PROPERTIES

Cyclosporin exists as white prismatic crystals.

Melting point

Cyclosporin melts in the range 148° to 151°.

Partition coefficient

Parr *et al*[1] cite the partition coefficient of cyclosporin in octanol/water as 120:1.

Solubility

Cyclosporin is insoluble or practically insoluble in water; soluble or very soluble in ethanol, in methanol, in acetone and in ether; very soluble in all organic solvents except *n*-hexane.

Effect of temperature
The solubility of cyclosporin was studied within the temperature range 5° to 37° in distilled water and in buffered media (disodium citrate with either hydrochloric acid 0.05M or sodium hydroxide 0.05M) chosen to represent the pH conditions in the stomach (pH 1.2) and small intestine (pH 6.6).[2] In all three aqueous media solubility was found to be inversely proportional to temperature, and an exothermic heat of solution was indicated. There was no difference in solubility behaviour of cyclosporin among the three media.

STABILITY

The oral dosage form of cyclosporin (100 mg/mL, Sandimmun, Sandoz USA) was stable when it was repackaged into plastic syringes[3] and stored for up to 28 days at 25°. Protection from light was not required to ensure stability during this period.

FURTHER INFORMATION. Kinetics of degradation of cyclosporin A in acidic aqueous solution and its implication in its oral absorption—Friis GJ, Bundgaard H. Int J Pharmaceutics 1992;82:79–83.

INCOMPATIBILITY/COMPATIBILITY

Intravenous vehicles and sorption to plastics

Cyclosporin (2 mg/mL, Sandoz, USA) was found to be stable at room temperature in: glucose 5% injection in glass containers or polyvinyl chloride minibags for 24 hours; and in sodium chloride 0.9% injection for 6 hours and 12 hours in polyvinyl chloride minibags and glass containers, respectively.[4] Exposure to room light did not affect the stability of cyclosporin in either vehicle. When samples were infused through 70-inch polyvinyl chloride infusion tubing at a rate of 0.67 mL/min over 75 minutes, about 10% of initial drug concentration was lost. It was suggested that loss of cyclosporin may be due to sorption to the tubing or degradation by plasticisers leached from the tubing.

Parr *et al*[1] demonstrated the stability of cyclosporin in both glucose 5% and sodium chloride 0.9% injections for up to 6 hours

in either glass or plastic containers. The addition of filters to the administration set caused a decrease in the amount of cyclosporin delivered.

Leaching

Leaching of diethylhexylphthalate from polyvinyl chloride bags into intravenous cyclosporin solutions (Sandoz, 3 mg/mL in glucose 5% injection) during storage at 24° for 48 hours was reported by Venkataramanan and others.[5] The nonionic surfactant Cremophor EL (polyethoxylated castor oil) present in the vehicle of the cyclosporin solution was thought to be responsible for the leaching process. The use of glass containers for the preparation of intravenous cyclosporin injections was recommended; however, if polyvinyl chloride bags are used the solutions should be administered immediately after preparation.

FURTHER INFORMATION. Compatibility of cyclosporine with fat emulsion—Jacobson PA, Maksym CJ, Landvey A, Weiner N, Whitmore R. Am J Hosp Pharm 1993;50:687–90.

FORMULATION

Excipients

Excipients that have been used in presentations of cyclosporin include:
Oral solutions: ethanol; olive oil; polyethoxylated oleic glycerides.
Intravenous infusions: Cremophor EL (polyethoxylated castor oil); ethanol; nitrogen.

Effect of vehicle on bioavailability

Johnston *et al*[6] found that dispersion of an oil-based oral formulation of cyclosporin in milk, chocolate milk, or orange juice had no effect on its oral absorption following single-dose administration in 12 healthy volunteers; measurements were by radioimmunoassay in whole blood.

Takada and others,[7] in a study using *rats*, demonstrated an approximately 1.5-fold increase in systemic availability of cyclosporin (administered as oral solutions) from a solubilised formulation containing a polyoxy 60 castor oil solution compared to that from an olive oil formulation.

Solid solutions

The preparation of solid surfactant solutions of cyclosporin (used as a model drug) with water-soluble sugar esters to yield a free-flowing powder which can be mixed with lubricants (for example, magnesium stearate) or with other excipients was reported by Hahn and Sucker.[8] Such solid solutions prepared from sucrose monolaurate and cyclosporin are reported to be suitable for direct tableting or for handling in liquid form (as suspensions in liquid paraffin) for filling hard gelatin capsules. The bioavailability of cyclosporin in *rats* was greater from the solid surfactant solution than from the commercially available oral solution. Solubilising capacities of sucrose monolaurate for cyclosporin at room temperature were presented.

Intravenous liposomal formulations

Intravenous liposomal formulations of cyclosporin with dimyristoylphosphatidylcholine (DMPC):stearylamine, molar ratio 7:1(A) and cyclosporin with DMPC:dimyristoylphosphatidylglycerol, molar ratio 4:1(B) were developed by Vadiei *et al*[9] and assessed in *rats*. Formulation A demonstrated a similar blood concentration-time profile (without significant reduction in glomerular filtration rate) to that of a commercially available intravenous formulation. Further investigation *in vitro* by the same authors[10] revealed that both liposomal formulations had greater immunosuppressive potency compared to that of the commercially available intravenous cyclosporin formulation.

Cyclosporin solutions containing Cremophor EL (polyethoxylated castor oil) have been associated with the onset of anaphylactic reactions; these solutions have also been reported to leach through silicone tubing thus reducing its tensile strength and causing pump dysfunction during drug delivery. In order to circumvent these problems Gruber et al[11] developed a liposomal formulation and compared its bioavailability with that of Sandimmun IV (Sandoz), a cyclosporin emulsion, and an ethanolic cyclosporin solution in *dogs*. Although systemic distribution of cyclosporin from the ethanolic solution and from the liposomal formulation were similar, *dogs* that received the latter showed no detectable adverse reactions.

Topical application

A topical preparation of cyclosporin (2% w/v in ethanol:olive oil, 1:2) was evaluated by Thomson et al[12] as a potential inhibitor of contact hypersensitivity in *guinea-pig* skin.
The standard formulation of cyclosporin (100 mg/mL) for oral administration was used as a mouthwash in the effective treatment of oral lichen planus.[13]

Enemas

A retention enema of cyclosporin (as infusion 50 mg/mL) was formulated with sorbitol and carmellose sodium dissolved in sterile water. This hydrophilic solution was clinically effective in a trial involving eight outpatients suffering from refractory ulcerative colitis.[14]

Modified-release preparations

D'Souza[15] describes the development of a modified-release microsphere formulation of cyclosporin (50%, 25%, and 5% drug loadings) with ethylene vinyl acetate co-polymer dissolved in methylene chloride (10% w/v). Microspheres containing 25% cyclosporin retained a good shape. Over a period of 144 hours, 96.3%, 83.9%, and 39.4% of the drug was released in sodium chloride 0.9% from the microspheres containing 50%, 25%, and 5% cyclosporin, respectively.

FURTHER INFORMATION. Bioavailability and patient acceptance of cyclosporine soft gelatin capsules in renal allograft recipients—Min DI, Hwang GC, Bergstrom S, Madras PM, Shaffer D, Sahyoun AI et al. Ann Pharmacother 1992;26:175–9. Enhancement of the oral absorption of cyclosporin in man—Drewe J, Meier R, Vonderscher J, Kiss D, Posanski U, Kissel T et al. Br J Clin Pharmacol 1992;34:60–4. Cyclosporin ointment for psoriasis and atopic dermatitis—Mizoguchi M, Kawaguchi K, Ohsuga Y, Ikari Y, Yanagawa A, Mizushima Y. Lancet 1992;339:1120. Adsorption of water on cyclosporin A, from zero to finite surface coverage—Djordjevic NM, Rohr G, Hinterleitner M, Schreiber B. Int J Pharmaceutics 1992;81:21–9. Prodrugs of peptides. 16. Isocyclosporin A as a potential prodrug of cyclosporin A—Bundgaard H, Friis GJ. Int J Pharmaceutics 1992;82:85–90.

REFERENCES

1. Parr MD, Barton SD, Haver VM, Porter WH [letter]. Drug Intell Clin Pharm 1988;22:173–4.
2. Ismailos G, Reppas C, Dressman JB, Macheras P. J Pharm Pharmacol 1991;43:287–9.
3. Ptachcinski RJ, Walker S, Burckart GJ, Venkataramanan R. Am J Hosp Pharm 1986;43:692–4.
4. Ptachcinski RJ, Logue LW, Burckart GJ, Venkataramanan R. Am J Hosp Pharm 1986;43:94–7.
5. Venkataramanan R, Burckart GJ, Ptachcinski RJ, Blaha R, Logue LW, Bahnson A et al . Am J Hosp Pharm 1986;43:2800–2.
6. Johnston A, Marsden JT, Hela KK, Henry JA, Holt DW. Br J Clin Pharmacol 1986;21:331–3.
7. Takada K, Furuya Y, Yoshikawa H, Muranishi S, Yasumura T, Oka T.Int J Pharmaceutics 1988;44:107–16.
8. Hahn L, Sucker H. Pharm Res 1989;6(11):958–60.
9. Vadiei K, Perez-Soler R, Lopez-Berestein G, Luke DR. Int J Pharmaceutics 1989;57:125–31.
10. Vadiei K, Lopez-Berestein G, Perez-Soler R, Luke DR. Int J Pharmaceutics 1989;57:133–8.
11. Gruber SA, Venkataram S, Canafax DM, Cipolle RJ, Bowers L, Elsberry D et al. Pharm Res 1989;6(7):601–7.
12. Thomson AW, Payne SNL, Winfield AJ [letter]. Lancet 1988;1:1000.
13. Eisen D, Griffiths CEM, Ellis CN, Nickoloff BJ, Voorhees JJ [letter]. Lancet 1990;1:535–6.
14. Brynskov J, Freund L, Thomsen O, Andersen CB, Rasmussen SN, Binder V [letter]. Lancet 1989;I:721–2.
15. D'Souza MJ. Drug Dev Ind Pharm 1988;14(10):1351–7.

Dapsone (BAN, USAN, rINN)　　　　　*Antileprotic*

DDS; diaphenylsulfane; DADPS
Bis(4-aminophenyl)sulphone; 4,4′-sulphonylbisbenzenamine; 4,4′-sulfonyldianiline
$C_{12}H_{12}N_2O_2S = 248.3$
CAS—80-08-0

Pharmacopoeial status

BP, USP

Preparations

Compendial
Dapsone Tablets BP. Tablets containing, in each, 50 mg and 100 mg are usually available.
Dapsone Tablets USP.

FURTHER INFORMATION. Dapsone: Dispensing confusion; current uses. Pharm J 1981;227:401.

Compound preparations
Tablets containing dapsone 100 mg and pyrimethamine 12.5 mg are available from Wellcome (Maloprim).

Containers and storage

Solid state
Dapsone BP should be protected from light.
Dapsone USP should be preserved in well-closed, light-resistant containers.

Dosage forms
Dapsone Tablets USP should be preserved in well-closed, light-resistant containers.

PHYSICAL PROPERTIES

Dapsone is a white or creamy white, crystalline powder; slightly bitter taste.

Melting point

Dapsone melts in the range 175° to 181°.

Dissociation constants

pK_a 1.3, 2.5

Solubility

Dapsone is very slightly soluble in water; soluble 1 in 30 of ethanol; freely soluble in acetone.

It is soluble in dilute mineral acids, for example 1 g dissolves in about 10 mL of 1M hydrochloric acid. It is reported to be soluble at room temperature in chloroform (3 mg/mL) and in benzene (0.5 mg/mL).

Dissolution

The USP specifies that for Dapsone Tablets USP not less than 75% of the labelled amount of $C_{12}H_{12}N_2O_2S$ is dissolved in 60 minutes. Dissolution medium: 1000 mL of dilute hydrochloric acid (2 in 100); Apparatus 1 at 100 rpm.

STABILITY

Dapsone becomes discoloured on exposure to light; however, discoloration is not accompanied by significant decomposition. It absorbs insignificant amounts of water when stored under ordinary conditions.

Dapsone becomes insoluble in water when oxidised by exposure to air.

Suspension

A suspension of dapsone (30 mg/5 mL), prepared by workers in Torquay[1] using crushed tablets, was chemically stable (ultraviolet assay) at ambient temperature for 3 months. The formulation consisted of: dapsone 600 mg (from tablets); methyl hydroxybenzoate 150 mg; propyl hydroxybenzoate 15 mg; carmellose sodium 1 g; sucrose 20 g; water to 100 mL.

Stabilisation

Dapsone in the solid state or in solution is stabilised in air by the addition of 10% of sodium bicarbonate.

FORMULATION

A formulation is given in the BPC 1973 for a suspension of dapsone that may be administered intramuscularly in certain circumstances. It contains 1.0 g to 1.2 g of dapsone in 5 mL of a sterile vehicle such as arachis oil, chaulmoogra oil, or ethyl esters of hydnocarpus oil. The injections are reported to be painful and may cause abscess formation. The dapsone is required to be in very fine powder.

Excipients

Excipients that have been used in presentations of dapsone include:
Tablets: colloidal silica; magnesium stearate; maize starch; microcrystalline cellulose.

Intramuscular injections

A formulation for an intramuscular injection solution of dapsone in a water-miscible vehicle was presented by French (University College Hospital).[2] It contained dapsone 5 g, ethanol 40 mL, benzyl alcohol 5 mL, and propylene glycol to 100 mL. Following filtration and filling into 2-mL ampoules, the solution was sterilised by autoclaving. There was no loss of potency of the solution after storage in the dark for nine months, although some discoloration occurred.

Modified-release preparations

Attempts were made to develop a modified-release intramuscular injection of dapsone by the preparation of solid dispersions comprising the parent compound with each of two less soluble derivatives; the monolauryl derivative (*N*-dodecanoyl-4,4'-sulfonylbisbenzamine) was identified as the more suitable carrier for reducing the dissolution rate of dapsone from solid dispersion.[3] In further work on sustained-release delivery systems, Swarbrick *et al*[4] assessed the feasibility of the chemical formation of a derivative or derivatives, of low solubility, on the surface of drug particles. Compression and precipitation techniques were used to prepare the 'surface-reacted' particles. As the size range of compressed particles increased from 114 micrometres to 323 micrometres, the fraction of dapsone converted to the derivatives of low solubility, monoacetyldapsone and diacetyldapsone, decreased. As an external layer of the derivatives built up around the dapsone core, the diameter of the unreacted core decreased. Approximately 30% diacetyldapsone had to be formed before there was a significant decrease in dapsone dissolution.

FURTHER INFORMATION. Design and *in vitro* evaluation of dapsone-loaded micropellets of ethylcellulose [determination of release and formulation variables]—Roy S, Das SK, Pal M, Gupta BK. Pharm Res 1989;6:945–8.

PROCESSING

Sterilisation

Dapsone is prepared as a sterile powder.
Oily suspensions are sterilised by dry heat at 150° for one hour.

REFERENCES

1. Middleton K. Yorkshire Regional Health Authority (YRHA). Quality Control Information Bulletin 1982;No.3(Nov):2
2. French TM. Lep Rev 1968;39(3):171.
3. Yang T-T, Swarbrick J. J Pharm Sci 1986;75(1):53–6.
4. Swarbrick J, Prakongpan S, Suzuki K. Int J Pharmaceutics 1986;32:21–9.

Dexamethasone (BAN, rINN)   *Corticosteroid*

Desamethasone; 9α-fluoro-16α-methylprednisolone
9α-Fluoro-11β,17α,21-trihydroxy-16α-methylpregna-1,4-diene-3,20-dione
$C_{22}H_{29}FO_5 = 392.5$

Dexamethasone Acetate (BANM, USAN, rINNM)
Dexamethasone 21-acetate
$C_{24}H_{31}FO_6 = 434.5$

Dexamethasone Isonicotinate (BANM, rINNM)
Dexamethasone 21-isonicotinate
$C_{28}H_{32}FNO_6 = 497.6$

Dexamethasone Phosphate (BANM, rINNM)
Dexamethasone 21-(dihydrogen phosphate)
$C_{22}H_{30}FO_8P = 472.45$

Dexamethasone Sodium Metasulphobenzoate (BANM)
Dexamethasone Sodium Metasulfobenzoate (rINNM); dexamethasone 21-(sodium m-sulphobenzoate)
$C_{29}H_{32}FNaO_9S = 598.6$

Dexamethasone Sodium Phosphate (BANM, rINNM)
Sodium 9α-fluoro-16α-methylprednisolone 21-phosphate
$C_{22}H_{28}FNa_2O_8P = 516.4$
CAS—50-02-2 (dexamethasone); 1177-87-3 (dexamethasone acetate, anhydrous); 55812-90-3 (dexamethasone acetate, mono-hydrate); 2265-64-7 (dexamethasone isonicotinate); 3936-02-5 (dexamethasone sodium metasulphobenzoate); 2392-39-4 (dexamethasone sodium phosphate)

Pharmacopoeial status
BP, USP (dexamethasone, dexamethasone acetate, dexamethasone sodium phosphate)

Preparations
Compendial
Dexamethasone Tablets BP. Tablets containing, in each, 500 micrograms and 2 mg are usually available.
Dexamethasone Tablets USP.
Dexamethasone Elixir USP.
Dexamethasone Sodium Phosphate Cream USP.
Dexamethasone Gel USP.
Dexamethasone Topical Aerosol USP.
Dexamethasone Ophthalmic Suspension USP.
Dexamethasone Sodium Phosphate Ophthalmic Ointment USP.
Dexamethasone Sodium Phosphate Ophthalmic Solution USP.
Dexamethasone Sodium Phosphate Inhalation Aerosol USP.
Sterile Dexamethasone Acetate Suspension USP. For parenteral use. pH 5.0 to 7.5.
Dexamethasone Sodium Phosphate Injection USP. pH 7.0 to 8.5.

Non-compendial
Decadron (MSD). *Tablets*, dexamethasone 500 micrograms.
Injection, dexamethasone sodium phosphate 4.17 mg/mL (equivalent to dexamethasone 3.33 mg/mL, dexamethasone phosphate 4 mg/mL). *Diluents*: sodium chloride 0.9% injection, glucose 5% injection.
Decadron Shock-Pak (MSD). *Injection*, dexamethasone 20 mg/mL (equivalent to dexamethasone sodium phosphate 25 mg/mL). *Diluents*: sodium chloride 0.9% injection, glucose 5% injection.
Dexamethasone (Organon). *Tablets*, dexamethasone 500 micrograms and 2 mg.
Injection, dexamethasone sodium phosphate 5 mg/mL (equivalent to dexamethasone 4 mg/mL, dexamethasone phosphate 4.8 mg/mL). The injection is compatible with sodium chloride 0.9% injection, anhydrous glucose 5% injection, invert sugar 10%, sorbitol 5%, compound sodium chloride injection, com-

pound sodium lactate injection, Rheomacrodex, and Haemaccel for at least 24 hours at room temperature in daylight.
Maxidex (Alcon). *Eye drops*, dexamethasone 0.1%, hypromellose 0.5%.

Containers and storage
Solid state
Dexamethasone BP and Dexamethasone Acetate BP should be kept in well-closed containers and protected from light. Dexamethasone Sodium Phosphate BP should be kept in an airtight container and protected from light.
Dexamethasone USP and Dexamethasone Acetate USP should be preserved in well-closed containers.
Dexamethasone Sodium Phosphate USP should be preserved in tight containers.

Dosage forms
Dexamethasone Tablets BP should be protected from light.
Dexamethasone Tablets USP should be preserved in well-closed containers.
Dexamethasone Elixir USP and Dexamethasone Ophthalmic Suspension USP should be preserved in tight containers.
Dexamethasone Sodium Phosphate Cream USP should be preserved in collapsible tubes or in tight containers.
Dexamethasone Gel USP should be preserved in tightly closed, collapsible tubes; avoid exposure to temperatures exceeding 30°.
Dexamethasone Topical Aerosol USP should be preserved in pressurised containers; avoid exposure to excessive heat.
Dexamethasone Sodium Phosphate Ophthalmic Ointment USP should be preserved in collapsible ophthalmic ointment tubes.
Dexamethasone Sodium Phosphate Ophthalmic Solution USP should be preserved in tight, light-resistant containers.
Dexamethasone Sodium Phosphate Inhalation Aerosol USP should be preserved in tight, pressurised containers; avoid exposure to excessive heat.
Sterile Dexamethasone Acetate Suspension USP and Dexamethasone Sodium Phosphate Injection USP should be preserved in single-dose or in multiple-dose containers, preferably of Type I glass; the latter preparation should be protected from light.
Decadron tablets should be stored in a well-closed container, in a cool place, protected from light.
Decadron injection and injection 'shock-pak' are sensitive to heat and should not be autoclaved to sterilise the outside of the vial. The injection should be stored below 25° protected from light, and the injection 'shock-pak' should be kept in a cool place; both preparations should be protected from freezing.
Dexamethasone preparations manufactured by Organon should be protected from light. The injection should be stored below 25°.
Maxidex eye drops should be stored in a cool place, away from direct sunlight. The container should be kept tightly closed.

PHYSICAL PROPERTIES

Dexamethasone is a white or almost white crystalline powder.
Dexamethasone acetate is a white or almost white crystalline powder.
Dexamethasone sodium phosphate is a white or slightly yellow crystalline powder; very hygroscopic.

Melting point
Dexamethasone melts at about 250° to 255°, with decomposition.
Dexamethasone acetate melts at about 225°, with decomposition.

pH

The BP states that a 1% w/v solution of *dexamethasone sodium phosphate* has a pH of 7.5 to 9.5; the USP lists the pH range for the same solution as 7.5 to 10.5.

Solubility

Dexamethasone is practically insoluble in water; soluble 1 in 42 of ethanol and 1 in 165 of chloroform; sparingly soluble in acetone, in methanol, and in dioxan; very slightly soluble in ether.
Dexamethasone acetate is practically insoluble in water; freely soluble in ethanol, in acetone, in dioxan, and in methanol; soluble 1 in 33 of chloroform, and 1 in 1000 of ether.
Dexamethasone sodium phosphate is soluble 1 in 2 of water; slightly soluble in ethanol; practically insoluble in chloroform and in ether; very slightly soluble in dioxan.

Dissolution

The USP specifies that for Dexamethasone Tablets USP not less than 70% of the labelled amount of $C_{22}H_{29}FO_5$ is dissolved in 45 minutes. Dissolution medium: 500 mL of dilute hydrochloric acid (1 in 100); Apparatus 1 at 100 rpm.

Crystal and molecular structure

Polymorphs

Two polymorphic crystalline forms of dexamethasone palmitate have been obtained from acetone (Form A) and *n*-heptane (Form B)[1] and characterised by infrared spectrophotometry and X-ray powder patterns.

STABILITY

Dexamethasone in the solid state is stable in air but should be protected from light. Oxidation of the C-17 α-ketol side-chain has been reported to occur in the presence of a base catalyst. A loss of dexamethasone concentration was observed in four different tablet formulations stored at elevated temperatures. Storage at high levels of relative humidity also had deleterious effects on the stability of the tablets. However, at 25° and 60% relative humidity (in a formulation containing dexamethasone 500 micrograms, lactose, starch, talc, and magnesium stearate, and granulated with 20% povidone in ethanol) dexamethasone had a half-life of 542 days.[2]
Analyses of 21 samples of sterile dexamethasone acetate suspensions (from two manufacturers in the USA) indicated apparent stability of the drug during storage 'under actual marketplace conditions'; however, 18 of 114 samples of dexamethasone sodium phosphate injection (from eleven manufacturers) showed evidence of oxidative degradation.[3] One vial of dexamethasone sodium phosphate injection, in which a white precipitate was present, was shown by TLC and HPLC to contain a mixture of the oxidation products 16α- and 16β-methyl-17-ketone. A previous identification of these compounds in a similar precipitate was reported by Juenge and Brower.[4]

INCOMPATIBILITY/COMPATIBILITY

Dexamethasone 21-phosphate (Decadron phosphate, MSD, 1 mL/5mL in distilled water) has been reported to be incompatible with 1 mL of prochlorperazine edisylate (SK&F) or vancomycin hydrochloride (Lilly); particulate matter was observed within two hours of admixture.[5] Patel *et al*[6] reported similar incompatibility with prochlorperazine maleate.
Immediate precipitation occurred at room temperature in solutions containing equal volumes of dexamethasone sodium phosphate 10 mg/mL (David Bull, Canada) and hydromorphone hydrochloride 40 mg/mL (Dilaudid, Knoll, Canada) or diphenhydramine hydrochloride (50 mg/mL, Benadryl, PD, Canada).[7] Precipitation also occurred when the latter preparation was mixed with dexamethasone sodium phosphate 4 mg/mL (Sabex, Canada). However, in some admixtures with low concentrations of both components dexamethasone sodium phosphate was visually compatible for up to 24 hours with diphenhydramine hydrochloride or hydromorphone hydrochloride; more than 90% of the initial concentration of both drugs remained in these admixtures.
The observed interaction (turbidity) between dexamethasone sodium phosphate and polymyxin B sulphate in ophthalmic solutions, in the pH range 5 to 7, was suggested to be due to formation of an insoluble complex between the cationic form of polymyxin and the negatively-charged dexamethasone phosphate ions.[8] The interaction was suppressed at pH values outside this range and by the addition of citrate and phosphate buffers.
In aqueous solution, dexamethasone phosphate is susceptible to reversible sodium bisulphite addition resulting in the formation of an A-ring substituted sulphonic acid salt, sodium 16α-methyl-9α-fluorohydrocortisone-1-sulphonate-21-phosphate.[9] In this second-order reaction, the major participants were identified as the di-anionic sulphite (active nucleophile) and the mono-anionic dexamethasone phosphate.
When samples of dexamethasone sodium phosphate injection (4 mg/mL, Quad, USA) were packaged in 3-mL polypropylene syringes from three different manufacturers, the loss of drug concentration during storage for 24 hours was rapid and marked; about 12% to 20% was lost at 25°, about 5% to 20% at 4°, and about 5% to 17% at −20°. There was no evidence (gas chromatographic-mass spectroscopic analysis) of leaching of organic substances into the solutions after storage at −20°, 4°, or 25° for periods ranging from 6 hours to 30 days.[10]

FORMULATION

Excipients

Excipients that have been used in presentations of dexamethasone include:
Tablets, dexamethasone: allura red AC (E122); brilliant blue FCF (133); calcium hydrogen phosphate; iron oxide; lactose; magnesium stearate; quinoline yellow (E104); starch; sunset yellow FCF (E110).
Dexamethasone acetate: gelatin; lactose; magnesium stearate; starch, potato; sucrose; talc.
Oral solutions, dexamethasone: benzoic acid solution; chloroform water; ethanol.
Aerosols, dexamethasone: butane; isobutane; isopropyl myristate.
Dexamethasone isonicotinate: dichlorodifluoromethane; dichlorotetrafluoroethane; sorbitan trioleate; trichlorofluoromethane.
Dexamethasone sodium phosphate: ethanol; fluorochlorohydrocarbons.
Creams, dexamethasone sodium phosphate: cetyl alcohol; creatinine; disodium edetate; liquid paraffin; methyl hydroxybenzoate; methyl polysilicone emulsion; sodium citrate; sodium hydroxide; sorbic acid; sorbitol solution; stearyl alcohol.
Ophthalmic drops, dexamethasone: benzalkonium chloride; citric acid; disodium edetate; hypromellose; polysorbate 80; sodium acid phosphate; sodium chloride; sodium phosphate.
Dexamethasone sodium metasulphobenzoate: carmellose sodium; glucose; phenylmercuric nitrate.
Dexamethasone sodium phosphate: boric acid; dextran; phenylmercuric nitrate; sodium borate.

Ophthalmic ointments, dexamethasone sodium phosphate: liquid paraffin; white soft paraffin.

Injections, dexamethasone acetate (not for intravenous use): benzyl alcohol; carmellose sodium; creatinine; disodium edetate; sodium bisulphite; sodium chloride; sodium hydroxide; polysorbate 80.

Dexamethasone sodium phosphate: creatinine; disodium edetate; glycerol; methyl and propyl hydroxybenzoates; sodium bisulphite; sodium citrate; sodium hydroxide.

Absorption

The importance of particle size on the absorption of ^{3}H-dexamethasone from aqueous ophthalmic suspension (containing sodium chloride 0.9%, polysorbate 80, and water for injections) was demonstrated in *rabbits*.[11] Measurement of dexamethasone concentrations in aqueous humour and in the cornea showed a significant rank-order correlation between increasing drug concentration and decreasing particle size.

In-vitro release

Workers in Egypt[12] reported that the *in-vitro* release rate of dexamethasone 0.1% w/w (through a semi-permeable Fischer cellulose membrane) was greater from a water-soluble basis (macrogol 400 with Veegum and water) and an oil-in-water emulsion basis than from an oleaginous basis, an absorption basis, or a water-in-oil emulsion basis.

In a study of the *in-vitro* release of ^{3}H-dexamethasone (into sodium chloride 0.9% at $37° \pm 5°$) from different polymeric inserts, the base polymer was found to influence the rate (but not the mechanism) of release; the greater the difference in the solubility of the drug and base polymer, the greater the release from the film.[13] Base polymers studied were gelatin, ethylcellulose, cellacephate, Eudragit RL100/RS100, Eudragit RSPM, and Eudragit E.

Novel dosage forms

A non-aqueous topical aerosol formulation that contained dexamethasone, macrogol 200, povidone, olive oil, ethanol, isopropanol, and propellant 12/11 (40/60) was prepared by Ali and Sharma.[14] The dosage form was stable when stored in glass containers at 37° and in metal (anodised aluminium) containers at 40° for 40 days.

Kassem *et al*[15] conducted an *in-vitro* evaluation of the effect of different surfactants on the permeation of ^{3}H-dexamethasone through an ophthalmic film delivery system (ocular inserts) at 37°; the surfactants used were benzalkonium chloride, polysorbate 20, Span 20, and cholesterol. The base polymers were ethylcellulose, polyvinyl alcohol, gelatin, Eudragit E, Eudragit RL 100/RS100, and Eudragit RSPM. The plasticisers were triacetin, dibutyl phthalate, macrogol 400, and glycerol/formalin. The effect of different surfactants as solubility modifiers was found to differ in different films, depending on the base polymer. The pharmacokinetic characteristics of dexamethasone in *dogs* following intravenous administration as a dexamethasone/hydroxypropyl-β-cyclodextrin (HPCD) inclusion complex and as dexamethasone sodium phosphate alone have been compared.[16] Values for the area under the plasma concentration versus time curve (during the first hour) and renal clearance were significantly greater following administration of the HPCD inclusion complex, although there were no significant differences between other pharmacokinetic parameters.

FURTHER INFORMATION. Fibrin based drug delivery systems [for sustained release of dexamethasone]—Senderoff RI, Sheu M-T, Sokoloski TD. J Parenter Sci Technol 1991;45(1):2–6. Development and evaluation of an intracutaneous depot formulation of corticosteroids using Transcutol as a cosolvent; *in-vitro, ex-vivo*, and *in-vivo rat* studies—Panchagnula R, Ritschel WA. J Pharm Pharmacol 1991;43:609–14. Liposome-incorporated dexamethasone palmitate: chemical and physical properties—Benameur H, De Gand G, Brasseur R, Van Vooren JP, Legros FJ. Int J Pharmaceutics 1993;89:157–67.

REFERENCES

1. Doi M, Ishida T, Sugio S, Imagawa T, Inoue M. J Pharm Sci 1989;78(5):417–22.
2. Wahba SK, Amin SW, Rofael N. J Pharm Sci 1968;57(7):1231–3.
3. Coffman HD, Crabbs WC, Joachims GL, Kolinski RE, Page DP. Am J Hosp Pharm 1983;40:2165–9.
4. Juenge EC, Brower JF. J Pharm Sci 1979;68(5):551–4.
5. Misgen R. Am J Hosp Pharm 1965;22:92–4.
6. Patel JA, Phillips GL. Am J Hosp Pharm 1966;23:409–11.
7. Walker SE, De Angelis C, Iazzetta J, Eppel JG. Am J Hosp Pharm 1991;48:2161–6.
8. Aggag M, Saleh AH. Mfg Chem 1977;48:43–4.
9. Smith GB, Weinstock LM, Roberts FE, Brenner GS, Hoinowski AM, Arison BH *et al*. J Pharm Sci 1972;61(5):708–16.
10. Speaker TJ, Turco SJ, Nardone DA, Miripol JE. J Parenter Sci Technol 1991;45(5):212–17.
11. Schoenwald RD, Stewart P. J Pharm Sci 1980;69(4):391–4.
12. Habib FS, El-Shanawany SM. Bull Pharm Sci Assiut Univ 1989;12:90–102.
13. Kassem MA, Attia MA, Safwat SM. J Pharm Belg 1986;41(2):106–10.
14. Ali A, Sharma SN. Indian J Pharm Sci 1988;50(4):221–4.
15. Kassem MA, Attia MA, Safwat SM. STP Pharma 1986;2(13):106–9.
16. Dietzel K, Estes KS, Brewster ME, Bodor NS, Derendorf H. Int J Pharmaceutics 1990;59:225–30.

Diamorphine (BAN)   *Opioid analgesic*

Acetomorphine; diacetylmorphine; heroin
4,5-Epoxy-17-methylmorphinan-3,6-diyl diacetate; 7,8-didehydro-4, 5-epoxy-17-methyl-(5α,6α)-morphinan-3,6-diol diacetate (ester); 3,6-*O*-diacetylmorphine
$C_{21}H_{23}NO_5 = 369.4$

Diamorphine Hydrochloride (BANM)

$C_{21}H_{23}NO_5, HCl, H_2O = 423.9$
CAS—561-27-3 (diamorphine); 1502-95-0 (diamorphine hydrochloride, anhydrous)

Pharmacopoeial status

BP (diamorphine hydrochloride)

Preparations

Compendial
Diamorphine Injection BP (Diamorphine Hydrochloride for Injection). A sterile solution of diamorphine hydrochloride in

water for injections. It is prepared by dissolving diamorphine hydrochloride for injection in the requisite amount of water for injections immediately before use. Sealed containers each containing 5, 10, 30, 100, and 500 mg are usually available.

Non-compendial
Diamorphine hydrochloride 10 mg tablets are usually available. Diamorphine hydrochloride injections are available from Evans, Napp (Diaphine).

Containers and storage

Solid state
Diamorphine Hydrochloride BP should be kept in a well-closed container and protected from light.

Dosage forms
Sealed containers of Diamorphine Injection BP should be protected from light. The injection deteriorates on storage and should be used immediately after preparation.

PHYSICAL PROPERTIES

Diamorphine exists as white crystals.
Diamorphine hydrochloride is an almost white, crystalline powder; odourless when freshly prepared, but an odour characteristic of acetic acid is produced on storage.

Melting point

Diamorphine melts at about 170°.
Diamorphine hydrochloride melts at 229° to 233°.

Dissociation constant

pK_a 7.6 (23°)

Partition coefficient

Log P (ether/pH 7.0), 0.2

Solubility

Diamorphine is soluble 1 in 1700 of water, 1 in 31 of ethanol, 1 in 1.5 of chloroform, and 1 in 100 of ether.
Diamorphine hydrochloride is soluble 1 in 1.6 of water, 1 in 12 of ethanol, and 1 in 1.6 of chloroform; practically insoluble in ether.

Crystal and molecular structure

Polymorphs
Diamorphine is thought to exist in two polymorphic forms. The higher melting (172° to 173°) crystalline material consists of rods, oblique plates, and needles. The form which melts at about 168° appears as spherical crystals and is readily converted into the alternative form.[1]

STABILITY

Diamorphine is rapidly hydrolysed by alkalis. In aqueous solution, diamorphine hydrolyses to 3-*O*-monoacetylmorphine and 6-*O*-monoacetylmorphine and then to morphine. Hydrolysis is catalysed by hydrogen ions and hydroxide ions. Solutions stored at 25° are most stable at about pH 4. At this pH, 10% degradation occurs in about 5 days at 25°, in 5 weeks at 4°, and in 7 weeks at 0°.
In 0.5M sodium carbonate, diamorphine undergoes hydrolysis to 6-*O*-monoacetylmorphine with a half-life of 4.2 minutes. The subsequent hydrolysis to morphine has a half-life of 55.5 minutes.[2] In phosphate buffer at pH 7.4 the estimated half-life for hydrolysis of diamorphine is 415 min.[3]

Poochikian and Cradock[4] calculated the times for 10% degradation of diamorphine hydrochloride 0.02% aqueous solutions at various pH values with phosphate buffers; their results are listed below:

pH	$t_{10\%}$ (days)
3.0	2.5
3.5	6
4.5	8
5.2	5
5.9	2
7.0	0.83
8.6	0.5

In a study of the hydrolysis of diamorphine in aqueous solution Davey and Murray[5] prepared solutions (with pH values ranging from 3.5 to 5.4) of diamorphine (0.5 g/10 mL) and maintained them at 25° and 50°. The pH of maximum stability in buffered solution was found to be about pH 4; a $t_{10\%}$ of 35 days at 4° was calculated. When an unbuffered solution stored at 25° had degraded by 7%, it yielded a precipitate of 6-monoacetylmorphine; the $t_{10\%}$ of the solution was estimated to be 10 days.
When aqueous solutions of diamorphine hydrochloride (0.98 mg/mL to 250 mg/mL) were stored for 8 weeks in sterile brown glass ampoules, protected from light, at −20°, 4°, 21°, and 37°, several observations were made:[6] degradation occurred in all solutions kept at 4° or above, and was greater at higher temperatures; pH fell in all solutions and an odour characteristic of acetic acid was apparent; the degradation products detected (by HPLC) were 6-monoacetylmorphine and morphine; and in solutions of diamorphine hydrochloride at 15.6 mg/mL or above, precipitates and white turbidity were apparent after 2 weeks.
Poochikian et al[7] investigated the effect of various excipients on the stability of diamorphine (as the hydrochloride) in aqueous solution. It was found that phosphate buffers catalysed diamorphine degradation to a greater extent than acetate buffers and diamorphine degradation was slower in unbuffered solution. No physical incompatibility was observed between diamorphine (concentration 10% w/v or below) and sodium chloride (0.9% w/v). Neither povidone (1%) nor mannitol (0.01, 0.1, or 0.5M) had any significant effect on the degradation of diamorphine. Lyophilised, unbuffered diamorphine formulations with or without lactose were stable both chemically and physically; three days after reconstitution of these formulations, with either bacteriostatic water for injections or bacteriostatic sodium chloride injection, at least 98% of the initial diamorphine concentration remained. The effects of buffer concentration, ionic strength, and excipients on the stability of diamorphine in aqueous solution were also examined.

Solutions in chloroform water

Beaumont[8] prepared a series of diamorphine hydrochloride 0.1% w/v solutions by adding various concentrations of McIlvaine's buffer (pH range 2.2 to 8.0) to diamorphine hydrochloride in double-strength chloroform water. These buffered solutions, plus unbuffered diamorphine solutions in chloroform water, and samples of Diamorphine Elixir BPC and of diamorphine hydrochloride 0.1% w/v in equal parts brandy and syrup, were found to be more stable at refrigerated temperatures than at room temperature. The pH of maximum stability was determined to be 3.8 to 4.4 and stability was greatest when no buffer was present. Ionic strength had a considerably greater effect than pH on diamorphine stability. Diamorphine hydrochloride was found to degrade by 10% in 39 days when presented in unbuffered chloroform water, pH 6.3 to 6.9, at 20°.

The stability of diamorphine in chloroform water, stored in amber screw cap bottles at 4° to 70°, was studied by Cooper *et al*.[9] The $t_{10\%}$ values at 4° and 20° were calculated to be 113 days and 31 days, respectively. It was suggested that solutions of diamorphine 1% in chloroform water should be used within three weeks of preparation when stored at room temperature.

Containers

Results of tests on the stability of solutions of diamorphine hydrochloride (in sodium chloride injection) when stored in polyvinyl chloride bags (Viaflex, Baxter), disposable glass syringes (Solopak Laboratories), and in two disposable infusion devices (Intermate 200, Infusion Systems and Infusor, Baxter) are presented in the following table.[10] Physical changes or pH changes in the test solutions were not substantial under any of the study conditions.

Container/ device	Concentration of diamorphine hydrochloride (mg/mL)	Temperature (°)	Stability period (<10% loss of initial concentration) (days)
Polyvinyl chloride bag	1	4, 23–25	at least 15
	20	4, 23–25	at least 15
Disposable glass syringe	1	4	15
	1	23–25	7
	20	4	15
	20	23–25	12
Intermate 200	1	4, 23–25	15
	1	31	2
	20	4, 23–25	15
	20	31	15
Infusor	1	4, 23–25, 31	at least 15
	20	4, 23–25, 31	at least 15

FURTHER INFORMATION. Stability of Brompton Mixtures: determination of heroin (diacetylmorphine) and cocaine in the presence of their hydrolysis products—Poochikian GK, Cradock JC. J Pharm Sci 1980;69:637–9. [Stability of] Diamorphine and cocaine elixir BPC 1973—Twycross RG. Pharm J 1974;212:153–4. Stability of elixir of diamorphine and cocaine—Gold EW. J Hosp Pharm 1973;31:12–15.

INCOMPATIBILITY/COMPATIBILITY

Diamorphine hydrochloride is incompatible with mineral acids and alkalis.

Allwood[11] studied the stability of diamorphine (200 mg/20 mL) mixed with anti-emetic drugs in plastic syringes. After 24 hours storage, the diamorphine content was not less than 90% of the initial concentration in mixtures with metoclopramide, haloperidol, hyoscine, prochlorperazine, and cyclizine. Similar results were obtained when the diamorphine concentration was increased to 500 mg/20 mL and 1 g/20 mL. Allwood later stated[12] that although cyclizine and haloperidol are incompatible with high concentrations of diamorphine hydrochloride, up to 200 mg diamorphine hydrochloride was compatible with cyclizine lactate injection 100 mg in 10 mL and up to 1 g diamorphine hydrochloride was compatible with haloperidol 7.5 mg in 10 mL; mixtures were prepared in plastic syringes, stored

for 24 hours at 5° and, under simulated conditions, 'administered' over 24 hours using a syringe pump.

Regnard *et al*[13] investigated the compatibility of diamorphine hydrochloride with metoclopramide, hyoscine hydrobromide, hyoscine butylbromide, haloperidol, and cyclizine lactate in plastic syringes. Cyclizine/diamorphine mixtures often crystallised out at cyclizine concentrations between 10 and 20 mg/mL. Precipitation was more likely above a cyclizine concentration of 25 mg/mL and especially if the diamorphine concentration also exceeded 25 mg/mL. Hyoscine/diamorphine mixtures appeared to be compatible over the one-week test period. Metoclopramide hydrochloride (5 mg/mL)/diamorphine hydrochloride (50 mg/mL and 150 mg/mL) mixtures (1:1) showed an 8% loss of metoclopramide and a 9% loss of diamorphine with a slight discoloration of the solution after one week at room temperature. Haloperidol 5 mg/mL gave an immediate precipitate when mixed with diamorphine hydrochloride 50 mg/mL or 150 mg/mL solutions, whereas haloperidol 2 mg/mL showed crystallisation after one week at room temperature when mixed with diamorphine hydrochloride 20 mg/mL. The authors recommended that all diamorphine/anti-emetic admixtures be protected from light and that cyclizine/diamorphine or haloperidol/diamorphine mixtures should not be used in slow infusion pumps. If the use of metoclopramide/diamorphine mixtures is required, the mixtures should be closely monitored for signs of instability.

Collins *et al*[14] reported that diamorphine (50 or 100 mg/8 mL) and haloperidol (2.5 mg/8 mL) were compatible when kept in polypropylene syringes at room temperature (22° to 24°) for 24 hours, or under refrigeration (4° to 8°) for 7 days. No loss of haloperidol was detected under these conditions, and no discoloration or precipitation was evident. A 1.5% loss of diamorphine was observed over the 7 days at refrigerated temperatures. Diamorphine hydrochloride has been reported to be incompatible in solution with sodium chloride. Poochikian *et al*[7] investigated the effect of the addition of sodium chloride to solutions of diamorphine hydrochloride (pH approximately 5.4). They did not observe any precipitate in solutions containing ≤ 10% w/v diamorphine and 0.9% w/v sodium chloride.

Kirk and Hain[15] prepared solutions of diamorphine hydrochloride (at concentrations of 0.02, 0.1, 0.2, and 0.4% w/v) in 0.9, 1.8, 3.6, and 7.2% w/v sodium chloride. Solutions of concentrations up to 0.2% diamorphine had a pH of between 6.05 and 6.6; whereas more concentrated solutions ranged in pH from 5.65 to 5.9. There was no visible precipitate in any of the solutions after storage for 24 hours at 23°. No precipitate was observed in a 5% w/v solution of diamorphine hydrochloride with a pH of 4.9 under the same conditions, but an identical solution with the pH adjusted to 6.6 with sodium hydroxide showed crystal formation after 24 hours.

FORMULATION

DIAMORPHINE AND COCAINE ELIXIR
The following formula was given in the *British Pharmaceutical Codex 1973*:

Diamorphine hydrochloride	1 g
Cocaine hydrochloride	1 g
Ethanol (90%)	125 mL
Syrup	250 mL
Chloroform water	to 1000 mL

It should be freshly prepared and protected from light. The proportion of diamorphine hydrochloride may be altered when specified by the prescriber.

DIAMORPHINE, COCAINE, AND CHLORPROMAZINE ELIXIR

The following formula was given in the *British Pharmaceutical Codex 1973*:

Diamorphine hydrochloride	1 g
Cocaine hydrochloride	1 g
Ethanol (90%)	125 mL
Chlorpromazine elixir	250 mL
Chloroform water	to 1000 mL

It should be freshly prepared and protected from light. The proportion of diamorphine hydrochloride may be altered when specified by the prescriber.

DIAMORPHINE LINCTUS

The following formula was given in the *British Pharmaceutical Codex 1973*:

Diamorphine hydrochloride	0.6 g
Compound tartrazine solution	12 mL
Glycerol	250 mL
Oxymel	250 mL
Syrup	to 1000 mL

It should be recently prepared. Diluent: syrup.

Suppositories

A displacement value of 1.5 for diamorphine in Witepsol has been reported.

REFERENCES

1. Borka L. Acta Pharm Suec 1977;14:210–12.
2. Nakamura GR, Thornton JI, Noguchi TT. J Chromatogr 1975;110:81–9.
3. Garrett ER, Gürkan T. J Pharm Sci 1979;68:26–32.
4. Poochikian GK, Cradock JC. J Chromatogr 1979;171:371–6.
5. Davey EA, Murray JB. Pharm J 1969;203:737.
6. Omar OA, Hoskin PJ, Johnston A, Hanks GW, Turner P. J Pharm Pharmacol 1989;41:275–7.
7. Poochikian GK, Cradock JC, Davignon JP. Int J Pharmaceutics 1983;13:219–26.
8. Beaumont IM. Pharm J 1982;229:39–41.
9. Cooper H, Mehta AC, Calvert RT. Pharm J 1981;226:682–3.
10. Kleinberg ML, Duafala ME, Nacov C, Flora KP, Hines J, Davis K *et al.* Am J Hosp Pharm 1990;47:377–81.
11. Allwood MC. Br J Pharm Pract 1984;6:88,90.
12. Allwood MC. Int Pharm J 1991;5(3):120.
13. Regnard C, Pashley S, Westrope F. Br J Pharm Pract 1986;8:218–20.
14. Collins AJ, Abethell JA, Holmes SG, Bain R. J Pharm Pharmacol 1986;38(Suppl):51P.
15. Kirk B, Hain WR [letter]. Pharm J 1985;233:171.

Diazepam (BAN, USAN, rINN)   *Anxiolytic*

7-Chloro-1,3-dihydro-1-methyl-5-phenyl-1,4-benzodiazepin-2-one; 7-chloro-1,3-dihydro-1-methyl-5-phenyl-2H-1,4-benzodiazepin-2-one

$C_{16}H_{13}ClN_2O = 284.7$

CAS —439-14-5

Pharmacopoeial status

BP, USP

Preparations

Compendial

Diazepam Capsules BP. Capsules containing, in each, 2 mg, and 5 mg are usually available.

Diazepam Tablets BP. Tablets containing, in each, 2 mg, 5 mg, and 10 mg are usually available.

Diazepam Oral Solution BP (Diazepam Elixir). A solution of diazepam in a suitable flavoured vehicle. An oral solution containing 2 mg in 5 mL is usually available. pH 4.7 to 5.4.

Diazepam Injection BP. A sterile solution of diazepam in water for injections or other suitable solvent. Injections containing 10 mg in 2 mL and 20 mg in 4 mL are usually available. pH 6.2 to 7.0.

Diazepam Capsules USP.

Diazepam Extended-release Capsules USP.

Diazepam Tablets USP.

Diazepam Injection USP. pH 6.2 to 6.9.

Non-compendial

Diazemuls (Dumex). *Injection* (emulsion), ampoules containing diazepam 10 mg in 2 mL; for intravenous injection or infusion. Diazemuls should be drawn up into the syringe immediately before administration. Diazemuls should only be mixed in the same container or syringe with glucose 5% or 10% solution or Intralipid 10% or 20%. The ampoule contents should not be mixed with any drugs other than infusion solutions specified by the manufacturer. Adsorption to plastic infusion equipment may occur.

Stesolid (CP). *Rectal tubes*, rectal solutions containing diazepam 2 mg/mL or 4 mg/mL.

Valium Roche (Roche). *Tablets*, diazepam 2 mg, 5 mg, and 10 mg.

Syrup, diazepam 2 mg in 5 mL. *Diluents*: sorbitol solution or syrup.

Injection, ampoules containing diazepam 10 mg in 2 mL. Solution is greenish-yellow. The ampoule solution should not normally be diluted except when given slowly in large intravenous infusions of sodium chloride injection or glucose. Not more than 40 mg (8 mL ampoule solution) should be added to 500 mL of infusion solution; the solution should be freshly made and used within six hours of dilution. Other drugs should not be mixed with the ampoule solution in the same infusion or in the syringe. Plastic containers should not be used for infusion solutions.

Diazepam tablets are also available, in various strengths, from APS, Berk (Atensine), Cox, DDSA (Tensium), Evans, Kerfoot, Rima (Rimapam).

Diazepam oral solution is also available from Cox, Lagap. Diazepam strong oral solution is available from Lagap.
Diazepam injection is also available from CP.
Diazepam suppositories are also available from Sinclair.

Containers and storage

Solid state

Diazepam BP should be kept in a well-closed container and protected from light.
Diazepam USP should be preserved in tight, light-resistant containers.

Dosage forms

All Diazepam BP preparations should be protected from light.
Diazepam Oral Solution BP should be stored at a temperature not exceeding 25°.
Diazepam Capsules USP, Diazepam Extended-release Capsules USP, and Diazepam Tablets USP should be preserved in tight, light-resistant containers.
Diazepam Injection USP should be preserved in single-dose or in multiple-dose containers, preferably of Type I glass, protected from light.
Diazemuls injection should be stored at room temperature and should not be frozen.
Stesolid rectal tubes should be stored in a cool place, preferably under refrigeration.
All Valium Roche preparations should be protected from light.
Valium Roche syrup and injection ampoules should be stored at a temperature not exceeding 30°.

PHYSICAL PROPERTIES

Diazepam is a white or yellow crystalline powder; odourless or almost odourless.

Melting point

Diazepam melts in the range 131° to 135°.

Dissociation constant

pK_a 3.3 (20°)
Changes in ultraviolet absorption spectra of diazepam in solution over a range of pH values led Barrett *et al*[1] to attribute the pK_a value of 3.3 for diazepam to the probable protonation of the nitrogen atom at position 4 in the diazepine ring.

Partition coefficient

Log *P* (octanol/pH 7.4), 2.7

Solubility

Diazepam is very slightly soluble in water (1 in 333); it is soluble 1 in 25 of ethanol, 1 in 8 of acetone, 1 in 39 of ether and 1 in 60 of propylene glycol; freely soluble in chloroform (1 in 2).
Solubility values for diazepam, after equilibration at 25°, in water for injections and in three common infusion solutions (glucose 5% injection, sodium chloride 0.9% injection, and compound sodium lactate injection) were determined by Newton *et al.*[2] Solubilities of diazepam added either as an alcoholic solution or as a commercial injection solution (Valium, Roche) were in the range 0.04 mg/mL to 0.05 mg/mL at 25°. A 1 in 100 dilution of the injection in intravenous infusions was proposed for admixtures, with an expiry period of up to 24 hours.

Effect of cosolvents

An equation was derived to predict solubility values for diazepam in binary mixtures of water with propylene glycol, 1,3-butanediol, glycerol, sorbitol (70% w/w), macrogols (200 or 400), ethanol, or methanol.[3] Experimental results showed that, in general, solubility increased linearly with increasing cosolvent concentration, although there was some deviation from the predicted values. These deviations were attributed primarily to interactions between the cosolvents and water.
The solubility of diazepam at 30° has been found to increase with increasing concentration of bile salts (sodium cholate, sodium deoxycholate, sodium taurocholate, sodium glycocholate, and sodium dehydrocholate) in solution.[4] Mixed micellar solutions of sodium cholate and lecithin also enhanced the solubility of diazepam but solubilising efficiency varied with the lecithin content.
The potential of human serum albumin (5% or 25%, and containing caprylate and tryptophan stabilisers) as a cosolvent for diazepam has been investigated in *mice*.[5] Solubility values for diazepam in 25% human serum albumin at 20° to 22° were about 768 micrograms/mL or 0.85 mole/mole albumin.

FURTHER INFORMATION. Solubility of diazepam and prazepam in aqueous non-ionic surfactants—Moro ME, Velazquez MM, Cachaza JM, Rodriguez LJ. J Pharm Pharmacol 1986;38:294–6. Statistical techniques applied to solubility predictions and pharmaceutical formulations: an approach to problem solving using mixture response surface methodology—Belloto RJ, Dean AM, Moustafa MA, Molokhia AM, Gouda MW, Sokoloski TD. Int J Pharmaceutics 1985;23:195–207.

Dissolution

The USP specifies that for Diazepam Capsules USP not less than 85% of the labelled amount of $C_{16}H_{13}ClN_2O$ is dissolved in 45 minutes. Dissolution medium: 900 mL of 0.1N hydrochloric acid; Apparatus 1 at 100 rpm.
The USP specifies that for Diazepam Extended-release Capsules USP, 15 to 27%, 49 to 66%, 76 to 96%, and 85 to 115% of the labelled amount of $C_{16}H_{13}ClN_2O$ is dissolved in 0.042D, 0.167D, 0.333D, and 0.500D hours respectively, where D represents the labelled dosing interval. Dissolution medium: 900 mL of simulated gastric fluid TS, prepared without enzymes; Apparatus 1 at 100 rpm.
The USP specifies that for Diazepam Tablets USP not less than 85% of the labelled amount of $C_{16}H_{13}ClN_2O$ is dissolved in 30 minutes. Dissolution medium: 900 mL of 0.1N hydrochloric acid; Apparatus 1 at 100 rpm.
Italian workers[6] who studied the effects of varying pH on the dissolution, partition coefficient, and diffusion rate constant of diazepam observed that the dissolution rate decreased as pH increased and that the influence of pH on dissolution was most marked for values below or equal to pK_a.
Enhanced dissolution of diazepam has been demonstrated[7] when in the presence of cellulose ethers (methylcellulose and hydroxyethylcellulose) in physical mixtures and residue after evaporation from organic solvents.

STABILITY

Diazepam degrades in aqueous solution by hydrolysis of the 4,5-azomethine bond (ring opening) resulting in the formation of an intermediate which undergoes further hydrolysis to produce 2-methylamino-5-chlorobenzophenone and a glycine derivative. The reaction is reversible and pH-dependent. Nakano *et al*[8] reported that in acid solutions, even at body temperature, the initial hydrolysis occurs at an 'appreciable' rate, the open-ring compound being in equilibrium with the protonated diazepam. On increasing the pH of the medium, diazepam is reformed.
Diazepam has maximum stability around pH 5. At room temperature, the rate constant for diazepam hydrolysis, k, is 1.41×10^{-5}/s at pH 0.93 and 2.95×10^{-8}/s at pH 10.18 (corre-

sponding to half-lives of 0.57 and 272 days, respectively). For a mixed solvent system, similar in composition to the commercial parenteral formulation, $k = 5.55 \times 10^{-11}/s$. Diazepam also appears to be susceptible to photochemical decomposition. After extended storage, diazepam tablets and suppositories with low moisture content show minimal decomposition.

Degradation products of diazepam described by Emery and Kowtko[9] are 3-amino-6-chloro-1-methyl-4-phenylcarbostyril and 2-methylamino-5-chlorobenzophenone. A manufacturing precursor of diazepam is 7-chloro-1,3-dihydro-5-phenyl-2H-1,4-benzodiazepin-2-one.

Photochemical decomposition

After the irradiation of diazepam (in methanolic solvent) under ultraviolet light at 254 nm, breakdown products found by Cornelissen et al[10] were benzophenones, 4-phenylquinazolinones, 4-phenylquinazolines, and glycine.

Repackaging

When diazepam injection (Valium, Hoffmann-La Roche, USA) was repackaged in disposable glass unit-dose syringes there was evidence of sorption of diazepam and the decomposition product 2-methylamino-5-chloro-benzophenone to the polymeric rubber stopper (mainly a halo-butyl-isoprene blend).[11] After storage of the syringes (in light-resistant bags) for 90 days at 30° and 4°, the original diazepam concentration decreased by 7.6% and 2.6%, respectively. Refrigeration of the prepackaged syringes was recommended, as was the avoidance of rubber and plastic materials when filling the syringes.

Stabilisation

To minimise hydrolysis, solid dosage forms and suppositories should have low moisture contents. In aqueous systems, maximum stability is in the range pH 4 to 8. Both stability and solubility are enhanced when diazepam is dissolved in propylene glycol or macrogol, with ethanol, benzyl alcohol, and buffers to pH 6.2 to 6.9. Containers should be of glass, polyethylene, or polypropylene; they should be protected from light. Some commercial injections are filled under nitrogen. See also Incompatibility/compatibility below.

Experimental pseudo-first-order rate constants for the acid hydrolysis of diazepam in aqueous solution at 25° decreased as the concentration of hydrochloric acid was increased.[12] The presence of micellar aggregates of nonionic (polyoxyethylene-23-dodecanol, Brij 35) or cationic (cetyltrimethyl ammonium bromide) surfactants had no appreciable effects on the rate of hydrolysis of diazepam. However, the inclusion of micelles of an anionic surfactant (sodium dodecyl sulphate) resulted in a reduction in the rate constant; this effect increased as the concentration of surfactant was increased.

FURTHER INFORMATION. Long-term stability of diazepam injections—Fyllingen G, Kristiansen F, Roksvaag PO. Pharm Acta Helv 1991;66:44–6.

INCOMPATIBILITY/COMPATIBILITY

Dilution with intravenous fluids

Morris[13] examined the compatibility and stability of diazepam injection (5 mg/mL, Valium, Hoffmann-La Roche, Canada) after dilution with four different intravenous fluids. Sodium chloride 0.9% injection, glucose 5% injection, compound sodium lactate injection, and compound sodium chloride injection were all suitable diluents for diazepam injection provided that dilution (in glass beakers) was greater than 1:20 (5 mg in 20 mL). At dilutions of 1:20 and 1:40, acceptable potency (90% of original) was maintained for 4 hours and 6 to 8 hours, respectively, whereas at higher dilutions (1:50, 1:75, and 1:100) potency and compatibility were maintained for 24 hours. Cloyd[14] recommended that all dilutions should be prepared by adding the intravenous solution to the diazepam injection in the volume-control set. Addition of diazepam injection to the diluent resulted in the rapid formation of a yellow precipitate. The nature of the precipitate formed in admixtures with diazepam injection (Valium, Roche) has been the subject of controversy. Raymond and Huber[15] confirmed that the precipitate is solely diazepam.

Other recommendations on the dilution of diazepam injection before intravenous administration have been made by Whyatt and Hu[16] and by Maloney.[17] Methods of preparing intravenous infusions of diazepam and the incidence of thrombophlebitis following diazepam infusion have been reviewed.[18,19]

Sorption to plastics

Sorption of diazepam to infusion fluid containers and administration sets composed of different plastics has been studied by various workers.[20-32] In general, when stored in glass or polyethylene containers, intravenous solutions of diazepam maintain their initial concentration; however, in polyvinyl chloride bags, diazepam is rapidly and extensively lost from solution. Considerable sorption of diazepam to polyvinyl chloride administration sets has been found.[22] Losses were increased by the addition of a cellulose propionate burette to the system. No loss of potency was observed when diazepam was infused through polybutadiene tubing with a methacrylate butadiene styrene burette.[22] Infusion of diazepam through a polyethylene-lined (non-polyvinyl chloride) administration set was superior to administration through polyvinyl chloride sets in terms of diazepam recovery.[28] Various parameters which affect sorption of diazepam to polyvinyl chloride containers and administration sets have been examined: sorption increases with increasing tube length or decreasing flow rate;[29-31] the rate of sorption increases as temperature rises;[26,30] fractional loss is greater at small volumes (in constant volume containers);[30] pH and initial concentration were not found to affect sorption to polyvinyl chloride containers.[25,30] In-line filters caused no reduction in potency[24] but end-line filters have been found to reduce the amount of drug delivered during the initial stages of infusion.[32] Solubility, permeability, and partitioning data for diazepam in aqueous systems and plastic materials have been examined by several workers.[25-27]

FURTHER INFORMATION. A study of the interaction of selected drugs and plastic syringes [influence of short-term storage at −20° to 25° on injection solutions or on syringes]—Speaker TJ, Turco SJ, Nardone DA, Miripol JE. J Parenter Sci Technol 1991;45(5):212–17.

FORMULATION

Excipients

Excipients that have been used in presentations of diazepam include:

Tablets: calcium stearate; indigo carmine (E132); iron oxide; lactose; magnesium stearate; microcrystalline cellulose; povidone; starch; sunset yellow FCF (E110); tartrazine (E102).

Oral liquids: aluminium magnesium silicate; carbomer; erythrosine (E127); glycerol; lactic acid; polyoxyethylene monostearate; sodium benzoate; sodium hydroxide; sorbitol.

Injections and injectable emulsions: benzoic acid; benzyl alcohol; ethanol; propylene glycol; sodium benzoate; sodium hydroxide.

Suppositories: macrogols; theobroma oil.

Rectal solutions: benzoic acid; benzyl alcohol; Cremophor EL; ethanol; glycofurol; propylene glycol; sodium benzoate; sodium hydroxide.

Bioavailability

Rates and extents of absorption of diazepam when administered by various routes to nine healthy volunteers were compared by Moolenaar et al.[33] Results following single doses of 10 mg diazepam (Stesolid, Dumex, Denmark) are summarised below:

Route of administration	Absorption	Time to reach mean peak plasma concentration
Oral (tablets)	rapid	within 60 minutes
Intramuscular (injection)	slow	95 minutes
Rectal (micro-enema)	very rapid	17 minutes
Rectal (suppositories)	slow	82 minutes

After administration by the oral route, there was considerable variation in absorption rate constants between subjects. After 24 hours, bioavailability from the micro-enema was almost complete, but from the suppositories it was incomplete and lower than that of the other dosage forms. The authors concluded that in single-dose therapy with diazepam, if a rapid therapeutic effect is required, only rectal administration of diazepam in solution form may be considered as an alternative route of administration for routine medication.

When diazepam preparations were administered rectally, a parenteral solution (Valium, Roche) gave peak plasma concentrations significantly higher than those from either a suppository (Valium, Roche) or a parenteral emulsion (Diazemuls, Dumex). The time to reach peak plasma concentration was also significantly less for the solution than for the other preparations but there was no significant difference between the area under plasma concentration versus time curves.[34]

Bioequivalence

Two diazepam 10 mg tablet preparations were not considered to be bioequivalent following a single-dose crossover study with 26 healthy subjects.[35] Significantly slower absorption of diazepam occurred from a generic preparation (NeoCalme, NeoLab, Canada) than from Valium (Roche, USA).

Tablets

When spray-dried from aqueous ethanol, an inclusion complex formed between diazepam and β-cyclodextrin but not between diazepam and lactose.[36] Intrinsic dissolution rates for diazepam were enhanced from the β-cyclodextrin complex at high diazepam concentrations but complex formation was less important than drug processing or the nature of the excipients in determining dissolution rate. In solid dosage forms, *in-vitro* release and *in-vivo* absorption were greater from the spray-dried products than from physical mixtures, irrespective of whether they contained lactose or β-cyclodextrin.

The capacity of directly compressible excipients to adsorb diazepam decreased in the order: activated charcoal (control) > Sta-Rx 1500 (compressible starch) > Avicel (microcrystalline cellulose) > Compactrol (dibasic calcium sulphate) > Emcompress (calcium hydrogen phosphate dihydrate). Adsorption to excipients was greater in distilled water than in buffer solutions (of pH 2.1 or 7.2). The authors observed no correlation between the adsorption data and the physicochemical characteristics of the tablets produced.[37]

Granulates containing solid dispersions of diazepam with macrogols of high molecular weight were compressed into tablets by Kinget and Kemel.[38] Macrogol 6000 was the most efficient carrier. A combination of magnesium stearate (0.5%) and cross-linked povidone (Polyplasdone 3%), added to the granules, produced tablets with shortest disintegration times.

Suspensions

A suspension 1 mg/mL containing crushed diazepam (10 mg) tablets was developed by Strom and Kalu.[39] After storage in amber glass bottles at 5°, 22°, and 40° for 60 days there was essentially no reduction in diazepam concentration and test suspensions remained homogeneous. When redispersed, suspensions were easily poured. There were minor increases in pH (initially 4.2) to 4.5 and to 5.1 in samples stored at 22° and at 40°, respectively.

A xanthan gum (Keltrol 0.5%) was used[40] in a hydroxybenzoate-preserved, flavoured vehicle to suspend diazepam (5 mg/5 mL) as crushed tablets or powder. Suspensions were reported to be physically and chemically stable for 12 weeks at room temperature.

Skin permeation

When investigating the permeation of diazepam from various solvent systems across *mouse* skin, Touitou[41] found that the inclusion of Azone (laurocapram) 5% in a propylene glycol-ethanol-water system greatly increased the permeation flux *in vitro*.

An enhancement of up to 5-fold in the cumulative permeation of diazepam (over 24 hours) across *rat* skin from a 1% w/v solution in *n*-methylpyrrolidone was achieved by the inclusion of 5% v/v *n*-alkane of chain length between 8 and 16. Flux of diazepam across hairless *mouse* skin from a 1% w/v solution in ethanol was enhanced by 10% v/v *n*-nonane but not by *n*-nonanol. Similarly, monoterpenes that were 'purely hydrocarbon' enhanced penetration of diazepam while monoterpenes with 'hydrogen-bonding ability' (such as menthol or menthone) were less effective.[42]

Suppositories, rectal solutions, and enemas

A new double-layer suppository formulated by Deshmukh and Thwaites[43] comprised a drug-free core of macrogol 6000 thinly coated with a layer of macrogol 1000 within which the diazepam was dissolved. In a dissolution cell, diazepam release from the novel suppositories was compared with that from three conventional suppository formulations with macrogol bases. The most rapid release was achieved from the double-layer suppository.

Watson[44] prepared a rectal solution of diazepam (pH 6.4 to 6.5) by dilution of a commercially available diazepam injection with equal parts propylene glycol and sterile water to a final strength of 1 mg/mL. After storage in glass bottles for 14 months below 25°, and protected from light, there was no significant reduction in potency and no evidence of anaerobic or aerobic bacterial contamination. An expiry date of one year after manufacture was allocated.

Frijlink et al[45] investigated the absorption *in vivo* of diazepam from inclusion complexes formed between diazepam and β-cyclodextrin. Solubility of diazepam was increased by complexation. When micro-enemas containing diazepam 2 mg alone or with β-cyclodextrin 230 mg were administered rectally to eight healthy volunteers in a crossover study, the absorption rate was greater from the micro-enemas that contained β-cyclodextrin. This enhancement was attributed mainly to displacement of diazepam from the complex by lipids in rectal mucus. Neither β-cyclodextrin nor the complex were absorbed rectally.

Injections

Parenteral formulations of diazepam were developed in which propylene glycol was partially or completely replaced by macrogol 400; the properties of these formulations were compared to those of a commercial diazepam injection (Valium, Hoffmann-La Roche, Canada).[46] The prepared injections (pH 4.5) had higher viscosity than the commercial injection (pH 6.7 to 7.3). Although all formulations developed a yellow discoloration during 15 days storage at room temperature under exposure to light, no decrease in diazepam content was detected. Bioequivalence of the test injections with Valium injection was concluded following intramuscular administration to three *dogs* in a randomised, crossover study.

In an assessment of Pluronic surfactants (poloxamers) as potential vehicles for diazepam injection, Lin and Kawashima[47] found that the aqueous solubility of diazepam increased as Pluronic concentration increased; solubilising effect was greatest with Pluronic F-108. Incorporation of Pluronics (5%) into commercial diazepam injection reduced both the turbidity in admixtures with commonly used transfusion fluids and the sorption of diazepam to polyvinyl chloride bags.

When administered into the ear veins of *rabbits*,[48] a dilution of diazepam injection containing poloxamer 188 (Pluronic F-68) produced fewer thrombotic and inflammatory effects than a diazepam injection without poloxamer 188.

As the concentration of sodium salicylate in an aqueous solution increased from 0% to 30%, the solubility of diazepam in the solution increased 200-fold.[49] Autoclaving of a 5 mg/mL solution in 30% sodium salicylate produced a slight discoloration but no reduction in diazepam content.

To prevent crystallisation of diazepam in injection solutions, Aquino *et al*[50] proposed the incorporation of hydroxypropyl β-cyclodextrin in the infusion vehicle before dilution of the diazepam injection solution (solvent system contained ethanol 4% w/w, propylene glycol 20.7% w/w, macrogol 300 60% w/w, and water 15.3% w/w). After five days at room temperature, more than 95% of diazepam remained in solution in dilutions of 1 in 63 when the diluent was sodium chloride 0.9% or hydroxypropyl β-cyclodextrin 6% w/v in sodium chloride 0.9%; in dilutions of 1 in 21 with the same two diluents, 33% and more than 97% of diazepam remained in solution, respectively.

Injectable emulsions

Levy and Benita[51] investigated the effects of pH, temperature, phase volume ratio, and the concentrations of nonionic emulsifier, phospholipids, and diazepam on the physicochemical properties of a submicronised parenteral emulsion (o/w) containing diazepam. Various emulsification and homogenisation techniques were examined. A typical formulation (% w/w) was: diazepam 0.5, oily phase 20.0, purified fractionated egg yolk phospholipids 1.2, poloxamer (Pluronic F-68) 2.0, glycerol 2.25, α-tocopherol 0.02, methyl and butyl *p*-hydroxybenzoic esters 0.2 and 0.075 respectively, and double-distilled water to 100.0. Sodium hydroxide (10%) solution was used to adjust pH to between 2 and 8. In further short-term and long-term stability studies[52] of this 'submicron emulsion', diazepam was stable in the emulsion at 4° and 25° for up to 25 months and 16 months respectively, but was less stable at 37°. The emulsion was stable to conventional steam sterilisation and to mechanical stress conditions. If the preparation contained less than 25% w/w oily phase, stability was apparent for 12 months at 25°, but emulsion stability was dependent on the concentration of poloxamer and phospholipid. By adjustment of the initial pH of the emulsion to 7.4 or 8.0, decreases in emulsion pH that had been observed during storage were 'significantly diminished'.

Solid dispersions

Solid dispersions of diazepam with macrogol 6000, prepared by either melting or solvent (ethanol) methods, were characterised as a simple eutectic mixture with a proposed eutectic composition of diazepam 13% and macrogol 6000 87%. A linear increase in the solubility of diazepam was observed as the concentration of macrogol 6000 was increased (at 27° and 37°).[53] In further work,[54] faster dissolution of diazepam (into artificial gastric fluid at 37°) was observed from such solid dispersions prepared by fusion methods ('melting' and 'melting carrier' methods) than from solid dispersions prepared by a solvent method or from physical mixtures of diazepam with macrogol 6000.

Earlier studies of physical mixtures and melts of diazepam with macrogol 6000 had reported problems associated with the accurate determination of the eutectic composition of the melts; the eutectic mixture contained less than 30% diazepam.[55] Inclusion of 1% or 5% polysorbate 80 or 1% stearic acid in the melts caused further increases in dissolution rates of diazepam (in water at 37°) above the enhancement achieved by the macrogol 6000. Changes induced by storage were investigated.

FURTHER INFORMATION. The effect of formulation on the plasma binding and blood/plasma concentration ratio of diazepam—McClean E, Collier PS, Fee JPH. Int J Pharmaceutics 1990;60:35–9. Optimisation of the composition of the granular material for the preparation of a diazepam-containing suspension—Dimitrova I, Welikova E, Iontschev H [German]. Pharmazie 1989;44:49–50. Diazepam oral suspension—Allen LV. US Pharm 1989;14:64–5. Physico-chemical aspects of the complexation of some drugs with cyclodextrins—Menard AC, Dedhiya MG, Rhodes CT. Drug Dev Ind Pharm 1990;16(1):91–113. Drug release from submicronised o/w emulsion: a new *in vitro* kinetic evaluation model—Levy MY, Benita S. Int J Pharmaceutics 1990;66:29–37. Absorption of diazepam and lorazepam following intranasal administration—Lau SWJ, Slattery JT. Int J Pharmaceutics 1989;54:171–4. [See also Lorazepam monograph—Formulation]. Preparation and investigation of products containing diazepam and dimethyl-β-cyclodextrin—Kata M, Schauer M, Selmeczi B. Acta Pharm Hung 1991;61:136–41.

PROCESSING

Sterilisation

Diazepam injection can be sterilised by filtration.

REFERENCES

1. Barrett J, Franklin Smyth W, Davidson IE. J Pharm Pharmacol 1973;25:387–93.
2. Newton DW, Driscoll DF, Goudreau JL, Ratanamaneichatara S. Am J Hosp Pharm 1981;38:179–82.
3. Rubino JT, Yalkowsky SH. J Parenter Sci Technol 1985;39:106.
4. Rosoff M, Serajuddin ATM. Int J Pharmaceutics 1980;6:137–46
5. Olson WP, Faith MR. J Parenter Sci Technol 1988;42:82.

6. Mura P, Liguori A, Bramanti G [French]. Pharm Acta Helv 1987;62(3):88–92.
7. Keipert S, Alde D [German]. Pharmazie 1986;41:845–7.
8. Nakano M, Inotsume N, Kohri N, Arita T. Int J Pharmaceutics 1979;3:195–204.
9. Emery M, Kowtko J. J Pharm Sci 1979;68(9):1185–97.
10. Cornelissen PJG, Beijersbergen van Henegouwen GMJ, Gerritsma KW. Int J Pharmaceutics 1978;1:173–81.
11. Smith FM, Nuessle NO. Am J Hosp Pharm 1982;39:1687–90.
12. Moro ME, Novillo-Fertrell J, Velazquez MM, Rodriguez LJ. J Pharm Sci 1991;80(5):459–68.
13. Morris ME. Am J Hosp Pharm 1978;35:669–72.
14. Cloyd JC [letter]. Am J Hosp Pharm 1981;38:32.
15. Raymond G, Huber JW [letter]. Drug Intell Clin Pharm 1979;13:612.
16. Whyatt J, Hu A [letter]. Aust J Hosp Pharm 1983;13(4):151.
17. Maloney TJ [letter]. Aust J Hosp Pharm 1983;13(2):79.
18. Michael KA, Lehman ME, Amerson AB. Drug Intell Clin Pharm 1984;18:214.
19. Robinson K. Aust J Hosp Pharm 1984;14(3):127.
20. Yliruusi JK, Sothmann AG, Laine RH, Rajasilta RA, Kristoffersson ER. Am J Hosp Pharm 1982;39:1018–21.
21. Smith A, Bird G. J Clin Hosp Pharm 1982;7:181–6.
22. Lee MG. Am J Hosp Pharm 1986;43:1945–50.
23. Cloyd JC, Vezeau C, Miller KW. Am J Hosp Pharm 1980;37:492–6.
24. Parker WA, MacCara ME. Am J Hosp Pharm 1980;37:496–500.
25. Yliruusi JK. Acta Pharm Fenn 1986;95:129–39.
26. Yliruusi JK. Acta Pharm Fenn 1986;95:151–65.
27. Mason NA, Cline S, Hyneck ML, Berardi RR, Ho NFH, Flynn GL. Am J Hosp Pharm 1981;38:1449–54.
28. Hancock BG, Black CD. Am J Hosp Pharm 1985;42:335–9.
29. Yliruusi JK, Uotila JA, Kristoffersson ER. Am J Hosp Pharm 1986;43:2789–94.
30. Kowaluk EA, Roberts MS, Polack AE. Am J Hosp Pharm 1983;40:417–23.
31. Yliruusi JK, Uotila JA, Kristoffersson ER. Am J Hosp Pharm 1986;43:2795–9.
32. De Muynck C, De Vroe C, Remon JP, Colardyn F. J Clin Pharm Ther 1988;13:335–40.
33. Moolenaar F, Bakker S, Visser J, Huizinga T. Int J Pharmaceutics 1980;5:127.
34. Walker R, Newman P, Candlish P, Hiller C, Seviour J. J Pharm Pharmacol 1982;34:33P.
35. Locniskar A, Greenblatt DJ, Harmatz JS, Shader RI. Biopharm Drug Dispos 1989;10:597–605.
36. Bootsma HPR, Frijlink HW, Eissens A, Proost JH, Van Doorne H, Lerk CF. Int J Pharmaceutics 1989;51:213–23.
37. Aboutaleb AE, Abdel Rahman AA, Saleh SI, Ahmed MO. STP Pharma 1986;2(12):23–7.
38. Kinget R, Kemel R. Pharmazie 1985;40:475–7.
39. Strom JG, Kalu AU. Am J Hosp Pharm 1986;43:1489–91.
40. Pharm J 1986;237:665.
41. Touitou E. Int J Pharmaceutics 1986;33:37–43.
42. Hori M, Satoh S, Maibach HI, Guy RH. J Pharm Sci 1991;80(1):32–5.
43. Deshmukh AA, Thwaites PM. Drug Dev Ind Pharm 1989;15(8):1289–307.
44. Watson HR. Aust J Hosp Pharm 1988;18(5):333–9.
45. Frijlink HW, Eissens AC, Schoonen AJM, Lerk CF. Int J Pharmaceutics 1990;64:195–205.
46. Shah AK, Simons KJ, Briggs CJ. Drug Dev Ind Pharm 1991;17(12):1635–54.
47. Lin S-Y, Kawashima Y. J Parenter Sci Technol 1987;41(3):83–7.
48. Prancan AV, Ecanou B, Bernardoni RJ, Sadove MS. J Pharm Sci 1980;69(8):970–1.
49. Saleh AM, Khalil SA, El-Khordagui LK. Int J Pharmaceutics 1980;5:161–4.
50. Aquino S, Quach N, Richardson C, McDonald C [letter]. J Parenter Sci Technol 1990;44(2):48–9.
51. Levy MY, Benita S. Int J Pharmaceutics 1989;54:103–12.
52. Levy MY, Benita S. J Parenter Sci Technol 1991;45(2):101–7.
53. Ginés JM, Sánchez-Soto PJ, Justo A, Vela MT, Rabasco AM. Drug Dev Ind Pharm 1990;16(15):2283–301.
54. Rabasco AM, Ginés JM, Fernández-Arévalo M, Holgado MA. Int J Pharmaceutics 1991;67:201–5.
55. Fernandez J, Vila-Jato JL, Blanco J, Ford JL. Drug Dev Ind Pharm 1989;15(14-16):2491–513.

Diclofenac (BAN, rINN) *Analgesic; Anti-inflammatory*

Diclophenac
[2-(2,6-Dichloroanilino)phenyl]acetic acid
$C_{14}H_{11}Cl_2NO_2 = 296.2$

Diclofenac Sodium (BANM, USAN, rINNM)

Diclophenac sodium
$C_{14}H_{10}Cl_2NNaO_2 = 318.1$
CAS—15307-86-5 (diclofenac); 15307-79-6 (diclofenac sodium)

Preparations

Non-compendial
Voltarol (Geigy). *Tablets*, enteric coated, diclofenac sodium 25 mg and 50 mg.
Dispersible tablets, diclofenac 46.5 mg (equivalent to diclofenac sodium 50 mg).
Suppositories, diclofenac sodium 12.5 mg and 100 mg.
Injection, diclofenac sodium 75 mg/3 mL. Ampoules should not be mixed with other injection solutions.
Voltarol Emulgel (Geigy). *Gel*, diclofenac diethylammonium salt 1.16% (equivalent to diclofenac sodium 1%) in a non-greasy emulsion in an aqueous gel.
Voltarol Ophtha (CIBA Vision). *Eye drops*, diclofenac sodium 0.1%.
Voltarol Retard (Geigy). *Tablets*, sustained release, diclofenac sodium 100 mg.
Voltarol 75 mg SR (Geigy). *Tablets*, sustained release, diclofenac sodium 75 mg.
Diclofenac tablets of various strengths are also available from APS, Ashbourne (Diclozip), Cox, Eastern (Volraman), Evans, Kerfoot, Lagap (Rhumalgan), Norton, Shire (Valenac), Sterwin.

Containers and storage

Dosage forms
Recommended storage conditions for Voltarol (Geigy) preparations:

Voltarol preparation	Protect from heat	Protect from moisture	Protect from light
Tablets	■	■	—
Dispersible tablets	■	■	—
Retard tablets	—	■	—
SR tablets*	■	■	—
Suppositories	■	—	—
Ampoules for injection	■	—	■
Emulgel	■		

* store below 30°

PHYSICAL PROPERTIES

Diclofenac exists as crystals.
Diclofenac sodium is reported to exist as crystals or as a white to off-white crystalline, odourless, slightly hygroscopic powder.[1]

Melting point

Diclofenac melts at 156° to 158°.
Diclofenac sodium melts at 283° to 285°.

Dissociation constant

To overcome problems associated with the determination of dissociation constants of poorly water-soluble drugs, including diclofenac, in water,[2] aqueous dimethyl sulphoxide (20:80 w/w) was used as a mixed solvent. For a range of carboxylic acids, experimental values of pK_a in the mixed solvent (by potentiometry at 25°) were linearly related to literature pK_a values in water. A derived equation was used to convert the experimental pK_a of 6.84 for diclofenac in aqueous dimethyl sulphoxide to a pK_a of 3.78 in water.
Maitani *et al*[3] demonstrated that pK_a values of diclofenac in water-ethanol mixtures increased linearly as the ethanol concentration was increased.
An estimated pK_a for diclofenac of 4.2 at 30° (by potentiometric titration) has been reported.[4]

Partition coefficient

Maitani *et al*[3] investigated apparent partition coefficients between *n*-octanol and water or buffers at various pH values. For both diclofenac and diclofenac sodium linear relationships were established between the concentration in octanol and in water at various pH values (diclofenac, pH 2.97 to 4.82 and diclofenac sodium, pH 6.03 to 8.03); however the apparent partition coefficients for both compounds were independent of drug concentration over the pH range 3 to 7. The presence of cations (sodium ions or potassium ions) markedly affected distribution between phases. Log *P* (octanol/water; 25°) values of 4.00 and 4.17 for diclofenac were calculated from water solubility data by means of derived equations.[5]

Solubility

Effects of pH and temperature
The aqueous solubility of diclofenac sodium is dependent on pH; solubility is poor at low values of pH but when the pH rises above the pK_a, rapid increases in solubility occur.[3,6] Herzfeldt and Kümmel[6] established a solubility for diclofenac sodium of less than 4×10^{-4}% w/v at pH 1.2 to 3, whereas in the pH range 4 to 7.5 solubilities were:

pH	Solubility (% w/v)
4.0	0.0021
5.0	0.0086
6.0	0.059
7.0	0.187
7.5	0.169

The solubilities of diclofenac in water (buffered to pH 2) or in octanol, at three temperatures, as determined by Fini *et al*[5] were as follows:

Temperature	Solubility in water (pH 2)	Solubility in octanol
5°	2.9×10^{-6}M	0.064M
25°	8.0×10^{-6}M	0.078M
37°	16.7×10^{-6}M	0.089M

At 25° and pH 2 the solubilities of diclofenac and diclofenac sodium have been reported to be 8.0×10^{-6}M and 1.5×10^{-5}M, respectively.[7]

Effects of additives
The presence of cations (sodium ions or potassium ions) markedly affects the solubility of diclofenac and diclofenac sodium.[3] Nishihata *et al*[8] reported solubilities for diclofenac sodium in 0.1M sodium phosphate buffer (pH 7.2) at room temperature and at 50° of 13.4 mM and 45.7 mM, respectively. The addition of ethanol 10% w/w to the buffer solution increased the solubility of diclofenac sodium to 51.4 mM at room temperature.
As the concentration of either hydroxypropyl-β-cyclodextrin or hydroxypropyl-γ-cyclodextrin was increased (up to about 70 mmol/L) the solubility of diclofenac sodium, in phosphate buffer pH 7.4 at 25°, also increased from 30 mmol/L to 85 mmol/L.[9]

Dissolution

Evidence for faster dissolution of diclofenac sodium compared to diclofenac in media at pH 2.0, 6.5, and 8.0 has been presented;[10] for either salt, dissolution rates decreased in the order: pH 8.0 > pH 6.5 > pH 2.0.
Dissolution rate studies of non-steroidal anti-inflammatory drugs showed that diclofenac sodium was completely dissolved after about 1 to 2 minutes in pH 7.5 buffer.[6]

STABILITY

Buffered solutions (pH 7.4) that contained diclofenac sodium (6.3×10^{-3}M) dissolved in 12.6×10^{-3}M of either β-cyclodextrin (β-CD) or hydroxypropyl-β-cyclodextrin (HP-β-CD) were prepared either in the presence or absence of oxygen and stored in the dark.[9] Solutions from which oxygen had been removed were claimed to be more stable than those with oxygen. Although precipitation was observed in solutions without β-CD or HP-β-CD during a short storage time at 21°, no loss of diclofenac sodium was reported after 520 days. At 71°, in solutions (without oxygen) that contained diclofenac sodium alone, or with β-CD, or with HP-β-CD, 24.7%, 30.4%, and 34.6% diclofenac remained, respectively, after 207 days.

FURTHER INFORMATION. A specific stability indicating HPLC method to determine diclofenac sodium in raw materials and pharmaceutical solid dosage forms—Kubala T, Gambhir B, Borst SI. Drug Dev Ind Pharm 1993;19(7):949–57.

FORMULATION

Excipients

Excipients that have been used in presentations of diclofenac include:

Tablets, diclofenac sodium: colloidal silica (purified); lactose; magnesium stearate; maize starch; microcrystalline cellulose; polyethoxylated castor oils; povidone; sodium starch glycollate.
Tablets (sustained release), diclofenac sodium: cetyl alcohol; colloidal silica (purified); ethylcellulose; magnesium stearate; povidone; sucrose; talc.
Tablets (dispersible), diclofenac: erythrosine (E127).
Suppositories, diclofenac sodium: mixtures of triglycerides of saturated fatty acids; semi-synthetic solid glycerides.
Gels, diclofenac diethylammonium salt: aromatic oils; benzyl alcohol; Carbopol; caprylic/capric acid fatty alcohol ester; cetomacrogol; diethylamine; liquid paraffin; isopropanol; propylene glycol; terpinyl acetate.
Injections, diclofenac sodium: benzyl alcohol; mannitol; propylene glycol; sodium hydroxide; sodium metabisulphite.

Bioequivalence

Bioequivalence of two enteric-coated diclofenac sodium 25 mg tablets (Anfenax 25, Instituto Biochimico Italiano and Voltaren 25, Ciba-Geigy, New Zealand) was established following a single-dose, randomised, crossover study involving eight healthy subjects.[11]

Modified-release preparations

(See also Suppositories, below)
Belgian workers[12] performed dissolution tests on two modified-release oral preparations of diclofenac sodium: hydrophobic matrix tablets based on a cetylalcohol skeleton (Voltaren, Ciba-Geigy) and hard gelatin capsules that contained pellets coated with Eudragit RL (polymethacrylates) and cellacephate (Eurand International). Both preparations demonstrated greater release of diclofenac sodium in media of higher pH. For example, no dissolution occurred in 0.1M hydrochloric acid (pH 1.0) and faster dissolution was demonstrated at pH 7.5 than at pH 6.8.

Bain *et al*[13] investigated the release characteristics of diclofenac sodium from two prepared modified-release tablets by observing their dissolution properties at pH 6.8 and 37°. The 'wax matrix' tablet contained diclofenac sodium 34.2%, sucrose 51.4%, povidone 2.06%, cetostearyl alcohol 10.3%, colloidal anhydrous silica (Aerosil) 1.02%, and magnesium stearate 1.02%; the 'hydrogel' tablet contained diclofenac sodium 24.9%, hypromellose 74.6%, and magnesium stearate 0.5%. Release of diclofenac sodium from the wax matrix tablet was attributed to diffusion through pores in the matrix, whereas release from hydrogel tablets was dependent on the extents of swelling and erosion of the hydrogel.

In a study with diclofenac sodium, indomethacin, and ibuprofen,[14] tablets of each were prepared that contained the drug in various ratios with a matrix that comprised an insoluble hydrophobic component (hydrogenated vegetable oil) and a hydrophilic gel-forming component (carbomer). (Sample formula: micronised diclofenac sodium, a matrix of hydrogenated vegetable oil (Emvelop):carbomer (Carbopol 934):microcrystalline cellulose (Avicel PH 101) in a 7:2:1 ratio, isopropanol, silica, and magnesium stearate). Release was examined in phosphate buffer at pH 6.5 with 0.02% Tween 80. Factors affecting dissolution, such as drug wettability, rate of matrix erosion, and interactions between matrix components were discussed.

Peña Romero *et al* developed a formula for a sustained-release oral tablet of diclofenac sodium. Following optimisation of tablet weight and composition (achieved by a factorial study for three independent variables: weight of tablet, ratio of the two inert polymers ethylcellulose:polyvinyl chloride, and concentration of talc) tablet properties were investigated; zero-order release of diclofenac sodium was apparent.[15] Further studies[16] were performed on optimised tablets (formulation: diclofenac sodium 25.0%, ethylcellulose 26.1%, polyvinyl chloride (Pevikon PE 737) 45.9%, talc 2.0%, magnesium stearate 1.0%) prepared by each of five processes (direct compression; double compression; compaction of five raw materials; separate compaction of diclofenac sodium and polyvinyl chloride; wet granulation). Measurement of penetration and uptake of water, and force development (forces within the compact caused by polymer swelling, or by interaction between polymer chains and penetrating liquid) revealed differences between tablets prepared by the different methods. These results were used to explain dissolution profiles and to investigate the 'microstructure' of tablets. See also Further Information, below. Prolonged release of diclofenac sodium has been achieved by formulation of tablets that contain the polymers chitosan[17] or chitin.[18] Tablets were prepared by direct compression of diclofenac sodium with lactose and chitosan or chitin, or by wet granulation of diclofenac sodium with a citric acid solution of chitosan. The hardness of tablets and the extent of release retardation increased as the polymer concentration was increased.

Topical preparations

The *in-vitro* release of diclofenac sodium from an oil-in-water emulsion-type ointment was greater than from either a commercial grade hydrophilic ointment or an absorption ointment.[19] The oil-in-water emulsion-type ointment consisted of diclofenac sodium 3% with 1,2,3-propanetriyl trioctanoate (caprylic acid glyceryl ester) and sugar wax as the oil phase and sugar ester as the emulsifier. In studies of emulsion stability at 40°, physical instability (separation of layers) was observed in the hydrophilic ointment and the absorption ointment after 10 days and 3 days, respectively, whereas the oil-in-water emulsion-type ointment showed no physical instability for at least 50 days.

Release of diclofenac sodium from aqueous gels of Pluronic F-127 (poloxamers) has been evaluated *in vitro* in a membraneless model system.[4] The apparent release rate increased as the initial concentration of diclofenac sodium increased (up to 0.465% w/v) and was dependent on pH (maximum at about pH 7). Release rates decreased with an increase in concentration of PF-127 (from 20% w/v to 30% w/v) and rates increased as temperature was increased (from 20° to 40°).

Topical application of diclofenac sodium (onto the skin of *rats*) as aqueous gels (prepared with hydrogenated soya phospholipid) produced significantly greater plasma concentrations of diclofenac than either an aqueous solution or an aqueous solution with ethanol 10% w/w.[8] The relative bioavailability of diclofenac sodium from one topical gel formulation (diclofenac sodium (2.25%), hydrogenated soya phospholipid (6.8%), triglyceride (6.8%), 0.1 M sodium phosphate buffer, pH 7 (74.15%), ethanol (10%)) was about 7% compared to that of rectal administration of a commercial diclofenac sodium suppository in one human subject.

Poor percutaneous absorption (in *rabbits*) of diclofenac sodium (1.43%) from a simple ointment, a hydrophilic (oil-in-water type) ointment, an absorption (water-in-oil type) ointment, a macrogols ointment (described in the Japanese Pharmacopoeia), and from carbomer as a gel ointment has been reported.[20] More favourable absorption of diclofenac sodium was demonstrated from a gel ointment prepared with methylcellulose or hypromellose as the basis and isopropyl myristate as the sorbefacient; preparations also contained propylene glycol, ethanol, and distilled water.

Vyas et al[21] developed a transdermal drug delivery system for diclofenac based on a polymeric pseudolatex dispersion. Preparations contained: diclofenac (3.4% w/w); Eudragit RL-100 polymer (10% to 6% w/w); povidone, hydrophilic polymer (0% to 4% w/w); liquid paraffin (2% w/w); dibutyl phthalate (4% w/w); Tween 80 (10% w/w). Factors evaluated were, physical and chemical characteristics, in-vitro release of diclofenac, in-vitro skin permeation, and in-vitro anti-inflammatory activity. A formulation that contained Eudragit RL-100:povidone (8:2) with an in-vitro skin permeation rate of 0.188 micrograms/hour/cm^2 was evaluated following topical administration to ten healthy subjects. The parameters were compared with those produced following oral administration of enteric-coated diclofenac 50 mg tablets (Voltarol 50, Ciba-Geigy, UK). The pseudolatex dispersion achieved constant (zero-order kinetics) and effective plasma concentrations of diclofenac over 24 hours, although inter-subject variation was marked.

Suppositories

Modified-release suppositories of diclofenac sodium were prepared by Nishihata et al[22]. The suppository basis consisted of a mixture of triglyceride (Witepsol H-15) and lecithin. As the concentration of lecithin in the basis increased, the apparent solubility of diclofenac sodium in the basis at 38° increased and the in-vitro rate of release (into sodium chloride 0.9% solution at 38°) decreased. Rectal bioavailability of diclofenac sodium (in three dogs) from suppositories with a triglyceride:lecithin (6.5:3.5) basis was similar to that from suppositories with a basis composed of triglyceride alone (65.6% to 90.2% and 68.8% to 92.0%, respectively, relative to intravenous administration of diclofenac sodium). However, effective plasma concentrations of diclofenac were maintained for 12 hours and 5 hours after administration of suppositories with and without lecithin, respectively.

Prolonged release of diclofenac sodium was achieved from suppositories prepared by absorption of a diclofenac sodium solution into a water absorbable polymer (Poys SA-20, Kao Co Ltd, Japan) followed by suspension of the dried polymer particles in a melted triglyceride basis[23]. In-vitro release of diclofenac sodium was five times slower from the modified-release suppositories than from conventional suppositories prepared with triglyceride basis alone. Further, absorption rates in vivo (in three dogs) were slower and more prolonged from sustained-release suppositories, with a reduction in the transient high plasma concentrations produced by conventional suppositories. Bioavailability of diclofenac sodium (25 mg) from the modified-release and conventional suppositories was 60.4% and 78.0%, respectively, compared to that produced following intravenous injection.

Release of diclofenac sodium 100 mg from five different suppositories was investigated in vitro and in vivo (in 8 to 12 subjects)[24]. Significant correlation was found between certain release parameters in vitro and absorption data in vivo.

FURTHER INFORMATION. Statistical optimisation of a controlled-release formulation of diclofenac sodium from inert matrices [ethylcellulose, polyvinyl chloride (Pevikon) and Eudragit RS]. Part 1. Aptitude for compression and preliminary tests—Peña Romero A, Poncet M, Jinot JC, Chulia D [French]. Pharm Acta Helv 1988;63(11):309–14. Statistical optimisation of a controlled-release formulation obtained by a double compression process: application of an Hadamard matrix and a factorial design—Peña Romero A, Costa JB, Castel-Maroteaux I, Chu-

lia D. Drug Dev Ind Pharm 1989;15:2419–40. Tablet formulation study of spray-dried sodium diclofenac enteric-coated microcapsules—Lin SY, Kao YH. Pharm Res 1991;8:919–24. In vitro and in vivo evaluation of sustained-release and enteric-coated microcapsules of diflocenac sodium—Hasan M, Najib N, Suleiman M, El-Sayed Y, Abdel-Hamid M. Drug Dev Ind Pharm 1992;18:1981–8. Dissolution of diclofenac sodium from matrix tablets—Sheu M-T, Chou H-L, Kao C-C, Liu C-H, Sokoloski TD. Int J Pharmaceutics 1992;85:57–63. Effect of ethanol in skin permeation of nonionised and ionised diclofenac—Obata Y, Takayama K, Maitani Y, Machida Y, Nagai T. Int J Pharmaceutics 1993;89:191–8.

REFERENCES

1. Adeyeye CM, Li P-K. In: Florey K, editor. Analytical profiles of drug substances; vol 19. London: Academic Press, 1990:123–45.
2. Fini A, DeMaria P, Guarnieri A, Varoli L. J Pharm Sci 1987;76(1):48–52.
3. Maitani Y, Nakagaki M, Nagai T. Int J Pharmaceutics 1991;74:105–16.
4. Tomida H, Shinohara M, Kuwada N, Kiryu S. Acta Pharm Suec 1987;24:263–72.
5. Fini A, Laus M, Orienti I, Zecchi V. J Pharm Sci 1986;75(1):23–5.
6. Herzfeldt CD, Kümmel R. Drug Dev Ind Pharm 1983;9(5):767–93.
7. Fini A, Zecchi V, Tartarini A. Pharm Acta Helv 1985;60(2):58–62.
8. Nishihata T, Kamada A, Sakai K, Takahashi K, Matsumoto K, Shinozaki K et al. Int J Pharmaceutics 1988;46:1–7.
9. Backensfeld T, Müller BW, Kolter K. Int J Pharmaceutics 1991;74:85–93.
10. Zecchi V, Rodriguez L, Tartarini A, Fini A. Arch Pharm (Weinheim) 1984;317:897–905.
11. Paton DM. Int J Clin Pharm Res 1987;7(4):239–42.
12. Van Wilder P, Detaevernier MR, Michotte Y. Drug Dev Ind Pharm 1991;17(1):141–8.
13. Bain JC, Tan SB, Ganderton D, Solomon MC. Drug Dev Ind Pharm 1991;17(2):215–32.
14. Malamataris S, Ganderton D. Int J Pharmaceutics 1991;70:69–75.
15. Peña Romero A, Poncet M, Jinot JC, Chulia D [French]. Pharm Acta Helv 1988;63(12):333–42.
16. Peña Romero A, Caramella C, Ronchi M, Ferrari F, Chulia D. Int J Pharmaceutics 1991;73:239–48.
17. Acarturk F. Pharmazie 1989;44(H8):547–9.
18. Acarturk F. Pharmazie 1989;44(H9):621–2.
19. Takamura A, Ishii F, Noro S, Koishi M. J Pharm Sci 1984;73(5):676–81.
20. Naito S-I, Tominaga H. Int J Pharmaceutics 1985;24:115–24.
21. Vyas SP, Gogoi PJ, Jain SK. Drug Dev Ind Pharm 1991;17(8):1041–58.
22. Nishihata T, Wada H, Kamada A. Int J Pharmaceutics 1985;27:245–53.
23. Nishihata T, Tsutsumi A, Ikawa C, Sakai K. Drug Dev Ind Pharm 1990;16(10):1675–86.
24. Terhaag B, le Petit G, Richter K, Rogner M. Pharmazie 1985;40(H11):784–6.

Diethylcarbamazine (BAN, rINN)

Anthelmintic (antifilarial)

N,N-Diethyl-4-methylpiperazine-1-carboxamide
$C_{10}H_{21}N_3O = 199.3$

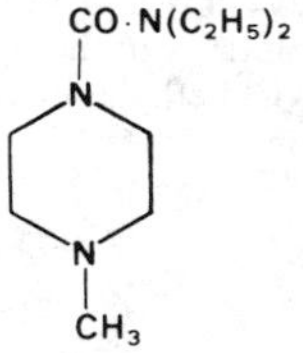

Diethylcarbamazine Citrate (BANM, rINNM)

$C_{10}H_{21}N_3O, C_6H_8O_7 = 391.4$
CAS—90-89-1 (diethylcarbamazine); 1642-54-2 (diethylcarbamazine citrate)

Pharmacopoeial status

BP, USP (diethylcarbamazine citrate)

Preparations

Compendial
Diethylcarbamazine Citrate Tablets USP.

Containers and storage

Solid state
Diethylcarbamazine Citrate BP should be kept in an airtight container.
Diethylcarbamazine Citrate USP should be preserved in tight containers.

Dosage forms
Diethylcarbamazine Citrate Tablets USP should be preserved in tight containers.

PHYSICAL PROPERTIES

Diethylcarbamazine exists as a crystalline powder.
Diethylcarbamazine citrate exists as a white crystalline powder; odourless or with a slight odour; slightly hygroscopic, with a bitter acid taste.

Melting point

Diethylcarbamazine melts at about 49°.
Diethylcarbamazine citrate melts between 136° and 141°, with decomposition.

Dissociation constant

pK_a 7.7 (20°)

Solubility

Diethylcarbamazine is soluble in water, in ethanol, in chloroform, and in ether.
Diethylcarbamazine citrate is very soluble in water, sparingly soluble in ethanol (1 in 35), and practically insoluble in acetone, in chloroform, and in ether.

Dissolution

The USP specifies that for Diethylcarbamazine Citrate Tablets USP not less than 75% of the labelled amount of $C_{10}H_{21}N_3O, C_6H_8O_7$ is dissolved in 45 minutes. Dissolution medium: 900 mL of water; Apparatus 2 at 50 rpm.

FORMULATION

Excipients

Excipients that have been used in presentations of diethylcarbamazine citrate include:
Tablets: lactose; magnesium stearate; silica (hydrated); starch.

Modified-release preparations

An experimental modified-release tablet of diethylcarbamazine as the salt with pamoic acid based on calcium hydrogen phosphate and granulated with ethylcellulose (in acetone) was stable and maintained release integrity over a 3-month period of storage under normal and elevated temperature and humidity conditions.[1] Release *in vitro* was almost uniform for 10 to 12 hours. Plots of urinary excretion (in normal volunteers) with time indicated that the product maintained steady-state levels for about 12 hours.
A mixture of Eudragit RS and Eudragit RL (polymethacrylates; 1% w/v in acetone) was used at an optimum ratio of 75:25 to coat tablets of diethylcarbamazine citrate (compressed with talc, lactose, and Eudragit RS 5%). The zero-order release rate was in linear relationship with the film thickness.[2] Uniform release over 11 hours was sustained at 4.5 mg/hour. An *in-vivo* comparison with standard commercial tablets involving healthy volunteers indicated that the test tablets maintained steady-state concentrations for about 12 hours.

FURTHER INFORMATION. Controlled clinical trial of oral and topical diethylcarbamazine in treatment of onchocerciasis [comparison of oral tablets and Nivea-based lotion (2%)]—Taylor HR, Greene BM, Langham ME. Lancet 1980;1:943–6.

PROCESSING

Sterilisation

Solutions of diethylcarbamazine citrate for injection are sterilised by autoclaving.

REFERENCES

1. Baveja SK, Ranga Rao KV, Kumar R, Padmalatha Devi K. Int J Pharmaceutics 1985;24:355–8.
2. Baveja SK, Ranga Rao KV, Singh A. Int J Pharmaceutics 1984;19:229–31.

Diethylpropion (BAN)

Appetite suppressant

Amfepramone (pINN)
α-Diethylaminopropiophenone;   2-(diethylamino)-1-phenyl-1-propanone
$C_{13}H_{19}NO = 205.3$

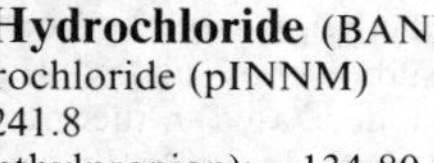

Diethylpropion Hydrochloride (BANM)

Amfepramone Hydrochloride (pINNM)
$C_{13}H_{19}NO, HCl = 241.8$
CAS—90-84-6 (diethylpropion); 134-80-5 (diethylpropion hydrochloride)

Pharmacopoeial status

BP, USP (diethylpropion hydrochloride)

Preparations

Compendial
Diethylpropion Hydrochloride Tablets USP.

Non-compendial
Tenuate Dospan (Merrell). *Tablets*, sustained release, diethylpropion hydrochloride 75 mg, in a hydrophilic colloid gum.

Containers and storage

Solid state
Diethylpropion Hydrochloride BP should be kept in a well-closed container, protected from light and stored at a temperature not exceeding 25°.
Diethylpropion Hydrochloride USP should be preserved in well-closed, light-resistant containers.

Dosage forms
Diethylpropion Hydrochloride Tablets USP should be preserved in well-closed containers.
Tenuate Dospan tablets should be stored in a cool, dry place.

PHYSICAL PROPERTIES

Diethylpropion hydrochloride is a white or almost white, fine crystalline powder; odourless or with a slight characteristic odour.

Melting point

Diethylpropion hydrochloride melts at about 175°, with decomposition.

Dissociation constant

pK_a 8.7

Solubility

Diethylpropion hydrochloride is freely soluble in water, in ethanol, and in chloroform; it is practically insoluble in ether.

Dissolution

The USP specifies that for Diethylpropion Hydrochloride Tablets USP not less than 75% of the labelled amount of $C_{13}H_{19}NO$, HCl is dissolved in 45 minutes. Dissolution medium: 900 mL of water; Apparatus 2 at 50 rpm.

FURTHER INFORMATION. Dissolution profiling of six modified-release oral solid dosage forms [includes one brand of diethylpropion hydrochloride tablets]—Baweja R. Drug Dev Ind Pharm 1986;12(14):2431–42.

STABILITY

Tartaric acid may be added as a stabilising agent to diethylpropion in the solid state; the BP permits 1%.
In aqueous solution diethylpropion hydrochloride degrades to form several products of which two have been attributed to hydrolysis and identified as diethylamine and 1-phenyl-1,2-propanedione; the latter is highly volatile.[1,2] Walters and Walters[1] identified and isolated the two compounds (by HPLC) from subpotent tablets of diethylpropion hydrochloride and demonstrated that the stability of diethylpropion hydrochloride, alone and as tablets, decreased in the presence of moisture. In further studies[2] of diethylpropion hydrochloride in aqueous solutions of various buffers at 45°, hydrolysis was demonstrated to be slow at pH below 3.5. As the pH was increased above 3.5 the rate increased markedly. A possible hydrolytic decomposition pathway which has been proposed involves enamine forma-tion and further complex rearrangement to diethylamine and several tautomeric species. Samples of six commercial tablets of diethylpropion hydrochloride (from five manufacturers) which were dispersed in water at 45° for 10 days revealed a greater stability in formulations that had pH values below 4. Photo-irradiation (at 254 nm) and radium-irradiation of aqueous and methanolic solutions of diethylpropion hydrochloride have been reported to yield ethylamine, diethylamine, acetaldehyde, and propiophenone.[3]

FORMULATION

Excipients

Excipients that have been used in presentations of diethylpropion hydrochloride include:
Capsules: maize starch; povidone; shellac; sucrose; talc; tartaric acid.
Tablets: lactose; magnesium stearate; maize starch; mannitol; pregelatinised maize starch; talc; tartaric acid.
Tablets (sustained release): carbomer 934P; lactose; mannitol; povidone; tartaric acid; zinc stearate.

REFERENCES

1. Walters MJ, Walters SM. J Pharm Sci 1977;66(2):198–201.
2. Walters SM. J Pharm Sci 1980;69(10):1206–9.
3. Weidman KG, Wolf A, Reisch J [German]. Arch Pharm 1973;306:954–8.

Digoxin (BAN, rINN)   *Cardiac glycoside*

Digoxosidum
3β-[O-2,6-Dideoxy-β-D-*ribo*-hexopyranosyl-(1 → 4)-O-2,6-dideoxy-β-D-*ribo*-hexopyranosyl-(1 → 4)-2,6-dideoxy-β-D-*ribo*-hexopyranosyl)-oxy]-12β,14β-dihydroxy-5β-card-20(22)-enolide; card-20(22)-enolide,3-[(O-2,6-dideoxy- β-D-*ribo*-hexopyranosyl-(1 → 4)-O-2,6-dideoxy-β-D-*ribo*-hexopyranosyl-(1 → 4)-2,6-dideoxy-β-D-*ribo*-hexopyranosyl)oxy]-12,14-dihydroxy-,(3β,5β,12β)-.
$C_{41}H_{64}O_{14}$ = 780.9
CAS—20830-75-5

Pharmacopoeial status

BP, USP

Preparations

Compendial

Digoxin Tablets BP. Tablets containing, in each, 62.5, 125, and 250 micrograms are usually available.

Paediatric Digoxin Oral Solution BP (Paediatric Digoxin Elixir). A solution containing 0.005% w/v of digoxin in a suitable flavoured vehicle. pH 6.8 to 7.2. It should not be diluted.

Digoxin Injection BP. pH 6.7 to 7.3. See Formulation, below.

Paediatric Digoxin Injection BP. pH 6.7 to 7.3. See Formulation, below.

Digoxin Tablets USP.

Digoxin Elixir USP.

Digoxin Injection USP.

Non-compendial

Lanoxin (Wellcome). *Tablets*, digoxin 125 and 250 micrograms. *Injection*, digoxin 250 micrograms/mL. The injection (250 micrograms/mL) is compatible when diluted (either under full aseptic conditions or immediately before use) with the following intravenous infusion solutions: sodium chloride 0.9% injection; glucose 5% injection; sodium chloride 0.18% and glucose 4% injection. Any unused solution should be discarded.

Lanoxin-PG (Wellcome). *Tablets*, digoxin 62.5 micrograms. *Elixir*, digoxin 50 micrograms/mL. Do not dilute, measure with pipette.

A paediatric injection of digoxin 100 micrograms/mL is available (hospital use only) from Boots.

Containers and storage

Solid state

Digoxin BP should be kept in a well-closed container and protected from light.

Digoxin USP should be preserved in tight containers.

Dosage forms

Paediatric Digoxin Oral Solution BP, Digoxin Injection BP, and Paediatric Digoxin Injection BP should all be protected from light. The Paediatric Oral Solution should be stored at a temperature not exceeding 25°.

Digoxin Tablets USP and Digoxin Elixir USP should be preserved in tight containers. Exposure of the elixir to excessive heat should be avoided. Digoxin Injection USP should be preserved in single-dose containers, preferably of Type I glass. Avoid exposure to excessive heat.

Lanoxin preparations should be stored below 25°. The injection should be protected from light.

PHYSICAL PROPERTIES

Digoxin exists as clear to white crystals or as a white or almost white powder; odourless.

Melting point

Digoxin melts, with decomposition, within the range 230° to 265°.

Chiou and Kyle[1] reported values ranging between 137° and 235° for the beginning and end of melting, respectively, of commercial samples of digoxin powders.

Solubility

Digoxin is practically insoluble in water, in acetone, in ether, and in ethyl acetate; slightly soluble in chloroform and in ethanol; at 20° it is soluble 1 in 122 of diluted ethanol (80%); freely soluble

in pyridine and in a mixture of equal volumes of chloroform and methanol.

Chiou and Kyle[1] determined that the solubilities of different untreated samples of digoxin in water at 37° (stirred at 200 rpm) ranged from 28.9 to 68.2 micrograms/mL. Recrystallisation from chloroform and from ethanol improved solubility although variation was evident between samples from different commercial sources. The effect of trituration of the powder was unpredictable and any enhancement of solubility as a result of milling or trituration was only temporary.

Dissolution

The BP states that, after following the specified dissolution test for Digoxin Tablets BP, the amount of digoxin per tablet in solution should not be less than 75% of the prescribed or stated amount.

The USP specifies that for Digoxin Tablets USP not less than 65% of the labelled amount of $C_{41}H_{64}O_{14}$ is dissolved in 60 minutes for not fewer than eleven-twelfths of the tablets tested, and no individual tablet tested is less than 55% dissolved in 60 minutes. Dissolution medium: as specified in USP monograph; Apparatus 1 at 120 rpm.

Dissolution properties

The dissolution and bioavailability of digoxin tablets from different sources were reviewed by Leach.[2] Aspects considered were the correlation of *in-vitro* and *in-vivo* data; batch to batch variation; dissolution procedures; and the relationship between particle size and dissolution rate. See also Bioavailability, below.

FURTHER INFORMATION. Observations on the use of compressed discs in dissolution studies [intrinsic dissolution rates]—Salole EG, Florence AT. Drug Dev Commun 1976;2(2):141–9.

STABILITY

Solid state

Digoxin powder is stable at room temperature and 75% relative humidity.

Solutions

In aqueous solutions of pH 1 to 4 at 37° digoxin hydrolysed[3] via a complex combination of parallel reactions to produce digoxigenin (unreactive), digoxigenin bisglycoside, and digoxigenin monoglycoside; both glycosides may undergo further hydrolysis. The hydrolysis followed pseudo-first-order kinetics and, at pH 1 and pH 2, the half-life of digoxin was 13.5 minutes and 131 minutes, respectively. Limited hydrolysis occurred at pH 7 over a period of 48 hours.

Half-life values for the hydrolysis of digoxin (0.0005 to 0.002% w/v) in acidic buffers and dissolution media ranged from 19.4 minutes (at pH 1.1) to 256.7 minutes (at pH 2.2). During one hour at pH 1.3, 27.5% hydrolysis occurred; there was no apparent hydrolysis in water over the same period.[4]

Dosage forms

Ninety-two samples of digoxin tablets from 44 different batches (three manufacturers) stored in hospitals throughout the USA were tested for content uniformity, potency, and dissolution properties. Most of the tablets tested were within 12 to 16 months of their expiry date. The authors concluded that digoxin tablets available from hospital pharmacies in the USA were stable in terms of uniformity, potency, and dissolution.[5]

In a factorially designed experiment, some of the digoxin tablets (0.25 mg) directly compressed with Emcompress (calcium hydrogen phosphate) and starch failed the dissolution test of the USP XXI after 9 months storage, but none degraded during 12 months.[6]

In general, dosage forms containing digoxin are stable when stored in well-closed containers and protected from light.

Stabilisation

The hydrolysis of digoxin during dissolution and a possible means of preventing digoxin degradation in acidic media were studied by Sonobe et al.[7] Equations representing dissolution and degradation behaviour were devised. Powders of digoxin mixed with either magnesium hydroxide-aluminium hydroxide, magnesium oxide, or aluminium silicate showed reduced decomposition under the USP XIX dissolution test conditions compared to a reference sample with no antacid.

Complexation of digoxin with α-cyclodextrin, β-cyclodextrin, and γ-cyclodextrin and the resultant effects on the rate of digoxin degradation and dissolution were studied by Uekama et al.[8] Digoxin hydrolysis was suppressed; the inhibitory effect of cyclodextrins decreasing in the order $\beta > \gamma > \alpha$.

INCOMPATIBILITY/COMPATIBILITY

Infusions

Digoxin injection (Burroughs Wellcome) was visually compatible when mixed with glucose 5% injection, sodium chloride 0.9% injection, compound sodium lactate injection, and glucose 5% in sodium chloride 0.45% with 20 mEq potassium chloride injection to provide 250 micrograms/100 mL solutions.[9] Radioimmunoassay indicated that all four admixtures were chemically stable for six hours. In addition digoxin was stable over a 48-hour study period in glucose 5% injection and in sodium chloride 0.9% injection.

Two admixtures which contained differing concentrations of milrinone and digoxin in glucose 5% injection were physically and chemically stable[10] after 4 hours at 22° to 23°.

Digoxin was included in a review of the compatibility of drugs in parenteral nutrition solutions.[11]

Adsorption

Adsorption of digoxin onto the clay montmorillonite (a major component of bentonite) was described by Porubcan et al.[12] At pH 6, over 90% of the initial digoxin concentration was adsorbed whereas at pH 2 an initial adsorption of 81% decreased to 22% over 5 hours. Adsorbed digoxin degraded at abnormally rapid rates (bisdigoxigenin was the main product) and it was suggested that the degradation rate increased owing to the ability of montmorillonite to concentrate digoxin molecules and protons on its surface, creating an acidic microenvironment in which digoxin hydrolysis was catalysed. The authors advised against the concomitant administration of drug products containing digoxin and montmorillonite.

FURTHER INFORMATION. The uptake of digoxin and digitoxin by some antacids—Khalil SAH. J Pharm Pharmacol 1974;26:961–7.

FORMULATION

DIGOXIN INJECTION BP

Digoxin	25 mg
Ethanol (80%)	12.5 mL
Propylene glycol	40 mL
Citric acid monohydrate	75 mg
Sodium phosphate	0.45 g
Water for injections sufficient to produce	100 mL

Dissolve the digoxin in the ethanol (80%) and add the propylene glycol, a solution of the citric acid monohydrate and the sodium phosphate in water for injections and sufficient water for injections to produce 100 mL.

PAEDIATRIC DIGOXIN INJECTION BP

Digoxin	10 mg
Ethanol (80%)	12.5 mL
Propylene glycol	40 mL
Citric acid monohydrate	75 mg
Sodium phosphate	0.45 g
Water for injections sufficient to produce	100 mL

Dissolve the digoxin in the ethanol (80%) and add the propylene glycol, a solution of the citric acid monohydrate and the sodium phosphate in water for injections and sufficient water for injections to produce 100 mL.

Excipients

Excipients that have been used in presentations of digoxin include:

Tablets: allura red AC (E129); D&C Green No.5; lactose; magnesium stearate; maize starch; potato starch; quinoline yellow (E104); stearic acid; sunset yellow FCF (E110); talc.

Paediatric oral solutions: citric acid; D&C Green No.5; ethanol; glycerol; methyl hydroxybenzoate; propylene glycol; quinoline yellow (E104); saccharin sodium; sodium phosphate; strawberry extract; sucrose.

Injections and paediatric injections: citric acid (anhydrous); ethanol; propylene glycol; sodium phosphate.

Bioavailability

The difference between the therapeutic and toxic blood concentrations of digoxin is very small and it is therefore essential to control the amount of bioavailable digoxin. It has been established that different formulations, and in some cases different batches of the same formulation, of digoxin tablets can vary considerably both in digoxin content and in bioavailability; a seven-fold variation in blood concentrations has been demonstrated between different formulations of the same labelled strength.

The differences in bioavailability have been shown to correspond very closely with variations in the dissolution rate. It has been suggested that differences in particle size and crystal form are mainly responsible for the variations in dissolution rate. See also Dissolution, above.

Tablets

To prepare rapidly dissolving digoxin tablets, potassium chloride or urea were used as directly compressible fillers; digoxin was incorporated either by simple blending or by deposition from solvent.[13] Tablets made using the solvent deposition method had faster dissolution rates and showed improved dissolution rate profiles over commercial tablets.

In a comparison of the pharmaceutical properties of two formulations of digoxin tablets,[14] both disintegrated within 10 minutes but dissolution rates differed markedly. It was suggested that this difference may be due either to variation of particle size or degree of crystallinity of the respective active principles or to the effect of povidone included as an excipient. Diffusion studies indicated that povidone lowered the diffusion rate of digoxin.

Capsules

A preparation of digoxin in soft gelatin capsules (Lanoxicaps, Burroughs Wellcome) is available in the USA. In young healthy volunteers, bioavailability from the capsules and from digoxin tablets (Lanoxin) was claimed to be 90% to 100% and 60% to 80%, respectively.[15] Drinka et al[16] noted an increase in the mean digoxin concentration in plasma when Lanoxin capsules were replaced by Lanoxin tablets in a study that lasted several months and involved 39 debilitated elderly patients. However, when workers in Holland[17] compared the bioavailability of the two preparations in elderly patients they concluded that the absorption of digoxin from tablets and capsules appeared to be similar.

FURTHER INFORMATION. Bioavailability of digoxin from rapidly dissolving preparations—Johnson BF, Lader S. Br J Clin Pharmacol 1974;1:329–33. Influence of soft gelatin on digoxin absorption—O'Grady J, Johnson BF, Bye C, Sabey GA. Br J Clin Pharmacol 1978;5:461–3.

PROCESSING

CAUTION. The USP states that digoxin should be handled with exceptional care, since it is extremely poisonous.

Sterilisation

Digoxin injection and digoxin paediatric injection can be sterilised by heating in an autoclave.

Comminution

Florence and Salole[18] examined the differences in physical properties of digoxin from various sources before and after comminution. Under a scanning electron microscope, normal samples appeared as either thin plates, mixtures of 'fines' and thick angular crystals, or as large crystals arranged in clusters. Equilibrium solubilities at 25°, powder dissolution rates, and melting behaviour differed between samples. Comminution by grinding or milling altered physical properties and the final common state was essentially characteristic of an amorphous material. Melting points were substantially lower than the originals and apparent equilibrium solubilities at 25° increased by 7% to 118% over those of the starting materials. Dissolution rates also increased but previously identified correlations between dissolution rate and solubility or surface area were no longer apparent. A powder dissolution test was recommended as a suitable technique for standardising polymorphic drugs of low solubility.

FURTHER INFORMATION. Estimation of the degree of crystallinity in digoxin by X-ray and infrared methods—Black DB, Lovering EG. J Pharm Pharmacol 1977;29:684–7.

REFERENCES

1. Chiou WL, Kyle LE. J Pharm Sci 1979;68(10):1224–9.
2. Leach RH. Proceedings of the Guild 1979;No.4:3–16.
3. Sternson LA, Shaffer RD. J Pharm Sci 1978;67(3):327–30.
4. Khalil SAH, El-Masry S. J Pharm Sci 1978;67(10):1358–60.
5. Belson JJ, Juhl YH, Moyer ES, Page DP, Shroff AP. Am J Hosp Pharm 1981;38:1903–7.
6. Vila-Jato JL, Concheiro A, Torres D. STP Pharma 1985;1:194–200.
7. Sonobe T, Hasumi S, Yoshino T, Kobayashi Y, Kawata H, Nagai T. J Pharm Sci 1980;69(4):410–13.
8. Uekama K, Fujinaga T, Hirayama F, Otagiri M, Kurono Y, Ikeda K. J Pharm Pharmacol 1982;34:627–30.
9. Shank WA, Coupal JJ. Am J Hosp Pharm 1982;39:844–6.
10. Riley CM. Am J Hosp Pharm 1988;45:2079–91.
11. Niemiec PW, Vanderveen TW. Am J Hosp Pharm 1984;41:893–911.
12. Porubcan LS, Born GS, White JL, Hem SL. J Pharm Sci 1979;68(3):358–61.
13. El Gholmy ZA, El-Khordagui LK, Hammouda Y. Drug Dev Ind Pharm 1988;14(11):1587–603.
14. Bramanti G, Mura P, Liguori A, Ceccarelli L, Santoni G, Grossi G, Torresi MC. Int J Pharmaceutics 1989;49:241–7.
15. Pharm J 1984;233:653.
16. Drinka PJ, Nickel DA, Schomisch GW, Depka CH, Deterville RJ. DICP Ann Pharmacother 1990;24:381–2.
17. Hooymans PM, Pouwels MJ, van der Aa GCHM, Gribnau FWJ. Pharm Weekbl (Sci) 1989;11(6):K4.
18. Florence AT, Salole EG. J Pharm Pharmacol 1976;28:637–42.

Dithranol (BAN, rINN)   *Antipsoriatic*

Anthralin; dioxyanthranol
1,8-Dihydroxyanthrone; 1,8-dihydroxy-9(10H)anthracenone
$C_{14}H_{10}O_3 = 226.2$

Dithranol Triacetate (BANM, rINNM)
Dithranol acetate
$C_{20}H_{16}O_6 = 352.3$
CAS—1143-38-0 (dithranol); 16203-97-7 (dithranol triacetate)

Pharmacopoeial status

BP (dithranol); USP (anthralin)

Preparations

Compendial

Dithranol Ointment BP. Contains dithranol, in fine powder, in a suitable hydrophobic basis. (See Formulation below). Ointments containing 0.1% to 1% w/w of dithranol are usually available.
Dithranol Paste BP. Contains dithranol in a suitable hydrophobic basis containing 24% w/w each of zinc oxide and starch and 2% w/w of salicylic acid. (See Formulation, below). Pastes containing 0.1% to 1% are usually available.
Anthralin Cream USP.
Anthralin Ointment USP.

Non-compendial

Alphodith (Stafford-Miller). *Ointment*, dithranol 0.4%, 1%, 2%, and 3% w/w.
Anthranol (Stiefel). *Ointment*, dithranol 0.4%, 1%, and 2% w/w.
Dithrocream (Dermal). *Cream* (aqueous), dithranol in a water-miscible basis, 0.1%, 0.25%, 0.5%, 1%, and 2% w/w.
Dithrolan (Dermal). *Ointment* (stiff), dithranol 0.5% w/w in equal quantities of hard and soft paraffin.
Exolan (Dermal). *Cream*, dithranol triacetate 1% w/w in a water-miscible basis.
Psoradrate (Norwich Eaton). *Cream*, dithranol 0.1% and 0.2% w/w in a powder-in-cream basis containing urea.
Psorin (Thames). *Ointment*, dithranol 0.11% w/w, crude coal tar 1% w/w, and salicylic acid 1.6% w/w in an emollient basis.

Containers and storage

Solid state

Dithranol BP should be kept in a well-closed container and protected from light.

Anthralin USP should be preserved in tight containers in a cool place and protected from light.

Dosage forms
Dithranol Ointment BP and Dithranol Paste BP. The labels of both state that the preparations should be protected from light. Alphodith ointment and Anthranol ointment should be stored in a cool place.
Anthralin Cream USP and Anthralin Ointment USP should be preserved in tight containers, in a cool place and protected from light.
Dithrocream and Exolan cream should be stored in a cool place and the cap replaced tightly after use.
Dithrolan ointment should be kept in a dark place and not exposed to direct heat. After use the cap must be replaced.
Psoradrate cream should be kept in a cool place. Psorin ointment should be kept in a cool place, away from light.

PHYSICAL PROPERTIES

Dithranol is a yellow to yellowish-brown, microcrystalline powder; odourless or almost odourless; tasteless.

Melting point

Dithranol melts in the range 175° to 181°.

pH

The filtrate from a suspension of *dithranol* in water is neutral to litmus.

Dissociation constant

pK_a 9.4[2]

Solubility

Dithranol is practically insoluble or insoluble in water; slightly soluble in ethanol, in ether, in glacial acetic acid, and in fixed oils; soluble in chloroform, in acetone, in benzene, and in alkali hydroxide solutions.

STABILITY

Degradation pathways

Dithranol is readily degraded in air by light and heat. In buffered solutions (made by dilution from concentrates in organic solvents) or in organic solvents alone, decomposition is rapid to a complex mixture of breakdown products. The major oxidation product is danthron (1,8-dihydroxy-9,10-anthraquinone) but oxidative dimerisation yields dianthrones, dimers of bi(1,8-dihydroxy-9-anthron-10-yl). By polymerisation or cross-linking insoluble coloured materials form (dithranol brown); as yet, these have not been identified.[1-3]
Degradation products are also common constituents of dithranol in the solid state. Both danthron and dianthrone (dimer) were identified and quantified in a commercial sample by Elsabbagh *et al*.[1]
Albert[4] determined dithranol and its degradation products (danthron and dianthrone) in eleven samples of bulk substances and in ten commercial ointments. Danthron (up to 2.6%) was found in ten bulk samples and (up to 7.4%) in four ointments. For dianthrone the contents were up to 6.2% in six bulk samples and up to 19.5% in three ointments.

Buffer-solvent systems

Taskinen *et al*[2] found that dithranol degraded rapidly in methanol (50%)-buffer solutions (pH 6.5 and 7.4) and in Hepes buffer

(pH 9.4). The decomposition rate increased with increasing pH; the half-life at pH 9.4 was 0.6 hours. The only decomposition product detected (by HPLC) was danthron which accounted for 50% of the decomposed dithranol at pH 9.4 after 90 minutes in the dark at room temperature.
Cavey *et al*[5] investigated the stability of dithranol (0.5 mg/mL) in acetone (1%)-Ringer's buffer (pH 7.5 at 37°, protected from light) and showed that complete decomposition occurred within 4 hours. The main decomposition product (40% of total) was identified as the 10,10-dimer but danthron was not detected. In simple acetone solution (0.5 mg/mL), exposed to light and air at 25°, dithranol decomposed completely within 4 days. Degradation was partly via the dimer as the intermediate, but the final solution, which had the characteristic colour of dithranol brown, contained danthron (20%). Similarly to the decomposed acetone (1%)-Ringer solutions of dithranol, the final solution completely inhibited the activity of glucose-6-phosphate dehydrogenase (a test system to indicate antipsoriatic activity).
Decomposition of dithranol has been shown to follow apparent first-order kinetics in aqueous ethanol-Tris buffer solution at 25° in the pH range 7.74 to 10.02 (ionic strength 0.5). From first-derivative absorbance spectra at 263 nm an Arrhenius plot was derived which demonstrated the temperature dependence of the decomposition, from 25° to 45°, and yielded an activation energy of 57.31 kJ/mol.[6]

Salt hydrolysis

Dithranol triacetate is hydrolysed in contact with water to form the active diacetyl compound, 1,8-diacetoxy-9-anthranol. It is claimed to be less staining and irritant to the skin than dithranol.

Ointments and pastes

In zinc oxide paste the chemical deterioration of dithranol has been shown[3] to be dependent on the interaction at the surface of the zinc oxide particles. The products of degradation remained on the zinc oxide surface. Deterioration could be greatly reduced by the addition of salicylic acid at the time of preparation. Studies of other solid surfaces indicated that both moisture and the adsorbent surface influence the decomposition of dithranol.
In a study of the clinical effects of components of dithranol paste[7] the development of a pink colour which became mauve, violet, and then dark brown was attributed to a reaction between zinc oxide and dithranol in the paste. The effectiveness of discoloured pastes was impaired in the treatment of psoriasis patients. Benzoic acid and salicylic acid were both found to be equally effective in the prevention and reversal of discoloration. Maloney[8] recommended the dispensing of dithranol in Lassar's paste (which includes salicylic acid 2%) rather than in compound zinc paste (with no salicylic acid) in order to avoid the rapid discoloration that occurs when the less effective zinc oxide-dithranol complex is formed. Dithranol products should be stored in well-filled, amber glass containers, sealed with a non-metallic cap to reduce decomposition by light and air.
Spectrophotometric analysis and quantification of colour changes of a stiff dithranol 0.5% ointment with added salicylic acid (0.3% to 2%) indicated that the optimum salicylic acid content ranged from 0.125% to 0.5%. In samples with salicylic acid 0.3%, colour change was inhibited for 2.25 years provided the ointment was protected from light and air. A double-blind clinical assessment of effectiveness was made in psoriatic patients.[9] Ointments which contained dithranol in concentrations of 0.05%, 0.1%, or 0.2%, with salicylic acid 0.5% and emulsifying ointment to 100% were found to be relatively unstable when

compared to ointments containing dithranol 0.5% to 1.0%, over a study period of 112 days.[10] The major degradation product detected was danthron. Over 56 days, stability of the ointment (dithranol 0.05%) was improved by the addition of 0.1% or 0.5% but not 1% ascorbyl palmitate.

Dithranol 0.05% w/w in an emulsifying ointment-based formulation with salicylic acid 0.5%, and containing ascorbyl palmitate 0.1%, was found to be stable (less than 10% dithranol content lost) when stored for 52 weeks at room temperature but less stable (57% of original dithranol content lost) when stored at 37°.[11] In contrast, dithranol 0.05% in Lassar's paste was stable for only 4 weeks at room temperature.

Lee[12] investigated the stability of dithranol, under dark and light conditions, when dissolved in methanol, in chloroform, or both, or dispersed in yellow soft paraffin, or in Zinc and Salicylic Acid Paste APF (Lassar's Paste). Methanolic solutions of dithranol 0.0015% w/v which contained salicylic acid were more stable than those without salicylic acid. Estimated shelf-lives for dithranol 4% w/v in chloroform, dithranol 1% w/w in yellow soft paraffin, and dithranol 0.5% w/w in Lassar's Paste were 101 days, 397 days, and 200 days, respectively, when protected from light.

FURTHER INFORMATION. Studies on the oxidation behaviour of dithranol—Schaltegger vA [German]. Arzneimittelforschung/Drug Res 1985;35(I)Nr4:666–8. The effect of surfactants on the solubility and stability of aqueous solutions of dithranol—Moody RR, Lubwika P. J Pharm Pharmacol 1992;44(Suppl):1051.

FORMULATION

Excipients

Excipients that have been used in presentations of dithranol include:

Ointments, dithranol: ascorbyl palmitate; butylated hydroxytoluene; cetyl alcohol; citric acid; cod liver oil; hard paraffin; lanolin; liquid paraffin; magnesium lauryl sulphate; maize starch; propylene glycol; salicylic acid; sodium lauryl sulphate; tocopherol; white soft paraffin; yellow beeswax; yellow soft paraffin; zinc oxide.

Creams, dithranol: aluminium distearate; ascorbic acid; ascorbyl palmitate; butylated hydroxyanisole; cetostearyl alcohol; chlorocresol; citric acid; disodium edetate; liquid paraffin; methyl and propyl hydroxybenzoates; octyldodecanol; polyglyceryl-4-oleate; polysorbate 40; salicylic acid; sodium bisulphite; sodium lauryl sulphate; tocopherol; white soft paraffin.

Dithranol triacetate: chlorocresol; emulsifying wax; liquid paraffin; white soft paraffin.

Ointments

A stiffened ointment evaluated by Seville[13] contained dithranol 0.5%, salicylic acid 0.5%, and chloroform 2.5%, in hard paraffin and white soft paraffin in equal quantities to 100%. The paraffins were heated until just melted, then triturated until smooth and brilliant white. Dithranol and salicylic acid dispersed in chloroform were added and triturated until cool. The ointment was rubbed down on a slab until smooth before being stored in the dark. The preparation appeared to have a shelf-life of more than one year and was claimed to be preferable to the paste for domiciliary treatment.

FURTHER INFORMATION. *In-vitro* and *in-vivo* comparison of creams containing dithranol 0.5%—Ros JJW, Van der Meer YG, De Hoop D, De Kort WJA, Van Andel P. Pharm Weekbl (Sci) 1991;13(5):210–4. A new diffusion cell—an automated method for measuring the pharmaceutical availability of topical dosage forms—Martin B, Watts O, Shroot B, Jamoulle JC. Int J Pharmaceutics 1989;49:63–8. Dithranol and related compounds. [A comprehensive historical review of dithranol development]. In: Polano MK, editor. Topical skin therapeutics. London: Churchill Livingstone, 1984:80–5.

PROCESSING

CAUTION. Dithranol is a powerful irritant and should be kept away from the eyes and tender parts of the skin.

REFERENCES

1. Elsabbagh HM, Whitworth CW, Schramm LC. J Pharm Sci 1979;68(3):388–90.
2. Taskinen J, Haarala J, Wartiovaara E, Halmekoski J. Arch Pharm (Weinheim) 1988;321:103–6.
3. Ponec-Waelsch M, Hulsebosch HJ. Arch Derm Forsch 1974;249:141–52.
4. Albert K [German]. Pharm Ztg 1985;130(41):2600–4.
5. Cavey D, Caron J-C, Shroot B. J Pharm Sci 1982;71(9):980–3.
6. Upadrashta SM, Wurster DE. Drug Dev Ind Pharm 1988;14(6):749–64.
7. Comaish S, Smith J, Seville RH. Br J Dermatol 1971;84:282–9.
8. Maloney TJ. Aust J Hosp Pharm 1977;7(3):120.
9. Bellis JD, Seville RH, Smith JF. J Clin Pharm 1978;3:7–11.
10. Middleton KR, Newman C. Proceedings of the Guild 1985;23:59–62.
11. Weller PJ, Newman CM, Middleton KR, Wicker SM. J Clin Pharm Ther 1990;15:419–23.
12. Lee RLH. Aust J Hosp Pharm 1987;17(4):254–8.
13. Seville RH. Br J Dermatol 1975;93:205–8.

Doxorubicin (BAN, USAN, rINN)   *Cytotoxic*

Adriamycin; 14-hydroxydaunorubicin; 3-hydroxyacetyldaunorubicin

8-Hydroxyacetyl (8*S*,10*S*)-10-[(3-amino-2,3,6-trideoxy-α-L-*lyxo*-hexopyranosyl)oxy]-6,8,11-trihydroxy-1-methoxy-7,8,9,10-tetrahydronaphthacene-5,12-dione; an anthracycline antibiotic produced by *Streptomyces peucetius*.

$C_{27}H_{29}NO_{11} = 543.5$

Doxorubicin Hydrochloride (BANM, rINNM)

$C_{27}H_{29}NO_{11}$, HCl = 580.0

CAS—23214-92-8 (doxorubicin); 25316-40-9 (doxorubicin hydrochloride)

Pharmacopoeial status

BP, USP (doxorubicin hydrochloride)

Preparations

Compendial
Doxorubicin Hydrochloride Injection USP. pH between 2.5 and 4.5.
Doxorubicin Hydrochloride for Injection USP. pH between 4.5 and 6.5, in the solution constituted as directed in the labelling, except that water is used as the diluent.

Non-compendial
Doxorubicin Rapid Dissolution (Farmitalia Carlo Erba). *Injection*, powder for reconstitution with water for injections or sodium chloride 0.9% injection, doxorubicin hydrochloride 10 mg per vial and 50 mg per vial.
Doxorubicin Solution for Injection (Farmitalia Carlo Erba). *Injection*, doxorubicin hydrochloride 2 mg/mL in sodium chloride 0.9% injection. Prolonged contact of Doxorubicin Rapid Dissolution and Doxorubicin Solution for Injection with any solution of alkaline pH should be avoided as it will result in hydrolysis of doxorubicin. The solutions should not be mixed with heparin, as precipitation may occur, and they are not recommended to be mixed with other drugs.

Containers and storage

Solid state
Doxorubicin Hydrochloride BP should be kept in an airtight container. If the substance is sterile the container should be sterile, tamper-evident and sealed so as to exclude micro-organisms. Doxorubicin Hydrochloride USP should be preserved in tight containers.

Dosage forms
Doxorubicin Hydrochloride Injection USP should be preserved in single-dose or in multiple-dose containers, preferably of Type I glass, protected from light. Store in a refrigerator. The injection may be packaged in multiple-dose containers not exceeding 100 mL in volume.
Doxorubicin Hydrochloride for Injection USP should be preserved in containers suitable for sterile solids, except that multiple-dose containers may provide for the withdrawal of not more than 100 mL when constituted as directed in the labelling.
Reconstituted solutions of Doxorubicin Rapid Dissolution should normally be stored at 2° to 8°, protected from light, and should be used within 24 hours; any unused solution should be discarded. The reconstituted solution is chemically stable for at least 24 hours at room temperature in strong sunlight.
Doxorubicin Solution for Injection should be stored at 2° to 8°.

PHYSICAL PROPERTIES

Doxorubicin hydrochloride is an orange-red, crystalline powder; it is hygroscopic.

Melting point

Doxorubicin hydrochloride melts at 204° to 205°, with decomposition.

pH

A 0.5% w/v solution of *doxorubicin hydrochloride* has a pH of 4.0 to 5.5.

Dissociation constants

pK_a 8.2, 10.2

FURTHER INFORMATION. Electronic absorption spectra and protolytic equilibria of doxorubicin: direct spectrophotometric determination of microconstants—Sturgeon RJ, Schulman SG. J Pharm Sci 1977;66(7):958–61.

Partition coefficient

Extraction of daunorubicin and doxorubicin and their hydroxyl metabolites: self-association in aqueous solution—Eksborg S. J Pharm Sci 1978;67(6):782–5.

Solubility

Doxorubicin hydrochloride is soluble in water and in methanol; soluble 1 in 75 of ethanol; practically insoluble in chloroform, in ether, and in other organic solvents.

STABILITY

Doxorubicin is very stable in the solid state. In solution, however, degradation of doxorubicin is dependent on a variety of factors such as pH, temperature, light, ionic strength, and drug concentration.

Effect of pH

Doxorubicin is stable in the pH range 3.0 to 6.5, with maximum stability[1] at about pH 4, but it decomposes at higher pH.
In acidic solution (pH less than 4), the initial degradation of doxorubicin is by hydrolysis to the red-coloured, water-insoluble aglycone, doxorubicinone, and the water-soluble amino sugar, daunosamine.[1,2]
In solution at pH greater than 4, the degradation pattern of doxorubicin is more complex. In alkaline media, decomposition is indicated by a colour change to deep purple. Beijnen *et al*[1] detected (by TLC) one pink-coloured major degradation product and minor quantities of fluorescent compounds. A possible mechanism for degradation was examined. Underberg and Beijnen[3] later reported that up to six decomposition products could be detected and characterised by various analytical methods.

Kinetics

Pseudo-first-order kinetics for the degradation of doxorubicin have been demonstrated at pH values up to 3.5[2] and also at pH 4, 6, 8, and 10[1] at constant pH, temperature, and ionic strength. In 0.01 to 0.5M hydrochloric acid solutions, pH 0.4 to 2.1 (in the temperature range 22° to 50°), the rate of hydrolysis exhibited a first-order dependency on the concentrations of hydrogen ions and of doxorubicin.[4] An activation energy of 92 kJ/mol was calculated.

Effect of doxorubicin concentration in solution

There is no concensus as to whether the initial concentration of doxorubicin influences the rate of decomposition in solution. Tavoloni *et al*[5] observed that the stability of doxorubicin in solutions stored in the dark was independent of concentration in the range 0.01 to 0.5 mg/mL whereas, on exposure to light, the degradation rate of similar solutions was inversely proportional to the drug concentration. In later studies,[1] the rate of degradation of doxorubicin at 50°, pH 8, was not determined to be dependent on concentration in the range 1 to 20 micrograms/mL, however precipitation was observed during degradation in solutions of higher concentrations (0.05, 0.1, and 0.5 mg/mL). In contrast, Janssen *et al*[6] found that decomposition of doxorubicin in buffer solution at pH 7.4 (at 37° and 61°) was faster in solutions with initial concentrations of 0.5 mg/mL than in those with initial concentration 0.05 mg/mL.

Effects of temperature, ionic strength, and buffers

The Arrhenius relationship was found to be obeyed when the degradation rate of doxorubicin was studied in 0.01M buffer solutions (ionic strength 0.3, pH range 4.0 to 10.0) over the temperature range 30° to 70°.[1] Activation energies were calculated (for example, 89.7 kJ/mol at pH 4, 105.5 kJ/mol at pH 7.4, and 67.3 kJ/mol at pH 10).

At constant pH (1.25), the degradation rate of doxorubicin increased with an increase in ionic strength; the logarithm of the observed rate constant was linearly related to the square root of the ionic strength.[2] However, at pH values greater than 4, the effect was negligible in the range of ionic strength 0.1 to 0.4.

Catalysis of degradation was demonstrated by acetate, phosphate, and carbonate buffers at pH values up to 9.5; at pH greater than or equal to 10 no buffer catalysis occurred.[1]

In a factorially designed study, Gupta et al[7] investigated the effects of temperature, light, media (organic/aqueous or aqueous), ionic strength, and pH on the stability of doxorubicin hydrochloride. Optimum stability was observed in non-aqueous media at low temperature and pH; a combination of darkness and low ionic strength also promoted stability. Significant two-way and three-way interactions were noted between temperature and pH, and between temperature, light, and ionic strength, respectively.

Janssen et al[6] investigated the kinetics of degradation of free doxorubicin hydrochloride (0.05 to 0.5 mg/mL) and of doxorubicin hydrochloride encapsulated in liposomes in aqueous media (Tris buffer, phosphate buffer, or cell culture media at pH 4 or 7.4) at 4° to 91°. For the doxorubicin hydrochloride (0.05 to 0.1 mg/mL) solutions at 4° to 61°, activation energies of 58 kJ/mol and 73 kJ/mol in Tris buffer and phosphate buffer, respectively, were calculated. Only at 37° in phosphate buffer at pH 7.4 did liposome encapsulation influence the degradation rate of doxorubicin hydrochloride; decomposition was accelerated. For either doxorubicin hydrochloride solution or liposome dispersions, optimum shelf-life conditions were pH 4 at 4°, protected from light.

Photodegradation

Doxorubicin is sensitive to light. Photodegradation under various light sources has been reported to follow first-order kinetics.[5,8,9] The rate of photodegradation was inversely proportional to the initial concentration of doxorubicin[5,8,9] and increased with an increase in pH, thus indicating a base-catalysed mechanism.[8,9] The importance of initial concentration on the stability of doxorubicin in solution has been discussed.[5,8] At concentrations less than or equal to 0.1 mg/mL photodegradation may be marked, whereas at concentrations of 0.5 mg/mL or greater special precautions aimed at protecting doxorubicin from light appeared to be unnecessary.

The light source also influences doxorubicin stability: Asker and Habib[9] demonstrated that fluorescent light was more detrimental to doxorubicin stability (in phosphate buffer at pH 7) than either shortwave or longwave ultraviolet irradiation; Tavoloni et al[5] calculated $t_{50\%}$ values for doxorubicin (0.01 mg/mL in distilled water) of 0.89 hours and 21.7 hours when exposed to intense fluorescent light and room fluorescent light, respectively. Three potential photodegradation products of doxorubicin were detected by HPLC following prolonged exposure of doxorubicin in aqueous solution at pH 6.1 and in Tris buffer at pH 7.2 and 8.0 to room fluorescent light (168 hours).[8]

The nature of solvent influences the rate of photodegradation. When doxorubicin (0.01 to 0.5 mg/mL) in various solvents was exposed to room or intense fluorescent light, the protective effect of the solvents decreased in rank order: fresh *rat* bile ≫ ethanol > sodium chloride 0.9% solution > distilled water > Ringer-Krebs bicarbonate.[5]

Vehicles and containers

When doxorubicin hydrochloride injection (Adriamycin, Adria, USA) was admixed in four infusion fluids (at a concentration of 0.02 mg/mL) and stored in glass flasks at 21° ± 0.5° under normal room fluorescent light, $t_{10\%}$ values were: 100 ± 10 hours in glucose 5% injection (pH 4.5); 63 ± 5.8 hours in sodium chloride 0.9% injection (pH 6.2); 28 ± 3.5 hours in compound sodium lactate injection (pH 6.3); and 24 ± 2.0 hours in Normosol-R (pH 7.4).[10] Doxorubicin was visually compatible with the fluids although there was visual evidence of partial adsorption of doxorubicin onto the glass surfaces.

Similarly, Beijnen et al[11] established that less than 5% decomposition of doxorubicin 0.1 mg/mL occurred when doxorubicin hydrochloride injection (Adriblastine, Bergel, The Netherlands) was admixed in glucose 5% injection (pH 4.7) or in glucose 3.3% with sodium chloride 0.3% injection (pH 4.4) and stored for 28 days in stoppered polypropylene test-tubes in the dark at 25° ± 2°. However, for similarly stored admixtures in compound sodium lactate injection (pH 6.8) or sodium chloride 0.9% injection (pH 7), $t_{10\%}$ values were 1.7 days and 6 days, respectively.

Doxorubicin (0.1 mg/mL) was reported to be stable (less than 10% decomposition) for at least 43 days at 4° and −20° when dissolved in glucose 5% injection (pH 4.36) or sodium chloride 0.9% injection (pH 6.47 and 5.20) in polyvinyl chloride minibags stored in the dark.[12] In sodium chloride 0.9% injection (pH 6.47), in similar packaging, stored in the dark at 25°, doxorubicin was stable for 24 days. Stability of doxorubicin was also maintained when reconstituted with water for injections and stored in polypropylene syringes at 4° for at least 43 days.

When admixtures of doxorubicin hydrochloride 0.5 mg/mL and 1.25 mg/mL in sodium chloride 0.9% injection or glucose 5% injection were stored in ethylene vinyl acetate portable infusion-pump reservoirs (protected from light), doxorubicin was considered to be stable for 14 days at 4° and 22° and for 7 days at 35°.[13]

The stability of doxorubicin injection (Adria) reconstituted with sodium chloride 0.9% injection and added to glucose 5% injection was examined in underfilled polyvinyl chloride bags and glass partial-fill bottles stored at room temperature, not protected from light.[14] In glass containers the $t_{10\%}$ for doxorubicin was 40 hours whereas no decrease in concentration of doxorubicin was apparent after 48 hours in polyvinyl chloride bags.

Refrigeration, freezing, and thawing

Hoffman et al[15] demonstrated that doxorubicin hydrochloride injection (Adriamycin, Adria) reconstituted with sterile water for injections (to 2 mg/mL) could be stored for up to 6 months when refrigerated at 4° and up to 30 days if frozen at −20°. Karlsen et al[16] showed that no significant reduction in concentration of doxorubicin occurred when doxorubicin hydrochloride (Farmitalia) 70 mg/50 mL in sodium chloride 0.9% injection (in polyvinyl chloride bags) was stored frozen at −20° for at least 30 days followed by rapid thawing in a microwave oven. Similarly,[17] no reduction in doxorubicin concentration was observed in solutions of doxorubicin hydrochloride (1 mg/mL) in sodium chloride 0.9% injection (in polyvinyl chloride bags) after storage frozen at −20° for 2 weeks and thawing for 150 minutes at room temperature or 3 minutes in a microwave oven. The effects of repeated freezing and thawing of the above solutions have been examined. Karlsen et al[16] observed that after four freeze-microwave thaw treatments, the concentration of doxorubicin had fallen by about 5%. After re-freezing and thawing solutions (in a microwave oven or at room temperature) after 5 weeks a small, but significant, decrease in concentration of doxorubicin was noted.[17] However, Hoffman et al[15] observed that subjecting aqueous solutions of doxorubicin hydrochloride to seven freeze-thaw procedures did not cause a significant loss of potency and Wood et al[12] noted that repeated freezing and thawing (at ambient temperature) did not cause degradation of doxorubicin in sodium chloride 0.9% injection in polyvinyl chloride minibags.

Although the stability of doxorubicin hydrochloride in frozen solutions has been demonstrated, Williamson and Luce[18] (Adria Laboratories) warned against the use of microwave ovens as a means of thawing such solutions; overheating (caused by uneven heat distribution in the microwave oven) may result in decomposition of doxorubicin or may cause plastic minibags to burst. The authors recommended thawing at room temperature only.

Stabilisation

Photostabilisation

The presence of glutathione in solutions of doxorubicin in phosphate buffer at pH 7 enhanced the photostability of doxorubicin under intense fluorescent light or normal laboratory light.[9] The half-life under normal laboratory light for doxorubicin solutions with glutathione was 462 hours in clear glass ampoules compared to half-lives of 61 hours and 38 hours in solutions without glutathione in amber glass and in clear glass ampoules, respectively.

The rate of photodegradation of doxorubicin hydrochloride (9.76×10^{-5}M) in phosphate buffer at pH 7 under fluorescent light was significantly reduced by the presence of 1% of p-aminobenzoic acid, urocanic acid, or sodium urate; thiourea, DL-methionine, or glycine also increased photostability but to a lesser extent. The presence of sodium thiosulphate, however, appeared to enhance the photodegradation of doxorubicin.[19]

Effects of cyclodextrins

The influence of cyclodextrins on the stability of doxorubicin in aqueous solutions has been investigated.[20-22] If complexation occurs neither the kinetics of decomposition of doxorubicin (pseudo-first-order) nor the decomposition mechanisms are changed. In acidic media (pH below 3.5) at 50° the degradation rate of doxorubicin was reduced in the presence of γ-cyclodextrin[20,21] and, to a lesser extent, in the presence of dimethyl-β-cyclodextrin.[20] In the pH range 4 to 10, however, the effect of γ-cyclodextrin was negligible, whereas in strongly alkaline solutions (at 50°) degradation of doxorubicin was enhanced by γ-cyclodextrin.[21] The presence of α-cyclodextrin or β-cyclodextrin in either acidic or alkaline media had negligible influence on stability.

Brewster et al[22] further demonstrated that modified cyclodextrins (such as hydroxypropyl-β-cyclodextrin and hydroxypropyl-γ-cyclodextrin) stabilised doxorubicin in aqueous solutions (pH 1.01, 1.84, 5.90, and 7.72) at 75°; the γ-cyclodextrin derivatives appeared to be more effective at all pH values except pH 7.72.

FURTHER INFORMATION. Stability of solutions of antineoplastic agents during preparation and storage for in vitro assays. II. Assay methods, adriamycin [doxorubicin] and other antitumour antibiotics—Bosanquet AG [review]. Cancer Chemother Pharmacol 1986;17:1–10. Anthracycline antitumour agents. A review of physicochemical, analytical and stability properties—Bouma J, Beijnen JH, Bult A, Underberg WJM. Pharm Weekbl (Sci) 1986;8:109–33.

INCOMPATIBILITY/COMPATIBILITY

Solutions of doxorubicin hydrochloride are incompatible with heparin sodium as evidenced by immediate precipitation.[23,24] Similarly, immediate precipitation has been observed in admixtures of doxorubicin hydrochloride with cephalothin sodium, diazepam, or hydrocortisone sodium succinate,[23] and also with frusemide.[24] When admixed with aminophylline or fluorouracil, solutions of doxorubicin darkened from red to blue-purple.[23] Admixtures[25] of doxorubicin hydrochloride (1.4 mg/mL, Adriablastina, Farmitalia, Italy) with vincristine sulphate (0.033 mg/mL, Oncovin, Eli Lilly, France) in sodium chloride 0.9% injection or in sodium chloride 0.45% with glucose 2.5% injection, were stable for at least seven days (more than 95% of initial concentration retained) when the admixtures were stored in polysiloxan bags protected from light at 25°, 30°, or 37°. However, in similar admixtures in sodium chloride 0.45% with Ringer's acetate injection degradation of both doxorubicin and vincristine was accelerated; about 28% and 9% decomposition, respectively, had occurred after 7 days at 25°, and about 40% and 15% decomposition, respectively, after 4 days at 37°. A reddish pink precipitate was apparent after 2 to 3 days at 37°. Cohen et al[24] observed that doxorubicin hydrochloride (2 mg/mL) was visually compatible with vincristine sulphate (1 mg/mL) and with vinblastine sulphate (1 mg/mL).

Sorption

Doxorubicin hydrochloride has been shown to adsorb to polytetrafluoroethylene, glass, and polyethylene containers, but not to polypropylene or siliconised glass containers.[26]

There is no concensus as to the adsorption of doxorubicin to filter materials. Binding of doxorubicin to filters may depend on the concentration of doxorubicin with more extensive binding apparent at concentrations lower than clinical concentrations. Hoffman et al[15] noted that filtration of doxorubicin hydrochloride 2 mg/mL in sterile water for injections through a sterile 0.22 micrometre Millex filter did not cause loss of doxorubicin from the solution. However, significant binding of doxorubicin hydrochloride to cellulose ester membranes and polytetrafluoroethylene filters has been reported.[27] Ennis et al[28] demonstrated that about 92% of the doxorubicin content was delivered when an injection (doxorubicin hydrochloride 30 mg/15 mL) was administered as a bolus through a 0.2 micrometre nylon, air-eliminating filter (Ultipor, Pall) and the filter was flushed with 10 mL of sodium chloride 0.9% solution.

Aluminium

Gardiner[29] noted that darkening of solutions of doxorubicin hydrochloride occurred when they were prepared in a syringe that had a standard needle with an aluminium hub or when pieces of aluminium were placed in vials containing the solution. The manufacturers reported further studies[30] in which a solution of doxorubicin hydrochloride (2 mg/mL in sodium chloride 0.9% injection or sterile water for injections) changed colour to a darker ruby red over 24 hours when pieces of aluminium were placed in the solution; the pH changed from 4.8 to 5.2. No colour or pH changes occurred in control solutions or in solutions containing stainless steel needles with steel or plastic hubs. Thus, doxorubicin did react with aluminium but the reaction was slow and did not result in a substantial loss of potency. It was recommended that syringes with reconstituted doxorubicin should not be capped with aluminium-hubbed needles for storage but that the solution may be injected through such needles.

Ogawa et al[31] later noted that when a needle that contained an aluminium-interlocking segment was immersed in a solution of doxorubicin hydrochloride 2 mg/mL (Adriamycin, Adria) the solution darkened to ruby red with formation of black patches on the aluminium surface after 12 to 24 hours.

FORMULATION

Excipient

Excipients that have been used in presentations of doxorubicin hydrochloride include:
Injections (powder for reconstitution): lactose; methyl hydroxybenzoate.
Injections: sodium chloride 0.9% injection.

Microemulsions

The behaviour of doxorubicin in various microemulsions has been examined.[32] Two oil-in-water microemulsions containing different proportions of isopropyl myristate, butanol, buffer (pH 6), and sodium bis-(2-ethylhexyl)sulphosuccinate or Tween 80 (as surfactants) and a water-in-oil microemulsion containing egg lecithin (as surfactant), water, hexanol, and ethyl oleate were subjected to repeated shaking and freeze-thaw cycles over six months; no changes in viscosity or turbidity were noted and the systems remained homogeneous with no phase separation. Distribution of doxorubicin between oily and aqueous phases and release from microemulsions was influenced by interactions with the surfactant. A 'reservoir effect' for doxorubicin in the water-in-oil microemulsion was indicated.

Novel delivery systems

Storm[33] reported that when doxorubicin was encapsulated into various types of liposomes and administered intravenously to *rats*, the toxicity of doxorubicin was reduced while antitumour activity was maintained in comparison to that of the free drug. This was attributed to a sustained-release mechanism from the liposomes.
Further to the stabilisation of doxorubicin in solution by the addition of hydroxypropyl-β-cyclodextrin or hydroxypropyl-γ-cyclodextrin, Brewster et al[22] demonstrated that dissolution of doxorubicin from lyophilised dosage forms of doxorubicin with either cyclodextrin derivative was faster than from commercially available doxorubicin/lactose preparations.
Jones et al reported that the *in-vitro* release of doxorubicin from biodegradable albumin microspheres into human plasma and sodium chloride 0.9% solution could be sustained for up to 10 days and release rates could be controlled by manipulation of the manufacturing conditions.[34] For example, when denaturation of the aqueous protein emulsion was achieved by thermal (at 110° to 135°) and chemical (in the presence of 1% or 2% glutaraldehyde) crosslinking methods, microspheres with slower release of doxorubicin were produced than when thermal methods alone were used.
Willmott et al[35] studied the incorporation of ^{14}C-doxorubicin within protease-sensitive casein microspheres and, from measurements of total drug and 'free' drug, suggested that most of the doxorubicin was incorporated via a covalent linkage to the matrix protein. Studies using tumour tissue indicated that antitumour activity was mediated mainly by the covalently bound doxorubicin and that biodegradation of the microsphere matrix was implicated in drug release and biological disposition and activity.
In an investigation of adsorption and release of doxorubicin incorporated into hydroxyapatite beads,[36] it was shown that although almost all the doxorubicin was released from solution-loaded wet beads, only 60% was released from the corresponding dry beads. This was thought to be due to strong irreversible binding between doxorubicin and the hydroxyapatite surface in the dry state.

FURTHER INFORMATION. Dissolution time, on reconstitution, of a new parenteral formulation of doxorubicin (Doxorubicin Rapid Dissolution)—Murphy A, Maltby S, Launchbury AP. Int J Pharmaceutics 1987;38:257–9. Stability of doxorubicin-liposomes [negatively-charged] on storage: as an aqueous dispersion, frozen or freeze-dried—Van Bommel EMG, Crommelin DJA. Int J Pharmaceutics 1984;22:229–310. Liposome encapsulation of doxorubicin: pharmaceutical [influence of lipid composition, physicochemical characteristics, stability of liposomes and drug] and therapeutic aspects [activity and toxicity in *rats*]—Storm G, van Bloois L, Steerenberg PA, van Etten E, de Groot G, Crommelin DJA. J Controlled Release 1989;9:215–29. Solid lipospheres of doxorubicin and idarubicin—Cavalli R, Caputo O, Gasco MR. Int J Pharmaceutics 1993;89:R9–R12. Binding mechanisms of doxorubicin in ion-exchange albumin microcapsules—Sawaya A, Benoit J-P, Benita S. J Pharm Sci 1987;7(6):475–80. Evaluation of drug delivery following the administration of magnetic albumin microspheres containing adriamycin [doxorubicin] to the *rat*—Gallo JM, Gupta PK, Hung CT, Perrier DG. J Pharm Sci 1989;78(3):190–4. *In-vitro* release of cytotoxic agents from ion exchange resins—Jones C, Burton MA, Gray BN, Hodgkin J. J Controlled Release 1989;8:251–7. The design and in vitro release characterisation of human cross-linked haemoglobin microcapsules containing doxorubicin for potential chemoembolisation use—Schutz M, Benita S. J Disper Sci Technol 1989;10(3):219–39. The distribution of doxorubicin in *mice* following administration in niosomes [large multilamellar nonionic surfactant vesicles prepared from a C_{16} triglyceryl ether with and without cholesterol]—Rogerson A, Cummings J, Willmott N, Florence AT. J Pharm Pharmacol 1988;40:337–42. Doxorubicin in cholesterol polyoxyethylene modified niosomes: evidence of enhancement of absorption in *mice*—Cable C, Cassidy J, Kaye SB, Florence AT. J Pharm Pharmacol 1988;40(Suppl):31P. Binding of doxorubicin to nonionic surfactant vesicles—Cable C, Florence AT, Cassidy J. J Pharm Pharmacol 1990;42(Suppl):51P. Uptake capacity and adsorption isotherms of doxorubicin on polymeric nanoparticles: effect of methods of preparation—Bapat N, Boroujerdi M. Drug Dev Ind Pharm 1992;18(1):65–77. *In vivo* kinetics of magnetically targeted low-dose doxorubicin—Senyei AE, Reich SD, Gonczy C, Widder KJ. J Pharm Sci 1981;70(4):389–91.

PROCESSING

Handling and disposal

CAUTION. Doxorubicin and doxorubicin hydrochloride are cytotoxic; avoid inhalation and contact with skin and mucous membranes.
Personnel handling doxorubicin preparations should wear protective clothing (goggles, gowns, and disposable gloves and masks). Reconstitution of doxorubicin injections should be performed in a designated area (preferably under a laminar flow system); the work surface should be protected by disposable, plastic-backed, absorbent paper. Care should be taken to avoid inhalation of any aerosol produced during reconstitution.
If accidental contact with skin occurs it should be treated immediately by washing with copious water, or soap and water, or sodium bicarbonate. Medical attention should be sought.
Chemical destruction or decontamination of doxorubicin (for example, of reconstituted solution, spillages, or leakages) is effected by treatment with dilute sodium hypochlorite (1%

available chlorine) solution, preferably by soaking, and then with copious water.[37]

Destruction of doxorubicin and of contaminated articles may be effected[37] by incineration at 700°.

General guidelines on handling and disposal are given in the chapter entitled Cytotoxic Drugs: Handling Precautions.

FURTHER INFORMATION. Visible-light system for detecting doxorubicin contamination on skin and surfaces—Van Raalte J, Rice C, Moss CE. Am J Hosp Pharm 1990;47:1067–74. Castegnaro M, Adams J, Armour MA, et al. IARC Scientific Publications No 73. Laboratory decontamination and destruction of carcinogens in laboratory wastes: some antineoplastic agents [includes method for destruction of doxorubicin waste using potassium permanganate/sulphuric acid]—London: International Agency for Research of Cancer, 1985.

REFERENCES

1. Beijnen JH, van der Houwen OAGJ, Underberg WJM. Int J Pharmaceutics 1986;32:123–31.
2. Beijnen JH, Wiese G, Underberg WJM. Pharm Weekbl (Sci) 1985;7:109–16.
3. Underberg WJM, Beijnen JH. Pharm Weekbl (Sci) 1987;9:146.
4. Wassermann K, Bundgaard H. Int J Pharmaceutics 1983;14:73–8.
5. Tavoloni N, Guarino AM, Berk PD. J Pharm Pharmacol 1980;32:860–2.
6. Janssen MJH, Crommelin DJA, Storm G, Hulshoff A. Int J Pharmaceutics 1985;23:1–11.
7. Gupta PK, Lam FC, Hung CT. Drug Dev Ind Pharm 1988;14(12):1657–71.
8. Wood MJ, Irwin WJ, Scott DK. J Clin Pharm Ther 1990;15:291–300.
9. Asker AF, Habib MJ. J Parenter Sci Technol 1988;42(5):153–6.
10. Poochikian GK, Cradock JC, Flora KP. Am J Hosp Pharm 1981;38:483–6.
11. Beijnen JH, Rosing H, de Vries PA, Underberg WJM. J Parenter Sci Technol 1985;39(6):220–2.
12. Wood MJ, Irwin WJ, Scott DK. J Clin Pharm Ther 1990;15:279–89.
13. Rochard EB, Barthes DM, Courtois PY. Am J Hosp Pharm 1992;49:619–23.
14. Benvenuto JA, Anderson RW, Kerkof K, Smith RG, Loo TL. Am J Hosp Pharm 1981;38:1914–18.
15. Hoffman DM, Grossano DD, Damin LA, Woodcock TM. Am J Hosp Pharm 1979;36:1536–8.
16. Karlsen J, Thønnesen HH, Olsen IR, Sollien AH, Skobba TJ. Nor Pharm Acta 1983;45:61–7.
17. Keusters L, Stolk LML, Umans R, Van Asten P. Pharm Weekbl (Sci) 1986;8:194–7.
18. Williamson M, Luce JK [letter]. Am J Hosp Pharm 1987;44:505,510.
19. Habib MJ, Asker AF. J Parenter Sci Technol 1989;43(6):259–61.
20. Bekers O, Beijnen JH, Bramel EHG, Otagiri M, Underberg WJM. Pharm Weekbl (Sci) 1988;10:207–12.
21. Bekers O, Beijnen JH, Vis BJ, Suenaga A, Otagiri M, Bult A et al. Int J Pharmaceutics 1991;72:123–30.
22. Brewster ME, Loftsson T, Estes KS, Lin J-L, Fridriksdóttir H, Bodor N. Int J Pharmaceutics 1992;79:289–99.
23. Dorr RT. Am J IV Ther 1979;6:42,45–6,52.
24. Cohen MH, Johnston-Early A, Hood MA, McKenzie M, Citron ML, Jaffe N et al. Cancer Treat Rep 1985;69:1325–7.
25. Beijnen JH, Neef C, Meuwissen OJAT, Rutten JJMH, Rosing H, Underberg WJM. Am J Hosp Pharm 1986;43:3022–7.
26. Tomlinson E, Malspeis L. J Pharm Sci 1982;71(10):1121–5.
27. Bosanquet AG. Cancer Chemother Pharmacol 1985;14:83–95.
28. Ennis CE, Merritt RJ, Neff DN. J Parenter Enter Nutr 1983;7(2):156–8.
29. Gardiner WA [letter]. Am J Hosp Pharm 1981;38:1276.
30. Williamson MJ, Luce JK, Hausmann WK [letter]. Am J Hosp Pharm 1983;40:214.
31. Ogawa GS, Young R, Munar M [letter]. Am J Hosp Pharm 1985;42:1042,1045.
32. Gasco MR, Pattarino F, Voltani I. Il Farmaco Ed Prat 1988;43(1):3–12.
33. Storm G. Pharm Weekbl (Sci) 1988;10:288–90.
34. Jones C, Burton MA, Gray BN. J Pharm Pharmacol 1989;41:813–16.
35. Willmott N, Magee GA, Cummings J, Halbert GW, Smyth JF. J Pharm Pharmacol 1992;44:472–5.
36. Yamamura K, Yotsuyanagi T. Int J Pharmaceutics 1992;79:R1–R3.
37. Garner S, Ross M, Wilson J. Pharm J 1988;241(Hosp Suppl):HS32.

Doxycycline (BAN, USAN, rINN)   *Antibacterial*

Doxycycline monohydrate

(4S,4aR,5S,5aR,6S,12aS)-4-Dimethylamino-1,4,4a,5,5a,6,11,12a-octahydro-3,5,10,12,12a-pentahydroxy-6-methyl-1,11-dioxo-naphthacene-2-carboxamide;   6-deoxy-5β-hydroxytetracycline monohydrate

$C_{22}H_{24}N_2O_8, H_2O = 462.5$

Doxycycline Calcium (BANM, rINNM)

Doxycycline Fosfatex (BAN, USAN)

$(C_{22}H_{24}N_2O_8)_3 (HPO_3)_3 NaPO_3 = 1675.2$

Doxycycline Hydrochloride (BANM)

Doxycycline Hyclate (rINNM)

$C_{22}H_{24}N_2O_8 HCl, \frac{1}{2}C_2H_5OH, \frac{1}{2}H_2O = 512.9$

CAS—564-25-0 (doxycycline, anhydrous); 17086-28-1 (doxycycline, monohydrate); 83038-87-3 (doxycycline fosfatex); 24390-14-5 (doxycycline hydrochloride)

Pharmacopoeial status

BP (doxycycline hydrochloride); USP (doxycycline, doxycycline hyclate)

Preparations

Compendial

Doxycycline Capsules BP. Capsules containing, in each, doxycycline hydrochloride equivalent to 50 mg and 100 mg of doxycycline are usually available.

Doxycycline Capsules USP.
Doxycycline Hyclate Capsules USP.
Doxycycline Hyclate Delayed-release Capsules USP.
Doxycycline Hyclate Tablets USP.
Doxycycline Hyclate for Injection USP.
Doxycycline for Oral Suspension USP.
Doxycycline Calcium Oral Suspension USP.
Sterile Doxycycline Hyclate USP. Suitable for parenteral use.

Non-compendial
Nordox (Panpharma). *Capsules*, doxycycline 100 mg (as hydro-chloride).
Vibramycin (Invicta). *Capsules*, doxycycline (as hydrochloride) 50 mg and 100 mg.
Vibramycin-D (Invicta). *Dispersible tablets*, doxycycline 100 mg (as monohydrate).
Doxycycline capsules are also available from APS, Ashbourne (Demix), Hillcross, Kerfoot, Lagap (Doxylar), Norton.

Containers and storage

Solid state
Doxycycline Hydrochloride BP should be stored in an airtight container, protected from light. If it is intended for use in the manufacture of a parenteral dosage form, the container should be sterile, tamper-evident, and sealed so as to exclude micro-organisms.
Doxycycline USP should be preserved in tight, light-resistant containers.
Doxycycline Hyclate USP should be preserved in tight contain-ers, protected from light.

Dosage forms
All Doxycycline USP and Doxycycline Hyclate USP prepara-tions should be preserved in tight, light-resistant containers.
Doxycycline Hyclate for Injection USP should be preserved in containers for sterile solids and protected from light.
Nordox capsules should be stored in a cool, dry place, protected from light. All Vibramycin preparations should be stored below 25°.

PHYSICAL PROPERTIES

Doxycycline is a yellow, crystalline powder.
Doxycycline hydrochloride is a yellow, crystalline, hygroscopic powder with an ethanolic odour and a bitter taste.

Melting point

Doxycycline hydrochloride is reported to melt about 200°, with decomposition.

pH

The pH of a 1% w/v aqueous suspension of *doxycycline* lies between 5.0 and 6.5.
The pH of a 1% w/v aqueous solution of *doxycycline hydrochlor-ide* lies between 2.0 and 3.0.

Dissociation constants

pK_a 3.5, 7.7, 9.5 (20°)
A pK_a value of 3.09 ± 0.09 was determined spectrophotometri-cally for the protonation of doxycycline (ionic strength 0.1 at 25°),[1] to form the monoprotonated species.

Partition coefficient

Log *P* (octanol/pH 7.5), −0.2

Solubility

Doxycycline is very slightly soluble in water; sparingly soluble in ethanol; practically insoluble in chloroform and in ether; freely soluble in dilute acids and alkali hydroxides.
Doxycycline hydrochloride is soluble 1 in 3 of water and 1 in 4 of methanol; sparingly soluble in ethanol; practically insoluble in chloroform and in ether. It dissolves in aqueous solutions of alkali hydroxides and carbonates.

Effect of pH and salts
The pH-solubility profile[1] for doxycycline monohydrate, in aqu-eous hydrochloric acid at 25° without added salt, reached a peak of 50 mg/mL at pH 2.16. A 65% increase in solubility was observed in 1M sodium nitrate compared to that in water. The strong positive salt effect was said to be related to the zwitterio-nic nature of doxycycline in aqueous solution.

Dissolution

The USP specifies that for Doxycycline Capsules USP and for Doxycycline Hyclate Tablets USP not less than 85% of the labelled amount of $C_{22}H_{24}N_2O_8$ is dissolved in 60 minutes and in 90 minutes, respectively. Dissolution medium: 900 mL of water; Apparatus 2 at 75 rpm.

FURTHER INFORMATION. Dissolution rates of doxycycline free base and hydrochloride salts [solubility in different media and effect of chloride ions].—Bogardus JB, Blackwood RK. J Pharm Sci 1979;68(9):1183–4.

STABILITY

Solutions

The degradation of doxycycline in aqueous solution follows first-order kinetics and is subject to general acid-base cataly-sis.[2] It has been shown to be most stable in strongly acid solu-tion; $t_{10\%}$ at pH 1.11 was 295 days.

Effect of relative humidity

Hard gelatin capsules containing doxycycline hydrochloride alone and in formulation with magnesium stearate, lactose, or both, were kept for up to 78 weeks at 40%, 60%, and 85% rela-tive humidities in desiccators protected from daylight.[3] The pre-sence of magnesium stearate or lactose increased doxycycline degradation at all levels of relative humidity. From formula-tions containing both lubricant and diluent, the loss of doxy-cycline at 40%, 60%, and 85% relative humidity was 9.28% by 78 weeks, 9.77% by 68 weeks, and 9.84% by 20 weeks, respectively.

Effect of freezing

Doxycycline hydrochloride for injection (Pfizer) was stored at −20° for up to 8 weeks following reconstitution in sterile water for injections (doxycycline 10 mg/mL; kept in original vials) or in glucose 5% (doxycycline 1 mg/mL; kept in flint-glass vials sealed with butyl stoppers).[4] No significant decomposition was detected by either ultraviolet spectrophotometry or by microbio-logical turbidimetric measurements. There were no visually per-ceptible changes in clarity or colour of the solutions and no significant changes in pH.

FURTHER INFORMATION. Quantitative estimation and separation of doxycycline HCl and its related products—Seth PW, Stamm A. Drug Dev Ind Pharm 1986;12(10):1469–75.

INCOMPATIBILITY/COMPATIBILITY

During simulated infusion there were no losses of doxycycline (Pfizer) in sodium chloride 0.9% solution due to sorption to polyvinyl chloride bags or tubing, polyethylene or Silastic tubing, or cellulose propionate burette chambers. In addition, no sorption occurred during storage of doxycycline in all-plastic syringes (polypropylene barrels and polyethylene plungers).[5,6]

FORMULATION

Excipients

Excipients that have been used in presentations of doxycycline include:

Capsules, doxycycline hydrochloride: indigo carmine (E132); lactose; magnesium stearate; maize starch; methacrylate polymer; microcrystalline cellulose; patent blue V(E131); povidone; quinoline yellow (E104); sodium lauryl sulphate; sucrose; talc; titanium dioxide (E171); yellow iron oxide (E172).

Doxycycline phosphate: lactose; magnesium stearate; silica; talc.

Tablets, doxycycline hydrochloride: colloidal silica; croscarmellose sodium type A; ethylcellulose; hydroxypropylcellulose; hypromellose; lactose; macrogol 400 and 10 000; magnesium stearate; methylcellulose; microcrystalline cellulose; povidone; propylene glycol; stearic acid; sodium lauryl sulphate; talc; titanium dioxide (E171); Yellow 6 lake.

Oral liquids, doxycycline calcium: aluminium magnesium silicate; butyl and propyl hydroxybenzoates; calcium chloride; carmine (E120); fruit flavours; glycerol; hydrochloric acid; povidone; propylene glycol; simethicone emulsion; sodium hydroxide; sodium metabisulphite; sorbitol.

Doxycycline monohydrate: carmellose sodium; Blue 1; methyl and propyl hydroxybenzoates; microcrystalline cellulose; raspberry flavour; Red 28; simethicone emulsion; sucrose.

Doxycycline hydrochloride: aluminium magnesium silicate; calcium chloride dihydrate; carmine (E120); glycerol; methyl and propyl hydroxybenzoates; concentrated hydrochloric acid; povidone; propylene glycol; saccharin sodium; sodium metabisulphite; sorbitol solution (70%).

Dosage form development

Crystallisation of doxycycline hydrochloride during lyophilisation of an aqueous solution was enhanced by the addition of glycine; 0.05 or 0.07 (mole fraction), and 0.1 (mole fraction) glycine induced 100% and 95% crystallinity of doxycycline hydrochloride, respectively.[7] No crystallinity was reported in doxycycline hydrochloride lyophilised in the absence of excipients.

Bioavailability/bioequivalence

The bioavailability of a pellet formulation of doxycycline hydrochloride (100 mg, Doryx, Faulding, Australia) was compared with that of Vibramycin (100 mg, Pfizer) in 24 healthy volunteers. Data suggested that the pellet formulation was bioequivalent to the Vibramycin capsule when taken in the absence of food.[8]

Three commercially available brands of doxycycline hydrochloride capsules (Vibramycin, Pfizer; Doxychell, Rachelle; Doxy II, USV Pharmaceutical Corp) were found by Antal and co-workers to be bioequivalent.[9] The time for 50% dissolution correlated with absorption rates *in vivo*. Subsequent *in-vivo* bioavailability studies comparing three different dosage forms (reconstituted doxycycline hydrochloride for injection (Vibramycin Intravenous) administered as an oral solution, the three brands of capsule, and Vibramycin monohydrate oral suspension) in six healthy volunteers revealed a significant difference in absorption rate between the capsules and the oral suspension but not between the capsules and the oral solution.

FURTHER INFORMATION. Doxycycline: *In vitro* release and bioavailability from 6 market preparations [soft and hard gelatin capsules and tablet]—Keller M, Bezler H [German]. Dtsch Apoth Ztg 1988;128:1565–71. Bioequivalence of an optimised doxycycline preparation—Lode H, Deppermann N, Schmidt V. Arzneimittelforschung 1989;39(II):1162-5. Studies on the bioavailability of doxycycline [bioequivalence of tablets]—Kees F, Dehner R, Dittrich W, Raasch W, Grobecker H [German]. Arzneimittelforschung 1990;40:1039-43. Bioequivalent [bioavailability] studies of doxycycline preparations: 100 mg tablets/capsules—Burhens KG, Berndt P, Harms J, Hilgenstock CM, Milbrandt T *et al* [German]. Dtsch Apoth Ztg 1990;130:1364–7.

REFERENCES

1. Bogardus JB, Blackwood RK. J Pharm Sci 1979;68(2):188–94.
2. Pawelczyk E, Plóciennik B [Polish]. Acta Polon Pharm 1985;XLII Nr 2:128–34.
3. Özol T. Acta Pharm Turcica 1984;26:41–5.
4. Petrick RJ, Woolleben JE, Vargas TA. Am J Hosp Pharm 1978;35:1386–7.
5. Kowaluk EA, Roberts MS, Blackburn HD, Polack AE. Am J Hosp Pharm 1981;38:1308–13.
6. Kowaluk EA, Roberts MS, Polack AE. Am J Hosp Pharm 1982;39:460–7.
7. Korey DJ, Schwartz JB. J Parenter Sci Technol 1989;43(2):80–3.
8. Williams DB, O'Reilly WJ, Boehm G, Story MJ. Biopharm Drug Dispos 1990;11:93-105.
9. Antal EJ, Jaffe JM, Poust RI, Colaizzi JL. J Pharm Sci 1975;64(12):2015-18.

Ergometrine (BAN, rINN)   *Oxytocic*

Ergonovine; ergobasine
9,10-Didehydro-*N*-[(*S*)-2-hydroxy-1-methylethyl]-6-methylergoline-8β-carboxamide;   *N*-[(*S*)-2-hydroxy-1-methylethyl]-D-lysergamide
$C_{19}H_{23}N_3O_2 = 325.4$

Ergometrine Maleate (BANM, rINNM)
Ergonovine maleate
$C_{19}H_{23}N_3O_2, C_4H_4O_4 = 441.5$

Ergometrine Tartrate (BANM, rINNM)
$(C_{19}H_{23}N_3O_2)_2, C_4H_6O_6 = 800.9$
CAS—60-79-7 (ergometrine); 129-51-1 (ergometrine maleate); 129-50-0 (ergometrine tartrate)

Pharmacopoeial status

BP (ergometrine maleate); USP (ergonovine maleate)

Preparations

Compendial

Ergometrine Tablets BP contain ergometrine maleate. Tablets containing, in each, 250 micrograms and 500 micrograms are usually available.

Ergometrine Injection BP is a sterile solution of ergometrine maleate in water for injections. The acidity of the solution is adjusted to pH 3 by the addition of maleic acid. An injection containing 500 micrograms in 1 mL is usually available. pH 2.7 to 3.5.

Ergometrine and Oxytocin Injection BP. pH 2.9 to 3.5.

Ergonovine Maleate Tablets USP.

Ergonovine Maleate Injection USP. pH 2.7 to 3.5.

Containers and storage

Solid state

Ergometrine Maleate BP should be kept in an airtight, glass container, protected from light and stored at a temperature of 2° to 8°.

Ergonovine Maleate USP should be preserved in tight, light-resistant containers, in a cold place.

Dosage forms

Ergometrine Injection BP should be protected from light and stored at a temperature of 2° to 8°.

Ergometrine and Oxytocin Injection BP should be protected from light and stored at a temperature of 2° to 8°. Under these conditions it may be expected to retain its potency for not less than three years.

Ergonovine Maleate Tablets USP should be preserved in well-closed containers.

Ergonovine Maleate Injection USP should be preserved in single-dose, light-resistant containers, preferably of Type I glass, and stored in a cold place.

PHYSICAL PROPERTIES

Ergometrine exists as colourless crystals.

Ergometrine maleate exists as a white or slightly yellow or grey crystalline powder; odourless and slightly hygroscopic; darkens with age and on exposure to light.

Ergometrine tartrate exists as white or slightly reddish-yellow, very light, matted masses of acicular crystals.

Melting point

Ergometrine melts at 162°.

Ergometrine maleate has been reported to melt at 167°, with decomposition.

pH

The pH of a 1% solution of *ergometrine maleate* is in the range 3.0 to 5.0.

Dissociation constant

pK_a 6.8 (20°)

Partition coefficient

Log *P* (ether), −0.9

Solubility

Ergometrine is slightly soluble in water (solutions give a blue fluorescence); more soluble in ethanol; sparingly soluble in chloroform; freely soluble in the lower alcohols, in ethyl acetate, and in acetone.

Ergometrine maleate is soluble 1 in 40 of water and 1 in 100 of ethanol; practically insoluble in ether and in chloroform.

Ergometrine tartrate is soluble in water and in ethanol; slightly soluble in chloroform and in ether.

Dissolution

The USP specifies that for Ergonovine Maleate Tablets USP not less than 75% of the labelled amount of $C_{19}H_{23}N_3O_2$, $C_4H_4O_4$ is dissolved in 45 minutes. Dissolution medium: 900 mL of water; Apparatus 1 at 100 rpm.

STABILITY

Ergometrine degrades by oxidation (and becomes darker); by reversible isomerisation (caused by heating under acid or alkaline conditions) to form ergometrinine; and by hydrolysis (under rigorous treatment with acid or alkali) to lysergic acid, isolysergic acid, and 2-amino-1-propanol. Ergometrine maleate is more stable than ergometrine base although it also undergoes oxidation. The stability of ergometrine in solution is improved by the presence of antoxidants. Irradiation of acidic solutions of ergometrine results in the formation of lumi- ergometrine products.

El-Masry developed a stability-indicating method suitable for a single-dose assay of ergometrine in pharmaceutical preparations.[1] Accelerated stability testing at 60° of a buffered solution of ergometrine maleate (pH 6.3) containing sodium metabisulphite 0.1% revealed 90% decomposition after 24 hours at 60°. In analyses of two batches of ergometrine maleate injection and one batch of tablets more decomposition was detected by the method under investigation than by the BP 1973 method.

The ergometrine content of ergometrine maleate injections was found to have decreased significantly (to 89.5%) when tested on arrival in Sudan from Europe.[2] The content further decreased (to 53%) during storage for 25 months at distribution centres. The colourless solutions began to darken within 12 months of storage and related alkaloid content increased to 20% (ten times the USP permitted limit). The supply of ergometrine maleate injection to tropical countries in the form of a dry powder with a separate solvent was suggested.

Of 24 samples of ergometrine maleate injection taken from 20 health centres in the tropics, only 9 complied with the BP and USP potency specifications, owing to prolonged storage at ambient temperatures.[3] Recommended storage of ergometrine maleate injection (in any country) is in a refrigerator, not above 8°, and protected from light.

An investigation of the stability of 80 ergometrine injection ampoules during shipment from Denmark to the tropics[4] revealed a mean loss of 5.8% of ergometrine. However, a large variation was found between samples; 18 ampoules lost more than 20% and 3 ampoules lost more than 40% of the stated content of ergometrine, although active content before shipment had not been determined.

Shelf-lives for ergometrine maleate injection reported in the literature are: 15 months at temperatures below 10° (Ergometrine injection, Antigen) and 1 to 2 years at temperatures below 10° (Phoenix).[5]

Ergometrine maleate injection (Lilly) is reported to be stable[6] at 15° to 30° and at temperatures[7] not exceeding 25° for up to 60 days and 2 months, respectively.

FORMULATION

Excipients

Excipients that have been used in presentations of ergometrine maleate include:

Injections: ethyl lactate; lactic acid; phenol.

PROCESSING

Sterilisation

Ergometrine Injection BP is sterilised by heating in an autoclave.

REFERENCES

1. El-Masry S. Mfg Chem 1978;49(9):53.
2. Abu-Reid IO, El-Samani SA, Hag Omer AI, Khalil NY, Mahgoub KM, Everitt G *et al.* Int Pharm J 1990;4(1):6–10.
3. Walker GJA, Hogerzeil HV, Hillgren U [letter]. Lancet 1988;2:393.
4. Hogerzeil HV, Battersby A, Srdanovic V, Stjernstrom NE. Br Med J 1992;304:210–12.
5. Longland PW, Rowbotham PC. Pharm J 1989;243;589–95.
6. Vogenberg FR, Souney PF. Am J Hosp Pharm 1983;40:101–2.
7. Wolfert RR, Cox RM. Am J Hosp Pharm 1975;32:585–7.

Ergotamine (BAN, rINN)

Vasoconstrictor; Analgesic (migraine)

(5′*S*)-5′-Benzyl-9,10-dihydro-12′-hydroxy-2′-methyl-3′,6′,18-trioxoergotaman; 12′-hydroxy-2′-methyl-5′α-benzylergotaman-3′,6′,18-trione

$C_{33}H_{35}N_5O_5 = 581.7$

Ergotamine Tartrate (BANM, rINNM)

$(C_{33}H_{35}N_5O_5)_2$, $C_4H_6O_6 = 1313.4$

CAS—113-15-5 (ergotamine); 379-79-3 (ergotamine tartrate)

Pharmacopoeial status

BP, USP (ergotamine tartrate)

Preparations

Compendial

Ergotamine Tablets BP. Tablets containing, in each, 1 mg ergotamine tartrate are usually available.

Ergotamine Injection BP is a sterile solution prepared by dissolving ergotamine tartrate in water for injections containing ethanol (96%), glycerol and sufficient tartaric acid to adjust the acidity of the solution to pH 3.3. An injection containing 500 micrograms in 1 mL is usually available. pH 2.8 to 3.8.

Ergotamine Tartrate Tablets USP.

Ergotamine Tartrate Injection USP. pH 3.5 to 4.0.

Ergotamine Tartrate Inhalation Aerosol USP.

Non-compendial

Lingraine (Sanofi Winthrop). *Tablets* (sublingual), ergotamine tartrate 2 mg.

Medihaler-Ergotamine (3M). *Aerosol inhalation* (oral), ergotamine tartrate 9 mg/mL (360 micrograms/metered inhalation).

Containers and storage

Solid state

Ergotamine Tartrate BP should be kept in an airtight, glass container, protected from light and stored at a temperature of 2° to 8°. Ergotamine Tartrate USP should be preserved in well-closed, light-resistant containers in a cold place.

Dosage forms

Ergotamine Injection BP should be protected from light.

Ergotamine Tartrate Tablets USP should be preserved in well-closed, light-resistant containers.

Ergotamine Tartrate Injection USP should be preserved in single-dose, light-resistant containers, preferably of Type I glass.

Ergotamine Tartrate Inhalation Aerosol USP should be preserved in small, non-reactive, light-resistant aerosol containers equipped with metered-dose valves and provided with oral inhalation actuators.

Medihaler-Ergotamine should be stored at 5° until dispensed. The pressurised container should not be punctured or burned.

PHYSICAL PROPERTIES

Ergotamine exists as hygroscopic crystals which darken and decompose on exposure to air, heat, and light.

Ergotamine tartrate exists as colourless crystals or a white or yellowish-white, crystalline powder; odourless and slightly hygroscopic.

Melting point

Ergotamine melts between 212° and 214°, with decomposition. *Ergotamine tartrate* melts around 180°, with decomposition.

pH

The pH of a 0.25% aqueous suspension of *ergotamine tartrate* lies between 4.0 and 5.5.

Dissociation constant

pK_a 6.4 (24°)

Solubility

Ergotamine is practically insoluble in water; soluble 1 in 300 of ethanol and 1 in 150 of acetone; freely soluble in chloroform.

Ergotamine tartrate is soluble in about 1 in 500 of water if a slight excess of tartaric acid is present to prevent the solution becoming turbid; it is slightly soluble in ethanol (1 in 500) and in chloroform; practically insoluble in ether.

The aqueous solubility of ergotamine tartrate in solutions of tartaric acid, citric acid, hydrochloric acid, and caffeine was found to be dependent upon pH, the concentration of the solvent, and the presence of chloride ions.[1]

Enhancement of solubility

Results of partitioning and pH studies (at pH 1.0 and 6.5) demonstrated that caffeine enhanced the solubility of ergotamine tartrate. Caffeine (5.0 g) was shown to enhance the dissolution rate of ergotamine tartrate (50 mg) by a factor of three at 'gastric pH' in 500 mL of 0.1N hydrochloric acid.[2] Maximum enhancement of solubility at pH 1.0, pH 5.5, and pH 6.5 was reached at 20:1, 30:1, and 800:1 molar ratios of caffeine to ergotamine tartrate, respectively.

Dissolution

The USP specifies that for Ergotamine Tartrate Tablets USP not less than 75% of the labelled amount of $(C_{33}H_{35}N_5O_5)_2,C_4H_6O_6$ is dissolved in 30 minutes. Dissolution medium : 1000 mL of tartaric acid solution (1 in 100); Apparatus 2 at 75 rpm.

Dissolution properties

The dissolution rate (in 0.1M hydrochloric acid) of ergotamine from 100-mg ergotamine tartrate disks was enhanced by 2.4 times when 0.15M citric acid was included in the medium, 6.5 times when 0.025M caffeine was included in the medium, and 7.0 times in the presence of both 0.15M citric acid and 0.025M caffeine.[1] The dissolution rate of ergotamine in a pH 5.0 acetate buffer was similar to that in 0.1M hydrochloric acid, whereas solubility was 20 times greater in the acetate buffer.

STABILITY

In aqueous acidic solution ergotamine degrades by reversible epimerisation to ergotaminine. In a study of the stability of ergotamine tartrate in aqueous solution, Kreilgård and Kisbye[3] propose heating for 85 minutes at 100° and pH 3.3 to 3.9 to promote sufficient epimerisation to achieve equilibrium and minimise other reactions. Degradation due to other processes was found to be minimal at pH 3.6. The epimerisation reaction was first-order at 30° to 60° with a calculated activation energy of 96.14 kJ/mol. In acidic solutions, ergotamine and ergotaminine invert to form aci-ergotamine and aci-ergotaminine. Degradation also occurs by hydrolysis to lysergic acid amide and isolysergic acid amide, by photolysis to various lumi-compounds and by oxidation. Protection from light and storage under inert gas has been shown to curb oxidation and formation of lumi-compounds.

It has been recommended[3] that injections of ergotamine tartrate should be formulated in water for injections that contains ethanol 5% w/v, glycerol 15% w/v, and enough tartaric acid to maintain an equilibrium mixture of the tartrates of ergotamine and ergotaminine at the pH of optimal stability (pH 3.6). It was claimed that this solution can be stored for an unlimited time when packaged with inert gas in ampoules, heated for 85 minutes at 100°, and kept in a cold place (3°), protected from light. The extent of ergotamine isomerism (to produce ergotaminine) in six preparations (1 capsule, 4 tablet and 1 parenteral solution) from five Australian manufacturers was examined by Heazlewood and Eadie.[4] Only a small trace of ergotaminine was detected in the capsules, but the ergotamine content ranged from less than 1% up to 12% in the tablet samples. The parenteral solution was found to contain 37% of ergotaminine tartrate and only 58% of the stated amount of ergotamine tartrate.

FURTHER INFORMATION. Stability of ergotamine tartrate in aqueous solution [degradation schemes for ergotamine are outlined]—Kreilgård B, Kisbye J. Arch Pharm Chemi (Sci) 1974;2:1–13.

FORMULATION

Excipients

Excipients that have been used in presentations of ergotamine tartrate include:
Tablets (sublingual): hydroxypropylcellulose; lactose; magnesium stearate; maize starch; mannitol; peppermint flavours, artificial; pregelatinised starch; saccharin sodium; sunset yellow FCF (E110), aluminium lake.
Aerosol inhaler: dichlorodifluoromethane; dichlorotetrafluoroethane; sorbitan trioleate; trichloromonofluoromethane.

PROCESSING

Sterilisation

Solutions of ergotamine tartrate for injection are sterilised by filtration. Oxidation can be minimised by replacing the air in containers by nitrogen or other suitable gas.

REFERENCES

1. Anderson JR, Pitman IH. J Pharm Sci 1980;69(7):832–5.
2. Zoglio MA, Maulding HV, Windheuser JJ. J Pharm Sci 1969;58(2):222–5.
3. Kreilgård B, Kisbye J. Arch Pharm Chemi Sci 1974;2:38–49.
4. Heazlewood RL, Eadie MJ. Aust J Pharm Sci 1980;9(3):90–1.

Erythromycin (BAN, rINN)   *Antibacterial*

Erythromycin A; eritromicina
(2R,3S,4S,5R,6R,8R,10R,11R,12S,13R)-5-(3-amino-3,4,6-tri-deoxy-N,N-dimethyl-β-D-*xylo*-hexopyranosyloxy)-3-(2,6-dideoxy-3-C,3-O-dimethyl-α-L-*ribo*-hexopyranosyloxy)-13-ethyl-6,11,12-trihydroxy-2,4,6,8,10,12-hexamethyl-9-oxotridecan-13-olide
$C_{37}H_{67}NO_{13} = 733.9$

Erythromycin Estolate (BAN, USAN, rINNM)
Erythromycin propionate lauryl sulphate; propionyl erythromycin lauryl sulphate
Erythromycin 2′-propionate dodecyl sulphate; erythromycin 2′-propanoate, dodecyl sulfate
$C_{40}H_{71}NO_{14}, C_{12}H_{26}O_4S = 1056.4$

Erythromycin Ethyl Succinate (BANM)
Erythromycin ethylsuccinate
Erythromycin 2′-(ethyl succinate); erythromycin 2′-(ethyl butanedioate)
$C_{43}H_{75}NO_{16} = 862.1$

Erythromycin Gluceptate (BANM, rINNM)
Erythromycin glucoheptonate
$C_{37}H_{67}NO_{13}, C_7H_{14}O_8 = 960.1$

Erythromycin Lactobionate (BANM)
Erythromycin mono(4-O-β-D-galactopyranosyl-D-gluconate)
$C_{37}H_{67}NO_{13}, C_{12}H_{22}O_{12} = 1092.2$

Erythromycin Propionate (BANM, USAN)
Erythromycin 2′-propanoate; erythromycin 2′-propionate
$C_{40}H_{71}NO_{14} = 790.0$

Erythromycin Stearate (BANM, rINNM)
The stearate of erythromycin with some uncombined stearic acid and sodium stearate.

$C_{37}H_{67}NO_{13}$, $C_{18}H_{36}O_2 = 1018.4$

CAS—114-07-8 (erythromycin); 3521-62-8 (erythromycin estolate); 41342-53-4, 1264-62-6 (erythromycin ethyl succinate); 304-63-2, 23067-13-2 (erythromycin gluceptate); 3847-29-8 (erythromycin lactobionate); 134-36-1 (erythromycin propionate); 643-22-1 (erythromycin stearate)

Pharmacopoeial status

BP (erythromycin, erythromycin estolate, erythromycin ethyl succinate, erythromycin lactobionate, erythromycin stearate); USP (erythromycin, erythromycin estolate, erythromycin ethylsuccinate, erythromycin stearate)

Preparations

Compendial
Erythromycin Tablets BP. Tablets containing in each, 250 mg and 500 mg are usually available. They are made gastro-resistant by enteric-coating or by other means.
Erythromycin Estolate Capsules BP. Capsules containing, in each, the equivalent of 250 mg of erythromycin are usually available.
Erythromycin Lactobionate Intravenous Infusion BP (Erythromycin Lactobionate for Intravenous Infusion). A sterile solution of erythromycin lactobionate in sodium chloride injection. It is prepared immediately before use by dissolving erythromycin lactobionate for intravenous infusion in the requisite amount of water for injections and diluting the resulting solution with the requisite amount of sodium chloride intravenous infusion. Sealed containers each containing the equivalent of 1 g of erythromycin are usually available.
Erythromycin Stearate Tablets BP. Tablets containing, in each, the equivalent of 250 mg and 500 mg of erythromycin are usually available.
Erythromycin Delayed-release Capsules USP.
Erythromycin Tablets USP.
Erythromycin Delayed-release Tablets USP.
Erythromycin Topical Solution USP.
Erythromycin Topical Gel USP.
Erythromycin Ointment USP.
Erythromycin Ophthalmic Ointment USP.
Erythromycin Pledgets USP.
Erythromycin Estolate Capsules USP.
Erythromycin Estolate Tablets USP.
Erythromycin Estolate Oral Suspension USP.
Erythromycin Estolate for Oral Suspension USP.
Erythromycin Ethylsuccinate Tablets USP.
Erythromycin Ethylsuccinate Oral Suspension USP.
Erythromycin Ethylsuccinate for Oral Suspension USP.
Erythromycin Ethylsuccinate Injection USP.
Sterile Erythromycin Ethylsuccinate USP.
Sterile Erythromycin Gluceptate USP. Suitable for parenteral use.
Erythromycin Lactobionate for Injection USP. pH between 6.5 and 7.5, in a solution containing the equivalent of 50 mg of erythromycin per mL; contains a suitable preservative.
Sterile Erythromycin Lactobionate USP. pH between 6.5 and 7.5, in a solution containing the equivalent of 50 mg of erythromycin per mL.
Erythromycin Stearate Tablets USP.
Erythromycin Stearate for Oral Suspension USP.

Non-compendial
Erycen (Berk). *Tablets*, enteric coated, erythromycin 250 mg and 500 mg.
Erymax (P-D). *Capsules*, containing enteric-coated pellets, erythromycin 250 mg.

Erythrocin (Abbott). *Tablets*, erythromycin (as stearate) 250 mg and 500 mg.
Erythrocin IV Lactobionate (Abbott). *Intravenous infusion*, powder for reconstitution, erythromycin 1 g (as lactobionate). For use specifically with the Abbott Add-Vantage flexible polyvinyl chloride container containing sodium chloride 0.9% injection.
Erythromid (Abbott). *Tablets*, enteric coated, erythromycin 250 mg and 500 mg (Erythromid DS).
Erythromycin Lactobionate (Abbott). *Intravenous infusion*, powder for reconstitution with water for injections, erythromycin 1 g (as lactobionate). *Diluents*: sodium chloride 0.9% injection or glucose 5% injection solution neutralised with sterile 8.4% w/v sodium bicarbonate solution.
Erythroped (Abbott). *Suspension PI*, erythromycin 125 mg (as ethyl succinate)/5 mL when reconstituted with water.
Suspension PI SF, sugar free, erythromycin 125 mg (as ethyl succinate)/5 mL when reconstituted with water.
Granules PI, erythromycin (as ethyl succinate) 125 mg/sachet.
Granules PI SF, erythromycin (as ethyl succinate) 125 mg/sachet.
Suspension, erythromycin 250 mg (as ethyl succinate)/5 mL when reconstituted with water.
Suspension SF, sugar free, erythromycin 250 mg (as ethyl succinate)/5 mL when reconstituted with water.
Granules, erythromycin (as ethyl succinate) 250 mg/sachet.
Granules SF, erythromycin (as ethyl succinate) 250 mg/sachet.
Suspension forte, erythromycin 500 mg (as ethyl succinate)/5 mL when reconstituted with water.
Granules forte, erythromycin (as ethyl succinate) 500 mg/sachet.
Erythroped A (Abbott). *Tablets*, sugar free, erythromycin 500 mg (as ethyl succinate).
Granules, erythromycin (as ethyl succinate) 1 g/sachet.
Ilosone (Dista). *Capsules*, erythromycin 250 mg (as estolate).
Tablets, erythromycin 500 mg (as estolate).
Suspension, erythromycin 125 mg (as estolate)/5 mL. *Diluent*: syrup, life of diluted suspension 14 days.
Suspension forte, erythromycin 250 mg (as estolate)/5 mL. *Diluent*: syrup, life of diluted suspension 14 days.
Stiemycin (Stiefel). *Topical solution*, erythromycin 2% in an alcoholic basis.
Erythromycin enteric-coated tablets of various strengths are also available from APS, Ashbourne (Rommix), Cox, CP, Evans, Kerfoot, Norton.
Erythromycin (as ethyl succinate) mixtures of various strengths are also available from APS, Ashbourne (Rommix), Berk, Cox, CP, Evans, Kerfoot, Norton, RP Drugs (Arpimycin).
Erythromycin lactobionate intravenous infusion (powder for reconstitution) is also available from David Bull.

Containers and storage

Solid state
Erythromycin BP and Erythromycin Stearate BP should be kept in well-closed containers, protected from light and stored at a temperature not exceeding 30°.
Erythromycin Estolate BP and Erythromycin Ethyl Succinate BP should be kept in airtight containers, protected from light and stored at a temperature not exceeding 30°.
Erythromycin Lactobionate BP should be kept in a well-closed container and stored at a temperature not exceeding 25°. If the substance is sterile, the container should be sterile, tamper-evident and sealed so as to exclude micro-organisms.
Erythromycin USP, Erythromycin Estolate USP, Erythromycin Ethylsuccinate USP, and Erythromycin Stearate USP should be preserved in tight containers.

Dosage forms

Erythromycin Lactobionate Intravenous Infusion BP, in the sealed container, should be stored at a temperature not exceeding 25°. It should be used immediately after preparation but, in any case, within the period recommended by the manufacturer when prepared and stored strictly in accordance with the manufacturer's instructions.

Erythromycin Stearate Tablets BP should be protected from light.

Erythromycin Delayed-release Capsules USP, Tablets USP, Delayed-release Tablets USP, Topical Solution USP, Topical Gel USP, and Pledgets USP should be stored in tight containers.

Erythromycin Ointment USP should be stored in collapsible tubes or in other tight containers, preferably at controlled room temperature.

Erythromycin Ophthalmic Ointment USP should be stored in collapsible ophthalmic ointment tubes.

Erythromycin Estolate Capsules USP, Erythromycin Estolate Tablets USP, and Erythromycin Estolate for Oral Suspension USP should all be preserved in tight containers. Erythromycin Estolate Oral Suspension USP should be preserved in tight containers, in a cold place.

Erythromycin Ethylsuccinate Tablets USP, Erythromycin Ethylsuccinate Oral Suspension USP, and Erythromycin Ethylsuccinate for Oral Suspension USP should all be preserved in tight containers. The oral suspension should be stored in a cold place.

Erythromycin Ethylsuccinate Injection USP should be preserved in single-dose or in multiple-dose containers, preferably of Type I glass.

Sterile Erythromycin Ethylsuccinate USP should be preserved in containers suitable for sterile solids.

Sterile Erythromycin Gluceptate USP should be preserved in containers suitable for sterile solids.

Erythromycin Lactobionate for Injection USP and Sterile Erythromycin Lactobionate USP should be stored in containers suitable for sterile solids.

Erythromycin Stearate Tablets USP and Erythromycin Stearate for Oral Suspension USP should be preserved in tight containers.

Erycen should be stored below 30° in a tightly closed container and protected from light.

Erymax should be stored below 25° and protected from moisture and light.

Erythrocin tablets should be stored in tightly closed bottles, protected from light, at a temperature below 25°.

Erythromid should be stored below 25° in a tightly closed container and protected from light.

Erythromycin Lactobionate (Abbott) powder for reconstitution is stable at room temperature. The reconstituted solution should be stored in a refrigerator at 2° to 8°.

Erythroped suspensions should be stored in a cool place and the containers kept tightly closed. The suspensions and sugar-free suspensions should be used within 14 days and 7 days of dispensing, respectively. Erythroped A preparations should be stored below 30°. Erythroped sugar-free preparations should be protected from heat.

Ilosone capsules, tablets, and suspensions should be stored in tightly closed containers. Ilosone suspensions should be protected from light.

Stiemycin should be stored in a cool place.

PHYSICAL PROPERTIES

Erythromycin exists as slightly yellow crystals or a white or slightly yellow powder; slightly hygroscopic; odourless or practically odourless with a bitter taste.

Erythromycin estolate is a white, crystalline powder.

Erythromycin ethyl succinate is a white or slightly yellow, odourless, almost tasteless, crystalline powder; hygroscopic.

Erythromycin gluceptate is a white powder; odourless or practically odourless; slightly hygroscopic.

Erythromycin lactobionate and *erythromycin propionate* are white powders.

Erythromycin stearate is a white or slightly yellow crystalline powder; odourless or may have a slight earthy odour with a slightly bitter taste.

Melting point

Crystals of *erythromycin* hydrated from water melt in the range 135° to 140°, followed by resolidification with a second melting point in the range 190° to 193°.

Erythromycin estolate melts in the range 135° to 138°.

Crystals of *erythromycin gluceptate* melt in the range 95° to 140°.

Erythromycin lactobionate melts in the range 145° to 150°.

Monohydrate crystals of *erythromycin propionate* formed by crystallisation from acetone and water melt in the range 122° to 126°.

The melting behaviour of crystalline erythromycin base was studied by Allen *et al*[1] using differential thermal analysis, thermal gravimetric analysis, X-ray diffractometry, and hot stage microscopy. A conversion of the monohydrate (requires either the presence of dimethicones or slow heating) and the dihydrate to the anhydrate (melting point 190° to 193°) via an amorphous intermediate was indicated. It was suggested that the melting range of 130° to 135° reported by other workers for the monohydrate and dihydrate represents the formation of an amorphous phase and that the true melting range is 190° to 193° corresponding to that of the anhydrate crystal form. In a later study, Fukumori *et al*[2] suggested that the monohydrate form identified by Allen *et al* was actually 'a desolvation product of the chloroform solvate with some degree of crystallinity'.

pH

The pH of a 0.067% w/v solution of *erythromycin* in carbon dioxide-free water is 8.0 to 10.5.

The BP states that when 0.4 g of *erythromycin estolate* is suspended in 10 mL of carbon dioxide-free water and the solution is shaken and allowed to stand, the pH of the clear supernatant liquid is 5.5 to 7.0.

The USP states that an aqueous suspension containing 10 mg/mL *erythromycin estolate* has a pH between 4.5 to 7.0.

The pH of a 1% w/v aqueous suspension of *erythromycin ethyl succinate* is in the range 6.0 to 8.5.

A 2.5% aqueous solution of *erythromycin gluceptate* has a pH of 6 to 8 and a 5% solution is neutral.

A 2% aqueous solution of *erythromycin lactobionate* has a pH of 6.0 to 7.5 and a 7.5% w/v solution has a pH of 6.5 to 7.5.

The pH of a 1% w/v suspension of *erythromycin stearate* is stated in the BP to be in the range 7.0 to 10.5; the USP specifies a pH range of 6.0 to 11.0 for a similar aqueous suspension.

Dissociation constants

pK_a values of 8.6, 8.7, 8.8, and 8.9 have been reported for *erythromycin*. In 66% dimethylformamide/34% water the pK_a is 8.6.

Erythromycin estolate: pK_a in 66% dimethylformamide/34% water, 6.9

Erythromycin ethyl succinate: pK_a 8.7

Erythromycin propionate: pK_a 6.9

Solubility

Erythromycin is soluble 1 in 1000 of water at 20° but is less soluble in hot water; soluble 1 in 5 of ethanol, 1 in 6 of chloroform, and 1 in 5 of ether; soluble in acetone and in methanol; it dissolves in 2M hydrochloric acid.

Erythromycin estolate is practically insoluble in water; soluble 1 in 2 of ethanol, 1 in 10 of chloroform, and 1 in 15 of acetone; practically insoluble in 2M hydrochloric acid.

Erythromycin ethyl succinate is very slightly soluble in water; freely soluble in ethanol, in acetone, in chloroform, in macrogol 400, and in methanol; soluble in ether.

Erythromycin gluceptate is freely soluble in water, in ethanol, in dioxan, in methanol, and in propylene glycol; slightly soluble in acetone and in chloroform; practically insoluble in benzene, in carbon tetrachloride, in ether, and in toluene.

Erythromycin lactobionate is freely soluble in water, in ethanol, and in methanol; slightly soluble in acetone and in chloroform; practically insoluble in ether.

Erythromycin propionate is slightly soluble in water; freely soluble in ethanol, in acetone, in chloroform, in dimethylformamide, in ethyl acetate, and in methanol.

Erythromycin stearate is practically insoluble in water; soluble in ethanol, in acetone, in chloroform, in methanol (solutions in these four solvents may be opalescent) and in ether.

Dissolution

The USP specifies that for Erythromycin Delayed-release Capsules USP, not less than 80% of the labelled amount of $C_{37}H_{67}NO_{13}$ is dissolved in 120 minutes. Dissolution medium: 900 mL of 0.06N hydrochloric acid (acid stage, 60 minutes) and 900 mL of pH 6.8 phosphate buffer (buffer stage, 60 minutes); Apparatus 1 at 50 rpm.

The USP specifies that for Erythromycin Tablets USP, not less than 70% of the labelled amount of $C_{37}H_{67}NO_{13}$ is dissolved in 60 minutes. Dissolution medium: 900 mL of 0.05M pH 6.8 phosphate buffer; Apparatus 2 at 50 rpm.

The USP specifies that for Erythromycin Ethylsuccinate Tablets USP not less than 75% of the labelled amount of $C_{37}H_{67}NO_{13}$ equivalent is dissolved in 45 minutes. Dissolution medium: 900 mL of 0.1N hydrochloric acid; Apparatus 2 at 50 rpm.

The USP specifies that for Erythromycin Stearate Tablets USP not less than 75% of the labelled amount of $C_{37}H_{67}NO_{13}$ is dissolved in 120 minutes. Dissolution medium: 900 mL of monobasic sodium phosphate buffer with 0.5% sodium lauryl sulphate; Apparatus 2 at 100 rpm.

Dissolution properties

Dissolution studies in aqueous solution[1] (0.01M phosphate buffer, pH 7.5) at 37° showed that the dihydrate form of erythromycin base dissolved at a significantly greater rate than the monohydrate and anhydrate. Differences in dissolution rates were attributed to particle-particle interactions and variations in the wettability of the different hydrates.

The crystalline form of erythromycin estolate had a more rapid dissolution rate (in phosphate buffer, pH 6, at 37°) than the amorphous form, which dissolved very slowly. Differences in the dissolution behaviour of the two forms may be related to their wettability.[3]

FURTHER INFORMATION. Characterisation of commercial lots of erythromycin base [a wide-ranging study of the thermal behaviour, crystal properties, solubility, dissolution properties, and wettability of erythromycin]—Murthy KS, Turner NA, Nesbitt RU, Fawzi MB. Drug Dev Ind Pharm 1986;12(5):665–90. Correlation of *in vivo* bioavailability of erythromycin stearate tablets with *in vitro* tests—Stavchansky S, Doluisio JT, Martin A, Martin C, Cabana B, Dighe S, Loper A. J Pharm Sci 1980;69(11):1307–10.

STABILITY

The stability of erythromycin base in aqueous solutions is affected by pH. Maximum stability occurs in the pH range 7.0 to 7.5.[4] Decomposition in both acid and alkaline media follows first-order kinetics. The activation energy for the hydrolysis of erythromycin at pH 7.0 has been reported to be 77.8 kJ/mol. Following treatment with weak acid (glacial acetic acid), erythromycin-6,9-hemiketal was produced and further treatment with a stronger acid (methanolic hydrochloric acid) yielded the 'spiroketal' anhydroerythromycin. Treatment with strong acid (hydrochloric acid, pH 2.0, 30 minutes) directly yielded the 'spiroketal' form following the loss of one molecule of water from the active erythromycin.[5] The reaction appeared to be irreversible. Further acid treatment of anhydroerythromycin produced erythralosamine and cladinose. Greater instability was demonstrated in acid media than in alkaline media. In an extensive review of the properties and degradation of erythromycin, Flynn[6] reported that, in alkaline media, erythromycin yielded an unidentified zwitterionic product that contained one extra molecule of water, compared with the base, and had an acidic group that had a pK_a of 4.3 and a basic group of pK_a 9.1. A 2,2-disubstituted-1,3-diketone was also suggested to be a possible degradation product. Workers in Belgium[7] identified the degradation products of erythromycin (at pH values greater than 8) as pseudoerythromycin enol ether and pseudoerythromycin hemiketal.

Erythromycin, in solid state and in solution (pH 4 and pH 8), is photostable.

Effect of buffers

Examination of decomposition in various buffer systems at different temperatures demonstrated that erythromycin base is more stable in sodium buffers than in potassium buffers, and citrate and phosphate buffers are preferable to acetate.[4]

Effect of metal ions

Amer and Takla[4] examined the effect of different metal ions on erythromycin stability in solution. Degradation was enhanced by the presence of Al^{3+}, Fe^{3+}, and Cu^{2+} ions whereas Co^{2+}, Zn^{2+}, Pb^{2+}, and Ni^{2+} had a stabilising effect (possibly due to chelate formation between the metal and erythromycin) and degradation was not affected by Ca^{2+}, Mg^{2+}, or Hg^{2+} ions.

Erythromycin salts

From an Arrhenius plot, the half-lives of four salts of erythromycin in 0.1M sodium citrate buffer (pH 7) at 25° were predicted as 18 days, 27 days, 33 days, and 36 days for the *lactobionate, gluceptate, ethylsuccinate*, and *estolate*, respectively.[4] *Erythromycin estolate* is acid-stable. *Erythromycin stearate* is not as susceptible to decomposition as some of the other erythromycin salts as it is the salt of the tertiary aliphatic amine and stearic acid and has low solubility.

Erythromycin lactobionate is most stable in the pH range 6 to 8 and stability decreases rapidly as the pH becomes more acidic.[8]

Effect of freezing and thawing

The stability of *erythromycin* (as *lactobionate*) infusions (Abbott) was not affected by storage for 12 months at −20°, followed by microwave thawing. The infusion solutions remained chemically and physically stable even when thawed after 6 months and subjected to three freeze-thaw cycles.[9]

Admixtures of *erythromycin gluceptate* (500 mg) in either sodium chloride 0.9% injection or glucose 5% in water (in Viaflex minibags) were stable for up to 30 days when frozen at $-20°$; samples that were thawed and stored for 21 hours at 5° to 6° were also stable.[10]

Ophthalmic preparation

Bialer *et al*[11] reported that erythromycin ophthalmic ointment (0.5%; Fougera, USA) was stable after being aseptically repackaged (in 0.2 mL aliquots) into 1-mL tuberculin syringes and stored at room temperature for up to 15 days. In addition, samples heated at 45° for 6 hours retained acceptable *in-vitro* activity.

Topical preparations

In a detailed study,[12] the stability of erythromycin 1.5% in an oil-in-water emulsion (cetyl alcohol, white beeswax, propylene glycol, sodium lauryl sulphate, methyl and propyl hydroxybenzoates, de-ionised water), a water-in-oil emulsion (white beeswax, spermaceti, cetiol V, sorbitan mono-oleate, methyl and propyl hydroxybenzoates, de-ionised water), an alcoholic solution, and an alcoholic gel, was observed to decrease with an increase in pH (from 6.3 to 8.5) and in temperature (from 4° to 25°). The emulsions and the gel were packaged in aluminium ointment tubes and the alcoholic solution was kept in a dark brown glass bottle. During storage of the emulsions at 4° and the alcoholic solution and gel at 25° for one month, acceptable stability (microbiological assay, over 90% of activity remaining) was apparent; emulsions of pH 8.5 lost about 60% activity after one month at 25°.

Rapid loss of erythromycin potency was reported from an ointment containing white soft paraffin with 5% to 10% white or yellow beeswax.

Stabilisation

Tablets containing erythromycin may be enteric coated to reduce rapid inactivation in the acidic gastric juice. The greater stability of the low solubility salts of erythromycin make them more suitable for the preparation of solid dosage forms. Preparations containing erythromycin in solution should have neutral pH.[4]

FURTHER INFORMATION. The influence of buffering on the stability of erythromycin injection in small-volume infusions—Allwood MC. Int J Pharmaceutics 1992;80:R7–R9. Stability of erythromycin in neutral and alkaline medium—Paesen J, Khan K, Roets E, Hoogmartens J. Pharm Weekbl (Sci) 1992;14(1):A7.

INCOMPATIBILITY/COMPATIBILITY

Erythromycin ethyl succinate is reported to be incompatible with ampicillin sodium and cloxacillin sodium.

Erythromycin lactobionate has been reported to be incompatible with aminophylline, ampicillin sodium, cephalothin sodium, chloramphenicol sodium succinate, colistin sulphomethate sodium, gentamicin sulphate, heparin sodium, metaraminol tartrate, tetracycline hydrochloride, and thiopentone sodium.

Injections and infusions

Erythromycin gluceptate (Ilotycin, Lilly) was included in a study of incompatibilities shown by 34 drugs. Incompatibility was identified between the salt and chloramphenicol sodium succinate (Chloromycetin), prochlorperazine edisylate (Compazine), phenytoin sodium (Dilantin) and phenobarbitone sodium (Luminal).[13] This salt is also reported to be incompatible with amikacin sulphate, cephalothin sodium, cephazolin sodium, heparin sodium, novobiocin, streptomycin, and tetracycline.

In a comparison of the stability of *erythromycin lactobionate* (Erythrocin IV, Abbott) and *erythromycin gluceptate* (Ilotycin, Lilly) either as the reconstituted injections or as intravenous admixtures in various infusion fluids in glass and plastic containers, no significant difference was apparent between the first-order rate constants for the degradation reactions or the times required for drug concentrations to decrease to 90% of their initial value ($t_{10\%}$). A table which lists the rate constants and $t_{10\%}$ values for erythromycin in acidic and alkaline solutions was also presented.[14] The addition of *erythromycin gluceptate* (Ilotycin, Lilly), in various concentrations to different volumes of either glucose 5% in water or glucose 5% in sodium chloride 0.9% caused the pH of the vehicles to increase by up to 1.7 units. As erythromycin gluceptate is stable only in the pH range 6.0 to 7.5, it was suggested that the pH of the injection be tested before its addition.[15]

Bergstrom and Fites[16] recommended that, following the addition of *erythromycin gluceptate* (Ilotycin, Lilly, USA), sodium chloride 0.9% and glucose 5% infusion solutions should be buffered to pH 7.0 to 8.0 with either phosphate-carbonate buffer or sodium bicarbonate 4% additive solution. Further studies led to the conclusion that the pH-dependent stability of erythromycin salts and esters is a function of the pH instability of the base.

Erythromycin lactobionate (Abbott, USA) was stable for 24 hours at room temperature in sodium chloride 0.9% injection with or without the inclusion of sodium bicarbonate 4%. However, the addition of buffer solution was necessary to ensure stability of the salt under similar storage conditions in glucose 5% injection.[17]

FORMULATION

Excipients

Excipients that have been used in presentations of erythromycin include:

Capsules, erythromycin: cellulose polymers; citrate ester; D&C Red No.30; lactose; magnesium stearate; povidone; quinoline yellow (E104); sunset yellow FCF (E110).

Tablets, erythromycin: allura red AC (E129); brilliant blue FCF (133); calcium phosphate; carmellose calcium; carnauba wax; cellacephate; cellulose; ponceau 4R (E124); D&C Red No.30; erythrosine (E127); hydroxypropylcellulose; hypromellose; iron oxide; lactose; liquid paraffin; macrogol; magnesium hydroxide; magnesium stearate; maize starch; microcrystalline cellulose; monoglycerides (diacetylated); ponceau 4R (E124); povidone; propylene glycol; silica; sodium citrate; sodium starch glycollate; sorbic acid; sorbitan mono-oleate; soybean derivatives; stearic acid; sucrose; sunset yellow FCF (E110); talc; titanium dioxide (E171); vanillin.

Erythromycin estolate: allura red AC (E129); cellulose; citric acid; D&C Red No.30; iron oxides; magnesium stearate; mannitol; povidone; quinoline yellow (E104); saccharin; sodium chloride; sodium citrate; starch (maize); stearic acid; sucrose; titanium dioxide (E171).

Erythromycin ethyl succinate: allura red AC (E129); aluminium magnesium silicate; Amberlite; calcium hydrogen phosphate; carmellose sodium; citric acid; D&C Red No.30; iron oxide; macrogol; magnesium stearate; mannitol; methyl and propyl hydroxybenzoates; polysorbate 60; propylene glycol; quinoline yellow (E104); saccharin sodium; sodium citrate; sodium starch glycollate; sorbic acid; sorbitan mono-oleate; starch; sucrose; sugar; sunset yellow FCF (E110); titanium dioxide (E171); vitamin E.

Erythromycin propionate: colloidal silica; glucose; magnesium stearate; microcrystalline cellulose; saccharin sodium; sorbitol; starch (maize); talc.

Erythromycin stearate: Amberlite; carmellose sodium; D&C Red No.7; erythrosine (E127); hydroxypropylcellulose; hypromellose; macrogol; magnesium hydroxide; magnesium stearate; methyl and propyl hydroxybenzoates; polacrilin potassium; potassium phosphate; povidone; propylene glycol; sodium citrate; sorbic acid; sorbitan mono-oleate; starch (maize); talc; titanium dioxide (E171); triethyl citrate; vanillin.

Oral liquids, erythromcyin estolate: allura red AC (E129); carmellose; cellulose; citric acid; butyl, methyl, and propyl hydroxybenzoates; silicone; sodium calcium edetate; sodium chloride; sodium citrate; sodium lauryl sulphate; sucrose; sunset yellow FCF (E110).

Erythromycin ethyl succinate: acid fuchsine D; allura red AC (E129); aluminium magnesium silicate; caramel; carmellose sodium; citric acid; erythrosine (E127); methyl and propyl hydroxybenzoates; polysorbate; quinoline yellow (E104); saccharin sodium; sodium chloride; sodium citrate; sucrose; Veegum; xanthan gum.

Granules, erythromycin ethyl succinate: acacia; aluminium magnesium silicate; ammoniated liquorice; beta carotene; carmellose sodium; colloidal silica (Aerosil); erythrosine (E127); mannitol; poloxamer 188; saccharin sodium; sodium citrate; sodium lauryl sulphate; sodium starch glycollate; sucrose; sunset yellow FCF (E110); Veegum.

Topical solutions, erythromycin: acetone; citric acid; ethanol; ethylene glycol monoethyl ether; hydroxypropylcellulose; Laureth 4; macrogol; propylene glycol.

Gels, erythromycin: butylated hydroxytoluene; ethanol; hydroxypropylcellulose.

Adsorption to sorbitol

In a study of the capacity of sorbitol to adsorb several different antibiotics (including *erythromycin ethyl succinate*), Nikolakakis and Newton[18] observed that 'instant' sorbitol had a greater adsorption capacity and binding strength than crystalline sorbitol.

Bioavailability

The bioavailabilities of different crystalline forms of erythromycin have been compared.[19] The anhydrate and dihyrate were identified as 'fast absorbing forms' and the amorphous form demonstrated slowest absorption. The bioavailability of the 'partially crystalline base' was lower than that of the other three forms.

Fraser[20] studied the bioavailabilities of erythromycin and three of its salts after oral administration, with particular reference to the effects of food and water volume in the stomach. The bioavailability of *erythromycin ethyl succinate* was affected by crystal structure and the degree of buffering in solid and liquid formulations. The presence of food improved the absorption of the *ethyl succinate* salt. When the bioavailabilities of various commercial products available in the USA (in 1980) were examined, only one enteric-coated *erythromycin base* tablet (E-Mycin, Upjohn) and one film-coated tablet (Erythrocin Filmtabs, Abbott, administered under fasting conditions) had acceptable bioavailability. When administered with water under fasting conditions, several commercial *erythromycin stearate* tablets had acceptable bioavailability (Erythrocin stearate, Abbott; Bristamycin, Bristol; Erypar, Parke Davis; and others marketed by Barr, Lederle, Mylan, and Purepac). Acceptable bioavailability was demonstrated by *erythromycin estolate* capsules and suspension (Ilosone).

Absorption of erythromycin was more complete after the administration of enteric-coated *base* pellets (base from Faulding, Australia) than from film-coated *stearate* tablets (Abbott, USA) and enteric-coated *base* tablets (Upjohn, USA).[21] Reduced bioavailability was apparent when the *stearate* tablets were administered immediately before meals.

Mather *et al*[22] compared the serum concentrations produced when enteric-coated *erythromycin base* capsules (Eryc, Faulding, Australia) were administered after meals with those produced by film-coated *erythromycin stearate* tablets (Erythrocin Filmtab, Abbott, USA) taken one hour before meals. The initial delay in absorption of *erythromycin base* was attributed to the effect of food; this contrasted with the findings of Rutland *et al*[23] that the bioavailability of erythromycin base (Eryc, Faulding) was apparently not affected by the presence of food. Once initiated, absorption of both preparations was rapid.[22] It was suggested that inter-subject variation in erythromycin absorption may be attributed to physiological rather than biopharmaceutical factors.

Bioequivalence was apparent between two test formulations of *erythromycin estolate* and their corresponding commercially available preparations. Absorption from the two capsule formulations was less uniform than from the two suspensions which also demonstrated approximately 15% greater bioavailability and a faster rate of absorption.[24]

Ointments

A formulation comprising erythromycin in an oleaginous basis (95% soft paraffin:5% hard paraffin) with 5% Span 80 was recommended by Kassem *et al*[25] following a study of the effect of additives on the stability of erythromycin in different ointment bases and on its release from the bases. When stored at room temperature ($20° \pm 5°$) for 15 months, the drug was stable in the oleaginous and water-soluble bases but the emulsion basis had a detrimental effect on drug stability. Inclusion of surfactants in the formulation greatly improved drug release from all the bases; and the inclusion of glycerol and ethanol increased release from the oleaginous basis. Incorporation of cholesterols, ethanol, glycerol, water, or beeswax all reduced erythromycin stability in the oleaginous and water-soluble bases.

FURTHER INFORMATION. Erythromycin [review article which discusses the bioavailability of erythromycin in general and details bioavailability studies in which commercial products were assessed and compared]—Nightingale CH. J Am Pharm Assoc 1976;NS16(4):203–6. Gastric acid inactivation of erythromycin stearate in solid dosage forms—Boggiano BG, Gleeson M. J Pharm Sci 1976;65(4):497–502. Bioavailability of erythromycin stearate: influence of food and fluid volume—Welling PG, Huang H, Hewitt PF, Lyons LL. J Pharm Sci 1978;67(6):764–6. Influence of food on the absorption of erythromycin from enteric-coated pellets and stearate tablets—Digranes A, Josefsson K, Schreiner A. Curr Ther Res 1984;35(3):313-20. Bioavailability of erythromycin acistrate from hard gelatin capsules containing sodium bicarbonate—Marvola M, Nykanen S, Nokelainen M. Pharm Res 1991;8:1056-8.

REFERENCES

1. Allen PV, Rahn PD, Sarapu AC, Vanderwielen AJ. J Pharm Sci 1978;67(8):1087–93.
2. Fukumori Y, Fukuda T, Yamamoto Y, Shigitani Y, Hanyu Y, Takeuchi Y *et al.* Chem Pharm Bull 1983;31(11):4029–39.
3. Piccolo J, Sakr A. Pharm Ind 1984;46:1277–9.
4. Amer MM, Takla KF. Bull Fac Pharm Cairo Univ 1978;15:325–39.

5. Atkins PJ, Herbert TO, Jones NB. Int J Pharmaceutics 1986;30:199–207.
6. Flynn EH, Sigal MV, Wiley PF, Gerzon K. J Am Chem Soc 1954;76:3121–31.
7. Van den Mooter G, Cachet T, Hauchecorne R, Vinckier C, Hoogmartens J. Pharm Weekbl (Sci) 1989;11(Suppl A):A11.
8. Parker EA. Am J Hosp Pharm 1969;26:412–13.
9. Sewell GJ, Palmer AJ. Int J Pharmaceutics 1991;72:57–63.
10. Dinel BA, Ayotte DL, Behme RJ, Black BL, Whitby JL. Drug Intell Clin Pharm 1977;11:542–8.
11. Bialer MG, Baron EJ, Harper RG. Antimicrob Agents Chemother 1987;31:354–5.
12. Vandenbossche GMR, Vanhaecke E, DeMuynck C, Remon JP. Int J Pharmaceutics 1991;67:195–9.
13. Misgen R. Am J Hosp Pharm 1965;22:92–4.
14. Pluta PL, Morgan PK [letter]. Am J Hosp Pharm 1986;43:2732, 2738.
15. Edward M. Am J Hosp Pharm 1967;24:440–9.
16. Bergstrom RF, Fites AL [letter]. Am J Hosp Pharm 1975;32:241.
17. Chow-Tung E, Gurwich EL, Sula JA, Kodack M. Drug Intell Clin Pharm 1980;14(12):848–50.
18. Nikolakakis I, Newton JM. J Pharm Pharmacol 1989;41:145–8.
19. Laine E, Kahela P, Rajala R, Heikkilä T, Saarnivaara K, Piippo I. Int J Pharmaceutics 1987;38:33–8.
20. Fraser DG. Am J Hosp Pharm 1980;37:1199–1202.
21. Josefsson K, Levitt MJ, Kann J, Bon C. Curr Ther Res 1986;39:131–42.
22. Mather LE, Austin KL, Philpot CR, McDonald PJ. Br J Clin Pharmacol 1981;12:131–40.
23. Rutland J, Berend N, Marlin GE. Br J Clin Pharmacol 1979;8:343–7.
24. Dugal R, Cooper SF, Bertrand M. Can J Pharm Sci 1976;11:92–5.
25. Kassem AA, Said SA, Shalaby S. Pharm Ind 1978;40:80–2.

Ethacrynic Acid (BAN, USAN)   *Diuretic*

Etacrynic Acid (rINN)

[(*E*)-2,3-Dichloro-4-(2-ethyl-acryloyl)phenoxy]acetic acid; [2,3-dichloro-4-(2-methylene-1-oxobutyl)phenoxy]acetic acid

$C_{13}H_{12}Cl_2O_4 = 303.1$

Sodium Ethacrynate (BANM)

Ethacrynate Sodium (USAN); Sodium Etacrynate (rINNM)

$C_{13}H_{11}Cl_2NaO_4 = 325.1$

CAS—58-54-8 (ethacrynic acid); 6500-81-8 (sodium ethacrynate)

Pharmacopoeial status

BP, USP (ethacrynic acid)

Preparations

Compendial

Ethacrynic Acid Tablets BP. Tablets containing, in each, 50 mg are usually available.

Sodium Ethacrynate Injection BP (Sodium Ethacrynate for Injection). A sterile solution of the sodium salt of ethacrynic acid in water for injections. It is prepared by dissolving sodium ethacrynate for injection in the requisite amount of the liquid stated on the label. Sealed containers each containing the equivalent of 50 mg of ethacrynic acid are usually available. pH 6.3 to 7.7 for a solution containing the equivalent of 0.1% w/v of ethacrynic acid.

Ethacrynate Tablets USP.

Ethacrynate Sodium for Injection USP. pH between 6.3 and 7.7.

Non-compendial

Edecrin (MSD). *Tablets*, ethacrynic acid 50 mg.

Injection, lyophilised powder for reconstitution, ethacrynic acid (as the sodium salt) 50 mg per vial. To be reconstituted with 50 mL of glucose 5% injection or sodium chloride 0.9% injection. If the pH of the glucose 5% injection is below 5, the resulting solution may be cloudy; use of such a solution is not recommended.

Containers and storage

Solid state

Ethacrynic Acid BP should be kept in a well-closed container.

Ethacrynic Acid USP should be preserved in well-closed containers.

Dosage forms

Sodium Ethacrynate Injection BP. The injection should be protected from light and used immediately after preparation but, in any case, within the period recommended by the manufacturer when prepared and stored strictly in accordance with the manufacturer's instructions.

Ethacrynic Acid Tablets USP should be preserved in well-closed containers.

Ethacrynate Sodium for Injection USP should be preserved in containers suitable for sterile solids.

Edecrin tablets and injection should be stored in a cool place, protected from light. The container for Edecrin tablets should be well closed. Unused reconstituted solutions of Edecrin injection should be discarded after 24 hours.

PHYSICAL PROPERTIES

Ethacrynic acid is a white or almost white, odourless or almost odourless, crystalline powder.

Melting point

Ethacrynic acid melts in the range 121° to 124°.

Dissociation constant

pK_a 3.5 (20°)

Solubility

Ethacrynic acid is very slightly soluble in water; it is freely soluble in ethanol (1 in 1.6), in chloroform (1 in 6) and in ether (1 in 3.5); it dissolves in ammonia and in dilute aqueous solutions of alkali hydroxides and carbonates.

Solubilisation of ethacrynic acid was achieved in the presence of polysorbates 20, 40, 60, or 80 at 20° at pH 2.8 to 4.0; a micellar solubilisation process was indicated as the solubility ratio was a linear function of the concentration of polysorbate surfactant.[1] Partition coefficients of the unionised ethacrynic acid between water and micelles were dependent on the length of the alkyl chain of the polysorbates.

Dissolution

The USP specifies that for Ethacrynic Acid Tablets USP not less than 75% of the labelled amount of $C_{13}H_{12}Cl_2O_4$ is dissolved in 45 minutes. Dissolution medium: 900 mL of 0.1M phosphate buffer, prepared by mixing 13.6 g of monobasic potassium phosphate and 96.2 mL of 0.1N sodium hydroxide with water to obtain 1000 mL of a solution having a pH of 8.0 ± 0.05; Apparatus 2 at 50 rpm.

STABILITY

Solutions of sodium ethacrynate at pH 7 are relatively stable at 25° for short periods of time, although stability is lower at higher pH or temperature.

The principal degradation product of ethacrynic acid has been reported to be a dimer, formed by a Diels-Alder type of condensation.[2] Formation of this dimer was demonstrated in the solid state and in aqueous slurries of ethacrynic acid (from tablets).[3] The dimer was reported to be [4-[2-[4-(carboxymethoxy)-2,3-dichlorobenzoyl]-3,4-dihydro-2,5-diethyl-2H-pyran-6-yl]-2,3-dichlorophenoxy]acetic acid. A rapid, reversed-phase HPLC method was used to investigate other degradation products. In the presence of water, hydration of the methylene double bond of ethacrynic acid to form [2,3-dichloro-4-(2-hydroxymethyl-1-oxobutyl)phenoxy]acetic acid was the initial reaction, which was dependent on temperature and pH, and the rate of reaction increased as the pH increased (pH 2 to 12). Rapid hydration also occurred in strongly alkaline solutions but loss of formaldehyde from the initial degradation product yielded [2,3-dichloro-4-(1-oxobutyl)phenoxy]acetic acid, which could subsequently undergo an addition reaction with ethacrynic acid. Solid dosage forms and lyophilised injections of ethacrynic acid were also analysed with similar results.

In highly acidic and in highly basic solution at 24° ethacrynic acid was very unstable (HPLC method), whereas in weakly acidic or neutral media greater stability was demonstrated.[4] Ammonium ions, unlike borate, phosphate, or sodium ions, caused rapid decomposition of ethacrynic acid in solution. Degradation in the presence of ammonium ions was thought to be a complex, reversible reaction, with formaldehyde as one of the products.

The extent of ethacrynic acid degradation in buffered aqueous solutions containing either sodium or ammonium ions was shown, by reversed-phase HPLC, to be dependent on the nature and concentration of the cation.[5] In solutions containing ammonium ions, the reported incompatibility was shown to involve the generation of an additional degradation product. In contrast to earlier work,[4] no evidence for the existence of equilibrium was found.

Ethacrynic acid (1 mg/mL, pH 7; in either sorbitol 50% or a mixture of sorbitol 50% with ethanol 10%) retained 80.6% and 85.3%, respectively, of its initial concentration[4] after 21 days at 65°, and 97.1% and 97.6%, respectively, after 62 days at 24°. Both solutions also contained 0.005% methyl hydroxybenzoate and 0.002% propyl hydroxybenzoate. In both solutions at either temperature decreases in pH were observed.

Das Gupta et al[6] prepared an oral liquid dosage form of ethacrynic acid (1 mg/mL) in an aqueous solution of ethanol and sorbitol; the formulation also contained methyl and propyl hydroxybenzoates. The pH of the final solution was adjusted to 7. Following storage in amber bottles at 24°, 100%, 97.6%,

and 95.6% of the initial concentration of ethacrynic acid remained after 21 days, 62 days, and 220 days, respectively. The pH of the final solution was 5.2; no physical changes were observed.

FURTHER INFORMATION. The kinetics of degradation of ethacrynic acid in aqueous solution—Yarwood RJ, Phillips AJ, Dickinson NA, Collett JH. Drug Dev Ind Pharm 1983;9:35–41.

INCOMPATIBILITY/COMPATIBILITY

Solutions of sodium ethacrynate are incompatible with solutions of pH below 5 and with whole blood or its derivatives.

Potential incompatibilities, as indicated by changes in ultraviolet absorption spectra, have been noted when sodium ethacrynate (Edecrin, MSD, USA) in sodium chloride injection was mixed with injections of hydralazine hydrochloride (Apresoline, Ciba, USA), procainamide hydrochloride (Pronestyl, ER Squibb, USA), or tolazoline hydrochloride (Priscoline, Ciba, USA) and stored for 8 hours at room temperature.[7] A white precipitate was observed when, under the same conditions, sodium ethacrynate injection was mixed with reserpine injection (Serpasil, Ciba, USA). Apparent compatibility was indicated between injections of sodium ethacrynate and chlorpromazine hydrochloride (Thorazine, SK&F, USA), prochlorperazine edisylate (Compazine, SK&F, USA), or promazine hydrochloride (Sparine, Wyeth, USA).

FORMULATION

Excipients

Excipients that have been used in presentations of ethacrynic acid include:

Tablets, ethacrynic acid: brilliant blue FCF (133); colloidal silica; lactose; magnesium stearate; quinoline yellow (E104); starch; sunset yellow FCF (E110); talc.

Oral solutions (of powdered ethacrynic acid): ethanol; methyl and propyl hydroxybenzoates; sodium hydroxide solution; sorbitol solution.

Oral suspensions (of powdered ethacrynic acid tablets): chloroform water; compound tragacanth powder; orange syrup.

Injections, sodium ethacrynate: mannitol; thiomersal.

PROCESSING

Handling precautions

CAUTION. Ethacrynic acid should be handled with care as it irritates the skin, eyes, and mucous membranes, especially when in the form of dust.

REFERENCES

1. Isamil S, Habib FS, Attia MA. Acta Pharm Fenn 1985;94:163–71.
2. Cohen EM. J Pharm Sci 1971;60(11):1702–4.
3. Yarwood RJ, Moore WD, Collett JH. J Pharm Sci 1985;74(2):220–3.
4. Das Gupta V. Drug Dev Ind Pharm 1982;8(6):869–82.
5. Yarwood RJ, Moore WD, Collett JH. J Pharm Biomed Anal 1987;5(4):369–78.
6. Das Gupta V, Gibbs CW, Ghanekar AG. Am J Hosp Pharm 1978;35:1382–5.
7. Catania PN, King JC. Am J Hosp Pharm 1972;29:141–6.

Ethambutol (BAN, rINN) *Antituberculous agent*

EMB
(*S,S*)-*N,N'*-Ethylenebis(2-aminobutan-1-ol)
$C_{10}H_{24}N_2O_2 = 204.3$

$$C_2H_5-\underset{\underset{CH_2OH}{|}}{\overset{\overset{H}{|}}{C}}-NH\cdot CH_2\cdot CH_2\cdot NH-\underset{\underset{H}{|}}{\overset{\overset{CH_2OH}{|}}{C}}-C_2H_5$$

Ethambutol Hydrochloride (BANM, USAN, rINNM)
$C_{10}H_{24}N_2O_2,2HCl = 277.2$
CAS—74-55-5 (ethambutol); 1270-11-7 (ethambutol hydrochloride)

Pharmacopoeial status
BP, USP (ethambutol hydrochloride)

Preparations
Compendial
Ethambutol Tablets BP. Tablets containing, in each, 100 mg and 400 mg of ethambutol hydrochloride are usually available.
Ethambutol Hydrochloride Tablets USP.

Non-compendial
Myambutol (Lederle). *Tablets*, ethambutol hydrochloride 100 mg and 400 mg.
Powder, ethambutol hydrochloride 50 g per bottle.
Details of a formulation for ethambutol syrup suitable for paediatric use are available on request from the manufacturer.

Containers and storage
Solid state
Ethambutol Hydrochloride BP should be stored in an airtight container.
Ethambutol Hydrochloride USP should be preserved in well-closed containers.

Dosage forms
Ethambutol Hydrochloride Tablets USP should be preserved in well-closed containers.
Myambutol should be stored at controlled room temperature (15° to 30°) in either the original pack or in containers that prevent access of moisture.

PHYSICAL PROPERTIES

Ethambutol hydrochloride is a white crystalline powder; odourless or almost odourless; hygroscopic when exposed to high relative humidities.

Melting point
Ethambutol melts at 88°.
Ethambutol hydrochloride melts in the range 199° to 204°.

pH
A 2% w/v solution of *ethambutol hydrochloride* has a pH of 3.7 to 4.0.

Dissociation constants
pK_a 6.3, 9.5 (20°)

Solubility
Ethambutol is sparingly soluble in water; very soluble in chloroform.

Ethambutol hydrochloride is soluble 1 in 1 of water, 1 in 4 of ethanol, 1 in 9 of methanol, and in dimethyl sulphoxide; slightly soluble in chloroform (1 in 850) and in ether.

Dissolution
The USP specifies that for Ethambutol Hydrochloride Tablets USP not less than 75% of the labelled amount of $C_{10}H_{24}N_2O_2, 2HCl$ is dissolved in 45 minutes. Dissolution medium: 900 mL of water; Apparatus 1 at 100 rpm.

STABILITY
Solutions of ethambutol hydrochloride are reported to be stable when heated at 121° for 10 minutes.

FORMULATION

Excipients
Excipients that have been used in presentations of ethambutol hydrochloride include:
Tablets: acacia; ethylcellulose; gelatin; hypromellose; magnesium stearate; shellac; sodium lauryl sulphate; sorbitol; starch; stearic acid; sucrose; talc; titanium dioxide (E171).
Oral liquids: acacia; chloroform; citric acid; hydroxybenzoate esters; methylcellulose; orange tincture; saccharin sodium; sodium benzoate; sorbitol; starch; sucrose; syrup; tragacanth.

Ethinyloestradiol (BAN) *Oestrogen*

Ethinyl estradiol; Ethinylestradiol (rINN)
19-Nor-17α-pregna-1,3,5 (10)-trien-20-yne-3,17β-diol
$C_{20}H_{24}O_2 = 296.4$
CAS—57-63-6

Pharmacopoeial status
BP (ethinyloestradiol); USP (ethinyl estradiol)

Preparations
Compendial
Ethinyloestradiol Tablets BP. Tablets containing, in each, 10, 20, 50, 100, and 1000 micrograms are usually available.
Ethinyl Estradiol Tablets USP.

Containers and storage
Solid state
Ethinyloestradiol BP should be kept in a well-closed container and protected from light.
Ethinyl Estradiol USP should be preserved in tight, non-metallic, light-resistant containers.

Dosage forms
Ethinyloestradiol Tablets BP should be protected from light.
Ethinyl Estradiol Tablets USP should be preserved in well-closed containers.

PHYSICAL PROPERTIES

Ethinyloestradiol is a white or slightly yellowish-white, odourless, crystalline powder.

Melting point

Ethinyloestradiol melts between 180° and 186°. It may also exist in a polymorphic modification melting between 141° to 146°.

Dissociation constant

A pK_a value of 10.4 ± 0.1 has been determined for *ethinyloestradiol* in aqueous solution (1.5×10^{-5}M) at room temperature.[1]

Solubility

Ethinyloestradiol is practically insoluble in water and soluble 1 in 6 of ethanol, 1 in 20 of chloroform, 1 in 4 of ether, and 1 in 5 of acetone. It is also soluble in vegetable oils and in dilute solutions of alkali hydroxides.

FURTHER INFORMATION. Simultaneous solubilisation of steroid hormones II: Androgens and oestrogens [extent of solubilisation of ethinyloestradiol by typical anionic, cationic and nonionic surfactants depended on order of addition]—Lundberg B, Lövgren T, Heikius B. J Pharm Sci 1979;68(5):542–5.

STABILITY

Lane and co-workers[2] reported no loss of ethinyloestradiol (solid state) after thermal stress at 37° for one year and after exposure to 80% relative humidity at 24° for 180 days.
Comparison of coloured and uncoloured tablets of ethinyloestradiol and norethisterone exposed to accelerated light conditions (approximately 1.076×10^4 lx) for 30 days[3] indicated that the presence of erythrosine (E127) could induce a decrease in content of ethinyloestradiol. Absence of this dye, or its replacement with sunset yellow FCF (E110), resulted in tablets in which the photostability of ethinyloestradiol was greater.

FORMULATION

Excipients

Excipients that have been used in presentations of ethinyloestradiol include:
Tablets: acacia; brilliant blue FCF (133); butyl hydroxybenzoate; calcium phosphate; calcium sulphate; carnauba wax; erythrosine (E127); gelatin; indigo carmine (E132) aluminium lake; lactose; magnesium stearate; maize starch; potato starch; sodium phosphate; sucrose; sunset yellow FCF (E110) aluminium lake; talc; tartrazine (E102); tartrazine (E102) aluminium lake; white beeswax.

Bioavailability

A comparison of the intravenous, nasal, and intraduodenal routes of administration of 17α-ethinyloestradiol, in *rats*, led Bawarshi-Nassar *et al*[4] to conclude that the nasal route was superior to the oral route in this species.

Bioequivalence

Bioequivalence of two oral contraceptive drugs containing norethindrone and ethinyl estradiol—Saperstein S, Edgren RA, Lee GJ-L, Jung D, Fratis A, Kusinsky S *et al.* Contraception 1989;40(5):581–90.

PROCESSING

CAUTION. Ethinyloestradiol is a powerful oestrogen. Contact with skin or inhalation should be avoided. Rubber gloves and a face mask should be worn when handling the powder.

REFERENCES

1. Hurwitz AR, Liu ST. J Pharm Sci 1977;66(5):624–7.
2. Lane PA, Mayberry DO, Young RW. J Pharm Sci 1987;76(1):44–7.
3. Kaminski EE, Cohn RM, McGuire JL, Carstensen JT. J Pharm Sci 1979;68(3):368–70.
4. Bawarshi-Nassar RN, Hussain A, Crooks PA. J Pharm Pharmacol 1989;41:214–15.

Fenoprofen (BAN, USAN, pINN)

Analgesic; Anti-inflammatory
(±)-2-(3-Phenoxyphenyl)propionic acid; (±)-α-methyl-3-phenoxybenzeneacetic acid
$C_{15}H_{14}O_3 = 242.3$

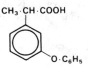

Fenoprofen Calcium (BANM, USAN, pINNM)

$(C_{15}H_{13}O_3)_2Ca, 2H_2O = 558.6$
CAS—31879-05-7 (fenoprofen);34597-40-5 (fenoprofen calcium, anhydrous); 53746-45-5 (fenoprofen calcium, dihydrate)

Pharmacopoeial status

BP, USP (fenoprofen calcium)

Preparations

Compendial
Fenoprofen Tablets BP (Fenoprofen Calcium Tablets). Tablets containing fenoprofen calcium. Tablets containing, in each, the equivalent of 200 mg, 300 mg, and 600 mg of fenoprofen are usually available.
Fenoprofen Calcium Capsules USP.
Fenoprofen Calcium Tablets USP.

Non-compendial
Fenopron (Dista). *Tablets,* fenoprofen calcium equivalent to 300 mg fenoprofen (Fenopron 300) and to 600 mg fenoprofen (Fenopron 600).
Progesic (Lilly). *Tablets,* fenoprofen calcium equivalent to 200 mg of fenoprofen.

Containers and storage

Solid state
Fenoprofen Calcium BP should be kept in a well-closed container.
Fenoprofen Calcium USP should be preserved in tight containers.

Dosage forms
Fenoprofen Calcium Capsules USP and Tablets USP should both be preserved in well-closed containers.
Progesic tablets should be stored at room temperature (15° to 25°).

PHYSICAL PROPERTIES

Fenoprofen is a viscous oil; boiling point 168° to 171°.
Fenoprofen calcium is a white or almost white, odourless or almost odourless, crystalline powder.

Melting point

Fenoprofen calcium melts in the range 105° to 110°.

Dissociation constant

pK_a 4.5 (25°)

Partition coefficient

Log *P* (octanol/pH 7.4), 0.8

Solubility

Fenoprofen calcium is slightly soluble in water (1 in 400 to 1 in 500); soluble 1 in 15 parts of ethanol; slightly soluble in chloroform (1 in 300), in *n*-hexanol, and in methanol.

Effect of pH

The aqueous solubility of fenoprofen calcium is low at low values of pH, but has been reported to increase rapidly at pH values approximately one unit greater than the pK_a value (4.5 in this study) and above.[1] Results were as in the table below. Variation in aqueous solubility (% w/v) of fenoprofen calcium with pH:

pH	1.2	3.0	4.0	5.0	6.0	7.0	7.5
Solubility (% w/v)	1.8×10^{-3}	5.8×10^{-3}	0.041	0.071	0.147	0.256	0.307

Dissolution

The USP states that for both Fenoprofen Calcium Capsules USP and Fenoprofen Calcium Tablets USP not less than 75% of the labelled amount of $C_{15}H_{14}O_3$ is dissolved in 60 minutes. Dissolution medium: 1000 mL of phosphate buffer pH 7.0; Apparatus 1 at 100 rpm.

Dissolution properties

Studies of the dissolution rates of non-steroidal anti-inflammatory drugs[1] indicated that, in pH 7.5 buffer, fenoprofen calcium was almost completely dissolved in 5 to 15 minutes (fenoprofen calcium 4.5×10^{-5} M in 900 mL buffer; USP XX Apparatus 1 at 100 rpm).

FURTHER INFORMATION. Characterisation of calcium fenoprofen. 2. Dissolution from formulated tablets and compressed rotating discs—Hendriksen BA, Williams JD. Int J Pharmaceutics 1991;69:175-80. Characterisation of calcium fenoprofen. 3. Mechanism of dissolution from rotating discs—Hendriksen BA. Int J Pharmaceutics 1991;75:63–72.

Crystal and molecular structure

Enantiomers

Fenoprofen exhibits stereoisomerism. Sallustio *et al*[2] have developed a quantitative enantiospecific HPLC method for the analysis of fenoprofen.

Crystallinity and polymorphism

Crystal forms of anhydrous and hydrated fenoprofen salts[3] were as follows:

Compound	Form
Fenoprofen calcium anhydrous	amorphous
Fenoprofen calcium monohydrate	amorphous
Fenoprofen calcium dihydrate	crystalline*
Fenoprofen sodium anhydrous	amorphous
Fenoprofen sodium dihydrate	crystalline

*only one crystal form observed

Hendriksen[4] found no evidence of polymorphic variation between samples of fenoprofen calcium crystals (prepared by several methods), during an assessment of powder dissolution rates and relative degrees of crystallinity.

FURTHER INFORMATION. Crystal morphology and structural changes in calcium fenoprofen—Stoddart CP, Agbada CO, York P, Shields L. J Pharm Pharmacol 1992;44(Suppl):1077.

STABILITY

Fenoprofen calcium in the solid state is quite stable to acid, base, and heat. In preformulation studies of several fenoprofen salts,[3] fenoprofen calcium dihydrate was found to be stable at relative humidities in the range 1% to 93% (25°) and retained its water of hydration up to 70°, whereas fenoprofen sodium dihydrate was unstable at 1% relative humidity (25°) and lost its water of hydration at about room temperature.

Significant photodegradation of fenoprofen sodium in solution under high intensity, short wavelength ultraviolet light has been reported.[3] Two isomeric hydroxybiphenylpropionic acids were the major degradation products formed following exposure of aqueous solutions of fenoprofen sodium (25 mg/mL) and solutions of fenoprofen acid in isopropanol (25 mg/mL) to a low pressure mercury lamp. Formation of hydroxybiphenylpropionic acids was attributed to Claisen rearrangement of fenoprofen. Minor degradation products were identified as *m*-phenoxyacetophenone and *m*-phenoxystyrene. The $t_{10\%}$ of the aqueous solution of fenoprofen sodium 25 mg/mL was 2 hours. Exposure of the solutions to a carbon arc lamp or to sunlight for one week, did not yield hydroxybiphenylpropionic acids, and *m*-phenoxyacetophenone was only detected in trace amounts on exposure to the carbon arc lamp.

INCOMPATIBILITY/COMPATIBILITY

In preformulation studies[3] fenoprofen calcium dihydrate was compatible, in the solid state, with propoxyphene hydrochloride, propoxyphene napsylate, and codeine sulphate pentahydrate. However, it was indicated that in the presence of water interaction may occur with propoxyphene salts. Fenoprofen sodium dihydrate was incompatible, in the solid state, with both the propoxyphene salts and the codeine salt.

FORMULATION

Excipients

Excipients that have been used in presentations of fenoprofen calcium dihydrate include:
Capsules: cellulose; gelatin; iron oxides; quinoline yellow (E104); silicone; sunset yellow FCF (E110); titanium dioxide (E171).
Tablets: Amberlite; calcium phosphate; hydroxypropylcellulose; magnesium stearate; maize starch; quinoline yellow (E104); stearic acid; sunset yellow FCF (E110).

Bioequivalence

Nash *et al*[5] prepared three capsule formulations of fenoprofen calcium (containing the equivalent of 60, 165, and 300 mg of fenoprofen) with various proportions of silicone fluid 350 centistokes, and microcrystalline cellulose with carmellose sodium (Avicel RC-591 MCC). Linear pharmacokinetics of fenoprofen calcium were shown in the range 70 to 350 mg when single doses of the three preparations were administered to three groups of healthy volunteers. Results from a bioavailability study in 13 healthy volunteers indicated that the three capsule preparations were bioequivalent.

REFERENCES

1. Herzfeldt CD, Kümmel R. Drug Dev Ind Pharm 1983;9(5):767–93.
2. Sallustio BC, Abas A, Hayball PJ, Purdie YJ, Meffin PJ. J Chromatogr Biomed Appl 1986;374:329–37.
3. Hirsch CA, Messenger RJ, Brannon JL. J Pharm Sci 1978;67(2):231–6.
4. Hendriksen BA. Int J Pharmaceutics 1990;60:243–52.
5. Nash JF, Bechtol LD, Bunde CA, Bopp RJ, Farid KZ, Spradlin CT. J Pharm Sci 1979;68(9):1087–90.

Ferrous Salts   *Haematinic*

Ferrous Fumarate

Iron (II) fumarate; 2-butenedioic acid, (*E*)-, iron(2+) salt
$C_4H_2FeO_4 = 169.9$

Ferrous Gluconate

Iron (II) di(D-gluconate); D-gluconic acid, iron(2+) salt (2:1), dihydrate
$C_{12}H_{22}FeO_{14}, 2H_2O = 482.2$

Ferrous Succinate

$C_4H_4FeO_4 = 171.9$

Ferrous Sulphate

Green vitriol; green copperas (crude ferrous sulphate)
Iron(2+) sulphate (1:1), heptahydrate; sulphuric acid, iron(2+) salt (1:1), heptahydrate
$FeSO_4, 7H_2O = 278.0$

Dried Ferrous Sulphate

Dried Ferrous Sulfate (USAN)
$FeSO_4, xH_2O = 151.9$ (anhydrous)
CAS—141-01-5 (ferrous fumarate); 299-29-6 (ferrous gluconate, anhydrous); 12389-15-0 (ferrous gluconate, dihydrate); 10030-90-7 (ferrous succinate); 7720-78-7 (ferrous sulphate, anhydrous); 7782-63-0 (ferrous sulphate, heptahydrate); 13463-43-9 (dried ferrous sulphate)

Pharmacopoeial status

BP (ferrous fumarate, ferrous gluconate, ferrous succinate, ferrous sulphate, dried ferrous sulphate); USP (ferrous fumarate, ferrous gluconate, ferrous sulfate, dried ferrous sulfate)

Preparations

Compendial
Ferrous Fumarate Tablets BP. Tablets containing, in each, 200 mg and 304 mg of ferrous fumarate, equivalent to 65 mg and 100 mg of ferrous iron respectively, are usually available.

Ferrous Fumarate Oral Suspension BP (Ferrous Fumarate Mixture). An oral suspension containing 140 mg of ferrous fumarate in 5 mL, equivalent to about 45 mg of ferrous iron, is usually available.
Ferrous Gluconate Tablets BP. Coated tablets containing, in each, 300 mg of ferrous gluconate, equivalent to 35 mg of ferrous iron, are usually available.
Ferrous Succinate Capsules BP. Capsules containing, in each, 100 mg of ferrous succinate are usually available.
Ferrous Succinate Tablets BP. Tablets containing, in each, 100 mg of ferrous succinate, equivalent to 35 mg of ferrous iron, are usually available.
Ferrous Sulphate Tablets BP contain dried ferrous sulphate. Coated tablets containing, in each, 200 mg and 300 mg, equivalent to 65 mg and 97 mg of ferrous iron respectively, are usually available.
Paediatric Ferrous Sulphate Oral Solution BP. A solution containing 1.2% w/v of ferrous sulphate and a suitable antioxidant in a suitable orange-flavoured vehicle.
Ferrous Fumarate Tablets USP.
Ferrous Gluconate Capsules USP.
Ferrous Gluconate Tablets USP.
Ferrous Gluconate Elixir USP.
Ferrous Sulfate Tablets USP.
Ferrous Sulfate Oral Solution USP.
Ferrous Sulfate Syrup USP.

Non-compendial
Feospan (SK&F). 'Spansules', sustained-release capsules, 150 mg dried ferrous sulphate (47 mg iron).
Fergon (Sanofi Winthrop). *Tablets*, ferrous gluconate 300 mg (35 mg iron).
Ferrocap (Consolidated). *Capsules*, slow release, ferrous fumarate 330 mg (110 mg iron).
Ferrocontin Continus (ASTA Medica). *Tablets*, controlled release, ferrous glycine sulphate equivalent to 100 mg iron.
Ferrograd (Abbott). 'Filmtabs', each containing 325 mg dried ferrous sulphate (105 mg iron) in a controlled-release form.
Ferromyn (Wellcome). *Elixir*, ferrous succinate 106 mg (37 mg iron)/5 mL.
Fersaday (Evans). *Tablets*, ferrous fumarate 304 mg (100 mg iron).
Fersamal (Evans). *Tablets*, ferrous fumarate 200 mg (65 mg iron).
Syrup, 140 mg ferrous fumarate (45 mg iron)/5 mL. *Diluent*: syrup.
Galfer (Galen). *Capsules*, ferrous fumarate 290 mg (100 mg iron).
Syrup, ferrous fumarate 140 mg (45 mg iron)/5 mL.
Plesmet (Napp). *Syrup*, ferrous glycine sulphate equivalent to 25 mg iron/5 mL.
Slow-Fe (Ciba). *Tablets*, 160 mg dried ferrous sulphate (50 mg iron) in a slow-release wax core.

Containers and storage

Solid state
Ferrous Gluconate BP, Ferrous Succinate BP, and Ferrous Sulphate BP should be kept in well-closed containers; Ferrous Gluconate BP should also be protected from light.
All USP Ferrous Salts should be kept in tight containers.

Dosage forms
Ferrous Fumarate Oral Suspension BP and Ferrous Succinate Capsules BP should be protected from light.
Ferrous Succinate Tablets BP should be stored at a temperature not exceeding 15° and protected from light.

All USP Ferrous Salt preparations should be preserved in well-closed or tight containers.

Ferrous Gluconate Elixir USP and Ferrous Sulfate Oral Solution USP should be preserved in light-resistant containers.

Fergon, Fersaday, and Fersamal tablets should be protected from light.

Ferrocontin Continus tablets should be kept in a cool, dry place, protected from light.

Ferromyn elixir should be stored below 25°, protected from light.

Feospan spansules should be stored below 25°, in a dry place.

Slow-Fe tablets should be protected from heat and moisture.

PHYSICAL PROPERTIES

Ferrous fumarate is a fine, red-orange to red-brown granular powder; almost odourless and with a faintly astringent taste.

Ferrous gluconate exists as a grey powder or granules with a green-yellow tint; slight odour of burnt sugar and taste which is saline at first then chalybeate.

Ferrous succinate is a brownish-yellow to brown amorphous powder; slight odour.

Ferrous sulphate exists as bluish-green crystals or light green crystalline powder; metallic, astringent taste. It is efflorescent in dry air. Oxidises in moist air to form basic ferric sulphate (brown in colour).

Dried ferrous sulphate is a greyish-white to buff-coloured powder.

pH

Ferrous gluconate (10% solution), pH 3.7 to 6.0. A pH of 4.0 to 5.5 has been reported for a 10% solution of ferrous gluconate in carbon dioxide-free water, 3 to 4 hours after preparation.

Ferrous sulphate (5% w/v solution), pH 3.0 to 4.0.

Solubility

Ferrous fumarate is slightly soluble in water; very slightly soluble in ethanol. Solubility in dilute hydrochloric acid is limited by the separation of fumaric acid.

Ferrous gluconate is slowly soluble 1 in 10 of water (giving a green-brown solution) and more readily soluble in hot water; practically insoluble in ethanol.

Ferrous sulphate is freely soluble in water (very soluble in boiling water); practically insoluble in ethanol.

Dissolution

The USP specifies that for Ferrous Gluconate Capsules USP not less than 75% of the labelled amount of $C_{12}H_{22}FeO_{14}, 2H_2O$ is dissolved in 45 minutes. Dissolution medium: 900 mL of 0.1 N hydrochloric acid; Apparatus 1 at 100 rpm.

The USP specifies that for Ferrous Gluconate Tablets USP not less than 80% of the labelled amount of $C_{12}H_{22}FeO_{14}, 2H_2O$ is dissolved in 80 minutes. Dissolution medium: 900 mL of simulated gastric fluid TS; Apparatus 2 at 150 rpm.

Dissolution properties

Comparative dissolution studies of iron tablets (Glubifer, Terapia, and Ferro-Gradumet, Galenika) were undertaken by Romanian workers[1] using a modified version of the USP XXI rotating basket apparatus at 37° in simulated gastric and intestinal fluids. The amount of iron (II) available decreased with increasing pH in a similar way for both drugs.

The dissolution rate and pH of 16 pharmaceutical products, including ferrous sulphate tablets (325 mg, Purity), were determined in an aqueous solution of synthetic saliva in order to determine their influence on drug-induced oesophageal injury.[2]

The pH after dissolution (under experimental conditions at 25°) was 5.96, and the dissolution time was 34 minutes.

STABILITY

Ferrous sulphate loses six molecules of water of crystallisation at 38°; at higher temperatures basic sulphates are produced. When exposed to moist air it is oxidised and becomes brown. Granular ferrous sulphate, prepared by precipitation with ethanol from a slightly acidic solution, is less liable to oxidation than crystalline powder.

Mitra and Matthews[3] investigated the oxidation of ferrous sulphate (10^{-4} M) to ferric ions in solutions containing various concentrations of phosphate buffer (0.005 to 0.0175M) over the pH range 6.6 to 7.1 at 25°. The reaction was dependent on both pH and phosphate concentration. At pH 6.9 the reaction kinetics were pseudo-first-order. The ferrous ion was more stable at pH values below 6.6 than at higher pH values. From measurements of the oxidation rates at 20°, 25°, 30°, and 35° in 0.01 M phosphate buffer at pH 6.7, the activation energy was determined to be 59.4 kJ/mol.

Ferrous Sulphate Mixture and Ferrous Sulphate Mixture, Paediatric BPC have been found to discolour on storage. It has been demonstrated that the stability of the mixtures is influenced by the hardness of the water used in their preparation, the amount of air in the container, and the ascorbic acid content. In partly-filled containers, ferrous sulphate mixtures showed discoloration within 5 to 10 days due to oxidation which could be retarded by increased ascorbic acid content. The recommended ascorbic acid content of the mixtures is 0.2%; a shelf-life of 4 weeks is recommended if kept in well-filled, tightly-closed containers at room temperature. Once the container has been opened, the mixtures should be used within one week.

FURTHER INFORMATION. The preparation and characterisation of ferrous sulphate hydrates [describes phase changes with temperature and relative humidity]—Mitchell AG. J Pharm Pharmacol 1984;36:506–10. The stability of aqueous solutions of ferrous gluconate—Johnson CA, Thomas JA. J Pharm Pharmacol 1954;6:1037–47.

FORMULATION

PAEDIATRIC FERROUS SULPHATE ORAL SOLUTION BP

Ferrous sulphate	12 g
Ascorbic acid	2 g
Orange syrup	100 mL
Double-strength chloroform water	500 mL
Water to	1000 mL

The mixture should be recently prepared. Darkening of the mixture and presence of a precipitate can be avoided if freshly boiled and cooled purified water is used in the preparation of the mixture. The clearest and 'brightest' mixture is obtained if the ascorbic acid is first dissolved in the chloroform water. Should dilution be necessary, either syrup or purified water (freshly boiled and cooled) can be used as diluent.

FERROUS SULPHATE MIXTURE

The following formula was given in the *British Pharmaceutical Codex 1973*:

Ferrous sulphate	30 g
Ascorbic acid	2 g
Orange syrup	50 mL
Double-strength chloroform water	500 mL
Water for preparations to	1000 mL

The mixture should be prepared as for the paediatric mixture, above. See also Stability above.

Excipients

Excipients that have been used in presentations of ferrous salts include:

Capsules, ferrous sulphate (dried): acid fuchsine D; allura red AC (E129); benzyl alcohol; brilliant blue FCF (133); cetylpyridinium chloride; erythrosine (E127); gelatin; glyceryl stearates; iron oxide; macrogol; povidone; quinoline yellow (E104); sodium lauryl sulphate; starch; sucrose; sunset yellow FCF (E110), aluminium lake; white beeswax.

Caplets, ferrous gluconate: benzyl alcohol; brilliant blue FCF (133); calcium stearate; D&C Red No.7; gelatin; glycerol; hydroxybenzoates; hydroxypropylcellulose; pharmaceutical glaze; povidone; sodium propionate; sucrose; talc.

Tablets, ferrous fumarate: docusate sodium; glycerol; hypromellose; maize starch; magnesium stearate; povidone; sodium starch glycollate.

Ferrous gluconate: acacia; brilliant blue FCF (133); calcium carbonate (precipitated); carmoisine (E122); carnauba wax; D&C Yellow No.6; gelatin; glucose; hydroxybenzoates; kaolin; magnesium stearate; ponceau 4R (E124); quinoline yellow (E104); sodium benzoate; starch; sucrose; talc; titanium dioxide (E171); yellow beeswax.

Ferrous succinate: dicalcium phosphate; magnesium stearate; maize starch; povidone.

Ferrous sulphate (dried): calcium sulphate; glucose; hypromellose; indigo carmine (E132); liquid paraffin; macrogol; quinoline yellow (E104); sodium lauryl sulphate; starch; stearic acid; talc; titanium dioxide (E171).

Oral liquids, ferrous gluconate: ethanol 7%; glycerol; liquid glucose; saccharin sodium.

Ferrous succinate: ascorbic acid; sorbitol.

Ferrous sulphate: citric acid; glucose; saccharin sodium; sucrose; sunset yellow FCF (E110).

Bioavailability

A gastric delivery system designed by Cook *et al*[4] for iron supplementation (as ferrous sulphate) comprised capsules containing hypromellose, hydrogenated vegetable oil, crospovidone, microcrystalline cellulose, xanthan gum, talc, magnesium stearate, and colloidal silica. Alteration of the capsule composition changed the dissolution rate of the preparations. Results of absorption studies in nine healthy volunteers showed a 3-fold to 4-fold increase in absorption of iron from the capsules when compared with that from a ferrous sulphate elixir.

Workers in Canada[5] evaluated the bioavailability of iron in five ferrous sulphate 300 mg preparations (an oral solution, two types of film-coated tablets, and two types of enteric-coated tablets) in ten healthy volunteers. Absorption was lower from the enteric-coated tablets than from the oral solution and film-coated tablets.

Modified-release preparations

Küttel *et al*[6] have described the manufacture and stability of a wax-coated, modified-release formulation of ferrous sulphate granules.

REFERENCES

1. Palivan C, Rughinis D, Tamas V, Cosofret VV. Pharmazie 1989;44:648.
2. Bailey RT, Bonavina L, Nwakama PE, De Meester TR, Shih-Chuan C. DICP Ann Pharmacother 1990;24:571–3.
3. Mitra AK, Matthews ML. Int J Pharmaceutics 1985;23:185–93.
4. Cook JD, Carriaga M, Kahn SG, Schalch W, Skikne BS. Lancet 1990;335:1136–9.
5. Walker SE, Paton TW, Cowan DH, Manuel MA, Dranitsaris G. Can Med Assoc J 1989;141:543–7.
6. Küttel S, Mezei J, Rácz I. Pharm Ind 1990;52:121–3.

Flucloxacillin (BAN, rINN)   *Antibacterial*

Floxacillin (USAN)

(6R)-6-[3-(2-Chloro-6-fluorophenyl)-5-methyl-1,2-oxazole-4-carboxamido]penicillanic acid; (6R)-6-[3-(2-chloro-6-fluorophenyl)-5-methylisoxazole-4-carboxamido]penicillanic acid; 6[3-(2-chloro-6-fluorophenyl)-5-methyl-4-isoxazolecarboxamido]-3,3-dimethyl-7-oxo-4-thia-1-azabicyclo [3.2.0]heptane-2-carboxylic acid

$C_{19}H_{17}ClFN_3O_5S = 453.9$

Flucloxacillin Magnesium (BANM, rINNM)

$(C_{19}H_{16}ClFN_3O_5S)_2Mg, 8H_2O = 1074.2$

Flucloxacillin Sodium (BANM, rINNM)

$C_{19}H_{16}ClFN_3NaO_5S, H_2O = 493.9$

CAS — 5250-39-5 (flucloxacillin); 58486-36-5 (flucloxacillin magnesium); 1847-24-1 (flucloxacillin sodium, anhydrous); 34214-51-2 (flucloxacillin sodium, monohydrate)

Pharmacopoeial status

BP (flucloxacillin magnesium, flucloxacillin sodium)

Preparations

Compendial

Flucloxacillin Capsules BP. Contain flucloxacillin sodium. Capsules containing, in each, the equivalent of 250 mg and 500 mg of flucloxacillin are usually available.

Flucloxacillin Oral Solution BP (Flucloxacillin Elixir; Flucloxacillin Syrup). A solution of flucloxacillin sodium in a suitable flavoured vehicle. It is prepared by dissolving the dry ingredients in the specified volume of water just before issue for use. If diluted, the diluted oral solution should be freshly prepared. pH 4.0 to 7.0.

Flucloxacillin Oral Suspension BP (Flucloxacillin Mixture). A suspension of flucloxacillin magnesium in a suitable flavoured vehicle. It is prepared by dispersing the dry ingredients in the specified volume of water just before issue for use. If diluted, the diluted oral suspension should be freshly prepared. pH 4.8 to 5.8.

Flucloxacillin Injection BP (Flucloxacillin Sodium for Injection). A sterile solution of flucloxacillin sodium in water for injections. It is prepared by dissolving flucloxacillin sodium for injection in the requisite volume of water for injections immediately before use. pH of a 10% w/v solution, 5.0 to 7.0. Sealed containers each containing the equivalent of 250 mg, 500 mg, and 1 g of flucloxacillin are usually available.

Non-compendial

Floxapen (Beecham). *Capsules*, flucloxacillin (as sodium salt) 250 mg and 500 mg.

Syrup, flucloxacillin 125 mg or 250 mg (as magnesium salt)/5 mL when powder is reconstituted with water. *Diluent*: syrup.

Injection, powder for reconstitution, vials containing 250 mg, 500 mg, and 1 g flucloxacillin (as sodium salt). Floxapen injection may be added to most intravenous fluids such as water for injections, sodium chloride 0.9% injection, glucose 5% injection, or sodium chloride 0.18% with glucose 4% injection. See also under Incompatibility/Compatibility, below. A solution for nebulisation can be prepared by dissolving 125 mg to 250 mg of the injection vial powder in 3 mL of sterile water. Flucloxacillin capsules of various strengths are also available from APS, Ashbourne (Fluclomix), Berk (Ladropen), Brocades (Stafoxil), Cox, CP, Evans, Galen (Galfloxin), Kerfoot. Flucloxacillin oral solutions are also available from APS, Cox, CP, Norton.

Flucloxacillin oral suspension and injection are available from Berk.

Compound preparations

Co-fluampicil is the British Approved Name for compound preparations containing a mixture of equal parts by mass of flucloxacillin and ampicillin. Preparation: Magnapen (Beecham). Co-fluampicil capsules are also available from Generics (Flu-Amp), Norton.

Containers and storage

Solid state

Flucloxacillin Magnesium BP should be kept in a well-closed container, protected from moisture. Store at a temperature not exceeding 25°.

Flucloxacillin Sodium BP should be kept in an airtight container and stored at a temperature not exceeding 25°. Protect from moisture. If the substance is sterile the container should be sterile, tamper-evident, and sealed so as to exclude micro-organisms.

Dosage forms

Flucloxacillin Oral Solution BP and Flucloxacillin Oral Suspension BP. The dry ingredients should be kept in a well-closed container and stored at a temperature not exceeding 25°. Reconstituted and diluted oral solutions and suspensions should be stored at the temperature and used within the period stated on the label.

Flucloxacillin Injection BP. The sealed container should be stored at a temperature not exceeding 25°. The injection should be stored in accordance with the manufacturer's instructions. It should be used immediately after preparation but, in any case, within the period recommended by the manufacturer.

Floxapen capsules in original packs and Floxapen syrups should be stored in a dry place. Floxapen capsules in reclosable containers and Floxapen vials for injection should be stored in a cool, dry place.

Once dispensed, Floxapen syrups remain stable for 14 days when kept in a cool place.

Floxapen solutions for intramuscular or direct intravenous injection should be administered within 30 minutes of preparation. Aqueous solutions of Floxapen injection retain their activity for up to 24 hours at 25° and up to 72 hours in a refrigerator (5°). Intravenous solutions of Floxapen for infusion, stored at 25°, should be used within 24 hours of preparation. If these extended storage periods are required, reconstitution and preparation should be carried out under appropriate aseptic conditions.

PHYSICAL PROPERTIES

Flucloxacillin magnesium is a white or almost white powder.
Flucloxacillin sodium is a white or almost white, crystalline powder with a bitter taste; hygroscopic.

pH

A 0.5% w/v solution of *flucloxacillin magnesium* has a pH of 4.5 to 6.5.
A 10% w/v solution of *flucloxacillin sodium* has a pH of 5.0 to 7.0.

Dissociation constant

pK_a 2.7
An apparent pK_a value for flucloxacillin of 2.76 at 37° was determined by potentiometric titration in ethanol-water mixtures and extrapolation of the results to 0% w/v ethanol.[1]

Partition coefficients

Using values of apparent partition coefficients for flucloxacillin, measured over a range of pH values, Tsuji *et al*[1] calculated the following intrinsic partition coefficients:
Log P (octanol/water) unionised species, 2.61 (37°)
Log P (octanol/water) ionised species, −0.82 (37°)

Solubility

Flucloxacillin magnesium is slightly soluble in water and in chloroform; soluble 1 in 1 of methanol.
Flucloxacillin sodium is soluble 1 in 1 of water, 1 in 8 of ethanol, 1 in 8 of acetone, and 1 in 2 of methanol. Flucloxacillin sodium is reported[2] to be insoluble in fixed oils and liquid paraffin.

Critical micelle concentration

With the use of light scattering methods, Attwood *et al*[3] studied micelle formation by flucloxacillin sodium in aqueous solutions. At 30°, the critical micelle concentration for flucloxacillin sodium was found to be 0.112 mol/kg (aggregation number 5) in water and 0.064 mol/kg (aggregation number 6) in 0.15M sodium chloride.

STABILITY

Flucloxacillin is susceptible to hydrolysis of the β-lactam ring by hydroxide ions or other nucleophiles to form the corresponding penicilloic acid or penicilloyl derivative.[4] It is resistant to most penicillinase enzymes (β-lactamases) which catalyse this reaction.

Solutions

In aqueous solutions of flucloxacillin sodium at the pH of maximum stability (approximately pH 6.5) decomposition is slow; such solutions lose only a small proportion of their potency when kept for several days at room temperature.

In a review of work on parenteral penicillins,[2] Lynn reported on the stability of aqueous solutions of flucloxacillin sodium (10% w/v), in the temperature range 20° to 25°, at several pH values. After 7 days, solutions at pH 6.0 (citrate buffer), pH 7.0 (phosphate buffer), and pH 8.0 (phosphate buffer) retained 92%, 97%, and 88% of their initial potency, respectively. Precipitation occurred within 3 days in the solution at pH 5.0 (citrate buffer) and within 7 days in the unbuffered solution.

In unbuffered aqueous solutions of flucloxacillin (2%), degradation products formed after 7 days at 37° were *N*-formylpenicillamine and penicillamine at maximum yields of 35% and 0.9%, respectively. The pH of the solutions decreased from 5.2 to 4.3. Possible degradation routes for flucloxacillin and other penicillins were presented.[5]

Effects of freezing

Reconstituted intravenous solutions of flucloxacillin sodium (1 g in 5 mL of sterile water) were added to sodium chloride 0.9% or glucose 5% solutions in 50-mL polyvinyl chloride minibags and stored frozen at $-27°$.[6] All samples removed after 1, 2, 3, 6, and 9 months, and thawed in a microwave oven for 2.5 minutes, retained at least 93% of their initial flucloxacillin potency. After storage of thawed solutions for 24 hours at 4°, at least 90% flucloxacillin potency was still retained. An unidentified yellow discoloration (attributed to reactions of the isoxazolyl group) was apparent in the solutions in glucose 5% stored for 6 and 9 months. The authors warn that these discoloured solutions would not be suitable for administration to patients.

INCOMPATIBILITY/COMPATIBILITY

Flucloxacillin sodium should not be mixed with blood products or other proteinaceous fluids (such as protein hydrolysates), or with intravenous lipid emulsions. It should not be mixed with aminoglycosides in the same syringe, intravenous fluid container, or giving set as precipitation may occur.

Flucloxacillin sodium injection (Floxapen, Beecham) was reported to be visually compatible with sodium chloride 0.9%, glucose 5%, glucose in sodium chloride, and sodium lactate 0.167M intravenous injection fluids.[2] Solutions of flucloxacillin sodium in these fluids retained at least 94% activity for up to 24 hours at room temperature.

Physical incompatibilities between flucloxacillin injection and solutions of other injectable drugs have been assessed by Beatson and Taylor[7] using the following criteria: colour change, precipitation, effervescence, cloudiness, and turbidity. Immediate visible incompatibilities were reported between flucloxacillin injection (Beecham Research) and amiodarone, calcium gluconate, chlorpromazine, dobutamine, erythromycin lactobionate, gentamicin sulphate, metoclopramide, papaveretum, pethidine hydrochloride, prochlorperazine, promethazine, tetracycline hydrochloride, and tobramycin sulphate. Reactions with other drugs, which were temperature dependent in some instances, became apparent with time.

Following admixture of ofloxacin injection (Hoechst, Netherlands) with flucloxacillin injection (Beecham), a precipitate was formed between 7 and 24 hours.[8]

Lignocaine hydrochloride and procaine hydrochloride are reported to be visually compatible with flucloxacillin sodium (Floxapen, Beecham) in solutions for intramuscular injection.[2]

FORMULATION

Excipients

Excipients that have been used in presentations of flucloxacillin include:

Syrups and unidose sachets (powder for reconstitution), flucloxacillin magnesium: sodium benzoate; sucrose.

REFERENCES

1. Tsuji A, Kubo O, Miyamoto E, Yamana T. J Pharm Sci 1977;66(12):1675–9.
2. Lynn B. J Hosp Pharm 1971;29:183–95.
3. Attwood D, Agarwal SP. J Pharm Pharmacol 1984;36:563–4.
4. Van Krimpen PC, Van Bennekom WP, Bult A [review article]. Pharm Weekbl (Sci) 1987;9:1–23.
5. Bird AE, Jennings KR, Marshall AC. J Pharm Pharmacol 1986;38:913–17.
6. Sanburg AL, Lyndon RC, Sunderland B. Aust J Hosp Pharm 1987;17(1):31–4.
7. Beatson C, Taylor A. Br J Pharm Pract 1987;9(7):223–6.
8. Janknegt R, Stratermans T, Cilissen J, Lohman JJHM, Hooymans PM. Pharm Weekbl (Sci) 1991;13(5):207–9.

Fludrocortisone (BAN, rINN)   *Corticosteroid*

9α-Fluorohydrocortisone
9α-Fluoro-11β,17α,21-trihydroxypregn-4-ene-3,20-dione
$C_{21}H_{29}FO_5 = 380.5$

Fludrocortisone Acetate (BANM, rINNM)

9α-fluorohydrocortisone 21-acetate
$C_{23}H_{31}FO_6 = 422.5$
CAS—127-31-1 (fludrocortisone); 514-36-3 (fludrocortisone acetate)

Pharmacopoeial status

BP, USP (fludrocortisone acetate)

Preparations

Compendial
Fludrocortisone Tablets BP. Contain fludrocortisone acetate. Tablets containing, in each, 100 micrograms are usually available.
Fludrocortisone Acetate Tablets USP.

Non-compendial
Florinef (Squibb). *Tablets*, fludrocortisone acetate 100 micrograms.

Containers and storage

Solid state
Fludrocortisone Acetate BP should be kept in a well-closed container.
Fludrocortisone Acetate USP should be preserved in well-closed containers, protected from light.

Dosage forms
Fludrocortisone Acetate Tablets USP should be preserved in well-closed containers.
Florinef tablets should be stored at room temperature.

PHYSICAL PROPERTIES

Fludrocortisone acetate is a white or almost white crystalline powder; odourless or almost odourless; hygroscopic.

Melting point

Fludrocortisone crystals decompose between 260° and 262°.
The melting point of *fludrocortisone acetate* depends upon its polymorphic form. Melting points of about 209°, about 225°, and 233° to 234° have been reported.

Solubility

Fludrocortisone is very soluble in water.

Fludrocortisone acetate is insoluble or practically insoluble in water; sparingly soluble in ethanol (1 in 50) and in chloroform (1 in 50); slightly soluble in ether (1 in 250).

Crystal and molecular structure

Polymorphs
Fludrocortisone acetate may exist in several (possibly as many as six) polymorphic forms.[1]

STABILITY

Fludrocortisone acetate in the solid state is reported to be very stable.[1] In aqueous and alcoholic solutions oxidative rearrangement of the α-ketol side-chain and degradation at alkaline pH values may occur.

FURTHER INFORMATION. Analysis of fludrocortisone acetate and its solid dosage forms by high-performance liquid chromatography [stability-indicating]—Ast TM, Abdou HM. J Pharm Sci 1979;68(4):421–3.

FORMULATION

Excipients

Excipients that have been used in presentations of fludrocortisone acetate include:
Tablets: dicalcium phosphate; erythrosine (E127); lactose; magnesium stearate; maize starch; sodium benzoate; talc.
Oral suspensions: chloroform water; compound tragacanth powder; syrup.
Eye drops: sodium chloride.

FURTHER INFORMATION. Dissolution of fludrocortisone from phospholipid coprecipitates—Vudathala GK, Rogers JA. J Pharm Sci 1992;81(3):282–6.

REFERENCE

1. Florey K. In: Florey K, editor. Analytical profiles of drug substances; vol 3. London: Academic Press, 1974:281–306.

Fluphenazine (BAN, rINN)   *Antipsychotic*

Triflumethazine
2-{4-[3-(2-Trifluoromethylphenothiazin-10-yl)propyl]piperazin-1-yl}ethanol
$C_{22}H_{26}F_3N_3OS = 437.5$

Fluphenazine Decanoate (BANM, rINNM)
$C_{32}H_{44}F_3N_3O_2S = 591.8$

Fluphenazine Enanthate (BANM)
Fluphenazine Enantate (rINNM); fluphenazine heptanoate
$C_{29}H_{38}F_3N_3O_2S = 549.7$

Fluphenazine Hydrochloride (BANM, rINNM)
$C_{22}H_{26}F_3N_3OS, 2HCl = 510.4$
CAS—69-23-8 (fluphenazine); 5002-47-1 (fluphenazine decanoate); 2746-81-8 (fluphenazine enanthate); 146-56-5 (fluphenazine hydrochloride)

Pharmacopoeial status

BP (fluphenazine decanoate, fluphenazine enanthate, fluphenazine hydrochloride); USP (fluphenazine decanoate, fluphenazine enanthate, fluphenazine hydrochloride)

Preparations

Compendial
Fluphenazine Tablets BP. Contain fluphenazine hydrochloride. Tablets containing, in each, 1 mg, 2.5 mg, and 5 mg are usually available.
Fluphenazine Decanoate Injection BP. A sterile solution of fluphenazine decanoate in sesame oil. Injections containing 12.5 mg and 50 mg in 0.5 mL, 25 mg and 100 mg in 1 mL, 50 mg in 2 mL, and 250 mg in 10 mL are usually available.
Fluphenazine Enanthate Injection BP. A sterile solution of fluphenazine enanthate in sesame oil. An injection containing 25 mg in 1 mL is usually available.
Fluphenazine Hydrochloride Tablets USP.
Fluphenazine Hydrochloride Elixir USP.
Fluphenazine Hydrochloride Oral Solution USP.
Fluphenazine Decanoate Injection USP.
Fluphenazine Enanthate Injection USP.
Fluphenazine Hydrochloride Injection USP. pH between 4.8 and 5.2.

Non-compendial
Modecate (Squibb). *Depot injection* (oily), fluphenazine decanoate 25 mg/mL.
Modecate Concentrate (Squibb). *Depot injection* (oily), fluphenazine decanoate 100 mg/mL.
Moditen (Squibb). *Tablets*, sugar coated, fluphenazine hydrochloride 1 mg, 2.5 mg, and 5 mg.

Containers and storage

Solid state
Fluphenazine Decanoate BP, Fluphenazine Enanthate BP, and Fluphenazine Hydrochloride BP should all be protected from light. Fluphenazine Hydrochloride BP should be kept in a well-closed container.
Fluphenazine Decanoate USP, Fluphenazine Enanthate USP, and Fluphenazine Hydrochloride USP should be preserved in tight, light-resistant containers.

Dosage forms
Fluphenazine Decanoate Injection BP and Fluphenazine Enanthate Injection BP should both be protected from light.
Fluphenazine Hydrochloride Tablets USP should be preserved in tight, light-resistant containers.
Fluphenazine Hydrochloride Elixir USP and Oral Solution USP should be preserved in tight containers, protected from light.
Fluphenazine Decanoate Injection USP and Fluphenazine Enanthate Injection USP should be preserved in single-dose or in multiple-dose containers, preferably of Type I (Fluphenazine Decanoate Injection) or Type I or Type III (Fluphenazine Enanthate Injection) glass, protected from light.
Fluphenazine Hydrochloride Injection USP should be preserved in single-dose or in multiple-dose containers, preferably of Type I glass, protected from light.
Modecate injection and Modecate Concentrate injection should be stored at room temperature and protected from direct sunlight.

The manufacturer warns against storage in a refrigerator, as it causes precipitation of triglycerides from the sesame oil. If precipitation does occur, the products can be warmed to 37° to dissolve the precipitate without harming the active ingredient. The 10-mL multidose vial of Modecate injection should be discarded 28 days after it is first used. Modecate and Modecate Concentrate should not be mixed in the same syringe.

Moditen tablets should be stored at room temperature.

PHYSICAL PROPERTIES

Fluphenazine is a dark brown viscous oil.

Fluphenazine decanoate is a pale yellow viscous liquid or a yellow crystalline oily solid; faint ester-like odour.

Fluphenazine enanthate is a pale yellow to yellow-orange, clear to slightly turbid, viscous liquid or a yellow crystalline oily solid; faint ester-like odour.

Fluphenazine hydrochloride is a white or almost white crystalline powder; odourless or almost odourless.

Melting point

Fluphenazine decanoate melts in the range 30° to 32°, and slowly crystallises at room temperature.

Fluphenazine hydrochloride melts at about 230°.

pH

pH of a 5% w/v solution of *fluphenazine hydrochloride*, 1.9 to 2.3.

Dissociation constants

pK_a 3.9, 8.1

For *fluphenazine enanthate*, pK_a and pK_{a2} values have been reported as 3.5 or 3.29 and 8.2 or 7.7, respectively.[1]

Sorby et al[2] established apparent pK_a values for the first and second basic groups of *fluphenazine hydrochloride* of 3.9 and 8.05, respectively, by titration.

A method based on the measurement of partition coefficients[3] of *fluphenazine hydrochloride* at various pH values was used to determine a pK_a of 7.98.

Partition coefficient

Log P (octanol/pH 7.0), 3.5

Solubility

Fluphenazine decanoate is practically insoluble in water; miscible with absolute ethanol, with chloroform, and with ether; dissolves in fixed oils.

Fluphenazine enanthate is practically insoluble in water; soluble 1 in less than 1 of absolute ethanol or of chloroform, and 1 in 2 of ether; dissolves in fixed oils.

Fluphenazine hydrochloride is freely soluble in water (1 in 10); slightly soluble in ethanol, in acetone, and in chloroform; practically insoluble in ether.

Dissolution

The USP specifies that for Fluphenazine Hydrochloride Tablets USP not less than 75% of the labelled amount of $C_{22}H_{26}F_3N_3OS,2HCl$ is dissolved in 45 minutes. Dissolution medium: 900 mL of 0.1N hydrochloric acid; Apparatus 1 at 100 rpm.

STABILITY

In alkaline media, fluphenazine enanthate and fluphenazine decanoate hydrolyse to fluphenazine.[1,4]

Fluphenazine hydrochloride in the solid state is hygroscopic, but in the absence of moisture, under air or nitrogen, it is reported to be stable at up to 50° for at least six months.[5]

Fluphenazine enanthate is unstable in strong light, but stable to air at room temperature.

Fluphenazine decanoate slowly crystallises at room temperature.

Fluphenazine decanoate, enanthate, and hydrochloride are all sensitive to light[1,4,5] and one of the products of photolysis is a sulphoxide.[4]

In aqueous solution,[5] degradation of fluphenazine hydrochloride on exposure to light occurred at a similar rate within the pH range 0.3 to 9, but was slower at pH values greater than 11. Light-catalysed degradation was not prevented by the exclusion of oxygen, but decomposition was claimed to be prevented or retarded by various solvents, for example methanol, ethanol, dimethylformamide, ethylene glycol, or ether.

FURTHER INFORMATION. High-performance liquid chromatographic separation of the N- and S-oxides of fluphenazine and fluphenazine decanoate—Heyes WF, Salmon JR, Marlow W. J Chromatogr 1980;194:416–20.

INCOMPATIBILITY/COMPATIBILITY

In aqueous solution at 20°, adsorption of fluphenazine hydrochloride by activated charcoal, kaolin, or talc was shown to be significant and to follow Langmuir plots.[2] The extent of adsorption by kaolin or talc was greater in media at pH 6.5 than at pH 2.5; adsorption by activated charcoal was less dependent on pH.

FORMULATION

Excipients

Excipients that have been used in presentations of fluphenazine include:

Tablets, fluphenazine hydrochloride: acacia powder; acid fuchsine D; allura red AC (E129); brilliant blue FCF (133); calcium carbonate; calcium phosphate; carnauba wax; castor oil; chalk; curcumin (E100); D&C Red No.27 lake; D&C Red No.30 lake; erythrosine (E127); ethylcellulose; gelatin; indigo carmine (E132); lactose; magnesium stearate; povidone; printing ink; semi-synthetic glycerides; shellac; sodium benzoate; starch (maize, potato, wheat); sucrose; sunset yellow FCF (E110); sunset yellow FCF (E110) lake; talc; tartrazine (E102); titanium dioxide (E171); white beeswax.

Oral liquids, fluphenazine hydrochloride: ethanol; glycerol; methyl and propyl hydroxybenzoates; polysorbate 40; sodium benzoate; sodium phosphate; sucrose; sunset yellow FCF (E110).

Injections, fluphenazine decanoate: benzyl alcohol; sesame oil.

Fluphenazine enanthate: benzyl alcohol; sesame oil.

Fluphenazine hydrochloride: hydrochloric acid; methyl and propyl hydroxybenzoates; sodium chloride; sodium hydroxide.

Bioequivalence

In a randomised, two-way crossover study, 21 'drug-free' psychiatric patients received single doses of fluphenazine dihydrochloride as 5-mg tablets from two manufacturers (Cord Laboratories and Prolixin, Squibb).[6] The two products were claimed to be bioequivalent.

Intramuscular injections

Injections of the decanoate ester and enanthate ester of ^{14}C-fluphenazine were prepared by dissolving 41 mg of the ester in

1.0 mL of sesame oil that contained 1.6% benzyl alcohol.[7] Following intramuscular injection (in *dogs*), maximum concentrations of radioactivity in plasma were greater and were reached more rapidly from ^{14}C-fluphenazine enanthate injections than from ^{14}C-fluphenazine decanoate injections. From measurements of total radioactivity the authors concluded that the release rate of the decanoate ester was less than half that of the enanthate ester.

FURTHER INFORMATION. Kinetics of fluphenazine after fluphenazine dihydrochloride, enanthate and decanoate administration to man [patients]—Curry SH, Whelpton R, de Schepper J, Vranckx S, Schiff AA. Br J Clin Pharmacol 1979;7:325–31.

PROCESSING

Sterilisation

Both fluphenazine decanoate injection and fluphenazine enanthate injection can be sterilised by filtration.

REFERENCES

1. Florey K. In: Florey K, editor. Analytical profiles of drug substances; vol 2. London: Academic Press, 1973:245–62.
2. Sorby DL, Plein EM, Benmaman JD. J Pharm Sci 1966;55(8):785–94.
3. Vezin WR, Florence AT. Int J Pharmaceutics 1979;3:231–7.
4. Clarke G. In: Florey K, editor. Analytical profiles of drug substances; vol 9. London: Academic Press, 1980:275–94.
5. Florey K. In: Florey K, editor. Analytical profiles of drug substances; vol 2. London: Academic Press, 1973:263–94.
6. Dreyfuss J, Ross JJ, Shaw JM, Miller I, Schreiber EC. J Pharm Sci 1976;65(4):502–7.
7. Midha KK, Chakraborty BS, Schwede R, Hawes EM, McKay G, Hubbard JW et al. J Pharm Sci 1990;79(1):3–8.

Folic Acid (BAN, rINN)   *Haematopoietic vitamin*

Folicin; folinsyre; pteroylglutamic acid; pteroylmonoglutamic acid
N-[4-(2-Amino-4-hydroxypteridin-6-ylmethylamino)benzoyl]-L-glutamic acid
$C_{19}H_{19}N_7O_6 = 441.4$
CAS—59-30-3

Pharmacopoeial status

BP, USP

Preparations

Compendial
Folic Acid Tablets BP. Tablets containing, in each, 100 micrograms and 5 mg are usually available.
Folic Acid Tablets USP.
Folic Acid Injection USP. pH between 8.0 and 11.0.

Non-compendial
Lexpec (RP Drugs). *Syrup*, sugar free, folic acid 2.5 mg/5 mL.

Containers and storage

Solid state
Folic Acid BP should be kept in a well-closed container and protected from light.
Folic Acid USP should be preserved in well-closed, light-resistant containers.

Dosage forms
Folic Acid Tablets BP should be protected from light.
Folic Acid Tablets USP should be preserved in well-closed containers.
Folic Acid Injection USP should be preserved in single-dose or in multiple-dose containers, preferably of Type I glass, protected from light.

PHYSICAL PROPERTIES

Folic acid is a yellow to orange microcrystalline powder; odourless or almost odourless; tasteless.

Melting point

Folic acid has no melting point but darkens and chars from about 250°.

pH

A suspension of *folic acid* 10% w/v in water has a pH of 4.0 to 4.8.

Dissociation constants

pK_a 4.7, 6.8, 9.0 (30°)

Solubility

Folic acid is practically insoluble in cold water and in ethanol; insoluble in most organic solvents. It dissolves in dilute acids and in dilute solutions of alkali hydroxides or carbonates.
The solubility of folic acid in aqueous solution (McIlvaine's buffers) increased in the pH range 3 to 7 at 30°. At a concentration of 1 mg/mL, folic acid was substantially undissolved at pH 3 to 4, incompletely dissolved at pH 5 and completely dissolved at about pH 5.6 or higher. Folic acid was completely dissolved over the entire pH range in a mixture of syrup with propylene glycol 75%. Solubility of folic acid in distilled water increased with temperature (from 25° to 95°) but precise values may depend on mixing time.[1]

STABILITY

Solid state

Degradation of folic acid in the solid state was observed to follow zero-order kinetics at 55°, 70°, and 85° and 30%, 50%, and 70% relative humidities over 18 months.[2] A decomposition rate of 1% per year was calculated at 20° and 65% relative humidity. A mixture of folic acid 50% in microcrystalline cellulose was more stable, but 10% and 5% dilutions in microcrystalline cellulose were less stable, than folic acid alone.

Solutions

Aqueous solutions of folic acid are partly or completely inactivated by heat or light, and rapid decomposition may also occur under certain conditions in the presence of riboflavine, thiamine, or heavy metals.

The pH of optimum stability has been reported by different workers to be 5 to 8, or about 7.8.

The stability of folic acid (1 mg/mL) was investigated in solution over the pH range 2.5 to 9.8 (in citrate-phosphate buffer with methyl and propyl hydroxybenzoates) during storage in the dark at 6°, 25°, and 45°.[1] In solution at pH 6.0 to 9.8, folic acid was shown to be stable for more than 12 months at 6° and 25°. At lower pH values (for example, pH 3 and 4) the small amount of folic acid that went into solution was unstable, whereas samples that contained undissolved folic acid at concentrations greater than its solubility showed good stability.

Effect of light, riboflavine, and other B vitamins

In a comprehensive study, Scheindlin et al[3] demonstrated that, individually, riboflavine and some intensities of light induced breakdown of folic acid in solution but that the combined effects of riboflavine and light are synergistic. Degradation of folic acid was attributed to oxidative cleavage to yield p-aminobenzoyl glutamic acid and a carbonyl compound that was assumed to be 2-amino-4-hydroxy-6-pteridine-carboxaldehyde; in the presence of riboflavine and light degradation was retarded, but not prevented, in the absence of air and was more rapid at pH 4 than at pH 6.5. Possible mechanisms are presented.

Biamonte and Schneller[1] comprehensively studied the stability of folic acid in the presence of components of the vitamin B complex (riboflavine, thiamine hydrochloride, pyridoxine hydrochloride, and pantothenyl alcohol) individually and together, in various aqueous media, pH 3 to 7, at 25° and 45°. In general, stability was dependent on pH and the extent of dissolution of folic acid. In solution, considerable degradation of folic acid was shown in the presence of riboflavine or thiamine hydrochloride; however, when folic acid was mainly undissolved (pH 3 to 4), it was stable in the presence of these vitamins. Pyridoxine hydrochloride, pantothenyl alcohol, or nicotinamide induced slight instability of folic acid at pH 6 to 7; the degree of instability was insignificant at pH 3 to 5. Of the vehicles studied, most degradation of folic acid in the presence of the multivitamin group occurred in a vehicle containing propylene glycol.

Total parenteral nutrition admixture

At concentrations of 0.25, 0.5, 0.75, or 1 mg/L, folic acid (as injection, Lederle, USA) was chemically stable (iodine-125 competitive binding radioassay) for up to 48 hours in a total parenteral nutrition (TPN) admixture that contained glucose 25%, amino acids 3.5%, and a multivitamin formulation (ascorbic acid, riboflavine 5-phosphate, thiamine hydrochloride, nicotinamide, pyridoxine hydrochloride, dexpanthenol, and vitamins A, D, and E).[4] Stability was unaffected by different temperatures (21° or 5° to 8°) or light conditions (fluorescent or dark) during storage. However, the authors noted that heavy metals in the form of electrolytes or trace elements commonly found in TPN solutions were not present and that preparation of the TPN solutions in air-evacuated containers may slow the oxidative cleavage rates of folic acid in the presence of riboflavine.

Barker et al[5] investigated the stability of folic acid when added, as folic acid injection USP, to several parenteral nutrition solutions to yield folic acid concentrations of 0.2, 10, and 20 mg/L and stored protected from light at 4° or 25° for 14 days. Chemi-

cal and physical stability was dependent on pH; folic acid, at 10 mg/L and 20 mg/L, was unstable in solutions of pH less than 5, for example in solutions that contained more than 20% glucose. In sodium chloride 0.9% or glucose 50% solutions degradation of folic acid was accompanied by precipitation, but above pH 5 folic acid remained in solution. Under similar storage conditions, folic acid (0.4 mg/L and 0.566 mg/L) was stable in total parenteral nutrition solutions of pH 5.6 to 6.0 that contained various concentrations and brands of an amino acid solution, an electrolyte and trace metal solution, a multivitamin solution (which included riboflavine, thiamine, sodium ascorbate, pyridoxine, and sodium pantothenate), glucose, potassium chloride, and sodium chloride.

In contrast to the stability results of Barker et al, Nordfjeld et al[6] calculated first-order degradation half-lives for folic acid 120 micrograms/L in a TPN mixture (which contained glucose, amino acids, electrolytes, and trace elements (pH 5.1)) with a multivitamin preparation (MVI 12 (USV Laboratories) which contained 12 vitamins including folic acid and riboflavine), stored in polyvinyl chloride bags, for about 2.7 hours at 24° in daylight, 5.36 hours at 24° protected from light, and 24.2 hours at 4° protected from light. In an isotonic sodium chloride solution half-lives of folic acid under these conditions were 56 hours, 135 hours, and 191 hours respectively.

Effect of reducing agents

Smith[7] assigned an arbitrary shelf-life of about six weeks at room temperature to solutions of folic acid 1 mg/mL in distilled water preserved with Nipa esters, adjusted to pH 8 to 8.5 and stored in brown glass bottles. Addition of ascorbic acid 0.1% w/v as a reducing agent caused 'an increase in the proportion of free amines'. Effects of sodium sulphite 0.1% w/v were also studied.

In an HPLC assay for folic acid in multivitamin-mineral tablets and capsules,[8] reduction of folic acid was observed under conditions (air and oxygen-enriched air but not a nitrogen-enriched atmosphere) that caused oxidation of ascorbic acid to form products that are strong reducing agents.

Stabilisation

Folic acid in solution in the presence of riboflavine and light can be stabilised by the addition of antioxidants, the exclusion of light and air, or the adjustment of the pH to a value that gives optimum stability.

FURTHER INFORMATION. Liquid chromatographic determination of folic acid in multivitamin preparations [stability-indicating assay]—Paveenbampen C, Lamontanaro D, Moody J, Zarembo J, Rehm C. J Pharm Sci 1986;75(12):1192–4.

INCOMPATIBILITY/COMPATIBILITY

Folic acid is incompatible with oxidising and reducing agents and heavy metal ions. In ethanolic solution, incompatibilities between folic acid and chloral hydrate, ferrous sulphate, sulphonamides, mucilage of acacia, acidic vitamin preparations, and cherry and raspberry syrups have been reported.

Scott et al[9] deduced that significant interaction between folic acid and calcium ions in solution can occur even if precipitate formation is not evident; for example, at low concentrations of folic acid (10 micrograms/mL Folvite intravenous solution, Lederle, diluted in 3.03% dibasic potassium phosphate) and calcium gluconate (0.5, 1, and 10 micrograms/mL injection 10%, Parke-Davis).

Sorption

There was no evidence for folic acid loss due to adsorption to 3-L polyvinyl chloride containers or administration sets from solutions of folic acid 13 micrograms/L in several total parenteral nutrition solutions (pH 5.6 to 6.0).[5] However Lee et al,[10] claimed that adsorption to polyvinyl chloride infusion bags contributed to variations in assay results for folic acid concentration in total parenteral nutrition solutions during the initial five days storage at room temperature in the light.

Negligible loss due to binding of folic acid was detected following an in-line filtration, at 120 mL/hour, of solutions of folic acid (Lederle) 0.5 mg in 1000 mL of either glucose 5% or sodium chloride 0.9% through an administration set (Venoset 60, Abbott Laboratories), a stainless steel stopcock, and a 0.22 micrometre filter membrane of nitrate and acetate esters of cellulose (Millipore Corp).[11]

Significant adsorption in vitro of folic acid onto magnesium trisilicate and onto edible clay in water and in 0.01M hydrochloric acid at 37° has been demonstrated.[12] In the presence of either adsorbent, dissolution of folic acid from tablets in 0.01M hydrochloric acid was retarded.

FORMULATION

Excipients

Excipients that have been used in presentations of folic acid include:
Tablets: magnesium stearate; starch; tricalcium citrate.

Bioavailability

Folic acid was well absorbed when administered in wines of high ethanol content (in which folic acid was readily soluble at 10 micrograms/mL) to six healthy volunteers.[13]

REFERENCES

1. Biamonte AR, Schneller GH. J Am Pharm Assoc (Sci) 1951;40(7):313-20.
2. Tripet FY, Kesselring UW [French]. Pharm Acta Helv 1975;50(10):318-22.
3. Scheindlin S, Lee A, Griffith I. J Am Pharm Assoc (Sci) 1952;41:420-7.
4. Louie N, Stennett DJ. J Parent Enter Nutr 1984;8(4):421-6.
5. Barker A, Hebron BS, Beck PR, Ellis B. J Parent Enter Nutr 1984;8(1):3-8.
6. Nordfjeld K, Lang Pedersen J, Rasmussen M, Gaunø Jensen V. J Clin Hosp Pharm 1984;9:293-301.
7. Smith SG. Pharm J 1976 Feb;216:108.
8. Tafolla WH, Sarapu AC, Dukes GR. J Pharm Sci 1981;70(11):1273-6.
9. Scott KR, Bell AF, Telang VG. J Pharm Sci 1980;69(2):234.
10. Lee DR, Ware I, Winsley BE. Br J Intraven Ther 1980;1:13-15.
11. Butler LD, Munson JM, DeLuca PP. Am J Hosp Pharm 1980;37:935-41.
12. Iwuagwu MA, Jideonwo A. Int J Pharmaceutics 1990;65:63-7.
13. Kaunitz JD, Lindenbaum J. Ann Intern Med 1977;87:542-5.

Frusemide (BAN)   *Diuretic*

Furosemide (USAN, rINN); fursemide
4-Chloro-*N*-furfuryl-5-sulphamoylanthranilic acid; 5-(aminosulfonyl)-4-chloro-2-[(2-furanylmethyl)-amino]-benzoic acid; 4-chloro-2-furfurylamino-5-sulphamoylbenzoic acid
$C_{12}H_{11}ClN_2O_5S = 330.7$
CAS—54-31-9

Pharmacopoeial status

BP (frusemide); USP (furosemide)

Preparations

Compendial
Frusemide Tablets BP. Tablets containing, in each, 20 mg, 40 mg, and 500 mg frusemide are usually available.
Frusemide Injection BP. A sterile solution of frusemide sodium, prepared by the interaction of frusemide with sodium hydroxide, in water for injections. Injections containing the equivalent of 20 mg of frusemide in 2 mL, 50 mg in 5 mL, and 250 mg in 25 mL are usually available. pH 8.0 to 9.3.
Furosemide Tablets USP.
Furosemide Injection USP. pH between 8.0 and 9.3.

Non-compendial
Dryptal (Berk). *Tablets*, frusemide 40 mg and 500 mg.
Injection, frusemide 250 mg/25 mL. Glucose solutions are not suitable infusion fluids for Dryptal injection and the injection solution should not be mixed with other drugs in the infusion bottle.
Lasix (Hoechst). *Tablets*, frusemide 20 mg, 40 mg, and 500 mg.
Paediatric liquid, sugar free, frusemide 1 mg/mL when reconstituted with purified water, freshly boiled and cooled.
Injection, frusemide 10 mg/mL in aqueous solution. Lasix injections should not be mixed with any other preparations. Frusemide may precipitate in solutions of low pH and therefore glucose solutions are not suitable infusion fluids for Lasix injections.
Rusyde (CP). *Tablets*, frusemide 20 mg and 40 mg.
Frusemide tablets are also available in various strengths from APS, Ashbourne (Frumax), Cox, Evans, Kerfoot, Norton.
Frusemide oral solutions are also available, on special order, from RP Drugs.
Frusemide injections are also available from IMS (Min-I-Jet), Evans.

Compound preparations
Co-amilofruse is the British Approved Name for compounded preparations of amiloride 5 parts and frusemide 40 parts. Preparations: Frumil (Rhône-Poulenc Rorer); Lasoride (Hoechst).

Containers and storage

Solid state
Frusemide BP should be protected from light.
Furosemide USP should be preserved in well-closed, light-resistant containers.

Dosage forms

Frusemide Injection BP should be protected from light.

Furosemide Tablets USP should be preserved in well-closed, light-resistant containers.

Furosemide Injection USP should be stored in single-dose or in multiple-dose, light-resistant containers, of Type I glass.

Rusyde, Dryptal, and Lasix tablets and Lasix injections should be stored in a cool dry place, protected from light. Lasix tablets should be kept in containers similar to those of the manufacturer. Dryptal ampoules should be stored in a cool place, protected from light. Opened injection ampoules should be used immediately and any remainder discarded.

Lasix paediatric liquid granulate should be stored in a cool dry place, protected from light, in the original container. When reconstituted, the liquid should be stored in a cool place, preferably in a refrigerator at 5°, protected from light, for up to 30 days, after which time any remaining solution should be discarded.

PHYSICAL PROPERTIES

Frusemide is a white to slightly yellow crystalline powder; odourless and practically tasteless.

Melting point

Frusemide melts within the range 203° to 210°, with decomposition.

Dissociation constant

pK_a 3.9 (20°)

Solubility

Frusemide is practically insoluble in water; sparingly soluble in ethanol (1 in 75); soluble in acetone (1 in 15), in methanol, and in dimethylformamide; slightly soluble in ether (1 in 850); very slightly soluble in chloroform. Frusemide is soluble in dilute aqueous solutions of alkali hydroxides.

When frusemide was recrystallised from either methanol or ethanol, a second, novel, crystal form (frusemide II) was identified.[1] Addition of water (5% to 20% v/v) to the recrystallising solvents caused the re-formation of the original crystal form (frusemide I). When recrystallised from methanol, frusemide II had a significantly higher solubility (at 37° in buffer at pH 4.95) compared to that of an untreated frusemide sample (57.13 mg/100 mL and 35.17 mg/100 mL, respectively); an increase of 58% in the intrinsic dissolution rate was also recorded.

Effect of surfactants and polymers

Shihab *et al*[2] compared the effect of macrogols 200, 4000, and 6000, sodium lauryl sulphate, and polysorbate 80 on the solubility of frusemide in water. An increase in solubility was observed in each case; sodium lauryl sulphate had the greatest effect, followed by polysorbate 80 and the macrogols. The solubilising effect of the macrogols increased as both their concentration and molecular weight increased. Solubility increased with higher temperature. The addition of electrolytes to frusemide in polysorbate 5% w/v increased the solubilising power of the surfactant.

Dissolution

The USP specifies that for Furosemide Tablets USP not less than 80% of the labelled amount of $C_{12}H_{11}ClN_2O_5S$ is dissolved in 60 minutes. Dissolution medium: 900 mL of phosphate buffer pH 5.8; Apparatus 2 at 50 rpm.

Dissolution properties

Doherty and York[3] have described the intrinsic dissolution behaviour (in acetate buffer pH 4.95) of frusemide from solid dispersions or mechanical mixtures with povidone. Dissolution rates were higher in dispersed systems. Peak dissolution in both the dispersed systems and the mixes was observed at frusemide contents of 40% w/w. In mix systems, peak dissolution was determined by the balance between dissolution-promoting effects (complex formation) and dissolution-retarding effects (viscosity related). Dissolution in solid dispersions was enhanced by the amorphous drug phase and retarded by viscosity related effects.

Enhancement of the dissolution of frusemide from solid dispersions with povidone, which was evident in constant surface area discs, was also demonstrated *in vitro* from formulations in hard gelatin capsules and in a bioavailability study in humans.[4]

FURTHER INFORMATION. Dissolution from ordered mixtures: The effect of stirring rate and particle characteristics on the dissolution rate [of frusemide]—De Villiers MM, van der Watt JG. Drug Dev Ind Pharm 1989;15(4):621–7. Relationship between the pH of the diffusion layer and the dissolution rate of [frusemide]—Marais AF, van der Watt JG. Drug Dev Ind Pharm 1991;17(12):1715–20.

Crystal and molecular structure

Polymorphs

Matsuda and Tatsumi[5] presented a detailed comparison of the results of their study of the polymorphism of frusemide (in which they characterised seven modifications) with those of Doherty and York[1] who investigated only two crystal forms (see Solubility, above).

FURTHER INFORMATION. Amorphism and physicochemical stability of spray-dried frusemide—Matsuda Y, Otsuka M, Onoe M, Tatsumi E. J Pharm Pharmacol 1992;44:627–33.

STABILITY

In acidic aqueous solution, frusemide undergoes hydrogen ion-catalysed hydrolysis which follows first-order kinetics. Frusemide is very stable in basic media. A suggested mechanism for the hydrolytic reaction involves protonation of the basic amino nitrogen followed by nucleophilic attack on the furfuryl carbon to give the hydrolysis product 4-chloro-5-sulphamoylanthranilic acid (saluamine) and furfuryl alcohol.[6] Frusemide is also susceptible to photodecomposition. Ultraviolet irradiation of frusemide in alkaline solution produces 4-chloro-5-sulphoanthranilic acid,[7] whereas in oxygen-free methanol solutions N-furfuryl-5-sulphamoylanthranilic acid is the main product[8] of a combination of reduction and substitution reactions.

Effect of pH

Cruz *et al*[6] undertook an *in-vitro* kinetic study of the hydrolysis of frusemide with respect to pH and temperature; the activation energy for the reaction was estimated as 98.32 kJ/mol. Under physiological conditions of the stomach (pH 1.0, 37°) the half-life of frusemide was estimated to be 2.97 hours. However, under similar conditions Bundgaard *et al*[8] predicted a half-life of 17.2 hours. Both studies suggest that acid-catalysed hydrolysis of frusemide in the stomach is not the main factor that affects its bioavailability following oral administration. At pH values above 7.2, the hydrolysis of frusemide is very slow.[6]

In acidic solution, the stability of frusemide esters was similar to that of the parent compound.[8] The single decomposition product of acid hydrolysis differed for each ester and was predicted to be the corresponding 4-chloro-5-sulphamoylanthranilic acid ester. In aqueous solutions of pH 8.8 to 9.7, the esters were hydrolysed to frusemide.

Effect of light

Bundgaard et al[8] found that at pH 8 to 10, buffered aqueous solutions of frusemide exposed to normal laboratory light or diffuse daylight showed no degradation over 24 hours but at pH 1.0 to 4.5 there was rapid photolytic degradation which followed first-order kinetics. The reaction rate of the unionised form was greatest at pH 1 to 2. Frusemide esters in aqueous solution are also susceptible to photodegradation when stored under artificial laboratory light or diffuse daylight.

Both hydrolysis and dechlorination reactions were reported[9] to occur as a result of the exposure of frusemide in methanolic solution to ultraviolet radiation (365 nm). The photohydrolysis reaction yielded saluamine whereas photoreduction produced N-furfuryl-5-sulphamoylanthranilic acid. Saturation with oxygen inhibited photolysis of frusemide in methanol but caused a slight increase in buffered aqueous systems.

Frusemide irradiated in degassed aqueous buffer (pH 10) which included either sodium metabisulphite (0.1%) or dry oxygen was examined by Rowbotham et al.[7] It was suggested that hydrolysis and photo-oxidation were involved in the photochemical degradation process.

Effect of moisture

Sorption of moisture by frusemide tablets at different temperatures and relative humidities occurred within the first four days of testing and followed first-order kinetics.[10] Effects of sorption and desorption on the physical properties of the tablets (hardness, disintegration time, dissolution rate) were substantial and tended to be irreversible.

Stability in formulations

Neil et al[11] developed a specific HPLC assay for the separation and quantification of frusemide and saluamine in intravenous solutions; the technique was used to determine the stability of frusemide in various solutions. Frusemide injection maintained acceptable stability (less than 10% saluamine in frusemide) following transfer from ampoules to polypropylene syringes and storage unprotected or protected from light for 24 hours at room temperature. Frusemide content in compound sodium lactate injection and sodium chloride 0.9% injection remained unchanged after storage in polypropylene syringes for 24 hours at room temperature unprotected from light. There was a mean loss of 9.7% frusemide in sodium chloride 0.9% injection when stored at 6° for 26 days. This loss may have been due to precipitation of frusemide free acid (at pH below 5.5) or adsorption to the polyvinyl chloride bag. Frusemide infusion (pH 7.7) was stable when autoclaved (pH 6.6) and remained so for 70 days when stored at room temperature and protected from light; storage of the autoclaved solution unprotected from light for 70 days resulted in the formation of a yellow to orange precipitate. The effects of different lighting conditions on the stability of frusemide (Lasix, Hoechst) in admixtures with sodium chloride 0.9% injection when stored in two different burette sets (Avon Medicals A200 or Amberset A2000 burettes) were examined.[12] In A200 burettes, both frusemide and saluamine were stable during exposure to diffuse daylight/fluorescent strip lighting for 48 hours but on exposure to sunlight, degradation above compendial limits was detected after only 30 minutes. The Amberset A2000 burettes, which were covered with a transparent yellow polyvinyl chloride sleeve, afforded protection from the photodegrading effects of sunlight.

Stabilisation

In aqueous solutions the incorporation of edetic acid and chlorbutol resulted in no improvement of frusemide stability. The effect of sodium metabisulphite varied according to its concentration and the amount of oxygen present. Solutions that contained propylene glycol were very stable. Shah et al[13] stated that the pH of frusemide solutions is the critical factor; solutions should be slightly basic and remain unchanged during storage. See also Formulation, below.

Among vehicles for oral liquid presentations of frusemide, greatest stability was found in basic media (about pH 8.5). Stability was reduced in the presence of sugars and was lowest in acidic media. Inclusion of ethanol (up to 20% v/v) enhanced the stability of vehicles which also contained sorbitol 50%.[14] See also Formulation, below.

FURTHER INFORMATION. Kinetic study of the solid-state photolytic degradation of two polymorphic forms of furosemide—De Villiers MM, van der Watt JG, Lötter AP. Int J Pharmaceutics 1992;88:275–83. Effect of cohesive behaviour of small particles on the solid-state photochemical degradation—De Villiers MM, van der Watt JG, Lötter AP. Drug Dev Ind Pharm 1993;19(3):383–94.

INCOMPATIBILITY/COMPATIBILITY

Christensen et al[15] studied the degradation of oral liquid forms of frusemide repackaged as 2-mL unit doses into polypropylene oral syringes or glass vials (stored at temperatures ranging between 4° and 76° and protected from light). Degradation was fastest in the solutions stored in polypropylene syringes. For both types of package, acceptable stability (retention of more than 90% of label claim) was demonstrated after 180 days at 4° and 25°. At higher temperatures degradation was more rapid.

After visual examination of samples during 72 hours, the following injectable drugs were reported[16] to be physically incompatible with frusemide injection (Lasix, Hoechst) when mixed under controlled conditions: amiodarone, benzylpenicillin, buprenorphine, chlorpromazine, diazepam, erythromycin lactobionate, gentamicin sulphate, metoclopramide, papaveretum, pethidine hydrochloride, prochlorperazine, promethazine, and verapamil hydrochloride.

A white precipitate (identified as frusemide) formed after admixture of frusemide injection (10 mg/mL) diluted in glucose 5% injection or sodium chloride 0.9% injection, with commercial injections of either gentamicin sulphate (Schering-Plough, USA) or netilmicin sulphate (Schering-Plough, USA). The precipitate redissolved when the pH of the mixture was adjusted to 5.9 by the addition of 1M sodium hydroxide.[17] The authors advised against the administration of aminoglycosides and frusemide in the same admixture.

A white cloudy precipitate was also observed on visual examination of admixtures of esmolol hydrochloride (American Critical Care, pH 4.9 to 5.1), with frusemide injection (Hoechst-Roussel, USA) in glucose 5% or sodium chloride 0.9% injections.[18]

Two admixtures containing different concentrations of milrinone and frusemide in glucose 5% both precipitated immediately. Separate administration of the two products was recommended.[19]

FORMULATION

Excipients

Excipients that have been used in presentations of frusemide include:

Capsules: aluminium hydroxide; maize starch; povidone; shellac; stearic acid; sucrose; talc.

Tablets: hydroxypropylcellulose; lactose; magnesium stearate; maize starch; microcrystalline cellulose; sodium bisulphite; stearic acid; sunset yellow FCF (E110); talc; ultra-amylopectin.

Oral solutions: citric acid; disodium edetate; ethanol; flavours; glycerol; methyl and propyl hydroxybenzoates; Nipasept sodium; quinoline yellow (E104); sodium hydroxide; sodium phosphate, anhydrous; sodium sulphite; sorbitol; sunset yellow FCF (E110); syrup.

Injections: mannitol; sodium chloride; sodium hydroxide.

Bioavailability

When solid dispersions of frusemide-povidone (amorphous and semi-crystalline dispersions) were compared *in vivo* (single-blind study in healthy males) with crystalline frusemide and with an oral solution of frusemide there were no significant differences in bioavailability (based on sodium and potassium excretion data). Absorption was more rapid from the amorphous dispersion than from the crystalline and semi-crystalline preparations.[20]

Bioequivalence

Kingsford *et al*[21] found a linear relationship between the extent of dissolution and relative bioavailability (compared to that of an oral solution) in four commercial and two experimental tablet formulations. Four tablets which were considered to be bioequivalent by McNamara and others[22] exhibited significantly different dissolution rates. Although seven tablet products satisfactorily met conventional bioequivalence parameters, because of inter-subject variability, only six were considered to be interchangeable.[23] A proprietary tablet and a generic tablet were not bioequivalent when compared in twelve volunteers.[24]

Aqueous solutions

Of two buffered systems containing frusemide with and without propylene glycol and antoxidants the most stable (at 24° and 50°) included propylene glycol (40% v/v), ethanol (10% v/v), and dibasic potassium phosphate (0.2M). During a 170-day period, frusemide losses were negligible and pH values in the range pH 8.0 to 8.4 remained constant in all samples.[13]

Following a stability study of frusemide in a variety of aqueous systems, Ghanekar *et al*[14] proposed the following formulation for a liquid dosage form of frusemide (1 mg/mL): sorbitol solution (50%) in water, ethanol (10% to 20% v/v), methyl and propyl hydroxybenzoates (0.005% and 0.002%, respectively), with pH adjustment to a minimum of 8.5 with an aqueous solution of 0.1N sodium hydroxide. The preparation had 'limited' stability.

Modified-release preparations

Workers in the Netherlands[25] formulated a sustained-release tablet of frusemide which was incorporated in a matrix of microporous polypropylene powder. In a bioavailability study in six males, the 60 mg matrix tablet, a 60 mg oral solution, and an intravenous bolus injection of 40 mg frusemide were compared. The test matrix tablet exhibited high diuretic efficacy but relatively low bioavailability.

Frusemide-povidone co-precipitates prepared by Akbuga *et al*[26] exhibited faster dissolution than physical mixtures or frusemide alone. A frusemide:povidone (molecular weight 49 000) ratio of 1:7 produced most favourable drug release. Direct compression was the method of choice for the preparation of tablets from frusemide:povidone solid dispersion systems.[27] Incorporation of

Kollidon CL (crospovidone) as disintegrant produced tablets that showed a 17-fold increase in drug release compared with that of tablets prepared by physical mixture. A further investigation[28] examined the effects of storage for 24 weeks at ambient temperature and relative humidities of 30%, 50%, and 75% on the stability of tablets (frusemide 40 mg, povidone 240 mg, Avicel PH101 70 mg, Kollidon CL 35 mg, talc 3.46 mg, magnesium stearate 0.385 mg) prepared from frusemide:povidone solid dispersions; little change in physical properties of the tablets due to ageing were shown, except in those stored at 75% relative humidity which demonstrated an alteration in crushing strength and disintegration times. Akbuga has also prepared controlled-release microspheres of frusemide using various types of acrylic polymer[29] or ethylcellulose[30] as the matrix. Microcapsules of frusemide:Eudragit-RL (polymethacrylate, prepared by phase separation) demonstrated sustained release of frusemide in phosphate buffer pH 7.4 compared with release from conventional capsules.[31] The $t_{50\%}$ values for release from conventional capsules and microcapsules with drug:polymer ratios of 1:1, 1:2, and 1:3 were 15, 30, 37, and 52 minutes, respectively. Diuretic efficacy of the microcapsules was investigated in human volunteers.

Stability of a solid dispersion

In an accelerated stability study of a frusemide:povidone solid dispersion (classified as X-ray powder diffraction amorphous) chemical stability of the drug was apparent during storage for 12 months at up to 45° and 40% relative humidity.[32] No marked changes in dissolution rate were observed during the study period.

FURTHER INFORMATION. Studies of furosemide [frusemide] tablets. II. Influence of wet-mixing time, binder volume and batch variation on dissolution rate—Akbuga J, Gursoy A. Drug Dev Ind Pharm 1987;13(14):2541–52. Influence of formulation on frusemide release from hydrophilic matrices of hydroxypropylmethylcellulose [hypromellose]—Meddeb F, Brossard C, Devissaguet JP [French]. STP Pharma 1986;2(18):623–9. Effect of microsphere size and formulation factors on drug release from controlled-release [frusemide] microspheres—Akbuga J. Drug Dev Ind Pharm 1991;17(4):593–607. Influence of substance properties on scaling up of [frusemide] tablet formulations [prepared by direct compression]—Nyqvist H. Drug Dev Ind Pharm 1989;15(6&7):957–64. [Frusemide] Prodrugs: synthesis, enzymatic hydrolysis and solubility of various [frusemide] esters—Mork N, Bundgaard H, Shalmi M, Christensen S. Int J Pharmaceutics 1990;60:163–9. Effect of surfactant [Pluronic F-68] treated diluents [lactose and calcium hydrogen phosphate] on the dissolution and bioavailability of frusemide from capsules and tablets—El-Shaboury MH. Acta Pharm Fenn 1989;98:253–9. Usefulness of certain varieties of Carbomer in the formulation of hydrophilic [frusemide] matrices—Perez-Marcos B, Gutierrez C, Gomez-Amoza JL, Martinez-Pacheco R, Souto C, Concheiro A. Int J Pharmaceutics 1991;67:113–21. Development of a novel [floating] dosage form for [frusemide]—Menon A, Ritschel WA, Sakr A. Pharm Weekbl (Sci) 1992;14(5) Suppl F:F55. Hygroscopic stability and dissolution properties of spray-dried solid dispersions of furosemide with Eudragit—Otsuka M, Onoe M, Matsuda Y. J Pharm Sci 1993;82(1):32–8.

PROCESSING

Sterilisation

Frusemide injection can be sterilised by heating in an autoclave.

REFERENCES

1. Doherty C, York P. Int J Pharmaceutics 1988;47:141–55.
2. Shihab FA, Ebian AR, Mustafa RM. Int J Pharmaceutics 1979;4:13–20.
3. Doherty C, York P. Int J Pharmaceutics 1987;34:197–205.
4. Doherty C, York P. J Pharm Pharmacol 1989;41:73–8.
5. Matsuda Y, Tatsumi E. Int J Pharmaceutics 1990;60:11–26.
6. Cruz JE, Maness DD, Yakatan GJ. Int J Pharmaceutics 1979;2:275–81.
7. Rowbotham PC, Stanford JB, Sugden JK. Pharm Acta Helv 1976;51(10):304–7.
8. Bundgaard H, Norgaard T, Nielsen NM. Int J Pharmaceutics 1988;42:217–24.
9. Moore DE, Sithipitaks V. J Pharm Pharmacol 1983;35:489–93.
10. Akbuga J, Gursoy A. Drug Dev Ind Pharm 1987;13:1827–45.
11. Neil JM, Fell AF, Smith G. Int J Pharmaceutics 1984;22:105–26.
12. Yahya AM, McElnay JC, D'Arcy PF. Int J Pharmaceutics 1986;31:65–8.
13. Shah KA, Das Gupta V, Stewart KR. J Pharm Sci 1980;69(5):594–6.
14. Ghanekar AG, Das Gupta V, Gibbs CW. J Pharm Sci 1978;67(6):808–11.
15. Christensen JM, Lee R-Y, Parrott KA. Am J Hosp Pharm 1983;40:612–15.
16. Beatson C, Taylor A. Br J Pharm Pract 1987;9:223–6.
17. Thomson DF, Allen LV, Desai SR, Rao PS. Am J Hosp Pharm 1985;42:116–19.
18. Thomson DF, Thomson GD. Am J Hosp Pharm 1987;44:2740.
19. Riley CM. Am J Hosp Pharm 1988;45:2079–91.
20. Doherty C, York P, Davidson R. J Pharm Pharmacol 1986;38:48P.
21. Kingsford M, Eggers NJ, Soteros G, Maling TJB, Shirkey RJ. J Pharm Pharmacol 1984;36:536–8.
22. McNamara PJ, Foster TS, Digenus GA, Patel RB, Craig WA, Welling PG et al. Pharm Res 1987;4(2):150–3.
23. Straughn AB, Wood GC, Raghow G, Meyer MC. Biopharm Drug Dispos 1986;7:113–20.
24. Martin BK, Uihlein M, Ings RMJ, Stevens LA, McEwen J. J Pharm Sci 1984;73(4):437–41.
25. Verhoeven J, Peschier LJC, Danhof M, Junginger HE. Int J Pharmaceutics 1988;45;65–77.
26. Akbuga J, Gursoy A, Kendi E. Drug Dev Ind Pharm 1988;14(10):1439–64.
27. Akbuga J, Gursoy A, Yetimoglu F. Drug Dev Ind Pharm 1988;14(15–17):2091–108.
28. Akbuga J, Gursoy A. Pharm Ind 1989;51(9):1046–8.
29. Akbuga J. Int J Pharmaceutics 1989;53:99–105.
30. Akbuga J. Int J Pharmaceutics 1991;76:193–8.
31. Al Gohary O, El Gamal S. Drug Dev Ind Pharm 1991;17(3):443–50.
32. Doherty C, York P. Drug Dev Ind Pharm 1989;15(12):1969–87.

Gentamicin (BAN, pINN)   *Antibacterial*

Gentamycin

Gentamicin consists of a complex mixture of three isomeric aminoglycoside antibiotics (gentamicin C_1, gentamicin C_{1A}, gentamicin C_2) produced by *Micromonospora purpurea*.

Gentamicin Sulphate (BANM, pINNM)
Gentamicin Sulfate (USAN)

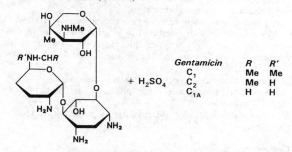

Gentamicin	R	R'
C_1	Me	Me
C_2	Me	H
C_{1A}	H	H

Gentamicin Hydrochloride (BANM, pINNM)

CAS—1403-66-3 (gentamicin); 1405-41-0 (gentamicin sulphate)

Pharmacopoeial status

BP (gentamicin sulphate); USP (gentamicin sulfate)

Preparations

Compendial

Gentamicin Cream BP. A viscous oil-in-water emulsion containing gentamicin sulphate dissolved in the aqueous phase; a cream containing the equivalent of 0.3% w/w of gentamicin is usually available.

Gentamicin Ointment BP. A dispersion of gentamicin sulphate in microfine powder in white soft paraffin or other suitable anhydrous greasy basis; an ointment containing the equivalent of 0.3% w/w of gentamicin is usually available.

Gentamicin Eye Drops BP. A sterile solution of gentamicin sulphate in purified water; eye drops containing the equivalent of 0.3% w/v of gentamicin are usually available.

Gentamicin Injection BP. A sterile solution of gentamicin sulphate in water for injections; injections containing the equivalent of 5 mg and 60 mg of gentamicin in 1 mL, 120 mg of gentamicin in 1.5 mL, and 10 mg and 80 mg in 2 mL are usually available. pH 3.0 to 5.0.

Gentamicin Sulfate Cream USP.

Gentamicin Sulfate Ointment USP.

Gentamicin Sulfate Ophthalmic Solution USP. pH between 6.5 and 7.5.

Gentamicin Sulfate Ophthalmic Ointment USP.

Gentamicin Sulfate Injection USP. pH between 3.0 and 5.5.

Non-compendial

Cidomycin (Roussel). *Cream*, gentamicin 0.3% (as sulphate) in a water-miscible basis. Do not dilute.

Ointment, gentamicin 0.3% (as sulphate) in a white soft paraffin basis. Do not dilute.

Eye/Ear drops, gentamicin 0.3% (as sulphate).

Eye ointment, gentamicin 0.3% (as sulphate) in Plastibase.

Injection, gentamicin 40 mg (as sulphate)/mL.

Paediatric injection, gentamicin 10 mg (as sulphate)/mL.

Intrathecal injection, gentamicin 5 mg (as sulphate)/mL.

Injectable preparations should not be mixed with other drugs, in particular penicillins, cephalosporins, erythromycin, heparins, and sodium bicarbonate.

Garamycin (Schering-Plough). *Eye/Ear drops*, gentamicin 0.3% (as sulphate).

Genticin (Nicholas). *Cream*, gentamicin 0.3% (as sulphate) in a water-miscible basis. Do not dilute.

Eye/Ear drops, gentamicin 0.3% (as sulphate).

Eye ointment, gentamicin 0.3% (as sulphate) in a greasy basis.

Injection, gentamicin 40 mg (as sulphate)/mL. Genticin Injectable should not be mixed with other drugs. In particular it is incompatible with penicillins, cephalosporins, erythromycin, heparins, and sodium bicarbonate.

Pure powder, gentamicin base 1 g (as gentamicin sulphate), sterile hygroscopic powder (sterilised by irradiation). May be dissolved in water or in sodium chloride 0.9% injection. The solution should be sterilised before use, preferably by membrane filtration.

Isotonic Gentamicin Injection (Baxter). *Intravenous infusion*, gentamicin 800 micrograms (as sulphate)/mL in sodium chloride 0.9% injection.

Minims Gentamicin (S&N Pharm). *Eye drops*, gentamicin 0.3% (as sulphate).

Containers and storage

Solid state

Gentamicin Sulphate BP should be kept in a well-closed container. If the substance is sterile, the container should be sterile, tamper-evident, and sealed so as to exclude microorganisms.

Gentamicin Sulfate USP should be preserved in tight containers.

Dosage forms

BP preparations of gentamicin should be labelled with the quantity of active ingredient stated in terms of the equivalent amount of gentamicin.

Gentamicin Sulfate Cream USP and Ointment USP should be preserved in collapsible tubes or in other tight containers; avoid exposure to excessive heat.

Gentamicin Sulfate Ophthalmic Ointment USP should be preserved in collapsible ophthalmic ointment tubes; exposure to excessive heat should be avoided.

Gentamicin Sulfate Injection USP should be preserved in single-dose or multiple-dose containers, preferably of Type I glass.

Gentamicin Sulfate Ophthalmic Solution USP should be preserved in tight containers, and exposure to excessive heat should be avoided.

Sterile Gentamicin Sulfate USP should be preserved in containers for sterile solids.

Cidomycin ointment and cream should be stored in a cool place. Cidomycin injection should not be frozen; refrigeration of the injection is not required. Cidomycin eye/ear drops should be stored below 25° and Cidomycin eye ointment should be stored below 30°.

Genticin cream, eye/ear drops, and eye ointment should be stored at room temperature; they should not be frozen. Genticin injectable should be stored at room temperature, refrigeration is not required. Genticin pure powder should be stored at room temperature.

Minims Gentamicin sulphate eye drops should be stored in a cool place; they should not be frozen. The eye drops should not be exposed to strong light.

PHYSICAL PROPERTIES

Gentamicin is a white, amorphous powder.

Gentamicin sulphate is a white or almost white powder; odourless.

Melting point

Gentamicin melts within the range 102° to 108°.

Gentamicin sulphate melts within the range 218° to 237°.

Gentamicin hydrochloride melts between 194° and 209°.

pH

A 4% w/v solution of *gentamicin sulphate* has a pH of 3.5 to 5.5.

Solubility

Gentamicin is freely soluble in water; sparingly soluble in ethanol; soluble in pyridine, in dimethylformamide, and in acidic media (with salt formation); sparingly soluble in methanol, in chloroform, and in acetone; practically insoluble in benzene and in halogenated hydrocarbons.

Gentamicin sulphate is freely soluble in water; insoluble or practically insoluble in ethanol; it is soluble in ethylene glycol and in formamide; insoluble or practically insoluble in chloroform, in ether, in acetone, and in benzene.

Gentamicin hydrochloride is freely soluble in water and methanol; slightly soluble in ether; practically insoluble in other organic solvents.

STABILITY

Solid state, solutions, and dosage forms

Gentamicin sulphate exhibits good stability as a raw material and in formulated products. In moderately acid to strongly alkaline aqueous solutions it is chemically stable and shows little decomposition in boiling aqueous buffers (pH 2 to 14). Decomposition can be induced by gamma irradiation. Freeman *et al*[1] obtained good recoveries of gentamicin from spiked injection vehicles subjected to adverse treatments (for example, 20 days at 85°). Injectable and topical preparations degraded by less than 10% following storage for 2.5 to 3 years at 37°. Gentamicin sulphate in aqueous solutions is described as moderately oxygen sensitive;[2] a commercial injection is protected from oxygen by gas barriers and by the inclusion of an antioxidant.

Repackaged dilutions

There was no loss of potency in gentamicin sulphate injections (Elkins-Sinn) that had been diluted from 40 mg/mL to 10 mg/mL with sodium chloride 0.9% injection and repackaged in glass syringes (Becton Dickinson) and stored at 4° for 12 weeks.[3]

Peritoneal dialysis solutions

In a study of the stability of diluted and undiluted solutions for peritoneal dialysis (Dianeal, Travenol) which contained different concentrations of gentamicin and glucose, no reduction in gentamicin concentration was observed in the diluted solutions over 24 hours. Small changes in gentamicin concentration in the undiluted solutions were not thought to be clinically significant.[4]

Roberts *et al*[5] demonstrated the stability of gentamicin sulphate 8 mg/L when combined with azlocillin 500 mg/L in one-litre bags of continuous ambulatory peritoneal dialysis fluid (Dianeal 1.36%) under simulated clinical conditions (at 37° over 8 hours). After storage at temperatures between 4° and 37° for 48 hours, gentamicin sulphate (8 mg/L) either alone or combined with cefazolin (75 mg/L and 150 mg/L) was stable in one-litre bags (Viaflex) of peritoneal dialysis solution that contained glucose (1.5%) and heparin (1000 Units/L).[6]

In a microbiological study conducted by Halstead *et al*[7] gentamicin (4 or 8 micrograms/mL, Elkins-Sinn, USA) maintained chemical and biological stability in 1.5% peritoneal dialysis solution (Dianeal, Travenol) for up to 72 hours, either alone or admixed with cefazolin (125 micrograms/mL, Eli Lilly, USA).

Ophthalmic solutions

Extemporaneously prepared ophthalmic solutions[8] of gentamicin sulphate comprising a mixture of an ophthalmic solution (Genoptic, Allergan, USA) and an injection solution (Lyphomed, USA) were shown to be stable for 90 days when packaged in plastic bottles and stored under refrigeration at 4° to 8°.

FURTHER INFORMATION. Stability and cost analysis of clindamycin-gentamicin admixtures given every eight hours—Mansur JM, Abramouitz PW, Lerner SA, Smith RB, Townsend RJ. Am J Hosp Pharm 1985;42:332–5.

INCOMPATIBILITY/COMPATIBILITY

Gentamicin sulphate injection has been reported to be incompatible in admixtures with aminophylline, amphotericin, cephalosporins, chloramphenicol, erythromycin, frusemide, heparin, penicillins, sodium bicarbonate, and sulphadiazine sodium.

When frusemide (10 mg/mL) was added to infusion admixtures containing gentamicin sulphate (1.6 mg/mL) in either sodium chloride 0.9% injection or glucose 5% injection, a white precipitate of frusemide was produced.[9]

Zbrozek et al[10] studied the compatibility and stability of admixtures of injections of gentamicin sulphate (80 mg/2 mL, Elkins-Sinn), clindamycin phosphate (900 mg/6 mL, Upjohn), and cefazolin sodium (1 g diluted with 5 mL sterile water, SKF) diluted to 100 mL with sodium chloride 0.9% or glucose 5% injections. Following storage in glass containers at room temperature under fluorescent light, gentamicin and clindamycin were stable (greater than 90% of initial concentration remaining) for 48 hours, but cefazolin was stable for only 12 hours and 4 hours in sodium chloride 0.9% injection and glucose 5% injection, respectively.

The stability of admixtures of gentamicin sulphate (Elkins-Sinn) and clindamycin phosphate (Upjohn) injections stored in various containers and diluted in different media has been studied by various workers.[10–12] Dilution of the admixture with sodium chloride 0.9% in a polypropylene syringe (Becton Dickinson) gave a product that was stable for 48 hours at constant room temperature under fluorescent lighting.[11] When added either individually or in combination to 50-mL plastic bags of sodium chloride 0.9% or glucose 5%, which were frozen at −20° for 28 days and thawed, both antibiotic components were found to be stable.[12]

Interactions with containers and administration sets

In a comprehensive study of interactions between intravenous infusions and the components of delivery systems,[13] no sorption of gentamicin sulphate was apparent during an experimental infusion using a cellulose propionate burette chamber and polyvinyl chloride, polyethylene, or Silastic tubing, or during 24 hours storage (in the dark at 15° to 20°) in single-use syringes with polypropylene barrels and polyethylene all-plastic plungers.

Weiner et al[14] used an agar diffusion bioassay to measure the potency of gentamicin sulphate injection (Garamycin, 40 mg/mL and 10 mg/mL, Schering) after it had been repackaged into disposable syringes of plastic (polypropylene, Monoject, Sherwood) or glass (Glaspak, Becton Dickinson). After 30 days at 4° and 25°, samples stored in plastic lost 16% of their original potency whereas those stored in glass lost less than 10%. Samples of concentrated injection (40 mg/mL) retained a

higher level of potency when repackaged in small volumes. A brown precipitate, which formed within 30 days in some plastic syringes and within 60 to 90 days in both glass and plastic syringes, contained plasticiser compounds (phthalic acid esters), methyl hydroxybenzoate, and sulphur amongst its constituents. Temperature had no effect on retained potency.

In response, Kresel et al[15] reported that, using an enzymatic assay, gentamicin sulphate (Garamycin, Schering) solutions repackaged into polypropylene syringes (Plastipak, Becton Dickinson) retained their initial concentration for a minimum of 30 days at 4° and at 25°. In reply,[16] the original workers emphasised that the plastic syringes used in the two studies were made by different manufacturers and that the assay methods also varied.

Chrai and Ambrosio[2] expressed concern about the exposure of gentamicin sulphate to air and moisture during the repackaging procedure adopted by Weiner et al.[14]

Gentamicin was not significantly adsorbed to either intravenous tubing or in-line filters during administration of small doses to neonates at slow infusion rates.[17]

FURTHER INFORMATION. Incompatibility of undiluted clindamycin and gentamicin sulfate [precipitation of a zinc-clindamycin complex]—Baker RP. [letter]. Am J Hosp Pharm 1992;49:2144. Aminoglycoside inactivation by penicillins and cephalosporins and its impact on drug-level monitoring—Tindula RJ, Ambrose PJ, Harralson AF. Drug Intell Clin Pharm 1983;17:906–8. Therapeutic implications of interaction of gentamicin and penicillins—Noone P, Pattison JR. Lancet 1971;2:575–8.

FORMULATION

Excipients

Excipients that have been used in presentations of gentamicin sulphate include:

Creams: cetomacrogol; cetostearyl alcohol; chlorocresol; hard paraffin; butyl and methyl hydroxybenzoates; isopropyl myristate; liquid paraffin; monosodium phosphate; polysorbate 40; propylene glycol; propylene glycol monostearate; sorbitol; stearic acid; white soft paraffin.

Ointments: methyl and propyl hydroxybenzoates; white soft paraffin.

Eye/Ear drops: benzalkonium chloride; disodium edetate; disodium phosphate; monosodium phosphate; sodium chloride; sodium metabisulphite.

Eye ointments: methyl and propyl hydroxybenzoates.

Injections: disodium edetate; methyl and propyl hydroxybenzoates; sodium bisulphite; sodium chloride; sodium metabisulphite.

Ophthalmic ointments

El-Shattawy[18] used microbiological growth inhibition on an agar plate to compare the release of gentamicin from 18 different ointment bases intended for ophthalmic use. An oleaginous gel comprising castor oil (85%) and hydrogenated castor oil (15%) with no wetting or spreading agent had the most favourable release properties. The basis that produced the least favourable results comprised cetyl alcohol (5%), liquid paraffin (19%), and yellow soft paraffin (76%). In another study El-Shattawy[19] examined the stability of gentamicin in the 18 ointment bases together with the effects of some additives on its antibacterial activity. All samples stored at 5° for 8 months demonstrated excellent stability and retained gentamicin activity. Of the best eight bases, six contained castor oil, gelled by hydrogenated castor oil or Aerosil; other ingredients included cetyl alcohol, Span

40, Span 80, and glyceryl monostearate as wetting and spreading agents. No significant effect on gentamicin activity was produced by the addition of methyl hydroxybenzoate, propyl hydroxybenzoate, or tocopheryl acetate.

Injections

After autoclaving a gentamicin injection prepared with gentamicin powder and freshly distilled water, a brown colour was produced. Tests on diluted samples of different combinations of the various excipients in the manufacturer's formula (sodium metabisulphite 3.2 mg/mL, methyl hydroxybenzoate 1.8 mg/mL, propyl hydroxybenzoate 0.2 mg/mL, and disodium edetate 0.1 mg/mL) demonstrated that sodium metabisulphite was essential to prevent the discoloration of samples autoclaved at 121° for 45 minutes. The author suggested that 0.08 mg/mL of sodium metabisulphite be used in injections prepared for intravenous administration to neonates.[20]

Novel dosage forms

Beads comprising gentamicin mixed with polymethylmethacrylate have been threaded on wire to form chains of 10 or 30 beads and used in pilot studies of prophylaxis against surgical wound infection.[21]

FURTHER INFORMATION. Biodegradable implants containing gentamicin: drug release and pharmacokinetics—Firsov AA, Nazarov AD, Fomina IP. Drug Dev Ind Pharm 1987;13:1651–74. Preparation and characterization of biodegradable poly(L-lactic acid) gentamicin delivery systems—Sampath SS, Garvin K, Robinson DH. Int J Pharmaceutics 1992;78:165–74. Preparation and characteristics of gentamicin-containing poly(lactide-co-glycolide) microspheres for lung targeting—Alpar HO, Malik A, Almeida A, Brown MRW. J Pharm Pharmacol 1992;44Suppl: 1082. Vaginal administration of gentamicin to *rats*. Pharmaceutical and morphological studies using absorption enhancers—Richardson JL, Minhas PS, Thomas NW, Illum L. Int J Pharmaceutics 1989;56:29–35. Biodegradable gentamicin-loaded controlled release implants made of beta-tricalcium phosphate ceramics. Part 2. Preparation and *in vitro* evaluation of gentamicin-loaded controlled release pellets—Thoma K, Alex R [German]. Pharmazie 1991;46:198–202.

PROCESSING

Sterilisation

Gentamicin injection can be sterilised by filtration. Irradiation has been used for sterilisation of the powder.

REFERENCES

1. Freeman M, Hawkins PA, Loran JS, Stead JA. J Liq Chromat 1979;2(9):1305–17.
2. Chrai SS, Ambrosio TJ [letter]. Am J Hosp Pharm 1977;34:920.
3. Nahata MC, Hipple TF, Strausbaugh SD. Hosp Pharm 1987;22:1131–2.
4. Matzke GR, Nance K. Drug Intell Clin Pharm 1981;15:480.
5. Roberts DE, Cross MD, Thomas PH, Walters TH. Br J Pharm Pract 1987;9:98–9.
6. Walker PC, Kaufmann RE, Massoud N. Drug Intell Clin Pharm 1986;20:697–700.
7. Halstead DC, Guzzo J, Giardina JA, Geshan AE. Antimicrob Agents Chemother 1989;33:1553–6.
8. McBride HA, Martinez DR, Trang JM, Lander RD, Helms HA. Am J Hosp Pharm 1991;48:507–9.
9. Thompson DF, Allen LV, Desai SR, Rao PS. Am J Hosp Pharm 1985;42:116–19.
10. Zbrozek AS, Marble DA, Bosso JA. Drug Intell Clin Pharm 1988;22:873–5.
11. Zbrozek AS, Marble DA, Bosso JA, Bair JN, Townsend RJ. Drug Intell Clin Pharm 1987;21:806–10.
12. Marble DA, Bosso JA, Townsend RJ. Drug Intell Clin Pharm 1986;20:960–3.
13. Kowaluk EA, Roberts MS, Polack AE. Am J Hosp Pharm 1982;39:460–7.
14. Weiner B, McNeely DJ, Kluge RM, Stewart RB. Am J Hosp Pharm 1976;33:1254–9.
15. Kresel JJ, Smith AL, Siber GR [letter]. Am J Hosp Pharm 1977;34:570.
16. McNeely DJ, Weiner B, Stewart RB, Kluge RM [letter]. Am J Hosp Pharm 1977;34:570–1.
17. Nazeravich DR, Otten NHH. Am J Hosp Pharm 1983;40:1961–4.
18. El-Shattawy HH. Drug Dev Ind Pharm 1982;8(5):617–29.
19. El-Shattawy HH. Drug Dev Ind Pharm 1982;8(4):487–96.
20. Sampson C [letter]. Pharm J 1976;216:229.
21. Aubrey DA, Jenkins NH, Morgan WP, Thomas M. Pharmatherapeutica 1986;4(8):536–40.

Glibenclamide (BAN, rINN)   *Antidiabetic*

Glyburide (USAN); glycbenzcyclamide
1-{4-[2-(5-Chloro-2-methoxybenzamido)ethyl]-benzenesulphonyl}-3-cyclohexylurea
$C_{23}H_{28}ClN_3O_5S = 494.0$
CAS—10238-21-8

Pharmacopoeial status

BP

Preparations

Compendial
Glibenclamide Tablets BP. Tablets containing, in each, 2.5 mg and 5 mg are usually available.

Non-compendial
Daonil (Hoechst). *Tablets*, glibenclamide 5 mg.
Euglucon (Roussel). *Tablets*, glibenclamide 2.5 mg and 5 mg.
Semi-Daonil (Hoechst). *Tablets*, glibenclamide 2.5 mg.
Glibenclamide tablets of various strengths are also available from APS (Libanil), Ashbourne (Diabetamide), Berk (Calabren), Cox, CP, Evans, Generics, Kerfoot, Lagap (Malix).

Containers and storage

Dosage forms
Daonil tablets should be stored in a cool, dry place protected from light and in containers similar to those of the manufacturer.

PHYSICAL PROPERTIES

Glibenclamide is a white or almost white, crystalline powder.

Melting point

Glibenclamide melts in the range 169° to 174°.

Dissociation constant

pK_a 5.3 (determined in solvent mixtures)

Solubility

Glibenclamide is practically insoluble in water and in ether; soluble 1 in 330 of ethanol, 1 in 250 of methanol, and 1 in 36 of chloroform. It dissolves in dilute solutions of alkali hydroxides.

Dissolution

Dissolution tests of glibenclamide samples of different particle sizes at 37° in 0.05M phosphate buffer (pH 7.6) with 0.02% w/v polysorbate 80 using the USP XXI paddle method have been reported.[1] Samples with median particle diameters of 2.0, 2.5, 7.5, and 27.5 micrometres had $t_{50\%}$ values for dissolution of 1.3, 2.2, 3.0, and 15 minutes, respectively. Equilibrium solubilities for the four samples were reported to be similar and to increase with pH in the range 5.8 to 9.0.

Crystal and molecular structure

Glass formation
Glibenclamide crystals were converted to an amorphous glassy state when the melt formed at 185° was solidified by cooling.[2] Analyses of the 'transparent and brittle mass' indicated that decomposition did not occur during glass formation. When the glass powder was stored for up to 4 months at room temperature no crystallisation was evident but after storage for 2 months at 50°, 60°, or 70°, partial transformation to crystalline glibenclamide was detected. Equilibrium solubilities of crystalline and glassy glibenclamide were 0.01 mg/mL and 0.1 mg/mL respectively in phosphate buffer (pH 7.4) at 37°. Solubility of the glass form decreased with storage time, to reach a plateau after 21 days. In the USP type 2 apparatus, dissolution of the glass form (in 500 mL of phosphate buffer, pH 7.4 at 37°) was complete in 45 minutes, whereas crystalline glibenclamide and Daonil (Hoechst) were less than 35% and 60% dissolved, respectively, after 90 minutes.

Polymorphs
Isolation and physicochemical characterisation of solid forms of glibenclamide [two polymorphs and two pseudo-polymorphs, crystallisation from solvents]—Suleiman MS, Najib NM. Int J Pharmaceutics 1989;50:103–9.

STABILITY

When glibenclamide is dissolved in methanol or chloroform:methanol (1:1), methyl N-4-[2-(5-chloro-2-methoxybenzamido)ethyl]phenylsulphonyl carbamate is reported to form at room temperature.[3] The ethyl carbamate analogue is a reaction product in ethanol or ethanol:chloroform solutions.

FURTHER INFORMATION. Takla PG. In: Florey K, editor. Analytical profiles of drug substances; vol 10. London: Academic Press, 1981:337–55 [From earlier studies Takla deduced cyclohexylamine and 4-[2-(5-chloro-2-methoxybenzamido)ethyl] benzenesulphonamide to be products of glibenclamide hydrolysis].

INCOMPATIBILITY/COMPATIBILITY

Adsorption to activated charcoal

More than 99% of a sample of glibenclamide (100 mg/L in sodium hydroxide/ethanol/phosphate buffer at pH 7.5) was adsorbed onto activated charcoal[4] when mixed (*in vitro* at 20° to 24°) in ratios of activated charcoal:glibenclamide of 5.3:1 to 16:1.

FORMULATION

Excipients

Excipients that have been used in presentations of glibenclamide include:
Tablets: allura red AC (E129); aluminium oxide; brilliant blue FCF (133); calcium hydrogen phosphate; colloidal anhydrous silica; lactose; magnesium stearate; maize starch; microcrystalline cellulose; quinoline yellow (E104); sodium alginate; talc.

Bioavailability

Australian workers[5] assessed the dissolution, bioavailability, and hypoglycaemic effect of glibenclamide (5 mg) from the following oral preparations: a solution (contents of an ampoule for parenteral use taken with water, Hoechst), branded tablets (Daonil, Hoechst) and two imported brands of tablets. Two methods of tablet dissolution (BP method in distilled water and Desaga flow-cell method in Sørensen buffer at pH 7.8) produced different rank orders of dissolution rates. Bioavailability, relative to the solution, (in 12 healthy volunteers) was 69% ± 21% for Daonil tablets and 49% ± 27% and 24% ± 13% respectively, for the other tablets. On comparison of the methods, bioavailability *in vivo* correlated with the rank order of therapeutic response but not with either dissolution method *in vitro*. In a single-dose, randomised, crossover study involving eight healthy subjects,[6] two commercial tablets of Finnish origin that contained 2.5 mg of non-micronised glibenclamide (Semi-Euglucon and Daonil) were compared with tablets that contained only 1.75 mg of a newer, micronised form of glibenclamide (Semi-Euglucon N and Daonil N). There were no significant differences in pharmacokinetics between the two micronised preparations, which were both absorbed and eliminated more rapidly than the non-micronised products. Without correction for dose, both micronised products produced mean areas under the plasma concentration versus time curves (AUC) similar to Semi-Euglucon. However, the greatest mean AUC was produced by Daonil tablets.
Dissolution rates (in phosphate buffer, pH 7.4 at 37°) of four tablets of glibenclamide 5 mg commercially available in Italy were found to be in the range between those produced by reference tablets of glibenclamide 5 mg in either micronised or non-micronised form.[7] In four healthy subjects, absorption from the reference tablet which contained micronised glibenclamide was faster and greater than absorption from the non-micronised product.

Tablets and suppositories

The stability, shelf-life, and dissolution profile of glibenclamide in experimentally prepared tablets and suppositories and in a tablet commercially available in India (Dionil) were studied under various storage conditions of light and humidity, and under ambient, refrigeration, and elevated temperatures.[8] Tablets contained glibenclamide, starch, talc, magnesium stearate with one of the following: dicalcium phosphate engranule (DCPE), Avicel PH 101 mixed 1:1 with DCPE, directly compressible lactose, or calcium hydrogen phosphate. Suppositories contained glibenclamide with the three macrogol suppository bases of the USP. Exposure to light or humidity slightly decreased stability of glibenclamide in tablets and suppositories. The most stable tablets were those made with direct compression bases followed by Dionil and the suppositories. Alteration of physical properties, dissolution *in vitro*, and bioavailability (in *rabbits*) was detected after 16 weeks storage at room temperature and at elevated temperatures.

Comparisons of tablet preparations

Shaheen *et al*[9] compared conventional glibenclamide 5-mg tablets (Daonil, Hoechst) with glibenclamide 3.5-mg tablets (Oramide, Al-Hikma) which contained macrogol (a water-soluble carrier) and tromethamine (as an alkalinising agent). The rate and extent of dissolution of glibenclamide (in 500 mL of phosphate buffer at pH 7.5 at 37°) was greater from Oramide than from Daonil tablets; complete dissolution from Oramide tablets occurred in less than 45 minutes, whereas from Daonil tablets only 60% dissolution had occurred in 90 minutes. Without correction for dose, similar plasma concentration versus time curves and bioavailabilities of glibenclamide were demonstrated from both tablets in a single-dose, randomised, crossover study involving six healthy subjects. Further, response curves for plasma concentrations of glucose and insulin were in close agreement after the administration of either tablet.

Using a wet granulation method, Singh and Singh[10] prepared tablets that contained glibenclamide, calcium hydrogen phosphate, povidone (10% w/v) in aqueous solution, Nymcel ZSB-16, talc, magnesium stearate and either sodium taurocholate or sodium tauroglycocholate as a surfactant. As the concentration of sodium tauroglycocholate was increased (6%, 8%, 10%, and 20% w/v) in tablets administered to *rabbits* absorption of glibenclamide increased. When sodium taurocholate was present at 10% or 20% w/v absorption of glibenclamide was lower than when the concentration was 6% or 8% w/v.

FURTHER INFORMATION. The effects of magnesium hydroxide on the absorption and efficacy of two glibenclamide preparations [enhancement of absorption from a non-micronised preparation but not from a micronised preparation]—Neuvonen PJ, Kivistö KT. Br J Clin Pharmacol 1991;32:215–20. On the bioavailability and pharmacodynamic activity of commercial glibenclamide preparations. Part 3. Bioequivalence study with volunteers under continuous infusion of glucose solution—Blume H, Ali SL, Stenzhorn G, Stuber W, Siewert M [German]. Pharm Ztg 1985;130:2605–10.

REFERENCES

1. Kaali RN, Rye RM, Wiseman D, York P. J Pharm Pharmacol 1987;39:44P.
2. Hassan MA, Najib NM, Suleiman MS. Int J Pharmaceutics 1991;67:131–7.
3. Poirier MA, Black DB, Lovering EG. Can J Pharm Sci 1980;15(1):8–9.
4. Kannisto H, Neuvonen PJ. J Pharm Sci 1984;73(2):253–6.
5. Chalk JB, Patterson M, Smith MT, Eadie MJ. Eur J Clin Pharmacol 1986;31:177–82.
6. Karttunen P, Uusitupa M, Nykänen S, Robinson JD, Sipilä J. Int J Clin Pharmacol Ther Toxicol 1985;23(12):642–6.
7. Ciranni Signoretti E, Dell'utri A, Cingolani E, Avico U, Zuccaro P, Campanari G *et al.* Farmaco (Prat) 1985;40:141–51.
8. Jayaswal SB, Srivastava HS. Drug Dev Ind Pharm 1987;13(3):529–46
9. Shaheen O, Othman S, Jalal I, Awidi A, Al-Turk W. Int J Pharmaceutics 1987;38:123–31.
10. Singh J, Singh S. Drug Dev Ind Pharm 1990;16(14):2193–8.

Glyceryl Trinitrate　　　　　*Vasodilator*

GTN; nitroglycerin; nitroglycerol; trinitrin; trinitroglycerin
Propane-1,2,3-triol trinitrate
$C_3H_5N_3O_9 = 227.1$
CAS—55-63-0

$$NO_2 \cdot O \cdot CH_2 \cdot \overset{\displaystyle O \cdot NO_2}{\overset{|}{CH}} \cdot CH_2 \cdot O \cdot NO_2$$

Pharmacopoeial status

BP (Concentrated Glyceryl Trinitrate Solution: a 9% to 11% solution of glyceryl trinitrate in ethanol); USP (Diluted Nitroglycerin: a mixture of approximately 10% glyceryl trinitrate with lactose, glucose, ethanol, propylene glycol, or other suitable inert excipient to permit safe handling).

Preparations

Compendial
Glyceryl Trinitrate Tablets BP (Trinitrin Tablets; Nitroglycerin Tablets). Contain mannitol and concentrated glyceryl trinitrate solution. Tablets containing, in each, 300 micrograms, 500 micrograms, and 600 micrograms of glyceryl trinitrate are usually available.
Nitroglycerin Tablets USP.
Nitroglycerin Ointment USP.
Nitroglycerin Injection USP. pH 3.0 to 6.5.

Non-compendial
Coro-Nitro Spray (Boehringer Mannheim). *Aerosol spray*, glyceryl trinitrate 400 micrograms/metered dose. Inflammable.
Deponit (Schwartz). *Transdermal '5' patch*, releases glyceryl trinitrate at a rate of 5 mg/24 hours when in contact with skin. Each patch contains 16 mg glyceryl trinitrate.
Transdermal '10' patch, releases glyceryl trinitrate at a rate of 10 mg/24 hours when in contact with skin. Each patch contains 32 mg glyceryl trinitrate.
Glytrin Spray (Sanofi Winthrop). *Aerosol spray*, glyceryl trinitrate 400 micrograms/metered dose. Inflammable.
GTN 300 mcg (Martindale). *Tablets* (sublingual), glyceryl trinitrate 300 micrograms.
Nitrocine (Schwartz). *Injection*, glyceryl trinitrate 1 mg/mL. To be given undiluted via syringe pump or diluted before admixture. *Diluents*: a suitable vehicle such as sodium chloride injection, glucose 5% injection. Open ampoules or bottles should be used immediately, and any unused drug discarded.
Nitrocontin Continus (ASTA Medica). *Tablets*, controlled release, glyceryl trinitrate 2.6 mg and 6.4 mg.
Nitro-Dur (Schering-Plough). *Transdermal patches*, releasing glyceryl trinitrate at rates of 2.5 mg/24 hours (Nitro-Dur 0.1 mg/h), 5 mg/24 hours (Nitro-Dur 0.2 mg/h), 10 mg/24 hours (Nitro-Dur 0.4 mg/h), and 15 mg/24 hours (Nitro-Dur 0.6 mg/h) when in contact with skin.
Nitrolingual Spray (Lipha). *Aerosol spray*, glyceryl trinitrate 400 micrograms/metered dose. Inflammable.
Nitronal (Lipha). *Injection*, glyceryl trinitrate 1 mg/mL. To be diluted before use or given undiluted with a syringe pump. *Diluents*: for example, glucose 5% injection, sodium chloride and glucose 5% injection, sodium chloride 0.9% injection or other protein-free infusion solution. Diluted solution should be admi-

nistered as soon as possible; it is stable up to 24 hours in recommended infusion system.

Percutol (Cusi). *Ointment*, glyceryl trinitrate 2%.

Suscard (Pharmax). *Tablets* (buccal), controlled release, glyceryl trinitrate 1 mg, 2 mg, 3 mg, and 5 mg.

Sustac (Pharmax). *Tablets*, prolonged release, glyceryl trinitrate 2.6 mg, 6.4 mg, and 10 mg.

Transiderm-Nitro (Ciba). *Transdermal '5' patch*, releases glyceryl trinitrate at a rate of 5 mg/24 hours when in contact with skin. Each patch contains 25 mg glyceryl trinitrate.

Transdermal '10' patch, releases glyceryl trinitrate 10 mg/24 hours when in contact with skin. Each patch contains 50 mg glyceryl trinitrate.

Tridil (Du Pont). *Injection*, glyceryl trinitrate 500 micrograms/mL. To be diluted before use. *Diluents*: see below.

Injection, glyceryl trinitrate 5 mg/mL. To be diluted before use. The drug should be administered at a constant infusion rate. *Diluents* (both injections): glucose 5% in water or sodium chloride 0.9%. Opened ampoules should be used immediately; unused diluted drug should be discarded.

Containers and storage

Solid state

Concentrated Glyceryl Trinitrate Solution BP should be kept in a well-closed container, protected from light and stored at a temperature of 8° to 15°.

CAUTION. Undiluted glyceryl trinitrate can be exploded by percussion or excessive heat. Appropriate precautions should be exercised and only exceedingly small amounts should be isolated.

Diluted Nitroglycerin USP should be preserved in tight, light-resistant containers and protected from exposure to excessive heat. A handling caution similar to that emphasised by the BP is recommended.

Dosage forms

Glyceryl Trinitrate Tablets BP should be protected from light and stored at a temperature not exceeding 25° in a glass container closed by means of a screw closure lined with aluminium or tin foil; additional packing that absorbs glyceryl trinitrate should be avoided. Glyceryl Trinitrate Tablets BP should be issued for patients in containers of not more than 100 tablets. The Council of the Royal Pharmaceutical Society of Great Britain recommends that Glyceryl Trinitrate Tablets BP be labelled with an indication that they should be discarded after eight weeks in use. This applies to either dispensed or over-the-counter preparations. Glyceryl trinitrate tablets should be dispensed only in glass containers, sealed with a foil-lined cap and containing no cotton wool wadding.

For parenteral preparations, the use of glass or polyethylene apparatus is preferable; loss of potency will occur if polyvinyl chloride is used.

Nitroglycerin Tablets USP should be preserved in tight containers, preferably of glass, at controlled room temperature. Each container holds not more than 100 tablets.

Nitroglycerin Ointment USP should be preserved in tight containers.

Nitroglycerin Injection USP should be preserved in single-dose or in multiple-dose containers, preferably of Type I or Type II glass.

Coro-Nitro spray should be kept away from direct sunlight or direct sources of heat. Glytrin spray should be stored below 25°, protected from frost and direct heat or sunlight. Nitrolingual spray should be stored below 25° and not exposed to sunlight or temperatures over 50°. The sprays are packaged in aerosol containers which should not be pierced, punctured or burnt.

Deponit (5 and 10) and Transiderm-Nitro (5 and 10) transdermal patches should be stored below 25°.

Nitrocontin Continus tablets should be stored in a cool, dry place, protected from light.

Nitrocine injection admixtures are stable for approximately 24 hours at room temperature in the recommended containers.

Nitro-Dur transdermal patches should be stored between 15° and 30° and should not be refrigerated.

Nitronal injection solution should be stored in a cool place, protected from light. The vial, for single dose only, should be stored in the carton until ready for use.

Percutol should be stored in a cool place (below 15°).

Suscard and Sustac tablets: storage at room temperature is recommended.

Tridil injection should be protected from strong light. It should not be used if discoloured.

FURTHER INFORMATION. Stability of nitroglycerin tablets in a unit of use pendant-type container—Shangraw RF, Dorsch B. Contemp Pharm Pract 1981;4(3):132–6. Personal nitroglycerin containers [letter]—Guernsey BG, Doutre WH, Ingrim NB, Hokanson JA, Dunn JK, Bryant SG. Drug Intell Clin Pharm 1983;17:754–5.

PHYSICAL PROPERTIES

Glyceryl trinitrate (undiluted) is a white to pale yellow, thick, inflammable liquid which explodes on rapid heating or percussion. When diluted with lactose it is a white, odourless powder. When diluted with propylene glycol or ethanol, it is a clear, colourless, or pale yellow liquid.

Solubility

Glyceryl trinitrate (undiluted) is slightly soluble in water; soluble in methanol, in ethanol, in carbon disulphide, in acetone, in chloroform, in ether, and in glacial acetic acid.

STABILITY

Glyceryl trinitrate is relatively stable in weakly acidic solution and in neutral solution but degrades very rapidly in the presence of strong alkali.

In a study by Aburawi et al,[1] glyceryl trinitrate was observed to decompose very slowly at pH 7.4, at a slightly faster rate in an acid environment (0.1M hydrochloric acid), and rapidly at pH values of 11 and 13, at 25°. Glyceryl trinitrate decomposed by denitration with formation of nitrate ions. Similar observations were made with the partially denitrated analogues 1,2-glyceryl dinitrate and 1,3-glyceryl dinitrate, the former being converted to the latter before undergoing denitration. The major decomposition products of glyceryl trinitrate were 1,2-glyceryl dinitrate, 1,3-glyceryl dinitrate, and inorganic nitrate. No inorganic nitrites were detected in this study. Calculated activation energies at pH 10 for decomposition of glyceryl trinitrate, 1,2-glyceryl dinitrate, and 1,3-glyceryl dinitrate were 87.7 kJ/mol, 91.2 kJ/mol, and 72.3 kJ/mol, respectively.

Sublingual tablets

Vaporisation of glyceryl trinitrate can lead to migration of the drug between tablets shortly after the tablets have been placed in the container; this process may result in poor uniformity of content of the tablets in a container. Inter-tablet migration of glyceryl trinitrate was shown to be due to capillary condensation, that is, the condensation of glyceryl trinitrate onto empty or partly filled small pores in the tablet structure.[2]

The evaporation rate of glyceryl trinitrate from the sublingual tablets Nitrostat (moulded), Nitrobaat (compressed) and two generic brands (compressed) by ACF and Pharbita, Netherlands, was found to be controlled by the vapour pressure and diffusion coefficient of the drug and by a matrix effect associated with the porous structure of the dosage form.[3] Storage in open containers (5 tablets/container, 3 months, room temperature) resulted in 2% loss of glyceryl trinitrate for the branded products and 7% and 10% for the generics from ACF and Pharbita, respectively. The moulded tablet had the lowest vapour pressure and was the most stable form. Potency loss (more pronounced at 37°) decreased when the number of tablets in the open container was increased, although no loss of glyceryl trinitrate was observed in tightly closed containers. Loss of glyceryl trinitrate from solid dosage forms is reduced by: storage in tightly closed containers, keeping a higher rather than lower number of tablets in each container, avoiding the use of absorbent stuffing material, avoiding high storage temperatures, and using narrow-necked containers.

In a further study by the same authors[4] release of glyceryl trinitrate, in vivo (healthy volunteers) and in vitro, from three compressed tablets was found to be strongly dependent upon the disintegration process of the dosage form. The moulded tablet did not disintegrate but dissolved completely. It was suggested that potency loss from correctly stored glyceryl trinitrate tablets may be a problem associated with release of the drug from the dosage form rather than a stability problem.

Repackaged tablets

Samples from two batches of commercially available glyceryl trinitrate tablets, repackaged in samples of 10 in amber glass bottles with tightly closed metal screw caps, were stable after storage at 37° (Nitrostat, PD, 0.6 mg) and 25° (Nitrostat, PD, 0.4 mg) for 4 months and then for a further month at room temperature.[5] Samples were compared with reference tablets which had been stored at 25° for 18 months and 37° for 17 months in their original containers. The results of the study cannot be applied to all glyceryl trinitrate tablets.

Effects of additives

Pikal et al[6] examined the effect of various glyceryl trinitrate-soluble excipients on moulded glyceryl trinitrate tablets. At additive:glyceryl trinitrate weight ratios near 1 most of the additives studied (povidone, macrogols 400, 4000, and 20 000, polyoxyethylene 23 lauryl ether, octoxinol, polysorbate 20, 60, and 80, ethylenediamine compounds, poloxamer 188, bis(2-ethylhexyl phthalate), and acetylated monoglycerides) caused sufficient lowering of the vapour pressure of glyceryl trinitrate to stabilise the content uniformity of the tablets. However, higher concentrations of most additives (additive:glyceryl trinitrate ratio near 2) except octoxinol and 100% acetylated monoglycerides led to reduced chemical stability of glyceryl trinitrate, especially at high temperatures (50°). Disintegration times for fresh tablets (except where povidone was the additive) were essentially the same as for tablets stored at 25° for 2 years.

The volatility of glyceryl trinitrate from compressed sublingual tablets was significantly reduced by the inclusion of povidone in the formulation.[7] The stability of the tablets increased with increasing concentration of povidone in the formulation (glyceryl trinitrate:povidone ratios up to 1:4 were examined). Inclusion of microcrystalline cellulose further stabilised glyceryl trinitrate. At the elevated temperatures of accelerated stability studies,[8] glyceryl trinitrate was found (by spectrophotometric assay) to be stable for at least 24 hours in povidone and in the solvents absolute ethanol, ethanol:water (1:1), propylene glycol, and glycerol, but not in macrogol 400. The observed $t_{10\%}$ of glyceryl trinitrate solution in macrogol 400 was approximately 10 days at 20° to 24°.

Intravenous solutions

Solutions of glyceryl trinitrate (0.2 mg/mL) for intravenous use were prepared in sodium chloride 0.9% or glucose 5% solutions using either sublingual tablets or a 10% glyceryl trinitrate-lactose adsorbate powder.[9] Stability studies were performed under various conditions. No significant reduction in concentration was found in stock solutions of glyceryl trinitrate (0.8 to 1.0 mg/mL) in sodium chloride 0.9% that had been stored at 6° in multidose vials for 6 months; but a 20% reduction in initial concentration was apparent after storage under fluorescent light at 22° to 30° for 87 days. When packaged in glass containers, the test intravenous glyceryl trinitrate solutions lost a maximum of 18% of their initial concentration during storage for 24 hours in the temperature range 6° to 38°. Their stability was not dependent on light, the vehicle, or the source of glyceryl trinitrate. However, solutions in contact with rubber stoppers or plastic exhibited marked decreases in glyceryl trinitrate concentration, possibly due to sorption.

FURTHER INFORMATION. Nitroglycerin stability: effects on bioavailability, assay and biological distribution—Sokoloski TD, Wu CC. J Clin Hosp Pharm 1981;6:227–32. Nitroglycerin intravenous infusion [review of stability and sterilisation]—Elliott GT, Quinn SL. Drug Intell Clin Pharm 1982;16:211–17. Stabilities of dobutamine, dopamine, nitroglycerin and sodium nitroprusside in disposable plastic syringes—Pramar Y, Das Gupta V, Gardner SN, Yau B. J Clin Pharm Ther 1991;16:203–7. Comment on intravenous nitroglycerin—Robinson LA, Wright BT [letter]. Drug Intell Clin Pharm 1983;17:49. Diminished activity of glyceryl trinitrate [the importance of recommended storage conditions]—O'Hanrahan M, McGarry K, Kelly JG, Horgan J, O'Malley K. Br Med J 1982;284:1183–4.

INCOMPATIBILITY/COMPATIBILITY

Sorption to plastics and rubber

There are many reports in the literature of sorption of glyceryl trinitrate to plastic containers and tubing,[10–18] in particular to polyvinyl chloride but also, to a lesser extent, to cellulose propionate and polystyrol-butadiene giving sets and burettes[10] or to polyethylene containers.[13] There appears to be little or no sorption of glyceryl trinitrate to glass containers[10,11,13,14] or to high density polyethylene tubing.[10,11] Baumgartner et al[19] reported negligible adsorption of glyceryl trinitrate to nylon and Posidyne 0.2 micrometre filters 15 minutes after the start of an infusion of glyceryl trinitrate 0.01% in glucose 5% injection; however, some adsorption to the Posidyne filter material was observed at 180 minutes.

Sokoloski et al[15] observed an increase in the degree of adsorption of glyceryl trinitrate from sodium chloride 0.9% solution to polyvinyl chloride tubing concomitant with increasing temperature (in the range 6.5° to 21°). Adsorption can be reduced[13] by pre-rinsing the infusion system with infusion fluid and increasing the flow-rate. Roberts et al[16] reported that loss of glyceryl trinitrate was related more to the surface area of plastic in contact with the solution and to the volume of solution than to the concentration of glyceryl trinitrate.

Adsorption of glyceryl trinitrate to rubber stoppers or closures of vials containing solutions or intravenous infusions of glyceryl trinitrate has been reported.[9,12] Greater losses of glyceryl trinitrate from solutions in larger, partially-filled glass containers has also been noted.[12]

The degree of sorption of glyceryl trinitrate from moulded tablets onto various thermoplastic polymer components of unit-dose strip packaging was shown to decrease in the rank order: vinyls ≫ low density polyethylene > ionomers > high density polyethylene.[20]

During a period of 24 hours, glyceryl trinitrate was shown[21] to be compatible (at concentrations 200 and 400 micrograms/mL) with the following infusion fluids in both glass and polyolefin containers at room temperature in ambient light and intense light, and at 5° and 40° in darkness: sodium chloride 0.9%, sodium chloride 0.45%, glucose 5%, glucose 5% and sodium chloride 0.9%, glucose 5% and sodium chloride 0.45%, glucose 5% and compound sodium lactate injection, and sodium lactate injection (0.167M). However, Ludwig and Ueda[22] reported significant losses of glyceryl trinitrate, during a 5-hour period, from solutions prepared with glucose 5% in water in both glass and plastic containers at room temperature with and without protection from light. Losses from solutions kept at 4° (refrigeration temperature) were smaller.

FURTHER INFORMATION. Effect of infusion administration set on the delivery rate and plasma concentration of nitroglycerin in dogs—McNiff EF, Lai CM, Look ZM, Yacobi A, Fung H-L. J Pharm Sci 1985;74(7):774–6. Intravenous nitroglycerin delivery: dynamics and cost considerations—Nix DE, Tharpe WN, Francisco GE. Hosp Pharm 1985;20:230–2. Pharmaceutical considerations of nitroglycerin [comprehensive review article; tables of incompatibilities; includes sorption to plastics]—Yacobi A, Amann AH, Baaske DM. Drug Intell Clin Pharm 1983;17:255–63. A study of the interaction of selected drugs and plastic syringes—Speaker TJ, Turco SJ, Nardone DA, Miripol JE. J Parenter Sci Technol 1991;45(5):212–17.

FORMULATION

Excipients

Excipients that have been used in presentations of glyceryl trinitrate include:

Capsules (modified release): brilliant blue FCF (133); calcium stearate; carmoisine (E122); colophony; ethylcellulose; gelatin; indigo carmine (E132); lactose; magnesium stearate; maize starch; pharmaceutical glaze; povidone; quinoline yellow (E104); shellac; silica gel; stearic acid; sucrose; sunset yellow FCF (E110); sodium bisulphite; talc; titanium dioxide (E171).

Tablets: carmine (E120); cellacephate; dextrin; diethyl phthalate; erythrosine (E127); lactose; magnesium stearate; spermaceti; sucrose; talc; white beeswax.

Tablets (sublingual): lactose; macrogol 3350; sucrose.

Transdermal patches/systems: acrylic adhesive; Aerosil 200; aluminium foil laminate; colloidal silica; di-(2-ethylhexyl) phthalate; glycerol; isopropyl palmitate; lactose; liquid paraffin; macrogol; polyethylene foam; polyvinyl alcohol; polyvinyl chloride/polyvinyl acetate copolymer; povidone; silicone fluid; silicone rubber; sodium citrate.

Sprays (lingual aerosols): caprylic/capric/diglyceryl succinate; dichlorodifluoromethane; dichlorotetrafluoroethane; ether; menthol; paraffin oil.

Ointments: hydrous wool fat; lactose; white soft paraffin.

Intravenous solutions: ethanol; glucose; lactose; macrogol 400; sodium acid phosphate; propylene glycol.

Sublingual tablets

Stable directly-compressed sublingual glyceryl trinitrate tablets were developed,[23] incorporating povidone to retard volatilisation of the drug, according to the following formulation: glyceryl trinitrate-lactose powder (10% w/w of glyceryl trinitrate) qs; sodium starch glycollate 1%; magnesium stearate 2%; povidone type I 10%; povidone type II 10%; lactose monohydrate to 100%. The tablets were claimed to be pharmaceutically elegant with low friability. Over 80% of the initial concentration of glyceryl trinitrate remained in the tablets after exposure to the atmosphere at room temperature for two months.

Intravenous solutions

The preparation of a glyceryl trinitrate 1% solution for infusion (in a stock solution prepared with dehydrated ethanol) from commercial sublingual tablets or from glyceryl trinitrate 10% w/w in lactose (ICI, USA) was detailed by Ward et al.[24] The solution was diluted to 0.1% with water for injections or sodium chloride 0.9% injection. Tablets were not recommended as a source of glyceryl trinitrate for the solution owing to the wide variation in drug content between tablets. The solution was sterilised by filtration; tests showed that the solution was free from pyrogens. The final 0.1% solution was diluted to the required concentration for infusion before administration.

Transdermal patches

Berner et al[25] demonstrated that the solution properties of an aqueous ethanol donor solution caused a flux enhancement of glyceryl trinitrate through porous and non-porous polymer membranes. Their findings led to the design of a 'mutually enhanced transdermal therapeutic system'.[26] A model that simulated skin permeation by glyceryl trinitrate from ethanol:water mixtures was presented. It was suggested that an aqueous ethanol reservoir saturated with glyceryl trinitrate and excess lactose, with an ethanol volume fraction less than or equal to 0.7, produced a flux of glyceryl trinitrate across skin *in vitro* that was proportional to the ethanol flux.

Absorption

The manufacturer of Susadrin (Forest, USA), an oral transmucosal, controlled-release tablet containing glyceryl trinitrate in a Synchron base (composed of a range of polymers made from naturally-occurring materials), reported superior absorption of the buccal tablet in healthy volunteers compared to that from a glyceryl trinitrate patch or ointment.[27] Absorption was similar to that of an intravenous infusion or of a sublingual tablet (0.8 mg). Synchron base was reported to stabilise glyceryl trinitrate and the recommended shelf-life for Susadrin tablets was three years at room temperature.

A transdermal glyceryl trinitrate patch (Minitran 54 mg in 20 cm,[2] 3M Riker, USA) delivered approximately 1.6 times more drug per square centimetre of surface area than a glyceryl trinitrate ointment (16 mg in 1 inch, Nitro-Bid, Marian Labs, USA) in a crossover study involving 24 healthy male volunteers.[28] An average of 15 mg glyceryl trinitrate/24 hours was released by the patch.

The area of application of a glyceryl trinitrate ointment (16 mg over either 25 cm^2 or 100 cm^2) was found to significantly influence the pharmacokinetics of glyceryl trinitrate in a study involving three healthy volunteers.[29]

Bioequivalence

Adesitrin (Farmitalia Carlo Erba, Italy) and NitroDur (Key Pharmaceuticals, USA) are both matrix transdermal delivery systems of glyceryl trinitrate. They were found to be bioequivalent (on the basis of pharmacokinetic parameters) with Nitroderm (Ciba-Geigy, USA), a reservoir/rate controlling membrane system, when tested in twelve healthy volunteers in a single-dose, three-way randomised crossover study.[30]

FURTHER INFORMATION. Improvement in transdermal bioavailability of nitroglycerin by formulation design—Huang YC, Keshavy PR, Chien YW, Moniot S, Goodhart FW. Drug Dev Ind Pharm 1985;11(6&7):1255–70. Comparative controlled skin permeation [hairless *mouse* skin] of nitroglycerin from marketed transdermal delivery systems—Chien YW, Keshavy PR, Huang YC, Sarpotdar PP [letter]. J Pharm Sci 1983;72(8):968–70. Development of biphasic transdermal nitroglycerin delivery systems [*in vitro* and *in vivo* (humans)]—Hadgraft J, Wolff M, Bonn R, Cordes G. Int J Pharmaceutics 1990;64:187–94. *In vitro* assessments of transdermal devices containing nitroglycerin [five commercial preparations]—Hadgraft J, Lewis D, Beutner D, Wolff HM. Int J Pharmaceutics 1991;73:125–30. *In vivo-in vitro* comparisons in the transdermal delivery of nitroglycerin—Hadgraft J, Beutner D, Wolff HM. Int J Pharmaceutics 1993;89:R1–R4. *In vitro* release of nitroglycerin from topical products by use of artificial membranes—Wu ST, Shiu GK, Simmons JE, Bronaugh RL, Skelly JP. J Pharm Sci 1992;81(12):1153–6. Controlled release nitroglycerin capsules [*in vitro* and *in vivo*]—Bhatt HR, Gurnasinghani ML, Dattani KK, Lalla JK. J Controlled Release 1989(June);9:43–55. Rectal absorption of nitroglycerin in the *rat*: avoidance of first-pass metabolism as a function of rectal length exposure—Kamiya A, Ogata H, Fung H-L. J Pharm Sci 1982;71(6):621–4.

PROCESSING

Glyceryl trinitrate is safe and stable in fatty or oily solution, but in alcoholic solution the substance must be handled with extreme caution.
See also Containers and Storage, above.

REFERENCES

1. Aburawi S, Curry SH, Whelpton R. Int J Pharmaceutics 1984;22:327–36.
2. Pikal MJ, Lukes AL, Ellis LF. J Pharm Sci 1976;65(9):1278–84.
3. Lagas M, Duchateau AMJA. Pharm Weekbl (Sci) 1988;10:246–53.
4. Lagas M, Duchateau AMJA. Pharm Weekbl (Sci) 1988;10:254–8.
5. Di Matteo FP, Sami A, Flack HL. Hosp Pharm 1974;9(8):299–302.
6. Pikal MJ, Lukes AL, Conine JW. J Pharm Sci 1984;73(11):1608–12.
7. Gucluyildiz M, Goodhart FW, Ninger FC. J Pharm Sci 1977;66(2):265-6.
8. Suphajettra P, Strohl JH, Lim JK. J Pharm Sci 1978;67(10):1394–6.
9. Scheife AH, Grisafe JA, Shargel L. J Pharm Sci 1982;71(1):55–9.
10. De Rudder D, Remon JP, Neyt EN. J Pharm Pharmacol 1987;39:556–8.
11. Cossum PA, Roberts MS, Galbraith AJ, Boyd GW. Lancet 1978;2:349–50.
12. Sturek JK, Sokoloski TD, Winsley WT, Stach PE. Am J Hosp Pharm 1978;35:537–40.
13. Christiansen H, Skobba TJ, Andersen R, Saugen JN. J Clin Hosp Pharm 1980;5:209–15.
14. Yuen L-H, Denman SL, Sokoloski TD, Burkman AM. J Pharm Sci 1979;68(9):1163–6.
15. Sokoloski TD, Wu C-C, Burkman AM. Int J Pharmaceutics 1980;6:63–76.
16. Roberts MS, Cossum PA, Galbraith AJ, Boyd GW. J Pharm Pharmacol 1980;32:237–44.
17. Hans P, Paris P, Mathot F. Intensive Care Med 1982;8:93–5.
18. Crouthamel WG, Dorsh B, Shangraw R [letter]. New Eng J Med 1978;296:262.
19. Baumgartner TG, Curry SH, Shaw MA, Russell WL. Am J IV Ther Clin Nutr 1984;11:7–13.
20. Pikal MJ, Bibler DA, Rutherford B. J Pharm Sci 1977;66(9):1293–7.
21. Wagenknecht DM, Baaske DM, Alam AS, Carter JE, Shah J. Am J Hosp Pharm 1984;41:1807–11.
22. Ludwig DJ, Ueda CT. Am J Hosp Pharm 1978;35:541–4.
23. Fung H-L, Yap SK, Rhodes CT. J Pharm Sci 1976;65(4):558–60.
24. Ward JW, Sandler AI, Tucker SV. Drug Intell Clin Pharm 1979;13(1):14–16.
25. Berner B, Otte JH, Mazzenga GC, Steffens RJ, Ebert CD. J Pharm Sci 1989;78(4):314–18.
26. Berner B, Mazzenga GC, Otte JH, Steffens RJ, Juang R-H, Ebert CD. J Pharm Sci 1989;78(5):402–7.
27. Schor JM, Davis SS, Nigalaye A, Bolton S. Drug Dev Ind Pharm 1983;9(7):1359–77.
28. Riedel DJ, Wick KA, Hawkinson RW, Kolars CA, Crowley JK, Armstrong KE, *et al.* Clin Ther 1989;11(2):225–31.
29. Sved S, McLean WM, McGilveray IJ. J Pharm Sci 1981;70(12):1368–9.
30. De Ponti F, Luca C, Pamparana F, Bianco L, D'Angelo L, Caravaggi M, *et al.* Curr Ther Res 1989;46(1):111–20.

Griseofulvin (BAN, rINN)   *Antifungal*

Curling Factor
(2S,4'R)-7-Chloro-2',4,6-trimethoxy-4'-methylspiro
[benzofuran-2(3H),3'-cyclohexene]-3,6'-dione
$C_{17}H_{17}ClO_6 = 352.8$
CAS—126-07-8

Pharmacopoeial status

BP, USP

Preparations

Compendial
Griseofulvin Tablets BP. Tablets containing, in each, 125 mg and 500 mg are usually available.
Griseofulvin Capsules USP.
Griseofulvin Tablets USP.
Griseofulvin Oral Suspension USP.
Ultramicrosize Griseofulvin Tablets USP. Composed of ultramicrosize crystals of griseofulvin dispersed in macrogol 6000 or dispersed by other suitable means.

Non-compendial
Fulcin (ICI). *Tablets*, griseofulvin 125 mg (Fulcin 125) and 500 mg (Fulcin 500).
Oral suspension, aqueous suspension, griseofulvin 125 mg/5 mL.
Diluent: syrup preserved with methyl hydroxybenzoate, life of diluted suspension 14 days.
Grisovin (Glaxo). *Tablets*, griseofulvin 125 mg and 500 mg.

Containers and storage

Solid state
Griseofulvin BP should be kept in a well-closed container.
Griseofulvin USP should be preserved in tight containers.

Dosage forms
Griseofulvin Capsules USP, Tablets USP and Oral Suspension
USP should be preserved in tight containers.
Ultramicrosize Griseofulvin Tablets USP should be preserved in
well-closed containers.
All Fulcin preparations should be stored at room temperature;
Fulcin tablets should be protected from moisture.

PHYSICAL PROPERTIES

Griseofulvin is a white to yellowish-white, crystalline powder;
tasteless; odourless or almost odourless.
The BP specifies that particles of the powder are generally up to
5 micrometres in maximum dimension, although larger particles, which may occasionally exceed 30 micrometres, may be present. The USP specifies that particles of the order of 4
micrometres in diameter predominate.

Melting point

Griseofulvin melts in the range 217° to 224°.

Solubility

At 20°, *griseofulvin* is very slightly soluble in water; slightly soluble in ethanol; soluble 1 in 300 of absolute ethanol, 1 in 250 of
methanol, 1 in 20 of acetone, 1 in 25 of chloroform, and 1 in 3
of 1,1,2,2-tetrachloroethane; freely soluble in dimethylformamide.
Ritschel and Hussain[1] determined the solubilities of griseofulvin
in various solvents, at 30°, to be as follows: 0.008 mg/mL in
water, 1.81 mg/mL in propylene glycol, 82.64 mg/mL in
dimethyl sulphoxide, 46.91 mg/mL in dimethyl acetamide,
33.42 mg/mL in N,N-diethyl-m-toluamide, and 13.71 mg/mL in
diethyleneglycol monoethylether.
At 37°, 3.2 mg of griseofulvin was found to dissolve in 1 mL of
70% macrogol 300 (equilibrium solubility).[2]
A moderate increase in solubility of micronised griseofulvin
occurred with an increase in concentration of macrogol 6000
in the range 0% w/v to 10% w/v in water.[3] The authors calculated that 555 molecules of macrogol 6000 were required to solubilise 1 molecule of griseofulvin.
During investigations into the dissolution kinetics of griseofulvin (as a model drug) in aqueous solutions of sodium dodecyl-
sulphate (SDS)[4] or sodium cholate or sodium taurocholate
(bile salts),[5] the solubility of griseofulvin was shown to increase
linearly with increasing concentration of SDS (above the critical
micelle concentration of SDS of 6.8 mmol/L at 37°) or bile salt.
The aqueous solubility of griseofulvin increased in a non-linear
manner in the presence of increasing concentrations of nicotinamide; the solubility increased from 2.2×10^{-5}M in water alone
to 2.6×10^{-3}M in the presence of nicotinamide 3.3M.[6] The
mechanisms of solubilisation were investigated.
FURTHER INFORMATION. Solubility and complexation behaviour
of griseofulvin in fatty acid-isooctane mixtures—Mehdizadeh
M, Grant DJW. J Pharm Sci 1984;73(9):1195–203. Solubility
behaviour of griseofulvin in solvents of relatively low polarity
[glyceride solvents]—Grant DJW, Abougela IKA. Labo Pharm
Probl Tech 1984 Mar;32:193–6.

Dissolution

The USP specifies that for Griseofulvin Capsules USP not less
than 80% of the labelled amount of $C_{17}H_{17}ClO_6$ is dissolved
in 30 minutes. Dissolution medium: 1000 mL of water contain-

ing 5.4 mg of sodium lauryl sulphate per mL; Apparatus 2 at
100 rpm.
The USP specifies that for Griseofulvin Tablets USP not less
than 70% of the labelled amount of $C_{17}H_{17}ClO_6$ is dissolved
in 60 minutes. Dissolution medium: 1000 mL of water containing 40.0 mg of sodium lauryl sulphate per mL; Apparatus 2 at
100 rpm.
The USP specifies that for Ultramicrosize Griseofulvin Tablets
USP not less than 85% of the labelled amount of $C_{17}H_{17}ClO_6$
is dissolved in 60 minutes. Dissolution medium: 1000 mL of
water containing 5.4 mg of sodium lauryl sulphate per mL.
Apparatus 2 at 100 rpm.

Dissolution properties

In a study on three experimental griseofulvin tablets, correlation
was shown between dissolution rates *in vitro* and absorption
in vivo (in *rabbits* and in humans).[7] Each tablet contained micronised griseofulvin (125 mg), carmellose calcium, lactose, magnesium stearate, and one of three grades of polyvinyl alcohol.
Dissolution rates in distilled water at 37° were significantly different between tablets; those that contained polyvinyl alcohol
of lowest viscosity exhibited the fastest dissolution rates. A
crossover study involving four healthy volunteers revealed that
bioavailability of griseofulvin from the tablets correlated with
dissolution rates.

Crystal and molecular structure

Griseofulvin exists as octahedral or rhombic crystals.
Analysis of a resolidified melt of griseofulvin by X-ray diffraction revealed that it existed in an amorphous form; conversion
to a crystalline form was thought to occur following comminution.[3]

STABILITY

Griseofulvin is reported to be a stable substance.
No photodegradation of griseofulvin was detected[8] when a solution of griseofulvin in methanol was irradiated with a xenon
lamp (to emit light that had a similar intensity and wavelength
to that of natural sunlight) for 20 hours; no changes in fluorescence or ultraviolet spectra of griseofulvin were measured.

FORMULATION

Excipients

Excipients that have been used in presentations of griseofulvin
include:
Capsules: allura red AC (E129); black iron oxide (E172); erythrosine (E127); gelatin; indigo carmine (E132); lactose; magnesium stearate; quinoline yellow (E104); sunset yellow FCF
(E110); talc; titanium dioxide (E171).
Tablets: calcium hydrogen phosphate; calcium stearate; carmellose calcium; colloidal silica; D&C Red No.36; ethylcellulose;
gelatin; gluten; glycerol; hypromellose; lactose; macrogols 400,
6000, and 8000; magnesium stearate; maize starch; methyl
hydroxybenzoate; microcrystalline cellulose; poloxomer 188;
polymethacrylate potassium; potato starch; povidone; rice
starch; silica; sodium lauryl sulphate; sodium starch glycollate;
stearic acid; talc; titanium dioxide (E171).
Oral suspensions: allura red AC (E129); aluminium magnesium
sulphate; calcium chloride; carmellose sodium; chocolate flavour; cocoa powder; docusate sodium; ethanol 0.008%;
menthol; methyl and propyl hydroxybenzoates; peppermint
oil; propylene glycol; saccharin sodium; simethicone emulsion;
sodium alginate; sodium citrate; sucrose; vanillin.
Ointments: glycerol.

Bioavailability

The absorption of griseofulvin is dependent upon particle size, dissolution rate, and inter-subject and intra-subject variations. The use of a small particle size (about 5 micrometres) has improved bioavailability but it is still poorly absorbed with only about 50% reaching the circulation in 30 to 40 hours. Various methods have been attempted to improve absorption; the use of dispersions in macrogol and in a mixture with microcrystalline cellulose have been successful.

In a comparison of tablets that contained griseofulvin of mean particle diameter 2.7 micrometres or 10 micrometres, blood-griseofulvin concentration following oral administration to healthy volunteers was two-fold greater from tablets prepared with griseofulvin of smaller particle size.[9]

Carrigan and Bates[10] assessed oral bioavailability, in *rats*, of griseofulvin from an aqueous suspension, a maize oil suspension, and an oil-in-water emulsion (see formulae below). The fraction of a 50 mg/kg single dose absorbed from the emulsion was 2.5-fold and 1.6-fold higher than from the aqueous and oily suspensions, respectively; mean peak plasma levels were also significantly higher. No significant difference in the extent of absorption was apparent between the two suspensions. The formulations of griseofulvin administered orally to *rats* were as follows:

Constituents	Aqueous suspension	Formulation Maize oil suspension	Maize oil-in-water emulsion
Micronised griseofulvin	10 mg	25 mg	10 mg
Polysorbate 60 (Tween 60)	10 mg	25 mg	10 mg
Mono and di glycerides of edible fats (Atmul 84)	—	—	10 mg
Maize oil	—	to 1 mL	0.4 mL
Distilled water	to 1 mL	—	to 1 mL

In a subsequent randomised, crossover study,[11] five healthy volunteers received a single 500 mg dose of griseofulvin in the form of commercially available tablets (Grifulvin V and Fulvicin-U/F), an aqueous suspension and a maize oil-in-water emulsion (both preparations contained 300 mg polysorbate 60 and 500 mg suspended griseofulvin in 30 g). Bioavailability of micronised griseofulvin from the emulsion was 2.34-fold, 2-fold, and 1.7-fold greater than from the aqueous suspension, Grifulvin V, and Fulvicin-U/F tablets, respectively. No significant differences in the extent of absorption were apparent among the aqueous suspension, Grifulvin V tablets, and Fulvicin-U/F tablets. Inter-patient variation in the extent of absorption of griseofulvin was less marked after administration of the emulsion than that following the administration of tablet preparations. Furthermore, the emulsion produced greater enhancement of griseofulvin absorption than a maize oil suspension, at doses that contained equivalent amounts of lipid. The significant enhancement of the extent and uniformity of absorption of griseofulvin that occurred following administration of a single dose of the maize oil-in-water emulsion was also apparent, although to a smaller extent, following administration at 12-hour intervals of five 50 mg/kg doses in *rats*.[12]

The pharmacokinetics of griseofulvin were studied following its administration as an intravenous injection (griseofulvin 30 mg/mL) in macrogol 300 to five healthy volunteers.[13] When the same subjects each received an oral tablet (0.5 g micronised griseofulvin), 27% to 72% of the dose was absorbed.

In a double-blind, multidose, crossover study involving 17 healthy volunteers,[14] the bioavailability of griseofulvin from tablets of micronised griseofulvin (250 mg) in macrogol 6000 basis ('ultramicrosize tablets') was compared with that from commercial tablets of micronised griseofulvin (500 mg, 'microsize tablets'). From steady-state plasma concentrations of griseofulvin, the authors concluded that the bioavailability of the ultramicrosize tablets (250 mg twice daily) was equivalent to that of the microsize tablets (500 mg twice daily).

Oral liquids

Interaction between griseofulvin and phenobarbitone following oral administration was shown to be dependent on the formulation of griseofulvin.[2] When *rats* that had been pretreated with phenobarbitone received griseofulvin orally in 0.5% and 2% polysorbate 80 suspensions, a 50% and 31% reduction in maximum plasma concentration of griseofulvin was noted, respectively, when compared with concentrations in control *rats* (which were not pretreated with barbiturate). No difference in absorption of griseofulvin occurred between pretreated and control *rats* when griseofulvin was administered in aqueous solution in 70% macrogol 300 or 100% macrogol 600.

Topical formulations

Permeation of griseofulvin through *rat* skin *in vitro* from solutions of griseofulvin 0.5% w/v in various solvents was studied.[1] Absorption from the solvents decreased in the order: dimethyl sulphoxide > dimethylacetamide > N,N-diethyl-m-toluamide > diethylene glycol monoethylether.

Release of griseofulvin was 1.4 times greater from macrogol-based ointments than from carbopol 940-based ointments.[15] The addition of surfactants increased the release from the macrogol-based ointments.

Solid dispersions and co-precipitates

Macrogols

Solid dispersions of microsized griseofulvin 1%, 2%, 4%, 10%, and 20% w/w in macrogol 3000 have been prepared by fusion and solvent methods.[16] Solid dispersions prepared by the fusion method had faster dissolution rates (in sodium chloride 0.9% solutions with 0.01% polysorbate 80 at 21°) and smaller mean particle sizes of griseofulvin than those prepared by the solvent method. Furthermore, increasing the concentration of griseofulvin resulted in a reduction of the dissolution rates of solid dispersions prepared by both methods.

The rate and extent of release of griseofulvin from a co-precipitate (prepared by a solvent method) of griseofulvin at 95% w/w with macrogol 4000 were not significantly different from the dissolution properties of griseofulvin itself.[17]

Two human subjects each received, on separate occasions, capsules and non-disintegrating tablets prepared from griseofulvin:macrogol 6000 (1:9 w/w) solid dispersions, and tablets of micronised griseofulvin (Grifulvin V, McNeil).[18] Urinary excretion data indicated that oral absorption of griseofulvin from the solid dispersion preparations was rapid and complete, whereas irregular, incomplete absorption occurred from the commercial tablets.

In an extensive study, Sakr et al[19] detailed the preparation of beads, moulded tablets, and compressed tablets that contained solid dispersions of griseofulvin with macrogols 4000, 6000, or 20 000. An increase in molecular weight of macrogol produced an increase in the hardness and friability of all preparations, but a decrease in dissolution rates. However, beads showed faster dissolution rates than the corresponding moulded or compressed tablets. Correlation was found, for all preparations, between the dissolution rate and bioavailability of griseofulvin in 12 healthy volunteers. Oral bioavailability of griseofulvin from the preparations, at a given molecular weight of macrogol, decreased in the order: beads > moulded tablets = compressed tablets > compressed physical mixtures.

Chiou and Riegelman[20] prepared fast-dissolving solid dispersions of griseofulvin with the following water-soluble carriers: macrogols 4000, 6000, and 20 000, pentaerythritol, pentaerythrityl tetraacetate, and citric acid. Partial degradation of griseofulvin was noted with anhydrous citric acid during the fusion process but not with the other carriers. When the griseofulvin-citric acid mixture was stored at 37° for several days a 'glass solution', which exhibited a high dissolution rate of griseofulvin, was formed.

After storage for 12 weeks at 4°, 25°, or 37°, the dissolution rates of griseofulvin from solid dispersions of griseofulvin 5%, 10%, and 15% in macrogol 6000, were found to have decreased by more than 90% compared to fresh solid dispersions, at all combinations of concentration and temperature.[21]

Lecithin
Co-precipitates of griseofulvin with 5% and 40% of dimyristoyl phosphatidylcholine (lecithin)[22] showed a 3.5-fold and 5-fold enhancement of dissolution rate respectively, compared to griseofulvin itself, and an increase in the amount of griseofulvin in solution (pH 2) after 60 minutes at 37°. The amount of griseofulvin dissolved from co-precipitates was more than double that from corresponding physical mixtures. Physical studies indicated that the griseofulvin:lecithin systems did not involve formation of a complex, or eutectic or solid solution formation.

When different physical forms of griseofulvin were administered as aqueous oral suspensions to *rats*, the resulting availability of griseofulvin was found to decrease in the order: griseofulvin:lecithin co-precipitates (19:1 and 4:1 w/w) > chloroform-solvated griseofulvin > physical mixture of griseofulvin:lecithin (4:1 w/w) > micronised griseofulvin.[23] No significant differences in bioavailability of the two co-precipitates were reported. Correlations were found between dissolution parameters (pH 2 at 37°) and absorption parameters.

Lipids
Enhanced dissolution of griseofulvin has been shown from co-precipitates with hydrogenated soya phospholipids[24] and with phosphatidylcholines (griseofulvin 80% w/w and 95% w/w) but not from co-precipitates with cholesterol.[17] Inclusion of lactose or calcium phosphate in the hydrogenated soya phospholipid co-precipitates further improved dissolution.[24] Co-precipitates prepared with chloroform as the solvent[17] showed enhanced release of griseofulvin, whereas ethanol or methylene chloride provided no such enhancement.

Effervescent solid dispersions
The release properties of effervescent solid dispersions of griseofulvin with various mixed carriers have been studied.[25] Of the mixed carriers examined, succinic acid with sodium bicarbonate was superior to citric acid with sodium bicarbonate, or tartaric acid with sodium bicarbonate, on the basis of promoting release of griseofulvin. Dissolution rates of solid dispersions increased with an increase in the proportion of sodium bicarbonate present.

Solvent deposition systems
Systems have been developed in which micronised griseofulvin in a solvent (acetone) was deposited on the surface of particles of disintegrants. The disintegrants used were modified starch (Primojel), unmodified wheat starch (Mobile Starch), and modified cellulose (Nymcel).[26] Dissolution of griseofulvin from the 'solvent deposition systems' was superior to that from physical mixtures or dissolution of micronised griseofulvin itself. Tablets prepared using griseofulvin (40%) deposited on Primojel (60%) had the fastest disintegration rates.

Ordered mixtures, interactive powder mixtures, and ground mixtures
The rate and extent of dissolution of micronised griseofulvin (agglomerates at 500 to 710 micrometres), in sodium chloride 0.9% w/w in distilled water at 23°, were improved by the addition of polysorbate 80 (Tween 80) 0.01% w/w or 0.001% w/w to the dissolution medium.[27] Ordered mixtures of griseofulvin with sodium chloride as carrier showed greater rates and extents of dissolution than micronised griseofulvin itself; addition of polysorbate 80 to the medium did not significantly affect dissolution of ordered mixtures.

Release of griseofulvin from ordered mixtures (0.153 g micronised griseofulvin:50 g carrier) was investigated[28] under sink conditions in sodium chloride 0.9% w/w solution with 0.01% w/w Tween 80. Carriers that had high solubility in the dissolution medium (sodium chloride, anhydrous lactose, or tricalcium dicitrate) released griseofulvin more readily than practically insoluble carriers (glass beads or Emcompress). Dissolution rates from all ordered mixtures studied (except when the carrier was paraffin granules) were greater than that from agglomerates of griseofulvin.

Extensive studies of 'interactive powder mixtures',[29, 30] showed that dissolution of griseofulvin (as a model drug) was improved by formulation with soluble excipients, with smaller particle size fractions of a given excipient, or with excipients that have smooth particle surfaces rather than indentations.

In comparison with micronised griseofulvin, in a crossover study involving 5 healthy volunteers, a mixture of griseofulvin ground in the ratio 1:9 with microcrystalline cellulose demonstrated faster dissolution and correspondingly greater oral bioavailability of griseofulvin.[31] 'Simple blends' of griseofulvin with microcrystalline or amorphous cellulose had similar dissolution profiles at one hour and similar bioavailabilities to that of micronised griseofulvin. The grinding process caused no apparent decomposition of griseofulvin.

Lyophilised mixtures
Enhanced dissolution rates were demonstrated by lyophilised formulations prepared from solutions of griseofulvin or mixtures of griseofulvin and mannitol in dioxan or dioxan:water (1:1) mixtures.[32] The rate of freezing influenced the physical properties and stability of the lyophilised formulations.

FURTHER INFORMATION. The use of a comparative analysis [computer predictions and laboratory data] of sedimentation and Brownian motion as a guide to suspension formulation [of griseofulvin]—Matthews BA, Rhodes CT. Pharm Acta Helv 1970;45:52–9. Distribution of griseofulvin in the rat: comparison of the oral and topical route of administration—Nimni ME, Ertl D, Oakes RA. J Pharm Pharmacol 1990;42:729–31. Development and *in vitro* evaluation of griseofulvin gels using Franz diffusion cells—Vlachou MD, Rekkas DM, Dallas PP, Choulis NH. Int J Pharmaceutics 1992;82:47–52. Dissolution rate of griseofulvin from solid dispersions with poly(vinylmethylether/maleic anhydride)—Flego C, Lovrecich M, Rubessa F. Drug Dev Ind Pharm 1988;14(9):1185–1202. Effect of cholesterol on the aging of griseofulvin-phospholipid [dimyristoyl phosphatidylcholine and egg phosphatidylcholine] co-precipitates—Vudathala GK, Rogers JA. Int J Pharmaceutics

1991;69:13–19. Oral bioavailability of griseofulvin from aged griseofulvin:lipid coprecipitates: *in vivo* studies in *rats*— Vudathala GK, Rogers JA. J Pharm Sci 1992;81(12):1166–9. Chemometric modelling of dissolution rates of griseofulvin from solid dispersions with [27] polymers [factors that influence the release rate of griseofulvin]—Bonelli D, Clementi S, Ebert C, Lovrecich M, Rubessa F. Drug Dev Ind Pharm 1989;15(9):1375–91. Physicochemical aspects of drug release. XIV. The effects of some ionic and non-ionic surfactants on properties of a sparingly soluble drug in solid dispersions [with macrogol 3000]—Sjökvist E, Nyström C, Alden M, Caram-Lelham N. Int J Pharmaceutics 1992;79:123–33. Structure of solid dispersions in the system polyethylene glycol-griseofulvin with additions of sodium dodecyl sulphate—Aldén M, Tegenfeldt J, Sjökvist E. Int J Pharmaceutics 1992;83:47–52. Effect of polystyrene beads on dissolution behaviour of drugs—Canal T, Lovrecich M, de Nardo M, Rubessa F. Pharm Acta Helv 1988;63(9-10):271–7. Dissolution characteristics of interactive powder mixtures. 4. Effects of additives on the dissolution of griseofulvin from Emcompress carrier—Sallam E, Ibrahim H, Takieddin M, Baghal T, Saket M, Awad R, Arafat T. Int J Pharmaceutics 1991;67:247–57. Physicochemical aspects of drug release XVII. The effect of drug surface area coverage to carrier materials on drug dissolution from ordered mixtures—Westerberg M, Nyström C. Int J Pharmaceutics 1993;90:1–17.

REFERENCES

1. Ritschel WA, Hussain AS. Pharm Ind 1988;50(4):483–6.
2. Jamali F, Axelson JE. J Pharm Sci 1978;67(4):466–70.
3. Chiou WL. J Pharm Sci 1977;66(7):989–91.
4. De Smidt JH, Offringa JCA, Crommelin DJA. J Pharm Sci 1987;76(9):711–14.
5. De Smidt JH, Offringa JCA, Crommelin DJA. J Pharm Sci 1991;80(4):399–401.
6. Rasool AA, Hussain AA, Ditter LW. J Pharm Sci 1991;80(4):387–93.
7. Maeda T, Takenaka H, Yamahira Y, Noguchi T. J Pharm Sci 1979;68(10):1286–9.
8. Neely WC, McDuffie JR. J Assoc Off Anal Chem 1972;55(6):1300–4.
9. Atkinson RM, Bedford A, Child KJ, Tomich EG. Nature 1962;193:588–9.
10. Carrigan PJ, Bates TR. J Pharm Sci 1973;62(9):1477–9.
11. Bates TR, Sequeira JA. J Pharm Sci 1975;64(5):793–7.
12. Bates TR, Carrigan PJ. J Pharm Sci 1975;64(9):1475–81.
13. Rowland M, Riegelman S, Epstein WL. J Pharm Sci 1968;57(6):984–9.
14. Barrett WE, Hanigan JJ. Curr Ther Res Clin Exp 1975;18(3):491–500.
15. Gritsaenko IS, Eres I, Ugri-Hunyadvary E [Russian]. Farmatsiya 1985;34:25–9.
16. Sjökvist E, Nyström C. Int J Pharmaceutics 1988;47:51–66.
17. Venkataram S, Rogers JA. Drug Dev Ind Pharm 1985;11:223–38.
18. Chiou WL, Riegelman S. J Pharm Sci 1971;60(9):1376–80.
19. Sakr FM, Abd El-Gawad AH, Zin El-Din EE. Bull Pharm Sci Assiut Univ 1988;11:1–17.
20. Chiou WL, Riegelman S. J Pharm Sci 1969;58(12):1505–9.
21. Dubois JL, Chaumeil JC, Ford JL. STP Pharma 1985;1(8):711–14.
22. Venkataram S, Rogers JA. J Pharm Sci 1984;73(6):757–61.
23. Venkataram S, Rogers JA. J Pharm Sci 1988;77(11):933–6.
24. Nishihata T, Chigawa Y, Kamada A, Sakai K, Mastumoto K, Shinozaki K *et al.* Drug Dev Ind Pharm 1988;14(9):1137–54.
25. Desai S, Allen LV, Greenwood R, Stiles ML, Parker D. J Pharm Sci 1987;76(11):N03-W-06, S254.
26. Law SL, Chiang CH. Drug Dev Ind Pharm 1990;16(1):137–47.
27. Nyström C, Westerberg M. J Pharm Pharmacol 1986;38:161–5.
28. Westerberg M, Jonsson B, Nyström C. Int J Pharmaceutics 1986;28:23–31.
29. Ibrahim H, Sallam E, Takieddin M, Abu Shamat M. Drug Dev Ind Pharm 1988;14(9):1249–76.
30. Sallam E, Ibrahim H, Takieddin M, Abu Shamat M, Baghal T. Drug Dev Ind Pharm 1988;14(9):1277–302.
31. Yamamoto K, Nakano M, Arita T, Nakai Y. J Pharmacokin Biopharm 1974;2(6):487–93.
32. Frömming Von K-H, Grote U, Lange A, Hosemann R [German]. Pharm Ind 1986;48(3):283–8.

Haloperidol (BAN, USAN, rINN)   *Antipsychotic*

4-[4-(4-Chlorophenyl)-4-hydroxypiperidino]-4'-fluorobutyrophenone
$C_{21}H_{23}ClFNO_2 = 375.9$

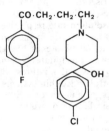

Haloperidol Decanoate (BANM, USAN, rINNM)
$C_{31}H_{41}ClFNO_3 = 530.1$
CAS—52-86-8 (haloperidol); 74050-97-8 (haloperidol decanoate)

Pharmacopoeial status

BP, USP (haloperidol)

Preparations

Compendial

Haloperidol Tablets BP. Tablets containing, in each, 0.5, 1.5, 5, 10, and 20 mg are usually available.

Haloperidol Oral Solution BP (Haloperidol Oral Drops; Haloperidol Solution). A clear, colourless, aqueous solution containing not more than 0.2% w/v of haloperidol. pH 2.5 to 3.5. Oral solutions containing 0.1% w/v and 0.2% w/v are usually available. If the oral solution is prescribed or demanded and no strength is stated, an oral solution containing 0.2% w/v haloperidol shall be dispensed or supplied.

Strong Haloperidol Oral Solution BP. (Strong Haloperidol Oral Drops). A clear, colourless, aqueous solution containing 1% w/v of haloperidol. It is intended to be diluted before use. pH 3.5 to 4.5.

Haloperidol Injection BP. A sterile solution of haloperidol in lactic acid diluted with water for injections. pH 2.8 to 3.6. Injections containing 5 mg in 1 mL, 10 mg in 2 mL, and 20 mg in 2 mL are usually available.

Haloperidol Tablets USP.

Haloperidol Oral Solution USP.

Haloperidol Injection USP. pH between 3.0 and 3.8.

Non-compendial

Dozic (RP Drugs). *Oral liquid*, sugar free, haloperidol 1 mg/mL (with pipette) and 2 mg/mL (with pipette).

Haldol (Janssen). *Tablets*, haloperidol 5 mg and 10 mg.

Oral liquid, sugar free, haloperidol 2 mg/mL (with pipette).

Oral liquid concentrate, sugar free, haloperidol 10 mg/mL for dilution. *Diluent*: an aqueous solution of methyl hydroxybenzoate 0.5 mg/mL and propyl hydroxybenzoate 0.05 mg/mL is recommended, life of diluted concentrate up to 2 months. Water should not be used as a diluent.

Injection, haloperidol 5 mg/mL.

Haldol Decanoate (Janssen). *Injection (oily)*, haloperidol (as decanoate ester) 50 mg/mL and 100 mg/mL.

Serenace (Baker Norton). *Capsules*, haloperidol 500 micrograms.

Tablets, haloperidol 1.5 mg, 5 mg, 10 mg, and 20 mg.

Oral liquid, sugar free, haloperidol 2 mg/mL.

Injection, haloperidol 5 mg/mL and 10 mg/mL.

Containers and storage

Solid state

Haloperidol BP should be kept in an airtight container and protected from light.

Haloperidol USP should be preserved in tight, light-resistant containers.

Dosage forms

Haloperidol Oral Solution BP and Strong Haloperidol Oral Solution BP should be protected from light and stored at a temperature of 15° to 25°.

Haloperidol Injection BP should be protected from light.

Haloperidol Tablets USP and Haloperidol Oral Solution USP should be preserved in tight, light-resistant containers.

Haloperidol Injection USP should be preserved in single-dose or in multiple-dose containers, preferably of Type I glass, protected from light.

Haldol tablets should be stored in a cool, dry place. Haldol oral liquid concentrate and oral liquid should be stored at room temperature. Diluted Haldol oral liquid concentrate should be stored in amber glass, screw-cap bottles.

Haldol Decanoate injection (oily) should be protected from light and stored at room temperature; it should not be stored below room temperature. If stored for long periods in the cold, precipitation may occur which may clear on storage at room temperature. If the precipitate does not clear, the injection should be discarded.

PHYSICAL PROPERTIES

Haloperidol is a white or slightly yellowish powder; amorphous or microcrystalline.

Melting point

Haloperidol melts at about 150°.

pH

Saturated solutions of *haloperidol* are neutral to litmus.

Dissociation constant

pK_a 8.3 (potentiometric titration in methanol-water)

Partition coefficient

Log *P* (octanol/pH 7.4), 4.3

Solubility

Haloperidol is practically insoluble in water, in dilute mineral acids and in alkali hydroxides; sparingly soluble in ethanol, in dichloromethane, and in methanol; soluble in chloroform; slightly soluble in ether.

A solubility of 0.374 mg/mL was determined[1] for haloperidol in water at 37°. Solubility values established for haloperidol in 1% solutions of lactic acid, tartaric acid, hydrochloric acid, and polysorbate 80 were 4.08 mg/mL, 3.8 mg/mL, 1.34 mg/mL, and 0.43 mg/mL, respectively.

Demoen[2] reported that stable solutions containing up to 2% w/v haloperidol can be prepared in the presence of 1% lactic acid or tartaric acid.

Solubility values[3] for haloperidol in several oils (with potential as vehicles for intramuscular depot injections) ranged from zero and 0.6 mg/mL in sesame oil and maize oil respectively, to 7.3 mg/mL in propyl oleate, at 25°. Solubilisation of haloperidol in the oils (to more than 40 mg/mL in most instances) was achieved by the addition of each of six aliphatic acids at 0.5M. On the addition of sodium chloride 0.9% solution to acid/oil solutions of haloperidol 40 mg/mL, there was immediate precipitation of haloperidol except when oleic or linoleic acid was present.

Dissolution

The USP specifies that for Haloperidol Tablets USP not less than 80% of the labelled amount of $C_{21}H_{23}ClFNO_2$ is dissolved in 60 minutes. Dissolution medium: 900 mL of simulated gastric fluid TS (without the enzyme); Apparatus 1 at 100 rpm.

STABILITY

Solid state

Haloperidol in the solid state is a relatively stable compound. Samples stored at room temperature in amber glass containers were reported to be stable for up to five years.[4] However, slow discoloration of haloperidol occurs on exposure to light[2] and to sunlight.[4]

Solutions

Solutions of haloperidol in lactic acid, at above pH 3, have been reported to be stable for up to two years and up to five years at 40° and room temperature respectively;[4] discoloration and degradation were noted on exposure to natural sunlight.

Solutions of haloperidol (0.5 mg/mL) were prepared in lactic acid 1% solution with or without methyl hydroxybenzoate 0.1% and were stored in glass and plastic containers under various conditions of temperature, light, and oxygen concentration for nine months.[1] Degradation of halperidol was not substantial but was accelerated by oxygen and light and was greater in plastic containers than in glass. Values for $t_{10\%}$ at 25° and 110° were calculated to be 1860 days to 1941 days, and 42 days to 50 days, respectively. Two degradation products were detected in small quantities by TLC but could not be identified.

Aqueous solutions of haloperidol (10 mg/100 mL) at pH 2 or pH 7 were stored in glass containers at 25°, 60° and 115° in the dark and at 25° in the presence of light.[5] Degradation of haloperidol was not apparent (HPLC analysis) after 14 days at 25° in the dark but was detected in samples stored in the presence of light after 14 days and 7 days at pH 2 and pH 7, respectively. At 60° degradation was apparent after 24 hours and 48 hours at pH 2 and pH 7 respectively, and at 115° decomposition occurred after 6 hours at both pH values.

Dosage forms

Haloperidol was concluded to be stable in the form of a compressed tablet, an oral solution, and a solution for injection for up to 18 months at 4°, 22°, and 45°; the solutions were stored in amber containers but the tablet container was not specified.[2] However, when haloperidol solutions were stored in clear glass containers and exposed to sunlight, discoloration was observed after a few hours and precipitation after several weeks.

Irradiation

When haloperidol (isolated from tablets) as a model drug was irradiated with a sterilising dose of gamma radiation (2.5 Mrad), the maximum loss of haloperidol was 9%.[6] The degradation products acrolein, chlorobenzene, p-fluorobenzaldehyde, p-fluoroacetophenone, and p-fluorophenyl propenyl ketone were detected in various quantities.

INCOMPATIBILITY/COMPATIBILITY

Admixture solutions

No instability or incompatibility of haloperidol was apparent when haloperidol injection (McNeil, USA) was diluted to 10 mg/100 mL in glucose 5% injection and stored in amber glass bottles or in polyvinyl chloride bags at 24° for 38 days.[7] At 21°, haloperidol lactate injection (Haldol, McNeil, USA) was visually compatible, at 0.1 mg/mL and 0.5 mg/mL, with sodium chloride 0.9% injection during 8 hours in glass vials under fluorescent light.[8] However, under the same conditions, an immediate precipitate was observed at and above a haloperidol concentration of 1 mg/mL. In further studies with ten other drugs, visual incompatibility was only apparent when 5 mL of haloperidol lactate injection 5 mg/mL (undiluted) was mixed with 5 mL of sodium nitroprusside injection (Abbott, 0.2 mg/mL in sterile water). However, haloperidol lactate injection diluted to 0.5 mg/mL in glucose 5% injection was visually compatible with the sodium nitroprusside solution for 24 hours.

Solomon and Nasinnyk[9] prepared admixtures of heparin sodium injection (Organon, USA) at two concentrations (100 units/mL and 200 units/mL) in sodium chloride 0.9% or glucose 5% in intravenous administration sets. On injection of a 1 mL bolus of undiluted haloperidol lactate (5 mg) injection (Haldol, McNeil, USA) into the sets, an immediate milky white precipitate (which varied in appearance depending on the vehicle) was observed, with a concomitant fall in pH.

No visual incompatibilities or significant losses of initial concentrations of drugs were reported when solutions of diamorphine hydrochloride (50 mg/8 mL or 100 mg/8 mL) were mixed with solutions of haloperidol (2.5 mg/8 mL) and stored in polypropylene syringes at room temperature (22° to 24°) protected and unprotected from light, or under refrigeration (4° to 8°) for 24 hours.[10]

Interaction with beverages

Incompatibility in vitro, as demonstrated by formation of precipitates, has been observed when solutions of haloperidol were mixed with the following drinks: coffee, tea, cocoa, milk, or lime-flower (tilia) tea.[1,11,12]

FORMULATION

Excipients

Excipients that have been used in presentations of haloperidol include:

Tablets, haloperidol: acid fuchsine D; alginic acid; allura red AC (E129); brilliant blue FCF (133); calcium hydrogen phosphate; calcium phosphate; calcium stearate; cellulose; colloidal silica; erythrosine (E127); indigo carmine (E132); lactose; magnesium stearate; maize starch; microcrystalline cellulose; quinoline yellow (E104); rice starch; sucrose; talc; tartrazine (E102).

Oral solutions and concentrates, haloperidol: lactic acid; methyl and propyl hydroxybenzoates.
Injections, haloperidol: lactic acid; methyl and propyl hydroxybenzoates.
Haloperidol decanoate: benzyl alcohol; sesame oil.

Bioequivalence

A bioavailability of 93% to 98% was calculated (from plasma concentration data) for a haloperidol 5 mg tablet (Cord) relative to two lots of a haloperidol 5 mg reference tablet (Haldol, McNeil), following a single-dose, three-way crossover study involving 28 healthy volunteers.[13] Considerable inter-subject differences were noted for all pharmacokinetic parameters.

Oily solutions

Release of haloperidol in vitro from several oleic acid/oil and linoleic acid/oil solutions into sodium chloride 0.9% at 37° was investigated.[3] The slowest rates of release, from solutions of oleic acid with maize oil, sesame oil, neutral oil (Miglyol 812), or myristate esters, were three to four times faster than release of haloperidol decanoate from a formulation, in clinical use, comprising sesame oil with benzyl alcohol. See also Solubility above.

FURTHER INFORMATION. Pharmacokinetic studies of haloperidol in man [intravenous and oral administration]—Forsman A, Öhman R. Curr Ther Res 1976;20(3):319–36.

PROCESSING

Sterilisation

Haloperidol injection can be sterilised by heating in an autoclave.

REFERENCES

1. Ölçer M, Hakyemez G. J Clin Pharm Ther 1988;13:341–9.
2. Demoen PJAW. J Pharm Sci 1961;50(4):350–3.
3. Radd BL, Newman AC, Fegely BJ, Chrzanowski FA, Lichten JL, Walkling WD. J Parenter Sci Technol 1985;39(1):48–50.
4. Janicki CA, Ko CY. In: Florey KF, editor. Analytical profiles of drug substances; vol 9. London: Academic Press, 1980;342–69.
5. Panaggio A, Greene DS. Drug Dev Ind Pharm 1983;9(3):485–92.
6. Booker J. Pharmazie 1988;43(H1):31–2.
7. Das Gupta V, Stewart KR. Am J Hosp Pharm 1982;39:292–4.
8. Outman WR, Monolakis J. Am J Hosp Pharm 1991;48:1539–41.
9. Solomon DA, Nasinnyk KK. Am J Hosp Pharm 1982;39:843–4.
10. Collins AJ, Abethell JA, Holmes SG, Bain R. J Pharm Pharmacol 1986;36:51P.
11. Lasswell WL, Weber SS, Wilkins JM. J Pharm Sci 1984;73(8):1056–8.
12. Kulhanek F, Linde OK, Meisenberg G [letter]. Lancet 1979;2:1130–1.
13. Midha KK, Chakraborty BS, Schwede R, Hawes EM, Hubbard JW, McKay G. J Pharm Sci 1989;78(6):443–7.

Heparin (BAN)   *Anticoagulant*

Heparinic acid
A heterogeneous mixture of variably sulphated polysaccharide chains composed of repeating units of D-glucosamine and either L-iduronic acid or D-glucuronic acids. Molecular weight ranges from 6000 to 30 000 Da. It may be obtained from ox lung or the intestinal mucosa of oxen, pigs, or sheep.

Heparin Calcium (BANM)
Calcium heparinate

Heparin Sodium (BANM, rINN)
Sodium heparin; soluble heparin
CAS—9005-49-6 (heparin); 37270-89-6 (heparin calcium); 9041-08-1 (heparin sodium)

Pharmacopoeial status

BP, USP (heparin calcium, heparin sodium)

Preparations

Compendial
Heparin Injection BP. A sterile solution of heparin calcium or heparin sodium in water for injections; the pH of the solution may be adjusted by the addition of a suitable alkali. An injection of heparin calcium containing 5000 units in 0.2 mL is usually available. Injections of heparin sodium containing 5000 units in 0.2 mL; 5000 units in 0.5 mL; 1000, 5000, and 25 000 units in 1 mL; 5000, 25 000, and 125 000 units in 5 mL; and 20 000 units in 20 mL are usually available.
Anticoagulant Heparin Solution USP. pH 5.0 to 7.5.
Heparin Lock Flush Solution USP. pH 5.0 to 7.5.
Heparin Calcium Injection USP. pH 5.0 to 7.5.
Heparin Sodium Injection USP. pH 5.0 to 7.5.
The USP states that the USP Heparin Units and International Units are not equivalent.

Non-compendial
Calciparine (Sanofi Winthrop). *Injection*, subcutaneous, heparin calcium 25 000 units/mL. Other preparations should not be mixed with Calciparine.
Hep-Flush (Leo). *Solution*, heparin sodium 100 units/mL in sodium chloride 0.9%. Not for therapeutic use. Preserved with chlorbutol 0.5%.
Heplok (Leo). *Solution*, heparin sodium 10 units/mL in sodium chloride 0.9%. Not for therapeutic use.
Hepsal (CP). *Solution*, heparin sodium (mucous) 10 units/mL in sodium chloride 0.9% injection. Not for therapeutic use.
Minihep (Leo). *Injection*, subcutaneous, heparin sodium (mucous) 25 000 units/mL.
Minihep Calcium (Leo). *Injection*, subcutaneous, heparin calcium (mucous) 25 000 units/mL.
Monoparin (CP). *Injection*, subcutaneous, heparin sodium (mucous) 25 000 units/mL.
Injection, heparin sodium (mucous) 1000 units/mL, 5000 units/mL, and 25 000 units/mL.
Monoparin Calcium (CP). *Injection*, subcutaneous, heparin calcium (mucous) 25 000 units/mL.
Multiparin (CP). *Injection*, heparin sodium (mucous) 1000 units/mL, 5000 units/mL, and 25 000 units/mL.
Pump-Hep (Leo). *Intravenous infusion*, heparin sodium (mucous) 1000 units/mL.
Unihep (Leo). *Injection*, heparin sodium (mucous) 1000 units/mL, 5000 units/mL, 10 000 units/mL, and 25 000 units/mL.
Uniparin (CP). *Injection*, subcutaneous, heparin sodium (mucous) 25 000 units/mL.

Uniparin Calcium (CP). *Injection*, subcutaneous, heparin calcium (mucous) 25 000 units/mL.
Other preparations should not be mixed with Uniparin or Uniparin Calcium.

Containers and storage

Solid state
Heparin Calcium BP and Heparin Sodium BP should be kept in airtight containers. If the contents are sterile, the container should also be sterile and tamper-evident.
Heparin Calcium USP should be preserved in tight containers.
Heparin Sodium USP should be preserved in tight containers and stored below 40°, preferably between 15° and 30°, unless otherwise specified by the manufacturer.

Dosage forms
Heparin Injection BP should be stored at a temperature not exceeding 25° and should preferably be kept in a container sealed by fusion of the glass.
Anticoagulant Heparin Solution USP should be preserved in single-dose containers of colourless, transparent, Type I or Type II glass, or of a suitable plastic material.
Heparin Lock Flush Solution USP should be preserved in single-dose, pre-filled syringes or containers, or in multiple-dose containers, preferably of Type I glass.
Heparin Calcium Injection USP and Heparin Sodium Injection USP should be preserved in single-dose or in multiple-dose containers, preferably of Type I glass.
Calciparine, Hep-Flush, Heplok, Minihep preparations, Pump-Hep, and Unihep preparations should be stored below 25°. Calciparine should not be frozen.
Hepsal, Monoparin, Multiparin, and Uniparin preparations should be stored below 25°. They should not be frozen; the manufacturer of these heparin preparations states that they should be protected from light.

PHYSICAL PROPERTIES

Heparin calcium is a white or almost white powder; moderately hygroscopic.
Heparin sodium is a white or almost white powder; moderately hygroscopic; odourless or practically odourless.

pH

A 1% w/v solution of either *heparin calcium* or *heparin sodium* has a pH of 5.5 to 8.0.

Solubility

Heparin calcium is soluble 1 in less than 5 of water.
Heparin sodium is soluble 1 in 2.5 of water.

STABILITY

In aqueous solution, stability of heparin is markedly reduced if the pH falls below 5.
Heparin sodium (20 and 40 units/mL) was found to be stable[1] in sodium chloride 0.9% at room temperature for 48 hours.
Preparations of heparin (1 unit/mL) in sodium chloride 0.9% injection, sterilised by autoclaving and stored at room temperature in daylight, remained stable for 12 months.[2]

Glucose solutions

Opinions vary regarding the stability of heparin in intravenous infusions containing glucose or lactates. Some workers claim that rapid inactivation occurs,[3] whereas others assert that there is no detectable loss in activity[1,4,5] for at least 24 or 48 hours after preparation. The stability of heparin sodium in glucose solutions has been reviewed by Trissel.[6]

A study comparing glucose 5% and sorbitol 5% injections showed that neither diluent impaired the potency of heparin.[7] Anderson and Harthill[8] described variations in the activity of heparin in autoclaved and non-autoclaved glucose-containing solutions. They concluded that no real degradation of heparin occurred and the fluctuations in heparin activity could be attributed to certain variables including pH, heparin concentration, salt concentration, glucose degradation products caused by autoclaving, heparin molecular weight distribution in the product, differences between proprietary glucose products, and container effects.

Effects of temperature and autoclaving

Pritchard[3] indicated that little loss of potency occurred when heparin solutions (containing 0.15% chlorocresol) at pH 5.5 to 8.5 were autoclaved at 69 kPa (115°) for 10 minutes. However, a marked reduction in potency was noted in solutions of pH less than 5.0. A solution of pH 7.5 remained stable when heated for 8 hours at 100° whereas degradation at acidic pH was marked. Gauthier et al[9] subsequently reaffirmed the influence of pH on heparin inactivation. A plot of activity against temperature demonstrated that a 'precipitous' loss in activity occurred within one hour at 68° (pH 1) and at 78° (pH 2) compared to only slight loss at lower temperatures. A more gradual decrease in activity in one hour occurred at 88° to 98° (pH 3) with very little effect observed at 100° (pH 4 to 7) in one hour. When preservative-free heparin solutions in ampoules (25 000 BP units/mL) were autoclaved at 115° or 121° for 50 minutes, no decrease in activity was observed by either the BP assay or the activated partial thromboplastin time (APTT) method.[10] However, at 126° or 130° a reduction in activity was noted. A maximum decrease in activity of 18% was observed using the BP assay after autoclaving at 130° for 50 minutes; no decrease was demonstrated by the APTT method. Autoclaving was associated with depolymerisation (analysis by HPLC); however, the integrity of the anionic sites on heparin was maintained.

Aggregation

Racey et al[11] reported a change in aggregation state during storage of five commercial heparin samples containing heparin sodium 10 000 to 25 000 USP units/mL, and heparin calcium 10 000 to 25 000 USP units/mL. Aggregation appeared to be greater, in both size and number, for samples that were stored for longer periods (up to 50 days). Once formed, the aggregates appeared to remain stable over time.

FURTHER INFORMATION. The macroanionic activity of heparins in the presence of dextrose [glucose] and calcium ion—Anderson W, Harthill JE. J Pharm Pharmacol 1982;34:631–7. New electromechanical method for the assay of heparin in vitro [stability to autoclaving and high energy electron irradiation]—Seip WF, Carski TR, Kramer DN. J Pharm Sci 1967;56(10):1304–8. Response to 'Aggregates in Heparin'—Racey TJ, Rochon P, Awang DVC, Neville GA [letter]. J Pharm Sci 1988;77(9):820.

INCOMPATIBILITY/COMPATIBILITY

Heparin (calcium or sodium salt) has been reported to be incompatible with amikacin sulphate, amiodarone, cephaloridine, ciprofloxacin lactate, daunorubicin hydrochloride, dobutamine hydrochloride, doxorubicin hydrochloride, erythromycin gluceptate, erythromycin lactobionate, gentamicin sulphate, haloperidol lactate, hyaluronidase, hydroxyzine hydrochloride, hydrocortisone sodium succinate, kanamycin sulphate, novo-biocin sodium, opioid analgesics, polymyxin B sulphate, prochlorperazine, promazine hydrochloride, promethazine hydrochloride, streptomycin sulphate, tobramycin sulphate, viomycin sulphate, and, depending on the diluent, with cephalothin sodium and vancomycin hydrochloride. Glucose can have variable effects. Incompatibility has also been reported with fat emulsions.

Conflicting evidence has been presented on the compatibility and incompatibility between heparin salts and ampicillin sodium, benzylpenicillin, dimenhydrinate, methicillin sodium, oxytetracycline hydrochloride, sulphafurazole diethanolamine, and tetracycline hydrochloride.

Heparin sodium injection is also known to be incompatible with chlordiazepoxide, chlorpromazine hydrochloride, and codeine phosphate.

Effect of concentration and diluents

Morphine sulphate and heparin sodium 100 or 200 USP units/mL in de-ionised water (from heparin sodium injection 10 000 USP units/mL, Wyeth, USA) were incompatible (characterised by precipitate formation) at morphine concentrations greater than 5 mg/mL.[12] The incompatibility was prevented when sodium chloride 0.9% was used as the admixture diluent. Precipitation occurred when vancomycin hydrochloride injection (Eli Lilly, Canada) 6900 to 14 300 mg/L was admixed with heparin sodium (Organon, Canada) 500 to 14 300 units/L in two peritoneal dialysis solutions.[13] However, no turbidity, effervescence, or colour change was noted (for up to 24 hours) in any sample containing heparin and vancomycin hydrochloride 15 to 5300 mg/L.

Nelson et al[14] reported the immediate formation of a white flocculent precipitate when intravenous tubing containing an admixture of dacarbazine (DTIC-Dome, Miles Laboratories) 25 mg/mL in sodium chloride 0.9% injection was flushed with heparin sodium 100 USP units/mL (Wyeth). Subsequent tests with less concentrated admixtures of dacarbazine (10 mg/mL) did not result in any noticeable precipitation.

Microcalorimetric investigation of the interaction between dopamine hydrochloride and heparin sodium[15] indicated a strong reaction between the drugs (as powder) in water and (as powder and injection) in glucose 5% injection but not in sodium chloride 0.9% injection.

The same authors identified a similar interaction between dobutamine hydrochloride injection (Dobutrex, Eli Lilly, USA) and heparin sodium injection (Lyphomed, USA) diluted with water or glucose 5% injection but not with sodium chloride 0.9% injection.[16] This result confirmed a previous report of precipitate formation within three minutes of addition of heparin sodium injection (Elkins-Sinn, USA) 100 USP units/mL in glucose 5% injection to an equal volume of dobutamine hydrochloride injection (Dobutrex, Eli Lilly, USA) 2 mg/mL in glucose 5% injection.[17] No precipitation was observed when sodium chloride 0.9% injection was the diluent. However, no precipitation was observed when undiluted heparin injection was added to dobutamine hydrochloride injection in glucose 5% injection.

Effect of containers

A study of 50 mL of a heparin solution 500 USP unit/mL in sodium chloride 0.9% injection, packaged in 50-mL polypropylene syringes, revealed an overall trend to lower activity (about 8% loss) after storage for three weeks at room temperature or at 0° to 4°. When this heparin solution was diluted into either a glass container or a polypropylene syringe, significantly less heparin activity was noted in the glass container. Although adsorption to glass surfaces was suggested it was not conclusively demonstrated.[18]

FORMULATION

Excipients

Excipients that have been used in presentations of heparin include:

Creams, heparin: methyl and propyl hydroxybenzoates; mixture of stearic esters of glycerol and of macrogol; sorbic acid.

Injections, heparin: methyl and propyl hydroxybenzoates; sodium chloride; sodium metabisulphite.

Heparin calcium: chlorocresol; hydrochloric acid; sodium hydroxide.

Heparin sodium: benzyl alcohol; chlorbutol; chlorocresol; hydrochloric acid; methyl and propyl hydroxybenzoates; sodium citrate; sodium chloride; sodium hydroxide.

FURTHER INFORMATION. Chemical composition, particle size range, and biological activity of some low molecular weight heparin derivatives—Neville GA, Mori F, Racey TJ, Rochon P, Holme KR, Perlin AS. J Pharm Sci 1990;79(4):339–43. Penetration enhancer effects on *in vitro* percutaneous absorption of heparin sodium salt—Bonina FP, Montenegro L. Int J Pharmaceutics 1992;82:171–7. Examination of a possible role for dermatan sulphate in the aggregation of commercial heparin samples—Racey TJ, Rochon P, Mori F, Neville GA. J Pharm Sci 1989;78(3):214–18.

REFERENCES

1. Mitchell JF, Barger RC, Cantwell L. Am J Hosp Pharm 1976;33:540–2.
2. Bowie HM, Haylor V. J Clin Pharm 1978;3:211–14.
3. Pritchard J. J Pharm Pharmacol 1964;16:487–9.
4. Moyle RS [letter]. Aust J Hosp Pharm 1983;13(3):124.
5. Joy RT, Hyneck ML, Berardi RR, Ho NFH. Am J Hosp Pharm 1979;36:618–21.
6. Trissel LA. Handbook on injectable drugs. 6th ed. Bethesda: American Society of Hospital Pharmacists, 1990:369.
7. Chessells JM, Braithwaite TA, Chamberlain DA. Br Med J 1972;2:81–2.
8. Anderson W, Harthill JE. J Pharm Pharmacol 1982;34:90–6.
9. Gauthier PB, Sawa T, Kenyon AJ. Arch Biochem Biophys 1969;130:690–2.
10. Menzies AR, Benoliel DM, Edwards HE. J Pharm Pharmacol 1989;41:512–16.
11. Racey TJ, Rochon P, Awang DVC, Neville GA. J Pharm Sci 1987;76(4):314–18.
12. Baker DE, Yost GS, Craig VL, Campbell RK. Am J Hosp Pharm 1985;42:1352–5.
13. Strong DK, Ho W, Nairn JG. Am J Hosp Pharm 1989;46:1832–3.
14. Nelson RW, Young R, Lamnin M [letter]. Am J Hosp Pharm 1987;44:2028.
15. Pereira-Rosario R, Utamura T, Perrin JH. Am J Hosp Pharm 1988;45:1350–2.
16. Perrin JH, Pereira-Rosario R, Utamura T. Drug Dev Ind Pharm 1988;14(11):1617–22.
17. Hasegawa GR, Eder JF [letter]. Am J Hosp Pharm 1984;41:2588,2590.
18. Tunbridge LJ, Lloyd JV, Penhall RK, Wise AL, Maloney T. Am J Hosp Pharm 1981;38:1001–4.

Hydralazine (BAN, rINN)

Antihypertensive; Vasodilator

Hydrallazine

Phthalazin-1-ylhydrazine; 1-hydrazinophthalazine

$C_8H_8N_4 = 160.2$

Hydralazine Hydrochloride (BANM, rINNM)

$C_8H_8N_4, HCl = 196.6$

CAS—86-54-4 (hydralazine); 304-20-1 (hydralazine hydrochloride)

Pharmacopoeial status

BP, USP (hydralazine hydrochloride)

Preparations

Compendial

Hydralazine Tablets BP (Hydralazine Hydrochloride Tablets). Tablets containing, in each, 25 mg and 50 mg hydralazine hydrochloride are usually available.

Hydralazine Injection BP (Hydralazine Hydrochloride for Injection). A sterile solution of hydralazine hydrochloride in water for injections. It is prepared by dissolving hydralazine hydrochloride for injection in the requisite amount of water for injections immediately before use. For intravenous infusion, hydralazine hydrochloride for injection should be dissolved in and then diluted with an appropriate volume of suitable diluent. Sealed containers each containing 20 mg are usually available. pH of a 2% w/v solution, 3.5 to 4.2. The label of the sealed container of Hydralazine Injection BP states that solutions containing glucose should not be used in the preparation of the intravenous infusion.

Hydralazine Hydrochloride Tablets USP.

Hydralazine Hydrochloride Injection USP. pH between 3.4 and 4.4.

Non-compendial

Apresoline (Ciba). *Tablets*, sugar coated, hydralazine hydrochloride 25 mg and 50 mg.

Injection, powder for reconstitution in water for injections, hydralazine hydrochloride 20 mg per ampoule. The reconstituted preparation should be further diluted with sodium chloride 0.9% injection. The injection must be given immediately and any remainder discarded. Mixtures for intravenous infusion should be made immediately before administration and should not be stored. Apresoline for infusion can also be used with 5% sorbitol infusion or isotonic inorganic infusion solutions such as compound sodium chloride infusion. The use of solutions that contain glucose is inadvisable as glucose causes hydralazine to be rapidly broken down.

Containers and storage

Solid state

Hydralazine Hydrochloride BP should be kept in a well-closed container.

Hydralazine Hydrochloride USP should be preserved in tight containers.

Dosage forms

Hydralazine Tablets BP and sealed containers of Hydralazine Injection BP should be protected from light and stored at a temperature not exceeding 25°. Hydralazine Injection BP deteriorates on storage and should be used immediately after preparation.

Hydralazine Hydrochloride Tablets USP should be preserved in tight, light-resistant containers.

Hydralazine Hydrochloride Injection USP should be preserved in single-dose or in multiple-dose containers, preferably of Type I glass.

Apresoline tablets should be protected from heat and moisture. Apresoline ampoules should be protected from heat and light.

PHYSICAL PROPERTIES

Hydralazine exists as yellow crystals.

Hydralazine hydrochloride is a white or almost white, odourless or almost odourless crystalline powder, with a bitter saline taste.

Melting point

Hydralazine melts at about 172° to 173°.

Hydralazine hydrochloride melts at about 275°, with decomposition.

pH

pH of a 2% w/v solution of *hydralazine hydrochloride*, 3.5 to 4.2.

Dissociation constants

pK_a 0.5, 7.1

Hydralazine is dibasic and pK_a values of 0.5 and 6.9 or 7.1 have been reported.[1]

Solubility

Hydralazine hydrochloride is soluble 1 in 25 of water; slightly soluble in ethanol (1 in 500) and in methanol; practically insoluble in chloroform and in ether.

Dissolution

The USP specifies that for Hydralazine Hydrochloride Tablets USP not less than 60% of the labelled amount of $C_8H_8N_4$, HCl is dissolved in 30 minutes. Dissolution medium: 900 mL of 0.1N hydrochloric acid; Apparatus 1 at 100 rpm.

STABILITY

Hydralazine hydrochloride is quite stable in the solid state.

Solutions

The effects of pH, temperature, and buffers on the kinetics of hydrolysis of hydralazine hydrochloride in buffered aqueous solutions (1.78×10^{-3} M) have been studied.[2] Hydrolysis was reported to yield phthalazine and other unidentified products and decomposition increased on exposure to light, oxygen, and increased pH. Maximum stability of hydralazine hydrochloride was demonstrated at about pH 3.5 and the rate of hydrolysis increased with an increase in pH. Negligible degradation was detected in solutions at pH 3.5 stored for 14 days protected from light at refrigeration or room temperatures. A rate constant of 7.71×10^{-6}/hour and $t_{10\%}$ of 1.56 years were calculated for hydrolysis at 25° and pH 3.5.

Intravenous fluids

Solutions of hydralazine injection (Apresoline, Ciba, reconstituted in distilled water) were mixed with glucose 5% injection, sodium chloride 0.9% injection, compound sodium lactate injection, or with a solution that contained glucose 3.3%, sodium, potassium, calcium, magnesium, and chloride ions.[3] Spectro-

photometric analysis revealed that in sodium chloride 0.9% or compound sodium lactate injections, negligible degradation of hydralazine had occurred after 4 days and 2 to 3 hours, respectively. In glucose 5% injection and in the other glucose-containing solution, reductions in concentration of hydralazine of about 4% and 5% respectively in 2 hours, and 19% and 25% respectively in 72 hours were measured. Furthermore, in both solutions containing glucose, yellow discoloration was observed within one hour of mixing with hydralazine.

Similarly, hydralazine hydrochloride was shown to be more stable in sodium chloride 0.9% injection than in glucose 5% injection at ambient temperature;[4] improved stability in both solutions was reported when they were protected from light.

Oral liquids

In studies of the stability of hydralazine hydrochloride in aqueous vehicles for oral liquids,[5] compatibility was demonstrated between hydralazine hydrochloride (1 mg/mL) and mannitol (0.28M) or sorbitol (0.28M and 0.56M); less than 10% of the initial concentration of hydralazine hydrochloride degraded in 21 days. In solutions that contained glucose, fructose, lactose, or maltose, extensive decomposition occurred in 24 hours. Sucrose did not interact with hydralazine hydrochloride but degradation occurred if products of the hydrolysis of sucrose (glucose and fructose) were present. Hence, rapid degradation of hydralazine hydrochloride was detected in solutions of sucrose with citric acid and in syrup or strawberry syrup (which both contained citric acid).

Formation of hydrazine

It has been deduced that hydrazine is a degradation product of hydralazine hydrochloride.[6] Hydrazine was not detected in raw material samples of hydralazine hydrochloride and only trace amounts were found in tablets of hydralazine hydrochloride, although following storage of tablets at 37° and 75% relative humidity for 221 days small amounts of hydrazine were detected. However, injections of hydralazine hydrochloride (20 mg/mL) contained hydrazine at levels between 0.0215% and 0.0327%, which increased to 0.1083% following storage at 37° for 221 days. The same workers[7] also found that at room temperature and 37° hydralazine hydrochloride tablets were stable for up to 24 months but an increase in the hydrazine content of injections was apparent after 16 months. It was noted that hydrazine may be used in the synthesis of hydralazine.

FURTHER INFORMATION. Stability of hydralazine hydrochloride syrup compounded from tablets—Alexander KS, Pudipeddi M, Parker GA. Am J Hosp Pharm 1993;50:683–6.

INCOMPATIBILITY/COMPATIBILITY

Enderlin[8] reported pink discoloration in hydralazine hydrochloride injection solutions (Apresoline, Ciba-Geigy), stored in syringes for up to 12 hours, when the solution had been drawn through needles that had stainless steel filters. It was stated that such a reaction may not be specific to any one metal.

Sorption

When solutions of hydralazine hydrochloride 27 micrograms/mL or 15 micrograms/mL in sodium chloride 0.9% injection were stored in Viaflex (polyvinyl chloride) infusion bags in the dark at 15° to 20°, significant losses due to sorption of hydralazine hydrochloride (at least 10%) occurred within one week.[9] However, in a further study,[10] negligible losses of hydralazine hydrochloride (in sodium chloride 0.9% injection) occurred during a seven-hour simulated infusion from glass bottles through a cellulose propionate burette chamber and polyvinyl chloride tubing, or during a one-hour simulated infusion through a syringe-pump system (polyethylene or Silastic tubing and glass syringe). No sorption was noted when solutions were stored in single-use, all-plastic syringes (polypropylene barrels and polyethylene plungers) in the dark at room temperature for 24 hours.

FORMULATION

Excipients

Excipients that have been used in presentations of hydralazine hydrochloride include:
Tablets: acacia; brilliant blue FCF (133); erythrosine (E127); gluten (wheat starch); lactose; macrogol; magnesium stearate; mannitol; quinoline yellow (E104); sodium starch glycollate; starch; stearic acid; sucrose; sunset yellow FCF (E110); tartrazine (E102).
Oral liquids: citric acid; sorbitol 70%; tragacanth mucilage.
Injections: methyl and propyl hydroxybenzoates; propylene glycol.

Bioavailability

In a double blind, crossover study involving healthy volunteers (who had similar acetylation rates), no significant difference in oral bioavailability was apparent between a standard tablet (Apresoline) and a sugar-coated tablet of hydralazine 25 mg.[11]

Modified-release preparations

Sustained-release oral dosage forms that consisted of an ethyl cellulose-coated hydralazine:ion exchange resin complex (Pennkinetic System) were prepared by Ludden *et al*[12] at various coating thicknesses. In studies involving 36 healthy, slow-acetylator volunteers, the sustained-release preparations provided lower peak plasma concentrations of hydralazine and more extended plasma concentration versus time graphs than conventional hydralazine hydrochloride tablets (Apresoline) or an oral solution of hydralazine hydrochloride (Apresoline parenteral solution in water).

REFERENCES

1. Naik DV, Davis BR, Minnet KM, Schulman SG. J Pharm Sci 1976;65(2):274–6.
2. Halasi S, Nairn JG. J Parenter Sci Technol 1990;44(1):30–4.
3. Clayton SK. J Clin Pharm 1978;2:247–56.
4. Halasi S, Nairn JG. Can J Hosp Pharm 1990;43:237–41.
5. Das Gupta V, Stewart KR, Bethea C. J Clin Hosp Pharm 1986;11:215–23.
6. Matsui F, Robertson DL, Lovering EG. J Pharm Sci 1983;72(8):948–51.
7. Lovering EG, Matsui F, Curran NM, Robertson DL, Sears RW. J Pharm Sci 1983;72(8):965–7.
8. Enderlin G [letter]. Am J Hosp Pharm 1984;41:634.
9. Kowaluk EA, Roberts MS, Blackburn HD, Polack AE. Am J Hosp Pharm 1981;38:1308–14.
10. Kowaluk EA, Roberts MS, Polack AE. Am J Hosp Pharm 1982;39:460–7.
11. Hawksworth GM, Morrice M, Petrie JC, Scott AK. Br J Clin Pharmacol 1980;9(1):111P.
12. Ludden TM, Rotenberg KS, Ludden LK, Shepherd AMM, Woodworth JR. J Pharm Sci 1988;77(12):1026–31.

Hydrochlorothiazide (BAN, rINN)   *Diuretic*

Chlorosulthiadil
6-Chloro-3,4-dihydro-2*H*-1,2,4-benzothiadiazine-7-sulphonamide 1,1-dioxide
$C_7H_8ClN_3O_4S_2 = 297.7$
CAS—58-93-5

Pharmacopoeial status

BP, USP

Preparations

Co-amilozide is the British Approved Name for compounded preparations of amiloride hydrochloride 1 part and hydrochlorothiazide 10 parts.
Co-triamterzide is the British Approved Name for compounded preparations of triamterene and hydrochlorothiazide in the proportions, by weight, 2 parts to 1 part, respectively.

Compendial
Hydrochlorothiazide Tablets BP. Tablets containing, in each, 25 mg and 50 mg are usually available.
Co-amilozide Tablets BP (Amiloride and Hydrochlorothiazide Tablets). Tablets containing, in each, the equivalent of 5 mg of anhydrous amiloride hydrochloride with 50 mg of hydrochlorothiazide and the equivalent of 2.5 mg of anhydrous amiloride hydrochloride with 25 mg of hydrochlorothiazide are usually available.
Co-amilozide Oral Solution BP (Amiloride and Hydrochlorothiazide Oral Solution). An oral solution containing the equivalent of 5 mg of anhydrous amiloride hydrochloride and 50 mg of hydrochlorothiazide in 5 mL is usually available. pH 2.8 to 3.2.
Hydrochlorothiazide Tablets USP.

Non-compendial
Esidrex (Ciba). *Tablets*, hydrochlorothiazide 25 mg and 50 mg.
HydroSaluric (MSD). *Tablets*, hydrochlorothiazide 25 mg and 50 mg.

Compound preparations
Co-amilozide preparations: Moduret 25 (Morson); Moduretic (Du Pont). Preparations are also available from APS, Ashbourne (Amilimax), Cox, Kerfoot, Norton (Amilco), Shire (Vasetic), Schwarz (Hypertane 50).
Co-triamterzide preparations: Dyazide (SK&F); Triamax Co (Ashbourne); Triamco (Norton).

Containers and storage

Solid state
Hydrochlorothiazide USP should be preserved in well-closed containers.

Dosage forms
Co-amilozide Tablets BP should be kept in a well-closed container, protected from light and stored at a temperature not exceeding 25°.
Hydrochlorothiazide Tablets USP should be preserved in well-closed containers.
Esidrex tablets should be protected from moisture and preferably dispensed in moisture-proof containers.

HydroSaluric tablets should be kept in a tightly closed container, stored in a cool place and protected from light.

PHYSICAL PROPERTIES

Hydrochlorothiazide is a white or almost white, odourless or almost odourless crystalline powder, with a slightly bitter taste.

Melting point

Hydrochlorothiazide melts at about 268°.

Dissociation constants

pK_a 7.9, 9.2
Mollica et al[1] determined the pK_a of hydrochlorothiazide by potentiometric titration using a radiometer titrator and a thermostated titration cell at 60°. Values of 8.6 and 9.9 were recorded. Spectrophotometric measurements yielded only one pK_a value of 8.7.

Partition coefficient

Log P (octanol/water), 0.00; log P (octanol/water), −0.07

Solubility

Hydrochlorothiazide is very slightly soluble in water; slightly soluble in ethanol (1 in 200); soluble 1 in 20 of acetone; sparingly soluble in methanol; insoluble in chloroform, in ether, and in dilute mineral acids; freely soluble in dimethylformamide, in dilute solutions of alkali hydroxides, and in *n*-butylamine.

The saturation solubility of hydrochlorothiazide in milk samples with varying fat content, in soluble casein (2.6%) solution, and in 0.2M phosphate buffer (pH 6.5) at different temperatures was assessed by Greek workers.[2] Solubility in the other media was greater than in the buffer solution. At 5° and 15° results showed slightly altered aqueous solubility in milk compared with that in buffer. At 25° and 37°, solubility of hydrochlorothiazide in phosphate buffer (pH 6.5) was 0.57 mg/mL and 1.02 mg/mL, respectively. The mechanism of the change in intrinsic solubility could not be fully explained.

Millar and Corrigan[3] prepared systems comprising hydrochlorothiazide and sodium caseinate by physical mixing and by lyophilisation. A significant increase in solubility of hydrochlorothiazide at 37° in phosphate buffer (pH 7.4) and in distilled water was measured as the concentration of sodium caseinate was increased (from zero to 30 mg/mL). Enhancement of intrinsic dissolution rates was demonstrated by the lyophilised systems.

Dissolution

The USP specifies that for Hydrochlorothiazide Tablets USP not less than 60% of the labelled amount of $C_7H_8ClN_3O_4S_2$ is dissolved in 60 minutes. Dissolution medium: 900 mL of 0.1N hydrochloric acid; Apparatus 1 at 100 rpm.

Dissolution properties

Correlation was found between dissolution rates and the bioavailability (in six volunteers) of four hydrochlorothiazide tablet formulations.[4] Of the three dissolution test procedures (USP basket, flask, and magnetic basket), that proposed for the prediction of *in-vivo* urinary excretion (50% hydrochlorothiazide dissolved in 10 minutes with the USP basket method at 150 rpm) was the best predictor of urinary hydrochlorothiazide excretion.

The dissolution behaviour of hydrochlorothiazide-adsorbent (Aerosil 200, Avicel PH 101, Veegum HV, and modified maize starch) triturations containing 25%, 50%, 75%, and 90% adsorbent, prepared by solvent deposition or simple blending, was studied by Boraie et al[5] using the USP paddle method at 37° and 50 rpm. Hydrochlorothiazide tablets that were prepared from their solvent-deposited triturations by direct compression triturations had the highest dissolution rates. Dissolution at 10 minutes from these formulations containing 25% Aerosil 200, 25% Avicel PH 101, 75% Veegum HV and 18.4% starch was 70%, 85%, 100%, and 99%, respectively, but the commercial preparation released only 50% of its content. At 30 minutes, 100% dissolution was achieved by all test formulations compared with 70% release from the commercial tablet.

STABILITY

Hydrochlorothiazide in aqueous solution hydrolyses to form formaldehyde and 6-chloro-2,4-disulphamoylaniline in a reversible, specific acid-catalysed and specific base-catalysed equilibrium process. At constant pH the hydrolysis reaction is pseudo-first-order. Hydrochlorothiazide is also subject to photolytic decomposition with near-ultraviolet light. No degradation of solid state hydrochlorothiazide was found after storage at room temperature for five years. A yellowish discoloration was observed after heating at 230° for two hours. Although stable in normal daylight, it should not be exposed to intense light.

Mollica et al[1] produced evidence to support the hypothesis that hydrolysis of hydrochlorothiazide is reversible; the reaction attained a state of equilibrium that was invariant with pH. Only limited buffer catalysis was demonstrated and variation of ionic strength (from 0.2 to 1.3) had no effect on reaction rate. The rate constant-pH profile was bell-shaped with a maximum at pH 7; a decomposition mechanism was postulated. Activation energies at pH 1.47 and pH 4.01 were 105.8 kJ and 128.0 kJ, respectively. The predicted pseudo-first-order rate constant at 25° and pH 4 was approximately 4×10^{-5}/hour. Between 45° and 70° the extent of the reaction did not increase markedly.

When hydrochlorothiazide tablets, formulated with three different granulating agents, were stored for up to 4 weeks at 37°, 50°, and 80°, the physical properties of those granulated with starch or povidone did not change significantly, while those that contained acacia increased in hardness, disintegration time, and dissolution time.[6] Findings in tablets stored at room temperature for one year were similar to those in the short-term study.

An examination of the photolytic decomposition of hydrochlorothiazide (0.5 mM) in oxygen-free methanol and in oxygen-free water with 5% methanol, revealed that hydrolysis and dechlorination of the thiadiazine ring occur simultaneously[7] and within about 6 hours in light at above 310 nm. Major degradation products identified were 5-chloro-2,4-disulphonamidoaniline, methoxyhydrothiazide, and 2,4-disulphonamidoaniline. Decomposition was inhibited when the methanol solutions were saturated with oxygen before irradiation. A photodegradation mechanism was proposed.

FURTHER INFORMATION. Stability studies of hydrochlorothiazide injection solution—Hennig B, Scholz F, Peinhardt G [German]. Pharmazie 1986;41:565–6. Stability of hydrochlorothiazide injections. II—Hennig B, Scholz F, Wolf G [German]. Pharmazie 1987;42:162–4. Chemical and physical stability of pediatric hydrochlorothiazide suspension—Tötterman AM, Riukka L, Rasilainen M, Järviluoma E, Kristoffersson E. Pharm Weekbl (Sci) 1992;14(4) Suppl E:E14.

FORMULATION

Excipients

Excipients that have been used in presentations of hydrochlorothiazide include:

Tablets: calcium stearate; colloidal silica; gluten; hydroxypropylcellulose; lactose; magnesium stearate; maize starch; microcrystalline cellulose; talc.
Suspensions: methylcellulose; sodium benzoate; syrup.

Bioavailability

The effect of the diluent on the bioavailability of hydrochlorothiazide from pellets was investigated in six healthy volunteers.[8] In a crossover study each subject was given hydrochlorothiazide 50 mg on three occasions, as a conventional tablet and as a gelatin capsule containing either type I or type II pellets in a defined size fraction. Pellets made by granulation, extrusion, and spheronisation, contained 25% hydrochlorothiazide. The matrix of type I pellets was microcrystalline cellulose; type II contained microcrystalline cellulose and carmellose sodium. Dissolution tests were performed in water and various media; release of hydrochlorothiazide was slower from both pellet formulations in simulated intestinal fluid than from the conventional tablet. Bioavailability of the conventional tablet was higher than that of either pellet formulation.
Plasma and urinary data for hydrochlorothiazide provided Patel *et al*[9] with a measure of its bioavailability following administration of single doses (25 to 200 mg) of tablets and a suspension (of crushed tablets) to 12 healthy volunteers. Rapid absorption, with uniform peak plasma concentrations after approximately 2 hours, was found at all doses. The authors concluded that the absorption efficiency of oral hydrochlorothiazide was independent of dose. Small differences observed between the two dosage forms were significant only at 0.5 hours.
Bioadhesive and non-adhesive suspensions of hydrochlorothiazide prepared with Carbopol 934 (5%) and with hydroxyethylcellulose (1.5%) respectively, were found to exhibit identical bioavailabilities when compared in *rats*.[10]

Formulation and processing factors affecting release

Dissolution of the slightly soluble hydrochlorothiazide was used to assess the effects of operating variables (number of tamps and tamping force) and formulation factors (soluble and insoluble fillers and with or without disintegrants) on capsules filled on an instrumented dosing-disk type of filling machine.[11] Multiple tamping, irrespective of compression force, caused slower drug release, especially when insoluble calcium hydrogen phosphate was the filler. Tamping effects were negated by the inclusion (with both fillers) of 4% croscarmellose sodium as disintegrant. At higher compression forces dissolution rates increased in capsules prepared with anhydrous lactose (soluble filler), but were impaired in preparations containing calcium hydrogen phosphate, except in the presence of the disintegrant.
The influence of lubricants (magnesium stearate or colloidal silica), fillers (lactose or microcrystalline cellulose), and a surfactant (polysorbate 80) on the dissolution of hydrochlorothiazide from hard gelatin capsules was investigated[12] in a study (2^3 factorial design) in 0.1M hydrochloric acid at 37°. The lubricant was the most important factor in determining the dissolution efficiency and the greatest effect on release of hydrochlorothiazide was produced by the excipients with greatest hydrophilicity.

FURTHER INFORMATION. Bioavailability of hydrochlorothiazide suspension [influence of excipients: agar, Veegum HV, hydrophilic Aerosil, Carbopol 934 and bentonite]—EL-Assay AEI,

Hamza YE, Halawa AEA. Drug Dev Ind Pharm 1985;11(1):65–81. A study of the influence of formulation factors and processing techniques on the dissolution rates of hydrochlorothiazide tablets [includes measurement of dissolution behaviour by Langenbucher's flow-cell method]—Seth P. Pharm Acta Helv 1972;47:457–65. Formulation of enteral hydrochlorothiazide suspension intended for premature infants—Luukkonen P, Tötterman AM, Rasilainen M, Järviluoma E, Kristoffersson E. Pharm Weekbl (Sci) 1992;14(4) Suppl E:E14.

REFERENCES

1. Mollica JA, Rehm CR, Smith JB, Govan HK. J Pharm Sci 1971;60(9):1380–4.
2. Macheras EP, Koupparis MA, Antimisiaris SG. J Pharm Sci 1989;78(1):933–6.
3. Millar FC, Corrigan OI. Drug Dev Ind Pharm 1991;17(12):1593–1607.
4. Shah KA, Needham TE. J Pharm Sci 1979;68(12):1486–90.
5. Boraie NA, El-Fattah SA, Hassan HM. Pharm Ind 1986;48:1202–6.
6. Alam AS, Parrott EL. J Pharm Sci 1971;60:263–6.
7. Tamat SR, Moore DE. J Pharm Sci 1983;72:180–3.
8. Herman J, Remon JP, Lefebvre R, Bogaert M, Klinger GH, Schwartz JB. J Pharm Pharmacol 1988;40:157–60.
9. Patel RB, Patel UR, Rogge MC, Shah VP, Prasad VK, Selen A *et al*. J Pharm Sci 1984;73:359–61.
10. Harris D, Fell JT, Taylor DC, Lynch J, Sharma HL. Int J Pharmaceutics 1989;56:97–102.
11. Shah KB, Augsburger LL, Marshall K. J Pharm Sci 1987;76(8):639–45.
12. Petrovick PR, Jacob M, Gaudy D, Bassani VL, Guterres SS. Int J Pharmaceutics 1991;76:49–53.

Hydrocortisone (BAN, rINN)   *Corticosteroid*

Cortisol; compound F; 17-hydroxycorticosterone
11β,17α,21-Trihydroxypregn-4-ene-3,20-dione
$C_{21}H_{30}O_5 = 362.5$

Hydrocortisone Acetate (BANM, rINNM)
Hydrocortisone 21-acetate
$C_{23}H_{32}O_6 = 404.5$

Hydrocortisone Butyrate (BANM, USAN, rINNM)
Hydrocortisone 17α-butyrate
$C_{25}H_{36}O_6 = 432.6$

Hydrocortisone Cypionate (BANM)
Hydrocortisone Cipionate (rINNM)
$C_{29}H_{42}O_6 = 486.65$

Hydrocortisone Hydrogen Succinate (BANM)

Hydrocortisone Hemisuccinate (rINNM)
$C_{25}H_{34}O_8 = 462.5$

Hydrocortisone Sodium Phosphate (BANM, rINNM)

Hydrocortisone 21-(disodium orthophosphate)
$C_{21}H_{29}Na_2O_8P = 486.4$

Hydrocortisone Sodium Succinate (BANM, rINNM)

Hydrocortisone 21-(sodium succinate)
$C_{25}H_{35}NaO_8 = 484.5$

Hydrocortisone Valerate (BANM, USAN, rINNM)

Hydrocortisone 17-valerate
$C_{26}H_{38}O_6 = 446.6$
CAS—50-23-7 (hydrocortisone); 50-03-3 (hydrocortisone acetate); 13609-67-1 (hydrocortisone butyrate); 508-99-6 (hydrocortisone cypionate); 2203-97-6 (hydrocortisone hydrogen succinate, anhydrous); 83784-20-7 (hydrocortisone hydrogen succinate, monohydrate); 6000-74-4 (hydrocortisone sodium phosphate); 125-04-2 (hydrocortisone sodium succinate); 57524-89-7 (hydrocortisone valerate)

Pharmacopoeial status

BP (hydrocortisone, hydrocortisone acetate, hydrocortisone hydrogen succinate, hydrocortisone sodium phosphate); USP (hydrocortisone, hydrocortisone acetate, hydrocortisone butyrate, hydrocortisone cypionate, hydrocortisone hemisuccinate, hydrocortisone sodium phosphate, hydrocortisone sodium succinate, hydrocortisone valerate)

Preparations

Compendial
Hydrocortisone Cream BP. Creams containing 0.1, 0.125, 0.5, 1.0, and 2.5% w/w are usually available.
Hydrocortisone Ointment BP. Ointments containing 0.5, 1.0, and 2.5% w/w are usually available.
Hydrocortisone Acetate Cream BP. A cream containing 1% w/w is usually available.
Hydrocortisone Acetate Ointment BP. An ointment containing 1% w/w is usually available.
Hydrocortisone Acetate Injection BP. A sterile suspension of hydrocortisone acetate in water for injections. Injections containing 25 mg in 1 mL and 125 mg in 5 mL are usually available.
Hydrocortisone Sodium Phosphate Injection BP. A sterile solution of hydrocortisone sodium phosphate in water for injections. pH 7.5 to 8.5. Injections containing the equivalent of 100 mg of hydrocortisone in 1 mL and 500 mg in 5 mL are usually available.
Hydrocortisone Sodium Succinate Injection BP (Hydrocortisone Sodium Succinate for Injection). A sterile solution of hydrocortisone sodium succinate in water for injections. It is prepared by dissolving hydrocortisone sodium succinate for injection in the requisite amount of water for injections immediately before use. The pH of a solution containing the equivalent of 5% w/v of hydrocortisone is 6.5 to 8.0. Sealed containers each containing the equivalent of 100 mg and 500 mg of hydrocortisone are usually available.
Hydrocortisone and Neomycin Cream BP. A cream containing 0.5% w/w of hydrocortisone and 3500 units of neomycin sulphate per gram is usually available.
Hydrocortisone Acetate and Clioquinol Cream BP. A cream containing 0.5% w/w of hydrocortisone acetate and 3.0% w/w of clioquinol is usually available.

Hydrocortisone and Clioquinol Ointment BP. An ointment containing 3% w/w of clioquinol and 1% w/w of hydrocortisone is usually available.
Hydrocortisone Acetate and Neomycin Eye Drops BP. A sterile suspension of hydrocortisone acetate in a solution of neomycin sulphate in purified water. Drops containing 0.5% w/v of hydrocortisone acetate and 3500 units of neomycin sulphate per mL and containing 1.5% w/v of hydrocortisone acetate and 3500 units of neomycin sulphate per mL are usually available.
Hydrocortisone Acetate and Neomycin Ear Drops BP. A suspension of hydrocortisone acetate in a solution of neomycin sulphate in purified water. Ear drops containing 0.5% w/v of hydrocortisone acetate and 3500 units of neomycin sulphate per mL and containing 1.5% w/v of hydrocortisone acetate and 3500 units of neomycin sulphate per mL are usually available.
Hydrocortisone and Neomycin Eye Ointment BP. An eye ointment containing 1.5% w/w of hydrocortisone acetate and 3500 units of neomycin sulphate per gram is usually available.
Hydrocortisone Tablets USP.
Hydrocortisone Cream USP.
Hydrocortisone Gel USP.
Hydrocortisone Lotion USP.
Hydrocortisone Ointment USP.
Hydrocortisone Enema USP.
Sterile Hydrocortisone Suspension USP. pH 5.0 to 7.0.
Hydrocortisone Acetate Cream USP.
Hydrocortisone Acetate Lotion USP.
Hydrocortisone Acetate Ointment USP.
Hydrocortisone Acetate Ophthalmic Ointment USP.
Hydrocortisone Acetate Ophthalmic Suspension USP.
Sterile Hydrocortisone Acetate Suspension USP. pH 5.0 to 7.0.
Hydrocortisone Butyrate Cream USP.
Hydrocortisone Cypionate Oral Suspension USP.
Hydrocortisone Sodium Phosphate Injection USP. pH 7.5 to 8.5.
Hydrocortisone Sodium Succinate for Injection USP. pH 7.0 to 8.0.
Hydrocortisone Valerate Cream USP.

Non-compendial
Colifoam (Stafford-Miller). *Foam*, aerosol, hydrocortisone acetate 10%.
Corlan (Evans). *Pellets* (lozenges), hydrocortisone 2.5 mg (as sodium succinate).
Dioderm (Dermal). *Cream*, hydrocortisone 0.1%.
Efcortelan (Glaxo). *Cream*, hydrocortisone 0.5%, 1%, or 2.5% in a water-miscible basis.
Ointment, hydrocortisone 0.5%, 1%, or 2.5% in a paraffin basis.
Efcortelan Soluble (Glaxo). *Injection*, powder for reconstitution with water for injections, hydrocortisone (as sodium succinate) 100 mg per vial.
Efcortesol (Glaxo). *Injection*, hydrocortisone 100 mg (as sodium phosphate)/mL.
Hydrocortistab (Boots). *Tablets*, hydrocortisone 20 mg.
Cream, hydrocortisone acetate 1%.
Ointment, hydrocortisone 1%.
Injection, aqueous suspension, hydrocortisone acetate 25 mg/mL.
Hydrocortisyl (Roussel). *Cream*, hydrocortisone 1%.
Ointment, hydrocortisone 1%.
Hydrocortone (MSD). *Tablets*, hydrocortisone 10 mg and 20 mg.
Locoid (Brocades). *Cream*, hydrocortisone butyrate 0.1%.
Lipocream, hydrocortisone butyrate 0.1%.
Ointment, hydrocortisone butyrate 0.1%.

Scalp lotion, hydrocortisone butyrate 0.1% in an aqueous iso-propanol basis.

Mildison (Brocades). *Lipocream,* hydrocortisone 1%.

Solu-Cortef (Upjohn). *Injection,* powder for reconstitution, hydrocortisone (as sodium succinate) 100 mg per vial. For reconstitution with sterile water for injections. *Diluents:* glucose 5% in water, sodium chloride 0.9% solution, or glucose 5% in sodium chloride 0.9% solution. No diluents other than those referred to are recommended. Parenteral products should be inspected visually for particulate matter and discoloration before administration.

Containers and storage

Solid state

Hydrocortisone BP, Hydrocortisone Acetate BP, and Hydro-cortisone Sodium Phosphate BP should be kept in well-closed containers and protected from light.

Hydrocortisone Hydrogen Succinate BP should be protected from light.

Hydrocortisone USP, Hydrocortisone Acetate USP, Hydrocor-tisone Butyrate USP, and Hydrocortisone Valerate USP should be preserved in well-closed containers.

Hydrocortisone Cypionate USP should be preserved in tight containers, and stored in a cold place, protected from light.

Hydrocortisone Hemisuccinate USP and Hydrocortisone Sodium Phosphate USP should be preserved in tight containers.

Hydrocortisone Sodium Succinate USP should be preserved in tight, light-resistant containers.

Dosage forms

Hydrocortisone Ointment BP and Hydrocortisone Acetate Ointment BP should be protected from light.

Hydrocortisone Acetate Injection BP and Hydrocortisone Sodium Phosphate Injection BP should be protected from light; the latter should also be stored at a temperature not exceeding 25° and should not be allowed to freeze.

Hydrocortisone Sodium Succinate Injection BP deteriorates on storage and should be used immediately after preparation.

Hydrocortisone Cream USP, Hydrocortisone Enema USP, Hydrocortisone Gel USP, Hydrocortisone Lotion USP, Hydro-cortisone Acetate Lotion USP, and Hydrocortisone Acetate Ophthalmic Suspension USP should be preserved in tight con-tainers.

Hydrocortisone Tablets USP, Hydrocortisone Ointment USP, Hydrocortisone Acetate Cream USP, Hydrocortisone Acetate Ointment USP, Hydrocortisone Butyrate Cream USP, and Hydrocortisone Valerate Cream USP should be preserved in well-closed containers.

Sterile Hydrocortisone Suspension USP, Sterile Hydrocortisone Acetate Suspension USP, and Hydrocortisone Sodium Phos-phate Injection USP should be preserved in single-dose or in multiple-dose containers, preferably of Type I glass.

Hydrocortisone Cypionate Oral Suspension USP should be pre-served in tight, light-resistant containers.

Hydrocortisone Acetate Ophthalmic Ointment USP should be preserved in collapsible ophthalmic ointment tubes.

Hydrocortisone Sodium Succinate for Injection USP should be preserved in containers suitable for sterile solids.

Colifoam is packaged in a pressurised container, which should be protected from sunlight and not exposed to temperatures above 50°. Do not pierce, burn, or refrigerate.

Corlan pellets should be kept in a firmly closed container.

Dioderm cream should be stored in a cool place and the cap tightly replaced after use.

Efcortelan Soluble and Efcortesol injection should be protected from light.

Hydrocortistab tablets should be stored in a cool, dry place. Hydrocortistab cream and ointment should be stored below 25°. Hydrocortistab injection should be stored between 15° to 20° and protected from light.

Hydrocortone tablets should be kept in a well-closed container, stored in a cool place, and protected from light.

Mildison lipocream and Locoid preparations should be stored at room temperature (15° to 25°).

Solu-Cortef should be stored at controlled room temperature (15° to 30°). Reconstituted solutions should be used immedi-ately.

PHYSICAL PROPERTIES

Hydrocortisone is a white or almost white crystalline powder.

Hydrocortisone acetate is a white or almost white crystalline powder.

Hydrocortisone butyrate is a white or almost white, practically odourless, crystalline powder.

Hydrocortisone cypionate is a white or almost white crystalline powder; odourless or with a slight odour.

Hydrocortisone hydrogen succinate is a white or almost white crystalline powder; odourless or almost odourless.

Hydrocortisone sodium phosphate is a white or light yellow, hygroscopic, odourless or almost odourless powder.

Hydrocortisone sodium succinate is a white or almost white, hygroscopic, crystalline powder or amorphous solid.

Melting point

Hydrocortisone melts at about 214°, with decomposition.

Hydrocortisone acetate melts at about 220°, with decomposition.

Hydrocortisone hydrogen succinate melts at about 168°; it may also occur in a form which melts at about 200°.

Hydrocortisone sodium succinate melts at 169° to 171°.

pH

A 0.5% w/v solution of *hydrocortisone sodium phosphate* in water has a pH of 7.5 to 9.0.

Dissociation constant

pK_a 5.1 (hydrocortisone sodium succinate)

Partition coefficients

Values of log *P* for hydrocortisone and some of its esters were determined in octanol/pH 7.4 aqueous buffer systems:[1] hydro-cortisone, 1.50; hydrocortisone 21-acetate, 2.21; hydrocortisone 17-butyrate, 3.18; hydrocortisone 17-valerate, 3.79.

Solubility

Hydrocortisone is practically insoluble in water; soluble 1 in 40 of ethanol and 1 in 80 of acetone; slightly soluble in chloro-form; very slightly soluble in ether.

Hydrocortisone acetate is practically insoluble in water; slightly soluble in ethanol (1 in 230) and in chloroform; practically inso-luble in ether.

Hydrocortisone butyrate is practically insoluble in water; soluble in methanol, in ethanol, and in acetone; freely soluble in chloro-form; slightly soluble in ether.

Hydrocortisone cypionate is insoluble or practically insoluble in water; soluble in ethanol; very soluble in chloroform; slightly soluble in ether.

Hydrocortisone hydrogen succinate is practically insoluble in water; soluble 1 in 40 of ethanol, 1 in 7 of absolute ethanol, and 1 in 25 of sodium hydrogen carbonate solution. It dis-solves, with decomposition, in 5M sodium hydroxide.

Hydrocortisone sodium phosphate is freely soluble in water (1 in 4); slightly soluble in ethanol; practically insoluble in absolute ethanol, in chloroform, in dioxan, and in ether.
Hydrocortisone sodium succinate is soluble 1 in 3 of water, and 1 in 34 of ethanol; practically insoluble in chloroform and in ether.

FURTHER INFORMATION. Solubility of hydrocortisone in organic and aqueous media: evidence for regular solution behaviour in apolar solvents—Hagen TA, Flynn GL. J Pharm Sci 1983;72(4):409–14.

Dissolution

The USP specifies that for Hydrocortisone Tablets USP not less than 70% of the labelled amount of $C_{21}H_{30}O_5$ is dissolved in 30 minutes. Dissolution medium: 900 mL of water; Apparatus 2 at 50 rpm.

STABILITY

In the solid state, hydrocortisone is very stable. However, in common with other corticosteroids, in aqueous solution over a wide pH range it degrades by both oxidative and non-oxidative reactions of the C-17 dihydroxyacetone side-chain. The main degradation products are reported to be steroid glyoxals, glycolic acids, etienic acid, and a 17-oxo-steroid. At strongly acid pH (less than 2) the main product is the 17-deoxy glyoxal derivative. At weakly acidic and neutral pH, degradation involves parallel non-oxidative and oxidative reactions; the main products are the 17-deoxy glyoxal and 21-dehydrohydrocortisone. At alkaline pH, degradation is more complex. The rate of degradation exhibits first-order dependence on hydrogen ions and hydroxide ions.

In an extensive and detailed study,[2–5] Hansen and Bundgaard examined the kinetics and pathways of hydrocortisone degradation in aqueous solution over a wide pH range. Oxidative degradation of the C-17 side-chain in neutral and basic solutions was catalysed by acetate and citrate ions from buffer solutions and by trace metal impurities (particularly iron III, nickel II, and copper II ions). Under similar conditions, oxidative degradation of the 21-alcohol group to an aldehyde group giving 21-dehydrohydrocortisone was also dependent on trace metal impurities. However, the accelerated degradation of hydrocortisone in phosphate, carbonate, and borate buffers was diminished by the addition of disodium edetate. At pH less than 2, the degradation rate was independent of trace metal impurities.[4,5] Maximum stability occurred[2] at pH 3.5 to 4.5.

The rate of the non-oxidative degradation reaction (which yielded the 17-deoxy glyoxal) was not affected by the addition of ethanol, 2-propanol, glycerol, or propylene glycol in increasing amounts to alkaline aqueous solutions of hydrocortisone, whereas the rate of the oxidation reaction was decreased.[5]

Major degradation products of hydrocortisone in aqueous solution over a wide pH range, identified by HPLC,[3] were the 21-aldehyde, 21-aldehyde-17-deoxy, 17-oxo, 17-carboxylic acid, 21-carboxylic acid, and 17-deoxy derivatives.

Decomposition in alkaline aqueous solution was more complex[4] with identification of several products at pH 9 to 11. In a 0.1M carbonate buffer solution, pH 10.21, in the absence of disodium edetate, the major products of decomposition were etienic acid and a glycolic acid, although minor amounts of the 17-ketosteroid and another glycolic acid were formed; these four products accounted for almost 90% of the total degradation.

Stability of esters

Hydrocortisone phosphate and hydrocortisone succinate are susceptible to pH-dependent degradation by hydrolysis in neutral or in alkaline solutions, to yield free hydrocortisone and phosphoric acid or succinic acid, respectively. Reported activation energies are 71.5 kJ/mol and 82.8 kJ/mol, respectively.

The degradation rate of hydrocortisone 21-acetate (as a 0.8 mg/mL methanolic solution mixed with buffer solutions) at 30° was shown to be pH-dependent and to be first-order down to 25% residual hydrocortisone 21-acetate.[6] Maximum stability occurred at pH 4.5. At pH 9.1 the minor degradation product hydrocortisone-17-acetate exists in equilibrium with the 21-acetate, but hydrolysis to hydrocortisone (the major degradation product) probably occurs directly from the 21-acetate.

Effect of vehicles and additives

The concentration of hydrocortisone sodium succinate (Solu-Cortef, Upjohn) in admixture with cytarabine and methotrexate sodium[7] fell to 86.5% and 94% of the initial concentrations (15 mg/12 mL and 25 mg/12 mL, respectively) following storage at 25° for 24 hours in Elliot's B infusion solution, pH 7.1. Decomposition was faster in Elliot's B solution than in compound sodium lactate injection, sodium chloride 0.9% injection, or glucose 5% injection. It was suggested that higher pH and lower initial drug concentration may decrease hydrocortisone stability. The stability of hydrocortisone was not affected by the presence of the other two drugs.

Similarly, dependence on pH and initial concentration was shown by Anderson and Latiolais[8] in a study of the compatibility of metaraminol bitartrate (Aramine) and hydrocortisone sodium succinate (Solu-Cortef) alone or in combination at various pH values in glucose 5% and in sodium chloride 0.9% intravenous solution. It was indicated that hydrocortisone stability decreased with increasing concentration.

Spectrophotometric and microscopic investigation of the stability of hydrocortisone sodium succinate in glucose 5% or in glucose 10% injections revealed the formation of crystals of hydrocortisone succinate during storage.[9] The extent of crystallisation depended on the pH of the glucose solutions and the length of storage time.

An investigation of the stability of hydrocortisone in various vehicles and the effect of inactive ingredients (by HPLC) revealed that hydrocortisone was unstable in water and in a water-miscible (macrogol) ointment basis.[10] The addition of ethanol 50% or glycerol 10% to water had a stabilising effect. Hydrocortisone in alcoholic solution, was extremely unstable under basic conditions at room temperature, only 25.1% remaining after 72 hours, although decomposition occurred under highly acidic conditions at room temperature over a period of 140 hours. Stability was not affected by the presence of iodochlorhydroxyquin, menthol, or phenol.

Timmins and Gray[11] reported poor stability of hydrocortisone (0.1% w/w) in an extemporaneous topical formulation (pH 8.76) prepared from a zinc oxide lotion and Hydrocortisone Lotion BPC. First-order decomposition, at 50° and at room temperature (20° ± 2°), yielded the 21-dehydrohydrocortisone as the major degradation product, although other products (such as the 17-keto steroid at 50°) were identified by HPLC.

The stability of hydrocortisone in aqueous solutions at 50° and 60° containing 20% ethanol, 50% glycerol, or 50% propylene glycol was not affected by the addition of the antioxidants ascorbic acid, propyl gallate, or sodium bisulphite.[12] Cysteine hydrochloride or sodium lauryl sulphate adversely affected stability whereas polysorbate 80 had a stabilising effect on hydrocortisone in an aqueous buffered solution (pH 3.5) at room temperature. At 60°, hydrocortisone was more stable in propylene glycol than in glycerol.

The degradation of hydrocortisone sodium succinate 1 mg/mL was faster in Elliot's B solution (an artificial cerebrospinal fluid, Travenol) than in either compound sodium lactate injection or sodium chloride 0.9% injection when stored in sealed glass ampoules at room temperature or at $30° \pm 0.1°$ under fluorescent light for seven days.[13]

Hydrocortisone butyrate 0.1% w/w in a carbomer gel formulated with 48% w/w aqueous solution of propylene glycol underwent base-catalysed, pH-dependent, reversible isomerisation to the C-21 ester of butyric acid.[14] The ester subsequently hydrolysed to hydrocortisone, followed by metal-catalysed degradation to other (unspecified) compounds.

Inclusion complexes

The presence of β-cyclodextrin in alkaline aqueous solution increased the rate of degradation of hydrocortisone (about 3-fold).[15] However, inclusion complexation had no effect on the stability of the steroid in neutral or acidic solutions. The rate-accelerating effect was attributed to a cyclodextrin-induced shift of the keto-enol equilibrium of the C-17 dihydroxyacetone side-chain to the more reactive enol form.

Radiolytic degradation

Hydrocortisone, hydrocortisone acetate, and hydrocortisone sodium succinate were degraded by ^{60}Co-irradiation at a rate of 1.0, 0.3, and 1.4 %/Mrad, respectively.[16] A common product of decomposition was 11β-hydroxy-4-androstene-3,17-dione; other products were cortisone, cortisone acetate, and cortisone sodium succinate.

Stabilisation

As discussed above, disodium edetate (a chelating agent) can reduce the catalytic effect of trace metals on the oxidation of the C-17 side chain to steroid glyoxals. The storage time of hydrocortisone sodium phosphate and hydrocortisone sodium succinate can be lengthened in the absence of water.

Bansal et al[17] reported significant improvement in hydrocortisone stability at 37°, 47°, and 57° in buffered (pH 7.4, 8.4, and 9.4), aqueous solutions containing a 25M excess of D-fructose. No similar improvement was observed at 37° in hydrocortisone solutions (pH 7.4) containing glucose, lactose, sucrose, sorbitol, propylene glycol, or glycerol.

FURTHER INFORMATION. The possible implication of steroid-glyoxal degradation products in allergic reactions to corticosteroids—Bundgaard H. Arch Pharm Chemi Sci 1980;8:83–90. Stability of hydrocortisone in polyethylene glycol [macrogol] ointment base—Allen AE, Das Gupta V. J Pharm Sci 1974;63(1):107–9. Nonisothermal kinetics applied to drugs in pharmaceutical suspensions—Waltersson J-O, Lundgren P. Acta Pharm Suec 1983;20:145–54. Sterilisation of corticosteroids by ^{60}Co-irradiation—Bussey DM, Kane MP, Tsuji K. J Parenter Sci Technol 1983;37(2):51–4.

INCOMPATIBILITY/COMPATIBILITY

Benzalkonium chloride can be adsorbed and partially inactivated by the hydrocortisone acetate in a sterile suspension for ophthalmic use containing 1% hydrocortisone acetate. These effects should be recognised in the selection of a suitable preservative system for eye drop formulations.

In aqueous suspension, hydrocortisone acetate powder adsorbed hydroxyethylcellulose and polysorbate 80, but not glucose, sucrose, or carmellose sodium.[18] In the presence of polysorbate 80, hydroxyethylcellulose was not adsorbed. In additive-free aqueous suspension, hydrocortisone acetate was still flocculated and free-flowing after two weeks storage, whereas low volume sediments formed in aqueous suspensions with polysorbate 80 or hydroxyethylcellulose.

Hydrocortisone degraded rapidly, in the presence of attapulgite, in suspension at pH 8.4 and 23°, whereas the hydrocortisone content of an aqueous solution at pH 8.4 remained constant over a two-day study period.[19] Kinetic and adsorption studies suggested that hydrocortisone is adsorbed weakly by attapulgite and undergoes oxidative degradation, catalysed by iron oxides or hydroxides and ferric iron contained in the clay minerals. Hydrocortisone sodium succinate has been reported to be incompatible with amylobarbitone sodium, chloramphenicol sodium succinate, colistin sulphomethate sodium, dimenhydrinate, diphenhydramine hydrochloride, ephedrine sulphate, heparin, hydralazine hydrochloride, kanamycin sulphate, metaraminol tartrate, methicillin sodium, nafcillin sodium, novobiocin sodium, oxytetracycline hydrochloride, pentobarbitone sodium, phenobarbitone sodium, prochlorperazine, promazine hydrochloride, promethazine hydrochloride, quinalbarbitone sodium, tetracycline hydrochloride, and vancomycin hydrochloride.

FORMULATION

HYDROCORTISONE LOTION

The following formula was given in the *British Pharmaceutical Codex 1973*:

Hydrocortisone, in sufficiently fine powder to meet the requirements of the standard	10.0 g
Chlorocresol	0.5 g
Self-emulsifying monostearin	40.0 g
Glycerol	63.0 g
Purified water, freshly boiled and cooled to	1000.0 g

Dissolve the chlorocresol in 850 mL of the water with the aid of gentle heat, add the self-emulsifying monostearin, heat to 60°, and stir until completely dispersed. Triturate the hydrocortisone with the glycerol, incorporate, with constant stirring, in the warm basis, allow to cool slowly, stirring until cold, add sufficient of the water to produce the required weight, and mix. Hydrocortisone Lotion BPC may be prepared using any other suitable basis.

Excipients

Excipients that have been used in presentations of hydrocortisone include:

Tablets, hydrocortisone: gelatin; lactose; magnesium stearate; potato starch; sucrose; talc.

Creams, hydrocortisone: benzyl alcohol; cetyl alcohol; citric acid, anhydrous; chlorocresol; dibasic sodium phosphate, dried; emulsifying ointment; glyceryl monostearate; hydrous wool fat; isopropyl myristate; isopropyl palmitate; liquid paraffin; macrogol monostearate; methyl and propyl hydroxybenzoates; polysorbate 60; polyoxyl 40 stearate; propylene glycol; sodium chloride; sodium lauryl sulphate; sorbic acid; sorbitan monostearate; stearyl alcohol; urea.

Hydrocortisone acetate: butylated hydroxyanisole; butylated hydroxytoluene; cetomacrogol 1000; chlorocresol; disodium edetate; esters of fatty acids, saturated; glycerol; liquid paraffin; menthol; methyl and propyl hydroxybenzoates; polysorbate 40; stearyl alcohol; white soft paraffin.

Hydrocortisone butyrate: cetomacrogol; cetostearyl alcohol; citric acid; liquid paraffin; methyl hydroxybenzoates; sodium citrate; white soft paraffin.

Ointments, hydrocortisone: cetyl alcohol; cholesterol; glycerol; liquid paraffin; methyl and propyl hydroxybenzoates; polysorbate

80; propylene glycol; sodium lauryl sulphate; stearyl alcohol; white soft paraffin.

Hydrocortisone butyrate: liquid paraffin; polyethylene.

Lotions, hydrocortisone: carbomer 940; ceteareth-20; cetyl alcohol; chlorocresol; dehydroacetic acid; glycerol; glyceryl stearate; isopropyl palmitate; lactic acid; light liquid paraffin; macrogol 100 stearate; myristl lactate; self-emulsifying monostearin; sodium hydroxide; stearyl alcohol.

Hydrocortisone butyrate: citric acid; glycerol; isopropanol; povidone; sodium citrate.

Topical aerosol sprays, hydrocortisone: butane; isopropyl myristate.

Enemas and rectal mousses, hydrocortisone: carbomer; methyl hydroxybenzoate; polysorbate 80.

Hydrocortisone acetate: cetostearyl alcohol; cetyl alcohol; colloidal silica; dichlorodifluoromethane/dichlorotetrafluoroethane; glycerol; methyl and propyl hydroxybenzoates; polysorbate 80; propylene glycol; triethanolamine; polyoxyl-10 stearyl ether.

Injections (powder for reconstitution), hydrocortisone acetate: benzyl alcohol; carmellose sodium; sodium chloride; Tween 80.

Hydrocortisone hydrogen succinate: monosodium phosphate dihydrate; sodium bicarbonate; sodium phosphate dodecahydrate.

Hydrocortisone sodium succinate: sodium acid phosphate; sodium phosphate.

Bioavailability

Maximum concentrations of hydrocortisone in plasma were reached two hours after rectal administration of a hydrocortisone acetate foam (100 mg, Colifoam, Trommsdorff, Germany) and were ten-fold lower than those obtained after oral administration of a 20-mg dose (Hydrocortisone, Hoechst) in the same eight healthy subjects.[20] The mean absolute rectal bioavailability was calculated to be 2% ± 1%.

Newrick et al[21] reported that administration of hydrocortisone (200 mg) by rectal suppository to ten healthy volunteers led to mean plasma-hydrocortisone concentrations that were as high as those obtained by intramuscular injection of hydrocortisone (200 mg) to twelve healthy volunteers.

Dispersion systems

Hydrocortisone dispersion systems were formulated by the fusion method with either 50% sucrose/50% mannitol, 50% sorbitol/50% mannitol, sorbitol, or mannitol and compared with those containing macrogol 6000. The dissolution rates in de-ionised water at 25° decreased in the following order: mannitol > sorbitol/mannitol > sucrose/mannitol > sorbitol > macrogol 6000. No decomposition of hydrocortisone was detected (by ultraviolet spectrophotometry) during preparation of the dispersion systems or direct compression of tablets.[22]

Ho and Hajratwala[23] prepared hydrocortisone dispersions in macrogol 4000 by fusion and solvent methods. Decomposition (indicated by discoloration) occurred in all dispersions prepared by the fusion method. Hydrocortisone dispersions prepared in povidone by the solvent method[24] remained stable. Those dispersions containing more than 40% hydrocortisone exhibited increasing crystalline structure as was evident from X-ray diffraction patterns and scanning electron micrographs. Further investigation at 5-day intervals, of dissolution characteristics of macrogol dispersions and povidone dispersions, containing 40% hydrocortisone, stored at 25° for 30 days, revealed no change in the former but increased dissolution rates in the latter.[25]

In-vitro release from topical formulations

The release of hydrocortisone butyrate propionate from an oil-in-water cream or an aqueous gel containing propylene glycol, to a silicone rubber model of human skin (at 35°, 75% relative humidity) under open conditions correlated closely with that of in-vivo vasoconstrictor activity in human volunteers.[26] In comparison to open conditions, release under closed conditions was higher, except when ethanol was incorporated in the aqueous gel, in which case release was markedly higher under open conditions. The variations in the release patterns of the formulations under open and closed conditions were linked to the changes in the thermodynamic activity of hydrocortisone butyrate propionate in the vehicle during the release period.

The viscosity of suspension-type ointment bases comprising homogeneous mixtures of yellow soft paraffin with liquid paraffin 6%, 12%, or 18% w/w and containing hydrocortisone 4% w/w (as a model drug) inversely influenced the initial release rate of the drug and the cumulative amount of drug released.[27]

In-vitro release of hydrocortisone and hydrocortisone acetate from Carbopol (carbomer) 940 hydrogels to a propylene glycol sink was retarded with increasing concentrations of gelling agent.[28] In comparison with hydrocortisone, release of hydrocortisone acetate was slower and the effect of Carbopol concentration on release rate was less. The inclusion of propylene glycol in gel formulations had no significant effect on the release of the acetate ester but caused an increase in the release of hydrocortisone. Turakka and Ala-Fossi[29] used propylene glycol as a cosolvent in the aqueous liquid phase of Carbopol gel containing hydrocortisone or hydrocortisone acetate. Hydrocortisone was completely dissolved in hydrogels containing more than propylene glycol 60% in the liquid phase. Hydrocortisone acetate was partly soluble or almost insoluble in all the gels studied. The optimum concentration of propylene glycol (60%) for the release of hydrocortisone corresponded to the solubility limit of hydrocortisone.

The in-vitro release rate of hydrocortisone from Pluronic F-127 aqueous gels increased with an increase in drug concentration up to 0.125% w/v and an increase in temperature (20°, 30°, and 40°), but decreased with an increase in Pluronic F-127 (poloxamer) concentration (20% w/v, 25% w/v, and 30% w/v).[30] No pH dependency was observed.

Shah et al[31] developed a method for the determination of the in-vitro release of hydrocortisone from creams (hydrocortisone 2.5%: Synacort, Syntex; Hytone, Dermik), using the Franz diffusion cell and synthetic membranes (Triton-free cellulose, pure cellulose acetate, cellulose acetate with a wetting agent, polysulfone, and glass fibre). Drug release was slightly faster from Hytone cream than from Synacort cream. The rate was not affected by the polymeric membranes but the glass fibre membrane retarded the release rate.

The concentration of hydrocortisone 17-valerate 0.2% cream (pH 4.8, Westcort) decreased by about 10% immediately when extemporaneously compounded with urea 10% (HPLC analysis).[32] When compounded with salicylic acid 2%, physical separation of the cream occurred after one month at ambient temperature; however, this could be easily redispersed. In-vitro human skin penetration of hydrocortisone 17-valerate, using adapted Franz diffusion cells, was enhanced three-fold by salicylic acid 2%, but was not affected by compounding with an admixture of camphor, menthol and phenol, coal tar 5% solution, or urea 10%.

Percutaneous absorption

Sarpotdar and Zatz[33] examined the influence of low concentrations of nonionic surfactants (polysorbates 20, 40, and 60) on hydrocortisone penetration through hairless *mouse* skin *in vitro*. Inclusion of a surfactant increased the permeation rate of hydrocortisone when the vehicle contained a high concentration of propylene glycol (over 40%). Permeation was slower from aqueous media without propylene glycol but with surfactant.

In an investigation of several potential penetration enhancers, Barry and Bennett[34] established that hydrocortisone (as a model drug) penetrated human cadaver skin mainly by a lipid route. Increased permeation from acetone-deposited films due to the addition of water and propylene glycol together with decylmethyl sulphoxide was relatively small. Propylene glycol increased the amount penetrated in 60 hours by a factor of 30 and the duration of effect by a factor of 50. Hydrocortisone permeation of the skin was also enhanced by 2-pyrrolidone, *N*-methyl-2-pyrrolidone, *N*-methylformamide, an admixture of propylene glycol and Azone (laurocapram), and an admixture of propylene glycol and oleic acid.

The flux of hydrocortisone through *mouse* skin from solutions containing propylene glycol as cosolvent varied inversely with propylene glycol concentration,[35] whereas the flux from aqueous solutions containing 2-propanol was higher and independent of concentration. An increase in flux was produced by the addition of low concentrations of the surfactant polysorbate 80 to the 2-propanol solutions. The penetration flux from gels prepared with hydroxyethylcellulose was similar to that from the solutions.

FURTHER INFORMATION. Effect of supersaturation on membrane transport. 1. Hydrocortisone acetate [potential application in topical drug delivery]—Davis AF, Hadgraft J. Int J Pharmaceutics 1991;76:1–8. Release of hydrocortisone from topical semisolid preparations using three different *in vitro* methods—Tuomi A, Turakka L, Räty T, Lehmussaari K. Acta Pharm Fenn 1989;98:93–9. Microemulsions: evolving technology for cosmetic applications [as a drug delivery system for hydrocortisone]—Jayakrishran A, Kalaiarasi K, Shah DO. J Soc Cosmet Chem 1983;34:335–50. The effect of sodium lauryl sulphate on the electrophoretic mobility of hydrocortisone acetate—Djuric Z, Jovanovic M. Acta Polon Pharm 1985;42(4):389–95. Development and evaluation of an intracutaneous depot formulation of corticosteroids using Transcutol as a cosolvent: *in-vitro*, *ex-vivo*, and *in-vivo rat* studies—Panchagnula R, Ritschel WA. J Pharm Pharmacol 1991;43:609–14. Enzymic and non-enzymic hydrolysis of a polymeric prodrug: hydrocortisone esters of hyaluronic acid—Rajewski LG, Stinnett AA, Stella VJ, Topp EM. Int J Pharmaceutics 1992;82:205–13.

PROCESSING

Sterilisation

Hydrocortisone sodium phosphate injection can be sterilised by filtration.

Hydrocortisone acetate injection can be prepared using aseptic technique.

The particle size distribution of hydrocortisone and hydrocortisone acetate was not affected by sterilisation by gamma or electron irradiation at 4.5 Mrad and 15 Mrad.[36] However, a significant decrease of 22% in the specific surface area of hydrocortisone acetate was observed after prolonged gamma irradiation at 15 Mrad.

REFERENCES

1. Ponec M, Kempenaar J, Shroot B, Caron J-C. J Pharm Sci 1986;75(10):973–5.
2. Hansen J, Bundgaard H. Arch Pharm Chemi Sci 1979;7:135–46.
3. Hansen J, Bundgaard H. Arch Pharm Chemi Sci 1980;8:91–9.
4. Hansen J, Bundgaard H. Int J Pharmaceutics 1980;6:307–19.
5. Hansen J, Bundgaard H. Arch Pharm Chemi Sci 1981;9:55–60.
6. Adam PS, Cripps AL. J Pharm Pharmacol 1980;32:47P.
7. Cheung Y-W, Vishnuvajjala BR, Flora KP. Am J Hosp Pharm 1984;41:1802–6.
8. Anderson RW, Latiolais CJ. Am J Hosp Pharm 1970;27:540–7.
9. Siedlecka E, Zakrzewski Z [Polish]. Farm Pol 1985;41(7):378–81.
10. Das Gupta V. J Pharm Sci 1978;67(3):299–302.
11. Timmins P, Gray EA. J Clin Hosp Pharm 1983;8:79–85.
12. Das Gupta V. Drug Dev Ind Pharm 1985;11(12):2083–97.
13. Cradock JC, Kleinman LM, Rahman A. Am J Hosp Pharm 1978;35:402–6.
14. Yip YW, Li Wan Po A, Irwin WJ. J Pharm Sci 1983;72(7):776–81.
15. Andersen FM, Bundgaard H. Arch Pharm Chemi Sci 1983;11:61–6.
16. Kane MP, Tsuji K. J Pharm Sci 1983;72(1):30–5.
17. Bansal NP, Holleran EM, Jarowski CI. J Pharm Sci 1983;72(9):1079–82.
18. Chapman JH, Neustadter EL. J Pharm Pharmacol 1965;17:138S.
19. Cornejo J, Hermosin MC, White JL, Peck GE, Hem SL. J Pharm Sci 1980;69(8):945–8.
20. Möllmann H, Barth J, Möllmann C, Tunn S, Krieg M, Derendorf H. J Pharm Sci 1991;80(9):835–6.
21. Newrick PG, Braatvedt G, Hancock J, Corrall RJM. Lancet 1990;335:212–13.
22. Allen LV, Levinson RS, Martono DD. J Pharm Sci 1978;67(7):979–81.
23. Ho DSS, Hajratwala BR. Aust J Pharm Sci 1981;10(3):65–9.
24. Hajratwala BR, Ho DSS. Aust J Pharm Sci 1981;10(3):70–3.
25. Hajratwala BR, Ho DSS. J Pharm Sci 1984;73(11):1539–41.
26. Tanaka S, Takashima Y, Murayama H, Tsuchiya S. Int J Pharmaceutics 1985;27:29–38.
27. Purwar S, Prasad KPP, Lim JK. Pharm Ind 1990;52(12):1553–6.
28. Turakka L. Acta Pharm Fenn 1985;94:17–21.
29. Turakka L, Ala-Fossi N. Acta Pharm Fenn 1987;96:15–21.
30. Tomida H, Shinohara M, Kuwada N, Kiryu S. Acta Pharm Suec 1987;24:263–72.
31. Shah VP, Elkins J, Lam S-Y, Skelly JP. Int J Pharmaceutics 1989;53:53–9.
32. Krochmal L, Wang JCT, Patel B, Rodgers J. J Acad Dermatol 1989;21(5):979–84.
33. Sarpotdar PP, Zatz JL. Drug Dev Ind Pharm 1987;13(1):15–37.
34. Barry BW, Bennett SL. J Pharm Pharmacol 1987;39:535–46.
35. Shahi V, Zatz JL. J Pharm Sci 1978;67(6):789–92.
36. Illum L, Møller N. Arch Pharm Chemi Sci 1974;2:167–74.

Ibuprofen (BAN, USAN, rINN)

Analgesic; Anti-inflammatory

2-(4-Isobutylphenyl)propionic acid; α-methyl-4-(2-methylpropyl)benzeneacetic acid

$C_{13}H_{18}O_2 = 206.3$

CAS—15687-27-1

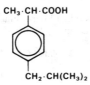

$CH_3 \cdot CH \cdot COOH$

$CH_2 \cdot CH(CH_3)_2$

Pharmacopoeial status

BP, USP

Preparations

Compendial

Ibuprofen Tablets BP. Coated tablets containing, in each, 200 mg, 400 mg, and 600 mg of ibuprofen are usually available. Ibuprofen Tablets USP.

Non-compendial

Apsifen (APS). *Tablets*, ibuprofen 200 mg and 400 mg.
Apsifen-F (APS). *Tablets*, ibuprofen 200 mg, 400 mg, and 600 mg.
Brufen (Boots). *Tablets*, ibuprofen 200 mg, 400 mg, and 600 mg.
Syrup, ibuprofen 100 mg/5 mL.
Granules, effervescent, ibuprofen 600 mg/sachet.
Brufen Retard (Boots). *Tablets*, sustained release, ibuprofen 800 mg.
Fenbid (SK&F). *Spansules* (*sustained-release capsules*), ibuprofen 300 mg.
Junifen (Boots). *Liquid*, sugar free, ibuprofen 100 mg/5 mL.
Ibugel (Dermal). *Gel*, ibuprofen 5% w/w.
Lidifen (Berk). *Tablets*, ibuprofen 200 mg, 400 mg, and 600 mg.
Motrin (Upjohn). *Tablets*, ibuprofen 200 mg, 400 mg, 600 mg, and 800 mg.
Proflex (Zyma). *Cream*, ibuprofen 5% w/w.
Ibuprofen tablets are also available, in various strengths, from Ashbourne (Arthrofen), Cox, DDSA (Ebufac), Evans, Kerfoot, Lagap (Ibular), Norton, Rima (Rimafen).
Ibuprofen gel is also available from DDD (Ibuleve).

Containers and storage

Solid state

Ibuprofen BP should be kept in a well-closed container.
Ibuprofen USP should be preserved in tight containers.

Dosage forms

Ibuprofen Tablets USP should be preserved in well-closed containers.
Apsifen, Apsifen-F, and Lidifen tablets should be stored at room temperature in a dry place and protected from light.
Brufen 600 mg tablets, Brufen granules, Brufen syrup, Brufen Retard tablets, and Junifen liquid should be stored below 25°.
Brufen syrup should be protected from light.
Fenbid spansules should be stored in a dry place, at a temperature not exceeding 30°, protected from light.
Ibugel gel should be stored at a temperature not exceeding 25° with the cap tightly replaced.
Motrin tablets should be stored at room temperature (15° to 30°) in a well-closed container.

Proflex cream should be protected from heat and stored below 30°.

PHYSICAL PROPERTIES

Ibuprofen exists as a white crystalline powder or colourless crystals.

Melting point

Ibuprofen melts in the range 75° to 78°.

Dissociation constant

pK_a^1 5.3
pK_a (ethanol 60%),[2] 5.2

Solubility

Ibuprofen is practically insoluble in water; soluble 1 in 1.5 of ethanol, 1 in 2 of ether, 1 in 1 of chloroform, and 1 in 1.5 of acetone. Ibuprofen is readily soluble in most organic solvents and is soluble in aqueous solutions of alkali hydroxides and carbonates. It is freely soluble in dichloromethane.

Effect of pH

A profile of ibuprofen solubility in water versus pH for the pH range 1.2 to 7.5 has been presented by Herzfeldt and Kümmel;[1] solubility increased rapidly at pH values higher than the pK_a. The approximate solubilities at pH 4, pH 6, and pH 7 were given as 1 in 35000, 1 in 1900, and 1 in 410 respectively.

Effect of temperature

Solubility of ibuprofen in aqueous buffer at pH 2 and in octanol as a function of temperature:[3]

	5°	25°	37°
Aqueous buffer, pH 2.0	$3.34 \times 10^{-5}M$	$4.3 \times 10^{-5}M$	$5.21 \times 10^{-5}M$
Octanol	0.059M	0.091M	0.122M

Dissolution

The USP specifies that for Ibuprofen Tablets USP not less than 70% of the labelled amount of $C_{13}H_{18}O_2$ is dissolved in 30 minutes. Dissolution medium: 900 mL of phosphate buffer pH 7.2; Apparatus 1 at 150 rpm.

Crystal and molecular structure

Ibuprofen has a chiral centre and can exist in two enantiomeric forms.
According to Hutt and Caldwell,[4] on administration of the racemic mixture, the pharmacologically inactive $R(-)$-enantiomer is converted to the active $S(+)$-enantiomer. A stereoselective assay is therefore necessary for pharmacokinetic studies and suitable methods have been developed by Maître et al[5] (HPLC) and Young et al[6] (GC-MS).

FURTHER INFORMATION. Characterisation of different crystal forms of ibuprofen, tinidazole and lorazepam—Udupa N. Drug Dev Ind Pharm 1990;16(9):1591–6. Studies on some crystalline forms of ibuprofen—Labhasetwar V, Deshmukh SV, Dorle AK. Drug Dev Ind Pharm 1993;19(6):631–41. Ibuprofen racemate and enantiomers: phase diagram, solubility and thermodynamic studies—Dwivedi SK, Sattari S, Jamali F, Mitchell AG. Int J Pharmaceutics 1992;87:95–104. Stereochemical aspects of the molecular pharmaceutics of ibuprofen—Romero AJ, Rhodes T. J Pharm Pharmacol 1993;45:258–62. Effects of crystallinity on absorption and excretion patterns of ibuprofen, tinidazole and lorazepam—Udupa N. Drug Dev Ind Pharm 1987;13(15):2749–69. Approaches to stereospecific preformulation of ibuprofen [studies of the racemate and the $S(+)$-isomer]—Romero AJ, Rhodes CT. Drug Dev Ind Pharm 1991;17(5):777–92. Comparative human study of ibuprofen enantiomer plasma concentrations produced by two commercially available ibuprofen tablets [tablets were not bioequivalent with respect to either enantiomer]—Cox SR, Brown MA, Squires DJ, Murrill EA, Lednicer D, Knuth DW. Biopharm Drug Dispos 1988;9:539-49. Disposition of ibuprofen enantiomers following the oral administration of a novel controlled release formulation [of the racemate] to healthy volunteers—Avgerinos A, Noormohammadi A, Hutt AJ. Int J Pharmaceutics 1991;68:97–103. The relationship between the pharmacokinetics of ibuprofen enantiomers and the dose of racemic ibuprofen in humans—Evans AM, Nation RL, Sansom LN, Bochner F, Somogyi AA. Biopharm Drug Dispos 1990;11:507–18.

STABILITY

Dondoni et al[7] used TLC and GLC to identify several products of the oxidative degradation of ibuprofen. In the absence of oxygen, ibuprofen was found to be stable, even at high temperatures (105° to 110°), for at least four days.

INCOMPATIBILITY/COMPATIBILITY

Interactions between ibuprofen and stearic acid, stearyl alcohol, calcium stearate, and magnesium stearate have been investigated by Gordon and co-workers.[8] Using differential scanning calorimetry, mixtures were heated at a rate of 1.5° per minute over the temperature range 30° to 110°. The formation of a simple eutectic mixture in each case indicated the incompatibility of the stearates with ibuprofen. The effect of these interactions on the chemical stability of ibuprofen was not determined.

Investigations of solid-state mixtures of ibuprofen and magnesium oxide stored at 55° and 40° indicated formation of the magnesium salt of ibuprofen.[9] No significant interaction was noted at 30° for up to 80 days. Ibuprofen showed no chemical degradation in the presence of magnesium oxide at 55°. Solid-state interactions (at 55°) were also reported between ibuprofen and magnesium hydroxide, sodium bicarbonate, potassium carbonate, or calcium oxide, but not between ibuprofen and magnesium chloride or aluminium hydroxide.

FORMULATION

Excipients

Excipients that have been used in presentations of ibuprofen include:

Capsules (spansules): sucrose.

Tablets: acacia; acetylated monoglycerides; black ink; brilliant blue FCF (133); calcium carbonate; calcium phosphate; calcium sulphate; carmellose sodium; carnauba wax; cellulose; colloidal silica; dimethicone; erythrosine (E127); gelatin; glucose; glyceryl triacetate; hydroxypropylcellulose; hypromellose; iron oxide; lecithin; macrogols 400 and 6000; magnesium stearate; maize starch; microcrystalline cellulose; pharmaceutical glaze; polysorbate 80; povidone; pregelatinised starch; propylene glycol; quinoline yellow (E104); sesame oil; shellac; silica; sodium benzoate; sodium lauryl sulphate; sodium starch glycollate; stearic acid; sucrose; sunset yellow FCF (E110); talc; titanium dioxide (E171); white beeswax.

Granules: sucrose.

Oral liquids: methyl and propyl hydroxybenzoates; sodium benzoate; sucrose; sunset yellow FCF (E110).

Suppositories: polysorbate 60; semi-synthetic glycerides.

Creams: fractionated coconut oil; glyceryl stearate and macrogol 100 stearate; lavender oil; macrogol 5 glyceryl stearate; propylene glycol; medium-chain triglycerides; sodium methyl hydroxybenzoate; xanthan gum.

Gels: carbomer; diethylamine; industrial methylated spirit; propylene glycol.

Bioavailability

Determination of the bioavailability of rectally administered ibuprofen sodium solution and aluminium ibuprofen suspension, relative to oral administration of the same compounds, showed that the suspension was less bioavailable than the solution irrespective of the route of administration (as measured by areas under plasma concentration versus time curves in eight healthy subjects).[10] The solution was approximately 13% less available when administered rectally.

Capsules

From a study of the effects of excipients (diluent, disintegrant, and glidant) on the pharmaceutical properties of ibuprofen hard gelatin capsule formulations, Hannula et al[11] concluded that formulations consisting of only ibuprofen and either lactose or calcium hydrogen phosphate as diluent possessed suitable properties for manual filling, whereas those formulations that contained ibuprofen with either lactose, spray-dried lactose, microcrystalline cellulose, or calcium hydrogen phosphate were suited to mechanical filling. The addition of a disintegrant (maize starch or carmellose sodium) and a glidant (talc) adversely affected dissolution of ibuprofen and content uniformity, respectively. The addition of sodium bicarbonate (as a disintegrant) to the diluent-based formulations did not markedly alter the dissolution rate of ibuprofen.[12] In a further study,[13] the disintegrants sodium starch glycollate (Explotab) or croscarmellose sodium (Ac-Di-Sol) were most effective in formulations containing calcium hydrogen phosphate. Both disintegrants also enhanced ibuprofen dissolution from sucrose-based capsules.

Injections

The solubility of ibuprofen[14] was increased 68-fold when it was dissolved in sodium benzoate 35% w/v solution at 35°. An aqueous solution formulated for parenteral use (ibuprofen 200 mg, 5 mL of sodium benzoate 30% w/v or 35% w/v, sodium metabisulphite 0.1%, and disodium edetate 0.01%) was sterilised by filtration. It had retained 93% of its initial ibuprofen concentration after 28 days storage at 8°. After storage for 22 days at 37°, 89.5% of the original ibuprofen concentration remained in the solution.

Ointments

The *in-vitro* release rate of ibuprofen from various topical bases decreased in the rank order: water-washable basis > hydrophilic basis > Canadian formulary basis > gel > macrogol water-washable basis > emulsion > cream > University of California basis.[15] The *in-vivo* bioavailability of ibuprofen (in *rabbits*) was significantly higher from the water-washable basis than from the other bases. Formulae for the ointments are presented.

Suspensions

When Law[16] compared the effects of nonionic water-soluble cellulose polymers (hypromellose and hydroxyethylcellulose) on the settling of ibuprofen particles, the results suggested that multilayer adsorption of polymer occurs with increasing polymer concentrations. Earlier work[17] indicated that particle stability is affected by steric stabilisation or flocculation depending on the concentration of polymer present. In a further study,[18] the same workers evaluated the same polymers and also hydroxypropyl-cellulose as suspending agents for ibuprofen dispersed in solutions adjusted to pH 4. Suspensions were flocculated at low polymer concentrations and deflocculated at high polymer concentrations, whichever polymer was used. However, flocculation was observed at high polymer concentrations in the suspensions that contained hydroxyethylcellulose.

Suppositories

Ibuprofen suppositories formulated by Ali and co-workers[19] contained one of the following bases; theobroma oil, Witepsol H-15, or macrogol 1540. The USP XX tablet dissolution apparatus (rotating basket, 100 rpm) and a cellophane dialysing membrane were used to obtain dissolution profiles in phosphate buffer at pH 8 and 37°. Release of ibuprofen by both in-vitro procedures occurred in the following rank order: macrogol 1540 > Witespol H-15 > theobroma oil. Bioavailability, based on serum concentrations in rabbits, was less from suppositories than from an oral suspension. Following rectal administration, the in-vivo bioavailability of ibuprofen was in general agreement with the results of in-vitro dissolution studies. The rapid release of ibuprofen in vitro from suppositories containing macrogol 1540 was attributed to the water solubility of the basis and the free solubility of ibuprofen at pH 8; a soluble complex may be formed between macrogol 1540 and ibuprofen. Ibuprofen decreased the melting range of suppositories made from Witepsol H-15 and theobroma oil. Suppositories containing Witepsol H-15 were the most brittle of the three formulations. A similar study by Ibrahim et al[20] concluded that in-vitro permeation (at pH 7.4) of ibuprofen from suppository bases occurred in the rank order: theobroma oil ≫ macrogol A > macrogol C > Witepsol E75 > macrogol D > macrogol B where,
    macrogol A = macrogol 1500:macrogol 4000 (3:1)
    macrogol B = macrogol 1500:macrogol 4000 (9:1)
    macrogol C = macrogol 1540:macrogol 6000 (7:3)
    macrogol D = macrogol 1540:macrogol 6000 (1:1).
Dissolution rates (in phosphate buffer) from the bases decreased in the rank order: theobroma oil > macrogol A > macrogol B > macrogol C = macrogol D > Witepsol E75.

Co-precipitates, complexes, and solid dispersions

There are many accounts in the literature of attempts to enhance the dissolution properties of ibuprofen by co-precipitation with Eudragits (polymethacrylates)[21] or urea,[22] by complexation with β-cyclodextrin,[23] or by dispersion in water-soluble polymer matrices, for example povidone[24,25] and macrogols.[26-29]

Modified-release preparations

Ibuprofen-loaded microspheres, prepared with cellulose acetate butyrate (CAB) or low molecular weight cellulose propionate (CPL) were formulated[30] with 0.5% w/v methylcellulose as stable suspensions buffered at pH 3.5. The suspensions of CAB and CPL microspheres showed less than 5% (pH independent) release, and approximately 8% (pH dependent) release of ibuprofen, respectively, after 30 days. There was no evidence of non-dispersible sedimentation, and uniform dose withdrawal was possible over the six-month study period. Ibuprofen blood concentrations (in rats) were sustained for longer by the suspension that contained CAB microspheres.
Kawashima et al[31] developed a controlled-release suspension of microspheres of ibuprofen with the acrylic polymer Eudragit RS-PM. Long-term uniform dispersibility in the suspension was achieved in a viscous acidic medium of carmellose sodium

by the addition of D-sorbitol which increased the amount of carmellose sodium adsorbed onto the microspheres. Without D-sorbitol, the suspensions could not be stabilised by carmellose sodium alone. During storage for six months, no leakage of ibuprofen from the microspheres was observed in the suspension.

FURTHER INFORMATION. Dissolution testing of ibuprofen tablets—Romero AJ, Grady LT, Rhodes CT. Drug Dev Ind Pharm 1988;14(11):1549–86. Predicting the dissolution rate of ibuprofen-acidic excipient compressed mixtures in reactive media—Healy AM, Corrigan OI. Int J Pharmaceutics 1992;84:167–73. The filling of molten ibuprofen into hard gelatin capsules [effect of low quantities of excipients]—Smith A, Lampard JF, Carruthers KM, Regan P. Int J Pharmaceutics 1990;59:115–19. Percutaneous absorption of ibuprofen: vehicle [propylene glycol] effects of transport through rat skin—Irwin WJ, Sanderson FD, Li Wan Po A. Int J Pharmaceutics 1990;66:193–200. Physico-chemical aspects of the complexation of some drugs [including ibuprofen] with cyclodextrins—Menard FA, Dedhiya MG, Rhodes CT. Drug Dev Ind Pharm 1990;16(1):91–113. Rapidly absorbed solid oral formulations of ibuprofen using water-soluble gelatin—Imai T, Kimura S, Iijima T, Miyoshi T, Ueno M, Otagiri M. J Pharm Pharmacol 1990;42:615–19. Pharmaceutical evaluation of ibuprofen fast-absorbed syrup containing low-molecular-weight gelatin—Kimura S, Imai T, Ueno M, Otagiri M. J Pharm Sci 1992;81(2):141–8. A new ibuprofen pulsed release oral dosage form [three-layer tablet, in vitro/in vivo correlation]—Conte U, Colombo P, La Manna A, Gazzaniga A, Sangalli ME, Guinchedi P. Drug Dev Ind Pharm 1989;15(14-16):2583–96. Ibuprofen-loaded ethylcellulose microspheres: analysis of the matrix structure by thermal analysis—Dubernet C, Rouland JC, Benoit JP. J Pharm Sci 1991;80(11):1029–33. Preparation of controlled-release microspheres of ibuprofen with acrylic polymers by a novel quasi-emulsion solvent diffusion method—Kawashima Y, Niwa T, Handa T, Takeuchi H, Iwamato T, Itoh K. J Pharm Sci 1989;78(1):68–72.
Uniform and improved bioavailability of newly developed rapid and sustained release suspensions of ibuprofen microspheres—Kawashima Y, Iwamoto T, Niwa T, Takeuchi H, Hino T. Int J Pharmaceutics 1993;89:9–17. Preparation and characterisation of sustained-release ibuprofen-cetostearyl alcohol spheres—Wong LP, Gilligan CA, Li Wan Po A. Int J Pharmaceutics 1992;83:95–114. Development and evaluation of sustained-release ibuprofen-wax microspheres. Part 1. Effect of formulation variables on physical characteristics—Adeyeye CM, Price JC. Pharm Res 1991;8:1377–83. Bimodal release of ibuprofen in a sustained-release formulation: a scintigraphic and pharmacokinetic open study in healthy volunteers under different conditions of food intake—Wilson CG, Washington N, Greaves JL, Kamali F, Rees JA, Sempik AK, et al. Int J Pharmaceutics 1989;50:155–61. Sustained release from matrix system comprising hydrophobic and hydrophilic (gel-forming) parts—Malamataris S, Ganderton D. Int J Pharmaceutics 1991;70:69–75. Evaluation of ethylcellulose as a matrix for prolonged release formulations. II. Sparingly water-soluble drugs: ibuprofen and indomethacin [solid dispersions of ibuprofen and ethylcellulose with 0.5% Primogel and 0.5% magnesium stearate]—Shaikh NA, Abidi SE, Block LH. Drug Dev Ind Pharm 1987;13(14):2495–518.

PROCESSING

Compacts

Marshall et al[32] have shown that both the applied pressure and the duration of compression influence the axial recovery of compacts of ibuprofen recrystallised from methanol. It has been suggested that with increasing compression time there is a change in the utilisation of compaction energy from reversible to irreversible deformation; this change results in reduced recovery of a compact at a given pressure. Similar trends were observed for samples of ibuprofen recrystallised from different solvents.

FURTHER INFORMATION. Fluid bed granulation of ibuprofen—Haldar R, Gangadharan B, Martin D, Mehta A. Drug Dev Ind Pharm 1989;15(14–16):2675–9. Determination of ibuprofen vapour pressure [9×10^{-6} mm Hg at 25°] at temperatures of pharmaceutical interest—Ertel KD, Heasley RA, Koegel C, Chakrabarti A, Carstensen JT [letter]. J Pharm Sci 1990;79(6):552.

REFERENCES

1. Herzfeldt CD, Kümmel R. Drug Dev Ind Pharm 1983;9:767–93.
2. Davis LJ. Drug Intell Clin Pharm 1975;9:501–3.
3. Fini A, Laus M, Orienti I, Zecchi V. J Pharm Sci 1986;75:23–5.
4. Hutt AJ, Caldwell J. J Pharm Pharmacol 1983;35:693–704.
5. Maître JM, Boss G, Testa B. J Chromatogr 1984;299:397–403.
6. Young MA, Aarons L, Davidson EM, Toon S. J Pharm Pharmacol 1986;38:60P.
7. Dondoni A, Dall'Occo T, Fantin G, Medici A, Pedrini P. Il Farmaco Ed Prat 1986;41:237–44.
8. Gordon RE, VanKoevering CL, Reits DJ. Int J Pharmaceutics 1984;21:99–105.
9. Kararli TT, Needham TE, Seul CJ, Finnegan PM. Pharm Res 1989;6(9):804–8.
10. Eller MG, Wright III C, Della-Coletta AA. Biopharm Drug Dispos 1989;10:269–78.
11. Hannula AM, Marvola M, Kopra T. Acta Pharm Fenn 1989;98:11–20.
12. Hannula AM, Marvola M, Aho E. Acta Pharm Fenn 1989;98:131–4.
13. Hannula AM, Marvola M, Jöns M. Acta Pharm Fenn 1989;98:189–96.
14. Jain NK, Jahagirdar A. Pharmazie 1989;44:727–8.
15. Muktadir A, Babar A, Cutie AJ, Plakogiannis FM. Drug Dev Ind Pharm 1986;12(14):2521–40.
16. Law SL. Drug Dev Ind Pharm 1985;11:2137–41.
17. Law SL, Kayes JB. Int J Pharmaceutics 1983;15:251–60.
18. Law SL, Kayes JB. Drug Dev Ind Pharm 1984;10:1049–69.
19. Ali A, Kazmi S, Deutsch T, Plakogiannis FM. Drug Dev Ind Pharm 1982;8:411–28.
20. Ibrahim SA, El-Faham TH, Tous SS, Mostafa EM. Int J Pharmaceutics 1990;61:1–7.
21. Kislalioglu MS, Khan MA, Blount C, Goettsch RW, Bolton S. J Pharm Sci 1991;80(8):799–804.
22. Mura P, Liguori A, Bramanti G. Il Farmaco Ed Prat 1986;41(12):378–87.
23. Chow DND, Karara AH. Int J Pharmaceutics 1986;26:95–101.
24. El-Hinnawi MA, Najib NM. Int J Pharmaceutics 1987;37:175–7.
25. Najib NM, El-Hinnawi MA, Suleiman MS. Int J Pharmaceutics 1988;45:139–44.
26. Mohamed MS, Ghazy FS, Mahdy MA. Pharm Ind 1985;47(12):1293–5.
27. Mura P, Liguori A, Bramanti G, Poggi L. Il Farmaco Ed Prat 1987;42:157–64.
28. Najib NM, Salem MAS. Drug Dev Ind Pharm 1987;13(12):2263–75.
29. Mura P, Liguori A, Bramanti G. Il Farmaco Ed Prat 1987;42:149–56.
30. Dalal PS, Narurkar MM. Int J Pharmaceutics 1991;73:157–62.
31. Kawashima Y, Iwamoto T, Niwa T, Takeuchi H, Itoh Y. Int J Pharmaceutics 1991;75:25–36.
32. Marshall PV, York P, Richardson R. J Pharm Pharmacol 1986;38:47P.

Imipramine (BAN, rINN)   *Tricyclic antidepressant*

3-(10,11-Dihydro-5*H*-dibenz[*b,f*]azepin-5-yl)propyldimethyl-amine; 10,11-dihydro-*N,N*-dimethyl-5*H*-dibenz[*b,f*]azepine-5-propanamine
$C_{19}H_{24}N_2 = 280.4$

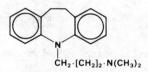

Imipramine Embonate (BANM, rINNM)
Imipramine pamoate
$(C_{19}H_{24}N_2)_2, C_{23}H_{16}O_6 = 949.2$

Imipramine Hydrochloride (BANM, rINNM)
Imizine
$C_{19}H_{24}N_2, HCl = 316.9$
CAS—50-49-7 (imipramine); 10075-24-8 (imipramine embonate); 113-52-0 (imipramine hydrochloride)

Pharmacopoeial status

BP, USP (imipramine hydrochloride)

Preparations

Compendial
Imipramine Tablets BP. Contain imipramine hydrochloride. Coated tablets containing, in each, 10 mg and 25 mg are usually available.
Imipramine Hydrochloride Tablets USP.
Imipramine Hydrochloride Injection USP. pH between 4.0 and 5.0.

Non-compendial
Tofranil (Geigy). *Tablets*, imipramine hydrochloride 10 mg and 25 mg.
Syrup, imipramine hydrochloride 25 mg/5 mL. *Diluents*: for dilutions down to 15 mg/5 mL, boiled, distilled or de-ionised water can be used; for dilutions below 15 mg/5 mL the recommended diluent is equal parts syrup and tragacanth mucilage (freshly prepared). The diluted syrup should be used within a few days.

Containers and storage

Solid state
Imipramine Hydrochloride BP should be kept in a well-closed container and protected from light.
Imipramine Hydrochloride USP should be preserved in tight containers.

Dosage forms
Imipramine Hydrochloride Tablets USP should be preserved in tight containers.
Imipramine Hydrochloride Injection USP should be preserved in single-dose containers, preferably of Type I glass.
Tofranil tablets should be protected from moisture.
Tofranil syrup should be protected from heat and containers kept tightly closed.

PHYSICAL PROPERTIES

Imipramine hydrochloride is a white or slightly yellow crystalline powder; odourless or almost odourless; it has a bitter taste followed by a sensation of numbness.
Imipramine hydrochloride absorbs insignificant amounts of moisture at 23° at relative humidities up to about 60%; under more humid conditions it absorbs significant amounts.
Imipramine embonate is a yellow powder.

Melting point

Imipramine hydrochloride melts in the range 170° to 174°.

pH

A 10% solution of *imipramine hydrochloride* has a pH of about 4.7.

Dissociation constant

pK_a 9.5 (24°)
From the relationship between hydrogen ion concentration and total solubility values for imipramine Green[1] determined a pK_a of 9.5 at 24°.

Partition coefficient

Log *P* (octanol/pH 7.4), 2.5
Partition of imipramine between isotonic phosphate buffer at pH 7.4 and several organic solvents (chloroform, *n*-hexane, ether, and 1,2-dichloroethane) has been investigated.[2] After equilibration, more than 98% of the imipramine was present in the organic phases.

Solubility

Imipramine hydrochloride is soluble 1 in 2 of water, 1 in 1.5 of ethanol, and 1 in 1.5 of chloroform; it is soluble in acetone, practically insoluble in ether, and insoluble in benzene.
Imipramine embonate is insoluble in water; soluble in ethanol, in chloroform, and in ether.
The solubility of imipramine free base in water has been determined[1] as 6.5×10^{-5} M at 24°.

Dissolution

The USP specifies that for Imipramine Hydrochloride Tablets USP not less than 75% of the labelled amount of $C_{19}H_{24}N_2$, HCl is dissolved in 45 minutes. Dissolution medium: 900 mL of 0.1 N hydrochloric acid; Apparatus 1 at 100 rpm.

STABILITY

Imipramine hydrochloride in the solid state is stable for several years when stored at room temperature provided that moisture is absent and that it is protected from light. Solutions of imipramine hydrochloride in water are stable when oxygen is absent and the solutions are protected from light.
Degradation occurs in the presence of water and oxygen and is accelerated by light and by an increase in temperature. Among the reactions which may occur are loss of the basic alkyl chain

with the formation of iminodibenzyl, hydroxylation followed by dehydration to the iminostilbene derivative, and ring contraction with the formation of the highly fluorescent acridine and acridone derivatives.
Iminodibenzyl is a starting material in the synthesis of imipramine hydrochloride but its presence as one of several impurities in commercial imipramine and in tablets is a possible decomposition product of imipramine.[3,4]

Solutions

Solutions of imipramine hydrochloride (5 mg/mL) in chloroform water in half-filled glass ampoules were stored for 28 days either exposed to light or in the dark at ambient temperature; samples were also kept in a refrigerator (4°) together with other solutions in purified water. A reddish-brown discoloration was observed in solutions exposed to light at ambient temperature.[5] Chromatograms (TLC) of solutions stored in the dark or in a refrigerator were identical to those of freshly prepared solutions; they all revealed five impurities, one of which was identified as iminodibenzyl. No significant decrease of imipramine hydrochloride concentration was detected in solutions (in either chloroform water or purified water) stored under any of the above conditions.
The manufacturers of Tofranil injection (Geigy, USA) state that, upon storage, minute crystals may form in some ampoules but this does not affect the therapeutic efficacy of the preparation. The crystals redissolve when the affected ampoules are immersed in hot tap water for one minute.

FURTHER INFORMATION. GLC method for iminodibenzyl and desipramine impurities in imipramine hydrochloride [solid state] and its formulated products—Thompson DW. J Pharm Sci 1982;71(5):536–8.

FORMULATION

Excipients

Excipients that have been used in presentations of imipramine include:
Capsules, imipramine embonate: brilliant blue FCF (133); disodium calcium edetate; erythrosine (E127); gelatin; hydroxybenzoates; magnesium stearate; sodium lauryl sulphate; sodium propionate; starch; sunset yellow FCF (E110); talc; tartrazine (E102); titanium dioxide (E171).
Tablets, imipramine hydrochloride: calcium phosphate; cellulose compounds; colloidal silica; docusate sodium; glycerol; iron oxides (E172); lactose; macrogol; magnesium stearate; maize starch; povidone; sodium starch glycollate; stearic acid; sucrose; talc; titanium dioxide (E171).
Oral liquids, imipramine hydrochloride: methyl and propyl hydroxybenzoates; sucrose; wild cherry syrup.
Injections (intramuscular), imipramine hydrochloride: ascorbic acid; sodium bisulphite; sodium sulphite, anhydrous.

Suppositories

A preliminary investigation of the partitioning of imipramine hydrochloride between purified water and a lipid phase and of its diffusion across a lipid-impregnated cellulose membrane indicated that the rectal route might be a suitable means of administration.[6] Suppositories of imipramine hydrochloride 75 mg in 2 g of a semi-synthetic glyceride basis (Suppocire NAI 10) were prepared. When suppositories were assessed (initially, and after 7 days of storage at 30°) their physicochemical properties exhibited changes only in spreading area; no degradation was evident. Studies of the kinetics of release measurements (rotating basket) gave dissolution $t_{10\%}$ values of 9 ± 1 minutes for imipramine hydrochloride. In *rabbits*, the relative bioavailability of imipramine hydrochloride (10 mg) administered as suppositories was 25% compared to an intravenous injection (Tofranil, Ciba Geigy).

Buccal absorption

Bickel and Weder[2] showed that buccal absorption of imipramine hydrochloride, administered to four subjects as mouthrinse solutions in several buffers at pH 4.5 to 9.0, increased as the pH of the solution increased. See also Dissociation constant and Partition coefficient, above.

Novel dosage forms

Ramsey *et al*[7] have prepared gel-precipitated spheres of aluminium hydroxide that contained imipramine hydrochloride (formula included: imipramine hydrochloride 1.6 g, Wisprofloc P [a water-soluble starch] 10 g in 150 mL, and aluminium chlorohydrate solution 80 mL). Release of imipramine hydrochloride from the spheres into media at 37° was a complex process controlled either by dissolution of, or diffusion through, the aluminium hydroxide gel matrix. Spheres heated at 90° for four hours showed a greater release rate of imipramine hydrochloride than unheated spheres. For both heated and unheated spheres (unwashed), an increase in the pH of the dissolution medium caused a decrease in the rate of release.

FURTHER INFORMATION. Drug partitioning and release characteristics of tricyclic antidepressant drugs using a series of related hydrophilic-hydrophobic copolymers [made from polyethylene oxide and a polydimethylsiloxane derivative]—Sung C, Raeder JE, Merrill EW. J Pharm Sci 1990;79(9):829–34.

REFERENCES

1. Green AL. J Pharm Pharmacol 1967;19:10–16.
2. Bickel MH, Weder HJ. J Pharm Pharmacol 1969;21:160–8.
3. Adank K, Hammerschmidt W. Chimia 1964;18:361–3.
4. McErlane KM, Curran NM, Lovering EG. J Pharm Sci 1977;66(7):1015–18.
5. Buckles J, Walters V. J Clin Pharm 1976;1:113–18.
6. Chaumeil JC, Khoury JM, Zuber M, Courteille F, Piraube C, Gard C. Drug Dev Ind Pharm 1988;14(15-17):2225–39.
7. Ramsey MP, Newton JM, Shaw GG, Sammon DC, Lane ES. J Pharm Pharmacol 1987;37:1–4.

Indomethacin (BAN, USAN)

Anti-inflammatory; Analgesic

Indometacin (rINN)
1-(4-Chlorobenzoyl)-5-methoxy-2-methylindol-3-ylacetic acid; 1-(4-chlorobenzoyl)-5-methoxy-2-methyl-1*H*-indole-3-acetic acid
$C_{19}H_{16}ClNO_4 = 357.8$

Indomethacin Sodium (BANM, USAN)
Indometacin Sodium (rINNM)
$C_{19}H_{15}ClNNaO_4, 3H_2O = 433.8$

CAS—53-86-1 (indomethacin); 74252-25-8 (indomethacin sodium)

Pharmacopoeial status

BP (indomethacin); USP (indomethacin, indomethacin sodium)

Preparations

Compendial
Indomethacin Capsules BP. Capsules containing, in each, 25 mg and 50 mg are usually available.
Indomethacin Suppositories BP. Suppositories containing, in each, 100 mg indomethacin in a suitable suppository basis are usually available.
Indomethacin Capsules USP.
Indomethacin Extended-release Capsules USP.
Indomethacin Oral Suspension USP.
Indomethacin Suppositories USP.
Sterile Indomethacin Sodium USP.

Non-compendial
Flexin (Napp). *Tablets*, controlled release, indomethacin 25 mg (Flexin-25 Continus), 50 mg (Flexin-LS Continus), and 75 mg (Flexin Continus).
Imbrilon (Berk). *Capsules*, indomethacin 25 mg and 50 mg.
Suppositories, indomethacin 100 mg in a macrogol basis.
Indocid (Morson). *Capsules*, indomethacin 25 mg and 50 mg.
Capsules (Indocid R), sustained release, indomethacin 75 mg.
Suspension, sugar free, indomethacin 25 mg/5 mL. Should not be diluted. Indocid Suspension is unstable in alkaline media and, therefore, should not be mixed with an antacid; the two preparations should be administered separately.
Suppositories, indomethacin 100 mg in macrogol basis.
Injection (Indocid PDA), lyophilised powder for reconstitution, unbuffered, indomethacin (as sodium trihydrate) 1 mg/vial. Should be reconstituted by the addition of either 1 or 2 mL of water for injections or sodium chloride 0.9% injection immediately before use. Glucose injection should not be used for reconstitution. Reconstitution at pH levels below 6 may cause precipitation of insoluble indomethacin. Further dilution with intravenous infusion solutions is not recommended.
Indolar SR (Lagap). *Capsules*, sustained release, indomethacin 75 mg.
Indomax 75 SR (Ashbourne). *Capsules*, modified release, indomethacin 75 mg.
Indomod (Kabi Pharmacia). *Capsules*, modified release with enteric-coated pellets, indomethacin 25 mg and 75 mg.
Rheumacin SR (CP). *Capsules*, modified release, indomethacin 75 mg.
Slo-Indo (Generics). *Capsules*, modified release, indomethacin 75 mg.
Indomethacin capsules in various strengths are also available from APS, Ashbourne (Indomax), Cox, DDSA (Artracin), Evans, Galen (Mobilan), Kerfoot, Rima (Rimacid).
Indomethacin suppositories are also available from Cox, Evans, Norton.

Containers and storage

Solid state
Indomethacin BP should be stored in well-closed containers, protected from light.
Indomethacin USP and Indomethacin Sodium USP should be preserved in well-closed, light-resistant containers.

Dosage forms
Indomethacin Capsules USP and Indomethacin Extended-release Capsules USP should be preserved in well-closed containers.

Indomethacin Oral Suspension USP should be preserved in tight, light-resistant containers.

Indomethacin Suppositories USP should be stored in well-closed containers, at controlled room temperature.

Sterile Indomethacin Sodium USP should be preserved in containers suitable for sterile solids.

Flexin Continus tablets should be stored at or below 20°.

Imbrilon preparations should be stored in a cool place, protected from light.

Indocid capsules, sustained-release capsules (Indocid R), suspension, and suppositories should be stored in well-closed containers in a dry place below 25°, and protected from light. Indocid suspension should be protected from freezing.

Indolar SR capsules should be stored in a cool, dry place, protected from light.

PHYSICAL PROPERTIES

Indomethacin is a white to brownish-yellow, odourless or almost odourless, crystalline powder.

Indomethacin sodium is a pale yellow crystalline powder.

Melting point

Indomethacin is generally reported to melt in the range 158° to 162°. Melting points have been cited for various polymorphic forms (see Crystal and molecular structure, below).

pH

A 1% solution of *indomethacin sodium* in water has a pH of 8.4.

Dissociation constant

pK_a 4.5 (carboxyl group)

Partition coefficient

Log P (octanol/pH 7.4), -1.0

Solubility

Indomethacin is practically insoluble in water; soluble in ethanol (1 in 50), in acetone, in chloroform (1 in 30), in ether (1 in 40 to 45), and in castor oil; dissolves in dilute mineral acids. The solubility of indomethacin in methanol at 25° is 32 mg/g.[1]

Indomethacin sodium is soluble in water and in ethanol; very slightly soluble in chloroform and in acetone; very soluble in methanol.

Dissolution

The USP specifies that for Indomethacin Capsules USP not less than 80% of the labelled amount of $C_{19}H_{16}ClNO_4$ is dissolved in 20 minutes. Dissolution medium: 750 mL of a mixture of phosphate buffer, pH 7.2, 1 volume and water 4 volumes; Apparatus 1 at 100 rpm.

The USP specifies that for Indomethacin Extended-release Capsules USP 10% to 32%, 20% to 52%, 35% to 80%, not less than 60%, and not less than 80% of the labelled amount of $C_{19}H_{16}ClNO_4$ is dissolved in 0.083D, 0.167D, 0.333D, 1.000D, and 2.000D hours, respectively, where D represents the labelled dosing interval in hours. Dissolution medium: 900 mL of phosphate buffer, pH 6.2; Apparatus 1 at 75 rpm.

The USP specifies that for Indomethacin Oral Suspension USP not less than 80% of the labelled amount of $C_{19}H_{16}ClNO_4$ is dissolved in 20 minutes. Dissolution medium: 900 mL of 0.01M phosphate buffer, pH 7.2, prepared by dissolving 1.36 g of monobasic potassium phosphate in 1 litre of water and adjusting with 0.1N sodium hydroxide to a pH of 7.2 ± 0.1; Apparatus 2 at 50 rpm.

The USP specifies that for Indomethacin Suppositories USP not less than 75% of the labelled amount of $C_{19}H_{16}ClNO_4$ is dissolved in 60 minutes. Dissolution medium: 900 mL of 0.1M phosphate buffer, pH 7.2: Apparatus 2 at 50 rpm.

FURTHER INFORMATION. Automated dissolution testing of indomethacin capsules and tablets [novel method]—Herzfeldt CD. Pharmaceut Technol 1984;8(70):73–6.

Crystal and molecular structure

Polymorphs

Borka[2] characterised four polymorphic forms of indomethacin, Form I (m.p. 160° to 161°), Form II (m.p. 154°), Form III (m.p. 148° to 149°), and Form IV (m.p. 133° to 134°). A solvent-containing 'pseudopolymorphic' modification (m.p. 90° to 100°) and an amorphous form (m.p. 55° to 57°) were also described. Transition of indomethacin from amorphous form to crystalline form has been found to follow first-order kinetics at 20°, 30°, and 40° with half-lives calculated to be 8.12, 3.12, and 0.70 days, respectively.[3]

FURTHER INFORMATION. Preparations of agglomerated crystals of polymorphic mixtures and a new complex of indomethacin-epirizole by the spherical crystallization technique—Kawashima Y, Lin SY, Ogawa M, Handa T, Takenaka H. J Pharm Sci 1985;74:1152–6. Isolation and solid-state characteristics of a new crystal form of indomethacin—Lin S-Y. J Pharm Sci 1992;81(6):572–6.

STABILITY

Indomethacin undergoes hydrolytic degradation with the formation of *p*-chlorobenzoate and 2-methyl-5-methoxy-indol-3-acetate. Hydrolysis is generally base-catalysed although at pH values less than 3, acid catalysis occurs. Base-catalysed hydrolysis of indomethacin has been shown to follow first-order kinetics. Values have been cited[1] for the degradation half-life of indomethacin at room temperature to be about 200 hours in pH 8 buffer, and about 90 minutes in pH 10 buffer. Li Wan Po *et al*[4] reported activation energy values for the base-catalysed hydrolysis of indomethacin of 65.4 kJ/mol and 68.4 kJ/mol for non-isothermal and isothermal methods, respectively.

Indomethacin is unstable to light, both in the solid state and in aqueous solution. Discoloration (darkening) of indomethacin solutions may occur on exposure to sunlight.

Indomethacin solution 50 micrograms/mL in pH 7.2 buffer, prepared for the purposes of a research study, was found to be chemically stable for 3 months when stored at 5° in glass containers or in plastic syringes.[5]

Stabilisation

Several workers have studied micellar solubilisation by the addition of surfactants as a method of stabilising indomethacin solutions. Surfactants included: ethoxylated lanolin, polysorbate 80, cetrimonium bromide;[6] polysorbates;[7] anionic and cationic surfactants;[8] and Pluronics (poloxamers).[9]

Backensfeld *et al* examined the effects of a number of cyclodextrins and cyclodextrin derivatives on the stability of indomethacin in aqueous solution. Beta-cyclodextrin was observed[10] to have the most favourable ring size for the stabilisation of indomethacin at pH 7.4. The derivatives studied (in particular, those of either *γ*- or *β*-cyclodextrin) also reduced the extent of hydrolysis, especially the derivatives that had lipophilic (for example, methyl or ethyl) substituents. The stabilising effect was greater as more hydroxyl groups of the glucose moiety were substituted.

FURTHER INFORMATION. Kinetics and mechanism of the basic hydrolysis of indomethacin and related compounds: a re-evaluation—Cipiciani A, Ebert C, Linda P, Rubessa F, Savelli G. J Pharm Sci 1983;72:1075–6. Nucleophilic aminoalcohol-catalyzed degradation of indomethacin in aqueous solution—Tomida H, Kuwada N, Tsuruta Y, Kohashi K, Kiryu S. Pharm Acta Helv 1989;64(11):312–15. Effect of zinc-ion on indomethacin degradation in alkaline aqueous solutions—Singla AK, Babber P, Pathak K. Drug Dev Ind Pharm 1991;17(10):1411–18. Photostability of indomethacin in crystalline form. Part 2.—Ekiz-Gucer N, Reisch J [German]. Pharm Acta Helv 1991;66(3):66–7. Kinetics of alkaline hydrolysis of indomethacin in the presence of surfactants and cosolvents—Suleiman MS, Najib NM. Drug Dev Ind Pharm 1990;16(4):695–706. Hydrolysis of indomethacin in Pluronic F-127 gels—Tomida H, Kuwada N, Kiryu S. Acta Pharm Suec 1988;25:87–96.

INCOMPATIBILITY/COMPATIBILITY

Incompatibility between indomethacin and benzalkonium chloride has been reported in eye drop formulations with ion-pair formation causing precipitation.[11]

FURTHER INFORMATION. Incompatibility of injectable indomethacin with gentamicin sulfate or tobramycin sulfate—Thompson DE, Heflin NR [letter]. Am J Hosp Pharm 1992;49:836, 838.

FORMULATION

INDOMETHACIN MIXTURE
The following description was given in the *British Pharmaceutical Codex 1973*: a suspension containing indomethacin in a suitable coloured vehicle; may contain a preservative; pH 4.3 to 4.7. The mixture should be stored in a cool place but should not be allowed to freeze. It should not be diluted.

Excipients

Excipients that have been used in presentations of indomethacin include:

Capsules, indomethacin: allura red AC (E129); brilliant blue FCF (133); cellulose; colloidal silica; confectioner's sugar; erythrosine (E127); fast green FC; gelatin; hydrogenated vegetable oil; hypromellose; indigo carmine (E132); lactose; lecithin; magnesium stearate; microcrystalline cellulose; polysorbate 80; polyvinyl acetate; polyvinyl acetate-crotonic acid copolymer; povidone; quinoline yellow (E104); sodium lauryl sulphate; starch; sucrose; tartrazine (E102); titanium dioxide (E171).
Suspensions, indomethacin: antifoam AF emulsion; chloroform water; ethanol; glycerol; hydrochloric acid; methyl and propyl hydroxybenzoates; raspberry syrup; sodium hydroxide; sorbic acid; sorbitol; syrup; tragacanth.
Eye drops (solutions), indomethacin: borax; boric acid; dextran; disodium edetate; macrogol 400.
Eye drops (suspensions), indomethacin: benzalkonium chloride; benzyl alcohol; disodium edetate; hydroxyethylcellulose; lecithin; phenethyl alcohol; polysorbate 80; sodium acid sulphite; sodium chloride; sorbitol.
Suppositories, indomethacin: acrylic polymers; butylated hydroxyanisole; butylated hydroxytoluene; edetic acid; glycerol; macrogols, including macrogol 3350, 4000, 6000, and 8000; povidone; sodium chloride.
Injections, indomethacin sodium: sodium acid phosphate; sodium hydroxide.

Bioequivalence

In a three-way, crossover study involving twelve healthy subjects over a seven day period, the bioavailabilities of Imbrilon (Berk) and Indocid (Morson) capsules (25 mg three times daily) did not differ significantly. However, the area under the plasma concentration versus time curve for Indocid R (sustained-release capsule, 75 mg twice daily), when normalised for dose, was significantly greater than that of Imbrilon but not significantly different to that of Indocid.[12]
McElnay *et al*[13] did not determine any marked differences between the *in-vivo* release properties of Indocid (Morson) and Imbrilon (Berk) suppositories (100 mg indomethacin) in twelve healthy volunteers.
The pharmacokinetic properties of commercially available suppositories comprising indomethacin in either an emulsifying basis (Suppocire-AP) or a water-soluble basis (macrogols 4000 and 6000) have been compared by Dutch workers.[14] From plasma indomethacin profiles in ten volunteers, following single doses, the authors concluded that the products were bioequivalent.

Paediatric preparations

Paediatric suspensions of indomethacin (2 mg/mL) extemporaneously prepared from indomethacin powder or from capsules and dispersed in syrup (containing 10% ethanol) had pH values of 5.2 and 5.6, respectively. After storage at 24° in amber-coloured containers for up to 224 days, less than 6% decomposition was determined (by ultraviolet spectroscopy); there was negligible change in pH.[15]
Of six extemporaneously prepared indomethacin formulations for paediatric use in Australia[16] (0.25 mg/mL to 5 mg/mL), five were suspensions (of pH between 4.95 and 5.8) and the other was a buffered solution (phosphate buffer to pH 8.15). Tragacanth was the suspending agent in two instances and the vehicles were either water, glycerol, or syrup (with and without sorbitol). The preservatives were chloroform or hydroxybenzoates (with and without ethanol). In samples stored at 20°, 35°, 55°, and ambient temperature, in amber or clear bottles, chemical decomposition was greater than 10% within 4 weeks for four of the preparations, and was approaching 10% after about 12 weeks for two. Under refrigeration, only a low-concentration suspension (0.25 mg/mL) degraded by more than 10% in less than 12 weeks. Decomposition rates at all temperatures were faster in the two suspensions of lower concentration and fastest in the buffered solution of the same concentration (possibly due to catalysis by hydroxide ions). With the exception of the solution, the pH of all samples decreased during storage. Effects caused by exposure to sunlight were not marked but slight discoloration was evident in samples kept in clear bottles. Caking was severe in the glycerol-based suspension and moderate in the syrup-containing products. With one exception (the syrup/sorbitol/tragacanth formulation), viscosity values remained constant throughout the 12 weeks.

Ophthalmic preparations

Following accelerated stability studies (at 85° to 100°), Vulovic *et al*[17] reported 'satisfactory' stability of indomethacin in suspensions (buffered to pH 5.6) that contained the preservative phenylmercuric nitrate and either hypromellose 0.5% or polyvinyl alcohol 1.4% to increase viscosity. Under ambient conditions $t_{10\%}$ was approximately 280 days and an activation energy of 106.2 kJ/mol was calculated for the indomethacin suspension containing polyvinyl alcohol. The particle size distribution of indomethacin in suspension was greatly affected by heating at 100° for 30 minutes. Inclusion of polyvinyl alcohol

1.4% or hypromellose 0.5% in the suspension protected indomethacin against significant changes in particle size distribution. In a further study of similar suspensions for ophthalmic use (buffered to pH 5.6), the same group[18] reported that benzalkonium chloride was an unsuitable preservative for indomethacin 1% w/v; precipitation was observed. The authors suggested phenylmercuric nitrate 0.002% w/v as a suitable preservative for indomethacin suspensions despite the observation that 90% of the preservative was adsorbed to indomethacin powder.

Suppositories

Apparent decomposition rate constants at 100° for indomethacin in macrogols (300, 4000, and 6000) alone and mixed with ethylene glycol have been presented. A preliminary study of macrogol-based suppositories of commercial origin led Finnish workers[19] to recommend a shelf-life of less than five years. Subsequently, workers from the same Finnish group[20] identified the triethylene glycol ester of indomethacin in commercial indomethacin suppositories (Inmetsin 100 mg) from 23 batches stored at room temperature for up to three years. Maximum ester concentration was approximately 4.5% of the original indomethacin content.

Data from a comparative study of a continuous flow-through bead bed dissolution technique and the USP XXI rotating paddle dissolution method indicated that the release rate of indomethacin was faster from water-soluble macrogol suppository bases than from fatty bases.[21] The release rate from fatty bases increased significantly in the presence of a surfactant.

The extent of release *in vitro* of indomethacin from suppositories prepared by the fusion method with several different bases decreased in the rank order: macrogols > glycerinated gelatin with macrogol and water > theobroma oil = Witepsol.[22] A significant increase in the proportion of indomethacin released from fatty bases and a small increase from water-soluble bases was noted following the addition of polysorbate 80 to the formulation.

Ointments and pertucaneous absorption

Kazmi *et al*[23] compared and correlated the *in-vitro* release and *in-vivo* absorption (through *rabbit* skin) of indomethacin (1%, 3%, and 5%) from ointment bases of two types. Release and bioavailability of indomethacin were greater from the absorption basis than from the hydrophilic basis.

The rate of absorption of indomethacin from aqueous solution through excised hairless *mouse* skin increased with a decrease in the pH of the solution.[24] The *in-vitro* absorption rate was enhanced by the addition of sodium lauryl sulphate or sodium cholate. Indomethacin patches containing sodium lauryl sulphate 4% or sodium cholate 4% and 6% produced greater and faster drug penetration than that from patches containing indomethacin alone. *In-vivo* studies in *rabbits* also demonstrated a greater rate and extent of absorption of indomethacin from a patch containing sodium cholate 6% compared to that from a patch containing indomethacin alone. An optimal pH of about 5 was suggested for the preparation of a transdermal delivery system for indomethacin.

Modified-release preparations

From a review of the literature in 1984, Green[25] was unable to support the development of sustained-release preparations of indomethacin; improved efficacy or a reduction of side-effects compared to conventional preparations could not be demonstrated.

Two groups of workers have developed sustained-release solid dispersions of indomethacin (as a model drug) using Eudragit

RS and Eudragit RL,[26] or Eudragit E[27] (polymethacrylates) as carriers. The Italian group[27] noted fast dissolution of indomethacin in solid dispersion with Eudragit E in media at pH 1.2, but a marked delay in dissolution in media at pH 7.5. The kinetics of drug release could be modified at pH 5.8 by varying the drug:polymer ratio.

Hadzija *et al*[28] examined the relative bioavailabilities of indomethacin in a controlled-release pellet formulation (CR Indomethacin Pellets, Temmler Werke, FRG) and an immediate-release capsule (Indocin, MSD) in a randomised crossover study involving eight healthy volunteers. A comparison of coating levels on the pellets revealed different *in-vivo* release characteristics. The relative bioavailability of the controlled-release formulation (75 mg once daily) compared to that of the immediate-release capsules (25 mg three times daily) during a study period of 24 hours was 1.077.

Morimoto *et al*[29] used a polyvinyl alcohol hydrogel as a controlled-release delivery system for the rectal administration of indomethacin. Although plasma concentrations of indomethacin were low, sustained plateau concentrations were observed over a longer time following rectal administration of the hydrogel formulation to *rats* compared to levels obtained after administration of a Witepsol-based suppository. An increase in plasma concentration of indomethacin corresponded with an increase in the pH of the hydrogel formulation and correlated with *in-vitro* predictions. Bioavailability of the hydrogel relative to the suppository was approximately 70% in *dogs*.

In physical mixtures of indomethacin with microcrystalline cellulose prepared by Laakso *et al*,[30] macrogol decreased the rate of indomethacin release. An increase in the amount of macrogol (4% to 8%) further reduced the dissolution rate from capsules and tablets prepared from the mixtures. The addition of polysorbate 80 to the mixtures did not compensate the inhibiting effect of macrogol on indomethacin release.

Laakso and Eerikäinen[31] demonstrated that the release of indomethacin (as a model drug) from film-coated granules was dependent on the water solubility and 'swellability' of the filler. Release was enhanced when maize starch was used as filler. The structures of granules containing sodium indomethacin trihydrate with various fillers (lactose, glucose, microcrystalline cellulose, maize starch, and calcium hydrogen phosphate) were subsequently investigated[32] as were the effects of these fillers on the release rates (in phosphate buffer pH 7.2 at 37°) of sodium indomethacin trihydrate from uncoated and film-coated granules. The results indicated 100% release from uncoated granules within ten minutes. Rates of release were similar from all granules except from those prepared with maize starch or calcium hydrogen phosphate, which gave slower release rates. Release was not markedly affected by the porosity of the ethylcellulose/hypromellose film except when maize starch was included.

Similar experiments with the same fillers in spheronised granules led to the conclusion that spheronisation produced granules with different indomethacin release rates.[33]

Further studies[34] identified indomethacin and calcium to be constituents of the precipitate formed during a reaction between sodium indomethacin and calcium hydrogen phosphate in aqueous solution at pH 7.2. It was suggested that the precipitate was the calcium salt of indomethacin.

Granules containing solid dispersions of indomethacin and macrogol 6000 were prepared by various techniques and compressed into tablets by Ford.[35] None of the techniques produced tablets with the enhanced dissolution rates previously shown by unformulated solid dispersions.

The potential of cyclodextrin polymer (CDP) as a disintegrant and its effect on the physical properties of indomethacin tablets were investigated by Turkish workers.[36] The dissolution rates of the tablets were increased and CDP was described as a good disintegrating agent.

Novel drug delivery systems

Oral drug delivery systems based on osmotic pumps that controlled the rate of drug release were developed in the early 1980s. Elementary or mini-osmotic pumps were designed to deliver their contents in solution at a constant rate, thus preventing large fluctuations in plasma-drug concentration. *Osmosin* was an elementary osmotic pump that contained indomethacin; however, it was recalled shortly after its introduction in Europe because of an unacceptable incidence of damage to the gastrointestinal wall.

Solubilisation

Najib and Suleiman[37] determined that the aqueous solubility of indomethacin (based on free energy change values at 25°) was most enhanced by sodium lauryl sulphate (1%) followed, in descending rank order, by polysorbate 80 (1%), macrogol 6000 (5%), and povidone (5%).

The bile salts cholic acid and deoxycholic acid, when conjugated with tripeptides, were shown[38] to enhance the solubility and dissolution rate of indomethacin in phosphate buffer pH 7.2 at 25°.

FURTHER INFORMATION. The effect of bases and formulation on the release of indomethacin from suppositories—*in vitro*—Othman S, Muti H. Drug Dev Ind Pharm 1986;12:1813–31. Kinetics of indomethacin release from suppositories. *In vitro-in vivo* correlation—Aiache J, Islasse M, Beyssac E, Aiache S, Renoux R, Kantelip J. Int J Pharmaceutics 1987;39:235–42. Study on the release of indomethacin from suppositories: *in vitro-in vivo* correlation—Lootvoet G, Beyssac E, Shiu GK, Aiache J-M, Ritschel WA. Int J Pharmaceutics 1992;85:113–20. Influence of fat composition on the melting behaviour and on the *in vitro* release of indomethacin suppositories—De Muynck C, Remon JP. Int J Pharmaceutics 1992;85:103–12. 1-Alkylazacycloalkan-2-one esters as prodrugs of indomethacin for improved delivery through human skin—Bonina FP, Montenegro L, De Caprans P, Bousquet E, Tirendi S. Int J Pharmaceutics 1991;77:21–9. Formulation design of indomethacin gel ointment containing *d*-limonene using computer optimisation methodology—Takayama K, Okabe H, Obata Y, Nagai T. Int J Pharmaceutics 1990;61:225–34. Novel approach for preparation of pH-sensitive hydrogels for enteric drug delivery—Dong L, Hoffman AS. J Controlled Release 1991;15:141–52. Release rate of indomethacin from coated granules—Sarisuta N, Sirithunyalug J. Drug Dev Ind Pharm 1988;14:683–7. Preparation and *in vitro* evaluation of controlled-release dosage form of indomethacin [micropellets]—Sa B, Roy S, Das SK. Drug Dev Ind Pharm 1987;13:1267–78. Sustained release of indomethacin from chitosan granules in beagle *dogs*—Miyazaki S, Yamaguchi H, Yockouchi C, Takada M, Hou W. J Pharm Pharmacol 1988;40:642–3.

Sustained release [of indomethacin] from matrix system comprising hydrophobic [hydrogenated vegetable oil] and hydrophilic [carboxypolymethylene] (gel-forming) parts—Malamataris S, Ganderton D. Int J Pharmaceutics 1991;70:69–75. An osmotically controlled delivery system for the treatment of arthritis [review]—Young JH. Br J Pharm Pract 1983;5(7):24–31. Targeting drugs to the enterohepatic circulation; a potential drug delivery system designed to enhance the bioavailability of indomethacin [effect of enteric coating and of exogenous addition of bile acids]—Cole SK, Story MJ, Laudanksi T, Dwyer M, Attwood D, Robertson J *et al.* Int J Pharmaceutics 1992;80:63–73. The properties of solid dispersions of indomethacin or phenylbutasone in polyethylene glycol [macrogol]—Ford JL, Stewart AF, Dubois JL. Int J Pharmaceutics 1986;28:11–22. The effect of storage on the dissolution rate of some drug-polyethylene glycol [macrogol] 6000 solid dispersions—Dubois JL, Chaumeil JC, Ford JL. STP Pharma 1985;1(8):711–14. A study of indomethacin-nicotinamide solid dispersions—Eshra AG, Naggar VF, Boraie NA. Pharm Ind 1986;48(12):1557–60. Improved dissolution of indomethacin in coprecipitates with phospholipids-I—Habib MJ, Akogyeram C, Ahmadi B. Drug Dev Ind Pharm 1993;19(4):499–505. Indomethacin delivery from matrix controlled release indomethacin [in macrogol 6000 in a Eudragit RS matrix] tablets—Gurnasinghari ML, Bhatt HR, Lalla JK. J Controlled Release 1989;8:211–22. Preparation of a controlled release drug delivery system of indomethacin: effect of process equipment, particle size of indomethacin, and size of the nonpareil seeds—Li SP, Feld KM, Kowarski CR. Drug Dev Ind Pharm 1989;15(8):1137–59. *In vitro* release of selected nonsteroidal anti-inflammatory analgesics (NSAIA) from reservoir-type transdermal formulations—Berba J, Goranson S, Langle J, Banakar UV. Drug Dev Ind Pharm 1991;17(1):55–65. Encapsulation and *in vitro* release of indomethacin [blended with semi-synthetic glycerides] from semi-solid matrix [hard shell gelatin] capsules—Naidoo NT. Int J Pharmaceutics 1989;55:53–7. Interaction of indomethacin with low molecular weight chitosan, and improvements of some pharmaceutical properties of indomethacin by low molecular weight chitosans—Imai T, Shiraishi S, Saito H, Otagiri M. Int J Pharmaceutics 1991;67:11–20. Modelling drug release from hydrophobic matrices [two indomethacin formulations containing acrylic/methacrylic copolymer] by use of thermodynamic activation parameters—Efentakis M, Buckton G. Int J Pharmaceutics 1990;60:229–34. [Reduced] bioavailability of indomethacin from zinc-indomethacin complex—Singla AK, Mediratta DK, Pathak K. Int J Pharmaceutics 1990;60:27–33. Indomethacin and cyclodextrin complexes [preparation and characterisation]—Lin S-Z, Wouessidjewe D, Poelman M-C, Duchêne D. Int J Pharmaceutics 1991;69:211–19. High-field nuclear magnetic resonance techniques for the investigation of a β-cyclodextrin:indomethacin inclusion complex—Djedaini F, Lin S-Z, Perly B, Wouessidjewe D. J Pharm Sci 1990;79(7):643–6. Stability of indomethacin-containing liposomes on long-term storage—Gürsoy A, Akbuga J. J Controlled Release 1988;8:127–31. *In vitro* release kinetic pattern of indomethacin from poly(D,L-lactide) nanocapsules—Ammoury N, Fessi H, De Vissaguet JP, Puisieux F, Benita S. J Pharm Sci 1990;79(9):763–7. Indomethacin polymeric nanosuspensions prepared by microfluidisation—Bodmeier R, Chen H. J Controlled Release 1990;12:223–33. Evaluation of indomethacin nanocapsules for their physical stability and inhibitory activity on inflammation and platelet aggregation—Gürsoy A, Eroglu L, Ulutin S, Tasyürek M, Fessi H, Puisieux F *et al.* Int J Pharmaceutics 1989;52:101–8.

The influence of three poly(oxyethylene)poly(oxypropylene) surface-active block copolymers [Pluronics] on the solubility behaviour of indomethacin—Lin S-Y, Kawashima Y. Pharm Acta Helv 1985;60(12):339–43. Solubilisation of indomethacin by polysorbate 80 in mixed water-sorbitol solvents—Attwood D, Ktistis G, McCormick Y, Story MJ. J Pharm Pharmacol 1989;41:83–6.

REFERENCES

1. O'Brien M, McCauley J, Cohen E. In: Florey K, editor. Analytical profiles of drug substances; vol 13. London: Academic Press, 1984:211–38.

2. Borka L. Acta Pharm Suec 1974;11:295–303.
3. Imaizumi H, Nambu N, Nagai T. Chem Pharm Bull 1980;28:2565–9.
4. Li Wan Po A, Elias AN, Irwin WJ. Acta Pharm Suec 1983;20:277–86.
5. Carter MA, Lewis CW [letter]. Pharm J 1982;228:569.
6. Dawson JE, Hajratwala BR, Taylor H. J Pharm Sci 1977;66:1259–63.
7. Krasowska H. Int J Pharmaceutics 1979;4:89–97.
8. Cipiciani A, Ebert C, Germani R, Linda P, Lovrecich M, Rubessa F et al. J Pharm Sci 1985;74:1184–7.
9. Lin S-Y, Kawashima Y. Pharm Acta Helv 1985;60(10):345–50.
10. Backensfeld T, Müller BW, Wiese M, Seydel JK. Pharm Res 1990;7(5):484–90.
11. Dreijer-van der Glas SM, Bult A. Pharm Weekbl (Sci) 1987;9:29–32.
12. Farrar K, Calvert R, Bird H, Metha A. Pharm J 1986;237:767.
13. McElnay JC, Taggart AJ, Kerr B, Passmore P. Int J Pharmaceutics 1986;33:195–9.
14. Jonkman JHG, van der Boon WJV, Schoenmaker R, Holtkamp A. Drug Res 1984;34(I)(4):523–5.
15. Das Gupta V, Gibbs CW, Ghanekar AG. Am J Hosp Pharm 1978;35:1382–5.
16 Stewart PJ, Doherty PG, Bostock JM, Petrie AF. Aust J Hosp Pharm 1985;15(1):55–60.
17. Vulovic N, Primorac M, Stupar M, Ford JL. Int J Pharmaceutics 1989;55:123–8.
18. Vulovic N, Primorac M, Stupar M, Brown MW, Ford JL. Pharmazie 1990;45(H9):678–9.
19. Kahela P, Liponkoski L, Hurmerinta T. Acta Pharm Fenn 1979;88:113–16.
20. Ekman R, Liponkoski L, Kahela P. Acta Pharm Suec 1982;19(4):241–6.
21. Archondikis A, Papaioannou G. Int J Pharmaceutics 1989;55:217–20.
22. Suleiman MS, Najib NM. Drug Dev Ind Pharm 1990;16(4):707–17.
23. Kazmi S, Kennon L, Sideman M, Plakogiannis FM. Drug Dev Ind Pharm 1984;10(7):1071–83.
24. Chiang C-H, Lai J-S, Yang K-H. Drug Dev Ind Pharm 1991;17(1):91–111.
25. Green JA. Drug Intell Clin Pharm 1984;18:1004–7.
26. Oth MP, Moës AJ. Int J Pharmaceutics 1989;55:157–64.
27. De Filippis P, Boscolo M, Gibellini M, Rupena P, Rubessa F, Moneghini M. Drug Dev Ind Pharm 1991;17(14):2017–28.
28. Hadzija BW, Obeng EK, Ruddy SB, Noormohammadi A, Beckett AH. Int J Pharmaceutics 1991;67:185–94.
29. Morimoto K, Nagayasu A, Fukanoki S, Morisaka K, Hyan S-H, Ikada Y. Pharm Res 1989;6(4):338–41.
30. Laakso R, Järveläinen O, Kristofferson E. Acta Pharm Fenn 1988;97:175–80.
31. Laakso R, Eerikäinen S. Int J Pharmaceutics 1991;67:79–88.
32. Eerikäinen S, Yliruusi J, Laakso R. Int J Pharmaceutics 1991;71:201–11.
33. Eerikäinen S, Lindqvist A-S. Int J Pharmaceutics 1991;75:181–92.
34. Eerikäinen S, Muttonen G, Yliruusi J. Int J Pharmaceutics 1992;80:259–61.
35. Ford JL. Pharm Acta Helv 1983;58(4):101–8.
36. Tarimci N, Celebi N. Pharmazie 1988;43:323–5.
37. Najib NM, Suleiman MS. Int J Pharmaceutics 1985;24:165–71.
38. Tripathi M, Kohli DV, Uppadhyay RK. Int J Pharmaceutics 1991;67:207–9.

Insulin   *Hypoglycaemic*

'Insulin' is the natural antidiabetic hormone from the pancreas of either the *pig* or the *ox*, appropriately purified. It consists of two chains of amino acids, the A and B chains, connected by two disulphide bridges.

'Human insulin' is a protein with the structure of the natural antidiabetic hormone produced by the human pancreas. Human insulin (emp) is produced by the enzymatic modification of insulin obtained from the porcine pancreas. Human insulin (crb) is produced by the chemical combination of A and B chains which have been obtained from bacteria genetically modified by recombinant DNA technology. Human insulin (prb) is produced from proinsulin obtained from bacteria genetically modified by recombinant DNA technology. Human insulin (pyr) is insulin produced from a precursor obtained from a yeast genetically modified by recombinant DNA technology.

Porcine insulin : $C_{256}H_{381}N_{65}O_{76}S_6 = 5777.6$
Bovine insulin : $C_{254}H_{377}N_{65}O_{75}S_6 = 5733.54$
Human insulin : $C_{257}H_{383}N_{65}O_{77}S_6 = 5807.6$

CAS—9004-10-8 (insulin; neutral insulin); 11070-73-8 (bovine insulin); 12584-58-6 (porcine insulin); 11061-68-0 (human insulin); 8063-29-4 (biphasic insulin); 9004-21-1 (globin zinc insulin); 8049-62-5 (insulin zinc suspensions); 53027-39-7 (isophane insulin); 9004-17-5 (protamine zinc insulin); 9004-12-0 (dalanated insulin); 51798-72-2 (bovine insulin defalan); 11091-62-6 (porcine insulin defalan)

Pharmacopoeial status

BP (insulin, human insulin); USP (insulin, insulin human)

Preparations

Compendial
For all the following BP preparations, injections containing 100 units/mL are usually available:

Biphasic Insulin Injection BP (Biphasic Insulin). A sterile suspension of crystals containing insulin (beef) in a solution of insulin (pork). pH 6.6 to 7.2. It is a white suspension; when examined under a microscope, the majority of the particles are seen as rhombohedral crystals, with a maximum dimension, when measured from corner to corner through the crystal, greater than 10 micrometres but rarely exceeding 40 micrometres.

Biphasic Isophane Insulin Injection BP (Biphasic Isophane Insulin). It is either a sterile buffered suspension of insulin (pork), complexed with protamine sulphate or another suitable protamine, in a solution of insulin (pork) or a sterile buffered suspension of human insulin, complexed with protamine sulphate or other suitable protamine, in a solution of human insulin. pH 6.9 to 7.5. It is a white suspension which on standing deposits a white sediment and leaves a colourless or almost colourless supernatant liquid. The sediment is readily resuspended by gentle shaking. When examined under a microscope, the particles in the sediment are seen to be rod-shaped crystals the majority having a dimension not less than 1 micrometre and rarely exceeding 60 micrometres, free from large aggregates.

Insulin Injection BP (Neutral Insulin; Neutral Insulin Injection; Soluble Insulin). A sterile solution of insulin or of human insulin. pH 6.6 to 8.0. It is a colourless liquid free from turbidity and foreign matter; during storage traces of a very fine sediment may be deposited.

Insulin Zinc Suspension BP (IZS; Insulin Zinc Suspension, Mixed). A sterile, neutral suspension of insulin or of human insulin in the form of a complex obtained by the addition of a suitable zinc salt; the insulin is in a form insoluble in water. When prepared from insulin it contains either beef or pork insulin or a mixture of beef and pork insulin. pH 6.9 to 7.5. It is a white suspension which on standing deposits a white sediment and leaves a colourless or almost colourless supernatant liquid. The sediment is readily resuspended by gentle shaking. When examined under a microscope, the majority of the particles are seen as rhombohedral crystals with a maximum dimension, when measured from corner to corner through the crystal, greater than 10 micrometres but rarely exceeding 40 micrometres; a considerable proportion of the particles can be seen under high power magnification to have no uniform shape and not to exceed 2 micrometres in maximum dimension.

Insulin Zinc Suspension (Amorphous) BP (Amorph. IZS). A sterile, neutral suspension of insulin (beef or pork) in the form of a complex obtained by the addition of a suitable zinc salt; the insulin is in a form insoluble in water. pH 6.9 to 7.5. It is a white suspension which on standing deposits a white sediment and leaves a colourless or almost colourless supernatant liquid. The sediment is readily resuspended by gentle shaking. When examined under a microscope, the particles are seen to have no uniform shape and rarely exceed 2 micrometres in maximum dimension.

Insulin Zinc Suspension (Crystalline) BP (Cryst. IZS). A sterile, neutral suspension of insulin (beef) or of human insulin in the form of a complex obtained by the addition of a suitable zinc salt; the insulin is in the form of crystals insoluble in water. pH 6.9 to 7.5. It is a white suspension which on standing deposits a white sediment and leaves a colourless or almost colourless supernatant liquid. The sediment is readily resuspended by gentle shaking. When examined under a microscope, the particles are seen to be rhombohedral crystals, the majority having a maximum dimension, when measured from corner to corner through the crystal, greater than 10 micrometres but rarely exceeding 40 micrometres.

Isophane Insulin Injection BP (Isophane Protamine Insulin Injection; Isophane Insulin; Isophane Insulin, NPH). A sterile suspension of insulin or of human insulin in the form of a complex obtained by the addition of protamine sulphate or another suitable protamine. pH 6.9 to 7.5. It is a white suspension which on standing deposits a white sediment and leaves a colourless or almost colourless supernatant liquid. The sediment is readily resuspended by gentle shaking. When examined under a microscope, the particles in the sediment are seen to be rod-shaped crystals the majority having a dimension not less than 1 micrometre and rarely exceeding 60 micrometres, free from large aggregates.

Insulin Injection USP. pH between 2.5 and 3.5, determined potentiometrically, for acidified Insulin Injection; pH between 7.0 and 7.8, determined potentiometrically, for neutral Insulin Injection.

Insulin Human Injection USP. pH between 7.0 and 7.8, determined potentiometrically.

Isophane Insulin Suspension USP. pH between 7.0 and 7.8, determined potentiometrically.

Insulin Zinc Suspension USP. pH between 7.0 and 7.8, determined potentiometrically.

Extended Insulin Zinc Suspension USP. pH between 7.0 and 7.8, determined potentiometrically.

Prompt Insulin Zinc Suspension USP. pH between 7.0 and 7.8, determined potentiometrically.

Protamine Zinc Insulin Suspension USP. pH between 7.1 and 7.4, determined potentiometrically.

Non-compendial
Human Actraphane 30/70 (Novo Nordisk). *Injection*, biphasic isophane insulin (human, pyr), 30% soluble, 70% isophane, 100 units/mL (*excipients*: glycerol, sodium phosphate, *m*-cresol, phenol).

Human Actrapid and Human Actrapid Penfill (Novo Nordisk). *Injections*, soluble insulin (human, pyr) 100 units/mL (*excipients*: glycerol, *m*-cresol).

Human Initard 50/50 (Novo Nordisk Wellcome). *Injection*, biphasic isophane insulin (human, emp), 50% soluble, 50% isophane, 100 units/mL (*excipients*: sodium phosphate, *m*-cresol, phenol).

Human Insulatard (Novo Nordisk Wellcome). *Injection*, isophane insulin (human, emp) 100 units/mL (*excipients*: sodium phosphate, *m*-cresol, phenol).

Human Mixtard 30/70 (Novo Nordisk Wellcome). *Injection*, biphasic isophane insulin (human, emp), 30% soluble, 70% isophane, 100 units/mL (*excipients*: sodium phosphate, *m*-cresol, phenol).

Human Monotard (Novo Nordisk). *Injection*, insulin zinc suspension (human, pyr), 30% amorphous, 70% crystalline, 100 units/mL (*excipients*: sodium chloride, sodium acetate, methyl hydroxybenzoate).

Human Protaphane and Human Protaphane Penfill (Novo Nordisk). *Injections*, isophane insulin (human, pyr) 100 units/mL (*excipients*: glycerol, sodium phosphate, *m*-cresol, phenol).

Human Ultratard (Novo Nordisk). *Injection*, insulin zinc suspension, crystalline (human, pyr) 100 units/mL (*excipients*: sodium chloride, sodium acetate, methyl hydroxybenzoate).

Human Velosulin (Novo Nordisk Wellcome). *Injection*, soluble insulin (human, emp) 100 units/mL (*excipients*: sodium phosphate, *m*-cresol).

Humulin I (Lilly). *Injection*, isophane insulin (human, prb) 100 units/mL (*excipients*: phosphate buffer, *m*-cresol, phenol).

Humulin Lente (Lilly). *Injection*, insulin zinc suspension (human, prb), 30% amorphous, 70% crystalline, 100 units/mL (*excipients*: methyl hydroxybenzoate).

Humulin M1, Humulin M2, Humulin M3, Humulin M4 (Lilly). *Injections*, biphasic isophane insulin (human, prb); 10% soluble, 90% isophane (M1); 20% soluble, 80% isophane (M2); 30% soluble, 70% isophane (M3); 40% soluble, 60% isophane (M4). Each contains 100 units/mL (*excipients*: *m*-cresol, phenol).

Humulin S (Lilly). *Injection*, soluble insulin (human, prb) 100 units/mL (*excipients*: *m*-cresol).

Humulin Zn (Lilly). *Injection*, insulin zinc suspension, crystalline (human, prb) 100 units/mL (*excipients*: methyl hydroxybenzoate).

Hypurin Isophane (CP). *Injection*, isophane insulin (bovine, highly purified) 100 units/mL (*excipients*: glycerol, phosphate buffer, *m*-cresol, phenol).

Hypurin Lente (CP). *Injection*, insulin zinc suspension (bovine, highly purified), 30% amorphous, 70% crystalline, 100 units/mL (*excipients*: acetate buffer, methyl hydroxybenzoate).

Hypurin Neutral (CP). *Injection*, soluble insulin (bovine, highly purified) 100 units/mL (*excipients*: phosphate buffer, *m*-cresol, phenol).

Hypurin Protamine Zinc (CP). *Injection*, protamine zinc insulin (bovine, highly purified) 100 units/mL (*excipients*: phosphate buffer, glycerol, phenol).

Initard 50/50 (Novo Nordisk Wellcome). *Injection*, biphasic isophane insulin (porcine, highly purified), 50% soluble, 50% isophane, 100 units/mL (*excipients*: sodium phosphate, *m*-cresol, phenol).

Insulatard (Novo Nordisk Wellcome). *Injection*, isophane insulin (porcine, highly purified) 100 units/mL (*excipients*: sodium phosphate, *m*-cresol, phenol).

Lentard MC (Novo Nordisk). *Injection*, insulin zinc suspension (bovine, highly purified, 70% and porcine, highly purified, 30%) 100 units/mL (*excipients*: sodium chloride, sodium acetate, methyl hydroxybenzoate).

Mixtard 30/70 (Novo Nordisk Wellcome). *Injection*, biphasic isophane insulin (porcine, highly purified), 30% soluble, 70% isophane, 100 units/mL (*excipients*: sodium phosphate, *m*-cresol, phenol).

PenMix 10/90 Penfill, PenMix 20/80 Penfill, PenMix 30/70 Penfill, PenMix 40/60 Penfill, PenMix 50/50 Penfill (Novo Nordisk). *Injections*, biphasic isophane insulin (human, pyr): 10% soluble, 90% isophane (10/90); 20% soluble, 80% isophane (20/80); 30% soluble, 70% isophane (30/70); 40% soluble, 60% isophane (40/60); 50% soluble, 50% isophane (50/50). Each contains 100 units/mL (*excipients* 30/70: glycerol, sodium phosphate, *m*-cresol, phenol).

PenMix 30/70 (Novo Nordisk). *Injection*, device containing biphasic isophane insulin (human, pyr), 30% soluble, 70% isophane, 100 units/mL.

Pur-In Isophane (CP). *Injection*, isophane insulin (human, emp) 100 units/mL (*excipients*: zinc chloride, glycerol, sodium acid phosphate, phenol, *m*-cresol).

Pur-In Neutral (CP). *Injection*, soluble insulin (human, emp) 100 units/mL (*excipients*: glycerol, sodium acid phosphate, *m*-cresol).

Pur-In Mix 15/85, Pur-In Mix 25/75, Pur-In Mix 50/50 (CP). *Injections*, biphasic isophane insulin (human, emp): 15% soluble, 85% isophane (15/18); 25% soluble, 75% isophane (25/75); 50% soluble, 50% isophane (50/50). Each contains 100 units/mL.

Rapitard MC (Novo Nordisk). *Injection*, biphasic insulin (bovine, highly purified, 75% and porcine, highly purified, 25%) 100 units/mL (*excipients*: sodium chloride, sodium acetate, methyl hydroxybenzoate).

Semitard MC (Novo Nordisk). *Injection*, insulin zinc suspension, amorphous (porcine, highly purified) 100 units/mL (*excipients*: sodium chloride, sodium acetate, methyl hydroxybenzoate).

Velosulin (Novo Nordisk Wellcome). *Injection*, soluble insulin (porcine, highly purified) 100 units/mL (*excipients*: sodium phosphate, *m*-cresol).

Humulin M1, M2, M3, and M4 (Lilly) cartridges are for use with B-D pens (Becton Dickinson).

Penfill (Novo Nordisk) cartridges are for use with Novopen devices (Novo Nordisk).

Pur-In (CP) cartridges are for use with Pur-In pens (CP).

Manufacturers' data sheets should be consulted for specific details of the correct appearance of solutions and suspensions before administration and for information about methods of resuspension and mixing of preparations.

Containers and storage

Solid state

Insulin BP and Human Insulin BP should be kept in airtight containers, protected from light and stored at a temperature not exceeding −20°.

Insulin USP should be preserved in tight containers, protected from light, in a cold place.

Insulin Human USP should be preserved in tight containers, in a cold place.

Dosage forms

All BP insulin preparations should be stored at a temperature of 2° to 8°; they should not be allowed to freeze. Under these conditions they may be expected to retain their potency for not less than two years.

Insulin Injection USP should be preserved in a refrigerator; avoid freezing. It should be dispensed in the unopened, multiple-dose container in which it was placed by the manufacturer. The container for Insulin Injection, up to 100 USP units/mL, is of approximately 10-mL capacity and contains not less than 10 mL of the injection; the container for Insulin Injection, 500 USP units/mL, is of approximately 20-mL capacity and contains not less than 20 mL of the injection.

Insulin Human Injection USP should be preserved in a refrigerator; avoid freezing. The container for Insulin Human Injection, 40 or 100 USP units/mL, is of approximately 10-mL capacity and contains not less than 10 mL of the injection; and the container for Insulin Human Injection, 500 USP units/mL, is of approximately 20-mL capacity and contains not less than 20 mL of the injection.

Isophane Insulin Suspension USP, Insulin Zinc Suspension USP, Extended Insulin Zinc Suspension USP, Prompt Insulin Zinc Suspension USP, and Protamine Zinc Insulin Suspension USP should all be preserved in a refrigerator; avoid freezing. They should be dispensed in the unopened, multiple-dose containers in which they were placed by the manufacturers. Containers are of approximately 10-mL capacity and contain not less than 10 mL of the specified preparation.

Human Actraphane 30/70, Human Actrapid, Human Monotard, Human Protaphane, Human Ultratard, Lentard MC, Rapitard MC, and Semitard MC injections should be stored between 2° and 8° and should not be exposed to excessive heat or sunlight or allowed to freeze. Vials in use may be kept at room temperature (maximum 25°) for up to four weeks.

Human Initard 50/50, Human Insulatard, Human Mixtard 30/70, Human Velosulin, Initard 50/50, Insulatard 30/70, Mixtard 30/70, and Velosulin injections should be stored between 2° and 8°, protected from sunlight and not allowed to freeze; insulin that has been frozen should not be used.

Humulin preparations should be stored in a refrigerator between 2° and 8°, and should not be frozen or exposed to excessive heat or sunlight. Vials in use may be kept at room temperature (up to 25°) for one month if refrigeration is not possible. Cartridges in use should be kept at room temperature (15° to 25°) and should not be refrigerated; the in-use maximum storage period is 21 days for all Humulins except Humulin S, for which it is 28 days.

Hypurin preparations should be stored between 2° and 8°, and should not be frozen.

Penfill cartridge preparations should be stored between 2° and 8°, and should not be frozen. Cartridges in use must not be stored in a refrigerator but may be kept at ambient temperature for up to one month; exposure to excessive heat or sunlight should be avoided.

Pur-In preparations should not be frozen or exposed to extremes of heat or cold; human insulin that has been frozen should not be used. When stored between 2° and 8° the shelf-life is two years; when stored at ambient temperature the shelf-life is three weeks.

PHYSICAL PROPERTIES

Insulin is a white or almost white crystalline powder.
Human insulin is a white or almost white powder.
Details of the physical properties of BP insulin preparations are given under the relevant entries; see Preparations, above.

Solubility

Insulin and *human insulin* are practically insoluble in water, in ethanol, in chloroform, and in ether; they dissolve in dilute solutions of mineral acids and, with degradation, in solutions of alkali hydroxides.

Effect of excipients

Quinn and Andrade[1] reported that the solubility of insulin may be enhanced by the addition of small amounts of lysine, aspartic acid, glutamic acid, edetic acid, Tris buffer, or bicarbonate buffer; such excipients may also inhibit reaggregation and precipitation of insulin.

The solubility of porcine insulin at 37° was increased by the addition of sodium salicylate, from 80 micrograms/mL in water to 630 mg/mL in 1.5M sodium salicylate.[2] The sodium salicylate was thought to cause a reduction in molecular self-association of insulin.

STABILITY

Insulin can degrade by deamidation and polymerisation, both in the solid state and in injections; deamidated insulin is reported to possess full or almost full biological potency and neither the desamido insulin nor the polymerised insulin were reported to be significantly immunogenic in *rabbits*.[3,4]

Activation energies for the degradation of purified crystalline bovine insulin in the solid state were calculated to be 66 kJ/mol for polymerisation and 45 kJ/mol for deamidation.[5] Studies at various temperatures (−20° to 60°) revealed that, in the solid state, insulin of this type should be stored at −20°.

Injections

In general, formulations at an acidic pH are less stable than those at neutral pH and shorter-acting insulins are less stable than longer-acting insulins.

Pingel and Volund[6] examined, by bioassay, the influence of temperature on the stability of insulin in seven types of insulin preparations during storage for various periods in the dark. Losses in biological potency for all the insulin preparations were predicted to be less than 10% after storage at 5° for 69 years, at 15° for 10 years, at 25° for 20 months, at 35° for 3 months, or at 45° for 10 days. Activation energies for the insulin preparations ranged from about 117 kJ/mol to about 180 kJ/mol.

Storage under incorrect conditions leads to damage of insulin preparations: for example,[7] white flakes, which cannot be resuspended, may be formed in crystalline insulin that has been frozen; granular deposits may appear on the sides of vials of crystalline insulin that has been subject to excess heat; or a brown discoloration may appear in insulin that has been exposed to bright sunlight. Ultraviolet light has been reported to break down histadyl residues within the insulin molecule resulting in discoloration and a loss of potency.[4]

The effect of a single freezing and thawing process on insulin suspensions (isophane insulin, protamine zinc insulin, and crystalline and amorphous insulin zinc suspensions) was investigated by Graham and Pomeroy.[8] Insulin preparations were frozen at −17° for 45 hours and then thawed (at 21° or 37°); this treatment caused the particles in the suspensions to agglomerate forming a coarser suspension that sedimented rapidly and some crystal damage was observed (microscopic examination). However, no chemical change (analysis by paper electrophoresis and immuno reactivity) or pH change occurred, and biological activity was similar to that of preparations that had not been frozen.

Tarr et al[9] investigated the effects of storage conditions on the stability and sterility of biosynthetic human insulin preparations (all Eli Lilly, USA): regular, Humulin R; isophane, Humulin N; combination, Humulin N/R (70/30); and an extemporaneous combination of these three preparations. Potency and sterility of the preparations were maintained during storage for 28 days in 1-mL polypropylene syringes and 1-mL propylene/ethylene copolymer syringes at 4° and 23°. Although no microbial growth occurred, the concentrations of the preservatives present in the formulations (*m*-cresol or phenol) decreased, particularly in preparations stored at 23°.

Aggregation and gelling

Sato et al[10] noted that in some insulin infusion devices, shear rates which accelerate self-association of insulin monomers may be generated. Addition of urea (1 mg/mL to 3 mg/mL) to insulin solutions (bovine-zinc insulin, 0.1 mg/mL) reduced self-association whereas higher concentrations of urea led to denaturation of insulin and accelerated self-association. See also Solubility, above.

Prolonged gentle agitation of solutions of crystalline bovine insulin (100 units), with or without buffer, and containing *m*-cresol and phenol either alone or in combination, resulted in formation of a cross-linked gel network.[11] Rheological studies indicated that the extents of gelling and aggregation (and increases in viscosity) that occur depend on the magnitude of shear rates applied to the insulin solutions.

FURTHER INFORMATION. The effectiveness of preservatives in [commercial] insulin injections [stored in syringes at 2° to 6°]—Allwood MC. Pharm J 1982;229:340. Sterility of insulin in prefilled disposable syringes—Jackson EA, Gallo BM. Am J Hosp Pharm 1990;47:2508–10. Insulin aggregation in aqueous media and its effect on alpha-chymotrypsin-mediated proteolytic degradation—Liu F, Kildsig DO, Mitra AK. Pharm Res 1991;8:925–9. The influence of gamma-irradiation upon the chemical and biological properties of insulin [bovine and porcine]—Salemink PJM, Kolkman-Roodbeen JC, Gribnau TCJ, Janssen PSL, Van der Veen AJ. Pharm Weekbl (Sci) 1987;9:172–8.

INCOMPATIBILITY/COMPATIBILITY

Mixtures of insulins

Adams et al[12] investigated the miscibility and stability of mixtures of short-acting and long-acting human, porcine, and bovine insulins (from various manufacturers). Mixtures were prepared in disposable plastic syringes (Plastipak, Becton Dickinson) by the addition of soluble insulin from one manufacturer in various ratios to a longer-acting insoluble insulin (zinc or isophane) from the same manufacturer. The amount of detectable soluble insulin decreased rapidly (losses of up to 50% or more in less than 2 minutes) when mixed with either zinc or isophane insulin although the loss was dependent on the ratio of the mixture, the type and origin of the insulin, and the excipients in the preparations. In soluble:zinc insulin mixtures, insulin loss decreased in the order: porcine > human > bovine. In soluble:isophane insulin mixtures, insulin loss decreased in the order: bovine > porcine > human.

In previous work,[13] there was a similar significant decrease in the detectable soluble insulin component of mixtures of soluble insulin and isophane insulin, stored in plastic syringes at room temperature, although the total content of insulin was unchanged. In some instances, when porcine soluble insulin was mixed with insulin zinc suspension no soluble insulin could be detected after 75 to 80 seconds, whereas in some similar bovine insulin mixtures 100% of the soluble insulin remained after one hour.

Following a study involving 16 healthy volunteers, Mühlhauser et al[14] commented on potential differences in hypoglycaemic effect produced by a mixture of human ultralente insulin (Ultratard HM, Novo, Denmark) with a regular insulin (Actrapid HM) compared to a mixture of bovine ultralente insulin (Ultratard MC, Novo) with a regular insulin (Actrapid MC).

The manufacturers of Semitard MC and Lentard MC (Novo Nordisk) warn that mixing phosphate-containing insulin preparations with insulin zinc preparations should be avoided.

Admixtures with other drugs

There was loss of clarity when intravenous solutions of insulin (aqueous) were mixed with those of amylobarbitone sodium, chlorothiazide sodium, nitrofurantoin sodium, novobiocin sodium, pentobarbitone sodium, phenobarbitone sodium, phenytoin sodium, sodium bicarbonate, sulphadiazine sodium, sulfafurazole diethanolamine, or thiopentone sodium.[15] Incompatibility with aminophylline may also occur.

Regular insulin (Eli Lilly, USA) was admixed with dobutamine hydrochloride (Dobutrex, Eli Lilly, USA) which had been reconstituted with sterile water for injections and diluted in either glucose 5% injection or sodium chloride 0.9% injection; concentrations of each drug were 50 units/mL and 1 mg/mL, respectively.[16] A white precipitate was noted immediately and at 30 minutes when the diluent was glucose 5% injection and sodium chloride 0.9% injection, respectively, at 21° under fluorescent light.

Formation of a precipitate was noted when 1 mL of a solution of regular human insulin (Humulin R, Lilly, USA) 50 units in 250 mL of sodium chloride 0.9% injection was mixed with 1 mL of nafcillin (as the sodium salt, Baxter) 20 mg/mL or 40 mg/mL at 25° under fluorescent light.[17]

Rosen[18] commented on a potential interaction between human insulin and octreotide in total parenteral nutrition solutions.

Physical compatibility, with little change in pH, was observed when regular insulin (Eli Lilly, USA) 20 to 100 units/L was admixed in parenteral nutrition solutions composed of 590 mL of protein hydrolysate 7% with 410 mL of glucose 50%; the parenteral nutrition solutions also contained calcium gluconate, potassium phosphate, magnesium sulphate, phytomenadione, cyanocobalamin, folic acid, and a multivitamin infusion (USV) or Solu B Forte (Upjohn, USA).[19]

Silicone

Chantelau and Berger[20] identified the potential risks of contamination of insulin solutions with silicone oil from disposable plastic syringes. In response, Collier and Dawson[21] outlined studies in which no loss of insulin 'potency' was shown in either samples of insulin from single-use syringes or experimental silicone-contaminated insulins.

Sorption to containers and administration sets

Insulin may be strongly sorbed to the surfaces of many materials including glass and plastics. Since insulin is not a lipophilic substance, adsorption to the surface of a plastic is unlikely to be followed by absorption into the matrix of the material. The extent of adsorption is, however, difficult to predict as it is dependent on many factors including the type of material. Methods to reduce the extent of binding may be employed.

Extensive sorption of insulin to various types of glass,[22–24] polyvinyl chloride,[23–27] polyolefin,[25] and ethyl vinyl acetate[26] containers and administration sets has been observed. Some studies have suggested that polyvinyl chloride binds greater amounts of insulin than glass; for example, losses of about 52% and 45% of insulin concentrations occurred from similar solutions in polyvinyl chloride and glass containers, respectively.[24] However, Whalen et al[23] found no difference in the extent of binding of insulin to comparable glass and polyvinyl chloride containers.

The presence of in-line filters (for example, composed of a cellulose ester membrane) can further increase losses of insulin because of sorption onto the membrane during intravenous administration.[24, 28]

McElnay et al[29] found that administration sets consisting of methacrylate butadiene styrene burettes with polybutadiene tubing (A2001, Avon Medicals, UK) bound insulin more extensively than sets comprising cellulose propionate burettes with polyvinyl chloride tubing (A200 and A2000, Avon Medicals, UK). Whalen et al[23] compared the extent of binding of insulin (in various solutions) to eight administration sets.

Twardowski et al[30] examined the nature of binding of insulin to plastic bags and concluded that it 'primarily followed the physical laws of adsorption'. Hirsch et al[27] evaluated the adsorption of insulin to polyvinyl chloride intravenous delivery systems and concluded that all systems obeyed the Langmuir isotherm.

Zell and Paone[31] demonstrated that insulin 100 units/mL (Iletin, Eli Lilly, USA) was stable for at least 14 days (analysis by radioimmunoassay) when stored under refrigeration in polypropylene syringes.

Factors affecting adsorption

Factors that may influence the extent of adsorption of insulin to various materials have been extensively investigated and are summarised below.

Type of insulin

Tol et al[32] could find no significant differences between porcine and human insulins in respect of their adsorption to polyvinyl chloride or polyethylene tubing.

Vehicles

The reported effects of vehicles on adsorption of insulin vary. Binding of insulin to polyvinyl chloride delivery systems was greater from sodium chloride 0.9% solutions than from glucose 5% solutions.[27] Mitrano and Newton[22] demonstrated that more insulin was sorbed to Type I glass from glucose 5% solutions (pH 4.3) than from sodium chloride 0.9% solutions (pH 6.0). However, Whalen et al[23] concluded that the relative effects of glucose 5%, sodium chloride 0.9%, glucose 5% in sodium chloride 0.45%, and compound sodium lactate solutions on adsorption of insulin varied significantly with the type and brand of administration set used.

Concentration of insulin

In general, the amount of insulin adsorbed from a solution decreases with higher initial concentrations of insulin, although the magnitude of this decrease will depend on the vehicle and the material from which the container is made.[22–24, 33]

Effects of time and flow rate

Adsorption of insulin is rapid during the first stages of delivery through administration sets; this is followed by a gradual increase in the amount of insulin delivered, until a plateau concentration is attained.[23, 24, 32] For example, in various vehicles and administration sets, the greatest insulin adsorption was apparent during the first 30 minutes of infusion.[23] The time to reach the plateau phase was affected by the flow rate, but the flow rate did not significantly influence the total amount of insulin delivered during an eight-hour period.[23]

Temperature

Greater amounts of insulin were adsorbed to peritoneal dialysis bags (containing glucose 1.5%) at 37° than at 25° at all concentrations of insulin studied (40 units to 280 units).[33] Barrera et al[34] reported that adsorption of insulin to polyvinyl chloride bags, ethyl vinyl acetate bags, and glass bottles was greater at 20° than at 4°.

Surface area and fill volume

In general, there is a direct relationship between the surface area of the container and the amount of insulin adsorbed; larger containers adsorb greater amounts of insulin. Mitrano and Newton[22] showed that the amount of insulin adsorbed (to Type I glass) increased as the ratio of fluid volume to container capacity was decreased.

Reduction of sorption

Several methods aimed at minimising the sorption of insulin have been investigated, although there is no consensus as to the extent of effects or clinical usefulness of such methods.

The addition of albumin to solutions of insulin inhibits the binding of insulin to containers and administration sets.[24,35,36] For example, loss of insulin by adsorption to glass containers was reduced by the addition of human serum albumin or plasma protein fraction (Plasmanate) to a compound sodium lactate vehicle.[35] Similarly, the addition of polygeline (a polymer of degraded gelatin) was found to reduce losses of insulin.[36,37] Kraegen et al[37] concluded that a polygeline 3.5% solution was a suitable alternative to the use of human serum albumin with sodium chloride 0.9% solution to reduce sorption of insulin. Barrera et al[34] observed that the presence of lipids or hydrolysed gelatin increased the amount of insulin recovered from stored solutions.

A reduction in the adsorption of insulin to the components of an infusion system was also demonstrated by the addition of whole blood to low-dose insulin intravenous infusions.[38]

The presence of amino acids in total parenteral nutrition solutions may affect the extent of insulin adsorption; Weber et al[24] examined the effects of amino acid or polypeptide sources (fibrin hydrolysate, casein hydrolysate or crystalline amino acids). Other components of parenteral nutrition solutions can also influence such effects; the addition of electrolytes and vitamins to solutions of insulin in a glucose solution that contained amino acids and protein hydrolysates caused a decrease in the loss of insulin.

Mitrano and Newton[22] demonstrated that the addition of potassium chloride (1 to 60 mEq/L) significantly reduced the extent of insulin adsorbed to Type I glass containers when the vehicle was glucose 5% solution; however, reduction in the extent of binding was not significant when the vehicle was sodium chloride 0.9% solution.

The addition of urea (1 to 3 mg/mL) to solutions of insulin (0.1 mg/mL) reduced the adsorption of insulin to various polymer surfaces although higher concentrations of urea led to insulin denaturation and accelerated self-association.[10]

Clinical relevance of adsorption

The clinical relevance of the binding of insulin to various materials is unclear but, in general, there should be an awareness that the dose of insulin administered may vary under different conditions, and that therapeutic response may vary depending on the type of administration set used.

Hirsch et al[27] reported that at low therapeutic concentrations insulin adsorption to polyvinyl chloride intravenous administration sets would be clinically significant.

Insulin has been shown to be active in the adsorbed state;[39] almost full biological activity was retained after adsorption to glass surfaces for three months.

FURTHER INFORMATION. Insulin adsorption to parenteral infusion systems: case report and review of the literature—Seres DS. Nutr Clin Pract 1990;5:111–17. Drug interactions with medical plastics—D'Arcy PF. Drug Intell Clin Pharm 1983;17:726–31. Binding of insulin to a continuous ambulatory peritoneal dialysis system—Kane M, Jay M, DeLuca PP. Am J Hosp Pharm 1986;43:81–8. Insulin adsorption to three-litre ethylene vinyl acetate bags during 24-hour infusion—Doglietto GB, Bellantone R, Bossola M, Perri V, Crucitti F, et al. J Parenter Enter Nutr 1989;13:539–41. Insulin adsorption to an air-eliminating inline filter—Wingert TD, Levin SR. Am J Hosp Pharm 1981;38:382–3. Insulin binding to plastic [peritoneal dialysis] bags: a methodologic study—Twardowski ZJ, Nolph KD, McGary TJ, Moore HL, Collin P, Ausman RK et al. Am J Hosp Pharm 1983;40:575–9. Effect of pretreatment with 0.9% sodium chloride or insulin solutions on the delivery of insulin from an infusion system—Furberg H, Jensen AK, Salbu B. Am J Hosp Pharm 1986;43:2209–13. Insulin adsorbance to polyvinyl chloride surfaces with implications for constant-infusion therapy [effect of albumin; clinical note]—Peterson L, Caldwell J, Hoffman J. Diabetes 1976;25(1):72–4.

FORMULATION

Excipients

Excipients that have been used in presentations of insulin are listed under the individual preparations of insulin; see Preparations, above.

Oral administration

Cho and Flynn[40] developed a water-in-oil microemulsion that contained insulin. They reported that the formulation successfully lowered concentrations of glucose in blood when administered orally to three diabetic patients in single-dose and multidose studies.

Preliminary studies of binding interactions between human insulin and diethylaminoethyl dextran in solution[41] revealed that the fraction of bound insulin increased with temperature (in the range 25° to 45°) and that, among the pH values studied (pH 6.9, 7.4, and 8.0), maximum binding occurred at pH 7.4. Ionic strength did not influence the binding capacity, and lyophilisation of the insulin-diethylaminoethyl dextran complex did not appear to change the integrity of bound and unbound insulin. Further detailed studies[42] using normal and diabetic *rats* indicated that potential drug delivery systems (oral administration and by injection into the colon and duodenum) for insulin could be achieved by entrapment of insulin-diethylaminoethyl dextran complexes in liposomes. Liposomal systems (neutral, positive, or negative) were prepared from a hydrogenated soy lecithin and cholesterol, and either stearylamine (positive liposomes) or dicetyl phosphate (negative liposomes). Samples of the complex entrapped in the liposomes were lyophilised and reconstituted in phosphate buffer (pH 7.4) before administration.

Weingarten et al[43] demonstrated that when insulin was associated with or entrapped in positively charged liposomes *in vitro*, it was protected from degradation by the digestive enzymes pepsin, α-chymotrypsin, and trypsin; the protective role of the liposomes was dependent on the molar proportion of phospholipid:insulin. A dosage form designed to target insulin delivery to the colon was prepared[44] by filling 100 mg of a formulation of porcine insulin (8 units) and surfactant mixture (sodium laurate:cetyl alcohol, 2:8) 20 mg in arachis oil into soft gelatin capsules that were coated with mixtures of various ratios of polyacrylic polymers (Eudragits RS, L, and S). Release of insulin *in vitro* was dependent on pH. Two formulations, which showed greatest release between pH 7.5 and 8.0 produced significant hypoglycaemic effects when administered orally to *rats*, although the relative bioavailability was low compared to intraperitoneal administration of neutral insulin.

Nasal administration

In *rats*, nasal absorption of insulin has been shown to be promoted by the inclusion of various surfactants, such as nonionic ethers, anionic surfactants, amphoteric surfactants, bile acid salts, saponin, and surfactin.[45] Among the nonionic surfactants, greatest absorption promoting effects were achieved when the HLB (hydrophile-lipophile balance) value was between 8 and 14. When administered as a solution at pH 3.1 without a promoter, absolute bioavailability of insulin (hypoglycaemic effect) was 5%; this increased to about 30% following the addition of, for example, sodium glycocholate 1% or polyoxyethylene-9-lauryl ether 1%.

Several workers have shown that sodium taurodihydrofusidate enhances the absorption of insulin through the nasal mucosa of *sheep*[46–48] and of humans.[48] In volunteers, when insulin (0.35 units/kg of body weight) with sodium taurodihydrofusidate 1% was administered intranasally, the mean bioavailability was 11.4% of that of intravenous insulin.[48]

In *sheep*, intranasal absorption of sodium insulin in water was not significantly different to that of zinc insulin in water, either in the presence or absence of sodium taurodihydrofusidate.[46] An intranasal aerosol spray of insulin that contained the surfactant laureth-9 was assessed *in vivo*;[49] insulin was rapidly absorbed intranasally and lowering of plasma-glucose concentrations in fasting controls and in diabetic patients was dependent on the concentration of insulin and surfactant in the formulation. Nasal irritation, which varied between subjects, was related to surfactant concentration.

Degradable starch microspheres (DSM) with a mean diameter of 45 micrometres increased nasal absorption when co-administered with insulin in *rats*.[50] When the insulin (0.75 units/kg and 1.7 units/kg)/DSM preparations were administered nasally as a dry powder, the absolute bioavailability compared to intravenous insulin (0.25 units/kg) was 30% and 33%, respectively, for the two doses. Intranasally administered soluble insulin or DSM alone had no effects on blood-glucose or serum-insulin concentrations.

Subcutaneous administration

When injected subcutaneously, insulin is partially 'biotransformed' at the injection site before absorption into the systemic circulation.[51] Several studies have examined compounds that enhance the absorption and bioavailability of subcutaneously administered insulin. Such compounds include benzyloxycarbonyl-Gly-Pro-Leu-Gly (in *rats*),[52] collagen (in *rats* and healthy volunteers),[51] and cholic acid or aprotinin (in *rats*).[53] Several of the compounds appeared to act by inhibition of insulin degradation at the injection site although other mechanisms may also be involved. Hyaluronidase did not increase the bioavailability of subcutaneous insulin.[53]

Wang[54] demonstrated that the release of bovine insulin (zinc salt) administered subcutaneously as implantable pellet discs (to diabetic *rats*) could be sustained over several weeks when a lipid excipient was compressed in the discs. Trilaurin, trimyristin, tripalmitin, or stearic acid showed promising results but the best results were achieved with palmitic acid.

Double-layered implants were prepared that contained a polymer matrix layer of low molecular weight poly(DL-lactic acid) with insulin and a poly(DL-lactic acid) coating layer.[55] Dissolution rates of insulin *in vitro* (into phosphate buffer with 0.001% methylcellulose, pH 7.4, at 37°) were controlled by the amount of poly(DL-lactic acid) in the polymer layer. When implanted subcutaneously in diabetic animals, the implants were biodegradable and provided sustained release of insulin over a period of 19 days.

Rectal preparations

The development of formulations that enhance absorption of insulin by the rectal route has been extensively investigated. Shichiri et al[56] prepared suppositories comprising crystalline porcine insulin suspended in an oily basis (maize oil) that contained a nonionic surfactant (polyoxyethylene-9-lauryl ether 2% w/w to 4% w/w). Significant reductions in plasma-glucose concentrations were achieved following administration of suppositories containing insulin doses of 2 units/kg or greater, and absorption of insulin was more rapid than from an intramuscular injection (Insulin Actrapid) in normal and depancreatised *dogs*. Further work revealed that the inclusion of an enamine derivative (DL-phenylalanine-ethylacetoacetate[57] or sodium phenylalanine enamine of ethylacetoacetate[58]) in triglyceride-based suppositories (Witepsol H-15) was more effective in promoting rectal absorption of insulin than inclusion of polyoxyethylene-9-lauryl ether, in normal and depancreatised *dogs*. Although insulin release and absorption *in vivo* were rapid, in depancreatised *dogs* maintenance of clinically effective concentrations of insulin in serum was achieved by administration of a suppository of enamine alone following administration of the insulin/enamine suppository.[58]

A significant decrease in plasma-glucose concentrations was observed when insulin was administered rectally, to normal *rats* and depancreatised *dogs*, in three formulations that contained an enamine derived from ethylacetoacetate and DL-phenylalanine.[59] When insulin was dispersed and dissolved in a gelatin 4% micro-enema, bioavailability was greater than from an aqueous micro-enema of insulin or from a crystalline suspension of insulin in a glyceride suppository basis; all formulations contained 100 mg of enamine. Dissolution of insulin *in vitro* was also more rapid from the gelatin micro-enema than from the glyceride suppository.

In further work involving six healthy volunteers,[60] insulin suppositories that contained enamine (L-phenylalanine enamine ethylacetoacetate) or sodium salicylate increased serum immunoreactive insulin concentrations significantly. The suppositories contained porcine insulin dissolved in citric acid and mixed in a Witepsol H-15 basis with either adjuvant. However, in order to decrease serum concentrations of glucose significantly, the use of sodium salicylate was preferable to enamine. Nishihata et al[61] demonstrated that triglyceride-based suppositories, which contained a solid dispersion of insulin (incorporated as a solution in citric acid) with sodium salicylate or mannitol, released insulin rapidly *in vitro* and produced significant decreases in plasma-glucose concentrations (in normal *dogs*). The addition of lecithin 10% w/w to 20% w/w to the formulations promoted the release of insulin and sodium salicylate *in vitro*. However, the addition of lecithin 30% to the suppository basis prolonged the effect of sodium salicylate (*in vivo*) due to slow release of the salicylate.

The two types of suppositories (comprising a triglyceride suppository basis with lecithin 10% and either sodium salicylate powder and insulin solution[60] or a solid dispersion of sodium salicylate powder with insulin[61]), which were found to facilitate dissolution of insulin, controlled postprandial hyperglycaemia in diabetic patients.[62] However, the use of suppositories that contained insulin as a solid dispersion effectively reduced the dose of insulin required.

Rectal absorption of insulin in *rats* was enhanced by the inclusion of the bile salt derivative sodium tauro-24,25-dihydrofusidate in solution. Compared to intravenous administration, rectal bioavailability of insulin from a solution containing 0% w/v, 1% w/v, or 4% w/v was 0.2 ± 0.2%, 4.2 ± 3.2%, or 6.7 ± 2.1%, respectively[63] (analysis by radioimmunoassay).

Further increases in bioavailability and hypoglycaemic response were achieved by co-administration of sodium tauro-24,25-dihydrofusidate with disodium edetate 0.25% w/v.

Enhancement of absorption

In *rats* the efficacy of insulin following buccal administration as a solution (pH 7.4, containing zinc 0.5%) was less than 4% of that following intramuscular administration of insulin.[64] Inclusion of an 'absorption promoter' in the buccal solution improved absorption. Promoters included steroidal detergents, laureth-9, sodium fusidate, sodium lauryl sulphate, sodium laurate, palmitoyl carnitine, and a lauric acid/propylene glycol vehicle. The pH and concentrations at which the 'promoters' were most effective varied.

Aungst et al[65] reported that, when administered to *rats* as a solution without an absorption enhancer, the efficacy of insulin was greater by the rectal route than by the nasal, buccal, or sublingual routes. Efficacy was improved by the inclusion of 5% sodium glycocholate (rank order of insulin efficacy: nasal > rectal > buccal > sublingual), although the efficacy by each route was low compared to intramuscular insulin.

When administered as a 1% solution to the eye (of *rabbits*), systemic absorption of insulin was enhanced by the inclusion of the following compounds (concentration 1%)[66] in the rank order: saponin > fusidic acid > polyoxyethylene-9-lauryl ether = edetic acid > glycocholate = decamethonium > Tween 20.

Bioerodible dosage forms

The major component of a bioerodible insulin delivery device developed by Heller et al[67] was a pH-sensitive poly(ortho ester) that could release insulin at varying rates in response to small changes in the surrounding pH.

Ishihara[68] also reported the development of polymer membranes that regulated release of insulin in response to changes in plasma-glucose concentration.

FURTHER INFORMATION. Nasal administration of insulin using bioadhesive microspheres as a delivery system—Farraj NF, Johansen BR, Davis SS, Illum L. J Controlled Release 1990;13:253–61. Intranasal delivery of insulin: deoxycholate helps it work—Am Pharm 1985;NS25(1):28, 30. Influence of bile salts on the permeability through the nasal mucosa of *rabbits* of insulin in comparison with dextran derivatives—Uchida N, Maitani Y, Machida Y, Nakagaki M, Nagai T. Drug Dev Ind Pharm 1991;17(12):1625–34. Thermogelling polymers as vehicles for nasal delivery of insulin to rats—Ryden L, Edman P. Pharm Weekbl (Sci) 1992;14(5) Suppl F:F40. Insulin and didecanoyl-L-α-phosphatidylcholine: *in vitro* study of the transport through *rabbit* nasal mucosal tissue—Bechgaard E, Jørgensen L, Larsen R, Gizurarson S, Carstensen J, Hvass A. Int J Pharmaceutics 1993;89:147–53. Continuous subcutaneous insulin infusion—Hughes J. Pharm J 1986;236:672. One-year trial of a remote-controlled implantable insulin infusion system in type I diabetic patients—Lancet 1988;2:866–9. A preliminary trial of the programmable implantable medication system for insulin delivery—Saudek CD, Selam J-L, Pitt HA, Waxman K, Rubio M, Jeandidier N et al. New Eng J Med 1989;321(9):574–9. Intratracheal delivery of insulin: Absorption from solution and aerosol by *rat* lung—Okumura K, Iwakawa S, Yoshida T, Seki T, Komada F. Int J Pharmaceutics 1992;88:63–73. A new approach for insulin delivery via the pulmonary route: Design and pharmacokinetics in non-diabetic *rabbits*—Sakr FM. Int J Pharmaceutics 1992;86:1–7.

Biological activity of insulin in microemulsion in *mice*—Patel DG, Ritchel WA, Chalasani P, Rao S [letter]. J Pharm Sci 1991;80(6):613–14. Effect of rectal suppository formulation on the release of insulin and on the glucose plasma levels in *dogs* [effect of acetic acid and suppository size]—Liversidge GG, Nishihata T, Engle KK, Higuchi T. Int J Pharmaceutics 1985;23:87–95. The influence of concentration of two salicylate derivatives [3,5-diiodosalicylate sodium and 5-methoxysalicylate sodium] on rectal insulin absorption enhancement—Hauss DJ, Ando HY. J Pharm Pharmacol 1988;40:659–61. Insulin administration via liposomes [review: oral and subcutaneous routes, and hepatic targeting]—Spangler RS. Diabetes Care 1990;13(9):911–22. Thermodynamic characteristics of a human insulin-DEAE-dextran complex entrapped in liposomes—Manosroi A, Blume A, Manosroi J, Bauer KH. Drug Dev Ind Pharm 1990;16(5):837–54. Effect of lipid composition on insulin-mediated fusion of small unilamellar liposomes: a kinetic study—Lai JY, Chow DD, Hwang KJ. J Pharm Sci 1988;77(5):432–7. Enteral insulin delivery by microspheres in 3 different formulations using Eudragit L100 and S100—Morishita I, Morishita M, Takayama K, Machida Y, Nagai T. Int J Pharmaceutics 1993;91:29–37. Insulin retard forms by matrix inclusion or complexation [with polamide gel, dextran, Sephadrex, or agar]—Losse G, Müller F, Raddatz H, Naumann W, Kossowicz J [German]. Pharmazie 1988;43(H5):355–7. Facilitated transdermal transport of insulin [iontophoresis; hairless *rat* model]—Siddiqui O, Sun Y, Liu J-C, Chien YW. J Pharm Sci 1987;76(4):341–5. Blood glucose control in diabetic *rats* by transdermal iontophotetic delivery of insulin—Liu J-C, Sun Y, Siddiqui O, Chien YW, Shi W-M, Li J. Int J Pharmaceutics 1988;44:197–204.

Jet injection of insulin—Lancet 1985;1:1140. Insulin delivery by a diffusion-controlled micropump in pancreatectomized *dogs*: phase 1—Sefton MV, Horvarth V, Zingg W. J Controllled Release 1990;12:1–12. An insulin suspension for controlled delivery with an insulin micropump—Vlahos E, Sefton MV. J Controlled Release 1990;12:13–23. NovoSol Basal: pharmacokinetics of a novel soluble long acting insulin analogue. Jorgensen S, Vaag A, Langkjaer L, Hougaard P, Markussen J. Br Med J 1989;299:415–19. A self-regulating insulin delivery system. I. Characterisation of a synthetic glycosylated insulin derivative—Seminoff LA, Olsen GB, Kim SW. Int J Pharmaceutics 1989;54:241–9. A self-regulating insulin delivery system. II. *In vivo* [*rabbits*] characteristics of a synthetic glycosylated insulin—Seminoff LA, Gleeson JM, Zheng J, Olsen GB, Holmberg D, Mohammad SF et al. Int J Pharmaceutics 1989;44:251–7. Devices for insulin administration [review]—Selam J-L, Charles MA. Diabetes Care 1990;13:955–79.

REFERENCES

1. Quinn R, Andrade JD. J Pharm Sci 1983;72(12):1472–3.
2. Touitou E, Alhaique F, Fisher P, Memoli A, Riccieri FM, Santucci E. J Pharm Sci 1987;76(10):791–3.
3. Connors KA, Amidon GL, Stella VJ, editors. Chemical stability of pharmaceuticals: a handbook for pharmacists. 2nd ed. New York: John Wiley & Sons, 1986:517–23.
4. Blakeman K. Pharm J 1983;231:711–12.
5. Fisher BV, Porter PB. J Pharm Pharmacol 1981;33:203–6.
6. Pingel M, Volund A. Diabetes 1972;21:805–13.
7. Hannon MF [letter]. Pharm J 1987;239:114.
8. Graham DT, Pomeroy AR. Int J Pharmaceutics 1978;1:315–22.
9. Tarr BD, Campbell RK, Workman TM. Am J Hosp Pharm 1991;48:2631–4.
10. Sato S, Ebert CD, Kim SW. J Pharm Sci 1983;72(3):228–32.
11. Hutchison KG. J Pharm Pharmacol 1985;37:528–31.

12. Adams PS, Haines-Nutt RF, Town R. J Pharm Pharmacol 1987;39:158–63.
13. Town R, Haines-Nutt RF, Adams P. Proceedings of the Guild 1987;23:63–7.
14. Mühlhauser I, Broermann C, Tsotsalas M, Berger M. Br Med J 1984;289:1656–7.
15. Patel JA, Phillips GL. Am J Hosp Pharm 1966;23:409–11.
16. Hasegawa GR, Eder JF. Am J Hosp Pharm 1984;41:949–51.
17. Smythe M, Malouf E. Am J Hosp Pharm 1991;48:125–6.
18. Rosen GH [letter]. Am J Hosp Pharm 1989;46:1128.
19. Kobayashi NH, King JC. Am J Hosp Pharm 1977;34:589–94.
20. Chantelau EA, Berger M [letter]. Lancet 1985;1:1459.
21. Collier FC, Dawson AD [letter]. Lancet 1985;2:611.
22. Mitrano FP, Newton DW. Am J Hosp Pharm 1982;39:1491–5.
23. Whalen FJ, LeCain WK, Latiolais CJ. Am J Hosp Pharm 1979;36:330–7.
24. Weber SS, Wood WA, Jackson EA. Am J Hosp Pharm 1977;34:353–7.
25. Hirsch JI, Wood JH, Thomas RB. Am J Hosp Pharm 1981;38:995–7.
26. Bolton D. Proceedings of the Guild 1982;14:45–6.
27. Hirsch JI, Fratkin MJ, Wood JH, Thomas RB. Am J Hosp Pharm 1977;34:583–8.
28. Butler LD, Munson JM, DeLuca PP. Am J Hosp Pharm 1980;37:935–41.
29. McElnay JC, Elliot DS, D'Arcy PF. Int J Pharmaceutics 1987;36:199–203.
30. Twardowski ZJ, Nolph KD, McGary TJ, Moore HL. Am J Hosp Pharm 1983;40:579–82.
31. Zell M, Paone RP. Am J Hosp Pharm 1983;40:637–8.
32. Tol A, Quik RFP, Thyssen JHH. Pharm Weekbl (Sci) 1988;10:213–16.
33. Twardowski ZJ, Nolph KD, McGary TJ, Moore HL. Am J Hosp Pharm 1983;40:583–6.
34. Barrera JC, Paloma FJB, Garcia de Pesquera F, Rios IP, Fernández MA [Spanish]. Rev Assoc Esp Farm 1988;12:251–4.
35. Petty C, Cunningham NL. Anesthesiology 1974;40(4):400–4.
36. Semple P, Ratcliffe JG, Manderson WG [letter]. Br Med J 1975;4:228–9.
37. Kraegen EW, Lazarus L, Meler H, Campbell L, Chia YO. Br Med J 1975;3:464–6.
38. Kerchner J, Colaluca DM, Juhl RP. Am J Hosp Pharm 1980;37:1323–5.
39. Mizutani T. J Pharm Sci 1980;69(3):279–81.
40. Cho YW, Flynn M [letter]. Lancet 1989;2:1518–19.
41. Manosroi A, Bauer KH. Drug Dev Ind Pharm 1990;16(5):807–19.
42. Manosroi A, Bauer KH. Drug Dev Ind Pharm 1990;16(9):1521–38.
43. Weingarten C, Moufti A, Delattre J, Puisieux F, Couvreur P. Int J Pharmaceutics 1985;26:251–7.
44. Touitou E, Rubinstein A. Int J Pharmaceutics 1986;30:95–9.
45. Hirai S, Yashiki T, Mima H. Int J Pharmaceutics 1981;9:165–72.
46. Longenecker JP, Moses AC, Flier JS, Silve RD, Carey MC, Dubovi EJ. J Pharm Sci 1987;76(5):351–5.
47. Lee WA, Narog BA, Patapoff TW, Wang YJ. J Pharm Sci 1991;80(8):725–9.
48. Moses AC. Pharm Weekbl (Sci) 1988;10:45–6.
49. Salzman R, Manson JE, Griffing GT, Kimmerle R, Ruderman N, McCall A et al. New Eng J Med 1985;312(17):1078–84.
50. Björk E, Edman P. Int J Pharmaceutics 1988;47:233–8.
51. Hori R, Komada F, Iwakawa S, Seino Y, Okumura K. Pharm Res 1989;6(9):813–16.
52. Hori R, Komada F, Okumura K. J Pharm Sci 1983;72(4):435–9.
53. Zhou XH, Li Wan Po A. Int J Pharmaceutics 1991;69:29–41.
54. Wang PY. Int J Pharmaceutics 1989;54:223–30.
55. Yamakawa I, Kawahara M, Watanabe S, Miyake Y. J Pharm Sci 1990;79(6):505–9.
56. Shichiri M, Yamasaki Y, Kawamori R, Kikuchi M, Hakui N, Abe H. J Pharm Pharmacol 1978;30:806–7.
57. Yagi T, Hakui N, Yamasaki Y, Kawamori R, Shichiri M, Abe H et al. J Pharm Pharmacol 1983;35:177–8.
58. Nishihata T, Okamura Y, Kamada A, Higuchi T, Yagi T, Kawamori R et al. J Pharm Pharmacol 1985;37:22–6.
59. Kim S, Nishihata T, Kawabe S, Okamura Y, Kamada A, Yaki T et al. Int J Pharmaceutics 1984;21:179–86.
60. Nishihata T, Okamura Y, Inagaki H, Sudoh M, Kamada A, Yagi T et al. Int J Pharmaceutics 1986;34:157–61.
61. Nishihata T, Sudoh M, Inagaki H, Kamada A, Yagi T, Kawamori R et al. Int J Pharmaceutics 1987;38:83–90.
62. Nishihata T, Kamada A, Sakai K, Yagi T, Kawamori R, Shichiri M. J Pharm Pharmacol 1989;41:799–801.
63. Van Hoogdalem EJ, Heijligers-Feijen CD, Verhoef JC, de Boer AG, Breimer DD. Pharm Res 1990;7(2):180–3.
64. Aungst BJ, Rogers NJ. Int J Pharmaceutics 1989;53:227–35.
65. Aungst BJ, Rogers NJ, Shefter E. J Pharm Sci 1987;76(11):N 03-W-11.
66. Chiou GCY, Chuang CY. J Pharm Sci 1989;78(10):815–18.
67. Heller J, Chang AC, Rodd G, Grodsky GM. J Controlled Release 1990;13:295–302.
68. Ishihara K. Int Pharm J 1989;3(Supp I):S5.

Ipecacuanha
Expectorant; Emetic

Ipecac; ipecacuanha root; ipecacuanha radix

Ipecacuanha contains the isoquinoline alkaloids emetine and cephaeline (dimethylemetine) and small proportions of psychotrine (dehydrocephaeline), methylpsychotrine, and emetamine. The root contains, in addition, ipecacuanhic acid, and the glycoside ipecacuanhin, a saponin, and about 30% to 40% of starch.

CAS—8012-96-2

Pharmacopoeial status

BP (ipecacuanha, powdered ipecacuanha, prepared ipecacuanha); USP (ipecac, powdered ipecac)

Ipecacuanha consists of the dried underground organs of *Cephaelis ipecacuanha* (Brot.) A. Rich, known in commerce as Matto Grosso Ipecacuanha, or of *Cephaelis acuminata* Karsten, known in commerce as Costa Rica Ipecacuanha, or of a mixture of both species. It contains not less than 2% of total alkaloids of ipecacuanha, calculated as emetine and with reference to the material dried at 100° to 105°.

Preparations

When Ipecacuanha BP, Ipecacuanha Root BP, or Powdered Ipecacuanha BP is prescribed, Prepared Ipecacuanha BP shall be dispensed.

Compendial

Ipecacuanha Liquid Extract BP. Contains the total alkaloids of ipecacuanha and may be prepared in a sufficient quantity of ethanol 80%. (see Formulation below).

Ipecacuanha Tincture BP. Prepared from Ipecacuanha Liquid Extract BP (see Formulation below). When ipecacuanha wine is prescribed or demanded, Ipecacuanha Tincture shall be dispensed or supplied.

Paediatric Ipecacuanha Emetic Mixture BP (Paediatric Ipecacuanha Emetic). Prepared from Ipecacuanha Liquid Extract BP (see Formulation below).

Ammonia and Ipecacuanha Mixture BP (Ammonia and Ipecacuanha Oral Solution) (see Formulation below).

Ipecac Syrup USP.

Containers and storage

Solid state

Ipecacuanha BP, Powdered Ipecacuanha BP, and Prepared Ipecacuanha BP should be kept in well-closed containers and protected from light.

Powdered Ipecac USP should be preserved in tight containers.

Dosage forms

Ipecac Syrup USP should be preserved in tight containers, preferably at a temperature not exceeding 25°.

PHYSICAL PROPERTIES

Powdered ipecacuanha is a light grey to yellowish-brown powder possessing the diagnostic microscopical characters, odour, and taste of the unground drug; faint odour; bitter taste.

STABILITY

Effect of heat and light

The rate of thermochemical and photochemical decomposition of emetine, one of the principal alkaloids in ipecacuanha, was described by Schuyt and others.[1] In aqueous solution at 120°, the rate of decomposition of emetine hydrochloride at a concentration of 3×10^{-2}M was dependent on oxygen concentration and buffer type, whereas at an emetine hydrochloride concentration of 3×10^{-4}M the rate of decomposition was pH-dependent. Greatest thermostability occurred at pH 2.0. At higher emetine concentrations thermal decomposition was decreased by the presence of lead ions but enhanced by the presence of copper ions. Analyses of emetine hydrochloride (3×10^{-6}M) solution exposed to light of wavelength 254 nm, showed that the rate of photodecomposition was dependent on pH but not on oxygen concentration. Photostability decreased at pH values below 3.0 and above 7.0.

The thermochemical and photochemical decomposition products of emetine, elucidated in a further study by Schuijt *et al*[2] were didehydroemetine, *O*-methylpsychotrine, tetrahydroemetine, rubremetine, and emetamine. Other products of photodecomposition were detected and identified. The photodecomposition rate decreased with increasing wavelength. However, degradation pathways of photochemical and thermochemical decomposition differed.

Syrups

The chemical stability of the alkaloid content of Ipecacuanha Syrup APF stored at 22° to 24° for up to 32 months was investigated by Australian workers.[3] Results of these studies and further data demonstrated that emetine and cephaeline did not decompose appreciably even after storage for up to 71 months under practical conditions. An expiry date of 3 years was recommended for the syrup.

Data collected on 200 children treated with expired ipecac syrup and 200 treated with unexpired syrup indicated a similar time between administration and emesis in both groups.[4] The oldest syrup used in the study was over 16 years old.

Although similar times between administration and emesis in children were also demonstrated for control samples and outdated samples of ipecacuanha syrup from various American manufacturers, Hornfeldt *et al*[5] identified signs of subpotency and physical deterioration (increase in viscosity) in some of the outdated samples. A total of 60% of samples did not meet the USP standards for potency.

Cooney[6] produced *in-vitro* evidence for the inactivation of emetine hydrochloride by adsorption onto activated charcoal in simulated gastric fluid, pH 1.2.

Stabilisation

The ability of the ipecacuanha alkaloids emetine and cephaeline in solution to withstand heating at 65° or ultraviolet irradiation at 100 micro W/cm² was reported[7] to improve 2-fold to 4-fold by the addition of β-cyclodextrin at pH 5.0. Emetine was reported to transform to cephaeline and other alkaloids on exposure to heat or light.

FURTHER INFORMATION. Effectiveness of ipecacuanha syrup as an emetic [stability of two formulations with different organoleptic properties]—Espinosa GM, Roca MM, Codina JC, Ribas SJM, Nogué S, Marqués J [Spanish]. Farm Clin (Spain) 1987;4(6):466–73.

FORMULATION

IPECACUANHA LIQUID EXTRACT BP

Ipecacuanha, in fine powder	1000 g
Ethanol (80%)	a sufficient quantity

Exhaust the ipecacuanha by percolation with the ethanol, reserving the first 750 mL of the percolate. Remove the ethanol from the remainder of the percolate by evaporation under reduced pressure at a temperature not exceeding 60° and dissolve the residual extract. Determine the proportion of alkaloids in the liquid thus obtained and to the remainder of the liquid add sufficient ethanol (80%) to produce an ipecacuanha liquid extract of the required strength. Allow to stand for not less than 24 hours, and filter.

IPECACUANHA TINCTURE BP

Ipecacuanha liquid extract	100 mL
Acetic acid (6%)	16.5 mL
Ethanol (90%)	210 mL
Glycerol	200 mL
Purified water	to 1000 mL

Mix the ethanol and the acetic acid with the glycerol and 450 mL of the purified water; add the ipecacuanha liquid extract and sufficient purified water to produce 1000 mL. Allow to stand for not less than 24 hours, and filter.

PAEDIATRIC IPECACUANHA EMETIC MIXTURE BP

Ipecacuanha liquid extract	70 mL
Hydrochloric acid	2.5 mL
Glycerol	100 mL
Syrup to	1000 mL

AMMONIA AND IPECACUANHA MIXTURE BP

Ammonium bicarbonate	20 g
Ipecacuanha tincture	30 mL
Concentrated anise water	5 mL
Concentrated camphor water	10 mL
Liquorice liquid extract	50 mL
Chloroform water, double-strength	500 mL
Water	to 1000 mL

The mixture should be recently prepared.

IPECACUANHA AND MORPHINE MIXTURE

The following formula was given in the *British Pharmacopoeia 1980*:

Ipecacuanha tincture	20 mL
Chloroform and morphine tincture	40 mL
Liquorice liquid extract	100 mL
Water	to 1000 mL

The mixture should be recently prepared.

PAEDIATRIC BELLADONNA AND IPECACUANHA MIXTURE

The following formula was given in the *British Pharmaceutical Codex 1973*:

Belladonna tincture	30 mL
Ipecacuanha tincture	20 mL
Sodium bicarbonate	20 g
Tolu syrup	200 mL
Chloroform water, double-strength	500 mL
Water	to 1000 mL

The mixture must be freshly prepared.

PAEDIATRIC IPECACUANHA AND AMMONIA MIXTURE

The following formula was given in the *British Pharmaceutical Codex 1973*:

Ipecacuanha tincture	20 mL
Ammonium bicarbonate	6 g
Sodium bicarbonate	20 g
Tolu syrup	100 mL
Chloroform water, double-strength	500 mL
Water for preparations	to 1000 mL

The mixture should be recently prepared.

PAEDIATRIC IPECACUANHA AND SQUILL LINCTUS

The following formula was given in the *British Pharmaceutical Codex 1973*:

Ipecacuanha tincture	20 mL
Squill tincture	30 mL
Compound orange spirit	1.5 mL
Blackcurrant syrup	500 mL
Syrup to	1000 mL

IPECACUANHA AND OPIUM POWDER

(Dover's Powder; Compound Ipecacuanha Powder)
The following formula was given in the *British Pharmaceutical Codex 1973*:

Prepared ipecacuanha	10 g
Powdered opium	10 g
Lactose	80 g
Content of anhydrous morphine	0.9% to 1.1%

PAEDIATRIC OPIATE IPECACUANHA MIXTURE

The following formula was given in the *British Pharmaceutical Codex 1973*:

Ipecacuanha tincture	20 mL
Camphorated opium tincture	30 mL
Sodium bicarbonate	20 g
Tolu syrup	200 mL
Chloroform water, double-strength	500 mL
Water	to 1000 mL

The mixture should be recently prepared.

Excipients

Excipients that have been used in presentations of ipecacuanha include:
Syrups: acetic acid (dilute); glycerol; syrup.

REFERENCES

1. Schuyt C, Beijersbergen Van Henegouwen GMJ, Gerritsma KW. Pharm Weekbl 1977;112:1125–31.
2. Schuijt C, Beijersbergen Van Henegouwen GMJ, Gerritsma KW. Pharm Weekbl (Sci) 1979;114:186–95.
3. Ilett KF, Tjokrosetio R, Unsworth RW. Aust J Hosp Pharm 1983;13(3):121–3.
4. Grbcich PA, Lacouture PG, Kresel JJ, Russell MT, Lovejoy FH. Pediatrics 1986;78(6):1085–9.
5. Hornfeldt CS, Rogers AA, Breutzmann DA, Suess MJ, Ling LJ. Vet Hum Toxicol 1987;29(3):254–6.
6. Cooney DO. J Pharm Sci 1978;67(3):426–7.
7. Teshima D, Yoshikawa M, Aoyama T. J Pharm Sci 1987;76(11):N 07-W–15.

Isoniazid (BAN, pINN)   *Antituberculous agent*

INAH; INH; isonicotinic acid hydrazide; isonicotinoylhydrazine; isonicotinylhydrazide; isonicotinylhydrazine; tubazid Isonicotinohydrazide; 4-pyridinecarboxylic acid hydrazide
$C_6H_7N_3O = 137.1$

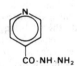

Isoniazid Aminosalicylate

Pasiniazid (pINN)
$C_6H_7N_3O, C_7H_7NO_3 = 290.3$
CAS—54-85-3 (isoniazid); 2066-89-9 (isoniazid aminosalicylate)

Pharmacopoeial status

BP, USP

Preparations

Compendial
Isoniazid Tablets BP. Tablets containing, in each, 50 mg and 100 mg are usually available.
Isoniazid Injection BP. A sterile solution of isoniazid in water for injections. pH 5.6 to 6.0. An injection containing 50 mg/2 mL is usually available.
Isoniazid Tablets USP.
Isoniazid Syrup USP.
Isoniazid Injection USP. pH 6.0 to 7.0.

Non-compendial
Rimifon (Cambridge). *Injection*, isoniazid 25 mg/mL.
Isoniazid oral solution (isoniazid 50 mg/5 mL) is available from Penn, RP Drugs.

Containers and storage

Solid state
Isoniazid USP should be preserved in tight, light-resistant containers.

Isoniazid Tablets BP should be protected from light.
Isoniazid Tablets USP should be preserved in well-closed, light-resistant containers.
Isoniazid Syrup USP should be preserved in tight, light-resistant containers.
Isoniazid Injection USP should be preserved in single-dose or multiple-dose containers, preferably of Type I glass, protected from light. If crystallisation occurs on storage, it is recommended that the injection should be warmed to redissolve the crystals before use.

PHYSICAL PROPERTIES

Isoniazid exists as colourless or white crystals or as a white crystalline powder; odourless; slowly affected by exposure to air and light; initial sweet taste that turns bitter.
Isoniazid aminosalicylate exists as yellow crystals.

Melting point

Isoniazid melts in the range 170° to 174°.
Isoniazid aminosalicylate melts between 140° to 142°.

pH

The BP specifies that a 5% solution of *isoniazid* in water has a pH of 6.0 to 8.0; the USP specifies that a 10% solution has a pH of 6.0 to 7.5; a 1% solution has been reported to have a pH of 5.5 to 6.5.

Dissociation constants

pK_a 1.8 (hydrazine nitrogen); 3.5 (pyridine nitrogen); 10.8 (acidic group)[1]

Partition coefficient

Log P (octanol/pH 7.4), −1.1

Solubility

Isoniazid is soluble 1 in 8 of water, 1 in about 45 of ethanol, and 1 in 1000 of chloroform; very slightly soluble in ether and in benzene.
Isoniazid aminosalicylate is soluble in water and in methanol.

Dissolution

The USP specifies that for Isoniazid Tablets USP not less than 80% of the labelled amount of $C_6H_7N_3O$ is dissolved in 45 minutes. Dissolution medium: 900 mL of 0.1N hydrochloric acid; Apparatus 1 at 100 rpm.

STABILITY

Many workers have examined the stability of isoniazid in solid state, in solution, and in dosage forms. Degradation reactions include both hydrolysis and oxidation but the route and the resultant degradation products depend on the conditions under which the reaction occurs.

Degradation kinetics and decomposition products

Hydrolysis

Products of the hydrolysis of isoniazid in alkaline solution have been recorded.[2] Under aerobic conditions, products were isonicotinic acid, isonicotinamide, and 1,2-diisonicotinoylhydrazine, plus small amounts of unidentified substances; under anaerobic conditions the predominant products were isonicotinic acid and 1,2-diisonicotinoylhydrazine.
In acid solution (pH 3.1) under anaerobic conditions the initial product of pseudo-first-order hydrolysis was isonicotinic acid.[2]

Oxidation

The oxidation and complexation products of isoniazid in aqueous solutions that contained copper (II) ions were isonicotinic acid, isonicotinamide, 1,2-diisonicotinoylhydrazine, isonicotine-carboxaldehyde, and isonicotinoyl hydrazone.[2] Degradation of the copper chelates followed first-order kinetics, the rate being dependent on the relative concentration of the chelated species.

Effect of pH

Under aerobic conditions,[2] isoniazid 1% solution was 37 times more stable at pH 6 than at pH 3.

Effect of heat and chelating agents

When buffered isoniazid solutions of pH 8.8 and pH 6.5 had been autoclaved for 15 minutes at 121°, Lewin and Hirsch[3] found that decomposition was 90% and 80% respectively, whereas a solution of pH 4.8 was decomposed by about 10%. When disodium edetate was added to buffered isoniazid solution (pH 6.7) there was no loss of isoniazid during autoclaving. Under autoclave conditions, copper (II) and manganese (II) ions were the most active of several metal cations in enhancing isoniazid degradation.
Ammar et al[4] investigated the effect of chelating agents on the stability of isoniazid (1%) in buffered (pH 5.65) injection solutions autoclaved at 116° for 30 minutes. Stabilising effects were concentration dependent and efficiency decreased in the order DTPA (diethylenetriaminepentaacetic acid, 3 or 5 mmol/L) > HEDTA (β-hydroxyethylethylenediaminetriacetic acid) > edetic acid (1 mmol/L) > NTA (nitrilotriacetic acid, 1 mmol/L).

Effect of sugars

In aqueous solutions of sucrose, in the presence of glucose and fructose (hydrolysis products of sucrose), isoniazid rapidly degrades by a complex condensation reaction that also involves oxidation, hydrolysis, and inversion.[5] The product is the isonicotinoyl hydrazone corresponding to the reducing sugar. Addition of sodium citrate (0.3%) reduces the rate of the hydrolysis of sucrose and consequently increases stability. Condensation of isoniazid does not occur in aqueous solutions of sorbitol, which is not hydrolysed to oxohexoses.
Devani et al[6] found that isoniazid only reacted with glucose or lactose at acidic pH values (1.0 to 6.0). The extent of formation of the isonicotinoyl hydrazone was greatest at pH 3.1. The reversible reaction followed second-order kinetics to form the hydrazone; the reverse hydrolysis was pseudo-first-order. At 37° in simulated gastric juice (pH 1.8), as the concentration of glucose and lactose increased, formation of the corresponding hydrazones also increased.
Wu et al[7] commented that the browning reaction involving the interaction of isoniazid with lactose may become significant during wet granulation or under tropical or subtropical conditions. Isoniazid also reacts rapidly with the lactose degradation product, hydroxymethylfurfural.
In commercial isoniazid tablets that contained lactose, between 10% and 22% isoniazid was present as lactose isonicotinoyl hydrazone.[8] When tablets were freshly prepared from lactose-containing granules, interaction between isoniazid and lactose was only 1% to 3%.
Matsui et al[9] quoted evidence that in laboratory animals hydrazine has carcinogenic and mutagenic properties; control of its content in pharmaceutical products is therefore imperative. A trace of hydrazine was detected in one lot of isoniazid raw material and in some tablets. In a previous study, isoniazid tablets

(100 mg) stored for 5 months at 60° and 70% relative humidity were found to contain 1.5% hydrazine.[10]

INCOMPATIBILITY/COMPATIBILITY

Isoniazid is incompatible with aldehydes and ketones; its reaction with reducing sugars produces isonicotinoyl hydrazones. Following a study of the kinetics of the interaction between isoniazid and excess reducing sugars *in vitro*, Devani et al[6] proposed that after oral administration, isoniazid bioavailability could be impaired because the hydrazones are not hydrolysed in alkaline media and are poorly absorbed from the gastrointestinal tract.

Isoniazid has also been reported to be incompatible with chloral, iodine, hypochlorites, ferric salts, and oxidising agents.

Evidence of chemisorption, and possibly physical adsorption, of isoniazid in the solid state to the surface of magnesium oxide has been presented by Wu *et al*.[7]

FORMULATION

ISONIAZID ELIXIR
(Isoniazid Syrup)
The following formula was given in the *British Pharmaceutical Codex 1973*:

Isoniazid	10.0 g
Citric acid monohydrate	2.5 g
Sodium citrate	12.0 g
Concentrated anise water	10 mL
Compound tartrazine solution	10 mL
Glycerol	200 mL
Chloroform water, double-strength	400 mL
Water for preparations	to 1000 mL

Dissolve the sodium citrate, citric acid, and isoniazid in 300 mL of the water, add the double-strength chloroform water, glycerol, compound tartrazine solution, and concentrated anise water, mix, and add sufficient water to produce the required volume. See also Containers and storage, above.

Alternatively, the double-strength chloroform water may be omitted and the preparation preserved with methyl hydroxybenzoate, 0.1%, together with propyl hydroxybenzoate, 0.02%. Dissolve these substances in 600 mL of the water with the aid of heat, cool, and dissolve the sodium citrate, citric acid, and the isoniazid in the solution; add the glycerol, compound tartrazine solution, and concentrated anise water, mix and add sufficient water to produce the required volume.

The elixir may be diluted with chloroform water. The diluted elixir must be freshly prepared. Life of diluted elixir 14 days. Syrup must not be used as diluent as isoniazid is unstable in the presence of sugars.

Isoniazid Elixir BPC 1973 should be protected from light. When stored in filled unopened containers at a temperature not exceeding 25°, it may be expected to retain its potency for one year. When dispensed, each container should be filled and the contents should represent not more than a one month supply.

Excipients

Excipients that have been used in presentations of isoniazid include:

Tablets: cellulose compounds; colloidal silica; lactose; magnesium stearate; sodium starch glycollate; starch; stearic acid.
Elixirs: chloroform water (double-strength); citric acid monohydrate; compound tartrazine solution; concentrated anise water; glycerol; sodium citrate.

Injections: hydrochloric acid; methyl and propyl hydroxybenzoates.

Bioavailability and bioequivalence

Mishra *et al*[11] found content uniformity, hardness, friability, disintegration times, and dissolution rates of isoniazid (100 mg) tablets from five commercial sources in India to be within compendial limits. However, *in-vivo* studies of cumulative urinary dose excreted, biological half-life, absorption rate constant, and bioavailability produced results that differed significantly, leading to the conclusion that the products were not bioequivalent.

Workers in Canada[12] compared the bioavailability of isoniazid (100 mg) tablets of Canadian origin in nine volunteers (slow acetylators). All three preparations met the *in-vitro* standards of the USP and there were no significant differences between their relative rates or extents of bioavailability.

Oral liquids

Glucose, fructose, and sucrose should not be included in liquid formulations of isoniazid because isoniazid forms isonicotinyl hydrazone in the presence of reducing sugars and may not be available for absorption.[13]

PROCESSING

Sterilisation

Isoniazid injection can be sterilised by heating in an autoclave.

REFERENCES

1. Albert A. Experientia 1953;IX/10:370.
2. Brewer GA. In: Florey K, editor. Analytical profiles of drug substances; vol 6. London: Academic Press, 1977:184–258.
3. Lewin E, Hirsch JG. Am Rev Tuberc Pulm Dis 1955;71(5):732–42.
4. Ammar HO, Ibrahim SA, Abdel-Mohsen MG. Pharmazie 1982;37:270–1.
5. Hald JG. Dansk Tidsskr Farm 1969;43:156–9.
6. Devani MB, Shishoo CJ, Doshi KJ, Patel HB. J Pharm Sci 1985;74(4):427–32.
7. Wu W-H, Chin TF, Lach JL. J Pharm Sci 1970;59(9):1234–42.
8. Devani MB, Shishoo CJ, Patel MA, Bhalara DD. J Pharm Sci 1978;67(5):661–3.
9. Matsui F, Robertson DL, Lovering EG. J Pharm Sci 1983;72(8):948–51.
10. Matsui F, McErlane KM, Lovering EG, Robertson DL. Can J Pharm Sci 1978;13(3):71–2.
11. Mishra AK, Saluja AK, Saini TR. East Pharm 1985;28:207–10.
12. Sved S, McGilveray IJ, Beaudoin N. J Pharm Sci 1977;66(12):1761–4.
13. Blake MI, Bode D, Rhodes HJ. J Pharm Sci 1974;63(8):1303–6.

Isosorbide (BAN, USAN, rINN) *Diuretic*

1,4:3,6-Dianhydro-D-glucitol
$C_6H_{10}O_4 = 146.14$

Isosorbide Dinitrate (BAN, USAN, rINN) *Vasodilator*
Sorbide nitrate
1,4:3,6-Dianhydro-D-glucitol 2,5-dinitrate
$C_6H_8N_2O_8 = 236.14$

Isosorbide Mononitrate (BAN, USAN, rINN) *Vasodilator*
Isosorbide-5-mononitrate
1,4:3,6-Dianhydro-D-glucitol 5-nitrate
$C_6H_9NO_6 = 191.1$
CAS—652-67-5 (isosorbide); 87-33-2 (isosorbide dinitrate); 16051-77-7 (isosorbide mononitrate)

Pharmacopoeial status

BP (diluted isosorbide dinitrate); USP (isosorbide concentrate, diluted isosorbide dinitrate)
Diluted Isosorbide Dinitrate BP is a dry mixture of isosorbide dinitrate with lactose, mannitol, or other suitable inert diluent; it may contain a suitable stabiliser.

Preparations

Compendial
Isosorbide Dinitrate Tablets BP (Sorbide Nitrate Tablets). Contain diluted isosorbide dinitrate. Tablets containing, in each, 5, 10, 20, and 30 mg of isosorbide dinitrate are usually available.
Isosorbide Oral Solution USP.
Isosorbide Dinitrate Extended-release Capsules USP.
Isosorbide Dinitrate Tablets USP.
Isosorbide Dinitrate Chewable Tablets USP.
Isosorbide Dinitrate Extended-release Tablets USP.
Isosorbide Dinitrate Sublingual Tablets USP.

Non-compendial
Cedocard (Tillotts). *Tablets*, sublingual, isosorbide dinitrate 5 mg (Cedocard-5).
Tablets, isosorbide dinitrate 10 mg (Cedocard-10), 20 mg (Cedocard-20), and 40 mg (Cedocard-40).
Tablets, sustained release, isosorbide dinitrate 20 mg (Cedocard Retard-20) and 40 mg (Cedocard Retard-40).
Injection, isosorbide dinitrate 1 mg/mL (Cedocard IV). To be diluted before use with sodium chloride 0.9% injection or glucose 5% to 30% injection. The dilution for infusion is stable for up to 24 hours. Diluted solutions must be well mixed before use. Bottles of Cedocard IV should be used once only and discarded. NOTE. Glass or polyethylene infusion apparatus is preferable; loss of potency occurs if polyvinyl chloride is used.
Elantan (Schwartz). *Capsules*, slow release, isosorbide mononitrate 25 mg (Elantan LA 25) and 50 mg (Elantan LA 50).
Tablets, isosorbide mononitrate 10 mg (Elantan 10), 20 mg (Elantan 20), 40 mg (Elantan 40).
Imdur (Astra). *Durules* (sustained-release tablets), isosorbide mononitrate 60 mg.
Imtack Spray (Astra). *Aerosol spray*, isosorbide dinitrate 1.25 mg/metered dose.
Ismo (Boehringer Mannheim). *Tablets*, isosorbide mononitrate 10 mg (Ismo 10), 20 mg (Ismo 20), and 40 mg (Ismo 40).

Tablets, sustained release, isosorbide mononitrate 40 mg (Ismo Retard).
Isoket (Schwartz). *Injection 0.05%*, isosorbide dinitrate 500 micrograms/mL. To be diluted before use or given undiluted using a syringe pump.
Injection 0.1%, isosorbide dinitrate 1 mg/mL. To be diluted before use. Bottles of Isoket are for single use only. Compatible with commonly employed infusion solutions. Incompatible with infusion bags and administration sets made from polyvinyl chloride; a loss of activity of up to 30% can occur after one hour. Glass or polyethylene infusion apparatus is compatible with Isoket.
Isoket Retard (Schwartz). *Tablets*, sustained release, isosorbide dinitrate 20 mg (Isoket Retard-20) and 40 mg (Isoket Retard-40).
Isordil (Monmouth). *Tablets*, sublingual, isosorbide dinitrate 5 mg.
Tablets, isosorbide dinitrae 10 mg and 30 mg.
Isordil Tembids (Monmouth). *Capsules*, sustained release, isosorbide dinitrate 40 mg.
Isotrate (Bioglan). *Tablets*, isosorbide mononitrate 20 mg.
Monit (Stuart). *Tablets*, isosorbide mononitrate 10 mg (Monit LS) and 20 mg.
Tablets, sustained release, isosorbide mononitrate 40 mg (Monit SR).
Mono-Cedocard (Tillotts). *Capsules*, slow release, isosorbide mononitrate 50 mg (MCR-50, Mono-Cedocard Retard-50).
Tablets, isosorbide mononitrate 10 mg (Mono-Cedocard 10), 20 mg (Mono-Cedocard 20), and 40 mg (Mono-Cedocard 40).
Soni-Slo (Lipha). *Capsules*, timed release, isosorbide dinitrate 20 mg and 40 mg.
Sorbichew (Stuart). *Tablets*, chewable, isosorbide dinitrate 5 mg.
Sorbid-20 SA (Stuart). *Capsules*, sustained release, isosorbide dinitrate 20 mg.
Sorbid-40 SA (Stuart). *Capsules*, sustained release, isosorbide dinitrate 40 mg.
Sorbitrate (Stuart). *Tablets*, isosorbide dinitrate 10 mg and 20 mg.
Vascardin (Nicholas). *Tablets*, isosorbide dinitrate (as diluted isosorbide dinitrate) 10 mg.
Tablets containing isosorbide dinitrate, of various strengths, are also available from Cox, Evans, Hillcross, Kerfoot, Norton.
Tablets containing isosorbide mononitrate, of various strengths, are available from APS, Ashbourne (Isib), Cox, CP, Evans, Kerfoot, Lagap, Norton.

Containers and storage

Isosorbide Concentrate USP should be preserved in tight, light-resistant containers.

Solid state
Diluted Isosorbide Dinitrate BP should be kept in a well-closed container, protected from light, and stored at a temperature not exceeding 15°.
Diluted Isosorbide Dinitrate USP should be preserved in tight containers.

Dosage forms
Isosorbide Oral Solution USP should be preserved in tight containers.
All Isosorbide Dinitrate USP preparations should be preserved in well-closed containers.
All Cedocard tablet preparations should be protected from heat and moisture.
Cedocard IV infusion solution should be protected from exposure to excessive heat.

Ismo tablets and Ismo Retard tablets should be kept in a cool, dry place.

Isotrate tablets should be stored at room temperature and protected from moisture.

Monit, Monit LS, and Monit SR tablets should be stored at room temperature and protected from moisture. Monit SR tablets should be protected from light.

All Mono-Cedocard tablet preparations should be protected from heat and moisture.

Soni-Slo capsules should be stored in a cool, dry place protected from light, in a tightly closed container.

Sorbid-20 SA and Sorbid-40 SA capsules should be stored at room temperature, protected from light and moisture.

Sorbichew and Sorbitrate tablets should be stored at room temperature and protected from moisture.

Vascardin tablets should be stored at room temperature (15° to 25°).

PHYSICAL PROPERTIES

Isosorbide concentrate is a colourless to slightly yellow liquid.
Diluted isosorbide dinitrate is a fine, white, crystalline powder; odourless or almost odourless.
Undiluted isosorbide dinitrate exists as white crystalline rosettes.
Isosorbide mononitrate exists as colourless, prismatic crystals.

Melting point

Isosorbide crystals melt in the range 61° to 64°.
Isosorbide dinitrate melts at about 70°.
Isosorbide mononitrate melts in the range 89° to 91°.

Solubility

Isosorbide concentrate is soluble in water and in ethanol.
Isosorbide dinitrate (undiluted) is very slightly soluble in water; sparingly soluble in ethanol; very soluble in acetone; freely soluble in chloroform.
Isosorbide mononitrate is soluble in water, in ethanol, in acetone, and in methanol; slightly soluble in chloroform and in ether.

Dissolution

The USP specifies that for Isosorbide Dinitrate Tablets USP not less than 70% of the labelled amount of $C_6H_8N_2O_8$ is dissolved in 45 minutes. Dissolution medium: 1000 mL of water; Apparatus 2 at 75 rpm.

The USP specifies that for Isosorbide Dinitrate Sublingual Tablets USP not less than 50% of the labelled amount of $C_6H_8N_2O_8$ is dissolved in 15 minutes, and not less than 70% of the labelled amount of $C_6H_8N_2O_8$ is dissolved in 30 minutes. Dissolution medium: 900 mL of water; Apparatus 2 at 50 rpm.

STABILITY

In the solid state, isosorbide dinitrate has been reported to be stable at 45° for 12 months and at room temperature for 60 months.

Under acidic conditions isosorbide dinitrate hydrolyses to form the intermediate products isosorbide-2-mononitrate and isosorbide-5-mononitrate, which in turn hydrolyse to form isosorbide and inorganic nitrate.

Workers in Japan[1] found isosorbide dinitrate to be stable in aqueous solution between pH 1.2 and 10 at 37° for 48 hours but it was unstable above pH 12. The hydrolysis of the nitrate groups of isosorbide-2-mononitrate, isosorbide-5-mononitrate, and isosorbide dinitrate in hydrochloric acid 0.1M and in sodium hydroxide 0.1M at 100° followed first-order kinetics.

Stabilisation

Isosorbide mononitrate was stabilised by the formation of a 1:1 inclusion complex with β-cyclodextrin.[2] Samples of isosorbide mononitrate powder stored at 75% relative humidity at both 60° and 45° for 30 days were shown to have only 8% and 63% of their initial isosorbide mononitrate concentration remaining, respectively. In contrast, complexed isosorbide mononitrate showed no significant decomposition over the same period at 60° and 75% relative humidity.

INCOMPATIBILITY/COMPATIBILITY

Sorption onto plastics

Losses of isosorbide dinitrate from solutions of the powder (Graesser Laboratories) and the diluted injection solution (Cedocard IV, Tillotts) by sorption to the polyvinyl chloride tubing in administration sets were influenced by the length of the extension line but not by the diluent (water for injection, sodium chloride 0.9% or glucose 5%).[3] Losses due to sorption to polypropylene syringes and polyethylene tubing were not significant; however, up to 80% of isosorbide dinitrate was sorbed onto the polyvinyl chloride matrix of an extension set tubing. An increase in the concentration of ethanol in the vehicle from 20% to 50% reduced sorption by 30% to 40%.

Cossum and Roberts[4] demonstrated that the loss of isosorbide dinitrate during simulated infusions at 20° to 24° through plastic giving sets from plastic infusion bags was flow-rate dependent. After storage for 300 hours in plastic infusion bags only half of the original drug concentration remained. Negligible loss occurred when glass syringes and high density polyethylene tubing were used.

Solutions of isosorbide dinitrate (275 micrograms/mL), isosorbide-2-mononitrate (150 micrograms/mL), and isosorbide-5-mononitrate (150 micrograms/mL) were stored in polyvinyl chloride infusion bags at 4°, room temperature (20° to 24°), 37°, 45°, and 60° for 1000 hours and in cellulose propionate burette chambers at room temperature for 150 hours.[5] No loss of either mononitrate form was detected in either container at room temperature; however, losses of the dinitrate were observed and were attributed to temperature-dependent sorption into the plastic matrix.

Lee and Fenton-May[6] showed that isosorbide dinitrate was sorbed onto polyvinyl chloride bags and administration sets (resulting in substantial losses in potency) but was not sorbed by glass or polypropylene.

During simulated infusion, Herbert[7] reported loss of up to 90% of the initial concentration of isosorbide dinitrate from the solution by sorption to polyvinyl chloride tubing. The extent of sorption varied markedly with changes in flow-rate and time but was consistently less with polyethylene tubing.

Isosorbide dinitrate showed no loss by sorption to polybutadiene intravenous administration sets;[8] however, loss to polyvinyl chloride sets was 15% to 35%.

De Muynck et al[9] presented evidence that sorption of isosorbide dinitrate to polyvinyl chloride tubing occurs to a greater extent when diluted in sodium chloride 0.9% than when diluted in glucose 10% solution. However, no sorption occurred when glass containers, methacrylate butadiene styrene burettes, and polybutadiene giving sets were used. There was no sorption to polypropylene syringes when glucose 10% was used as diluent.

Similarly,[10] when solutions of isosorbide dinitrate (250 micrograms/mL) in sodium chloride 0.9% injection or in glucose 10% injection were administered in a simulated infusion at 20 mL/hour through polybutadiene tubing (composed of various molecular weights of polybutadiene), the extent of sorption was similar to that when administered through polyethylene tubing (less than 2.5% in 5 hours). However, when polybutadiene/polyvinyl chloride laminates were used, sorption was significantly greater. Increased sorption was associated with low molecular weight polybutadiene and lower hardness (Shore hardness measurements) of the polyvinyl chloride. The type of plasticiser used did not influence sorption.

A maximal loss of 10% of isosorbide mononitrate due to sorption to a variety of plastics in giving sets was detected[11] following simulated infusion in sodium chloride 0.9% and also in glucose 10%.

FURTHER INFORMATION. Sorption of isosorbide dinitrate to central venous catheters—De Muynck C, Vandenbossche GMR, Colardyn F, Remon JP. J Pharm Pharmacol 1993;45:139–41.

FORMULATION

Excipients

Excipients that have been used in presentations of isosorbide include:

Capsules, isosorbide mononitrate: erythrosine (E127); indigo carmine (E132); lactose; quinoline yellow (E104); shellac; talc.
Isosorbide dinitrate: confectioner's sugar; erythrosine (E127); ethanol; gelatin; iron oxide; lactose; macrogol 4000; maize starch; methacrylic polymer; povidone; quinoline yellow (E104); starch; stearic acid; shellac; sucrose; talc.
Tablets, isosorbide mononitrate: colloidal silica; Eudragit E; glucose; kaolin; lactose; macrogol; magnesium stearate; microcrystalline cellulose; montanic acid/ethylene glycol ester; povidone; silica; sodium starch glycollate; sucrose; talc; titanium dioxide (E171).
Isosorbide dinitrate: brilliant blue FCF (133); carbomer 934P; carmellose sodium; cellulose; erythrosine (E127); hydrogenated vegetable oil; icing sugar; lactose; macrogol; magnesium stearate; maize starch; mannitol; microcrystalline cellulose; povidone; quinoline yellow (E104); Red 7; saccharin sodium; sodium silicoaluminate; sodium starch glycollate; starch; sunset yellow FCF (E110); talc.

Bioavailability

Chasseaud *et al*[12] compared the oral bioavailability in 12 healthy volunteers of isosorbide dinitrate from tablet formulations containing 5, 10, and 20 mg and an oral solution containing 10 mg with that of a sublingual tablet containing 5 mg. Relative bioavailabilities of the oral formulations were not significantly different over the dose range studied, but were equivalent to only half that of the sublingual form.
Workers in Italy[13] compared the pharmacokinetic parameters of a sustained-release preparation containing 40 mg isosorbide mononitrate (Ismo Diffutab, Boehringer Biochemia Robin S.p.A. Milan, Italy) with that of the conventional preparation Ismo 20, from the same manufacturer, in a multidose study involving five healthy volunteers. The sustained-release preparation allowed a reduction in the number of daily administrations and produced effective plasma concentrations lasting more than 12 hours.

Oral mixture

A mixture containing isosorbide 50% w/v and sorbitol 5% w/v formulated and used in a hospital in Sheffield was given a shelf-life of 12 months following evaluation of chemical and microbiological stability by Brown *et al*.[14] Excipients included saccharin sodium, sodium citrate, potassium citrate, malic acid, potassium sorbate, ethyl alcohol, vanillin, peppermint oil, burnt sugar solution, and distilled water.

FURTHER INFORMATION. Bioavailability of sustained release and non-sustained release isosorbide-5-mononitrate—Muck B, Bonn R, Reitbrock N [German]. Arzneimittelforschung 1989;39(II),Nr.10:1274–6. Assessment of bioavailability of organic nitrates: comparative bioavailability study of sustained-release isosorbide dinitrate preparations—Scheidel B, Blume H, Stenzhorn G, Siewert M, Babej-Dolle RM [German]. Arzneimittelforschung 1991;41(3):212–18. A new multiple-unit oral floating dosage system. II: *In vivo* evaluation of floating and sustained-release characteristics with *p*-aminobenzoic acid and isosorbide dinitrate as model drugs—Ichikawa M, Kato T, Kawahara M, Watanabe S, Kayano M. J Pharm Sci 1991;80(12):1153–6.

PROCESSING

Handling precautions

CAUTION. Both undiluted isosorbide dinitrate and isosorbide mononitrate can be exploded by percussion or excessive heat. Appropriate precautions should be exercised and only exceedingly small amounts of these substances should be isolated.

REFERENCES

1. Mizuno N, Shimizu C, Morita E. J Chromatogr 1983;264:159–63.
2. Vekama K, Oh K, Irie T, Otagiri M, Nishimiya Y, Nara T. Int J Pharmaceutics 1985;25:339–46.
3. Allwood MC. Int J Pharmaceutics 1987;39:183–8.
4. Cossum PA, Roberts MS. Eur J Clin Pharmacol 1981;19:181–5.
5. Roberts MS, Cossum PA, Kowaluk EA, Polack AE. Int J Pharmaceutics 1983;17:145–59.
6. Lee MG, Fenton-May V. J Clin Hosp Pharm 1981;6:209–11.
7. Herbert MC. Proc Guild Hosp Pharm 1990;28:10–14.
8. Lee MG. Am J Hosp Pharm 1986;43:1945–9.
9. De Muynck C, Remon JP, Colardyn F. J Pharm Pharmacol 1988;40:601–4.
10. De Muynck C, Colardyn F, Remon JP. J Pharm Pharmacol 1991;43:601–4.
11. De Muynck C, Colardyn F, Remon JP. J Pharm Pharmacol 1990;42:433–4.
12. Chasseaud LF, Darragh A, Doyle E, Lambe RF, Taylor T. J Pharm Sci 1984;73(5):699–701.
13. Gandini R, Cunietti E, Assereto R, Castoldi D, Tofanetti O, Baggio G. Arzneimittelforschung 1987;37(II),Nr.7:835–9.
14. Brown AF, Fisher B, Harvey DA, Hoddinott DJ. J Clin Hosp Pharm 1983;8:339–44.

Ketoprofen (BAN, USAN, rINN)

Analgesic; Anti-inflammatory
2-(3-Benzoylphenyl)propionic acid; 3-benzoyl-α-methylbenzeneacetic acid
$C_{16}H_{14}O_3 = 254.3$

CAS—22071-15-4

Pharmacopoeial status

BP

Preparations

Compendial
Ketoprofen Capsules BP. Capsules containing, in each, 50 mg and 100 mg are usually available.

Non-compendial
Alrheumat (Bayer). *Capsules*, ketoprofen 50 mg.
Orudis (Rhône-Poulenc Rorer). *Capsules*, ketoprofen 50 mg and 100 mg.
Suppositories, ketoprofen 100 mg.
Oruvail (Rhône-Poulenc Rorer). *Capsules*, pH-sensitive controlled-release delivery system, ketoprofen 100 mg (Oruvail 100) and 200 mg (Oruvail 200).
Gel, ketoprofen 2.5%. It should not be diluted.
Injection, aqueous solution, ketoprofen 50 mg/mL (Oruvail IM).

Containers and storage

Dosage forms
Orudis and Oruvail capsules and injection should be stored in a dry place, below 25°. Oruvail gel should be stored at room temperature (22° ± 4°) and kept away from naked flames. It should not be incinerated.

PHYSICAL PROPERTIES

Ketoprofen is a white or almost white, odourless, crystalline powder.

Melting point

Ketoprofen melts in the range 93° to 96°.

Dissociation constant

To overcome the problems associated with the determination of dissociation constants of poorly water-soluble drugs, including ketoprofen, in water,[1] aqueous dimethyl sulphoxide (20:80 w/w) was used as a mixed solvent. For a range of carboxylic acids, experimental values of pK_a in the mixed solvent (by potentiometry at 25°) were linearly related to literature pK_a values determined in water. A derived equation was used to convert the experimental pK_a of 7.84 for ketoprofen in aqueous dimethyl sulphoxide (20:80 w/w) to a pK_a of 4.45 in water.

Partition coefficient

Log P (octanol/pH 7.4), 0

Solubility

Ketoprofen is practically insoluble in water; freely soluble in ethanol, in chloroform, in ether, and in acetone; soluble in benzene.

Crystal and molecular structure

Enantiomers
Ketoprofen possesses a chiral centre; it is used as the racemate.

FURTHER INFORMATION. Pharmacokinetics of ketoprofen enantiomers in healthy subjects following single and multiple doses—Foster RT, Jamali F, Russell AS, Aballa SR. J Pharm Sci 1988;77(1):70–3. Ketoprofen pharmacokinetics in humans: evidence of enantiomeric inversion and lack of interaction—Jamali F, Russell AS, Foster RT, Lemko C. J Pharm Sci 1990;79(5):460–1. Ketoprofen enantiomers in synovial fluid—Foster RT, Jamali F, Russell AS [letter]. J Pharm Sci 1989;78(10):881–2.

STABILITY

Exposure of aqueous solutions of ketoprofen (as the sodium salt) to ultraviolet light at 254 nm or daylight, for one hour at room temperature, was reported to yield (3-benzoylphenyl)ethane which was subsequently converted to (3-benzoylphenyl)ethanol and (3-benzoylphenyl)ethanone (analysis by TLC and HPLC).[2] Samples that were protected from light showed negligible decomposition over 24 months.

INCOMPATIBILITY/COMPATIBILITY

Compatibility of ketoprofen in 1:1 physical mixtures with various tablet excipients has been investigated using differential scanning calorimetry.[3] No interactions were shown between ketoprofen and starch, Sta-Rx 1500 (directly compressible starch), Primojel (sodium starch glycollate), Avicel PH 101 (microcrystalline cellulose), Elcema G250 (microfine cellulose), Ac-Di-Sol (a cross-linked form of carmellose sodium), and Sterotex (hydrogenated cotton seed oil). Results were observed that might be attributed to interactions (the nature of which were not determined) between ketoprofen and Precirol Ato 5 (glyceryl palmito stearate), magnesium stearate, Emcompress (calcium hydrogen phosphate), povidone, crospovidone, and lactose.
Evidence of adsorption *in vitro* of ketoprofen onto aluminium hydroxide and dihydroxyaluminium sodium carbonate but not onto magnesium trisilicate or light kaolin has been presented.[4] The authors recommended that co-administration of aluminium-containing antacids with ketoprofen be viewed with caution.

FORMULATION

Excipients

Excipients that have been used in presentations of ketoprofen include:
Capsules: brilliant blue FCF (133); gelatin; lactose; magnesium stearate; quinoline yellow (E104); sucrose; sunset yellow FCF (E110); titanium dioxide (E171).
Tablets: calcium hydrogen phosphate; gelatin; hydroxyethylcellulose; lactose; magnesium stearate; maize starch.
Oral suspensions: chloroform water; compound tragacanth powder; peppermint water (concentrated); saccharin sodium 1% solution.
Gels: carbomer; ethanol; lavender oil; triethanolamine.
Suppositories: semi-synthetic glycerides.
Intramuscular injections (solutions and powder for reconstitution): arginine; benzyl alcohol; citric acid; glycine; sodium hydroxide.

Absorption and bioavailability

Ketoprofen is well absorbed after parenteral, rectal, or oral administration.
Suppositories were prepared that contained micronised ketoprofen suspended in semi-synthetic glycerides (Massa Estarinum A, Massa Estarinum B, or Massa Estarinum 299).[5] In *dogs*, bioavailability following rectal administration of the suppositories or an aqueous solution of ketoprofen with macrogol 400 was about 20% less than the bioavailability of an orally administered solution. No differences in bioavailability were observed between the three suppository formulations. Oral absorption of the solution was complete relative to the solution given intravenously.
In a crossover study involving nine healthy volunteers,[6] bioavailability of ketoprofen (single 200 mg doses) from encapsulated

sustained-release pellets (Oruvail, M&B) was found to be equivalent to that from conventional-release capsules (Orudis, M&B).

Modified-release preparations

Giunchedi et al[7] prepared extended-release multiple-unit oral formulations of ketoprofen in which four hydrophilic matrix units (each containing ketoprofen 50 mg, hypromellose 37.5 mg, mannitol 20 mg, povidone 7.5 mg, magnesium stearate 0.5 mg, and colloidal silica 0.2 mg) were placed in a gelatin capsule. In a crossover study with 12 healthy subjects, 'pulsatile plasma levels' (characterised by two peaks) were produced following the administration of single doses of the multiple-unit formulation, whereas a single plasma concentration peak was produced after the administration of ketoprofen 200 mg capsules (Oruvail). These in-vivo results could not be predicted by in-vitro studies as release in simulated intestinal fluid at pH 7.5 (without enzyme) at 37° occurred at a 'fairly constant rate'. Release of ketoprofen was faster from Oruvail capsules than from the multiple-unit preparation; 80% dissolution occurred after 6 hours and 10 hours, respectively.

Dissolution rates of ketoprofen at pH 2.2 and 37° were greater from 'rapid-release capsules' that contained a water-miscible formulation of ketoprofen dispersed in Gelucire 44/14 and Amberlite resin, than from Orudis capsules (Rhône-Poulenc).[8] Sustained-release capsules that contained a slowly hydrating formulation of ketoprofen in Gelucire 50/13, Gelucire 50/02, and Amberlite resin, produced dissolution rates similar to Oruvail capsules (Rhône-Poulenc). However, when the two experimental preparations were administered to seven healthy volunteers, absorption data did not correlate with dissolution data. Bioavailability of the sustained-release capsules was 61.2% relative to that of rapid-release capsules. Further, following storage for 28 days at 30°, the time for 50% release of ketoprofen from the sustained-release capsules was 161 minutes compared to 253 minutes for freshly prepared capsules; however, no significant differences in absorption were observed between fresh and stored capsules.

Release of ketoprofen in vitro from 'matrix tablets', which contained ketoprofen with hypromellose, followed zero-order kinetics and was independent of pH.[9] When glyceryl monostearate (Precirol) was incorporated in the matrix no reduction in the rate of release of ketoprofen was apparent, but partial coating of the matrix tablets with cellacephate did provide prolonged release. However, pan-spray coating of matrix tablets with a mixture of Eudragit E30 D and macrogol 400 was considered to be the most efficient technique for retarding the release of ketoprofen; a release profile similar to that from commercial sustained-release capsules (Orudis Retard) was shown at a one-coat thickness.

Modified-release beads containing ketoprofen were prepared by Bianchini and Vecchio.[10] Sugar seeds were sprayed, in a coating pan, with an aqueous dispersion of ketoprofen and the beads were then sealed with an aqueous polymer coat. Sealed beads were coated with either an 'enteric-coating' formulation of hypromellose phthalate in an organic solution or a 'controlled-release' formulation of ethylcellulose, hypromellose phthalate, and diethyl phthalate in an organic solution. Details of formulations, production processes, dissolution, and physical properties of the beads were presented.

Conte et al[11] prepared a zero-order delivery system for ketoprofen as an 'active core' coated by a polymeric membrane of polyvinyl alcohol. In-vitro release was affected by core composition, membrane layer thickness, and the exposed surface area of the systems.

Topical preparations

Takayama and Nagai[12] used a simultaneous optimisation technique to design a formulation for a gel ointment: ketoprofen was dissolved in ethanol with d-limonene (as absorption enhancers), and mixed with a solution of a carbomer and triethanolamine in distilled water. Experimental absorption results in rats correlated with mathematical predictions.

Release of ketoprofen from topical gels with poloxamer 407 (Pluronic F-127) as the gel basis has been investigated in a diffusion cell (no membrane).[13] Gels consisted of ketoprofen (0.2% w/w to 3% w/w), poloxamer 407 (20% w/w to 30% w/w), ethanol (0% w/w to 20% w/w), and buffer (pH 3 to 6) or water to 100% w/w. With an increase of poloxamer 407 concentration, release of ketoprofen decreased exponentially. Enhanced release was shown in the presence of ethanol and on increasing pH from 3 to 6. Effects of temperature and initial ketoprofen concentration were also examined. All the gels were 'elegant in appearance' and, when applied to skin, formed smooth films that were easily removed with water.

Potential 'transdermal delivery reservoir formulations' were assessed for their ability to release ketoprofen across a semipermeable membrane through which ketoprofen had been shown to penetrate.[14] From a water-soluble basis (Macrogol Ointment USP) or an oil-in-water basis (Acid Mantle Creme), release of ketoprofen was superior to that from oleagenous bases (Eucerin or Vaseline) or a water-in-oil basis (cold cream).

Suppositories

Liversidge and Grant[15] investigated interactions between ketoprofen and the triglyceride constituents of fatty suppository bases. Results of partition chromatography experiments, designed to assess interaction between ketoprofen and individual triglycerides (tricaprin, trimyristin, trilaurin, tripalmitin, tristearin) correlated in inverse rank order with solubility values for ketoprofen in the triglycerides. Melting points and disintegration times were determined for suppositories prepared with triglycerides (in different proportions) and semi-synthetic glyceride bases (Witepsol and Suppocire).

FURTHER INFORMATION. Chemical properties—dissolution relationship of NSAIDs. III. Release from monoliths [excipients: acrylic resins, ethylcellulose, or polytetrafluoroethylene polymer] in a three phase system—Fini A, Orienti I, Zecchi V. Arch Pharm (Weinheim) 1988;321:209–11. Factors affecting the dissolution of ketoprofen from solid dispersions in various [17] water-soluble polymers—Takayama K, Nambu N, Nagai T. Chem Pharm Bull 1982;30(8):3013-16. Influence of physicochemical interactions on the properties of suppositories. V. The in vitro release of ketoprofen and metronidazole from various fatty suppository bases [commercial bases and binary mixtures of pure triglycerides] and correlations with in vivo plasma levels [in rats]—Grant DJW, Liversidge GG, Bell J. Int J Pharmaceutics 1983;14:251–62. Anti-inflammatory activity of ketoprofen gel on carrageenan-induced paw edema in rats [a 1% ketoprofen gel in 20% Pluronic F-127]—Chi S-C, Jun HW. J Pharm Sci 1990;79(11):974-7.

REFERENCES

1. Fini A, DeMaria P, Guarnieri A, Varoli L. J Pharm Sci 1987;76(1):48-52.
2. Pietta P, Manera E, Ceva P. J Chromatog 1987;390(2):454–7.
3. Botha SA, Lötter AP. Drug Dev Ind Pharm 1989;15(3):415–26.
4. Ismail FA, Khalafallah N, Khalil SA. Int J Pharmaceutics 1987;34:189–96.

5. Schmitt M, Guentert TW. J Pharm Sci 1990;79(7):614–16.
6. Houghton GW, Dennis MJ, Rigler ED. Biopharm Drug Dispos 1984;5:203–9.
7. Guinchedi P, Maggi L, Conte U, Caramella C. Int J Pharmaceutics 1991;77:177–81.
8. Dennis AB, Farr SJ, Kellaway IW, Taylor G, Davidson R. Int J Pharmaceutics 1990;65:85–100.
9. Mura P, Bramanti G, Fabbri L, Valleri M. Drug Dev Ind Pharm 1989;15:2695–706.
10. Bianchini R, Vecchio C. Boll Chim Farm 1987;126(Nov):441–8.
11. Conte U, Colombo P, Caramella C, La Manna A. Il Farmaco (Ed Prat) 1984;39(3):68–75.
12. Takayama K, Nagai T. Int J Pharmaceutics 1991;74:115–26.
13. Chi SC, Jun HW. J Pharm Sci 1991;80(3):280–3.
14. Berba J, Goranson S, Langle J, Banakar UV. Drug Dev Ind Pharm 1991;17(1):55–65.
15. Liversidge GG, Grant DJW. Drug Dev Ind Pharm 1983;9(1&2):223–46.

Levodopa (BAN, USAN, rINN)

Antiparkinsonian; Dopaminergic

Dihydroxyphenylalanine; dopa; L-dopa
3-(3,4-Dihydroxyphenyl)-L-alanine; (−)-3-(3,4-dihydroxyphenyl)-L-alanine; 3-hydroxy-L-tyrosine
$C_9H_{11}NO_4 = 197.2$
CAS—59-92-7

Pharmacopoeial status

BP, USP

Preparations

Compendial
Levodopa Capsules BP. Capsules containing, in each, 125 mg, 250 mg, and 500 mg are usually available.
Levodopa Tablets BP. Tablets containing, in each, 500 mg are usually available.
Levodopa and Carbidopa Tablets BP. Tablets containing, in each, 100 mg of levodopa with 10 mg of anhydrous carbidopa, 100 mg of levodopa with 25 mg of anhydrous carbidopa, and 250 mg of levodopa with 25 mg of anhydrous carbidopa are usually available.
Levodopa Capsules USP.
Levodopa Tablets USP.
Carbidopa and Levodopa Tablets USP.

Non-compendial
Brocadopa (Brocades). *Capsules*, levodopa 125 mg, 250 mg, and 500 mg.
Larodopa (Cambridge). *Tablets*, levodopa 500 mg.

Compound preparations
Co-beneldopa is the British Approved Name for a mixture of benserazide hydrochloride and levodopa in mass proportions corresponding to 1 part of benserazide and 4 parts of levodopa. Preparations: Madopar and Madopar CR (Roche).
Co-careldopa is the British Approved Name for a mixture of carbidopa and levodopa; the proportions are expressed in the form *X/Y* where *X* and *Y* are the strengths in milligrams of carbidopa and levodopa respectively. Preparations: Sinemet, Sinemet LS, Sinemet-Plus, and Sinemet CR (Du Pont).

Containers and storage

Solid state
Levodopa BP should be kept in a well-closed container and protected from light.
Levodopa USP should be preserved in tight, light-resistant containers, in a dry place; exposure to excessive heat should be prevented.

Dosage forms
All Levodopa USP preparations should be preserved in tight, light-resistant containers, in a dry place; exposure to excessive heat should be prevented.

PHYSICAL PROPERTIES

Levodopa is a white or slightly cream, odourless, almost tasteless crystalline powder.

Melting point

Levodopa melts above 270°, with decomposition.

pH

The pH of a 1% aqueous suspension of *levodopa* lies between 4.5 and 7.0.

Dissociation constants

pK_a 2.3, 8.7, 9.7, 13.4 at 25°

Solubility

Levodopa is slightly soluble in water; practically insoluble in ethanol, in chloroform, and in ether. It is freely soluble in 1M hydrochloric acid but sparingly soluble in 0.1M hydrochloric acid; soluble in aqueous solutions of alkali carbonates.

Dissolution

The USP specifies that for Levodopa Capsules and Tablets USP, not less than 75% of the labelled amount of $C_9H_{11}NO_4$ is dissolved in 30 minutes. Dissolution medium: 900 mL of 0.1N hydrochloric acid; Apparatus 1 at 100 rpm.

STABILITY

In the presence of moisture, oxidation of levodopa by atmospheric oxygen causes rapid discoloration. Solid state levodopa showed marked discoloration (which increased with heating time) after storage at 105° for 24 hours. However, no decomposition could be detected by thin-layer chromatography. In alkaline solution, oxidation of levodopa results in the formation of melanin and related intermediates.

Effect of pH and temperature

Solutions of levodopa (1 mg/mL) in glucose 5% injection, adjusted to pH 5 or 6 with sodium acetate injection or sodium phosphate injection, respectively, were stored at 4°, 25°, and 45° (pH 5) and 25° (pH 6) for 21 days.[1] Solutions buffered to pH 5 and stored at 25° and 45° showed discoloration within 12 hours and 14 days, respectively; solutions at 45° were black at 7 days. Solutions buffered to pH 6 (25°) began to discolour at

36 hours and were black at 14 days. All solutions maintained at least 90% of their initial levodopa concentration for 7 days.

In a brief report den Hartigh et al[2] investigated the stability of both an injection concentrate of levodopa 1 mg/mL in water for injection (pH 3.7) stored in the dark at 0° to 4°, and a 'ready-to-use' infusion solution (with ascorbic acid as a stabiliser) stored at room temperature, protected from light. It was concluded that the injection concentrate could be stored for at least 3 months under the conditions studied and the infusion was stable for at least 24 hours.

FORMULATION

Excipients

Excipients that have been used in presentations of levodopa include:

Capsules: ethylcellulose; magnesium stearate; maize starch; microcrystalline cellulose; talc.
Tablets: citric acid, anhydrous; D&C Red No.7 lake; magnesium stearate; methylhydroxyethylcellulose; microcrystalline cellulose; povidone; sodium bicarbonate; starch; talc.
Suspensions: syrup.

Bioavailability

Administration of levodopa radiolabelled with carbon-14 to *dogs* demonstrated that oral bioavailability was about 50% of that following intravenous or hepatoportal administration.[3]

Extemporaneous formulations

Two extemporaneous suspensions of levodopa formulated by Allwood,[4] one containing a citrate buffer, were compared after storage for 35, 42, and 84 days at ambient temperature in amber glass bottles. Methylcellulose was rejected and was replaced by 0.4% w/v Keltrol as a suspending agent for levodopa. In the unbuffered and buffered suspensions 99.6% and 96.9% of levodopa concentration was retained, respectively, after 84 days. The author concluded that to maintain stability of levodopa in the suspensions buffering was unnecessary. The following formulation was recommended:

Brocadopa (125 mg, Brocades)	20 capsules
Keltrol	0.4 g
Syrup, preservative-free	25 mL
Chloroform spirit	5 mL
Water	to 100 mL

Levodopa is stated to be stable in this formulation for at least 4 weeks.

FURTHER INFORMATION. Bioavailability and acceptability of a dispersible formulation of levodopa-benserazide in Parkinsonian patients with and without dysphagia [in comparison with the standard capsule]—Bayer AJ, Day JJ, Finucane P, Pathy MSJ. J Clin Pharm Ther 1988;13:191–4. L-Dopa esters as potential prodrugs: behavioural activity in experimental models of Parkinson's disease—Cooper DR, Marrel C, van de Waterbeemd H, Testa B, Jenner P, Marsden CD. J Pharm Pharmacol 1987;39:627–35.

REFERENCES

1. Stennett DJ, Christensen JM, Anderson JL, Parrott KA. Am J Hosp Pharm 1986;43:1726–8.
2. den Hartigh J, Twiss I, Vermeij P. Pharm Weekbl (Sci) 1991;13(5):J3.
3. Cotler S, Holazo A, Boxenbaum HG, Kaplan SA. J Pharm Sci 1976;65(6):822–7.
4. Allwood MC. Br J Pharm Pract 1987;9(Feb):34–6.

Lignocaine (BAN)   *Local anaesthetic; Anti-arrhythmic*

Lidocaine (rINN)
2-Diethylaminoaceto-2',6'-xylidide
$C_{14}H_{22}N_2O = 234.3$

Lignocaine Hydrochloride (BANM)

Lidocaine Hydrochloride (rINNM)
$C_{14}H_{22}N_2O, HCl, H_2O = 288.8$
CAS—137-58-6 (lignocaine); 73-78-9 (lignocaine hydrochloride, anhydrous); 6108-05-0 (lignocaine hydrochloride, monohydrate)

Pharmacopoeial status

BP (lignocaine, lignocaine hydrochloride); USP (lidocaine, lidocaine hydrochloride)

Preparations

Compendial
Lignocaine Gel BP (Lignocaine Hydrochloride Gel). A sterile solution of lignocaine hydrochloride in a suitable, water-miscible basis. Gels containing the equivalent of 1% and 2% w/v of anhydrous lignocaine hydrochloride are usually available.
Lignocaine Injection BP (Lignocaine Hydrochloride Injection). A sterile solution of lignocaine hydrochloride in water for injections. Injections containing 0.5% w/v of lignocaine hydrochloride in 10, 20, and 50-mL containers; 1.0% w/v in 0.5, 2, 10, 20, and 50-mL containers; 1.5% w/v in 25-mL containers; and 2% w/v in 0.5, 2, 20, and 50-mL containers are usually available.
Lignocaine and Chlorhexidine Gel BP (Lignocaine Hydrochloride and Chlorhexidine Gluconate Gel). A sterile solution of lignocaine hydrochloride containing 0.25% v/v of chlorhexidine gluconate solution in a suitable water-miscible basis. A gel containing the equivalent of 2% w/v of anhydrous lignocaine hydrochloride and 0.25% v/v of chlorhexidine gluconate solution is usually available.
Lignocaine and Adrenaline Injection BP. A sterile solution of lignocaine hydrochloride and adrenaline acid tartrate in water for injections. The following injections are usually available: 2% w/v of lignocaine hydrochloride with both 1 in 100 000 and 1 in 80 000 of adrenaline, each in 1.8-mL and 2-mL containers; 1 in 200 000 of adrenaline with 0.5, 1.0, and 2.0% w/v of lignocaine hydrochloride, each in 20-mL and 50-mL containers; 1 in 200 000 of adrenaline with 1% w/v of lignocaine hydrochloride in 10-mL containers. pH 3.0 to 4.5.
Lidocaine Topical Aerosol USP.
Lidocaine Ointment USP.
Lidocaine Oral Topical Solution USP.
Lidocaine Hydrochloride Jelly USP.
Lidocaine Hydrochloride Oral Topical Solution USP.
Lidocaine Hydrochloride Topical Solution USP.
Lidocaine Hydrochloride Injection USP. pH 5.0 to 7.0.
Sterile Lidocaine Hydrochloride USP. Suitable for parenteral use.

Non-compendial

Lignostab (Astra). *Aqueous solution*, lignocaine hydrochloride 2%. For use with dental-type syringes.

Lignostab A (Astra). *Aqueous solution*, lignocaine hydrochloride 2% with adrenaline 1:80 000. For use with dental-type syringes.

Min-I-Jet Lignocaine (IMS). *Injection*, lignocaine hydrochloride 1% (10 mg/mL), 2% (20 mg/mL).

Min-I-Jet Lignocaine Hydrochloride with Adrenaline (IMS). *Injection*, lignocaine hydrochloride 5 mg/mL, adrenaline 1 in 200 000.

Select-A-Jet Lignocaine (IMS). *Injection*, lignocaine hydrochloride 20% (200 mg/mL). Dilute before use.

Xylocaine (Astra). *Gel*, anhydrous lignocaine hydrochloride 2% in a sterile lubricant water-miscible basis.

Ointment, lignocaine 5% in a water-miscible basis.

Spray (pump spray), lignocaine 10% (100 mg/g), 10 mg/dose.

Topical 4%, anhydrous lignocaine hydrochloride 40 mg/mL.

Injection 0.5%, lignocaine hydrochloride equivalent to anhydrous lignocaine hydrochloride 5 mg/mL.

Injection 0.5% with adrenaline 1 in 200 000, anhydrous lignocaine hydrochloride 5 mg/mL, adrenaline 1 in 200 000.

Injection 1%, lignocaine hydrochloride equivalent to anhydrous lignocaine hydrochloride 10 mg/mL.

Injection 1% with adrenaline 1 in 200 000, anhydrous lignocaine hydrochloride 10 mg/mL, adrenaline 1 in 200 000.

Injection 1.5%, lignocaine hydrochloride equivalent to anhydrous lignocaine hydrochloride 15 mg/mL.

Injection 2%, lignocaine hydrochloride equivalent to anhydrous lignocaine hydrochloride 20 mg/mL.

Injection 2% with adrenaline 1 in 200 000, anhydrous lignocaine hydrochloride 20 mg/mL, adrenaline 1 in 200 000.

Xylocard (Astra). *Injection 100 mg*, lignocaine hydrochloride (anhydrous) 20 mg/mL.

Intravenous infusion, lignocaine hydrochloride (anhydrous) 200 mg/mL. Dilute before use.

Injections of lignocaine hydrochloride 0.1% (1 mg/mL) or 0.2% (2 mg/mL) in glucose 5% injection are available from Baxter.

Containers and storage

Solid state

Lignocaine BP should be kept in a well-closed container.

Lignocaine Hydrochloride BP should be kept in a well-closed container and protected from light.

Lidocaine USP and Lidocaine Hydrochloride USP should be preserved in well-closed containers.

Dosage forms

Lignocaine Gel BP and Lignocaine and Chlorhexidine Gel BP should be kept in suitable tamper-evident containers holding sufficient of the gel for use on one occasion and should be stored at a temperature of 8° to 15°.

Lignocaine and Adrenaline Injection BP should be protected from light.

Lidocaine Topical Aerosol USP should be preserved in non-reactive aerosol containers equipped with metered-dose valves.

Lidocaine Ointment USP, Lidocaine Oral Topical Solution USP, Lidocaine Hydrochloride Jelly USP, Lidocaine Hydrochloride Oral Topical Solution USP, and Lidocaine Hydrochloride Topical Solution USP should all be preserved in tight containers.

Lidocaine Hydrochloride Injection USP should be preserved in single-dose or in multiple-dose containers, preferably of Type I glass.

Sterile Lidocaine Hydrochloride USP should be preserved in containers suitable for sterile solids.

Lignostab preparations should be stored at 2° to 25°, protected from light.

Xylocaine ointment, spray, topical 4%, and injection solutions should all be stored at room temperature.

Xylocard injection solutions should be stored in a cool place.

PHYSICAL PROPERTIES

Lignocaine is a white to slightly yellow crystalline powder with a characteristic odour.

Lignocaine hydrochloride is a white crystalline powder, odourless or almost odourless, with a slightly bitter taste.

Melting point

Lignocaine melts at 66° to 69°.

Lignocaine hydrochloride melts at 74° to 79°.

pH

The pH of a 0.5% w/v solution of *lignocaine hydrochloride* lies between 4.0 and 5.5.

Dissociation constant

pK_a 7.9 (25°)

Partition coefficient

Log P (octanol/water),[1] 3.4

Solubility

Lignocaine is practically insoluble in water; very soluble in ethanol, in dichloromethane, and in chloroform; freely soluble in benzene and in ether.

Lignocaine hydrochloride is soluble 1 in 0.7 of water, 1 in 1.5 of ethanol, and 1 in 40 of chloroform; practically insoluble in ether.

Effect of pH

The solubility of lignocaine,[2] at 25°, was 22.9 ± 0.1 mM in 0.5M phosphate buffer, pH 7.4, and 16.3 ± 0.1 mM in 1 to 4mM sodium hydroxide, pH in the range 10.4 to 11.9.

Effect of temperature

The solubility of lignocaine base in 0.5M phosphate buffer, pH 7.4, decreased with increasing temperature[2] from 30.3 ± 1.4 mM at 14.5° to 16.5mM at 37°.

STABILITY

Lignocaine hydrochloride is extremely stable in the solid state and in solution. Even at extreme pH values and high temperatures, hydrolysis to 2,6-xylidine and *N,N*-diethylglycine is very slow. It does not degrade by oxidation.

In aqueous solution, lignocaine base is generally stable to both acid and alkali, and to heat; if decomposition occurs it is more readily hydrolysed by acid than by alkali.

The potential of lignocaine, bupivacaine, and mepivacaine bases to precipitate from their hydrochloride salts in phosphate buffer at sites of injection[2] was indicated by increasing the pH of the solution to the tissue pH or by lowering the free base solubility at body temperature relative to ambient temperature.

Bonhomme *et al*[3] demonstrated that pH-adjusted solutions of lignocaine (lignocaine 2%, pH 7.2; lignocaine 2%, adrenaline, pH 6.5; lignocaine 2%, adrenaline, pH 7.05) were stable for at least six hours after preparation.

FURTHER INFORMATION. Stability-indicating high-performance liquid chromatographic analysis of lignocaine hydrochloride and lignocaine hydrochloride with epinephrine [adrenaline] injectable solutions—Waraszkiewicz SM, Milano EA, Di Rubio R. J Pharm Sci 1981;70(11):1215–18. Stability of sterile aqueous lidocaine [lignocaine] hydrochloride and epinephrine [adrenaline] injections submitted by US hospitals—Kirchhoefer RD, Allgire JF, Juenge EC. Am J Hosp Pharm 1986;43:1736–41.

INCOMPATIBILITY/COMPATIBILITY

Lignocaine base may be precipitated from alkaline solutions of lignocaine hydrochloride at concentrations greater than 4 mg/mL.

Lignocaine hydrochloride injection may present incompatibility problems with certain acid-stable drugs such as noradrenaline and isoprenaline; its buffering action may raise the pH of intravenous admixtures above 5.5, causing rapid deterioration of the other drugs.

Immediate precipitation was observed when lignocaine hydrochloride (2 g/L) in glucose 5% injection was admixed with methohexitone sodium (2 g/L), and a crystalline precipitate occurred when admixed with sulphadiazine sodium (4 g/L).[4]

Admixtures of lignocaine hydrochloride (2 mg/mL) were visually and chemically stable (in both glass and polyvinyl chloride containers) during storage at 25° for 14 days in the following solutions: glucose 5% injection, sodium chloride 0.9% injection, compound sodium lactate injection, glucose 5% in compound sodium lactate injection, and sodium chloride 0.45% and glucose 5% injection.[5] During a period of 24 hours, lignocaine hydrochloride in either glucose 5% injection, sodium chloride 0.9% injection, or compound sodium lactate injection was visually compatible with aminophylline, bretylium tosylate, calcium gluconate, digoxin, dopamine hydrochloride, soluble insulin, and procainamide hydrochloride. However, incompatibility between lignocaine hydrochloride and phenytoin sodium was noted in all three infusion solutions and was manifest by an immediate cloudy white precipitate.

Lignocaine hydrochloride and phenylephrine hydrochloride admixed in aqueous solution were chemically and visually stable for at least 66 days at room temperature.[6] The solution pH decreased slightly during this time but remained within the optimum pH range for both drugs.

Sorption onto plastics

Lignocaine hydrochloride injection (Elkins-Sinn, USA) 4 mg/mL in glucose 5% injection was stable for up to 120 days when stored at either 30° or 4° in plastic infusion bags (Viaflex, Travenol, USA); there was no substantial loss of lignocaine by sorption or degradation.[7]

No significant sorption of lignocaine hydrochloride from solutions containing 6 mg/mL and 30 mg/mL occurred during storage in soda glass tubes, borosilicate glass volumetric flasks, or soda glass microlitre syringes at 4° or 25°. However, contact between lignocaine solutions and rubber stoppers for extended periods of time led to a 4% decrease in concentration at 240 minutes for the 6 mg/mL solution and a 14% decrease at 420 minutes for the 30 mg/mL solution. No sorption was demonstrated during infusion through polyvinyl chloride or polyethylene catheters.[8]

However, in a slightly alkaline (pH 8) cardioplegic solution containing lignocaine hydrochloride 450 mg/L (Elkins-Sinn, USA), the percentage of unionised lignocaine base increased to 58% (compared to 1.7% and 2.7% in glucose 5% injection and sodium chloride 0.9% injection, respectively, at about pH 6.0).[9] Storage of the cardioplegic solutions in 500-mL and 250-mL polyvinyl chloride bags, at 22°, resulted in a 12% to 19% loss of lignocaine in 2 days, and a 65% to 74% loss in 21 days, believed to be due to sorption to the plastic; it was suggested that the lipid-soluble unionised form may have inter-

acted with the polyvinyl chloride. Losses were unlikely to be due to degradation as storage of the control solutions, in glass containers under similar conditions, showed no loss of lignocaine concentration. Refrigeration of the polyvinyl chloride bags at 4° slowed the loss of lignocaine to 9% or less in 21 days. The greatest loss of lignocaine from the cardioplegic solution occurred in 'underfilled' polyvinyl chloride bags.

Suspensions

Meier and Wendt[10] reported that no interaction or complex formation took place between lignocaine hydrochloride and carmellose sodium when the two were incorporated in a hydrocortisone suspension.

FURTHER INFORMATION. Interactions between lignocaine and caffeine, theophylline and theobromine—Martinez L, Gutierrez P, Hernandez A, Martinez PJ, Thomas J [Spanish]. An Real Acad Farm 1986;52:505–16.

FORMULATION

Excipients

Excipients that have been used in presentations of lignocaine include:

Topical solutions, lignocaine hydrochloride: calcium sorbate; carmellose sodium; hydrochloric acid; methyl and propyl hydroxybenzoates; sodium hydroxide; sodium saccharin.

Aerosols, lignocaine: cetylpyridinium chloride; cineole; ethanol; macrogol; menthol; propylene glycol; saccharin; trichlorofluoromethane/dichlorodifluoromethane.

Ointments, lignocaine: macrogols 1500 and 4000; peppermint oil; propylene glycol; sodium saccharin; spearmint oil.

Gels, lignocaine hydrochloride: carbomer; carmellose; hydrochloric acid; hypromellose; methyl and propyl hydroxybenzoates; sodium cyclamate; sodium hydroxide; sodium methyl hydroxybenzoate; sodium propyl hydroxybenzoate.

Lollipops, lignocaine hydrochloride: amaranth (E123); lemon essence, soluble.

Injections, lignocaine hydrochloride: disodium edetate; glucose; methyl hydroxybenzoate; sodium chloride; sodium hydroxide; sodium metabisulphite.

Eye drops, lignocaine hydrochloride: chlorhexidine acetate.

Bioavailability

The absolute oral and rectal bioavailability of lignocaine hydrochloride solution (20 mg) was determined in *rats*, by two methods, and compared to that following intra-arterial administration.[11] Values for bioavailability were $7.7 \pm 2.3\%$ and $7.1 \pm 2.3\%$ (oral), and $105.6 \pm 43.3\%$ and $83.1 \pm 22.3\%$ (rectal).

The systemic availability of a slow-release rectal preparation of lignocaine hydrochloride (a gelatin capsule containing lignocaine hydrochloride, 300 mg in a wax/cellulose matrix) was found to be 38% to 78% of that of an intravenous infusion (lignocaine hydrochloride 200 mg, Xylocaine 2% solution, Astra) in a study involving six healthy volunteers.[12]

The absorption of lignocaine hydrochloride (100 mg) was variable and incomplete (less than 50% compared to that of an intravenous infusion) when it was administered intranasally as a gel[13] to six healthy subjects in a single-dose, two-way crossover study.

Percutaneous absorption

The percutaneous absorption of lignocaine hydrochloride 1% in the presence of two nonionic surfactants (1% w/w polysorbate 20 and 1% and 3% w/w polysorbate 60) in vehicles containing various proportions of propylene glycol and water was investigated using excised hairless *mouse* skin.[14] The lignocaine penetration flux was enhanced by the surfactants at high concentrations of propylene glycol (60% w/w or above, in both infinite and finite dose experiments) although penetration behaviour was complicated by changes in vehicle composition and temperature changes due to evaporation or moisture uptake following application.

The permeability coefficient for unionised radiolabelled lignocaine (from a 5% suspension in propylene glycol 40% w/w, gelled with hydroxypropylcellulose 1.0% w/w and preserved with chlorbutol 0.25% w/w) through hairless *mouse* skin and human epidermis was 15 times and 50 times greater than for the ionised form, respectively.[15] The authors concluded that hairless *mouse* skin is not an adequate *in-vitro* substitute for human skin when investigating lignocaine penetration.

Effect of additives

Release of lignocaine hydrochloride from films of cellulose acetate butyrate containing dimethyl phthalate and diethyl phthalate as plasticisers (into phosphate buffer pH 6.8, at 37°) increased as the plasticiser concentration increased (to a maximum at 20%).[16] However, release from films containing propylene glycol and castor oil as plasticisers was slower than from unplasticised films. An increase in lignocaine concentration also resulted in an increased release rate.

FURTHER INFORMATION. Temperature and cosurfactant effects on [lignocaine] release from submicron oil in water emulsions—Lostritto RT, Silvestri SL. J Parenter Sci Technol 1987;41(6):220–5. Phonophoresis of lignocaine and prilocaine from Emla cream—Benson HAE, McElnay JC, Harland R. Int J Pharmaceutics 1988;44:65–9. Buffered [lignocaine] in local anaesthesia—Tran S, Middleton RK. DICP Ann Pharmacother 1990;24:1180–1. Formulation of sustained-release products: dissolution and diffusion-controlled release from gelatin films [incorporating lignocaine]—Li Wan Po A, Mhando JR. Int J Pharmaceutics 1984;20:87–98. Effect of some ophthalmic vehicles on *in vivo* performance of xylocaine hydrochloride in *rabbits* eye—Mohamed AA, Ismail S. Pharm Ind 1990;52(12):1556–8. *In vitro* and *in vivo* studies on ophthalmic preparations [aqueous or micellar solutions; o/w or w/o/w emulsions] of xylocaine hydrochloride—Ismail S, Mohamed AA, Hasan SA. Bull Pharm Sci Assiut Univ 1989;12:68–89.

PROCESSING

Sterilisation

Lignocaine gel, lignocaine and chlorhexidine gel, lignocaine injection, and lignocaine and adrenaline injection can be sterilised by heating in an autoclave.

REFERENCES

1. Grouls R, Ackerman E, Machielsen E, Casparie R, Korsten H. Pharm Weekbl (Sci) 1992;14(5) Suppl F:F27.
2. Nakano NI [letter]. J Pharm Sci 1979;68(5):667–8.
3. Bonhomme L, Postaire E, Touratier S, Benhamou D, Martre-Sauvageon H, Preaux N. J Clin Pharm Ther 1988;13:257–61.
4. Riley BB. J Hosp Pharm 1970;28:228–40.
5. Kirschenbaum HL, Aronoff W, Perentesis GP, Plitz GW, Cutie AJ. Am J Hosp Pharm 1982;39:1013–15.
6. Das Gupta V, Stewart KR. J Clin Hosp Pharm 1986;11:449–52.
7. Smith FM, Nuessle NO. Am J Hosp Pharm 1981;38:1745–7.
8. Upton RN, Mather LE, Runciman WB. J Pharm Pharmacol 1987;39:485–7.
9. Lackner TE, Baldus D, Butler CD, Amyx C, Kessler G. Am J Hosp Pharm 1983;40:97–101.
10. Meler J, Wendt L. Pharmazie 1990;45(H9):692–3.
11. de Boer AG, Breimer DD, Pronk J, Gubbens-Stibbe JM. J Pharm Sci 1980;69(7):804–7.
12. Beckett AH, Burgess CD, Johnston A, Warrington SJ. Br J Clin Pharmacol 1978;6:442P–443P.
13. Scavone JM, Greenblatt DJ, Fraser DG. Br J Clin Pharmacol 1989;28:722–4.
14. Sarpotdar PP, Zatz JL. J Pharm Sci 1986;75(2):176–81.
15. Kushla GP, Zatz JL. Int J Pharmaceutics 1991;71:167–73.
16. Safwat SM, Hafez E, El-Monem HA, Ibrahim EA. Bull Pharm Sci Assiut Univ 1989;12:152–72.

Lithium Salts

Treatment and prophylaxis of affective disorders

Lithium Carbonate (USAN)

$Li_2CO_3 = 73.9$

Lithium Citrate

Trilithium 2-hydroxypropane-1,2,3-tricarboxylate tetrahydrate
$C_6H_5Li_3O_7, 4H_2O = 282.0$
CAS—554-13-2 (lithium carbonate); 6080-58-6 (lithium citrate, tetrahydrate); 919-16-4 (lithium citrate, anhydrate)

Pharmacopoeial status

BP, USP (lithium carbonate, lithium citrate)

Preparations

Compendial
Lithium Carbonate Tablets BP. Tablets containing, in each, 250 mg are usually available.
Lithium Carbonate Capsules USP.
Lithium Carbonate Tablets USP.
Lithium Carbonate Extended-release Tablets USP.
Lithium Citrate Syrup USP. Prepared from lithium citrate or lithium hydroxide to which an excess of citric acid has been added. Lithium Hydroxide (USAN) is the subject of a USP monograph.

Non-compendial
Camcolit (Norgine). *Tablets*, Camcolit 250, lithium carbonate 250 mg (6.8 mmol Li⁺).
Tablets, Camcolit 400, controlled release, lithium carbonate 400 mg (10.8 mmol Li⁺).
Li-Liquid (RP Drugs). *Oral solution*, sugar free, lithium citrate 509 mg/5 mL (5.4 mmol Li⁺/5 mL) and 1.018 g/5 mL (10.8 mmol Li⁺/5 mL).
Liskonum (SK&F). *Tablets*, controlled release, lithium carbonate 450 mg (12.2 mmol Li⁺).
Litarex (CP). *Tablets*, controlled release, lithium citrate 564 mg (6 mmol Li⁺).
Phasal (Lagap). *Tablets*, sustained release, lithium carbonate 300 mg (8.1 mmol Li⁺).
Priadel (Delandale). *Tablets*, controlled release, lithium carbonate 200 mg (5.4 mmol Li⁺) and 400 mg (10.8 mmol Li⁺).
Liquid, sugar free, lithium citrate 520 mg/5 mL (approximately 5.4 mmol Li⁺/5 mL). Dilution is not recommended.

Containers and storage

Solid state

Lithium Citrate BP should be kept in an airtight container.

Lithium Carbonate USP should be preserved in well-closed containers.

Lithium Citrate USP should be preserved in tight containers.

Dosage forms

Lithium Carbonate Capsules USP and Lithium Carbonate Tablets USP should be preserved in well-closed containers.

Lithium Citrate Syrup USP should be preserved in tight containers.

Camcolit tablets, Litarex tablets, Phasal tablets, and Priadel tablets should be stored in a cool, dry place; Priadel tablets should be dispensed in airtight containers.

Liskonum tablets should be stored in a dry place.

Priadel Liquid should be stored in a cool place and protected from direct sunlight.

PHYSICAL PROPERTIES

Lithium carbonate is a white, granular, odourless powder.

Lithium citrate is a white or almost white, fine crystalline powder; odourless and with a faintly alkaline taste; deliquesces on exposure to moist air.

Melting point

Melting points ranging from 618° to 720° have been reported for lithium carbonate.

pH

A saturated solution of lithium carbonate is alkaline to litmus. The pH of a 1 in 20 solution of lithium citrate is in the range 7.0 to 10.0.

Solubility

Lithium carbonate is soluble 1 in 100 of water and 1 in 140 of boiling water; practically insoluble in ethanol; soluble, with effervescence, in dilute mineral acids.

Lithium citrate is soluble 1 in 2 of water; slightly soluble in ethanol and in ether.

Dissolution

The USP specifies that for Lithium Carbonate Capsules USP and Lithium Carbonate Tablets USP not less than 60% of the labelled amount of Li_2CO_3 is dissolved in 30 minutes. Dissolution medium: 900 mL of water; Apparatus 1 at 100 rpm.

Dissolution properties

Wall et al[1] established linear intrinsic dissolution rate profiles for lithium carbonate (from lithium carbonate discs) in simulated gastric fluid without pepsin, in Tris buffer or in water. However, in simulated intestinal fluid that contained phosphate, but without pancreatin, precipitation of trilithium phosphate onto the surface of the discs was detected. The authors suggested that dissolution studies of dosage forms of lithium carbonate may not be valid in media that contain a phosphate buffer.

Dissolution studies of lithium carbonate powder, four brands of lithium carbonate tablets, and three brands of lithium carbonate capsules by three methods using potassium biphthalate buffer, pH 3.0 at 37°, revealed no significant differences in drug release, after a lag time for capsules.[2] Significant correlation was shown between dissolution rates under certain conditions and saliva concentrations (in a crossover study with seven healthy volunteers) after two hours. Inter-subject variation in concentrations of lithium carbonate in saliva was significant.

Workers in Australia[3] compared four conventional oral dosage forms of lithium carbonate, two sustained-release forms of lithium carbonate, and a sustained-release form of lithium sulphate, in eight volunteers, with respect to dissolution in simulated intestinal fluid and in simulated gastric fluid and, for some of these products, salivary concentrations of lithium. Selected products produced in-vivo results in keeping with in-vitro predictions.

FURTHER INFORMATION. Dissolution of some lithium dosage forms [one sustained-release and six conventional-release products] and correlation with Enslin number—Ritschel WA, Parab P. Drug Dev Ind Pharm 1985;11(1):147–67.

STABILITY

It has been reported that lithium carbonate decomposes in acidic solution to yield the lithium salt of the acid, bicarbonate, carbonic acid, and subsequently carbon dioxide.[4]

INCOMPATIBILITY/COMPATIBILITY

Lithium carbonate in solution is reported to be incompatible with cations (such as calcium or barium) and anions (such as phosphate). Carbonate salts of such cations and lithium salts of such anions are less soluble than lithium carbonate.[4]

McGee et al[5] reported the formation of a precipitate when lithium citrate syrup (Lithonate-S) was mixed with trifluoperazine hydrochloride concentrate (Stelazine).

Immediate visual incompatibility (opaque turbidity or separation into two immiscible liquid phases) was observed[6] when 5 mL or 10 mL of lithium citrate syrup (Philips Roxane Labs and Rowell Labs, 1.6 mEq Li^+/mL) was mixed with various volumes of each of the following neuroleptics, as solutions or concentrates: chlorpromazine hydrochloride (Lederle, or Thorazine, SK&F, 100 mg/mL); haloperidol lactate (Haldol, McNeil, 2 mg/mL); thioridazine hydrochloride (Melleril, Sandoz, 100 mg/mL); trifluoperazine hydrochloride (Stelazine, SK&F, 10 mg/mL). Samples were prepared by both orders of mixing and were stored at 4° and 25°.

FORMULATION

Excipients

Excipients that have been used in presentations of lithium salts include:

Capsules, lithium carbonate: allura red AC (E129); gelatin; talc; titanium dioxide (E171).

Tablets, lithium carbonate: brilliant blue FCF (133), lake; calcium hydrogen phosphate; calcium stearate; macrogol; magnesium stearate; maize starch; microcrystalline cellulose; potato starch; povidone; sodium lauryl sulphate; sodium starch glycollate; tartrazine (E102), lake.

Slow-release tablets, lithium carbonate: brilliant blue FCF (133), aluminium lake; calcium stearate; carnauba wax; cellulose compounds; erythrosine (E127), aluminium lake; lactose; hydroxybenzoates; povidone; propylene glycol; sodium chloride; sodium lauryl sulphate; sodium starch glycollate; sorbitol; sunset yellow FCF (E110), aluminium lake; titanium dioxide (E171).

Syrups, lithium citrate: citric acid; ethanol (0.3% v/v); raspberry flavour; sodium benzoate; sodium saccharin; sorbitol.

Bioequivalence

Bioequivalence of two capsule preparations of lithium carbonate 300 mg (Pfi-Lithium, Pfizer and Eskalith, SK&F) was indicated following a single-dose, crossover study involving 18 healthy volunteers.[7]

Modified-release preparations

Sustained-release tablets of lithium carbonate 400 mg in a fat matrix were prepared; tablets contained glyceryl palmito-stearate (Precirol Ato; 260, 300, or 340 mg), carbomer (Carbopol 940; 22, 31, or 40 mg), magnesium stearate (12 mg), and talc (26 mg), and several compression forces were used.[8] Zero-order release of lithium in vitro at about 10^{-3} M/hour was demonstrated. For one preparation, a crossover study with six healthy subjects revealed a bioavailability of 75% relative to that of an immediate-release capsule of lithium carbonate with the same excipients.

Directly compressed tablets

Dedhiya et al[9] investigated relationships between physical properties of directly compressed tablets of lithium carbonate (with maize starch, calcium hydrogen phosphate, macrogol, magnesium stearate, and sodium lauryl sulphate as excipients) and the compression force used in preparation of the tablets. There was a linear correlation between the maximum compression force (in the range 4000 to 7020 lb) and tablet hardness. Dissolution rates of lithium carbonate from tablets, but not disintegration times of tablets, were also related to compression force.

Syrups

In studies involving five manic-depressive patients who were stabilised on lithium carbonate,[10] a single dose of lithium carbonate, as tablets, was replaced by an equivalent dose of lithium citrate syrup. No differences in peak plasma-lithium concentration or bioavailability (area under plasma concentration versus time curves) were detected between preparations, although lithium was absorbed more rapidly from the syrup.

Ointments

Skinner[11] has reported that use of an ointment comprising lithium succinate 8%, zinc sulphate 0.05%, and DL-α-tocopherol 0.1% in a wool fat basis achieved symptomatic relief and decreased viral excretion in genital herpes treatment. An ointment (water-in-oil emulsion) of lithium succinate 8% w/w and zinc sulphate 0.05% w/w (Efalith, Scotia) is marketed for treatment of seborrhoeic dermatitis. It also contains wool alcohols and hard, soft, and liquid paraffins.

Lubricants and surfactants

Dissolution of lithium from capsules that contained lithium carbonate and spray-dried lactose was affected by the presence of various lubricants and surfactants.[12] Dissolution in hydrochloric acid 0.3% was slow from preparations that contained magnesium stearate (lubricant), owing to a 'water-proofing' effect, whereas dissolution was rapid from preparations with sodium lauryl sulphate (surfactant-lubricant) but these capsules showed poor 'weight control'. Rapid dissolution and satisfactory weight control were shown by capsules prepared with sodium lauryl sulphate and magnesium stearate. Sodium lauryl sulphate was more effective at promoting dissolution of lithium when added to the formulation than when added to the dissolution medium. Studies of lithium carbonate capsules formulated with magnesium stearate established a direct relationship between the dissolution of magnesium and of lithium.

FURTHER INFORMATION. Steady-state pharmacokinetics of lithium carbonate in healthy volunteers [differences in single and multiple dose lithium pharmacokinetics]—Hunter R. Br J Clin Pharmacol 1988;25:375–80. Serum concentrations of lithium after three proprietary preparations of lithium carbonate (Priadel, Phasal, and Camcolit) [in patients]—Bennie EH, Manzoor AKM, Scott AM, Fell GS. Br J Clin Pharmacol 1977;4:479–83. Gastro-intestinal bioavailability assessment [in ten healthy subjects] of commercially prepared sustained-release lithium tablets using a deconvolution technique—Llabrés M, Fariña JB. Drug Dev Ind Pharm 1989;15(11):1827–41. Influence of the kind of pore-creating agent [wheat starch, microcrystalline cellulose, crospovidone] on the diffusion rate of lithium acetate from a gastro-intestinal diffusion system—Janicki S, Jedras Z [Polish]. Farm Pol 1989;45:447–51. In vitro and in vivo release of lithium from a lithium sulphate gastrointestinal diffusion system [a soluble tablet coated with a membrane of cellulose acetate with a pore-creating agent, gum arabic]—Jedras Z, Jakitowicz J, Nowicki Z, Galuszko P, Janicki S. J Controlled Release 1989;9:13–19. Lithium acetate gastrointestinal diffusion system. Part 2. Lithium acetate multi-unit gastro-intestinal diffusion system: preparation and release rate studies—Jedras Z, Janicki S. Pharmazie 1990;45:116–18. Libération in vitro du sulfate de lithium incorporé à des matrices hydrophiles—Ventouras K, Buri P [French]. Pharm Acta Helv 1976;51(7/8):212–18.

REFERENCES

1. Wall BP, Parkin JE, Sunderland VB. J Pharm Pharmacol 1985;37:338–40.
2. Needham TE, Javid D, Brown W. J Pharm Sci 1979;68(8):952–4.
3. Wall BP, Parkin JE, Sunderland VB, Zorbas A. J Pharm Pharmacol 1982;34:601–3.
4. Stober HC. In: Florey K, editor. Analytical profiles of drug substances; vol 15. London: Academic Press, 1986:367–91.
5. McGee JL, Alexander B, Perry PJ [letter]. Am J Hosp Pharm 1980;37:1052.
6. Theesen KA, Wilson JE, Newton DW, Ueda CT. Am J Hosp Pharm 1981;38:1750–3.
7. Foster TS, Crass RE, Bustrack JA, Smith RB, Munson JW. Am J Hosp Pharm 1980;37:1528–31.
8. Llabrés M, Fariña JB. J Pharm Sci 1991;80(11):1012–16.
9. Dedhiya MG, Woodruff CW, Menard FA, Rhodes CT. Drug Dev Ind Pharm 1988;14(1):53–61.
10. Hunter R, Taylor A. Br J Pharm Pract 1989;11(4):146–9.
11. Skinner GRB [letter]. Lancet 1983;2:288.
12. Caldwell HC. J Pharm Sci 1974;63(5):770–3.

Lorazepam (BAN, USAN, rINN)   *Anxiolytic*

7-Chloro-5-(2-chlorophenyl)-1,3-dihydro-3-hydroxy-1,4-benzodiazepin-2-one
$C_{15}H_{10}Cl_2N_2O_2 = 321.2$
CAS—846-49-1

Pharmacopoeial status
BP, USP

Preparations

Compendial

Lorazepam Tablets BP. Tablets containing, in each, 0.5 mg, 1 mg, and 2.5 mg are usually available.

Lorazepam Injection BP. A sterile solution of lorazepam in a suitable solvent. An injection containing 4 mg in 1 mL is usually available.

Lorazepam Tablets USP.

Lorazepam Injection USP.

Non-compendial

Ativan (Wyeth). *Tablets*, lorazepam 1 mg and 2.5 mg.

Injection, lorazepam 4 mg/mL. The solution is clear and colourless. To facilitate injection the solution may be diluted with an equal volume of water for injections or sodium chloride 0.9% injection immediately before administration. For intramuscular injection it must be diluted. Ativan injection should not be mixed with other drugs in the same syringe.

Lorazepam tablets of various strengths are also available from APS, Cox, CP, Evans, Kerfoot, Lagap, Norton, Wyeth.

Containers and storage

Solid state

Lorazepam BP should be kept in a well-closed container and protected from light.

Lorazepam USP should be preserved in tight, light-resistant containers.

Dosage forms

Lorazepam Tablets BP should be protected from light and stored at a temperature not exceeding 25°.

Lorazepam Injection BP should be protected from light and stored at a temperature of 2° to 8°.

Lorazepam Tablets USP should be preserved in tight, light-resistant containers.

Lorazepam Injection USP should be preserved in single-dose or in multiple-dose containers, preferably of Type I glass, protected from light.

Ativan tablets should be stored in a cool, dry place.

Ativan injection should be stored in a refrigerator between 0° and 4°. Protect from light.

PHYSICAL PROPERTIES

Lorazepam is a white or almost white crystalline powder; odourless or almost odourless.

Melting point

Lorazepam melts in the range 166° to 168°.

Dissociation constants

pK_a 1.3, 11.5 (20°)

The pK_a values for lorazepam of 1.3 and 11.5 were determined spectrophotometrically.[1] The neutral species can act as a base by undergoing protonation in acid (pK_a 1.3), or as an acid by undergoing deprotonation within the pH range 7 to 12 (pK_a 11.5). The site of protonation was predicted to be the nitrogen atom at position 4 in the diazepine ring. Deprotonation was concluded to occur most probably at the hydroxyl group at position 3 in the diazepine ring.

Partition coefficient

Log P (octanol/pH 7.4), 2.4

Solubility

Lorazepam is practically insoluble in water; sparingly soluble in ethanol, in ethyl acetate, and in propylene glycol; slightly soluble in chloroform and in ether.

As part of a wider study of the sorption of lorazepam from intravenous admixtures, Newton et al[2] investigated its solubility in water and in three aqueous intravenous solutions. Results were as follows:

Solution	pH	Solubility (mg/mL)
Glucose 5% injection	4.4	0.062
Sodium chloride 0.9% injection	6.3	0.027
De-ionised water	7.1	0.054
Compound sodium lactate injection	7.2	0.055

The dependence of solubility on pH was explained by the ampholytic nature of lorazepam. Glucose 5% injection was considered to be the most suitable diluent for lorazepam intended for intravenous infusion.

Non-aqueous solvents were evaluated to determine their suitability as vehicles for the intranasal administration of lorazepam.[3] Solely on solubility criteria (capability to dissolve 4 mg in less than 0.25 mL), triacetin, dimethyl sulphoxide, macrogol 400, Lipal-9-LA [laureth-9(polyoxyethylene-9 lauryl ether)], Cremophor EL (polyoxyethylated castor oil), isopropyl adipate, and azone 1-dodecylazacycloheptane-2-one were suitable. Only Cremophor EL was acceptable on grounds of freedom from irritancy (on two human subjects). See Formulation–Bioavailability.

Dissolution

The USP specifies that for Lorazepam Tablets USP not less than 60% of the labelled amount of $C_{15}H_{10}Cl_2N_2O_2$ is dissolved in 30 minutes and not less than 80% in 60 minutes. Dissolution medium: 500 mL of water; Apparatus 1 at 100 rpm.

Dissolution properties

In a study where lorazepam was recrystallised from water or aqueous solutions of surfactants or polymers,[4] the crystals collected from an ethanolic solution of lorazepam (1%) mixed with an aqueous solution of povidone 44000 (2.5%) had the fastest dissolution rate; the authors suggested that this may be due to adsorption of povidone to the surface of lorazepam crystals.

Crystal and molecular structure

In a physicochemical study of lorazepam[5] no evidence of polymorphism was found; however, recrystallisation from various solvents yielded solvate forms which were then characterised. Similarly, by cooling and precipitation methods, Udupa[6] prepared crystal forms of lorazepam and examined stability, dissolution, and diffusion rates.

STABILITY

Loss of a molecule of water from lorazepam and rearrangement produces 6-chloro-4-(2-chlorophenyl)-2-quinolinecarboxaldehyde. This can further disproportionate and either oxidise to the corresponding quinazolinecarboxylic acid or reduce to the quinazoline alcohol.

Lorazepam is susceptible to acid hydrolysis to form 2-amino-2′,5-dichlorobenzophenone. In alkaline solution, lorazepam rearranges to form 7-chloro-5-(2-chlorophenyl)-4,5-dihydro-2H-1,4-benzodiazepin-2,3(1H)-dione.

The effects of elevated temperature and humidity on the stability of lorazepam in the solid state and as tablets have been investigated.[7] Samples were stored at room temperature, 37°, and 60°, in air and at 80% relative humidity, for periods up to one year. The degradation product in all instances was 6-chloro-4-(2-chlorophenyl)-2-quinazolinecarboxaldehyde. Further compounds were detected following storage of lorazepam at 60° and tablets at 37° and 60°; these included the corresponding quinazolinecarboxylic acid and the quinazolinone.

A kinetic model for lorazepam degradation[8] was constructed by analogue-hybrid simulation of experimental data obtained for the stability of a lorazepam solution (1.0×10^{-5}M in buffer pH 7) at 40° and 50°. Application of the model led to the deduction that, under the stated conditions, the lorazepam degradation reaction to form 6-chloro-4-(2-chlorophenyl)-2-quinazolinecarboxaldehyde followed first-order kinetics.

FURTHER INFORMATION. Stability of lorazepam diluted in bacteriostatic water for injection at two temperatures—Nahata MC, Morosco RS, Hipple TF. J Clin Pharm Ther 1993;18(1):69–71.

INCOMPATIBILITY/COMPATIBILITY

In injection solutions, lorazepam has been reported to be incompatible with buprenorphine hydrochloride.

No visual effects were reported during a four-hour period when 1 mL of lorazepam 2 mg/mL (Wyeth) was mixed with 2 mL of cimetidine hydrochloride 300 mg/2 mL (SKF).[9] Layer formation, which disappeared after vortex mixing, was reported during a one-hour study period when 1 mL of lorazepam 4 mg/mL (Wyeth) was added to 2 mL of ranitidine hydrochloride 50 mg/2 mL (Glaxo).[10]

Sorption to polyvinyl chloride

Loss of lorazepam to flexible polyvinyl chloride bags and delivery tubing from intravenous admixtures (40 micrograms/mL) with glucose 5% infusions, under static storage conditions, was initially rapid (attributed to diffusion partitioning of lorazepam to the plasticiser), followed by a slower loss due to sorption.[2] During storage at 23° ± 1°, solutions of 50 mL or 100 mL in bags of 50-mL, 100-mL, and 250-mL capacity contained not less than 90% of the initial lorazepam concentration after 5 hours or after 2 hours, depending on the surface area:volume ratio. Under continuous flow (100, 200, and 600 mL/h) through tube lengths of 180 cm and 350 cm, the maximum loss of lorazepam recorded was 5% to the 350 cm tube at a flow rate of 100 mL/h. The authors concluded that up to 5 hours is a suitable period for the intravenous infusion of admixtures of lorazepam in glucose 5%.

FORMULATION

Excipients

Excipients that have been used in presentations of lorazepam include:
Tablets: aluminium hydroxide; colloidal silica; dibutyl phthalate; lactose; macrogol; magnesium stearate; microcrystalline cellulose; talc.
Injections: benzyl alcohol; macrogol 400; propylene glycol.

Bioavailability

In a crossover study with six healthy volunteers,[11] six single doses of 2 mg or 4 mg lorazepam were administered by the intravenous, intramuscular, and oral routes at intervals of one week.

Dose-dependence was not indicated by the absorption kinetics of either intramuscular or oral lorazepam. Apparent systemic availability of oral lorazepam ranged between 89% and 95% and that of intramuscular lorazepam between 84% and 100%.

Sublingual tablets

Greenblatt *et al*[12] compared the pharmacokinetics of lorazepam administered by the sublingual, intravenous, intramuscular, and oral routes. In a crossover study, ten healthy volunteers received single doses of lorazepam 2 mg on five occasions at intervals of not less than one week. During sublingual administration, the tablets were held under the tongue for 15 minutes. There was no significant difference in bioavailability between routes and the rate and extent of absorption of sublingual lorazepam was similar to that of oral administration. The authors concluded that sublingual lorazepam had an acceptable absorption profile, but that formulations with more rapid dissolution rates may provide more rapid sublingual absorption.

Suppositories

In a study in *dogs*, Singh *et al*[13] evaluated the physical properties, dissolution behaviour, pharmacokinetics, and bioavailability of lorazepam suppositories prepared with fatty bases (theobroma oil alone and with sodium lauryl sulphate or Tween 80) and water-soluble bases (combinations of macrogols). Absorption following rectal administration of the 1 g suppositories, which contained lorazepam 2 mg, was compared to that following oral administration of a solution of lorazepam 2 mg in a vehicle of ethanol 20%, glycerol 20%, and propylene glycol 60%. Bioavailability of lorazepam from the fatty-based suppositories ranged from 75% (theobroma oil alone) to 92% (theobroma oil:Tween 80, 8:2) of that of the oral solution. Bioavailability of lorazepam from the water-based suppositories ranged from 81% (macrogol 4000:macrogol 6000:water, 33:47:20) to 102% (macrogol 1540:macrogol 6000:water, 33:47:20). All the suppository formulations had slower rates of absorption than the oral solution.

Nasal drops

The bioavailability of lorazepam after intranasal administration was evaluated by Lau and Slattery[3] in a crossover study with five healthy volunteers. Single doses of lorazepam 4 mg in Cremophor EL 0.1 mL (see Solubility, above) were administered as nasal drops. Times to peak plasma concentration ranged from 0.5 to 4 hours (mean 2.5 hours), with bioavailability ranging from 35% to 63% (mean 51%) of that following intravenous administration of a 2 mg dose. Intranasal absorption is slow for emergency treatments but it was suggested that it has potential for non-acute treatment. In the same study, intranasal administration of the more lipophilic diazepam had a shorter peak time and greater extent of absorption than lorazepam.

Tablets

Effect of surfactants

When a surfactant (sodium lauryl sulphate, Tween 80, sodium taurocholate, or sodium tauroglycocholate) was included in tablets of lorazepam, *in-vitro* dissolution rates and *in-vitro* permeation through *rabbit* jejunal sac were increased with increasing concentration of surfactant.[14] Tablets also contained lactose, starch paste, potato starch, talc, and magnesium stearate.

PROCESSING

Sterilisation

Lorazepam injection can be sterilised by filtration.

REFERENCES

1. Barrett J, Franklin Smyth W, Davidson IE. J Pharm Pharmacol 1973;25:387–93.
2. Newton DW, Narducci WA, Leet WA, Ueda CT. Am J Hosp Pharm 1983;40:424–7.
3. Lau SWJ, Slattery JT. Int J Pharmaceutics 1989;54:171–4.
4. Shawky S, Mesiha MS. STP Pharma 1988;4(4):270–4.
5. Rambaud J, Pauvert B, Maury L, Delarbe JL, Dubourg A. Il Farmaco 1989;44(5):519–29.
6. Udupa N. Drug Dev Ind Pharm 1990;16(9):1591–6.
7. Dabas PC, Ergüven H, Carducci CN. Drug Dev Ind Pharm 1988;14(1):133–41.
8. Kmetec V, Mrhar A, Karba R, Kozjek F. Int J Pharmaceutics 1984;21:211–18.
9. Souney PF, Solomon MA, Stancher D. Am J Hosp Pharm 1984;41:1840–1.
10. Parker WA. Can J Hosp Pharm 1985;38(6):160–1.
11. Greenblatt JR, Shader RI, Franke K, MacLauchlin DS, Harmatz JS, Divoll Allen M *et al.* J Pharm Sci 1979;68(1):57–63.
12. Greenblatt DJ, Divoll M, Harmatz JS, Shader RI. J Pharm Sci 1982;71(2):248–52.
13. Singh J, Jayaswal SB. Pharm Ind 1985;47:664–8.
14. Singh J, Singh S. Drug Dev Ind Pharm 1990;16(10):1717–23.

Meprobamate (BAN, rINN)   *Anxiolytic*

Meprotanum
2-Methyl-2-propyltrimethylene dicarbamate; 2-methyl-2-propyl-1,3-propanediol dicarbamate
$C_9H_{18}N_2O_4 = 218.3$
CAS—57-53-4

$$CH_2 \cdot O \cdot CO \cdot NH_2$$
$$CH_3 \cdot C \cdot [CH_2]_2 \cdot CH_3$$
$$CH_2 \cdot O \cdot CO \cdot NH_2$$

Pharmacopoeial status

BP, USP

Preparations

Compendial
Meprobamate Tablets USP.
Meprobamate Oral Suspension USP.

Non-compendial
Equanil (Wyeth). *Tablets*, meprobamate 200 mg and 400 mg.

Containers and storage

Solid state
Meprobamate USP should be preserved in tight containers.

Dosage forms
Meprobamate Tablets USP should be preserved in well-closed containers.
Meprobamate Oral Suspension USP should be preserved in tight containers.

PHYSICAL PROPERTIES

Meprobamate exists as a white crystalline powder or as colourless crystals with a characteristic bitter taste.

Melting point

In the BP, the melting range of *meprobamate* is 104° to 108°. *Meprobamate* of the USP melts between 103° and 107°; between the beginning and ending of melting the range does not exceed 2°.

pH

Aqueous solutions of *meprobamate* are neutral.

Partition coefficient

Log *P* (octanol), 0.7

Solubility

Meprobamate is slightly soluble in water (1 in 240); freely soluble in ethanol (1 in 7) and in acetone; sparingly soluble in ether (1 in 70) and in chloroform (1 in 80).

Dissolution

The USP specifies that for Meprobamate Tablets USP not less than 60% of the labelled amount of $C_9H_{18}N_2O_4$ is dissolved in 30 minutes. Dissolution medium: 900 mL of de-aerated water; Apparatus 1 at 100 rpm.

Crystal and molecular structure

Clements and Popli[1] prepared a crystal modification of meprobamate by recrystallisation from distilled water (Form I) and then obtained a second crystal modification (Form II) by melting Form I (at 110°) and supercooling the fused mass. The two forms showed different physicochemical properties; for Form I and Form II melting ranges were 103° to 106° and 94° to 96°, respectively, and aqueous solubilities at 25° were 3.3 mg/mL and 6.2 mg/mL, respectively. In water, Form II reverted to Form I after about 168 hours at 25° or after about 28 hours at 40°.

FURTHER INFORMATION. The polymorphic drugs of the Ph.Eur.,II: IR-spectroscopic and thermodynamic investigations of three polymorphs of meprobamate—Burger A, Schulte K [German]. Arch Pharm (Weinheim) 1981;314:398–408. Study of different polymorphic forms of meprobamate—Lefebvre C, Guillaume F, Bouche R, Bouaziz R, Guyot JC [French]. Pharm Acta Helv 1991;66:90–6.

STABILITY

Meprobamate in the solid state is very stable. It is reported to be stable in dilute acid and dilute alkali and is therefore not degraded by gastric or intestinal juices.
When meprobamate was refluxed with hydrochloric acid 25% w/v for 2 hours as part of an assay method, complete hydrolysis to its monocarbamate and subsequently to 2-methyl-2-propyl-1,3-propanediol was achieved.[2] Both these compounds further decomposed to yield ammonia.

FURTHER INFORMATION. Impurities in drugs V: Meprobamate [identified in one lot of raw material and 28 lots of tablets]—Lawrence RC, Lovering EG, Poivier MA, Watson JR. J Pharm Sci 1980;69:1444–5.

FORMULATION

Excipients

Excipients that have been used in presentations of meprobamate include:
Capsules: brilliant blue FCF (133); gelatin; maize starch; sucrose; sunset yellow FCF (E110).

Tablets: acacia; alginic acid; calcium carbonate; carnauba wax; castor oil; ethylcellulose; gelatin; hypromellose; macrogol 6000; magnesium carbonate; magnesium stearate; methylcellulose; patent blue V (E131); potassium polymethylacrylate; sodium lauryl sulphate; stearic acid, purified; starch; sugar; talc; titanium dioxide (E171); white beeswax.
Injections: benzyl alcohol; macrogol 400.

Bioequivalence

In a study of the relative bioavailability of meprobamate 400 mg tablets from eleven different manufacturers, two groups of six healthy volunteers received single doses of a reference tablet and five test tablets.[3] Bioequivalence of the tablets was concluded following analysis of plasma concentration versus time curves. Considerable intra-subject variation in absorption of meprobamate was reported.

REFERENCES

1. Clements JA, Popli SD. Can J Pharm Sci 1973;8(3):88–92.
2. Dreijer-Van Der Glas SM, Dingjan HA. Pharm Weekbl (Sci) 1983;5:186–8.
3. Meyer MC, Melikian AP, Straughn AB. J Pharm Sci 1978;67(9):1290–3.

Mesalazine (BAN, rINN)

Treatment of ulcerative colitis
NOTE. Distinguish from 4-aminosalicylic acid (Aminosalicylic Acid), which is used in the treatment of tuberculosis.
5-Aminosalicylic acid; 5-ASA; fisalamine; Mesalamine (USAN)
5-Amino-2-salicylic acid
$C_7H_7NO_3 = 153.1$
CAS—89-57-6

Preparations

Non-compendial
Asacol (SK&F). *Tablets*, enteric coated with an acrylic-based resin (Eudragit S), mesalazine 400 mg.
Suppositories, mesalazine 250 mg and 500 mg.
Pentasa (Brocades). *Tablets*, slow release, mesalazine 250 mg.
Retention enema, mesalazine 1 g in 100-mL single-dose bottle.
Salofalk (Thames). *Tablets*, enteric coated, mesalazine 250 mg.

Containers and storage

Dosage forms
Asacol tablets should be stored in a dry place, below 25°, and protected from direct sunlight. Asacol suppositories should be stored below 25°, protected from light.
Pentasa slow-release tablets should be stored at room temperature and protected from sunlight. Pentasa enema should be stored at room temperature, protected from light, and used immediately after opening the individual foil pack.
Salofalk tablets should be stored at room temperature protected from direct light.

PHYSICAL PROPERTIES

Mesalazine exists as white to pink crystals.

Melting point

Mesalazine decomposes at about 280°.

Dissociation constants

The pK_a values of mesalazine were determined by Allgayer et al[1] to be 3.0 (−COOH), 6.0 (−NH$_3^+$), and 13.9 (−OH).

Solubility

Mesalazine is slightly soluble in cold water and in ethanol; more soluble in hot water; soluble in hydrochloric acid.

STABILITY

At least 90% of the initial concentration of mesalazine in an extemporaneously prepared suspension (for use as an enema) with tragacanth remained (HPLC assay) after storage in amber glass medicine bottles at room temperature or refrigeration temperature for 90 days.[2] The suspension also contained dibasic sodium phosphate, monobasic sodium phosphate, sodium chloride, sodium ascorbate, methyl and propyl hydroxybenzoates, propylene glycol, and water.
A combination enema that contained beclomethasone dipropionate (2 mg/40 mL) and mesalazine (1 g/40 mL) suspended in a carbomer-water gel was stored at 4°, 20°, and 37° for 44 days in brown glass bottles.[3] Although only very slight discoloration was observed at 4°, the enema suspension became progressively darker during storage at 20° and 37°, possibly owing to the presence of mesalazine degradation products. However, no change in mesalazine content could be detected by reversed-phase HPLC after storage for two weeks at 37°.

FURTHER INFORMATION. Identification of major degradation products of [mesalazine] 5-aminosalicylic acid formed in aqueous solutions and in pharmaceuticals—Jensen J, Cornett C, Olsen CE, Tjornelund J, Hansen SH. Int J Pharmaceutics 1992;88:177–87.

FORMULATION

Excipients

Excipients that have been used in presentations of mesalazine include:
Tablets: lactose.
Suppositories: Witepsol W45.

Modified-release preparations

Following ingestion of a single delayed-release tablet of mesalazine 400 mg within an acrylic resin coat (Eudragit S), by eight ileostomy subjects, 88% of the dose appeared unchanged in the ileostomy effluent during the subsequent 12 hours.[4] Drug release was pH dependent. Coat dissolution *in vitro* was rapid above pH 7.0, but was slow between pH 6.0 and 7.0; the coat did not dissolve at pH 2.0 to 4.0.
The *in-vitro* release of mesalazine from three controlled-release tablet formulations commercially available in the Netherlands[5] (Pentasa 250 mg, Gist-Brocades; Asacol 400 mg, Cedona; and Salofalk 250 mg, Tramedico; containing coatings of ethylcellulose, Eudragit S, and ethylcellulose plus Eudragit S, respectively) was examined at pH 1.0, 6.0, and 7.5. Intra-brand and inter-brand differences in dissolution profiles were demonstrated.

An emulsification-solvent evaporation technique was used to produce mesalazine:Eudragit RS (acrylate-methacrylate copolymer) microspheres with one of two emulsifiers, sodium dodecyl sulphate or Tween 20 (polysorbate 20), at a range of concentrations.[6] The yield of microspheres was greatest when Tween 20 was used. The rate of drug release was enhanced with increased surfactant concentration; microspheres made without surfactant showed greatest retardation in drug release.

FURTHER INFORMATION. pH influence on *in-vitro* release of 5-ASA (mesalazine)—Duchateau A, Philipse R, van der Hoek E, Conemans J. Pharm Weekbl (Sci) 1989;11(Suppl):E10. 5-Aminosalicylate suppositories for the therapy of inflammatory colon disorders [production, assay, and stability]—Vollmer P [German]. Krankenhauspharmazie 1982;3:47–8.

REFERENCES

1. Allgayer H, Sonnenbichler J, Kruis W, Paumgartner G. Arzneimittelforschung 1985;35(II),Nr9:1457–9.
2. Montgomery HA, Smith FM, Scott BE, White SJ, Gerald KB. Am J Hosp Pharm 1986;43:118–20.
3. Stolk LML, Gerrits M, Wiltink EHH, Mulder CJJ, Tytgat GNJ. Pharm Weekbl (Sci) 1989;11(1):20–2.
4. Riley SA, Tavares IA, Bennett A, Mani V. Br J Clin Pharmacol 1988;26:173–7.
5. Stolk LML, Rietbroek R, Wiltink EH, Tukker JJ. Pharm Weekbl (Sci) 1990;12(5):200–4.
6. Watts PJ, Davies MC, Melia CD. J Controlled Release 1991;16:311–18.

Methadone (BAN, pINN)   *Opioid analgesic*

Amidine; amidone; phenadone
6-Dimethylamino-4,4-diphenylheptan-3-one
$C_{21}H_{27}NO = 309.5$

$$CH_3 \cdot CH_2 \cdot CO \cdot \overset{\overset{\displaystyle C_6H_5}{|}}{\underset{\underset{\displaystyle C_6H_5}{|}}{C}} \cdot CH_2 \cdot \overset{\overset{\displaystyle CH_3}{|}}{CH} \cdot N(CH_3)_2$$

Methadone Hydrochloride (BANM, pINNM)

$C_{21}H_{27}NO,HCl = 345.9$
CAS—76-99-3 (methadone); 297-88-1 (methadone, ±); 1095-90-5 (methadone hydrochloride); 125-56-4 (methadone hydrochloride, ±)

Pharmacopoeial status

BP, USP (methadone hydrochloride)

Preparations

Compendial
Methadone Tablets BP. Contain methadone hydrochloride. Tablets containing, in each, 5 mg are usually available.
Methadone Linctus BP. A solution containing 0.04% w/v of methadone hydrochloride in a suitable vehicle with a tolu flavour.
Methadone Injection BP. A sterile solution of methadone hydrochloride in water for injections. An injection containing 10 mg in 1 mL is usually available.
Methadone Hydrochloride Tablets USP.
Methadone Hydrochloride Oral Concentrate USP.
Methadone Hydrochloride Oral Solution USP.

Methadone Hydrochloride Injection USP. pH between 3.0 and 6.5.

Non-compendial
Physeptone (Wellcome). *Tablets*, methadone hydrochloride 5 mg.
Injection, methadone hydrochloride 10 mg/mL.
Methadone Mixture 1 mg/mL is also available from Martindale, and Penn (special order).

Containers and storage

Solid state
Methadone Hydrochloride BP should be kept in a well-closed container and protected from light.
Methadone Hydrochloride USP should be preserved in tight, light-resistant containers.

Dosage forms
In 1992, the Council of the Royal Pharmaceutical Society of Great Britain recommended that child resistant containers should be used for methadone mixture.
Methadone Hydrochloride Tablets USP should be preserved in well-closed containers.
Methadone Hydrochloride Oral Concentrate USP and Methadone Hydrochloride Oral Solution USP should be preserved in tight containers, protected from light, at controlled room temperature.
Methadone Hydrochloride Injection USP should be preserved in single-dose or in multiple-dose, light-resistant containers, preferably of Type I glass.
Physeptone tablets and injection should be stored below 25°; the injection should be protected from light.

PHYSICAL PROPERTIES

Methadone hydrochloride exists as colourless crystals or as a white crystalline powder.

Melting point

Methadone hydrochloride melts in the range 233° to 236°.

pH

A 1% solution of *methadone hydrochloride* has a pH in the range 4.5 to 6.5.

Dissociation constant

pK_a 8.3 (20°)

Partition coefficient

Log P (octanol/pH 7.4), 2.1

Solubility

Methadone hydrochloride is soluble in water; freely soluble in ethanol and in chloroform; practically insoluble in ether and in glycerol.

Dissolution

The USP specifies that for Methadone Hydrochloride Tablets USP (that are intended to be swallowed) not less than 75% of the labelled amount of $C_{21}H_{27}NO,HCl$ is dissolved in 45 minutes. Dissolution medium: 500 mL of water; Apparatus 1 at 100 rpm.

STABILITY

The carbonyl group of methadone is relatively unreactive and methadone is stated to be stable to acid.[1]

In aqueous solutions of methadone hydrochloride, the free base is precipitated from solutions of pH higher than 6. Aqueous solutions can be autoclaved at 120° for 1 hour without loss of potency. However, photolysis and radiolysis of methadone hydrochloride in solution are reported to yield 3,3-diphenyl-2-ethylidene-5-methyltetrahydrofuran and 3-dimethylamino-1,1-diphenylbutene, respectively.[1]

Less than 10% of the initial concentration of methadone hydrochloride was lost during a 4-week study period when solutions of methadone hydrochloride (1 mg/mL, 2 mg/mL, and 5 mg/mL) were prepared in single-dose, flexible polyvinyl chloride containers of sodium chloride 0.9% injection and stored at room temperature, exposed to room light.[3]

Lauriault et al[4] prepared solutions of methadone hydrochloride (0.2 mg/mL, 0.8 mg/mL, and 1.5 mg/mL) in each of four proprietary drink solutions (pH 2.7 to 3.5, which contained either sucrose or aspartame) and in one drink solution to which sodium benzoate had been added. Over 95% of the initial concentration of methadone hydrochloride was maintained for periods ranging from 8 days to 17 days when stored at 20° to 25° (unprotected from light) and for periods ranging from 34 days to 55 days in a refrigerator at 5°. However, unacceptable levels of microbial contamination were apparent after about 2 weeks at 20° to 25° in the solutions that did not contain sodium benzoate.

FURTHER INFORMATION. IR-spectroscopic investigation of the photostability of crystalline drugs—Reisch J, Ulbrich R, Reisch G [German]. Dtsch Apoth Ztg 1980;120(48):2385–90. Influence of pH on the stability of methadone hydrochloride in oral solutions—Nuez AB, Orgega BA, Trillo CF, Del Pozo Carrascosa A [Spanish]. Farm Clin (Spain) 1989;6:616, 618–22.

INCOMPATIBILITY/COMPATIBILITY

Methadone hydrochloride has been reported to be incompatible with alkalis, chlorocresol, oxidising agents, iodides, mercury salts, and saccharin sodium, with some dyes such as amaranth and bordeaux B, and with wild cherry syrup.

Methadone hydrochloride was found to be physically incompatible with aminophylline, ammonium chloride, amylobarbitone sodium, chlorothiazide sodium, heparin sodium, methicillin sodium, pentobarbitone sodium, phenobarbitone sodium, phenytoin sodium, quinalbarbitone sodium, sodium bicarbonate, sodium iodide, and thiopentone sodium.[5]

Physical incompatibility (turbidity or precipitation) was evident when Methadone Linctus BPC 1973 was prepared or diluted with syrup preserved with 0.05% of a combination of hydroxybenzoate esters (Nipastat) or with syrup preserved with a combination of methyl hydroxybenzoate 0.03% and propyl hydroxybenzoate 0.015%.[6] Similar incompatibility was observed when syrup preserved with 0.05% of a combination of hydroxybenzoate esters was used to prepare methadone mixture DTF[7] (see Formulation, below).

Ching et al[8] prepared a methadone hydrochloride (50 mg/10 mL) mixture that contained methyl hydroxybenzoate 0.1%. No significant decomposition of methadone hydrochloride (HPLC analysis) and no physical or microbial deterioration was detected after storage in clear glass containers at 20° to 25° for 113 days. The mixture also contained lemon spirit, citric acid monohydrate, syrup, glycerol, and purified water.

Australian workers[9] reported that the chemical stability of methadone hydrochloride (2.5 mg/30 mL to 80 mg/30 mL) mixtures was within shelf-life requirements for a three-year period when stored in plastic, 'unit-of-use' containers at 23° ± 2° in the absence of light. Excipients in the mixtures were: methyl hydroxybenzoate, citric acid, glycerol, and purified water.

More than 90% of the initial concentration of methadone hydrochloride remained after two weeks when an admixture of methadone hydrochloride 10 mg (Dolophine hydrochloride injection, Eli Lilly, USA) and hydroxyzine hydrochloride 25 mg (Vistaril pamoate, Pfizer, USA) in Cherry Syrup NF was stored at refrigerated or room temperature.[10]

FORMULATION

METHADONE MIXTURE
(Previously: Drug Tariff Formula)

Methadone hydrochloride	500 mg
Syrup	250 mL
Green S and tartrazine solution	1 mL
Tartrazine compound solution	4 mL
Chloroform water, double strength to	500 mL

Excipients

Excipients that have been used in presentations of methadone hydrochloride include:

Tablets: acacia; cellulose; lactose; magnesium stearate; maize starch; microcrystalline cellulose; potassium phosphate; silica; stearic acid; sucrose; sunset yellow FCF (E110); talc.

Oral liquids: allura red AC (E129); chloroform water; compound tartrazine solution; ethanol; glycerol; green S and tartrazine solution; sodium methyl hydroxybenzoate; sodium propyl hydroxybenzoate; sorbitol; syrup; tolu syrup.

Injections: chlorbutol; hydrochloric acid; sodium chloride; sodium hydroxide.

Absorption

In a crossover study involving six healthy volunteers[11] rectal absorption of methadone hydrochloride was investigated from the following preparations, each containing 10 mg of methadone hydrochloride: a 5 mL solution, distilled water pH 6; a 5 mL solution, glycofurol:water (1:1), pH 8; a 5 mL solution, glycofurol:water (1:4), pH 8; fatty suppositories (Witepsol H15); and macrogol 1540 suppositories. A reference oral solution of methadone hydrochloride 10 mg/50 mL in water was also administered. Among the rectal solutions (administered as micro-enemas), the glycofurol:water (1:4) solution produced the fastest initial absorption rate of methadone hydrochloride. Compared with the oral solution, rectal absorption from the fatty suppository was slow and incomplete, whereas the absorption rate and bioavailability (24 hours after administration) from the macrogol suppositories were similar to those from the oral solution.

Modified-release preparations

Choulis et al[12] developed a three-layer, slow-eroding tablet that contained various proportions of methadone hydrochloride, cellacephate, and carbomer in each layer; several methods of manufacture were investigated. The *in-vitro* release rate increased as the proportion of carbomer decreased. Limited studies in *rats* indicated that the sustained-release tablets had longer durations of action and no apparent adverse effects in comparison with intravenous and oral solutions.

FURTHER INFORMATION. The development of an addiction treatment service [use of a methadone hydrochloride oral solution formulated with sorbitol]—Cherry P, Tredree R, Streeter H, Brain K. Pharm J 1986;236:329-31. Methadone mixture formulation [with sorbitol syrup]—Baltzars JE [letter]. Pharm J 1986;237:678.

PROCESSING

Sterilisation

Methadone injection can be sterilised by heating in an autoclave.

REFERENCES

1. Eggers NJ. Aust J Hosp Pharm 1978;8(3):91–2.
2. Bishara RH. In: Florey K, editor. Analytical profiles of drug substances; vol 3. London: Academic Press, 1974:366–439.
3. Denson DD, Crews JC, Grummich KW, Stirm EJ, Sue CA. Am J Hosp Pharm 1991;48:515–17.
4. Lauriault G, LeBelle MJ, Lodge BA, Savard C. Am J Hosp Pharm 1991;48:1252–6.
5. Patel JA, Phillips GL. Am J Hosp Pharm 1966;23:409–11.
6. *PSGB Lab report P/79/2*, 1979.
7. *PSGB Lab report P/80/1*, 1980.
8. Ching MS, Stead CK, Shilson AD. Aust J Hosp Pharm 1989;19(3):159–61.
9. Fellows L, Sunderland VB [letter]. Aust J Hosp Pharm 1990;20(5):468–9.
10. Little TL, Tielke VM, Carlson RK. Am J Hosp Pharm 1982;39:646–7.
11. Moolenaar F, Kaufmann BG, Visser J, Meijer DKF. Int J Pharmaceutics 1986;33:249–52.
12. Choulis NH, Papadopoulos H, Choulis M. Pharmazie 1976;31(H7):466–70.

Methotrexate (BAN, USAN, rINN)   *Cytotoxic*

Amethopterin; 4-amino-10-methylfolic acid
4-Amino-4-deoxy-10-methylpteroyl-L-glutamic acid; *N*-{4-[(2,4-diaminopteridin-6-ylmethyl)methylamino]benzoyl}-L-glutamic acid
$C_{20}H_{22}N_8O_5 = 454.4$

Methotrexate Sodium (BANM, rINNM)

Methotrexate disodium
$C_{20}H_{20}N_8Na_2O_5 = 498.4$
CAS—59-05-2 (methotrexate); 7413-34-5 (methotrexate disodium); 15475-56-6 (methotrexate sodium, *x*Na)

Pharmacopoeial status

BP, USP

Preparations

Compendial
Methotrexate Tablets BP. Tablets containing, in each, 2.5 mg and 10 mg are usually available.
Methotrexate Injection BP. A sterile solution of methotrexate in water for injections containing sodium hydroxide. pH 7.5 to 9.0. Injections containing 2.5 mg and 25 mg in 1 mL, 5 mg and 50 mg in 2 mL, 100 mg in 4 mL, 200 mg in 8 mL, 250 mg and 1 g in 10 mL, 1 g in 40 mL, 5 g in 50 mL, and 500 mg and 5 g in 200 mL are usually available.

Methotrexate Tablets USP.
Methotrexate Sodium Injection USP. pH 7.0 to 9.0.
Methotrexate Sodium for Injection USP.

Non-compendial
Arthitrex (Lederle). *Tablets*, methotrexate (as sodium salt) 2.5 mg.
Maxtrex (Farmitalia Carlo Erba). *Tablets*, methotrexate 2.5 mg and 10 mg.
Methotrexate (Lederle). *Tablets*, methotrexate (as sodium salt) 2.5 mg.
Injection, methotrexate 25 mg (as sodium salt)/mL.
Injection, lyophilised powder for reconstitution with water for injections immediately before use, methotrexate as sodium salt, equivalent to 500 mg methotrexate.
Neither the injection nor the lyophilised powder for injection contain an antimicrobial preservative.
Parenteral methotrexate preparations are stable for 24 hours when diluted with the following intravenous infusion fluids: sodium chloride 0.9%, glucose, sodium chloride and glucose, compound sodium chloride, compound sodium lactate.

Containers and storage

Solid state
Methotrexate BP should be kept in an airtight container, and protected from light.
Methotrexate USP should be preserved in a tight, light-resistant container.
Methotrexate is irritant and care should be taken to avoid contact with skin and mucous membranes.

Dosage forms
Methotrexate Tablets BP and Methotrexate Injection BP should be protected from light.
Methotrexate Tablets USP should be preserved in well-closed containers.
Methotrexate Sodium Injection USP and Methotrexate Sodium for Injection USP should be preserved in containers suitable for sterile solids, the latter protected from light.
Maxtrex tablets should be stored at room temperature protected from light.
Arthitrex and Methotrexate (Lederle) preparations should be stored at controlled room temperature (15° to 30°) and protected from direct sunlight. Other drugs should not be mixed with methotrexate in the same infusion container.

PHYSICAL PROPERTIES

Methotrexate is a yellow to orange-brown crystalline powder.

Melting point

Methotrexate melts in the range 182° to 189°.

Dissociation constants

pK_a 3.8, 4.8, 5.6

Partition coefficients

Wallace *et al*[1] determined partition coefficient values between octanol and water to be 0.034 at pH 3.5, 0.021 at pH 5.3 (buffered suspensions), and 0.005 at pH 8.2 (solution in 0.5% bicarbonate).

Solubility

Methotrexate is practically insoluble in water, in ethanol, in chloroform, in 1,2-dichloro-ethane, and in ether. It dissolves in solutions of mineral acids and in dilute solutions of alkali hydroxides and carbonates. It is slightly soluble in 6M hydrochloric acid.

FURTHER INFORMATION. Solubility and stability characteristics of [methotrexate and] a series of methotrexate dialkyl esters—Fort JJ, Mitra AK. Int J Pharmaceutics 1990;59:271–9.

Dissolution

The USP specifies that for Methotrexate Tablets USP not less than 75% of the labelled amount of $C_{20}H_{22}N_8O_5$ is dissolved in 45 minutes. Dissolution medium: 900 mL of 0.1N hydrochloric acid. Apparatus 2 at 50 rpm.

Crystal and molecular structure

Polymorphs

Methotrexate: Existence of different types of solid [preparation and characterisation of two stable and metastable pseudopolymorphs and an amorphous form of methotrexate]—Chan H-K, Gonda I. Int J Pharmaceutics 1991;68:179–90.

STABILITY

Degradation pathways and kinetics

Methotrexate, in solution, is subject to photolytic and thermal degradation. In alkaline solutions (pH above 8.0) at 85°, first-order hydrolysis yielded the decomposition product N^{10}-methyl-folic acid (methopterin).[2] When methotrexate solutions (pH 8.3) were kept under laboratory fluorescent light at room temperature the major degradation products were identified by ultraviolet spectrophotometry and HPLC as 2,4-diamino-6-pteridinecarbaldehyde, 2,4-diamino-6-pteridinecarboxylic acid, and p-aminobenzoylglutamic acid. The photolytic reaction followed zero-order kinetics with respect to methotrexate concentration and was catalysed by bicarbonate ions.

Hansen et al[3] studied the degradation of methotrexate ($2 \times 10^{-5}M$) in aqueous buffer solution at pH up to 12 at 85°, ionic strength 0.5. The route of degradation was complex below pH 6.5. Above pH 6.5 only one degradation product, methopterin, was formed in quantitative amounts. Maximum stability was shown at about pH 7. Degradation was subject to general acid-base catalysis by various buffers. The temperature dependence of methotrexate degradation was examined in isotonic buffer-free solution (initially pH 8.5) over the range 65° to 95°, and an activation energy of 96.8 kJ/mol was established. The $t_{10\%}$ of this solution (initial pH 8.5) at 25° and at 4° was predicted to be 4.5 years and 88.7 years, respectively.

Effect of temperature, light, and containers

Thermal degradation of methotrexate in clear glass ampoules, characterised by hydrolysis to methopterin, followed apparent zero-order kinetics.[4] Storage of methotrexate injection in glass ampoules for longer than 20 days at 75° resulted in formation of an orange precipitate. Storage in a range of sealed plastic disposable syringes at 64° and 75° also resulted in apparent zero-order degradation of methotrexate.

Methotrexate injection (Lederle, powder for injection, reconstituted with water for injections to 50 mg/mL), stored in the absence of light at a temperature not exceeding 25°, was stable for up to eight months in Plastipak (Becton Dickinson) or Monoject (Sherwood) plastic syringes, both with polypropylene barrels.[4] However, repackaging in Sabre (styrene acrylonitrile, Gillette) or Steriseal (polypropylene, Needle Industries) plastic syringes limited the stability of the solution to 70 days. The degradation process was influenced by the light-absorbing properties of the plastics and to a lesser extent by permeability of the syringes to water vapour. Polypropylene and styrene acrylonitrile syringes provided better light protection than glass ampoules. In an attempt to obviate the problems of sorption and photodegradation of methotrexate intravenous solutions in plastic burette administration sets, McElnay et al[5] compared a standard set (cellulose propionate burette and polyvinyl chloride tubing, A200, Avon UK) with a similar set that had an amber pigment (Amberset A2000, Avon UK) and a set consisting of a methacrylate butadiene styrene burette and polybutadiene tubing (Sureset A2001, Avon UK). The solution was prepared by reconstitution of methotrexate injection (Lederle) in water for injections and dilution in sodium chloride 0.9% to 0.5 mg/mL. An 11% decrease in methotrexate concentration occurred in the standard sets after exposure to sunlight for 7 hours. Drug loss after 48 hours was 65.52% and 79.13% in the unprotected polyvinyl chloride tubing of the standard set and the polybutadiene tubing of the Sureset, respectively; and 16.38% and 12.07% in the polyvinyl chloride tubing of Amberset and light-protected Sureset, respectively. Wrapping the standard sets in foil also prevented photodegradation.

The concentration of methotrexate (0.75 mg/mL) in glucose 5% with sodium bicarbonate (0.05 mEq/mL) decreased by 1.4% and 6.1% after 3 days and 7 days, respectively, in samples stored at 4° to 5° protected from light. In samples stored at room temperature and exposed to light methotrexate concentrations decreased by 6.2% and 14.9% over the same time intervals, respectively.[6] Solutions of methotrexate (0.1, 1, and 20 mg/mL) in admixture with sodium chloride 0.9% in Viaflex (polyvinyl chloride) minibags were microwave-thawed after storage at $-20°$ for 5 weeks and 12 weeks.[7] No significant reduction in either methotrexate content or pH was reported. The polyvinyl chloride bags were thought to afford some protection to methotrexate from photodegradation when solutions were exposed to light.

Effect of concentration

Methotrexate solutions (1.25 to 12.5 mg/mL in sodium chloride 0.9% injection) were physically and chemically stable for up to 15 weeks of refrigerated storage followed by an additional week at room temperature in polyvinyl chloride (Viaflex) or glass containers, protected from light.[8] The limiting factor for long-term stability was a progressive increase in drug concentration due to evaporation of water from the polyvinyl chloride containers.

INCOMPATIBILITY/COMPATIBILITY

Intravenous admixtures

Admixtures of methotrexate sodium with cytarabine (Cytosar-U, Upjohn, USA) and hydrocortisone sodium succinate (Solu-Cortef, Upjohn, USA) were stable in each of four infusion fluids (Elliot's B solution, sodium chloride 0.9% injection, glucose 5% injection, and compound sodium lactate injection) during storage in disposable syringes for at least 10 hours at 25°. However, storage for several days resulted in precipitation.[9] These results were similar to those obtained by Cradock et al[10] who examined the stability of methotrexate, in each of the four vehicles, in glass ampoules at 30° for up to 7 days under fluorescent light.

Methotrexate sodium (Lederle, 200 micrograms/mL) in glucose 5% injection was found (by ultraviolet absorption spectrophotometry) to be incompatible at room temperature with 5-fluorouracil (Roche, 250 micrograms/mL), prednisolone sodium phosphate (Hydeltrasol, MSD, USA, 200 micrograms/mL), and cytarabine (Oncovin, Eli Lilly, USA, 400 micrograms/mL).[11]

Sorption

Chen and Chiou[12] demonstrated the adsorption of about 23% or 7% methotrexate (at concentration 1 microgram/mL) to a glass flask when in solutions of methanol or ethanol (80%), respectively. No adsorption was noted from a solution in water. The extent of adsorption was dependent upon the solvent used and the drug concentration; it was reduced at lower pH (2 to 4) and at higher pH (8 to 9) values, and decreased as the concentration of methotrexate increased up to 100 micrograms/mL.

During a simulated infusion (in sodium chloride 0.9%) at 80 mL/hour, negligible sorption of methotrexate (David Bull Laboratories) to a PALL ELD 96 filter containing a 0.2 micrometre nylon 66 (Posidyne) end-line filter was apparent.[13]

FURTHER INFORMATION. Apparent compatibility of methotrexate and vancomycin—Seay R, Bostrom B [letter]. Am J Hosp Pharm 1990;47:2657–8. Identification and quantitation of impurities in methotrexate—Chatterji DC, Frazier AG, Gallelli JF. J Pharm Sci 1978;67(5):622–4.

FORMULATION

Excipients

Excipients that have been used in presentations of methotrexate include:

Tablets, methotrexate: magnesium stearate; wheat starch.
Methotrexate sodium: lactose; magnesium stearate; maize starch; modified food starch.
Oral solutions, methotrexate: chloroform water; sodium bicarbonate; syrup.
Injections, methotrexate: methyl and propyl hydroxybenzoates; sodium chloride; sodium hydroxide.
Methotrexate sodium: benzyl alcohol; hydrochloric acid; sodium chloride; sodium hydroxide.

Novel dosage forms

In a study in *rats*, Law and Lin[14] investigated the *in-vitro* and *in-vivo* release characteristics of methotrexate from microsphere-in-oil-in-water emulsions. Rapid and slow biphasic drug release was demonstrated. A similar but slower release rate of methotrexate was observed following the addition of phosphatidylcholine to the emulsions.

A monoclonal antibody to methotrexate was produced by Pimm and others;[15] the distribution of methotrexate and methotrexate-antibody complexes compared in *mice* were markedly different.

Halbert *et al*[16] investigated and prepared methotrexate-bovine serum albumin conjugates, which may have the potential to reduce the toxicity of antineoplastic drugs. Release *in vitro* was biphasic and the rate was dependent on both the quantity of methotrexate in the conjugate and the pH of the release medium. Activity in tissue cultures was influenced by a combination of several factors.

Percutaneous absorption

The effects of pH, solubility, and vehicle composition on the percutaneous absorption of methotrexate were examined.[17] Results of skin diffusion studies *in vitro*, using saturated solutions of methotrexate in 50% v/v propylene glycol-water vehicles of pH 1.98 to 6.34, identified a solution with pH between 4.0 and 5.0 as providing the optimum environment for passive diffusion through human cadaver skin.

FURTHER INFORMATION. The influence of Azone on the percutaneous absorption of methotrexate [enhancement of penetration *in vitro*]—Brain KR, Hadgraft J, Lewis D, Allan G. Int J Pharmaceutics 1991;71:R9–R11. Topical methotrexate therapy for psoriasis [enhancement by Azone]—Weinstein GD, McCullough JL, Olsen E. Arch Dermatol 1989;125:227–30. Synthesis of methotrexate-dimyristoylphosphatidylethanolamine analogs and characterization of methotrexate release *in vitro*—Williams AS, Love WG, Williams BD. Int J Pharmaceutics 1992;85:189–97.

PROCESSING

Sterilisation

Methotrexate injection can be sterilised by filtration.

Handling precautions

Methotrexate powder for injection should be reconstituted in a designated area by trained personnel wearing protective gloves and goggles. The work surface should be covered with disposable plastic-backed absorbent paper. Any spillage, waste, or other contaminated materials may be disposed of by incineration. In the case of accidental contamination, if there is any danger of systemic absorption of significant quantities of methotrexate, by any route, the administration of calcium folinate should be considered, to counteract the folate antagonist action of methotrexate.

Polyvinyl chloride glove membranes (Travenol) were shown to be less permeable to methotrexate injection (Lederle) than latex glove membranes.[18] Although only microgram amounts of the drug appeared to permeate the gloves, considerable variation was apparent between samples of gloves from the same batch. The authors recommended double gloving with routine glove changes every 30 minutes to minimise the potential exposure of personnel to methotrexate.

General guidelines on the handling and disposal of cytotoxic drugs are given in the chapter entitled Cytotoxic Drugs: Handling Precautions.

REFERENCES

1. Wallace SM, Runikis JO, Stewart WD. Can J Pharm Sci 1978;13(3):66–8.
2. Chatterji DC, Gallelli JF. J Pharm Sci 1978;67(4):526–31.
3. Hansen J, Kreilgård B, Nielsen O, Veje J. Int J Pharmaceutics 1983;16:141–52.
4. Wright MP, Newton JM. Int J Pharmaceutics 1988;45:237–44.
5. McElnay JC, Elliott DS, Cartwright-Shamoon J, D'Arcy PF. Int J Pharmaceutics 1988;47:239–47.
6. Humphreys A, Marty JJ, Gooey SL, Bourne DWF. Aust J Hosp Pharm 1978;8(2):66–7.
7. Dyvik O, Grislingaas A-L, Tønnesen HH, Karlsen J. J Clin Hosp Pharm 1986;11:343–8.
8. Vincke BJ, Verstraeten AE, El Eini DID, McCarthy TM. Int J Pharmaceutics 1989;54:181–9.
9. Cheung Y-W, Vishnuvajjala BR, Flora KP. Am J Hosp Pharm 1984;41:1802–6.
10. Cradock JC, Kleinman LM, Rahman A. Am J Hosp Pharm 1978;35:402–6.
11. McRae MP, King JC. Am J Hosp Pharm 1976;33:1010–13.
12. Chen M-L, Chiou WL. J Pharm Sci 1982;71(1):129–31.
13. Stevens RF, Wilkins KM. J Clin Pharm Ther 1989;14:475–9.
14. Law SL, Lin FM. Drug Dev Ind Pharm 1991;17(7):919–30.
15. Pimm MV, Caten JE, Clegg JA, Jacobs E, Baldwin RW. J Pharm Pharmacol 1987;39:764–7.

16. Halbert GW, Florence AT, Stuart JFB. J Pharm Pharmacol 1987;39:871–6.
17. Vaidyanathan R, Chaubul MG, Vasavada RC. Int J Pharmaceutics 1985;25:85–93.
18. Stoikes ME, Carlson JD, Farris FF, Walker PR. Am J Hosp Pharm 1987;44:1341–6.

Methyldopa (BAN, USAN, rINN)

Antihypertensive

Alpha-methyldopa; metildopa
(−)-3-(3,4-Dihydroxyphenyl)-2-methyl-L-alanine sesquihydrate
$C_{10}H_{13}NO_4$, $1\frac{1}{2}H_2O = 238.2$

Methyldopate Hydrochloride (BANM, USAN)

The hydrochloride of the ethyl ester of anhydrous methyldopa
$C_{12}H_{17}NO_4$, HCl = 275.7
CAS—555-30-6 (methyldopa, anhydrous); 41372-08-1 (methyldopa, sesquihydrate); 2544-09-4 (methyldopate); 2508-79-4 (methyldopate hydrochloride)

Pharmacopoeial status

BP, USP (methyldopa, methyldopate hydrochloride)

Preparations

Compendial
Methyldopa Tablets BP. Coated tablets containing, in each, the equivalent of 125 mg, 250 mg, and 500 mg of anhydrous methyldopa are usually available.
Methyldopate Injection BP. A sterile solution prepared by dissolving methyldopate hydrochloride in water for injections. An injection containing 250 mg in 5 mL is usually available. pH 3.5 to 4.2.
Methyldopa Tablets USP.
Methyldopa Oral Suspension USP.
Methyldopate Hydrochloride Injection USP. pH 3.0 to 4.2.

Non-compendial
Aldomet (MSD). *Tablets*, methyldopa, equivalent to anhydrous methyldopa 125 mg, 250 mg, and 500 mg.
Suspension, methyldopa 250 mg/5 mL. Do not dilute.
Injection, methyldopate hydrochloride 50 mg/mL. *Diluent*: glucose 5% injection.
Dopamet (Berk). *Tablets*, methyldopa, equivalent to anhydrous methyldopa 125 mg, 250 mg, and 500 mg.
Methyldopa tablets of various strengths are also available from APS, Ashbourne (Metalpha), Cox, CP, Evans, Kerfoot.

Containers and storage

Solid state
Methyldopa BP should be kept in a well-closed container and protected from light.
Methyldopate Hydrochloride BP should be protected from light.

Methyldopa USP should be preserved in well-closed, light-resistant containers.
Methyldopate Hydrochloride USP should be preserved in well-closed containers.

Dosage forms
Methyldopa Tablets BP and Methyldopate Injection BP should be protected from light.
Methyldopa Tablets USP should be preserved in well-closed containers.
Methyldopa Oral Suspension USP should be preserved in tight, light-resistant containers at a temperature not exceeding 26°.
Methyldopate Hydrochloride Injection USP should be preserved in single-dose containers, preferably of Type I glass.
Aldomet preparations should be kept in well-closed containers and tablets and suspension should be stored below 25°, protected from light. The injection should also be protected from freezing.
Dopamet tablets should be stored in a cool, dry place, protected from light.

PHYSICAL PROPERTIES

Methyldopa exists as colourless, or almost colourless, crystals or as a white to yellowish-white fine powder which may contain friable lumps.
Methyldopate hydrochloride is a white or almost white, odourless, crystalline powder.

Melting point

Melting points for *methyldopa* ranging between 290° and 310° have been reported.

pH

The pH of a 1% w/v solution of *methyldopate hydrochloride* is 3.0 to 5.0.

Dissociation constants

pK_a 2.2 (—COOH), 9.2 (—OH), 10.6 (—NH₂), 12.0 (—OH) at 25°

Solubility

Methyldopa is soluble 1 in 100 of water and 1 in 400 of ethanol; practically insoluble in chloroform and in ether; it dissolves in dilute mineral acids.
Methyldopate hydrochloride is soluble 1 in 1 of water, 1 in 3 of ethanol, and 1 in 2 of methanol; it is slightly soluble in chloroform and practically insoluble in ether.

Dissolution

The USP specifies that for Methyldopa Tablets USP not less than 80% of the labelled amount of $C_{10}H_{13}NO_4$ is dissolved in 20 minutes. Dissolution medium: 900 mL of 0.1N hydrochloric acid. Apparatus 2 at 50 rpm.

STABILITY

Methyldopa is unstable in aqueous solution because of the susceptibility of the catechol ring to oxidation. The reaction is catalysed by heavy metal ions. The rate of degradation increases with an increase in pH and oxygen supply and a decrease in the initial reactant concentration. Degraded solutions develop a red coloration (a manifestation of the relatively stable intermediate α-methyldopa chrome) and becomes progressively darker with the eventual formation of a black precipitate, an insoluble α-methylmelanin polymer.

Solutions of methyldopate hydrochloride (25 mg/mL) extemporaneously prepared with syrup from either the injection or from the powder (with and without antoxidant, sodium metabisulphite, and chelating agent, disodium edetate) were stable for at least 168 days when stored at 24° in amber-coloured bottles.[1] The solution of methyldopate hydrochloride prepared from the powder without antoxidant or chelating agent became discoloured after 98 days.

No differences in stability of methyldopa (50 mg/mL) were detected when extemporaneous preparations of triturated methyldopa tablets (MSD) in simple syrup (unpreserved, final solution pH 3.7) and in simple syrup containing 0.02N hydrochloric acid and citric acid (final solution pH 1.8) were compared at 5° and 25° in the dark for up to 14 days.[2]

Stabilisation

Solutions of methyldopa can be stabilised by the addition of chelating agents and antoxidants. Oxidation is inhibited by borate ions.

INCOMPATIBILITY/COMPATIBILITY

Crystals were formed when methyldopate hydrochloride (1 g/L) was in admixture with methohexitone sodium (200 mg/L) or sulphadiazine sodium (4 g/L) in sodium chloride 0.9% injection and with sulphadiazine sodium (4 g/L) or tetracycline hydrochloride (1 g/L) in glucose 5% injection.[3] A haze developed over 3 hours when methyldopate hydrochloride (1 g/L) was admixed with either amphotericin (200 mg/L) or methohexitone sodium (200 mg/L) in glucose 5% injection.

FORMULATION

Excipients

Excipients that have been used in presentations of methyldopa include:

Tablets, methyldopa: calcium disodium edetate; candelilla wax; carnauba wax; cellulose; citric acid; colloidal silica; ethylcellulose; diethyl phthalate; guar gum; hypromellose; hydroxypropylcellulose; iron oxide; macrogol 3350; magnesium stearate; methyl and propyl hydroxybenzoates; microcrystalline cellulose; micronised silica; pregelatinised starch; propylene glycol; quinoline yellow (E104); stearic acid; talc; tartrazine (E102); titanium dioxide (E171); white beeswax.

Oral liquids, methyldopa: benzoic acid; carmellose sodium; cellulose; citric acid; confectioner's sugar; disodium edetate; ethanol; glycerol; hydrochloric acid; polysorbate; syrup; sodium bisulphite; sodium metabisulphite.

Methyldopate hydrochloride: disodium edetate; syrup; sodium benzoate; sodium metabisulphite.

Injections, methyldopate hydrochloride: citric acid, anhydrous; disodium edetate; methyl and propyl hydroxybenzoates; monothioglycerol; sodium bisulphite; sodium hydroxide; sodium metabisulphite.

Dry suspensions

A sustained-release dry suspension of methyldopa prepared with a styrene-ethyl-glycol copolymer matrix was shown to release the drug in a prolonged, controlled manner over 12 hours in simulated gastric fluid at various pH values.[4]

FURTHER INFORMATION. The effect of pH and concentration on α-methyldopa absorption in man—Merfield AE, Mlodozeniec AR, Cortese MA, Rhodes JB, Dressman JB, Amidon GL. J Pharm Pharmacol 1986;38:815–22.

PROCESSING

Sterilisation

Methyldopate injection can be sterilised by filtration.

REFERENCES

1. Das Gupta V, Gibbs CW, Ghanekar AG. Am J Hosp Pharm 1978;35:1382–5.
2. Newton DR, Rogers AG, Becker CH, Torosian G. Am J Hosp Pharm 1975;32:817–21.
3. Riley BB. J Hosp Pharm 1970;28:228–40.
4. Katare OP, Jain SK, Vyas SP. Indian J Pharm Sci 1988;50(1):19–22.

Methylprednisolone (BAN, rINN) *Corticosteroid*

6α-Methylprednisolone
11β,17α,21-Trihydroxy-6α-methylpregna-1,4-diene-3,20-dione
$C_{22}H_{30}O_5 = 374.5$

Methylprednisolone Acetate (BANM, rINNM)
Methylprednisolone 21-acetate
$C_{24}H_{32}O_6 = 416.5$

Methylprednisolone Hemisuccinate (BANM, rINNM)
Methylprednisolone hydrogen succinate
$C_{26}H_{34}O_8 = 474.5$

Methylprednisolone Sodium Succinate (BANM, rINNM)
$C_{26}H_{33}NaO_8 = 496.5$
CAS—83-43-2 (methylprednisolone); 53-36-1 (methylprednisolone acetate); 2921-57-5 (methylprednisolone hemisuccinate); 2375-03-3 (methylprednisolone sodium succinate)

Pharmacopoeial status

BP (methylprednisolone, methylprednisolone acetate); USP (methylprednisolone, methylprednisolone acetate, methylprednisolone hemisuccinate, methylprednisolone sodium succinate)

Preparations

Compendial
Methylprednisolone Tablets BP. Tablets containing, in each, 2 mg, 4 mg, and 16 mg are usually available.
Methylprednisolone Acetate Injection BP. A sterile suspension of methylprednisolone acetate in water for injections. Injections containing 40 mg in 1 mL, 80 mg in 2 mL, and 200 mg in 5 mL are usually available. pH 3.5 to 7.0.
Methylprednisolone Tablets USP.
Methylprednisolone Acetate Cream USP.
Methylprednisolone Acetate for Enema USP.
Sterile Methylprednisolone Acetate Suspension USP. pH 3.5 to 7.0.

Methylprednisolone Sodium Succinate for Injection USP. A solution containing about 50 mg/mL of methylprednisolone sodium succinate. pH between 7.0 and 8.0.
Neomycin Sulfate and Methylprednisolone Acetate Cream USP.

Non-compendial
Depo-Medrone (Upjohn). *Injection*, aqueous suspension, methylprednisolone acetate 40 mg/mL. Depo-Medrone should not be mixed with any other fluid. Vials are intended for single dose use.
Medrone (Upjohn). *Tablets*, methylprednisolone 2 mg, 4 mg, 16 mg, and 100 mg.
Solu-Medrone (Upjohn). *Injection*, powder for reconstitution, methylprednisolone (as sodium succinate, all with solvent), 40-mg, 125-mg, 500-mg, 1-g, and 2-g vials. The prepared solution may be diluted with glucose 5% in water, sodium chloride 0.9% solution, or glucose 5% in sodium chloride 0.9% solution. Solu-Medrone at dilute concentrations (250 micrograms/mL or less) in these infusion fluids is physically and chemically stable for 24 hours and, at higher concentrations, is physically and chemically stable for at least 6 hours. Solu-Medrone should be diluted only in the solutions mentioned and administered separately from other drugs to avoid potential incompatibilities. Methylprednisolone Sodium Succinate powder for reconstitution is also available from Evans.

Containers and storage

Solid state
Methylprednisolone BP and Methylprednisolone Acetate BP should both be kept in well-closed containers and protected from light.
Methylprednisolone USP, Methylprednisolone Acetate USP, and Methylprednisolone Sodium Succinate USP should all be preserved in tight, light-resistant containers.
Methylprednisolone Hemisuccinate USP should be preserved in tight containers.

Dosage forms
Methylprednisolone Tablets BP should be protected from light.
Methylprednisolone Acetate Injection BP should be protected from light and stored at a temperature not exceeding 30°. It should not be frozen.
Methylprednisolone Tablets USP should be preserved in tight containers.
Methylprednisolone Acetate Cream USP should be preserved in collapsible tubes or in tight containers, protected from light.
Methylprednisolone Acetate for Enema USP should be preserved in well-closed containers.
Sterile Methylprednisolone Acetate Suspension USP should be preserved in single-dose or in multiple-dose containers, preferably of Type I glass.
Methylprednisolone Sodium Succinate for Injection USP should be preserved in containers suitable for sterile solids.
Depo-Medrone should be protected from freezing. Discard any remaining suspension after use.
Medrone tablets (100 mg) should be stored at controlled room temperature, 15° to 30°.
Solu-Medrone should be stored at controlled room temperature (15° to 30°). Solutions prepared using sterile water for injections should be used immediately.

PHYSICAL PROPERTIES

Methylprednisolone is a white or almost white, odourless, crystalline powder.

Methylprednisolone acetate is a white or almost white, odourless or almost odourless, crystalline powder.
Methylprednisolone hemisuccinate is a white or nearly white, odourless or nearly odourless, hygroscopic solid.
Methylprednisolone sodium succinate is a white or nearly white, odourless, hygroscopic, amorphous solid.

Melting point

Methylprednisolone melts, with decomposition, at about 243° (BP) or about 240° (USP).
Methylprednisolone acetate melts at about 225°, with decomposition.

Partition coefficient

Al-Habet and Rogers[1] refer to work in which an octanol/phosphate buffer (pH 7.4) partition coefficient of 238.18 for methylprednisolone was obtained.

Solubility

Methylprednisolone is practically insoluble in water; sparingly soluble in ethanol (1 in 100), in dioxan, and in methanol; slightly soluble in acetone, in chloroform, and in ether.
Methylprednisolone acetate is practically insoluble in water; slightly soluble in ethanol; very slightly soluble in ether; sparingly soluble in acetone, in chloroform, and in methanol; soluble in dioxan.
Methylprednisolone hemisuccinate is very slightly soluble in water; freely soluble in ethanol; soluble in acetone.
Methylprednisolone sodium succinate is very soluble in water and in ethanol; very slightly soluble in acetone; insoluble or practically insoluble in chloroform; practically insoluble in ether.

Dissolution

The USP specifies that for Methylprednisolone Tablets USP not less than 50% of the labelled amount of $C_{22}H_{30}O_5$ is dissolved in 30 minutes. Dissolution medium: 900 mL of water; Apparatus 1 at 100 rpm.

Crystal and molecular structure

Polymorphs
Hamlin *et al*[2] examined the dissolution rates of constant surface pellets of two polymorphic forms of methylprednisolone *in vitro* by four methods and *in vivo* following implantation in *rats*.

STABILITY

Degradation of methylprednisolone 21-succinate sodium initially follows two parallel first-order reactions: hydrolysis and reversible acyl migration of the succinate side-chain from the 21-hydroxyl group to the 17-hydroxyl group. Products include free methylprednisolone, succinate ions, and methylprednisolone 17-succinate sodium. Kinetics of degradation of methylprednisolone 21-hemisuccinate (as the sodium salt, methylprednisolone sodium succinate, Solu-Medrol, Upjohn) were studied[3] by measurement of the initial rates of product formation as a function of pH at 25°. Both reactions were first-order with respect to methylprednisolone 21-hemisuccinate. Within the pH range 3.6 to 7.4 reversible acyl migration was the dominant reaction. The 21-hemisuccinate was stated to be thermodynamically more stable, although it hydrolysed more rapidly than the 17-hemisuccinate. Potential mechanisms and roles of acid and base catalysis were discussed.

Photodegradation

Hamlin *et al*[4] observed the photolytic degradation of methylprednisolone in alcoholic solution during storage of solutions of methylprednisolone (Medrol, Upjohn) 40 mg/mL in 95% ethanol under normal fluorescent light at about 25°; a $t_{50\%}$ of 21.7 days was calculated.

Irradiation

Solid-state methylprednisolone and methylprednisolone acetate were irradiated with a cobalt-60 source. Degradation rates were 0.7%/Mrad and 0.6%/Mrad, respectively.[5] Major degradation products were formed by loss of the C-17 side-chain to yield the C-17 ketone (6α-methyl-11β-hydroxy-1,4-androstadiene-3,17-dione in both instances) and by oxidation of the C-11 alcohol to the C-11 ketone (methylprednisone and methylprednisone acetate, respectively). Minor degradation products were identified as 11β,17α-dihydroxy-6α-methyl-1,4-androstadiene-3-one and 11β,17α-dihydroxy-6α-methyl-1,4-pregnadiene-3,20-dione, respectively.

Intravenous vehicles

The visual compatibility of methylprednisolone sodium succinate injection (Solu-Medrol, Upjohn, of strength 125 mg to 3000 mg) when reconstituted and added to 50 mL and 100 mL of sodium chloride 0.9% or glucose 5% injections was investigated;[6] a nephrometer was used to quantify haze formation. Durations of visual clarity varied at different concentrations and volumes; at each dose, a volume of diluent could be chosen to provide a haze-free solution that lasted over 12 hours. Haze formation was attributed to precipitation of free methylprednisolone; an increase of 1.4% to 3.2% in the free methylprednisolone concentration secondary to hydrolysis was observed during the 24-hour test period.

In a later study,[7] the stability of methylprednisolone sodium succinate (A-methaPred Abbott, USA) was investigated by observation and measurement of turbidity, at initial concentrations of free methylprednisolone of 1% w/w or 5% w/w, in glucose 5% injection and in sodium chloride 0.9% injection at pH 7.2 and 8.0. Greater turbidity was observed in glucose 5% than in sodium chloride 0.9% solutions. Initial free methylprednisolone concentrations and pH also affected the extent of turbidity that occurred. In further work, at a given concentration of the drug at 25°, greater turbidity was again detected in glucose 5% solutions, but only minor differences were observed between the amount of free methylprednisolone formed in each diluent. In both diluents, higher turbidity values were recorded at intermediate concentrations of the drug (2.5 mg/mL to 15 mg/mL) than at lower (0.3 mg/mL) or higher (20 mg/mL) concentrations.

Freezing and microwave thawing

Infusions of methylprednisolone sodium succinate (Solu-Medrone, Upjohn) were prepared in polyvinyl chloride (Viaflex) bags; they were reconstituted with the diluent supplied by the manufacturer and diluted with sodium chloride 0.9% injection to yield a concentration of methylprednisolone 500 mg/108 mL. Following storage frozen at −20° for 24 hours, 1 month, 6 months, and 12 months, infusions were thawed by microwave radiation; no loss of drug concentration was detected by a stability-indicating HPLC assay.[8] After thawing, the infusions were clear and colourless although small changes in pH, infusion weight, and sub-visual particulate concentrations were observed.

Solutions

The degradation of methylprednisolone (sterile, micronised) in aqueous formulations was reduced by alteration of both the pH and the amount of polysorbate 80 present as a solubiliser.[9]

The formulations contained methylprednisolone (0.525, 0.55, or 0.575 mg/mL), polysorbate 80 (35.8, 37.0, or 41.0 mg/mL), disodium edetate (0.5 mg/mL), neomycin base (22.0 mg/mL), lincomycin base (22.0 mg/mL), hydrochloric acid, sodium hydroxide 30% solution, and purified water. The kinetics of the apparent first-order thermal degradation (attributed to auto-xidation of the alcohol group at C-21) of methylprednisolone were examined. Apparent activation energies were calculated to be about 76.2 kJ/mol and 96.6 kJ/mol in formulations that contained, respectively: 0.55 mg/mL methylprednisolone with 35.8 mg/mL polysorbate 80 (pH 5.0), and 0.575 mg/mL methylprednisolone with 41.0 mg/mL polysorbate 80 (pH 4.6). The concentration of oxygen present was found to influence the degradation rate.

Stabilisation

In a comprehensive study of the self-association of methylprednisolone 21-succinate (as the sodium salt, Solu-Medrol, Upjohn) in aqueous solution at about pH 8.5 at 25°, increased stability was observed when the concentration was increased;[10] this apparent stabilisation was associated with dimer formation and micelle formation at higher concentrations of the drug.

INCOMPATIBILITY/COMPATIBILITY

Formation of a haze was noted[11] after 4 hours at room temperature, when methylprednisolone sodium succinate (40 mg/mL, Solu-Medrol, Upjohn, USA) was added at the Y-injection site of administration sets (in a 1:1 ratio as a 'secondary additive') to the following admixtures: vitamin B complex with C (Berocca-C, Roche) 10 mL/L in compound sodium lactate injection; potassium chloride (Eli Lilly) 40 mEq/L in sodium chloride 0.9% injection (immediate haze) or in compound sodium lactate injection; heparin sodium (Lipo-Hepin, Riker) 1000 units/L with hydrocortisone sodium succinate (Solu-Cortef, Upjohn) 100 mg/L in sodium chloride 0.9% injection or in compound sodium lactate injection.

No visual changes were observed[12] when methylprednisolone sodium succinate injection (Solu-Medrol, Upjohn, USA), initial pH 7.57 to 7.7, was added to each of two concentrations of theophylline in glucose 5% injection (0.4 mg/mL and 4 mg/mL, Abbott, USA), initial pH 4.5 to 4.68, to yield final concentrations of methylprednisolone sodium succinate equivalent to methylprednisolone alcohol 0.5 mg/mL and 2 mg/mL. Admixtures were stored in glass containers under fluorescent light for 24 hours at room temperature. Immediately after admixture, there was a fall in pH of the solutions to within the range 6.34 to 7.33; however, pH values did not vary significantly thereafter. Significant decreases in concentration were measured in admixtures of methylprednisolone sodium succinate 0.5 mg/mL and 2 mg/mL with theophylline 0.4 mg/mL (after 24 hours), and of 2 mg/mL with theophylline 4 mg/mL (after 12 hours). In admixtures of methylprednisolone sodium succinate 2 mg/mL, the molar decrease in drug concentration was not significantly different from the concomitant increase in concentration of methylprednisolone alcohol (detected after 3 hours and 12 hours with theophylline 4 mg/mL and 0.4 mg/mL, respectively).

Methylprednisolone sodium succinate injection (Solu-Medrol, Upjohn, USA), reconstituted with bacteriostatic water for injections that contained benzyl alcohol as preservative, was mixed with glucose 5% solutions in polyvinyl chloride containers to yield final concentrations equivalent to methylprednisolone 0.4 mg/mL and 1.25 mg/mL.[13] On addition of cimetidine 300 mg, as the hydrochloride (Tagamet, SKF, USA), the pH of solutions fell. However, the two drugs were concluded to be visually compatible and chemically stable in the admixtures tested following storage for 24 hours at 24°.

FORMULATION

Excipients

Excipients that have been used in presentations of methylprednisolone include:

Tablets, methylprednisolone: brilliant blue FCF (133); calcium stearate; erythrosine sodium; lactose; liquid paraffin; magnesium stearate; maize starch; sorbic acid; sucrose; sunset yellow FCF (E110); tartrazine (E102).

Creams, methylprednisolone: butylated hydroxyanisole; butylated hydroxytoluene; cetyl alcohol; cholesterol; glycerol; liquid paraffin; maize oil; oleic acid; polyoxyethylene stearate; sorbitan mono-oleate; spermaceti; squalene; stearic acid; stearyl alcohol; α-tocopherol acetate.

Injections, methylprednisolone acetate: hydrochloric acid; macrogols 3350 and 4000; myristyl-gamma-picolinium chloride; sodium chloride; sodium hydroxide.

Methylprednisolone sodium hemisuccinate: lactose; sodium acid phosphate; sodium phosphate.

Methylprednisolone sodium succinate: benzyl alcohol; dibasic sodium phosphate, dried; hydrochloric acid; lactose, anhydrous; lactose, hydrous; monobasic sodium biphosphate, anhydrous; monobasic sodium phosphate, anhydrous; sodium hydroxide; sodium phosphate, anhydrous.

Bioavailability

An oral bioavailability of $82 \pm 11\%$ for methylprednisolone from tablets (methylprednisolone 5 mg, Medrone, Upjohn) was determined[1] during a pharmacokinetic investigation in which five healthy volunteers received 20 mg, 40 mg, and 80 mg of methylprednisolone sodium succinate intravenously (Solu-Medrone, Upjohn) and 20 mg methylprednisolone orally (as 4×5 mg tablets).

Sugar glass dispersions

Allen *et al*[14] prepared hygroscopic, solid glass dispersions of methylprednisolone acetate (6 mg) with glucose, galactose, or sucrose (200 mg) as carriers, by a fusion method. In de-ionised water, the dissolution rate of methylprednisolone acetate from glass dispersions was markedly greater than that of methylprednisolone acetate itself. After storage for 30 days at 25° in a desiccator, no changes in dissolution rates or ultraviolet spectra of the dispersions were measured and no decomposition products of methylprednisolone acetate were detected by TLC.

FURTHER INFORMATION. Bioavailability and nonlinear disposition of methylprednisolone and methylprednisone in the *rat*— Haughey DB, Jusko WJ. J Pharm Sci 1992;81(2):117–21.

REFERENCES

1. Al-Habet SMH, Rogers HJ. Br J Clin Pharmacol 1989;27:285–90.
2. Hamlin WE, Nelson E, Ballard BE, Wagner JG. J Pharm Sci 1962;51(5):432–5.
3. Anderson BD, Taphouse V. J Pharm Sci 1981;70(2):181–5.
4. Hamlin WE, Chulski T, Johnson RH, Wagner JG. J Am Pharm Assoc (Sci) 1960;49(4):253–5.
5. Kane MP, Tsuji K. J Pharm Sci 1983;72(1):30–5.
6. Townsend RJ, Puchala AH, Nail SL. Am J Hosp Pharm 1981;38:1319–22.
7. Pyter RA, Hsu LCC, Buddenhagen JD. Am J Hosp Pharm 1983;40:1329–33.
8. Sewell GJ, Palmer AJ. Int J Pharmaceutics 1991;72:57–63.
9. Amin MI, Bryan JT. J Pharm Sci 1973;62(11):1768–71.
10. Anderson BD, Conradi RA, Johnson K. J Pharm Sci 1983;72(4):448–54.
11. Allen LV, Levinson RS, Phisutsinthop D. Am J Hosp Pharm 1977;34:939–43.
12. Johnson CE, Cohen IA, Michelini TJ, McMahon RE. Am J Hosp Pharm 1987;44:1620–4.
13. Strom JG, Miller SW. Am J Hosp Pharm 1991;48:1237–41.
14. Allen LV, Yanchick VA, Maness DD. J Pharm Sci 1977;66(4):494–6.

Metoclopramide (BAN, rINN)

Anti-emetic; Antispasmodic

4-Amino-5-chloro-*N*-(2-diethylaminoethyl)-2-methoxybenz-amide; 4-amino-5-chloro-*N*-[2-(diethylamino)ethyl]-*o*-anisamide
$C_{14}H_{22}ClN_3O_2 = 299.8$

Metoclopramide Hydrochloride (BANM, USAN, rINNM)

$C_{14}H_{22}ClN_3O_2,HCl,H_2O = 354.3$

CAS—364-62-5 (metoclopramide); 7232-21-5 (metoclopramide hydrochloride, anhydrous); 54143-57-6 (metoclopramide hydrochloride); 2576-84-3 (metoclopramide dihydrochloride, anhydrous)

Pharmacopoeial status

BP, USP (metoclopramide hydrochloride)

Preparations

Compendial

Metoclopramide Tablets BP. Contain metoclopramide hydrochloride. Tablets containing, in each, the equivalent of 10 mg of anhydrous metoclopramide hydrochloride are usually available.

Metoclopramide Injection BP. A sterile solution of metoclopramide hydrochloride in water for injections free from dissolved air. pH 3.0 to 5.0. Injections containing the equivalent of 10 mg in 2 mL and 100 mg in 20 mL of anhydrous metoclopramide hydrochloride are usually available.

Metoclopramide Tablets USP. Contain metoclopramide hydrochloride.

Metoclopramide Oral Solution USP. Contains metoclopramide hydrochloride.

Metoclopramide Injection USP. A sterile solution of metoclopramide hydrochloride in water for injection, pH 2.5 to 6.5.

Non-compendial

Gastrobid Continus (Napp). *Tablets*, controlled release, metoclopramide hydrochloride 15 mg.

Gastromax (Farmitalia Carlo Erba). *Capsules*, controlled release, metoclopramide hydrochloride 30 mg.

Maxolon (Beecham). *Capsules* (Maxolon SR), sustained release, metoclopramide hydrochloride 15 mg.

Tablets, metoclopramide hydrochloride 10 mg.

Syrup, sugar free, metoclopramide hydrochloride 5 mg/5 mL. *Diluent*: purified water to half strength, life of diluted syrup one month.

Paediatric liquid, sugar free, metoclopramide hydrochloride 1 mg/mL. Life of dispensed liquid 14 days.

Injection, metoclopramide hydrochloride 10 mg/2 mL.

Intravenous infusion (Maxolon High Dose), metoclopramide hydrochloride 100 mg/20 mL. It should be diluted before use. May be diluted with glucose 5%, sodium chloride 0.9%, sodium chloride 0.18% with glucose 4%, or compound sodium lactate. Although it is preferable to prepare infusions immediately before administration, the above solutions are reported to be stable for at least 48 hours at room temperature when administered in polyvinyl chloride infusion bags following preparation under appropriate aseptic conditions. It is compatible at certain concentrations with cisplatin, cyclophosphamide, doxorubicin hydrochloride, morphine hydrochloride, and diamorphine hydrochloride, when stored under specified conditions.

Primperan (Berk). *Tablets*, metoclopramide hydrochloride 10 mg.

Syrup, sugar free, metoclopramide hydrochloride 5 mg/5 mL. *Diluent*: purified water.

Injection, metoclopramide hydrochloride 10 mg /2 mL.

Metoclopramide tablets are also available from APS, Ashbourne (Gastroflux), Cox, CP, Evans, Kerfoot, Lagap (Parmid), Nicholas (Metramid), Norton.

Metoclopramide oral solution is also available from Lagap (Parmid, sugar free).

Containers and storage

Solid state

Metoclopramide Hydrochloride BP should be protected from light.

Metoclopramide Hydrochloride USP should be preserved in tight, light-resistant containers.

Dosage forms

Metoclopramide Tablets BP and Metoclopramide Injection BP should be protected from light.

Metoclopramide Tablets USP should be preserved in tight, light-resistant containers.

Metoclopramide Oral Solution USP should be stored in tight, light-resistant containers at controlled room temperature. Protect from freezing.

Metoclopramide Injection USP should be preserved in single-dose or multiple-dose containers, preferably of Type I glass; protection from light is required if the injection does not contain an antioxidant.

Gastrobid Continus tablets should be stored at or below 25°.

Maxolon SR capsules should be protected from direct light.

Maxolon syrup should be protected from light and dispensed in amber glass bottles.

If ampoules of Maxolon injection or Maxolon High Dose infusion are removed from their carton, they should be stored away from light and ampoules showing signs of discoloration following inadvertent exposure should be discarded.

Primperan preparations should be protected from light and stored in a cool place.

PHYSICAL PROPERTIES

Metoclopramide is a white crystalline powder.

Metoclopramide hydrochloride is a white or almost white, odourless or almost odourless, crystalline powder.

Melting point

Metoclopramide base melts at about 148°.

Metoclopramide hydrochloride melts in the range 182° to 185°.

pH

A 10% w/v solution of *metoclopramide hydrochloride* has a pH of 4.5 to 6.5.

Dissociation constants

Dissociation constants determined (spectrophotometrically at 25°) by Hanocq *et al*[1] for two functional groups of metoclopramide were 9.71 (aliphatic amine) and 0.48 (aromatic amine). Other values reported in the literature are 0.6 (base); 7.3; 9.0 (base); and 9.3 (base).

Partition coefficient

Log *P* (octanol/pH 7.4),[2] 2.62

Solubility

Metoclopramide is practically insoluble in water; soluble 1 in 45 of ethanol and 1 in 15 of chloroform.

Metoclopramide hydrochloride is soluble 1 in 0.7 of water, 1 in 3 of ethanol, and 1 in 55 of chloroform; practically insoluble in ether.

Dissolution

The USP specifies that for Metoclopramide Tablets USP not less than 75% of the labelled amount of $C_{14}H_{22}ClN_3O_2$ is dissolved in 30 minutes. Dissolution medium: 900 mL of water; Apparatus 1 at 50 rpm.

Crystal and molecular structure

Polymorphs

Thermal analyses of metoclopramide base and metoclopramide hydrochloride have been carried out by Mitchell[3] in order to identify their polymorphic forms. Metoclopramide base was found to exist as two enantiotropic polymorphs; one form, which was stable at room temperature, quickly underwent transition at 125° to a second form which was stable at high temperatures and had a melting point of 147°. Reverse transition back to the first form took one month at room temperature. Dehydration of metoclopramide hydrochloride led to the formation of two anhydrous monotropic polymorphs, a stable and a metastable form, melting at about 187° and 155°, respectively. The stable form also formed on recrystallisation of the melt of the metastable form.

STABILITY

Metoclopramide undergoes hydrolysis with the formation of 2-diethylaminoethylamine and other decomposition products.

Metoclopramide solutions become discoloured following exposure to light.

Solutions of metoclopramide hydrochloride for injection are reported to be stable within the pH range 2 to 9.

Loss of up to 40% potency has been reported following the storage of metoclopramide hydrochloride infusion in glucose 5% in polyvinyl chloride bags for 4 weeks at −20°; metoclopramide hydrochloride infusion in sodium chloride 0.9% remained stable when stored under the same conditions.

INCOMPATIBILITY/COMPATIBILITY

Preparations of metoclopramide have been reported to be incompatible with cephalothin sodium, chloramphenicol sodium succinate, and sodium bicarbonate. Possible incompatibility has also been reported with ampicillin sodium, benzylpenicillin potassium, calcium gluconate, cisplatin, erythromycin lactobionate, frusemide, methotrexate sodium, sodium bicarbonate, and tetracycline hydrochloride. Maxolon High Dose intravenous infusion (Beecham, UK) is specially formulated to ensure compatibility in solution with cisplatin (see Preparations, above).

FORMULATION

Excipients

Excipients that have been used in presentations of metoclopramide include:
Capsules, metoclopramide hydrochloride: polymethacrylate; starch; stearic acid; sucrose; talc.
Tablets, metoclopramide hydrochloride: brilliant blue FCF (133), aluminium lake; cetostearyl alcohol; erythrosine (E127), aluminium lake; ethylcellulose; guar gum; hydroxyethylcellulose; lactose; magnesium stearate; mannitol; methylcellulose; microcrystalline cellulose; quinoline yellow (E104), lake; silica; starch; stearic acid; sunset yellow FCF (E110), aluminium lake; talc.
Oral drops, metoclopramide dihydrochloride: benzoic acid; methyl and propyl hydroxybenzoates; propylene glycol; saccharin sodium; sodium metabisulphite.
Oral liquids, metoclopramide as the hydrochloride or dihydrochloride: citric acid; glycerol; hydroxyethylcellulose; methyl and propyl hydroxybenzoates; saccharin sodium; sodium cyclamate; sorbitol; sunset yellow FCF (E110).
Suppositories, metoclopramide: semi-synthetic glycerides.
Injections, metoclopramide as the hydrochloride or dihydrochloride: benzyl alcohol; hydrochloric acid; sodium chloride; sodium hydroxide; sodium metabisulphite.

Bioavailability

Metoclopramide 20 mg was administered to 10 healthy subjects by mouth as a retarded-release capsule (Paspertin retard, Kali-Chemie, Germany). Compared with the same dose given as conventional tablets (Reglan, Alkaloid, Yugoslavia), the retarded-release preparation produced higher and later peak serum concentrations and a larger area under the serum concentration versus time curve.[4]
The bioavailability of metoclopramide hydrochloride 30 mg was compared after oral administration of a controlled-release capsule (Gastro-Timelets, Temmler-Werke, Germany) and an oral solution to four healthy volunteers in a single-dose, crossover study.[5] The products were found to be equivalent in terms of extents of absorption. In a subsequent multidose, crossover study,[6] lower and later peak plasma concentrations of metoclopramide were produced by the controlled-release capsules than by the solution. However, the areas under the plasma concentration versus time curves indicated that the products were bioequivalent.

Intranasal preparations

Absolute bioavailability following the intranasal administration of metoclopramide 5 mg in 0.5 mL of sterile water was $50.5 \pm 29.5\%$ compared to intravenous administration; this value, determined in six healthy volunteers, was lower than that previously reported for absolute bioavailability following oral administration of an aqueous solution.[7]

Suppositories

Suppositories containing metoclopramide 150 mg in Witepsol H15 basis showed similar bioavailability to the same dose administered intravenously;[8] in three patients in an oncology unit who received metoclopramide by both routes, the systemic availability of the suppository appeared to be complete.
A comparison of the bioavailability and pharmacokinetics of two rectally administered metoclopramide (20 mg) preparations (Gastrosil, Heuman Pharma GmbH, Germany and a reference suppository) and an intravenous injection (17.8 mg) in twelve healthy subjects was carried out by Vergin *et al.*[9] Absolute bioavailabilities for Gastrosil and the reference suppositories were $66.0 \pm 16.8\%$ and $71.7 \pm 20.9\%$, respectively, and the suppositories were concluded to be bioequivalent. The absolute bioavailabilities of the suppositories were stated to correspond approximately to the absolute systemic availability of metoclopramide following oral administration.

Modified-release preparations

Naggar and Samaha[10] demonstrated the potential of polycarbophil (a loosely cross-linked hydrophilic resin) as a support matrix for the sustained release of metoclopramide hydrochloride. Adsorption of metoclopramide hydrochloride onto polycarbophil from water and 0.1M hydrochloric acid was studied at 37°. Tablets were prepared by direct compression; dissolution studies in 0.1M hydrochloric acid and in phosphate buffer (pH 7.2) demonstrated sustained zero-order drug release.

FURTHER INFORMATION. A single dose pharmacokinetic study of Gastrobid Continus and Maxolon in the perioperative period—Madej TH, Ellis FR, Tring I. Br J Clin Pharmacol 1988;26:747–51.

PROCESSING

Sterilisation

Metoclopramide injection can be sterilised by heating in an autoclave.

REFERENCES

1. Hanocq M, Topart J, van Damme M, Molle L [French]. J Pharm Belg 1973;28:649–62.
2. Verbiese-Génard N, Hanocq M, van Damme M, Molle L. Int J Pharmaceutics 1981;9:295–303.
3. Mitchell AG. J Pharm Pharmacol 1985;37:601–4.
4. Wolf-Coporda A, Vrhovac B, Manojlovic Z, Plavsic F. Acta Pharm Jugosl 1988;38:213–21.
5. Beckett AH, Behrendt WA, Hadzija BW. Arzneimittelforschung 1987;37(I)Nr2:221–4.
6. Beckett AH, Behrendt WA, Hadzija BW. Arzneimittelforschung 1987;37(I)Nr2:224–8.
7. Ward MJ, Buss DC, Ellershaw J, Nash A, Routledge PA. Br J Clin Pharmacol 1989;28:616–18.
8. Hardy F, Warrington PS, MacPherson JS, Hudson SA, Jefferson GC, Smyth JF. J Clin Pharm Ther 1990;15:21–4.
9. Vergin H, Krammer R, Nitsche V, Miczka M, Strobel K, Schimmel H. Arzneimittelforschung 1990;40(I)Nr 6:679–83.
10. Naggar VFB, Samaha MW. Pharm Ind 1989;51(5):543–6.

Metronidazole (BAN, USAN, rINN)

Antibacterial; Antiprotozoal

2-(2-Methyl-5-nitroimidazol-1-yl)ethanol;   1-(2-hydroxyethyl)-2-methyl-5-nitroimidazole

$C_6H_9N_3O_3 = 171.2$

Metronidazole Benzoate (BAN)

$C_{13}H_{13}N_3O_4 = 275.3$

Metronidazole Hydrochloride (BANM, USAN, rINNM)

$C_6H_9N_3O_3, HCl = 207.6$

Metronidazole Phosphate (BANM, USAN, rINNM)

$C_6H_{10}N_3O_6P = 251.14$

CAS—443-48-1 (metronidazole); 13182-89-3 (metronidazole benzoate); 69198-10-3 (metronidazole hydrochloride); 73334-05-1 (metronidazole phosphate).

Pharmacopoeial status

BP, USP (metronidazole)

Preparations

Compendial

Metronidazole Tablets BP. Tablets containing, in each, 200 mg, 250 mg, and 400 mg metronidazole are usually available.

Metronidazole Suppositories BP. Contain metronidazole in a suitable suppository basis. Suppositories containing, in each, 0.5 g and 1 g metronidazole are usually available.

Metronidazole Tablets USP.

Metronidazole Gel USP.

Metronidazole Injection USP. pH between 4.5 and 7.0.

Non-compendial

Flagyl (Rhône-Poulenc Rorer). *Tablets,* metronidazole 200 mg and 400 mg.

Suspension (Flagyl-S), metronidazole 200 mg (as benzoate)/5 mL. *Diluent:* syrup, life of diluted suspension 14 days.

Suppositories, metronidazole 0.5 g or 1 g.

Injection (for intravenous infusion), metronidazole 5 mg/mL in 100-mL bottles, 100-mL Viaflex containers or 20-mL ampoules. As the injection does not contain preservative the 100-mL bottles are not intended for multidose use. *Diluents:* sodium chloride 0.9% injection; sodium chloride and glucose injection; glucose 5% injection; potassium chloride (20 and 40 mmol/L) injection. It must not be mixed with cefamandole nafate, cefoxitin sodium, glucose 10% injection, compound sodium lactate injection, benzylpenicillin potassium, or any other substance except for specified diluents (see Incompatibility below).

Metrogel (Sandoz). *Gel,* metronidazole 0.75%.

Metrolyl (Lagap). *Tablets,* metronidazole 200 mg and 400 mg.

Suppositories, metronidazole 0.5 g or 1 g.

Injection (for intravenous infusion), metronidazole 5 mg/mL in 100-mL polyvinyl chloride minibags. The injection is not intended for multidose use. *Diluents:* sodium chloride 0.9% injection; sodium chloride and glucose injection; glucose 5% injection; potassium chloride (20 mmol or 40 mmol) injection.

Metrotop (Farmitalia Carlo Erba). *Gel,* metronidazole 0.8% in an aqueous basis.

Zadstat (Lederle). *Tablets,* metronidazole 200 mg.

Suppositories, metronidazole 0.5 g or 1 g.

Metronidazole tablets of various strengths are also available from APS, Cox, CP, DDSA (Vaginyl), Evans, Kerfoot, Norton. An intravenous infusion is also available from David Bull.

Containers and storage

Solid state

Metronidazole BP should be kept in a well-closed container and protected from light.

Metronidazole USP should be preserved in well-closed, light-resistant containers.

Dosage forms

Metronidazole Suppositories BP should be protected from light.

Metronidazole Tablets USP should be preserved in well-closed, light-resistant containers.

Metronidazole Gel USP should be preserved in laminated collapsible tubes at controlled room temperature.

Metronidazole Injection USP should be preserved in single-dose containers of Type I or Type II glass, or in suitable plastic containers, protected from light.

Metrolyl preparations should be stored in a cool, dry place, protected from light.

Metrotop gel should be stored at 15° to 25°.

Flagyl-S suspension and Flagyl injection in 100-mL Viaflex containers should be stored below 25°. Flagyl suppositories should be stored below 20°. All Flagyl preparations should be protected from light.

Zadstat preparations should be protected from light.

PHYSICAL PROPERTIES

Metronidazole is a white to pale yellow crystalline powder; odourless or almost odourless.

Melting point

Metronidazole melts in the range 159° to 163°.

pH

A saturated aqueous solution of *metronidazole* has a pH of 5.8.

Dissociation constant

pK_a 2.5

Partition coefficient

Log *P* (octanol/pH 7.4), −0.1

Solubility

Metronidazole is soluble 1 in 100 of water, 1 in 200 of ethanol, and 1 in 250 of chloroform; very slightly soluble in ether; slightly soluble in acetone and in dichloromethane; sparingly soluble in dimethylformamide; soluble in dilute acids.

In aqueous sodium chloride 0.6% w/v the solubility of metronidazole is reported[1] to be 0.81% w/v at 20°.

The solubility of metronidazole at 37° in an ascending homologous series of triglycerides decreased in the order: tricaprin > trilaurin > trimyristin > tripalmitin > tristearin.[2]

Effect of temperature

Hughes *et al*[1] determined the aqueous solubility of metronidazole at 20°, 26°, and 30° to be 0.83% w/v, 0.99% w/v, and 1.14% w/v, respectively.

Effect of cosolvents

Aqueous solubility of metronidazole was improved by the addition of one or more water-miscible cosolvents.[3] Solubility increased exponentially with an increase in volume fraction of the cosolvents; examples are given below.

Solvent/additive	Cosolvent mixture					
	1	2	3	4	5	6
Water	100	24.1	32.6	27.7	21.5	26.5
Ethanol	—	75.9	47.4	42.3	48.5	51.5
N,N-Dimethyl acetamide	—	—	20	30	20	20
Propylene glycol	—	—	—	—	10	—
Nicotinamide	—	—	—	—	—	2
Solubility (mg/mL) of metronidazole	10	42.1	45.7	65.4	59.2	59.8

The authors further determined that increasing concentrations of nicotinamide, ascorbic acid, and pyridoxine hydrochloride linearly increased the aqueous solubility of metronidazole.

Dissolution

The USP specifies that for Metronidazole Tablets USP not less than 85% of the labelled amount of $C_6H_9N_3O_3$ is dissolved in 60 minutes. Dissolution medium: 900 mL of 0.1N hydrochloric acid; Apparatus 1 at 100 rpm.

Crystal and molecular structure

Crystalline forms of metronidazole benzoate in aqueous suspension can exist as the anhydrate or as the monohydrate.[4] In water, at temperatures below 8°, a commercial sample of the anhydrate form converted to the thermodynamically stable monohydrate. Crystals of the monohydrate were less soluble and considerably larger than the anhydrate; they rapidly became yellow on exposure to light. The transition temperature for the hydrate-anhydrate system was 38°. Further investigation revealed that the anhydrate exhibits polymorphism; an anhydrate Form II was occasionally crystallised from the monohydrate in isopropanol-water at room temperature.

STABILITY

Metronidazole in the solid state is stable in air but darkens on exposure to light.

Solutions

Metronidazole undergoes hydrolysis in aqueous solution; maximum stability is reported[5] to occur at pH 5.
Under alkaline conditions, hydrolysis of metronidazole was observed[6] to yield ammonia, acetic acid, and an unidentified compound that produced a pink to violet colour with ninhydrin reagent.

Photodegradation

Aqueous solutions of metronidazole 0.5% in citrate:phosphate buffer at pH 5 became bright yellow after exposure to daylight for 18 months,[7] but this discoloration disappeared after exposure for a further 21 months. Analysis by HPLC revealed that an initial degradation product (characterised as a yellow oil) further decomposed to yield at least two colourless compounds. Solutions that were stored in the dark showed no degradation after 18 months.
Yellow discoloration occurred[8] in solutions of metronidazole (for topical use) that had been subjected to ultraviolet-A light (320 nm to 400 nm) for 1 to 4 hours; the discoloration disappeared within 2 to 48 hours. Exposure to sunlight and ultraviolet-B light (290 nm to 320 nm) did not produce discoloration of the solutions. Solutions contained metronidazole 0.5% in water or metronidazole 1% in a solution of lactic acid 1.5% in distilled water. The extent of photodecomposition of metronidazole solutions (in phosphate buffer, pH 7) under different light sources decreased in the order: fluorescent light > artificial sunlight

(ultraviolet-B) > ultraviolet-A.[9] A catalytic effect by buffers, at pH 7, on this photodegradation decreased in the order: citrate > acetate > phosphate. With increasing pH (above pH 7 in phosphate buffers) the stability of metronidazole under ultraviolet-B light decreased. Addition of sodium urate to solutions of metronidazole retarded the rate (under fluorescent and ultraviolet-B light) and reduced the extent of photodecomposition; photostabilisation was attributed to formation of a complex between metronidazole and sodium urate.
Kendall et al[10] investigated the decomposition of metronidazole in buffer solution (pH 9.2) on exposure to light and sonic energy. At 360 nm there was rapid photolysis at 20°, 48°, and 63°. During sonication of the solution, however, no degradation occurred below 40° and only slow degradation occurred at 70°. In all instances, the addition of hydrogen peroxide solutions increased the rates of decomposition. The order of the decomposition reaction appeared to be dependent on temperature. During assessment of an analytical method for metronidazole in the presence of possible degradation products, the pseudo-first-order photodegradation of metronidazole was claimed to increase with temperature, pH, and intensity of radiation; to decrease with increase in drug concentration; and to be dependent on the solvent (water, chloroform, methanol, or isopropanol).[11]

Esters of metronidazole

Products of the hydrolysis of metronidazole benzoate in solution were metronidazole and benzoic acid, detected by reversed-phase HPLC.[12] In the pH range 4.0 to 8.4 at 80° metronidazole benzoate was most stable at pH 4.0.
In aqueous buffer, maximum stability of metronidazole monosuccinate was reported[13] to occur in the pH range 3 to 6 (60°). Hydrolysis followed first-order kinetics and was subject to specific acid-base catalysis.

FURTHER INFORMATION. Degradation kinetics of metronidazole in solution—Wang D-P, Yeh M-K. J Pharm Sci 1993;82(1):95–8. Influence of production and storage conditions on the stability of metronidazole infusion solutions—Theuer H [German]. Pharm Ztg 1983;128:2919–23. Comparative stability of intravenous metronidazole products [protection from light—two US manufacturers' recommendations]—McDonald JE [letter]. Am J Hosp Pharm 1983;40:772. A comparison of the chemical stability and the enzymatic hydrolysis of a series of aliphatic and aromatic ester derivatives of metronidazole [including metronidazole benzoate]—Johansen M, Larsen C. Int J Pharmaceutics 1985;26:227–41. Macromolecular prodrugs. IV. Kinetics of hydrolysis of metronidazole monosuccinate dextran ester conjugates in aqueous solution and in plasma—sequential release of metronidazole from the conjugates at physiological pH—Larsen C, Johansen M. Int J Pharmaceutics 1987;35:39–45. Hydrolysis of dextran metronidazole monosuccinate ester prodrugs. Evidence for participation of intramolecularly catalysed hydrolysis of the [conjugate ester] by neighbouring dextran hydroxy groups—Larsen C. Acta Pharm Suec 1986;23:279–88.

INCOMPATIBILITY/COMPATIBILITY

It is generally recommended that other drugs should not be added to intravenous solutions of metronidazole or its hydrochloride. However, the manufacturers of Flagyl injection state that it is physically and chemically *compatible* with cefuroxime sodium and physically *compatible* (with respect to pH and appearance) over normal administration periods with: amikacin sulphate, ampicillin sodium, carbenicillin sodium, cephazolin sodium, cefotaxime sodium, cephalothin sodium, chloramphenicol sodium succinate, clindamycin phosphate, gentamicin sulphate, hydrocortisone sodium succinate, latamoxef disodium, netilmicin sulphate, and tobramycin sulphate.

Some incompatibilities with metronidazole in intravenous admixtures are detailed below.

Stability of metronidazole in admixture solutions:

Preparations of metronidazole	Additive	Results	Reference
(a) Metronidazole solution 5 mg/mL for intravenous infusion (Flagyl, Rhône-Poulenc), in 100-mL minibags	ampicillin sodium 2000 mg as Penbritin (Ayerst Labs) injection in sterile water	significant initial fall in pH on admixing then pH constant on storage for 72 hours at 23°	14
(b) Metronidazole injection 5 mg/mL (Searle), 100 mL	ampicillin sodium (as powder, Bristol Myers) 2% in admixture	ampicillin decomposed by about 10% in 1 day at 25° and 12 days at 5°—metronidazole stable over 3 days at 25° and 12 days at 5°	15
As (a) above	benzylpenicillin potassium 1.2 × 10^6 units (Ayerst Labs) injection in sterile water	continuous fall in pH of admixture over 14 days at 23°	14
As (b) above	benzylpenicillin potassium (as powder, Pfizer) 1% in admixture	chemical compatibility for 3 days at 25° and 12 days at 5°	15
As (a) above	cefamandole nafate 2000 mg, as Mandol (Eli Lilly) injection in sterile water	continuous fall in pH of admixture over 14 days at 23° but not significant fall at 4°	14
Metronidazole injection solution 5 mg/mL (Searle, USA)	cefamandole nafate solution (Lilly, USA), 2%	metronidazole decomposed by about 9% in under 2 hours at 25° and in under 6 hours at 5°	16
As (a) above	cefoxitin sodium 3000 mg as Mefoxin (CE Frosst) injection in sterile water	continuous rise in pH of admixture over 14 days at 23° and 4°	14
As (b) above	cefoxitin sodium (as powder, MSD) 3% in admixture	chemical compatibility for 2 days at 25° and 12 days at 5°	15
As (a) above	cephalothin sodium 2000 mg as Keflin (Eli Lilly) injection in sterile water	significant initial fall in pH on admixing	14
As (b) above	cephalothin sodium (as powder, Lilly) 2% in admixture	cephalothin decomposed by more than 10% after 1 day at 25° but stable for at least 12 days at 5°. Metronidazole stable over 3 days at 25° and 12 days at 5°	15
Metronidazole injection (500 mg in 100-mL polyvinyl chloride bags)	cefuroxime sodium 750 mg as Zinacef (Glaxo) injection	cefuroxime degraded, calculated $t_{10\%}$ values: 36 hours at 25° and 20 days at 4°. Stable with respect to metronidazole. Admixture assigned a 7-day storage period at 4°	17
As (a) above	hydrocortisone sodium succinate 1000 mg as Solu-Cortef (Upjohn) injection in sterile water	significant initial fall in pH on admixing then pH constant on storage for 14 days at 23°	14
As (b) above	hydrocortisone sodium succinate (as powder, Elkins-Sinn) 1% in admixture	chemical stability over 7 days at 25° and 12 days at 5°	15

Visual compatibility and chemical stability were demonstrated[18] between metronidazole injection 500 mg/100 mL (Flagyl, Searle) and gentamicin sulphate injection 80 mg/100 mL and 120 mg/100 mL (Garamycin, Schering Plough) in polyvinyl chloride bags during storage for 2 days at 18° (ambient light) and for 7 days at 7° (in a dark refrigerator).

Metronidazole injection, ready-to-use, (Abbott, USA) and cefotaxime sodium (Claforan, Hoechst-Roussel, USA) in sodium chloride 0.9% injection were chemically stable in admixture in water (at concentrations of 5 mg/mL and 10 mg/mL, respectively) when stored in glass vials for up to 72 hours at 8°.[19]

Vervloet et al[20] demonstrated that admixtures of metronidazole 500 mg with netilmicin sulphate 100 mg in 100 mL sodium chloride 0.9% injection were chemically stable in glass bottles for 24 hours at room temperature.

Aluminium

Metronidazole hydrochloride solutions for injection have been reported to interact with aluminium.[21] A precipitate and reddish-brown discoloration occurred after 6 hours and 24 hours, respectively, in solutions in contact with needles that contained aluminium.

Sorption

Negligible loss of metronidazole was reported[22] when a solution of metronidazole (M&B, Australia) 3 mg/100 mL in sodium chloride 0.9% injection was stored in polyvinyl chloride infusion bags or glass vials in the dark for one week at 15° to 20°.

In a further comprehensive study of interactions between drugs in intravenous infusions and components of delivery systems, Kowaluk et al[23] found negligible reduction in metronidazole concentration during simulated infusion (in sodium chloride 0.9% injection) through a cellulose propionate burette chamber and polyvinyl chloride tubing, or through polyethylene or Silastic tubing attached to glass syringes on syringe pumps. No sorption of metronidazole was evident after storage of the infusion in the dark at 15° to 20° for 24 hours in single-use syringes with polypropylene barrels and polyethylene all-plastic plungers.

During simulated continuous infusion over 60 minutes, no significant adsorption of metronidazole (Flagyl, Specia, France; 5 mg/mL in sodium chloride 0.9% or in glucose 5% solutions) to cellulose ester membrane filters or to an intravenous administration set occurred.[24]

FURTHER INFORMATION. Compatibility of magnesium sulfate solutions with various antibiotics during simulated Y-site injection [visual compatibility with metronidazole injection (Flagyl RTU) confirmed]—Souney PF, Colucci RD, Mariani G, Campbell D. Am J Hosp Pharm 1984;41:323–4. Stability of metronidazole [in water] and ten antibiotics when mixed with magnesium sulphate solutions—Das Gupta V, Stewart KR. J Clin Hosp Pharm 1985;10:67–72.

FORMULATION

Excipients

Excipients that have been used in presentations of metronidazole include:

Tablets, metronidazole: cellulose; hydroxypropylcellulose; hypromellose; indigo carmine (E132) lake; lactose; macrogol; magnesium stearate; microcrystalline cellulose; povidone; sodium starch glycollate; stearic acid; titanium dioxide (E171); wheat starch.

Suspensions, metronidazole benzoate: ethanol; methyl and propyl hydroxybenzoates; monosodium phosphate dihydrate; oil of lemon (concentrated); saccharin sodium; sugars.

Metronidazole: Cologel; cherry syrup; syrup.
Mixtures, metronidazole: anise oil; ethanol; glycerol.
Gels, metronidazole: benzalkonium chloride; hypromellose; propylene glycol.
Suppositories, metronidazole: Witepsol.
Ovules, metronidazole: semi-synthetic glycerides.
Injections, metronidazole: citric acid; sodium chloride; sodium phosphate.
Injections (lyophilised powder for reconstitution), metronidazole hydrochloride: mannitol.

Bioavailability

In a single-dose, crossover study,[25] nine healthy female volunteers received 500 mg metronidazole as 2½ metronidazole 200 mg tablets (Flagyl) orally and as an intravenous infusion 500 mg/100 mL (Flagyl) administered over 20 minutes. No differences in systemic availability between the routes were observed.

Compared with the intravenous route, the apparent oral bioavailability of metronidazole was 111% in a crossover study[26] in which five healthy subjects received an intravenous infusion of metronidazole 500 mg (Flagyl, 5 mg/mL, Rhône-Poulenc) over 20 minutes and one 500 mg metronidazole tablet (Elyzol, Dumex) orally. In further studies, two groups of six healthy volunteers received either a rectal suppository (metronidazole 1000 mg, Flagyl, Rhône-Poulenc) or a pessary (metronidazole 500 mg, Flagyl); compared to the oral route, average absorption by the rectal and vaginal routes was 53% (corrected for dose) and 25%, respectively.

Rectal absorption of metronidazole has been examined in a crossover study in seven healthy volunteers.[27] Rectal preparations were: an aqueous suspension of metronidazole 500 mg in 10 mL of 0.5% methylcellulose 400 cP in distilled water; a fatty suppository of metronidazole 500 mg in a triglyceride basis (Elysol, Dumex); and suppositories of metronidazole 500 mg in the water-soluble vehicles macrogol 1000, macrogol 6000, and macrogol 1000:macrogol 6000 (1:1). Rectal bioavailabilities relative to the oral bioavailability (100%) of a solution of metronidazole 500 mg in 50 mL water were determined over 24 hours. Results are given below.

Relative bioavailabilities of rectal preparations of metronidazole:[27]

Preparations (each containing metronidazole 500 mg)	Average relative bioavailability %	Additional information
Oral solution	100	
Aqueous suspension (rectal)	55 ± 20	absorption showed marked interpatient variability
Fatty suppository	55 ± 7	relatively slow rate of absorption
Suppository– macrogol 1000	69 ± 8	*
Suppository– macrogol 6000	74 ± 10	*
Suppository– macrogol 1000: macrogol 6000 (1:1)	78 ± 13	*

* no significant differences in absorption data between these three preparations.

Meijer *et al*[28] prepared suppositories of metronidazole 500 mg in Witepsol H15. Steady-state plasma-metronidazole concentrations in eight female patients were measured after multiple-dose administration of an intravenous infusion (metronidazole 500 mg/100 mL) and of the suppositories. Compared to intravenous availability, an average rectal bioavailability of 75.7% was calculated for the suppositories.

In a randomised, crossover study involving ten healthy subjects, Bergan and Arnold[29] compared the pharmacokinetics of oral tablets of metronidazole (Elyzol, Dumex) with those of rectal suppositories of metronidazole in a 'pure fat' basis. At doses of 500 mg and 1000 mg, bioavailability of the suppositories was 86.2% and 88.5%, respectively, compared to that of the tablets.

Metronidazole was poorly absorbed following vaginal administration of metronidazole 500 mg pessaries (Flagyl, Rhône-Poulenc) as single and repeated doses.[30] However, steady-state plasma concentrations were claimed to exceed the minimum inhibitory concentrations for metronidazole against anaerobic *Streptococci* and *Clostridium tetani*.

Bioequivalence

Two brands of metronidazole 200 mg tablets (May & Baker and Servipharm, both New Zealand) were observed to be bioequivalent in eight healthy volunteers.[31]

Suspensions

Among various suspending agents investigated at several concentrations,[32] mucilages of carmellose sodium (1.5% w/v) or methylcellulose (1.0% w/v) provided the best 'suspendability' (highest sedimentation volumes) and ease of redispersion of metronidazole benzoate (300 mg/10 mL) suspensions following storage at 28° for 6 months. Suspensions also contained Tween 20 solution (0.1% w/v) as a wetting agent.

Transdermal delivery

Rates of hydrolysis of aliphatic esters of metronidazole to regenerate metronidazole (by first-order kinetics at 37°) were greater in the presence of a homogenate of human skin (0.91% w/v in phosphate buffer at pH 7.4) than in phosphate buffer pH 7.4 alone.[33] In the skin homogenate, hydrolysis rates of the esters increased in the order: acetate < propionate < butyrate < valerate ≈ caproate. Comparison of permeation of metronidazole itself and the esters (each in a vehicle of ethanol and propylene glycol) through human skin *in vitro* revealed that the use of the esters produced a slight enhancement in the percentage of metronidazole transported.

For further information about prodrugs, see Stability–Esters of metronidazole, above.

Topical preparations

Thomas and Hay[34] prepared a topical preparation of metronidazole 0.8% w/v in Scherisorb gel (Smith and Nephew) that contained a modified copolymer derived from maize starch with water and propylene glycol. In this preparation, metronidazole retained its antimicrobial potency for at least 28 days at room temperature. Antimicrobial properties of the preparation and also of Metrotop gel (Farmitalia Carlo Erba) were investigated *in vitro*, although Morgan and Oppenheim[35] later warned about indiscriminate use of topical metronidazole.

A metronidazole solution 1% w/v in sodium chloride 0.6% solution used in a hospital as a topical lotion[36] was sterilised by heating in an autoclave for 20 minutes at 121°.

Suppositories

Displacement value of metronidazole in fatty bases, 1.7.
Meijer *et al*[28] established that 500 mg of powdered metronidazole displaced 220 mg of Witepsol H15.

Suppositories that contained metronidazole 250 mg were reported to have been prepared with each of five bases: Massupol, Novata B, theobroma oil (which melt at body temperature), macrogols 400:4000 (20:80), and glycogelatin (which dissolve in rectal secretions).[37] In dissolution studies release of metronidazole from the suppositories and from Flagyl (M&B) suppositories decreased in the order: glycogelatin > macrogols > Novata B > Massupol > Flagyl suppositories > theobroma oil. Liversidge and Grant[2] investigated interactions between metronidazole and the triglycerides that are constituents of fatty suppository bases. Results of partition chromatography experiments designed to assess the interaction between metronidazole and individual triglycerides did not correlate with solubility values for metronidazole in the triglycerides. Melting points and disintegration times were determined for suppositories that contained triglycerides (in different proportions), Witepsol or Suppocire bases. See also Solubility, above.

Modified-release preparations

Jones et al[38] studied polymer films of Eudragit (polymethacrylate) retard resins alone and in combination for their potential to control the release of metronidazole. Preparations consisted of solutions of the polymer granules in dichloromethane, with a plasticiser (dibutyl phthalate) and metronidazole. Films that contained 50% Eudragit RL100 with 50% Eudragit RS100 produced slower release of metronidazole in vitro than films with 100% Eudragit RL100.

Metronidazole has been used as a model drug in the study in vitro of bioadhesive, controlled-release tablets.[39] Tablets were prepared by compression of metronidazole 50% w/w with a swellable system that consisted of hypromellose and poly(acrylic acid) (Carbopol 934) in various proportions. The amount of metronidazole released from the tablets increased as the proportion of poly(acrylic acid) increased (dissolution medium: 0.1N hydrochloric acid, pH 1.0 at 37°).

Mechanical properties of tablets

In a 2^3 factorially designed experiment, Itiola and Pilpel[40] examined the effect of the type and concentration of binder (povidone or methylcellulose) and physical nature of the formulation (powdered or granular) on tensile strength and susceptibility of metronidazole tablets to fracture. Methylcellulose 20 exhibited stronger binding properties than povidone (mol. wt. 44 000).

FURTHER INFORMATION. Influence of physicochemical interactions on the properties of suppositories. V. The in vitro release of ketoprofen and metronidazole from various fatty suppository bases [commercial bases and binary mixtures of pure triglycerides] and correlations with in vivo plasma levels [in rats]— Grant DJW, Liversidge GG, Bell J. Int J Pharmaceutics 1983;14:251–62. Influence of polyisobutylene on microencapsulation of metronidazole—Chemtob C, Gruber T, Chaumeil JC. Drug Dev Ind Pharm 1989;15(8):1161–74. Nanoparticles—colloidal drug delivery system for primaquine and metronidazole [preliminary investigation of nanoparticles of gelatin, albumin, polyglutaraldehyde, and acrylamide]—Labhasetwar VD, Dorle AK. J Controlled Release 1990;12:113–19. Vehicle effect on topical drug delivery. III. Effect of Azone on the cutaneous permeation of metronidazole and propylene glycol—Wotton PK, Møllgaard B, Hadgraft J, Hoelgaard A. Int J Pharmaceutics 1985;24:19–26. Vehicle effect on topical drug delivery. IV. Effect of N-methylpyrrolidone and polar lipids on percutaneous drug transport—Hoelgaard A, Møllgaard B, Baker E. Int J Pharmaceutics 1988;43:233–40. Design of a water-soluble, solution-stable and biolabile prodrug of metronidazole for parenteral administration: N-substituted aminomethylbenzoate

esters—Jensen E, Bundgaard H, Falch E. Int J Pharmaceutics 1990;58:143–53. In vitro antitrichomonal activity of water-soluble prodrug esters of metronidazole [metronidazole bound to dextran by a 'spacer arm'—phenylalanine, leucine, glycine, or succinic acid]—Vermeersch H, Remon JP, Permentier D, Schacht E. Int J Pharmaceutics 1990;60:253–60. Fundamental properties of metronidazole formulations in relation to tableting [effects of the binding agents: povidone, gelatin, and methylcellulose]—Itiola OA, Pilpel N. J Pharm Pharmacol 1987;39:644–7.

REFERENCES

1. Hughes J, Tenni P, McDonald C, Sunderland VB. Aust J Hosp Pharm 1982;12(3):58.
2. Liversidge GG, Grant DJW. Drug Dev Ind Pharm 1983;9:223–46.
3. Chien YW. J Parenter Sci Technol 1984;38(1):32–6.
4. Hoelgaard A, Møller N. Int J Pharmaceutics 1983;15:213–21.
5. Baveja SK, Rao AVR. Indian J Technol 1973;11:311–12.
6. Baveja SK, Khosla HK. Indian J Technol 1975;13:528–9.
7. Godfrey R, Edwards R. J Pharm Sci 1991;80(3):212–18.
8. Gamborg Nielsen P. Arch Pharm Chemi (Sci) 1986;14:119–23.
9. Habib MJ, Asker AF. Pharm Res 1989;6(1):58–61.
10. Kendall AT, Stark E, Sugden JK. Int J Pharmaceutics 1989;57:217–21.
11. A/Karim EI, Ibrahim KE, Adam ME. Int J Pharmaceutics 1991;76:261–4.
12. Sa'sa' SI, Khalil HS, Jalal IM. J Liq Chromatogr 1986;9(16):3617–31.
13. Johansen M, Larsen C. Int J Pharmaceutics 1984;21:201–9.
14. Bisaillon S, Sarrazin R. J Parenter Sci Technol 1983;37(4):129–32.
15. Das Gupta V, Stewart KR. J Parenter Sci Technol 1985;39(3):145–8.
16. Das Gupta V, Stewart KR, Dela Torre M. J Clin Hosp Pharm 1985;10:379–83.
17. Barnes AR. J Clin Pharm Ther 1990;15:187–96.
18. Rovers JP, Meneilly G, Souney PF, Rekhi GS, Drum D. Can J Hosp Pharm 1989;42(4):143–6.
19. Rivers TE, McBride A, Trang JM. Am J Hosp Pharm 1991;48:2638–40.
20. Vervloet E, Lammers J, Tan LSL, Van Mourik CH, Rots M [letter]. DICP Ann Pharmacother 1990;24(4):440–2.
21. Schell KH, Copeland JR [letter]. Am J Hosp Pharm 1985;42:1040–2.
22. Kowaluk EA, Roberts MS, Blackburn HD, Polack AE. Am J Hosp Pharm 1981;38:1308–14.
23. Kowaluk EA, Roberts MS, Polack AE. Am J Hosp Pharm 1982;39:460–7.
24. Khue NV, Jung L. STP Pharma 1985;1(3):201–7.
25. Houghton GW, Thorne PS, Smith J, Templeton R, Collier J. Br J Clin Pharmacol 1979;8:337–41.
26. Mattila J, Männistö PT, Mäntylä R, Nykänen S, Lamminsivu U. Antimicrob Agents Chemother 1983;23(5):721–5.
27. Vromans H, Moolenaar F, Visser J, Meijer DKF. Pharm Weekbl (Sci) 1984;6:18–20.
28. Meijer RTW, Oostinga J, Schwietert HR, Scholtanus J, Van Schoonhoven JC. Pharm Weekbl 1984;119:351–5.
29. Bergan T, Arnold E. Chemotherapy 1980;26:231–41.
30. Salas-Herrera IG, Lawson M, Johnston A, Turner P, Gott GM, Dennis MJ. Br J Clin Pharmacol 1991;32:621–3.
31. Paton DM, Webster DR. Int J Clin Pharmacol Res 1988;8(4):227–9.

32. Chowdary KPR, Kumar KTR. East Pharm 1985;28:125–7.
33. Johansen M, Møllgaard B, Wotton PK, Larsen C, Hoel-gaard A. Int J Pharmaceutics 1986;32:199–206.
34. Thomas S, Hay NP. Pharm J 1991;246:264–6.
35. Morgan DA, Oppenheim B [letter]. Pharm J 1991;246:353.
36. Jones PH, Willis AT, Ferguson IR [letter]. Lancet 1978;1:214.
37. Chin CLS, Roller L [letter]. Aust J Hosp Pharm 1986;16(4):217.
38. Jones CE, Newton JM, O'Neill RC. J Pharm Pharmacol 1987;39:42P.
39. Ponchel G, Touchard F, Wouessidjewe D, Duchêne D, Peppas NA. Int J Pharmaceutics 1987;38:65–70.
40. Itiola OA, Pilpel N. J Pharm Pharmacol 1991;43:145–7.

Miconazole (BAN, rINN)   *Antifungal*

1-[2,4-Dichloro-β-(2,4-dichlorobenzyloxy)phenethyl]imidazole;
1-[2-(2,4-dichlorophenyl)-2-[(2,4-dichlorophenyl)methoxy]
ethyl]-1H-imidazole
$C_{18}H_{14}Cl_4N_2O = 416.1$

Miconazole Nitrate (BANM, USAN, rINNM)

$C_{18}H_{14}Cl_4N_2O,HNO_3 = 479.1$
CAS—22916-47-8 (miconazole); 22832-87-7 (miconazole nitrate)

Pharmacopoeial status

BP (miconazole nitrate); USP (miconazole, miconazole nitrate)

Preparations

Compendial
Miconazole Cream BP (Miconazole Nitrate Cream). A cream containing miconazole nitrate in a suitable basis. A cream containing 2% w/w is usually available.
Miconazole Nitrate Cream USP.
Miconazole Nitrate Topical Powder USP.
Miconazole Nitrate Vaginal Suppositories USP.
Miconazole Injection USP. A sterile solution of miconazole in water for injections. pH between 3.7 and 5.7.

Non-compendial
Daktarin (Janssen). *Tablets*, miconazole 250 mg.
Cream, miconazole nitrate 2% w/w in a water-miscible cream.
Dusting powder, contains miconazole nitrate 2% w/w.
Spray powder, miconazole nitrate 0.16%, in an aerosol basis.
Oral gel, miconazole 2% w/w (25 mg/mL) in a sugar-free oral gel.
Intravenous solution, miconazole 10 mg/mL in a sterile solution for dilution and administration as an infusion. *Diluents*: solution must be diluted with either sodium chloride 0.9% injection or glucose 5% injection.
Femeron (Janssen). *Cream*, miconazole nitrate 2%.

Soft pessary, miconazole nitrate 1.2 g.
Gyno-Daktarin (Janssen). *Intravaginal cream*, miconazole nitrate 2% w/w in a water-miscible cream.
Pessaries, contain miconazole nitrate 100 mg.
Tampons, each coated with miconazole nitrate 100 mg.
Ovule, vaginal capsule, (Gyno-Daktarin 1), a soft Scherer capsule containing miconazole nitrate 1200 mg in a fatty basis.
Miconazole nitrate cream (2%) is also available from Hillcross.

Containers and storage

Solid state
Miconazole Nitrate BP should be kept in a well-closed container and protected from light.
Miconazole USP and Miconazole Nitrate USP should be preserved in well-closed containers, protected from light.

Dosage forms
Miconazole Cream BP: if the cream is kept in aluminium tubes, their inner surfaces should be coated with a suitable lacquer.
Miconazole Injection USP should be preserved in single-dose containers, preferably of Type I glass, at controlled room temperature.
Miconazole Nitrate Cream USP should be preserved in collapsible tubes or in tight containers.
Miconazole Nitrate Topical Powder USP should be preserved in well-closed containers.
Miconazole Nitrate Vaginal Suppositories USP should be preserved in tight containers, at controlled room temperature.
Daktarin cream should be stored away from direct heat and Daktarin powder stored at room temperature. Daktarin intravenous solution should be stored at room temperature.
All Gyno-Daktarin preparations should be stored in a cool place.

PHYSICAL PROPERTIES

Miconazole is a white to pale cream, crystalline powder.
Miconazole nitrate is a white or nearly white, odourless or nearly odourless, crystalline or microcrystalline powder.

Melting point

Miconazole melts in the range 78° to 82°.
Miconazole nitrate melts in the range 178° to 184°, with decomposition.

Dissociation constant

pK_a 6.7

Solubility

Solubilities of miconazole and miconazole nitrate in various solvents are as follows:

Solvent	Miconazole	Miconazole nitrate
Water	insoluble	very slightly soluble
Ethanol	freely soluble	slightly soluble (1 in 40 parts)
Chloroform	freely soluble	slightly soluble
Ether	soluble	very slightly soluble
Acetone	freely soluble	—
Dimethyl formamide	freely soluble	soluble
Dimethyl sulphoxide	—	freely soluble
Isopropanol	freely soluble	very slightly soluble
Methanol	freely soluble	sparingly soluble
Propylene glycol	freely soluble	slightly soluble

Enhancement of solubility

Van Doorne et al[1] reported that in the presence of β-cyclodextrin (18 mg/mL) there was a 5-fold increase in the aqueous solubility of miconazole nitrate.

Macrogol 6000 and urea have been found to increase the aqueous solubility of miconazole nitrate.[2] See also Formulation.

Effect of pH

As part of a study of chewing gum as a drug delivery system,[3] workers in Denmark determined the equilibrium solubilities of miconazole and miconazole nitrate in citrate buffer at pH 3 to be 0.794 mg/mL and 0.451 mg/mL, respectively; in phosphate buffer at pH 7.9, the solubility of both drugs was less than 5×10^{-4} mg/mL.

STABILITY

Non-commercial eye drop formulations of miconazole (1 g) in 100 mL of either arachis oil or castor oil were sterilised by dry heat at 160° for 90 minutes.[4] Miconazole remained stable in both oils under these conditions and no subsequent loss of drug occurred when the sterilised samples were stored for 3 months at ambient temperature. Samples of arachis and castor oils that did not contain miconazole darkened slightly when heated at 160° for 90 minutes.

INCOMPATIBILITY/COMPATIBILITY

Intravenous solutions of miconazole (Daktarin, Janssen) in sodium chloride 0.9% injection showed losses of 4% to 5% of their initial drug content when stored for 24 hours at room temperature in plastic infusion bags.[5] During continuous flow studies through intravenous administration sets (from three manufacturers) for up to 257 minutes, losses of miconazole ranged from 1.06% to 10.39% (average 4.76%). There was no correlation between percentage loss and the time required for the solution to flow through the set.

FORMULATION

Solutions of miconazole 1% w/v and 2% w/v in arachis oil have been prepared and used as eye drops in an Australian hospital.[4] See Stability above.

Excipients

Excipients that have been used in presentations of miconazole include:

Tablets, miconazole: lactose; magnesium stearate; potato starch; povidone; sodium lauryl sulphate; sucrose.
Creams, miconazole nitrate: benzoic acid; butylated hydroxyanisole; glycol stearate; liquid paraffin; macrogol stearate; peglicol oleate.
Powders, miconazole nitrate: colloidal silica; talc; zinc oxide.
Oral gels, miconazole: ethanol; glycerol; pregelatinised starch; polysorbate 20; saccharin sodium.
Vaginal suppositories (ovules), miconazole nitrate: gelatin; glycerol; hydrogenated vegetable oil; liquid paraffin; potassium sorbate; sodium ethyl hydroxybenzoate; sodium propyl hydroxybenzoate; titanium dioxide (E171).
Intravenous solution, miconazole: lactic acid; methyl and propyl hydroxybenzoates; polyethoxylated castor oil.

Bioavailability

Absorption of miconazole after oral administration as a 5% microsuspension was 27% of that after intravenous administration of a solution of miconazole in Cremophor EL, in a single-dose study involving four healthy volunteers.[6]

Solid dispersions

Solid dispersions of miconazole nitrate with macrogol 6000, urea, or povidone 10000 (prepared by fusion and co-precipitation) have been studied *in vitro*.[2] Fused dispersions with urea and co-precipitated dispersions with macrogol 6000 showed an approximately seven-fold increase in dissolution rate at 30 minutes, when compared to miconazole nitrate alone; dispersions with povidone 10000 produced an approximately two-fold increase. Physical mixtures of miconazole nitrate with each of the test excipients did not show significant enhancement of the dissolution rate of miconazole nitrate. Solubilisation and wetting of miconazole nitrate by macrogol 6000 were greater than by povidone 10000. The authors concluded that solubilisation and wetting had more effect than particle size reduction in the enhancement of dissolution of miconazole nitrate.

Pedersen and Rassing[3] investigated the release of miconazole and miconazole nitrate from chewing gum. Both substances were incorporated in the gum as solid dispersions with either macrogol 6000, povidone 40000, urea, or xylitol. No correlation was found between dissolution rates of the solid dispersions *in vitro* and release of drug when the gums were subjected to simulated chewing *in vitro*. Only the solid dispersion of miconazole:macrogol 6000 (20:80) had a greater release rate from gum than miconazole itself during simulated chewing at pH 7.9 (approximately salivary pH).

The same workers also studied[7] the *in-vivo* release of miconazole from chewing gum when incorporated as a solid dispersion, which comprised miconazole:macrogol 6000 (20:80). Enhancement of *in-vitro* release of miconazole correlated with increased salivary concentrations of miconazole in six healthy volunteers; the authors claimed that therapeutic concentrations were achieved. Results from the same study showed that lecithin also enhanced the release of miconazole from chewing gum *in vivo*. Lecithin, which has no antifungal activity, antagonised the antifungal activity of miconazole at pH 5.3 but not at pH 7.2.

REFERENCES

1. Van Doorne H, Bosch EH, Lerk CF. Pharm Weekbl (Sci) 1988;10:80–5.
2. Jafari MR, Danti AG, Ahmed I. Int J Pharmaceutics 1988;48:207–15.
3. Pedersen M, Rassing MR. Drug Dev Ind Pharm 1990;16(13):1995–2013.
4. Lee RLH. Aust J Hosp Pharm 1985;15(4):233–4.
5. McGookin AG, Millership JS, Scott EM. J Clin Pharm Ther 1987;12:433–7.
6. Boelaert J, Daneels R, Van Landuyt H, Symoens J. In: Williams JD, Geddes AM, editors. Chemotherapy; vol 6. New York: Plenum Press, 1976:165–9.
7. Pedersen M, Rassing MR. Drug Dev Ind Pharm 1990;16(13):2015–30.

Morphine (BAN)   *Opioid analgesic*

Morphia
7,8-Didehydro-4,5-epoxy-17-methylmorphinan-3,6-diol;   7,8-
didehydro-4,5-epoxy-17-methyl-(5α,6α)-morphinan-3,6-diol;
(4a*R*,5*S*,7a*R*,8*R*,9c*S*)-4a,5,7a,8,9,9c-hexahydro-12-methyl-8,9c-
iminoethanophenanthro[4,5-*bcd*]furan-3,5-diol monohydrate
$C_{17}H_{19}NO_3,H_2O = 303.4$

Morphine Acetate (BANM)
$C_{17}H_{19}NO_3,C_2H_4O_2,3H_2O = 399.4$

Morphine Hydrochloride (BANM)
$C_{17}H_{19}NO_3,HCl,3H_2O = 375.8$

Morphine Sulphate (BANM)
Morphine sulfate
$(C_{17}H_{19}NO_3)_2,H_2SO_4,5H_2O = 758.8$

Morphine Tartrate (BANM)
$(C_{17}H_{19}NO_3)_2,C_4H_6O_6,3H_2O = 774.8$
CAS—57-27-2 (morphine, anhydrous); 6009-81-0 (morphine,
monohydrate); 596-15-6 (morphine acetate, anhydrous); 5974-
11-8 (morphine acetate, trihydrate); 52-26-6 (morphine hydrochloride, anhydrous); 6055-06-7 (morphine hydrochloride, trihydrate); 64-31-3 (morphine sulphate, anhydrous); 6211-15-0
(morphine sulphate, pentahydrate); 302-31-8 (morphine tartrate, anhydrous); 6032-59-3 (morphine tartrate, trihydrate)

Pharmacopoeial status

BP (morphine hydrochloride, morphine sulphate); USP (morphine sulfate)

Preparations

Compendial
Morphine Tablets BP (Morphine Sulphate Tablets). Contain
morphine sulphate.
Morphine Suppositories BP. Contain morphine hydrochloride
or morphine sulphate in a suitable suppository basis. Suppositories containing, in each, 15 mg and 30 mg of either morphine
hydrochloride or morphine sulphate are usually available.
Morphine Sulphate Injection BP. A sterile solution of morphine
sulphate in water for injections. Injections containing 10, 15, 20,
and 30 mg in 1 mL and 20, 30, 40, and 60 mg in 2 mL are usually
available.
Morphine and Atropine Injection BP. A sterile isotonic solution
containing morphine sulphate 1% w/v and atropine sulphate
0.06% w/v in water for injections.
Morphine Sulfate Injection USP. pH 2.5 to 6.5.
Ammonium Chloride and Morphine Mixture BP (Ammonium
Chloride and Morphine Oral Solution). See the monograph
for Ammonium Chloride.
Kaolin and Morphine Mixture BP (Kaolin and Morphine Oral
Suspension). The mixture contains light kaolin or light kaolin
(natural) 20% w/v, sodium bicarbonate 5% w/v, and chloro-

form and morphine tincture 4% v/v in a suitable vehicle. For
extemporaneous preparation see Formulation.
Chloroform and Morphine Tincture BP (Chlorodyne). See Formulation, below.

Non-compendial
Min-I-Jet Morphine Sulphate (IMS). *Injection*, morphine sul-
phate 10 mg/mL.
MST Continus (Napp). *Tablets*, controlled release, morphine
sulphate 5, 10, 15, 30, 60, 100, and 200 mg.
Suspension, controlled release, morphine sulphate 20 mg and
30 mg. Granules for reconstitution with water.
Oramorph (Boehringer Ingelheim). *Oral solution*, morphine sul-
phate 10 mg/5 mL.
Concentrated oral solution, sugar free, morphine sulphate
100 mg/5 mL.
Oral vials (Unit Dose Vials), morphine sulphate 10 mg/5 mL,
30 mg/5 mL, and 100 mg/5 mL.
Sevredol (Napp). *Tablets*, morphine sulphate 10 mg and 20 mg.
Suppositories, morphine sulphate 10 mg, 20 mg, and 30 mg.
SRM-Rhotard (Farmitalia Carlo Erba). *Tablets*, sustained
release, morphine sulphate 10, 30, 60, and 100 mg.
Morphine suppositories (morphine hydrochloride or morphine
sulphate) of various strengths are also available from Evans,
Martindale.

Containers and storage

Solid state
Morphine Hydrochloride BP and Morphine Sulphate BP should
be kept in well-closed containers and protected from light.
Morphine Sulfate USP should be preserved in tight, light-resistant containers.

Dosage forms
Morphine Tablets BP, Morphine Sulphate Injection BP, and
Morphine and Atropine Injection BP should be protected
from light.
Kaolin and Morphine Mixture BP should be stored in well-
filled, well-closed glass containers, and Chloroform and Morphine Tincture BP should be kept in an airtight container.
Morphine Sulfate Injection USP should be preserved in single-
dose or in multiple-dose containers, preferably of Type I glass,
protected from light. Preserve injection labelled 'preservative-
free' in single-dose containers.
MST Continus tablets and suspension should be stored at or
below 25°.
Oramorph oral solution and concentrated oral solution should
be stored at room temperature and protected from light. Oramorph Unit Dose Vials should be stored below 25°, protected
from light. Discard any unused solution after administration.
Sevredol tablets should be stored at or below 30°. Sevredol suppositories should be stored at or below 25°.
SRM-Rhotard tablets should be stored in a cool dry place, protected from light.

PHYSICAL PROPERTIES

Morphine appears as a white crystalline powder or as colourless
or white acicular crystals.
Morphine acetate is a white amorphous or crystalline powder.
Morphine hydrochloride appears as colourless, silky crystals,
cubical masses, or as a white or almost white, crystalline powder.
Morphine sulphate appears as white, acicular crystals or cubical
masses, or a white crystalline powder; odourless or almost
odourless. Darkens on prolonged exposure to light; gradually
loses water of crystallisation on exposure to air.

Morphine tartrate appears as minute, colourless, acicular, efflorescent crystals.

Melting point

Morphine melts between 254° and 256°.
Morphine hydrochloride melts at about 200°, with decomposition.
Morphine sulphate melts at 250°, with decomposition.

pH

A saturated solution of *morphine* has a pH of 8.5.

Dissociation constants

pK_a 8.0, 9.9 (20°)

Partition coefficient

Log P (octanol/pH 7.4), −0.1
Drustrup *et al*[1] determined a log P (octanol/phosphate buffer, pH 7.4) value for morphine of −0.06 at 21°.

Solubility

Solubility of morphine and morphine salts:

	Water	Ethanol	Chloroform	Ether	Glycerol
Morphine*	1 in 5000	1 in 250	1 in 1500	practically insoluble	1 in 125
Morphine acetate	1 in 2.5	1 in 100	—	practically insoluble	1 in 5
Morphine hydrochloride	1 in 24	1 in 100 (at 15°)	practically insoluble	practically insoluble	1 in 10
Morphine sulphate	1 in 21	1 in 1000	practically insoluble	practically insoluble	—
Morphine tartrate	1 in 10	1 in 1000	practically insoluble	practically insoluble	—

* Solubility can vary according to the method of preparation and crystalline state.

Morphine is moderately soluble in mixtures of chloroform and alcohols.
At 25° *morphine* is freely soluble in solutions of fixed alkali and alkaline earth hydroxides, phenol, and cresols; slightly soluble in amyl alcohol (1 in 114), in ammonia, and in benzene; very slightly soluble in ethyl acetate (1 in 525).

FURTHER INFORMATION. Solubility behaviour of narcotic analgesics in aqueous media: solubilities and dissociation constants of morphine, fentanyl and sufentanil—Roy SD, Flynn GL. Pharm Res 1989;6:147–51.

STABILITY

Decomposition of morphine is due to an oxidation reaction that results in the formation of pseudomorphine and morphine *N*-oxide in the ratio 9:1 with a small amount of the base methylamine.[2] The oxidation and condensation of morphine to pseudomorphine involves the phenolic group in the same manner as the formation of dimolecular compounds from naphthols. Degradation of morphine is catalysed by oxygen, sunlight, ultraviolet radiation, iron, and organic impurities. Yeh and Lach[2] determined the rate constants for the oxidative degradation of morphine at various pH values. The results are shown in the table below. The stability of morphine in aqueous solution is largely dependent on the hydrogen ion concentration. Acidic solutions are reasonably stable, but under alkaline or neutral conditions, morphine degrades rapidly at room temperature.
Rate constants for morphine degradation:

pH	$k \times 10^3/h$ observed	$k \times 10^3/h$ calculated
2.5	1.76	1.77
4.0	1.95	1.90
4.5	2.16	2.19
5.0	2.99	3.08
5.5	5.61	5.77
6.0	13.78	13.17
6.5	29.36	29.23
7.0	48.70	51.20

Oral solutions

Beaumont[3] prepared a range of morphine hydrochloride 1 mg/mL solutions in buffers (McIlvaine's citric acid-sodium phosphate system) ranging in pH from 2.2 to 8.0. All solutions were found to be stable with no breakdown products detected after storage at room temperature for three months. When a simple solution of morphine hydrochloride in unbuffered chloroform water (pH 6.5) was stored at room temperature for three months, no breakdown products were detected. A limiting factor in the stability of such solutions is the efficacy of the antimicrobial preservative. The recommended shelf-life for a morphine hydrochloride solution in chloroform water was three months unopened and one month in use.
Four aqueous solutions of morphine hydrochloride were prepared: one contained morphine hydrochloride 10 mg/mL with ethanol 22.5% in an acidic medium (hydrochloric acid 36%, 0.55 mL in 100 mL, pH 1 to 2); the others contained morphine hydrochloride 1 mg/mL, 40 mg/mL, or 50 mg/mL in the same medium, with ethanol 1%, glycerol 10% or 20% and methyl and propyl hydroxybenzoates (total hydroxybenzoates, 0.1% w/v).[4] In all solutions, more than 90% of the initial morphine concentration remained after storage for 52 weeks, protected from light, at 25° to 27°. However, only about 65% to 67% of the initial concentration of the hydroxybenzoates remained after this time.
Helliwell and Jennings[5] determined the anhydrous morphine content of samples of Ammonium Chloride and Morphine Mixture BP. From a 2000-mL batch of the mixture (anhydrous morphine content 0.0052% w/v), twelve samples were prepared in 300-mL bottles. Four fill volumes (300 mL, 200 mL, 100 mL, and 50 mL) were used. Plastic caps with Steran-faced wads were the closures selected. The bottles were stored undisturbed in the dark at room temperature. One bottle from each group was assayed after five weeks. A further bottle from each group was assayed at 15 weeks and the final four samples at 25 weeks. Bottles filled to capacity retained their morphine content, while those containing 200 mL, 100 mL, and 50 mL of mixture showed 5%, 40%, and 70% losses in morphine content, respectively, over the 25-week period. A similar study involved Kaolin and Morphine Mixture BP. Assays were undertaken at 1 month, 3 months, and 6 months. During the 6 months, the morphine content of the filled bottles was virtually constant. However, the partially filled bottles had losses ranging from 10% to 60% for the 200-mL and 50-mL fill volumes, respectively.[6]

Injection solutions

Morphine hydrochloride 10 mg/mL in sodium chloride 0.9% solution, pH 5.3 (isobaric solution), and 5 mg/mL in glucose 7% solution, pH 5.5 (hyperbaric solution), was stable when stored in 1-mL ampoules at 4° and 37° for at least two months;[7] no precipitation, discoloration, or degradation was detected.

The pH of morphine injection is important for stability. However, at low pH (range 2 to 4), Roksvaag *et al*[8] determined that the level of degradation in morphine hydrochloride injections, which had been stored for between 1 and 43 years, was more dependent on the volume of air in the container than on the formulation.

Thörn and Ågren[9] examined morphine hydrochloride 2% solutions after two years storage and found no detectable decrease in morphine concentration. The solutions were liable to discoloration, which could be decreased by adding small amounts of acid.

Sterilisation by autoclave

Deeks *et al*[10] investigated the stability of intrathecal morphine sulphate injection to repeated autoclave cycles and long-term storage. After storage for 48 weeks, none of the samples kept at room temperature showed greater than 10% degradation to pseudomorphine; the unautoclaved samples showed less than 5% degradation to pseudomorphine. Repeated autoclaving of the injection resulted in a progressive build up of pseudomorphine in the ampoules. Samples stored at 32° showed greater than 10% degradation to pseudomorphine after 32 weeks. There appeared to be no correlation between small differences in oxygen content or pH in paired ampoules and the degree of degradation in these ampoules. A shelf-life of one year was recommended for a 2 mg/10 mL injection (autoclaved once) stored at a temperature not exceeding 15°.

Brown discoloration was reported following autoclaving of solutions of morphine sulphate 1 mg/mL in sodium chloride 0.9% injection in 1-litre bottles.[11]

According to Turner and Potter[12] an injection of morphine sulphate 2 mg in 10 mL of sodium chloride 0.9% can be packed under nitrogen and autoclaved at 115° for 20 minutes. They suggest that it is unwise to subject morphine sulphate injection to more than one sterilisation by autoclaving.

Morphine injection preserved with hydroxybenzoates was subjected to three sterilisation cycles at 120° to 121° for 30 minutes by Austin and Mather.[13] No degradation of the active ingredient was detected.

Taylor and Sherwood[14] stated that if oxygen is excluded during the manufacture, filling, and sealing of ampoules of intrathecal morphine sulphate injection 2 mg/10 mL, it could be allocated a shelf-life of two years and be re-autoclaved at 115° for 30 minutes at least twice before there was significant build up of pseudomorphine. Ampoules should not be re-autoclaved within six months of their expiry date.

Similarly, Bunn and Hobbs[15] stated that an epidural morphine sulphate injection containing morphine sulphate 2 mg in 10 mL of sodium chloride 0.9% could be satisfactorily prepared by bubbling oxygen-free nitrogen through the solution immediately before sealing the ampoules and autoclaving the product at 115° for 30 minutes. No degradation of morphine was detected after storage for four months at ambient room temperature.

Containers and infusion devices

Samples of aqueous solutions of morphine sulphate 2 mg/mL (without preservative or antioxidant) and solutions of morphine sulphate 5 mg/mL containing chlorocresol 0.2% w/v and sodium metabisulphite 0.1% w/v were filled into two types of plastic disposable syringes and stored for 12 weeks at 22°± 2° (under light and dark conditions) or in a refrigerator at 3°. In solutions with and without additives, degradation at 22° in the presence of light was less than 2% and less than 3%, respectively, while in the dark, or at 3°, degradation was much lower. The major degradation product was pseudomorphine, although a minor unidentified product was detected in solutions without additives after 4 weeks in the light.[16]

The stability of injections of morphine sulphate (1, 5, 15, and 25 mg/mL, from three manufacturers) was determined by storing 30-mL samples in portable pump reservoirs in the dark at 5° for 30 days.[17] The concentration of morphine sulphate increased by up to 6%; this was attributed to evaporation of water. An increase of up to 16% was observed in similar solutions stored at 25° in the dark. No significant changes in concentration of morphine sulphate occurred after connection of the pump reservoirs to portable infusion pumps and simulation of infusion at 0.4 mL/hour for 3 days at 37°.

Similarly,[18] more than 90% of the initial concentration remained in solutions of morphine sulphate 25 mg/mL and 50 mg/mL (Sabex International) and 10 mg/mL in either sodium chloride 0.9% or glucose 5% solution, following storage in portable infusion pump cassettes (Pharmacia) at 4° and 23° for 31 days. No visual changes or changes in pH were observed. The presence of sodium metabisulphite had no significant effect on the stability of morphine sulphate. (See also Stabilisation, below).

Morphine sulphate 15 mg/mL (injection with preservative, Eli Lilly, USA) was stable (more than 90% of the initial concentration remained) after storage at 4° and 23° to 25° in polyvinyl chloride containers (Viaflex, Baxter, USA), in disposable glass syringes (Hypod, Solopak, USA), and in two disposable infusion devices (Intermate 200, Infusion Systems, USA and Infusor, Baxter, USA) for at least 12 days.[19] Stability was also demonstrated at 31° in both infusion devices for at least 12 days. Solutions of morphine sulphate 0.5, 15, 30 and 60 mg/mL in sodium chloride 0.9% solution were filtered through membrane filters (Millipore, USA) into 100-mL Cormed III (Kalex, CR Bard, USA) intravenous bags.[20] In all solutions morphine sulphate was stable for 14 days at 37°, and in all except the 60 mg/mL solution, stability was demonstrated for 14 days at 5°. After 9 days at 5° only 57% of the initial concentration of the 60 mg/mL solution remained, with concomitant production of a white precipitate. A brown discoloration in all solutions after 5 days was not associated with changes in concentration of morphine sulphate.

Lyophilisation

The stability of lyophilised formulations of morphine acetate was studied by Poochikian *et al*.[21] Samples were stored at 50°. A preparation containing 100 mg of morphine acetate and 15 mg of lactose, which was sealed under vacuum, lost less than 2% of its labelled content of morphine after 6 months at 50°. A solution of this product in sterile or bacteriostatic water for injection, was stable for 5 days at 25°. The pH of the solution was 5 to 6.

Stabilisation

From a knowledge of the reaction mechanism for the degradation of morphine, the factors that must be controlled in order to increase stability are oxygen content and pH.

Several authors have investigated the effect of including antioxidants in morphine injection formulations. Yeh and Lach[22] found that morphine sulphate solutions were stabilised by the inclusion of sodium bisulphite. Van Arkel and Van Waert[23] found that decomposition (1%) of a 1% solution of morphine hydrochloride sterilised in free-flowing steam for one hour (100°) was completely prevented by the inclusion of 0.05% sodium bisulphite. An examination of the effect of sodium metabisulphite (0.1%) on the stability of morphine sulphate injections stored in Clinbritic bottles was undertaken by Foster *et al*.[24] After nine months at room temperature, the samples that contained metabisulphite had developed a slight colour, but those without metabisulphite showed the greatest discoloration. Only small amounts of pseudomorphine were detected even in discoloured preparations; discoloration was not attributed to pseudomorphine. The effect of hydrogen ion concentration, disodium edetate, sodium metabisulphite, air, and nitrogen on the stability of autoclaved solutions of morphine sulphate was discussed by Coombe and Roxon.[25] An injection containing morphine sulphate (2.5%), disodium edetate (0.005%), sodium metabisulphite (0.1%), sodium chloride (0.12%), sodium phosphate (1.02%), citric acid (0.75%), and water for injection (carbon dioxide-free, to 100%), pH 3.4, in soda glass ampoules was stable to autoclaving, showing no colour change or decomposition after storage for 12 months at room temperature (15° to 25°).

FURTHER INFORMATION. Stability of morphine hydrochloride in a portable pump reservoir—Roos PJ, Glerum JH, Meilink JW. Pharm Weekbl (Sci) 1992;14(1):23–6. Stability of morphine sulfate in bacteriostatic 0.9% sodium chloride injection stored in glass vials at two temperatures—Nahata MC, Morosco RS, Hipple TF. Am J Hosp Pharm 1992;49:2785–6.

INCOMPATIBILITY/COMPATIBILITY

Morphine salts are reported to be incompatible with some barbiturates, pethidine, phenytoin, promethazine, and thiopentone. Morphine salts are also reported to be incompatible with alkalis, borax, bromides, chlorates, ferric chloride, gold salts, iodic acid, iodides, lead acetate, mercury bichloride, potassium permanganate, tannic acid, and solutions of ammonia, and with salts of iron, manganese, silver, copper, and zinc.

Admixtures of morphine sulphate and heparin sodium were prepared in de-ionised water or sodium chloride 0.9% solution and stored in glass vials. Concentrations of morphine sulphate were 1, 2, 5, and 10 mg/mL, and those of heparin were 100 and 200 units/mL. No precipitate was visible in any of the samples with a morphine concentration of 5 mg/mL or less and there was no significant loss of morphine in admixtures prepared with sodium chloride 0.9%. A precipitate was formed on addition of 5 mL samples of morphine sulphate 10 mg/mL in de-ionised water to solutions containing heparin sodium 100 and 200 units/mL in de-ionised water; morphine was assumed to be a component of the precipitate and the reaction was thought to be due to an ionic strength effect rather than to a pH change.[26] Visual compatibility for at least one hour was demonstrated[27] when 1 mL of morphine sulphate injection (1 mg/mL, Elkins-Sinn, USA) in sodium chloride 0.9% solution was admixed with 1 mL of heparin sodium injection (60 units/mL, Elkins-Sinn, USA) in glucose 5% injection.

Attention has been drawn to differences in compatibility between morphine sulphate and prochlorperazine edisylate injections from various manufacturers. Visible milky-white precipitates formed when either of two prochlorperazine edisylate injections (SKF and Elkins-Sinn, USA) were mixed in syringes with morphine sulphate injection (Winthrop-Breon).[28] Other reports of similar incompatibilities are stated. However, one manufacturer reported[29] that following reformulation of morphine sulphate injection (Wyeth) in 1984 to contain chlorbutol instead of phenol, admixtures with prochlorperazine edisylate injection (SKF) were physically compatible for 24 hours at about 25°.

When 1 mL of morphine sulphate injection (1 mg/mL, Abbott, USA) was mixed at 25° under fluorescent light with 1 mL of acyclovir sodium injection (5 mg/mL, Burroughs Wellcome, USA) or with 1 mL of frusemide injection (0.8, 2.4, or 10 mg/mL, Elkins-Sinn, USA) a white precipitate was formed after 2 hours or 1 hour, respectively.[30]

Parker and Shearer[31] admixed metoclopramide 10 mg/2 mL injection (Maxeran) with morphine sulphate 10 mg/mL injection (Allen & Hanburys) at room temperature in 5-mL plastic syringes. The mixture was visually stable over 15 minutes. No precipitation was evident when the admixture was examined microscopically (×100). Nieves-Cordero et al[32] reported on the visual compatibility of 32 antimicrobial agents with a solution of morphine sulphate 1 mg/mL (Winthrop, USA) in glucose 5% injection during simulated Y-site injection. The morphine solution was incompatible with minocycline hydrochloride (Lederle) and also with tetracycline hydrochloride (Lederle). During the 4-hour test period no other visual incompatibility was noted.

In addressing the problems associated with the administration of concurrent drug and nutritional therapy to cancer patients, Macias et al[33] investigated the compatibility, stability, and availability of morphine sulphate (Eli Lilly, USA) in a total parenteral nutrition (TPN) solution, glucose 5% injection, and sterile water for injection when stored in polyvinyl chloride bags. Morphine sulphate was visually and chemically compatible with TPN solution or glucose 5% injection and was also stable when stored for 36 hours at 21.5° with no protection from environmental light.

Less than 7% of the initial concentration of morphine sulphate was lost[34] when oral solutions of morphine sulphate (Roxanol, Roxane, USA) at concentrations of 0.5 mg/mL and 1 mg/mL in each of two enteral tube feeding products (Isocal, Mead Johnson, USA and Vivonex Standard, Norwich Eaton, USA) were stored for 24 hours at 25° in enteral feeding bags, or for 24 hours at 4° in glass containers, or for 24 hours at 4° followed by 24 hours storage at 25°.

Sorption to glass and plastics

Adsorption of morphine onto detergent-cleaned glassware can be a problem when extracting morphine from aqueous solutions and biological tissues. In a report by Bhargava,[35] it was concluded that loss of morphine sulphate by adsorption could be minimised by siliconisation of all glassware that comes into contact with the aqueous solution.

No significant losses of morphine hydrochloride occurred when morphine hydrochloride 75 mg/L in sodium chloride 0.9% was stored in polyvinyl chloride infusion bags at 15° to 20° in the dark for one week.[36] Similarly,[37] no significant losses were reported following a 7-hour simulated infusion through a set comprising a cellulose propionate burette chamber and polyvinyl chloride tubing, or following a simulated infusion for at least one hour at 0.08 mL/min through polyethylene tubing or Silastic tubing connected to a glass syringe on a syringe pump. No sorption of the solution to all-plastic (polypropylene and polyethylene) single-use syringes was apparent.

FURTHER INFORMATION. Effect of morphine sulphate concentration on flow rate of an implantable reservoir pump—Rippe ES, Kresel JJ, Coombs DW, Mroz WT, Smith CR. Am J Hosp Pharm 1984;41:496–500.

FORMULATION

CHLOROFORM AND MORPHINE TINCTURE BP

Chloroform	125 mL
Morphine hydrochloride	2.29 g
Peppermint oil	1 mL
Anaesthetic ether	30 mL
Purified water	50 mL
Ethanol (90%)	125 mL
Liquorice liquid extract	125 mL
Treacle, of commerce	125 mL
Syrup sufficient to produce	1000 mL

Dissolve the peppermint oil in the ethanol (90%), add the purified water, dissolve the morphine hydrochloride in the mixture and add the chloroform and the anaesthetic ether. Separately, mix the liquorice liquid extract and the treacle with 400 mL syrup. Mix the two solutions, add sufficient syrup to produce 1000 mL and mix.

KAOLIN AND MORPHINE MIXTURE BP

Light kaolin or light kaolin (natural)	200 g
Sodium bicarbonate	50 g
Chloroform and morphine tincture	40 mL
Water sufficient to produce	1000 mL

The mixture should be recently prepared unless the kaolin has been sterilised.

MORPHINE HYDROCHLORIDE SOLUTION

The following formula was given in the *British Pharmaceutical Codex 1973*:

Morphine hydrochloride	10 g
Dilute hydrochloric acid	20 mL
Ethanol (90%)	250 mL
Purified water, freshly boiled and cooled	to 1000 mL

Mix the alcohol with an equal volume of the water, add the dilute hydrochloric acid, dissolve the morphine hydrochloride in the mixture, add sufficient of the water to produce the required volume, and mix. This solution should be protected from light.

MORPHINE AND COCAINE ELIXIR

The following formula was given in the *British Pharmaceutical Codex 1973*:

Morphine hydrochloride	1 g
Cocaine hydrochloride	1 g
Ethanol (90%)	125 mL
Syrup	250 mL
Chloroform water	to 1000 mL

The elixir should be recently prepared and protected from light. The proportion of morphine hydrochloride may be altered when specified by the prescriber.

MORPHINE, COCAINE AND CHLORPROMAZINE ELIXIR

The following formula was given in the *British Pharmaceutical Codex 1973*:

Morphine hydrochloride	1 g
Cocaine hydrochloride	1 g
Ethanol (90%)	125 mL
Chlorpromazine elixir	250 mL
Chloroform water	to 1000 mL

The elixir should be recently prepared and protected from light. The proportion of morphine hydrochloride may be altered when specified by the prescriber.

Excipients

Excipients that have been used in presentations of morphine sulphate include:
Tablets: cetostearyl alcohol; diethyl phthalate; ethylcellulose; hydroxyethylcellulose; hypromellose; lactose (anhydrous); magnesium stearate; maize starch; methanol; talc.
Oral liquids: allura red AC (E129); disodium edetate; glycerol; invert sugar; sodium benzoate; sodium chloride; sucrose.
Injections: sodium chloride.

Bioavailability

Absolute bioavailabilities of morphine (as morphine sulphate 10 mg) from an oral aqueous solution, a controlled-release oral tablet (MST-Continus), and a controlled-release buccal tablet were approximately 23.9%, 22.4%, and 18.7%, respectively, compared to intravenous morphine sulphate, in six healthy subjects.[38]

When a solution of morphine hydrochloride in sodium chloride 0.9% solution was administered to *rats* via the oral and rectal routes, systemic bioavailability was estimated to be 10% and 90%, respectively, compared to that by the intravenous route.[39]

In a detailed study of the absorption properties of morphine via the ocular route,[40] a bioavailability of 44% relative to that by the intravenous route was calculated following single-dose conjunctival administration of a morphine acetate solution to *rabbits*.

Solid oral dosage forms

Pellets containing morphine sulphate 25% w/w in a polysiloxane polymer with and without a water-soluble carrier were prepared by McGinity *et al*.[41] Release rates were measured in phosphate buffer (0.13M, pH 7.4 at 37°). It was found that the drug was released only very slowly (9% in one week) when a carrier was not present. Gelatin, sodium lauryl sulphate, or lactose at a concentration of 10% increased the drug release rate to 20% release in one week. The inclusion of sodium alginate (10%) in the matrix produced a morphine sulphate release rate of 50% in one week. As the sodium alginate concentration was increased, the morphine release rate increased reaching a maximum at sodium alginate 20%.

Suppositories and rectal solutions

Displacement value: approximately 1.5 g of morphine hydrochloride or morphine sulphate displaces 1 g of theobroma oil.

A study by Harris *et al*[42] demonstrated that 12% to 61% of morphine, as a solution, was absorbed from the rectal mucosa, compared to the intramuscular route, in six female patients. In an attempt to formulate a suitable vehicle for the rectal delivery of morphine, the properties of hydrogels were examined. Release profiles *in vitro* for morphine from a hydrogel formulation and a morphine chloride solution were obtained. After three hours, the amount of morphine released from the gel was about 60% of the amount released from a morphine chloride solution of the same concentration.

A comparison between the *in-vivo* absorption of morphine hydrochloride (10 mg) from a fatty-based suppository and an oral solution was made by Moolenaar *et al*.[43] The suppositories were prepared by mixing morphine hydrochloride with lactose and incorporating this mixture into molten Witepsol H15. The oral liquid was a simple solution of morphine hydrochloride dissolved in water. It was concluded that rectal dosing with the suppositories resulted in plasma concentrations similar to those observed after dosing with the oral liquid, but a lag time in achieving peak plasma concentration was noted following administration of the suppositories. The presence of lactose in the suppository had little effect on *in-vivo* release characteristics when compared with a suppository without lactose.

Cole *et al*[44] investigated *in-vitro* and *in-vivo* properties of a sustained-release, hydrogel suppository of morphine sulphate. The hydrogel was prepared by polymerisation of macrogol 4000, dicyclohexylmethane 4,4'-diisocyanate and 1,2,6-hexane triol with anhydrous ferric chloride as a catalyst. Single-dose administration to five healthy volunteers produced steady-state plasma concentrations of morphine within two to four hours, which were maintained throughout the 12-hour study period.

Topical preparations

In studies of the rheological properties of a 20% poloxamer 407 solution (as a thermoreversible gel), the inclusion of morphine acetate in the preparation did not alter the thermoreversible properties.[45] Characteristics demonstrated *in vitro* indicated potential use of the preparation as a controlled-release system.

Prodrugs

Several aliphatic esters of morphine were prepared[1] (esterification at the 3-hydroxy or 6-hydroxy group in morphine) that had greater water and lipid solubilities and were more lipophilic (greater octanol/pH 7.4 phosphate buffer partition coefficients) than morphine. Enhanced penetration through skin *in vitro* was shown by the esters. The kinetics of the hydrolysis of the esters to morphine were investigated at 37° and 60°, over a wide pH range.

FURTHER INFORMATION. How MST Continus suspension works——Pharm J 1992;249:775. The Brompton Cocktail [morphine-cocaine elixir]—Lancet 1979;1:1221. A mathematical model for drug release from o/w emulsions: application to controlled-release morphine emulsions [stable submicronised emulsions of morphine sulphate]—Friedman D, Benita D. Drug Dev Ind Pharm 1987;13:2067–85.

PROCESSING

Sterilisation

Morphine sulphate injection can be sterilised by heating in an autoclave.

REFERENCES

1. Drustrup J, Fullerton A, Christrup L, Bundgaard H. Int J Pharmaceutics 1991;71:105–16.
2. Yeh S-Y, Lach JL. J Pharm Sci 1961;50:35–42.
3. Beaumont IM. Pharm J 1982;229:39–41.
4. Sullivan JA. Aust J Hosp Pharm 1989;19(2):74–6.
5. Helliwell K, Jennings P. Pharm J 1982;229:600–1.
6. Helliwell K, Game P. Pharm J 1981;227:128–9.
7. Caute B, Monsarrat B, Lazorthes Y, Cros J, Bastide R. J Pharm Pharmacol 1988;40:644–5.
8. Roksvaag PO, Fredrikson JB, Waaler T. Pharm Acta Helv 1980;55:198–202.
9. Thörn N, Ågren A [Swedish]. Sven Farm Tidskr 1951;55:61–7.
10. Deeks T, Davis S, Nash S. Pharm J 1983;230:495–7.
11. Campbell A, Nixon A [letter]. Pharm J 1991;247:456.
12. Turner S, Potter SR [letter]. Pharm J 1980;225:108.
13. Austin KL, Mather LE. J Pharm Sci 1978;67:1510–11.
14. Taylor JB, Sherwood MJ [letter]. Pharm J 1983;230:543.
15. Bunn RJ, Hobbs RM [letter]. Pharm J 1980;224:334–5.
16. Hung CT, Young M, Gupta PK. J Pharm Sci 1988;77(8):719–23.
17. Stiles ML, Tu Y-H, Allen LV. Am J Hosp Pharm 1989;46:1404–7.
18. Walker SE, Iazzetta J, Lau DWC. Can J Hosp Pharm 1989;42(5):195–200, 218–19.
19. Duafala ME, Kleinberg ML, Nacov C, Flora KP, Hines J, Davis K *et al.* Am J Hosp Pharm 1990;47:143–6.
20. Altman L, Hopkins RJ, Ahmed S, Bolton S. Am J Hosp Pharm 1990;47:2040–2.
21. Poochikian GK, Cradock JC, Davignon JP [letter]. JAMA 1980;244:1434.
22. Yeh S-Y, Lach JL. Am J Hosp Pharm 1960;17:101–3.
23. Van Arkel CG, Van Waert JH [Dutch]. Pharm Weekbl 1950;85:319–21.
24. Foster GE, Macdonald J, Whittet TD. J Pharm Pharmacol 1950;11:673–84.
25. Coombe RG, Roxon JJ. Australas J Pharm 1963;44:534–5.
26. Baker DE, Yost GS, Craig VL, Campbell RK. Am J Hosp Pharm 1985;42:1352–5.
27. Smythe MA, Patel MA, Gasloli RA. Am J Hosp Pharm 1990;47:819–20.
28. Stevenson JG, Patriarca C [letter]. Am J Hosp Pharm 1985;42:2651.
29. Zuber DEL [letter]. Am J Hosp Pharm 1987;44:67.
30. Pugh CB, Pabis DJ, Rodriguez C. Am J Hosp Pharm 1991;48:123–5.
31. Parker WA, Shearer CA [letter]. Can J Hosp Pharm 1979;32:38.
32. Nieves-Cordero AL, Luciw HM, Souney PF. Am J Hosp Pharm 1985;42:1108–9.
33. Macias JM, Martin WJ, Lloyd CW. Am J Hosp Pharm 1985;42:1087–94.
34. Michelini T, Bhargava VO, DuBé JE. Am J Hosp Pharm 1988;45:628–30.
35. Bhargava HN. J Pharm Sci 1977;66:1044–5.
36. Kowaluk EA, Roberts MS, Blackburn HD, Polack AE. Am J Hosp Pharm 1981;38:1308–14.
37. Kowaluk EA, Roberts MS, Polack AE. Am J Hosp Pharm 1982;39:460–7.
38. Hoskin PJ, Hanks GW, Aherne GW, Chapman D, Littlejohn P, Filshie J. Br J Clin Pharmacol 1989;27:499–505.
39. Katagiri Y, Itakura T, Naora K, Kanba Y, Iwamoto K. J Pharm Pharmacol 1988;40:879–81.
40. Chast F, Bardin C, Sauvageon-Martre H, Callaert S, Chaumeil J-C. J Pharm Sci 1991;80(10):911–17.
41. McGinity JW, Hunke LA, Combs AB. J Pharm Sci 1979;68:662–4.
42. Harris AS, Westerling D, Andersson K-E. Br J Pharm Pract 1982;21,23,26.
43. Moolenaar F, Visser J, Leuverman A, Schoonen BJM. Int J Pharmaceutics 1988;45:161–4.
44. Cole L, Hanning CD, Robertson S, Quinn K. Br J Clin Pharmacol 1990;30:781–6.
45. Dumortier G, Grossiord JL, Zuber M, Couarraze G, Chaumeil J-C. Drug Dev Ind Pharm 1991;17(9):1255–65.

Naproxen (BAN, USAN, rINN)

Analgesic; Anti-inflammatory

(*S*)-2-(6-Methoxy-2-naphthyl)-propionic acid; (+)-6-methoxy-α-methyl-2-naphthaleneacetic acid

$C_{14}H_{14}O_3 = 230.3$

Naproxen Sodium (BANM, USAN, rINNM)

$C_{14}H_{13}NaO_3 = 252.2$

CAS—22204-53-1 (naproxen); 26159-34-2 (naproxen sodium)

Pharmacopoeial status

BP (naproxen); USP (naproxen, naproxen sodium)

Preparations

Compendial

Naproxen Tablets BP. Tablets containing, in each, 250 mg and 500 mg naproxen are usually available.

Naproxen Oral Suspension BP. An aqueous suspension of naproxen in a suitable flavoured vehicle. An oral suspension containing 125 mg in 5 mL is usually available. pH 2.1 to 4.0.

Naproxen Suppositories BP. Suppositories containing naproxen in a suitable suppository basis. Suppositories containing, in each, 500 mg are usually available.

Naproxen Tablets USP.

Naproxen Sodium Tablets USP.

Non-compendial

Arthroxen (CP). *Tablets*, naproxen 250 mg and 500 mg.

Naprosyn (Syntex). *Tablets*, naproxen 250 mg, 375 mg, and 500 mg.

Suspension, naproxen 125 mg/5 mL.

Granules containing 500 mg naproxen per sachet. To be dispersed in water to form a white, flavoured suspension.

Suppositories, each containing naproxen 500 mg.

Naprosyn EC (Syntex). *Tablets*, enteric coated, naproxen 250 mg, 375 mg, and 500 mg.

Nycopren (Nycomed). *Tablets*, enteric coated, naproxen 250 mg and 500 mg.

Pranoxen Continus (Napp). *Tablets*, modified release, naproxen 375 mg and 500 mg.

Synflex (Syntex). *Tablets*, naproxen sodium 275 mg (equivalent to naproxen 250 mg).

Naproxen tablets of various strengths are available from Ashbourne (Arthrosin), BHR (Prosaid), Cox, Evans, Goldshield (Rheuflex), Kerfoot, Lagap (Laraflex), Shire (Valrox), Sterwin.

Containers and storage

Solid state

Naproxen BP should be kept in a well-closed container and protected from light.

Naproxen USP and Naproxen Sodium USP should be preserved in tight containers.

Dosage forms

Naproxen Tablets BP should be protected from light.

Naproxen Tablets USP and Naproxen Sodium Tablets USP should be preserved in well-closed containers.

Arthroxen tablets should be stored in a cool dry place and protected from light.

Naprosyn tablets, suspension, and granules, and Naprosyn EC tablets should be protected from light and stored below 30°.

Naprosyn suppositories should be stored in a dry place at not more than 15°.

Nycopren tablets should be stored in their original container at room temperature.

Synflex tablets should be protected from light and moisture.

PHYSICAL PROPERTIES

Naproxen is a white or almost white powder.

Naproxen sodium is a white to creamy crystalline powder.

Melting point

Naproxen melts at about 156°.

Naproxen sodium melts at about 255°, with decomposition.

pH

The pH of an aqueous solution of *naproxen sodium* 13.7% is reported[1] to be 9.65.

Dissociation constant

pK_a 4.2 (25°)

Reported experimental values for the pK_a of naproxen:[2-4] 4.1; 4.21, at 25°, ionic strength 0.01; 4.28, at 25°, ionic strength 0.1; and 4.57, at 25°, ionic strength 0.1.

To overcome the problems associated with the determination of dissociation constants of poorly water-soluble drugs (including naproxen) in water,[5] aqueous dimethyl sulphoxide (20:80 w/w) was used as a mixed solvent. For a range of carboxylic acids, experimental values of pK_a in the mixed solvent (determined by potentiometry at 25°) were linearly related to literature pK_a values in water. An equation was derived which was used to convert the experimental pK_a of 7.60 for naproxen in aqueous dimethyl sulphoxide (20:80 w/w) to a pK_a of 4.29 in water.

Partition coefficients

Unger et al[3] determined experimental values of log P (octanol/phosphate buffer pH 7.0; 25°) of 3.18 and 3.20 ± 0.01 by shake-flask and reversed-phase HPLC methods, respectively.

Log P (octanol/water; 25°) values of 3.22 and 3.48 were calculated, using derived equations, from water solubility data.[6]

Solubility

Naproxen is practically insoluble in water; it is soluble 1 in 25 of ethanol, 1 in 15 of chloroform, 1 in 40 of ether, and 1 in 20 of methanol.

Naproxen sodium is soluble in water; sparingly soluble in ethanol; soluble in methanol; very slightly soluble in acetone; practically insoluble in chloroform.

The solubility of naproxen free acid and its salts was found to increase in the order: naproxen free acid < calcium salt < magnesium salt < sodium salt < potassium salt.[7]

At 25° and pH 2.0 the solubilities of naproxen and naproxen sodium were reported to be 6.9×10^{-5}M and 1.0×10^{-4}M, respectively.[8]

Effect of pH

The aqueous solubility of naproxen is low at low values of pH, but marked increases in solubility have been reported[2] at pH values approximately one unit greater than the pK_a value (4.1 in this study) and above. The results of the investigation (at room temperature) by Herzfeldt and Kümmel are presented below:

pH	1.2	2.0	3.0	4.0	5.0	6.0	7.0	7.5
Solubility (% w/v)	1.3×10^{-3}	2.2×10^{-3}	1.5×10^{-3}	2.9×10^{-3}	3.5×10^{-3}	0.053	0.257	0.315

Effect of temperature

The solubilities of 500 mg naproxen in 10 mL of octanol or water at three temperatures[6] were as follows:

Temperature	Water (buffered at pH 2)	Octanol
5°	4.3×10^{-5}M	0.061M
25°	6.9×10^{-5}M	0.116M
37°	11.46×10^{-5}M	0.157M

Dissolution

The USP specifies that for Naproxen Tablets USP and Naproxen Sodium Tablets USP not less than 70% of the labelled amount of $C_{14}H_{14}O_3$ and $C_{14}H_{13}NaO_3$, respectively, is dissolved in 45 minutes. Dissolution medium: 900 mL of 0.1M, pH 7.4 phosphate buffer; Apparatus 2 at 50 rpm.

Dissolution properties

Dissolution rate studies of non-steroidal anti-inflammatory drugs showed that in pH 7.5 buffer, naproxen was completely dissolved after about 5 minutes.[2]

The extent of dissolution of salts of naproxen increased in the order: arginium < N-methylglucosammonium < N-(2-hydroxyethyl)piperazinium < sodium.[8]

For the effect of cyclodextrins and povidone on dissolution of naproxen see Formulation below.

Crystal and molecular structure

Enantiomeric purity of naproxen by liquid chromatographic analysis of its diastereomeric octyl esters—Johnson DM, Reuter A, Collins JM, Thompson GF. J Pharm Sci 1979;68(1):112–14.

STABILITY

Peswani and Lalla[1] studied the formulation and stability of naproxen sodium in parenteral dosage forms. Precipitation occurred in aqueous solutions of naproxen sodium (13.7%) stored overnight at 4° at pH 7.0, 7.5, 8.0, and 9.0. At pH 8 or greater, no precipitation occurred for up to 6 months in solutions of naproxen sodium (13.7%) in a propylene glycol:water (40:60) vehicle at 4°; however, at pH values below 8 precipitation occurred overnight. One formulation (naproxen sodium 13.626%, naproxen 0.062%, propylene glycol 40%, benzyl alcohol 0.5%; pH 8) was selected for accelerated stability studies. Thermal degradation of naproxen sodium was first-order (activation energy 33.1 kJ/mol) and the shelf-life was determined to be 4.2 years. The preparation was stable to autoclaving. Samples of the formulation that were packaged in ampoules and sealed under air had a faster thermal degradation rate than those packaged in ampoules sealed under nitrogen.

FURTHER INFORMATION. Oxidative decarboxylation of naproxen—Bosca F, Martinez-Manez R, Miranda MA, Primo J, Soto J, Vano L. J Pharm Sci 1992;81(5):479–82.

INCOMPATIBILITY/COMPATIBILITY

Compatibility of naproxen in 1:1 physical mixtures with various tablet excipients has been investigated using differential scanning calorimetry.[9] No interactions were shown between naproxen and starch, directly compressible starch (Sta-Rx 1500), sodium starch glycollate (Primojel, Explotab), microcrystalline cellulose (Avicel PH 101), microfine cellulose (Elcema G250), a cross-linked form of carmellose sodium (Ac-Di-Sol), or hydrogenated cotton seed oil (Sterotex). Effects that might be attributed to interactions were shown between naproxen and povidone, crospovidone, calcium hydrogen phosphate (Emcompress), stearic acid, magnesium stearate, and glyceryl palmito stearate (Precirol Ato 5).

FORMULATION

Excipients

Excipients that have been used in presentations of naproxen include:

Tablets, naproxen: croscarmellose sodium; lactose; magnesium stearate; maize starch; povidone; pregelatinised maize starch; quinoline yellow (E104); sunset yellow FCF (E110).

Naproxen sodium: ethanol; hydroxypropylcellulose; hypromellose; indigo carmine (E132); lactose; macrogol 8000; magnesium stearate; microcrystalline cellulose; povidone; sunset yellow FCF (E110); talc; titanium dioxide (E171).

Suspensions, naproxen: aluminium magnesium silicate; fumaric acid; methyl hydroxybenzoate; orange flavour; pineapple flavour; sodium chloride; sorbitol; sucrose; sunset yellow FCF (E110); syrup.

Suppositories, naproxen: semi-synthetic solid glycerides.

Formulation with cyclodextrins

Two groups of workers prepared inclusion complexes comprising naproxen with α-, β-, and γ-cyclodextrins[10] or with β-cyclodextrin alone and examined the effects on both the aqueous solubility of naproxen and its dissolution properties. Naproxen solubility in water increased linearly with concentration of cyclodextrin but the extent of the increase with β-cyclodextrin was 6.25 and 12.5 times greater than with γ-cyclodextrin and α-cyclodextrin, respectively.[10] Interaction between naproxen and β-cyclodextrin was attributed to a combination of binding forces. Solid state studies indicated that inclusion complexes formed when naproxen and β-cyclodextrin were co-evaporated or co-lyophilised, but not when they were physically mixed or ground together. The incorporation of naproxen in the inclusion complexes enhanced its dissolution rate. Similarly,[11] a solid inclusion complex prepared by a lyophilisation method (naproxen:β-cyclodextrin, 1:1 molar ratio) had superior solubility and dissolution properties to those of a physical mixture and of a solid complex prepared by a neutralisation method.

Otero-Espinar *et al*[12] concluded that naproxen, lyophilised naproxen, and a 1:1 inclusion complex of naproxen with β-cyclodextrin were bioequivalent following oral administration to 12 healthy subjects. Dissolution profiles in artificial gastric juice (pH 1.2 at 37°) indicated that the percentage of naproxen dissolved in five minutes decreased in the order: a 1:3 naproxen:β-cyclodextrin inclusion complex (99%) > a 1:1 naproxen:β-cyclodextrin inclusion complex (61%) > lyophilised naproxen (12%) > a 1:1 physical mixture (11%) > naproxen alone (5%).

Frijlink *et al*[13] investigated the rectal absorption of naproxen from inclusion complexes formed between naproxen and β-cyclodextrin. Micro-enemas containing naproxen 8 mg either alone or with β-cyclodextrin 200 mg (96% complexed) were administered rectally to four healthy volunteers in a crossover study. The extent of absorption of naproxen was greater from micro-enemas that contained β-cyclodextrin. The enhancement of absorption was attributed mainly to the displacement of naproxen from the complex by lipids in rectal mucus; neither β-cyclodextrin itself nor the complex were absorbed.

Formulation with povidone

Bettinetti *et al*[14] prepared solid dispersions containing various ratios of naproxen and povidone (mol. wt. 25 000). The aqueous solubility of naproxen increased linearly with the concentration of povidone in the dispersions. All the preparations studied had a higher dissolution rate (in water at 37°) than naproxen alone or in physical mixtures; the greatest dissolution rate occurred with solid dispersions containing 40% to 60% povidone.

Release from inert matrices

Factors affecting the release of naproxen from inert matrices have been investigated.[15] Naproxen and naproxen sodium (200 mg) were each directly compressed with 200 mg of polymeric materials: polytetrafluoroethylene, ethylcellulose, or acrylic resins. From all matrices, dissolution of naproxen sodium was greater than that of naproxen alone, but drug release was not significantly influenced by the choice of polymer. The amount of drug released increased with an increase in pH.

Modified-release preparations

Three compressed matrix tablet preparations of naproxen sodium were evaluated by Dahl et al,[16] in vitro and in vivo, as controlled-release systems. Naproxen sodium was mixed with hydrophilic polymers (hypromellose or hydroxypropylcellulose) and then granulated with either water or an aqueous dispersion of polymethacrylic acid ester copolymers. Experimental controlled-release tablet formulations were as follows:

Constituents *	Formulation		
	1	2	3
Hypromellose	25%	—	15%
Hydroxypropylcellulose	—	20%	—
Polymethacrylic acid ester copolymers	—	15%	15%

* tablets contained naproxen sodium 550 mg, distilled water, and magnesium stearate.

In a crossover study, six healthy volunteers received a single dose of preparations 1, 2, and 3 and conventional naproxen sodium tablets (two 275 mg tablets, Anaprox, Syntex). Although the controlled-release tablets had similar rates and extents of dissolution, the extents of absorption of preparations 1 and 3 were approximately 10% greater than that of preparation 2 after 48 hours. This difference was attributed to the presence of a higher polymer content in preparation 2 and to possible differences in the in vivo and in vitro properties of hydroxypropylcellulose. In comparison with conventional tablets, all three controlled-release tablets had a slower rate of absorption and a greater bioavailability (113%, 102%, and 113% for preparations 1, 2, and 3, respectively).

The relative bioavailability of a controlled-release tablet of naproxen 500 mg (Naprosyn CR, Syntex, Australia) was shown to be 96% of the standard (2 × 250 mg) Naprosyn tablets during a randomised, crossover study involving 15 healthy volunteers.[17]

Bioavailability of suppositories

Rectal administration of suppositories containing 125, 250, 500, and 750 mg naproxen in 'Stearinum B', to 30 healthy volunteers indicated dose-dependent kinetics that were nonlinear at doses greater than 500 mg.[18] Absorption was rapid and bioavailability of the suppositories ranged from 80% (250 mg dose) to 90% (500 mg dose) of that after intravenous administration. Similarly, naproxen was rapidly and well absorbed from naproxen 500 mg suppositories administered to 22 healthy volunteers.[19] However, when administered vaginally as suppositories[20] naproxen absorption was slow and effective therapeutic concentrations in blood were not achieved.

No difference in bioavailability was reported between naproxen sodium suppositories and naproxen tablets.[21] Rectal administration of naproxen sodium in a triglyceride basis (each suppository equivalent to 500 mg naproxen) was compared with oral administration of two naproxen 250 mg tablets, in a crossover study involving eleven healthy volunteers; the rate of absorption from the suppositories was greater than from the tablets although bioavailabilities were equivalent. Naproxen sodium suppositories were also compared with naproxen (free acid) suppositories; the in-vitro dissolution rate (pH 7.3) of the suppositories prepared with the sodium salt was faster (50% dissolved in 15 minutes) than that of the naproxen suppositories (15% dissolved in 80 minutes). When administered rectally to six healthy volunteers, naproxen sodium suppositories had a significantly greater bioavailability than naproxen suppositories.

Percutaneous absorption

In studies that compared the percutaneous absorption of naproxen through human, rabbit, and rat skin[22] the effect of the inclusion of surfactants in different formulations was investigated. From aqueous gel preparations (containing hydroxypropylcellulose or carboxyvinyl polymer) the relative flux of naproxen across human skin in vitro was not significantly affected by the incorporation of nonionic, cationic, or amphoteric surfactants. However, the anionic surfactants sodium lauryl sulphate 4% and sodium laurate 4% increased the relative flux by factors of 8.3 and 2.5, respectively. From oil-in-water creams the relative flux of naproxen was enhanced by anionic surfactants; the order for increasing effect was sodium lauryl sulphate 2% < sodium laurate 2% < methyldecyl sulphoxide 1%. Magnitudes and orders of effects did not correlate with those across rabbit or rat skins. The transcutaneous absorption of naproxen, as 5% w/w and 10% w/w gels, was reported to be slow, although it may be therapeutically effective.[23]

FURTHER INFORMATION. Interaction of naproxen with β-cyclodextrin in solution and in the solid state—Otero-Espinar FJ, Anguiano-Igea S, García-González N, Vila-Jato JL, Blanco-Méndez J. Int J Pharmaceutics 1992;79:149–57. Interaction of naproxen with β-cyclodextrin in ground mixture—Çelebi N, Erden N. Int J Pharmaceutics 1992;78:183–7. Influence of method of preparation on inclusion complexes of naproxen with different cyclodextrins—Blanco J, Vila-Jato JL, Otero-Espinar FJ. Drug Dev Ind Pharm 1991;17(7):943–57. Thermal behaviour and dissolution properties of naproxen in combinations with chemically modified β-cyclodextrins—Bettinetti G, Gazzaniga A, Mura P, Giordano F, Setti M. Drug Dev Ind Pharm 1992;18(1):39–53. Macromolecular prodrugs. XII. Kinetics of release of naproxen from various polysaccharides [dextran, soluble starch, and hydroxyethyl starch] ester prodrugs in neutral and alkaline solution—Larsen C. Int J Pharmaceutics 1989;51:233–40. Macromolecular prodrugs. XV. Colon-targeted delivery—bioavailability of naproxen from orally administered dextran-naproxen ester prodrugs varying in molecular size in pig—Harboe E, Larsen C, Johansen M, Olesen HP. Pharm Res 1989;6:919–23. Ester and amide prodrugs of ibuprofen and naproxen: synthesis, anti-inflammatory activity, and gastro-intestinal toxicity—Shanbhag VR, Crider AM, Gokhale R, Harpalani A, Dick RM. J Pharm Sci 1992;81(2):149–54. Studies on a bioerodible drug carrier system based on a polyphosphazene—Part II. Experiments in vitro [release of naproxen as a model drug]—Grolleman CWJ, de Visser AC, Wolke JGC. J Controlled Release 1986;4:119–31. Studies on a bioerodible drug carrier system based on a polyphosphazene—Part III. Experiments in vivo [naproxen as a model drug]—Grolleman CWJ, de Visser AC, Wolke JGC, Klein CPAT. J Controlled Release 1986;4:133–42. Medicament release from ointment bases. V. Naproxen, in vitro release and in vivo percutaneous absorption in rabbits [detailed study, including effects of additives (urea, ethanol, dimethyl sulphoxide and macrogol 400)]—Rahman MS, Babar A, Patel NK, Plakogiannis FM. Drug Dev Ind Pharm 1990;16(4):651–72. Evaluation of maltodextrins as excipients for direct compression tablets and their influence on the rate of dissolution—Papadimitriou E, Efentakis M, Choulis NH. Int J Pharmaceutics 1992;86:131–6. Naproxen microcapsules: preparation and in vitro characterization—Sveinsson SJ, Kristmundsdóttir T. Int J Pharmaceutics 1992;82:129–33.

REFERENCES

1　Peswani KS, Lalla JK. J Parenter Sci Technol 1990;44(6):336–42.

2. Herzfeldt CD, Kümmel R. Drug Dev Ind Pharm 1983;9(5):767–93.
3. Unger SH, Cook JR, Hollenberg JS. J Pharm Sci 1978;67(10):1364–6.
4. McNamara DP, Amidon GL. J Pharm Sci 1986;75(9):858–68.
5. Fini A, De Maria P, Guarnieri A, Varoli L. J Pharm Sci 1987;76(1):48–52.
6. Fini A, Laus M, Orienti I, Zecchi V. J Pharm Sci 1986;75(1):23–5.
7. Chowhan ZT. J Pharm Sci 1978;67(9):1257–60.
8. Fini A, Zecchi V, Tartarini A. Pharm Acta Helv 1985;60(Feb):58–62.
9. Botha SA, Lötter AP. Drug Dev Ind Pharm 1990;16(4):673–83.
10. Bettinetti GP, Mura P, Liguori A, Bramanti G, Giordano F. Farmaco 1989;44(Feb):195–213.
11. Erden N, Çelebi N. Int J Pharmaceutics 1988;48:83–9.
12. Otero-Espinar FJ, Anguiano-Igea S, García-González N, Vila-Jato JL, Blanco-Méndez J. Int J Pharmaceutics 1991;75:37–44.
13. Frijlink HW, Eissens AC, Schoonen AJM, Lerk CF. Int J Pharmaceutics 1990;64:195–205.
14. Bettinetti GP, Mura P, Liguori A, Bramanti G, Giordano F. Farmaco (Prat) 1988;43 (Nov): 331–43.
15. Zecchi V, Tartarini A, Conte U. Arch Pharm (Weinheim) 1985;318:615–20.
16. Dahl T, Ling T, Yee J, Bormeth A. J Pharm Sci 1990;79(5):389–92.
17. Wanwimolruk S, Lipschitz S, Roberts MS. Int J Pharmaceutics 1991;75:55–62.
18. Calvo MV, Lanao JM, Domínguez-Gil A. Int J Pharmaceutics 1987;38:117–22.
19. Guelen PJM, Janssen TJ, Brueren MM, Vree TB, Lipperts GJH. Int J Clin Pharmacol Ther Toxicol 1988;26(4):190–3.
20. Constantine G, Hale K, Brennan C, Eccleston D. J Clin Pharm Ther 1987;12:193–6.
21. Gamst ON, Vesje AK, Aarbakke J. Int J Clin Pharmacol Ther Toxicol 1984;22(2):99–103.
22. Chowhan ZT, Pritchard R. J Pharm Sci 1978;67(9):1272–4.
23. van den Ouweland FA, Eenhoorn PC, Tan Y, Gribnau FWJ. Pharm Weekbl (Sci) 1988;10:178.

Nifedipine (BAN, USAN, rINN)

Calcium-channel blocker

Dimethyl 1,4-dihydro-2,6-dimethyl-4-(2-nitrophenyl)pyridine-3,5-dicarboxylate; 1,4-dihydro-2,6-dimethyl-4-(2-nitrophenyl)-3,5-pyridinedicarboxylic acid dimethyl ester

$C_{17}H_{18}N_2O_6 = 346.3$

CAS—21829-25-4

Pharmacopoeial status

BP, USP

Preparations

Compendial

Nifedipine Capsules USP.

Non-compendial

Adalat (Bayer). *Capsules*, nifedipine 5 mg (Adalat 5) and 10 mg (Adalat).

Tablets, modified release, nifedipine 10 mg (Adalat Retard 10), 20 mg (Adalat Retard), 30 mg (Adalat LA 30), and 60 mg (Adalat LA 60).

Coronary Injection, nifedipine 100 micrograms/mL (Adalat IC). Use polyethylene catheters only.

Coracten (Evans). *Capsules*, sustained release, nifedipine 10 mg and 20 mg.

Nifensar XL (Rhône-Poulenc Rorer). *Tablets*, sustained release, nifedipine 20 mg.

Nifedipine capsules are also available from APS, Ashbourne (Angiopine), Cox, CP, Eastern (Calcilat), Evans, Kerfoot, Norton.

Containers and storage

Solid state

Nifedipine BP should be protected from light.

Nifedipine USP should be preserved in tight, light-resistant containers.

Dosage forms

Nifedipine Capsules USP should be preserved in tight, light-resistant containers at a temperature between 15° and 25°.

Adalat, Adalat 5, Adalat Retard, Adalat Retard 10, Adalat LA 30, and Adalat LA 60 should all be protected from strong light and stored in the manufacturer's original container.

Coracten capsules should be stored in the original pack at a temperature not exceeding 30° and protected from light.

Nifensar XL tablets should be stored in a cool, dry place, protected from strong light.

PHYSICAL PROPERTIES

Nifedipine is a yellow, crystalline powder.

Melting point

Nifedipine melts in the range 171° to 175°.

Dissociation constant

$pK_a > 10$

Partition coefficient

Diez et al[1] determined an apparent octanol-water partition coefficient of 1387.2 ± 145.7 for nifedipine at 37°.

Solubility

Nifedipine is practically insoluble in water; slightly soluble in ethanol; soluble in chloroform and 1 in 10 of acetone.

A solubility of 4.83 ± 0.04 mg/mL has been determined[1] for nifedipine in ethanol:water (50:50).

Enhancement of solubility

Jain et al[2] examined the effects of two hydrotropic agents, sodium benzoate and sodium salicylate, in enhancing the solubility of nifedipine. At low concentrations (5% to 10% w/v) there was a linear increase in the amount of drug dissolved, whereas beyond this concentration range there was a sharp increase in solubility. A range of different factors was suggested to be involved in the mechanism of solubility enhancement, including complexation (in dilute solutions) and aggregate formation.

Temperature effects were also studied. Sodium salicylate had a greater effect than sodium benzoate, indicating that a hydroxyl group in the aromatic ring enhances solubility.

Dissolution

The USP specifies that for Nifedipine Capsules USP not less than 80% of the labelled amount of $C_{17}H_{18}N_2O_6$ is dissolved in 20 minutes. Dissolution medium: 900 mL of simulated gastric fluid TS (without pepsin); Apparatus 2 at 50 rpm.

Dissolution properties

Co-precipitates of nifedipine in various carriers were prepared and the dissolution rate of the drug was markedly increased when either urea, macrogol (4000, 6000, or 10000), or povidone (K-25, K-30, or K-90) were used as carriers.[3] The increase in nifedipine dissolution rate was mainly attributed to reduced particle size. X-ray powder diffractometry and differential thermal analysis indicated that binary mixtures formed between nifedipine and urea, or the macrogols, may have been eutectic. The influence of carrier weight ratio, molecular weight, solvent, and particle size of the solid dispersions were examined; the gastro-intestinal absorption of the co-precipitates in *rats* was also investigated.

Improvements in the dissolution rate of nifedipine roll-mixed with povidone and mixed with either macrogol or an additional solvent (ethanol or water) compared favourably with improvements achieved by co-precipitation and physical mixing with povidone.[4]

FURTHER INFORMATION. Cross-linked sodium carboxymethylcellulose [carmellose sodium] as a carrier for dissolution rate improvement of drugs—Sangalli ME, Giunchedi P, Colombo P, *et al.* Boll Chim Farm 1989;128:242–7.

STABILITY

Nifedipine is a light-sensitive compound; when exposed to daylight and to artificial light of certain wavelengths, it readily converts to a nitrosophenylpyridine derivative. Exposure to ultraviolet light leads to formation of a nitrophenylpyridine derivative.

Solid state

Matsuda *et al*[5] undertook a preformulation study to examine the photostability of nifedipine. Following exposure to either a mercury vapour or a fluorescent lamp, four degradation products were identified: a nitroso-derivative, 4-(2-nitrosophenyl)-2,6-dimethyl-3,5-dimethoxycarbonylpyridine; a nitro-derivative, 4-(2-nitrophenyl)-2,6-dimethyl-3,5-dimethoxycarbonylpyridine; an azoxy derivative, 2,2'-bis-(2,6-dimethyl-3,5-dimethoxycarbonylpyridine-4-yl)azoxybenzene; and a fourth product whose structure could not be defined as it was present in only trace amounts. It was suggested that the solid-state photodegradation of nifedipine followed apparent first-order kinetics and degradation rate constants were determined. No temperature dependence was shown indicating that the activation energy required was negligible and that in the presence of light nifedipine will decompose even at very low temperatures. The extent of degradation was significantly affected by the wavelength of light to which the drug was exposed. The drug was easily decomposed by ultraviolet light and visible light below 500 nm; greatest decomposition occurred following exposure to ultraviolet light at 380 nm and no photodegradation was observed at wavelengths greater than 500 nm.

Sadana and Ghogare[6] also investigated degradation of nifedipine in the solid state under several light conditions. Half-lives for nifedipine under artificial room light and ultraviolet light were 58 days and 32 days, respectively. Degradation in the solid state was concluded to be slower than in solution but nevertheless significant.

Solutions

The BP recommends that solutions of nifedipine should be prepared immediately before use in the dark or under long-wavelength light (greater than 420 nm), and should be protected from light.

Various workers[7–9] have examined photodegradation of nifedipine in the liquid phase and found that, on exposure to daylight, the nitroso-derivative was formed whereas exposure to ultraviolet light resulted in the formation of the nitro-derivative.

The reaction kinetics and the effects of concentration, light intensity, and pH on the stability of nifedipine were examined by Majeed *et al.*[10] Following exposure of solutions of nifedipine in 95% ethanol to fluorescent light, it was deduced that the non-aromatic nitrophenyl-dihydropyridine form was converted to the aromatic nitrosophenylpyridine derivative. Exposure to monochromatic light within the wavelength range 400 to 700 nm caused no apparent photo-oxidation. Irradiation of 1×10^{-4}M solutions under fluorescent light indicated that decomposition followed zero-order kinetics. The rate of photo-decomposition increased with increasing nifedipine concentration in the range 2×10^{-5} to 6×10^{-5}M; within the range 6×10^{-5} to 1×10^{-4}M the reaction rate was independent of concentration. The rate of photo-oxidation decreased exponentially with decreasing light intensity. In aqueous solution, the rate of photo-oxidation was most rapid at pH 2 and slowest at pH 5. The same workers reported[11] that photodecomposition of nifedipine in ethanol, chloroform, and acetonitrile followed similar spectral patterns, whereas the spectrum produced by nifedipine in cyclohexane differed. After irradiation for 3 hours, spectral changes in aqueous solutions were similar to those in ethanol. Addition of different concentrations of sodium bisulphite (antioxidant) in solutions of 6×10^{-5}M nifedipine in phosphate buffer (0.2M) at pH 7, altered the absorption spectrum of the drug. When protected from light, nifedipine demonstrated very favourable stability.

Degradation of nifedipine under several light conditions was investigated by ^{1}H-NMR and ^{13}C-NMR to simultaneously determine nifedipine and the degradation products 4-(2-nitrosophenyl)pyridine and 4-(2-nitrophenyl)pyridine.[6] The effects of solvent polarity, light intensity, duration of irradiation, and initial concentration of nifedipine on the extent and mechanism of decomposition in solution were also examined.

Workers in Germany undertook a two-part investigation of the photostability of nifedipine. Initially, they studied the kinetics and mechanism of degradation,[12] followed by an examination of the effects of 'medium' conditions (wavelength and intensity of light exposure, solution concentration, solvent effects, quality of vials, temperature, pH, and ionic strength) on drug stability.[13]

Degradation in cardioplegic solutions

The stability of nifedipine (275 or 500 micrograms/L) in plastic (Viaflex) bags containing cardioplegic solutions has been studied.[14] A graph of log drug concentration against time was linear but was independent of nifedipine concentration. When protected from light, bags stored at 4° retained significantly more nifedipine than bags stored at 25°. Statistical evaluations suggested that the refrigerated solutions retained more than 90% of their original concentration for up to 6 hours after preparation. No photodegradation was apparent within clear polyvinyl chloride tubing following exposure to normal room or yellow light. It was concluded that cardioplegic solutions containing nifedipine should be prepared immediately before surgery.

Stabilisation

Sadana and Ghogare[6] reported that sodium benzoate (at concentrations less than 1×10^{-2}M) retarded photodecomposition of nifedipine in solution.

Teraoka et al[15] used titanium dioxide or tartrazine or both as colourants in film-coating systems to stabilise nifedipine. The thickness of the film and concentrations of the colourants were varied and greatest protection was achieved by using a binary film of 80 micrometre thickness, containing 0.7% of each colourant. Films containing no colourant offered minimal protection, whereas degradation was inhibited to a greater extent by inclusion of tartrazine than by titanium dioxide. A method for direct evaluation of the protective effect of the film coatings was also developed.

FURTHER INFORMATION. Ali SL. In; Florey K, editor. Analytical profiles of drug substances; vol 18. London: Academic Press, 1989:221–88 [comprehensive review of stability and bioavailability]. Analytical study of nifedipine and its photo-oxidised form—Al-Turk W, Othman S, Majeed I, Murray W, Newton D. Drug Dev Ind Pharm 1989;15(2):223–33. High-performance liquid chromatography of nifedipine, its metabolites and photochemical degradation products—Pietta P, Rava A, Biondi P. J Chromatogr 1981;210:516–21. Quantitative proton magnetic resonance spectroscopic determination of nifedipine and its photodecomposition products from pharmaceutical preparations—Sadana GS, Ghogare AB. J Pharm Sci 1991;80(9):895–8. Film coating: effect of titanium dioxide concentration and film thickness on the photostability of nifedipine—Béchard SR, Quraishi O, Kwong E. Int J Pharmaceutics 1992;87:133–9. Inhibitory effect of 2-hydroxypropyl-β-cyclodextrin on crystalgrowth of nifedipine during storage: superior dissolution and oral bioavailability compared with polyvinylpyrrolidone [povidone] K-30—Uekama K, Ikegami K, Wang Z, Horiuchi Y, Hirayama F. J Pharm Pharmacol 1992;44:73–8.

FORMULATION

Excipients

Excipients that have been used in presentations of nifedipine include:

Capsules: gelatin; glycerol; lactose; macrogol 400; mint oil; saccharin sodium; sunset yellow FCF (E110); titanium dioxide (E171).

Tablets: lactose; macrogol 4000; magnesium stearate; maize starch; microcrystalline cellulose; polysorbate 80; red iron oxide; titanium dioxide (E171).

Injections: ethanol; macrogol 400.

Bioavailability

Rietbrock et al[16] compared the absorption characteristics of nifedipine following oral administration (capsule swallowed whole) and sublingual administration (capsule bitten to release liquid contents) of a reference (Adalat, Bayer) capsule and a generic (Corotrend, Siegfried GmbH) capsule. Compared to those produced by oral administration, peak plasma concentrations after sublingual administration were reduced by 43% and 59% for the reference and generic preparations, respectively. There was also a significant difference between the plasma concentrations produced sublingually by the two products; it was suggested that this difference was due to the use of a double-concentrated nifedipine solution and a correspondingly smaller volume, in the generic capsule. A further study by workers in the Netherlands[17] concluded that sublingual absorption of nifedipine is negligible and in cardiovascular emergencies the patient should bite the capsule and swallow the contents with water.

The pharmacokinetics of a novel sublingual nifedipine spray (Unipack, Austria) were compared with those of sublingually administered standard nifedipine 5 mg capsules (Adalat, Bayer).[18] Significantly higher mean peak plasma concentrations were produced by the 5 mg spray although the bioavailability of nifedipine via both routes was similar.

In a study of the main pharmacokinetic parameters and bioavailability of three nifedipine formulations, a newly developed, sustained-release capsule (hard gelatin capsule with pellets) compared favourably with two marketed preparations.[19] The bioavailability of the new formulation was 27% greater than that of the existing sustained-release tablet and peak plasma concentrations were reached later with the new preparation.

In a randomised crossover study in Finland[20] twelve healthy volunteers received single and multiple doses of four different 'short-acting' commercial preparations of nifedipine (one capsule and three tablet preparations). One tablet, which showed poor dissolution characteristics *in vitro*, produced 27% to 40% lower bioavailability than the other preparations and was subsequently withdrawn from the market.

Modified-release preparations

Swanson and co-workers[21] reported on the development of a 'push-pull osmotic pump' as a once-daily oral dosage form for the controlled zero-order delivery of nifedipine. In bioavailability studies comparing the experimental form with standard nifedipine capsules, the absorption rate was equal to the *in-vitro* release rate during the delivery period.

Kohri et al[22] prepared two types of sustained-release granules: one with pH-dependent release (composed of nifedipine, hypromellose phthalate and ethylcellulose as binders, and microcrystalline cellulose as filler) and another with pH-independent release (containing nifedipine, hypromellose and ethylcellulose as binders, and maize starch as filler). Eight formulations were examined to identify any relationship that existed between the release rate of nifedipine from the granules and the drug concentration versus time profile in *rabbit* plasma. It was concluded that the granules with pH-independent release would be preferable for an oral sustained-release dosage form of nifedipine on the basis of prolonging effective plasma concentrations and minimising inter-subject variation.

Transdermal absorption

Diez et al[1] determined the permeability constant, lag time, and flux of nifedipine, across hairless *mouse* skin *in vitro*, as a measure of the intrinsic transdermal permeability of nifedipine.

Injections

Following their earlier work on hydrotropic enhancement of solubility of nifedipine (see Solubility above), Jain et al[23] demonstrated that the incorporation of sodium benzoate 30% w/v and sodium salicylate 30% w/v in an aqueous vehicle enabled the formulation of injections with final drug concentrations of 1 mg/5 mL and 1 mg/2 mL of nifedipine, respectively. Both formulations were stable to autoclaving. The inclusion of sodium benzoate or sodium salicylate did not protect the drug from photodecomposition; however, the degradation rate was less in amber-coloured containers than in colourless containers.

Suppositories

Kurosawa *et al*[24] prepared nifedipine suppositories using macrogols 400 and 4000 as the basis. The suppositories demonstrated acceptable physical properties. Following storage for 30 months (wrapped in aluminium foil within tightly closed, light-resistant containers) at 5° in a refrigerator, 92.4% of the original drug content remained. The bioavailability of the suppositories in healthy volunteers compared well with that of soft gelatin capsules for oral administration. The suppositories had adequate absorption characteristics for the treatment of hypertensive emergency. It was also suggested that the suppository may be useful as a sustained-release formulation for the treatment of essential hypertension.

While investigating alternatives to oral nifedipine administration, workers in the Netherlands[25] prepared suppositories (Estarine B as the basis) and enemas (glycerol and macrogol 400 as the vehicle). After investigation of single-dose pharmacokinetics, rectal administration of nifedipine was concluded to be a good alternative to the oral route; the enema would be most suitable when urgent treatment is required whereas the suppository could be used for longer-term treatment.

Co-precipitates

Following preparation of co-precipitates of nifedipine with urea, macrogol (4000, 6000, or 10 000) or povidone (K-25, K-30, or K-90), the stabilities of the various co-precipitates under different storage conditions were examined.[26] Nifedipine-urea co-precipitates were chemically unstable. Changes in drug dissolution behaviour were observed after 1:9 w/w nifedipine:povidone co-precipitates were stored at room temperature and 75% relative humidity. It was suggested that partial crystallisation of the drug in the povidone matrices had occurred. The author concluded that, of the co-precipitates studied, macrogols were the most suitable matrix materials for nifedipine.

The solubility and dissolution of co-precipitates of nifedipine with povidone or macrogol 6000 (prepared by different methods) were investigated before evaluation of the chemical and physical stability of nifedipine in the co-precipitates at various temperatures and humidities.[27]

FURTHER INFORMATION. The effect of some natural polymers on the solubility and dissolution characteristics of nifedipine— Acartürk F, Kislal Ö, Çelebi N. Int J Pharmaceutics 1992;85:1–6. Sustained release nifedipine formulations [of a nifedipine:povidone (1:3) co-precipitate with Gelucire as a wax matrix]: moment, modelling and simulation as pharmacokinetic approach [in *rabbits*]—Remunán C, Mrhar A, Primozic S, Karba R, Vila-Jato JL. Drug Dev Ind Pharm 1992;18(2):187–202. Accelerated stability study of sustained release nifedipine tablets prepared with Gelucire—Remunán C, Bretal MJ, Núnez A, Vila-Jato JL. Int J Pharmaceutics 1992;80:151–9. Polyacrylate (Eudragit Retard) microspheres for oral controlled release of nifedipine.I. Formulation design and process optimisation—Barkai A, Pathak YV, Benita S. Drug Dev Ind Pharm 1990;16(13):2057–75. Dissolution and absorption of nifedipine in polyethylene glycol [macrogol] solid dispersion containing phosphatidylcholine—Law SL, Lo WY, Lin FM, Chaing CH. Int J Pharmaceutics 1992;84:161–6. Studies on solid dispersions of nifedipine—Save T, Venkitachalam P. Drug Dev Ind Pharm 1992;18(15):1663–79. Subcutaneous administration of nifedipine—Krichbaum DW, Malone PM. Drug Intell Clin Pharm 1988;22:891–2. Bioavailability and bioequivalence of a new nifedipine preparation [capsule]—v.Achtert G, Wisotzki R, Lutz D, Jaegar H [German], Arzneimittelforschung 1987;37:1296–7. The bioavailability of two new nifedipine formulations [capsule and solution]—Herr-

mann R [German]. Pharm Ztg 1986;131:869–70. Proof of bioequivalence of two nifedipine preparations [hard and soft gelatin capsules]—Herrmann R, Rahlfs VW, Zimmermann H. Arzneimittelforschung 1989;39:1143–8. Bioavailability of nifedipine from different oral dosage forms in healthy volunteers [capsule, tablet, and sugar-coated tablet]—Leucuta SE, Vida-Simiti L, Caprioara MG, Fagarasan E, Vlaicu R et al. Pharmazie 1989;44:336–8. The influence of the 'Spansule' sustained release mechanism on the bioavailability of nifedipine at steady state—Hyman-Taylor P, Barton C, Curram J, Rubin P. Br J Clin Pharmacol 1993;35(1):76P.

REFERENCES

1. Diez I, Colom H, Moreno J, Obach R, Peraire C, Domenech J. J Pharm Sci 1991;80(10):931–4.
2. Jain NK, Patel VV, Taneja LN. Pharmazie 1988;43:194-6.
3. Sumnu M. STP Pharma 1986;2(14):214–20.
4. Nozawa Y, Mizumoto T, Higashide F. Pharm Acta Helv 1986;61:337–41.
5. Matsuda Y, Teraoka R, Sugimoto I. Int J Pharmaceutics 1989;54:211–21.
6. Sadana GS, Ghogare AB. Int J Pharmaceutics 1991;70:195–9.
7. Ebel VS, Schütz H, Hornitschek A [German]. Arzneimittelforschung 1978;28:2188–93.
8. Testa R, Dolfini E, Reschiotto C, Secchi C, Biondi PA. Farmaco 1979;34:463–73.
9. Jakobsen P, Pedersen OL, Mikkelsen E. J Chromatogr 1979;162:81–7.
10. Majeed IA, Murray WJ, Newton DW, Othman S, Al-Turk W. J Pharm Pharmacol 1987;39:1044–6.
11. Al-Turk WA, Majeed IA, Murray WJ, Newton DW, Othman S. Int J Pharmaceutics 1988;41:227–30.
12. Thoma K, Klimek R [German]. Pharm Ind 1985;47:207–15.
13. Thoma K, Klimek R [German]. Pharm Ind 1985;47:319–27.
14. Bottorff MB, Graves DA, McAllister RG, Batenhorst RL, Foster TS. Am J Hosp Pharm 1984;41:2068–70.
15. Teraoka R, Matsuda Y, Sugimoto I. J Pharm Pharmacol 1988;41:293–7.
16. Rietbrock N, Kausch M, Engelhardt M, Woodcock BG [letter]. Br J Clin Pharmacol 1987;23:589–90.
17. van Harten J, Burggraaf J, Danhof M, van Brummelen P, Breimer DD. Pharm Weekbl (Sci) 1987;9(6):334.
18. Eagle S, Acton G, Manchee K, Meineke I, De Mey C, Broom C. Br J Clin Pharmacol 1990;30(2):331P.
19. Pabst G, Lutz D, Molz KH, Dahmen W, Jaegar H. Arzneimittelforschung 1986;36:256–60.
20. Eränkö PO, Palva ES, Konnok, Venho VM. Pharm Med 1990;4:197–205.
21. Swanson DR, Barclay BL, Wong PSL, Theeuwes F. Am J Med 1987;83(Suppl 6B):3–9.
22. Kohri N, Mori K-I, Miyazaki K, Arita T. J Pharm Sci 1986;75(1):57–61.
23. Jain NK, Patel VV, Taneja LN. Pharmazie 1988;43:254–5.
24. Kurosawa N, Owada E, Ito K, Ueda K, Takahashi A, Kikuiri T. Int J Pharmaceutics 1985;27:81–8.
25. van Schaik BAM, Geers AB. Pharm Weekbl (Sci) 1989;11:Suppl H, H7.
26. Sumnu M. STP Pharma 1986;2(15):299–302.
27. Pezoa R, Jimenez J, Arancibia A, Gaete G [Spanish]. An Real Acad Farm 1988;54:589–603.

Nitrazepam (BAN, USAN, rINN)   *Hypnotic*

1,3-Dihydro-7-nitro-5-phenyl-1,4-benzodiazepin-2-one; 1,3-dihydro-7-nitro-5-phenyl-2*H*-1,4-benzodiazepin-2-one
$C_{15}H_{11}N_3O_3 = 281.3$
CAS—146-22-5

Pharmacopoeial status

BP

Preparations

Compendial
Nitrazepam Capsules BP. Capsules containing, in each, 5 mg are usually available.
Nitrazepam Tablets BP. Tablets containing, in each, 5 mg and 10 mg are usually available.
Nitrazepam Oral Suspension BP (Nitrazepam Mixture). A suspension of nitrazepam in a suitable flavoured vehicle. An oral suspension containing 2.5 mg in 5 mL is usually available.

Non-compendial
Mogadon (Roche). *Capsules*, nitrazepam 5 mg.
Tablets, nitrazepam 5 mg.
Somnite (Norgine). *Suspension*, nitrazepam 2.5 mg/5 mL. *Diluent*: syrup (preserved), life of diluted suspension 14 days (may be diluted to a maximum of 1 in 5).
Nitrazepam tablets are also available from APS, Cox, DDSA (Remnos), Evans, Kerfoot, Unigreg (Unisomnia).

Containers and storage

Solid state
Nitrazepam BP should be kept in a well-closed container and protected from light.

Dosage forms
Nitrazepam Tablets BP and Nitrazepam Oral Suspension BP should both be protected from light. The suspension should be stored at a temperature not exceeding 25°.
Mogadon tablets and capsules should be protected from light and the recommended maximum storage temperature is 30°.
Somnite suspension should be stored in a cool place, protected from light.

PHYSICAL PROPERTIES

Nitrazepam is a crystalline, yellow, odourless powder.

Melting point

Nitrazepam melts in the range 224° to 230°.

Dissociation constants

pK_a 3.2, 10.8 (20°)
Barrett *et al*[1] determined by spectrophotometry pK_a values of 3.2 and 10.8 for nitrazepam in solution (5×10^{-5}M). The values were associated with protonation in acid and deprotonation of the neutral molecule in alkaline media (pH 7 to 12).

Partition coefficient

Log *P* (octanol/pH 7.4), 2.1

Solubility

Nitrazepam is practically insoluble in water, in benzene, and in hexane; soluble 1 in 120 of ethanol, 1 in 900 of ether, and 1 in 45 of chloroform; soluble in acetone and in ethyl acetate.

Dissolution

Dissolution properties
Dissolution of nitrazepam improved after processing with methylcellulose and hydroxyethylcellulose to form either physical mixtures or 'evaporates' from volatile solvents. After trituration with methylcellulose, nitrazepam solubility increased. The binding of nitrazepam to methylcellulose was both concentration-dependent and temperature-dependent.[2]

STABILITY

Nitrazepam is relatively stable. After storage for 280 days under various storage conditions (45° and 60°, 47% and 87% relative humidity) no decomposition was detected.[3]
The lactam ring hydrolysis of nitrazepam follows two routes, which are dependent on the amount of water available; both reactions are pseudo-first-order. In aqueous solution, the main decomposition product is 2-amino-5-nitrobenzophenone, whereas in the solid state the major product is 3-amino-6-nitro-4-phenyl-2(1*H*)-quinolone.
Genton and Kesselring[4] reported that the stability of nitrazepam in the solid state as a 1% dilution in microcrystalline cellulose is affected by both temperature and relative humidity. Values given for $t_{10\%}$ were 62.8 years at 18° and 50% relative humidity and 12.9 years at 20° and 65% relative humidity.
The effects of calcium hydrogen phosphate and of colloidal silica on the decomposition of nitrazepam was examined by Loewe *et al.*[3] Under all combinations of temperature (45° and 60°) and relative humidity (47% and 87%), nitrazepam tablets that contained calcium hydrogen phosphate degraded predictably by pseudo-zero-order kinetics to the major decomposition products: 2-amino-5-nitrobenzophenone and 3-amino-nitrocarbostyril. The inclusion of colloidal silica in nitrazepam preparations increased the rate of degradation; the rate was greatly accelerated under conditions of increased temperature and relative humidity although the reaction did not follow zero-order, first-order, or second-order kinetics. From a model based on the sorption of nitrazepam to silica under conditions of high humidity, hypotheses were put forward to describe the decomposition processes and secondary reactions.
Solutions of nitrazepam in methanol and ethanol were reported[5] to be stable for several weeks; aqueous solutions are more likely to decompose, particularly under acidic and alkaline conditions. Han *et al*[6] examined the kinetics and mechanisms of hydrolysis of nitrazepam in buffered solutions.

Photostability

Irradiation of nitrazepam with light at 300 nm in an oxygen-poor medium led to photoreduction and photoreductive dimerisation whereas in an oxygen-rich medium (at 350 nm) nitrazepam was relatively photostable.[7]

FURTHER INFORMATION. Isolation and identification of an alkali-catalysed hydrolysis product of nitrazepam [intermediate product *N*-(α-2-amino-5-nitrophenyl)benzylidene glycine]—Davidson AG, Chee S-M, Miller FM, Watson D. Int J Pharmaceutics 1990;63:29–34. Isolation and characterisation of an acid-catalysed intermediate hydrolysis product [2-glycylamino-5-nitrobenzophenone] of nitrazepam—Davidson AG, Smail GA. Int J Pharmaceutics 1991;69:1–3.

FORMULATION

Excipients

Excipients that have been used in presentations of nitrazepam include:
Tablets: lactose; magnesium stearate; starch; talc.
Oral suspensions: amaranth solution; blackcurrant syrup; benzoic acid solution; chloroform spirit; compound tragacanth powder; methylcellulose; Nipasept; raspberry syrup; syrup.

REFERENCES

1. Barrett J, Smyth WF, Davidson IE. J Pharm Pharmacol 1973;25:387–93.
2. Keipert S, Alde D [German]. Pharmazie 1986;41:845–9.
3. Loewe W, Soliva M, Speiser PP. Drugs Made in Germany 1983;26:158–64.
4. Genton D, Kesselring UW. J Pharm Sci 1977;66(5):676–80.
5. Clifford JM, Smyth WF. Analyst 1974;99:241.
6. Han WW, Yakatan GJ, Maness DD. J Pharm Sci 1977;66:795–8.
7. Cornelissen PJG, Beyersbergen van Henegouwen GMJ. Pharm Weekbl (Sci) 1981;3:800–9.

Nitrofurantoin (BAN, rINN)   *Antibacterial*

Furadoninum
1-(5-Nitrofurfurylideneamino)hydantoin; 1-[[(5-nitro-2-furanyl)methylene]amino]-2,4-imidazolidinedione
$C_8H_6N_4O_5 = 238.2$

Nitrofurantoin Sodium (BANM, rINNM)

$C_8H_5N_4NaO_5 = 260.1$
CAS—67-20-9 (nitrofurantoin anhydrous); 17140-81-7 (nitrofurantoin monohydrate); 54-87-5 (nitrofurantoin sodium)

Pharmacopoeial status

BP, USP (nitrofurantoin)

Preparations

Compendial
Nitrofurantoin Tablets BP. Tablets containing, in each, 50 mg and 100 mg are usually available.
Nitrofurantoin Oral Suspension BP (Nitrofurantoin Mixture, Nitrofurantoin Suspension). An oral suspension containing 25 mg in 5 mL is usually available. Nitrofurantoin Oral Suspension should not be diluted.
Nitrofurantoin Capsules USP.
Nitrofurantoin Tablets USP.
Nitrofurantoin Oral Suspension USP.

Non-compendial
Furadantin (Procter & Gamble Pharm). *Tablets*, nitrofurantoin 50 mg and 100 mg.
Suspension, sugar free, nitrofurantoin 25 mg/5 mL. Do not dilute.
Macrobid (Procter & Gamble Pharm). *Capsules*, modified release, nitrofurantoin 100 mg (as nitrofurantoin macrocrystals and nitrofurantoin monohydrate).

Macrodantin (Procter & Gamble Pharm). *Capsules*, nitrofurantoin macrocrystals 50 mg and 100 mg.
Nitrofurantoin tablets are also available from Biorex.

Containers and storage

Solid state
Nitrofurantoin BP should be kept in a well-closed container, protected from light and stored at a temperature not exceeding 25°.
Nitrofurantoin USP should be preserved in tight, light-resistant containers.

Dosage forms
Nitrofurantoin Tablets BP and Nitrofurantoin Oral Suspension BP should be protected from light and stored at a temperature not exceeding 25°.
All Nitrofurantoin preparations USP should be preserved in tight, light-resistant containers.
Furadantin tablets should be stored at a temperature not exceeding 30°; they should be dispensed in light-proof, preferably moisture-resistant containers. Furadantin suspension should be stored and dispensed in amber bottles made of neutral glass as exposure to light will cause darkening of the active principle. It should be stored at a temperature not exceeding 30° and protected from freezing.
Macrodantin 50 mg and 100 mg capsules should be stored at a temperature not exceeding 30°. Macrodantin 100 mg capsules should be dispensed in light-proof and preferably moisture-resistant containers.

PHYSICAL PROPERTIES

Nitrofurantoin is a yellow, crystalline powder; odourless or almost odourless with a bitter aftertaste.

Melting point

Nitrofurantoin melts at about 271°.

Dissociation constant

pK_a 7.2 (25°)

Solubility

Nitrofurantoin is soluble 1 in 5000 of water, 1 in 2000 of ethanol, 1 in 200 of acetone, 1 in 16 of dimethylformamide, and 1 in 70 of macrogol 300.
The incorporation of low concentrations of urea (up to approximately 2%) enhanced the solubility of nitrofurantoin in aqueous solution at 30° and 37°; however, as the concentration of urea was increased, nitrofurantoin solubility decreased to levels that were lower than the actual solubility of nitrofurantoin in water.[1] The same workers demonstrated[2] enhanced solubility of nitrofurantoin in aqueous pyridoxine hydrochloride solutions (of concentration up to 20%), buffered to pH 3.0 or 5.0 at 37°. Solubility increased linearly with increasing concentration of pyridoxine.

Dissolution

The USP specifies that for Nitrofurantoin Tablets USP not less than 25% of the labelled amount of $C_8H_6N_4O_5$ is dissolved in 60 minutes and not less than 85% of the labelled amount of $C_8H_6N_4O_5$ is dissolved in 120 minutes. Dissolution medium: 900 mL of phosphate buffer pH 7.2; Apparatus 1 at 100 rpm.

FURTHER INFORMATION. *In vivo/in vitro* correlation regarding nitrofurantoin tablets—Munoz Carnago E, Porto EG. Pharmazie 1986;41(H4):290–1.

Crystal and molecular structure

Crystal size affects the absorption of nitrofurantoin (See Formulation—Bioavailability). Crystallisation of nitrofurantoin from formic acid and a formic acid:water (2:1) binary solvent resulted in long tabular crystals and needle-shaped crystals, respectively.[3–5] The latter formation was shown by thermal analyses[3] to be the monohydrate, which formed the stable anhydrate when dried at 125°. Differences in the crystal habit of the two forms were studied.[4]

Garti and Tibika[4] also examined the habit modifications of nitrofurantoin crystallised from formic acid with methanol, ethanol, or dioxan.

FURTHER INFORMATION. The compaction properties of nitrofurantoin samples crystallised from different solvents—Marshall PV, York P. Int J Pharmaceutics 1991;67:59–65.

STABILITY

Crystals and solutions of nitrofurantoin are discoloured by alkali and by exposure to light; they are decomposed upon contact with metals other than stainless steel and aluminium.

Hydrolysis of nitrofurantoin at the azomethine bond occurs in acid solution at 37° and was shown by Inotsume and Nakano[6] to be reversible, pH-dependent, and acid-catalysed. The degradation product 5-nitrofurfural was formed. Nitrofurantoin was stable within the pH range 5.4 to 9.9. At constant temperature and pH, hydrolysis followed first-order kinetics. The rate constants for the forward reaction in 0.1M hydrochloric acid at 25°, 37°, and 50° were 0.035 ± 0.009/h, 0.135 ± 0.026/h, and 0.462 ± 0.073/h, respectively; values for the reverse reaction at the same temperatures were 0.193 ± 0.009/h, 0.443 ± 0.026/h, and 0.834 ± 0.073/h. Activation energies were 79.1 kJ/mol for the forward reaction and 41.6 kJ/mol for the reverse reaction.

Effect of storage

Gouda and co-workers[7] examined the effects of storage, for two-week and ten-week periods, on the content and dissolution properties of nitrofurantoin capsules and tablets in blister packs, child-proof vials, or plastic bags at 40° and 79% relative humidity, 25° and 79% relative humidity, and 40° and 31% relative humidity. Under all conditions there was a marked decrease in the degree of dissolution (at 37°, pH 7.2) of nitrofurantoin from capsules that contained macrocrystalline nitrofurantoin, but not from capsules containing microcrystalline nitrofurantoin. There was no change in content uniformity of any of the dosage forms.

FURTHER INFORMATION. Physicochemical stability of nitrofurantoin anhydrate and monohydrate under various temperature and humidity conditions—Otsuka M, Teraoka R, Matsuda Y. Pharm Res 1991;8:1066–8.

INCOMPATIBILITY/COMPATIBILITY

Nitrofurantoin sodium forms a precipitate when added to aqueous solutions containing methyl and propyl hydroxybenzoates, phenol, or cresol.

Nitrofurantoin sodium for injection is reported to be incompatible with ammonium chloride, codeine phosphate, insulin, noradrenaline acid tartrate, methyl hydroxybenzoate, morphine sulphate, procaine hydrochloride, streptomycin sulphate, and vitamin B complex with C.

Several nitrofurantoin oral suspensions containing mixtures of citric acid, sodium citrate, and saccharin sodium were found by HPLC to contain 3-(5-nitrofurfurylideneamino)hydantoic acid generated by the reaction of nitrofurantoin with the citrate buffer.[8] The concentration of this degradation product in several lots of commercial oral suspensions ranged from 20 to 300 micrograms/mL.

FORMULATION

Excipients

Excipients that have been used in presentations of nitrofurantoin include:

Capsules, macrocrystalline and microcrystalline nitrofurantoin: edible black ink; ethylcellulose; gelatin; iron oxide; lactose; paraffin; quinoline yellow (E104); sodium bisulphite; starch; sunset yellow FCF (E110); talc; titanium dioxide (E171).

Tablets: calcium pyrophosphate; lactose; magnesium stearate; starch; sucrose.

Oral suspensions: aluminium magnesium silicate; carmellose sodium; citric acid; glycerol; methyl and propyl hydroxybenzoates; saccharin; sodium citrate; sorbitol.

Bioavailability and absorption

The absorption of nitrofurantoin is influenced by particle size; large (macro) crystals are more slowly absorbed than small (micro) crystals. In fasting patients, the bioavailabilities of the macro and micro forms are increased by 80% and 30%, respectively.

Kinetic data from studies of capsules (Macrodantin, Norwich Eaton) by Mason and Conklin,[9] showed low intra-lot and inter-lot variability in macrocrystalline nitrofurantoin bioavailability but relatively large inter-subject variation in the rate and extent of absorption.

The absorption of nitrofurantoin in six healthy volunteers was significantly enhanced from solid dispersions containing nitrofurantoin with either povidone 25 000, macrogol 6000, or mannitol.[10] These results correlated well with the *in-vitro* dissolution rates at 37° of the test formulations in solution at pH 7.4 and in 0.1M hydrochloric acid pH 1.2. Furadantin tablets were used as the control.

Oral nitrofurantoin therapy has been associated with nausea and vomiting. In a study by Parrott and Matheson,[11] oral administration of nitrofurantoin 400 mg capsules caused gastro-intestinal upset in four out of seven healthy volunteers. Various formulations of suppositories were prepared, each formulation contained 400 mg nitrofurantoin with one or a combination of the following excipients: theobroma oil; lecithin and dried whey (Leciflow); polyoxyethylene 4 sorbitan monostearate (Tween 61); glyceryl monolaurate (Aldo MLD); macrogols 1540, 6000, and 400 with sodium bicarbonate; macrogols 1540, 6000, and 400 with colloidal silica (Cab-O-Sil); and macrogols 1540, 6000, and 400 with polysorbate 80. Only the macrogol-polysorbate 80 and macrogol-silica suppository bases produced an adequate bacteriostatic concentration of nitrofurantoin in the urine. There were no reports of gastric upset associated with oral administration. Rectal absorption was less than oral absorption, hence the requirement for the large dose (400 mg) of nitrofurantoin.

Bioequivalence

A comparison of macrocrystalline nitrofurantoin products (Uvamin Retard, Mepha Ltd, Switzerland; Nitrofurantoin Retard, Ratiopharm GmbH, FRG; Furaben, Laboratorio Abeefe SA, Peru) 100 mg capsules against the innovator product (Macrodantin, Norwich Eaton, USA) in 24 healthy volunteers indicated that the test products all exhibited faster absorption and greater bioavailability than the reference product.[12] Within the first hour of dissolution testing, the test products dissolved more rapidly than Macrodantin.

Bioinequivalence of three nitrofurantoin products commercially available in Mexico was demonstrated[13] in relation to the innovator product (Furadantin) in studies involving 22 healthy volunteers. Widespread inter-lot and intra-lot variation was reflected in the results of disintegration, dissolution, and bioavailability tests.

Processing

The *in-vitro* dissolution of eight tablet formulations (prepared by wet granulation) containing micronised nitrofurantoin 50 mg was correlated by quadrant analysis with *in-vivo* absorption in 14 healthy volunteers.[14] The eight formulations contained equal amounts of wheat starch, lactose, and a glyceryl behenate (Compritol), but various amounts of binder: either Carbopol 934 (0.625 mg and 1.25 mg) or gelatin (0.21 mg and 4.2 mg). Four of the formulations were compressed at a higher force than the others. Results of urinary analyses indicated that the bioavailability of nitrofurantoin was unaffected (over the ranges studied) by either the type and proportion of binder or the compression force. In a further study,[15] the Carbopol 934-containing tablet formulations, freshly made, showed bioequivalence with capsules containing nitrofurantoin 50 mg; however, after storage for one year at 40° and 60% relative humidity, the tablet with the higher Carbopol 934 content exhibited reduced bioavailability when tested in 15 healthy volunteers. The hardness of both tablets decreased while disintegration times increased during the storage period.

Pezoa *et al*[16] found that the dissolution rate of capsule preparations containing microcrystalline nitrofurantoin was decreased by increasing the blending time with the excipients lactose and magnesium stearate, while that of the macrocrystalline preparations remained unaffected. *In-vivo* studies involving six healthy volunteers[17] showed that although the amount of nitrofurantoin excreted in urine was higher with the microcrystalline preparation, it was reduced when the blending time was prolonged beyond attainment of homogeneity with lactose and magnesium stearate.

Suspending agents

An increase in the viscosity of suspensions of nitrofurantoin containing the suspending agents carmellose sodium (Edifas 50), methylcellulose, or xanthan gum was shown to reduce the dissolution rate of nitrofurantoin and to cause a decrease in the amount of drug excreted in the urine of *rats*.[18] Complexation between nitrofurantoin and any of the suspending agents could not be detected.

However, a study by Soci and Parrott[19] demonstrated that the oral bioavailability of nitrofurantoin (200 mg) in eleven healthy volunteers was not affected by the apparent complexation between methylcellulose (Methocel 90) and nitrofurantoin and between carbomer (Carbopol 934) and nitrofurantoin in suspension formulations. Other suspending agents studied were sodium alginate (Kelgin MV), guar gum (Supercol GF), and colloidal aluminium magnesium silicate (Veegum); these showed no such interaction.

Modified-release preparations

Solid dispersions and physical mixtures of nitrofurantoin with macrogol 6000 released nitrofurantoin significantly faster than solid dispersions and physical mixtures with mannitol.[20] An increase in the concentration of the drug in the carrier caused a decrease in the release rate of nitrofurantoin. An optimum concentration of nitrofurantoin 30% in macrogol 6000 was established for tablet formulation. The solid dispersion of nitrofurantoin with macrogol 6000 exhibited better drug releasing properties from tablets than either the physical mixture prepared with macrogol 6000 or a formulation containing microcrystalline cellulose (Avicel PH 101).

Release of nitrofurantoin *in vitro* was delayed from gelatin-peptone microcapsules of larger particle size or microcapsules that had been hardened by exposure to formaldehyde vapour.[21] A later study by the same author demonstrated that release of nitrofurantoin from gelatin microcapsules was more rapid than from microcapsules formulated with ethylcellulose.[22] The dissolution rate of the microcapsules met the USP XX test specifications.

FURTHER INFORMATION. Effect of formulation and process variables on bioequivalency of nitrofurantoin I: preliminary studies—Mendes RW, Masih SZ, Kanumuri RR. J Pharm Sci 1978;67(11):1613–16. Effect of formulation and process variables on bioequivalency of nitrofurantoin II: *in vivo-in vitro* correlation—Mendes RW, Masih SZ, Kanumuri RR. J Pharm Sci 1978;67(11):1616–19. Electrophoretic study of nitrofurantoin in aqueous suspensions. Effect of the addition of a polymeric thickener [Carbopol 934]—Gallardo V, Delgado A, Parera A, Salcedo J. J Pharm Pharmacol 1990;42:225–9. Effect of the preservatives antipyrin [phenazone], benzoic acid and sodium metabisulfite on properties of the nitrofurantoin/solution interface—Gallardo V, Salcedo J, Parera A, Delgado A. Int J Pharmaceutics 1991;71:223–7. Preparation and *in vitro* dissolution tests of egg albumen micro-capsules of nitrofurantoin—Jun HW, Lai JW. Int J Pharmaceutics 1983;16:65–77. Fluid volume effects on tablet properties [and effects of compression force]—Shubair MS, Dingwall D. Mfg Chem 1977 Nov:52–9. *In vitro* and *in vivo* study [in *rats*] of nitrofurantoin with mixed carriers—Madhusudan V, Nasa SL. East Pharm 1988;31:129–30. Nitrofurantoin [microcrystalline and macrocrystalline preparations]—bioavailability and therapeutic equivalence—Cunha BA. Adv Therapy 1988;5:54–63.

REFERENCES

1. Cadwallader DE, Jun HW, Chen L-K [letter]. J Pharm Sci 1975;64(5):886–7.
2. Cadwallader DE, Lee BH, Ansel HC [letter]. J Pharm Sci 1977;66(9):1357–8.
3. Marshall PV, York P. Int J Pharmaceutics 1989;55:257–63.
4. Garti N, Tibika F. Drug Dev Ind Pharm 1980;6(4):379–98.
5. Marshall PV, York P. J Pharm Pharmacol 1987;39:88P.
6. Inotsume N, Nakano M. Int J Pharmaceutics 1981;8:111–19.
7. Gouda HW, Moustafa MA, Al-Shora HI. Int J Pharmaceutics 1984;18:213–15.
8. Juenge EC, Kreienbaum MA, Gurka DF. J Pharm Sci 1985;74(1):100–2.
9. Mason WD, Conklin JD, Hailey FJ. Pharm Res 1987;4(6):499–503.
10. Ali AA, Gorashi AS. Int J Pharmaceutics 1984;19:297–306.
11. Parrott EL, Matheson LE. J Pharm Sci 1977;66(7):955–8.
12. Mason WD, Conklin JD, Hailey FJ. Int J Pharmaceutics 1987;36:105–11.
13. Lopez AA, Molina MM, Jung HC, Dorantes AG, Espejo OO, Garcia CR. Int J Pharmaceutics 1986;28:167–75.
14. Concheiro A, Vila-Jato JL, Martinez-Pacheco R, Seijo B, Ramos T. Drug Dev Ind Pharm 1987;13(3):501–16.
15. Vila-Jato JL, Concheiro A, Seijo B. Drug Dev Ind Pharm 1987;13(8):1315–27.
16. Pezoa R, Morasso MI, Ludwig B, Arancibia A. Drug Dev Ind Pharm 1988;14(4):475–87.

17. Morasso MI, Pezoa R, Villanueva Y, Gai MN, Arancibia A. Il Farmaco 1990;45(1):123–30.
18. Barzegar-Jalali M, Richards JH. Int J Pharm Tech & Prod Mfr 1980;1(3):22–5.
19. Soci MM, Parrott EL. J Pharm Sci 1980;69(4):403–6.
20. Akade MA, Agrawal DK, Lauwo JAK. Pharmazie 1986;41,H12:849–51.
21. Chowdary KPR, Ramana Murthy KV. Indian J Pharm Sci 1985;47:158–9.
22. Chowdary KPR, Murty ASR. Indian J Pharm Sci 1985;47:161–2.

Norethisterone (BAN, pINN)   *Progestogen*

Norethindrone; ethinylnortestosterone; norpregneninolone
17β-Hydroxy-19-nor-17α-pregn-4-en-20-yn-3-one; 19-nor-17α-ethynyl-17β-hydroxy-4-androsten-3-one
$C_{20}H_{26}O_2 = 298.4$

Norethisterone Acetate (BANM, pINNM)
Norethindrone acetate
$C_{22}H_{28}O_3 = 340.5$

Norethisterone Enanthate (BANM)
Norethisterone Enantate (pINNM)
$C_{27}H_{38}O_3 = 410.6$
CAS—68-22-4 (norethisterone); 51-98-9 (norethisterone acetate); 3836-23-5 (norethisterone enanthate)

Pharmacopoeial status

BP (norethisterone, norethisterone acetate); USP (norethindrone, norethindrone acetate)

Preparations

Compendial
Norethisterone Tablets BP. Tablets containing, in each, 350 micrograms or 5 mg norethisterone are usually available.
Norethindrone Tablets USP.
Norethindrone Acetate Tablets USP.

Non-compendial
Menzol (Schwartz). *Tablets,* norethisterone 5 mg.
Micronor (Ortho). *Tablets,* norethisterone 350 micrograms.
Noriday (Syntex). *Tablets,* norethisterone 350 micrograms.
Noristerat (Schering Health Care). *Injection,* norethisterone enanthate 200 mg/mL in an oily solution for intramuscular administration.
Primolut N (Schering Health Care). *Tablets,* norethisterone 5 mg.
Utovlan (Syntex). *Tablets,* norethisterone 5 mg.

Containers and storage

Solid state
Norethisterone BP should be kept in a well-closed container and protected from light.
Norethisterone Acetate BP should be protected from light.

Norethindrone USP and Norethindrone Acetate USP should be preserved in well-closed containers.

Dosage forms
Norethisterone Tablets BP should be protected from light.
Norethindrone Tablets USP and Norethindrone Acetate Tablets USP should be preserved in well-closed containers.
Storage of proprietary norethisterone and norethisterone acetate and enanthate preparations:

Preparation	Manufacturers' recommendations
Menzol tablets	protect from heat, light, and moisture
Micronor tablets	protect from light
Noriday tablets	store in cool, dry place away from direct sunlight
Noristerat injection	store away from strong sunlight
Primolut N tablets	store in cool, dry conditions

PHYSICAL PROPERTIES

Norethisterone is a white or yellowish-white, odourless, crystalline powder.
Norethisterone acetate is a white or creamy-white, odourless, crystalline powder.

Melting point

Norethisterone melts in the range 201° to 208°.
Norethisterone acetate melts at about 163°.

Partition coefficient

In studies of the solution thermodynamics of norethisterone and seven of its derivatives, Lewis and Enever[1] measured and predicted partition coefficients between water and iso-octane; the measured partition coefficient of norethisterone acetate was $10^{2.4}$ at 25°.

Solubility

Norethisterone is practically insoluble in water; slightly soluble in ethanol (1 in 150) and in ether; soluble in chloroform (1 in 30) and in dioxan; freely soluble in pyridine (1 in 5); sparingly soluble in acetone (1 in 80); very slightly soluble in vegetable oils.
Norethisterone acetate is practically insoluble in water; soluble 1 in 12.5 of ethanol and 1 in 18 of ether; very soluble in chloroform (1 in less than 1); freely soluble in dioxan (1 in 2) and in acetone (1 in 4).
An aqueous solubility of norethisterone of 28.2 micromoles/L was determined[2] by equilibration of excess norethisterone for 24 hours at 37°.
Higuchi *et al*[3] reported aqueous solubilities of norethisterone and norethisterone acetate at 25° to be 2.36×10^{-5}M and 1.57×10^{-5}M, respectively. Solubilities in iso-octane were 6.9×10^{-5}M and 2.52×10^{-3}M, respectively, for norethisterone and the acetate.
By use of phase solubility analysis techniques, Lewis and Enever[1] measured and predicted solubilities of norethisterone, norethisterone acetate, and six other norethisterone derivatives in water and in iso-octane; solubilities at 25° correlated with values predicted from group thermodynamic data.

Dissolution

The USP specifies that for Norethindrone Acetate Tablets USP not less than 70% of the labelled amount of $C_{22}H_{28}O_3$ is dissolved in 60 minutes. Dissolution medium: 900 mL of dilute hydrochloric acid (1 in 100) containing 0.02% of sodium lauryl sulphate; Apparatus 1 at 100 rpm.

STABILITY

Photodegradation

When solutions of norethisterone, 0.167×10^{-3}M in aqueous phosphate buffer (pH 7.4) that contained 10% ethanol, were subjected to irradiation by ultraviolet-B light (280 nm to 300 nm) for 40 minutes at ambient temperature, 95% decomposition of norethisterone was observed.[4] Compounds in the solutions were isolated by TLC and identified using spectral data; approximately 25 compounds were detected, some of which may have been formed by the decomposition of the primary degradation products. Some of the major degradation products of norethisterone were 5α,17β-dihydroxy-19-nor-17α-pregn-20-yn-3-one, the corresponding 5β-isomer, norethisterone-4β,5β-epoxide, and the corresponding 4α,5α-epoxide. The authors concluded that photodecomposition of norethisterone in solution occurred by addition of solvent molecules across the 4,5 double bond, by oxidation, and by dimerisation.

When a solution of norethisterone (1.67×10^{-4}M in phosphate-buffered sodium chloride solution pH 7.4, with ethanol 10%) was irradiated with ultraviolet-B light (300 nm) at 37° for 30 minutes, norethisterone-4β,5β-epoxide was found to account for 23% of the degradation products.[5] After storage of the irradiated solutions in the dark for 4 hours at 37°, no further degradation of norethisterone was detected although the amount of epoxide present had increased; it was suggested that other photodegradation products of norethisterone had subsequently decomposed to form norethisterone-4β,5β-epoxide.

Effect of colourants in tablets
Accelerated light stability studies were performed[6] on combined norethisterone 0.5 mg/ethinyloestradiol 0.035 mg tablets that were either pink (containing erythrosine, E127), orange (containing sunset yellow FCF, E110), or white (no colourant). The light applied approximated to the energy spectrum of sunlight. After 30 days, greatest loss of norethisterone (6%) had occurred in the white tablets.

Hydrolysis of norethisterone acetate

During dissolution studies,[7] degradation of the norethisterone acetate component of combined norethisterone acetate/ethinyloestradiol tablets became apparent. The only hydrolysis product detected was norethisterone. In acidic media (0.1M hydrochloric acid with 0.02% sodium lauryl sulphate) 50% and 5% to 6% of the dissolved norethisterone acetate degraded at room temperature and at about 4°, respectively, in 48 hours.

INCOMPATIBILITY/COMPATIBILITY

Adsorption *in vitro* of norethisterone from solution onto magnesium trisilicate in suspension has been observed.[2]

FORMULATION

Excipients

Excipients that have been used in presentations of norethisterone include:
Tablets, norethisterone: acacia; confectioner's sugar; D&C Green No.5; hypromellose; lactose; magnesium stearate; maize starch; microcrystalline cellulose; povidone; propylene glycol; quinoline yellow (E104); sodium starch glycollate; starch; sunset yellow FCF, aluminium lake (E110); talc.
Norethisterone acetate: acacia; confectioner's sugar; D&C Red No.30, aluminium lake; lactose; light liquid paraffin; magne-

sium stearate; maize starch; microcrystalline cellulose; povidone; sunset yellow FCF (E110), aluminium lake; talc.
Injections, norethisterone enanthate: benzyl benzoate; castor oil.

Bioequivalence of two oral contraceptive drugs containing norethindrone and ethinyl estradiol. Saperstein S, Edgren RA, Lee G J-L, Jung D, Fratis A, Kushinsky S, Mroszczak E, Dorr A. Contraception 1989;40:581–90.

REFERENCES

1. Lewis GA, Enever RP. Int J Pharmaceutics 1979;3(6):319–33.
2. Khalil SAH, Iwuagwu M. J Pharm Sci 1978;67(2):287–9.
3. Higuchi T, Shih F-M L, Kimura T, Rytting JH. J Pharm Sci 1979;68(10):1267–72.
4. Sedee AGJ, Beijersbergen van Henegouwen GMJ, de Vries H, Guijt W, Hassnoot CAG. Pharm Weekbl (Sci) 1985;7(5):194–201.
5. Sedee AGJ, Beijersbergen van Henegouwen GMJ, Blaauwgeers HJA. Int J Pharmaceutics 1983;15:149–58.
6. Kaminski EE, Cohn RM, McGuire JL, Carstensen JT. J Pharm Sci 1979;68(3):368–70.
7. Nguyen HT, Shiu GK, Worsley WN, Skelly JP. J Pharm Sci 1990;79(2):163–7.

Nystatin (BAN, USAN, rINN)   *Antifungal*

Fungicidin; nistatina
A substance, or a mixture of two or more substances, produced by the growth of certain strains of *Streptomyces noursei*. It contains mainly tetraenes, the principal component being nystatin A1.
Approximate molecular formula: $C_{47}H_{75}NO_{17} = 926.1$
CAS—1400-61-9

Pharmacopoeial status

BP, USP

Preparations

Compendial
Nystatin Tablets BP. Coated tablets containing, in each, 500 000 units are usually available.
Nystatin Oral Suspension BP (Nystatin Mixture, Nystatin Oral Drops, Nystatin Suspension). A suspension of nystatin in a suitable flavoured vehicle. An oral suspension containing 100 000 units per mL is usually available. It should not be diluted.
Nystatin Ointment BP. A dispersion of nystatin in microfine powder in a suitable basis. An ointment containing 100 000 units per gram is usually available.
Nystatin Pessaries BP. Pessaries containing, in each, 100 000 units are usually available.
Nystatin Tablets USP.
Nystatin Oral Suspension USP.
Nystatin for Oral Suspension USP.
Nystatin Lozenges USP.
Nystatin Cream USP.
Nystatin Lotion USP.
Nystatin Ointment USP.
Nystatin Topical Powder USP.
Nystatin Vaginal Suppositories USP.
Nystatin Vaginal Tablets USP.

Non-compendial

Nystan (Squibb). *Tablets*, nystatin 500 000 units.

Suspension, nystatin 100 000 units/mL. Dilution is not recommended.

Suspension, powder for reconstitution with water, free from lactose, gluten, and sugar, nystatin 100 000 units/mL. Dilution is not recommended.

Pastilles, nystatin 100 000 units.

Cream, nystatin 100 000 units/g. Do not dilute.

Gel, nystatin 100 000 units/g. Do not dilute.

Ointment, nystatin 100 000 units/g in Plastibase (liquid paraffin and polyethylene resin). Do not dilute.

Vaginal cream, nystatin 100 000 units/4-g application. Dilution is not recommended.

Pessaries, nystatin 100 000 units.

Nystatin-Dome (Lagap). *Suspension*, nystatin 100 000 units/mL.

Containers and storage

Solid state

Nystatin BP should be kept in an airtight container, protected from light and stored at a temperature of 2° to 8°.

Nystatin USP should be preserved in tight, light-resistant containers.

Dosage forms

Nystatin Tablets BP and Nystatin Pessaries BP should be stored at a temperature not exceeding 25°.

Nystatin Oral Suspension BP should be protected from light and stored at a temperature not exceeding 15°.

Nystatin Tablets USP, Nystatin Oral Suspension USP, Nystatin Lozenges USP, Nystatin Vaginal Suppositories USP and Nystatin Vaginal Tablets USP should be preserved in tight, light-resistant containers. The vaginal suppositories should be preserved at controlled room temperature. Where so specified in the container label, the vaginal tablets should be stored in a refrigerator. Nystatin for Oral Suspension USP and Nystatin Lotion USP should be preserved in tight containers; the lotion should be kept at controlled room temperature.

Nystatin Cream USP should be preserved in collapsible tubes, or in other tight containers, and exposure to excessive heat should be avoided.

Nystatin Ointment USP and Nystatin Topical Power USP should be preserved in well-closed containers, the ointment preferably at controlled room temperature.

Nystan tablets, powder for suspension, pastilles, ointment, and pessaries should be stored at room temperature.

Nystan suspension, cream, and vaginal cream should be stored at room temperature; avoid freezing.

Nystan gel should be stored in a cool place; avoid freezing.

Reconstituted Nystan suspension is stated to remain suitable for use for 7 days or 10 days at room temperature or under refrigeration, respectively.

PHYSICAL PROPERTIES

Nystatin is a yellow or slightly brown, hygroscopic powder; it has an odour suggestive of cereals.

Melting point

Nystatin gradually decomposes above 160°, without melting by 250°.

pH

A 3% aqueous suspension of *nystatin* has a pH between 6.5 and 8.0.

Dissociation constants

Apparent pK_a values of 5.72 (carboxyl group) and 8.64 (amino group) have been reported.[1]

Solubility

Nystatin is very slightly soluble in water; sparingly to slightly soluble in ethanol; practically insoluble in chloroform, in ether, and in benzene; it is slightly to sparingly soluble in methanol; freely soluble in dimethylformamide and in formamide.

The solubility of nystatin will depend to a considerable extent on its purity and homogeneity, and the rate of solution will depend on its particle size. Michel[1] has comprehensively reviewed the solubility of nystatin in various solvent systems.

STABILITY

In the solid state and in solution or suspension, nystatin is sensitive to elevated temperatures, ultraviolet light, oxygen, extremes of pH, and moisture. The presence of a pH-sensitive ring lactone linkage and the unsaturated nature of nystatin are suggested to contribute to its degradation. Oxidative polymerisation and degradation of the polyene system are the most probable mechanisms.[1,2] However, stability data are often inconsistent; differences in experimental methods (spectrophotometric assays do not correlate with microbiological assays of nystatin),[3,4] variations in the origin and state of nystatin (crystalline and amorphous forms show different stabilities), as well as the possible occurrence of various decomposition reactions, all contribute to inconsistencies. Comprehensive reviews of the literature have been published.[1,2]

In general, solutions and aqueous suspensions or hydroalcoholic suspensions lose antimicrobial activity soon after preparation. Although nystatin is rapidly inactivated at pH ≥ 9 and at pH ≤ 2, it is stable in slightly alkaline conditions. Hamilton-Miller[5] demonstrated that maximum stability at 37° occurred at about pH 7, with an activation energy of 78 kJ/mol. At pH 3 and 4, decomposition of about 90% of nystatin occurred by 3 hours and 6 hours, respectively. Van Doorne and Bosch[3] later showed that solutions of nystatin (7 micrograms/mL) at four pH values at 20° were least stable at pH 5, with little difference between decomposition rates at pH 6, 7, or 8. However, as the initial concentration of the solutions at pH 6 and 7 was increased to 0.1 mg/mL, the degradation rates increased, but to a lesser extent at pH 7. The same workers also established that the solubility and stability of nystatin could be enhanced by γ-cyclodextrin.

Degradation of nystatin can be accelerated by the presence of polyvalent metal ions.

Nystatin was less stable in various suppository bases (theobroma oil; macrogol 1540:macrogol 4000, 60:40; Imhausen E; Imhausen H; Imhausen M:Imhausen H, 1:1) in comparison to the stability of nystatin powder alone.[4] After six months, however, the difference was less marked. Although nystatin powder was less stable at 25° than at 5°, its activity in the bases decreased more slowly at 25° than at 5°.

Trivedi and Shah[6] investigated the stability of nystatin (0.5, 0.75, and 1.0% w/w) in various ointment bases: oleaginous, absorption, water miscible, w/o creams, o/w creams, and hair creams at 37°. Ointments prepared with macrogol bases in the hydrous form with nonionic surfactants demonstrated good stability with a half-life for nystatin of about 60 days.

FURTHER INFORMATION. Evaluation of nystatin stability using tristimulus colorimetry—Fairbrother JE, Heyes WF, Clarke G, Wood PR. J Pharm Sci 1980;69:697–700. Determination of the stability of nystatin and natamycin by UV-spectrophotometry—Ruzickova J, Parrak V [German]. Arch Pharm (Weinheim) 1982;315:614–19.

FORMULATION

Excipients

Excipients that have been used in presentations of nystatin include:

Tablets: acacia; calcium carbonate; carnauba wax; castor oil; cellulose; chalk; erythrosine (E127); ethylcellulose; gelatin; indigo carmine (E132); iron oxide; lactose; maize starch; magnesium stearate; methylcellulose; povidone; semi-synthetic glycerides; shellac; stearic acid; sucrose; talc; titanium dioxide (E171); vanillin; white beeswax.

Oral suspensions: benzoic acid; carmellose sodium; cellulose (purified); disodium calcium edetate; ethanol; glycerol; hydrochloric acid; magnesium aluminium silicate; methyl and propyl hydroxybenzoates; polysorbate 80; povidone; saccharin; saccharin sodium; silica; sodium benzoate; sodium hydroxide; sodium phosphate; sucrose; wood cellulose.

Pastilles: anise oil; antifoam emulsion; cinnamon oil; gelatin; glucose monohydrate; hydrochloric acid; liquid glucose; potassium hydroxide; silicone; sucrose.

Creams: aluminium hydroxide (compressed or wet gel); antifoam emulsion; benzyl alcohol; cetostearyl alcohol; emulsifying wax; glycerol; glyceryl monostearate; hydrochloric acid; isopropyl myristate; lactic acid; macrogol ether; macrogol monostearate 400; methyl and propyl hydroxybenzoates; polyoxyl 40 stearate; polysorbate 60; propylene glycol; simethicone; sodium hydroxide; sorbic acid; sorbitol solution; titanium dioxide (E171); white soft paraffin.

Ointments: liquid paraffin; polyethylene resin.

Gels: Carbopol; chlorocresol; potassium phosphates; sodium hydroxide.

Topical powders: talc.

Pessaries: ethylcellulose; lactose; magnesium stearate; maize starch; microcrystalline cellulose; modified cellulose gum; povidone; sorbitol; stearic acid.

Eye drops: chlorhexidine acetate; sodium chloride.

Nebuliser solutions: ethanol.

Novel dosage forms

The preparation and use of frozen lollipops of nystatin as a means of disguising the unpleasant taste of nystatin and improving patient compliance have been reported.[7–9] Formulations consisted of, for example, a cherry-flavoured nystatin suspension mixed with sorbitol solution, banana flavouring, and distilled water; a small tongue depressor served as a stick.

Release of nystatin *in vitro* from chewing gum preparations was investigated[10] using a device that simulated mastication with phosphate buffer, pH 7.4, at 37° ± 1°. Inclusion of solubilising agents, at a nystatin:solubiliser ratio of 1:1, produced a 50-fold to 70-fold increase in release; during the first 10 minutes, release of 98% to 99% of the total amount of released nystatin occurred. The solubilisers were nonionic surfactants (polyoxyethylene glycol trihydroxy stearate 40, Cremophor RH 40; polysorbate 60, Tween 60) and an anionic surfactant (monoglyceride diacetyl tartrate, Panodan AB 90). These surfactants produced only a 3-fold to 7-fold increase in the solubility of nystatin at pH 7.4 at 22° ± 1°.

FURTHER INFORMATION. Pharmaceutical investigation of a bioerodible nystatin system [monolithic system with pectin]—Krusteva V, Lambov N, Velinov G [German]. Pharmazie

1990;45(H3):195–7. Antimycotic buccal and vaginal tablets [of nystatin] with chitosan [stability]—Knapczyk J. Int J Pharmaceutics 1992;88:9–14.

REFERENCES

1. Michel GW. In: Florey K, editor. Analytical profiles of drug substances; vol 6. London: Academic Press, 1977:341–421.
2. Youngberg C. In: Connors KA, Amidon GL, Stella VJ, editors. Chemical stability of pharmaceuticals. A handbook for pharmacists. 2nd ed. New York: John Wiley & Sons, 1986:631–6.
3. van Doorne H, Bosch EH. Int J Pharmaceutics 1991;73:43–9.
4. Elkouly AE, Elsayed NA, Motawi AM. Mfg Chem 1973;44(8):37–8.
5. Hamilton-Miller JMT. J Pharm Pharmacol 1973;25:401–7.
6. Trivedi BM, Shah NB. Indian J Pharm 1970;32(6):156–8.
7. Dobbins JC. Hosp Pharm 1983;18(9):452–3.
8. Br J Pharm Pract 1984;6(2):70.
9. Allen LV, Tu Y-H. US Pharm 1990;15(Feb):64–6.
10. Andersen T, Gram-Hansen M, Pedersen M, Rassing MR. Drug Dev Ind Pharm 1990;16(13):1985–94.

Orphenadrine (BAN, rINN)   *Antimuscarinic*

Mephenamine

NN-Dimethyl-2-(2-methylbenzhydryloxy)ethylamine;   *NN*-dimethyl-2-[(2-methylphenyl)phenylmethoxy]ethanamine

$C_{18}H_{23}NO = 269.4$

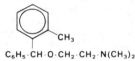

$C_6H_5 \cdot CH \cdot O \cdot CH_2 \cdot CH_2 \cdot N(CH_3)_2$

Orphenadrine Citrate (BANM, rINNM)

$C_{18}H_{23}NO, C_6H_8O_7 = 461.5$

Orphenadrine Hydrochloride (BANM, rINNM)

$C_{18}H_{23}NO, HCl = 305.8$

CAS—83-98-7 (orphenadrine); 4682-36-4 (orphenadrine citrate); 341-69-5 (orphenadrine hydrochloride)

Pharmacopoeial status

BP (orphenadrine citrate, orphenadrine hydrochloride); USP (orphenadrine citrate)

Preparations

Compendial

Orphenadrine Hydrochloride Tablets BP. Tablets containing, in each, 50 mg are usually available.

Orphenadrine Citrate Injection USP. pH between 5.0 and 6.0.

Non-compendial

Biorphen (Bioglan). *Elixir*, sugar free, orphenadrine hydrochloride 25 mg/5 mL.

Disipal (Brocades). *Tablets*, orphenadrine hydrochloride 50 mg.

Norflex (3M). *Injection*, orphenadrine citrate 30 mg/mL.

Containers and storage

Solid state

Orphenadrine Citrate BP and Orphenadrine Hydrochloride BP should be kept in well-closed containers and protected from light.

Orphenadrine Citrate USP should be preserved in tight, light-resistant containers.

Dosage forms

Orphenadrine Citrate Injection USP should be preserved in single-dose or in multiple-dose containers, preferably of Type I glass, protected from light.

Biorphen elixir should be stored at room temperature, protected from light.

Norflex injection should be stored in a cool, dry place.

PHYSICAL PROPERTIES

Orphenadrine is a liquid.

Orphenadrine citrate is a white or almost white, odourless or almost odourless, crystalline powder with a taste which is bitter and followed by a sensation of numbness.

Orphenadrine hydrochloride is a white or almost white, odourless or almost odourless, crystalline powder with a taste which is bitter and followed by a sensation of numbness.

Melting point

Orphenadrine citrate melts in the range 134° to 138°.
Orphenadrine hydrochloride melts in the range 159° to 162°.

pH

An aqueous solution of *orphenadrine hydrochloride* has a pH of about 5.5.

Dissociation constant

pK_a 8.4

Partition coefficient

Log *P* (heptane), 1.5

Solubility

Orphenadrine citrate is sparingly soluble in water; slightly soluble in ethanol; insoluble or practically insoluble in chloroform, in ether, and in benzene.

Orphenadrine hydrochloride is soluble 1 in 1 of water, 1 in 1 of ethanol, and 1 in 2 of chloroform; practically insoluble in ether.

STABILITY

In solution and oral liquids

Selkirk *et al*[1] reported that degradation of orphenadrine hydrochloride in 1% m/v aqueous solutions in the pH range 2 to 7 at 70° appeared to follow first-order kinetics; maximum stability was apparent at about pH 5. In an investigation (ion-pair, reversed-phase HPLC) of orphenadrine hydrochloride stability in a syrup formulation, *o*-methylbenzhydrol was found to be the major degradation product. In samples stored in amber glass bottles with unlined, polypropylene screw-caps, the extent of degradation after 99 days was 0.06% at 25° and 1.05% at 50°. The formulation (pH 5) contained orphenadrine hydrochloride (1 g), distilled water (10 mL), benzoic acid solution (2 mL), citric acid monohydrate (0.288 g), sodium citrate (1.068 g) and syrup, preservative-free (to 100 mL).

Walls *et al*[2] reported that the therapeutic efficacy of orphenadrine in an extemporaneously prepared suspension was decreased owing to instability during storage of the preparation for up to six weeks by a patient with Parkinson's disease. It was stated that orphenadrine could be suspended in an aqueous vehicle but would remain stable for only 14 days at a pH below 5.

FORMULATION

Excipients

Excipients that have been used in presentations of orphenadrine include:

Tablets, orphenadrine citrate: calcium stearate; ethylcellulose; lactose.

Orphenadrine hydrochloride: acacia; acetylated monoglycerides; amaranth (E123); brilliant blue FCF (133); colloidal anhydrous silica; ethylcellulose; hydroxypropylcellulose; hypromellose; indigo carmine (E132); kaolin; lactose; magnesium stearate; microcrystalline cellulose; quinoline yellow (E104); starch; stearic acid; sucrose; sunset yellow FCF (E110); talc; tartrazine (E102); titanium dioxide (E171).

Injections, orphenadrine citrate: sodium bisulphite; sodium chloride; sodium hydroxide.

Oral syrup

Bryant *et al*[3] described an analytical method (second derivative ultraviolet spectrophotometry) for the determination of orphenadrine hydrochloride in a hospital-formulated oral syrup of orphenadrine hydrochloride that contained chloroform emulsion BPC 1963, purified water BP, and raspberry syrup BPC. (See also Stability, above).

REFERENCES

1. Selkirk SM, Miller JHM, Smith G, Fell AF. J Pharm Pharmacol 1983;35:23P.
2. Walls TJ, Dick DJ, Fletcher J. Br Med J 1985;290:444–5.
3. Bryant SL, Neel AR, Sewell GJ. J Clin Hosp Pharm 1986;11:327–34.

Paracetamol (BAN, rINN)   *Analgesic; Antipyretic*

Acetaminophen; *N*-acetyl-*p*-aminophenol
4′-Hydroxyacetanilide; *N*-(4-hydroxyphenyl)acetamide
$C_8H_9NO_2 = 151.2$
CAS—103-90-2

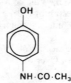

Pharmacopoeial status

BP (paracetamol); USP (acetaminophen)

Preparations

Co-codamol is the British Approved Name for compounded preparations of codeine phosphate and paracetamol in proportions expressed in the form x/y, where x and y are the strengths in milligrams of codeine phosphate and paracetamol, respectively.

Co-dydramol is the British Approved Name for compounded preparations of dihydrocodeine tartrate and paracetamol in the proportions, by weight, 1 part to 50 parts, respectively.

Co-proxamol is the British Approved Name for compounded preparations of dextropropoxyphene hydrochloride and paracetamol in the proportions, by weight, 1 part to 10 parts, respectively.

Paracetamol Tablets BP. Tablets containing, in each, 500 mg are usually available.

Paediatric Paracetamol Oral Solution BP (Paediatric Paracetamol Elixir). A solution containing 2.4% w/v of paracetamol in a suitable flavoured vehicle. The solution should not be diluted.

Paracetamol Oral Suspension BP. Oral suspensions containing, in each, 2.4% w/v and 5.0% w/v are usually available.

Co-codamol Tablets BP. Tablets containing codeine phosphate and paracetamol in the proportions, by weight, 2 parts to 125 parts.

Co-dydramol Tablets BP. Tablets containing dihydrocodeine tartrate and paracetamol in the proportions, by weight, 1 part to 50 parts.

Co-proxamol Tablets BP. Tablets containing dextropropoxyphene hydrochloride and paracetamol in the proportions, by weight, 1 part to 10 parts.

Acetaminophen Capsules USP.
Acetaminophen Tablets USP.
Acetaminophen Oral Solution USP.
Acetaminophen for Effervescent Oral Solution USP.
Acetaminophen Oral Suspension USP.
Acetaminophen Suppositories USP.

Non-compendial

Alvedon (Novex). *Suppositories*, paracetamol 125 mg.
Calpol (Wellcome). *Infant suspension*, paracetamol 120 mg/5 mL. *Diluent*: syrup.
Sugar-free Infant suspension, sugar free, paracetamol 120 mg/5 mL. *Diluents*: Sorbitol Solution BPC (non-crystallising) or glycerol. All dilutions should be freshly prepared and used within 28 days.
Six Plus suspension, paracetamol 250 mg/5 mL.
Disprol (R&C). *Paediatric suspension*, sugar free, paracetamol 120 mg/5 mL. *Diluent*: water, boiled and cooled.
Paracetamol tablets are available from APS, Cox, Evans, Kerfoot, Sterling Health (Panadol).
Soluble paracetamol tablets are available from Sanofi Winthrop (Panadol Soluble) and paediatric soluble tablets from R&C (Disprol Junior).
Paediatric paracetamol oral solutions are available from Berk, Evans, RP Drugs (Paldesic), Wallace Mfg (Salzone).
Oral suspensions of paracetamol 120 mg/5 mL are also available from Cupal (Cupanol Under 6 sugar free), Sterling Health (Panadol sugar free).
An oral suspension of paracetamol 250 mg/5 mL is also available from Cupal (Cupanol Over 6).

Compound preparations

Co-codamol tablets are available from APS, Cox, Evans, Galen (Parake), Kerfoot, Norton, Sterling Health (Panadeine). Dispersible or effervescent co-codamol tablets are available from Fisons (Paracodol), Sterwin, and co-codamol capsules from Fisons (Paracodol).
Co-dydramol tablets are available from APS, Cox, Evans, Galen (Galake), Kerfoot, Napp, Norton, Sterwin.
Co-proxamol tablets are available from APS, Cox (Cosalgesic), Dista (Distalgesic), Evans, Kerfoot, Sterwin.

Containers and storage

Solid state

Paracetamol BP should be kept in a well-closed container and protected from light.
Acetaminophen USP should be preserved in tight, light-resistant containers.

Dosage forms

Paracetamol Tablets BP, Paediatric Paracetamol Oral Solution BP, and Paracetamol Oral Suspension BP should all be protected from light.
Acetaminophen Capsules USP, Acetaminophen Tablets USP, Acetaminophen Oral Solution USP, Acetaminophen for Effervescent Oral Solution USP, and Acetaminophen Oral Suspension USP should all be preserved in tight containers.
Acetaminophen Suppositories USP should be preserved in well-closed containers, in a cool place.
Alvedon suppositories should be stored below 25°.
Disprol Paediatric suspension and Calpol preparations should be stored below 25° and protected from light. Disprol Paediatric suspension should not be frozen.

PHYSICAL PROPERTIES

Paracetamol is a white crystalline powder; odourless, with a slightly bitter taste.

Melting point

Paracetamol melts within the range 168° to 172°.

pH

A saturated solution of *paracetamol* has a pH between 5.3 and 6.5.

Dissociation constant

pK_a 9.5 (25°)

Solubility

Paracetamol is soluble 1 in 70 of cold water, 1 in 20 of boiling water, 1 in 7 of ethanol, 1 in 13 of acetone, 1 in 40 of glycerol, and 1 in 9 of propylene glycol. Paracetamol is also soluble in methanol, in dimethylformamide, in ethylene dichloride, in ethyl acetate, and in solutions of alkali hydroxides; very slightly soluble in ether and in chloroform.

Effect of cosolvents

Hamza and Paruta[1] examined the enhancing effect of two cosolvents (glycerol and propylene glycol) on paracetamol solubility, of various surfactants (Tween 20, Tween 80, Myrj 53 and 59, Brij 58 and 700), and of mixtures of Tween 20 with the two cosolvents. Paracetamol (at saturation concentration) decreased the dielectric constant of water (from 78.5 to 70.1) and changed the dielectric constants of the surfactant-water and cosolvent-water blends. With the exception of Brij 58, increasing concentration of surfactant increased paracetamol solubility to different degrees. Solubility values in propylene glycol and glycerol, with or without surfactant, were greater than those achieved in the surfactants alone. It was suggested that these cosolvents may suppress micelle formation. There was physical evidence of an apparent increase in the stability of paracetamol in the various systems.

At 20° and 37°, the solubility of paracetamol decreased with an increase in concentration of glucose, sucrose, or sorbitol (10% w/v to 70% w/v solutions); sorbitol exhibited the greatest effect followed by glucose then sucrose, with respect to the decrease in paracetamol solubility.[2] Thermodynamic parameters indicated differences in the mechanisms of solubility of paracetamol in the different sugar solutions, although it was suggested that hydrophobic interactions may have caused the reduction in solubility in each sugar solution.

Enhancement of solubility

In a preliminary study[3] of the enhancement of solubility of paracetamol, the hydrotropic agents sodium glycinate, sodium gentisate, sodium salicylate, and nicotinamide were all found to increase its aqueous solubility, in particular, sodium salicylate and nicotinamide. It was concluded that such effects involved only 'hydrotropy' and not an identifiable chemical interaction or complexation.

The antihistamines brompheniramine maleate, chlorpheniramine maleate, and pheniramine maleate solubilised paracetamol;[4] the aqueous solubility of paracetamol (initially 0.11M at 30°) increased about five-fold as the concentration of the antihistamine was increased from zero up to 0.8M.

Dissolution

The USP specifies that for Acetaminophen Tablets USP not less than 80% of the labelled amount of $C_8H_9NO_2$ is dissolved in 30 minutes. Dissolution medium: 900 mL of phosphate buffer pH 5.8; Apparatus 2 at 50 rpm.

The USP specifies that for Acetaminophen Capsules USP not less than 75% of the labelled amount of $C_8H_9NO_2$ is dissolved in 45 minutes. Dissolution medium: 900 mL of water; Apparatus 2 at 50 rpm.

Effect of additives

In a 2^3 factorial study,[5] the intrinsic dissolution rate of paracetamol (in McIlvaine's buffer, pH 6.8, at 37°) was reduced by the presence of glycine, taurine, or sorbitol (singly or in combination); this was attributed to an increase in the viscosity of the dissolution medium.

FURTHER INFORMATION. Irregular solution behaviour of paracetamol in binary solvents [ethyl acetate/methanol and water/normal alcohols; extended Hildebrand solubility approach]—Subrahmanyam CVS, Reddy MS, Rao JV, Rao PG. Int J Pharmaceutics 1992;78:17–24. Effects of granule size, compression force and lubricants on the dissolution time of paracetamol tablets—Muti HY, Papaioannou G, Choulis NH. Pharmazie 1985;40:552–3. Correlation between dissolution and disintegration rate constants for acetaminophen tablets—Najib N, Jalal I. Int J Pharmaceutics 1988;44:43–7.

STABILITY

Solutions

The degradation kinetics of paracetamol in aqueous solutions at various pH and temperature values were studied by Koshy and Lach.[6] The hydrolysis of paracetamol was both acid-catalysed and base-catalysed and was first-order with respect to paracetamol, hydrogen ion, and hydroxide ion concentration. The degradation rate was directly dependent on paracetamol concentration and was not related to ionic strength. Within the pH range 2 to 9, the activation energy for paracetamol degradation was about 73.22 kJ/mol. Hydrolysis was at a minimum at pH 5 to 7; at 25° the half-lives of paracetamol at pH 2, 5, 6, and 9 were 0.73, 19.8, 21.8, and 2.28 years, respectively.

Effects of light, heat, and oxygen

In solution, paracetamol requires protection from light. In the dry state pure paracetamol is stable at temperatures up to 45°. If the hydrolysis product of paracetamol, *p*-aminophenol, is present as a contaminant or as a result of exposure to humid conditions the *p*-aminophenol may degrade by oxidation to quinonimine and coloured products of pink, brown, and black. Paracetamol is relatively stable to oxidation.

Hygroscopicity

Paracetamol absorbs insignificant amounts of moisture at 25° at relative humidities up to about 90%.

Tablets

Sarisuta and Parrott[7] investigated the changes in hardness, disintegration, and dissolution of paracetamol tablets (prepared with povidone and pregelatinised starch) during storage for eight weeks at 40° and 52% relative humidity and at 40° and 94% relative humidity. The tablets that were wet-granulated with pregelatinised starch were less affected by high humidity than those made with povidone.

Aspirin-Paracetamol interaction

Koshy et al[8] investigated the interaction between aspirin and paracetamol in solid dosage forms. Reaction products were identified as diacetyl-*p*-aminophenol and salicylic acid; both were found in commercial products from retail outlets. Magnesium stearate increased the rate of formation of diacetyl-*p*-aminophenol in moistened mixtures of the two powders.

However, many of the findings of the above study were disputed by Kalatzis[9] who suggested that diacetyl-*p*-aminophenol is unstable, especially under accelerated storage conditions. The importance of minimising the moisture content of products containing paracetamol was emphasised.

INCOMPATIBILITY/COMPATIBILITY

Hydrogen bonding has been reported to be the mechanism whereby paracetamol is linked to the surfaces of nylon and rayon.

FURTHER INFORMATION. Adsorption of paracetamol and chloroquine phosphate by some antacids—Iwuagwu MA, Aloko KS. J Pharm Pharmacol 1992;44:655–8.

FORMULATION

PAEDIATRIC PARACETAMOL ELIXIR

The following formula was given in the *British Pharmacopoeia 1980*:

Paracetamol	24 g
Amaranth solution	2 mL
Chloroform spirit	20 mL
Concentrated raspberry juice	25 mL
Ethanol (96%)	100 mL
Propylene glycol	100 mL
Invert syrup	275 mL
Glycerol	to 1000 mL

Dissolve the paracetamol in a mixture of the ethanol, the propylene glycol, and the chloroform spirit; dilute the concentrated raspberry juice with the invert syrup and add this to the solution of paracetamol, add the amaranth solution, and sufficient glycerol to produce 1000 mL, and mix. This elixir should not be diluted and it should be protected from light.

Excipients

Excipients that have been used in presentations of paracetamol include:

Capsules: brilliant blue FCF (133); calcium stearate; carmellose sodium; cellulose; colloidal silica; croscarmellose sodium; D&C Red No.7; docusate sodium; erythrosine (E127); ethylcellulose; hypromellose; indigo carmine (E132); macrogol; magnesium stearate; maize starch; methylcellulose; microcrystalline cellulose; povidone; propylene glycol; sodium benzoate; sodium bisulphite; sodium lauryl sulphate; sodium metabisulphite; sodium starch glycollate; starch; stearic acid; talc; titanium dioxide (E171); yellow iron oxide.

Tablets: alginic acid; brilliant blue FCF (133); calcium carbonate, light; calcium stearate; carmellose sodium; cellulose, microfine and granulated; colloidal silica; croscarmellose sodium; docusate sodium; erythrosine (E127); hypromellose; lactose; macrogol 8000; magnesium stearate; magnesium trisilicate; mannitol; microcrystalline cellulose; povidone; pregelatinised starch; propylene glycol; sodium benzoate; sodium lauryl sulphate; sodium starch glycollate; starch (maize, potato); stearic acid; talc; titanium dioxide (E171).

Effervescent tablets: citric acid; docusate sodium; fumaric acid; glucose; L-leucine; mannitol; povidone; saccharin sodium; sodium benzoate; sodium bicarbonate; sodium carbonate; sorbitol.

Chewable tablets: activated dimethicone; allura red AC (E129); aspartame; cetyl alcohol; citric acid; colloidal silica; dibutyl sebacate; ethylcellulose; hydrogenated vegetable oil; hypromellose; magnesium stearate; mannitol; microcrystalline cellulose; starch; sucrose.

Oral solutions: acid fuchsine D; allura red AC (E129); amaranth (E123); benzoic acid; chloroform spirit; citric acid; disodium edetate; ethanol; glycerol; invert syrup; macrogol; methyl and propyl hydroxybenzoates; potassium sorbate; propylene glycol; raspberry juice, concentrated; saccharin sodium; sodium benzoate; sodium chloride; sodium hydroxide; sorbic acid; sorbitol; sucrose; trisodium citrate.

Oral suspensions: methyl and propyl hydroxybenzoates.

Suppositories: semi-synthetic glycerides.

Bioavailability

The pharmacokinetics of paracetamol were dose-dependent during a single-dose bioavailability study[10] in which 15 healthy volunteers received paracetamol 325 mg tablets (Tylenol, McNeil, USA) and 500 mg tablets (Tylenol Extra-Strength, McNeil, USA) in various combinations to achieve doses of 325, 500, 1000, 1500, or 2000 mg.

By use of an *in-vitro* dissolution-dialysis technique[11] (in 0.1M hydrochloric acid and in phosphate buffer pH 7.4), Razden and Verma established correlation between the dialysis rate constant and areas under salivary concentration versus time curves (AUC) of five commercial paracetamol tablets.[12] The single-dose bioavailability study of Latin square design involved six healthy volunteers. No similar correlations could be demonstrated between AUC values and disintegration times or dissolution rates of the tablets.

The absolute bioavailabilities of a paracetamol elixir and paracetamol tablets were determined in healthy volunteers by Ameer *et al*.[13] Drug absorption was rapid and there was no significant difference between the two preparations in the apparent half-life of absorption or lag time before the start of absorption. Although peak plasma concentrations were similar, the time to reach peak concentration was significantly shorter for the elixir (0.48 hours) than for the tablet (0.75 hours). The absolute availability of the elixir was significantly greater than that of the tablets (87% and 79%, respectively). Elimination half-lives were similar. A study of the comparative bioavailability of two commercially available brands of paracetamol tablets indicated therapeutic equivalence.

Three commercially available brands of paracetamol tablets and a reference oral solution were evaluated *in vitro* and *in vivo*.[14] Tablets were tested for weight variation, hardness, uniformity of thickness, friability, disintegration time, and dissolution behaviour; significant differences between brands were apparent. Relative bioavailabilities (in four volunteers) were 82%, 87%, and 92% compared to the reference. Statistical evaluation of the results indicated that absorption may be controlled by the rate of dissolution of the tablets.

In a comparison of three liquid/semi-liquid dosage forms in healthy volunteers, the bioavailability of paracetamol from a novel alcohol-free syrup was greater than that from an elixir, which in turn was greater than from a suspension.[15] The three formulations appeared to be equivalent in terms of their distribution and elimination profiles.

Intramuscular administration of 300 mg or 600 mg paracetamol (150 mg/mL, Apotel) was reported by Greek workers[16] to produce similar plasma concentrations but lower rates of absorption of paracetamol compared to those produced following oral administration of paracetamol at equivalent doses. In six healthy subjects, absorption rates varied with the site of injection (fat or muscle) and the volume of solution.

Relative bioavailabilities of paracetamol were considered to be equivalent from two solid dosage forms and two liquid dosage forms (each with 500 mg paracetamol) that were administered orally to twelve healthy subjects.[17] Similarly, bioequivalence between two rectal preparations was established, but there were differences between rectal and oral pharmacokinetic parameters.

Tablets

In an investigation of the capping tendencies of three paracetamol tablet formulations, Krycer *et al*[18] were unable to make predictions based solely on residual die wall pressure values. Results indicated that the extent of elastic deformation, plastic flow, and bonding determined the strength and capping tendency of tablets.

From analyses of the ratios of friability to tensile strength and of elastic to plastic properties in tablets prepared from mixtures of paracetamol and microcrystalline cellulose (Avicel), Yu *et al*[19] determined that a 50% w/w mixture of each produced the most pharmaceutically acceptable tablets.

In factorially designed experiments using a three-way analysis of variance,[20] paracetamol 500 mg tablets containing either povidone, gelatin, or tapioca starch as binder were evaluated. Binding effects of povidone and gelatin were similar and either was considered suitable for use in tablet formulations of paracetamol. Tapioca starch showed weaker binding properties, with higher concentrations being required to produce tablets of acceptable mechanical strength. An extension of the previous study involved measurement of the wettability of paracetamol tablets (prepared with the same three binders) and determination of any correlation between disintegration/dissolution properties and the adhesion tension of water on tablets.[21] A correlation was found to exist and it was concluded that the nature and quantity of binder affects the wettability of the tablet surfaces and hence their adhesion tension.

Tablets were prepared that contained paracetamol directly compressible granules with magnesium stearate as a lubricant; several commercial grades and a high-purity grade of magnesium stearate were investigated[22] for their lubricating properties. Compared to unlubricated tablets, release of paracetamol (in 0.1M hydrochloric acid at 37°) was slightly reduced from tablets with high-purity magnesium stearate but was appreciably reduced from those prepared with commercial grades of magnesium stearate.

Increased aqueous solubility was demonstrated by powders of paracetamol in the form of either physical mixtures or solid dispersions with β-cyclodextrin (1:1 w/w) compared to that of paracetamol itself.[23] Similarly, increased dissolution rates were demonstrated by tablets prepared from these powders compared to those that contained paracetamol with no cyclodextrin; tablets also contained Avicel PH101 (microcrystalline cellulose), Aerosol 200 (colloidal silica), Ac-Di-Sol (cross-linked carmellose sodium), and magnesium stearate.

Modified-release preparations

El-Said et al[24] prepared gelatin microspheres that contained paracetamol and were hardened with formaldehyde (10%, 20%, or 30% v/v) in isopropanol. In vitro, smaller microspheres (355 to 710 micrometres) released the drug at a faster rate than larger ones and variation in formaldehyde concentration resulted in different rates of release. Two phases of drug release were apparent; an initial rapid 'burst', followed by a period of sustained release. In an in-vivo study involving five healthy volunteers, paracetamol encapsulated in microspheres (prepared using formaldehyde 30% in isopropanol) had lower bioavailability than the free powder, when taken in capsules.

The use of powdered lipids (castor wax and Durkee 07) as granulating agents and as retardants in the formulation of sustained-release paracetamol tablets was examined by Kopcha and Lordi.[25] Lipids were incorporated as free-flowing powder prepared by spray drying an emulsion. Tablets made with Durkee 07 were more plastic and capped less often than those made with castor wax.

Phuapradit and Bolton[26] prepared low density bilayer compressed matrix (LDM) tablets, in which the upper layer contained excipients thought to yield carbon dioxide in an acidic environment and create a 'buoyant' dosage form, and similar high density matrix (HDM) tablets, which did not generate carbon dioxide. Both LDM and HDM tablets exhibited similar dissolution profiles in vitro (100% release in 12 hours in 0.1M hydrochloric acid at 37°). In six healthy volunteers under fasted conditions, the test tablets exhibited slower absorption compared to commercial paracetamol tablets (Tylenol), which demonstrated 95% release in 15 minutes in 0.1M hydrochloric acid at 37°. However, the relative bioavailability of the LDM tablets was not significantly different from that of Tylenol tablets but was significantly greater than that of the HDM tablets.

Suppositories

Displacement values for paracetamol in the following bases have been reported:

Macrogol 300:4000 (20:80% w/w) = 1.25
Massuppol = 1.54
Fatty basis = 1.5
Witepsol = 1.4

On investigation of the in-vitro release of paracetamol from different suppository bases, Abd Elbary et al[27] found that release from anhydrous and hydrous macrogols was greater than from hard fat bases. Drug release from the hard fat bases appeared to depend on the melting range and chemical composition of the basis and decreased in the order: Witepsol H15 > Witepsol H12 > theobroma oil > Witepsol E75 > Dehydag G 37/39. The addition of various nonionic surfactants to either Witepsol H15 or Witepsol H12 caused both increases and decreases in paracetamol release, depending on the chemical structure and HLB value of the surfactant; Myrj 52 and 53, Tween 61 and 65, Brij 35 and 53 all increased the amount released, whereas Span 60 decreased the amount released. The rate of paracetamol release from Witepsol H15 was reduced by incorporation of Aerosil (both hydrophilic and hydrophobic grades). Suggested formulae for maximal release were based on either Witepsol H15 or H12 with either Myrj 53 or Tween 61 in the ratio 85:5 (basis:surfactant).

Shangraw and Walkling[28] measured the rectal absorption of paracetamol in ten male adults from an aqueous suspension (buffered at pH 6, prepared in a 4% microcrystalline cellulose-carmellose gel), from a suspension in propylene glycol, and from a theobroma oil-based suppository. Four to six hours after administration, urinary excretion of paracetamol was significantly greater from an oral control solution and from the aqueous and theobroma oil vehicles than from the propylene glycol suspension. It was indicated that if the vehicle had a dielectric constant corresponding to high solubility of paracetamol, rectal absorption tended to be poor; in contrast, if the dielectric constant of the vehicle was too high or too low for good paracetamol solubility, then rectal absorption was relatively high.

Pagay et al[29] determined the paracetamol bioavailability of rectally administered dosage forms with macrogol bases of varying dielectric properties, and an aqueous solution, in six male subjects. The extent of rectal absorption of paracetamol was apparently related to its solubility-dielectric profile. As the dielectric values of the bases increased up to a value of 13.6, bioavailability was reduced; above this value, bioavailability appeared to increase but the relationship was less well defined.

The addition of insoluble povidone (Polyplasdone XL 1%, 5%, or 10%) to four formulations of paracetamol suppositories (based on blends of macrogols) increased the extent and rate of dissolution in three of the four formulations.[30] The increase was not linear with respect to povidone concentration.

Kahela et al[31] examined differences in the rate and extent of rectal absorption between paracetamol suppositories (in a fatty or a hydrous basis) that had either been freshly prepared or stored for four years. In a study involving ten volunteers, absorption was faster from freshly prepared suppositories with the fatty basis (Novata E, which consisted of a mixture of monoglycerides, diglycerides, and triglycerides of C_{12} to C_{18} fatty acids and 0.8% polysorbate) than from both sets of suppositories formulated with the water-soluble basis (mixture of carbowaxes 4000 and 6000 and glycerol in a ratio 8:1:1). After four years storage at room temperature, absorption from the water-soluble suppositories was virtually unaffected, but bioavailability of paracetamol from the fatty suppositories was lower than from the freshly prepared fatty suppositories. The rate of absorption of an oral solution used as a reference was significantly higher than that of all except the freshly made fatty basis suppositories.

From four bases evaluated for a paediatric suppository formulation, rapid paracetamol release was observed in vitro from glyco-gelatin and macrogol bases (100% release in 10 minutes and 35 minutes, respectively). After two hours, suppositories formulated using Massuppol or polysorbate bases had released only about 15% and 2% of their paracetamol content, respectively. Relative bioavailabilities (in four volunteers) ranged from 92.2% for the macrogol basis to 6.5% for the polysorbates. The macrogol basis (grades 400 and 4000 in 20:80 ratio) was recommended for paediatric paracetamol suppositories.[32]

Novel dosage forms

Torrado-Duran et al[33] developed micro-aggregated egg albumen particles, which contained paracetamol, by a micro-encapsulation method. The particles masked the bitter taste and improved the flow properties of paracetamol powder. Chewable and non-chewable tablets, prepared with the micro-encapsulated paracetamol (250 mg), had a bioavailability (calculated from urinary excretion data) of 99.5% and 92.5%, respectively, relative to a standard paracetamol tablet (Panadol, Sterling Winthrop) following a single-dose, randomised, crossover study with six healthy subjects. Comparison of in-vitro and in-vivo release data indicated that enzymes in vivo may enhance the dissolution rate of the micro-encapsulated particles.

The synthesis, structure, and physicochemical properties of N-[4-(acetyloxy)phenyl] acetamide, a prodrug of paracetamol, were investigated by Bhalla and Lalla.[34] Comprehensive preformulation studies of a chewable tablet of the prodrug were also performed.

A free-flowing, directly-compressible agglomerated form of paracetamol 95% with povidone 5% was prepared by use of a fluid-bed technique.[35] Detailed studies of the characteristics of the agglomerates, of their development into tablets, and the properties of such tablets were performed. Experimental tablets, which also contained magnesium stearate and microcrystalline cellulose:pregelatinised starch (70:30), showed similar in-vitro properties and in-vivo availability (urinary excretion data from a randomised, crossover study with five healthy subjects) compared to those of commercial paracetamol tablets (McNeil, USA).

FURTHER INFORMATION. *In vitro* and *in vivo* release studies [from tablets] of paracetamol crystals produced by solvent change method—Shahwan KS, Nath BS, Shahwan HK. Indian J Pharm Sci 1987;49(2):37–9. Tensile strength of paracetamol and Avicel powders and their mixtures—Bangudu AB, Pilpel N. J Pharm Pharmacol 1984;36:717–22. The influence of moisture content on the consolidation and compaction properties of paracetamol—Garr JSM, Rubinstein MH. Int J Pharmaceutics 1992;81:187–92. Dispersion availability of paracetamol. part 2. Influence of the porosity and the mechanical properties of dosage forms on the dissolution—Abebe A, Chulia D, Verain A [French]. Pharm Acta Helv 1991;66:83–7. Microencapsulation of paracetamol using polyacrylate resins (Eudragit Retard), kinetics of drug release and evaluation of kinetic model—Benita S, Hoffman A, Donbrow M. J Pharm Pharmacol 1985;37:391–5. Influence of dielectric constant of the base on the release of acetaminophen from suppositories—Stavchansky S, Garabedian M, Wu P, Martin A. Drug Dev Ind Pharm 1979;5(5):507–21. The influence of the addition of colloidal silica and of aluminium stearate on the properties of rectal suppositories formulations—Moës A [French]. J Pharm Belg 1976;31(4):355–65. Interaction of paracetamol with nonionic surfactants; influence on the rectal absorption from suppositories—Djimbo M, Moës AJ [French]. J Pharm Belg 1986;41(6):393–401. Studies relating to the content uniformity of suppositories. Part 1. Use of lactose as a drug carrier to hinder sedimentation—Sallam E, Ibrahim H, Takieddin M, Saket M, Awad R, Arafat T et al. Drug Dev Ind Pharm 1989;15:2653–73. Bioavailability of the granules of different species prepared from micronised paracetamol—Soininen A, Löppönen M. Acta Pharm Fenn 1980;89:139–45. Comparison of the *in vitro* and *in vivo* release characteristics of acetaminophen from gradient matrix systems—Van Bommel EM, Raghoebar M, Tukker JJ. Biopharm Drug Dispos 1991;12:367–73.

Effect of humidity on the formation and stability of acetaminophen-β-cyclodextrin inclusion complexes—Lin S-Y. Drug Dev Ind Pharm 1990;16:2221–41. Modification of acetaminophen crystals: influence of growth in aqueous solutions containing *p*-acetoxyacetanilide on crystal properties—Chow AH-L, Chow PKK, Zhongshan W, Grant DJW. Int J Pharmaceutics 1985;24:239–58. Modification of acetaminophen crystals. II. Influence of stirring rate during solution-phase growth on crystal properties in the presence and absence of *p*-acetoxyacetanilide—Chow AH-L, Grant DJW. Int J Pharmaceutics 1988;41:29–39. Modification of acetaminophen crystals. III. Influence of initial supersaturation during solution-phase growth on crystal properties in the presence and absence of *p*-acetoxyacetanilide—Chow AH-L, Grant DJW. Int J Pharmaceutics 1988;42:123–33. Influence of crystallisation conditions on the physical properties of acetaminophen crystals: evaluation of multiple linear regression—Chow AH-L, Grant DJW. Int J Pharmaceutics 1989;51:115–27.

PROCESSING

The characteristics of paracetamol granules prepared by fluidised bed granulation and by wet massing (using hydrolysed gelatin as binder) have been compared.[36] Wet-massed granules were regular in shape, with the drug particles contained within the binder matrix. Fluidised-bed granules were irregularly shaped and made up of intact drug crystals bonded together by crystalline bridges of paracetamol and a sponge-like network of fibrous gelatin; they were more porous than the wet-massed granules. In tablets compressed from each granule type there were small but significant differences in tensile strength, disintegration rates, and dissolution times.

FURTHER INFORMATION. Fluid volume effects on tablet properties [release *in vitro* affected by compressional force and amount of binder fluid]—Shubair MS, Dingwall D. Mfg Chem 1977;48:52,56,59. Influence of compression force on the physical characteristics of paracetamol tablets—Tasic LJ, Djuric Z, Jovanovic M. Pharmazie 1991;46:226–7. Influence of compaction on the intrinsic dissolution of modified acetaminophen and adipic acid crystals—Chan H-K, Grant DJW. Int J Pharmaceutics 1989;57:117–24. Compaction characterisation of paracetamol and Avicel mixtures—Yu HCM, Rubinstein MH, Jackson IM, Elsabbagh HM. Drug Dev Ind Pharm 1989;15(5):801–23. Effect of crospovidone on the wet granulation aspects of acetaminophen—Phadke DH, Anderson NR. Drug Dev Ind Pharm 1990;16:983–4.

REFERENCES

1. Hamza YE, Paruta AN. Drug Dev Ind Pharm 1985;11(1):187–206.
2. Etman MA, Naggar VF. Int J Pharmaceutics 1990;58:177–84.
3. Hamza YE, Paruta AN. Drug Dev Ind Pharm 1985;11(8):1577–96.
4. Shah SP, Flanagan DR. J Pharm Sci 1990;79:889–92.
5. Mahmud A, Li Wan Po A. Drug Dev Ind Pharm 1991;17(5):709–24.
6. Koshy KT, Lach JL. J Pharm Sci 1961;50(2):113–18.
7. Sarisuta N, Parrott EL. Drug Dev Ind Pharm 1988;14(13):1877–81.
8. Koshy KT, Troup AE, Duvall RN, Conwell RC, Shankle LL. J Pharm Sci 1967;56(9):1117–21.
9. Kalatzis E. J Pharm Sci 1970;59(2):193–6.
10. Borin MT, Ayres JW. Int J Pharmaceutics 1989;54:199–209.
11. Razdan B, Rastogi KC. STP Pharma 1990;6:242–6.
12. Razdan B, Verma PK. Int J Pharmaceutics 1992;79:83–8.
13. Ameer B, Divoll M, Abernethy DR, Greenblatt DJ, Shargel L. J Pharm Sci 1983;72(8):955–8.
14. Sotiropoulus JB, Deutsch T, Plakogiannis FM. J Pharm Sci 1981;70(4):422–5.
15. Ali HM, Homeida MMA, Ford J, Truman CA, Roberts CJC, Badwan AA. Int J Pharmaceutics 1988;42:155–9.
16. Macheras P, Parissi-Poulous M, Poulos L. Biopharm Drug Dispos 1989;10:101–5.
17. Walter-Sack I, Luckow V, Guserle R, Weber E [German]. Arzneimittelforschung 1989;39(I)Nr 6:719–24.
18. Krycer I, Pope DG, Hersey JA. J Pharm Pharmacol 1982;34:802–4.
19. Yu HCM, Rubinstein MH, Jackson IM, Elsabbagh HM. J Pharm Pharmacol 1988;40:669–73.
20. Zubair S, Esezobo S, Pilpel N. J Pharm Pharmacol 1988;40:278–81.

21. Esezobo S, Zubair S, Pilpel N. J Pharm Pharmacol 1989;41:7–10.
22. Hussain MSH, York P, Timmins P. Int J Pharmaceutics 1992;78:203–7.
23. Tasic LM, Jovanovic MD, Djuric ZR. J Pharm Pharmacol 1992;44:52–5.
24. El-Said Y, El-Helw AE, Hashern F. Acta Pharm Fenn 1987;96:175–81.
25. Kopcha M, Lordi NG. Drug Dev Ind Pharm 1988;14(10):1389–427.
26. Phuapradit W, Bolton S. Drug Dev Ind Pharm 1991;17(8):1097–107.
27. Abd Elbary A, Ibrahim SA, Elsorady H, Abd Elmonem H. Pharm Ind 1983;45(1):87–90.
28. Shangraw RF, Walkling WD. J Pharm Sci 1971;60(4):600–2.
29. Pagay SN, Poust RI, Colaizzi JL. J Pharm Sci 1974;63(1):45–7.
30. Palmieri A, Danson T, Groben W, Jukka R, Dummer C. Drug Dev Ind Pharm 1983;9:421–42.
31. Kahela P, Laine E, Anttila M. Drug Dev Ind Pharm 1987;13(2):213–24.
32. Roller L. Aust J Hosp Pharm 1977;7(3):97–101.
33. Torrado-Duran JJ, Torrado-Valeiras JJ, Cadorniga R. Drug Dev Ind Pharm 1991;17(10):1305–23.
34. Bhalla DV, Lalla JK. Drug Dev Ind Pharm 1990;16(1):115–35.
35. Patel NK, Poola NR, Babar A, Plakogiannis FM. Drug Dev Ind Pharm 1989;15(8):1175–98.
36. Gamlen MJ, Seager H, Warrack JK. Int J Pharm Tech & Prod Mfr 1982;3(4):108–14.

Pethidine (BAN, rINN)   *Opioid analgesic*

Meperidine
Ethyl 1-methyl-4-phenylpiperidine-4-carboxylate
$C_{15}H_{21}NO_2 = 247.3$

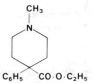

Pethidine Hydrochloride (BANM, rINNM)

Meperidine hydrochloride
$C_{15}H_{21}NO_2,HCl = 283.8$
CAS—57-42-1 (pethidine); 50-13-5 (pethidine hydrochloride)

Pharmacopoeial status

BP (pethidine hydrochloride); USP (meperidine hydrochloride)

Preparations

Compendial
Pethidine Tablets BP. Tablets containing, in each, 25 mg and 50 mg pethidine hydrochloride are usually available.
Pethidine Injection BP. A sterile solution of pethidine hydrochloride in water for injections. Injections containing 50 mg in 1 mL, 50 mg in 5 mL, 100 mg in 2 mL, and 100 mg in 10 mL are usually available.
Meperidine Hydrochloride Tablets USP.
Meperidine Hydrochloride Syrup USP.
Meperidine Hydrochloride Injection USP. pH 3.5 to 6.0.

Non-compendial
Pethidine Roche (Roche). *Tablets*, pethidine hydrochloride 50 mg. *Injection*, pethidine hydrochloride 10 mg/mL and 50 mg/mL. Ampoule solution may be diluted with water for injections. Stability cannot be guaranteed once the solution is diluted.

Containers and storage

Solid state
Pethidine Hydrochloride BP should be kept in an airtight container and protected from light.
Meperidine Hydrochloride USP should be preserved in well-closed, light-resistant containers.

Dosage forms
Meperidine Hydrochloride Tablets USP should be preserved in well-closed, light-resistant containers.
Meperidine Hydrochloride Syrup USP should be preserved in tight, light-resistant containers.
Meperidine Hydrochloride Injection USP should be preserved in single-dose or in multiple-dose containers, preferably of Type I glass.
Pethidine Roche tablets in blister packs should be stored in a dry place. The recommended maximum storage temperature is 35°.
Pethidine Roche ampoules should be stored at a temperature not greater than 30°.

PHYSICAL PROPERTIES

Pethidine is an oily liquid, which slowly crystallises.
Pethidine hydrochloride is a fine, white, crystalline powder; odourless, with a slightly bitter taste.

Melting point

Pethidine hydrochloride melts in the range 186° to 190°.

pH

The pH of a 2% solution of *pethidine hydrochloride* is in the range 4.5 to 5.5.

Dissociation constant

pK_a 8.7

Partition coefficient

Log P (octanol), 1.6
Chan *et al*[1] cite a value of 1.68 for the partition coefficient of pethidine in *n*-heptane/buffer at pH 7.4.

Solubility

Pethidine hydrochloride is very soluble in water; freely soluble in ethanol and in chloroform; practically insoluble in ether.

Dissolution

The USP specifies that for Meperidine Hydrochloride Tablets USP not less than 75% of the labelled amount of $C_{15}H_{21}NO_2,HCl$ is dissolved in 45 minutes. Dissolution medium: 500 mL of water; Apparatus 1 at 100 rpm.

STABILITY

Pethidine hydrochloride is stable in the solid state but hydrolyses in aqueous solution to yield pethidic acid and ethanol.
In dilute hydrochloric acid, the hydrolysis of pethidine hydrochloride was first-order with respect to drug concentration and was shown[2] to be specific hydronium-ion catalysed at constant temperature (70°). A positive, primary salt effect was noted in dilute acidic solution. Dihydrogen phosphate ions also catalysed decomposition. In aqueous buffer, pH 1 to 7, the pH-rate

profile for the hydrolysis reaction indicated maximum stability of pethidine hydrochloride at pH 4.0 to 5.0. Activation energies at pH 2, 3, 4 and 5, and 6 were calculated to be 57.48, 56.51, 86.12, and 78.51 kJ/mol, respectively.

INCOMPATIBILITY/COMPATIBILITY

Rhodes et al[3] found that a mixture comprising 1 mL volumes of pethidine hydrochloride (50 mg/mL), promethazine hydrochloride (25 mg/mL), and atropine sulphate (0.4 mg/mL) was chemically stable in plastic syringes for 24 hours at room temperature. An admixture of pethidine hydrochloride (Winthrop, USA, 25 mg/mL), hydroxyzine hydrochloride (Pfizer, USA, 12.5 mg/mL), and chlorpromazine hydrochloride (Elkins-Sinn, USA, 6.25 mg/mL) was stable[4] for 366 days in both glass and plastic (polypropylene) single-dose syringes at 4° or 25° but not at 44°. All samples stored at 44° turned yellow by day 30 and continued to darken throughout the study period with a concomitant rapid decrease in pH.

Admixtures of hydroxyzine hydrochloride (Pfizer, USA) and pethidine hydrochloride (Demerol, Winthrop, USA), 50 mg/2 mL each, and of these two drugs (50 mg/2.5 mL each) with atropine sulphate (Elkins-Sinn, USA, 0.4 mg/2.5 mL) in pre-filled glass and plastic syringes showed apparent compatibility and stability over a ten-day period at 3° or 25°. The authors[5] stressed that the results were exclusive to the particular materials and conditions of the study and could not be extrapolated. Pethidine hydrochloride was physically incompatible in intravenous admixture (manifested solely by the lack of clarity of the resulting solution admixture) with aminophylline, amylobarbitone, heparin sodium, methicillin sodium, morphine sulphate, nitrofurantoin sodium, pentobarbitone sodium, phenobarbitone sodium, phenytoin sodium, sodium bicarbonate, sodium iodide, sulphadiazine sodium, sulphafurazole diethanolamine, and thiopentone sodium.[6]

Smythe et al[7] reported immediate visual incompatibility of pethidine hydrochloride (Wyeth, USA, 100 mg/mL solution diluted to 10 mg/mL with sodium chloride 0.9% injection) and nafcillin sodium (Wyeth, USA, 20 mg/mL and 30 mg/mL in glucose 5% injection), which persisted throughout a one-hour observation period.

Pethidine hydrochloride (Abbott, 10 mg/mL) was also observed to be visually incompatible at 25° under fluorescent light in admixture with imipenem-cilastatin (MSD, USA, 5 mg/mL), acyclovir sodium (Burroughs-Wellcome, USA, 5 mg/mL), or frusemide (Elkins-Sinn, USA, 120 mg/50 mL and 10 mg/mL) under conditions that simulated Y-site injection.[8]

FORMULATION

Excipients

Excipients that have been used in presentations of pethidine hydrochloride include:
Tablets: calcium hydrogen phosphate; calcium sulphate; starch; stearic acid; talc.
Syrups: benzoic acid; banana flavour; liquid glucose; saccharin sodium.

Suppositories

A displacement value of 1.6 is given for pethidine hydrochloride in theobroma oil.

PROCESSING

Sterilisation

Pethidine injection can be sterilised by heating in an autoclave.

REFERENCES

1. Chan K, Murray GR, Ong GC. Br J Clin Pharmacol 1980;9(1):122P.
2. Patel RM, Chin T-F, Lach J-L. Am J Hosp Pharm 1968;25:256–61.
3. Rhodes RS, Rhodes PJ, McCurdy HH. Am J Hosp Pharm 1985;42:112–15.
4. Conklin CA, Kerege JF, Christensen JM. Am J Hosp Pharm 1985;42:339–42.
5. Stanaszek WF, Pan I-H. Am J Hosp Pharm 1978;35:1084–7.
6. Patel JA, Phillips GL. Am J Hosp Pharm 1966;23:409–11.
7. Smythe MA, Patel MA, Gasloli RA. Am J Hosp Pharm 1990;47:819–20.
8. Pugh CB, Pabis DJ, Rodriguez C. Am J Hosp Pharm 1991;48:123–5.

Phenobarbitone (BAN)   *Sedative; Anticonvulsant*

Phenobarbital (rINN); phenylethylbarbituric acid; phenylethyl-malonylurea
5-Ethyl-5-phenylbarbituric acid
$C_{12}H_{12}N_2O_3 = 232.2$

Phenobarbitone Sodium (BANM)

Phenobarbital Sodium (rINNM); soluble phenobarbitone
$C_{12}H_{11}N_2NaO_3 = 254.2$
CAS—50-06-6 (phenobarbitone); 57-30-7 (phenobarbitone sodium)

Pharmacopoeial status

BP (phenobarbitone, phenobarbitone sodium); USP (phenobarbital, phenobarbital sodium)

Preparations

Compendial
Phenobarbitone Tablets BP. Tablets containing, in each, 15, 30, 60, and 100 mg of phenobarbitone are usually available.
Phenobarbitone Sodium Tablets BP. Tablets containing, in each, 30 mg and 60 mg of phenobarbitone sodium are usually available.
Phenobarbitone Elixir BP (Phenobarbitone Oral Solution). A solution containing 0.3% w/v of phenobarbitone in a suitable flavoured vehicle containing a sufficient volume of ethanol or of an appropriate dilute ethanol to give a final concentration of 38% v/v of ethanol. If the elixir is diluted, the diluted elixir should be freshly prepared.
Phenobarbitone Injection BP (Phenobarbitone Sodium Injection). A sterile solution containing 20% w/v of phenobarbitone sodium in a mixture of nine volumes of propylene glycol and one volume of water for injections. pH 10.0 to 11.0.
Phenobarbital Tablets USP.
Phenobarbital Elixir USP.
Sterile Phenobarbital Sodium USP. Suitable for parenteral use.
Phenobarbital Sodium Injection USP. pH 9.2 to 10.2.

Non-compendial
Gardenal Sodium (Rhône-Poulenc Rorer). *Injection*, phenobarbitone sodium 200 mg/mL in a propylene glycol/water mixture.
Diluent: water for injections.

Injections of phenobarbitone sodium are also available from Martindale.

Containers and storage

Solid state
Phenobarbitone Sodium BP should be kept in an airtight container.
Phenobarbital USP should be preserved in well-closed containers.
Phenobarbital Sodium USP should be preserved in tight containers.

Dosage forms
Phenobarbitone Elixir BP should be protected from light.
Phenobarbital Tablets USP should be preserved in well-closed containers.
Phenobarbital Elixir USP should be preserved in tight, light-resistant containers.
Phenobarbital Sodium Injection USP should be preserved in single-dose or in multiple-dose containers, preferably of Type I glass.
Sterile Phenobarbital Sodium USP should be preserved in containers suitable for sterile solids.
Gardenal Sodium should be stored below 25° and protected from light.

PHYSICAL PROPERTIES

Phenobarbitone exists as colourless crystals or as a white, crystalline powder; it is odourless.
Phenobarbitone sodium exists as flaky crystals or as white crystalline granules, or as a white powder; it is odourless, hygroscopic, and has a bitter taste.

Melting point
Phenobarbitone melts at 174° to 178°, but the range between the beginning and end of melting does not exceed 2°.

pH
A saturated solution of *phenobarbitone* in water has a pH of approximately 5.
The pH of a 10% w/v solution of *phenobarbitone sodium* is not greater than 10.2.

Dissociation constant
pK_a 7.4 (25°)

Partition coefficient
Log P (octanol), 1.4

Solubility
Phenobarbitone is soluble 1 in 1000 of water, 1 in 10 of ethanol, 1 in 40 of chloroform, and 1 in 40 of ether. It dissolves in aqueous solutions of alkali hydroxides and carbonates and in aqueous ammonia.
Phenobarbitone sodium is freely soluble in carbon dioxide-free water (a small fraction may be insoluble); soluble 1 in 25 of ethanol; practically insoluble in chloroform, in dichloromethane, and in ether.
Phenobarbitone concentrations of up to 45 mg/mL (approximately ten times greater concentration than that of BPC or USP elixirs containing ethanol) were achieved in various binary and ternary propylene glycol-glycerol-water solvent systems.[1] Phenobarbitone solubility was increased to a greater extent by the presence of propylene glycol than by glycerol.

Phenobarbitone Elixir BP has a high ethanol content to ensure that the phenobarbitone remains in solution.

Effect of pH
Phenobarbitone may be precipitated from solutions of phenobarbitone sodium, depending on concentration and pH:

Concentration	pH at which precipitation occurs
3 mg/mL	7.5 or below
6 mg/mL	7.9 or below
10 mg/mL	8.3 or below
20 mg/mL	8.6 or below

Solubilisation
The degree of solubilisation of phenobarbitone by the nonionic surfactants polyoxyethylene-20-cetyl ether and polysorbate 80 was greater than that by the ionic surfactants cetrimide and sodium lauryl sulphate[2]. The apparent solubility of phenobarbitone increased linearly with increasing surfactant concentration, indicating micellar solubilisation. The capacity of each surfactant to solubilise phenobarbitone was related to its micellar size or molecular weight; compounds with high molecular weights had greater solubilising capacities. However, spectrophotometric measurements of the *in-vitro* 'availability' of phenobarbitone revealed that initial transport from the solubilised systems was slower than from standard aqueous solutions. In general, the higher the solubilising capacity of the surfactant, the slower was the 'availability' of phenobarbitone from its solubilised system.

FURTHER INFORMATION. Correlation between the solubility of phenobarbitone and the polarity of various solvent systems—Maher N, Sirois G [French]. Can J Pharm Sci 1971;6(3):55–8. Solubility of various barbiturates in buffered aqueous solutions. I. Test of a theoretical equation—Wang L-H, Paruta AN. Drug Dev Ind Pharm 1984;10(4):667–83. Thermodynamics of buffered aqueous solutions of various barbiturates. II. Effect of buffers, substituents and solute polarity—Wang L-H, Paruta AN. Drug Dev Ind Pharm 1984;10(6):861–71. Solubilisation of [phenobarbitone] in sodium paraffinsulfonate—Vaution C, Paris J, Puisieux F, Carstensen JT. Int J Pharmaceutics 1978;1:349–59. [Solubilisation of phenobarbitone with polyols]—Dominguez-Gil A, Cadorniga R, Llabres M [Spanish]. Cienc Ind Farm 1974;6:53–7.

Dissolution
The USP specifies that for Phenobarbital Tablets USP not less than 75% of the labelled amount of $C_{12}H_{12}N_2O_3$ is dissolved in 45 minutes. Dissolution medium: 900 mL of water; Apparatus 2 at 50 rpm.

Crystal and molecular structure

Polymorphs
Up to 13 polymorphic forms of phenobarbitone have been identified and examined by infrared spectroscopy, X-ray diffraction, and differential scanning calorimetry.[3] Conditions for interconversion between forms were investigated. Commercial phenobarbitone was identified as Form II, the most stable form at room temperature. The different polymorphs had different melting points.

FURTHER INFORMATION. Dimorphism of phenobarbitone sodium—Bosly J, Lapiere CL, Bouche R [French]. J Pharm Belg 1981;36(4):249–50. Characterisation of phenobarbitone samples—Riley GS. J Pharm Pharmacol 1974;26:919–20. Studies of the polymorphism of drugs in powders and tablets. Part 1: Preparation and characterisation of polymorphic modifications of [phenobarbitone]—Traue J, Kala H, Wenzel U, Wiegeleben A, Pintye-Hodi K, Szabo-Revesz P et al [German]. Pharmazie 1987;42(H2):86–9. Investigations about polymorphism of drugs in powders and tablets. Part 4: The influence of the polymorphism of drugs on the physical properties and drug release of phenobarbitone tablets—Szabo-Revesz P, Pintye-Hodi K, Miseta M, Selmeczi B, Kedvessy G, Traue J et al [German]. Pharmazie 1987;42(H3):179–81.

STABILITY

Phenobarbitone is stable in air, but in solution it is subject to hydrolysis, particularly at high pH, leading to cleavage of the barbituric acid ring at the 1,2-position or the 1,6-position to yield the diamide or the ureide, respectively. Further decomposition of the diamide and ureide can occur.

A 10% aqueous solution of phenobarbitone sodium, at 20°, showed the following decomposition pattern: 3% to 4% in 15 days, 6% to 8% in 30 days, and about 15% after 90 days. The apparent first-order rate constants for the decomposition of phenobarbitone 2 mg/mL at 80° in aqueous solution with 0.1M sodium hydroxide buffer (pH 11.5) or with 0.033M sodium hydroxide buffer (pH 10.99) were reported to be 3×10^{-4}/s and 1.5×10^{-4}/s, respectively.[4]

Liquid dosage forms

The stability of phenobarbitone sodium in liquid dosage forms is dependent on the vehicle. In comparison to the stability of phenobarbitone in water alone, ethanol had the maximum stabilising effect on phenobarbitone sodium 0.5 mg/mL solution followed by propylene glycol and glycerol.[5] Estimated half-lives (at 50°, pH approximately 8) were 78, 95, 109, and 127 days in water and in 20% aqueous solutions of glycerol, propylene glycol, and ethanol, respectively. The effects of phosphate buffer and ionic strength were negligible.

A rapid HPLC assay demonstrated that phenobarbitone (4 mg/mL) was stable in an emulsion (containing cholesterol, Span 85, maize oil, Sørensen buffer pH 5, propylene glycol, and Tween 85), in a propylene glycol solution (Sørensen buffer pH 5, propylene glycol), and in an elixir (Lilly, USA); however, it was not stable in an aqueous solution (the last three solutions were prepared using phenobarbitone sodium).[6] The $t_{50\%}$ values for first-order decomposition were 693 (± 240), 990 (± 163), 770 (± 27), and 130 (± 11) weeks for the propylene glycol emulsion, the elixir, the propylene glycol solution, and the aqueous solution, respectively.

The hydrolytic decomposition of phenobarbitone sodium 10% w/v in aqueous solution pH 9.8 or 9.9 was negligible after storage in the frozen state at −25° for 8 weeks. However, after 4 weeks at 20°, only 93% of the initial phenobarbitone sodium concentration remained.[7]

Phenobarbitone sodium injection (65 mg/mL), diluted to 10 mg/mL in sodium chloride 0.9% injection (unadjusted pH 8.5) was demonstrated by HPLC to be stable when stored for 4 weeks in a refrigerator at 4°, without the need for pH adjustment.[8] The diluted solution was considered to be potentially suitable for administration to infants.

Stabilisation

Propylene glycol, macrogol 400, ethanol, and, to a lesser extent, glycerol have a stabilising effect when added to aqueous solutions of phenobarbitone sodium.

FURTHER INFORMATION. Influence of pH and solubilising agents on the stability of phenobarbitone—Cadorniga R, Lastres JL, Ballesteros MP [Spanish]. Boll Chim Farm 1980;119:405–16. Stabilisation of phenobarbitone in injectable solution—Colombo BM, Primavera P, Lojodice D [Italian]. Il Farmaco Ed Pr 1970;25:241–7.

INCOMPATIBILITY/COMPATIBILITY

Phenobarbitone sodium is incompatible with ammonium salts, acids and acidic substances (for example, ammonium chloride and carbon dioxide), and with chloral hydrate. The precipitation of free barbiturates from mixtures containing their sodium derivatives usually depends on the concentration of barbiturates present and on the final pH of the mixture. If the mixture is obviously acid then the solubility of the barbiturate can be taken as that of the free acid. If the mixture is slightly alkaline precise determination of pH might be necessary. Precipitation of the free acid has been reported at pH 8.8.

Incompatibility of phenobarbitone sodium has also been reported with the following compounds: cephalothin sodium, chlorpromazine hydrochloride, clindamycin phosphate, dimenhydrinate, diphenhydramine hydrochloride, ephedrine sulphate, erythromycin glucepate, hydralazine hydrochloride, hydrocortisone sodium succinate, hydroxyzine hydrochloride, insulin, kanamycin sulphate, metaraminol tartrate, opioid salts, oxytetracycline hydrochloride, pentazocine lactate, phenytoin sodium, procaine hydrochloride, prochlorperazine salts, promazine hydrochloride, promethazine hydrochloride, propiomazine hydrochloride, streptomycin sulphate, suxamethonium chloride, tetracycline hydrochloride, thiamine hydrochloride, tripelennamine hydrochloride, and vancomycin hydrochloride; many of these incompatibilities may be explained on the basis of pH effects.

Phenobarbitone sodium injection is also reported to be incompatible with benzylpenicillin potassium, calcium chloride, codeine phosphate, codeine sulphate, magnesium sulphate, methyl and propyl hydroxybenzoates, para-aminobenzoic acid, sodium bicarbonate, suxamethonium chloride.

A poorly soluble precipitate is formed when papaverine hydrochloride is added to solutions of phenobarbitone sodium. However, when an aqueous solution of an inclusion complex of phenobarbitone sodium and β-cyclodextrin was mixed with papaverine hydrochloride, no precipitation was observed.[9]

When phenobarbitone sodium (261 mg) was added to diphenhydramine hydrochloride solution (10 mg/mL, pH 5.5), the mixture became turbid and crystals were formed.[10] The pH changed to 7.5.

A complex with reduced solubility is reported to form when phenobarbitone is mixed with macrogol 4000. Dissolution and absorption of phenobarbitone were reduced from tablets containing macrogol 4000.

FORMULATION

Excipients

Excipients that have been used in presentations of phenobarbitone include:

Tablets, phenobarbitone: alginic acid; calcium carbonate; dextrin; erythrosine (E127); lactose; magnesium stearate; microcrystalline cellulose; starch (potato, wheat); titanium dioxide (E171).

Elixirs, phenobarbitone: aromatic syrup; compound orange spirit; ethanol; glycerol; talc.

Mixtures, phenobarbitone sodium: compound hydroxybenzoate solution; concentrated chloroform water; glycerol; sorbitol.

Injections, phenobarbitone sodium: ethanol; 2-ethoxyethanol; glyceryl acetate; glycine; propylene glycol; sodium glycinate.

Bioavailability

The relative bioavailabilities of four different phenobarbitone 100 mg tablets (Parke-Davis, Lannett, West-Ward, and Wyeth) determined from areas under plasma concentration versus time curves following a three-way crossover study involving 24 healthy volunteers and compared with that of an elixir (Parke-Davis, 20 mg/5 mL) were all within 10% of each other.[11]

Although generic tablets of phenobarbitone from six different manufacturers met pharmacopoeial requirements (BP 1980), wide variations in disintegration and dissolution times were noted.[12]

Phenobarbitone sodium injection solution (Wyeth) was well absorbed following rectal administration to seven healthy volunteers;[13] mean bioavailability relative to the intramuscular route was 90%. Absorption was slower following rectal administration than after intramuscular injection.

Moolenaar et al[14] examined the rectal absorption (in six healthy volunteers) of phenobarbitone and its sodium salt following administration in micro-enemas (phenobarbitone sodium in aqueous solution containing methylcellulose, or a suspension of micronised phenobarbitone free acid in the same medium) or in fatty suppositories containing micronised phenobarbitone or coarse phenobarbitone sodium in Witepsol H15. Rectal administration of both types of micro-enema resulted in almost complete absorption; however, the rate of absorption was slower than that following oral administration of an aqueous solution of phenobarbitone sodium. The absorption rate from micro-enemas was similar whether the free acid or the sodium salt was used. The difference in in-vitro release rate between phenobarbitone and its sodium salt in a fatty suppository basis was reflected in in-vivo absorption profiles; a slower rate of absorption was observed when the free acid was used in the fatty suppository dosage form.

Oral liquids

The release rate of phenobarbitone from a 2% suspension in liquid paraffin into aqueous media was shown to increase with an increase in the pH (3.0, 7.4, and 10.0)[15] of the medium, especially when the pH was greater than the pK_a.

Suppositories

Workers in Japan[16] formulated a phenobarbitone suppository from a co-precipitate of phenobarbitone and a water-soluble carrier (such as hydroxypropylcellulose dispersed on lactose) in a novel three-component basis (an oleaginous basis, a water-soluble basis, and a polyoxyethylene-polyoxypropylene block copolymer, Unilube). An improvement in phenobarbitone absorption compared to that from a suppository containing phenobarbitone alone was noted in rabbits.

Effect of excipients

The apparent partition coefficient of phenobarbitone between chloroform and 0.05M Tris buffer, pH 5.9, decreased in the presence of polysorbate 80 (up to 0.01% w/v), reaching a minimum at the critical micelle concentration of polysorbate 80, then increased markedly at higher polysorbate 80 concentration (1% w/v).[17]

The influence of microcrystalline cellulose (as Avicel PH 101), microcrystalline cellulose and lactose, and microcrystalline cellulose and maize starch on the physical parameters of phenobarbitone tablets has been extensively investigated.[18-20]

The formation of a weak phenobarbitone:urea (1:2) compound has been demonstrated, using infrared spectroscopy, in physical and fused mixtures of phenobarbitone and urea.[21]

Solid dispersions

Solid dispersions of phenobarbitone have been prepared in sucrose and in sorbitol by the melting method, and in povidone by the solvent method.[22] Physicochemical determination (including infrared, ultraviolet, and X-ray diffraction studies) revealed that the dispersions in sucrose were interstitial and solid crystallised whereas the dispersions in sorbitol and povidone were amorphous and glassy.

FURTHER INFORMATION. Thermal characterisation of citric acid solid dispersions with benzoic acid and [phenobarbitone]— Timko RJ, Lordi NG. J Pharm Sci 1979;68(5):601–5. In vitro adsorption of [phenobarbitone] onto activated charcoal— Javaid KA, El-Mabrouk BH. J Pharm Sci 1983;72(1):82–4. Availability of [phenobarbitone] from suppository form— Puech A, Lasserre Y, Jacob M, Duru C [French]. J Pharm Belg 1981;36(5):332–6. Cinétique de libération des suppositoires à base de phénobarbital acide et sodique et de glycéride semi-synthétique (Witepsol H 15). I. Cas de suppositoires fraîchement préparés—Lasserre Y, Peneva B, Jacob M, Puech A [French]. Pharm Acta Helv 1984;59(3):77–9. II. Cas de suppositoires après conservation—Lasserre Y, Penevar B, Jacob M, Puech A, Sabatier R [French]. Pharm Acta Helv 1987;62(10–11):287–91. Effect of temperature of dissolution on the release kinetics of phenobarbitone from poly (DL-lactic acid) microcapsules: calculation of activation energy—Jalil R, Nixon JR. Drug Dev Ind Pharm 1990;16(15):2257–66.

PROCESSING

Fluid volume effects [of binder] on tablet properties [effect of compressional force]—Shubair MS, Dingwall D. Mfg Chem 1977;48(11):52,56,59.

REFERENCES

1. Moustafa MA, Molokhia AM, Gouda MW. J Pharm Sci 1981;70(10):1172–4.
2. Naggar VF, Moustafa MA, Khalil SA, Motawi MM. Can J Pharm Sci 1972;7(4):112–14.
3. Mesley RJ, Clements RL, Flaherty B, Goodhead K. J Pharm Pharmacol 1968;20:329–40.
4. Maulding HV, Polesuk J, Rosenbaum D. J Pharm Sci 1975;64(2):272–4.
5. Das Gupta V. J Pharm Sci 1984;73(11):1661–2.
6. Dietz NJ, Cascella PJ, Houglum JE, Chappell GS, Sieve RM. Pharm Res 1988;5(12):803–5.
7. Larsen SS, Jensen VG. Dansk Tidsskr Farm 1970;44:21–31.
8. Nahata MC, Hipple TF, Strausbaugh SD. Am J Hosp Pharm 1986;43:384–5.
9. Racz I, Plachy J, Szabon-Tabori M, Stadler-Szoke A, Vikmon M, Szejtli J [Hungarian]. Acta Pharm Hung 1984;54:154–9.
10. Dunker MFW, Sirois LM. J Pharm Sci 1982;71(8):962–3.
11. Meyer MC, Straughn AB, Raghow G, Schary WL, Rotenberg KS. J Pharm Sci 1984;73(4):485–8.
12. Bain R, Dixson SJ [letter]. Pharm J 1982;229:99.
13. Graves NM, Holmes GB, Kriel RL, Jones-Saete C, Ong B, Ehresman DJ. DICP Ann Pharmacother 1989;23:565–7.
14. Moolenaar F, Koning B, Huizinga T. Int J Pharmaceutics 1979;4(2):99–109.

15. Fokkens JG, De Blaey CJ. Pharm Weekbl (Sci) 1982;4:117–21.
16. Kitagawa A, Inotsume N, Iwaoku R, Nakano M. J Pharm Sci 1987;76(11):S277, N 04-W-27.
17. Hikal AH. Int J Pharmaceutics 1981;7:205–10.
18. Szabo-Revesz VP, Kamuti G, Pintye-Hodi K [German]. Pharm Ind 1985;47(12):1285–8.
19. Szabo-Revesz VP, Peto K, Pintye-Hodi K [German]. Pharm Ind 1986;48(3):289–91.
20. Pintye-Hodi K, Szabo-Revesz VP [German]. Pharm Ind 1986;48(9):1079–82.
21. Winfield AJ, Al Saidan SMH. Int J Pharmaceutics 1981;8:211–16.
22. Leucuta S, Neamtu M [French]. Ann Pharm Franc 1980;38(5):411–20.

Phenoxymethylpenicillin (BAN, rINN)

Antibacterial

Penicillin V (USAN)
6(R)-6-(2-Phenoxyacetamido)penicillanic acid; (2S,5R,6R)-3,3-dimethyl-7-oxo-6-(2-phenoxyacetamido)-4-thia-1-azabicyclo[3.2.0]heptane-2-carboxylic acid
$C_{16}H_{18}N_2O_5S = 350.4$

Penicillin V Benzathine (USAN)

$(C_{16}H_{18}N_2O_5S)_2,C_{16}H_{20}N_2 = 941.1$

Phenoxymethylpenicillin Calcium (BANM, rINNM)

$(C_{16}H_{17}N_2O_5S)_2Ca,2H_2O = 774.9$

Phenoxymethylpenicillin Potassium (BANM, rINNM)

Penicillin V Potassium (USAN)
$C_{16}H_{17}KN_2O_5S = 388.5$
CAS—87-08-1 (phenoxymethylpenicillin); 5928-84-7 (penicillin V benzathine); 147-48-8 (phenoxymethylpenicillin calcium, anhydrous); 132-98-9 (phenoxymethylpenicillin potassium)

Pharmacopoeial status

BP (phenoxymethylpenicillin, phenoxymethylpenicillin potassium); USP (penicillin V, penicillin V benzathine, penicillin V potassium)

Preparations

Compendial
Phenoxymethylpenicillin Capsules BP (Phenoxymethylpenicillin Potassium Capsules, Penicillin VK Capsules). Contain phenoxymethylpenicillin potassium. Capsules containing, in each, the equivalent of 250 mg of phenoxymethylpenicillin are usually available.
Phenoxymethylpenicillin Tablets BP (Penicillin VK Tablets). Contain phenoxymethylpenicillin potassium. Tablets containing, in each, the equivalent of 125 mg and 250 mg phenoxymethylpenicillin are usually available.
Phenoxymethylpenicillin Oral Solution BP (Phenoxymethylpenicillin Elixir, Phenoxymethylpenicillin Syrup). A solution of phenoxymethylpenicillin potassium in a suitable flavoured vehicle. It is prepared by dissolving the dry ingredients in the specified volume of water just before issue for use. If the oral solution is diluted, the diluted oral solution should be freshly prepared.
Penicillin V Tablets USP.
Penicillin V Potassium Tablets USP.
Penicillin V for Oral Suspension USP.
Penicillin V Benzathine Oral Suspension USP.
Penicillin V Potassium for Oral Solution USP.

Non-compendial
Apsin VK (APS). *Tablets*, phenoxymethylpenicillin (as potassium salt) 250 mg.
Syrup, granules for reconstitution with water, phenoxymethylpenicillin (as potassium salt) 125 mg/5 mL and 250 mg/5 mL. *Diluent:* syrup, dilutions must be freshly prepared.
Distaquaine V-K (Dista). *Tablets*, phenoxymethylpenicillin (as potassium salt) 250 mg.
Stabillin V-K (Boots). *Tablets*, phenoxymethylpenicillin (as potassium salt) 250 mg.
Elixir, granules for reconstitution with water, phenoxymethylpenicillin (as potassium salt) 125 mg/5 mL and 250 mg/5 mL.
Phenoxymethylpenicillin potassium tablets are also available from Berk, Cox, CP, Evans, Kerfoot.
Phenoxymethylpenicillin potassium oral solutions are also available from Cox, CP, Evans, Kerfoot.

Containers and storage

Solid state
Phenoxymethylpenicillin BP and Phenoxymethylpencillin Potassium BP should be kept in airtight containers.
Penicillin V USP, Penicillin V Benzathine USP, and Penicillin V Potassium USP should be preserved in tight containers.

Dosage forms
Phenoxymethylpenicillin Oral Solution BP. The dry ingredients should be kept in a well-closed container. The oral solution and the diluted oral solution should be stored at the temperature and used within the period stated on the label.
All Penicillin V, Penicillin V Benzathine, and Penicillin V Potassium preparations USP should be preserved in tight containers. Penicillin V Benzathine Oral Suspension USP should be stored in a refrigerator.
Apsin VK tablets and granules for syrup should be stored below 20° in a dry place, not in a refrigerator. The tablets should be dispensed in airtight containers. The reconstituted syrup should be used within seven days and will retain its potency for this period if stored below 15°.
Distaquaine V-K tablets should be protected from moisture.
Stabillin V-K elixir and reconstituted elixir should be stored in a cool place; the reconstituted elixir should be used within one week of preparation.

PHYSICAL PROPERTIES

Phenoxymethylpenicillin is a white crystalline powder.
Penicillin benzathine is a practically white powder with a characteristic odour.
Phenoxymethylpenicillin calcium is a white, finely crystalline powder; odourless or with a slight characteristic odour; slightly bitter taste.
Phenoxymethylpenicillin potassium is a white crystalline powder.

Melting point

Phenoxymethylpenicillin crystals decompose in the range 120° to 128°.

Phenoxymethylpenicillin potassium has been reported to melt in the range 263° to 265°, with decomposition.

pH

pH of a 0.5% w/v suspension of *phenoxymethylpenicillin*, 2.4 to 4.0.

pH of a 3% w/v suspension of *phenoxymethylpenicillin*, 2.5 to 4.0.

pH of a 3% w/v suspension of *penicillin V benzathine*, 4.0 to 6.5.

pH of a 0.5% w/v solution of *phenoxymethylpenicillin calcium*, 5.0 to 7.5.

pH of a 0.5% w/v solution of *phenoxymethylpenicillin potassium*, 5.5 to 7.5.

pH of a 3% w/v solution of *phenoxymethylpenicillin potassium*, 4.0 to 7.5.

Dissociation constant

pK_a 2.7 (25°)

Rapson and Bird[1] determined a pK_a value for phenoxymethylpenicillin of 2.73 or 2.74 in water at 25°.

An apparent pK_a value for phenoxymethylpenicillin of 2.79 has been determined by potentiometric titration at 37° in water.[2]

Partition coefficients

Values of log *P* (octanol/water) of 2.1 or 2.01 have been reported. Using values of apparent partition coefficients for phenoxymethylpenicillin measured over a range of pH and ionic strength, Tsuji *et al*[2] calculated the following intrinsic partition coefficients:

Log *P* (octanol/water) unionised species, 1.95 (37°)

Log *P* (octanol/water) ionised species, −1.65 (37°)

Solubility

Phenoxymethylpenicillin is very slightly soluble in water (1 in 1700); freely soluble in ethanol (1 in 7) and in acetone (1 in 6); soluble in chloroform; practically insoluble in fixed oils and in liquid paraffin.

Phenoxymethylpenicillin benzathine is very slightly soluble in water; slightly soluble in ethanol and in ether; sparingly soluble in chloroform.

Phenoxymethylpenicillin calcium is slowly soluble 1 in 120 of water; practically insoluble in fixed oils and in liquid paraffin.

Phenoxymethylpenicillin potassium is soluble 1 in 1.5 of water; slightly soluble in ethanol (1 in 150); practically insoluble in chloroform, in ether, in fixed oils and in liquid paraffin; insoluble in acetone.

Enhancement of solubility

A three-fold increase in the aqueous solubility of phenoxymethylpenicillin (at pH 2 and 35°) was reported in the presence of 10mM polyoxyethylene-23-lauryl ether.[3]

Dissolution

The USP specifies that for Penicillin V Tablets USP not less than 75% of the labelled amount of $C_{16}H_{18}N_2O_5S$ is dissolved in 45 minutes. Dissolution medium: 900 mL of water; Apparatus 2 at 50 rpm.

The USP specifies that for Penicillin V Potassium Tablets USP not less than 75% of the labelled amount of Penicillin V Units is dissolved in 45 minutes. Dissolution medium: 900 mL of pH 6.0 phosphate buffer; Apparatus 2 at 50 rpm.

STABILITY

The properties, stability, and degradation of phenoxymethylpenicillin have been extensively reviewed.[4-6] The β-lactam ring is susceptible to attack by nucleophiles and the penicillin nucleus is also susceptible to electrophilic attack. Enzymatic hydrolysis (by penicillinase enzymes) can also occur.

In acidic media, hydrolysis of phenoxymethylpenicillin yields phenoxymethylpenillic acid. In neutral solution, hydrolysis yields the penicilloic acid via the penicillenic acid. The major product of mild alkaline hydrolysis is the penicilloic acid, which subsequently forms the penilloic acid under acidic conditions.

In a study of unbuffered aqueous solutions of phenoxymethylpenicillin by Bird *et al*,[7] the degradation products under investigation, *N*-formylpenicillamine and penicillamine, were formed at maximum yields of 3% and 0.1%, respectively, after 7 days at 37°. The pH of solutions decreased from 6.3 to 5.1. Possible degradation routes were presented.

In acidic and neutral aqueous solutions (pH 3 to 7), phenoxymethylpenicillin potassium was hydrolysed to phenoxymethylpenicilloic acid and α- and β-phenoxymethylpenilloic acids.[8] In alkaline solutions, hydrolysis to the penicilloic acid only occurred. The pH-rate profile of the hydrolysis reaction had a minimum at pH 5.7.

Maximum stability of phenoxymethylpenicillin in aqueous solution is reported to occur at pH 6 to 7.

At 37° in 0.1M hydrochloric acid, phenoxymethylpenicillin degradation was found to be a pseudo-first-order process, with a half-life of 29 minutes (determined by microbiological assay).[9] A half-life of 160 minutes was reported[6] for phenoxymethylpenicillin in 50% aqueous ethanol at pH 1.3 and 35°; compared to benzylpenicillin, phenoxymethylpenicillin is considered to be relatively acid stable.

Complete degradation of phenoxymethylpenicillin occurred in the presence of 0.5M sodium hydroxide after 15 to 30 minutes at room temperature.[10]

Effect of sucrose

Degradation of phenoxymethylpenicillin potassium 0.01M in 0.06M citrate buffer pH 7.0 at 45° was accelerated in the presence of sucrose.[11] The degradation rate constant increased about 3-fold to 5-fold as the sucrose concentration was increased to 0.15M. Analysis of experimental data and a kinetic model indicated that a 1:1 molar complex formed between intact phenoxymethylpenicillin and sucrose. Complexed phenoxymethylpenicillin was claimed to degrade by the same pathway as uncomplexed drug.

Bundgaard and Larsen[12] demonstrated a linear relationship between the pseudo-first-order degradation rate constant of phenoxymethylpenicillin (in 0.1M carbonate buffer, pH 10.12 at 35°) and the concentration of sucrose (2% w/v to 10% w/v) in aqueous solution. The mechanisms by which sucrose promotes degradation of phenoxymethylpenicillin were investigated.

Effect of surfactants

Tsuji *et al*[3, 13] elucidated that acid-catalysed degradation of phenoxymethylpenicillin potassium (at 37°) was inhibited in the presence of a cationic or a nonionic surfactant (cetyltrimethylammonium bromide or polyoxyethylene-23-lauryl ether, respectively), but was promoted in the presence of an anionic surfactant (sodium lauryl sulphate). At surfactant concentrations above their critical micelle concentrations, rate constants for phenoxymethylpenicillin degradation approached constant values; this was attributed to the formation of penicillin-micelle complexes.

Reconstituted oral syrups and solutions

In a comprehensive study[14] Hempenstall *et al* investigated methods used for the reconstitution of granules to produce phenoxymethylpenicillin oral syrups (two brands, 125 mg/5 mL) and subsequent dilution (with water, water/syrup, or syrup) to produce half-strength preparations. Separation of dry granules into two 'equal' lots followed by reconstitution of each lot to 100 mL was shown to be unreliable as segregation of phenoxymethylpenicillin in the granules had occurred and final preparations contained variable concentrations of the penicillin. Dilution of the full-strength syrup affected the shelf-life of phenoxymethylpenicillin in the syrups; stability decreased as the sucrose content of the diluent increased.

Jaffe et al[15] investigated the stability of five brands of phenoxymethylpenicillin potassium for oral solution, reconstituted (250 mg/5 mL), and stored at 5°, 25°, and 35°. The initial concentration of phenoxymethylpenicillin potassium (as percentage of label claim) varied between products. The rank order of apparent first-order degradation rate constants of the products varied at different temperatures. After 14 days at 5° (manufacturers' recommended storage period) only one product (Lilly) contained more than 90% of the label claim for drug content, whereas after 7 days at room temperature none of the products contained more than 90% of their label claims.

Phenoxymethylpenicillin potassium for oral solution (Veetids 125, Squibb, USA) was reconstituted (125 mg/5 mL) with distilled water and 5-mL samples were stored in 6-mL plastic oral syringes (Monoject) at 4°, 25°, 41°, 60°, and 75°, protected from light.[16] First-order degradation rate constants for phenoxymethylpenicillin potassium in the repackaged solutions increased with increasing temperature. No significant differences were found between the results of microbiological and spectrophotometric assays. Shelf-lives of less than 6 days at 4° and less than 1 day at 25° were calculated for repackaged solutions; these shelf-lives were shorter than the recommended periods for storage in original containers.

When 5-mL samples of phenoxymethylpenicillin potassium reconstituted oral solution (250 mg/5 mL, V-Cillin K, Eli Lilly, USA) were stored at 25°, 5°, 0°, −10°, and −20° in 26-mL amber, screw-cap, glass vials, degradation (by apparent first-order kinetics) increased with increasing temperature.[17] At least 90% of the initial phenoxymethylpenicillin potassium concentration was retained for 60 days at −20°, −10°, and 0°. None of the samples stored at 5° or 25° were stable for 60 days.

FURTHER INFORMATION. Penicillins and cephalosporins. Physicochemical properties and analysis in pharmaceutical and biological matrices [includes review of degradation routes]—Van Krimpen PC, Van Bennekom WP, Bult A. Pharm Weekbl (Sci) 1987;9:1–23. Nonisothermal kinetics using a microcomputer: A derivative approach to the prediction of the stability of penicillin formulations—Hempenstall JM, Irwin WJ, Li Wan Po A, Andrews AH. J Pharm Sci 1983;72(6):668–73.

FORMULATION

Excipients

Excipients that have been used in presentations of phenoxymethylpenicillin include:

Tablets, phenoxymethylpenicillin: colloidal silica, anhydrous; lactose; magnesium stearate; talc; wheat starch.
Phenoxymethylpenicillin calcium: titanium dioxide (E171).
Phenoxymethylpenicillin potassium: carnauba wax; cellulose; clove oil; D&C Red No.30; lactose; macrogol; magnesium stearate; maize starch; microcrystalline cellulose; povidone; sodium lauryl sulphate; sunset yellow FCF (E110); talc.
Oral liquids (powder for reconstitution), phenoxymethylpenicillin: arginine; sucrose; vanilla essence.
Phenoxymethylpenicillin potassium: allura red AC (E129); aspartame; citric acid; ponceau 4R (E124); saccharin sodium; silica gel; sodium citrate; sodium phosphate; sodium propionate; sucrose; sunset yellow FCF (E110); tartrazine (E102); xanthan gum.

Dry powder syrups

Displacement values

To overcome the problems associated with accurate measurement of 'inconvenient volumes' of water for reconstitution of dry syrups, Gibbins and James[18] presented equations that allowed determination of a dry syrup composition and selection of a corresponding 'convenient' volume of water for reconstitution. Displacement values (the volume of water, in mL, displaced by 1 g of the solid) for powders of phenoxymethylpenicillin potassium (0.66 mL), sucrose (0.65 ± 0.03 mL), glucose (0.69 ± 0.02 mL), lactose (0.67 ± 0.08 mL), and compound tragacanth (0.70 ± 0.07 mL) were calculated using values for the densities of solutions. Examples were presented in which the necessary quantities of sweetening agents required to produce the desired dry powder composition were calculated.

REFERENCES

1. Rapson HDC, Bird AE. J Pharm Pharmacol 1963;15:222T–231T.
2. Tsuji A, Kubo O, Miyamoto E, Yamana T. J Pharm Sci 1977;66(12):1675–9.
3. Tsuji A, Miyamoto E, Matsuda M, Nishimura K, Yamana T. J Pharm Sci 1982;71(12):1313–18.
4. Dunham JM. In: Florey K, editor. Analytical profiles of drug substances; vol 1. London: Academic Press, 1972:249–300.
5. Sieh DH. In: Florey K, editor. Analytical profiles of drug substances; vol 17. London: Academic Press, 1988:677–748.
6. Doyle FP, Nayler JHC. Advan Drug Res 1964;1:1–69.
7. Bird AE, Jennings KR, Marshall AC. J Pharm Pharmacol 1986;38:913–17.
8. Hartmann VV, Rödiger M, Schnabel G [German]. Pharm Ind 1976;39(11):991–7.
9. Forist AA, Brown LW, Royer ME. J Pharm Sci 1965;54(3):476–7.
10. Parker G, Cox RJ, Richards D. J Pharm Pharmacol 1955;7:683–91.
11. Hem SL, Russo EJ, Bahal SM, Levi RS. J Pharm Sci 1973;62(2):267–70.
12. Bundgaard H, Larsen C. Int J Pharmaceutics 1978;1:95–104.
13. Tsuji A, Matsuda M, Miyamoto E, Yamana T. J Pharm Pharmacol 1978;30:442–4.
14. Hempenstall JM, Irwin WJ, Li Wan Po A, Andrews AH. Int J Pharmaceutics 1985;23:131–46.
15. Jaffe JM, Certo NM, Pirakitikuir P, Colaizzi JL. Am J Hosp Pharm 1976;33:1005–10.
16. Grogan LJ, Jensen BK, Makoid MC, Baldwin JN. Am J Hosp Pharm 1979;36:205–8.
17. Allen LV, Lo P. Am J Hosp Pharm 1979;36:209–11.
18. Gibbins LB, James KC. Int J Pharmaceutics 1980;4:353–5.

Phenytoin (BAN, USAN, rINN) *Anticonvulsant*

Diphenylhydantoin
5,5-Diphenylimidazolidine-2,4-dione
$C_{15}H_{12}N_2O_2 = 252.3$

Phenytoin Sodium (BANM, rINNM)

Soluble phenytoin
$C_{15}H_{11}N_2NaO_2 = 274.3$
CAS—57-41-0 (phenytoin); 630-93-3 (phenytoin sodium)

Pharmacopoeial status

BP, USP (phenytoin, phenytoin sodium)

Preparations

Compendial

Phenytoin Oral Suspension BP (Phenytoin Mixture). An oral suspension containing 30 mg in 5 mL is usually available.
Phenytoin Capsules BP (Phenytoin Sodium Capsules). Contain phenytoin sodium. Capsules containing, in each, 25 mg, 50 mg, and 100 mg are usually available.
Phenytoin Tablets BP (Phenytoin Sodium Tablets). Contain phenytoin sodium. Coated tablets containing, in each, 50 mg and 100 mg are usually available.
Phenytoin Injection BP (Phenytoin Sodium Injection) is a sterile solution containing 5% w/v of phenytoin sodium in a mixture of 40% v/v of propylene glycol and 10% v/v of ethanol in water for injections. pH 11.5 to 12.1.
Phenytoin Tablets USP.
Phenytoin Oral Suspension USP.
Extended Phenytoin Sodium Capsules USP.
Prompt Phenytoin Sodium Capsules USP.
Phenytoin Sodium Injection USP. pH 10.0 to 12.3.

Non-compendial

Epanutin (P-D). *Capsules*, phenytoin sodium 25 mg, 50 mg, 100 mg, and 300 mg.
Infatabs (chewable tablets), phenytoin 50 mg.
Suspension, phenytoin 30 mg/5 mL. *Diluent*: syrup, life of diluted suspension 14 days.
Injection, (Epanutin Ready Mixed Parenteral), phenytoin sodium 50 mg/mL. The injection should not be used if a precipitate or haziness develops in the solution in the ampoule. It should not be added to intravenous infusion fluids as this causes precipitation of the acid.
Capsules and tablets of phenytoin sodium are also available from APS, Cox, Kerfoot.

NOTE. For an equivalent therapeutic effect, phenytoin 90 mg as phenytoin suspension 90 mg in 15 mL ≡ phenytoin sodium 100 mg as capsules or tablets. The Medicines Control Agency now advises that there are no clinically relevant differences in bioavailability between available phenytoin sodium tablets and capsules.

Containers and storage

Solid state

Phenytoin BP should be kept in a well-closed container.
Phenytoin Sodium BP should be kept in an airtight container.
Phenytoin USP and Phenytoin Sodium USP should be preserved in tight containers.

Dosage forms

Phenytoin Injection BP should be protected from light and stored at a temperature not exceeding 25°. Solutions in which a haziness or precipitate develops should not be used. Phenytoin Tablets USP should be preserved in well-closed containers. Extended Phenytoin Sodium Capsules USP, Prompt Phenytoin Sodium Capsules USP, and Phenytoin Oral Suspension USP should all be preserved in tight containers. The suspension should not be frozen.
Phenytoin Sodium Injection USP should be preserved in single-dose or in multiple-dose containers, preferably of Type I glass, at controlled room temperature. The injection should not be used if it is hazy or contains a precipitate.
Epanutin capsules and infatabs should be stored at a temperature not exceeding 30°.
Epanutin suspension and Epanutin Ready Mixed Parenteral should be stored at room temperature, not exceeding 25°; the latter should be protected from light.

PHYSICAL PROPERTIES

Phenytoin is a white or almost white crystalline powder; odourless or almost odourless.
Phenytoin sodium is a white crystalline powder; odourless and slightly hygroscopic. It gradually absorbs carbon dioxide on exposure to air with the subsequent liberation of phenytoin.

Melting point

Phenytoin melts at about 295°, with decomposition.

Dissociation constant

pK_a 8.3 (25°)

FURTHER INFORMATION. Application of a second-order derivative spectroscopic technique: determination of the ionisation constants of phenytoin and phenobarbital—Rosenberg LS, Jackson JL. Drug Dev Ind Pharm 1989;15(3):373–86.

Partition coefficient

Pinal and Yalkowsky[1] calculated a value of log P (octanol/water) for *phenytoin* of 2.32 at 25°.

Solubility

Phenytoin is practically insoluble in water; sparingly soluble in ethanol (1 in 70); slightly soluble in chloroform and in ether; and soluble in solutions of alkali hydroxides.
Phenytoin sodium is soluble in water and in ethanol; and practically insoluble in dichloromethane and in ether. Aqueous solutions absorb carbon dioxide which liberates the free base and causes the solution to become turbid.
Schwartz *et al*[2] determined the solubility profile of phenytoin in phosphate buffers of pH 7.4 and pH 5.4, at 25°, 30°, 37°, 44°, and 50°. Solubility increased as temperature increased. The solubility of phenytoin in aqueous buffered solution (pH 4.8 to 8.4) at 25° was low although it was greater at higher pH values (for example, 18.4 micrograms/mL at pH 4.9; 56.8 micrograms/mL at pH 8.3). In buffered (pH 7.4) methanolic solutions at 25° and 37°, phenytoin solubility was shown to be enhanced as the concentration of methanol was increased (up to 4% w/v).

FURTHER INFORMATION. Prediction of phenytoin solubility in intravenous admixtures: physicochemical theory [a comprehensive review with data for aqueous solubility, effect of pH and storage]—Newton DW, Kluza RB. Am J Hosp Pharm 1980;37:1647–51. Solubilisation by cosolvents II: phenytoin in binary and tertiary solvents [ethanol, methanol, propylene glycol, macrogol 400, macrogol 200, glycerol, sorbitol 70%, 1,3 butanediol]—Rubino JT, Blanchard J, Yalkowsky SH. J Parenter Sci Technol 1984;38:215–21.

Dissolution

The USP specifies that for Extended Phenytoin Sodium Capsules USP, the percentage of the labelled amount of $C_{15}H_{11}N_2NaO_2$ dissolved is not more than 40% in 30 minutes, is 55% in 60 minutes and is not less than 70% in 120 minutes. Dissolution medium: 900 mL of water; Apparatus 1 at 50 rpm.

The USP specifies that for Prompt Phenytoin Sodium Capsules USP, not less than 85% of the labelled amount of $C_{15}H_{11}N_2NaO_2$ is dissolved in 30 minutes. Dissolution medium: 900 mL of water; Apparatus 1 at 50 rpm.

Dissolution properties
Eleven commercially available brands of phenytoin sodium capsules (100 mg) were subjected to dissolution studies in distilled water using the USP XX basket and paddle methods and the spin-filter method.[3] Results, when correlated with observed differences in *in-vivo* parameters, suggested the availability of two types of phenytoin sodium capsules on the market; those that dissolved slowly with only 50% to 60% dissolution in one hour, and those that dissolved rapidly with over 80% dissolution in 30 minutes.

Workers in South Africa[4] demonstrated an increased rate of dissolution of phenytoin from montmorillonite:phenytoin combinations (1:1, 1:4, and 1:9) than from pure phenytoin; the dissolution rate of the test mixtures were comparable to that of phenytoin sodium capsules. Bioavailability studies in four healthy volunteers revealed that more phenytoin was absorbed from the montmorillonite mixtures (except the 1:4 combination) than from a commercially available phenytoin sodium capsule (Lennon, Ltd: stated to have bioequivalence with Epanutin, P-D), although the rate of absorption was comparable.

FURTHER INFORMATION. Comparison of ultraviolet and liquid chromatographic methods for dissolution testing of sodium phenytoin capsules—Shah VP, Ogger KE. J Pharm Sci 1986;75(11):1113–15. The effects of aging on the dissolution of phenytoin sodium capsule formulations—Rubino JT, Halterlein LM, Blanchard J. Int J Pharmaceutics 1985;26:165–74.

Crystal and molecular structure

Enantiomers
Two crystalline forms of phenytoin were isolated by Chakrabarti *et al*.[5] The needle-shaped crystals exhibited a slower rate of dissolution than the more regular crystalline form.

STABILITY

Reports of phenytoin crystallisation in infusion solutions are numerous.

Greenblatt and Shader[6] observed slow and incomplete precipitation of phenytoin sodium 500 mg (as a ready-mixed intravenous solution) from solutions in glucose 5%. After 24 hours at room temperature, phenytoin concentration in the supernatant was 85% of that predicted.

Spectrophotometric analysis[7] of free phenytoin crystallisation demonstrated greater stability of intravenous phenytoin sodium solution in sodium chloride 0.9% and in compound sodium lactate than in glucose 5% or glucose 5% in sodium chloride 0.9%. The authors suggested that crystallisation was a pH-dependent phenomenon. This theory was supported by Sistare and Greene[8] who added increasing amounts of 0.1M

sodium hydroxide followed by phenytoin injection (P-D) to each of four bottles of glucose 5% and found that a pH value greater than 9.5 was critical for the prevention of phenytoin precipitation. The inclusion of 0.1M sodium hydroxide prevented precipitation for over 24 hours.

Phenytoin sodium injection (100 mg/2 mL, Dilantin P-D) was admixed with 25, 50, 100 or 150 mL of glucose 5% or of sodium chloride 0.9%, the resulting infusion solutions were observed over a one-hour period for pH changes and crystal formation.[9] Although pH decreased with increasing dilution, admixture pH did not vary significantly during the study period. Crystallisation occurred rapidly in glucose 5% admixtures (pH 9.44 to 10.15) but no precipitation was observed in sodium chloride 0.9% (pH 9.82 to 10.81). Following infusion of admixtures (100 mg/50 mL) at a rate of 1 mL/minute over one hour, the phenytoin concentration in glucose 5% was significantly lower than that in sodium chloride 0.9% solution. The inclusion of filters in administration sets had no significant effect on phenytoin concentration in solution.

In a study of admixtures of phenytoin sodium injection (Elkins-Sinn and P-D) at various concentrations, crystal formation with a concomitant rapid decrease in phenytoin concentration was observed in each of four glucose 5% injection solutions from different manufacturers.[10] Greater stability of phenytoin was demonstrated in sodium chloride 0.9% injection and in compound sodium lactate injection; both of these solutions maintained over 95% of their initial concentration for eight hours.

The tendency of three different phenytoin sodium injection solutions (Dilantin, P-D, USA and Phenhydan and Phenytoin Concentrate, Desitin-Werk Carl Klinke, West Germany) to crystallise was investigated by Giacona and others[11] using macroscopic, microscopic and spectrophotometric methods. The two European formulations contained glycofurol or propylene glycol as diluent and tromethamine (Tris buffer) and/or sodium hydroxide as stabiliser, whereas the US product contained propylene glycol as diluent and sodium hydroxide as stabiliser. After 24 hours, crystallisation was apparent in Dilantin admixtures in glucose 5% or sodium chloride 0.9% but not in Phenhydan or Phenytoin Concentrate admixtures. Phenhydan and Phenytoin Concentrate were stable in glucose 5% injection for at least 24 hours.

In a comparative study, undiluted Dilantin injection (P-D) was shown to have lower 'inter-lot' variability and significantly higher 'apparent' pH than any of three generic injections (Elkins-Sinn, Lyphomed, or Solopak) examined.[12] At both concentrations studied (9.2 mg/mL and 18.4 mg/mL), the mean apparent pH was significantly higher for Dilantin than for the generic products on admixture with sodium chloride 0.9% injection. Microscopic and macroscopic crystals were detected in each of the lots of generic admixtures that had lower apparent pH, but not in admixtures of Dilantin. No significant differences in phenytoin sodium concentrations were detected between products.

Salem *et al*[13] found no significant difference between initial concentrations (1.0, 2.5, 5.0, 7.5, and 10 mg/mL) of phenytoin sodium (Dilantin, P-D) admixed in sodium chloride 0.9%, and concentrations measured after storage for 24 hours at 6°; however, in all samples, there was a slight increase in phenytoin concentration at one hour. Although crystal formation was not visible in the first hour after dilution, colloidal solutions were observed. Unfiltered and filtered solutions (1 mg/mL and 10 mg/mL) formed crystals after 18 hours and 72 hours, respectively.

Concentrations of phenytoin (4.6 mg/mL, 9.2 mg/mL, and 18.4 mg/mL), obtained by admixture of phenytoin sodium injection (Dilantin, P-D, USA) with sodium chloride 0.45% injection or sodium chloride 0.9% injection, were maintained at ambient temperature (29° ± 1°) in both filtered and unfiltered samples over a 24-hour study period.[14] Concentrations of phenytoin showed greatest variability in glucose 5% and in compound sodium lactate injection. Crystallisation was observed in all samples at all concentrations.

Stabilisation

Prevention of crystallisation of phenytoin from solutions of phenytoin sodium in sodium chloride 0.9% by 0.1M sodium hydroxide has been observed.[15]

FURTHER INFORMATION. An evaluation of the stability and safety of phenytoin infusion [review]—Goldschmied S. NY State J Pharm 1987;7:45–7.

INCOMPATIBILITY/COMPATIBILITY

Phenytoin was found to be chemically stable at 24° for 24 hours in three enteral nutrient products when added either as the free acid from the oral suspension (Dilantin-125 Suspension, P-D, USA, 125 mg/5 mL) or as the sodium salt from capsules (Dilantin Kapseals, P-D, USA, 100 mg).[16] However, passage of the samples through ultrafiltration tubes showed binding of phenytoin to components (possibly fats) in the enteral nutrient formulae. The therapeutic activity of phenytoin has been reported to be reduced when given concurrently with nasogastric feeds.[17]
Some workers have found markedly reduced phenytoin recovery (undiluted Dilantin, P-D, 25 mg/mL) following nasogastric administration of the suspension in a simulated clinical setting; the loss was attributed to a binding interaction between phenytoin and the plastic tubing.[18] Significantly more phenytoin was recovered from diluted samples. Subsequent studies by Butler et al[19] with a polyethylene-lined tube and two polyvinyl chloride tubes indicated that this interaction was an unlikely cause of phenytoin loss if the tube was flushed with distilled water or other suitable fluid after administration of the suspension.
However, dilution of phenytoin suspension (Dilantin-125, P-D, 125 mg/5 mL) with de-ionised water before in-vitro administration through percutaneous endoscopic gastrostomy (PEG) latex Pezzer catheters, under three different temperature regimens, led to an appreciable reduction in recovery of phenytoin compared to that observed with an undiluted sample.[20] The authors concluded that more drug was solubilised following dilution and adsorbed to the latex tubing. A similar but lesser effect was noted following irrigation of the catheter with de-ionised water.
Phenytoin sodium is reported to be incompatible with amikacin sulphate, cefapirin sodium, and clindamycin phosphate.

FURTHER INFORMATION. Phenytoin admixture solutions: a review of the literature with recommendations—Koren JF, Taylor T. Hosp Pharm 1988;23:646–8. Compatibilities and incompatibilities of some intravenous solution admixtures—Misgen R. Am J Hosp Pharm 1965;22:92–4. A guide to physical compatibility of intravenous drug admixtures—Patel JA, Phillips GL. Am J Hosp Pharm 1966;23:409–11.

FORMULATION

Excipients

Excipients that have been used in presentations of phenytoin include:
Capsules, phenytoin sodium: lactose; sucrose; talc.
Tablets: lactose; magnesium stearate; mannitol; povidone; quinoline yellow (E104) aluminium lake; saccharin sodium; sucrose; sunset yellow FCF (E110) aluminium lake; talc; wheat starch.

Oral liquids: acid fuchsine D; allura red AC (E129); aluminium magnesium silicate; carmellose sodium; citric acid, anhydrous; glycerol; polysorbate 40; sodium benzoate; sucrose; sunset yellow FCF (E110); vanillin.
Gingival pastes, phenytoin sodium: aluminium magnesium silicate; calcium carbonate; carmellose sodium; glycerol; saccharin sodium; sodium stearate; tricalcium phosphate.
Suppositories: Witepsol H15.
Injections, phenytoin sodium: ethanol; propylene glycol; sodium hydroxide.

Bioavailability

The administration of different phenytoin preparations has resulted in subtherapeutic serum-phenytoin concentrations and poor seizure control.[21]
A study by McElnay et al[22] using everted rat intestine and spectrophotometric techniques revealed a reduction in phenytoin absorption in the presence of constituents of gastro-intestinal medications and calcium in the rank order: calcium citrate > activated dimethicone > light kaolin > magnesium trisilicate. Bismuth subcarbonate actually increased phenytoin absorption by 28.2% over the 100-minute test period.
A comparison of phenytoin bioavailability from an oral solution and from several rectal dosage forms (fatty suppositories, an aqueous suspension, and micro-enema solutions in various solvents) was performed in eight healthy volunteers.[23] Mean peak plasma concentrations of phenytoin were achieved within 4 hours of oral dosing but phenytoin could not be detected following rectal dosing with fatty suppositories (Witepsol H15) or the aqueous suspension. Following administration of the rectal solutions, absorption occurred only in the first 30 minutes with a glycofurol vehicle, whereas slow, continuous absorption occurred over at least 8 hours with a macrogol 600 vehicle.
No significant difference was indicated between the bioavailabilities produced from five commercial phenytoin formulations, available as 100 mg tablets from Boots, Evans, Kerfoot, and Cox and as 100 mg capsules from Parke-Davis, when given in doses of 300 mg to eight healthy volunteers.[24] Mean absolute bioavailability of the oral preparations was 68% to 74% compared to a single intravenous dose of Epanutin Ready Mixed Parenteral (P-D, 300 mg in 6 mL) administered to four volunteers as a slow infusion in 50 mL of sodium chloride 0.9% injection.
Spanish workers[25] developed two phenytoin oral suspensions, from Epanutin capsules containing phenytoin sodium 100 mg. The suspensions differed only in the viscosity-increasing agents they contained (carmellose sodium or sodium alginate). Absorption studies in four healthy volunteers demonstrated the 'safety and usefulness' of both suspensions.
Shah et al[26] correlated the relative bioavailabilities (in 24 epileptic patients) of an oral solution (P-D), a slow-dissolving capsule (P-D), and a fast-dissolving capsule (Zenith) of phenytoin sodium 100 mg with dissolution data. The relative bioavailability of the slow-dissolving product was 73% and 80% of that of the oral solution and fast-dissolving capsule respectively.

Complexes and solid dispersions

A pharmaceutically elegant oral suspension (100 mg/5 mL) and a tablet (50 mg) were formulated from a lyophilised complex of phenytoin and β-cyclodextrin.[27] The oral suspension contained the complex dispersed in a 1:1 v/v mixture of water and glycerol and physical stability was maintained during six months storage at ambient temperature. Although sedimentation volume was 60%, the preparation was easily redispersed. Tablets prepared from the complex by wet granulation met

USP dissolution and other physical standards. Both preparations were thought to offer potential for enhanced absorption *in vivo*, due mainly to the amorphous, fine-particle nature of the compound being more amenable to rapid dissolution after administration.

The dissolution and aqueous solubility of phenytoin as a model drug was shown to be improved when incorporated into complexes with α-, β-, and γ-cyclodextrin epichlorhydrin polymers.[28] These results were mirrored by absorption studies in *dogs*, which demonstrated that the area under the plasma concentration versus time curves of the complex (for up to 24 hours after oral administration) was about twice that from phenytoin alone.

Solid dispersions of phenytoin with macrogol 6000, urea, or povidone 160 000 or 25 000 (in ratio 1:9) showed higher solubility and dissolution rates of phenytoin in water at 37° than corresponding physical mixtures or the drug alone.[29] Dissolution was greatest from the dispersions that contained povidone. The phenytoin content of tablets containing solid dispersions remained stable for two years at 20°. Phenytoin was stable during the preparation of both the solid dispersions and the tablets.

Suppositories

A displacement value of 1.2 has been recorded for phenytoin in Witepsol H15.

South African workers[30] formulated suppositories containing phenytoin and phenytoin sodium in different combinations of macrogol bases using Myrj 59 (polyoxyl 59 stearate) as surfactant. The formulations with the optimal *in-vitro* release rate of phenytoin were the macrogol blend 1000:1500:4000 (1:2:1) and those with Myrj 59 concentration of 10% (phenytoin sodium:Myrj 59, 1:1). These were selected for *in-vivo* release studies in *rabbits* and absorption data confirmed the *in-vitro* results. It was noted that the sodium salt gave the fastest absorption.

Factors affecting release rate

Bastami and Groves[31] investigated factors affecting the release pattern of phenytoin as the acid or the sodium salt from tablet and capsule formulations in water at 37°. The use of the free acid reduced the rate of release as did an increase in the amount of diluent, replacement of lactose by maize starch or calcium sulphate dihydrate, or the addition of magnesium stearate. The addition of sodium lauryl sulphate accelerated release. The tablets (phenytoin sodium 50 mg, Kerfoot) released their contents more rapidly than the capsules (phenytoin sodium 50 mg, P-D) in water; the time for release of 50% of the drug was 12 minutes and 32 minutes, respectively.

FURTHER INFORMATION. Bioavailability and dissolution of proprietary and generic formulations of phenytoin—Soryal I, Richens A. J Neurol Neurosurg Psychiatry 1992;55:688–91. Studies of the effect of pH, temperature and ring size on the complexation of phenytoin with cyclodextrins—Menard A, Dedhiya MG, Rhodes CT. Pharm Acta Helv 1988;63(11):303–8. Effect of some excipients [lactose, microcrystalline cellulose, aluminium hydroxide, aluminium magnesium silicate, colloidal silica, magnesium carbonate, mannitol, calcium hydrogen phosphate] on the dissolution of phenytoin and acetazolamide from capsule formulations—Hashim F, El-Din EZ. Acta Pharm Fenn 1989;98:197–204. Effect of formulation factors [lactose, maize starch, calcium sulphate, sodium sulphate, magnesium stearate:talc (1:9), Aerosil] on the *in vitro* dissolution characteristics of phenytoin sodium capsules—Ari-Ulubelen A, Akbuga J, Bayraktar-Alpmen G, Gülhan S. Pharm Ind 1986;48:393–5. Influence of pH on release of phenytoin sodium from slow-release dosage forms—Serajuddin ATM, Jarowski CI. J Pharm Sci 1993;82(3):306–10. Phenytoin prodrugs III: water-soluble prodrugs for oral and/or parenteral use—Varia SA, Schuller S, Sloan KB, Stella VJ. J Pharm Sci 1984;73(8):1068–73. New highly water-soluble phenytoin prodrugs—Pozzo AD, Acquasaliente M. Int J Pharmaceutics 1992;81:263–5. The determination of the amphiphilic properties of a prodrug (DDMS) of phenytoin in aqueous media—Müller DG, Stella VJ, Lötter AP. Int J Pharmaceutics 1992;86:175–86.

PROCESSING

Sterilisation

Phenytoin injection can be sterilised by filtration.

REFERENCES

1. Pinal R, Yalkowsky SH. J Pharm Sci 1988;77(6):518–22.
2. Schwartz PA, Rhodes CT, Cooper JW. J Pharm Sci 1977;66(7):994–7.
3. Shah VP, Prasad VK, Alston T, Cabana BE, Gural RP, Meyer MC. J Pharm Sci 1983;72(3):306–8.
4. Koeleman HA, van Zyl R, Steyn N, Boneschans B, Steyn HS. Drug Dev Ind Pharm 1990;16(5):791–805.
5. Chakrabarti S, van Severen R, Braeckman P. Pharmazie 1977;33:338–9.
6. Greenblatt DJ, Shader RI [letter]. N Eng J Med 1976;295:1078.
7. Bauman JL, Siepler JK, Fitzloff J. Drug Intell Clin Pharm 1977;11(11):646–9.
8. Sistare F, Greene R [letter]. Drug Intell Clin Pharm 1978;12:120.
9. Carmichael RR, Mahoney CD, Jeffrey LP. Am J Hosp Pharm 1980;37:95–8.
10. Pfeifle CE, Adler DS, Gannaway WL. Am J Hosp Pharm 1981;38:358–62.
11. Giacona N, Bauman JL, Siepler JK. Am J Hosp Pharm 1982;39:630–4.
12. Markowsky SJ, Kohls PR, Ehresman D, Leppik I. Am J Hosp Pharm 1991;48:510–14.
13. Salem RB, Yost RL, Torosian G, Davis FT, Wilder BJ. Drug Intell Clin Pharm 1980;14(9):605–8.
14. Cloyd JC, Bosch DE, Sawchuk RJ. Am J Hosp Pharm 1978;35:45–8.
15. Salem RB [letter]. Drug Intell Clin Pharm 1979;13(3):169.
16. Miller SW, Strom JG. Am J Hosp Pharm 1988;45:2529–32.
17. Summers VM, Grant R [letter]. Pharm J 1989;243:181.
18. Cacek AT, DeVito JM, Koonce JR. Am J Hosp Pharm 1986;43:689–92.
19. Butler HE, Lyndon RC, McDonald C [letter]. Aust J Hosp Pharm 1987;17(2):91.
20. Splinter MY, Seifert CF, Bradberry JC, Allen LV, Tu Y-H, Welsh JD. Am J Hosp Pharm 1990;47:373–7.
21. Pharm J 1985;235:406.
22. McElnay JC, D'Arcy PF, Throne O. Int J Pharmaceutics 1980;7:83–8.
23. Moolenaar F, Jelsma RBH, Visser J, Meijer DKF. Pharm Weekbl (Sci) 1981;116(3):1051–6.
24. Hirji MR, Measuria H, Kuhn S, Mucklow JC. J Pharm Pharmacol 1987;37:570–2.
25. Selva-Otaolaurruchi J, Rius-Atarcó F [Spanish]. Rev Soc Esp Farm Hosp 1989;13:291–5.
26. Shah VP, Prasad VK, Freeman C, Skelly JP, Cabana BE. J Pharm Sci 1983;72(3):309–10.
27. Hegde RP, Rhodes CT. Pharm Acta Helv 1985;60(2):53–7.

28. Uekama K, Otagiri M, Irie T, Seo H, Tsuruoka M. Int J Pharmaceutics 1985;23:35–42.
29. Jachowicz R. Int J Pharmaceutics 1987;35:7–12.
30. Pienaar EW, Boneschans B, Koeleman HA. Drug Dev Ind Pharm 1991;17(10):1397–1404.
31. Bastami SM, Groves MJ. Int J Pharmaceutics 1978;1:15.

Pilocarpine (BAN)   *Parasympathomimetic*

(2S,3R)-α-Ethyl-β-(1-methyl-1H-imidazol-5-yl)-γ-butyrolactone;   (3S,4R)-3-ethyldihydro-4-[(1-methyl-1H-imidazol-5-yl)methyl]furan-2(3H)-one
$C_{11}H_{16}N_2O_2 = 208.3$

Pilocarpine Hydrochloride (BANM)
Pilocarpine monohydrochloride
$C_{11}H_{16}N_2O_2,HCl = 244.7$

Pilocarpine Nitrate (BANM)
Pilocarpine mononitrate
$C_{11}H_{16}N_2O_2,HNO_3 = 271.3$
CAS—92-13-7 (pilocarpine); 54-71-7 (pilocarpine hydrochloride); 148-72-1 (pilocarpine nitrate)

Pharmacopoeial status

BP (pilocarpine hydrochloride, pilocarpine nitrate); USP (pilocarpine, pilocarpine hydrochloride, pilocarpine nitrate)

Preparations

Compendial
Pilocarpine Eye Drops BP. A sterile solution of pilocarpine hydrochloride in purified water. Eye drops containing 0.5, 1, 2, 3, and 4% w/v are usually available.
Pilocarpine Ocular System USP. A sterile device containing pilocarpine intended to permit the gradual release of pilocarpine.
Pilocarpine Hydrochloride Ophthalmic Solution USP. pH between 3.5 and 5.5.
Pilocarpine Nitrate Ophthalmic Solution USP. pH between 4.0 and 5.5.

Non-compendial
Isopto Carpine (Alcon). *Eye drops*, pilocarpine hydrochloride 0.5%, 1%, 2%, 3%, and 4%.
Minims Pilocarpine Nitrate (S&N Pharm). *Eye drops (single use)*, pilocarpine nitrate 1%, 2%, and 4% w/v.
Ocusert (Cusi). *Ocular insert*, modified release, pilocarpine 20 micrograms released per hour for one week (Pilo-20) and pilocarpine 40 micrograms released per hour for one week (Pilo-40).
Sno Pilo (S&N Pharm). *Eye drops*, pilocarpine hydrochloride 1%, 2%, and 4% w/v in a viscous vehicle. Do not dilute.

Containers and storage

Solid state
Pilocarpine Hydrochloride BP should be kept in an airtight container and protected from light.
Pilocarpine Nitrate BP should be kept in a well-closed container and protected from light.
Pilocarpine USP should be preserved in tight, light-resistant containers, in a cold place.

Pilocarpine Hydrochloride USP and Pilocarpine Nitrate USP should be preserved in tight, light-resistant containers.

Dosage forms
Pilocarpine Ocular System USP should be preserved in single-dose containers, in a cold place.
Pilocarpine Hydrochloride Ophthalmic Solution USP should be preserved in tight containers and Pilocarpine Nitrate Ophthalmic Solution USP in tight, light-resistant containers.
Isopto Carpine should be stored in a cool place away from direct sunlight. The container (with screw-on cap) should be kept tightly closed.
Minims Pilocarpine Nitrate should be stored in a cool place (8° to 15°) and not exposed to strong sunlight.
Ocusert systems should be stored in a refrigerator at 2° to 8°. Do not freeze.
Sno Pilo should be stored in a cool place and should not be dispensed from any container other than the original bottle.

PHYSICAL PROPERTIES

Pilocarpine exists as a viscous, oily liquid or as crystals; it is exceedingly hygroscopic.
Pilocarpine hydrochloride exists as colourless crystals or as a white or almost white crystalline powder; odourless and hygroscopic.
Pilocarpine nitrate exists as colourless or shiny white crystals or as a white crystalline powder; odourless.

Melting point

Pilocarpine melts at about 34°.
Pilocarpine hydrochloride melts, within a range of not more than 3° from beginning to end of melting, between 199° and 205°.
Pilocarpine nitrate melts, within a range of not more than 3° from beginning to end of melting, between 171° and 176°, with decomposition.

pH

Solutions of *pilocarpine hydrochloride* and of *pilocarpine nitrate* are acid to litmus.
pH of a 5% w/v solution of *pilocarpine hydrochloride* in carbon dioxide-free water, 3.5 to 4.5.
pH of a 5% w/v solution of *pilocarpine nitrate*, 3.5 to 4.5.

Dissociation constants

pK_a 1.6, 7.1 (15°)
pK_a 6.88 (25°), 6.67 (34°)[1]

Partition coefficients

Observed partition coefficients for *pilocarpine* in octanol-aqueous buffer systems at 25° tended to increase with an increase in temperature and pH.[1] No detectable partitioning of *pilocarpine* into the octanol phase of an octanol-water system at pH 4.67 was observed; at this pH, over 99% of the molecules were thought to be ionised (cationic species). See Formulation, below.

Solubility

Pilocarpine is soluble in water, in ethanol, and in chloroform; sparingly soluble in ether and in benzene; practically insoluble in light petroleum.
Pilocarpine hydrochloride is very soluble in water (1 in less than 1 part); freely soluble in ethanol (1 in 3); slightly soluble in chloroform (1 in 360); practically insoluble or insoluble in ether.
Pilocarpine nitrate is freely soluble in water (1 in 8); sparingly soluble in ethanol; practically insoluble or insoluble in chloroform and in ether.

STABILITY

Degradation pathways and kinetics

In aqueous solution, degradation of pilocarpine proceeds by two processes: hydrolysis of the ester linkage of the lactone ring to yield pilocarpic acid, and epimerisation about the α-carbon to yield isopilocarpine which can subsequently hydrolyse to isopilocarpic acid. The hydrolysis[2] is proposed to be a cyclic equilibrium process that is catalysed by hydrogen ions and hydroxide ions. In neutral and basic aqueous solutions the equilibrium position shifts to pilocarpic acid whereas in acidic aqueous solutions it shifts to pilocarpine. Epimerisation occurs at alkaline pH and although some workers[3] reported that epimerisation of pilocarpine to isopilocarpine was irreversible, further work[4] has revealed the reversible nature of this reaction. At pH 10.9, and other alkaline pH values, the equilibrium was in favour of isopilocarpine. It was also shown that pilocarpine and isopilocarpine had similar hydrolysis rate constants (0.04/min and 0.044/min, respectively). Thus, in alkaline solution, pilocarpine undergoes concurrent epimerisation and hydrolysis. In general, preparation of pilocarpine solutions at pH 4 to 5 is recommended to ensure acceptable stability.

The kinetics of the overall degradation of pilocarpine (psuedo-first-order reaction[4]) and of the hydrolysis and epimerisation processes have been discussed.[2-4]

Effect of temperature

The relative importance of epimerisation to hydrolysis of pilocarpine in aqueous solution at pH 10.9 increased[4] with an increase in temperature, from 12% at 18° to 20% at 66°.

During storage at 2° or at 20° the major degradation product of pilocarpine hydrochloride eye drops was pilocarpic acid whereas during heating at 100° the major product was isopilocarpine.[5] Values for $t_{10\%}$ of 3.6 months, 1 month, and 1.7 hours at 2°, 20°, and 100°, respectively, were calculated. The eye drops (pH 6.5) contained pilocarpine hydrochloride 20 mg/mL, benzalkonium chloride 0.2 mg/mL, boric acid 7 mg/mL, borax 3.75 mg/mL, and disodium edetate 1 mg/mL, and were sterilised at 100° for 30 minutes.

Aqueous solutions of pilocarpine chloride 2% w/w, buffered with sodium phosphate to pH 6.9, were stabilised by storage at −5° in the frozen state.[6] Over a period of 28 weeks, 2% decomposition occurred at −5° compared with 9% at 4°, and 38% at 20°.

Buffers for eye drops

Conflicting views exist concerning the influence of different buffers on the degradation of pilocarpine. In general, phosphate and carbonate but not borate buffers are thought to catalyse decomposition. Riegelman and Vaughan[7] recommended that for patient comfort pilocarpine hydrochloride eye drops should be buffered to pH 6.8 with sodium acid phosphate and sodium phosphate although, at this pH, stability is less than in unbuffered solutions; Cadwallader[8] also considered that a mixture of these salts at pH 6.5 was suitable. However, Anderson and FitzGerald[9] noted that phosphates catalyse the degradation of pilocarpine and suggested that either sodium hydroxide or borax be used to adjust the pH to about 6.5. Other workers[10] have used a combination of glacial acetic acid and sodium hydroxide as the buffer system.

Brown et al[11] showed that Sørensen's phosphate buffer decreased the stability of a pilocarpine hydrochloride 1% solution (pH 6.2) but the addition of 0.5% methylcellulose 4000 cP significantly reduced this deleterious effect. In buffered solutions, benzalkonium chloride increased the rate of hydrolysis. However, in unbuffered solutions, methylcellulose or benzalkonium chloride 0.01% enhanced the stability of pilocarpine

hydrochloride. In the presence of combinations of these three additives, effects on pilocarpine stability were more complex.

Containers

Lime-glass containers have been noted to leach alkali, which can catalyse the hydrolysis of pilocarpine.[12] Pilocarpine solutions should be stored in glass or plastic containers that leach negligible alkali.

Autoclaving

Fagerström[13] demonstrated that aqueous solutions of pilocarpine hydrochloride 2% (with sodium chloride 0.4% and phenylmercuric nitrate 0.001%), of initial pH 4.2, withstood autoclaving at 110° for 30 minutes and remained stable for at least 12 months when stored at room temperature in the dark (final pH 3.5). At pH 5, about 5% loss of initial concentration of pilocarpine was detected[14] following autoclaving for 24 hours at 120°. Pilocarpine eye drops[10] buffered to pH 5 with acetic acid and sodium hydroxide were stable to autoclaving at 120° for 20 minutes and less than 10% decomposition was detected after storage for 5 years. At pH 6.8 however,[14] the half-life of pilocarpine was calculated as 34 minutes at 120° compared to 66 days at room temperature (25°).

FURTHER INFORMATION. Contribution á l'étude de la stabilité de la pilocarpine en milieu aqueux [Part 1–identification of decomposition products of pilocarpine]—Baeschlin K, Etter JC, Moll H [French]. Pharm Acta Helv 1969;44:301–9. [Part 2–kinetic study of the hydrolysis of pilocarpine]—Baeschlin K, Etter JC [French]. Pharm Acta Helv 1969;44:339–47. Quantitative analysis of degradation products in pilocarpine hydrochloride ophthalmic formulations—Neville GA, Hasan FB, Smith ICP. J Pharm Sci 1977;66(5):638–42. High-performance liquid chromatographic analysis of pilocarpine hydrochloride, isopilocarpine, pilocarpic acid and isopilocarpic acid in eye-drop preparations [commercially available in Australia]—Kennedy JM, McNamara PE. J Chromatogr 1981;212:331–8. Stability of pilocarpine hydrochloride and pilocarpine nitrate ophthalmic solutions submitted by US hospitals—Kreienbaum MA, Page DP. Am J Hosp Pharm 1986;43:109–17. [Study of the hydrolysis of pilocarpine in Carbopol hydrogels]—Testa B, Etter JC [French]. Can J Pharm Sci 1975;10(1):16–20.

INCOMPATIBILITY/COMPATIBILITY

Pilocarpine hydrochloride is incompatible with chlorhexidine acetate and phenylmercuric salts. Incompatibility is also reported with alkalis, iodine, silver salts, and mercurous chloride.

Pilocarpine nitrate is incompatible with chlorhexidine acetate and solutions containing more than 1% pilocarpine nitrate are incompatible with benzalkonium chloride. Incompatibility is also reported with silver nitrate, mercuric bichloride, iodides, gold salts, tannins, mercurous chloride, potassium permanganate, and alkalis.

FORMULATION

Excipients

Excipients that have been used in presentations of pilocarpine include:

Eye drops, pilocarpine hydrochloride: benzalkonium chloride; borax; boric acid; disodium edetate; hypromellose; sodium chloride; sodium citrate.

Pilocarpine nitrate: borax; boric acid; camphor; chlorbutol; citric acid; menthol; methylcellulose; methyl hydroxybenzoate;

phenol; phenylmercuric nitrate; polyvinyl alcohol; sodium acetate; sodium chloride; sodium nitrate.

Ocular absorption

Several physicochemical and physiological properties must be considered during the formulation of ophthalmic solutions of pilocarpine. Pilocarpine is most stable at acidic pH. However, ocular absorption is reduced at lower pH as most of the pilocarpine is in the less permeable, ionised form. Other factors that influence absorption include the buffer capacity and extent of production of tear fluid. These factors also influence the irritant properties of ophthalmic solutions; the further the pH is below physiological pH the more pain and irritation occurs.

Mitra and Mikkelson[1] investigated the *in-vitro* permeation of pilocarpine across *rabbit* corneal membrane as a function of the state of ionisation of pilocarpine. Although the permeability of the unionised species was about double that of the ionised species, there was evidence of transport of ionised pilocarpine under certain pH conditions. The corneal permeability of pilocarpine was linearly related to its octanol-water partition coefficient and both of these properties were linearly related to the degree of ionisation.

A comprehensive study of the effects of the vehicle on ocular penetration of pilocarpine in albino *rabbits* revealed that as the pH of an aqueous solution of pilocarpine was increased (isotonic Sørensen's phosphate buffer, from pH 5 to 8) corneal penetration of pilocarpine increased.[15] This was attributed to the solubility characteristics of pilocarpine as well as reduced irritation and lachrymation in the eye at neutral and alkaline pH, rather than specific pH-partition behaviour.

The magnitude and duration of the reduction in pH of tear film following administration of pilocarpine eye drops[16] was related to the contact time and acidic buffer capacity as well as to the solution pH. Administration of commercial eye drops or sprays (pH 4.4 to 5.5) of pilocarpine salts to *rabbits* lowered the tear film pH (initially pH 7.47) by 1.1 to 1.6 units whereas continuous administration of pilocarpine base as ocular therapeutic systems produced negligible effects on the tear film pH.

Patton[17] demonstrated that as the instilled volume of a pilocarpine nitrate solution was decreased, the fraction of the dose absorbed into the interior of the eye (of *rabbits*) was increased. For example, a 5-microlitre dose of 1.61×10^{-2}M pilocarpine nitrate was expected to yield the same area under the aqueous humour concentration versus time curve as a 25-microlitre dose of 1×10^{-2}M pilocarpine nitrate.

Effect of buffers

When aqueous isotonic pilocarpine nitrate 1% w/v solutions, buffered at pH 4.75 with 0.075M buffer, were instilled ocularly to *rabbits*, the pharmacological effect (miotic response) of the different formulations decreased in the order: unbuffered > acetate-buffered > phosphate-buffered > citrate-buffered.[18] Methods of predicting the relative ocular bioavailability of pilocarpine from such solutions as a function of concentration of these buffers were discussed. The same workers[19] had previously demonstrated that the pharmacological activity of pilocarpine in solution (as the nitrate) was dependent on the concentration of the buffer (citrate) in the formulation.

Ahmed and Chaudhuri[20] examined the influence of buffer capacity on the ocular absorption (in *rabbits*) of pilocarpine from solutions of pilocarpine nitrate 1% w/v at pH 4.0 that contained acetate, phosphate, or citrate buffers and inulin 0.2% w/v. Ocular absorption from the solutions (calculated by several methods) decreased in the order: unbuffered > acetate-buffered > phosphate-buffered > citrate-buffered. However, other factors such as excessive lachrymation and irritation can also affect absorption. Thus the concentration and type of buffer was found to influence the ocular absorption of pilocarpine. Earlier work[21] had claimed that for 'optimum ocular penetration of pilocarpine, the system should not reduce the tear film pH appreciably, and should allow rapid tear pH re-equilibration'.

Gels, inserts, and other ocular vehicles

Major approaches that have been investigated (*in vitro* and *in vivo*) during the development of sustained-release preparations of pilocarpine include the use of viscous gels, erodible or non-erodible matrices, and emulsion systems. Examples of these and other approaches are outlined below.

Pilocarpine-loaded gelatin or albumin microspheres,[22] and gels and films (erodible and non-erodible),[23] exhibited prolonged release of pilocarpine *in vitro*, and prolonged activity and enhanced miotic activity in *rabbits* when compared with aqueous or viscous solutions. Similarly, when pilocarpine nitrate was incorporated into a 25% poloxamer gel, enhanced activity (in *rabbits*) compared to that of an aqueous solution was demonstrated.[24]

The duration of miotic response (in albino *rabbits*)[25] produced by pilocarpine nitrate 2% w/v in Carbopol 940 or Carbopol 941 gels was greater than that of conventional eye drops of pilocarpine 2% w/v. Increasing the concentration of Carbopol 940 (1% w/v to 6% w/v) in the gel increased the duration of response. Addition of benzalkonium chloride, autoclaving (at 121° for 30 minutes), or gamma irradiation (2.5 Mrad) had no effect on response although irradiation produced a brittle gel. Addition of chlorbutol or disodium edetate to the gels decreased the response. Viscosities of these and other hydrogels were measured.

Rheological properties of hydrogels and hydrosols of pilocarpine based on carmellose sodium, povidone, or polyacrylic acids were investigated and diffusion coefficients measured as an indication of their potential for sustained release.[26] A lyophilised preparation of pilocarpine with an acrylic-methacrylic acid copolymer (Fluka-AG, Switzerland) showed superior stability compared to an aqueous solution of pilocarpine. Studies in *rabbits* and in humans[27] revealed that the miotic activity of pilocarpine was prolonged and intensified in preparations based on Carbopol 934 or on the acrylic-methacrylic acid copolymer compared with an aqueous solution. Further work[28] examined the optimisation of the formulation of a liquid preparation based on the latter copolymer *in vitro* and *in vivo* (in humans).

Schoenwald *et al*[29] investigated the effects of the viscosity of pilocarpine nitrate gels on miotic response in *rabbits*. Gels were prepared with ethylene maleic anhydride, carbomer (Carbopol 940), hydroxyethylcellulose, polyacrylamide, ethylhydroxyethylcellulose, hydroxypropylcellulose, and poly(methylvinyl ether-maleic anhydride).

Saettone *et al*[30] developed polymeric ophthalmic inserts, based on four types of polyvinyl alcohol and two types of hydroxypropylcellulose, that contained pilocarpine nitrate or a pilocarpine/polyacrylic acid salt. Mechanisms of release *in vitro* and chemical and physicochemical factors affecting release were studied. All inserts produced a significant increase in bioavailability (area under miosis versus time curves) in albino *rabbits* compared to a standard ophthalmic solution of pilocarpine nitrate. Preliminary studies *in vitro* of ophthalmic inserts of pilocarpine nitrate prepared with pepsin-treated telopeptide-poor foetal calf skin collagen as a carrier revealed zero-order kinetics for the release of pilocarpine following an initial 'boost release'.[31] Three types of collagen film (plain, cross-linked, and a collagen-hydrazide derivative) were used; alteration of the rate of release was achieved by modification of the collagen carrier. Increased amounts of pilocarpine were detected in the aqueous humour of *rabbits* following administration of a 10^{-2}M pilocarpine ointment, which consisted of a soft paraffin-based vehicle and 5% water, compared to an equivalent dose of an aqueous solution of pilocarpine.[15] The increase was attributed to a higher effective concentration of pilocarpine in the ointment and an increase in contact time.

Attia and Habib[32] measured the intra-ocular pressure and miotic responses in *rabbits* following administration of o/w, w/o, o/w/o, and w/o/w emulsions and an oil suspension, each containing pilocarpine hydrochloride 1%. Diffusion coefficients *in vitro* did not correlate with results *in vivo*.

FURTHER INFORMATION. Preliminary pharmacokinetic model of pilocarpine [nitrate] uptake and distribution in the eye [in *rabbits*]—Himmelstein KJ, Guvenir I, Patton TF. J Pharm Sci 1978;67(5):603–6. Quantitative evaluation of topically applied pilocarpine in the precorneal area [in *rabbits*]—Thombre AG, Himmelstein KJ. J Pharm Sci 1984;73(2):219–22. Mechanistic and quantitative evaluation of precorneal pilocarpine disposition in albino *rabbits* [influence of precorneal loss parameters on bioavailability]—Lee VH-L, Robinson JR. J Pharm Sci 1979;68(6):673–84. Pilocarpine release [*in vitro*] from hydroxypropylcellulose-polyvinylpyrrolidone matrices—Urtti A, Juslin M, Miinalainen O. Int J Pharmaceutics 1985;25:165–78. Systemic absorption of ocular pilocarpine [modified by polymer matrices—Urtti A, Salminen L, Miinalainen O. Int J Pharmaceutics 1985;23:147–61. Pilocarpine bioavailability [in *rabbits*] from a mucoadhesive liposomal ophthalmic drug delivery system [based on Carbopol 1342]—Durrani AM, Davies NM, Thomas M, Kellaway IW. Int J Pharmaceutics 1992;88:409–15. Controlled release of pilocarpine from coated polymeric ophthalmic inserts prepared by extrusion—Saettone MF, Torracca MT, Pagano A, Giannaccini B, Rodriguez L, Cini M. Int J Pharmaceutics 1992;86:159–66. Optimisation of pilocarpine loading onto nanoparticles by sorption procedures—Harmia T, Speiser P, Kreuter J. Int J Pharmaceutics 1986;31:45–54. Enhancement of the myotic response of *rabbits* with pilocarpine-loaded polybutylcyanoacrylate nanoparticles—Harmia T, Kreuter J, Speiser P, Boye T, Gurny R, Kubis A. Int J Pharmaceutics 1986;31:187–93. Vehicle effects on ocular drug bioavailability. III. Shear-facilitated [mechanical shearing or blinking] pilocarpine release from ointments [water-in-oil emulsion *in vitro* and in *rabbits*]—Sieg JW, Robinson JR. J Pharm Sci 1979;68(6):724–8. Stability-indicating assay method for pilocarpine nitrate in reservoirs used in the cystic fibrosis indictor system—Wong O, Anderson C, Allaben L, Pabmanabhan R, Lattin G. Int J Pharmaceutics 1991;76:171–5. Electrically controlled drug delivery system using polyelectrolyte gels. Sawahata K, Hara M, Yasunaga H, Osada Y. J Controlled Release 1990;14:253–62. Pilocarpine prodrugs. I. Synthesis, physicochemical properties and kinetics of lactonisation of pilocarpic acid [mono] esters—Bundgaard H, Falch E, Larsen C, Mikkelson TJ. J Pharm Sci 1986;75(1):36–43. Pilocarpine prodrugs. II. Synthesis, stability, bioconversion, and physicochemical properties of sequentially labile pilocarpine acid diesters—Bundgaard H, Falch E, Larsen C, Mosher GL, Mikkelson TJ. J Pharm Sci 1986;75(8):775–83. Ocular bioavailability of pilocarpic acid mono- and di-ester prodrugs as assessed by miotic activity in the *rabbit*—Mosher GL, Bundgaard H, Falch E, Larsen C, Mikkelson TJ. Int J Pharmaceutics 1987;39:113–20.

REFERENCES

1. Mitra AK, Mikkelson TJ. J Pharm Sci 1988;77(9):771–5.
2. Chung P-H, Chin T-F, Lach J-L. J Pharm Sci 1970;59(9):1300–5.
3. Nunes MA, Brochmann-Hanssen E. J Pharm Sci 1974;63(5):716–21.
4. Bundgaard H, Hansen SH. Int J Pharmaceutics 1982;10:281–9.
5. Kuks PFM, Weekers LEA, Goldhoorn PB. Pharm Weekbl (Sci) 1990;12(5):196–9.
6. Larsen SS. Dansk Tidsskr Farm 1971;45:317–19.
7. Riegelman S, Vaughan DG. J Am Pharm Assoc (Pract Pharm) 1958;19(8):474–7.
8. Cadwallader DE. Am J Hosp Pharm 1967;24:33–6.
9. Anderson RA, FitzGerald SD. Australas J Pharm 1967;48:S108–9.
10. Baeschlin K, Etter JC [French]. Pharm Acta Helv 1969;44:348–55.
11. Brown IR, Dyer AE, Elowe IN, Stauffer IE, Walker GC. Can J Pharm Sci 1966;1(May):22–6.
12. Gibbs IS, Tuckerman MM. J Pharm Sci 1974;63(2):276–9.
13. Fagerström R. J Pharm Pharmacol 1963;15:479–82.
14. Riegelman S, Vaughan DG. J Am Pharm Assoc (Pract Pharm) 1958;19(9):537–40.
15. Sieg JW, Robinson JR. J Pharm Sci 1977;66(9):1222–8.
16. Longwell A, Birss S, Keller N, Moore D. J Pharm Sci 1976;65(11):1654–7.
17. Patton TF. J Pharm Sci 1977;66(7):1058–9.
18. Mitra AK, Mikkelson TJ. Int J Pharmaceutics 1987;37:19–26.
19. Mitra AK, Mikkelson TJ. Int J Pharmaceutics 1982;10:219–29.
20. Ahmed I, Chaudhuri B. Int J Pharmaceutics 1988;44:97–105.
21. Ahmed I, Patton TF. Int J Pharmaceutics 1984;19:215–27.
22. Leucuta SE. Int J Pharmaceutics 1989;54:71–8.
23. Grass GM, Cobby J, Makoid MC. J Pharm Sci 1984;73(5):618–21.
24. Miller SC, Donovan MD. Int J Pharmaceutics 1982;12:147–52.
25. Deshpande SG, Shirolkar S. J Pharm Pharmacol 1989;41:197–200.
26. Pergande G, Keipert S [German]. Pharmazie 1990;45(H8):582–6.
27. Pergande G, Keipert S, Klatt A [German]. Pharmazie 1990;45(H8):587–91.
28. Keipert S, Siebenbrodt I [German]. Pharmazie 1990;45(H8):596–9.
29. Schoenwald RD, Ward RL, De Santis LM, Roehrs RE. J Pharm Sci 1978;67(9):1280–3.
30. Saettone MF, Giannaccini B, Chetoni P, Galli G, Chiellini E. J Pharm Pharmacol 1984;36:229–34.
31. Vasantha R, Sehgal PK, Rao KP. Int J Pharmaceutics 1988;47:95–102.
32. Attia MA, Habib FS. STP Pharma 1986;2(18):636–40.

Piperazine   *Anthelmintic*

Piperazine
$C_4H_{10}N_2 = 86.14$

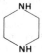

Piperazine Adipate
$C_4H_{10}N_2, C_6H_{10}O_4 = 232.3$

Piperazine Citrate
$(C_4H_{10}N_2)_3,2C_6H_8O_7,xH_2O = 642.7$ (anhydrous)

Piperazine Hydrate
$C_4H_{10}N_2,6H_2O = 194.2$

Piperazine Phosphate
$C_4H_{10}N_2,H_3PO_4,H_2O = 202.1$
CAS—110-85-0 (piperazine); 142-88-1 (piperazine adipate); 144-29-6 (piperazine citrate, anhydrous); 41372-10-5 (piperazine citrate, hydrate); 142-63-2 (piperazine hydrate); 14538-56-8 (piperazine phosphate, anhydrous); 18534-18-4 (piperazine phosphate)

Pharmacopoeial status

BP (piperazine adipate, piperazine citrate, piperazine hydrate, piperazine phosphate); USP (piperazine, piperazine citrate)

Preparations

Compendial
Piperazine Phosphate Tablets BP. Tablets containing, in each, 520 mg of piperazine phosphate are usually available. Piperazine phosphate 520 mg is approximately equivalent to 500 mg of piperazine hydrate.
Piperazine Citrate Elixir BP. A solution containing 18.75% w/v of piperazine citrate in a suitable flavoured vehicle. If the elixir is diluted, the diluted elixir should be freshly prepared. Piperazine citrate elixir contains, in 5 mL, the equivalent of about 750 mg of piperazine hydrate.
Piperazine Citrate Tablets USP.
Piperazine Citrate Syrup USP. The syrup is prepared from piperazine citrate or from piperazine to which an equivalent amount of citric acid has been added.

Non-compendial
Pripsen (R&C). *Oral powder*, piperazine phosphate 4 g and sennosides 15.3 mg/sachet.
An elixir of piperazine hydrate 750 mg/5 mL (as citrate) is available from Cupal (Expelix).

Containers and storage

Solid state
Piperazine Hydrate BP should be kept in an airtight container and protected from light.
Piperazine Adipate BP and Piperazine Citrate BP should be kept in well-closed containers.
Piperazine USP should be preserved in tight containers and protected from light.
Piperazine Citrate USP should be preserved in well-closed containers.

Dosage forms
Piperazine Citrate Elixir BP should be protected from light and stored at a temperature not exceeding 25°.
Piperazine Citrate Tablets USP and Piperazine Citrate Syrup USP should be preserved in tight containers.
Pripsen powder should be stored below 25° in a dry place. Any unused powder should be discarded.

PHYSICAL PROPERTIES

Piperazine appears as white to slightly off-white lumps or flakes with an ammoniacal odour.
Piperazine adipate is a white, crystalline powder.
Piperazine citrate is a white, granular powder.
Piperazine hydrate exists as colourless, deliquescent crystals.

Piperazine phosphate is a white crystalline powder; odourless or almost odourless.

Melting point

Piperazine melts in the range 109° to 113°.
Piperazine adipate melts at about 250°, with decomposition.
Piperazine citrate melts at about 190° (after drying at 100° to 105°).
Piperazine hydrate melts at about 43°.

pH

A 10% solution of *piperazine* has a pH of 10.8 to 11.8.
Aqueous solutions of *piperazine adipate* (0.2 to 0.01M) have a pH of 5.45.
A 10% solution of *piperazine citrate* has a pH of 5.0 to 6.0.
A 5% solution of *piperazine hydrate* has a pH of 10.5 to 12.0.
A 1% solution of *piperazine phosphate* has a pH of 6.0 to 6.5.

Dissociation constants

pK_a 5.7, 9.8 (20°)

Partition coefficient

Log *P* (octanol), −1.2

Solubility

	Water	Ethanol	Chloroform	Ether
Piperazine	soluble	soluble	—	insoluble
Piperazine adipate	1 in 18	practically insoluble	practically insoluble	practically insoluble
Piperazine citrate	1 in 1.5	practically insoluble	practically insoluble	practically insoluble
Piperazine hydrate	1 in 3	1 in 1	—	very slightly soluble
Piperazine phosphate	1 in 60	practically insoluble	practically insoluble	practically insoluble

Piperazine is freely soluble in glycerol and glycols.
Piperazine phosphate is soluble in dilute hydrochloric acid.

Effect of temperature
The approximate solubility of *piperazine adipate* in water at 30° is 1 in 15, and at 56.3° is 1 in 10.

Dissolution

The USP specifies that for Piperazine Citrate Tablets USP not less than 75% of the labelled amount of $C_4H_{10}N_2,6H_2O$ is dissolved in 45 minutes. Dissolution medium: 900 mL of water; Apparatus 2 at 50 rpm.

STABILITY

Piperazine adipate is stable to heat and air.
It was postulated by Nielsen and Reimer[1] that a reduction in the piperazine content of a syrup, containing piperazine citrate, over an 18-month period was due to an interaction between piperazine and glucose and fructose, which were produced by the hydrolysis of sucrose. Glucose may react with piperazine to form an aminofructose, which may in turn react with another piperazine molecule; a similar reaction can occur with fructose. A syrup containing sorbitol instead of sucrose was stable for 14 months when stored at 25°.

INCOMPATIBILITY/COMPATIBILITY

Piperazine is reported to be incompatible with glucose and fructose.[1]

FORMULATION

PIPERAZINE CITRATE ELIXIR
The following formula was given in the *British Pharmaceutical Codex 1973*:

Piperazine citrate		187.5 g
Peppermint spirit		5.0 mL
Green S and tartrazine solution		15.0 mL
Glycerol		100.0 mL
Syrup		500.0 mL
Water	to	1000.0 mL

Dissolve the piperazine citrate in part of the water and add the green S and tartrazine solution, glycerol, syrup, peppermint spirit, and sufficient water to produce the required volume, and mix. Diluent, syrup. The diluted elixir should be freshly prepared.

Excipients

Excipients that have been used in presentations of piperazine include:
Tablets, piperazine sebacate: lactose; macrogol 4000; magnesium stearate; maize starch; sucrose.
Effervescent granules, piperazine hydrate: citric acid; D-mannitol; monosodium carbonate; povidone; tartaric acid.
Syrups, piperazine hydrate: carmoisine (E122); citric acid; pomegranate oil; syrup.
Oral powders, piperazine phosphate: carmine (E120); saccharin.
Suppositories, piperazine sebacate: semi-synthetic glycerides.

REFERENCE

1. Nielsen A, Reimer P. Arch Pharm Chemi Sci 1975;3:73–8.

Piroxicam (BAN, USAN, rINN)

Analgesic; Anti-inflammatory
4-Hydroxy-2-methyl-*N*-2-pyridyl-2*H*-1,2-benzothiazine-3-carboxamide 1,1-dioxide
$C_{15}H_{13}N_3O_4S$ = 331.35
CAS—36322-90-4

Pharmacopoeial status

USP

Preparations

Compendial
Piroxicam Capsules USP.

Non-compendial
Feldene (Pfizer). *Capsules*, piroxicam 10 mg and 20 mg.
Tablets, dispersible, piroxicam 10 mg and 20 mg.
Melt tablets, piroxicam 20 mg.
Suppositories, piroxicam 20 mg.
Gel, piroxicam 0.5%.
Injection, intramuscular, piroxicam 20 mg/mL.

Piroxicam capsules of various strengths are also available from APS, Ashbourne (Pirozip), Cox, Evans, Kerfoot, Lagap, Norton.

Containers and storage

Solid state
Piroxicam USP should be preserved in tight, light-resistant containers.

Dosage forms
Piroxicam Capsules USP should be preserved in tight, light-resistant containers.
Feldene capsules, dispersible tablets, melt tablets, and gel should be stored below 30°. Feldene intramuscular injection and suppositories should be stored below 25° and the latter should not be refrigerated.

PHYSICAL PROPERTIES

Piroxicam is an off-white to light tan or light yellow, odourless powder. It forms a monohydrate that is yellow. It is reported to have a bitter taste.[1]

Melting point

Piroxicam melts in the range 198° to 200°.

Dissociation constant

A saturated solution of *piroxicam* in dioxan:water (2:1) has a pK_a of 6.3 (enolic hydroxyl group at C-4).[1]
Herzfeldt and Kümmel[2] reported a pK_a of 5.3 for *piroxicam*.

Partition coefficient

Piroxicam is reported[1] to have a partition coefficient of 1.8 between octanol and aqueous buffer pH 7.4.

Solubility

Piroxicam is very slightly soluble in water, in dilute acids, and in most organic solvents; slightly soluble in ethanol and in aqueous alkaline solutions.
The solubility of piroxicam was determined by Herzfeldt and Kümmel[2] to be very low up to pH 7.5; it was 2.3 mg/100 mL at pH 2.0, 7.6 mg/100 mL at pH 6.0, 57 mg/100 mL at pH 7.0, and 103 mg/100 mL at pH 7.5.

Dissolution

The USP specifies that for Piroxicam Capsules USP, not less than 75% of the labelled amount of $C_{15}H_{13}N_3O_4S$ is dissolved in 45 minutes. Dissolution medium: 900 mL of simulated gastric fluid TS, prepared without pepsin; Apparatus 1 at 50 rpm.

FURTHER INFORMATION. Comparative dissolution performance of internationally available piroxicam products [72% of 25 capsule brands and 80% of 5 tablet brands failed to meet the USP requirement for piroxicam capsules]—Barone JA, Lordi NG, Byerly WG, Colaizzi JL. Drug Intell Clin Pharm 1988;22:35–40.

Crystal and molecular structure

Polymorphs
It is reported[3] that piroxicam can exist in two interconvertible crystal polymorphic forms; the needle-shaped form melts in the range 196° to 198° and the cubic form melts in the range 199° to 201°. The two forms can be differentiated by infrared absorption and by X-ray powder diffraction techniques.
Vrecer *et al*[4] identified the existence of four polymorphic forms of piroxicam and at least one pseudo-polymorphic form; they were characterised by differential scanning calorimetry and infrared spectroscopy. The conditions under which different forms were produced and interconverted are detailed.

FURTHER INFORMATION. Physico-chemical properties and bioavailability of two crystal forms of piroxicam [needles, m.p. 198° and cubes, m.p. 202°]—Kozjek F, Golic L, Zupet P, Palka E, Vodopivek P, Japelj M. Acta Pharm Jugosl 1985;35:275–81. Effect of compressional forces on piroxicam polymorphs—Ghan GA, Lalla JK. J Pharm Pharmacol 1992;44:678–81.

STABILITY

Solid state

Piroxicam in the solid state was stable at 20° and at 40° for two years when kept in a coloured container in the dark.[1] There was no change in content of piroxicam or in shape, colour, smell, or taste of the crystals. When filled into colourless glass bottles and irradiated with light (300 nm to 830 nm) at 30°, piroxicam content was maintained for 72 hours.

Spanish workers[5] determined the shelf-lives ($t_{10\%}$) of piroxicam tablets formulated with Emcompress or with Celutab (for direct compression) to be about 1241 and 1302 days at 8°, 864 and 1144 days at 24°, and 413 and 476 days at 70°, respectively.

Solutions

Hydroxyalkylated cyclodextrin derivatives were found to reduce the stability of piroxicam (0.5 mg/mL) in solutions (pH 7.4) that contained a 10-fold excess of the cyclodextrin, stored at 21° to 71°. The order of destabilisation was hydroxypropyl-γ-cyclodextrin > β-cyclodextrin > hydroxypropyl-β-cyclodextrin.[6]

FURTHER INFORMATION. Determination of potential degradation products of piroxicam by HPTLC densitometry and HPLC [2-aminopyridine; 2-methyl-2H-1,2-benzothiazine-4(3H)-one 1,1-dioxide; N-methyl-N'-(2-pyridinyl)-ethane-diamide]—Tomankova H, Sabortova J. Chromatographia 1989;28(3/4):197–202.

FORMULATION

Excipients

Excipients that have been used in presentations of piroxicam include:
Capsules: erythrosine (E127); indigo carmine (E132); lactose; magnesium stearate; maize starch; sodium lauryl sulphate; titanium dioxide (E171).
Tablets: lactose.
Melt tablets: aspartame; citric acid, anhydrous; gelatin; mannitol.
Gels: benzyl alcohol; Carbopol 940; di-isopropanolamine; ethanol; hydroxyethylcellulose; propylene glycol.
Suppositories: microcrystalline wax; propyl gallate; solid semi-synthetic glycerides.
Injections (intramuscular): benzyl alcohol; ethanol; hydrochloric acid; nicotinamide; propylene glycol; sodium monophosphate, monohydrate; sodium hydroxide.

Bioavailability

The relative bioavailabilities of two commercially available piroxicam 20 mg suppositories (Felden, Pfizer and Lubor, Podravka-Belupo) in *dogs* were found to be similar and greater than the oral bioavailability of a piroxicam capsule (Lubor, Podravka-Belupo) following administration of single doses of the preparations.[7] Marked inter-individual and intra-individual differences in absorption were noted.

Capsules

The *in-vitro* dissolution of piroxicam (20 mg) from capsules was enhanced in the presence of the following excipients in the order:

Tween 80 > sodium lauryl sulphate > Primogel (sodium starch glycollate).[8]

Gels and ointments

Babar et al[9] prepared gels and ointment bases containing piroxicam 1% in order to study the *in-vitro* release of the drug. The gel contained hypromellose, propylene glycol, sodium hydroxide, methyl and propyl hydroxybenzoates, and purified water. The modified hydrophilic basis contained white soft paraffin, stearyl alcohol, sodium lauryl sulphate, propylene glycol, sodium hydroxide, methyl and propyl hydroxybenzoates, and purified water. The emulsion basis contained liquid paraffin, isopropyl lanolate, stearic acid TP, cetyl alcohol, self-emulsifying glyceryl monostearate, triethanolamine, glycerol, sodium hydroxide, methyl and propyl hydroxybenzoates, and purified water. The general rank order for *in-vitro* drug release through a cellulose membrane from all bases evaluated was: gel basis > hydrophilic basis > emulsion basis. Drug release was adversely affected by inclusion of ethanol or macrogol 400. The gel basis (containing also dimethyl sulphoxide) produced the best *in-vitro* drug release both through the cellulose membrane and hairless *mouse* skin. Tsai et al[10] found that the percutaneous absorption of piroxicam from an oil-in-water ointment basis (University of California Hospital basis containing 12% propylene glycol), in *rabbits*, was superior to that from three other USP ointments (simple ointment, macrogol ointment, and petrolatum rosewater ointment). When the water (pH 7.2) in the oil-in-water ointment basis was replaced by a sodium bicarbonate-buffered solution (pH 9.2), percutaneous absorption of piroxicam was increased. An optimal effect was attained with the addition of 5% urea.

FURTHER INFORMATION. The effect of pretreatment by penetration enhancers on the *in vivo* percutaneous absorption of piroxicam from its gel form in *rabbits*—Hsu L-R, Tsai Y-H, Huang Y-B. Int J Pharmaceutics 1991;71:193–200. Freeze drying process produces melt-in-the-mouth tablet—Pharm J 1992;249:442. Characterization of solid dispersions of piroxicam/polyethylene glycol [macrogol] 4000—Fernández M, Rodríguez IC, Margarit MV, Cerezo A. Int J Pharmaceutics 1992;84:197–202.

REFERENCES

1. Mihalic M, Hofman H, Kajfez F, Kuftinec J, Blazevic N, Zinic M. Acta Pharm Jugosl 1982;32:13–20.
2. Herzfeldt CD, Kümmel R. Drug Dev Ind Pharm 1983;9(5):767–93.
3. Mihalic M, Hofman H, Kuftinec J, Krile B, Caplar V, Kajfez F et al. In: Florey K, editor. Analytical profiles of drug substances; vol 15. London: Academic Press, 1986:500–31.
4. Vrecer F, Srcic S, Smid-Korbar J. Int J Pharmaceutics 1991;68:35–41.
5. Burson JLS, Rabasco AM, Faulí C [Spanish]. Cienc Ind Pharm 1987;6:401–4.
6. Backensfeld T, Müller BW, Kolter K. Int J Pharmaceutics 1991;74:85–93.
7. Skreblin M, Alebic-Kolbah T, Kuftinec J, Hofman H, Plavsic F. Acta Pharm Jugosl 1987;37:361–9.
8. Chowdhary KPR, Madhusudhan P. East Pharm 1990;33:143–4.
9. Babar A, Solanki UD, Cutie AJ, Plakogiannis F. Drug Dev Ind Pharm 1990;16(3):523–40.
10. Tsai Y-H, Hsu L-R, Naito S-I. Int J Pharmaceutics 1985;24:61–78.

Polymyxin B (BAN, rINN)   *Antibacterial*

Polymyxin B Sulphate (BANM, rINNM)
Polymyxin B sulfate

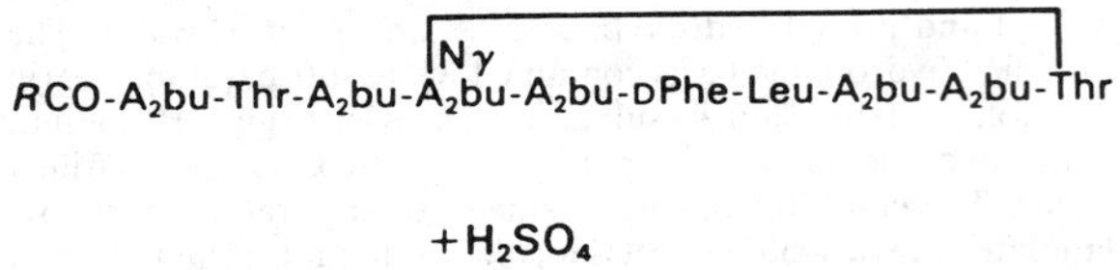

$$RCO\text{-}A_2bu\text{-}Thr\text{-}A_2bu\text{-}A_2bu\text{-}A_2bu\text{-}DPhe\text{-}Leu\text{-}A_2bu\text{-}A_2bu\text{-}Thr$$

(with $N\gamma$ bridge)

$$+\,H_2SO_4$$

Polymyxin	R
B_1	$-CH_2\cdot(CH_2)_5\cdot CHMe\cdot CH_3$
B_2	$-CH_2\cdot(CH_2)_4\cdot CHMe\cdot CH_3$

A mixture of the sulphates of polypeptides produced by the growth of certain strains of *Bacillus polymyxa* or obtained by other means.
CAS—1404-26-8 (polymyxin B); 1405-20-5 (polymyxin B sulphate)

Pharmacopoeial status

BP (polymyxin B sulphate); USP (polymyxin B sulfate)

Preparations

Compendial
Polymyxin and Bacitracin Eye Ointment BP (Polymyxin B Sulphate and Bacitracin Zinc Eye Ointment). A sterile preparation containing polymyxin B sulphate and bacitracin zinc in a suitable basis. An eye ointment containing 10 000 units of polymyxin B sulphate and 500 units of bacitracin zinc per gram is usually available.
Sterile Polymyxin B Sulfate USP. Suitable for parenteral use.

Containers and storage

Solid state
Polymyxin B Sulphate BP should be kept in an airtight container and protected from light. If it is intended for use in the manufacture of a parenteral dosage form the container should be sterile, tamper-evident, and sealed so as to exclude micro-organisms.
Polymyxin B Sulfate USP should be preserved in tight, light-resistant containers.

Dosage forms
Sterile Polymyxin B Sulfate USP should be preserved in containers suitable for sterile solids, protected from light.

PHYSICAL PROPERTIES

Polymyxin B sulphate is a white or almost white, almost odourless, hygroscopic powder.

pH

The pH of a 2% w/v solution of *polymyxin B sulphate* is 5.0 to 7.0 (BP); a 0.5% w/v solution has a pH of 5.0 to 7.5 (USP).

Dissociation constant
pK_a 8.9

Solubility

Polymyxin B sulphate is soluble or freely soluble in water; slightly soluble in ethanol.

STABILITY

Polymyxin B sulphate is extremely stable in the solid state. Stability is maintained in aqueous solutions for some months at room temperature and for longer periods under refrigeration. Maximum stability occurs at pH 3.0 to 5.0; alkaline solutions are less stable. Solutions of polymyxin B sulphate are rapidly inactivated by strong alkalis or strong acids, and by calcium, magnesium, cobalt, ferrous, or manganese ions.

INCOMPATIBILITY/COMPATIBILITY

Loss of activity, or incompatibility, of polymyxin B sulphate has been reported with the following compounds: amphotericin, ampicillin sodium, cephalothin sodium, cephazolin sodium, chloramphenicol sodium succinate, heparin sodium, nitrofurantoin sodium, prednisolone sodium phosphate, and tetracycline hydrochloride.
Potential incompatibility between polymyxin B sulphate and dexamethasone sodium phosphate in ophthalmic solutions has been investigated.[1] Turbidity developed when various volumes of both drugs at concentrations of 0.1% were mixed.

FORMULATION

Excipients

Excipients that have been used in presentations of polymyxin B sulphate include:
Ear drops: propylene glycol.
Eye drops: phenylmercuric nitrate; sodium chloride.

REFERENCE

1. Aggag M, Khahil SAH. Mfg Chem 1977;45(12):43–4.

Potassium Citrate   *Systemic alkalinising agent*

Kalii citras; Pot. Cit.
Tripotassium 2-hydroxypropane-1,2,3-tricarboxylate monohydrate
$C_6H_5K_3O_7,H_2O = 324.4$
CAS—866-84-2 (anhydrous); 6100-05-6 (monohydrate)

Pharmacopoeial status
BP, USP

Preparations

Compendial
Potassium Citrate Mixture BP (Potassium Citrate Oral Solution). A solution containing 30% w/v of potassium citrate and 5% w/v of citric acid monohydrate in a suitable vehicle with a

lemon flavour. It is intended to be diluted with water before use. For extemporaneous preparation see Formulation below.

Potassium Citrate Extended-release Tablets USP.
Potassium Citrate and Citric Acid Oral Solution USP.
Potassium Chloride, Potassium Bicarbonate, and Potassium Citrate Effervescent Tablets for Oral Solution USP.
Potassium Gluconate and Potassium Citrate Oral Solution USP.
Potassium Gluconate, Potassium Citrate, and Ammonium Chloride Oral Solution USP.

Non-compendial

Effercitrate (Typharm). *Tablets* (effervescent), contain the equivalent of 1.5 g of potassium citrate (13.9 mmol potassium ions) and 250 mg of citric acid. Each tablet contains the equivalent of the potassium citrate and citric acid content of 5 mL of Potassium Citrate Mixture.
Concentrates for preparation of Potassium Citrate Mixture are available from Evans, Hillcross.

Containers and storage

Solid state

Potassium Citrate BP should be kept in an airtight container. Potassium Citrate USP should be preserved in tight containers.

Dosage forms

Potassium Citrate Extended-release Tablets USP and Potassium Citrate and Citric Acid Oral Solution USP should be preserved in tight containers.
Effercitrate tablets should be stored in a cool, dry place below 20°. Because the tablets are hygroscopic they should be dispensed in the original containers, which include a desiccant, and should be kept closed.

PHYSICAL PROPERTIES

Potassium citrate exists as transparent crystals or as a white, granular powder; hygroscopic; odourless with a saline taste; deliquescent in moist air. It loses its monohydrate water at 180°.

pH

Aqueous solutions of *potassium citrate* are alkaline to litmus; pH about 8.5.

Solubility

Potassium citrate is soluble 1 in 1 of water; practically insoluble in ethanol.

Dissolution

The USP specifies that for Potassium Citrate Extended-release Tablets USP the percentages of the labelled amount of $C_6H_5K_3O_7$ dissolved are not more than 45% in 30 minutes, not more than 60% in 1 hour, and not less than 80% in 3 hours. Dissolution medium: 900 mL of water: Apparatus 2 at 50 rpm.

INCOMPATIBILITY/COMPATIBILITY

Evidence of physical incompatibility was shown when potassium citrate mixture (BPC 1973) was prepared or diluted with syrup preserved with 0.05% of a mixture of hydroxybenzoate esters (Nipastat); visible differences in turbidity were noted between samples made with preserved and unpreserved syrup after about 12 months.

FORMULATION

POTASSIUM CITRATE MIXTURE BP

Potassium citrate	300 g
Citric acid monohydrate	50 g
Lemon spirit	5 mL
Quillaia tincture	10 mL
Syrup	250 mL
Chloroform water, double-strength	300 mL
Water sufficient to produce	1000 mL

The mixture should be recently prepared and well diluted with water before use.

Excipients

Excipients that have been used in presentations of potassium citrate include:
Mixtures: citric acid monohydrate; concentrated chloroform water; lemon syrup; methyl hydroxybenzoate solution; quillaia tincture.

Bioavailability

Eighteen healthy volunteers received single doses of the following: a wax matrix placebo tablet; a wax matrix, sustained-release potassium citrate tablet (60 mEq, Urocit-K, Mission Pharmacal Co.); and a rapid-release liquid preparation of potassium citrate (60 mEq of powdered potassium citrate dissolved in distilled water) at intervals of at least 3 days.[1] Clinical effects over 24 hours, measured by urinary potassium and citrate excretion patterns and urinary pH, were similar between the potassium citrate tablet and liquid, although the tablet had a slightly more prolonged effect and the liquid a slightly more rapid onset.

REFERENCE

1. Harvey JA, Zobitz MM, Pak CYC. J Clin Pharmacol 1989;29:338–41.

Prednisolone (BAN, rINN)   *Corticosteroid*

1,2-Dehydrocortisone; deltahydrocortisone; metacortandralone
$11\beta,17\alpha,21$-Trihydroxypregna-1,4-diene-3,20-dione
$C_{21}H_{28}O_5 = 360.4$

Prednisolone Acetate (BANM, rINNM)
Prednisolone 21-acetate
$C_{23}H_{30}O_6 = 402.5$

Prednisolone Hemisuccinate (BANM, rINNM)
Prednisolone 21-(hydrogen succinate)
$C_{25}H_{32}O_8 = 460.5$

Prednisolone Hexanoate (BANM, rINNM)
Prednisolone caproate; prednisolone 21-hexanoate
$C_{27}H_{38}O_6 = 458.6$

Prednisolone Metasulphobenzoate Sodium (BANM)

Prednisolone Sodium Metasulphobenzoate (rINNM); prednisolone 21-(sodium *m*-sulphobenzoate)
$C_{28}H_{31}NaO_9S = 566.6$

Prednisolone Pivalate (BANM, rINNM)

Prednisolone 21-pivalate; prednisolone trimethylacetate
$C_{26}H_{36}O_6 = 444.6$

Prednisolone Sodium Phosphate (BANM, rINNM)

Prednisolone 21-(disodium orthophosphate)
$C_{21}H_{27}Na_2O_8P = 484.4$

Prednisolone Steaglate (BAN, rINN)

Prednisolone stearoylglycollate; prednisolone 21-stearoylglycollate
$C_{41}H_{64}O_8 = 685.0$

Prednisolone Tebutate (BANM, rINNM)

Prednisolone butylacetate; prednisolone 21-(3,3-dimethylbutyrate)
$C_{27}H_{38}O_6,H_2O = 476.6$
CAS—50-24-8 (prednisolone, anhydrous); 52438-85-4 (prednisolone, sesquihydrate); 52-21-1 (prednisolone acetate); 2920-86-7 (prednisolone hemisuccinate); 630-67-1 (prednisolone metasulphobenzoate sodium); 1107-99-9 (prednisolone pivalate); 125-02-0 (prednisolone sodium phosphate); 5060-55-9 (prednisolone steaglate); 7681-14-3 (prednisolone tebutate, anhydrous)

Pharmacopoeial status

BP (prednisolone, prednisolone acetate, prednisolone pivalate, prednisolone sodium phosphate); USP (prednisolone, prednisolone acetate, prednisolone hemisuccinate, prednisolone sodium phosphate, prednisolone tebutate)

Preparations

Compendial
Prednisolone Tablets BP. Tablets containing, in each, 1, 5, 25, and 50 mg of prednisolone are usually available.
Prednisolone Enema BP. A solution of prednisolone sodium phosphate in purified water.
Prednisolone Tablets USP.
Prednisolone Syrup USP.
Prednisolone Cream USP.
Prednisolone Acetate Ophthalmic Suspension USP. pH between 5.0 and 6.0.
Sterile Prednisolone Acetate Suspension USP. pH between 5.0 and 7.5.
Prednisolone Sodium Phosphate Ophthalmic Solution USP. pH between 6.2 and 8.2.
Prednisolone Sodium Phosphate Injection USP. pH between 7.0 and 8.0.
Prednisolone Sodium Succinate for Injection USP. pH between 6.7 and 8.0, determined in the solution constituted as directed in the labelling.
Sterile Prednisolone Tebutate Suspension USP. pH between 6.0 and 8.0.

Non-compendial
Deltacortril Enteric (Pfizer). *Tablets*, enteric coated, prednisolone 2.5 mg and 5 mg.
Deltastab (Boots). *Tablets*, prednisolone 1 mg and 5 mg.
Injection (aqueous suspension), prednisolone acetate 25 mg/mL.
Minims Prednisolone (S&N Pharm). *Eye drops* (single-use), prednisolone sodium phosphate 0.5% w/v.

Precortisyl (Roussel). *Tablets*, prednisolone 1 mg and 5 mg.
Precortisyl Forte (Roussel). *Tablets*, prednisolone 25 mg.
Pred Forte (Allergan). *Eye drops*, prednisolone acetate 1%.
Predenema (Pharmax). *Retention enema*, prednisolone 20 mg (as metasulphobenzoate sodium) in 100-mL single-dose disposable pack.
Predfoam (Pharmax). *Foam* (mucoadhesive), in an aerosol pack, prednisolone 20 mg (as metasulphobenzoate sodium) per metered application.
Prednesol (Glaxo). *Tablets*, soluble, prednisolone 5 mg (as sodium phosphate).
Predsol (Evans). *Drops* (for ear or eye), prednisolone sodium phosphate 0.5% w/v.
Retention enema, prednisolone 20 mg (as sodium phosphate) in 100-mL single-dose disposable pack.
Suppositories, prednisolone 5 mg (as sodium phosphate).
Prednisolone tablets and enteric-coated tablets are also available, in various strengths, from APS, Biorex, Cox, CP, Evans, Kerfoot.

Containers and storage

Solid state
Prednisolone BP, Prednisolone Acetate BP, Prednisolone Pivalate BP, and Prednisolone Sodium Phosphate BP should be kept in well-closed containers and protected from light.
Prednisolone USP and Prednisolone Acetate USP should be preserved in well-closed containers.
Prednisolone Hemisuccinate USP and Prednisolone Sodium Phosphate USP should be preserved in tight containers.
Prednisolone Tebutate USP should be preserved in tight containers sealed under sterile nitrogen, in a cool place.

Dosage forms
Prednisolone Tablets BP should be protected from light.
Requirements for the storage of USP preparations are as follows:

USP dosage form	Storage requirements
Prednisolone Tablets	well-closed containers
Prednisolone Syrup; Prednisolone Sodium Phosphate Ophthalmic Solution	tight, light-resistant containers
Prednisolone Cream	collapsible tubes or tight containers
Prednisolone Acetate Ophthalmic Suspension	tight containers
Sterile Prednisolone Acetate Suspension; Sterile Prednisolone Tebutate Suspension	single-dose or multiple-dose containers, preferably of Type I glass
Prednisolone Sodium Phosphate Injection	single-dose or multiple-dose containers, preferably of Type I glass, protected from light
Prednisolone Sodium Succinate for Injection	containers suitable for sterile solids

Deltacortril Enteric tablets and Predenema should be stored below 25°, the latter protected from light.
Deltastab injection should be stored at 15° to 20°. The injection and Deltastab tablets should be protected from light.
Minims prednisolone sodium phosphate should be stored in a cool place (8° to 15°) and not exposed to strong light.
Pred Forte should be protected from freezing.

Predfoam should be protected from sunlight and not exposed to temperatures above 50°. As the container is pressurised it should not be pierced or burned even after use.
Prednesol tablets and Predsol retention enema should be protected from light.

PHYSICAL PROPERTIES

Prednisolone is a white or almost white, crystalline powder; hygroscopic.
Prednisolone acetate is a white or almost white, crystalline powder.
Prednisolone hemisuccinate exists as a fine, creamy white powder with friable lumps; practically odourless.
Prednisolone pivalate is a white or almost white, crystalline powder.
Prednisolone sodium phosphate exists as white or slightly yellow friable granules or powder; odourless or with a slight odour; slightly hygroscopic.
Prednisolone tebutate exists as a white to slightly yellow, free-flowing powder; odourless or with a characteristic odour; hygroscopic.

Melting point

Prednisolone melts at about 230°, with decomposition.
Prednisolone acetate melts at about 235°, with decomposition.
Prednisolone hemisuccinate melts at about 205°, with decomposition.
Prednisolone pivalate melts at about 229°, with decomposition.

pH

A 1% solution of *prednisolone sodium phosphate* has a pH in the range 7.5 to 10.5.
A 5% solution of *prednisolone sodium phosphate* in carbon dioxide-free water has a pH in the range 7.5 to 9.0.

Partition coefficient

Log P (octanol/pH 7.4 aqueous buffer),[1] 1.58

Solubility

The solubilities of prednisolone and its salts and esters in various solvents have been recorded below:

Dissolution

The USP specifies that for Prednisolone Tablets USP, not less than 70% of the labelled amount of $C_{21}H_{28}O_5$ is dissolved in 30 minutes. Dissolution medium: 900 mL of water; Apparatus 2 at 50 rpm.

Crystal and molecular structure

Polymorphs
Veiga *et al*[2] prepared, isolated, and identified three forms of prednisolone. Characterisation by scanning electron microscopy, X-ray powder diffraction, and hot stage microscopy indicated that Forms I and III were 'true' polymorphs of prednisolone (anhydrous) and Form II (the 1.5 hydrate) was a 'twin'.

FURTHER INFORMATION. Study of the solubility coefficient and dissolution rates of several polymorphs of prednisolone—Veiga MD, Cadorniga R [Spanish]. Cienc Ind Farm 1988;7(7/8):201–5.

STABILITY

In studies of the anaerobic decomposition of prednisolone, Dekker identified the decomposition products of a suspension of prednisolone in aqueous buffers (pH 2 to 8) that was heated for 16 hours at 120°. Neutral products were 17-deoxyprednisolone,[3] 17-deoxy-21-dehydroprednisolone,[4] the 17-ketosteroid,[5] and the D-homosteroid.[6] Acidic compounds were thought to be 17-deoxy-17-carboxylic acid, and 17-deoxy-20-hydroxy-21-carboxylic acid of α and β configurations.[7]
Under anaerobic conditions at 100°, an aqueous solution of prednisolone (at pH 1.8 to 8.3 in 0.1M phosphate solutions containing disodium edetate 0.05% w/v) was most stable at pH 2.5. Decomposition was almost pH-independent between pH 5.0 and 6.0. Below pH 5.5, prednisolone decomposed to 17-deoxy-21-dehydroprednisolone. At higher pH values, a mixture of the decomposition products was observed.[8] Above pH 6, the 17-ketosteroid, 17-deoxyprednisolone, and the D-homosteroid were detected; the 17-ketosteroid was the most abundant. Decomposition was first-order with respect to prednisolone concentration at constant pH over the pH range 1.8 to 8.3. The presence of a yellow precipitate was detected, following complete decomposition, after 22 hours at pH 6.3 and after 4 hours at pH 8.3.
Anaerobic decomposition of prednisolone phosphate in aqueous solution at pH 8.3 and 120° yielded the major decomposition

	Prednisolone	Prednisolone acetate	Prednisolone hemi-succinate	Prednisolone pivalate	Prednisolone sodium phosphate	Prednisolone tebutate
Water	1 in 1300	practically insoluble	very slightly soluble	practically insoluble	1 in 3 or 4	very slightly soluble
Ethanol	1 in 30	1 in 120	1 in 6	1 in 150	very slightly soluble	sparingly soluble
Absolute ethanol	1 in 27	1 in 170	—	—	1 in 1000	—
Chloroform	1 in 180	1 in 150	—	1 in 16	slightly soluble	freely soluble
Methanol	soluble	—	—	—	1 in 13	sparingly soluble
Acetone	sparingly soluble	slightly soluble	soluble	—	very slightly soluble	soluble
Dioxan	soluble	—	—	—	very slightly soluble	freely soluble
Ether	—	—	1 in 250	—	—	—
Dichloromethane	—	—	—	soluble	—	—

product 17a-hydroxy-17a-hydroxymethyl-17-keto-D-homosteroid phosphate.[9]

Guttman and Meister[10] investigated the kinetics of the base-catalysed degradation of prednisolone. Degradation, which exhibited a first-order dependency on the concentration of prednisolone, was accompanied by the concomitant appearance of acidic and neutral steroidal compounds. In either the presence or absence of air, the rate of decomposition of prednisolone in aqueous solution increased as the concentration of hydroxide ions was increased; however, the rate was faster in the presence of air. It was suggested that three parallel pseudo-first-order reactions occurred, one of which was oxygen dependent.

Stroud et al[11] measured first-order rate constants for the degradation of prednisolone sodium phosphate (in sealed glass ampoules) at pH 8 as 1.13×10^{-3}/hour at 80°, 4.145×10^{-3}/hour at 90°, 1.271×10^{-2}/hour at 100°, and 3.323×10^{-2}/hour at 110°. The principal degradation pathway was thought to be hydrolysis of the phosphate ester group to yield prednisolone.

Effect of buffers and trace metals

Trace metal impurities present in buffer salts were shown to catalyse the decomposition of prednisolone in aqueous solution.[12] The rate of decomposition was dependent on the concentration of buffer (phosphate or borate) but incorporation of a sequestering agent (disodium edetate) eliminated this dependency. At pH values less than 5 and greater than 7, the rate of the apparent metal-catalysed reaction was independent of pH, but in the pH range 5 to 7 the reaction showed a first-order dependency on hydroxide ion concentration.

Irradiation

When prednisolone and prednisolone acetate were subjected to cobalt-60 irradiation the major degradation products identified were 11β-hydroxy-1,4-androstadiene-3,17-dione (from both compounds) and prednisone and prednisone acetate (from prednisolone and the acetate salt, respectively).[13] Rates of radiolytic degradation of prednisolone and prednisolone acetate were 0.7%/Mrad and 0.4%/Mrad, respectively.

FURTHER INFORMATION. A stability-indicating HPLC assay for prednisolone sodium phosphate [detection of prednisolone as a breakdown product] in implantable infusion pumps [stored at 37°]—Bachman WJ, Gambertoglio JG. Anal Lett 1990;23(5):893–900. On the stability-indicating properties of some spectrometric assays for corticosteroids—Bundgaard H, Hansen J. Pharm Weekbl (Sci) 1980;2:127–8. Surface area stability of micronised steroids [including prednisolone and prednisolone hydrate] sterilised by irradiation [electron and gamma]—Illum E, Møller N. Arch Pharm Chemi (Sci) 1974;2:167–74. [Stability study of an aqueous injection of prednisolone sodium phosphate]—Kuizenga AJ, De Vos HJ, Voorhuis MH [Dutch]. Pharm Weekbl 1973;108:809–14. Stability of betamethasone sodium phosphate, hydrocortisone sodium phosphate, and prednisolone sodium phosphate injections submitted by US hospitals—Kreienbaum MA. Am J Hosp Pharm 1986;43:1747–50. [Stability of prednisolone hemisuccinate eye drops]—Riedel H [German]. Krankenhauspharmazie 1986;7:432–3.

INCOMPATIBILITY/COMPATIBILITY

Prednisolone is incompatible with alkalis.

Particulate matter was observed within 2 hours when 1 mL of commercial prednisolone sodium phosphate injection was mixed with 5 mL of sterile water and 1 mL of any of the following commercial injection solutions: calcium gluconate, dimenhydrinate, prochlorperazine edisylate, promazine hydrochloride, and promethazine hydrochloride.[14]

Formation of a haze or precipitation was observed within an hour when prednisolone sodium phosphate (20 mg/100 mL) was mixed in glucose 5% injection with polymyxin B sulphate (20 mg/100 mL).[15]

When injections of prednisolone sodium phosphate (Hydeltrasol, MSD, USA) and methotrexate sodium (Lederle, USA) were mixed in glucose 5% injection (both drug concentrations 0.2 mg/mL), chemical incompatibility was indicated by changes in the ultraviolet spectra of both drugs within one hour at room temperature.[16]

Solid buffers

The effects of aqueous suspensions of antacids on prednisolone at 37.5° have been investigated.[17] Magnesium trisilicate (suspension pH 8.9) adsorbed intact prednisolone and magnesium oxide (suspension pH 10.4) caused an alkaline degradation of the side-chain. Aluminium hydroxide, calcium carbonate, and magnesium carbonate (suspension pH 7.4, 9.1, and 9.2, respectively) were without effect.

Plastics

Negligible losses due to sorption were detected when prednisolone (Sigma, USA) 9 mg/L in sodium chloride 0.9% injection was stored for one week in polyvinyl chloride bags at room temperature in the dark.[18]

Kowaluk et al[19] investigated interactions between prednisolone (Sigma, USA) 9 mg/L in sodium chloride 0.9% injection and various intravenous delivery equipment. No sorption was observed when the solution was infused at 1 mL/min through sets consisting of a cellulose propionate burette chamber and 170 cm polyvinyl chloride tubing during a seven-hour simulated infusion. During a one-hour simulated infusion (at 0.08 mL/min) of a similar solution through 20 cm of polyethylene tubing or 50 cm of Silastic tubing (attached to a glass syringe on a syringe pump) no sorption of prednisolone was detected. Similarly, no loss due to sorption occurred when the solution was stored in single-use plastic syringes composed of polypropylene barrels and polyethylene plungers for 24 hours in the dark at room temperature (15° to 20°).

FURTHER INFORMATION. [Prednisolone 21-hemisuccinate sodium: compatibility in different basic parenteral solutions]—Hehenberger H [German]. Krankenhauspharmazie 1986;7:128–32.

FORMULATION

Excipients

Excipients that have been used in presentations of prednisolone include:

Tablets, prednisolone: acacia; beeswax; calcium carbonate; carnauba wax; cellacephate; citroflex A-2; gelatin; iron oxide, brown and red (E172); kaolin; lactose; magnesium stearate; methyl hydroxybenzoate; ponceau 4R (E124); shellac; starch (maize; potato); sucrose; talc.

Prednisolone steaglate: lactose.

Soluble/effervescent tablets, prednisolone metasulphobenzoate sodium: citric acid; monosodium carbonate; silicone emulsion antimousse 30; sodium bicarbonate; sodium saccharin; sucrose; tartaric acid.

Oral liquids, prednisolone: ethanol; glycerol; sodium benzoate; sorbitol; sucrose.

Eye drops, prednisolone acetate: benzalkonium chloride; boric acid; disodium edetate; hypromellose; polysorbate 80; sodium acid phosphate; sodium chloride; sodium citrate; sodium phosphate.

Prednisolone sodium phosphate: benzalkonium chloride; disodium edetate; sodium acid phosphate; sodium chloride; sodium hydroxide.

Eye/ear drops, prednisolone sodium phosphate: benzalkonium chloride.

Eye ointments, prednisolone pivalate: cetyl alcohol; liquid paraffin; wool fat.

Enemas, prednisolone metasulphobenzoate sodium: disodium edetate; methyl, ethyl, and propyl hydroxybenzoates.

Aerosol foams, prednisolone metasulphobenzoate sodium: disodium edetate; hydroxybenzoates; phenoxyethanol.

Injections, prednisolone acetate: benzyl alcohol; carmellose sodium; polysorbate 80; sodium chloride.

Prednisolone sodium phosphate: disodium edetate; nicotinamide; phenol; sodium bisulphite; sodium hydroxide.

Prednisolone tebutate: benzyl alcohol; polysorbate 80; sodium citrate; sorbitol solution.

Bioavailability

No differences in the time to reach peak concentration and extent of absorption were detected (serum-prednisolone concentrations) when prednisolone 21-phosphate or prednisolone (as Prednesol, Glaxo or Precortisyl, Roussel, respectively) were administered orally as 5 mg tablets in water or as 1 mg and 5 mg tablets, respectively, to nine healthy volunteers.[20] In comparison with prednisolone 21-phosphate administered intravenously (Codelsol, MSD) absorption of the oral forms was considered to be complete (about 90% to 93% bioavailability). Data obtained during a two-way crossover study involving twelve healthy subjects[21] indicated that there was no significant difference between the bioavailabilities of two brands of prednisolone 5 mg tablets (Meticortelone, Schering and Sterane, Pfizer). Results from dissolution studies (at 37°) in 0.01% polysorbate 80/0.1M hydrochloric acid correlated better with the *in-vivo* data than when de-ionised water was used as the dissolution medium. Dissolution rates differed significantly both between the tablets and the media.

In a double-blind, crossover study involving six fasted or nonfasted healthy subjects, considerable inter-subject variation in plasma prednisolone concentrations was noted following administration of shellac-based, enteric-coated tablets (2.5 mg, Pfizer).[22] However, such variability was reduced when the formulation was altered and the enteric coating was based on cellacephate. The presence of food in the stomach affected neither the absorption pattern nor the bioavailability of enteric-coated prednisolone. Comparison of this study with a previous study of plain prednisolone tablets (in nine healthy volunteers) indicated that the bioavailability of the cellacephate-based formulation was similar to that of plain prednisolone.

Stability in vehicles

Christen *et al*[23] examined the stability of prednisolone and prednisolone acetate when they were triturated in seven semisolid vehicles and stored at 37° for 28 days. In general, prednisolone acetate was more stable than prednisolone. In a bentonite gel, stability of both compounds was poor with degradation of prednisolone occurring during the initial trituration. Amphiphilic vehicles (Cremophor RH 40 and Lanette N) affected mainly prednisolone with some decomposition occurring during trituration in Cremophor RH 40. Prednisolone was stable in a carbomer gel although prednisolone acetate hydrolysed slightly during trituration. The stability of the steroids was greatest in a hydroxypropylcellulose hydrogel. Prednisolone was examined

in two lipophilic bases (almond oil and white beeswax); stability was maintained for at least 28 days.

No significant decrease in the concentration of prednisolone was detected (by normal-phase and reversed-phase HPLC) following storage of a hydroalcoholic prednisolone mixture for 52 weeks at 22° to 24° in 100-mL amber glass bottles exposed to laboratory light.[24] The mixture contained prednisolone (500 mg), ethanol (27 mL), propylene glycol (20 mL), sucrose (20 g), orange tincture (2.4 mL), and water to 100 mL. Microbiological stability was not assessed.

Solid dispersions and co-precipitates

There was a marked increase in the dissolution rate (in deionised water) of prednisolone contained within solid glass dispersions (prepared by the fusion method) using glucose, galactose, and sucrose as carriers, compared to the dissolution rate of the plain prednisolone powder.[25]

Improved dissolution of prednisolone into water at 37° was obtained from solid dispersion systems prepared using macrogol 6000, povidone (25 000, 40 000, or 160 000), sorbitol, urea, mannitol, and Cremophor when compared with that of prednisolone alone or a physical mixture with carrier; maximum dissolution rates were achieved using dispersions containing prednisolone 10% w/w.[26]

In an attempt to improve the dissolution profile of prednisolone, Ahmed and Madan[27] prepared co-precipitates and physical mixtures of the drug with fructose, xylose, and polydextrose. Dissolution of the co-precipitates was rapid, with more than 90% released within 10 minutes. In physical mixtures, the ability of the carriers to improve dissolution followed the rank order: polydextrose > xylose > fructose.

Suspensions

Significant differences in dissolution rates, observed[28] for commercially available ophthalmic/otic suspensions of prednisolone acetate, were due, in part, to variations in particle size and to differences in formulation, notably the presence of hypromellose.

Modified-release preparations

The rate of release of prednisolone from two monolithic controlled-release block copolyurethane devices (hydrophobic urethane-urea 'domains' dispersed in a hydrophilic polyether matrix) was dependent on the method used to incorporate prednisolone into the device (solution casting or swelling in saturated solutions).[29] Intermolecular interactions between prednisolone and the urethane segment of the copolyurethane contributed to the lower rates of release from the solution-cast devices. Such interactions were absent in the devices loaded by swelling; these exhibited higher release rates.

FURTHER INFORMATION. Oral absorption of 21-corticosteroid esters: a function of aqueous stability and intestinal enzyme activity and distribution [prednisolone succinate and phosphate]—Fleisher D, Johnson KC, Stewart BH, Amidon GL. J Pharm Sci 1986;75(10):934–9. Absorption of enteric and non-enteric coated prednisolone tablets [in patients]—Hulme B, James VHT, Rault R. Br J Clin Pharmacol 1975;2:317–20. Plasma prednisolone levels in man following administration of plain and enteric-coated forms [similar bioavailability in patients]. Wilson CG, May CS, Paterson JW. Br J Clin Pharmacol 1977;4:351–5. A thermographic assessment of three intra-articular prednisolone analogues [prednisolone acetate, prednisolone pivalate, prednisolone tertiary butylacetate; effect of solubility] given in rheumatoid synovitis—Esselinckx W, Bacon PA, Ring EFJ, Crooke D, Collins AJ, Demottaz D. Br J Clin Pharmacol 1978;5:447–51. Ocular bioavailability of topical prednisolone [as acetate and sodium phosphate] preparations [absorption and penetration pharmacokinetics]—Olejnik O, Weisbecker CA. Clin Ther 1990;12(1):2–11. Dissolution performance related to particle size distribution for commercially available prednisolone acetate suspensions [parenteral]—Meyer Stout PJ, Khoury N, Howard SA, Mauger JW. Drug Dev Ind Pharm 1992;18(4):395–408. Suspending agent [hypromellose and carmellose sodium] effects on steroid [prednisolone acetate] suspension dissolution profiles—Howard SA, Mauger J, Hsieh JW, Amin K. J Pharm Sci 1979;68(12):1475–9. Influence of the drug [prednisolone] solubility and dissolution medium on the release from poly(2-hydroxyethyl methacrylate) microspheres—Robert CCR, Buri PA, Peppas NA. J Controlled Release 1987;5:151–7. Prednisolone-21-acetate poly(glycolic acid) microspheres: influence of matrix characteristics on release—Redmon MP, Hickey AJ. De Luca PP. J Controlled Release 1989;9:99–109.

REFERENCES

1. Ponec M, Kempenaar J, Shroot B, Caron J-C. J Pharm Sci 1986;75(10):973–5.
2. Veiga MD, Cadorniga R, Fonseca I, Garcia-Blanco S. Il Farmaco Ed Prat 1987;42(4):93–102.
3. Dekker D. Pharm Weekbl (Sci) 1979;1:112–19.
4. Dekker D. Pharm Weekbl (Sci) 1980;2:14–18.
5. Dekker D, Buijs DJ. Pharm Weekbl (Sci) 1980;2:54–9.
6. Dekker D. Pharm Weekbl (Sci) 1980;2:59–64.
7. Dekker D. Pharm Weekbl (Sci) 1980;2:87–95.
8. Dekker D, Beijnen JH. Pharm Weekbl (Sci) 1980;2:112–16.
9. Beijnen JH, Dekker D. Pharm Weekbl (Sci) 1984;6:1–6.
10. Guttman DE, Meister PD. J Am Pharm Assoc Sci Ed 1958;47:773–8.
11. Stroud N, Richardson NE, Davies DJG, Norton DA. Analyst 1980;105:455–61.
12. Oesterling TO, Guttman DE. J Pharm Sci 1964;53(10):1189–92.
13. Kane MP, Tsuji K. J Pharm Sci 1983;72(1):30–5.
14. Misgen R. Am J Hosp Pharm 1965;22:92–4.
15. Meisler JM, Skolaut MW. Am J Hosp Pharm 1966;23:557–63.
16. McRae MP, King JC. Am J Hosp Pharm 1976;33:1010–13.
17. Chulski T, Forest AA. J Am Pharm Assoc Sci Ed 1958;47:553–5.
18. Kowaluk EA, Roberts MS, Blackburn HD, Polack AE. Am J Hosp Pharm 1981;38:1308–14.
19. Kowaluk EA, Roberts MS, Polack AE. Am J Hosp Pharm 1982;39:460–7.
20. Olivesi A. Therapie 1985;40:1–4.
21. Sullivan TJ, Stoll RG, Sakmar E, Blair DC, Wagner JG. J Pharmacokinet Biopharm 1974;2:29–41.
22. Lee DAH, Taylor GM, Walker JG, James VHT. Br J Clin Pharmacol 1979;7:523–8.
23. Christen P, Kloeti F, Gander B. J Clin Pharm Ther 1990;15:325–9.
24. Sullivan JA. Aust J Hosp Pharm 1991;21:239–41.
25. Allen LV, Yanchick VA, Maness DD. J Pharm Sci 1977;66(4):494–6.
26. Jachowicz R. Int J Pharmaceutics 1987;35:1–5.
27. Ahmed SU, Madan PL. Drug Dev Ind Pharm 1989;15(8):1243–61.
28. Howard SA, Mauger JW, Phusanti L. J Pharm Sci 1977;66(4):557–9.
29. Sharma K, Knutson K, Kim SW. J Controlled Release 1988;7:197–205.

Primidone (BAN, rINN)   *Anticonvulsant*

Hexamidinum; primaclone
5-Ethylperhydro-5-phenylpyrimidine-4,6-dione;   5-ethyldihydro-5-phenyl-4,6-[1H,5H]-pyrimidinedione;   5-ethyl-5-phenyl-hexahydropyrimidine-4,6-dione
$C_{12}H_{14}N_2O_2 = 218.3$
CAS—125-33-7

Pharmacopoeial status

BP, USP

Preparations

Compendial
Primidone Tablets BP. Tablets containing, in each, 250 mg are usually available.
Primidone Oral Suspension BP (Primidone Mixture). A suspension of primidone in a suitable flavoured vehicle. An oral suspension containing 250 mg in 5 mL is usually available. See Formulation below.
Primidone Tablets USP.
Primidone Oral Suspension USP.

Non-compendial
Mysoline (ICI). *Tablets*, primidone 250 mg.
Oral suspension, primidone 250 mg/5 mL. *Diluent*: contains carmellose sodium (50 cP) 1% w/v, sucrose 20% w/v, methyl hydroxybenzoate 0.15% w/v, propyl hydroxybenzoate 0.015% w/v, in freshly boiled and cooled purified water to 100%.

Containers and storage

Solid state
Primidone USP should be preserved in well-closed containers.

Dosage forms
Primidone Tablets USP should be preserved in well-closed containers.
Primidone Oral Suspension USP should be preserved in tight, light-resistant containers.
Mysoline tablets and oral suspension should be stored at room temperature.

PHYSICAL PROPERTIES

Primidone is a white or almost white, crystalline powder; odourless or almost odourless with a slightly bitter taste.

Melting point

Primidone melts in the range 279° to 284°.

Solubility

Primidone is soluble 1 in 2000 of water and 1 in 170 to 200 of ethanol; practically insoluble in chloroform and in ether; very slightly soluble or practically insoluble in most other organic solvents.
Solubility in water at 37° is reported to be 60 mg/100 mL.

Enhancement of solubility
An equilibrium solubility of 56.4 mg/100 mL was determined[1] for primidone in distilled water, pH 5.5 at 37°. In the presence

of citric acid (500 mg/mL) the aqueous solubility of primidone was increased to 172.2 mg/100 mL.

In aqueous octoxinol 9 (Triton-X 100) solutions, at concentrations below its critical micelle concentration of 0.018% w/w, the solubility of micronised primidone[2] was 0.0384% w/w at 25°. In aqueous octoxinol 9 solutions in the concentration range 0.018% w/w to 0.408% w/w, the solubility of primidone increased to 0.048% w/w; using a derived equation, the authors deduced that 0.039% w/w primidone was dissolved in the aqueous phase and 0.009% w/w was solubilised in micelles of octoxinol 9.

Dissolution

The USP specifies that for Primidone Tablets USP not less than 75% of the labelled amount of $C_{12}H_{14}N_2O_2$ is dissolved in 60 minutes. Dissolution medium: 900 mL of water; Apparatus 2 at 50 rpm.

Crystal and molecular structure

Yeates and Palmer[3] determined the crystal structure of primidone; crystals of primidone (produced by evaporation from a solution in absolute ethanol) were classed as monoclinic prismatic crystals.

Polymorphs

The existence of two polymorphic forms of primidone has been reported.[1] No differences were recorded between either the solubility or dissolution rate of the two forms in distilled water, pH 5.5, at 37°.

FORMULATION

Excipients

Excipients that have been used in presentations of primidone include:

Tablets: carmellose calcium; gelatin; lactose; macrogol 8000; magnesium stearate; povidone; starch; stearic acid.

Oral suspensions: aluminium magnesium silicate; ammonia solution (diluted); carmellose sodium; cetostearyl alcohol/ethylene oxide condensate; citric acid; methylcellulose; methyl and propyl hydroxybenzoates; quinoline yellow (E104); saccharin sodium; sodium alginate; sodium benzoate; sodium citrate; sodium hypochlorite solution; sorbic acid; sorbitan monolaurate; sucrose; sunset yellow FCF (E110); syrup; vanilla flavouring.

Bioequivalence

It has been reported[4] that generic primidone tablets were not bioequivalent to Mysoline (Ayerst) tablets in one epileptic patient who had been stabilised on Mysoline; seizure frequency increased when Mysoline was replaced by the generic tablets (Bolar, USA). Low plasma-drug concentrations produced by the generic primidone led to the conclusion that the generic tablets were not absorbed to any significant degree.

Borst and Lockwood[5] found no significant difference between plasma concentrations of primidone or its metabolites when two commercial primidone tablets (from two Canadian manufacturers) were administered to two groups of nine epileptic patients over a period of 14 days.

When two batches of Mysoline (Ayerst) tablets (which had different *in-vitro* disintegration and dissolution times) were compared in a crossover study involving twelve epileptic patients, the two batches were not bioequivalent.[6] Significant differences in plasma concentrations of phenobarbitone (an active metabolite of primidone) were measured, although plasma concentrations of primidone produced by tablets from the two separate batches were not significantly different.

Solid dispersions

Solid dispersions containing primidone (1% to 32% w/w) were prepared by fusion with citric acid monohydrate followed by rapid cooling of the melt.[1] The solid dispersions were clear glasses and were unstable; devitrification of glasses that contained low concentrations of primidone was more rapid than that of those with higher concentrations. Phase studies revealed that the devitrified solid dispersions with primidone concentrations above 3% w/w were eutectic mixtures of primidone and citric acid. At 37°, in distilled water (pH 5.5), the dissolution rate of primidone from devitrified solid dispersions was greater than that from physical mixtures of primidone with citric acid or from primidone powder alone.

Desai *et al*[7] reported that among the effervescent solid dispersions of primidone prepared with various mixed carriers, greater release of primidone was promoted by citric acid with sodium bicarbonate than by either succinic acid with sodium bicarbonate or tartaric acid with sodium bicarbonate.

Adsorption

Adsorption of octoxinol 9 (Triton-X 100) from aqueous solution onto micronised solid primidone (at 25°) increased to reach saturation (5.76 mg octoxinol per gram primidone) at the critical micelle concentration of octoxinol 9 (0.018% w/w).[2] Adsorption was shown to be completely or almost completely reversible.

Deflocculation of suspensions

Sedimentation of micronised, solid primidone in aqueous solutions of surfactants (octoxinols) was dependent on the concentration and hydrophile-lipophile balance (HLB) value of the surfactant.[2] In primidone suspensions that contained octoxinol 9 (Triton-X 100) at concentrations at or above its critical micelle concentration of 0.018% w/w, sediments were almost completely deflocculated and sedimentation volumes were at a minimum (3% to 4% v/v). Sedimentation volumes increased with an increase in HLB value (and increase in polyoxyethylene chain length) of the octoxinol.

REFERENCES

1. Summers MP, Enever RP. J Pharm Sci 1976;65(11):1613–17.
2. Schott H, Royce AE. J Pharm Sci 1985;74(9):957–62.
3. Yeates DGR, Palmer RA. Acta Cryst 1975;B31:1077–82.
4. Wyllie E, Pippenger CE, Rothner AD. J Am Med Assoc 1987;258(9):1216–17.
5. Borst SI, Lockwood CH. Int J Clin Pharmacol Biopharm 1975;12:309–14.
6. Bielman P, Levac TH, Langlois Y, Tetreault L. Int J Clin Pharmacol Ther Toxicol 1974;9:132–7.
7. Desai S, Allen LV, Greenwood R, Stiles ML, Parker D. J Pharm Sci 1987;76(11):S254,N03-W-06.

Prochlorperazine (BAN, rINN)

Anti-emetic; Antipsychotic

Chlormeprazine; prochlorpemazine
2-Chloro-10-[3-(4-methylpiperazin-1-yl)propyl]phenothiazine
$C_{20}H_{24}ClN_3S = 373.9$

Prochlorperazine Edisylate (BANM)

Prochlorperazine Edisilate (rINNM); prochlorperazine ethane-disulphonate
$C_{20}H_{24}ClN_3S,C_2H_6O_6S_2 = 564.1$

Prochlorperazine Maleate (BANM, rINNM)

$C_{20}H_{24}ClN_3S,2C_4H_4O_4 = 606.1$

Prochlorperazine Mesylate (BANM)

Prochlorperazine Mesilate (rINNM); prochlorperazine dimethanesulphonate; prochlorperazine methanesulphonate
$C_{20}H_{24}ClN_3S,2CH_3SO_3H = 566.1$
CAS—58-38-8 (prochlorperazine); 1257-78-9 (prochlorperazine edisylate); 84-02-6 (prochlorperazine maleate); 5132-55-8 (prochlorperazine mesylate)

Pharmacopoeial status

BP (prochlorperazine maleate, prochlorperazine mesylate); USP (prochlorperazine, prochlorperazine edisylate, prochlorperazine maleate)

Preparations

Compendial
Prochlorperazine Tablets BP. Tablets containing, in each, prochlorperazine maleate 5 mg and 25 mg are usually available.
Prochlorperazine Injection BP. A sterile solution of prochlorperazine mesylate in water for injections free from dissolved air. Injections containing prochlorperazine mesylate 12.5 mg in 1 mL and 25 mg in 2 mL are usually available. pH of solution 5.5 to 6.5.
Prochlorperazine Maleate Tablets USP.
Prochlorperazine Edisylate Oral Solution USP.
Prochlorperazine Edisylate Syrup USP.
Prochlorperazine Suppositories USP.
Prochlorperazine Edisylate Injection USP. pH 4.2 to 6.2.

Non-compendial
Buccastem (R&C). *Buccal tablets*, prochlorperazine maleate 3 mg.
Stemetil (Rhône-Poulenc Rorer). *Tablets*, prochlorperazine maleate 5 mg and 25 mg.
Syrup, prochlorperazine mesylate 5 mg in 5 mL.
Suppositories, prochlorperazine base equivalent to 5 mg and 25 mg of prochlorperazine maleate.
Injection, prochlorperazine mesylate 12.5 mg/mL.
Stemetil Eff (Rhône-Poulenc Rorer). *Granules*, effervescent, sugar free, prochlorperazine mesylate 5 mg/sachet. To be dissolved in cold water.
Vertigon (SK&F). *Spansules*, sustained-release capsules, prochlorperazine (as maleate) 10 mg and 15 mg.

Containers and storage

Solid state
Prochlorperazine Maleate BP should be kept in a well-closed container and protected from light.
Prochlorperazine Mesylate BP should be protected from light.
Prochlorperazine USP, Prochlorperazine Edisylate USP, and Prochlorperazine Maleate USP should all be preserved in tight, light-resistant containers.

Dosage forms
Prochlorperazine Tablets BP and Prochlorperazine Injection BP should be protected from light.
Prochlorperazine Maleate Tablets USP should be preserved in well-closed containers, protected from light.
Prochlorperazine Edisylate Oral Solution USP and Prochlorperazine Edisylate Syrup USP should be preserved in tight, light-resistant containers.
Prochlorperazine Suppositories USP should be preserved in tight containers at a temperature below 37° and the unwrapped suppositories must not be exposed to sunlight.
Prochlorperazine Edisylate Injection USP should be preserved in single-dose or in multiple-dose containers, preferably of Type I glass and protected from light.
Buccastem tablets should be protected from light.
Stemetil preparations should be protected from light. The injection solution rapidly discolours on exposure to light; discoloured solutions should be discarded. Stemetil suppositories should be stored in a cool dark place.
Stemetil Eff granules should be kept in a cool place.
Vertigon Spansules should be stored below 25° in a dry place and protected from light.

PHYSICAL PROPERTIES

Prochlorperazine is a clear, pale yellow viscous liquid; sensitive to light.
Prochlorperazine edisylate is a white to very light yellow crystalline powder; odourless.
Prochlorperazine maleate is a white or pale yellow crystalline powder; almost odourless with a slightly bitter taste.
Prochlorperazine mesylate is a white or almost white powder; odourless or almost odourless; slightly bitter taste.

Melting point

Prochlorperazine maleate melts at about 200°.
Prochlorperazine mesylate melts at about 242°.

pH

Solutions of *prochlorperazine edisylate* in water are acidic to litmus.
Saturated solutions of *prochlorperazine maleate* have a pH of 3.0 to 4.0.
Solutions of *prochlorperazine mesylate* 2% w/v have a pH of 2.0 to 3.0.

Dissociation constants

Prochlorperazine is dibasic: pK_a 8.1, 3.73
Green[1] determined a pK_a of 8.1 (24°) based on the pH dependence of the water solubility of prochlorperazine. Vezin and Florence[2] determined a pK_a of 8.14 (20°) by measurement of partition coefficients between cyclohexane and aqueous buffer over a range of pH values.

Partition coefficient

Log *P* (octanol/pH 7), 2.4

Solubility

Prochlorperazine is very slightly soluble in water; it is freely soluble in ethanol, in chloroform, and in ether.

Prochlorperazine edisylate is freely soluble in water (1 in 2); very slightly soluble in ethanol (1 in 1500); practically insoluble in chloroform and in ether.

Prochlorperazine maleate is very slightly soluble in water and in ethanol; practically insoluble in ether and in chloroform, but slightly soluble in warm chloroform.

Prochlorperazine mesylate is soluble 1 in less than 0.5 of water; soluble 1 in 40 of ethanol; slightly soluble in chloroform; practically insoluble in ether.

Dissolution

The USP specifies that for Prochlorperazine Maleate Tablets USP not less than 75% of the labelled amount of prochlorperazine, $C_{20}H_{24}ClN_3S$, is dissolved in 60 minutes. Dissolution medium: 500 mL of 0.1N hydrochloric acid; Apparatus 2 at 75 rpm.

STABILITY

Solutions of prochlorperazine and its salts are light sensitive and will darken on exposure to light. Ravin et al[3] investigated the influence of light on the oxidation of prochlorperazine. Unbuffered aqueous solutions of prochlorperazine edisylate 5% were placed in a Warburg respirometer (to measure oxygen uptake) at 25° and exposed to a light source. After a lag time of six minutes, oxygen uptake increased linearly with time. When the light source was removed, oxygen uptake ceased, but resumed at the same rate when light was reapplied. Colour was noted in the solutions soon after initial exposure to light and, on continued exposure, the solutions darkened further.

INCOMPATIBILITY/COMPATIBILITY

Syrups and elixirs

Addition of prochlorperazine[4] (1.25 mg/10 mL) to diamorphine and cocaine elixir (BPC 1973 formula but cocaine hydrochloride 5 mg/10 mL) reduced the shelf-life (in terms of the $t_{10\%}$ of diamorphine) from eight weeks to two weeks, at 22°.

After reformulation of Stemetil syrup to contain citric acid and ascorbic acid, the manufacturer stated that the new formulation was incompatible with magnesium trisilicate mixture; effervescence was reported when the two preparations were mixed.[5]

Prochlorperazine edisylate syrup is compatible with syrups that are slightly acidic and with those that do not contain oxidising agents or tannins.

Infusion vehicles

Visual incompatibility (cloudiness in solution) was reported[6] when prochlorperazine edisylate injection 5 mg/mL (Compazine, SKF, USA) was diluted to 1 mg/mL with sodium chloride 0.9% injection that contained methyl and propyl hydroxybenzoates. However, no incompatibility occurred on similar dilution of prochlorperazine edisylate injection with sodium chloride 0.9% injection that contained benzyl alcohol or sodium chloride 0.9% injection without preservative.

Injections

Prochlorperazine mesylate

Riley[7] investigated the compatibility of prochlorperazine mesylate injection BP (100 mg/L) with each of 66 intravenous drugs in two infusion vehicles. Visible changes were recorded over three hours at 20°. Incompatibilities noted are given below.

Drug solutions visually incompatible with Prochlorperazine Mesylate Injection BP (100 mg/L) at 20°:

Vehicle	Immediate precipitate	Visible changes Haze formed over 3 hours
Sodium chloride 0.9%, pH 7.0	aminophylline (1 g/L)	benzylpenicillin (6 g/L)
	ampicillin sodium (2 g/L)	chloramphenicol (4 g/L)
	ethamivan (2 g/L) phenobarbitone sodium (800 mg/L) sulphadiazine sodium (4 g/L) sulphadimidine sodium (4 g/L)	chlorothiazide (2 g/L)
Glucose 5%, pH 4.3	aminophylline (1 g/L)	amphotericin (200 mg/L)
	ampicillin sodium (2 g/L)	methohexitone sodium (2 g/L)
	chlorothiazide (2 g/L)	phenobarbitone sodium (800 mg/L) sulphadiazine sodium (4 g/L) sulphadimidine sodium (4 g/L)

Prochlorperazine edisylate

The manufacturer recommends that prochlorperazine edisylate injection (SKF, USA) should not be mixed with other agents in the same syringe.

The potential for incompatibility between prochlorperazine edisylate and morphine sulphate injections has been noted.[8] Visible precipitates (milky-white) formed when two prochlorperazine edisylate injections (SKF and Elkins-Sinn, USA) were mixed with morphine sulphate injection (Winthrop) in syringes. However, a manufacturer reported[9] that following reformulation of morphine sulphate injection (Wyeth) in 1984 to contain chlorbutol instead of phenol, admixtures with prochlorperazine edisylate injection (SKF) were physically compatible for 24 hours at about 25°.

Visual incompatibility (particulate matter) was noted[10] between prochlorperazine edisylate injection (SKF) and commercial brands of the following injection solutions: aminophylline, benzylpenicillin potassium, chloramphenicol sodium succinate, dexamethasone sodium phosphate, dimenhydrinate, heparin sodium, methicillin sodium, phenobarbitone sodium, phenytoin sodium, prednisolone sodium phosphate, sulphafurazole diethanolamine, vitamin B complex with C.

However, prochlorperazine edisylate injection (SKF) 10 mg/1000 mL was reported to be physically compatible, in glucose 5% injection, for 24 hours with buffered benzylpenicillin potassium injection (pH 6.0 to 7.0, Squibb).[11]

Prochlorperazine edisylate injection has also been reported to be incompatible with chlorothiazide sodium, cyanocobalamin, erythromycin gluceptate, hydrocortisone sodium succinate, kanamycin sulphate, methicillin sodium, oxytetracycline hydrochloride, paraldehyde, pentobarbitone sodium, tetracycline hydrochloride, and vancomycin hydrochloride.

Sorption

No significant adsorption of prochlorperazine edisylate to cellulose membrane filters occurred during 'in-line filtration' (over 8 hours) of prochlorperazine edisylate infusion solutions (Compazine, SKF, USA) 5 mg/1000 mL in glucose 5% or sodium chloride 0.9% solutions.[12]

FORMULATION

Excipients

Excipients that have been used in presentations of prochlorperazine include:

Tablets, prochlorperazine maleate: acacia; brilliant blue FCF (133); calcium sulphate; D&C Green No. 5; gelatin; lactose; liquid paraffin; quinoline yellow (E104); starch; stearic acid; sucrose; sunset yellow FCF (E110); talc.

Spansules (sustained-release capsules), prochlorperazine maleate: allura red AC (E129); benzyl alcohol; brilliant blue FCF (133); cetylpyridinium chloride; D&C Green No.5; gelatin; glyceryl monostearate; quinoline yellow (E104); sodium lauryl sulphate; starch; sucrose; sunset yellow FCF (E110); wax.

Granules, prochlorperazine maleate: aspartame.

Oral liquids, prochlorperazine edisylate: sodium benzoate; sodium citrate; sucrose; sunset yellow FCF (E110).

Prochlorperazine mesylate: citric acid monohydrate; ethanol; ponceau 4R; propylene glycol; saccharin sodium; sodium benzoate; sodium metabisulphite; sodium sulphite; sugars (68% w/v).

Suppositories, prochlorperazine: glycerol; glyceryl monopalmitate; glyceryl monostearate; hydrogenated coconut oil fatty acids; hydrogenated palm kernel oil fatty acids.

Injections, prochlorperazine edisylate: benzyl alcohol; sodium biphosphate; sodium bisulphite; sodium phosphate; sodium saccharin; sodium sulphite; sodium tartrate.

Prochlorperazine mesylate: ethanolamine; sodium chloride; sodium metabisulphite; sodium sulphite.

Bioavailability

Prochlorperazine has been shown to have poor bioavailability following administration via the oral route. When administered orally as 25 mg single doses to eight healthy volunteers[13] prochlorperazine absorption was slow. Bioavailability ranged from 0% to 16% compared to that after intravenous administration. Detection of low concentrations of prochlorperazine in plasma was problematic. Similarly, in a comprehensive study of the pharmacokinetics and pharmacodynamics of prochlorperazine following single and repeated administration both orally and intravenously (to five healthy subjects), oral bioavailability was reported to be low.[14]

Hessell *et al*[15] reported that, in a crossover study using six healthy volunteers, the bioavailability of prochlorperazine maleate after administration of buccal tablets (which have a gelling polysaccharide matrix) was more than double that after oral administration.

PROCESSING

Sterilisation

Solutions of prochlorperazine mesylate for injection are sterilised by heating in an autoclave in an atmosphere of nitrogen or other suitable gas.

REFERENCES

1. Green AL. J Pharm Pharmacol 1967;19:10–16.
2. Vezin WR, Florence AT. Int J Pharmaceutics 1979;3:231–7.
3. Ravin LJ, Kennon L, Swintosky JV. J Am Pharm Assoc Sci Ed 1958;47:760.
4. Twycross RG, Gilhooley RA [letter]. Br Med J 1973;4:552.
5. Greig JR [letter]. Pharm J 1986;237:504.
6. Jett S, Eng SS, Milewski B [letter]. Am J Hosp Pharm 1983;40:210.
7. Riley BB. J Hosp Pharm 1970;28:228–40.
8. Stevenson JG, Patriarca C [letter]. Am J Hosp Pharm 1985;42:2651.
9. Zuber DEL [letter]. Am J Hosp Pharm 1987;44:67.
10. Misgen R. Am J Hosp Pharm 1965;22:92–4.
11. Parker EA. Am J Hosp Pharm 1969;26:543–4.
12. Styles ML, Allen LV. Infusion 1979;3:67–9.
13. Taylor WB, Bateman DN. Br J Clin Pharmacol 1987;23:137–42.
14. Isah AO, Rawlins MD, Bateman DN. Br J Clin Pharmacol 1991;32:677–82.
15. Hessell PG, Lloyd-Jones JG, Muir NC, Sugden K. J Pharm Pharmacol 1988 Dec;40:150P.

Promethazine (BAN, rINN)

Histamine H₁-receptor antagonist
Dimethyl(2-phenothiazin-10-ylpropyl)amine; 1,*N,N*-trimethyl-2-(phenothiazin-10-yl)ethylamine
$C_{17}H_{20}N_2S = 284.4$

Promethazine Hydrochloride (BANM, rINNM)

Diprazinum; proazamine chloride
$C_{17}H_{20}N_2S,HCl = 320.9$

Promethazine Theoclate (BAN)

Promethazine Teoclate (rINN). The promethazine salt of 8-chlorotheophylline
$C_{17}H_{20}N_2S,C_7H_7ClN_4O_2 = 499.0$
CAS—60-87-7 (promethazine); 58-33-3 (promethazine hydrochloride); 17693-51-5 (promethazine theoclate)

Pharmacopoeial status

BP (promethazine hydrochloride, promethazine theoclate); USP (promethazine hydrochloride)

Preparations

Compendial
Promethazine Hydrochloride Tablets BP. Coated tablets containing, in each, 10 mg, 20 mg, and 25 mg are usually available.
Promethazine Oral Solution BP (Promethazine Elixir, Promethazine Hydrochloride Elixir). A solution containing promethazine hydrochloride in a suitable flavoured vehicle; if the oral solution is diluted, the diluted oral solution should be freshly prepared. An oral solution containing 5 mg in 5 mL is usually available.
Promethazine Injection BP (Promethazine Hydrochloride Injection). A sterile solution of promethazine hydrochloride in water for injections free from dissolved air. pH 5.0 to 6.0. Injections containing 25 mg in 1 mL and 50 mg in 2 mL are usually available.
Promethazine Theoclate Tablets BP. Tablets containing, in each, 25 mg are usually available.
Promethazine Hydrochloride Tablets USP.

Promethazine Hydrochloride Syrup USP.
Promethazine Hydrochloride Suppositories USP.
Promethazine Hydrochloride Injection USP. pH between 4.0 and 5.5.

Non-compendial
Avomine (Rhône-Poulenc Rorer). *Tablets*, promethazine theoclate 25 mg.
Phenergan (Rhône-Poulenc Rorer). *Tablets*, promethazine hydrochloride 10 mg and 25 mg.
Elixir, sugar free, promethazine hydrochloride 5 mg/5 mL.
Injection, promethazine hydrochloride 25 mg/mL. *Diluent*: water for injections. Solutions of Phenergan are incompatible with alkaline substances, which precipitate the insoluble promethazine base.

Containers and storage
Solid state
Promethazine Hydrochloride BP and Promethazine Theoclate BP should be kept in well-closed containers and protected from light.

Dosage forms
Promethazine Oral Solution BP should be protected from light and stored at a temperature not exceeding 25°.
Promethazine Injection BP and Promethazine Theoclate Tablets BP should be protected from light.
Promethazine Hydrochloride Tablets USP, Promethazine Hydrochloride Syrup USP, and Promethazine Hydrochloride Suppositories USP should be preserved in tight, light-resistant containers. The suppositories should be stored in a cold place.
Promethazine Hydrochloride Injection USP should be preserved in single-dose or in multiple-dose containers, preferably of Type I glass, protected from light.
Avomine tablets and Phenergan preparations should be protected from light. Phenergan tablets should be stored below 30° and Phenergan elixir below 25°.

PHYSICAL PROPERTIES
Promethazine is a crystalline solid.
Promethazine hydrochloride is a white or faintly yellowish, crystalline powder; practically odourless. On prolonged exposure to air it is slowly oxidised, acquiring a blue colour.
Promethazine theoclate is a white or almost white, odourless or almost odourless powder.

Melting point
Promethazine melts at about 60°.
Promethazine hydrochloride melts at about 222°, with decomposition.

pH
Promethazine hydrochloride: pH 4.0 to 5.0 for a freshly prepared 10% w/v solution (BP) and a 1 in 20 solution (USP).

Dissociation constant
pK_a 9.1 (25°)

Partition coefficient
Log P (octanol/pH 7.4), 2.9

Solubility
Solubilities of salts of promethazine in various solvents are as follows:

	Promethazine hydrochloride	Promethazine theoclate
Water	1 in 0.6	very slightly soluble
Ethanol	1 in 9	1 in 70
Chloroform	1 in 2	1 in 2.5
Ether	practically insoluble	practically insoluble
Acetone	practically insoluble	—

Critical micelle concentration
In anoxic aqueous solution,[1] the critical micelle concentration of promethazine hydrochloride decreased with an increase in temperature from 1.33% at 25° to 0.82% at 70°.

FURTHER INFORMATION. Nuclear magnetic resonance studies on micelle formation by promethazine hydrochloride—Florence AT, Parfitt RT. J Pharm Pharmacol 1970;22:122S–125S.

Dissolution
The USP specifies that for Promethazine Hydrochloride Tablets USP not less than 75% of the labelled amount of $C_{17}H_{20}N_2S,HCl$ is dissolved in 45 minutes. Dissolution medium: 900 mL of 0.1N hydrochloric acid; Apparatus 1 at 100 rpm.

STABILITY
In aqueous solution, promethazine hydrochloride can undergo oxidation and photolysis. Metal ions, such as iron (III) or copper (II), accelerate the degradation rate. In general, the stability of promethazine hydrochloride increases with a decrease in pH. Micelle formation, which occurs at concentrations above 0.5% of promethazine hydrochloride, decreases the decomposition rate.

Degradation pathways and kinetics
When thermal degradation of promethazine hydrochloride (at 65°) in water was investigated in the presence of oxygen, in the dark, the following products were identified (by TLC) and isolated: 10-methylphenothiazine, phenothiazine, 3*H*-phenothiazine-3-one, phenothiazine 5-oxide, promethazine 5-oxide, 7-hydroxy-3*H*-phenothiazine-3-one, acetaldehyde, formaldehyde, and dimethylamine.[2]
In an oxygen-saturated solution, in the dark, degradation of promethazine hydrochloride[3] followed first-order kinetics in the temperature range 45° to 90° and the pH range 1.5 to 6.3. The rate constant increased with pH to a constant value at above pH 5.0. An activation energy of about 128 kJ/mol was calculated at pH 4.6. Of the metal ions investigated (at 65°), copper (II) and iron (III) ions, even in trace quantities, increased the degradation rate, although iron (III) only accelerated the initial rate. The decomposition products studied were 3*H*-phenothiazine-3-one, promethazine 5-oxide, and 7-hydroxy-3*H*-phenothiazine-3-one. Under anaerobic conditions, promethazine hydrochloride did not degrade, although in the presence of copper (II) or iron (III) ions some degradation occurred, with formation of 10-methyl phenothiazine, phenothiazine, and 3*H*-phenothiazine-3-one. Mechanisms of oxidative degradation were discussed.
First-order degradation was apparent in oxygenated solutions of promethazine hydrochloride (0.05% to 0.3%) in ethanol 50% with dibutyl phthalate 1%, pH 1.2 to 5.0 (citrate buffer with edetic acid 0.1%), maintained at 90° in the dark.[4] The pH of minimum stability was about 4.3. However, at pH 5.5 to 7.0, degradation was not first order at 60° and above; coacervation of promethazine was observed under such conditions.

Solutions of promethazine hydrochloride form micellar aggregates above the critical micelle concentration and this can influence the kinetics of degradation. Meakin et al[5] prepared solutions of promethazine hydrochloride in citrate buffer (pH 4.0, ionic strength 0.5) with edetic acid 0.1%. At 90° in the dark, decomposition followed first-order kinetics at concentrations of promethazine hydrochloride of up to 1.56×10^{-2}M (0.5%) and zero-order kinetics at concentrations of above 9.35×10^{-2}M (3%); half-lives at these two concentrations were 7.95 hours and 22.28 hours, respectively. Complex kinetics were followed at intermediate concentrations. These effects were correlated with micelle formation.

Photolytic degradation[6] of 0.05% promethazine hydrochloride-Sørensen buffer solutions at pH 2.98, 3.94, and 5.12 did not follow simple kinetics under intense ultraviolet light at 30°.

When 1-mL samples of promethazine hydrochloride injection (25 mg/mL, Fellows, USA) were repackaged in 3-mL amber glass syringes (Hy-Pod) and stored at 25°, a loss of about 5.4% of the initial concentration was measured after 360 days.[7] No significant changes in pH or physical appearance were noted. From accelerated studies at elevated temperature (40°, 50°, and 60°) a $t_{10\%}$ of 441 days at 25° was predicted.

Stabilisation

Under aerobic conditions (at 65° in the dark) the observed rate constant for decomposition of promethazine hydrochloride, pH 3.2, decreased in the presence of disodium edetate at 2×10^{-3}M and 1×10^{-2}M.[3] However, at pH 6.5 no reduction was observed. Similarly, the presence of edetic acid 0.1% reduced the rate of decomposition of solutions buffered to pH 3 and 4 (at 90° in the dark).[5]

Antoxidants had variable effects[3] on the stability of promethazine hydrochloride at pH 3.2 at 65°. Hydroquinone, at low concentrations, exerted a stabilising effect whereas at higher concentrations, decomposition was accelerated. Effects of ascorbic acid were unpredictable and sodium metabisulphite had no influence.

FURTHER INFORMATION. Oxidative degradation of pharmaceutically important phenothiazines. II. Quantitative determination of promethazine and some degradation products—Underberg WJM. J Pharm Sci 1978;67(8):1131–3. Kinetics and mechanism of oxidation of promazine and promethazine by ferric perchlorate—Gasco MR, Carlotti ME. J Pharm Sci 1978;67(2):168–71. Gas liquid chromatographic determination of promethazine hydrochloride in cocoa butter [theobroma oil]-white wax suppositories [in presence of thermal and photolytic degradation products]—Stavchansky S, Wu P, Wallace JE. Drug Dev Ind Pharm 1983;9(6):989–98.

INCOMPATIBILITY/COMPATIBILITY

Promethazine hydrochloride has been reported to be incompatible with: alkalis; barbiturates; benzylpenicillin salts; calcium gluconate; carbenicillin; chloramphenicol sodium succinate; chlordiazepoxide; codeine sulphate; heparin sodium; hydrocortisone sodium succinate; methylprednisolone; methicillin sodium; morphine sulphate; phenytoin sodium; sulphafurazole diethanolamine; vitamin B complex with C.

Immediate precipitation occurred when 1 mL of promethazine hydrochloride (100 mg/L) was admixed with 1 mL of aminophylline (1 g/L), chlorothiazide (2 g/L), ethamivan (2 g/L), methohexitone sodium (2 g/L), or sulphadimidine sodium (4 g/L); all solutions were prepared in either glucose 5% injection or sodium chloride 0.9% injection.[8] A haze developed over a 3-hour period in admixtures of promethazine hydrochloride (100 mg/L) with phenobarbitone sodium (800 mg/L) in glucose 5% injection whereas an immediate precipitate formed in admixtures in sodium chloride 0.9% injection.

A white precipitate was observed[9] when promethazine hydrochloride injection was administered after cefoperazone sodium injection through the same set of intravenous tubing; this was attributed to formation of an ionic complex between the two drugs.

About 5% of the initial concentration of promethazine hydrochloride was lost (attributed to sorption) when unbuffered (pH 5) promethazine hydrochloride injection 8 mg/L in sodium chloride 0.9% injection was stored in polyvinyl chloride infusion bags for one week in the dark at room temperature (15° to 20°).[10] However, when the solution was buffered to pH 7.4, about 59% of the initial concentration was lost (by sorption) under the same storage conditions.

In a further study,[11] the concentration of promethazine hydrochloride 8 mg/mL in sodium chloride 0.9% injection decreased by 22% during a seven-hour simulated infusion (at 1 mL/min) through a delivery system consisting of a cellulose propionate burette chamber and 170 cm of polyvinyl chloride tubing. During one-hour simulated infusions (at 0.08 mL/min) of similar solutions using a syringe pump system, which consisted of a 20-cm length of polyethylene tubing or a 50-cm length of Silastic tubing attached to a glass syringe on a syringe pump, 5% of the initial promethazine hydrochloride concentration was lost to the polyethylene tubing and 72% to the Silastic tubing. However, no loss due to sorption was detected when promethazine hydrochloride injection 8 mg/L in sodium chloride 0.9% injection was stored in all-plastic syringes consisting of polypropylene barrels and polyethylene plungers for 24 hours at room temperature in the dark.

FURTHER INFORMATION. An in vitro chemical interaction between promethazine hydrochloride and chloroquine phosphate - Abubakar AA, Mustapha A, Wambebe OC. Int Pharm J 1993;7:14–18.

FORMULATION

Excipients

Excipients that have been used in presentations of promethazine include:

Tablets, promethazine hydrochloride: erythrosine (E127); lactose; magnesium stearate; methylcellulose; saccharin sodium; sunset yellow FCF (E110).

Promethazine theoclate: lactose; sodium metabisulphite.

Oral liquids, promethazine hydrochloride: acid fuchsine D; brilliant blue FCF (133); chloroform water; citric acid; ethanol; glycerol; hydrogenated glucose; orange tincture; quinoline yellow (E104); saccharin sodium; sodium benzoate; sodium citrate; sodium metabisulphite; sodium sulphite; sodium propionate; sunset yellow FCF (E110).

Creams, promethazine: cholesterol; coumarin; glycerol; hydrous wool fat; lavender oil; methyl hydroxybenzoate; stearic acid; triethanolamine.

Suppositories, promethazine hydrochloride: ascorbyl palmitate; silica; theobroma oil; white beeswax.

Injections, promethazine hydrochloride: calcium chloride; disodium edetate; phenol; sodium acetate/acetic acid buffer; sodium metabisulphite; sodium sulphite.

Bioavailability

Stavchansky et al[12] undertook a three-way crossover study (involving 14 or 20 healthy volunteers) to compare the pharmacokinetic parameters of promethazine following single-dose administration of promethazine hydrochloride 50 mg as a macrogol suppository, a theobroma oil/white beeswax suppository, and an oral syrup (Phenergan syrup fortis, Wyeth, USA). Relative to the oral syrup, the bioavailabilities of the macrogol suppository and the theobroma oil/white beeswax suppository were 118.3% and 62.8%, respectively.

In a single-dose, crossover study with six healthy subjects,[13] absorption profiles of promethazine hydrochloride did not differ significantly when administered as an oral solution (25 mg in 50 mL of water) or a rectal solution (25 mg in 5 mL of buffer, pH 5). However, the relative bioavailability of a fatty suppository (promethazine hydrochloride 25 mg in Witepsol H15) was significantly less than that of the oral or rectal solutions. Although the suppository showed 'fast' release *in vitro* (85% released within 30 minutes at pH 5), a 'sustained' *in-vivo* absorption profile was observed.

In a crossover study,[14] 15 healthy subjects received single 50 mg doses of promethazine hydrochloride as an innovator tablet (Wyeth, USA), a generic tablet (Cord Laboratories, USA), and an oral solution (10.25 mg/mL in 2.5% v/v of ethanol 95%). Although there were no significant differences in the areas under plasma concentration versus time curves between the three products, the innovator product had a significantly lower peak plasma concentration and took longer to reach this concentration than the oral solution; the generic tablet did not exhibit such a delay. There was no significant difference between the dissolution rates of the two tablets *in vitro*. Intersubject variation was high for all parameters.

FURTHER INFORMATION. Pharmacokinetics of promethazine and its sulphoxide metabolite after intravenous and oral administration to man—Taylor G, Houston JB, Shaffer J, Mawer G. Br J Clin Pharmacol 1983;15:287–93. Mathematical modelling of drug [promethazine hydrochloride] release from hydroxypropyl-methylcellulose [hypromellose] matrices: Effect of temperature—Ford JL, Mitchell K, Rowe P, Armstrong DJ, Elliott PNC, Rostron C, *et al.* Int J Pharmaceutics 1991;71:95–104.

PROCESSING

Sterilisation

Promethazine injection can be sterilised by heating in an autoclave.

REFERENCES

1. Stevens J, Meakin BJ, Davies DJG. J Pharm Pharmacol 1973;25:119P.
2. Underberg WJM. J Pharm Sci 1978;67(8):1128–30.
3. Underberg WJM. J Pharm Sci 1978;67(8):1133–8.
4. Stevens J, Meakin BJ, Davies DJG. J Pharm Pharmacol 1972;24:133P.
5. Meakin BJ, Stevens J, Davies DJG. J Pharm Pharmacol 1978;30:75–80.
6. Stavchansky S, Wallace JE, Wu P. J Pharm Sci 1983;72(5):546–8.
7. Kleinberg ML, Stauffer GL, Latiolais CJ. Am J Hosp Pharm 1980;37:680–2.
8. Riley BB. J Hosp Pharm 1970;28:228–40.
9. Scott SM [letter]. Am J Hosp Pharm 1990;47:519.
10. Kowaluk EA, Roberts MS, Blackburn HD, Polack AE. Am J Hosp Pharm 1981;38:1308–14.
11. Kowaluk EA, Roberts MS, Polack AE. Am J Hosp Pharm 1982;39:460–7.
12. Stavchansky S, Wallace JE, Geary R, Hecht G, Robb CA, Wu P. J Pharm Sci 1987;76(6):441–5.
13. Moolenaar F, Ensing JG, Bolhius BG, Visser J. Int J Pharmaceutics 1981;9:353–7.
14. Zaman R, Honigberg IL, Francisco GE, Kotzan JA, Stewart JT, Brown WJ, *et al.* Biopharm Drug Dispos 1986;7:281–91.

Propranolol (BAN, rINN)

Beta-adrenoceptor antagonist

($\pm$)1-Isopropylamino-3-(1-naphthyloxy)propan-2-ol;   1-[(1-methylethyl)amino]-3-(1-naphthalenyloxy)-2-propanol

$C_{16}H_{21}NO_2 = 259.3$

Propranolol Hydrochloride (BANM, USAN, rINNM)

$C_{16}H_{21}NO_2,HCl = 295.8$

CAS—525-66-6,   13013-17-7($\pm$)   (propranolol);   318-98-9, 3506-09-0 ($\pm$) (propranolol hydrochloride)

Pharmacopoeial status

BP, USP (propranolol hydrochloride)

Preparations

Compendial

Propranolol Tablets BP. Tablets containing, in each, 10, 40, 80, and 160 mg of propranolol hydrochloride are usually available.
Propranolol Injection BP. A sterile solution of propranolol hydrochloride in water for injections containing anhydrous citric acid or citric acid monohydrate. pH 3.0 to 3.5. An injection containing 1 mg in 1 mL is usually available.
Propranolol Hydrochloride Extended-release Capsules USP.
Propranolol Hydrochloride Tablets USP.
Propranolol Hydrochloride Injection USP. pH between 2.8 and 4.0.

Non-compendial

Apsolol (APS). *Tablets*, propranolol hydrochloride 10, 40, 80, and 160 mg.
Berkolol (Berk). *Tablets*, propranolol hydrochloride 10, 40, 80, and 160 mg.
Cardinol (CP). *Tablets*, propranolol hydrochloride 10, 40, 80, and 160 mg.
Half-Inderal LA (ICI). *Capsules*, sustained release, propranolol hydrochloride 80 mg.
Inderal LA (ICI). *Capsules*, sustained release, propranolol hydrochloride 160 mg.
Inderal (ICI). *Tablets*, propranolol hydrochloride 10 mg, 40 mg, and 80 mg.
Injection, propranolol hydrochloride 1 mg/mL. Compatible with sodium chloride 0.9% injection and glucose 5% injection.
Propranolol tablets are also available in various strengths from Ashbourne (Propanix), Cox, DDSA (Angilol), Evans, Kerfoot, Norton.
Propranolol sustained-release capsules are also available from Ashbourne (Propanix SR), CP (Sloprolol), Lagap (Bedranol SR), Monmouth (Betadur CR, Half-Betadur CR), Tillomed (Beta-Prograne).

Containers and storage

Solid state

Propranolol Hydrochloride USP should be preserved in well-closed containers.

Dosage forms

Propranolol Hydrochloride Extended-release Capsules USP should be preserved in well-closed containers.
Propranolol Hydrochloride Tablets USP should be preserved in well-closed, light-resistant containers.
Propranolol Hydrochloride Injection USP should be preserved in single-dose, light-resistant containers, preferably of Type I glass.
Apsolol tablets and Berkolol tablets should be protected from light.
Cardinol tablets should be stored in a cool, dry place protected from light and moisture.
Inderal, Inderal LA, and Half-Inderal LA preparations should be stored at room temperature, protected from light and moisture. Inderal injection should be stored at room temperature, protected from light.

PHYSICAL PROPERTIES

Propranolol exists in the form of crystals.
Propranolol hydrochloride is a white or almost white powder; odourless, with a bitter taste. It absorbs less than 1% of water at 25° at relative humidity up to 80%.

Melting point

Propranolol melts in the range 94° to 96°.
Propranolol hydrochloride melts in the range 163° to 166°.

pH

The pH of a 1% solution of *propranolol hydrochloride* in water lies between 5.0 and 6.0.

Dissociation constant

pK_a 9.5 (24°)

Partition coefficients

Log P (octanol/pH 7.4), 1.2
A value for log P of 3.37 (octanol/water) for propranolol was cited by Burgot *et al*.[1]
Nieder *et al*[2] measured the partition coefficient of propranolol in octanol/phosphate buffer, pH 7.4, as 11.61 (log P, 1.06) after 2 hours and 13.41 (log P, 1.13) after 6 hours (at 37°) 'of equilibrium time'.

FURTHER INFORMATION. Ionisation constants by curve fitting: determination of partition and distribution coefficients of acids and bases and their ions—Clarke FH, Cahoon NM. J Pharm Sci 1987;76(8):611–19.

Solubility

Propranolol hydrochloride is soluble 1 in 20 of water and 1 in 20 of ethanol; slightly soluble in chloroform and practically insoluble in ether.

Critical micelle concentration

Elliot *et al*[3] reported that increasing concentration of electrolyte reduced the degree of ionisation and increased the aggregation number of propranolol hydrochloride in solution. The authors suggest that charged micelles of propranolol hydrochloride are formed in aqueous solutions. Critical micelle concentrations (mol/L) of 0.108, 0.098, 0.078, and 0.069 were established in

water (pH 4.06), 0.03M potassium chloride (KCl) (pH 4.52), 0.1M KCl (pH 4.62), and 0.2M KCl (pH 4.72), respectively.

Crystal and molecular structure

Enantiomers

Simultaneous determination of propranolol enantiomers in plasma by high-performance liquid chromatography with fluorescence detection—Prakash C, Koshakji RP, Wood AJJ, Blair IA. J Pharm Sci 1989;78(9):771–5.

STABILITY

Propranolol hydrochloride is affected by light. In aqueous solutions, it decomposes with oxidation of the isopropylamine side-chain, accompanied by reduction in the pH and discoloration of the solution. Solutions are most stable at pH 3.0 and decompose rapidly under alkaline conditions.

Extemporaneous liquid preparations

Brown and Kayes[4] found microbial contamination in suspensions of propranolol hydrochloride, prepared according to the manufacturer's formulation from crushed Inderal (ICI) tablets with and without methyl or propyl hydroxybenzoates as preservative, after storage at 20° in amber bottles for 5 days. Coagulation of the suspensions occurred at 40° and 60°. Ultraviolet spectrophotometric analysis of aqueous solutions of propranolol hydrochloride (0.05% w/v) containing either hydroxybenzoates or carmellose sodium suggested that the hydroxybenzoates interacted with propranolol and that this interaction could result in inactivation of the preservatives. In aqueous solutions, colour intensity was greater with increased storage time, corresponding to degradation of propranolol hydrochloride. An alternative formulation proposed by the authors (see under Formulation, below) was buffered to pH 3.0 with McIlvaine's buffer or citric acid. The chemical stability of these suspensions was greater than that of an unbuffered version of the same formulation (pH 7.0).

The chemical stability of propranolol hydrochloride in five extemporaneous paediatric formulations (and of the preservatives present in two of these formulations) was shown by workers in Australia[5] to be unaffected by storage at 4°, 30°, and 50° during a study period of 12 weeks. However, several physical instabilities and interactions were noted including pH changes, possible interaction of propranolol hydrochloride with some excipients, precipitation, turbidity and colour development, changes in viscosity, and fungal growth. None of the formulations tested (in common use in Australia) could be recommended unequivocally. No caking was evident in any of the formulae.

A suspension of propranolol hydrochloride (1 mg/mL) was formulated from 100 finely-powdered 10 mg tablets (Inderal, Ayerst) in a commercial vehicle (Roxanne Diluent, flavoured for oral use), containing ethanol 1% and saccharin 0.05% in a cherry-flavoured 33% macrogol 8000 basis.[6] After storage in amber glass bottles at 2° or 25° for 4 months, at least 90% of the initial concentration of propranolol remained, leading the authors to recommend a shelf-life of at least 120 days for this suspension at room and refrigeration temperatures. The pH of the samples remained constant and there was no visible evidence of microbial growth throughout the study period. Even after 4 months, settled suspensions could be easily resuspended. Other extemporaneous preparations of propranolol hydrochloride, formulated by Gupta and Stewart[7] using compounded 20 mg tablets (to form a suspension) or propranolol injection (to form a solution) with a syrup (sucrose 600 mg/mL in purified water with sodium benzoate 0.1% and citric acid), remained stable for at least 238 days at room temperature. However, Rooney and Creurer[8] pointed out that Gupta and Stewart's suspension contained an unspecified amount of citric acid in order to adjust the pH of the syrup closer to that of maximum stability for propranolol (pH 3.0). They warned that the stability data published by Gupta and Stewart cannot be applied to a suspension where the syrup has been prepared extemporaneously without such pH adjustment.

FURTHER INFORMATION. Oxidation of β-blocking agents. V. Light-influenced oxidation of propranolol and its glycol with *N*-bromosuccinamide—Salomies H. Acta Pharm Suec 1987;24:193–8.

INCOMPATIBILITY/COMPATIBILITY

Intravenous admixtures

Propranolol hydrochloride injection (Inderal Injectable Solution, Ayerst) was judged to be visually and chemically compatible for 24 hours with the following intravenous fluids (USP standard) at final propranolol hydrochloride concentrations of 0.5 and 20 micrograms/mL: glucose 5% injection, glucose 5% and sodium chloride 0.9% injection, glucose 5% and sodium chloride 0.45% injection, compound sodium lactate injection (lactated Ringer's injection), and sodium chloride 0.9% injection. The pH of the solutions remained unchanged during the 24-hour period. There was no sorption to polyvinyl chloride bags, polyolefin containers, or filters.[9]

Adsorption

There are reports in the literature of interactions between propranolol hydrochloride and various adsorbents, resulting in a possible alteration of the bioavailability of the drug.

Al-Gohary *et al*[10] studied the effect of pH and temperature on adsorption of propranolol hydrochloride by attapulgite, charcoal, kaolin, and magnesium trisilicate. Adsorption of propranolol occurred in the rank order charcoal > magnesium trisilicate > attapulgite > kaolin. Over the pH range 1.6 to 7.4 an eight-fold increase in adsorption of propranolol onto magnesium trisilicate was apparent but a lesser effect was noted with the other excipients. An increase in temperature (25° to 50°) caused an increase in adsorption of propranolol by charcoal (164.1 mg/g to 213.6 mg/g) but a decrease in adsorption of propranolol by kaolin and magnesium trisilicate.

In further work,[11] the same authors demonstrated that the adsorption of propranolol hydrochloride onto magnesium trisilicate in the presence of magnesium chloride, sodium chloride, or hypromellose (Methofas), in various solutions, was suppressed by these additives. The greater the ionic strength and cation valency of the additive, the greater was the suppression of adsorption.

Interaction between propranolol hydrochloride and antacids or excipients having adsorbent properties was examined by Çalis *et al*.[12] Magnesium trisilicate was found to have the highest adsorptive capacity for propranolol hydrochloride, followed by magnesium hydroxide, dihydroxyaluminium sodium carbonate and aluminium hydroxide. Magnesium carbonate and kaolin exhibited low adsorptive capacities. The authors suggest that co-administration of propranolol hydrochloride and the adsorbents listed could lead to a reduction in bioavailability of propranolol.

FORMULATION

Excipients

Excipients that have been used in presentations of propranolol include:

Tablets, propranolol: alginic acid; gelatin; magnesium stearate; mannitol; stearic acid.
Propranolol hydrochloride: alginic acid; brilliant blue FCF (133); carmellose calcium; carmine (E120); D&C Red No.30; erythrosine (E127); formocasein; gelatin; glycerol; hypromellose; lactose; magnesium carbonate; magnesium stearate; maize starch; mannitol; microcrystalline cellulose; povidone; quinoline yellow (E104); stearic acid; sunset yellow FCF (E110); synthetic iron oxide; titanium dioxide (E171).
Capsules, propranolol hydrochloride: brilliant blue FCF (133); erythrosine (E127); ethylcellulose; gelatin; glycerol; hypromellose; iron oxide (E172); microcrystalline cellulose; povidone; talc; titanium dioxide (E171).
Suspensions, propranolol hydrochloride: cherry syrup; Cologel; glycerol; Roxanne diluent; sodium benzoate; syrup.
Intravenous fluids, propranolol hydrochloride: citric acid.

Bioavailability and bioequivalence

The bioavailability of propranolol in six healthy volunteers was found by South American workers[13] to be 2.73-times greater following rectal administration of a suppository (80 mg propranolol) formulated in a Witepsol H-15 basis, than by the oral route (two propranolol 40 mg tablets).
After oral administration of 160 mg propranolol (Inderal, ICI) and 160 mg Long Acting propranolol (ICI) to ten healthy volunteers, plasma concentrations peaked at 2 hours and 10 hours, respectively.[14] At 24 hours, plasma concentrations were significantly higher after Long Acting propranolol.
In a comparative study in 24 healthy male volunteers, generic propranolol hydrochloride (Parke-Davis) tablets 10 mg, 40 mg, and 80 mg were found to be bioequivalent with Inderal (Ayerst) tablets 10 mg and 80 mg.[15]
No significant difference was apparent between the bioavailabilities of four brands of propranolol commercially available in India (Inderal, Ciplar, Corbeta, and Propal) following single and multiple dosing in six healthy male volunteers, although much inter-individual variation in the pharmacokinetics of propranolol was observed.[16]

Generic tablets

An *in-vitro* comparison of proprietary (Inderal, ICI, 40 mg) and generic (Antigen, Cox, Evans, Generics UK, Norton) tablets[17] revealed no major differences in physical characteristics and dissolution rates between any of the samples studied.

Oral liquids

Brown and Kayes[4] prepared a suspension of propranolol hydrochloride, adjusted to pH 3.0 with McIlvaine's buffer, using ethanol as preservative and suggested the following formulation as suitable for '14 days supply': propranolol hydrochloride (Inderal tablets) 0.05% w/v, ethanol (90%) 22.50% w/v, compound orange spirit 0.20% w/v, compound tartrazine solution 0.20% w/v, amaranth solution 0.05% w/v, cetomacrogol 1000 q.s., syrup 12.5% w/v, water to 100.0% w/v. See Stability above.
Ahmed *et al*[5] evaluated six extemporaneous oral liquid formulations of propranolol hydrochloride in common use in Australia (prepared using crushed Inderal 40 mg tablets). See Stability above.

Modified-release preparations

A sparingly soluble complex of propranolol hydrochloride and methacrylic acid copolymer (Eudragit L) was formed at saturation equilibrium and formulated into tablets, containing the equivalent of 100 mg propranolol base, with lactose, sodium starch glycollate (Explotab), magnesium stearate, and microcrystalline cellulose (Avicel).[18] Dissolution data indicated a five-fold decrease in the dissolution rate of the polymer complex compared with that of propranolol hydrochloride, in either 0.1M hydrochloric acid or pH 7.4 phosphate buffer.

The dissolution rate of propranolol hydrochloride from four tablet formulations containing magnesium stearate and Eudragit RS 100 or carmellose sodium, or both, at various concentrations, was found to be increased by an increase in dissolution apparatus stirring speed, pH (from 1.2 to 7.2), temperature (25° to 60°), and increased Eudragit RS 100 content.[19] The release rate of propranolol hydrochloride from tablets formulated with 17% Eudragit RS 100 and 50% carmellose sodium after storage at 60° for 100 days was slower than that of tablets stored at 25° for 100 days, whereas storage at 45° did not alter the rate of dissolution.

An experimental sustained-release tablet formulation of propranolol, containing Methocel, was reported to have a better *in-vitro* release profile than the marketed capsule.[20] The release rate was reported to be affected by molecular weight and concentration of polymer, 'drug loading', and pH.

The release rate of propranolol hydrochloride from matrix tablets into water was decreased when the anionic surfactant sodium dodecyl sulphate was included in the formulation, which also contained hypromellose and magnesium stearate; this effect was attributed to formation of propranolol dodecyl sulphate which formed lyotropic liquid crystals on contact with water. When the cationic surfactant cetrimide was included in the matrix tablets a slight increase in the dissolution rate of propranolol hydrochloride was observed. Interactions similar to those between propranolol hydrochloride and the anionic surfactant were not thought to occur.[21]

FURTHER INFORMATION. Bioavailability of propranolol following oral and transdermal administration in *rabbits* [transdermal delivery resulted in increased systemic bioavailability compared to oral delivery]—Corbo M, Liu J-C, Chien YW. J Pharm Sci 1990;79(7):584–7. Pharmacokinetic and pharmacodynamic studies with long-acting propranolol—McAinsh J, Baber NS, Smith R, Young J. Br J Clin Pharmacol 1978;6:115–21. Nasal absorption of propranolol from different dosage forms by *rats* and *dogs*—Hussain A, Hirai S, Bawarshi R. J Pharm Sci 1980;69(12):1411–13. Nasal absorption of propranolol in humans [nasal route produced bioavailability equivalent to intravenous route and superior to oral route]—Hussain A, Foster T, Hirai S, Kashihara T, Batenhorst R, Jones M [letter]. J Pharm Sci 1990;69(10):1240. Compatibility study between propranolol hydrochloride and tablet excipients using differential scanning calorimetry—Gerber JJ, Lötter AP. Drug Dev Ind Pharm 1993;19(5):623–9.

Evaluation of drug-containing polymer films prepared from aqueous latexes—Bodmeier R, Paeratakul O. Pharm Res 1989;6(8):725–30. Propranolol HCl release from acrylic films prepared from aqueous latexes—Bodmeier R, Paeratakul O. Int J Pharmaceutics 1990;59:197–204. Release and permeation studies of propranolol hydrochloride from hydrophilic polymeric matrices—Babar A, Pillai J, Plakogiannis FM. Drug Dev Ind Pharm 1992;18(16):1823–30. Formulation, *in-vitro* release and therapeutic effect of hydrogels based controlled release tablets of propranolol hydrochloride—Ganga S, Singh PN, Singh J. Drug Dev Ind Pharm 1992;18(19):2049–66. Adhesive and *in vitro* release characteristics of propranolol bioadhesive disc system—Chen W-G, Hwang GC-C. Int J Pharmaceutics 1992;82:61–6. Hollow fibres as an oral sustained-release delivery system using propranolol hydrochloride [*in vitro* and *in vivo* bioavailability in *dogs*]—Hussain MA, Di Luccio RC, Shefter E, Hurwitz AR. Pharm Res 1989;6(12):1052–5. Transdermal controlled delivery of propranolol from a multilaminate adhesive device—Corbo M, Liu J-C, Chien YW. Pharm Res 1989;6(9):753–8.

Enhancement of propranolol hydrochloride and diazepam skin absorption *in vitro*. II: Drug, vehicle, and enhancer penetration kinetics—Hori M, Maibach HI, Guy RH. J Pharm Sci 1992;81(4):330–3. Improved oral bioavailability of propranolol in healthy human volunteers using a liver bypass drug delivery system containing oleic acid—Barnwell SG, Laudanski T, Story MJ, Mallinson CB, Harris RJ, Cole SK et al. Int J Pharmaceutics 1992;88:423-32. The effect of Miglyol 812 oil on the oral absorption of propranolol in the *rat*—Palin KJ, Davis SS. J Pharm Pharmacol 1989;41:579–81. Solubilisation of liposomes by weak electrolyte drugs. Part I. Propranolol—Rogers JA, Betageri GV, Choi YW. Pharm Res 1990;7:957–61. Formulation, pharmacokinetic and pharmacodynamic evaluation of fast releasing compressed propranolol HCl suppositories—Sastry MSP, Satyanarayana NV, Diwan PV, Krishna DR. Drug Dev Ind Pharm 1993;19(9):1089–96.

Prodrugs of propranolol: hydrolysis and intramolecular aminolysis of various propranolol esters and an oxazolidin-2-one derivative—Buur A, Bundgaard H, Lee VHL. Int J Pharmaceutics 1988;42:51–60. Drug-delivery by ion-exchange. Part IV: coated resinate complexes of ester prodrugs of propranolol—Irwin WJ, Belaid KA, Alpar HO. Drug Dev Ind Pharm 1988;14(10):1307–25. Drug-delivery by ion-exchange. Stability of ester prodrugs of propranolol in surfactant and enzymatic systems—Irwin WJ, Belaid KA. Int J Pharmaceutics 1988;48:159–66. An *in-vitro* and *in-vivo* [in *dogs*] correlative approach to the evaluation of ester prodrugs to improve oral stability of propranolol—Shameem M, Imai T, Otagiri M. J Pharm Pharmacol 1993;45:246–52.

PROCESSING

Sterilisation

Propranolol injection can be sterilised by heating in an autoclave.

REFERENCES

1. Burgot G, Serrand P, Burgot J-L. Int J Pharmaceutics 1990;63:73–6.
2. Nieder M, Strösser W, Kappler J. Arzneimittelforschung 1987;37(1)Nr5:549–50.
3. Elliot DN, Elworthy PH, Attwood D. J Pharm Pharmacol 1973;25:118P.
4. Brown GC, Kayes JB. J Clin Pharm 1976;1:29–37.
5. Ahmed GH, Stewart PJ, Tucker IG. Aust J Hosp Pharm 1988;18(5):312–18.
6. Henry DW, Repta AJ, Smith FM, White SJ. Am J Hosp Pharm 1986;43:1492–5.
7. Gupta VD, Stewart KR. Am J Hosp Pharm 1987;44:360–1.
8. Rooney M, Creurer I [letter]. Am J Hosp Pharm 1988;45:530–1.
9. Cummings DS, Park MK, Howard AB. Am J Hosp Pharm 1982;39:1685–7.
10. Al-Gohary O, Lyall J, Murray JB. Pharm Acta Helv 1987;62(3):66–72.
11. Al-Gohary O, Lyall J, Murray JB. Pharm.Acta Helv 1987;62(10-11):313–16.
12. Çalis S, Sumnu M, Hincal AA. *In vitro* adsorption of propranolol hydrochloride by various antacids. In: MH Rubenstein, editor. Pharmaceutical technology: controlled drug release; vol 1. Chichester: Ellis Horwood, 1987:116–24.

13. Cid E, Mella F, Lucchini L, Carcamo M, Monasterio J [French]. Therapie 1985;40:447–9.
14. Leahey WJ, Neill JD, Varma MPS, Shanks RG. Br J Clin Pharmacol 1980;9:33–40.
15. Eldon MA, Kinkel AW, Daniel JE, Latts JR. Biopharm Drug Dispos 1989;10:69–76.
16. Biswas NR, Garg SK, Kumar N, Mukherjee S, Sharma PL. Int J Clin Pharmacol Ther Toxicol 1989;27(10):515–19.
17. Weller PJ. Br J Pharm Pract 1990;12:388–90.
18. Lee H-K, Hajdu J, McGoff P. J Pharm Sci 1991;80(2):178–80.
19. Al-Hmoud H, Efentakis M, Choulis NH. Int J Pharmaceutics 1991;68:R1–R3.
20. Parikh NH, Babar A, Patel NK, Plakogiannis FM. J Pharm Sci 1987;76(11):S292,N 06-W-11.
21. Ford JL, Mitchell K, Sawh D, Ramdour S, Armstrong DJ, Elliot PNC et al. Int J Pharmaceutics 1991;71:213–21.

Quinidine (BAN)   *Anti-arrhythmic*

Chinidinum; quinidina
(8R,9S)-6'-Methoxycinchonan-9-ol dihydrate; (+)-(αS)-α-(6-methoxy-4-quinolyl)-α-[(2R,4S,5R)-(5-vinylquinuclidin-2-yl)]-methanol dihydrate
$C_{20}H_{24}N_2O_2,2H_2O = 360.5$

Quinidine Bisulphate (BANM)
$C_{20}H_{24}N_2O_2,H_2SO_4 = 422.5$

Quinidine Gluconate (BANM)
$C_{20}H_{24}N_2O_2,C_6H_{12}O_7 = 520.6$

Quinidine Polygalacturonate
$C_{20}H_{24}N_2O_2,(C_6H_{10}O_7)_x,xH_2O$

Quinidine Sulphate (BANM)
Quinidine sulfate
$(C_{20}H_{24}N_2O_2)_2,H_2SO_4,2H_2O = 783.0$
CAS—56-54-2 (quinidine, anhydrous); 63717-04-4 (quinidine, dihydrate); 747-45-5 (quinidine bisulphate); 7054-25-3 (quinidine gluconate); 27555-34-6 (quinidine polygalacturonate, anhydrous); 65484-56-2 (polygalacturonate, hydrate); 50-54-4 (quinidine sulphate, anhydrous); 6591-63-5 (sulphate, dihydrate)

Pharmacopoeial status

BP (quinidine bisulphate, quinidine sulphate); USP (quinidine gluconate, quinidine sulfate)

Preparations

Compendial
Quinidine Sulphate Tablets BP. Tablets containing, in each, 200 mg and 300 mg are usually available.
Quinidine Sulfate Capsules USP.
Quinidine Gluconate Extended-release Tablets USP.
Quinidine Sulfate Tablets USP.
Quinidine Gluconate Injection USP.

Non-compendial
Kiditard (Delandale). *Capsules*, sustained release, quinidine bisulphate 250 mg (equivalent to quinidine sulphate 200 mg).
Kinidin Durules (Astra). *Tablets*, sustained release, quinidine bisulphate 250 mg (equivalent to quinidine sulphate 200 mg).
Quinidine sulphate tablets of various strengths are available from CP, Evans.

Containers and storage

Solid state
Quinidine Bisulphate BP and Quinidine Sulphate BP should be kept in well-closed containers and protected from light.
Quinidine Gluconate USP and Quinidine Sulfate USP should be preserved in well-closed, light-resistant containers.

Dosage forms
Quinidine Sulphate Tablets BP should be protected from light.
Quinidine Sulfate Capsules USP should be preserved in tight, light- resistant containers.
Quinidine Gluconate Extended-release Tablets USP and Quinidine Sulfate Tablets USP should be preserved in well-closed, light-resistant containers.
Quinidine Gluconate Injection USP should be preserved in single-dose or in multiple-dose containers, preferably of Type I glass.
Kiditard capsules are recommended to be protected from light and moisture.
Kinidin Durules should be stored in a cool dry place.

PHYSICAL PROPERTIES

Quinidine exists as a white amorphous powder or acicular crystals.
Quinidine bisulphate exists as colourless, odourless or almost odourless crystals, with an intensely bitter taste.
Quinidine gluconate is a white, odourless powder with a very bitter taste.
Quinidine sulphate exists as fine, white needles that frequently cohere in masses, or as a white or almost white, crystalline powder; odourless with a very bitter taste; darkens on exposure to light.

Melting point

Quinidine gluconate melts in the range 175° to 177°.
Quinidine sulphate melts at about 207°, with decomposition.

pH

pH of a 1% w/v aqueous solution of *quinidine bisulphate*, 2.6 to 3.6.
pH of a 1% w/v aqueous solution of *quinidine sulphate*, 6.0 to 6.8.

Dissociation constants

pK_a 4.2, 8.8 (20°)
An apparent ionisation constant of pK_a 8.79 was calculated following potentiometric titration in ethanol:water mixtures at various ratios, and extrapolation to ethanol-free solutions.[1]

Solubility

Quinidine is soluble 1 in 2000 of water and 1 in 70 of ether.
Quinidine bisulphate is soluble 1 in 8 of water and 1 in 3 of ethanol; practically insoluble in ether.

Quinidine gluconate is freely soluble in water (1 in 9); slightly soluble in ethanol.

Quinidine sulphate is slightly soluble in water but soluble in boiling water; soluble 1 in 10 of ethanol and 1 in 15 of chloroform; practically insoluble in acetone and in ether.

Dissolution

The USP specifies that for both Quinidine Sulfate Capsules USP and Quinidine Sulfate Tablets USP not less than 85% of the labelled amount of $(C_{20}H_{24}N_2O_2)_2,H_2SO_4,2H_2O$ is dissolved in 30 minutes. Dissolution medium: 900 mL of 0.1N hydrochloric acid; Apparatus 1 at 100 rpm.

Dissolution properties

Correlation was established between the dissolution parameters at pH 5.4 (acetate or phosphate buffers) and the bioavailability of two commercial quinidine gluconate controlled-release tablets (one with and one without FDA approval).[2] Differences in bioavailabilities (in 12 volunteers) of the two products reflected differences in their dissolution profiles.

FURTHER INFORMATION. The effects of pH, ionic concentration and ionic species of dissolution media on the release rates of quinidine gluconate sustained release dosage forms [disintegrating and non-disintegrating tablets]—Soltero R, Krailler R, Czeisler J. Drug Dev Ind Pharm 1991;17(1):113–40. Influence of dissolution rate and pH of oral medications on drug-induced esophageal injury—Bailey RT, Bonavina L, Nwakama PE, De Meester TR, Cheng S-C. DICP Ann Pharmacother 1990;24:571–3.

Crystal and molecular structure

Quinidine is an optical isomer of quinine.

Doherty *et al*[3] investigated the crystal structure of quinidine (crystallised from ethanol as the ethanolate) by X-ray diffraction.

STABILITY

Impurities

The BP specifies that samples of quinidine bisulphate contain not more than 15% of dihydroquinidine bisulphate.

The USP specifies that samples of quinidine gluconate contain not more than 20% of dihydroquinidine gluconate and samples of quinidine sulfate contain not more than 20% of dihydroquinidine sulfate.

FURTHER INFORMATION. Dihydroquinidine contamination of quinidine raw materials and dosage forms: rapid estimation by high-performance liquid chromatography—Narang PK, Crouthamel WG. J Pharm Sci 1979;68(7):917– 9.

INCOMPATIBILITY/COMPATIBILITY

Quinidine sulphate is reported to be incompatible with alkalis, iodides, and tannic acid.

Intravenous admixtures

Campbell *et al*[4] investigated the compatibility of amiodarone hydrochloride 900 mg (Cordarone, Labaz, France) with quinidine gluconate 500 mg (Eli Lilly) in 500 mL of either glucose 5% or sodium chloride 0.9% injections, stored in either polyvinyl chloride or polyolefin containers for 24 hours at 24°. In polyvinyl chloride containers, amiodarone hydrochloride concentration in both admixtures fell by over 12% whereas in polyolefin containers no loss of amiodarone hydrochloride in either admixture was detected. However, a milky precipitate was observed immediately following addition of amiodarone hydro-

chloride to solutions of quinidine gluconate in glucose 5% in either type of container and remained during the study period. The precipitate was not identified.

When admixtures of milrinone and quinidine gluconate, in glucose 5% solution, were stored in glass containers at 22° to 23° under fluorescent light, no reduction in the initial concentration of either drug was detected; no visible changes or pH shifts were observed.[5]

Sorption

Negligible loss of quinidine sulphate was reported[6] when a 0.45 mg/100 mL solution in sodium chloride 0.9% injection was stored in Viaflex (polyvinyl chloride) infusion bags or glass vials in the dark for up to three months at 15° to 20°.

In a further study, Kowaluk *et al*[7] detected negligible reduction in quinidine sulphate concentration during simulated infusion in sodium chloride 0.9% injection through a cellulose propionate burette chamber and polyvinyl chloride tubing, or through polyethylene or Silastic tubing attached to glass syringes on syringe pumps. No sorption of quinidine sulphate was evident after storage of the infusion in the dark at 15° to 20° for 24 hours in single-use syringes with polypropylene barrels and polyethylene all-plastic plungers.

Adsorption of quinidine sulphate onto kaolin in aqueous solution (ionic strength 0.1M) at 37° was demonstrated by Bucci *et al*;[8] the amount of quinidine sulphate adsorbed increased as pH increased (pH 2.4, 5.5, 6.5, and 7.5). Monolayer adsorption onto kaolin was indicated at pH 2.4 and multilayer adsorption at the higher pH values. Interaction of quinidine sulphate with pectin (in solution at ionic strength 0.1M and 37°) was greater in water than in phosphate buffer pH 6.5; this interaction was attributed to complexation. In control solutions, no sorption of quinidine sulphate to glassware was detected.

Adsorption *in vitro* of quinidine sulphate in solution, at 37° and pH 2.2, onto Kaopectate (a kaolin-pectin suspension, Upjohn), or onto magnesium trisilicate was greater than onto Simeco tablets (co-dried aluminium hydroxide and magnesium carbonate with magnesium hydroxide and simethicone, Wyeth) or onto bismuth subnitrate.[9] Adsorption followed Freundlich and Langmuir isotherms. Further, when four healthy volunteers received 30 mL of Kaopectate before 100 mg of quinidine sulphate, there was a significant decrease in bioavailability of quinidine (salivary concentration data), but not in the rate of absorption, compared to that following administration of quinidine sulphate alone.

FORMULATION

Excipients

Excipients that have been used in presentations of quinidine include:

Tablets, quinidine bisulphate: hypromellose; macrogol 8000; magnesium stearate; polyvinyl acetate; polyvinyl chloride; titanium dioxide (E171).

Quinidine gluconate: calcium hydrogen phosphate; confectioner's sugar; magnesium stearate; maize starch; povidone; silica gel; stearic acid.

Quinidine polygalacturonate: lactose; magnesium stearate; maize starch; povidone; talc.

Quinidine sulphate: acacia; allura red AC (E129), aluminium lake; acetylated monoglycerides; calcium sulphate; carnauba wax; edible ink; indigo carmine (E132); gelatin; guar gum; lactose; magnesium oxide; magnesium stearate; polysorbates; shellac; sucrose; sunset yellow FCF (E110), aluminium lake; titanium dioxide (E171); white beeswax.

Oral solutions, quinidine sulphate: citric acid; ethanol; syrup.
Injections, quinidine gluconate: disodium edetate; phenol.

Bioavailability

In a study involving ten healthy volunteers, the mean oral bioavailability of quinidine sulphate from a 1% aqueous solution was 70% ± 17% compared to that of an intravenous injection of quinidine gluconate in sodium chloride 0.9% solution (both formulations administered as doses of quinidine base 3.74 mg/kg).[10]

Large intra-subject and inter-subject variability in plasma-quinidine concentration was observed when 13 healthy volunteers received quinidine sulphate as tablets, capsules, or an oral solution and quinidine gluconate as an intramuscular injection, in a single-dose, randomised, crossover study.[11] No differences in rates of absorption from the preparations were apparent. Bioavailability of quinidine was not significantly different between the three oral preparations. However, in relation to quinidine gluconate administered intramuscularly, bioavailability from the quinidine sulphate tablet was lower. Studies that compared bioavailability from intramuscular injection with that from the capsule or oral solution were inconclusive; the results depended on the method of data evaluation.

Eleven healthy volunteers who participated in a single-dose, crossover study received quinidine (as different salts) on four occasions by three routes.[12] Apparent systemic availabilities of quinidine lactate intramuscular injection, quinidine sulphate tablets (Parke Davis), and quinidine gluconate tablets (Cooper) were 85% to 90%, about 80%, and about 70%, respectively, compared to a quinidine lactate infusion in glucose 5%.

Absorption of oral quinidine preparations commercially available in Canada was investigated in a single-dose study involving 24 healthy volunteers.[13] Eight different quinidine sulphate tablets, one quinidine gluconate tablet, and one quinidine polygalacturonate tablet had similar bioavailabilities although another quinidine gluconate tablet showed lower bioavailability. Wide inter-subject variation and, to a lesser extent, intrasubject variation was apparent. No correlation was established between absorption and dissolution rates *in vitro* (which varied greatly), except that slowest dissolution was shown by the quinidine gluconate tablet with low bioavailability.

Modified-release preparations
Results of a single-dose, crossover bioavailability study involving twelve healthy volunteers[14] led to a Class I recall (by the US Food and Drug Administration) of a generic prolonged-release quinidine gluconate tablet (Bolar, USA); the extent of absorption of quinidine from this product was about 50% less than that from another marketed sustained-release product, Quinaglute DuraTabs (Berlex, USA), which contained the same amount of quinidine gluconate.

In a single-dose study of Latin square design,[15] eight healthy volunteers received the following preparations: quinidine sulphate tablets 200 mg (Chinidina solfato Erba, Carlo Erba, Italy); quinidine polygalacturonate tablets (Ritmocor, Malesci, Italy); quinidine bisulphate tablets 250 mg (Kinidin Durules, AB, Hässle, Sweden); quinidine arabogalactansulphate capsules 275 mg (Longacor, Nativelle, France). No significant difference in areas under the plasma-concentration versus time curves was found between preparations of quinidine sulphate, quinidine polygalacturonate, and quinidine arabogalactansulphate (after correction of results to account for different doses); the area under the plasma-concentration versus time curve for quinidine bisulphate tablets was significantly lower. Quinidine bisulphate and quinidine arabogalactansulphate preparations had significantly lower absorption rate constants than the other two preparations.

Canadian workers showed that the rate of absorption of quinidine from different sustained-release preparations may vary.[16] In a multidose, randomised, crossover study, twelve healthy volunteers received Quinidex 300 mg (AH Robins, Canada), Biquin Durules 250 mg (Astra Pharmaceuticals, Canada), and Quinaglute DuraTabs 324 mg (Pentagone Pharma Inc, Canada). After 'normalisation' of data for anhydrous quinidine content, similar extents of absorption were shown by the preparations, but differences in rates of absorption were evident.

Bioequivalence

No significant differences in the extent of absorption of quinidine from four brands of quinidine sulphate 200 mg tablets were detected following administration of two tablets of each brand to eleven healthy volunteers in a randomised, crossover study.[17] However, significant differences in absorption rate constants, times to reach peak concentration, and mean serum concentrations (at 30 minutes and 60 minutes) were measured between tablets; these absorption data correlated in rank order with disintegration times of tablets (USP XIX method at 37°). In further work,[18] times to reach 50% dissolution of the same tablets (in 0.1M hydrochloric acid at 37°) were substantially different and were found to correlate in rank order with disintegration times and absorption parameters described previously.

Sustained-release tablets

Admixtures of quinidine gluconate and glycerol palmito-stearate (Precirol) at drug:Precirol ratios of 1:1, 1:9, and 3:7, prepared by granulation or hot fusion techniques, were formed into tablets.[19] For both tablet preparations, an increase in the content of Precirol produced a decrease in release of quinidine gluconate (dissolution studies in 0.1M hydrochloric acid). Dissolution from tablets produced by the granulation method was more rapid than that from tablets prepared by hot fusion.

Novel dosage forms

Bodmeier *et al*[20] prepared biodegradable films and microspheres that contained quinidine (as a model drug) with poly(DL-lactide)(PLA); blends of low and high molecular weight (2000 and 120 000, respectively) PLA were used in various ratios. Release of quinidine into phosphate buffer, pH 7.4 at 37°, from films and microspheres was dependent on the polymer ratio. Negligible release occurred from films with high molecular weight PLA alone; inclusion of low molecular weight PLA enhanced release. No overall relationships between release and the amounts of quinidine and PLA present, in any system, were established; it was suggested that interactions between quinidine and the carboxyl groups of PLA may occur.

FURTHER INFORMATION. Bioavailability of three commercial sustained-release tablets of quinidine in maintenance therapy—Huynh-Ngoc T, Chabot M, Sirois G. J Pharm Sci 1978;67(10):1456–9.

REFERENCES

1. Voigt W, Mannhold R, Limberg J, Blaschke G. J Pharm Sci 1988;77(12):1018–20.
2. Prasad VK, Shah VP, Knight P, Malinowski H, Cabana BE, Meyer MC. Int J Pharmaceutics 1983;13:1–7.
3. Doherty R, Benson WR, Maienthal M, Stewart JM. J Pharm Sci 1978;67(12):1698–700.
4. Campbell S, Nolan PE, Bliss M, Wood R, Mayersohn M. Am J Hosp Pharm 1986;43:917–21.

5. Riley CM. Am J Hosp Pharm 1988;45:2079–91.
6. Kowaluk EA, Roberts MS, Blackburn HD, Polack AE. Am J Hosp Pharm 1981;38:1308–14.
7. Kowaluk EA, Roberts MS, Polack AE. Am J Hosp Pharm 1982;39:460–7.
8. Bucci AJ, Myre SA, Tan SI, Shenouda LS. J Pharm Sci 1981;70(9):999–1002.
9. Moustafa MA, Al-Shora HI, Gaber M, Gouda MW. Int J Pharmaceutics 1987;34:207–11.
10. Guentert TW, Holford NHG, Coates PE, Upton RA, Riegelman S. J Pharmacokinet Biopharm 1979;7(4):315–30.
11. Mason WD, Covinsky JO, Valentine JL, Kelly KL, Weddle OH, Martz BL. J Pharm Sci 1976;65(9):1325–8.
12. Greenblatt DJ, Pfeifer HJ, Ochs HR, Franke K, MacLaughlin DS, Smith TW *et al.* J Pharmacol Exp Ther 1977;202(2):365–78.
13. McGilvery IJ, Midha KK, Rowe M, Beaudoin N, Charette C. J Pharm Sci 1981;70(5):524–9.
14. Meyer MC, Straughn AB, Lieberman P, Jacob J. J Clin Pharmacol 1982;22:131–4.
15. Frigo GM, Perucca E, Teggia-Droghi M, Gatti G, Mussini A, Salerno J. Br J Clin Pharmacol 1977;4:449–54.
16. Mahon WA, Leeder JS, Brill-Edwards MM, Correia J, MacLeod SM. Clin Pharmacokinet 1987;13:118–24.
17. Strum JD, Colaizzi JL, Jaffe JM, Martineau PC, Poust RI. J Pharm Sci 1977;66(4):539–42.
18. Strum JD, Ebersole JW, Jaffe JM, Colaizzi JL, Poust RI. J Pharm Sci 1978;67(4):568–9.
19. Saraiya D, Bolton S. Drug Dev Ind Pharm 1990;16(13):1963–9.
20. Bodmeier R, Oh KH, Chen H. Int J Pharmaceutics 1989;51:1–8.

Quinine (BAN)

Antimalarial

Chininum

(8*S*,9*R*)-6′-Methoxycinchonan-9-ol; (α*R*)-α-(6-methoxy-4-quinolyl)-α-[(2*S*,4*S*,5*R*)-(5-vinylquinuclidin-2-yl)]methanol

$C_{20}H_{24}N_2O_2 = 324.4$

Quinine Bisulphate (BANM)

$C_{20}H_{24}N_2O_2,H_2SO_4,7H_2O = 548.6$

Quinine Dihydrobromide (BANM)

$C_{20}H_{24}N_2O_2,2HBr,3H_2O = 540.3$

Quinine Dihydrochloride (BANM)

$C_{20}H_{24}N_2O_2,2HCl = 397.3$

Quinine Ethyl Carbonate

$C_{23}H_{28}N_2O_4 = 396.5$

Quinine Hydrobromide (BANM)

$C_{20}H_{24}N_2O_2,HBr,2H_2O = 441.4$

Quinine Hydrochloride (BANM)

$C_{20}H_{24}N_2O_2,HCl,2H_2O = 396.9$

Quinine Salicylate (BANM)

$C_{20}H_{24}N_2O_2,C_7H_6O_3,H_2O = 480.6$

Quinine Sulphate (BANM)

Quinine sulfate

$(C_{20}H_{24}N_2O_2)_2,H_2SO_4,2H_2O = 782.9$

CAS—130-95-0 (quinine, anhydrous); 549-56-4 (quinine bisulphate, anhydrous); 549-47-3 (quinine dihydrobromide, anhydrous); 60-93-5 (quinine dihydrochloride); 83-75-0 (quinine ethyl carbonate); 549-49-5 (quinine hydrobromide, anhydrous); 130-89-2 (quinine hydrochloride, anhydrous); 6119-47-7 (quinine hydrochloride, dihydrate); 750-90-3 (quinine salicylate, anhydrous); 804-63-7 (quinine sulphate, anhydrous); 6119-70-6 (quinine sulphate, dihydrate).

Pharmacopoeial status

BP (quinine bisulphate, quinine dihydrochloride, quinine hydrochloride, quinine sulphate); USP (quinine sulfate)

Preparations

Compendial

Quinine Bisulphate Tablets BP (Quinine Acid Sulphate Tablets). Tablets containing, in each, 200 mg and 300 mg are usually available. They are coated.

Quinine Sulphate Tablets BP. Tablets containing, in each, 125 mg, 200 mg, and 300 mg are usually available. They are coated.

Quinine Sulfate Capsules USP.

Quinine Sulfate Tablets USP.

Non-compendial

An injection of quinine dihydrochloride 300 mg/mL for dilution with sodium chloride 0.9% injection and use as an infusion is available from 'specials' manufacturers or specialist malarial centres.

Containers and storage

Solid state

Quinine Bisulphate BP, Quinine Dihydrochloride BP, Quinine Hydrochloride BP, and Quinine Sulphate BP should all be kept in well-closed containers and protected from light.

Quinine Sulfate USP should be preserved in well-closed, light-resistant containers.

Dosage forms

Quinine Bisulphate Tablets BP that are not sugar coated and Quinine Sulphate Tablets BP that are not sugar coated should be protected from light.

Quinine Sulfate Capsules USP should be preserved in tight containers.

Quinine Sulfate Tablets USP should be preserved in well-closed containers.

PHYSICAL PROPERTIES

Quinine is a white, granular or microcrystalline powder; slightly efflorescent in dry air.

Quinine bisulphate exists as colourless crystals or a white, crystalline powder; odourless or almost odourless; effloresces in dry air and becomes yellow on exposure to light; bitter taste.

Quinine dihydrobromide exists as white to yellowish crystals or powder; odourless.

Quinine dihydrochloride is a white or almost white powder; odourless or almost odourless with a very bitter taste.

Quinine ethyl carbonate exists as white masses of silky, almost tasteless crystals which darken on exposure to light.

Quinine hydrobromide exists as white, silky, needle crystals which darken on exposure to light. Crystals are odourless and bitter; efflorescent in dry air.

Quinine hydrochloride exists as fine, colourless or white, silky, acicular needles, often grouped in clusters; odourless and with a very bitter taste. The dihydrate effloresces in dry air and on exposure to light it gradually becomes yellowish.

Quinine salicylate exists as white silky crystals or as a crystalline powder; it becomes pink on storage; odourless with a bitter taste.

Quinine sulphate exists as a white or almost white, crystalline powder or fine, colourless, acicular needles; odourless with a very bitter taste; becomes brown on exposure to light.

Melting point

Quinine melts at about 173°.
Quinine ethyl carbonate melts in the range 91° to 95°.

pH

pH of a saturated aqueous solution of *quinine*, 8.8.
pH of a 1% w/v solution of *quinine bisulphate*, 2.8 to 3.4.
pH of a 3% w/v solution of *quinine dihydrochloride*, 2.0 to 3.0.
pH of a 1% w/v solution of *quinine hydrochloride*, 6.0 to 6.8.
pH of a 1% w/v suspension of *quinine sulphate*, 5.7 to 6.6.

Dissociation constants

pK_a 4.1, 8.5 (20°)

Solubility

Solubility (in parts) of quinine and its salts:

	Water	Ethanol	Chloroform	Ether	Additional information
Quinine	very slightly soluble	1 in 1	1 in 3	1 in 4 parts of ether saturated with water	—
Quinine bisulphate	1 in 8	1 in 50	1 in 625	—	solution in water gives a blue fluorescence
Quinine dihydrobromide	1 in 7	soluble	—	practically insoluble	—
Quinine dihydrochloride	1 in 0.5	1 in 14	1 in 7	practically insoluble	—
Quinine ethyl carbonate	very slightly soluble	1 in 2	1 in 1	1 in 10	—
Quinine hydrobromide	1 in 55	1 in 0.7	1 in 1	—	solution in chloroform is turbid owing to separation of water
Quinine hydrochloride	1 in 23	1 in 0.9	freely soluble (1 in 2)	very slightly soluble	solution in chloroform may not be clear owing to formation of droplets of water
Quinine salicylate	very slightly soluble	1 in 24	1 in 25	—	—
Quinine sulphate	slightly soluble (1 in 810); sparingly soluble in boiling water	sparingly soluble (1 in 95)	very slightly soluble	practically insoluble	soluble in a 2:1 mixture of chloroform and absolute ethanol

Dissolution

The USP specifies that for Quinine Sulfate Capsules USP and Quinine Sulfate Tablets USP not less than 75% of the labelled amount of $(C_{20}H_{24}N_2O_2)_2,H_2SO_4,2H_2O$ is dissolved in 45 minutes. Dissolution medium: 900 mL of 0.1N hydrochloric acid; Apparatus 1 at 100 rpm.

Crystal and molecular structure

Quinine is an optical isomer of quinidine.

INCOMPATIBILITY/COMPATIBILITY

Quinine sulphate solutions precipitate quinine in the presence of alkalis and their carbonates. Quinine salts are also reported to be incompatible with acetates, benzoates, citrates, iodides, salicylates, and tartrates.

The extent to which quinine hydrochloride 2% was bound by several hydrocolloids in solution decreased in the order: carrageenan > carmellose sodium > furcellaran > sodium alginate > pectin > gum tragacanth > locust bean gum > gum acacia.[1] The amount of quinine hydrochloride bound was measured by equilibrium dialysis, colorimetry, and spectrophotometry.

FURTHER INFORMATION. Interaction of carrageenan and other hydrocolloids with alkaloids I. Precipitation studies—Graham HD, Thomas LB. J Pharm Sci 1961;50:483–6.

FORMULATION

Excipients

Excipients that have been used in presentations of quinine include:

Tablets, quinine hydrochloride: magnesium stearate; maize starch; talc; wheat starch.

Quinine sulphate: maize starch; pregelatinised starch; sodium starch glycollate; sucrose; zinc stearate.

Suspensions, quinine sulphate: cocoa powder; compound tragacanth powder; methyl and propyl hydroxybenzoates; syrup; vanilla essence.

Suppositories, quinine hydrochloride: theobroma oil.

Displacement value of quinine hydrochloride in theobroma oil: 1.1.

Absorption

Quinine dihydrochloride, quinine hydrochloride and quinine sulphate are readily absorbed after oral administration; rectally administered doses are poorly absorbed and intramuscular or subcutaneous doses of quinine salts are slowly absorbed.

In a single-dose, crossover study,[2] nine healthy volunteers received oral tablets of quinine hydrochloride, quinine sulphate, and quinine ethyl carbonate (each equivalent to 600 mg of quinine base). No significant differences in the rate or extent of absorption of quinine were demonstrated between the preparations. However, marked inter-subject and intra-subject variations in absorption parameters were noted.

Palatability

Of several official syrups and imitation flavoured syrups evaluated by a taste panel of 15 persons, Cacao Syrup USP (cocoa syrup) was the most successful means of disguising the bitter taste of quinine hydrochloride in solution.[3] Other syrups were less effective but better than water or reconstituted skimmed milk. The following procedures were found to improve the ability of flavoured syrups to mask the taste of quinine: doubling the flavour concentration; increasing the sweetness (sugar content); adding sodium chloride to some flavoured syrups; adding excess citric acid to fruit-flavoured syrups; and increasing the viscosity of solutions.

Modified-release preparations

Dissolution of quinine sulphate was investigated from 'slowly eroding timed-release' tablets that contained different proportions of carbomer (Carbopol 934), and cellulose acetate hydrogen phthalate as the diluent.[4] Release rates of quinine sulphate increased as the proportion of carbomer decreased (from 75% to 20%) at a fixed level of quinine sulphate (25%). Alteration of the proportion of quinine sulphate (10%, 20%, 40%, 50% parts) present when carbomer levels were fixed (at 25% or 40%) did not affect the release rate.

FURTHER INFORMATION. Elaboration, evaluation and study of the stability of saline solutions of quinine hydrochloride—Garcia RMC, Rueda GME, Saiz GS, Lopez RA, Mila YJI et al. Farmacia Hosp 1991;15:149–52. Some properties of chloroquine phosphate and quinine hydrochloride microcapsules—Chukwu A, Agarwal SP, Adikwu MU. STP Pharma Sci 1991;1:117–20.

REFERENCES

1. Graham HD, Thomas LB. J Pharm Sci 1962;51(10):988–92.
2. Jamaludin A, Mohamad M, Navaratnam V, Selliah K, Tan SC, Wernsdorfer WH et al. Br J Clin Pharmacol 1988;25:261–3.
3. Entrekin DN, Becker CH. J Am Pharm Assoc (Sci) 1954;43(11):693–7.
4. Choulis NH, Papadopoulos H. J Pharm Sci 1975;64(6):1033–5.

Ranitidine (BAN, rINN)

Histamine H$_2$-receptor antagonist

N,N-Dimethyl-5[2-(1-methylamino-2-nitrovinylamino)-ethyl-thiomethyl]furfurylamine; N-[2-[[[-5-[(dimethylamino)methyl]-2-furanyl]methyl]thio]ethyl]-N'-methyl-2-nitro-1,1-ethenediamine

$C_{13}H_{22}N_4O_3S = 314.4$

Ranitidine Hydrochloride (BANM, rINNM)

$C_{13}H_{22}N_4O_3S,HCl = 350.9$

CAS—66357-35-5 (ranitidine); 71130-06-8 (ranitidine hydrochloride)

Pharmacopoeial status

USP (ranitidine hydrochloride)

Preparations

Compendial
Ranitidine Tablets USP. Contain ranitidine hydrochloride.
Ranitidine Oral Solution USP. Contains ranitidine hydrochloride.
Ranitidine Injection USP. Contains ranitidine hydrochloride. pH between 6.7 and 7.3.
Ranitidine in Sodium Chloride Injection USP. Contains ranitidine hydrochloride. pH between 6.7 and 7.3.

Non-compendial
Zantac (Glaxo). *Tablets*, ranitidine (as hydrochloride) 150 mg and 300 mg.
Dispersible tablets, sugar free, ranitidine (as hydrochloride) 150 mg.
Effervescent tablets, ranitidine (as hydrochloride) 150 mg and 300 mg.
Syrup, sugar free, ranitidine (as hydrochloride) 75 mg/5 mL. Should not be diluted or admixed with other liquid preparations.
Effervescent granules, for reconstitution with water, ranitidine (as hydrochloride) 150 mg and 300 mg per sachet.
Injection, ranitidine 25 mg (as hydrochloride)/mL. Compatible with the following intravenous infusion fluids: sodium chloride 0.9%, glucose 5%, sodium chloride 0.18% and glucose 4%, sodium bicarbonate 4.2% and compound sodium lactate. Compatibility studies were performed in polyvinyl chloride infusion bags, with the exception of sodium bicarbonate 4.2% which was packaged in glass containers. Unused admixtures of Zantac injection with infusion fluids should be discarded 24 hours after preparation.

Containers and storage

Solid state
Ranitidine Hydrochloride USP should be preserved in tight, light-resistant containers.

Dosage forms
Ranitidine Tablets USP should be preserved in tight, light-resistant containers.
Ranitidine Oral Solution USP should be preserved in tight, light-resistant containers, below 25°. Do not freeze.
Ranitidine Injection USP should be preserved in single-dose or in multiple-dose containers of Type I glass, protected from light, below 30°. Do not freeze.
Ranitidine in Sodium Chloride Injection USP should be preserved in intact flexible containers (that meet specified USP general requirements), protected from light, at room temperature. Do not freeze.
Zantac Syrup should be stored at a temperature not exceeding 25°.
Effervescent Zantac products should be stored below 30° in a dry place.
Zantac Injection should be stored below 25°, protected from light. It should not be autoclaved.

PHYSICAL PROPERTIES

Ranitidine is a white solid.
Ranitidine hydrochloride is a white to pale yellow crystalline, practically odourless powder.

Melting point

Ranitidine melts at about 70°.
The melting point of *ranitidine hydrochloride* depends on its crystalline form. Reported ranges are: about 140°, with decomposition; about 130°; and 133° to 134°.

pH

A 1% solution of *ranitidine hydrochloride* has a pH between 4.5 and 6.0.

Dissociation constants

pK_a 2.3, 8.2

Solubility

Ranitidine hydrochloride is very soluble in water; moderately soluble in ethanol; sparingly soluble in chloroform.

Dissolution

The USP specifies that for Ranitidine Tablets USP not less than 80% of the labelled amount of $C_{13}H_{22}N_4O_3S$ is dissolved in 45 minutes. Dissolution medium: 900 mL of water; Apparatus 2 at 50 rpm.

FURTHER INFORMATION. Dissolution studies [rotating basket apparatus; pH 1 and 6.5] of drug formulations using ion-selective electrodes as sensors in an air-segmented continuous flow analyzer—Mitsana-Papazoglou A, Christopoulos TK, Diamandis EP, Koupparis MA. J Pharm Sci 1987;76(9):724–30.

STABILITY

Ranitidine hydrochloride is sensitive to light and moisture.
When 3 mL of a ranitidine hydrochloride 0.1% aqueous solution was boiled for 20 minutes with 1 mL of either 1N sulphuric acid or 1N sodium hydroxide, 15% and 84.4% of the initial ranitidine concentration were lost, respectively.[1] Storage of 3 mL of a ranitidine hydrochloride 0.1% aqueous solution with 3 mL of hydrogen peroxide 3% at room temperature for 20 minutes resulted in a 37.8% loss. A stability-indicating, reversed-phase HPLC assay was developed to quantify ranitidine hydrochloride in tablets and injections.
In an accelerated degradation study, Walker and Kirby[2] deduced a half-life of about 60 minutes for the first-order decline of ranitidine hydrochloride concentration in solution at pH 11 at 66° over 4 hours.

Intravenous solutions

Ranitidine hydrochloride has been shown to be less stable in glucose 5% injection than in sodium chloride 0.9% injection.[3] When solutions of ranitidine hydrochloride 1 mg/mL in sodium chloride 0.9% injection and in glucose 5% injection were stored in Viaflex plastic bags, losses of initial concentration of 0% and 7.9%, respectively (after 18 days at 25°) and of 0.2% and 3.5%, respectively (after 66 days at 5°) were noted. The pH of solutions in glucose 5% injection stored at 25° fell from 6.8 to 3.4 over a period of 18 days.
The stability of ranitidine 0.05 mg/mL was evaluated in five intravenous infusion solutions.[4] After 48 hours at 20° to 25° under continuous fluorescent light and ambient humidity, the stability of ranitidine (as the hydrochloride, Zantac injection, Glaxo, USA) in the infusion fluids in 150-mL polyvinyl chloride bags decreased in the order: sodium chloride 0.9% > glucose 5% > glucose 5% with sodium chloride 0.45% > glucose 10% > glucose 5% with compound sodium lactate. No visual or pH changes were noted in any solution. More than 90% of the initial concentration of ranitidine remained after 48 hours in all solutions except glucose 5% with compound sodium lactate. At concentrations of 0.05 mg/mL, 0.5 mg/mL, 1 mg/mL, and 2 mg/mL, ranitidine hydrochloride was stable in sodium chloride 0.9% injection for 28 days under the same storage conditions but stability in glucose 5% injection was dependent on concentration; stability over 28 days improved as the initial concentration was increased to 2 mg/mL.
In a further study with the same vehicles, Stewart et al[5] demonstrated that over 90% of the initial concentration was retained when solutions of ranitidine 0.5 mg/mL, 1 mg/mL, and 2 mg/ mL (as the hydrochloride, Zantac injection, Glaxo, USA) were stored in polyvinyl chloride bags for 7 days at room temperature in light or for 30 days at 4°. Furthermore, at all concentra-

tions, ranitidine hydrochloride was stable in admixtures stored for 60 days at −20° followed by storage for 7 days at room temperature in the light or during storage for 14 days at 4° in all vehicles except the glucose 5% with compound sodium lactate; storage of ranitidine hydrochloride in this vehicle frozen at −20° was not recommended.
Lampasona et al[6] had previously demonstrated that solutions of ranitidine hydrochloride 1 mg/mL mixed with sodium chloride 0.9% injection or glucose 5% injection in polyvinyl chloride minibags could be stored for 10 days at 4° with negligible loss of the initial concentration of ranitidine. In addition, more than 90% of the initial concentration remained when solutions of ranitidine hydrochloride 0.5 mg/mL, 1 mg/mL, or 2 mg/mL in either vehicle in polyvinyl chloride minibags were stored frozen at −30° for 30 days followed by refrigeration at 4° for 14 days. No visual or pH changes were noted.
Ranitidine hydrochloride (Zantac Injection, Glaxo) 1 mg/mL in sodium chloride 0.9% or glucose 5% solutions was visually and chemically stable (stability-indicating HPLC assay) at 4° in polyvinyl chloride minibags for 92 days.[2] Although low concentrations of at least one degradation product were detected (to a greater extent in the admixture in glucose 5%), no significant change in ranitidine concentration was observed.

Tablets

At least 92% of the initial concentration of ranitidine hydrochloride remained in tablets (which also contained Avicel PH101, anhydrous lactose, maize starch, magnesium stearate, talc, and povidone or ethylcellulose), prepared by direct compression or wet granulation, that had been stored at relative humidities of 30%, 50%, or 75%, or ambient conditions, for 120 days.[7]

FURTHER INFORMATION. High-performance liquid chromatographic methods for the determination of ranitidine and related substances [synthetic intermediates and 'degradation products'] in raw materials and tablets—Beaulieu N, Lacroix PM, Sears RW, Lovering EG. J Pharm Sci 1988;77(10):889–92.

INCOMPATIBILITY/COMPATIBILITY

Injections

A white turbidity, haze, or precipitate formed immediately when 2 mL of ranitidine hydrochloride injection (50 mg/2 mL, Glaxo) was mixed with 1 mL of injections of methotrimeprazine (25 mg/ mL, Rhône-Poulenc), opium alkaloids (20 mg/mL, Roche), or phenobarbitone sodium (120 mg/mL, Abbott) at 25° under fluorescent light.[8] When the ranitidine hydrochloride solution was mixed with 1 mL of injections of diazepam (10 mg/mL, Roche), hydroxyzine hydrochloride (50 mg/mL, Pfizer), or lorazepam (4 mg/mL, Wyeth) a transient haze layering, which disappeared during vortex mixing, was observed. Nineteen other drugs, including morphine sulphate (10 mg/mL, A&H), were physically compatible with the ranitidine hydrochloride solution over a period of one hour.

Total parenteral nutrition solutions

The stability and compatibility of ranitidine hydrochloride in total parenteral nutrition (TPN) solutions has been investigated.[9–12] Walker and Bayliff[9] demonstrated that about 10% of the initial concentration of ranitidine hydrochloride was lost in 48 hours from an admixture of ranitidine hydrochloride (phenol free, Zantac 25 mg/mL, Glaxo, Canada) in a TPN solution that contained glucose 25%, amino acids 4.25%, electrolytes, trace elements, heparin, and multivitamins (MVI-12, USV, Canada) at 23°. The rate of loss was independent of the initial concentration of ranitidine hydrochloride (100, 200, and

300 mg/1200 mL). However, Bullock et al[10] concluded that admixtures of ranitidine hydrochloride (Zantac injection, Glaxo) 50 and 100 micrograms/mL in nutrient solutions (which contained glucose 25%, crystalline amino acids 4.25% or 2.125%, electrolytes, trace elements, vitamins and heparin sodium) were stable for 24 hours at room temperature.

Later work[11] suggested that at least 90% of the initial concentration of ranitidine hydrochloride was retained after 48 hours when admixtures in two solutions were stored at 4° or room temperature, either protected from or exposed to fluorescent light. The solutions comprised ranitidine hydrochloride 50 or 100 micrograms/mL (Zantac 25 mg/mL, Glaxo, USA) in either a TPN solution (glucose 22.7%, crystalline amino acids 4.5%, and electrolytes) or in a 10% lipid emulsion. In the same study, however, similar admixtures of ranitidine hydrochloride in a TPN solution (glucose 18.5%, crystalline amino acids 3.7%, and electrolytes), which also contained 3.7% lipid emulsion, retained 86% to 91.4% of the initial concentration of ranitidine hydrochloride after 48 hours in ethylene vinyl acetate bags. An earlier study[12] demonstrated the loss of about 10% of the initial ranitidine hydrochloride concentration in 12 hours when solutions of 50 and 100 micrograms/mL in TPN solutions (glucose 12.5%, amino acids, electrolytes, trace elements and vitamins), which also contained 5% lipid emulsion, were stored in ethylene vinyl acetate bags at room temperature (23° ± 2°) under fluorescent light.

Infusion solutions

Galante et al[13] demonstrated the compatibility of ranitidine hydrochloride (Zantac injection, Glaxo, USA) at 0.05 mg/mL and 2.0 mg/mL in sodium chloride 0.9% injection or glucose 5% injection, in admixture with various concentrations of potassium chloride (LyphoMed, USA), heparin sodium, aminophylline, dopamine hydrochloride (all Elkins-Sinn, USA), lignocaine hydrochloride (Astra, USA), dobutamine hydrochloride (Eli Lilly, USA), sodium nitroprusside (Roche, USA), or noradrenaline acid tartrate (Winthrop, USA), in polyvinyl chloride bags. More than 90% of the initial concentration of ranitidine remained in all admixtures for up to 48 hours; stability of the additive drugs was not determined.

Admixtures of netilmicin sulphate 100 mg with ranitidine hydrochloride 50 mg in 100 mL sodium chloride 0.9% injection, in glass bottles, were chemically stable (less than 5% of either drug was lost) and physically compatible for 24 hours at room temperatures.[14]

Visual compatibility over a period of 24 hours has been reported[15] between 1 mL of ranitidine hydrochloride injection (0.5 mg/mL, Glaxo, USA) and 1 mL of aminophylline, bretylium tosylate, heparin sodium (all LyphoMed), dobutamine hydrochloride (Lilly), dopamine hydrochloride (Elkins-Sinn), glyceryl trinitrate (SoloPak), or procainamide hydrochloride (Baxter), in glucose 5% injection, in clear glass vials.

Similarly, mixtures of 1 mL of ranitidine hydrochloride injection (0.5 mg/mL, Glaxo) with 1 mL of either labetalol hydrochloride injection[16] (Normodyne, Schering, USA) 1 mg/mL in glucose 5% injection or esmolol hydrochloride injection[17] (DuPont Critical Care, USA) 10 mg/mL in glucose 5% injection were physically stable (no visual changes) over 24 hours at 18° or 22° respectively, under fluorescent light.

Visual compatibility over a period of 4 hours was observed when 1 mL of zidovudine[18] (Retrovir, Burroughs Wellcome, USA) 4 mg/mL in glucose 5% injection or acyclovir sodium[19] (Burroughs Wellcome, USA) 5 mg/mL in glucose 5% injection were mixed with 1 mL of ranitidine hydrochloride (1 mg/mL, Glaxo) and stored at 25° under fluorescent light.

FURTHER INFORMATION. Stability of ranitidine hydrochloride with aztreonam, ceftazidime, or piperacillin sodium during simulated Y-site administration—Inagaki K, Gill MA, Okamoto MP, Takagi J. Am J Hosp Pharm 1992;49:2769–72. [Compatibility of ranitidine hydrochloride with other injectable pharmaceuticals (26) in common use]—Marti E, Cervera P [Spanish]. Rev Soc Esp Farm Hosp 1985;9:169–72. [H₂ histamine antagonists and total parenteral nutrition]—Salvador-Collado MP, Montoro-Ronsano J, Cano-Marrón SM [Spanish]. Rev Soc Esp Farm Hosp 1989;13:307–11.

FORMULATION

Excipients

Excipients that have been used in presentations of ranitidine hydrochloride include:
Tablets: carmellose sodium; croscarmellose sodium; hydroxypropyl cellulose; hypromellose; magnesium stearate; microcrystalline cellulose; quinoline yellow (E104); titanium dioxide (E171).
Effervescent tablets and granules: aspartame.
Syrups: ethanol.
Suspensions: concentrated anise water BPC; syrup.
Injections: sodium phosphate; disodium phosphate anhydrous; monobasic potassium phosphate; phenol; sodium chloride.

Bioavailability and absorption

An absolute oral bioavailability for ranitidine of 60% ± 17% was calculated from pharmacokinetic data following a single-dose study in which five healthy subjects received 150 mg of ranitidine as a tablet or an intravenous injection.[20]

In an evaluation of the pharmacokinetics of ranitidine, the oral bioavailability of ranitidine was 56% or 58% (treatment of data by two methods) of that of the intravenous route.[21] Doses of 20 mg, 40 mg, and 80 mg were administered to six subjects. It was noted that following oral or parenteral administration, a secondary peak in the blood concentration versus time curve was produced.

Concentrations of ranitidine in plasma that were considered to be 'effective and quite constant' at steady state were achieved when an aqueous solution of ranitidine hydrochloride 267 mg/mL was administered rectally to six healthy subjects via an osmotic delivery system (Osmet, ALZA, USA) that delivered 20 mg of ranitidine hydrochloride per hour for eight hours.[22] Zero-order release of ranitidine at a rate of 75 microlitres per hour had been established *in vitro*. However, inter-subject differences in mean absorption times were noted.

Bioequivalence

Two brands of ranitidine 150 mg tablets (Zantac, Glaxo, UK and Ranidine, Jordanian Pharmaceutical Manufacturing Company, Jordan) were considered to have comparable *in-vitro* dissolution and disintegration properties and to be bioequivalent following a single-dose, randomised, two-way crossover study with ten healthy volunteers.[23] Inter-subject and intra-subject variations were not statistically significant. Similarly, bioequivalence between Zantac tablets (Glaxo, UK) and Antagonin tablets (Arab Pharmaceutical Manufacturing Company, Jordan)[24] and between Gastran tablets (Toro, Iceland) and another commercially available formulation[25] has been demonstrated in single-dose, crossover studies. All tablets contained 150 mg of ranitidine. Antagonin and Zantac tablets were comparable based on *in-vitro* characterisation.[24]

Suspensions

An extemporaneous suspension of ranitidine 150 mg/10 mL was prepared by the suspension of 36 powdered tablets of ranitidine 150 mg (Glaxo, USA) in 180 mL of distilled water and dilution with syrup to 360 mL.[26] Sonication of the suspension was claimed to improve the uniformity of ranitidine concentration in the formulation. Despite rapid settling of particles, 22% to 64% of the total sedimentation occurring within the first minute after cessation of mechanical shaking, the suspensions could be easily redispersed. A significant decrease in concentration (to about 82% to 96% of the original) of ranitidine occurred during storage at 25° for 14 days (in amber bottles); the authors concluded that the suspension was stable for 7 days after preparation, about 91% to 99% of the initial concentration was retained during this period.

FURTHER INFORMATION. Ranitidine hydrochloride [review of pharmacokinetics, pharmacology, clinical efficacy and safety]—Gaginella TS, Bauman JH. Drug Intell Clin Pharm 1983;17:873–85.

REFERENCES

1. Das Gupta V. Drug Dev Ind Pharm 1988;14(12):1647–55.
2. Walker SE, Kirby K. Can J Hosp Pharm 1988;41(3):105–8.
3. Das Gupta V, Parasrampuria J, Bethea C. J Clin Pharm Ther 1988;13:329–34.
4. Galante LJ, Stewart JT, Warren FW, Johnson SM, Duncan R. Am J Hosp Pharm 1990;47:1580–4.
5. Stewart JT, Warren FW, Johnson SM, Galante LJ. Am J Hosp Pharm 1990;47:2043–6.
6. Lampasona V, Mullins RE, Parks RB. Am J Hosp Pharm 1986;43:921–5.
7. Uzunarslan K, Akbuga J. Drug Dev Ind Pharm 1991;17(8):1067–81.
8. Parker WA. Can J Hosp Pharm 1985;38(6):160–1.
9. Walker SE, Bayliff CD. Am J Hosp Pharm 1985;42:590–2.
10. Bullock L, Parks RB, Lampasona V, Mullins RE. Am J Hosp Pharm 1985;42:2683–7.
11. Williams MF, Hak LJ, Dukes G. Am J Hosp Pharm 1990;47:1574–9.
12. Cano SM, Montoro JB, Pastor C, Pou L, Sabin P. Am J Hosp Pharm 1988;45:1100–2.
13. Galante LJ, Stewart JT, Warren FW, Edgar JW, Huff AJ. Am J Hosp Pharm 1990;47:1606–10.
14. Vervloet E, Lammers J, Tan LSL, Van Mourik CH, Rots M [letter]. DICP Ann Pharmacother 1990;24:440–2.
15. Chilvers MR, Lysne JM [letter]. Am J Hosp Pharm 1989;46:2057–8.
16. Colucci RD, Cobuzzi LE, Halpern NA. Am J Hosp Pharm 1988;45:1357–8.
17. Colucci RD, Cobuzzi LE, Halpern NA. Am J Hosp Pharm 1988;45:630–2.
18. Bashaw ED, Amantea MA, Minor JR, Gallelli JF. Am J Hosp Pharm 1988;45:2532–3.
19. Forman JK, Lachs JR, Souney PF. Am J Hosp Pharm 1987;44:1408–9.
20. Van Hecken AM, Tjandramaga TB, Mullie A, Verbesselt R, DeScheper PJ. Br J Clin Pharmacol 1982;14:195–200.
21. Miller R. J Pharm Sci 1984;73:1376–9.
22. De Bree H, De Boer AG. Pharm Weekbl (Sci) 1987;9:179–81.
23. Alkaysi HN, Sheikh Salem MA, Gharaibeh AM, El-Sayed YM, Ali-Gharaibeh KI, Badwan AA. J Clin Pharm Ther 1989;14:111–17.
24. Saket M, Arafat T, Awad R, Ibrahim H, Saleh M, Sallam E et al. Curr Ther Res 1989;46(5):924–31.
25. Hilgenstock C, Schmiedel G, Bührens K-G. Arzneimittelforschung 1987;37(II)Nr 8:974–6.
26. Karnes TH, Harris SR, Garnett WR, March C. Am J Hosp Pharm 1989;46:304–7.

Riboflavine (BAN)   *Vitamin*

Lactoflavin; Riboflavin (rINN); vitamin B_2; vitamin G
3,10-Dihydro-7,8-dimethyl-10-[(2S,3S,4R)-2,3,4,5-tetrahydroxypentyl]benzopteridine-2,4-dione; 7,8-dimethyl-10-(1-D-ribityl)isoalloxazine
$C_{17}H_{20}N_4O_6 = 376.4$

Riboflavine Sodium Phosphate (BANM)

Riboflavin 5′-phosphate sodium; Riboflavin Sodium Phosphate (rINNM)
$C_{17}H_{20}N_4NaO_9P,2H_2O = 514.4$
CAS—83-88-5 (riboflavine); 130-40-5 (riboflavine sodium phosphate, anhydrous)

Pharmacopoeial status

BP (riboflavine, riboflavine sodium phosphate); USP (riboflavin, riboflavin 5′-phosphate sodium)

Preparations

Compendial
Riboflavin Tablets USP.
Riboflavin Injection USP. pH 4.5 to 7.0.

Non-compendial
Riboflavine is an ingredient of compound vitamin B tablets, of compound vitamin B tablets strong, and of vitamin capsules.

Containers and storage

Solid state
Riboflavine BP should be kept in an airtight container and protected from light. Solutions, especially in the presence of alkali, deteriorate on exposure to light.
Riboflavine Sodium Phosphate BP should be kept in a well-closed container and protected from light.
Riboflavin USP and Riboflavin 5′-Phosphate Sodium USP should be preserved in tight, light-resistant containers.

Dosage forms
Riboflavin Tablets USP should be preserved in tight, light-resistant containers.
Riboflavin Injection USP should be preserved in light-resistant, single-dose or multiple-dose containers, preferably of Type I glass.

PHYSICAL PROPERTIES

Riboflavine is a yellow to orange-yellow crystalline powder with a slight odour and a persistent bitter taste.
Riboflavine sodium phosphate is a yellow to orange-yellow crystalline powder; odourless or almost odourless; hygroscopic.

Melting point

Riboflavine melts at about 280°, with decomposition.

pH

The pH of a saturated solution of *riboflavine* lies between 5.5 and 7.2. A saturated solution (USP) is neutral to litmus.
The pH of a 2% w/v solution of *riboflavine sodium phosphate* lies between 4.0 and 6.3 (BP). The pH of a 1% solution is 5.0 to 6.5 (USP).

Dissociation constants

pK_a 1.9, 10.2 (20°)

Partition coefficient

Log *P* (hexanol), −0.92

Solubility

Riboflavine is soluble 1 in 3000 to 1 in 20 000 of water. The variation in solubility is attributed to the existence of three crystal forms with different internal structures. It is more soluble in solutions of sodium chloride 0.9% and of urea 10% than in water. It is practically insoluble in ethanol, in acetone, in chloroform and in ether. It is very soluble in dilute solutions of alkali hydroxides.
Riboflavine sodium phosphate is soluble in 20 parts of water; very slightly soluble in ethanol; practically insoluble in chloroform and in ether.

Solubility enhancers
Substances which enhance the solubility of riboflavine in water include benzyl alcohol, nicotinamide, propylene glycol, tryptophan, urea, and urethane.

STABILITY

Under normal storage conditions riboflavine and riboflavin 5′-phosphate sodium, in the dry state, are unaffected by diffused light; when in solution both are subject to rapid photodegradation. In the presence of light, especially in alkaline solution, riboflavine degrades rapidly to form lumiflavine, a fluorescent decomposition product with no biological activity. Acid solutions of riboflavine are more stable to heat than alkaline solutions but following irradiation riboflavine degrades to the biologically inactive blue product lumichrome. The photolytic mechanism is attributed to the intramolecular transfer of hydrogen from the ribityl side-chain; the product depends on the alkalinity of the solution.
Values for the pH of maximum stability for riboflavine and the more soluble phosphate in buffered vehicles are pH 5 and pH 4, respectively.
Reduction of riboflavine to the leuco form may be effected under anaerobic conditions or by strong reducing agents. Leucoriboflavine is colourless and non-fluorescent and is readily reoxidised in air.

Infusion solutions

Workers in Japan[1] demonstrated the photodecomposition of riboflavine sodium phosphate 10 mg (on exposure to 2000 lux indoors for three hours) when mixed with various infusion solutions. Lumichrome was identified as a main degradation product. Decomposition was inhibited in infusion solutions of amino acids and by the addition of ascorbic acid.
The stability of riboflavine sodium phosphate in Parentrovite IVHP (Bencard) when admixed with five common infusion fluids was greater in sodium chloride 0.9% than in glucose 5% and in other glucose-containing fluids after seven hours at ambient temperature in the presence of light.[2]
Allwood[3] reported that light-induced losses of riboflavine from a total parenteral nutrition infusion can amount to 40% after eight hours and 55% after a typical 24-hour administration period. Passage through the administration set can lead to a further 2% loss.

Thermostability

Waltersson and Lundgren[4] applied an accelerated non-isothermal method to the determination of riboflavine thermostability using a linear temperature programme. Activation energies calculated for the base-catalysed, first-order degradation reaction (in 0.05M sodium hydroxide at 20° to 50°), were in good agreement with a literature value (87.7 kJ/mol) derived from isothermal tests.

Stabilisation

Casini and co-workers[5] reported that low concentrations of methyl and propyl hydroxybenzoates retarded the photodegradation of riboflavine in aqueous buffer solutions.
Buffered riboflavine phosphate solutions exposed to fluorescent light were stabilised by the following compounds in descending rank order: disodium edetate > thiourea > methyl hydroxybenzoate > DL-methionine > sodium thiosulphate. The rate of photodegradation was influenced by the pH and buffer species of the solutions[6] in the presence and the absence of disodium edetate.
In liposomes, the stability of riboflavine (in solution as the sodium phosphate) to fluorescent light increased in neutral and negatively charged liposomes but decreased in positively charged liposomes.[7] Greatest stabilisation was shown when the dimyristoyl-phosphatidylcholine content of liposomes was increased. Photodegradation followed first-order kinetics and was influenced by pH but not by the ionic strength of the solution.

INCOMPATIBILITY/COMPATIBILITY

Sorption to plastics

Among the plastic devices to which no significant sorption of riboflavine has been reported (from infusion solutions usually protected from light during test periods which ranged from seven hours to seven days) are: polyvinyl chloride bags; polyvinyl chloride tubing; cellulose propionate burette chamber; polyethylene tubing; Silastic tubing; and polypropylene and polyethylene syringe components.

FURTHER INFORMATION. Riboflavin enhances photo-oxidation of amino acids under simulated clinical conditions—Bhatia J, Stegink LD, Ziegler EE. J Parenter Enter Nutr 1983;7(3):277–9.

FORMULATION

Bioavailability

Levy and Rao[8] demonstrated that the oral absorption of riboflavine-5′-phosphate in five healthy volunteers increased by 50% when the vitamin was administered in a viscous, thixotropic solution of sodium alginate 2% instead of the usual aqueous vehicle.

The bioavailability of riboflavine, in 25 mg capsules administered orally to nine healthy volunteers,[9] remained unaffected (when measured microbiologically) when the capsules also contained physical mixtures of the vitamin (1:2) with either povidone 25 000 or dextran 40 000.

Adsorbents

Khalil et al[10] examined the *in-vitro* adsorption of riboflavine by kaolin (light, natural and white fine), attapulgite, magnesium trisilicate, and Veegum (aluminium magnesium trisilicate) under simulated *in-vivo* conditions over the pH range 2.1 to 7.0 (adjusted not buffered). Other variable parameters were: volume of adsorption medium and the presence of electrolytes, a surfactant, and a hydrocolloid. Under all conditions, riboflavine adsorption in the presence of an adsorbent decreased in the order: Veegum > attapulgite > kaolin > magnesium trisilicate. Dissolution tests of riboflavine from capsules revealed a decrease in its concentration in solution in the presence of either Veegum or kaolin. In all the systems examined only partial desorption of riboflavine was found after four hours at 37°.

Reductions in both the rate and extent of absorption of riboflavine when orally ingested concomitantly with various grades of attapulgite were detected by Khalil et al during a randomised crossover trial in six healthy volunteers.[11] The extent of reduction in the amount excreted was about 50% or 40% when 10 mg riboflavine (in solution) was co-administered either with 2 g suspended attapulgite or with 30 mL of a commercial antidiarrhoeal suspension (Quintess, Eli Lilly, USA; containing activated attapulgite 10% and colloidal attapulgite 3%). There was no significant effect on absorption when the adsorbent was administered two hours before the riboflavine.

FURTHER INFORMATION. Effect of ageing on dissolution rates and bioavailability of riboflavine in sugar-coated tablets—Khalil SA, Barakat NS, Boraie NA. STP Pharm 1991;1:189–94.

REFERENCES

1. Yamaji A, Ueno T, Fujii Y, Kurata Y, Kishi H, Hiraoka E [Japanese]. Jap J Hosp Pharm 1981;7(5):279–84.
2. Buxton PC, Conduit SM, Hathaway J. Br J Intraven Ther 1983;4:5,12.
3. Allwood MC. J Clin Hosp Pharm 1984;9:181–98.
4. Waltersson J-O, Lundgren P. Acta Pharm Suec 1982;19:127–36.
5. Casini G, De Laurentis N, Maggi N, Ottolino S [Italian]. Farmaco (Prat) 1981;36:553–8.
6. Asker AF, Habib MJ. Drug Dev Ind Pharm 1990;16(1):149–56.
7. Habib MJ, Asker AF. J Parenter Sci Technol 1991;45(3):124–7.
8. Levy G, Rao BK. J Pharm Sci 1972;61(2):279–80.
9. Geneidi AS, Kassem AA, Elbayoumy TE, Ibrahim EA. J Drug Res Egypt 1989;18:29–36.
10. Khalil SAH, Mortada LM, Shams-Eldeen MA, El-Khawas MM. Drug Dev Ind Pharm 1987;13(3):547–63.
11. Khalil SAH, Mortada LM, Shams-Eldeen MA, El-Khawas MM. Drug Dev Ind Pharm 1987;13(2):369–82.

Rifampicin (BAN, rINN)   *Antituberculous agent*

Rifaldazine; Rifampin (USAN); rifamycin AMP
(12*Z*,14*E*,24*E*)-(2*S*,16*S*,17*S*,18*R*,19*R*,20*R*,21*S*,22*R*,23*S*)-1,2-Dihydro-5,6,9,17,19-pentahydroxy-23-methoxy-2,4,12,16,-18,20,22-heptamethyl-8-(4-methylpiperazin-1-yliminomethyl)-1,11-dioxo-2,7-(epoxypentadeca-1,11,13-trienoimino)
naphtho[2,1-b]furan-21-yl   acetate;   3-(4-methylpiperazin-1-yl-iminomethyl)rifamycin SV; 3-{[(4-methyl-1-piperazinyl) imino] methyl}-rifamycin
$C_{43}H_{58}N_4O_{12} = 823.0$
CAS—13292-46-1

Pharmacopoeial status

BP (rifampicin); USP (rifampin)

Preparations

Compendial

Rifampicin Capsules BP. Capsules containing, in each, 150 mg and 300 mg are usually available.

Rifampicin Oral Suspension BP. A suspension containing rifampicin powder of suitable fineness in a suitably flavoured vehicle; a suspension containing 100 mg in 5 mL is usually available. pH 4.2 to 4.8.

Rifampin Capsules USP.

Rifampin and Isoniazid Capsules USP.

Rifampin for Injection USP. pH between 7.8 and 8.8, in a solution containing rifampin 6%.

Non-compendial

Rifadin (Merrell). *Capsules*, rifampicin 150 mg and 300 mg.
Syrup, rifampicin 100 mg/5 mL. The preparation should not be diluted.
Intravenous infusion, lyophilised powder for reconstitution, rifampicin 600 mg with 10-mL ampoule of solvent (pyrogen-free water with polysorbate 81). On reconstitution, the solution should be immediately diluted with 500 mL of glucose 5% injection or with one of the following recommended infusion fluids: compound sodium lactate; fructose 5% and 10%; glucose 10%; Macrodex with glucose; Macrodex with sodium chloride 0.9%; mannitol 10% and 20%; Rheomacrodex; Ringer acetate; sodium bicarbonate 1.4%; sodium chloride 0.9%. Infusions should be used within 6 hours. Incompatible with the

following infusion fluids: Perfudex; sodium bicarbonate 5%; sodium lactate 0.167M; Ringer acetate with glucose.

Rimactane(Ciba). *Capsules*, rifampicin 150 mg and 300 mg.

Syrup, rifampicin 100 mg/5 mL. The preparation should not be diluted.

Intravenous infusion, lyophilised powder for reconstitution, rifampicin 300 mg in a vial containing sodium formaldehyde sulphoxylate (pyrogen-free) with 5-mL ampoule of solvent (water for injections). On reconstitution, the solution should be immediately diluted with 250 mL of glucose 5% injection or with one of the following recommended infusion fluids: compound sodium lactate; fructose 5% and 10%; glucose 10%; Macrodex with glucose; Macrodex with sodium chloride 0.9%; mannitol 10% and 20%; Rheomacrodex; Ringer acetate; sodium bicarbonate 1.4%; sodium chloride 0.9%. Infusions should be used within 6 hours. Incompatible with the following infusion fluids: sodium bicarbonate 5%; Ringer acetate with glucose; Perfudex; sodium lactate 0.167M. When diluted in glucose injections or in sodium chloride 0.9% injection Rimactane infusion is incompatible with cephamandole, tetracycline, rolitetracycline, or doxycycline. If there is a possibility of precipitation, it should not be mixed with other drugs.

Rifampicin capsules are also available from Generics.

Containers and storage

Solid state

Rifampicin BP should be kept in airtight containers under an atmosphere of nitrogen; it should be protected from light and stored at a temperature not exceeding 15°.

Rifampin USP should be preserved in tight, light-resistant containers; it should be protected from excessive heat.

Dosage forms

Rifampin Capsules USP and Rifampin and Isoniazed Capsules USP should be preserved in tight, light-resistant containers; they should not be exposed to excessive heat.

Rifampin for Injection USP should be preserved in containers suitable for sterile solids.

Rifadin capsules should be protected from light and moisture and stored below 25°. Rifadin syrup should be dispensed in clear or amber glass bottles. Rifadin infusion should be freshly prepared. Rimactane capsules and syrup should be protected from heat and moisture; the syrup should be stored below 25°. Vials of Rimactane infusion should be protected from heat and light. The infusion should be freshly prepared.

PHYSICAL PROPERTIES

Rifampicin is a practically odourless, brick-red to reddish-brown crystalline powder.

Melting point

Rifampicin melts at about 185°, with decomposition.

pH

A 1% w/v suspension of *rifampicin* has a pH of 4.5 to 6.5.

Dissociation constants

pK_a 1.7 (naphthalene hydroxy groups), 7.9 (piperazine nitrogen)

Partition coefficient

Log P (octanol/pH 7.4),[1] 1.2

Solubility

Rifampicin is slightly soluble in water, in ethanol, in acetone, in carbon tetrachloride, and in ether; practically insoluble in buta-

nol, in cyclohexane, in glycerol, and in propylene glycol; soluble in ethyl acetate, in methanol, and in tetrahydrofuran; freely soluble in chloroform and in dimethyl sulphoxide.

Effect of pH

Rifampicin solubility is greater at low pH values. At 37°, it is soluble 1 in approximately 100 of phosphate buffer, pH 7.4, and 1 in 5 of 0.1M hydrochloric acid.[1] At 25° rifampicin is soluble 1 in approximately 10, 250, and 360 of water at pH 2.0, 5.3, and 7.5, respectively.[2]

Dissolution

The USP specifies that for Rifampin Capsules USP not less than 75% of the labelled amount of $C_{43}H_{58}N_4O_{12}$ is dissolved in 45 minutes. Dissolution medium: 900 mL of 0.1N hydrochloric acid; Apparatus 1 at 50 rpm.

Crystal and molecular structure

Although rifampicin contains nine asymmetric centres and three double bonds, it exists in only one isomeric form.

STABILITY

In the solid state, rifampicin is stable for at least five years at 25°. In aqueous solution, rifampicin degradation is both acid-catalysed and base-catalysed; decomposition is slower in neutral media. Under acidic conditions (pH 2.3), rifampicin is hydrolysed to 1-amino-4-methyl-piperazine and to 3-formyl rifamycin SV, which is prone to precipitation.[3] The activation energy for the degradation of rifampicin in 0.1M hydrochloric acid was calculated by Seydel[1] to be 80.3 kJ/mol. Decomposition is reported to be catalysed by phosphate buffer.[1]

In basic media (pH 8.0) and in the presence of atmospheric oxygen, rifampicin was oxidised to a quinone derivative[3] at 20° to 22°. At higher temperatures (90° to 95°), at pH 8.2, various 25-desacetyl derivatives were formed.[4]

In aqueous solution at 37°, maximum stability of rifampicin is demonstrated[5] at about pH 5. The degradation of rifampicin at pH 1 to 5 at 37°, in the presence of ascorbic acid as antoxidant, was attributed to rapid reversible hydrolysis of its azomethine bond, followed by one or more slower secondary reactions.[6] The overall loss of rifampicin from solution was dependent on its initial concentration. Below pH 4.3, a complex pH-rate profile was observed.

Rifampicin is stable for at least eight months[7] in solutions of dimethyl sulphoxide at 15°, and for six hours[8] in sodium chloride 0.9% injection and in glucose 5% injection at 25°.

Suspensions of rifampicin (prepared using the contents of rifampicin capsules, Rifadin, Merrell Dow, USA) 1% w/v in various syrup formulations (some containing preservatives and flavours) were found to be stable for four weeks when stored in amber glass bottles at room temperature or in a refrigerator.[9]

Stabilisation

The oxidation of rifampicin in basic media may be prevented by the addition of ascorbic acid. Chelating agents have also been shown to inhibit this reaction indicating that the oxidative pathway may be catalysed by trace metal impurities.[5]

FURTHER INFORMATION. Stability and compatibility of minocycline hydrochloride and [rifampicin] in intravenous solutions at various temperatures—Pearson SD, Trissel LA. Am J Hosp Pharm 1993;50:698–702.

INCOMPATIBILITY/COMPATIBILITY

Bentonite should not be included in rifampicin formulations as the clay may adsorb the drug.

FORMULATION

Excipients

Excipients that have been used in presentations of rifampicin include:

Capsules: allura red AC (E129); brilliant blue FCF (133); calcium stearate; erythrosine (E127); gelatin; indigo carmine (E132); lactose; magnesium stearate; red ferric oxide; phloxine B; silica; sodium lauryl sulphate; starch; sunset yellow FCF(E110); talc; titanium dioxide (E171).

Oral liquids: agar; carmellose; citric acid; diethanolamine; glycerol; methylcellulose; methyl and propyl hydroxybenzoates; potassium metabisulphite; potassium sorbate; polysorbate 80; saccharin; silicone anti-foaming agent; sodium benzoate; sodium metabisulphite; sucrose.

Intravenous infusions: polysorbate 81; sodium formaldehyde sulphoxylate; sodium hydroxide.

Solid dispersions

Solid dispersions of rifampicin with either macrogol 4000 (50:50 and 30:70) or urea (30:70) showed faster dissolution in simulated gastric fluid at $37° \pm 2°$ than either simple rifampicin or five rifampicin capsules marketed in India.[10] *In-vivo* studies indicated that superior bioavailability was shown by the rifampicin:macrogol 4000, 30:70 solid dispersions in comparison with the capsules, in a crossover study involving six subjects.

FURTHER INFORMATION. Formulation of rifampicin suppositories—Abdel-Monem Sayed H, Ismail S, Mohamed AA. Bull Pharm Sci Assiut Univ 1990;13:97–102. Solid dispersion systems as a means for enhancing rifampicin release from ointments. Clinical evaluation of the proposed formulation—Youssef MK, El-Sayed ED, Fouda MA. Drug Dev Ind Pharm 1988;14:2667–85. Rifampicin microspheres:formulation and *in vitro* release characteristics—Iseri E, Kas HS, Hincal AA. Chim Oggi 1989;7:15–16.

PROCESSING

Sterilisation

Crippa *et al*[11] reported that rifampicin appears to be stable to sterilising doses of gamma radiation.

REFERENCES

1. Seydel JK. Antibiotica Chemother 1970;16:380–91.
2. Kenny MT, Strates B. Drug Metab Rev 1981;12:159–218.
3. Maggi N, Pasqualucci CR, Ballotta P, Sensi P. Chemotherapia 1966;11:285–92.
4. Maggi N, Vigevani A, Gallo GG, Pasqualucci CR. J Med Chem 1968;11:936–9.
5. Awata N, Iwane I, Nakagawa H, Sugimoto I [Japanese]. Yakuzaigaku 1978;38:145–50.
6. Prankerd RJ, Walters JM, Parnes JH. Int J Pharmaceutics 1992;78:59–67.
7. Karlson AG, Ulrich JA. Appl Microbiol 1969;18:692–3.
8. Fletcher NR, Fletcher P, Yates RJ. Br J Pharm Pract 1988;10:442,444,448,453.
9. Krukenberg CC, Mischler PG, Massad EN, Moore LA, Chandler AD. Am J Hosp Pharm 1986;43:2225–8.
10. Vadav SK, Pande S, Dixit VK. East Pharm 1990 Apr;33:129–31.
11. Crippa PR, Tedeschi R, Vecli A. Farmaco (Prat) 1972;28:226–32.

Salbutamol (BAN, rINN)

Bronchodilator; Beta-adrenoceptor agonist

Albuterol (USAN)

1-(4-Hydroxy-3-hydroxymethylphenyl)-2-(*tert*-butylamino)ethanol

$C_{13}H_{21}NO_3 = 239.3$

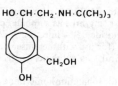

Salbutamol Sulphate (BANM, rINNM)

Albuterol Sulfate (USAN)

$(C_{13}H_{21}NO_3)_2,H_2SO_4 = 576.7$

CAS—18559-94-9 (salbutamol); 51022-70-9 (salbutamol sulphate)

Pharmacopoeial status

BP (salbutamol, salbutamol sulphate); USP (albuterol, albuterol sulfate)

Preparations

Compendial

Salbutamol Tablets BP contain salbutamol sulphate. Tablets containing, in each, the equivalent of 2 mg and 4 mg of salbutamol are usually available.

Salbutamol Pressurised Inhalation BP (Salbutamol Aerosol Inhalation). A suspension of salbutamol in a suitable liquid in a suitable pressurised container. Pressurised inhalations delivering 100 micrograms of salbutamol per actuation of the valve are usually available.

Salbutamol Injection BP is a sterile solution of salbutamol sulphate in water for injections. Injections containing the equivalent of 0.5 mg of salbutamol in 1 mL, and 0.25 mg in 5 mL are usually available. pH 3.4 to 5.0. A sterile solution for intravenous infusion containing the equivalent of 5 mg of salbutamol in 5 mL is also usually available.

Non-compendial

Aerolin Autohaler (3M). *Aerosol inhalation*, salbutamol 100 micrograms (as sulphate)/metered inhalation.

Asmaven (Berk). *Tablets*, salbutamol (as sulphate) 2 mg and 4 mg.

Aerosol inhalation, salbutamol 100 micrograms/metered inhalation.

Salbulin (3M). *Aerosol inhalation*, salbutamol 100 micrograms/metered inhalation.

Ventodisks (A&H). *Powder for inhalation*, disks containing microfine salbutamol (as sulphate) 200 micrograms/blister and 400 micrograms/blister.

Ventolin (A&H). *Tablets*, salbutamol (as sulphate) 2 mg and 4 mg.

Syrup, sugar free, salbutamol (as sulphate) 2 mg/5 mL. *Diluent*: purified water, freshly boiled and cooled. Precipitation of the cellulose thickening agent may result if the preparation is diluted with syrup or sorbitol solution.

Injection, salbutamol (as sulphate) 50 micrograms/mL and 500 micrograms/mL.

Solution for intravenous infusion, salbutamol (as sulphate) 1 mg/mL. Dilute before use to a maximum concentration of 500 micrograms/mL.

Ventolin parenteral preparations may be diluted with water for injections, sodium chloride 0.9% injection, sodium chloride and glucose injection, or glucose 5% injection. They should not be administered in the same syringe or infusion as any other medication. All unused admixtures of Ventolin parenteral preparations should be discarded 24 hours after preparation.

Aerosol inhalation, salbutamol 100 micrograms/metered inhalation.

Nebules (for use with nebuliser), salbutamol 0.1% (1 mg/mL) as sulphate and 0.2% (2 mg/mL) as sulphate. pH of solution, 4.0. *Diluent*: sodium chloride 0.9% injection.

Respirator solution (for use with nebuliser or ventilator), salbutamol 0.5% (5 mg/mL) as sulphate. *Diluent*: sodium chloride 0.9% injection.

Rotacaps (powder for inhalation), microfine salbutamol (as sulphate) 200 micrograms and 400 micrograms.

Volmax (DF). *Tablets*, controlled release, salbutamol (as sulphate) 4 mg and 8 mg.

Salbutamol tablets are also available in various strengths from Cox, CP, Evans, Kerfoot, Norton, Tillotts (Salbuvent).

Salbutamol syrup is also available from Tillotts (Salbuvent).

Salbutamol aerosol inhalation is also available from Ashbourne (Maxivent), Cox, CP, Evans, Kerfoot, Norton, Tillotts (Salbuvent).

Salbutamol 0.1% (1 mg/mL, as sulphate) is also available for nebulisation in 2.5-mL unit doses as Steri-Neb Salamol (Baker Norton).

Salbutamol capsules containing 200 or 400 micrograms salbutamol (as sulphate) as dry powder for inhalation are also available as Salbutamol Cyclocaps (Du Pont); only for use with a Cyclohaler.

Containers and storage

Solid state

Salbutamol BP and Salbutamol Sulphate BP should be kept in well-closed containers and protected from light.

Albuterol USP and Albuterol Sulfate USP should be preserved in well-closed, light-resistant containers.

Dosage forms

Asmaven tablets should be stored below 25°, protected from light.

Ventodisks, Ventolin tablets, Ventolin Rotacaps and Volmax tablets should be stored at a temperature below or not exceeding 30°. Ventolin Rotacaps and Ventodisks should not be exposed to extremes of temperature. Ventolin tablets and Rotacaps should be stored in a dry place.

Ventolin syrup should be kept at a temperature not exceeding 30°, protected from light.

Ventolin parenteral presentations should be protected from light and stored below 30°.

Aerosol preparations of salbutamol should be stored in a cool place (Ventolin below 30°) protected from frost, direct heat, and sunlight. The pressurised canister should not be punctured, broken, or burnt.

Ventolin nebules should be stored below 25° and protected from light. Solutions in nebulisers should be replaced daily.

Ventolin respirator solution should be stored below 25°, protected from light, and the contents of the opened bottles discarded after one month. Solutions in nebulisers should be replaced daily.

PHYSICAL PROPERTIES

Salbutamol base is a white or almost white crystalline powder. *Salbutamol sulphate* is a white or almost white crystalline powder.

Melting point

Salbutamol melts at about 156°, with decomposition.

Dissociation constant

pK_a 9.3 (amino group), 10.3 (phenolic group)

Solubility

Salbutamol is soluble 1 in 70 of water, 1 in 25 of ethanol; slightly soluble in ether.

Salbutamol sulphate is soluble 1 in 4 of water; slightly soluble in ethanol, in chloroform, and in ether.

Solubility studies of the inclusion complex formed between the clathrate of salbutamol and β-cyclodextrin showed that salbutamol solubility increased with increasing β-cyclodextrin concentration up to the saturation solubility of the latter.[1]

STABILITY

Solutions

Kinetic data for salbutamol sulphate in aqueous solutions showed that degradation was first order and that the rate was dependent on temperature, pH, and drug concentration.[2] The activation energy for a 0.5% solution (pH 9.0) over the temperature range 50° to 75° was 101 kJ/mol. The stability-indicating HPLC assay emphasised the inaccuracy of the BPC indoaniline colorimetric assay, which overestimated the salbutamol content of degraded systems.

The same authors[3] showed that decomposition of salbutamol sulphate solution at 70° was accelerated in a concentration-dependent manner by both glucose and sucrose at pH 3.5, but only by glucose at pH 7. The effect of fructose was similar to that of glucose.

Degradation of salbutamol sulphate at 55° to 85° in buffered aqueous solutions protected from light was shown[4] to follow apparent first-order kinetics with maximum stability at pH 3.5. At pH 1.9, 3.5, and 7.1 at 65°, the $t_{10\%}$ values of a 0.036M solution were 37.1 days, 91.7 days, and 1.7 days, respectively. For a salbutamol sulphate 1% solution at pH 8.8 (temperature 55° to 85°), the activation energy was 132 kJ/mol. Assuming an unaltered reaction mechanism, the rate constant and shelf-life for the same solution at 25° were calculated to be 7.14×10^{-6}/h and 1.7 years, respectively. Four major and several minor decomposition products were detected by thin layer chromatography; they were phenolic in character but their structures were not identified. Decomposition rate was enhanced by increased drug concentration and elevated temperature. The decomposed solutions changed colour from yellow to brownish-red, depending upon alkalinity.

Effect of antioxidants

Sodium metabisulphite was found to decompose rapidly in an aqueous solution of salbutamol sulphate under anaerobic conditions.[5] Thiourea was suggested as a possible alternative stabilising agent.

Thiourea was shown to exhibit superior antioxidant properties to sodium metabisulphite by Valdés Santurio and Vega Eguino[6] while investigating the stability of salbutamol sulphate nebuliser solution. They recommend, for their formulation (salbutamol sulphate 0.5%, thiourea 0.05%, also containing propylene glycol and polysorbate 80), a shelf-life of one year at a temperature not greater than 30°, or two years at 25°.

FORMULATION

Excipients

Excipients that have been used in presentations of salbutamol sulphate include:

Tablets: calcium phosphate; calcium sulphate dihydrate; erythrosine (E127); lactose; magnesium stearate; maize starch; patent blue V (E131); pregelatinised starch.

Syrups: citric acid monohydrate; fruit flavours; methyl and propyl hydroxybenzoates; hypromellose; saccharin sodium; sodium benzoate; sodium chloride; sodium citrate; sorbitol; sugar-free syrup; sunset yellow FCF (E110).

Suppositories: semi-synthetic glycerides; Witepsol H15.

Injections and infusions: sodium chloride; sulphuric acid.

Inhaler solutions: benzalkonium chloride; sulphuric acid.

Powders for inhalation: lactose (larger particle).

Aerosol inhalations, salbutamol or salbutamol sulphate: dichlorodifluoromethane; oleic acid; propellants 11, 12, and 114; sorbitan trioleate; trichloromonofluoromethane.

Bioavailability

Administration of salbutamol as a powder inhalation (400 micrograms via Rotahaler) and as tablets (4 mg) produced peak expiratory flow rates which measured 75% and 61% (at 15 minutes), respectively, compared with nebulised salbutamol (4 mg).[7] In a double-blind, triple-dummy study which involved 17 asthmatic children, nebulised salbutamol gave the largest bronchodilation effect while tablets produced the most prolonged effect.

Comparison of sublingual, oral, and inhaled doses of salbutamol in a randomised, crossover, placebo-controlled trial with seven asthmatic subjects showed no clinical advantage for the sublingual route.[8]

Modified-release preparations

Experimental controlled-release tablets of salbutamol sulphate (10.6 mg/tablet) included the polymers Eudragit RS-100 (polymethacrylate; low permeability) or Methocel K-100 M (methylcellulose; fast hydrating) as matrix formers.[9] The effect of several water-insoluble diluents on dissolution was examined using the USP XIX basket method with distilled water and buffers. The only diluents which significantly retarded drug diffusion from preparations containing Eudragit RS-100 were magnesium oxide and calcium hydroxide. Drug release from both matrices followed first-order kinetics and was retarded when the Eudragit concentration increased from 10% to 30% w/w. Stability studies at 30°, 45°, and 60°, and at 85% relative humidity (30°) revealed no change in the appearance, hardness, friability, or mean drug content of the Methocel matrix tablets. Calculated $t_{50\%}$ and $t_{10\%}$ values at 30° for Methocel:calcium hydrogen phosphate (40:55) preparations were 2.1 hours and 10.2 hours, respectively.

Transdermal delivery

In Franz diffusion cells, the penetration of salbutamol 1% into excised hairless *mouse* dorsal skin (in 93 hours) was 2.45 mg/cm^2 from aqueous cream and 0.02 mg/cm^2 from white soft paraffin.[10] When 5-mg amounts of salbutamol in a variety of bases were applied to the forearm skin of volunteer subjects, percutaneous absorption (from measurements of induced erythema) decreased in the rank order: aqueous cream > cetomacrogol cream > Aquadrate > white soft paraffin.

In a transdermal delivery system developed by Jain *et al*,[11] release of salbutamol was controlled by an osmo-regulatory mechanism with sodium chloride and macrogol 4000 in a laminated matrix containing cellulose acetate. Release followed zero-order kinetics depending upon the macrogol 4000 concentration in the transdermal patch; an increase from 2% to 10% resulted in an increased drug release rate from 212.5 to 412.5 micrograms/h/cm.^{2} The reservoir patch that showed optimal skin permeation *in vitro* was compared in twelve asthmatic patients with conventional oral 4 mg tablets (Asthaline, Cipla India). Although peak plasma concentrations (and correlated forced expiratory volume values) measured for the transdermal route were not achieved as rapidly as by the oral route, they remained constant over 24 hours.

Bannon *et al*[12] demonstrated transport of salbutamol from a hydrogel matrix across a cellophane membrane *in vitro* and transdermally. In the cellophane membranes the rate of passive diffusion was matrix controlled; by application of iontophoresis, enhanced transport was achieved in proportion to current intensity. Passive transport across the stratum corneum *in vitro* was negligible but transport was significant when induced iontophoretically. In two normal volunteers passive transport again was neglible but about 10% of salbutamol applied in 2 mg and 4 mg patches was calculated to have reached the systemic circulation.

FURTHER INFORMATION. *In vitro* and *in vivo* studies of sustained-release floating dosage forms containing salbutamol sulfate—Babu VB, Khar RK. Pharmazie 1990;45:268–70. Sustained-release formulation [tablets prepared by wax matrix granulation] of salbutamol sulphate [*in vitro* and in *dogs*]—Murthy RSR, Malhotra M, Miglani BD. Drug Dev Ind Pharm 1991;17(10):1373–80. Micro-encapsulation of salbutamol sulphate using multiple emulsion technique—Lata M, Nasa SL, Murthy RSR. East Pharm 1987;30:137–8. Metabolic effects of salbutamol: comparison of aerosol and intravenous administration—Neville A, Palmer JBD, Gaddie J, May CS, Palmer KNV, Murchison LE. Br Med J 1977;1:413–14. Determination of the relative bioavailability of salbutamol to the lung following inhalation—Hindle M, Chrystyn H. Br J Clin Pharmacol 1992;34:311–15. Pharmacokinetics of intravenous and oral salbutamol and its sulphate conjugate—Morgan DJ, Paull JD, Richmond BH, Wilson-Evered E, Ziccone SP. Br J Clin Pharmacol 1986;22:587–93. Comparison of intravenous and aerosol salbutamol—Hetzel MR, Clark TJH. Br Med J 1976;2:919. Paradoxical deterioration in lung function after nebulised salbutamol in wheezy infants [contains a warning concerning the acidification of nebulised salbutamol solutions]—O'Callaghan C, Milner AD, Swarbrick A. Lancet 1986;2:1424–5. Spray dried salbutamol sulphate for use in dry powder aerosol formulations—Chawla A, Taylor KMG, Newton JM, Johnson MCR. J Pharm Pharmacol 1992;44(Suppl):1069. Transdermal drug delivery systems of albuterol [salbutamol]: *in vitro* and *in vivo* studies—Gokhale R, Schmidt C, Alcorn L, Stolzenbach J, Schoenhard G, Farhadieh B. J Pharm Sci 1992;81(10):996–9.

PROCESSING

Sterilisation

Salbutamol injection can be sterilised by heating in an autoclave.

REFERENCES

1. Cabral Marques HM, Pugh WJ, Hadgraft J, Kellaway IW. J Pharm Pharmacol 1989;41:62P.
2. Hakes LB, Corby TC, Meakin BJ. J Pharm Pharmacol 1979;31:25P.

3. Hakes LB, Meakin BJ, Winterborn IK. J Pharm Pharmacol 1980;32:49P.
4. Mälkki L, Tammilehto S. Int J Pharmaceutics 1990;63:17–22.
5. Valdés Santurio JR, Vega Eguino E [Spanish]. Rev Cubana Farm 1985;19:156–72.
6. Valdés Santurio JR, Vega Eguino E [Spanish]. Rev Cubana Farm 1986;20:28–34.
7. Grimwood K, Johnson-Barrett JJ, Taylor B. Br Med J 1981;282:105–6.
8. Lipworth BJ, Clark RA, Dhillon DP, Moreland TA, Struthers AD, Clark GA et al. Eur J Clin Pharmacol 1989;37:567–71.
9. Sanghavi NM, Bijlani CP, Kamath PR, Sarwade VB [letter]. Drug Dev Ind Pharm 1990;16(12):1955–61.
10. Green KL, Sapra M. J Pharm Pharmacol 1988;40:102P.
11. Jain SK, Vyas SP, Dixit V. Drug Dev Ind Pharm 1990;16(9):1565–77.
12. Bannon YB, Corish J, Corrigan OI, Masterson JG. Drug Dev Ind Pharm 1988;14(15-17):2151–66.

Sodium Nitroprusside

Vasodilator

Sodium nitroprussiate; sodium nitroferricyanide dihydrate
Sodium pentacyanonitrosylferrate (III) dihydrate
$Na_2Fe(CN)_5NO,2H_2O = 298.0$
CAS—14402-89-2 (anhydrous); 13755-38-9 (dihydrate)

Pharmacopoeial status

BP, USP

Preparations

Compendial
Sodium Nitroprusside Intravenous Infusion BP is a sterile solution of sodium nitroprusside in glucose injection containing 50 g of anhydrous glucose per litre. It is prepared immediately before use by dissolving sodium nitroprusside for injection in the requisite amount of glucose injection (50 g per litre) and diluting the resulting solution with 250 to 500 times its volume of glucose injection (50 g per litre). Sodium nitroprusside for injection is a material obtained from a solution of sodium nitroprusside by freeze-drying. Sealed containers each containing the equivalent of 50 mg of sodium nitroprusside dihydrate are usually available.
Sterile Sodium Nitroprusside USP. For parenteral use.

Non-compendial
Nipride (Roche). *Infusion*, ampoules containing the equivalent of 50 mg sodium nitroprusside for reconstitution with glucose 5% injection. The resulting solution should be diluted in 250 mL to 1000 mL of glucose 5% injection, sodium chloride 0.9% injection, compound sodium lactate injection, compound sodium chloride injection, or sorbitol 5% injection. The initial solution should be prepared immediately before use and any unused portion discarded. The freshly prepared infusion solution has a faint orange-brownish tint. If highly coloured it should not be used. The infusion solution should not be used after a period of 24 hours from the time of preparation. No preparations other than those recommended should be added to the Nipride ampoule or mixed with the Nipride infusion solutions. In aqueous solution Nipride yields the nitroprusside ion which reacts with minute quantities of a wide variety of inorganic or organic substances to form reaction products which may be highly coloured.

Sodium nitroprusside intravenous solutions are available from David Bull, CP.

Containers and storage

Solid state
Sodium Nitroprusside BP should be kept in a well-closed container and protected from light.
Sodium Nitroprusside USP should be preserved in tight, light-resistant containers.

Dosage forms
Sodium Nitroprusside Intravenous Infusion BP should be used immediately after preparation. The label of the sealed container states that the diluted solution must be protected from light during infusion.
Sterile Sodium Nitroprusside USP should be preserved, protected from light, in containers suitable for sterile solids.
Nipride ampoules and infusion should be protected from light. When the infusion solution is prepared, the container should be wrapped in aluminium foil or other opaque material.

PHYSICAL PROPERTIES

Sodium nitroprusside exists as reddish-brown crystals or powder.

Solubility

Sodium nitroprusside is freely soluble in water; slightly soluble in ethanol; very slightly soluble in chloroform; insoluble in benzene.

STABILITY

Sodium nitroprusside, slightly light-sensitive in the dry solid state, becomes extremely photosensitive when in solution.[1] Irradiated diluted solutions are reported to decompose more readily than concentrated solutions.[2] See also Photoprotection, below.

Degradation mechanisms and products

There is a lack of consensus in the literature concerning the exact nature of the pathways of photodegradation. However, it is generally agreed that, upon exposure to light, sodium nitroprusside solution shows increased absorbance at 394 nm and 395 nm; the maxima represent sodium nitroprusside, photo-excited sodium nitroprusside, and several degradation products including aquopentacyanoferrate (APCF) III. The primary degradation reactions are independent of the effects of pH and irradiation wavelength, unlike the secondary reactions which are dependent on these factors.
Various workers have used spectroscopy to determine the products and extent of photodegradation in solution.[2–5] During photolysis, the pH of a 4 mg/mL solution of sodium nitroprusside decreased[2] from about neutral to about 3.5, due to cleavage of the NO moiety and formation of nitrate, or nitrite and nitrate ions in the presence of oxygen. APCF II was formed and was rapidly converted to APCF III; this reaction was catalysed by ferrous ions. The APCF II or III formed ferrocyanide or ferricyanide, and ferrous and ferric ions. Prussian blue was the product under such conditions.[2] Hydrogen cyanide and nitric oxide are also possible products of photodecomposition.[5,6] Hargrave[6] recommended that the solution be discarded once it turned blue. However, Sewell[7] noted that development of a blue colour in an infusion of 0.5 mg/mL in glucose 5% injection in a non-wrapped polypropylene syringe was only apparent after 8 hours in daylight and laboratory light, by which time 17% of the original sodium nitroprusside content had degraded. Simultaneously, a marked increase in the concentration of the toxic degradation

product, free cyanide, to exceed 2.0 micrograms/mL was measured.

The stability of sodium nitroprusside was reported[8,9] to be greater in acidic than in alkaline solutions.

Decomposition of sodium nitroprusside in solution was observed by several authors to be greater in direct sunlight than in artificial light.[3,10,11]

Aqueous solutions of sodium nitroprusside (20 mg/mL) were observed to be stable for 13 days at room temperature.[9] Chelation with various agents in aqueous solutions resulted in enhanced stability, for example: sorbitol (50%), 32 days; macrogol 300 (20%), 24 days; disodium edetate (0.01%), more than 39 days; or sodium citrate (5%), more than 800 days.

Photoprotection

Physical methods

When protected from light, aqueous solutions of sodium nitroprusside have been reported to be stable for up to six months at room temperature.[3,4]

Protected from light, an undiluted injection solution of sodium nitroprusside (10 g/L) was stable for more than two years[10] at room temperature and at 4°. Infusion solutions (approximately 200 mg/L) in sodium chloride 0.9% or in glucose 5% were stable for at least seven days when stored in foil-wrapped bottles, but decomposed on exposure to light. It was recommended that infusion solutions should be prepared in glucose 5%.

Davidson and Lyall[11] established the efficacy of a light-protective administration set (Amberset) in maintaining the stability of sodium nitroprusside 0.1% w/v reconstituted in glucose 5% injection under fluorescent light but not direct sunlight. The manufacturers of sodium nitroprusside (David Bull Laboratories) continue to stress the importance of foil wrapping of final infusion solutions in areas of high light energy and where specialised light-protective administration sets are not available.[12]

Sodium nitroprusside 1 mg/mL (Nipride, Roche, USA) was found[13] to be stable in glucose 5% in disposable aluminium-wrapped plastic syringes for 24 hours at 25°. The pH of solutions in unwrapped syringes fell from 4.2 to 3.5; the solutions had discoloured (to pale yellow) after 12 hours and a 22% loss of sodium nitroprusside was noted.

Mahoney et al[14] detected no appreciable degradation of sodium nitroprusside (50 or 100 micrograms/mL) in either glucose 5%, sodium chloride 0.9%, or compound sodium lactate injections in glass or plastic containers, wrapped in aluminium foil, and exposed to fluorescent light for 48 hours. There was no decrease in the delivered potency of sodium nitroprusside solutions during simulated infusions at 10 mL/hour, through polyvinyl chloride tubing exposed to light for up to 24 hours. These results contrast with those of Frank et al[5] who found an increased rate of degradation of sodium nitroprusside 0.01% in glucose 5% infusion under fluorescent light in polyvinyl chloride containers but not in glass (Pyrex) containers.

Chemical methods

Dimethyl sulphoxide (DMSO) in various buffers was found to enhance the stability of 50 mg/100 mL solutions of sodium nitroprusside;[15] however, its photoprotective action was influenced by the pH of the medium and its buffer species. The effect of DMSO 10% v/v with phosphate buffer was greater at pH 7.0 than at pH 7.9 or pH 4.65.

A photoprotective effect was exerted by dimethyl sulphoxide (DMSO) 10% v/v on a 50 mg/100 mL solution of sodium nitroprusside under fluorescent light in the presence of sodium chloride 0.9%, glucose 5%, sodium edetate 0.2%, citric acid 0.2%, methyl hydroxybenzoate 0.01%, sodium sulphite 0.1%, macrogol 300 (30% w/v), or Tween 80 (0.5%).[16] In the absence of DMSO the photostability of sodium nitroprusside was slightly enhanced by macrogol 300, citric acid, or sodium edetate and diminished by sodium sulphite.

Leeuwenkamp et al,[17] using ion-pair reversed-phase chromatography, found that the photostability of sodium nitroprusside 50 micrograms/mL in glucose 5% solution was not improved by the addition of citric acid or disodium edetate. However, cyanocobalamin 1 mg/mL did exert a photostabilising effect on exposure of sodium nitroprusside solutions in glucose 5% to light at 350 nm.

Intravenous admixtures

It has been noted that sterile water for injection containing preservative (such as benzyl alcohol) should not be used as diluent for reconstitution of sodium nitroprusside injection since benzyl alcohol reacts with sodium nitroprusside, increasing the decomposition rate of the latter.[18]

FURTHER INFORMATION. Injectable preparations of sodium nitroprusside. Galenical and analytical development—Chabrel B, Mollet M, Puisieux F, Thao TX, Canivet P, Assamoi L et al [French]. Ann Pharm Fr 1980;38(4):307–14. Two methods for monitoring the photodecomposition of sodium nitroprusside in aqueous and glucose solutions—Hartley TF, Philcox JC, Willoughby J. J Pharm Sci 1985;74(6):668–71.

INCOMPATIBILITY/COMPATIBILITY

Sodium nitroprusside solution should not be mixed with any other drug or preservative as it reacts with minute quantities of organic and inorganic substances forming highly coloured products. If this occurs, the solution should be discarded.

An admixture of sodium nitroprusside (Nipride, Roche, USA 200 micrograms/mL) and esmolol hydrochloride (Brevibloc, Dupont, USA, 10 mg/mL) in glucose 5% injection was shown to be stable when protected from light for up to 24 hours at room temperature (15° to 30°).[19]

PROCESSING

Sterilisation

Sterilisation of solutions of sodium nitroprusside (1%) by heating in an autoclave at 115° for up to two hours caused some degradation[3] (manifested by increased absorbance values at 395 nm); sterilisation by filtration was recommended, provided that adequate protection from light was ensured.

In another study,[17] analysis of solutions of sodium nitroprusside 50 micrograms/mL (autoclaved for 15 minutes at 121°) showed that the initial concentration of sodium nitroprusside in glucose 5% solution was reduced by 40% during autoclaving.

REFERENCES

1. Leeuwenkamp OR, Van Bennekom WP, Van Der Mark EJ, Bult A. Pharm Weekbl (Sci) 1984;6:129–40.
2. Van Loenen AC, Hofs-Kemper W. Pharm Weekbl (Sci) 1979;I(114):424–36.
3. Anderson RA, Rae W. Aust J Pharm Sci 1972;NS1(2):45–6.
4. Patel JA. Am J Hosp Pharm 1969;26:51–3.
5. Frank MJ, Johnson JB, Rubin SH. J Pharm Sci 1976;65(1):44–8.
6. Hargrave RE. J Hosp Pharm 1974;32:188–91.

7. Sewell GJ, Forbes DR, Munton TJ. J Clin Hosp Pharm 1985;10:351–60.
8. Challen RG [letter]. Australas J Pharm 1967;48(574):S110.
9. Schumacher GE. Am J Hosp Pharm 1966;23:533.
10. Vesey CJ, Batistoni GA. J Clin Pharm 1977;2:105–17.
11. Davidson SW, Lyall D. Pharm J 1987;239:599–601.
12. Hatton IN [letter]. Pharm J 1988;240:5.
13. Pramar Y, Das Gupta V, Gardner SN, Yau B. J Clin Pharm Ther 1991;16:203–7.
14. Mahony C, Brown JE, Stargel WW, Verghese CP, Bjornsson TD. J Pharm Sci 1984;73(6):838–9.
15. Asker AF, Gragg R. Drug Dev Ind Pharm 1983;9(5):837–48.
16. Asker AF, Canady D. Drug Dev Ind Pharm 1984;10(7):1025–39.
17. Leeuwenkamp OR, van der Mark EJ, van Bennekom WP, Bult A. Int J Pharmaceutics 1985;24:27–41.
18. Vrabel RB, Amerson AB [letter]. Am J Hosp Pharm 1975;32:140–1.
19. Karnatz NN, Wong J, Baaske DM, Johnson JH, Speicher ER, Herbranson DE. Am J Hosp Pharm 1989;46:101–4.

Sodium Valproate (BANM, rINNM)

Anticonvulsant

Valproate Sodium (USAN)
Sodium 2-propylpentanoate; sodium 2-propylvalerate
$C_8H_{15}NaO_2 = 166.2$

$$CH_3 \cdot CH_2 \cdot CH_2 \cdot \underset{\underset{CH_2 \cdot CH_2 \cdot CH_3}{|}}{CH} \cdot COONa$$

Valproic Acid (BAN, USAN, rINN)

2-Propylpentanoic acid; 2-propylvaleric acid
$C_8H_{16}O_2 = 144.2$
CAS—1069-66-5 (sodium valproate; valproate sodium); 99-66-1 (valproic acid)

Pharmacopoeial status

BP (sodium valproate); USP (valproic acid)

Preparations

Compendial
Sodium Valproate Tablets BP. Tablets containing, in each, 100 mg are usually available.
Sodium Valproate Enteric-coated Tablets BP.
Sodium Valproate Oral Solution BP (Sodium Valproate Elixir). A solution of sodium valproate in a suitable flavoured vehicle. An oral solution containing 200 mg in 5 mL is usually available.
Valproic Acid Capsules USP.
Valproic Acid Syrup USP.

Non-compendial
Epilim (Sanofi Winthrop). *Tablets*, sodium valproate 100 mg. *Tablets*, enteric coated, sodium valproate 200 mg and 500 mg. *Liquid*, sugar free, sodium valproate 200 mg/5 mL; do not dilute. *Syrup*, sodium valproate 200 mg/5 mL. *Diluent*: syrup (without sulphur dioxide as a preservative), life of diluted syrup 14 days.
Epilim Intravenous (Sanofi Winthrop). *Injection*, powder for reconstitution, sodium valproate 400-mg vials; supplied with an ampoule of 4 mL of solvent (water for injections). The intravenous solution is compatible with polyvinyl chloride, polyethylene, and glass containers but should not be administered via the same intravenous line as other intravenous additives.

Various tablets of sodium valproate are available from Cox, CP(Orlept), Hillcross, Norton.
Sodium valproate (200 mg/5 mL) sugar-free oral solution is also available from Norton.

Containers and storage

Solid state
Sodium Valproate BP should be kept in an airtight container. Valproic Acid USP should be preserved in tight, glass or stainless steel containers.

Dosage forms
Valproic Acid Capsules USP should be preserved in tight containers, at controlled room temperature.
Valproic Acid Syrup USP should be preserved in tight containers.
Due to their hygroscopicity, Epilim tablets must remain in their protective foil until they are taken or administered. They should be stored in a dry place below 30°. Epilim syrup and Epilim liquid should be stored below 30° and away from direct sunlight. Epilim Intravenous lyophilised powder should be stored below 25°. Reconstituted solutions should be stored at 2° to 8° and any solution remaining after 24 hours should be discarded.

PHYSICAL PROPERTIES

Sodium valproate is a white or almost white, crystalline, hygroscopic powder.
Valproic acid is a clear, colourless to pale yellow, slightly viscous liquid with a characteristic odour.

Dissociation constant

Values of 4.8 and 4.5 have been recorded for the pK_a of *sodium valproate*.
Values of 4.6 and 5.0 have been recorded for the pK_a of *valproic acid*.

Solubility

Sodium valproate is soluble 1 in 5 of water, 1 in 5 of ethanol, and 1 in 5 of methanol; practically insoluble in benzene, in chloroform, in ether, and in *n*-heptane.
Valproic acid is very slightly soluble in water; freely soluble in ethanol, in acetone, in chloroform, in ether, and in methanol.

STABILITY

Sodium valproate is stable in water, acid, and alkali. It is also heat stable.
Valproic acid is stable to heat, light, and strong aqueous alkali and acid.
Sodium valproate is hygroscopic. Following a World Health Organization (WHO) study of the stability of sodium valproate tablets it was reported that 'in a water saturated atmosphere the tablets became humid and their appearance completely changed, therefore they are considered degradable'.[1]

INCOMPATIBILITY/COMPATIBILITY

The stability of sodium valproate syrup, 250 mg/5 mL (of valproic acid) repackaged in three types of unit-dose containers and stored at 4°, 25°, or 60° (± 1°) in enclosed compartments for various time intervals was studied by Sartnurak and Christensen.[2] The results were analysed by factorial experimental design. Measurements were based on valproic acid concentrations as the assay method involved the instantaneous conversion of sodium valproate to valproic acid. As storage temperature increased, greater losses of valproic acid from the repackaged samples were observed. Samples stored in glass oral syringes and glass vials at 4° and 25° for 180 days retained 95% of their original concentration. Samples stored in polypropylene oral syringes for 20 days at 25° retained 88.5% of their label claim; however, samples stored at 4° retained 90% of their label claim for at least 90 days. Desorption experiments on the polypropylene oral syringes stored at 4° and 25° for 180 days resulted in the recovery of 80% to 92% of drug lost from the syringes.

FORMULATION

Excipients

Excipients that have been used in presentations of sodium valproate and valproic acid include:

Capsules, valproic acid: gelatin; glycerol; maize oil; methyl and propyl hydroxybenzoates; iron oxide; sunset yellow FCF (E110); titanium dioxide (E171).

Tablets, sodium valproate: amaranth (E123); calcium silicate; cellacephate; diethyl phthalate; macrogol 400; magnesium stearate; maize starch; povidone; talc; titanium dioxide (E171); yellow iron oxide.

Oral solutions, sodium valproate: hydroxybenzoates; ponceau 4R (E124); sodium hydroxide; sorbitol; urea.

Syrups, sodium valproate: allura red AC (E129); erythrosine (E127); flavours; glycerol; hydrochloric acid, concentrated; methyl and propyl hydroxybenzoates; ponceau 4R (E124); sodium hydroxide; sorbitol; sucrose.

Bioavailability

Workers in Finland[3] undertook a single-dose, crossover study in 12 healthy volunteers to compare the absorption and bioavailability of three enteric-coated dosage forms (one valproic acid 300-mg capsule, Convulex, Leiras, and two sodium valproate 300-mg tablets, Deprakine, Orion and Orfiril, Rhône-Poulenc). No significant difference was identified between the bioavailabilities of the three preparations but no correlation was found between dissolution rates and *in-vivo* absorption rates.

In a comparison of the rectal absorption of sodium valproate with oral and intravenous absorption in *rats*, rectal dosage forms prepared with a Witepsol basis (lipophilic) had considerably higher bioavailability than those prepared with macrogol as basis (hydrophilic).[4] Bioavailability following administration of the suppository with the lipophilic basis was higher than that following oral administration.

Hygroscopicity

Workers in Japan[5] examined the effect of various water-insoluble carriers incorporated in solid dispersions on the moisture absorption of sodium valproate. Saturated fatty acids, such as stearic acid, inhibited moisture absorption, whereas incorporation of ethylcellulose, stearyl alcohol, or tristearin did not inhibit hygroscopicity.

Suppositories

An evaluation of excipients for use in rectal formulations of sodium valproate[6] revealed that the presence of sodium valproate affected the rheological properties of two melted fatty bases (Suppocire AS₂ and Witepsol H-15), determined with a Brookfield Synchro-Lectric LVT viscometer. These bases alone appeared to exhibit dilatant flow at 39° but the addition of sodium valproate resulted in a change to plastic flow with thixotropy and a marked rise in viscosity.

Margarit *et al*[7] prepared suppositories of sodium valproate with the basis Suppocire AS₂ alone (formula A), or the basis with Aerosil R972 (formula B), or with Span 80 (formula C). The extents and rates of first-order release *in vitro* through cellulose membranes were lower from formula B and C than from formula A. Similarly, in *rabbits*, formulae B and C took longer to produce peak plasma concentrations of sodium valproate, but relative bioavailabilities, compared to that of an oral aqueous solution of sodium valproate, were about 106.5%, 167.7%, and 139.1% for formulae A, B, and C, respectively.

FURTHER INFORMATION. Pharmacokinetic evaluation of novel sustained-release dosage forms of valproic acid [as sodium valproate] in humans—Bialer M, Friedman M, Dubrovsky J. Biopharm Drug Disposit 1985;6:410–11. Myrj 51 as a suppository excipient: Influence on pharmaceutical availability and bioavailability of sodium valproate—Margarit MV, Rodriguez IC, Cerezo A. Int J Pharmaceutics 1992;81:67–73.

REFERENCES

1. World Health Organization. WHO/PHARM/86.531. Accelerated stability studies of drugs in pharmaceutical forms under simulated tropical conditions. Geneva: The Organization, 1986.
2. Sartnurak S, Christensen JM. Am J Hosp Pharm 1982;39:627–9.
3. Palva ES, Eränkö O, Konno K, Venho VMK. Acta Pharm Fenn 1986;95:97–100.
4. Sugioka N, Okada K, Ihara N, Nosaka K, Mizuno M [Japanese]. Yakuzaigaku 1987;47:38–41.
5. Hasegawa A, Kawamura R, Sugimoto I, Matsuda Y [Japanese]. Yakuzaigaku 1987;47:86–92. From: Int Pharm Abstrs 1989;26(2):2600933.
6. Margarit MV, Rodríguez IC, Cerezo A. Drug Dev Ind Pharm 1992;18(1):79–92.
7. Margarit MV, Rodriguez IC, Cerezo A. J Pharm Pharmacol 1991;43:721–5.

Spironolactone (BAN, rINN)   *Diuretic*

Espironolactona; spirolactone
7α-Acetylthio-3-oxo-17α-pregn-4-ene-21,   17β-carbolactone; (7α,17α)-7-(acetylthio)-17-hydroxy-3-oxo-pregn-4-ene-21-carboxylic acid γ-lactone
$C_{24}H_{32}O_4S = 416.6$
CAS—52-01-7

Pharmacopoeial status

BP, USP

Preparations

Compendial

Spironolactone Tablets BP. Tablets containing, in each, 25 mg, 50 mg, and 100 mg are usually available.

Spironolactone Tablets USP.

Non-compendial

Aldactone (Searle). *Tablets*, spironolactone 25 mg, 50 mg, and 100 mg.

Spiroctan (Boehringer Mannheim). *Tablets*, spironolactone 25 mg and 50 mg.

Capsules, spironolactone 100 mg.

Spirolone (Berk). *Tablets*, spironolactone 25 mg and 100 mg.

Spironolactone tablets of various strengths are also available from APS, Ashbourne (Spirospare), Cox, CP, Evans, Kerfoot, Lagap (Laractone), Norton.

Spironolactone sugar-free oral suspension is available by special order from RP Drugs.

Compound preparations

Co-flumactone is the British Approved Name for compounded preparations of hydroflumethiazide and spironolactone in equal proportions by weight. Preparations: Aldactide 25, Aldactide 50 (Gold Cross).

Containers and storage

Solid state

Spironolactone BP should be protected from light.

Spironolactone USP should be preserved in well-closed containers.

Dosage forms

Spironolactone Tablets BP should be protected from light.

Spironolactone Tablets USP should be preserved in tight, light-resistant containers.

Aldactone tablets should be stored in a dry place below 30°.

Spiroctan tablets and capsules should be stored in a cool, dry place.

Spirolone tablets should be stored below 25° and protected from light.

PHYSICAL PROPERTIES

Spironolactone is a white to cream powder; odourless or with a slight odour of thioacetic acid.

Melting point

Spironolactone melts in the range 198° to 207°.

Partition coefficient

Log P (heptane/water), 0.54 (25°)[1]

Solubility

Spironolactone is practically insoluble in water; soluble 1 in 80 of ethanol, 1 in 3 of chloroform, and 1 in 100 of ether; soluble in ethyl acetate; slightly soluble in methanol and in fixed oils.

Complexation with cyclodextrin

Complexation of spironolactone with β-cyclodextrin in a 1:3 stoichiometric ratio caused an approximate ten-fold increase in its aqueous solubility[2] at 25° and 37°.

FURTHER INFORMATION. Cyclodextrin-spironolactone complexes—*in vitro* dissolution and *in vivo* bioavailability—Yusuff NT, York P, Chrystyn H, Swallow RD, Bramley PN, Losowsky MS. J Pharm Pharmacol 1991;42(Suppl):8P.

Dissolution

The USP specifies that for Spironolactone Tablets USP not less than 75% of the labelled amount of $C_{24}H_{32}O_4S$ is dissolved in 60 minutes. Dissolution medium: 1000 mL of 0.1N hydrochloric acid containing 0.1% sodium lauryl sulphate; Apparatus 2 at 75 rpm.

Dissolution properties

See Formulation below.

Crystal and molecular structure

Polymorphs

Salole and Al-Sarraj[3] obtained three polymorphic and five solvated crystalline forms of spironolactone using different solvents and conditions for crystallisation. Dissolution rate and solubility of the eight forms differed.

Similarly, Agafonov *et al*[4] obtained and examined the characteristics of single crystals of two polymorphic and four solvated crystalline forms of spironolactone.

STABILITY

During the development of a stability-indicating HPLC method for the quantitative determination of spironolactone, Das Gupta and Ghanekar[5] observed that the decomposition of spironolactone in water followed pseudo-first-order kinetics. At 65°, the rate constant was 0.0253/day.

Pramar and Das Gupta[6] conducted preformulation studies on spironolactone in 20% aqueous ethanol solution (0.25 mg/mL) using a stability-indicating HPLC assay. A pH-rate curve indicated the pH of maximum stability to be about 4.5. Decomposition of spironolactone was enhanced by increased buffer concentration but was unaffected by ionic strength. Decomposition followed first-order kinetics at 40°, 50°, and 60°. Activation energies were 78.8 kJ/mol and 96.0 kJ/mol at pH 4.3 and pH 5.3, respectively. Unionised spironolactone was subject to general acid-base catalysis.

The stability of spironolactone when prepared as a suspension in simple syrup (preserved with sodium benzoate 0.1%) with ethanol 10% was determined by Das Gupta *et al*[7] using HPLC. After storage for 160 days at 24° in amber-coloured bottles, the percentage of the initial spironolactone concentration remaining was 97.4%.

FORMULATION

Excipients

Excipients that have been used in presentations of spironolactone include:

Capsules: colloidal silica; lactose; magnesium stearate; microcrystalline cellulose; polyoxyl stearate; sodium carboxylamylopectin; sodium lauryl sulphate; starch (maize); talc.

Tablets: calcium stearate; calcium sulphate; copolymerised dimethylaminoethylmethacrylate and neutral esters of methacrylic acids; Eudragit E; hydroxypropylcellulose; hypromellose; indigo carmine (E132); iron oxide; lactose; macrogol; magnesium stearate; microcrystalline cellulose; pregelatinised starch; polysorbate 80; potassium polymethylacrylate; povidone; quinoline yellow (E104); starch (maize and rice); sodium lauryl sulphate; sucrose; sunset yellow FCF (E110); talc; tartrazine (E102); titanium dioxide (E171).

Oral suspensions: carmellose; cherry syrup; chloroform water (double strength); Cologel; glycerol; Nipasept; simple syrup; sodium benzoate; tragacanth mucilage.

Bioequivalence

The bioavailability and dissolution properties of ten spironolactone tablet formulations were determined by Clarke *et al*.[8] Formulation variables were: weight of spironolactone per tablet, weight of tablet, source of spironolactone, site of manufacture of tablet, principal excipient, and type of spironolactone powder (micronised or unmicronised). The results indicated that spironolactone bioavailability can be variable and that the amount of spironolactone absorbed is related to the dissolution characteristics of the tablets. However, differences in bioavailability cannot be fully explained by dissolution properties. Factors such as tablet weight, site of manufacture of bulk drug and tablet, and quantity of spironolactone per tablet had little influence on bioavailability; but the excipient used and micronisation of the bulk drug could be responsible for the differences in behaviour observed between two of the tablet formulations. The only tablet formulated using calcium hydrogen phosphate as the principal excipient exhibited good bioavailability, but low *in-vitro* dissolution. The tablet prepared with micronised spironolactone also showed a higher bioavailability than would be suggested by the *in-vitro* dissolution results.

Asbury *et al*[9] determined that tablets prepared using micronised spironolactone exhibited greater bioavailability when compared with a standard spironolactone tablet formulation and a formulation designed to exhibit a high dissolution rate. This effect was attributed to the reduced particle size of the micronised drug.

It was determined by Concheiro *et al*[10] that the inclusion of gelatin in a spironolactone tablet formulation, prepared with micronised spironolactone, had a significant effect on tablet dissolution. Dissolution behaviour was modified in such tablets by the inclusion of different quantities of talc, but varying the magnesium stearate content did not exert a significant effect. Despite the observed differences in dissolution properties, bioequivalence was maintained, and it was concluded that the factors that were identified as causing differences in dissolution had no effect on bioavailability at the concentrations studied.

Suspensions

Mathur and Wickman[11] found no appreciable loss of spironolactone from suspensions prepared using spironolactone tablets (Searle, USA) in Purified Water USP with Cherry Syrup NF when samples were stored in amber glass bottles at 5°, 20° to 24°, or 30° under intense fluorescent light for up to four weeks. No substantial visual or microbiological deterioration was detected.

A suspension of spironolactone 2.5 mg/mL can be prepared in simple syrup. The mixture is reported to be stable for 30 days when stored in a refrigerator.[12]

A xanthan gum, Keltrol (Kelco International, UK) has been successfully used to prepare a spironolactone suspension 5 mg/5 mL. A Keltrol 1% solution containing hydroxybenzoates is prepared in advance and diluted to 0.5% with water (with addition of a flavouring agent if necessary) before making the suspension using crushed tablets or powder. The product is physically and chemically stable for 12 weeks at room temperature.[13]

FURTHER INFORMATION. Development of a stable oral liquid dosage form of spironolactone—Pramar Y, Das Gupta V, Bethea C. J Clin Pharm Ther 1992;17:245–8.

REFERENCES

1. Sutter JL, Lau EPK. In: Florey K, editor. Analytical profiles of drug substances; vol 4. London: Academic Press, 1975:431–51.
2. Yusuff NT, York P. J Pharm Pharmacol 1988;40(Suppl):2P.
3. Salole EG, Al-Sarraj FA. Drug Dev Ind Pharm 1985;11:855–64.
4. Agafonov V, Legendre B, Rodier N, Wouessidjewe D, Cense J-M. J Pharm Sci 1991;80(2):181–5.
5. Das Gupta V, Ghanekar AG. J Pharm Sci 1978;67:889–91.
6. Pramar Y, Das Gupta V. J Pharm Sci 1991;80(6):551–3.
7. Das Gupta V, Gibbs CW, Ghanekar AG. Am J Hosp Pharm 1978;35:1382–5.
8. Clarke JM, Ramsay LE, Shelton JR, Tidd MJ, Murray S, Palmer RF. J Pharm Sci 1977;66:1429–32.
9. Asbury MJ, McInnes GT, Ramsay LE, Shelton JR. Br J Clin Pharmacol 1981;12(Suppl):270P.
10. Concheiro A, Llabres M, Vila-Jato JL, Martinez R, Blanco J. Drug Dev Ind Pharm 1987;13:2301–14.
11. Mathur LK, Wickman A. Am J Hosp Pharm 1989;46:2040–2.
12. Rappaport P. Can J Hosp Pharm 1983;36:66–70,74.
13. Pharm J 1986;239:665.

Sulphadimidine (BAN)   *Antibacterial*

Sulfadimidine (rINN); sulfamethazine
N^1-(4,6-Dimethylpyrimidin-2-yl)sulphanilamide; 4-amino-N-(4,6-dimethyl-2-pyrimidinyl)benzenesulphonamide
$C_{12}H_{14}N_4O_2S = 278.3$

Sulphadimidine Sodium (BANM)

Soluble sulphadimidine; soluble sulphamethazine
$C_{12}H_{13}N_4NaO_2S = 300.3$
CAS—57-68-1 (sulphadimidine); 1981-58-4 (sulphadimidine sodium)

Pharmacopoeial status

BP (sulphadimidine, sulphadimidine sodium); USP (sulfamethazine)

Preparations

Compendial
Sulphadimidine Tablets BP. Tablets containing, in each, 500 mg sulphadimidine are usually available.
Paediatric Sulphadimidine Oral Suspension BP (Paediatric Sulphadimidine Mixture). A pink suspension containing 10% w/v of sulphadimidine in a suitable flavoured vehicle.
Sulphadimidine Injection BP. A sterile solution of sulphadimidine sodium in water for injections free from dissolved air. It is prepared either from sulphadimidine sodium or by the interaction of sulphadimidine and sodium hydroxide. An injection containing 1 g of sulphadimidine sodium in 3 mL is usually available. pH 10.0 to 11.0.

Non-compendial
Sulphadimidine tablets are available from CP.

Containers and storage

Solid state
Sulphadimidine BP should be kept in a well-closed container and protected from light.
Sulphadimidine Sodium BP should be protected from light.
Sulfamethazine USP should be preserved in well-closed, light-resistant containers.

Dosage forms
Sulphadimidine Tablets BP and Sulphadimidine Injection BP should be protected from light.

PHYSICAL PROPERTIES

Sulphadimidine exists as white to yellowish-white crystals or powder; practically odourless with a slightly bitter taste. It may darken on exposure to light.
Sulphadimidine sodium exists as white or creamy-white hygroscopic crystals or powder; odourless or almost odourless with a bitter alkaline taste.

Melting point

Sulphadimidine melts in the range 197° to 200°.

pH

The pH of a 10% solution of *sulphadimidine sodium* is 10.0 to 11.0.

Dissociation constant

pK_a 7.4 (25°)

Partition coefficient

Log *P* (octanol), 0.3

Solubility

Sulphadimidine is very slightly soluble in water; soluble 1 in 120 of ethanol, 1 in 600 of chloroform, and 1 in 30 of acetone; very slightly soluble to practically insoluble in ether; it is soluble in dilute mineral acids and in aqueous solutions of alkali hydroxides and carbonates.
Sulphadimidine sodium is soluble 1 in 2.5 of water and 1 in 60 of ethanol. On exposure to air it absorbs carbon dioxide and becomes less soluble in water.

FURTHER INFORMATION. Solubility studies of silver sulfonamides [solubility and ionisation properties of silver sulphadimidine included]—Nesbitt RU, Sandmann BJ. J Pharm Sci 1978;67(7):1012–17.

STABILITY

Sulphadimidine, in the solid state, darkens on exposure to light. On exposure to air, solutions of sulphadimidine sodium absorb carbon dioxide and precipitate sulphadimidine; a fall in pH below 10 also results in precipitation of sulphadimidine. Heating 10 g of sulphadimidine in 135 mL of 2M hydrochloric acid for 6 hours under reflux conditions was reported to yield the decomposition products sulphanilic acid and 2-amino-4,6-dimethylpyrimidine.[1]

INCOMPATIBILITY/COMPATIBILITY

Sulphadimidine sodium is incompatible with acids, iron salts, and salts of heavy metals.
Riley[2] reported sulphadimidine sodium (4 g/L) to be visually incompatible with amiphenazole hydrochloride, a haze developing within three hours of admixture in sodium chloride 0.9% injection. Immediate precipitation in sodium chloride 0.9% injection was noted when sulphadimidine sodium (4 g/L) was added to chlorpromazine hydrochloride, prochlorperazine mesylate, promazine hydrochloride, or promethazine hydrochloride; and within three hours when it was added to hydralazine hydrochloride. Precipitation in admixture with the above drugs also occurred in glucose 5% injection, with the exception of admixture with prochlorperazine mesylate, which resulted in the development of a haze within three hours.

FORMULATION

PAEDIATRIC SULPHADIMIDINE MIXTURE

The following formula was given in the *British Pharmaceutical Codex 1973*:

Sulphadimidine, in fine powder	100 g
Compound tragacanth powder	40 g
Amaranth solution	10 mL
Benzoic acid solution	20 mL
Raspberry syrup	200 mL
Chloroform water, double-strength	500 mL
Water for preparations	to 1000 mL

Triturate the compound tragacanth powder and the sulphadimidine with the raspberry syrup to form a smooth paste; add gradually, with constant stirring, the benzoic acid solution and the amaranth solution diluted with the double-strength chloroform water, and sufficient water to produce the required volume. It must be recently prepared.
The compound tragacanth powder may be replaced by 10 g of carmellose sodium (50) and 20 g of maize starch, and the double-strength chloroform water by 50 mL of chloroform spirit for each 1000 mL of mixture. The mixture is prepared as follows: stir a suspension of the starch in 125 mL of water into about 350 mL of boiling water. Maintain the temperature until the mixture becomes translucent, and cool rapidly. Triturate the carmellose sodium (50) and the sulphadimidine with the raspberry syrup to form a smooth paste; add gradually, with constant stirring, the starch mucilage, the benzoic acid solution, the amaranth solution, the chloroform spirit, and sufficient water to produce the required volume.

Excipients

Excipients that have been used in presentations of sulphadimidine include:
Oral liquids: benzoic acid solution; chloroform water (concentrated); raspberry syrup; compound tragacanth powder.

Bioavailability

Differences in binding agents, compression and formulation of sulphadimidine tablets may result in variation in dissolution rate and also in absorption.

Suspensions

Results of studies by Kellaway and Najib[3] showed that povidone, acid gelatins, and alkaline gelatins were more effective (at relatively high polymer concentrations) as steric stabilisers than as flocculants of suspended sulphadimidine particles. Addition of carmellose sodium resulted in increased flocculation of sulphadimidine suspensions. Relationships between electrophoretic mobility and sedimentation volume of the suspended particles were investigated.
An assessment of Carbopol 934 as a suspending agent for sulphadimidine suspensions (10% w/v)[4] indicated that at a concentration of 0.3% to 3% the readily pourable, non-sedimenting suspensions maintained uniformity over a period of six months at 20°.
Sulphadimidine in suspension with kaolin was adsorbed to the extent of 160 mg/g of kaolin but was adsorbed to a lesser extent when in a mixed suspension with ampicillin and kaolin.[5] The amount of available sulphadimidine from the simple suspension with kaolin increased when any of the following additives were present: sorbitol 70%, propylene glycol, syrup, glycerol, absolute

ethanol, tragacanth, acacia, macrogol 600, povidone, or Gifford's buffer (pH 5.2 or 8.6). All additives, except gum acacia, improved the physical properties of the mixed suspensions (for example, sedimentation volume and redispersibility).

PROCESSING

Sterilisation

When required in a sterile condition for local application, sulphadimidine may be sterilised by dry heat. The material is first reduced to a fine powder and dried at 100°, then sterilised by dry heat in the final sealed containers. The sterilised powder should show only slight discoloration.

Sulphadimidine injection can be sterilised by heating in an autoclave.

REFERENCES

1. Venturella VS. J Pharm Sci 1968;57(7):1151–7.
2. Riley BB. J Hosp Pharm 1970;28:228–40.
3. Kellaway IW, Najib NM. Int J Pharmaceutics 1981;9:59–66.
4. Berney M, Deasy PB. Int J Pharmaceutics 1979;3:73–80.
5. Hosny EA, Kassem A, El-Shattawy HH. Drug Dev Ind Pharm 1988;14(6):779–89.

Sulphamethoxazole (BAN)   *Antibacterial*

Sulfamethoxazole (USAN, rINN); sulfisomezole
N^1-(5-Methylisoxazol-3-yl)sulphanilamide;   4-amino-N-(5-methyl-3-isoxazolyl)-benzenesulphonamide
$C_{10}H_{11}N_3O_3S = 253.3$
CAS—723-46-6 (sulphamethoxazole); 8064-90-2 (co-trimoxazole)

Pharmacopoeial status

BP, USP

Preparations

Co-trimoxazole is the British Approved Name for compounded preparations of trimethoprim 1 part and sulphamethoxazole 5 parts.

Compendial
Co-trimoxazole Tablets BP. Tablets containing, in each, sulphamethoxazole 400 mg with trimethoprim 80 mg and sulphamethoxazole 800 mg with trimethoprim 160 mg are usually available.
Dispersible Co-trimoxazole Tablets BP. Tablets containing, in each, sulphamethoxazole 400 mg with trimethoprim 80 mg and sulphamethoxazole 800 mg with trimethoprim 160 mg, in a suitable dispersible basis, are usually available.
Paediatric Co-trimoxazole Tablets BP. Tablets containing, in each, sulphamethoxazole 100 mg with trimethoprim 20 mg.

Co-trimoxazole Oral Suspension BP (Co-trimoxazole Mixture). A suspension containing sulphamethoxazole 400 mg and trimethoprim 80 mg in each 5 mL of a suitable flavoured vehicle.
Paediatric Co-trimoxazole Oral Suspension BP (Paediatric Co-trimoxazole Mixture). A suspension containing sulphamethoxazole 200 mg and trimethoprim 40 mg in each 5 mL of a suitable flavoured vehicle.
Co-trimoxazole Intravenous Infusion BP. A sterile solution containing the sodium derivative of sulphamethoxazole and trimethoprim, prepared immediately before use by the dilution of sterile co-trimoxazole concentrate with 25 to 35 times its volume of either glucose 5% injection or sodium chloride 0.9% injection. Sterile co-trimoxazole concentrate is a sterile solution of trimethoprim and sulphamethoxazole sodium prepared by the interaction of sulphamethoxazole and sodium hydroxide, and trimethoprim in water for injections containing propylene glycol 40% to 45% v/v. A concentrated solution containing sulphamethoxazole 400 mg and trimethoprim 80 mg in 5 mL to be diluted before use is usually available. pH 9.5 to 11.0.
Sulfamethoxazole Tablets USP.
Sulfamethoxazole Oral Suspension USP.
Sulfamethoxazole and Trimethoprim Tablets USP.
Sulfamethoxazole and Trimethoprim Oral Suspension USP.
Sulfamethoxazole and Trimethoprim Injection for Concentrate USP. pH 9.5 to 10.5.

Non-compendial
Bactrim (Roche). *Tablets* (Drapsules), co-trimoxazole 480 mg.
Tablets (dispersible), co-trimoxazole 480 mg.
Tablets (double strength), co-trimoxazole 960 mg.
Suspension (adult), co-trimoxazole 480 mg/5 mL. Dilution not recommended.
Syrup (paediatric), sugar free, co-trimoxazole 240 mg/5 mL. Dilution not recommended.
Septrin (Wellcome). *Tablets*, co-trimoxazole 480 mg.
Tablets (dispersible), sugar free, co-trimoxazole 480 mg.
Tablets (forte), co-trimoxazole 960 mg.
Suspension (adult), co-trimoxazole 480 mg/5 mL. *Diluent*: syrup, 1:1, life of diluted suspension 14 days.
Suspension (paediatric), sugar free, co-trimoxazole 240 mg/5 mL. *Diluent*: syrup or sorbitol solution (70%), non-crystallising grade, 1:1, life of diluted suspension 14 days.
Intramuscular injection, co-trimoxazole 320 mg/mL. pH 9.0 to 10.5.
Intravenous infusion, co-trimoxazole 96 mg/mL. pH approximately 10. It must be diluted. Dilution should be carried out immediately before use with one of the following infusion solutions: glucose 5% or 10%; sodium chloride 0.9%; compound sodium chloride injection BPC 1959; dextran 40 injection 6% in glucose 5% or sodium chloride 0.9%; or dextran 70 injection 10% in glucose 5% or sodium chloride 0.9%. Usually one, two, or three 5-mL ampoules should be added to 125, 250, or 500 mL of infusion solution, respectively, and thoroughly mixed by shaking. No other substance should be mixed with the infusion.
Co-trimoxazole tablets of various strengths are also available from APS, Ashbourne (Comixco), Cox, CP, DDSA (Fectrim, Fectrim Forte), Evans, Kerfoot, Lagap (Laratrim), Norton.
Co-trimoxazole dispersible tablets are also available from APS, Ashbourne (Comixco Disp), Kerfoot, Norton (Comox).
Co-trimoxazole oral suspension is also available from APS, CP, Evans, Lagap (Laratrim).
Co-trimoxazole paediatric oral suspension is also available from APS, Ashbourne (Comixco), CP, Lagap (Laratrim), Norton, RP Drugs (Chemotrim).
A co-trimoxazole strong sterile solution for dilution and use as an intramuscular injection is also available from David Bull.

Containers and storage

Solid state

Sulphamethoxazole BP should be stored in well-closed containers, protected from light.
Sulfamethoxazole USP should be preserved in well-closed, light-resistant containers.

Dosage forms

Co-trimoxazole Oral Suspension BP and Paediatric Co-trimoxazole Oral Suspension BP should be stored at a temperature not greater than 30°, protected from light.
Strong Sterile Co-trimoxazole Solution for the preparation of Co-trimoxazole Intravenous Infusion BP should be protected from light.
Sulfamethoxazole Tablets USP and Sulfamethoxazole and Trimethoprim Tablets USP should be preserved in well-closed, light-resistant containers.
Sulfamethoxazole Oral Suspension USP and Sulfamethoxazole and Trimethoprim Oral Suspension USP should be preserved in tight, light-resistant containers.
Sulfamethoxazole and Trimethoprim Concentrate for Injection USP should be preserved in single-dose, light-resistant containers, preferably of Type I glass.
Bactrim adult suspension and paediatric syrup should be stored at a temperature not exceeding 30°.
Septrin for intravenous infusion should be stored below 30°, protected from light. All other Septrin preparations should be stored at a temperature not exceeding 25° and protected from light. Septrin dispersible tablets should be kept dry and Septrin intramuscular injection should not be frozen. Diluted Septrin suspensions should be stored below 25°.
Septrin intramuscular injection should not be used if precipitation is visible or the solution is cloudy and mixtures of Septrin for intravenous infusion should be discarded if visible turbidity or crystallisation is apparent.

PHYSICAL PROPERTIES

Sulphamethoxazole is a white or almost white, crystalline powder.

Melting point

Sulphamethoxazole melts in the range 167° to 172°.

pH

A 10% suspension of *sulphamethoxazole* has a pH of 4 to 6.

Dissociation constant

pK_a 5.6 (25°)

Solubility

Sulphamethoxazole is practically insoluble in water; soluble 1 in 50 of ethanol and 1 in 3 of acetone; slightly soluble in chloroform and in ether; dissolves in dilute solutions of sodium hydroxide.

Effect of pH

Dahlan et al[1] studied the influence of pH on the solubilities and dissolution rates of sulphamethoxazole and trimethoprim. Sulphamethoxazole solubility decreased with decreasing pH to reach a minimum at pH 3.22 and 25° in glycine buffer; at lower pH values solubility increased rapidly, reflecting its amphoteric properties. The dissolution rate of sulphamethoxazole in buffer solutions at 25° was studied at pH values ranging from 1.23 to 7.60. Dissolution rate decreased with increasing pH, then increased at pH 7.60.

Effect of temperature

The solubility of sulphamethoxazole in aqueous buffers has been found to increase[1] with increasing temperature in the range 25° to 37°.

Solubilisation

McDonald and Faridah[2] found that solubility of trimethoprim increased linearly in the presence of hydroxypropyl β-cyclodextrin (HPCD) at pH values from 7.0 to 9.9 (attributed to formation of 1:1 complexes) and similarly for sulphamethoxazole at pH 7.0. However, the influence of HPCD on solubility was negligible at pH 7.5. In the presence of sulphamethoxazole in HPCD solutions at pH 7.0, the solubility of trimethoprim was markedly reduced while that of sulphamethoxazole was slightly reduced. The presence of HPCD 10% w/v in trimethoprim/sulphamethoxazole injection in phosphate buffer at pH 7.8 delayed but did not prevent the precipitation (attributed mainly to trimethoprim) observed in solutions without HPCD. When the injection was admixed with sodium chloride 0.9%, the addition of HPCD 10% w/v prevented crystallisation of either drug over a 5-day period.
In respect of the enhancement of sulphamethoxazole solubility, povidone 0.1% and methylcellulose 0.1% were equally effective,[3] whereas macrogol 4000 was ineffective. As the temperature was increased (from 25° to 55°) the solubility of sulphamethoxazole in water and in polymer solutions was increased.

Dissolution

The USP specifies that for Sulfamethoxazole Tablets USP not less than 50% of the labelled amount of $C_{10}H_{11}N_3O_3S$ is dissolved in 20 minutes. Dissolution medium: 900 mL of dilute hydrochloric acid (7 in 100); Apparatus 1 at 100 rpm.
The USP specifies that for Sulfamethoxazole and Trimethoprim Tablets USP not less than 70% of the labelled amounts of $C_{10}H_{11}N_3O_3S$ and $C_{14}H_{18}N_4O_3$ are dissolved in 60 minutes. Dissolution medium: 900 mL of 0.1N hydrochloric acid; Apparatus 2 at 75 rpm.

Dissolution properties

See Effect of pH, above, and also Formulation, below.

STABILITY

Sulphamethoxazole has been reported to be stable for 5 days at 110°. Refluxing in 0.4M hydrochloric acid promotes its degradation to sulphanilic acid and 5-methyl-3-amino-isoxazole. Continued heating in hydrochloric acid leads to the production of three additional products. Studies have indicated that sulphamethoxazole is relatively stable under alkaline conditions.[4]
Investigations by Graf et al[5] have shown the physical instability of sulphamethoxazole in aqueous suspension to be due to the formation of a semihydrate. The reaction was accelerated in the presence of carmellose sodium, but retarded by methylcellulose, povidone, and sucrose.

FURTHER INFORMATION. Stability of undiluted trimethoprim-sulfamethoxazole for injection in plastic syringes—Kaufman MB, Scavone JM, Foley JJ. Am J Hosp Pharm 1992;49:2782–3.

INCOMPATIBILITY/COMPATIBILITY

Sulphamethoxazole (weakly acidic) and trimethoprim (weakly basic) are incompatible in aqueous solution. To prevent precipitation, propylene glycol 40% is added as a cosolvent to commercial solutions for intravenous infusion.
Lesko et al[6] reported that co-trimoxazole injection, diluted to 3.84 mg/mL with glucose 5% injection or sodium chloride

0.9% injection and stored at $22° \pm 1°$ was stable for up to four hours. Co-trimoxazole injection, diluted to 9.6 mg/mL with glucose 5% injection and stored at the same temperature, was stable for up to two hours. A study by Deans et al[7] indicated that co-trimoxazole solutions with concentrations of 3.84, 4.8, 6.4, and 9.6 mg/mL were stable for at least 12 hours when stored in glass containers at 23° to 25° in glucose 5%, sodium chloride 0.45%, sodium chloride 0.9%, glucose 5% and sodium chloride 0.45%, or compound sodium lactate injections.

However, Jarosinski et al[8] reported that when sulphamethoxazole/trimethoprim as Bactrim (Roche) or Septra (Burroughs Wellcome) was admixed with glucose 5% injection or sodium chloride 0.9% injection, trimethoprim stability was dependent on concentration and vehicle. The authors concluded that concentrated solutions of sulphamethoxazole/trimethoprim should be prepared in glucose 5% injection, infused within one hour of preparation and visually inspected for precipitation at all times.

The formation of a precipitate following the addition of an admixture of co-trimoxazole and verapamil hydrochloride to infusions of sodium chloride 0.9% or glucose 5% was reported.[9]

Baumgartner and Russell[10] reported precipitation of co-trimoxazole in intravenous infusion set tubing; the authors recommended thorough flushing or replacement of the tubing after administration of the dose.

FORMULATION

Excipients

Excipients that have been used in presentations of sulphamethoxazole include:

Tablets, sulphamethoxazole: brilliant blue FCF (133); magnesium stearate; maize starch; polyvinyl acetate; polyvinyl alcohol; pregelatinised starch; quinoline yellow (E104), lake; sodium starch glycollate; sunset yellow FCF (E110), lake.

Co-trimoxazole: allura red AC (E129); brilliant blue FCF (133); carmellose calcium; docusate sodium; gelatin; hydroxyethylmethylcellulose; hypromellose; magnesium stearate; maize starch; povidone; pregelatinised starch; quinoline yellow (E104); sodium chloride; sodium starch glycollate; sunset yellow FCF (E110); talc; triacetin.

Suspensions, sulphamethoxazole: allura red AC (E129); carbomer; citric acid; disodium edetate; methylcellulose; saccharin; saccharin sodium; simethicone; sodium benzoate; sodium citrate; sodium hydroxide; sodium lauryl sulphate; sorbitol; sucrose.

Co-trimoxazole: activated dimethicone; allura red AC (E129); ammoniated liquorice; anise oil; bentonite; carmellose sodium; citric acid; disodium edetate; dispersible cellulose; ethanol; glucose syrup; glycerol; lactic acid; methyl and propyl hydroxybenzoates; microcrystalline cellulose; polysorbate 80; potassium chloride; potassium sorbate; saccharin; saccharin sodium; sodium benzoate; sodium methyl hydroxybenzoate; sodium propyl hydroxybenzoate; sorbitol solution; sucrose; sunset yellow FCF (E110); vanilla.

Intramuscular injections, co-trimoxazole: benzyl alcohol; ethanolamine; glycofurol; sodium metabisulphite.

Intravenous infusions, co-trimoxazole: benzyl alcohol; diethanolamine; ethanol; propylene glycol; sodium hydroxide; sodium metabisulphite.

Bioavailability

The relative bioavailability of a co-trimoxazole suspension (Belocid-Suspension, VEB Berlin-Chemie, Germany) was the same as that of another commonly used, commercially available co-trimoxazole suspension and was also comparable to that of co-trimoxazole tablets when tested in eight healthy subjects.[11]

Hutt et al[12] compared the pharmacokinetics and bioavailability of a trimethoprim/sulphamethoxazole tablet (Kepinol forte) with those of another commercially available tablet in a randomised, two-way crossover study involving 24 healthy volunteers. Results showed that the preparations were bioequivalent.

Suspensions

Agglomeration of sulphamethoxazole with white beeswax or ethylcellulose to produce spherical matrices led to prolongation of drug release from aqueous suspension.[13]

The dissolution rate of sulphamethoxazole from aqueous suspensions was reported to be enhanced by the addition of erythrosine dye, probably due to its selective adsorption onto drug particles. Enhancement of the dissolution rate of sulphamethoxazole from suspensions was also observed following the addition of hydroxybenzoic acid and its methyl and propyl esters. Addition of benzoic acid, however, led to an inhibition of dissolution rate.[14]

Tablets

Agrawal and Prakasam[15] have investigated the effect of five different binders on various properties of sulphamethoxazole tablets. Starch was the binder of choice; its inclusion in tablets promoted good overall granulation and dissolution properties. Granules made using ethylcellulose produced acceptable tablets, those prepared with povidone showed favourable flow properties, and those containing acacia were hard and dense and did not dissolve easily, despite ready disintegration. Carmellose sodium produced granules with poor cohesion properties and could not be compressed satisfactorily.

Ointments

Diffusion of sulphamethoxazole from various ointment bases through excised *mouse* skin occurred in the order: water-soluble basis > oil-in-water emulsion > water-in-oil emulsion = oleaginous basis = hydrophilic basis.[16] The addition of a surfactant to the basis or an increase in the concentration of sulphamethoxazole was found to increase the diffusion rate.

Suppositories

Workers in Egypt[17] formulated suppositories of sulphamethoxazole with trimethoprim in three bases and evaluated release *in vitro* and *in vivo* (in six healthy subjects). For both drugs, the extent of release from the bases decreased in the order: Witepsol H15 with 10% Tween 60 > macrogol mixture > Witepsol H15.

FURTHER INFORMATION. Studies on a new technique of microencapsulation by ethylcellulose—Chowdary KPR, Rao GN. Indian J Pharm Sci 1984;46:213–15. Effect of wall thickness on drug release from ethylcellulose microcapsules—Chowdary KPR, Rao GN. East Pharm 1985;28:185–6. Polymorphism of spray-dried microencapsulated sulphamethoxazole with cellulose acetate phthalate and colloidal silica, montmorillonite, or talc—Takenaka H, Kawashima Y, Lin SY. J Pharm Sci 1981;70(11):1256–60. Polymorphism and drug release behaviour of spray-dried microcapsules of sulphamethoxazole with polysaccharide gum and colloidal silica—Kawashima Y, Lin SY, Takenaka H. Drug Dev Ind Pharm 1983;9(8):1445–63. Dissolution of sulphamethoxazole from polyethylene glycols [macrogols] and polyvinylpyrrolidone [povidone] solid dispersions—Singla AK, Vijan T. Drug Dev Ind Pharm 1990;16(5):875–82. Development of sulphamethoxazole-trimethoprim spheroidal granules: factors affecting drug release *in vitro*—Athanassiou GC, Rekkas DM, Choulis NH. Int J

Pharmaceutics 1991;72:141–7. Correlation of *in vitro* dissolution data with *in vivo* plasma concentrations, for three, orally administered, formulations of sulphamethoxazole-trimethoprim, by statistical moments analysis—Athanassiou GC, Rekkas DM, Choulis NH. Int J Pharmaceutics 1993;90:51–8.

PROCESSING

Sterilisation

Sterile co-trimoxazole concentrate can be sterilised by heating in an autoclave.

Complexation

Sulphamethoxazole and trimethoprim in [co-trimoxazole] tablets and suspension interact under certain conditions to form a molecular complex. Bettinetti *et al*[18] observed that, during tablet production, interaction was induced by the wetting medium during granulation and by heat and humidity; interaction could be avoided by using a direct compression method. Inclusion of microcrystalline cellulose and silica in the formulation appeared to inhibit interaction due to humidity effects. In a later study on the influence of complex formation on suspension stability, La Manna[19] found that in some suspensions, crystals of the sulphamethoxazole-trimethoprim complex remained suspended while sulphamethoxazole itself formed a sediment that caked and was difficult to redisperse.

REFERENCES

1. Dahlan R, McDonald C, Sunderland VB. J Pharm Pharmacol 1987;39:246–51.
2. McDonald C, Faridah. J Parenter Sci Technol 1991;45(3):147–51.
3. Doganay T, Ataberk ZP. Gazi Univ Eczacilik Fak Derg 1988;5(2):185–93.
4. Rudy BC, Senkowski BZ. In: Florey K, editor. Analytical profiles of drug substances; vol 2. London: Academic Press, 1973:467–86.
5. Graf E, Beyer C, Abdallah O. Pharm Ind 1982;44:1071–4.
6. Lesko LJ, Marion A, Ericson J, Siber GR. Am J Hosp Pharm 1981;38:1004–6.
7. Deans KW, Lang JR, Smith DE. Am J Hosp Pharm 1982;39:1681–4.
8. Jarosinski PF, Kennedy PE, Gallelli JF. Am J Hosp Pharm 1989;46:732–7.
9. Cutie MR. Am J Hosp Pharm 1983;40:1205–7.
10. Baumgartner TG, Russell WL. Am J IV Ther Clin Nutr 1983;10:14–15.
11. Gunther C, Truckenbrodt J, Traeger A [German]. Pharmazie 1987;42(H6):397–9.
12. Hutt VV, Klingmann I, Pabst GU, Salama Z, Nieder M, Jaeger H [German]. Arzneimittelforschung 1988;38(II), Nr 9:1347–50.
13. Kawashima Y, Ohno H, Takenaka H. J Pharm Sci 1981;70:913–16.
14. Rao YM, Rambhau D. Indian J Pharm Sci 1983;45:161–4.
15. Agrawal YK, Prakasam K. J Pharm Sci 1988;77:885–8.
16. Ezzedeen FW, Shihab FA, Husain EJ. Pharmazie 1990;45:512–14.
17. Abd El-Gawad AH, Ramadan E, Nouh AT. Pharm Ind 1988;50:257–60.
18. Bettinetti GP, Giordano F, Caramella C, Colombo P, Conte U, La Manna A. Farmaco (Prat) 1983;38:259–64.
19. La Manna A. STP Pharma 1985;1:425–33.

Suxamethonium Chloride (BAN, pINN)

Skeletal muscle relaxant

Succinylcholine chloride
2,2′-Succinyldioxybis(ethyltrimethylammonium)dichloride;
2,2′-[(l,4-dioxo-1,4-butanediyl)bis(oxy)]-bis[*N*,*N*,*N*-trimethyle-thanaminnium]dichloride
$C_{14}H_{30}Cl_2N_2O_4,2H_2O = 397.3$

$$[(CH_3)_3N^+\cdot[CH_2]_2\cdot O\cdot CO\cdot[CH_2]_2\cdot CO\cdot O\cdot[CH_2]_2\cdot N^+(CH_3)_3] \quad 2Cl^-, 2H_2O$$

Suxamethonium Bromide (BAN)

$C_{14}H_{30}Br_2N_2O_4,2H_2O = 486.2$
CAS—306-40-1 (suxamethonium); 55-94-7 (suxamethonium bromide); 71-27-2 (suxamethonium chloride, anhydrous); 6101-15-1 (suxamethonium chloride, dihydrate)

Pharmacopoeial status

BP (suxamethonium chloride); USP (succinylcholine chloride)

Preparations

Compendial
Suxamethonium Chloride Injection BP (Succinylcholine Chloride Injection). A sterile solution of suxamethonium chloride in water for injections. Injections containing 100 mg in 2 mL and 500 mg in 10 mL are usually available. pH 3.0 to 5.0.
Succinylcholine Chloride Injection USP. pH 3.0 to 4.5.
Sterile Succinylcholine Chloride USP.

Non-compendial
Anectine (Wellcome). *Injection*, suxamethonium chloride 50 mg/mL. pH 3.0 to 5.0. It should not be mixed in the same syringe with any other agent, especially thiopentone. *Diluents*: glucose 5% injection, sodium chloride 0.9% injection.
Scoline (Evans). *Injection*, suxamethonium chloride 50 mg/mL. It should not be mixed in the syringe with any other drug, in particular, short-acting barbiturates such as thiopentone or methohexitone. *Diluents*: glucose 5% injection, sodium chloride 0.9% injection.

Containers and storage

Solid state
Suxamethonium Chloride BP should be kept in a well-closed container and protected from light.
Succinylcholine Chloride USP should be preserved in tight containers.

Dosage forms
Suxamethonium Chloride Injection BP should be stored at a temperature as low as possible above its freezing point and not exceeding 4°. Under these conditions, it may be expected to meet monograph specifications for not less than 18 months after the date of preparation.
Succinylcholine Chloride Injection USP should be preserved in single-dose or in multiple-dose containers, preferably of Type I or Type II glass, in a refrigerator.
Sterile Succinylcholine Chloride USP should be preserved in containers suitable for sterile solids.
Anectine should be stored below 4° and protected from light. It should not be frozen or resterilised.
Scoline should be stored at a temperature as low as possible above its freezing point and not exceeding 4°. The injection should not be autoclaved.

PHYSICAL PROPERTIES

Suxamethonium chloride is a white or almost white crystalline powder; almost odourless; hygroscopic; slightly salty taste.

Melting point

Suxamethonium chloride anhydrate melts at about 190°.
Suxamethonium chloride dihydrate melts at about 160°.

pH

The pH of a 0.5% w/v solution of *suxamethonium chloride* is 4.0 to 5.0.

Solubility

Suxamethonium chloride is soluble 1 in 1 of water; slightly soluble in ethanol (1 in 350); practically insoluble in chloroform and in ether; sparingly soluble in benzene; soluble in methanol.

STABILITY

Suxamethonium chloride is stable in the crystalline form. It is unstable in alkaline solutions but relatively stable in acidic solutions. Degradation in aqueous solution occurs by hydrolysis (which is dependent on pH, temperature, and concentration) to succinylmonocholine chloride which is further hydrolysed to form succinic acid and choline.

Suzuki[1] predicted rates of reaction for hydrolysis of suxamethonium chloride in buffered solution at various pH values (pH 0.9 to 8.5) and temperatures. Decomposition was first-order, at a given pH, with respect to suxamethonium chloride. Rate constants and extents of acid and base catalysis were reported to vary depending on the pH and on the type and concentration of buffer used.

Unbuffered injection solutions of suxamethonium chloride (Burroughs Wellcome, USA 20 mg/mL, pH range 3.0 to 4.5) decomposed at a greater rate[2] when stored at 40° than when stored at 25°. The loss in potency (measured by HPLC) after one week at pH 3.5 was 3.2% and 1% at 40° and 25°, respectively. The pH range of maximum stability was 3.75 to 4.5. The reaction followed apparent zero-order kinetics,[2] although the underlying hydrolysis mechanism followed first-order kinetics with respect to concentration of suxamethonium chloride.[1] The authors recommended storage under refrigeration, or if necessary, at room temperature for not longer than four weeks.

During storage at 37° and at room temperature, the extents of hydrolysis of suxamethonium chloride (injection, 50 mg/mL) after 25 weeks were 50% and 8.1%, respectively; and after 52 weeks, the extents of hydrolysis were 100% and 22%, respectively.[3]

Significant degradation of suxamethonium chloride in injection solution was observed following transportation from Europe to Sudan.[4] The pH was reported to have fallen well below the BP limit. The content of hydrolysis products increased rapidly during subsequent storage.

Stabilisation

The extent of hydrolysis of suxamethonium chloride may be minimised by avoidance of water (by using sterile reconstitutable powder for injection), by refrigeration of the aqueous solutions, and by avoidance of the use of buffers (which may accelerate hydrolysis of suxamethonium chloride[1]).

FURTHER INFORMATION. Suxamethonium—a review. Part I. Physico-chemical properties and fate in the body—Gibb DB. Anaesth Intens Care 1972;I(2):109–18.

INCOMPATIBILITY/COMPATIBILITY

Suxamethonium chloride is rapidly destroyed by alkalis and should not be mixed with alkaline injections such as thiopentone sodium.

FORMULATION

Excipients

Excipients that have been used in presentations of suxamethonium chloride include:
Injections: hydrochloric acid; methyl hydroxybenzoate; sodium chloride; sodium hydroxide.

PROCESSING

Sterilisation

Suxamethonium chloride injection can be sterilised by heating in an autoclave.

REFERENCES

1. Suzuki T. Chem Pharm Bull 1962;10:912–21.
2. Boehm JJ, Dutton DM, Poust RI. Am J Hosp Pharm 1984;41:300–2.
3. Earles MP, Foster GE, Hardstone BL, Stewart GA. J Pharm Pharmacol 1954;6:773–9.
4. Abu-Reid IO, El-Samani SA, Hag Omer AI, Khalil NY, Mahgoub KM, Everitt G *et al.* Int Pharm J 1990;4(1):6–10.

Tamoxifen (BAN, rINN)   *Anti-oestrogen*

(*Z*)-2-[*p*-(1,2-Diphenylbut-1-enyl)phenoxy]ethyldimethylamine;
(*Z*)-2-[4-(1,2-diphenyl-1-butenyl)-phenoxy]-*N*,*N*-dimethylethanamine
$C_{26}H_{29}NO = 371.5$

Tamoxifen Citrate (BANM, USAN, rINNM)

$C_{26}H_{29}NO,C_6H_8O_7 = 563.6$
CAS—10540-29-1 (tamoxifen); 54965-24-1 (tamoxifen citrate)

Pharmacopoeial status

BP, USP (tamoxifen citrate)

Preparations

Compendial

Tamoxifen Tablets BP (Tamoxifen Citrate Tablets). Tablets containing, in each, tamoxifen citrate equivalent to 10, 20, and 40 mg of tamoxifen are usually available.
Tamoxifen Citrate Tablets USP.

Non-compendial

Emblon (Berk). *Tablets*, tamoxifen (as citrate) 10 mg and 20 mg.
Noltam (Lederle). *Tablets*, tamoxifen (as citrate) 10 mg and 20 mg.
Nolvadex (ICI). *Tablets*, tamoxifen (as citrate) 10 mg, 20 mg (Nolvadex-D), and 40 mg (Nolvadex Forte).
Tamofen (Tillotts). *Tablets*, tamoxifen (as citrate) 10 mg, 20 mg, and 40 mg. Tamoxifen tablets of various strengths are also available from APS, Ashbourne (Oestrifen), Cox, CP, Evans, Farmitalia Carlo Erba, Kerfoot.

Containers and storage

Solid state

Tamoxifen Citrate USP should be preserved in well-closed, light-resistant containers.

Dosage forms

Tamoxifen Tablets BP should be protected from light.
Tamoxifen Citrate Tablets USP should be preserved in well-closed, light-resistant containers.
Recommended storage conditions for tamoxifen citrate preparations:

Preparation	Manufacturers' recommended storage
Emblon	protect from heat and light
Noltam	protect from light and store at controlled room temperature (15°–30°)
Nolvadex Nolvadex-D Nolvadex-Forte	store at room temperature protected from light
Tamofen* Tamofen-20 Tamofen-40*	protect from moisture and heat; *store below 25°

PHYSICAL PROPERTIES

Tamoxifen citrate is a white or almost white, fine, crystalline powder.

Melting point

Tamoxifen citrate melts at about 140° to 142°, with decomposition.

Dissociation constant

pK_a 8.85

Solubility

Tamoxifen citrate is slightly soluble in water and in acetone; it is very slightly soluble in ethanol and in chloroform; it is soluble in methanol.
The equilibrium solubility of tamoxifen citrate at 37° in water is 0.5 mg/mL, and in 0.02M hydrochloric acid it is 0.2 mg/mL.
Tukker *et al*[1] observed that the aqueous solubility of tamoxifen citrate (344 ± 8 mg/L in demineralised water at 37°) decreased with the addition of increasing concentrations of sodium chloride (26 ± 2 mg/L in sodium chloride 0.9% solution at 37°).

Dissolution

The USP specifies that for Tamoxifen Citrate Tablets USP not less than 75% of the labelled amount of tamoxifen, $C_{26}H_{29}NO$, is dissolved in 30 minutes. Dissolution medium: 1000 mL of 0.02N hydrochloric acid; Apparatus 1 at 100 rpm.

Crystal and molecular structure

Enantiomers

Tamoxifen citrate exhibits geometric isomerism (around the ethylenic double bond) and exists as the *E* (cis) and *Z* (trans) isomers.[2] The *trans* isomer is the active form, possessing antioestrogenic properties whereas the *cis* isomer exhibits oestrogenic activity.[3]
The BP and USP have requirements for the content of *E*-isomer in tamoxifen citrate in the solid state (BP, USP) and in tablets (BP). Assay methods (by HPLC) are specified.
Jalonen[2] developed an HPLC method for the separation and assay of *Z*-tamoxifen citrate and the *E*-isomer impurity, in the solid state and in tablets. Several advantages over pharmacopoeial methods are claimed. The HPLC method described can also give an indication of the stability of tamoxifen citrate (see Stability below).

Polymorphs

Tamoxifen citrate is thought to exist in two polymorphic forms (A and B). Goldberg and Becker[4] characterised the crystal and molecular structure of polymorph B, a stable form, but were unable to elucidate the structure of polymorph A. It was suggested that polymorph A is a metastable form of tamoxifen citrate. In a suspension of ethanol at room temperature, Form A was found to convert spontaneously to Form B.

FURTHER INFORMATION. Separation of tamoxifen geometric isomers and metabolites by bonded-phase ß-cyclodextrin chromatography—Armstrong RD, Ward TJ, Pattabiraman N, Benz C, Armstrong DW. J Chromatogr 1987;414:192–6.

STABILITY

Tamoxifen citrate is reported to be sensitive to ultraviolet light and to oxidising agents. As part of a study of tamoxifen citrate isomers,[2] an aqueous methanolic solution of tamoxifen citrate was irradiated with ultraviolet light (at 254 nm). After five days, the content of active tamoxifen citrate (*Z*-isomer) had decreased to 90% of its initial concentration, while that of the *E*-isomer (impurity) had increased from less than 0.1% to 7.5%. Another compound detected was suggested to be a phenanthrene derivative. When tamoxifen citrate was stored for 24 hours in a 3% aqueous methanolic solution of hydrogen peroxide, a degradation product that had the same retention time as tamoxifen *N*-oxide was detected by HPLC.

INCOMPATIBILITY/COMPATIBILITY

Tamoxifen has been reported to be incompatible with a brand of xanthan gum (Keltrol, Kelco International) used as a suspending agent.[5]

FORMULATION

Excipients

Excipients that have been used in presentations of tamoxifen citrate include:
Tablets: carmellose calcium; colloidal silica, anhydrous; croscarmellose sodium; gelatin; hypromellose; lactose; macrogol; magnesium stearate; maize starch; mannitol; povidone; talc; titanium dioxide (E171).

Bioequivalence

Bioequivalence between tamoxifen citrate tablets (containing the equivalent of 10 mg tamoxifen), from two manufacturers (Nolvadex, ICI and generic, Berk) has been shown in a single-dose, crossover study with twelve healthy male volunteers.[6]

Suppositories

Rectal administration of tamoxifen citrate in suppositories has been studied by Tukker et al.[1] Suppositories that contained tamoxifen (as citrate) 40 mg were prepared with one of two bases: Witepsol H15 or Suppocire AML (which contains lecithin 2% as a surfactant). Release in vitro of tamoxifen from both preparations was rapid but incomplete (65% release to water in one hour). In a crossover study, six healthy volunteers received two tamoxifen citrate tablets orally (Nolvadex-20, each equivalent to 20 mg tamoxifen) and one of each suppository preparation rectally. Relative bioavailabilities of the suppositories compared to the tablets were 28% ± 11% and 13% ± 4% for the Witepsol-based and Suppocire-based preparations respectively. Low rectal availability was attributed to several factors, including poor solubility in iso-osmotic rectal fluids (see Solubility above).

REFERENCES

1. Tukker JJ, Blankenstein MA, Nortier JWR. J Pharm Pharmacol 1986;38:888–92.
2. Jalonen HG. J Pharm Sci 1988;77(9):810–13.
3. Harper MJK, Walpole AL. Nature 1966;212-:87.
4. Goldberg I, Becker Y. J Pharm Sci 1987;76(3):259–64.
5. UKCPA Symposium, Pharm J 1986;237:665.
6. Stevenson D, Briggs R, Mould GP. J Pharm Biomed Anal 1986;4(2):191–6.

Temazepam (BAN, USAN, rINN)   *Hypnotic*

3-Hydroxydiazepam
7-Chloro-1,3-dihydro-3-hydroxy-1-methyl-5-phenyl-2H-1,4-benzodiazepin-2-one
$C_{16}H_{13}ClN_2O_2 = 300.7$
CAS—846-50-4

Pharmacopoeial status

BP

Preparations

Compendial
Temazepam Oral Solution BP. pH 7.3 to 8.3. An oral solution containing 10 mg in 5 mL is usually available.

Non-compendial
Gel-filled capsules (soft gelatin) containing temazepam 10 mg, 15 mg, 20 mg, and 30 mg are available from APS, Berk, Cox, CP, Evans, Farmitalia Carlo Erba (Temazepam Gelthix), Kerfoot, Norton, Wyeth.

NOTE. Gel-filled capsules, in particular, may be subject to abuse.

Normison (Wyeth). *Capsules*, soft gelatin, temazepam 10 mg and 20 mg.
Tablets containing temazepam 10 mg and 20 mg are available from Wyeth.

A sugar-free elixir containing temazepam 10 mg/5 mL is available from Farmitalia Carlo Erba. *Diluent* (if required): glycerol.

Containers and storage

Solid state
Temazepam BP should be kept in a well-closed container and protected from light.

Dosage forms
Temazepam Oral Solution BP should be protected from light. Temazepam capsules (Wyeth) and Normison capsules should be stored in a dry place between 15° and 25°, protected from light. They should be dispensed into well-closed amber glass or amber/opaque plastic containers.
Temazepam elixir (Farmitalia Carlo Erba) should be stored below 25° and protected from direct light.
Temazepam tablets (Wyeth) should be stored in a cool, dry place.

PHYSICAL PROPERTIES

Temazepam is a white or almost white, crystalline powder; odourless or almost odourless.

Melting point

Temazepam melts in the range 156° to 159°.

Dissociation constant

pK_a 1.6

Solubility

Temazepam is practically insoluble in water; sparingly soluble in ethanol; freely soluble in chloroform.
Solubilisation of temazepam was demonstrated by each of various surfactants present at concentrations greater than their critical micelle concentration.[1] Among the nonionic surfactants studied (polysorbates, Emulgins, Brijs, Myrjs, and cetomacrogol), polysorbate 80 was the most efficient solubiliser and Myrj 59 was the least efficient. The anionic surfactant sodium lauryl sulphate was more efficient than the cationic surfactant cetrimide. In general, the amount of temazepam solubilised increased with an increase in temperature. The thermal process of micellar solubilisation was investigated by use of calculated thermodynamic parameters.

FURTHER INFORMATION. Determination of three-component partial solubility parameters for temazepam and the effects of change in partial molal volume on the thermodynamics of drug solubility [in 29 solvents]—Richardson PJ, McCafferty DF, Woolfson AD. Int J Pharmaceutics 1992;78:189–98. Solubility and thermodynamics of aqueous solutions of benzodiazepines—Regosz A, Krzykowska Z, Weclawska K, Chmielewska A. Pharmazie 1990;45(H11):867–8.

STABILITY

Gordon et al[2] described a method (isocratic reversed-phase HPLC) by which temazepam and its major degradation products (diazepam and 7-chloro-1-methyl-5-phenyl-4,5-dihydro-2H-1,4-benzodiazepin-2,3-9-(H)-dione) could be determined in the contents of soft gelatin capsules.
Similarly, Fatmi and Hickson[3] performed reversed-phase HPLC analyses in which temazepam in capsules could be quantified and separated from a synthetic precursor and two possible degradation products, which were reported to be 7-chloro-1-methyl-5-phenyl-4,5-dihydro-2H-1,4-benzodiazepin-2,3-one and 5-chloro-2-methylaminobenzophenone.

McCafferty et al[4] examined the stability of temazepam 5 mg/mL in various mixtures of propylene glycol:water (containing at least 80% w/w propylene glycol) during storage in borosilicate glass ampoules at 4°, 25°, 37°, and 55° for 190 days. Yellow discoloration was observed in all formulations; discoloration appeared more rapidly as the temperature was increased. No detectable loss of temazepam was noted (by HPLC) in samples stored at 4° and 25°, although a 3% and 20% loss was detected in samples stored at 37° and 55°, respectively. Mixtures with propylene glycol 80% w/w had approximate $t_{10\%}$ values for temazepam of 7.93 years, 1.86 years, and 0.26 years at 25°, 37°, and 55°, respectively. After autoclaving at 121° for 40 minutes, slight discoloration was observed but there was no detectable loss of temazepam from any of the formulations.

In a comparison of the suitability of propylene glycol and macrogol 400 as cosolvents for temazepam in aqueous solution, temazepam was stable at all concentrations of propylene glycol whereas at concentrations of macrogol 400 of less than 60%, a decrease in stability was reported.[5] There was little difference in solubility of temazepam in either glycol at cosolvent concentrations up to about 60% w/w but above this concentration macrogol 400 was more effective.

Woolfson et al[6] prepared an aqueous solution that contained temazepam 20 mg/mL, sodium salicylate 400 mg/mL, and lactose 100 mg/mL in water for injections; sodium salicylate was included as a hydrotropic complexing ligand to increase the solubility of temazepam. Although solutions were stable for at least 24 hours at room temperature and one week when refrigerated, a deep yellow discoloration occurred within one week at room temperature. However, when the solution was lyophilised no loss of temazepam was detected after storage of the lyophilised product for a six-month period at 4°, 25°, or 40° followed by reconstitution in water for injections immediately before analysis.

FURTHER INFORMATION. Review article. Degradation of 1,4-benzodiazepines—Selkämaa R. Acta Pharm Fenn 1988;97:37–44.

FORMULATION

Excipients

Excipients that have been used in presentations of temazepam include:
Capsules: benzyl alcohol; brilliant blue FCF (133); butyl, methyl, and propyl hydroxybenzoates; erythrosine (E127); gelatin; glycerol; lactose; macrogol 400; magnesium stearate; red ferric oxide, synthetic; silica; sodium bisulphite; sodium calciumedetate; sodium lauryl sulphate; sodium propionate; titanium dioxide (E171).

Bioavailability

In a single-dose, crossover study involving ten healthy volunteers,[7] no significant differences were apparent between the extents of absorption of temazepam (20 mg) from a soft gelatin capsule (Euhypnos Forte) and from an elixir. It was suggested that absorption of temazepam was more rapid (higher plasma concentrations after 20 minutes) from the elixir.

A comparison of the relative bioavailability of temazepam administered to six healthy subjects as two 10-mg hard gelatin capsules (Levanxol, Carlo Erba) and two 10-mg soft gelatin capsules (Euhypnos, Montedison) revealed no significant differences in areas under plasma concentration versus time curves or peak plasma concentrations.[8] However, there was a significant difference in the mean time to reach peak plasma concentrations of temazepam: about 50 minutes and 86 minutes for the soft and hard capsules, respectively.

Further discussions have been reported about differences in the rate of absorption and in therapeutic effects of temazepam from soft gelatin (liquid filled) and hard gelatin (powder filled) capsules, despite their similar eventual bioavailabilities.[9, 10]

No significant differences were reported between the pharmacokinetic parameters (monitored over a 12-hour period) of a tablet and a soft gelatin capsule of temazepam.[11]

Interactions with excipients

Botha and Lötter[12] used differential scanning calorimetry to show that temazepam was compatible with starch, Sta-Rx 1500 (directly compressible starch), Primojel and Explotab (both sodium starch glycollate), Elcema G 250 (microfine cellulose), Sterotex (hydrogenated cotton seed oil), and lactose. Interactions that may be indicative of incompatibilities were noted between temazepam and povidone, crospovidone, Precirol Ato 5 (glyceryl palmitostearate), stearic acid, magnesium stearate, Emcompress (calcium hydrogen phosphate), and possibly Avicel PH101 (microcrystalline cellulose) and Ac-Di-Sol (cross-linked carmellose sodium).

Solid dispersions of temazepam were prepared in macrogols or in Gelucire 44/14 and phase interactions were investigated by differential thermal analysis and hot stage microscopy.[13] Temazepam showed partial solubility in the carriers. Enhanced *in-vitro* release rates of temazepam were shown from the solid dispersions; the release rate was dependent on the temazepam:carrier ratio. Increased dissolution rates from the solid dispersions were also demonstrated and were attributed to a reduction in the particle size of temazepam. Furthermore, dissolution rates of temazepam from capsules that contained solid dispersions with Gelucire 44/14 or lower molecular weight macrogols (for example, macrogols 1000 or 1500) were faster, and solid dispersions were more stable, than when higher molecular weight macrogols were used as carriers.

The interaction between temazepam and macrogols 2000, 4000, and 6000 in physical mixtures and co-precipitates and the dissolution rates from such binary systems were investigated.[14] Phase diagrams from differential scanning calorimetry and hot stage microscopy revealed that the systems were monotectic. No evidence of complexation between temazepam and the carrier in the solid state was apparent (using infrared spectrometry) and no decomposition of temazepam occurred during the preparation of the co-precipitates.

Gel-filled capsules

Launchbury et al[15] outlined the formulation and process development of a commercially available gel-filled capsule of temazepam, with the overall aim of reducing the abuse potential of the temazepam preparation. The formulation contained a macrogol combination that was semi-solid at room temperature but 'mobile' enough to be encapsulated at elevated temperatures. It was reported that, at ambient temperature, the gel formulation could not be drawn up into a syringe and could not be injected through a 25 G needle. It has been noted that the gel contents of such capsules are soluble in water,[16, 17] although precipitation has been reported to occur on the addition of water to the formulation.[15]

Griffiths and Rothwell[16] examined the physical appearance of the gel contents of two brands of temazepam capsules (Wyeth and Farmitalia) at various temperatures (rising and falling). As the temperature was increased the gel changed from a solid at 22°, to a softening gel at 32°, to a free-flowing liquid at 40°; as the temperature was decreased from 40° the free-flowing liquid formed a gel at 33°.

FURTHER INFORMATION. Interaction of 1,4-benzodiazepines with certain macromolecules. Part 1. Effect of nonionic surfactants on the dissolution rate of temazepam—Mulley BA, Aboutaleb AE, Abdel Rahman AA, Ahmed SM. Bull Pharm Sci Assiut Univ 1985;8(2):158–70. Part 2. Crystallisation of temazepam in presence of hydrophilic macromolecules—Mulley BA, Aboutaleb AE, Abdel Rahman AA, Ahmed SM. Bull Pharm Assiut Univ 1985;8(2):171–85. Preformulation studies on directly compressed tablets of temazepam [effects of combinations of directly compressible excipients]—Aboutaleb AE, Abdel Rahman AA, Ahmed MO. Bull Pharm Sci Assiut Univ 1986;9(2):172–86. A comparison of the soft gelatin capsule and the tablet form of temazepam [pharmacodynamic assessment]—Salonen M, Aantaa E, Aaltonen L, Hovi-Viander M, Kanto J. Acta Pharm Toxicol 1986;58:49–54. The influence of particle size on the bioavailability of inhaled temazepam—Fee JPH, Collier PS, Launchbury AP, Clarke RSJ. Br J Clin Pharmacol 1992;33:641–4.

REFERENCES

1. Mulley BA, Aboutaleb AE, Abdel Rahman AA, Ahmed SM. Bull Pharm Sci Assiut Univ 1988;11:70–87.
2. Gordon SM, Freeston LK, Collins AJ. J Chromatogr 1986;368(1):180–3.
3. Fatmi AA, Hickson EA. J Pharm Sci 1988;77(1):87–9.
4. McCafferty DF, Woolfson AD, Launchbury AP. Int J Pharmaceutics 1986;31:9–13.
5. McCafferty DF, Woolfson AD, Richardson P, Launchbury AP. J Pharm Pharmacol 1989;41:103P.
6. Woolfson AD, McCafferty DF, Launchbury AP. Int J Pharmaceutics 1986;34:17–22.
7. Pickup ME, Rogers MS, Launchbury AP. Int J Pharmaceutics 1984;22:311–19.
8. Fucella LM, Bolcioni G, Tamassia V, Ferrario L, Tognoni G. Eur J Clin Pharmacol 1977;12:383–6.
9. Launchbury AP [letter]. Lancet 1988;1:833–4.
10. Godfrey H, Launchbury AP, Priest RG, Hindmarch I [letters]. Lancet 1988;1:1113–14.
11. Woolfe AJ [letter]. Pharm J 1990;244:611.
12. Botha SA, Lötter AP. Drug Dev Ind Pharm 1990;16(2):331–45.
13. Dordunoo SK, Ford JL, Rubinstein MH. Drug Dev Ind Pharm 1991;17(12):1685–1713.
14. Mulley BA, Aboutaleb AE, Abdel Rahman AA, Ahmed SM. Bull Pharm Sci Assiut Univ 1988;11:50–69.
15. Launchbury AP, Morton FSS, Lacy JE. Mfg Chem 1989 Dec;60:38–40.
16. Griffiths SJ, Rothwell JG [letter]. Pharm J 1990;244:675.
17. Liston DJ [letter]. Pharm J 1990;244:715.

Testosterone (BAN, rINN)

Androgen; Anabolic steroid

17β-Hydroxyandrost-4-en-3-one
$C_{19}H_{28}O_2 = 288.4$

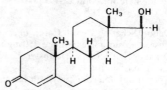

Testosterone Acetate (BANM, rINNM)
$C_{21}H_{30}O_3 = 330.5$

Testosterone Cypionate (BANM)
Testosterone Cipionate (rINNM); testosterone cyclopentylpropionate
$C_{27}H_{40}O_3 = 412.6$

Testosterone Decanoate (BANM, rINNM)
$C_{29}H_{46}O_3 = 442.7$

Testosterone Enanthate (BANM)
Testosterone Enantate (rINNM); testosterone heptanoate
$C_{26}H_{40}O_3 = 400.6$

Testosterone Isocaproate (BANM, rINNM)
Testosterone isohexanoate
$C_{25}H_{38}O_3 = 386.6$

Testosterone Phenylpropionate (BANM, rINNM)
$C_{28}H_{36}O_3 = 420.6$

Testosterone Propionate (BANM, rINNM)
$C_{22}H_{32}O_3 = 344.5$

Testosterone Undecanoate (BANM, rINNM)
$C_{30}H_{48}O_3 = 456.7$
CAS—58-22-0 (testosterone); 1045-69-8 (testosterone acetate); 58-20-8 (testosterone cypionate); 5721-91-5 (testosterone decanoate); 315-37-7 (testosterone enanthate); 15262-86-9 (testosterone isocaproate); 1255-49-8 (testosterone phenylpropionate); 57-85-2 (testosterone propionate)

Pharmacopoeial status

BP (testosterone, testosterone decanoate, testosterone enanthate, testosterone isocaproate, testosterone propionate); USP (testosterone, testosterone cypionate, testosterone enanthate, testosterone propionate).

Preparations

Compendial
Testosterone Implants BP. Sterile cylinders prepared by the fusion or heavy compression of testosterone without the addition of any other substance. Implants containing 100 mg and 200 mg are usually available.
Testosterone Propionate Injection BP. A sterile solution of testosterone propionate in ethyl oleate or other suitable ester, in a suitable fixed oil or in any mixture of these. Injections containing 10 mg, 25 mg, and 50 mg in 1 mL are usually available.

Testosterone Pellets USP.
Sterile Testosterone Suspension USP. pH between 4.0 and 7.5.
Testosterone Cypionate Injection USP.
Testosterone Enanthate Injection USP.
Testosterone Propionate Injection USP.

Non-compendial
Primoteston Depot (Schering Health Care). *Injection* (oily), for intramuscular use, testosterone enanthate 250 mg/mL.
Restandol (Organon). *Capsules*, testosterone undecanoate 40 mg in oleic acid (oily solution).
Sustanon 100 (Organon). *Injection* (oily), for intramuscular use, 1 mL contains testosterone propionate 20 mg, testosterone phenylpropionate 40 mg, and testosterone isocaproate 40 mg.
Sustanon 250 (Organon). *Injection* (oily), for intramuscular use, 1 mL contains testosterone propionate 30 mg, testosterone phenylpropionate 60 mg, testosterone isocaproate 60 mg, and testosterone decanoate 100 mg.
Testosterone (Organon). *Implant*, testosterone 100 mg and 200 mg.
Virormone (Paines & Byrne). *Injection*, for intramuscular use, testosterone propionate 50 mg/mL in ethyl oleate.

Containers and storage

Solid state
Testosterone BP should be protected from light.
Testosterone Decanoate BP, Testosterone Enanthate BP, and Testosterone Isocaproate BP should all be kept in well-closed containers, protected from light and stored at a temperature not exceeding 15°.
Testosterone Propionate BP should be kept in a well-closed container and protected from light.
Testosterone USP and Testosterone Enanthate USP should be preserved in well-closed containers. Testosterone Enanthate USP should be kept in a cool place.
Testosterone Cypionate USP and Testosterone Propionate USP should be preserved in well-closed, light-resistant containers.

Dosage forms
Testosterone Implants BP and Testosterone Propionate Injection BP should be protected from light.
Testosterone Pellets USP should be preserved in tight containers each holding one pellet and suitable for maintaining sterile contents.
Sterile Testosterone Suspension USP, Testosterone Cypionate Injection USP, Testosterone Enanthate Injection USP, and Testosterone Propionate Injection USP should be preserved in single-dose or in multiple-dose containers, preferably of Type I glass. Testosterone Cypionate Injection USP should be protected from light.
Primoteston Depot injection should be stored in cool, dry conditions away from strong sunlight.
Restandol capsules and Virormone injection should be protected from light. Restandol capsules should be stored in a cool, dry place (at 6° to 15°).
Sustanon preparations should be protected from light and stored at room temperature (15° to 25°). Storage at lower temperatures may result in precipitation of the arachis oil vehicle; this precipitate can be dissolved by heating at 100° for a few minutes or at 40° for one hour. Neither precipitation nor rewarming will affect the activity of the preparations.

PHYSICAL PROPERTIES

The appearances of testosterone and its salts and esters have been recorded as follows:

Compound	Properties
Testosterone	white or creamy-white crystals or crystalline powder; odourless or almost odourless
Testosterone cypionate	white or creamy-white crystalline powder; odourless or with a slight odour
Testosterone decanoate	white or creamy-white crystals or crystalline powder
Testosterone enanthate	white or creamy-white crystalline powder; odourless or with a faint odour characteristic of heptanoic acid
Testosterone isocaproate	white or creamy-white crystals or crystalline powder
Testosterone phenylpropionate	white or almost white crystalline powder with a characteristic odour
Testosterone propionate	white or creamy-white crystalline powder, or colourless or white to creamy-white crystals; odourless

Melting point
The melting points of testosterone and its salts and esters have been recorded as follows:

Compound	Melting point
Testosterone	152° to 157°
Testosterone acetate	140° to 141°
Testosterone cypionate	98° to 104°
Testosterone decanoate	about 50° or 55°
Testosterone enanthate	about 37°
Testosterone isocaproate	about 80°
Testosterone phenylpropionate	114° to 117°
Testosterone propionate	118° to 123°

Partition coefficient

Log P (octanol/water), 3.32

Solubility

Testosterone is practically insoluble in water; soluble 1 in 5 of ethanol, 1 in 2 of chloroform, and 1 in 100 of ether; soluble in dioxan and in vegetable oils; slightly soluble in ethyl oleate.
Testosterone cypionate is insoluble in water; freely soluble in ethanol, in chloroform, in ether, and in dioxan; soluble in vegetable oils.
Testosterone decanoate is practically insoluble in water; very soluble in ethanol and in chloroform.
Testosterone enanthate is practically insoluble in water; soluble 1 in 0.3 of ethanol; very soluble in ether; freely soluble in fixed oils.
Testosterone isocaproate is practically insoluble in water; very soluble in ethanol and in chloroform.
Testosterone phenylpropionate is practically insoluble in water; soluble 1 in 40 of ethanol.
Testosterone propionate is practically insoluble in water; soluble 1 in 6 of ethanol and 1 in 4 of acetone; very soluble in chloroform; freely soluble in ether, methanol, dioxan, and fixed oils; soluble in vegetable oils.
The simultaneous solubilisation of testosterone and of oestradiol were independent of each other in tetradecyltrimethylammonium bromide (at 20°), polysorbate 40 (at 20°), and sodium lauryl sulphate (at 40°). However, solubilisation of testosterone and of ethinyloestradiol in the same association colloids depended on their order of addition.[1]

An increase in the solubility of testosterone from 0.026 mg/mL in water to 38.0 mg/mL in hydroxypropyl-β-cyclodextrin 40% in water has been reported; the effectiveness of several other solubility enhancers was also investigated.[2]

FURTHER INFORMATION. The correlation of polymer-water and octanol-water partition coefficients: estimation of drug solubilities in polymers—Pitt CG, Bao YT, Andrady AL, Samuel PNK. Int J Pharmaceutics 1988;4:1–11. Transport of micelle-solubilised steroids [in Brij 35, Triton X 100 and sodium dodecyl sulphate] across microporous membranes—Johnson KA, Westermann-Clark GB, Shah DO. J Pharm Sci 1987;76(4):277–85.

Crystal and molecular structure

Polymorphs

Six polymorphic forms of testosterone have been prepared and investigated by infrared spectroscopy and differential scanning calorimetry.[3] Polymorph I was obtained when any other form was heated to 117°.

STABILITY

Although testosterone and its esters are reasonably stable in the solid state, photodegradation can occur in the presence of light. Irradiation of testosterone is reported to yield 4-androstene-3,17-dione and 5α-androstane-3,17-dione.[4] Photodegradation may also occur in solution.

INCOMPATIBILITY/COMPATIBILITY

Testosterone and testosterone propionate are reported to be incompatible with oxidising agents; the latter is also incompatible with alkalis.

FORMULATION

Excipients

Excipients that have been used in presentations of testosterone include:

Capsules, testosterone undecanoate: oleic acid; sodium ethyl hydroxybenzoate; sodium propyl hydroxybenzoate.
Intramuscular injections, testosterone cypionate: benzyl alcohol; benzyl benzoate; cottonseed oil.
Testosterone enanthate: benzyl benzoate; castor oil; sesame oil.
Testosterone propionate: ethyl oleate.
Testosterone decanoate, isocaproate, phenylpropionate, propionate: arachis oil; benzyl alcohol.

Absorption and bioavailability

Absolute systemic bioavailabilities of free testosterone (in twelve female volunteers) following oral administration of capsules containing testosterone dissolved in paraffin oil (Miglyol 810) or capsules containing testosterone undecanoate (Andriol, Organon) were calculated to be 3.66% ± 2.45% and 6.83% ± 3.32%, respectively, compared to that of an intravenous solution of testosterone in propylene glycol/water administered to another six female volunteers.[5] Inter-subject variation between the two oral preparations was marked.

When testosterone was combined with 5α-dihydrocholesterol, in the proportions at which a solid solution was formed (25:75% w/w), an increase in intestinal absorption, compared to that of testosterone propionate in arachis oil, was apparent following oral administration to female volunteers.[6]

In an investigation of the influence of the solvent (ethyl oleate, octanol, isopropyl myristate, or light liquid paraffin) on the availability of ^{14}C-testosterone propionate from oily intramuscular injections in *rats*,[7] the rate of disappearance from the injection site was rectilinearly related to partition coefficients determined *in vitro* (between solvent and water at 37°). However, delayed elimination from the body was independent of the solvent used and was influenced by biliary recycling of testosterone.

Chien[8] developed disk-shaped devices (based on microsealed drug delivery systems) that released testosterone at a constant rate *in vitro*. A controlled rate of delivery of testosterone *in vivo* and an enhanced systemic bioavailability for at least one month were achieved when bandage-type delivery systems of the disks were administered to the navels of rhesus *monkeys*. In another study,[9] transdermal absorption of testosterone was faster when administered, as ^{14}C-testosterone in acetone, via the navel area of *monkeys* than via the forearm area. Relative bioavailabilities of testosterone, compared to intravenous administration, following navel and forearm administration were 79.9% and 49.9%, respectively (plasma concentration data); and 78.9% and 57.9%, respectively (urinary recovery data).

Topical preparations

Ointments of testosterone were prepared by a fusion method in three bases: a water-miscible basis, a modified hydrophilic ointment USP (o/w), and a modified Beller's basis (o/w).[10] Release *in vitro* through a semi-permeable Cellophane membrane into phosphate buffer, pH 6 at 37°, was faster and more extensive from the water-miscible basis. Inclusion of either urea or macrogol 400, both at concentrations of 10%, to the water-miscible basis further enhanced testosterone release; however, at concentrations of 3% and 5% of these excipients no such enhancement was observed. Diffusion, permeability, partition coefficients, and release rate constants were also measured.

In-vitro release of testosterone from several bases (containing testosterone 2%) through a cellulose membrane into distilled water at 37° decreased in the general rank order: water-miscible basis > hydrophilic basis > University of California basis > gel basis > cream basis > water-soluble basis > emulsion basis.[11] The inclusion of various additives (ethanol, dimethyl sulphoxide, and macrogol 400) at 5%, 10%, and 15% had negligible effects on release; with the exception of the water-miscible basis, which demonstrated an increase in the extent of release following the addition of 15% macrogol 400. However, topical administration to the forearm of one healthy subject revealed greater absorption of testosterone from the water-washable basis on its own than when it was applied in combination with 15% macrogol 400. Comparison of urinary excretion data following administration of testosterone 50 mg orally or topically indicated that more free testosterone was available in the body following topical administration because of a reduced incidence of presystemic inactivation.

Complexation with cyclodextrins

Pitha and Pitha[12] prepared amorphous, water-soluble derivatives of cyclodextrins (α, β, and γ) by condensation with epoxides. Enhanced solubility of testosterone by the derivatives was demonstrated and when the solutions were lyophilised, solids that could be compressed into tablets with rapid dissolution properties were obtained. Administration of buccal/sublingual tablets containing complexes of testosterone with condensation products of β-cyclodextrin (such as hydroxypropyl-β-cyclodextrin and poly-β-cyclodextrin) led to effective absorption in two patients.[13]

Later work[14] established that although a crystalline complex of testosterone with γ-cyclodextrin showed a lower solubility and dissolution rate than complexes of testosterone with amorphous derivatives of cyclodextrins, tablets of the crystalline complex could be prepared; the tablets demonstrated slow dissolution when administered sublingually to one patient, but absorption of testosterone was considered to be 'efficient'. Administration of similar complexes with β-cyclodextrin was 'ineffective'.

FURTHER INFORMATION. The effect of drug lipophilicity and lipid vehicles on the lymphatic absorption of various testosterone esters—Noguchi T, Charman WNA, Stella VJ. Int J Pharmaceutics 1985;24:173–84. Diffusive characteristics of testosterone in novel gels [of propylene glycol dipelargonate and silicic acid in contact with a microporous polytetrafluoroethylene membrane]—Conrath G, Falson-Reig F, Besnard M, Peppas NA. J Controlled Release 1988;5:285–91. Transdermal dual-controlled delivery of testosterone and estradiol: (I) Impact of system design, (II) Enhanced skin permeability and membrane-moderated delivery—Yu J-W, Chien T-Y, Chien YW. Drug Dev Ind Pharm 1991;17(14):1883–1904,1905–30.

REFERENCES

1. Lundberg B, Lövgren T, Heikius B. J Pharm Sci 1979;68(5):542–5.
2. Pitha J, Milecki J, Fales H, Pannell L, Uekama K. Int J Pharmaceutics 1986;29:73–82.
3. Kang IPS. Aust J Pharm Sci 1974;NS3(2):55–8.
4. Reisch J, Ekiz N, Takács M [German]. Arch Pharm (Weinheim) 1989;322:173–5.
5. Täuber U, Schröder K, Düsterberg B, Matthes H. Eur J Drug Metab Pharmacokinet 1986;11(2):145–9.
6 Kincl FA. Arch Pharm (Weinheim) 1986;319:615–24.
7. Al-Hindawi MK, James KC, Nicholls PJ. J Pharm Pharmacol 1987;39:90–5.
8. Chien YW. J Pharm Sci 1984;73(8):1064–7.
9. Chien YW [letter]. J Pharm Sci 1984;73(2):283–5.
10. Parikh NH, Babar A, Plakogiannis FM. Drug Dev Ind Pharm 1986;12(14):2493–509.
11. Babar A, Khaleque RA, Cutie AJ, Plakogiannis FM. Drug Dev Ind Pharm 1989;15(9):1405–22.
12. Pitha J, Pitha J. J Pharm Sci 1985;74(9):987–90.
13. Pitha J, Harman SM, Michel ME. J Pharm Sci 1986;75(2):165–7.
14. Pitha J, Anaissie EJ, Uekama K. J Pharm Sci 1987;76(10):788–90.

Tetracycline (BAN, rINN)   *Antibacterial*

4S,4aS,5aS,6S,12aS-4-Dimethylamino-1,4,4a,5,5a,6,11,12a-octahydro-3,6,10,12,12a-pentahydroxy-6-methyl-1,11-dioxonaphthacene-2-carboxamide
It contains a variable quantity of water.
$C_{22}H_{24}N_2O_8 = 444.4$

Tetracycline Hydrochloride (BANM, rINNM)
$C_{22}H_{24}N_2O_8,HCl = 480.9$

Tetracycline Phosphate Complex (BAN)
CAS—60-54-8 (tetracycline, anhydrous); 6416-04-2 (tetracycline, trihydrate); 64-75-5 (tetracycline hydrochloride); 1336-20-5 (tetracycline phosphate complex)

Pharmacopoeial status

BP (tetracycline, tetracycline hydrochloride); USP (tetracycline, tetracycline hydrochloride, tetracycline phosphate complex)

Preparations

Compendial
Tetracycline Capsules BP. Contain tetracycline hydrochloride. Capsules containing, in each, 250 mg are usually available.
Tetracycline Tablets BP. Contain tetracycline hydrochloride. Coated tablets containing, in each, 250 mg are usually available.
Tetracycline Oral Suspension BP (Tetracycline Mixture). A suspension of tetracycline in a suitable flavoured vehicle. If the suspension is diluted the diluted suspension should be freshly prepared. pH 3.5 to 6.0.
Tetracycline Intravenous Infusion BP (Tetracycline Hydrochloride for Intravenous Infusion). A sterile solution of tetracycline hydrochloride in water for injections. It is prepared by dissolving tetracycline hydrochloride for intravenous infusion in the requisite amount of water for injections and diluting the resulting solution with a suitable diluent in accordance with the manufacturer's instructions immediately before use. Sealed containers each containing 250 mg and 500 mg of tetracycline hydrochloride are usually available. pH of a 10% w/v solution, 2.0 to 3.0.
Sterile Tetracycline Hydrochloride USP.
Sterile Tetracycline Phosphate Complex USP.
Tetracycline Hydrochloride Capsules USP.
Tetracycline Phosphate Complex Capsules USP.
Tetracycline Hydrochloride Tablets USP.
Tetracycline Oral Suspension USP. Contains tetracycline.
Tetracycline Hydrochloride Ointment USP.
Tetracycline Hydrochloride Ophthalmic Ointment USP.
Tetracycline Hydrochloride for Topical Solution USP. Also contains epitetracycline.
Tetracycline Hydrochloride Ophthalmic Suspension USP. Contains sterile tetracycline hydrochloride.
Tetracycline Hydrochloride for Injection USP. Contains sterile tetracycline hydrochloride. pH between 2.0 and 3.0 in a solution containing 10 mg/mL.
Tetracycline Phosphate Complex for Injection USP. Contains sterile tetracycline phosphate complex. pH between 2.0 and 3.0, in a solution containing 10 mg/mL.

Non-compendial
Achromycin (Lederle). *Capsules*, tetracycline hydrochloride 250 mg.
Tablets, tetracycline hydrochloride 250 mg.
Ointment, tetracycline hydrochloride 3% in a wool fat and white soft paraffin basis. Dilution is not recommended.
Eye and ear ointment, tetracycline hydrochloride 1% in a white soft paraffin and wool fat basis. Dilution is not recommended.
Intravenous/intrapleural infusion, powder for reconstitution in water for injections; each vial contains tetracycline hydrochloride 250 mg or 500 mg. It should be diluted immediately before administration by intravenous infusion. The reconstituted infusion is compatible with sodium chloride 0.9% injection, glucose 5% injection, sodium chloride and glucose injection, and compound sodium lactate injection. Although solutions that contain calcium should not be used unless necessary since precipitation tends to occur, particularly in neutral to alkaline solution, compound sodium lactate injection may be used with

caution; the calcium ion content of this diluent does not normally precipitate tetracycline in an acid medium. The following compounds should not be administered in the same drip as Achromycin injection: aminophylline, amphotericin, barbiturates, cephalothin, chloramphenicol, chlorothiazide, chlorpromazine, cyanocobalamin, dimenhydrinate, erythromycin, heparin, hydrocortisone, methicillin, methohexitone, methyldopa, nitrofurantoin, novobiocin, penicillins, phenytoin, polymyxin B, prochlorperazine, riboflavine, sodium bicarbonate, sulphadiazine, sulphafurazole, thiopentone sodium, vitamin B complex, warfarin, various inorganic ions (calcium, magnesium, aluminium, manganese, iron) and donor blood.

Intramuscular injection, powder for reconstitution in water for injections; each vial contains tetracycline hydrochloride 100 mg and procaine hydrochloride 40 mg.

Achromycin Intramuscular and Achromycin Intravenous/Intrapleural should be reconstituted immediately before use. The brown appearance of vials is produced when the powders for reconstitution for injections are sterilised by irradiation and does not indicate any degradation.

Sustamycin (Boehringer Mannheim). *Capsules*, sustained release, tetracycline hydrochloride 250 mg.

Tetrabid-Organon (Organon). *Capsules*, sustained release, tetracycline hydrochloride 250 mg.

Tetrachel (Berk). *Capsules*, tetracycline hydrochloride 250 mg. *Tablets*, tetracycline hydrochloride 250 mg.

Topicycline (Procter & Gamble). *Solution*, powder for reconstitution, tetracycline hydrochloride 154 mg and 4-epitetracycline 230 mg. Provides tetracycline hydrochloride 2.2 mg/mL when reconstituted with solvent that contains *n*-decyl methyl sulphoxide and citric acid in a 40% ethanol solution. Use within 8 weeks of reconstitution. Any unused material should be discarded.

Containers and storage

Solid state

Tetracycline BP and Tetracycline Hydrochloride BP should be kept in well-closed containers and protected from light. If Tetracycline Hydrochloride BP is intended for use in the manufacture of a parenteral dosage form the container should be sterile, tamper-evident and sealed so as to exclude micro-organisms.

Tetracycline USP, Tetracycline Hydrochloride USP, and Tetracycline Phosphate Complex USP should be preserved in tight, light-resistant containers. Sterile Tetracycline Hydrochloride USP and Sterile Tetracycline Phosphate Complex USP should be preserved in containers suitable for sterile solids and protected from light.

Dosage forms

Tetracycline Oral Suspension BP should be kept in a well-closed container, protected from light and stored at a temperature not exceeding 15°.

Tetracycline Intravenous Infusion BP: the sealed container should be protected from light. The infusion deteriorates on storage and should be used immediately after preparation.

Tetracycline Oral Suspension USP, Tetracycline Hydrochloride Capsules USP, Tetracycline Hydrochloride Tablets USP, Tetracycline Hydrochloride for Topical Solution USP, and Tetracycline Phosphate Complex Capsules USP should be preserved in tight, light-resistant containers.

Tetracycline Hydrochloride Ointment USP should be preserved in well-closed containers, preferably at controlled room temperature.

Tetracycline Hydrochloride Ophthalmic Ointment USP should be preserved in collapsible ophthalmic ointment tubes.

Tetracycline Hydrochloride Ophthalmic Suspension USP should be preserved in tight, light-resistant containers of glass or plastic, containing not more than 15 mL. The containers or individual cartons are sealed and tamper-proof so that sterility is assured at time of first use.

Tetracycline Hydrochloride for Injection USP and Tetracycline Phosphate Complex for Injection USP should be preserved in containers suitable for sterile solids and protected from light.

Achromycin capsules, tablets, intramuscular injection, and intravenous/intrapleural infusion should be stored at controlled room temperature (15° to 30°). Achromycin intramuscular injection and intravenous/intrapleural infusion should be protected from light. Achromycin ointment and eye/ear ointment should be stored in a cool place (8° to 15° and 8° to 25°, respectively). All Achromycin preparations should be stored in the original containers.

Sustamycin and Tetrabid-Organon capsules should be stored below 30°, the former in well-closed containers.

Tetrachel capsules and tablets should be stored in a cool place. Topicycline should be stored at a temperature not exceeding 25° before reconstitution, and at or below 25° after reconstitution.

PHYSICAL PROPERTIES

Tetracycline is a yellow, odourless crystalline powder.
Tetracycline hydrochloride is a yellow. hygroscopic crystalline powder; odourless with a bitter taste.
Tetracycline phosphate complex is a yellow, crystalline powder with a faint, characteristic odour.

Melting point

Tetracycline hydrochloride melts at about 214°, with decomposition.

pH

pH of a 1% w/v aqueous suspension of *tetracycline* (BP), 3.5 to 6.0.
pH of a 1% w/v aqueous suspension of *tetracycline* (USP), 3.0 to 7.0.
pH of a 1% w/v aqueous solution of *tetracycline hydrochloride*, 1.8 to 2.8.
pH of a 1% w/v aqueous suspension of *tetracycline phosphate complex*, 2.0 to 4.0.

Dissociation constants

pK_a 3.3 (acidic), 7.7 (acidic), 9.7 (basic) at 25°
Apparent macroscopic ionisation constants of tetracycline (5×10^{-4}M aqueous solution at 60°) were reported;[1] pK_a values were 3.74 ± 0.01, 6.97 ± 0.07, and 8.46 ± 0.1.

Partition coefficient

Log P (octanol/pH 7.4), −1.4

Solubility

Tetracycline is soluble 1 in 2500 of water; sparingly soluble in ethanol (1 in 50) and in acetone; practically insoluble in chloroform and in ether; it is freely soluble in dilute acids and, with decomposition, in solutions of alkali hydroxides.
Tetracycline hydrochloride is freely soluble in water (1 in 10); slightly soluble in ethanol (1 in 100); practically insoluble in acetone, in chloroform, and in ether; it is soluble in methanol and in aqueous solutions of carbonates or alkali hydroxides, although it is rapidly destroyed by alkali hydroxides. Solutions in water become turbid on standing due to precipitation of tetracycline.
Tetracycline phosphate complex is sparingly soluble in water; slightly soluble in methanol; very slightly soluble in acetone.

Dissolution

The USP specifies that for Tetracycline Hydrochloride Capsules USP not less than 70% of the labelled amount of $C_{22}H_{24}N_2O_8$,HCl is dissolved in 60 minutes. Dissolution medium: 900 mL of water; Apparatus 2 at 75 rpm.

Dissolution properties

Considerable differences in both disintegration rates and dissolution rates (at pH 7 or in simulated gastric fluid) were apparent among 13 different commercial brands of tetracycline (250 mg) tablets.[2] Following administration of six preparations (in a single-dose, crossover study with 15 healthy volunteers), bioavailability of tetracycline (from serum concentration data) showed rank correlation with dissolution rates in water at pH 7 but not in simulated gastric fluid. However, assessment of all 13 preparations in a double-blind, single-dose, crossover study involving 42 volunteers revealed marked inter-patient variation in bioavailability (from urinary excretion data) and limited correlation with dissolution rates.

STABILITY

The mechanisms and kinetics of degradation of tetracycline have been extensively studied and reported.

Degradation pathways

Tetracycline is rapidly inactivated at pH less than 2 and is slowly destroyed at pH 7 and above. In aqueous solution, tetracycline and its hydrochloride degrade by epimerisation and dehydration to yield 4-epitetracycline (low antimicrobial activity) and anhydrotetracycline, respectively, which subsequently dehydrate and epimerise, respectively, to yield the toxic product 4-epianhydrotetracycline. Epimerisation[1] is a reversible, first-order reaction that occurs between pH 2.5 and 6, whereas dehydration,[1,3] at carbons 5a and 6, occurs at very low pH. Tetracycline can also degrade by oxidation.[1,4]

Solid state

In the form of powder or crystals, tetracycline and tetracycline hydrochloride darken in strong sunlight in a moist atmosphere. In the solid state, no degradation of tetracycline was detected (by HPLC) during storage in well-closed containers at 37° and 50° for 27 months and 16 months, respectively.[5] At 70° a decrease in tetracycline content was noted with a slight increase in the amount of anhydrotetracycline present but there was no change in amounts of epitetracycline or epianhydrotetracycline. A $t_{10\%}$ of 19 months at 70° was predicted. Walton et al[6] demonstrated that after storage of tetracycline hydrochloride powder at 37° and 66% relative humidity, about 10% of the initial potency was lost in 70 days. Under the same conditions, tetracycline hydrochloride powder from capsules, either alone or with added citric acid, lost 0% and 93% of the initial potency, respectively, in 70 days; large amounts of anhydrotetracycline and epianhydrotetracycline were detected in the sample with citric acid.
At room temperature, $t_{10\%}$ values for tetracycline hydrochloride nongranulated or granulated with the solvents ethanol, methanol, or acetone were between 994 days and 1074 days.[7]
Microbiological analysis of samples of tetracycline hydrochloride, stored for eight weeks at 37° or 20°, indicated that 9% and 7%, respectively, had decomposed.[8] However, spectrophotometric analysis of the same samples, at three wavelengths, did not reveal any decomposition and was not recommended by the authors as a dependable method.

Kinetics

The degradation kinetics of tetracycline hydrochloride in aqueous solution at 60°, over the pH range 0.5 to 12.6 (in various buffers) were investigated by ultraviolet spectroscopy and HPLC.[1] At pH below 2, dehydration to form anhydrotetracycline occurred, whereas in the pH range 2.5 to 5, reversible first-order epimerisation to 4-epitetracycline predominated. In the pH range 7.1 to 8.6, oxidation was suggested to occur as deoxygenation of solutions by the addition of nitrogen improved stability, although formation of 4-epitetracycline was also detected. Specific base catalysis was demonstrated above pH 11 and isotetracycline was reported to be a product of this reaction. Further, in the pH range 3.5 to 10.0, acetate, phosphate, and borate buffers caused general acid-base catalysis of tetracycline hydrochloride degradation. Maximum stability was concluded to occur at about pH 3.
Yuen and Sokoloski[9] examined the kinetics of simultaneous degradation reactions of tetracycline hydrochloride in phosphate buffer (pH 1.5) in the temperature range 60° to 80°. Activation energies for epimerisation and dehydration of tetracycline hydrochloride were 85.7 kJ/mol and 81.15 kJ/mol, respectively, and for epimerisation of anhydrotetracycline and dehydration of epitetracycline were 58.9 kJ/mol and 111.2 kJ/mol, respectively.
Taylor et al[10] studied the kinetics of each individual reaction involved in the degradation of tetracycline, by use of an initial rate method. The rate constant for the overall degradation increased with a decrease in pH from 8.0 to 2.3 (at 75°) and with an increase in temperature from 40° to 70° (at pH 7.0). Kinetics and mechanisms of dehydration of epitetracycline[3] at pH 2 and epimerisation of anhydrotetracycline[11] at pH 4.2 have been studied.

Effect of riboflavine

When aqueous solutions of tetracycline hydrochloride (0.8 mg/mL and buffered to pH 4.5) were mixed with riboflavine and stored for 24 hours at 26.7° under fluorescent light and in the presence of air, the extent of degradation of tetracycline hydrochloride increased to a maximum in the concentration range of riboflavine 0.1 to 10 mg/mL.[4] Degradation was attributed to oxidation and epimerisation; no dehydration products were detected. Although decomposition of tetracycline hydrochloride alone did not demonstrate light-dependence (at 37°), the degradation-promoting effect of riboflavine was dependent on light. In the presence of light and air, ascorbic acid (2.5 mg/mL) prevented the promotion of degradation by riboflavine, although slight loss of tetracycline hydrochloride was attributed to the effects of ascorbic acid.

Photodegradation

Photo-oxidation of tetracycline in aerated aqueous solution was studied by measurement of oxygen uptake during irradiation with ultraviolet light.[12] Below pH 8, oxygen uptake was insignificant. At pH 9, uptake of oxygen (of 1:1 stoichiometry with tetracycline) was accompanied by a yellow to pink, red, or brown discoloration. Anhydrotetracycline, epianhydrotetracycline, and peroxides were not detected. Addition of disodium edetate did not affect the rate of photo-oxidation, but addition of copper(II) ions caused a reduction in the rate. The reaction was concluded to occur by a sensitised photo-oxygenation mechanism. When air-saturated aqueous solutions of tetracycline hydrochloride (5×10^{-5}M) buffered to pH 9 were irradiated with ultraviolet-A light, differential pulse polarographic studies indicated that a product of photodegradation was a quinone.[13]

The ability of compounds (at a concentration of 0.2%) to stabilise tetracycline hydrochloride (0.04%) in solution, buffered to pH 7 with phosphate buffer, under fluorescent light, decreased in the order: reduced glutathione > *p*-aminobenzoic acid > disodium edetate > DL-cysteine > thiourea > sodium thiosulphate > DL-methionine.[14] In kinetic studies with and without reduced glutathione, the rate of photodegradation of tetracycline hydrochloride (at pH 7) was greater under fluorescent light than under ultraviolet-A or ultraviolet-B light and the rate increased with increasing pH. At pH 4.5, the reaction rate was faster in the presence of acetate buffer than in the presence of phosphate or citrate buffers.

Suspensions

Workers in Belgium[15] investigated the stabilities of tetracycline and its hydrochloride in several modified suspensions from Dutch and Belgian National Formularies which included, respectively: syrup, tragacanth, and methyl hydroxybenzoate; and syrup, tragacanth, and glycerol. Suspensions of tetracycline hydrochloride buffered to pH 4.0 or 5.4 with acetate, citrate, or phosphate buffers were stable for at least 12 weeks at 5° or 20°. Extensive degradation of tetracycline hydrochloride occurred in suspensions buffered to pH 2.8 or unbuffered (pH 1.9 and 2.0) during 12 weeks at 20°. An unbuffered suspension of tetracycline base (pH 4.0) remained stable under the same conditions.

Topical preparations

Tetracycline hydrochloride in methylcellulose gels had $t_{10\%}$ values at room temperature and at 4° of 2.1 days and 7.1 days, respectively.[7]

In India, a tetracycline hydrochloride 1% ointment in white soft paraffin (5 g in a collapsible tube) retained its antimicrobial activity, had acceptable physical characteristics, and showed no local conjunctival toxicity in *rabbits* or humans during storage for up to 44 months.[16]

FURTHER INFORMATION. Tetracycline degradation products in commercially available tetracycline-7-^{3}H—Lanman RC, Ludden TM, Schanker LS. J Pharm Sci 1973;62(9):1461–3. Differential pulse polarography of some degradation products of tetracycline—Jochsberger T, Cutie AJ, Wang H-Y, Mary NY. J Pharm Sci 1982;71(11):1284–5. Quality assessment of the tetracyclines. Part 4. Accelerated stability test of solid formulations—Siewert M [German]. Pharm Ztg 1985;130:434–9. Evaluation of the quality of tetracyclines. Part 5. Accelerated stability tests of tetracycline and oxytetracycline capsule formulations—Siewert M, Wenzel B, Blume H [German]. Pharm Ztg 1986;131:495–500. Effect of solubilisers on the stability of tetracycline [stabilisation by macrogol 6000, polysorbate 20, thiourea, and urea]—Nagar V, Daabis NA, Motawi MM. Pharmazie 1974;29(H2):126–9. Photodecomposition of sulfonamides and tetracyclines at oil-water interfaces—Sanniez WHK, Pilpel N. J Pharm Sci 1980;69(1):5–8.

INCOMPATIBILITY/COMPATIBILITY

Tetracycline hydrochloride has been reported to be incompatible with solutions containing: alkalis, amikacin sulphate, aminophylline, amphotericin, ampicillin sodium, soluble barbiturates, benzylpenicillin, calcium chloride, calcium gluconate, carbenicillin sodium, cefapirin sodium, cephaloridine, cephalothin sodium, cephazolin sodium, chlorothiazide sodium, cloxacillin sodium, corticotrophin, dimenhydrinate, erythromycin salts, heparin, hydrocortisone sodium succinate, hyaluronidase, methicillin sodium, nafcillin sodium, nitrofurantoin sodium, novobiocin sodium, oxacillin sodium, phenytoin sodium,

sodium bicarbonate, streptomycin sulphate, sulphadiazine sodium, sulphafurazole diethanolamine, and warfarin sodium. See also Preparations, Non-compendial, above.

Intravenous solutions and admixtures

When Achromycin Intravenous injection was reconstituted with bacteriostatic water for injection and mixed with compound sodium lactate injection (with potassium chloride 40 mEq) the pH of solutions was about 3 to 4; chemical and visual compatibility was reported over 24 hours and 48 hours under ambient and refrigerated conditions, respectively.[17]

Tetracycline hydrochloride (Achromycin 500 mg/L) was stable for up to 6 hours in the following intravenous solutions: glucose 5% in sodium chloride 0.9%, glucose 5% in water, sodium chloride 0.9%, or water for injection (all at pH 3), or in a multiple electrolyte solution (at pH 5).[18] However, losses of between 7.7% and 11.6% of the initial concentration occurred over a longer period of 24 hours.

Visual incompatibility was apparent within one hour when 1 mL of tetracycline hydrochloride injection 2.5 mg/mL (Lederle) was mixed (under conditions that simulated Y-site injection at 25°) with 1 mL of morphine sulphate 1 mg/mL (Winthrop), pethidine hydrochloride 10 mg/mL (Wyeth), or hydromorphone 0.2 mg/mL (Wyeth) solutions in glucose 5% injection; solutions changed from pale yellow to light green.[19]

Chelation with metal ions

Diffusion rates of tetracycline hydrochloride (1×10^{-4}M) in various buffers through a semipermeable membrane were studied in the presence of metal ions (tetracycline:metal ions, molar ratio 1:1).[20] No changes in the ultraviolet absorption spectrum or diffusion rate occurred in the presence of aluminium or copper ions (at pH 1) or calcium, magnesium, or cobalt ions (at pH 1 and 5.5). However, at pH 5.5, aluminium or copper ions produced spectral shifts and decreases in the diffusion rate. At pH 8, magnesium or calcium ions produced no spectral changes but induced decreases in the diffusion rate, which was further reduced by a ten-fold increase in concentration of these ions.

FURTHER INFORMATION. Differential pulse polarography of tetracycline: determination of complexing tendencies of tetracycline analogs in the presence of cations [ferrous, ferric, and aluminium ions]—Jochsberger T, Cutie A, Mills J. J Pharm Sci 1979;68(8):1061–3. Mechanism of adsorption of clindamycin and tetracycline by montmorillonite [effect of pH]—Porubcan LS, Serna CJ, White JL, Hem SL. J Pharm Sci 1978;67(8):1081–7. Decreased tetracycline bioavailability caused by a bismuth subsalicylate antidiarrhoeal mixture. Albert KS, Welch RD, De Sante KA, DiSanto AR. J Pharm Sci 1979;68(5):586–8.

FORMULATION

Excipients

Excipients that have been used in presentations of tetracycline hydrochloride include:

Capsules: Aerosil; brilliant blue FCF (133); colloidal silica; erythrosine (E127); fumaric acid; gelatin; lactose; liquid paraffin; magnesium stearate; maize starch; patent blue V (E131); povidone; Red 28; shellac; sodium metaphosphate; sunset yellow FCF (E110); talc (purified); titanium dioxide (E171); Yellow 10.

Tablets: acacia; D&C Red No.30; glycerol; kaolin (heavy); hypromellose; lactose; magnesium stearate; maize starch; microcrystalline cellulose; povidone; pregelatinised starch; stearic acid; sunset yellow FCF (E110); talc; titanium dioxide (E171).

Oral liquids: aluminium magnesium silicate; Blue 1; calcium disodium edetate; citric acid; methyl and propyl hydroxybenzoates; polysorbate 80; potassium citrate; potassium metaphosphate; quinoline yellow (E104); Red 40; saccharin sodium; sodium benzoate; sodium citrate; sodium metabisulphite; sorbitol solution; sucrose; tragacanth.

Ointment: methyl and propyl hydroxybenzoates; white soft paraffin; wool fat.

Eye/Ear ointments: white soft paraffin; wool fat.

Ophthalmic suspensions: light liquid paraffin; Plastibase 50 W; sesame oil.

Injections (powder for reconstitution): ascorbic acid; magnesium chloride; procaine hydrochloride.

Bioavailability and absorption

In a crossover study,[21] twelve healthy volunteers received tetracycline either intravenously or orally as a syrup or as two different capsules. Absolute bioavailability of tetracycline was 57% from the syrup, and 58% and 50% from the two capsules.

Absorption of tetracycline hydrochloride in solution across everted *rat* intestinal sacs *in vitro* was increased by inclusion of polysorbate 80 with or without calcium chloride.[22] However, calcium chloride decreased absorption of tetracycline hydrochloride in the absence of polysorbate 80.

Bioequivalence

The bioequivalence of two batches of tetracycline hydrochloride capsules (fresh or stored for 42 months at ambient temperature) was reported following a randomised study involving six healthy volunteers.[23] Dissolution kinetics were also studied.

Modified-release preparations

Beads that consisted of tetracycline hydrochloride, succinic acid, microcrystalline cellulose, and povidone were coated with a mixture of magnesium stearate, dibutyl phthalate, and either Eudragit RS 100, Eudragit RL 100, or Eudragit RS 100:Eudragit RL 100 (1:1); coated beads were then filled into capsules.[24] Dissolution studies (at 37° and pH 1.2 to 7.5) revealed that release of tetracycline hydrochloride decreased as the amount of coating increased. Effectiveness of coatings to prolong release decreased in the order: Eudragit RS 100 > 1:1 mixture > Eudragit RL 100. In a crossover study involving four healthy volunteers, the controlled-release capsules had significantly greater bioavailabilities than conventional tetracycline hydrochloride capsules. Following storage of capsules that contained beads coated with Eudragit RS 100:RL 100 (1:1) at various temperatures and relative humidities, a shelf-life of over 18 months was predicted. Zero-order diffusion (at 37°) of tetracycline was demonstrated *in vitro* from trilaminate disk delivery devices.[25] Devices consisted of a core of tetracycline with 2-hydroxyethyl methacrylate:methyl methacrylate (63:37) which was coated with a membrane of the copolymer at the ratio 2:98 or 22:78. The rate of release of tetracycline was controlled by varying either the amount of tetracycline present, the composition and thickness of the membrane, or the geometry of the device. The zero-order release of tetracycline was also shown following intraperitoneal implantation of the trilaminate devices into *rats*;[26] two groups of ten *rats* received disks coated with 2-hydroxyethyl methacrylate:methyl methacrylate in the ratio 2:98 or 22:78. Plasma concentrations of tetracycline reached steady state after 2 to 4 days. At steady state, release rates *in vivo* correlated with excretion rates of tetracycline.

Release of tetracycline *in vitro* from ethyl cellulose films that contained macrogol was dependent on the amount of tetracycline (20% w/w to 50% w/w) embedded in the film and

increased with an increase in concentration of macrogol (up to 5% w/w) present in the film.[27]

Sustained-release tablets were prepared that contained either granules of tetracycline hydrochloride, succinic acid, and other excipients coated with glyceryl distearate, or uncoated granules that comprised tetracycline hydrochloride, Eudragit RSPM, succinic acid, and other excipients.[28] Tablets coated with glyceryl distearate were more difficult to prepare. When stored at room temperature in amber bottles, both sets of tablets remained stable with respect to drug concentration and release patterns for at least 18 months.

Preparations for periodontal treatment

Strips, for insertion into periodontal pockets, which consisted of tetracycline hydrochloride in a biodegradable polymer matrix of polyhydroxybutyric acid (drug:matrix, 25:75 and 10:90) were evaluated *in vitro* and *in vivo*.[29] In 100 mL of McIlvaine's buffer, pH 6.6 at 37°, the strips remained intact, but lost mechanical strength, during dissolution of tetracycline hydrochloride over 5 days. The strips were tolerated by patients and an acceptable clinical response was shown in patients with advanced periodontal disease.

Collins *et al*[30] prepared controlled-release compacts that contained tetracycline hydrochloride and polyhydroxybutyric acid. The effects of compaction pressure, drug loading, molecular weight of polyhydroxybutyric acid, copolymerisation of polyhydroxybutyric acid with polyhydroxyvalerate, and the diameter of compacts on the *in-vitro* release of tetracycline hydrochloride were evaluated. In studies, compacts were acceptable to twelve patients and clinical improvement was apparent.

FURTHER INFORMATION. Intrapleural tetracycline: new formulation—Batty KT. Aust J Hosp Pharm 1989;19:145–6.

PROCESSING

Sterilisation

High-energy gamma radiation has been used to sterilise aqueous solutions of tetracycline hydrochloride 0.01 mg/mL.[31] No significant loss of tetracycline hydrochloride was detected by spectrophotometry following 1 Mrad or 2.5 Mrad doses, although traces of products that may be due to radiolysis were detected following 15 Mrad doses. Samples that had been deliberately contaminated initially with 10^5 *Bacillis pumilus* spores showed no growth following irradiation, whereas growth occurred in solutions that had not been irradiated.

Mixing

The dissolution rate of tetracycline hydrochloride from hard gelatin capsules was demonstrated to increase as the time of mixing with magnesium stearate and the amount of magnesium stearate present were decreased.[32]

FURTHER INFORMATION. Radiosterilized tetracycline ophthalmic ointment [review of background to sterilisation of Achromycin (Lederle)]—Nash RA. Bull Parent Drug Assoc 1974;28(4):181–7.

REFERENCES

1. Vej-Hansen B, Bundgaard H. Arch Pharm Chemi Sci 1978;6:201–14.
2. Barnett DB, Smith RN, Greenwood ND, Hetherington C. Br J Clin Pharmacol 1974;1:319–23.
3. Hoener B-A, Sokoloski TD, Mitscher LA, Malspeis L. J Pharm Sci 1974;63(12):1901–4.

4. Leeson LJ, Weidenheimer JF. J Pharm Sci 1969;58(3):355–7.
5. Dihuidi K, Roets E, Hoogmartens J, Vanderhaeghe H. J Chromatogr 1982;246:350–5.
6. Walton VC, Howlett MR, Selzer GB. J Pharm Sci 1970;59(8):1160–4.
7. Kubis A, Dybek K, Krutul H. Pharmazie 1987;42(H8):519–20.
8. Shrestha B, Frier M. Br J Pharm Pract 1986;8:122–4.
9. Yuen PH, Sokoloski TD. J Pharm Sci 1977;66(11):1648–50.
10. Taylor RB, Durham DG, Shivji ASH. Int J Pharmaceutics 1985;26:259–66.
11. Sokoloski TD, Mitscher LA, Yuen PH, Juvarkar JV, Hoener B. J Pharm Sci 1977;66(8):1159–65.
12. Wiebe JA, Moore DE. J Pharm Sci 1977;66(2):186–9.
13. Moore DE, Fallon MP, Burt CD. Int J Pharmaceutics 1983;14:133–42.
14. Asker AF, Habib MJ. J Parenter Sci Technol 1991;45(2):113–15.
15. Grobben-Verpoorten A, Dihuidi K, Roets E, Hoogmartens J. Vanderhaeghe H. Pharm Weekbl (Sci) 1985;7:104–7.
16. Gupta SK, Mohan M, Mahajan VM. East Pharm 1985;28(334):125–8.
17. Roach M [letter]. Pharm J 1978;220:143.
18. Parker EA. Am J Hosp Pharm 1967;24:435–9.
19. Nieves-Cordero A, Luciw HM, Souney PF. Am J Hosp Pharm 1985;42:1108–9.
20. Chin T-F, Lach JL. Am J Hosp Pharm 1975;32:625–9.
21. Saux MC, Fourtillan JB, Lefebvre MA, Crockett R [French]. J Pharm Clin 1985;4(3):401–13.
22. Allen LV, Levinson RS, Robinson C, Lau A. J Pharm Sci 1981;70(3):269–71.
23. Mohamad H, Renoux R, Aiache S, Aiache J-M, Kantelip J-P [French]. STP Pharma 1986;2(18):630–5.
24. Jain NK, Misra AN. Drug Dev Ind Pharm 1989;15(5):825–44.
25. Olanoff L, Koinis T, Anderson JM. J Pharm Sci 1979;68(9):1147–50.
26. Olanoff L, Anderson JM. J Pharm Sci 1979;68(9):1151–5.
27. Azoury R, Elkayam R, Friedman M. J Pharm Sci 1988;77(5):428–31.
28. Jain NK, Misra AN. Indian J Pharm Sci 1985;47(4):148–50.
29. Deasy PB, Collins AEM, MacCarthy DJ, Russell RJ. J Pharm Pharmacol 1989;41:694–9.
30. Collins AEM, Deasy PB, MacCarthy DJ, Shanley DB. Int J Pharmaceutics 1989;51:103–14.
31. Jacobs GP. Pharm Acta Helv 1977;52(12):302–4.
32. Sickmüller A [German]. Acta Pharm Technol 1984;30(1)44–9.

Theophylline (BAN)   *Xanthine bronchodilator*

Anhydrous theophylline
3,7-Dihydro-1,3-dimethylpurine-2,6(1H)-dione;   1,3-dimethyl-purine- 2,6(3H,1H)-dione; 1,3-dimethylxanthine
$C_7H_8N_4O_2 = 180.2$

Aminophylline (BAN, pINN)
$(C_7H_8N_4O_2)_2,C_2H_4(NH_2)_2,2H_2O = 456.5$
(This compound is the subject of a separate monograph)

Choline Theophyllinate (BAN, rINN)
Oxtriphylline
$C_{12}H_{21}N_5O_3 = 283.3$

Theophylline Hydrate (BANM)
$C_7H_8N_4O_2,H_2O = 198.2$

Theophylline Monoethanolamine
$C_7H_8N_4O_2,C_2H_7NO = 241.2$

Theophylline Sodium Glycinate
An equilibrium mixture of theophylline sodium ($C_7H_7N_4NaO_2 = 202.1$) and glycine ($C_2H_5NO_2 = 75.07$) in approximately equimolecular proportions, buffered with an additional mole of glycine.
CAS—58-55-9 (theophylline); 4499-40-5 (choline theophyllinate); 5967-84-0 (theophylline hydrate); 573-41-1 (theophylline monoethanolamine); 8000-10-0 (theophylline sodium glycinate)

Pharmacopoeial status

BP (choline theophyllinate, theophylline hydrate); USP (oxtriphylline, theophylline [hydrous or anhydrous], theophylline sodium glycinate)

Preparations

Compendial

NOTE. For BP preparations containing theophylline refer to the Aminophylline monograph.
Choline Theophyllinate Tablets BP. Coated tablets containing, in each, 100 mg and 200 mg are usually available.
Oxtriphylline Delayed-release Tablets USP.
Oxtriphylline Elixir USP.
Theophylline Capsules USP.
Theophylline Extended-release Capsules USP.
Theophylline Tablets USP.
Theophylline Sodium Glycinate Tablets USP.
Theophylline Sodium Glycinate Elixir USP.
Theophylline in Dextrose Injection USP.

Non-compendial
Biophylline (Delandale). *Tablets*, controlled release, theophylline 350 mg and 500 mg.
Syrup, sugar free, theophylline hydrate 125 mg (as sodium glycinate)/5mL. Dilution not recommended.
Choledyl (P-D). *Tablets*, choline theophyllinate 100 mg and 200 mg.
Syrup, choline theophyllinate 62.5 mg/5 mL.
Labophylline (LAB). *Injection*, theophylline 20 mg/mL, lysine 12.2 mg/mL. *Diluents*: glucose 5% injection or sodium chloride 0.9% injection. Incompatible in infusion fluids with fructose, insulin, cimetidine, hydralazine, isoprenaline, noradrenaline, phenytoin sodium, vitamin B and C injection, and many antibiotics including benzylpenicillin, cephalothin, clindamycin, gentamicin, methicillin, tetracycline, and vancomycin.
Lasma (Pharmax). *Tablets*, sustained release, theophylline 300 mg.
Nuelin (3M). *Tablets*, microcrystalline theophylline 125 mg.
Liquid, theophylline 60 mg (as sodium glycinate)/5 mL.
Nuelin-SA (3M). *Tablets*, slow release, theophylline 175 mg.
Nuelin SA 250 (3M). *Tablets*, slow release, theophylline 250 mg.
Sabidal SR 270 (Zyma). *Tablets*, sustained release, choline theophyllinate 424 mg.

Slo-Phyllin (Lipha). *Capsules*, timed release, theophylline 60 mg, 125 mg, and 250 mg.
Theo-Dur (Astra). *Tablets*, slow release, theophylline 200 mg and 300 mg.
Uniphyllin Continus (Napp). *Tablets*, controlled release, theophylline 300 mg and 400 mg.
Paediatric tablets, controlled release, theophylline 200 mg.

Containers and storage

Solid state
Choline Theophylline BP should be kept in a well-closed container, protected from light and stored at a temperature not exceeding 25°.
Theophylline USP should be preserved in well-closed containers.
Theophylline Sodium Glycinate USP should be preserved in tight containers.
Oxtriphylline USP should be preserved in tight containers.

Dosage forms
Choline Theophyllinate Tablets BP should be protected from light and stored at a temperature not exceeding 25°.
Theophylline Capsules USP, Theophylline Extended-release Capsules USP, Theophylline Tablets USP, and Theophylline Sodium Glycinate Tablets USP should be preserved in well-closed containers.
Theophylline Sodium Glycinate Elixir USP should be preserved in tight containers.
Theophylline in Dextrose Injection USP should be preserved in single-dose containers, preferably of Type I or Type II glass, or of a suitable plastic material.
Oxtriphylline Delayed-release Tablets USP and Oxtriphylline Elixir USP should be preserved in tight containers.
Biophylline tablets should be stored in a cool, dry place. The syrup should be stored in a cool place, protected from direct sunlight.
Choledyl tablets and syrup should be stored in a dry place, protected from light and at a temperature that does not exceed 25°.
Labophylline injection should be stored below 25° and should not be frozen.
Nuelin preparations should be stored in a cool, dry place.
Slo-Phyllin capsules should be stored below 25° in a dry place.
Uniphyllin Continus tablets should be stored at room temperature in a dry place and protected from light.

PHYSICAL PROPERTIES

Theophylline is a white crystalline powder; odourless, with a bitter taste.
Choline theophyllinate is a white crystalline powder; odourless or with a faint amine-like odour.
Theophylline hydrate is a white crystalline powder; odourless.
Theophylline monoethanolamine is a white crystalline powder.
Theophylline sodium glycinate is a white crystalline powder; it has a slight ammoniacal odour and a bitter taste.

Melting point

Theophylline melts in the range 270° to 274°.
Choline theophyllinate melts in the range 185° to 192°.
Theophylline hydrate melts at about 272°, after drying.

pH

A saturated solution of *theophylline sodium glycinate* has a pH of 8.5 to 9.5.

Dissociation constants

$pK_a < 1$, 8.6 (theophylline at 25°)

Partition coefficient

Log P (octanol), 0.0 (theophylline)

Solubility

Theophylline is soluble 1 in 120 of water (it is more soluble in hot water), 1 in 80 of ethanol, 1 in 200 of chloroform; very slightly soluble in ether. Theophylline dissolves in solutions of alkali hydroxides, in aqueous ammonia, and in mineral acids.
Choline theophyllinate is soluble 1 in less than 1 of water and 1 in 10 of ethanol; very slightly soluble in chloroform and in ether.
Theophylline hydrate is soluble 1 in 120 of water and 1 in 80 of ethanol; slightly soluble in chloroform; very slightly soluble in ether. It dissolves in solutions of alkali hydroxides, in aqueous ammonia, and in mineral acids.
Theophylline monoethanolamine is soluble 1 in 20 of water.
Theophylline sodium glycinate is soluble 1 in 6 of water; very slightly soluble in ethanol; practically insoluble in chloroform.

Effect of cosolvents
In binary aqueous systems containing either ethanol or propylene glycol, solubility profiles demonstrated that theophylline solubility (at 30°) was greatest at cosolvent concentrations of 60% and 75%, respectively; profiles for macrogol 400 and dimethylformamide were also produced.[1] The solubility of theophylline decreased following hydrate formation. According to the amount of cosolvent in the system, the solid phase of theophylline was either the anhydrous or the monohydrate form.

Dissolution

The USP specifies that for Theophylline Capsules USP not less than 80% of the labelled amount of $C_7H_8N_4O_2$ is dissolved in 60 minutes. Dissolution medium: 900 mL of water; Apparatus 2 at 50 rpm.
The USP specifies that for Theophylline Tablets USP not less than 80% of the labelled amount of $C_7H_8N_4O_2$ is dissolved in 45 minutes. Dissolution medium: 900 mL of water; Apparatus 2 at 50 rpm.
The USP specifies that for Theophylline Sodium Glycinate Tablets USP not less than 75% of the labelled amount of anhydrous $C_7H_8N_4O_2$ is dissolved in 45 minutes. Dissolution medium: 900 mL of water; Apparatus 1 at 100 rpm.

Dissolution properties
Dissolution studies in simulated gastric and intestinal fluids showed that drug release from halved sustained-release theophylline 100 mg tablets (Theo-Dur, Astra, Canada) was significantly greater than from whole tablets. However, in bioavailability studies (in seven healthy volunteers) there were no significant differences between the areas under serum concentration versus time curves, or between mean serum concentrations.[2] Although significant differences were apparent between some of the dissolution profiles of whole versus halved theophylline 300 mg controlled-release tablets (eight brands tested), Shah et al[3] concluded that the differences were not sufficient to necessitate bioavailability studies on the halved tablets. Significant differences were observed between the profiles produced in the two test media (simulated gastric fluid and simulated intestinal fluid) and brand to brand variation was also apparent.
Marked variation was observed[4] between the dissolution profiles of five controlled-release theophylline dosage forms when tested in buffered media at pH 2.6 and 6.0. The dissolution rates of Theo-grad (Abbott) and Uniphyllin Continus (Napp) were independent of pH; Pro-Vent (Wellcome) showed slight

pH-dependency; the release of both Nuelin (Riker) and Theo-Dur (Fisons) was pH-dependent. The apparent first-order rate constants for theophylline release from each preparation were calculated.

Kinetic equations were applied to characterise the dissolution behaviour of eight marketed controlled-release theophylline dosage forms.[5] In phosphate buffer (pH 7.5) or 0.1M hydrochloric acid (pH 1) drug release followed apparent first-order kinetics and was controlled by both diffusion and dissolution. The first-order equation and the Hixon-Crowell cube root law were suggested to characterise most suitably the dissolution of controlled-release preparations of theophylline.

FURTHER INFORMATION. Dissolution of theophylline monohydrate and anhydrous theophylline in buffer solutions—de Smidt JH, Fokkens JG, Grijseels H, Crommelin DJA. J Pharm Sci 1986;75(5):497–501. Dissolution kinetics of theophylline [model drug] in aqueous polymer solutions [hypromellose and povidone as model polymers]—de Smidt JH, Offringa JCA, Crommelin DJA. Int J Pharmaceutics 1991;77:255–9. Dissolution of theophylline from sustained-release dosage forms and correlation with saliva bioavailability parameters—Chung B-H, Shim C-K. J Pharm Sci 1987;76(10):784–7. Effect of pH on the *in vitro* dissolution and *in vivo* absorption of controlled-release theophylline in dogs—Vashi VI, Meyer MC. J Pharm Sci 1988;77(9):760–4. Dissolution profiling of six modified-release oral solid dosage forms—Baweja R. Drug Dev Ind Pharm 1986;12(14):2431–42. *In vitro* testing of controlled release theophylline preparations: Theolair, Theograd and Theolin [comparison of three methods of dissolution testing]—Crombeen JP, De Blaey CJ. Pharm Weekbl (Sci) 1983;5:65–9. Validation of the *in vitro* dissolution method used for a new sustained-release theophylline pellet formulation—Dietrich R, Brausse R, Bautz A, Diletti E. Arzneimittelforschung 1988;38(II)Nr 8a:1220–8. A novel approach to the specification of *in vitro* dissolution boundaries based on regulatory requirements for bioequivalence—Steinijans VW, Dietrich R, Trautmann H, Sauter R, Benedikt G. Arzneimittelforschung 1988;38(II)Nr 8a:1238–40. *In vitro* dissolution behaviour of some sustained-release theophylline dosage forms—Lin S-Y, Yang J-C. Pharm Acta Helv 1989;64(8):236–40.

Crystal and molecular structure

Phase transition and heterogeneous/epitaxial nucleation of hydrated and anhydrous theophylline crystals—Rodríguez-Hornedo N, Lechuga-Ballesteros D, Wu H-J. Int J Pharmaceutics 1992;85:149–62.

STABILITY

Theophylline base is sensitive to light, with the appearance of a yellow discoloration following extended exposure; it is stable in air.

Solutions

Solutions of theophylline are stable over a wide range of pH although they may decompose at low and high pH values.
There was no decrease in theophylline concentration after aqueous solutions of theophylline 0.1% with pH values of 3, 5, 6.5, and 7 were autoclaved at 120° for 20 minutes.[6]

Crystal growth in tablets

During storage at 90% relative humidity, growth of theophylline hydrate crystals was observed on the surface of two anhydrous theophylline tablet formulations that contained either magnesium chloride or potassium acetate (both hygroscopic materials).[7] No crystal growth was seen in a third formulation

that did not contain either of these excipients or in any samples stored at lower relative humidity values (59% and 75%).

FURTHER INFORMATION. Effect of surface characteristics of theophylline anhydrate powder on hygroscopic stability—Otsuka M, Kaneniwa N, Kawakami K, Umezawa O. J Pharm Pharmacol 1990;42:606–10. Effect of moisture on crystallization of theophylline in tablets—Ando H, Ishii M, Kayano M, Ozawa H. Drug Dev Ind Pharm 1992;18:453–67. Effect of humidity and packaging on the long-term aging of commercial sustained-release theophylline tablets—Sánchez E, Evora CM, Llabrés M. Int J Pharmaceutics 1992;83:59–63.

INCOMPATIBILITY/COMPATIBILITY

Plastics

Unit doses of theophylline oral liquid (Elixophyllin, Berlex, USA) repackaged in polypropylene syringes and capped glass vials were stable during storage for 180 days at 4° and 25° under constant moisture conditions, protected from light.[8] In samples stored at higher temperatures, in both syringes and vials, volume reduction was observed after 60 days and a reduction in alcohol content of the elixir resulted in theophylline precipitation.

After storage at 24° ± 1° under fluorescent lighting for 180 days, samples of an alcohol-free liquid theophylline preparation, repackaged in both clear and amber disposable polypropylene unit-dose syringes, retained at least 96% of their mean initial concentration.[9] Reductions in the volume of the liquid preparation and increases in theophylline concentration were statistically insignificant.

Intravenous admixtures

Following the addition of verapamil hydrochloride injection to premixed solutions of theophylline (Abbott) 0.4 mg/mL and 4.0 mg/mL in glucose 5% injection (final verapamil concentrations of 0.1 mg/mL and 0.4 mg/mL) and storage in glass flasks at 24° ± 1° under fluorescent light for 24 hours, macroscopic and microscopic examination demonstrated all solutions to be stable, indicating chemical compatibility.[10]

Johnson *et al*[11] prepared admixtures of premixed theophylline (Abbott) 4.0 mg/mL and 0.4 mg/mL in glucose 5% injection and methylprednisolone sodium succinate (Solu-Medrol, Upjohn) with final concentration equivalent to 2.0 mg/mL or 0.5 mg/mL of the active methylprednisolone alcohol. The solutions were stored in glass flasks at room temperature (stated to be 37°) under fluorescent light for 24 hours. Although theophylline was stable in all the test solutions, methylprednisolone sodium succinate had limited stability in the presence of the lower concentration of theophylline in glucose solution. In solutions that initially contained methylprednisolone sodium succinate 2.0 mg/mL and either theophylline 4.0 mg/mL or 0.4 mg/mL an increase in the concentration of methylprednisolone alcohol was detected after 3 and 12 hours, respectively. It was concluded that the two test solutions can be mixed (at concentrations that do not exceed the experimental values) providing that they are administered within 24 hours of admixture.

FURTHER INFORMATION. Interactions between lignocaine and caffeine, theophylline and theobromine—Martinez L, Gutierrez P, Hernandez A, Martinez PJY, Thomas J [Spanish]. An R Acad Farm 1986;52:505–16.

FORMULATION

Excipients

Excipients that have been used in presentations of theophylline include:

Capsules, theophylline: calcium stearate; Eudragit L and S; maize starch; povidone; shellac; stearic acid; sucrose; talc; triacetin.

Tablets, theophylline: carmellose sodium; cellacephate; lactose; magnesium stearate; talc.

Theophylline hydrate: acacia; butyl stearate; cellacephate; colloidal silica; glucose; gluten; hypromellose; lactose; magnesium stearate; patent blue V (E131); quinoline yellow (E104); shellac; sucrose.

Theophylline monoethanolamine: acacia; gelatin; kaolin; magnesium stearate; maize starch; shellac; sucrose; titanium dioxide (E171).

Oral liquids, theophylline: ammoniated liquorice; ethanol; glycerol; methyl hydroxybenzoate; orange flower water; potassium anisate; potassium hydroxide; sucrose.

Theophylline sodium glycinate: sodium butyl hydroxybenzoate; sucrose.

Suppositories, theophylline hydrate: chlorophyll; semi-synthetic glycerides.

Injections, theophylline hydrate: disodium phosphate.

Bioavailability

The bioavailability and release characteristics of two theophylline and two aminophylline sustained-release preparations and a standard theophylline solution were compared in seven healthy subjects.[12] Differences in formulation methods between older and more recently introduced products were thought to explain partly the marked variation in the extents of bioavailability observed (mean $\pm$ SD; 78% $\pm$ 40% to 123% $\pm$ 23%). The role of modern technology in the production of sustained-release theophylline preparations was discussed.

No statistical difference was observed between the bioavailabilities (in eight healthy volunteers) of Somophyllin-CRT capsules (Fisons), which contained theophylline 250 mg, and Theo-Dur tablets (Key Pharmaceuticals) which contained 300 mg theophylline.[13] The tablets were absorbed at a more variable rate than the capsules. Absorption profiles produced by the two preparations differed markedly between individual subjects.

In multidose studies (in 18 healthy fasted and non-fasted adults) bioavailability of Austyn sustained-release capsules (200 mg and 300 mg; Faulding Australia) containing theophylline as sustained-release pellets, compared well with that of reference rapid-release Nuelin tablets (50 mg and 125 mg; Riker, Australia) and Theo-Dur sustained-release tablets (200 mg and 300 mg; Astra, Australia).[14]

At steady state, bioequivalence was evident between a once-daily theophylline capsule (Euphylong, Byk Gulden, Germany) and the twice-daily administration of theophylline tablets (Theo-Dur, Key Pharmaceuticals, USA).[15] The study (in 18 adults) indicated that absorption from the once-daily product was slightly less and peak to trough fluctuations greater when compared with those of the twice-daily tablet.

When the contents of a sustained-release theophylline capsule (Slo-Phyllin 250 Gyrocap, Dooner Laboratories) were mixed with two teaspoonfuls of apple sauce and administered to 12 healthy adults, the resulting theophylline bioavailability was comparable to that produced by an intact sustained-release theophylline capsule (Slo-Phyllin 250 Gyrocap, Dooner Laboratories) and also a liquid preparation (Slo-Phyllin-80 syrup, Dooner Laboratories). The test preparation also retained the sustained-release properties of the original capsule.[16]

In a comparison of a fast-dissolving tablet (Oxyphyllin, Draco, Sweden) and a sustained-release tablet (Theo-Dur, Draco, Sweden) in healthy adults, no significant difference in bioavailability of theophylline was evident between the two products.[17] The extent of absorption was similar for both products although, as expected, the rates of absorption differed considerably; absorption was completed within 2 hours for the fast-dissolving tablets and continued over 12 hours for the sustained-release preparation.

Bioequivalence

Al-Angary *et al*[18] demonstrated differences in the dissolution behaviour (in a dissolution medium of simulated gastric fluid pH 1.2 for one hour followed by simulated intestinal fluid pH 7.5) of two commercially available sustained-release theophylline 300 mg tablets (Quibron, Mead Johnson, USA and Theodur, Recordati, Italy); $t_{50\%}$ values were 40 minutes and 6.5 hours, respectively. They observed pH-dependent dissolution in the case of Theodur, but not of Quibron. Bioavailability data in six healthy volunteers (measured by salivary concentration) indicated bioequivalence of the products. A direct correlation was perceived between the percent absorbed *in vivo* and the percent dissolved *in vitro* for each product.

Intravenous infusion

The formulation for an intravenous infusion used clinically in Norway consisted of theophylline monohydrate 1 g, glucose (anhydrous, for parenteral use) 50 g, and water for injections 969 g to produce a final volume of 1000 mL. When autoclaved at 120° for 20 minutes, no reduction in theophylline or glucose concentration was detected,[6] although the pH of the solution fell from 6.30 to 4.45.

Percutaneous absorption

Touitou *et al*[19] measured the permeation of theophylline, through hairless *mouse* skin, from different types of basis (macrogol; water-in-oil cream; Carbopol hydroalcoholic gel; ointment), with and without the inclusion of penetration enhancers, using Franz diffusion cells. The water-in-oil cream basis had the highest theophylline skin/carrier partition coefficient and this was reflected by the observation that it produced the greatest permeation flux. However, the most efficient basis studied consisted of a mixture of macrogols 400 and 4000 with a combination of oleic acid 10% and diethylene glycol monoethyl ether 20% (Transcutol) as permeation enhancers.

Hydrogel discs prepared by cross-linking poly-2-hydroxyethylmethacrylate 90% w/w with polytetramethylene oxide 10% w/w were loaded (by swelling in a saturated solution) with choline theophyllinate.[20] Following repeated application of the discs to the skin of five preterm infants, therapeutic serum concentrations were reached and maintained for several days. The authors concluded that transdermal delivery resulted in a therapeutic response similar to that achieved following oral or intravenous theophylline to preterm infants.

Evans *et al*[21] prepared a gel comprising theophylline sodium glycinate 15% w/v in hydroxymethylcellulose 5%. Percutaneous administration under an occlusive dressing (of doses equivalent to 17 mg anhydrous theophylline) to 13 premature infants (aged 1 to 20 days) produced therapeutic drug concentrations (4 to 12 mg/L) within 30 hours of application in all except 2 infants; blood concentrations remained in the therapeutic range for up to 72 hours. When the gel was administered to 12 infants who had previously received intravenous aminophylline therapy, blood-theophylline concentrations were maintained or increased compared to those produced by the infusion.

Suppositories

With the aim of formulating a suppository vehicle from which theophylline would be rapidly released, Moës[22] prepared two fatty bases (containing Witepsol H12 and W25) and three water-soluble bases (consisting of mixtures of macrogols 400, 1500, 4000, and 6000 to give average molecular weights of 2380, 2570, and 4500). Suppositories containing, in each, anhydrous theophylline 375 mg were prepared in 2-gram moulds; soft gelatin rectal capsules were also included in the study. Measurements included intrinsic dissolution rates, solubility, partition coefficients, and in-vitro release characteristics. Faster release rates were observed from suppositories with water-soluble bases and experimental data indicated that mixtures of high molecular weight macrogols, with low dielectric constant values, should be used to prepare the vehicle. The suppository that incorporated theophylline in the macrogol blend of molecular weight 2570 was recommended for in-vivo studies in humans. An in-vitro study of five formulations of theophylline suppositories indicated that, among the bases studied, Suppocire AP (Gattefoss Est) followed by Suppocire AM were the two most favoured vehicles.[23] The suppositories were stored at 4° or 30° for 8 days and subjected to a number of physicochemical tests. The release kinetics of suppositories stored at 4° were examined in a dissolution medium of purified water at 36.5° ± 0.5°.

Modified-release preparations

The choice of filler included in theophylline 300 mg controlled-release tablets had a marked effect on the dissolution profiles of various formulations.[24] Each dosage form contained theophylline 60%, Eudragit S100 10% (an acrylic resin release retardant), fumed silica 1.5%, magnesium stearate 0.5%, and the chosen filler 28% (either microcrystalline cellulose, lactose, glucose, sucrose, or calcium sulphate). Drug release was most rapid from tablets prepared with microcrystalline cellulose. Calcium sulphate was the filler that produced tablets with slowest drug release. In acidic media, inclusion of the acrylic resin decreased the dissolution rate whereas in phosphate buffer (pH 7.4) the rate was increased.

Ritschel and Gangadharan[25] examined various formulations based on the hydrophilic matrix principle with the aim of developing a theophylline dosage form with controlled, zero-order release over a 12-hour period. A formulation composed of anhydrous theophylline 200 mg/unit, hypromellose 120 mg/unit, distilled water 0.11 mg/unit and talc 8.3 mg/unit produced the most favourable results in in-vitro tests.

A sustained-release theophylline tablet formulation with a matrix base containing Precirol (glycerol palmito-stearate, Gattefosse Corp, NY) and lactose was prepared.[26] Dissolution tests in 0.1M hydrochloric acid and in phosphate buffer (pH 7.4) indicated that the rate of theophylline release was greater from tablets containing Precirol 5% than from those containing either 7.5% or 10% of the excipient. All preparations released 100% of the drug within 24 hours and release from the tablets containing Precirol 10% was independent of pH.

Workers in Germany[27] demonstrated that the relative bioavailability of an oral theophylline depot preparation, as microcapsules, was 92% of that of an aqueous solution following a single administration to seven volunteers.

The release in vitro of theophylline from sustained-release or controlled-release preparations commercially available in the UK was examined by Li Wan Po et al[28] using 'drug-release' models. The release of drug from all products studied (Lasma, Nuelin SA 250, Phyllocontin, Pro-Vent, Sabidal, Slo-Phyllin, Theo-Dur, Theograd, and Uniphyllin) showed varying degrees of pH dependency. Changes in ionic strength also had a marked effect on drug release from some products. The authors considered that theophylline sustained-release products are not clinically interchangeable without dose readjustment to achieve steady-state blood concentrations.

Effects of excipients

Diluents

Herman et al[29] undertook a comprehensive study to identify the causes of variations in the dissolution and drug release rates of formulations that contained anhydrous theophylline and microcrystalline cellulose. Four formulations were examined: two containing anhydrous theophylline and Avicel PH 101 (microcrystalline cellulose); one with theophylline monohydrate and Avicel PH 101; and one containing anhydrous theophylline and Sta RX-1500. Simulated pellets and tablets were prepared and stored under different conditions of relative humidity and packaging; they were then subjected to dissolution, X-ray diffraction, and weight-determination tests. Variations in drug release following storage were not attributed to the interconversion between polymorphs (anhydrous theophylline and the monohydrate), which was known to occur. It was suggested that storage in a humid environment promoted the formation of additional bindings between theophylline and microcrystalline cellulose, which resulted in a decrease in drug release rate. Processing by wet granulation also reduced drug release rate. The use of an alternative diluent, such as Sta RX-1500 (directly compressible starch), overcame the stability problems associated with microcrystalline cellulose in theophylline preparations.

Lubricants

The effects of incorporating different hydrophobic (magnesium stearate or powdered hydrogenated vegetable oil (Sterotex)) and hydrophilic (sodium lauryl sulphate or macrogol 6000) lubricants in directly compressed tablets containing anhydrous theophylline (200 mg), glucose (Emdex), and talc have been examined.[30] Good compaction properties were observed with the hydrophobic lubricants but the extents of disintegration and dissolution were low. The hydrophilic lubricants produced tablets with faster disintegration and dissolution rates, but sodium lauryl sulphate had poor lubricating properties. A combination of magnesium stearate and sodium lauryl sulphate resulted in tablets with enhanced drug release compared with those formulated with magnesium stearate alone and superior compaction properties to those tablets that contained only sodium lauryl sulphate.

Disintegrants

The disintegrant properties of a hydrogel were comparable to those of microcrystalline cellulose (Avicel PH 101), Ac-Di-Sol (a cross-linked form of carmellose sodium), maize starch, and Primojel (sodium starch glycollate) in directly compressed tablets containing anhydrous theophylline as the active drug.[31]

Coatings

Calcium hydrogen phosphate was incorporated in a tablet coating (as a pore former) by dispersion in an aqueous latex composed of poly(ethylacrylate-methylmethacrylate).[32] Core tablets containing theophylline, lactose, and magnesium stearate were coated with the microporous membrane and dissolution studies indicated a constant release rate of theophylline from the tablets. With increasing concentrations of pore former, the lag time before release decreased and the amount and rate of drug release increased. Increasing the membrane thickness retarded theophylline release; alteration of the rate of agitation had minimal effect.

Munday and Fassihi[33] prepared 'mini-tablets' containing anhydrous theophylline, carmellose sodium (as a 5% w/v aqueous paste), and magnesium stearate 0.5% w/w and examined the coating properties of several water-insoluble and water-soluble polymers and their effect on drug release from the dosage forms. The composition and thickness of the polymer film and the choice of dissolution medium affected the *in-vitro* drug release profiles obtained. The authors concluded that a set number of 'mini-tablets' with different coating thicknesses could be enclosed in a hard gelatin capsule to produce the required rate of theophylline release.

FURTHER INFORMATION. Influence of formulation on bioavailability of theophylline. Welling PG, Domoradzki J, Sims JA, Reed CE. J Clin Pharmacol 1976;16:43–50. Comparison of theophylline blood levels after oral administration of two different galenic forms to asthmatic children—Albuquerque MM, Gaudy D, Castel J, Durand H, Jacob M, Duru C [French]. J Pharmacol Clin 1988;7(2):281–93. Enhanced permeation of theophylline through the skin [from a macrogol base with oleic acid and Transcutol] and its effect on fibroblast proliferation—Touitou E, Levi-Schaffer F, Shaco-Ezra N, Ben-Yossef R, Fabin B. Int J Pharmaceutics 1991;70:159–66. Influence of surfactants, polymers, and concentration of the water phase on *in vitro* drug release from emulsion-type suppositories—Noro S, Komatsu Y, Uesugi T. Chem Pharm Bull 1982;30(8):2912–18. Influence of adjuvants of polyethylene glycol suppositories on the physical characteristics and drug bioavailability in *rabbits* [comprehensive study of theophylline suppositories formulated with macrogol bases with various additives]. Fassihi AR, Dowse R, Daya S. Drug Dev Ind Pharm 1989;15(2):235–51. Design and formulation of sustained release theophylline dosage forms [comprehensive review of design, formulation, and manufacture of sustained-release products]—Shangraw RF. Drug Dev Ind Pharm 1988;14(2&3):319–35. A new sustained-release theophylline suspension for asthmatic children: evaluation of serum theophylline concentrations—Boner AL, Vallone G, Valletta E, Bernocchi D, Plebani M. Int J Clin Pharmacol Res 1987;VII(5):345–50. Sustained release from inert matrices. I. Effect of microcrystalline cellulose on aminophylline and theophylline release—Said S, Al-Shora H. Int J Pharmaceutics 1980;6:11–18. *In vitro* and *in vivo* evaluation of a controlled release preparation of theophylline [multilayer model containing anhydrous theophylline, Eudragit RS, ethylcellulose, Emcompress, lactose, talc, and magnesium stearate]—Fassihi AR. J Pharm Pharmacol 1988;40:32P. Galenical development of a new sustained-release theophylline pellet formulation for once-daily administration [characteristics of *in-vitro* drug release from a 'micro-osmotic system' are examined, leading to prediction of the effect of varying membrane porosity and thickness on *in-vivo* absorption]—Benedikt G, Steinijans VW, Dietrich R. Arzneimittelforschung 1988;38(II)Nr 8a:1203–9.
Sustained-release from Precirol (glycerol palmito-stearate) matrix. Effect of mannitol and hydroxypropyl methylcellulose [hypromellose] on the release of theophylline—Parab PV, Oh CK, Ritschel WA. Drug Dev Ind Pharm 1986;12(8&9):1309–27. Modified starches as hydrophilic matrices for controlled oral delivery. III. Evaluation of sustained-release theophylline formulations based on thermal modified starch matrices in *dogs*—Herman J, Remon JP. Int J Pharmaceutics 1990;63:201–5. Performance of a modified starch hydrophilic matrix for the sustained release of theophylline in healthy volunteers—Vandenbossche GMR, Lefebvre RA, De Wilde GA, Remon J-P. J Pharm Sci 1992;81(3):245–8. *In vitro* controlled release of theophylline from tablets containing a silicone elastomer latex—Li LC. Int J Pharmaceutics 1992;87:117–24. Development of a new controlled-release theophylline tablet: *in-vitro* and *in-vivo* studies [evaluation of three carriers and influence of filler choice on dissolution rate; *in-vitro* comparison with Theodur]—Georgarakis M, Panagopoulou A, Hatzipantou P, Iliopoulos T, Kondylis M, Grekas D. Drug Dev Ind Pharm 1990;16(2):315–29. Eudragit RL and RS pseudolatices: proper-

ties and performance in pharmaceutical coating as a controlled release membrane for theophylline pellets—Chang R-K, Hsiao C. Drug Dev Ind Pharm 1989;15(2):187–96. Effect of drug (core) particle size on the dissolution of theophylline from microspheres made from low molecular weight cellulose acetate propionate—Shukla AJ, Price JC. Pharm Res 1989;6(5):418–21. Effect of drug loading and molecular weight of cellulose acetate propionate on the release characteristics of theophylline microspheres—Shukla AJ, Price JC. Pharm Res 1991;8:1396–1400. Development and *in-vitro* evaluation of a multiparticulate sustained release theophylline formulation—Yuen KH, Deshmukh AA, Newton JM. Drug Dev Ind Pharm 1993;19(8):855–74. Formulation parameters affecting the preparation and properties of microencapsulated ion-exchange resins containing theophylline [microencapsulation with ethylcellulose]—Moldenhauer MG, Nairn JG. J Pharm Sci 1990;79(8):659–66.
Effect of excipients on tablet properties and dissolution behaviour of theophylline-tabletted microcapsules under different compression forces—Lin S-Y. J Pharm Sci 1988;77(3):229–32. Bioavailability studies [in *rats*] of theophylline ethylcellulose microcapsules prepared by using ethylene-vinyl acetate copolymer as a coacervation-inducing agent [favourable sustained-release behaviour and *in-vitro/in-vivo* correlation]—Lin S-Y, Yang J-C. J Pharm Sci 1987;76(3):219–23. Formation and *in vitro* evaluation of theophylline-loaded poly(methyl methacrylate) microspheres—Pongpaibul Y, Maruyama K, Iwatsuni M. J Pharm Pharmacol 1988;40:530–3. Modelling of theophylline compound release from hard gelatin capsules containing gelucire matrix granules—Brossard C, Ratsimbazafy V, Lefort des Ylouses D. Drug Dev Ind Pharm 1991;17(10)1267–77. Controlled theophylline release from microcapsules of acrylic and methacrylic acid ester copolymer—Chattaraj SC, Das SK, Karthikeyan M, Ghosal SK, Gupta BK. Drug Dev Ind Pharm 1991;17(4):551–60. Changes in drug release rate: effect of stress storage conditions on film-coated mini-tablets—Munday DL, Fassihi AR. Drug Dev Ind Pharm 1991;17(15):2135–43. Xanthan gum and alginate based controlled-release theophylline formulations—Fu Lu M, Woodward L, Borodkin S. Drug Dev Ind Pharm 1991;17(14):1987–2004. Development of a new controlled—release theophylline tablet: *in vitro* and *in vivo* studies—Georgarakis M, Panagopoulou A, Hatzipantou P, Iliopoulos T, Kandylis M, Grekas D. Drug Dev Ind Pharm 1990;16(2):315–29. The effect of film-coating additives on the *in vitro* dissolution release rate of ethylcellulose-coated theophylline granules—Li SP, Mehta GN, Buehler JD, Grim WM, Harwood RJ. Pharmaceut Technol 1990;14:20–4. Bioavailability and pharmacokinetics of new sustained-release theophylline microcapsules after single and multiple oral administration—Lin SY, Wang SR, Chang HN. Curr Ther Res 1990;48:524–34. Release control of theophylline by β-cyclodextrin derivatives: hybridizing effect of hydrophilic, hydrophobic and ionizable β-cyclodextrin complexes—Horiuchi Y, Abe K, Hirayama F, Uekama K. J Controlled Release 1991;15:177–83.

PROCESSING

Effect of tableting pressure on hydration kinetics of theophylline anhydrate tablets—Otsuka M, Kaneniwa N, Kawakami K, Umezawa O. J Pharm Pharmacol 1991;43:226–31. Effect of tableting pressure and geometrical factor of tablet on dehydration kinetics of theophylline monohydrate tablets—Otsuka M, Kaneniwa N, Otsuka K, Kawakami K, Umezawa O. Drug Dev Ind Pharm 1993;19(5):541–57. Preparation of coated particles using a spray drying process with an aqueous system—Wan LSC, Heng PWS, Chia CGH. Int J Pharmaceutics 1991;77:183–91.

REFERENCES

1. Gould PL, Howard JR, Oldershaw GA. Int J Pharmaceutics 1989;51:195–202.
2. Simons JK, Frith EM, Simons FER. J Pharm Sci 1982;71(5):505–11.
3. Shah VP, Yamamoto LA, Schuirman D, Elkins J, Skelly JP. Pharm Res 1987;4(5):416–19.
4. Buckton G, Ganderton D, Shah R. Int J Pharmaceutics 1988;42:35–9.
5. Jalal I, Zmaily E, Najib N. Int J Pharmaceutics 1989;52:63–70.
6. Askerud L, Finholt P, Karlsen J, Kure R. Medd Norsk Farm Selsk 1981;43:17–24.
7. Ando H, Ohwaki T, Ishii M, Watanabe S, Miyake Y. Int J Pharmaceutics 1986;34:153–6.
8. Christensen JM, Lee R-Y, Parrott KA. Am J Hosp Pharm 1983;40:612–15.
9. Johnson CE, Drabik BT. Am J Hosp Pharm 1989;46:980–1.
10. Johnson CE, Lloyd CW, Aviles AI, Rybarz KL. Am J Hosp Pharm 1988;45:609–12.
11. Johnson CE, Cohen IA, Michelini TJ, McMahon RE. Am J Hosp Pharm 1987;44:1620–4.
12. Summers RS, Summers B, Rawnsley S. Int J Pharmaceutics 1986;30:83-8.
13. Ferrari M, Olivieri M, Barozzi E, Ramponi C. Clin Ther 1986;8(6):646–54.
14. West RJ, Boehm G, Dwyer M, Williams DB, Sansom LN, Penna AC. Biopharm Drug Dispos 1990;11:165–77.
15. Jonkman JNG, Steinijans VW, Beier W, Yska JP, Kerkhof FA, de Noord OE, Grasmeyer G. Int J Pharmaceutics 1988;43:139–43.
16. Green ER, Green AW, Lanc R, Slaughter R, Middleton E. J Pediatr 1981;98(5):832–4.
17. Fagerström PO, Mellstrand T, Svedmyr N. Int J Clin Pharmacol Ther Toxicol 1981;19(3):131–8.
18. Al-Angary AA, Khidr SH, Mahrous GM, Gouda MW. Int J Pharmaceutics 1990;65:R5–R8.
19. Touitou E, Levi-Schaffer F, Shaco-Ezra N, Ben-Yossef R, Fabin B. Int J Pharmaceutics 1991;70:159–66.
20. Cartwright RG, Cartlidge PHT, Rutter N, Melia CD, Davis SS. Br J Clin Pharmacol 1990;29:533–9.
21. Evans NJ, Rutter N, Hadgraft J, Parr G. J Pediatr 1985;107(2):307–11.
22. Moës AJ. Pharm Acta Helv 1981;56(1):21–5.
23. Zuber M, Pellion B, Arnauld P, Chaumeil JC. Int J Pharmaceutics 1988;47:31–6.
24. Cameron CG, McGinity JW. Drug Dev Ind Pharm 1987;13(2):303–18.
25. Ritschel WA, Gangadharan B. Pharm Ind 1988;50(3):355–9.
26. Saraiya D, Bolton S. Drug Dev Ind Pharm 1990;16(13):1963–9.
27. Lippold VBC, Förster H [German]. Arzneimittelforschung 1984;34(II)Nr 7:824–927.
28. Li Wan Po A, Wong LP, Gilligan CA. Int J Pharmaceutics 1990;66:111–30.
29. Herman J, Visavarungroj N, Remon JP. Int J Pharmaceutics 1989;55:143–6.
30. Naidoo NT, Beare MA, Kanfer I, Sparrow N. S Afr Pharm J 1986;53:100–3.
31. Fassihi AR. J Pharm Pharmacol 1989;41:853–5.
32. Bodmeier R, Paeratakul O. J Pharm Sci 1990;79(10):925–8.
33. Munday DL, Fassihi AR. Int J Pharmaceutics 1989;52:109–14.

Thyroxine (BAN)   *Thyroid hormone*

Levothyroxine; L-thyroxine
O^4-(4-Hydroxy-3,5-di-iodophenyl)-3,5-di-iodo-L-tyrosine
$C_{15}H_{10}I_4NO_4 = 776.9$

Thyroxine Sodium (BANM)

Levothyroxine Sodium (rINN)
$C_{15}H_{10}I_4NNaO_4, xH_2O = 798.9$ (anhydrous)
CAS—51-48-9 (thyroxine); 55-03-8 (thyroxine sodium, anhydrous); 25416-65-3 (thyroxine sodium, hydrate)

Pharmacopoeial status

BP (thyroxine sodium); USP (levothyroxine sodium)

Preparations

Compendial
Thyroxine Tablets BP. Tablets containing, in each, the equivalent of 25, 50, and 100 micrograms of anhydrous thyroxine sodium are usually available.
Levothyroxine Sodium Tablets USP.

Non-compendial
Eltroxin (Evans). *Tablets*, thyroxine sodium 50 and 100 micrograms.
Various strengths of thyroxine sodium tablets are also available from APS, Cox, CP, Evans, Kerfoot.

Containers and storage

Solid state
Thyroxine Sodium BP should be kept in a well-closed container and protected from light.
Levothyroxine Sodium USP should be preserved in tight containers, protected from light.

Dosage forms
Thyroxine Tablets BP should be protected from light.
Levothyroxine Sodium Tablets USP should be preserved in tight, light-resistant containers.
Eltroxin tablets should be protected from light.
The USP directs that all containers that are in contact with solutions of thyroxine sodium should be composed of glass.

PHYSICAL PROPERTIES

Thyroxine sodium appears as an almost white or slightly brownish-yellow powder or a fine, slightly coloured, crystalline powder; odourless and tasteless; hygroscopic. It may take on a slight pink colour on exposure to light.

Melting point

Thyroxine crystals melt at 235° to 236°, with decomposition.

pH

A saturated aqueous solution of *thyroxine sodium* has a pH of about 8.9.

Dissociation constants

pK_a 2.2, 6.7, 10.1

Solubility

Thyroxine sodium is very slightly soluble in water; slightly soluble in ethanol; practically insoluble in acetone, in chloroform, and in ether. It is soluble in solutions of alkali hydroxides, in hot solutions of alkali carbonates, and in mineral acids.

Effect of pH

The solubility of thyroxine sodium decreases as pH falls. The solubility is increased when the pH is increased above pH 7.4.

Dissolution

The USP specifies that for Levothyroxine Sodium Tablets USP not less than 55% of the labelled amount of $C_{15}H_{10}I_4NNaO_4$ is dissolved in 80 minutes. Dissolution medium: 500 mL of 0.05M phosphate buffer, pH 7.4; Apparatus 2 at 100 rpm.

STABILITY

Thyroxine sodium is stable in dry air, but it may turn pink on exposure to light.
Exposure of thyroxine, in dilute aqueous solution, to high energy gamma radiation causes de-iodination and transformation into other iodinated organic molecules.[1]
Brower *et al*[2] found that when bulk samples of thyroxine sodium were subject to drying at 60° in a vacuum over phosphorus pentoxide, decomposition in the order of 10% to 15% in 4 hours occurred if the vacuum was not maintained below 10 mm of mercury. However, thyroxine sodium solutions in 0.01M methanolic sodium hydroxide were stable over a 6-month period when stored at 5°.

Tablets

Following extraction of thyroxine from thyroxine sodium tablets (during a stability-indicating HPLC analysis), results indicated that the 200 microgram pink tablets from one manufacturer contained an excipient or excipients that accelerated degradation of thyroxine.[3] This catalytic effect was suggested to require the presence of light.

FURTHER INFORMATION. Stability-indicating assay, dissolution, and content uniformity of [thyroxine] sodium in tablets—Richheimer SL, Amer TM. J Pharm Sci 1983;72:1349–51.

INCOMPATIBILITY/COMPATIBILITY

Apparent leaching of diethyl phthalate, present as a plasticiser in the desiccant, into one brand of thyroxine sodium tablets was detected in bottles containing 100 tablets, but not in bottles containing 1000 tablets; no leaching was detected in three other brands.[4]

FORMULATION

Excipients

Excipients that have been used in presentations of thyroxine sodium include:

Tablets: calcium hydrogen phosphate; cellulose; citric acid, anhydrous; lactose; magnesium stearate; maize starch; microcrystalline cellulose; ponceau 4R (E124); sodium starch glycollate; sunset yellow FCF (E110); talc.
Oral drops: ethanol; propylene glycol.
Injections: sodium hydroxide.

Bioequivalence

It was postulated by Dong *et al*[5] that the variability in thyroxine sodium content of tablets, which caused bioinequivalence between tablets with the same labelled content, was in part due to inadequate assay procedures; introduction of a more accurate HPLC assay method could result in greater uniformity. In conjunction with a clinical study that indicated bioequivalence in hypothyroid patients, Curry *et al*[6] concluded that two brands of thyroxine sodium tablets were bioequivalent because they were chemically equivalent, because micronised thyroxine sodium powder had been used to produce the tablets, and because of stringent quality control procedures during the production process. These factors contributed to the production of tablets with thyroxine sodium contents within 5% of the label claim.
Two thyroxine sodium tablets (Levothroid and Synthroid) were deemed therapeutically interchangeable after long-term therapy although the area under the plasma-thyroxine concentration versus time curve was significantly greater following administration of Levothroid than after Synthroid (in 18 patients).[7]

REFERENCES

1. Tata J. Clin Chim Acta 1959;4:427–37.
2. Brower JF, Toler DY, Reepmeyer JC. J Pharm Sci 1984;73:1315–17.
3. Das Gupta V, Odom C, Bethea C, Plattenburg J. J Clin Pharm Ther 1990;15:331–6.
4. Cafmeyer NR, Wolfson BB. Am J Hosp Pharm 1991;48:735–9.
5. Dong BJ, Young VR, Rapaport B [letter]. Drug Intell Clin Pharm 1986;20:77–8.
6. Curry SH, Gums JG, Williams LL, Curry RW, Wolfson BB. Drug Intell Clin Pharm 1988;22:589–91.
7. Blouin RA, Clifton GD, Adams MA, Foster TS, Flueck J. Clin Pharm 1989;8:588–92.

Timolol (BAN, USAN, rINN)

Beta-adrenoceptor antagonist
(*S*)-1-*tert*-Butylamino-3-(4-morpholino-1,2,5-thiadiazol-3-yl-oxy)propan-2-ol; (*S*)-1-[(1,1-dimethylethyl)amino]-3-[[4-(4-morpholinyl)-1,2,5-thiadiazol-3-yl]oxy]-2-propanol
$C_{13}H_{24}N_4O_3S = 316.4$

Timolol Maleate (BANM, USAN, rINNM)

$C_{13}H_{24}N_4O_3S,C_4H_4O_4 = 432.5$
CAS—26839-75-8 (timolol); 26921-17-5 (timolol maleate)

Pharmacopoeial status

BP, USP (timolol maleate)

Preparations

Compendial

Timolol Tablets BP (Timolol Maleate Tablets). Contain timolol maleate. Tablets containing, in each, 10 mg are usually available.
Timolol Eye Drops BP (Timolol Maleate Eye Drops). A sterile solution of timolol maleate in purified water. pH 6.5 to 7.5. Eye drops containing the equivalent of 0.25% w/v and 0.5% w/v of timolol are usually available.
Timolol Maleate Tablets USP.
Timolol Maleate Ophthalmic Solution USP. pH 6.5 to 7.5.
Timolol Maleate and Hydrochlorothiazide Tablets USP.

Non-compendial

Betim (Leo). *Tablets*, timolol maleate 10 mg.
Blocadren (MSD). *Tablets*, timolol maleate 10 mg.
Timoptol (MSD). *Eye drops*, timolol (as maleate) 0.25% w/v and 0.5% w/v.
Eye drops, preservative free, timolol (as maleate) 0.25% w/v and 0.5% w/v.

Containers and storage

Solid state

Timolol Maleate BP should be kept in a well-closed container and protected from light.
Timolol Maleate USP should be preserved in well-closed containers.

Dosage forms

Timolol Maleate Tablets USP should be preserved in well-closed containers.
Timolol Maleate Ophthalmic Solution USP should be preserved in tight, light-resistant containers.
The container for Blocadren tablets should be kept well closed. Storage should be in a cool place, protected from light.
Timoptol eye drops should be protected from light. They are stable at room temperature.

PHYSICAL PROPERTIES

Timolol maleate exists as a white or almost white crystalline powder or as colourless crystals.

Melting point

Timolol maleate melts at about 199°, with decomposition.

pH

pH of a 2% w/v solution of *timolol maleate*, 3.8 to 4.3.

Dissociation constant

pK_a 8.8
pK_a values of 9.03[1] and 9.21[2] have been determined by potentiometric titration at 20° and 35°, respectively.

Partition coefficient

Log P (water/octanol),[3] 1.98
An octanol-water partition coefficient of 82.0 (log P, 1.91) was calculated[2] at pH 7.4 at 35°.

Solubility

Timolol maleate is soluble 1 in 15 of water, 1 in 21 of ethanol, and in methanol; it is sparingly soluble in chloroform (1 in 40) and in propylene glycol; it is practically insoluble or insoluble in ether and in cyclohexane.

Dissolution

The USP specifies that for Timolol Maleate Tablets USP not less than 80% of the labelled amount of timolol maleate ($C_{13}H_{24}N_4O_3S,C_4H_4O_4$) is dissolved in 20 minutes. Dissolution medium: 500 mL of 0.1N hydrochloric acid; Apparatus 1 at 100 rpm.

STABILITY

Timolol maleate is reported[4] to be extremely stable at room temperature both in the solid state and in aqueous solutions (the latter protected from light). However, in solution, decomposition can occur on exposure to elevated temperatures or intense ultraviolet irradiation; the pH of maximum stability is about pH 4. Several degradation products (including isotimolol, 4-hydroxy-3-morpholino-1,2,5-thiadiazole, and 4-hydroxy-3-morpholino-1,2,5-thiadiazole 1-oxide) have been isolated. In the solid state, a 5% loss of timolol maleate was reported when it was heated at 95° for 3 weeks (100% relative humidity), whereas no decomposition was noted on exposure to intense ultraviolet irradiation, although surface discoloration was observed.
Eye drop solutions of timolol maleate 0.2% w/v at pH 2.6, 6.8, 9.7, and 11.8 were sterilised either by autoclaving at 110° for 30 minutes or by sterile filtration;[5] accelerated stability tests at 40°, 60°, and 80° were then undertaken. Optimum stability of timolol maleate was indicated at pH 6.8.

INCOMPATIBILITY/COMPATIBILITY

Adsorption of timolol onto various adsorbents was shown to decrease in the order: charcoal > magnesium trisilicate > regular attapulgite = colloidal attapulgite > kaolin.[6] In general, the extent of adsorption increased as the pH (range 0.5 to 8.5, at 37°) was increased whereas negligible change in the degree of adsorption occurred with increase in temperature (range 37° to 50°).

FORMULATION

Excipients

Excipients that have been used in presentations of timolol maleate include:
Tablets: indigo carmine (E132); magnesium stearate; microcrystalline cellulose; starch.
Eye drops: benzalkonium chloride; sodium acid phosphate; sodium hydroxide; sodium phosphate.

Bioavailability

The oral bioavailability of timolol relative to the intravenous route has been calculated as 75.8% and 61% ± 6% in studies involving five[7] and ten[8] healthy volunteers, respectively.

Transdermal delivery

Skin permeation *in vitro* of timolol maleate from a 10 mg/mL solution in buffer (pH 7.4) through human cadaver skin was significantly enhanced by the addition of lauryl chloride.[9] An increase in the concentration of lauryl chloride from 6% v/v to 10% v/v increased the total timolol maleate permeation, as did an increase in the duration of application. Dimethyl sulphoxide 10% v/v and oleic acid 10% v/v also enhanced permeation, although to a lesser extent.
Permeation of timolol through hairless *mouse* skin *in vitro* was studied from several reservoirs with or without a rate-controlling membrane (Silastic, polyethylene vinyl acetate, or microporous polypropylene).[1] The reservoirs were hydrophilic (4% carmellose sodium in purified water or 1% Carbopol 934 in purified water, adjusted to pH 7) or hydrophobic (4% Aerosil 200 in silicone fluid or Plastibase).

Ocular delivery

The release rate of timolol *in vitro* from a Gelrite (a polysaccharide, low-acetyl gellan gum) 0.6% solution was similar to that from a hydroxyethylcellulose 0.5% solution; both solutions contained timolol maleate 0.34% and mannitol (to achieve isotonicity).[10] However, in *rabbits*, greater ocular concentrations of timolol were measured from the Gelrite solution at all times during the study period.

In further work,[11] the ocular bioavailability of timolol (areas under concentration versus time curves over four hours in cornea, aqueous humour, and iris/ciliary body, in *rabbits*) was greater from solutions with 0.6% polyacrilic acid ('bioadhesive' polymer) and with polyvinyl alcohol ('non-mucoadhesive' polymer) than from the reference solution (Timoptol 0.5%).

The suitability of alkyl monoesters of poly(vinyl methyl ether-maleic anhydride) as bioerodible acidic polymers for topical controlled-release delivery of timolol maleate has been investigated *in vitro* and *in vivo*.[12–16] Mechanisms of release were elucidated and methods to improve the ocular:systemic absorption ratio were studied in *rabbits*.

FURTHER INFORMATION. Interpretation and prediction of the kinetics of transdermal drug delivery: oestradiol, hyoscine and timolol—Guy RH, Hadgraft J. Int J Pharmaceutics 1986;32:159–63. Finite dose percutaneous drug absorption: theory and its application to *in vitro* timolol permeation—Kubota K, Yamada T. J Pharm Sci 1990;79(11):1015–19. Effects of epinephrine pretreatment and solution pH on ocular and systemic absorption of ocularly applied timolol in *rabbits*—Kyyrönen K, Urtti A. J Pharm Sci 1990;79(8):688–91. Prodrugs of timolol for improved ocular delivery: synthesis, hydrolysis kinetics and lipophilicity of various timolol esters [*O*-acetyl, propionyl, butyryl and pivaloyl]—Bundgaard H, Buur A, Chang S-C, Lee VHL. Int J Pharmaceutics 1986;33:15–26. Timolol prodrugs: synthesis, stability and lipophilicity of various alkyl, cycloalkyl and aromatic esters of timolol—Bundgaard H, Buur A, Chang S-C, Lee VHL. Int J Pharmaceutics 1988;46:77–88. Nanoencapsulation of timolol by suspension and micelle polymerisation [successful preparation by micelle polymerisation (encapsulation of 50% of timolol) using nonionic surfactants and various stabilisers]—Harmia-Pulkkinen T, Ihantola A, Tuomi A, Kristoffersson E. Acta Pharm Fenn 1986;95(2):89–96. Preparation of biodegradable poly(lactic-co-glycolic) acid microspheres and their *in vitro* release of timolol maleate—Sturesson C, Carlfors J, Edsman K, Anderson M. Int J Pharmaceutics 1993;89:235–44. Controlled drug delivery devices for experimental ocular studies with timolol. 1. In vitro release studies—Urtti A, Pipkin JD, Rork G, Repta AJ. Int J Pharmaceutics 1990;61:235–40. 2. Ocular and systemic absorption in *rabbits*—Urtti A, Pipkin JD, Rork G, Sendo T, Finne U, Repta AJ. Int J Pharmaceutics 1990;61:241–9.

REFERENCES

1. O'Neill CT, Deasy PB. Int J Pharmaceutics 1988;48:247–54.
2. Schoenwald RD, Huang H-S. J Pharm Sci 1983;72(11):1266–72.
3. Burgot G, Serrand P, Burgot J-L. Int J Pharmaceutics 1990;63:73–6.
4. Mazzo DJ, Loper AE. In: Florey K, editor. Analytical profiles of drug substances; vol 16. London: Academic Press, 1987:641–92.
5. Güvener B, Cevher E. Acta Pharm Turcica 1989;31(4):169–76.
6. Al-Gohary O, Lyal J, Murray JB. Pharm Acta Helv 1988;63(1):13–18.
7. Else OF, Sorenson H, Edwards IR. Eur J Clin Pharmacol 1978;14:431–4.
8. Wilson TW, Firor WB, Johnson GE, Holmes GI, Tsianco MC, Huber PB *et al.* Clin Pharmacol Ther 1982;32(6):676–85.
9. Soni S, Jain SK, Jain NK. Drug Dev Ind Pharm 1992;18(10):1127–35.
10. Rozier A, Mazuel C, Grove J, Plazonnet B. Int J Pharmaceutics 1989;57:163–8.
11. Thermes F, Rozier A, Plazonnet B, Grove J. Int J Pharmaceutics 1992;81:59–65.
12. Finne U, Kyyrönen K, Urtti A. J Controlled Release 1989;10:189–94.
13. Finne U, Väisänen V, Urtti A. Int J Pharmaceutics 1990;65:19–27.
14. Finne U, Rönkkö KM, Urtti A. J Pharm Sci 1991;80(7):670–3.
15. Finne U, Hannus M, Urtti A. Int J Pharmaceutics 1992;78:237–41.
16. Finne U, Salivirta J, Urtti A. Int J Pharmaceutics 1991;75:R1–R4.

Tolbutamide (BAN, rINN)   *Antidiabetic*

Butamidum; tolglybutamide
1-Butyl-3-tosylurea; benzenesulfonamide, *N*-[(butylamino)carbonyl]-4-methyl-; 1-butyl-3-*p*-tolylsulphonylurea
$C_{12}H_{18}N_2O_3S = 270.35$

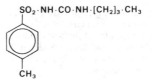

Tolbutamide Sodium (BANM, rINNM)
$C_{12}H_{17}N_2NaO_3S = 292.3$
CAS—64-77-7 (tolbutamide); 473-41-6 (sodium salt)

Pharmacopoeial status

BP, USP

Preparations

Compendial
Tolbutamide Tablets BP. Tablets containing, in each, 500 mg tolbutamide are usually available.
Tolbutamide Tablets USP.
Sterile Tolbutamide Sodium USP, prepared from tolbutamide with the aid of sodium hydroxide; it is suitable for parenteral use. pH between 8.0 and 9.8, in a solution containing 50 mg/mL.

Non-compendial
Rastinon (Hoescht). *Tablets*, tolbutamide 500 mg.
Tolbutamide tablets (50 mg) are also available from APS, Cox, CP, Evans, Kerfoot.

Containers and storage

Solid state
Tolbutamide BP should be kept in well-closed containers.
Tolbutamide USP should be preserved in well-closed containers.

Dosage forms
Sterile Tolbutamide Sodium USP should be kept in containers suitable for sterile solids.

Rastinon tablets should be stored at ambient temperature in a dry place, protected from light, in the original container or in containers similar to those of the manufacturer.

PHYSICAL PROPERTIES

Tolbutamide is a white or almost white, almost odourless, crystalline powder with a slightly bitter taste.
Sterile Tolbutamide Sodium is a white to off-white, practically odourless, crystalline powder, with a slightly bitter taste.

Melting point

Tolbutamide melts in the range 126° to 130°.
Tolbutamide sodium (anhydrous) melts in the range 130° to 133°.

Dissociation constant

pK_a 5.3 (20°)
Other reported values are 5.32 (37.5°) and 5.43 (25°).

Partition coefficient

Log P (octanol), 2.34

Solubility

Tolbutamide is practically insoluble in water; soluble 1 in 10 of ethanol, and 1 in 3 of acetone; soluble in chloroform; slightly soluble in ether. It forms water-soluble salts with alkalis and dissolves in dilute mineral acids.
Tolbutamide sodium is freely soluble in water; soluble in ethanol and in chloroform; slightly soluble in ether.

Effect of cosolvents
The solubility, flowability, and dissolution rate of tolbutamide[1] were improved after crystals of the drug had been modified by a spherical crystallisation method (a combination of crystallisation and agglomeration) in the presence of soluble polymers and surfactants including hypromellose, carmellose sodium, hydrogenated castor oil 60, and polyoxyl 40 stearate.

Dissolution

The USP specifies that for Tolbutamide Tablets USP not less than 70% of the labelled amount of $C_{12}H_{18}N_2O_3S$ is dissolved in 30 minutes. Dissolution medium: 900 mL of pH 7.4 phosphate buffer; Apparatus 2 at 75 rpm.

Dissolution properties
Workers in America[2] demonstrated that after formation of an inclusion complex with β-cyclodextrin, the solubility of tolbutamide was increased 2.5 fold. The dissolution rate of tolbutamide measured by USP XX method 2 at 60 rpm, pH 1.2 buffer at 37°, was considerably enhanced. The amount of tolbutamide dissolved after 20 minutes was 12% and 93% for tolbutamide alone and for the complex, respectively. Phase solubility studies indicated that at high concentrations of β-cyclodextrin, an insoluble microcrystalline complex precipitated which had a stoichiometry of 1:2 (tolbutamide:β-cyclodextrin). The inclusion complex[3] had a faster dissolution rate (USP XXI method, apparatus 2 at 75 rpm at 37°, pH 2) than either tolbutamide alone or in solid dispersion with macrogol 6000 prepared by co-precipitation or co-melting. The percentage of tolbutamide dissolved after 20 minutes was 19%, 33%, 38%, and 100% for the powdered drug, co-precipitate, co-melt, and inclusion complex, respectively. Partly pregelatinised maize starch (disintegrant) was mixed with tolbutamide and subjected to a novel spray-drying method to yield particles that enhanced the dissolution rate of poorly soluble tolbutamide.[4] Dissolution was more rapid than from either powdered tolbutamide alone or from a mixture of tolbutamide powder with either low-substituted hydroxypropylcellulose or maize starch. Rapid dissolution was noted from tablets prepared with spray-dried particles, although the rate was dependent on the drug-to-disintegrant ratio.

Crystal and molecular structure

Polymorphs
Two polymorphic forms of tolbutamide were isolated and characterised by Simmons and others[5] using recrystallisation techniques. Form A was obtained either by crystallisation from benzene-hexane or by precipitation from ammoniacal aqueous medium by treatment with acetic acid. Form B was crystallised from ethanol-water. At elevated temperatures (above 110°), Form B readily reverted to Form A. No significant differences were found in dissolution rate *in vitro* or absorption rate between the two forms in *dogs*.
The existence of two stable polymorphs of tolbutamide, with similar melting points (126° to 128°), was established by Leary *et al*,[6] using X-ray powder photography, infrared spectroscopy, and differential scanning calorimetry. Form A converted almost completely to Form B after repeated heating and cooling, but there was no tendency to convert from one form to the other at room temperature.

FURTHER INFORMATION. Examination of the compressibility of tolbutamide crystals. Kása Pintye-Hodi K, Szabo-Révész P, Miseta M, Selmeczi B, Traue J, Wenzel [German]. Pharmazie 1989;44:47–8. Preparation, characterisation and study of the polymorphs of tolbutamide—Georgarakis M [German]. Pharmazie 1989;44:209–10.

STABILITY

Decomposition of tolbutamide has been reported to occur by various routes, including hydrolysis and thermal dissociation. Products of the hydrolytic decomposition of tolbutamide tablets detected by Kaistha and French[7] were *n*-butylamine and *p*-toluenesulphonamide. A potential product, dibutyl urea was not detected in the tablets examined.
Following an earlier finding that the concentration of tolbutamide decreased significantly when it was dissolved in oil at 70° to 80°, Bottari *et al*[8] measured the extent of dissociation in 2 hours at 80° in mixtures with 12 primary aliphatic alcohols and with macrogol 400. In anhydrous mixture at equilibrium, about 40% of the tolbutamide dissociated to butylamine and *p*-toluenesulphonyl isocyanate. In mixtures where the solvent contained 2% water, *p*-toluenesulphonamide was also detected. When tolbutamide was heated[9] in water, alcohols (ethanol and *n*-octadecyl alcohol), and amines (aniline and cyclohexylamine) at relatively low temperatures, the resultant products supported the hypothesis that the reaction mechanism was dissociation.

Solid dispersions

The stability of tolbutamide, as the commercial powder, when co-precipitated as a solid dispersion with macrogols 6000 or 20 000 (up to 20% w/w), was investigated by Alonso and others.[10] During storage for 12 months at 25° no changes were found by differential scanning and by dissolution testing. When plasma-glucose concentrations produced by the powdered dispersion were compared with those of tolbutamide alone in *rabbits*, the lowest concentrations were obtained most rapidly with the orally-administered solid dispersion. In samples of this solid dispersion stored for one year at 25° there were no significant changes in either the rate or the extent of the therapeutic response.

Tablets

The stability of tolbutamide tablets from five different commercial sources was investigated[11] during storage in opened amber tablet bottles at ambient temperature, 45°, or 60° and either zero or 75% relative humidity. During 390 days at ambient temperature and at 45° and either 0% or 75% relative humidity, all five formulations were stable. After 131 days at 60° and 75% relative humidity, the breakdown product p-toluenesulphonamide was detected in two formulations (which contained povidone) and in a further two formulations after 211 days.

FORMULATION

Excipients

Excipients that have been used in presentations of tolbutamide include:
Tablets: aluminium hydroxide; aluminium magnesium silicate; colloidal silica; croscarmellose sodium; calcium hydrogen phosphate; magnesium stearate; pregelatinised starch; rice starch; talc.

Bioavailability

Complexation of tolbutamide with macrogol 6000 or povidone 40 000 was shown by workers in Egypt to enhance its bioavailability in *rats*.[12] Macrogol had a greater effect than povidone. *In-vivo* analysis of plasma-glucose concentrations in *rabbits*[10] following oral administration of tolbutamide alone or in solid dispersion with macrogols 6000 or 20 000 (freshly prepared or aged for 6, 9, and 12 months) revealed that the co-precipitate dosage form improved bioavailability of tolbutamide.

REFERENCES

1. Sano A, Kuriki T, Handa T, Takeuchi H, Kawashima Y. J Pharm Sci 1987;76(6):471–4.
2. Gandhi RB, Karara AH. Drug Dev Ind Pharm 1988;14(5):657–82.
3. Kedzierewicz F, Hoffman M, Maincent P. Int J Pharmaceutics 1990;58:221–7.
4. Takeuchi H, Handa T, Kawashima Y. J Pharm Pharmacol 1987;39:769–73.
5. Simmons DL, Ranz RJ, Gyanchandani ND, Picotte P. Can J Pharm Sci 1972;7(4):121–3.
6. Leary JR, Ross SD, Thomas MJK. Pharm Weekbl (Sci) 1981;3:62–6.
7. Kaistha KK, French WN. J Pharm Sci 1968;57(3):459–64.
8. Bottari F, Mannelli M, Saettone MF. J Pharm Sci 1970;59(11):1663–6.
9. Bottari F, Giannaccini B, Nannipieri E, Saettone MF. J Pharm Sci 1972;61(4):602–6.
10. Alonso MJ, Maincent P, Garcia-Arias T, Vila-Jato JL. Int J Pharmaceutics 1988;42:27–33.
11. Matsui F, Curran NM, Lovering EG, Robertson DL. Can J Pharm Sci 1981;16(1):11–13.
12. Said SA, Saad SF. Aust J Pharm Sci 1975;NS4(4):121–2.

Triamcinolone (BAN, rINN)   *Corticosteroid*

9α-Fluoro-16α-hydroxyprednisolone; fluoxiprednisolonum
9α-Fluoro-11β,16α,17α,21-tetrahydroxypregna-1,4-diene-3,20-dione
$C_{21}H_{27}FO_6 = 394.4$

Triamcinolone Acetonide (BANM, rINNM)
$C_{24}H_{31}FO_6 = 434.5$

Triamcinolone Diacetate (BANM, rINNM)
$C_{25}H_{31}FO_8 = 478.5$

Triamcinolone Hexacetonide (BAN, USAN, rINN)
Triamcinolone acetonide 21-(3,3-dimethylbutyrate)
$C_{30}H_{41}FO_7 = 532.6$
CAS—124-94-7 (triamcinolone); 76-25-5 (triamcinolone acetonide); 67-78-7 (triamcinolone diacetate); 5611-51-8 (triamcinolone hexacetonide)

Pharmacopoeial status

BP (triamcinolone, triamcinolone acetonide); USP (triamcinolone, triamcinolone acetonide, triamcinolone diacetate, triamcinolone hexacetonide)

Preparations

Compendial
Triamcinolone Tablets BP. Tablets containing, in each, 2 mg and 4 mg triamcinolone are usually available.
Triamcinolone Cream BP (Triamcinolone Acetonide Cream). A cream containing 0.1% w/w is usually available.
Triamcinolone Ointment BP (Triamcinolone Acetonide Ointment). An ointment containing 0.1% w/w is usually available.
Triamcinolone Dental Paste BP (Triamcinolone Acetonide Dental Paste). A dental paste containing 0.1% w/w is usually available.
Triamcinolone Tablets USP.
Triamcinolone Acetonide Topical Aerosol USP.
Triamcinolone Acetonide Lotion USP.
Triamcinolone Acetonide Ointment USP.
Triamcinolone Acetonide Dental Paste USP.
Sterile Triamcinolone Acetonide Suspension USP. Injection, pH 5.0 to 7.5.
Triamcinolone Diacetate Syrup USP.
Sterile Triamcinolone Diacetate Suspension USP. Injection, pH 4.5 to 7.5.
Sterile Triamcinolone Hexacetonide Suspension USP. Injection, pH 4.0 to 8.0.

Non-compendial
Adcortyl (Squibb). *Cream*, triamcinolone acetonide 0.1%. *Diluents*: cetomacrogol cream (formula B) or aqueous cream. Preservative efficacy may be reduced depending on the diluent. Store diluted creams below 25° and discard 14 days after dilution.
Ointment, triamcinolone acetonide 0.1%. *Diluent*: white soft paraffin.

Oral paste (Adcortyl in Orabase), triamcinolone acetonide 0.1% in an adhesive basis. The oral paste should not be diluted.
Injection (Adcortyl Intra-articular/Intradermal), aqueous suspension, triamcinolone acetonide 10 mg/mL.
Kenalog Intra-articular/Intramuscular (Squibb). *Injection*, aqueous suspension, triamcinolone acetonide 40 mg/mL.
Ledercort (Lederle). *Tablets*, triamcinolone 2 mg and 4 mg.
Cream, triamcinolone acetonide 0.1%, in a water-miscible basis. May be diluted with aqueous cream. The diluted cream must be freshly prepared and not used more than one month after issue.
Lederspan (Lederle). *Injection*, aqueous suspension, micronised triamcinolone hexacetonide 5 mg/mL (for intralesional or sublesional injection) and 20 mg/mL (for intra-articular or intrasynovial injection). May be diluted immediately before injection with water for injections, sodium chloride injection, sodium chloride and glucose injection or lignocaine hydrochloride injection. Fluids that contain methyl or propyl hydroxybenzoates or phenol should be avoided, as flocculation of the steroid may result.

Containers and storage

Solid state
Triamcinolone BP should be kept in a well-closed container.
Triamcinolone Acetonide BP should be kept in a well-closed container and protected from light.
Triamcinolone USP, Triamcinolone Acetonide USP, Triamcinolone Diacetate USP, and Triamcinolone Hexacetonide USP should all be preserved in well-closed containers.

Dosage forms
Triamcinolone Tablets USP and Triamcinolone Acetonide Ointment USP should be preserved in well-closed containers.
Triamcinolone Acetonide Cream USP, Triamcinolone Acetonide Lotion USP, and Triamcinolone Acetonide Dental Paste USP should be preserved in tight containers.
Triamcinolone Acetonide Topical Aerosol USP should be preserved in pressurised containers, and exposure to excessive heat avoided.
Triamcinolone Diacetate Syrup USP should be preserved in tight, light-resistant containers.
Sterile Triamcinolone Acetate Suspension USP, Sterile Triamcinolone Diacetate Suspension USP, and Sterile Triamcinolone Hexacetonide Suspension USP should all be preserved in single-dose or in multiple-dose containers, preferably of Type I glass. Sterile Triamcinolone Acetonide Suspension USP should be protected from light.
Adcortyl cream, Adcortyl ointment, and Adcortyl in Orabase should be stored at room temperature. Avoid freezing the cream.
Adcortyl Intra-articular/Intradermal suspension should be stored in an upright position at room temperature. Avoid freezing.
Kenalog Intra-articular/Intramuscular and Lederspan injections should be stored at room temperature and freezing should be avoided.
Ledercort tablets should be stored at controlled room temperature (15° to 30°) in either the original pack or in containers that prevent access of moisture.
Ledercort cream should be stored in a cool place (8° to 15°) in either the original packs or in containers with complete closure.

PHYSICAL PROPERTIES

Triamcinolone is a white or almost white, crystalline powder; odourless; slightly hygroscopic.
Triamcinolone acetonide is a white or almost white, crystalline powder, with not more than a slight odour.
Triamcinolone diacetate is a fine, white or almost white, crystalline powder, with not more than a slight odour.

Triamcinolone hexacetonide is a white to cream-coloured powder.

Melting point

Triamcinolone,[1] *triamcinolone acetonide*[2] and *triamcinolone diacetate*[3,4] do not have sharp melting points; some melting temperature ranges (which may depend, for example, on polymorphic or solvate forms or rate of heating) are reported as:
Triamcinolone: 248° to 250°; 260° to 262°; about 266°; 269° to 271°.
Triamcinolone acetonide: about 277°; 292° to 294°.
Triamcinolone diacetate: 151°; 186° to 188° with effervescence; 235° after drying.
Triamcinolone hexacetonide has been reported[5] to melt, with decomposition, at 271° to 272° and at 295° to 296°.
See also Polymorphism, below.

Partition coefficients

Log *P* values determined by an HPLC method in 1-octanol saturated with phosphate buffer (pH 7) were 1.02 and 2.27 for *triamcinolone* and *triamcinolone acetonide*, respectively.[6]
From octanol-water partition coefficients established at 25° by Tomida *et al*[7] for *triamcinolone* (10.8), *triamcinolone acetonide* (205) and *triamcinolone diacetate* (83.7), Yalkowsky and Valvani[8] derived an equation in which log *P* values (1.03, 2.31, and 1.92, respectively) and melting points were used to estimate aqueous solubilities.

Solubility

Triamcinolone. BP solubilities: slightly soluble in water; soluble 1 in 40 of ethanol. USP solubilities: very slightly soluble in water; slightly soluble in ethanol. It is very slightly soluble in chloroform and in ether; slightly soluble in methanol.
Triamcinolone acetonide is practically insoluble in water; sparingly soluble in ethanol, in chloroform, and in methanol; very slightly soluble in ether.
Triamcinolone diacetate is practically insoluble in water; slightly soluble in ether; sparingly soluble in methanol (1 in 40). USP solubilities: sparingly soluble in ethanol; soluble in chloroform. It is also reported to be soluble 1 in 13 of ethanol and 1 in 80 of chloroform.
Triamcinolone hexacetonide is practically insoluble in water; soluble in chloroform; slightly soluble in methanol.
Aqueous solubilities, at 25°, of triamcinolone, triamcinolone acetonide, and triamcinolone diacetate were measured as 2.07×10^{-4} M, 4.95×10^{-5} M, and 7.41×10^{-5} M, respectively.[7] Solubilisation of these and 16 other steroid hormones by polyoxyethylene lauryl ether was reported.
Solubilities[9] of triamcinolone acetonide (mg/mL) were determined[9] in the following compounds at 22° and 37°: propylene glycol, 8.04 ± 0.19 and 12.09 ± 0.18; cetyl alcohol, 0.92 ± 0.3 and 1.25 ± 0.05; wool alcohol, 0.13 ± 0.01 and 0.41 ± 0.01.

Effect of temperature and ionic strength
The solubility of triamcinolone acetonide in distilled water was 21.0 micrograms/mL at 28°, 25.5 micrograms/mL at 37° and 33.6 micrograms/mL at 50°, as measured by a colorimetric method.[10] However, a radioisotopic method[11] revealed lower solubilities (for ^{14}C-triamcinolone acetonide) of 17.5 micrograms/mL at 28°, 20.7 micrograms/mL at 37° and 26.5 micrograms/mL at 50°. In both studies, solubilities and dissolution rates at each temperature were lower in potassium chloride solutions and decreased as the concentration of potassium chloride was increased from 0.2M to 1M.

Dissolution

The USP specifies that for Triamcinolone Tablets USP not less than 75% of the labelled amount of $C_{21}H_{27}FO_6$ is dissolved in 45 minutes. Dissolution medium; 900 mL of 0.1N hydrochloric acid: Apparatus 1 at 100 rpm.

Crystal and molecular structure

Polymorphs

Triamcinolone may exist in two polymorphic forms, depending on the solvent of crystallisation, as shown by infrared spectra and powder X-ray diffraction data. Polymorph I (or A) has been obtained from pyridine and aqueous pyridine,[12] and aqueous isopropanol 60% and potassium tetraborate-water.[1] Polymorph II (or B) has been obtained from methanol and aqueous methanol[12] and dimethylacetamide-water.[1] Melting points of the polymorphs differ.

Evidence for the possible existence of two polymorphs of triamcinolone acetonide has been found using powder X-ray diffraction; infrared spectroscopy or differential scanning calorimetry could not differentiate between the polymorphs.[13]

Smith and Halwer[12] identified and characterised two polymorphs of triamcinolone diacetate, one form (from methylene chloride or chloroform) and another form (from acetone); they had melting ranges of 185° to 232° and 145° to 236°, respectively. Borka and Shefter[4] prepared three forms of triamcinolone diacetate with distinct infrared spectra: polymorphic forms I and II and an N,N-dimethylacetamide (DMA) solvate. Melting points were reported to be 186° to 188°, 151°, and 103°, respectively. Conditions for transformation between forms were discussed. Of two batches of triamcinolone diacetate 40 mg/mL suspension for injection (Aristocort, Lederle), one batch contained pure Form II whereas the other also contained 10% of Form I.

Polymorphism of triamcinolone hexacetonide has not been established under conditions used to demonstrate polymorphism of triamcinolone or triamcinolone diacetate.[4, 5]

STABILITY

Solid state

Triamcinolone, triamcinolone acetonide, triamcinolone diacetate, and triamcinolone hexacetonide are all reported to be very stable in the solid state.[1–3, 5]

Solutions

In aqueous and alcoholic solutions, at alkaline pH, the α-ketol side-chain of triamcinolone and triamcinolone acetonide is susceptible to oxidative rearrangement and degradation.[1, 2]

The results of a detailed investigation[14] indicated that isomerism of triamcinolone in solution yielded a D-homo-analogue, 9α-fluoro-11β,16α,17aα-trihydroxy-17aβ-hydroxymethyl-1,4-D-homoandrostadiene-3,17-dione. Isomerism of triamcinolone can occur under various conditions, for example: in alkaline solution; in certain solvents (such as warm dimethylformamide or some commercial reagent methanol solutions); or in the presence of certain metal cations (such as ferric ions). Under conditions that promote acid hydrolysis of triamcinolone 16α,17α-acetonide, no isomerism was detected.

The 21-acetate group of triamcinolone diacetate was easily removed in mildly alkaline solution.[3]

The major decomposition products of triamcinolone acetonide in aqueous solution of hydrochloric acid with ethanol 25% v/v (pH 1.6) were triamcinolone and acetone.[15]

Kinetics and effect of pH

Timmins and Gray[16] compared the first-order decomposition of triamcinolone and triamcinolone acetonide in aqueous buffers, which contained disodium edetate 0.05% w/v to retard metal-ion catalysed oxidation, at 50°. Triamcinolone acetonide degradation demonstrated specific acid catalysis at pH 1 to 3, specific base catalysis at pH 4 to 7 and pH 9 to 12, and was pH-independent at pH 7 to 9; maximum stability was at about pH 4. Rate constants were calculated as 0.161/day at pH 1.4, 2.12×10^{-3}/day at pH 4.2, 7.58×10^{-2}/day at pH 9.3, and 2.13/day at pH 11.17. Triamcinolone degradation demonstrated specific base catalysis above pH 4; maximum stability was at about pH 3.5. Decomposition products, formed mainly from degradation of the C-17 side-chain, differed between the steroids; a major decomposition product of triamcinolone in alkaline media, the D-homologue, was not observed to be a prominent decomposition product of triamcinolone acetonide. It was concluded that, in neutral and alkaline solutions, the cyclic ketal group in triamcinolone acetonide stabilises the molecule.

Decomposition of triamcinolone acetonide 0.025% in aqueous solutions that contained ethanol 25% v/v followed pseudo-first-order kinetics and showed a minimum at about pH 3.4 at 50°, in amber bottles.[15] At 25°, solutions were estimated to remain stable for 9-times longer than at 50°. Triamcinolone acetonide was subject to general acid-base catalysis and, at above pH 7, decomposition decreased when ionic strength was increased. An observed degradation rate constant of 0.008/day was estimated for triamcinolone acetonide (40 mg) in macrogol ointment basis (polyethylene glycol ointment base USP, 19.96 g) at 50° in opaque white glass jars.[15]

FURTHER INFORMATION. Triamcinolone—Sieh DH. In: Florey K, editor. Analytical profiles of drug substances; vol 11. London: Academic Press, 1982:593–614. Triamcinolone diacetate—Sieh DH. ibid:651–61.

FORMULATION

Excipients

Excipients that have been used in presentations of triamcinolone include:

Tablets, triamcinolone: calcium hydrogen phosphate; docusate sodium; lactose; magnesium stearate; maize starch; microcrystalline cellulose; Red 30; sodium benzoate; sodium starch glycollate; Yellow 10.

Syrups, triamcinolone diacetate: aluminium magnesium silicate; kaolin; methyl and propyl hydroxybenzoates; Red 33; Red 40; sodium acid phosphate; sodium phosphate.

Creams, triamcinolone acetonide: benzyl alcohol; butylated hydroxyanisole; cetyl alcohol; cetyl esters wax; citric acid; diglycerides; emulsifying wax; glycerol; glyceryl monostearate; isopropyl palmitate; lactic acid; methyl and propyl hydroxybenzoates; monoglycerides; polyoxyl 40 stearate; polysorbate 60; polysorbate 80; potassium sorbate; propylene glycol; propyl gallate; simethicone; sorbic acid; sorbitol solution; squalene; stearyl alcohol; white soft paraffin.

Lotions, triamcinolone acetonide: cetyl alcohol; methyl and propyl hydroxybenzoates; polysorbate 20; propylene glycol; simethicone; sorbitan monopalmitate; stearyl alcohol.

Ointments, triamcinolone acetonide: butylated hydroxyanisole; citric acid; emulsifying wax; lactic acid; methyl and propyl hydroxybenzoates; Plastibase (liquid paraffin and polyethylene resin); propyl gallate; propylene glycol; white soft paraffin.

Topical aerosols, triamcinolone acetonide: dehydrated ethanol; isobutane propellant; isopropyl palmitate.

Dental pastes, triamcinolone acetonide: carmellose sodium; gelatin; liquid paraffin; pectin; polyethylene resin.

Inhalers, triamcinolone acetonide: dehydrated ethanol; dichlorodifluoromethane.

Injections (not intravenous), triamcinolone acetonide: benzyl alcohol; carmellose sodium; hydrochloric acid; polysorbate 80; sodium chloride; sodium hydroxide.

Triamcinolone diacetate: benzyl alcohol; cetyl pyridinium chloride; hydrochloric acid; macrogols 3350 and 4000; polysorbate 80; sodium chloride.

Triamcinolone hexacetonide: benzyl alcohol; hydrochloric acid; polysorbate 80; sodium hydroxide; sorbitol solution.

Bioavailability

No significant differences in the absorption parameters of triamcinolone were identified between a group of ten healthy subjects who received two 8 mg triamcinolone tablets and five healthy subjects who received 16 mg crystalline triamcinolone diacetate suspended in 150 mL of water.[17]

Topical preparations

No physical incompatibilities were observed[18] when triamcinolone acetonide 0.1% cream (Kenalog) at pH 6.2 was mixed with each of the following additives and stored in amber glass jars under ambient conditions for two months: salicylic acid 2%; urea 10%; Coal Tar Solution USP 5%; or a camphor 0.25%, menthol 0.25%, and phenol 0.25% mixture. Initial pH values of compounded creams were 2.6, 8.0, 6.4, and 6.2, respectively. After mixing with the urea 10%, the concentration of triamcinolone acetonide decreased by more than 10% immediately and by 45% in two months. The penetration rate of triamcinolone acetonide through human skin was twice as rapid from creams with salicylic acid 2% or urea 10% than from the other compounded creams or from triamcinolone acetonide cream itself.

Wiechers *et al*[19] presented evidence that inclusion of 1-dodecylazacycloheptan-2-one (laurocapram; Azone, Nelson Research, USA) 1.6% w/w in triamcinolone acetonide 0.05% w/w creams enhanced the rate and extent of percutaneous absorption of triamcinolone acetonide when applied topically under occlusion in single and multiple doses to healthy volunteers.

Jackson *et al*[20] evaluated six brands of triamcinolone acetonide 0.1% creams (Aristocort, Fougera, Kenalog, My K, NMC, and Rugby) by a quantitative vasoconstrictor assay in a double-blind study with twelve subjects. All creams produced less vasoconstriction as the area of application was increased.

Iyer and Vasavada[9] evaluated the ability of wool alcohol to form films; the 'integrity' of films was improved by inclusion of ethylcellulose, and incorporation of propylene glycol or cetyl alcohol further improved the hardness and modulus of elasticity of the films. Release kinetics of triamcinolone acetonide from such films were investigated.

Iyer and Vasavada[21] later demonstrated that the release of triamcinolone acetonide from wool alcohol/ethylcellulose films, which contained propylene glycol or hexadecyl alcohol as a 'solvent-plasticiser', was the rate-limiting step for percutaneous absorption *in vitro* through human abdominal skin. Films were applied in isopropanolic solutions. Maximum release was apparent from systems containing wool alcohol:ethylcellulose:propylene glycol in the ratio 6.5:1.5:2.0. No differences in rates of penetration of triamcinolone acetonide were observed between systems containing propylene glycol or hexadecyl alcohol.

From the results of skin blanching assays in ten healthy subjects,[22] a hydrocolloid patch (consisting of pectin, carmellose sodium, and gelatin, in a polyisobutylene-based adhesive) that was impregnated with triamcinolone acetonide was suggested to be a 'viable proposition' as a transdermal delivery system.

Adsorbents

The adsorption of triamcinolone onto various antacids or other adsorbents (percentage adsorbed per gram of adsorbent) decreased in the order: charcoal > magnesium trisilicate > bismuth subcarbonate > kaolin > talc > aluminium hydroxide > magnesium oxide. Magnesium carbonate and calcium carbonate showed no adsorbent properties.[23]

FURTHER INFORMATION. Delivery of triamcinolone acetonide [from hydroalcoholic tinctures] through human epidermis: effect of Actiderm, a new hydrocolloid dermatological patch [consisting of a powder mixture of pectin, gelatin, and carmellose sodium dispersed in a pressure-sensitive adhesive]—Kadir R, Barry BW, Fairbrother JE, Hollingsbee DA. Int J Pharmaceutics 1990;60:139–45. Development of a triamcinolone acetonide formulation. Sterile suspension—Fernandez R, Callava H, Selmar E, Diaz M, Corrales C, Leyva Z [Spanish]. Rev Cub Farm 1985;19:27–36.

REFERENCES

1. Florey K. In: Florey K, editor. Analytical profiles of drug substances; vol 1. London: Academic Press, 1972:367–96.
2. Florey K. *ibid*:397–421.
3. Florey K. *ibid*:423–42.
4. Borka L, Shefta E. Int J Pharmaceutics 1983;16:93–6.
5. Zbinovsky V, Chrekian GP. In: Florey K, editor. Analytical profiles of drug substances; vol 6. London: Academic Press, 1977:579–95.
6. Caron JC, Shroot B. J Pharm Sci 1984;73(12):1703–6.
7. Tomida H, Yotsuyanagi T, Ikeda K. Chem Pharm Bull 1978;26(9):2832–7.
8. Yalkowsky SH, Valvani SC. J Pharm Sci 1980;69(8):912–22.
9. Iyer BV, Vasavada RC. J Pharm Sci 1979;68(6):782–7.
10. Block LH, Patel RN. J Pharm Sci 1973;62(4):617–21.
11. Behl CR, Block LH, Borke ML. J Pharm Sci 1976;65(3):429–30.
12. Smith LL, Halwer M. J Am Pharm Assoc (Sci) 1959;48:348–52.
13. Sieh DH. In: Florey K, editor. Analytical profiles of drug substances; vol 11. London: Academic Press, 1982:615–49.
14. Smith LL, Marx M, Garbarini JJ, Foell T, Origoni VE, Goodman JJ. J Am Chem Soc 1960;82:4616–23.
15. Das Gupta V. J Pharm Sci 1983;72(12):1453–6.
16. Timmins P, Gray EA. J Pharm Pharmacol 1983;35:175–7.
17. Hochhaus G, Pörtner M, Barth J, Möllmann H, Rohdewald P. Pharm Res 1990;7(5):558–60.
18. Krochmal L, Wang JCT, Patel B, Rodgers J. J Am Acad Dermatol 1989;21(5):979–84.
19. Wiechers JW, Drenth BFH, Jonkman JHG, de Zeeuw RA. Int J Pharmaceutics 1990;66:53–62.
20. Jackson DB, Thompson C, McCormack JR, Guin JD. J Am Acad Dermatol 1989;20(5):791–6.
21. Iyer BV, Vasavada RC. Int J Pharmaceutics 1979;3:247–60.
22. Monger L, Martin GP, Marriott C, Hollingsbee D, Fairbrother JE. J Pharm Pharmacol 1991;43(Suppl):57P.
23. Naggar VF, Gouda MW, Khalil SA. Pharmazie 1977;32(2):778–81.

Trimethoprim (BAN, USAN, rINN) *Antibacterial*

Trimethoxyprim
5-(3,4,5-Trimethoxybenzyl)pyrimidine-2,4-diyldiamine;
5-[(3,4,5- trimethoxyphenyl)methyl]-2,4-pyrimidinediamine
$C_{14}H_{18}N_4O_3 = 290.3$
CAS—738-70-5

Pharmacopoeial status

BP, USP

Preparations

Co-trimoxazole is the British Approved Name for compounded preparations of trimethoprim 1 part and sulphamethoxazole 5 parts.
For compendial and non-compendial preparations containing co-trimoxazole refer to the Sulphamethoxazole monograph.

Compendial
Trimethoprim Tablets BP. Tablets containing, in each, 100 mg, 200 mg, and 300 mg are usually available.
Trimethoprim Tablets USP.

Non-compendial
Ipral (Squibb). *Tablets*, trimethoprim 100 mg and 200 mg.
Monotrim (Duphar). *Tablets*, trimethoprim 100 mg and 200 mg.
Suspension, sugar free, trimethoprim 50 mg/5 mL. *Diluents*: sorbitol solution or water, life of diluted suspension 14 days.
Injection, trimethoprim 20 mg (as lactate)/mL, pH 4.0. *Diluents*: glucose 5%, compound sodium chloride, sodium chloride 0.9%, sodium chloride 0.45% and glucose 2.5%, sodium lactate, compound sodium lactate, fructose 5%, dextran 40 10% in sodium chloride 0.9%, or dextran 70 6% in sodium chloride 0.9% injections. It is incompatible with solutions of sulphonamides.
Trimopan (Berk). *Tablets*, trimethoprim 100 mg and 200 mg.
Suspension, sugar free, trimethoprim 50 mg/5 mL. *Diluents*: water or sorbitol solution.
Trimethoprim tablets of various strengths are also available from APS, Cox, CP, Evans, Kerfoot, Lagap (Trimogal), Norton.

Containers and storage

Solid state
Trimethoprim USP should be preserved in tight, light-resistant containers.

Dosage forms
Trimethoprim Tablets USP should be preserved in tight, light-resistant containers.
Ipral tablets should be stored in closed containers at room temperature.
Monotrim injection and suspension should be stored below 25°.
The injection should be protected from light.
Trimopan suspension should be protected from light.
For directions on the storage of co-trimoxazole and its preparations refer to the Sulphamethoxazole monograph.

PHYSICAL PROPERTIES

Trimethoprim exists as white or yellowish-white, odourless or almost odourless crystals or crystalline powder.

Melting point

Trimethoprim melts in the range 199° to 203°.

pH

A 1% aqueous suspension of *trimethoprim* has a pH of about 8.2.

Dissociation constant

pK_a 7.2

Solubility

Trimethoprim is soluble 1 in 2500 of water, 1 in 300 of ethanol, 1 in 55 of chloroform, and 1 in 80 of methanol; it is slightly soluble in acetone; soluble in benzyl alcohol; practically insoluble in carbon tetrachloride and in ether.

Effect of pH
Dahlan *et al*[1] studied the influence of pH on the solubilities and dissolution rates of sulphamethoxazole and trimethoprim. Trimethoprim solubility increased with decreasing pH, but decreased at pH values below 2, owing to the common ion effect. Maximum solubility occurred at pH 5.5 and 32° in either water or hydrochloric acid. The dissolution rate of trimethoprim in hydrochloric acid solutions at 32° was studied at pH values ranging from 1.48 to 6.00. Zero-order dissolution was observed at pH 2.93 and 6.00; at the other pH values dissolution was found to be non-linear with time. In general, the dissolution rate of trimethoprim increased with decreasing pH, except at pH 1.48, owing to the common ion effect.

Effect of temperature
The solubility of trimethoprim in various buffer solutions has been found to increase with increase in temperature.[1]

Dissolution

The USP specifies that for Trimethoprim Tablets USP not less than 75% of the labelled amount of $C_{14}H_{18}N_4O_3$ is dissolved in 45 minutes. Dissolution medium: 900 mL of 0.01 N hydrochloric acid; Apparatus 2 at 50 rpm.
The dissolution test for Sulphamethoxazole and Trimethoprim Tablets USP is described in the Sulphamethoxazole monograph.

Crystal and molecular structure

Polymorphs
Bettinetti *et al*[2] identified two polymorphs of trimethoprim. A triclinic form was found most frequently and was obtained by recrystallisation from various solvents. A monoclinic form was identified following recrystallisation from toluene or methylisobutylketone.

STABILITY

The degradation of trimethoprim in acidic and alkaline media at elevated temperature and in direct sunlight was examined by Bergh *et al*.[3] Five decomposition products were identified, all of which were dimethoxybenzylpyrimidines or trimethoxybenzylpyrimidines. The main routes of degradation were found to be hydrolysis of the amino groups and oxidation of the benzylic methylene group. Hydrolysis of the *p*-methoxy group was also observed with the formation of a sixth, unidentified, product.

Tu *et al*[4] reported a loss of less than 10% trimethoprim from a 5% solution containing 52% *N,N*-dimethylacetamide and 48% propylene glycol following storage at 80° for 45 days. Trimethoprim degradation appeared to exhibit zero-order kinetics at 25° at a rate of 0.0113%/day; this gave an extrapolated value for $t_{10\%}$ of 885 days.

For reference to studies on the stability and incompatibility of co-trimoxazole injection, refer to the Sulphamethoxazole monograph.

FORMULATION

Excipients

Excipients that have been used in presentations of trimethoprim include:

Tablets: gelatin; lactose; magnesium stearate; maize starch; pregelatinised starch; quinoline yellow (E104); sodium starch glycollate; talc.

Suspensions: methyl and propyl hydroxybenzoates; sorbitol.

For excipients used in presentations of co-trimoxazole refer to the Sulphamethoxazole monograph.

Solid dispersions

The dissolution rate of trimethoprim was enhanced from co-precipitates of trimethoprim with macrogols 4000, 6000, or 9000, or with povidone (mol. wt. 40 000); most rapid release was apparent from the macrogol 6000 co-precipitate. These results correlated well with absorption studies in six healthy volunteers.[5]

FURTHER INFORMATION. Biodegradable microspheres VI: Lysosomal release of covalently bound antiparasitic drugs from starch microparticles. [Covalent coupling of trimethoprim to polyacryl starch microparticles as a drug carrier complex]— Laakso T, Stjärnkvist P, Sjöholm I. J Pharm Sci 1987;76:134–40.

PROCESSING

For reference to studies of the interaction between trimethoprim and sulphamethoxazole in co-trimoxazole preparations under certain conditions, refer to the Sulphamethoxazole monograph.

REFERENCES

1. Dahlan R, McDonald C, Sunderland VB. J Pharm Pharmacol 1987;39:246–51.
2. Bettinetti GP, Giordano F, La Manna A, Giuseppetti G. J Pharm Pharmacol 1976;28:87–8.
3. Bergh JJ, Breytenbach JC, Wessels PL. J Pharm Sci 1989;78:348–50.
4. Tu Y-H, Wang D-P, Allen LV. Am J Hosp Pharm 1989;46:301–4.
5. Gupta RL, Kumar R, Singla AK. Drug Dev Ind Pharm 1991;17(3):463–8.

Verapamil (BAN, USAN, rINN)

Calcium-channel blocker

Iproveratril

5-[*N*-(3,4-Dimethoxyphenethyl)methylamino]-2-(3,4-dimethoxyphenyl)-2-isopropylvaleronitrile; α-[3-[[2-(3,4-dimethoxyphenyl)ethyl]methylamino]propyl]-3,4-dimethoxy-α-(1-methylethyl)-benzeneacetonitrile

$C_{27}H_{38}N_2O_4 = 454.6$

Verapamil Hydrochloride (BANM, USAN, rINNM)

$C_{27}H_{38}N_2O_4,HCl = 491.1$

CAS—52-53-9 (verapamil); 152-11-4 (verapamil hydrochloride)

Pharmacopoeial status

BP, USP (verapamil hydrochloride)

Preparations

Compendial

Verapamil Tablets BP. Coated tablets containing in each, 40, 80, 120, and 160 mg verapamil hydrochloride are usually available.

Verapamil Injection BP. A solution of verapamil hydrochloride in water for injections. An injection containing 5 mg in 2 mL is usually available. pH 4.5 to 6.0.

Verapamil Tablets USP.

Verapamil Injection USP. pH between 4.0 and 6.5.

Non-compendial

Berkatens (Berk). *Tablets*, verapamil hydrochloride 40, 80, 120, and 160 mg.

Cordilox (Baker Norton). *Tablets*, verapamil hydrochloride 40, 80, 120, and 160 mg.

Injection, verapamil hydrochloride 2.5 mg/mL.

Securon (Knoll). *Tablets*, verapamil hydrochloride 40, 80, 120, and 160 mg.

Tablets (Securon SR), sustained release, verapamil hydrochloride 240 mg.

Tablets (Half Securon SR), sustained release, verapamil hydrochloride 120 mg.

Injection (Securon IV), verapamil hydrochloride 2.5 mg/mL. Incompatible with alkaline solutions.

Univer (Rhône-Poulenc Rorer). *Capsules*, sustained release, verapamil hydrochloride 120 mg, 180 mg, and 240 mg.

Verapamil hydrochloride tablets of various strengths are also available from APS, Cox, CP, Cusi (Geangin), Evans, Kerfoot, Norton.

A sugar-free oral solution of verapamil hydrochloride 40 mg/5 mL is available by special order from RP Drugs.

Containers and storage

Solid state

Verapamil Hydrochloride BP should be kept in a well-closed container and protected from light.

Verapamil Hydrochloride USP should be preserved in tight, light-resistant containers.

Dosage forms
Verapamil Injection BP should be protected from light.
Verapamil Tablets USP should be preserved in tight, light-resistant containers.
Verapamil Injection USP should be preserved in single-dose containers, preferably of Type I glass, protected from light.
Securon tablets and Securon SR tablets should be stored in a dry place at room temperature. Half Securon SR tablets should be stored in a dry place, below 25°. Securon IV injection should be stored at room temperature and protected from light.
Univer capsules should be stored in a cool, dry place.

PHYSICAL PROPERTIES

Verapamil is a pale yellow viscous oil.
Verapamil hydrochloride is a white crystalline powder; practically odourless; bitter taste.

Melting point

Verapamil hydrochloride melts in the range 140° to 144°.

pH

A 5% w/v solution of *verapamil hydrochloride*, prepared with the aid of heat, has a pH in the range 4.5 to 6.5. A 7% w/w solution of *verapamil hydrochloride* is reported to have a pH of 4.24.

Dissociation constant

Determination of dissociation constants by spectrophotometric and potentiometric methods does not produce reliable values, because of the low solubility of verapamil in aqueous media. Values obtained by alternative methods are: 8.9 (at 25° by partitioning between aqueous buffers and non-polar solvents: *n*-heptane, *n*-hexane, or *n*-pentane);[1] 8.6 (by titration with 0.1N potassium hydroxide in methanol/water); 8.9.[2]

Partition coefficient

Partition and transport of verapamil and nicotine through artificial membranes—Santi P, Catellani PL, Colombo P, Ringard-Lefebvre C, Barthélémy C, Guyot-Hermann A-M. Int J Pharmaceutics 1991;68:43–9.

Solubility

Verapamil is practically insoluble in water; soluble in ethanol, in chloroform, and in ether.
Verapamil hydrochloride is soluble 1 in 20 of water; sparingly soluble in ethanol; soluble 1 in 1.5 of chloroform; practically insoluble in ether.

Dissolution

The USP specifies that for Verapamil Tablets USP not less than 75% of the labelled amount of $C_{27}H_{38}N_2O_4$,HCl is dissolved in 30 minutes. Dissolution medium: 900 mL of 0.1N hydrochloric acid; Apparatus 2 at 50 rpm.

STABILITY

Verapamil hydrochloride, in the solid state, is both thermally and photochemically stable, although it should be stored under protection from light. It is also stable in neutral, acidic, and basic solution. A solution of verapamil hydrochloride in methanol decomposed by 52% during exposure to ultraviolet light for 2 hours.
Aqueous solutions of verapamil hydrochloride (0.5 mg/mL) were stable for 105 days at 50° (corresponding to about 4.5 years at 25°). Maximum stability was shown in the pH range 3.2 to 5.6. The inclusion of phosphate buffer in the solutions and variation of their ionic strengths had minimal effect on stability.[3]

INCOMPATIBILITY/COMPATIBILITY

Verapamil hydrochloride injection 40 mg/mL (Isoptin, Knoll) was visually and chemically compatible with ten parenteral solutions when stored at 25° for 48 hours.[4] Glucose-containing admixtures produced slightly elevated spectrophotometric readings, possibly due to the presence of glucose degradation products formed during sterilisation. No adsorption to glass, polyvinyl chloride, or polyolefin packaging materials was apparent.
Visual compatibility during a 48-hour period, with the exception of a transient precipitate apparent with aminophylline, was observed when verapamil hydrochloride injection (Knoll) was mixed with nine parenteral drug products in 500 mL of either sodium chloride 0.9% injection or glucose 5% injection.[5] In a more extensive study, verapamil hydrochloride injection, 80 mg/mL (Knoll), was shown to be visually compatible with a further 68 secondary additives in the same two large-volume parenteral solutions, with the exceptions of mixtures that contained albumin, amphotericin, dobutamine hydrochloride, hydralazine hydrochloride, and trimethoprim with sulphamethoxazole.[6]
Verapamil hydrochloride 160 micrograms/mL (Isoptin, Knoll) and dobutamine hydrochloride 250 micrograms/mL (Dobutrex, Lilly) were found to be compatible when mixed together in either sodium chloride 0.9% injection or glucose 5% injection, despite the formation of a light-pink coloration (which later disappeared in the glucose solutions) within 24 hours of mixing. When stored in plastic intravenous bags and in amber glass bottles, the solutions appeared stable for 48 hours and seven days when stored at 24° and 5°, respectively. No variation in pH was apparent in the sodium chloride solutions, but a reduction from pH 4.0 to 3.1 occurred in the glucose solutions stored at 24° for seven days.[7]
When verapamil hydrochloride (10 mg/4 mL) was added to admixtures of eleven penicillins in minibags of either glucose 5% injection or sodium chloride 0.9% injection, an initial cloudiness which cleared on agitation was observed with nafcillin sodium, oxacillin sodium, ampicillin sodium, and mezlocillin sodium following visual and microscopic examination (at time 0, 15 minutes, and 24 hours). A reduction in pH occurred in all the admixtures.[8] As part of the same study, these four penicillins were mixed in a 1:1 ratio with verapamil hydrochloride injection under simulated conditions of Y-site injection. A milky-white precipitate formed (at time 0 and 15 minutes), accompanied by a reduction in verapamil hydrochloride concentration but no change in pH. Separate intravenous administration of verapamil hydrochloride, or alternatively, thorough flushing of the intravenous line before and after injection of verapamil hydrochloride was recommended.
Precipitate formation in an intravenous line following simultaneous infusion of verapamil hydrochloride and nafcillin sodium was reported earlier by Tucker and Gentile.[9]
Following the addition of verapamil hydrochloride solutions (final concentrations 0.4 and 0.1 mg/mL) to admixtures of glucose 5% injection with theophylline (4.0 and 0.4 mg/mL), no precipitation was observed under visual and microscopic examination and no chemical decomposition was apparent during a 24-hour study period.[10] However, in a similar study,[11] a 99% reduction in initial verapamil concentrations (0.1 and 0.4 mg/mL) and precipitate formation were observed directly after its

addition to admixtures of aminophylline (0.1 mg/mL) in glucose 5% injection. Precipitation of verapamil hydrochloride was related to the pH of the solutions.

Two admixtures that contained differing concentrations of milrinone and verapamil in glucose 5% injection were physically and chemically stable[12] after 4 hours at 22° to 23°.

Precipitation of verapamil hydrochloride was observed[13] after administration into an intravenous line containing sodium bicarbonate solution in sodium chloride 0.9%. It was suggested[14] that the formation of the precipitate was due to the high pH of the solution.

FORMULATION

Excipients

Excipients that have been used in presentations of verapamil and verapamil hydrochloride include:

Capsules, verapamil: lactose; magnesium stearate; silicic acid; talc.

Tablets, verapamil: acacia; Aerosil; calcium carbonate; carmellose sodium; yellow iron oxide (E172); lactose; magnesium stearate; povidone; starch (maize or potato); sugar; talc; titanium dioxide (E171).

Verapamil hydrochloride: calcium hydrogen phosphate; carmellose sodium; cellulose; colloidal silica; gelatin; hydroxypropylcellulose; hypromellose; iron oxide; lactose; macrogol; magnesium stearate; maize starch; microcrystalline cellulose; polysorbate 80; povidone; propylene glycol; sodium alginate; talc; titanium dioxide (E171).

Sustained-release tablets, verapamil hydrochloride: cellulose; hypromellose; indigo carmine (E132) lake; macrogol 400; macrogol 6000; magnesium stearate; microcrystalline cellulose; povidone; quinoline yellow (E104) lake; sodium alginate; titanium dioxide (E171).

Suspensions: Cologel; cherry syrup; chloroform water; glycerol; natural anisette; syrup; tragacanth mucilage.

Injections, verapamil hydrochloride: hydrochloric acid; sodium chloride; sodium hydroxide.

Bioequivalence

The bioequivalence of a verapamil sustained-release tablet (Securon SR, Knoll) administered in multiple doses of 240 mg as either a whole tablet or as two halves has been studied in eleven healthy male volunteers.[15] There was no significant difference between plasma concentrations produced by the two modes of administration. The sustained-release formulation consisted of the incorporation of verapamil into the hydrocolloid matrix of alginate.

Devane et al[16] compared the dissolution behaviour and the single-dose pharmacokinetic characteristics of two sustained-release verapamil tablets (Verelan, Elan Pharma and Isoptin SR, Knoll). *In-vitro* dissolution studies demonstrated that drug release from Verelan was slower than from Isoptin SR (after 8 hours, 50% and 90% release, respectively). This observation was reflected in the *in-vivo* results; the time to reach peak plasma concentration being 7.3 hours (Verelan) and 5 hours (Isoptin SR), respectively. In terms of degree of absorption, the two preparations were bioequivalent.

FURTHER INFORMATION. Permeation of verapamil hydrochloride through skin—Ritschel WA, Agrawala P. Acta Pharm Tech 1988;34(3):156–9. Transdermal controlled delivery of verapamil: characterization of *in vitro* skin permeation—Shah HS, Tojo K, Chien YW. Int J Pharmaceutics 1992;86:167–73. Enhancement of *in vitro* skin permeation of verapamil—Shah HS, Tojo K, Chien YW. Drug Dev Ind Pharm

1992;18(13):1461–76. A novel technique to determine verapamil HCl diffusion coefficients through hydroxypropyl methylcellulose gels—Bain JC, Ganderton D, Solomon MC. J Pharm Pharmacol 1990;42(Suppl):27P. Verelan [verapamil hydrochloride]: critical appraisal [a review of differences and advantages of a controlled-absorption oral system in comparison with that of previous formulations]—Pool PE. Adv Ther 1990;7:257–63. Pharmacokinetics and pharmacodynamics of verapamil following sublingual and oral administration to healthy volunteers—John DN, Fort S, Lewis MJ, Luscombe DK. Br J Clin Pharmacol 1992;23:623–7. Formulation and *in-vitro* evaluation of verapamil hydrochloride suppositories—Hammouda YE, Kasim NA, Nada AH. Int J Pharmaceutics 1993;89:111–18.

PROCESSING

Sterilisation

Solutions of verapamil hydrochloride can be sterilised by heating in an autoclave.

REFERENCES

1. Hasegawa J, Fujita T, Hayashi Y, Iwamoto K, Watanabe J. J Pharm Sci 1984;73(4):442–5.
2. Giacomini KM, Massoud N, Wong FM, Giacomini JC. J Cardiovasc Pharmacol 1984;6:924–8.
3. Das Gupta V. Drug Dev Ind Pharm 1985;11(8):1497–506.
4. Cutie MR, Lordi NG. Am J Hosp Pharm 1980;37:675–6.
5. Cutie MR. Am J Hosp Pharm 1981;38:231.
6. Cutie MR. Am J Hosp Pharm 1983;40:1205–7.
7. Das Gupta V, Stewart KR. Am J Hosp Pharm 1984;41:686–9.
8. Thomson DF, Stiles ML, Allen LV, Tu Y-H. Am J Hosp Pharm 1988;45:142–5.
9. Tucker R, Gentile JF [letter]. Am J Hosp Pharm 1984;41:2588.
10. Johnson CE, Lloyd CW, Aviles AI, Rybarz KL. Am J Hosp Pharm 1988;45:609–12.
11. Johnson CE, Lloyd CW, Mesaros JL, Rubley GJ. Am J Hosp Pharm 1989;46:97–100.
12. Riley CM. Am J Hosp Pharm 1988;45:2079–91.
13. Bar-Or D, Kulig K, Marx JA, Rosen P [letter]. Ann Intern Med 1982;97:619.
14. Cutie MR [letter]. Ann Intern Med 1983;98:672.
15. Moreland TA, McMurdo MET, McEwen J. Biopharm Drug Dispos 1989;10:311–19.
16. Devane JG, Kelly JG, Geoghegan B. Drug Dev Ind Pharm 1990;16(7):1233–48.

Vinblastine (BAN, rINN)   *Cytotoxic*

Vincaleucoblastine; vincaleukoblastine
An alkaloid extracted from *Vinca rosea (Catharanthus roseus)*
(Apocynaceae)
$C_{46}H_{58}N_4O_9 = 811.0$

Vinblastine Sulphate (BANM, rINNM)
Vinblastine Sulfate (USAN)
$C_{46}H_{58}N_4O_9,H_2SO_4 = 909.1$

CAS—865-21-4 (vinblastine); 143-67-9 (vinblastine sulphate)

Pharmacopoeial status

BP (vinblastine sulphate); USP (vinblastine sulfate)

Preparations

Compendial
Vinblastine Injection BP (Vinblastine Sulphate for Injection). A
sterile solution of viblastine sulphate in water for injections. It is
prepared by dissolving vinblastine sulphate for injection in the
requisite amount of sodium chloride 0.9% injection. pH of a
0.15% w/v solution, 3.5 to 5.0. Sealed containers each containing the equivalent of 10 mg of anhydrous vinblastine sulphate
are usually available.
Sterile Vinblastine Sulfate USP. Vinblastine sulfate suitable for
parenteral use.

Non-compendial
Velbe (Lilly). *Powder for reconstitution*, vinblastine sulphate
10 mg per vial. *Diluent* (included), 10 mL vial containing 90 mg
sodium chloride, with 2% benzyl alcohol. Velbe should never
be mixed with any other drug and should not be diluted with
solvents that raise or lower the pH from between 3.5 and 5.0.
Vinblastine Injection 10 mg (Lederle). *Powder for reconstitution*,
vinblastine sulphate. *Diluent* (included): 10 mL of sodium chloride 0.9% injection with 2% benzyl alcohol.
An injection of vinblastine sulphate 1 mg/mL and vinblastine
sulphate powder for reconstitution are also available from
David Bull.

Containers and storage

Solid state
Vinblastine Sulphate BP should be kept in an airtight, glass container, protected from light and stored at a temperature of −20°.
If the substance is sterile it should be kept in a sterile, tamper-
evident, glass container sealed so as to exclude micro-organisms.

Vinblastine Sulfate USP should be preserved in tight, light-resistant containers, in a freezer.

Dosage forms
Vinblastine Injection BP. The sealed container should be stored
at a temperature of 2° to 8°. Vinblastine Injection should be used
immediately after preparation but, in any case, within the period
recommended by the manufacturer when prepared and stored
strictly in accordance with the manufacturer's instructions.
Sterile Vinblastine Sulfate USP should be preserved in containers suitable for sterile solids, in a refrigerator.
Velbe (vials) should be stored in a refrigerator between 2° and 8°.
Following reconstitution, once a portion of the solution has
been removed from the vial, the remainder of the contents of
the vial may be stored in a refrigerator for further use for 30
days without significant loss of potency. When the reconstituted
vial of Velbe is to be stored for more than 48 hours, the accompanying diluting solutions or a diluent that contains a preservative must be used for reconstitution.
Vinblastine Injection 10 mg (Lederle) should be stored in a
refrigerator (2° to 8°). Injections reconstituted with the diluting
solution provided (which contains an antimicrobial preservative) may be kept in a refrigerator for 30 days without significant loss of potency.

PHYSICAL PROPERTIES

Vinblastine exists as crystals.
Vinblastine sulphate is a white to slightly yellow, very hygroscopic, crystalline powder.

Melting point

Vinblastine melts between 211° and 216°.
Vinblastine sulphate melts at about 284°, with decomposition.

pH

The pH of a 0.15% solution of *vinblastine sulphate* in water is 3.5
to 5.0.

Dissociation constants

pK_a 5.4, 7.4

Solubility

Vinblastine sulphate is soluble 1 in 10 of water and 1 in 50 of
chloroform; soluble in methanol; practically insoluble in ethanol and in ether.

Effect of pH
Vinblastine base can precipitate from solutions of vinblastine
sulphate at pH values greater than 6.

STABILITY

Vinblastine sulphate lyophilised powder is relatively stable to
heat when protected from the atmosphere.
Heating an aqueous solution of vinblastine sulphate at 50° for 16
hours at pH 2 caused 80% to 90% degradation; the primary
hydrolytic degradation product was desacetylvinblastine.
The degradation kinetics of vinblastine sulphate were studied at
80° over a wide pH range using a stability-indicating HPLC
assay.[1] The degradation pathway was complex; the major
degradation product, desacetylvinblastine, was formed at pH
values below 1.5 and above 10.5. Between pH 2.5 and 7.5, the
amount formed was negligible and several other (unidentified)
products were detected. The decomposition reaction followed

pseudo-first-order kinetics at constant pH. Activation energies calculated from Arrhenius plots were 66, 71, and 106 kJ/mol at pH 0.9, 5.1, and 8.7, respectively. Maximum stability of vinblastine in aqueous solution occurred between pH 2.0 and 4.0. At pH 3.0, 90% of the initial concentration of vinblastine remained after storage for 39 days at 20°. The degradation process was unaffected by either the addition of phosphate buffer (0.005 to 0.05M) or an increase in ionic strength from 0.1 to 0.4 by the addition of sodium chloride.

Aqueous solutions of vinblastine sulphate (1 mg/mL, pH 4.5 to 5.0) were sealed into glass ampoules, protected from light, and maintained at one of six different temperatures (55°, 37°, 25°, 5°, −5°, or −25°) for 84 days.[2] Data obtained by HPLC led to the detection of eight different degradation products. The two major products of early heat degradation were tentatively identified by mass spectrometry as a C19′-oxidation product (19′-oxovinblastine) and an isomer of vinblastine. Later degradation products were thought to include 19′-hydroxy-3′,4′-dehydrovinblastine or 3′,4′-dehydrovinblastine-6′-N-oxide. Photodegradation, at room temperature, elicited a different sequence of appearance of the same degradation products. The $t_{10\%}$ values for samples stored, protected from light, at 25°, 37°, and 55° were estimated to be 150 days, 16.6 days, and 2.4 days, respectively. No degradation at −25°, −5°, or 5° was detected over 84 days.

Photodegradation

Decomposition of vinblastine sulphate was observed[3] after 8 days and after 14 days when solutions (1.197 mg/mL, pH 5.0) were exposed to direct intermittent light (25°) and to direct continuous incandescent light (30°), respectively; an amber tint developed by the end of the 70-day study period. Samples exposed to indirect incandescent light (shielded samples) remained stable, optically clear and colourless over 70 days. Samples subjected to direct, continuous incandescent light, at 30°, lost 10% of their initial vinblastine sulphate concentration after slightly more than one day.

During stability studies, little degradation of vinblastine sulphate injection was observed after 2 months at room temperature.[4] The product was still within pharmacopoeial specifications (USP XXII) after 2 months at 40° and 2 weeks at 55°.

An aqueous solution of vinblastine (1 mg/mL) was stable[5] during storage for 3 weeks in a glass container in the dark at 4°. Stability of vinblastine was maintained (less than 5% decomposition) when stored at 4° and 25° for 3 weeks in the dark in sealed polypropylene test-tubes at a concentration of 20 micrograms/mL in either glucose 5% injection, sodium chloride 0.9% injection, or compound sodium lactate injection. Reconstituted injections of vinblastine sulphate (1 mg/mL) were chemically stable for at least 30 days when stored in polypropylene syringes at either room temperature (21°) in the dark or in a refrigerator (6° to 9°).[6]

INCOMPATIBILITY/COMPATIBILITY

Vinblastine sulphate (3 micrograms/mL) in glucose 5% injection was stable during storage in methacrylate butadiene styrene burette administration sets (A2001, Sureset, Avon); a 5.14% loss was recorded after 48 hours, which was reduced to 2.25% when the set was protected from light.[7] However, when the standard (A200, Avon) and the Amberset (A2000, Avon) administration sets were used, adsorption of vinblastine to components constructed from cellulose propionate led to losses of 14.47% and 20.58%, respectively after 48 hours. Adsorption

to the polyvinyl chloride tubing from both these sets caused a reduction in vinblastine concentration of 42.16% and 44.12% respectively, whereas only 6% loss to polybutadiene was detected (Sureset).

In contrast, no significant loss of vinblastine sulphate (40 micrograms/mL) was observed during simulated infusions in either glucose 5% or sodium chloride 0.9% injections for 2 hours, at ambient temperatures, using polyvinyl chloride infusion bags and administration sets.[8] Vinblastine sulphate (100 micrograms/mL) was also found to be stable, in either glucose 5% or sodium chloride 0.9% injections, when stored in polyvinyl chloride infusion bags for 7 days at 4°, protected from light.

Vinblastine sulphate in glucose 5% or sodium chloride 0.9% injections showed no binding to an in-line intravenous filter containing a cellulose ester (nitrate and acetate esters) membrane.[9] Vinblastine sulphate (1 mg/mL)[10] in sodium chloride 0.9% injection (with preservative) lost 24% of its initial concentration when kept in an implantable infusion device (Infusaid Pump model 400) at 37° for 24 hours; after 12 days, loss was 48%. No loss occurred when similar solutions were stored in amber glass vials at 37° for 24 hours although 20% was lost after 12 days.

PROCESSING

Handling precautions

CAUTION. Vinblastine sulphate should be handled with great care as it is a potent cytotoxic agent.

Vinblastine is irritant, especially to the eyes and skin. Protective clothing, masks, goggles, and latex rubber gloves should be worn by trained personnel during reconstitution and administration of the drug. Any contamination must be thoroughly washed with copious amounts of water. Reconstitution should be performed in a designated area where the work surface should be covered with disposable, plastic-backed, absorbent paper. Any spillage or contaminated waste materials may be disposed of by incineration at 1000°.

In addition to the above guidelines, the manufacturer of Velbe (Lilly) recommended the use of Luer-lock fittings on all syringes and administration sets. The use of large bore needles is recommended to minimise pressure and aerosol formation. A venting needle may also be used to prevent aerosol formation.

General guidelines on the handling and disposal of cytotoxic drugs are given in the chapter entitled Cytotoxic Drugs: Handling Precautions.

REFERENCES

1. Vendrig DEMM, Smeets BPGM, Beijnen JH, van der Houwen OAGJ, Holthuis JJM. Int J Pharmaceutics 1988;43:131–8.
2. Black J, Buechter DD, Chinn JW, Gard J, Thurston DE. J Pharm Sci 1988;77(7):630–4.
3. Black J, Buechter DD, Thurston DE [letter]. Drug Intell Clin Pharm 1988;22:634–5.
4. Steffeck R, Alam A, Pai S. ASHP Midyear Clinical Meeting 1991;26:P-394R.
5. Beijnen JH, Vendrig DEMM, Underberg WJM. J Parenter Sci Technol 1989;43:84–7.
6. Weir PJ, Ireland DS. Br J Pharm Pract 1990;12(2):53–4,60.
7. McElnay JC, Elliott DS, Cartwright-Shamoon J, D'Arcy PF. Int J Pharmaceutics 1988;47:239–47.
8. Dine T, Luyckx M, Cazin JC, Brunet C, Cazin M, Goudaliez F et al. Int J Pharmaceutics 1991;77:279–85.

9. Butler LD, Munson JM, De Luca PP. Am J Hosp Pharm 1980;37:935–41.
10. Keller JH, Ensminger WD. Am J Hosp Pharm 1982;39:1321–3.

Vincristine (BAN, rINN)   *Cytotoxic*

Leurocristine
22-Oxovincaleukoblastine
An alkaloid obtained from *Vinca rosea* (*Catharanthus roseus*) (Apocynaceae)
$C_{46}H_{56}N_4O_{10} = 825.0$

Vincristine Sulphate (BANM, rINNM)
Vincristine Sulfate (USAN)
$C_{46}H_{56}N_4O_{10},H_2SO_4 = 923.0$

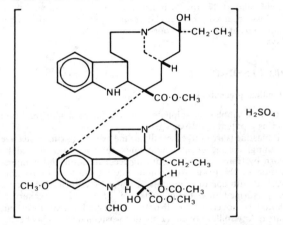

CAS—57-22-7 (vincristine); 2068-78-2 (vincristine sulphate)

Pharmacopoeial status

BP (vincristine sulphate); USP (vincristine sulfate)

Preparations

Compendial
Vincristine Injection BP (Vincristine Sulphate for Injection). A sterile solution of a mixture of one part by weight of vincristine sulphate and ten parts by weight of lactose in water for injections. It is prepared by dissolving vincristine sulphate for injection in the requisite amount of sodium chloride 0.9% injection. Sealed containers each containing the equivalent of 1 mg, 2 mg, and 5 mg of anhydrous vincristine sulphate are usually available.
Vincristine Sulfate Injection USP. pH 3.5 to 5.5.
Vincristine Sulfate for Injection USP.

Non-compendial
Oncovin (Lilly). *Injection*, vincristine sulphate 1 mg/mL. Oncovin should never be mixed with any other drug and should not be diluted with solutions that raise or lower the pH outside the range 3.5 to 5.5.
Vincristine Injection 1 mg, 2 mg, 5 mg (Lederle). *Powder for reconstitution*, in a vial containing 1 mg, 2 mg, or 5 mg vincristine sulphate with 10 mg, 20 mg, or 50 mg of lactose respectively. *Diluent* (included): 10 mL sodium chloride 0.9% injection with 2% benzyl alcohol.

An injection of vincristine sulphate 1 mg/mL and vincristine sulphate powder for reconstitution are also available from David Bull.

Containers and storage

Solid state
Vincristine Sulphate BP should be kept in an airtight, glass container, protected from light and stored at a temperature of −20°. If the substance is sterile it should be kept in a sterile, tamper-evident, glass container sealed so as to exclude micro-organisms. Vincristine Sulfate USP should be preserved in tight, light-resistant containers, in a freezer.

Dosage forms
Vincristine Injection BP. The sealed container should be stored at a temperature of 2° to 8°. The injection should be used immediately after preparation but, in any case, within the period recommended by the manufacturer when prepared and stored strictly in accordance with the manufacturer's instructions.
Vincristine Sulfate Injection USP should be preserved in light-resistant, glass containers, in a refrigerator.
Vincristine Sulfate for Injection USP should be preserved in containers suitable for sterile solids, in a refrigerator.
Oncovin solution should be stored in a refrigerator (2° to 8°). Protect from light.
Vincristine Injection 1 mg, 2 mg, and 5 mg (Lederle) should be stored in a refrigerator at 2° to 8°. After reconstitution with the diluting solution provided (which contains an antimicrobial preservative) the injection may be kept in a refrigerator for 14 days without significant loss of potency.

PHYSICAL PROPERTIES

Vincristine exists as crystals.
Vincristine sulphate is a white to slightly yellow, very hygroscopic, crystalline powder.

Melting point

Vincristine melts at 218° to 220°.
Vincristine sulphate melts at about 277°.

pH

A 0.1% w/v solution of *vincristine sulphate* in water has a pH of 3.5 to 4.5.

Dissociation constants

pK_a 5.0, 7.4

Solubility

Vincristine base is insoluble in water.
Vincristine sulphate is soluble 1 in 2 of water, 1 in 600 of ethanol, and 1 in 30 of chloroform; soluble in methanol; practically insoluble in ether.

Effect of pH
Precipitation of vincristine sulphate solutions can occur above pH 6.0.

STABILITY

When dried vincristine sulphate was heated in sealed containers at 100° for up to 16 hours, very slight degradation occurred. However, when treated similarly but open to the atmosphere, 50% of the drug decomposed.
Although aqueous solutions of vincristine sulphate at about pH 4.5 are reasonably stable for up to 3 hours at 90°, a decrease in the pH results in an increase in decomposition.

The pseudo-first-order degradation[1] of vincristine sulphate (elucidated by stability-indicating HPLC at 80°) yielded the product desacetylvincristine in minor quantities at pH values up to 11, but mainly at pH > 9. Other degradation products were formed but not identified. Vincristine in aqueous solution was most stable between pH 3.5 and 5.6; optimum stability was established at pH 4.8. The rate of decomposition was not affected by either ionic strength (0.1 to 0.4) or phosphate buffer (0.005M to 0.05M). Activation energies at pH 1.2, 5.2, and 8.2 were calculated to be 62, 73, and 116 kJ/mol, respectively.

The stability of an aqueous solution of vincristine sulphate (1 mg/mL) was maintained for 21 days at 4° when stored in glass containers, in the dark.[2] The same reversed-phase, stability-indicating HPLC assay was used to ascertain the stability of vincristine sulphate 20 micrograms/mL for three weeks at 4° and 25° in either glucose 5%, sodium chloride 0.9%, or compound sodium lactate injections in sealed polypropylene test-tubes; more than 95% of the initial concentration remained in each of the infusion fluids.

When protected from light, the stability of vincristine sulphate injection[3] remained within US pharmacopoeial limits (USP XXII) after one month at room temperature but for only two weeks at 40°, and three days at 55°.

INCOMPATIBILITY/COMPATIBILITY

Vincristine was visually and chemically stable for seven days when admixed with mitozantrone in glucose 5% injection and stored, protected from light, at room temperature.[4]

In aseptically prepared admixtures of vincristine sulphate (Oncovin, Lilly, France) (0.033 mg/mL or 0.053 mg/mL) and doxorubicin, in either sodium chloride 0.9% injection or sodium chloride 0.45% and glucose 2.5% injection, more than 90% of vincristine concentration was retained for 14 days at 25°, 30°, and 37° when stored in polysiloxane bags and protected from light.[5] Under similar conditions, vincristine degradation was most rapid in admixture in sodium chloride 0.45% and Ringer's acetate injection; more than 10% degradation occurred after 8 days, 5 days, and 3 days at 25°, 30°, and 37°, respectively.

Sorption

Butler et al[6] demonstrated measurable binding of vincristine sulphate (1 mg/50 mL) to a cellulose ester (nitrate and acetate esters) membrane during in-line filtration; 12.1% and 6.5% losses occurred from solutions in sodium chloride 0.9% injection and glucose 5% injection, respectively. In equilibrium binding studies, the saturation concentration was approximately 1.5 micrograms vincristine sulphate per mg filter material.

No significant sorption to polyvinyl chloride (from either glucose 5% injection or sodium chloride 0.9% injection) was observed either after storage of vincristine sulphate 20 micrograms/mL for seven days in infusion bags at 4°, protected from light, or during simulated infusion of vincristine sulphate 8 micrograms/mL solution for two hours at ambient temperature, protected from light.[7]

FORMULATION

Excipients

Excipients that have been used in presentations of vincristine sulphate include:
Injections, (powder for reconstitution): lactose.
Injection solutions: acetic acid; glycine; mannitol; methyl and propyl hydroxybenzoates; phosphate buffer; sodium acetate.

PROCESSING

Handling precautions

CAUTION. Vincristine sulphate should be handled with great care as it is a potent cytotoxic agent.
Vincristine is irritant, particularly to the eyes and skin. Adequate protective clothing, masks, latex rubber gloves, and goggles should be worn by trained personnel during reconstitution and administration of the drug. Any contamination should be thoroughly washed with copious amounts of water. Reconstitution should be performed in a designated area and the work surface should be covered with disposable, plastic-backed, absorbent paper. Any spillage, waste, or other contaminated materials may be disposed of by incineration at 1000°. Chemical destruction can be effected by use of 5% sodium hypochlorite for 24 hours.

In addition to the above guidelines, the manufacturer of Oncovin (Lilly) recommend the use of Luer-lock fittings on all syringes and administration sets. The use of large bore needles is recommended to minimise pressure and aerosol formation. A venting needle may also be used to prevent aerosol formation. General guidelines on the handling and disposal of cytotoxic drugs are given in the chapter entitled Cytotoxic Drugs: Handling Precautions.

REFERENCES

1. Vendrig DEMM, Beijnen JH, van der Houwen OAGJ, Holthuis JJM. Int J Pharmaceutics 1989;50:189–96.
2. Beijnen JH, Vendrig DEMM, Underberg WJM. J Parenter Sci Technol 1989;43:84–7.
3. Steffeck R, Alam A, Pai S. ASHP Midyear Clinical Meeting 1991;26:P-394R through Int Pharm Abstr 1992;29(1):2900594.
4. Cacek T, Weber R. ASHP Midyear Clinical Meeting 1990;25:P-470E.
5. Beijnen JH, Neef C, Meuwissen OJAT, Rutten JJMH, Rosing H, Underberg WJM. Am J Hosp Pharm 1986;43:3022–7.
6. Butler LD, Munson JM, De Luca PP. Am J Hosp Pharm 1980;37:935–41.
7. Dine T, Luyckx M, Cazin JC, Brunet C, Cazin M, Goudaliez F *et al.* Int J Pharmaceutics 1991;77:279–85.

Warfarin (BAN, rINN)   *Anticoagulant*

4-Hydroxy-3-(3-oxo-1-phenylbutyl)coumarin;   4-hydroxy-3-(3-oxo-1-phenylbutyl)-2*H*-1-benzopyran-2-one
$C_{19}H_{16}O_4 = 308.3$

Warfarin Potassium (BANM, rINNM)
$C_{19}H_{15}KO_4 = 346.4$

Warfarin Sodium (BANM, rINNM)
$C_{19}H_{15}NaO_4 = 330.3$

Warfarin Sodium Clathrate
The clathrate of warfarin sodium with isopropanol in the molecular proportions of 2 to 1, respectively.

NOTE. Until 1991, the BP and the USP allowed the use of warfarin sodium or warfarin sodium clathrate in their definition of warfarin sodium.

CAS—81-81-2 (warfarin); 2610-86-8 (warfarin potassium); 129-06-6 (warfarin sodium)

Pharmacopoeial status

BP (warfarin sodium, warfarin sodium clathrate); USP (warfarin sodium or its clathrate with isopropanol)

Preparations

Compendial
Warfarin Tablets BP. Contain warfarin sodium or warfarin sodium clathrate. Tablets containing, in each, the equivalent of 1, 3, 5, and 10 mg of anhydrous and isopropanol-free warfarin sodium are usually available.
Warfarin Sodium Tablets USP.
Warfarin Sodium for Injection USP.

Non-compendial
Marevan (Evans). *Tablets*, warfarin sodium 1 mg, 3 mg, and 5 mg.
Warfarin WBP (Boehringer Ingelheim). *Tablets*, warfarin sodium 1 mg, 3 mg, and 5 mg.

Containers and storage

Solid state
Warfarin Sodium BP and Warfarin Sodium Clathrate BP should be kept in airtight containers and protected from light.
Warfarin Sodium USP should be preserved in well-closed, light-resistant containers.

Dosage forms
Warfarin Tablets BP should be protected from light.
Warfarin Sodium Tablets USP should be preserved in tight, light-resistant containers.
Warfarin Sodium for Injection USP should be preserved in light-resistant containers suitable for sterile solids.
Marevan tablets should be protected from light.
Warfarin WBP tablets should be protected from heat, light and moisture.

PHYSICAL PROPERTIES

Warfarin occurs as colourless crystals.
Warfarin potassium is a white, crystalline powder; odourless; it discolours on exposure to light.
Warfarin sodium is a white, amorphous or crystalline powder; odourless or almost odourless; it discolours on exposure to light.
Warfarin sodium clathrate is a white powder.

Melting point

Warfarin (purified) melts in the range 159° to 160°; the technical grade melts at 157°.

pH

A 1% w/v solution of *warfarin potassium* or *warfarin sodium* in water has a pH of 7.2 to 8.3.

Dissociation constant

pK_a 5.0 (20°)

Partition coefficient

Log P (octanol/pH 8.0), 0.0

Solubility

Warfarin is practically insoluble in water; soluble in acetone and in dioxan; moderately soluble in methanol, in ethanol and in some oils; freely soluble in aqueous alkaline solutions.
Warfarin potassium is soluble 1 in 1.5 of water and 1 in 1.9 of ethanol; very slightly soluble in chloroform and in ether.
Warfarin sodium is soluble 1 in less than 1 of water and 1 in less than 1 of ethanol; slightly soluble in chloroform and in ether.
Warfarin sodium clathrate is very soluble in water; freely soluble in ethanol; soluble in acetone; very slightly soluble in dichloromethane and in ether.
For reference to a study of the solubility and dissolution of warfarin in combination with cyclodextrins, see Dissolution below.

Dissolution

The USP specifies that for Warfarin Sodium Tablets USP not less than 80% of the labelled amount of $C_{19}H_{15}NaO_4$ is dissolved in 30 minutes. Dissolution medium: 900 mL of water; Apparatus 2 at 50 rpm.

Dissolution properties
Lin and Yang[1] studied the solubility and dissolution of warfarin alone and in combination with α-cyclodextrin and β-cyclodextrin. The solubility of warfarin, when complexed with cyclodextrins to form an inclusion complex, increased rapidly with increasing β-cyclodextrin concentration although only a small increase in solubility was observed with increasing α-cyclodextrin concentration. Results from dissolution studies using various forms of warfarin-cyclodextrin mixtures compressed into tablets showed that physical mixtures of warfarin and cyclodextrins, both lyophilised, dissolved faster than non-lyophilised mixtures. Dissolution of warfarin from lyophilised solid inclusion complexes with cyclodextrins was much faster than from pure warfarin or from physical mixtures of warfarin and cyclodextrins, and lyophilised warfarin dissolved about 30 times faster than pure warfarin. Warfarin dissolution from the lyophilised warfarin complex with α-cyclodextrin and with β-cyclodextrin was 1200 and 550 times faster, respectively, than pure warfarin.

STABILITY

Goding and West[2] reported that during 48 hours at 150° and pH 9, warfarin underwent hydrolysis and decarboxylation reactions to form 3-(*O*-hydroxyphenyl)-5-phenyl-2-cyclohexen-1-one.
In aqueous solution, warfarin may hydrolyse to form *cis*-coumarinic acid. However, the molecule could be protected from lactone hydrolysis by ionisation of the enol.
At pH values of less than 8, there may be precipitation due to formation of the insoluble enol form.[3]
Experiments carried out by Benya and Wagner[4] using thin layer chromatography and ultraviolet spectrophotometry suggested that warfarin was sensitive to air and light.
Results from studies carried out by Hiskey and Melnitchenko[5] on the nature of clathrate complexes of warfarin sodium showed that as the amount of water in the crystalline clathrate increased, the crystal size decreased, and the clathrate structure deteriorated.
An indirect indication of the instability of warfarin sodium in aqueous solution came from the manufacturers of a lyophilised amorphous warfarin sodium preparation for injection (Coumadin, Du Pont, USA) who recommended that it should be used immediately after reconstitution.[6]

Stabilisation

Precipitation of free warfarin from aqueous solutions of its salts may be prevented by pH adjustment, for instance by the addition of sodium hydroxide.

INCOMPATIBILITY/COMPATIBILITY

Warfarin sodium is reported to be incompatible with adrenaline hydrochloride, amikacin sulphate, cyanocobalamin, metaraminol tartrate, oxytocin, promazine hydrochloride, tetracycline hydrochloride, vancomycin hydrochloride, and vitamin B complex with vitamin C. However, the manufacturers of Coumadin (warfarin sodium for injection, Du Pont, USA) stated that warfarin sodium and heparin may be admixed in the same syringe. Warfarin sodium has also been reported to be incompatible with solutions of the following: ammonium chloride, fructose, glucose 5%, compound sodium lactate injection, and invert sugar.[7]

Sorption to plastics

Moorhatch and Chiou[7] reported the sorption of warfarin sodium from aqueous solution onto polyvinyl chloride strips. There was increased sorption when glucose 5% injection was used as the vehicle; an increase in sorption was not observed with sodium chloride 0.9%. In a later study, Illum and Bundgaard[8] found that the unionised form of warfarin was sorbed from aqueous solutions of warfarin sodium onto 100-mL polyvinyl chloride infusion bags. A decrease in pH to 2 or 4 led to an increase in sorption. Negligible sorption of warfarin occurred when 300-mL polypropylene infusion bags were used.

FORMULATION

Excipients

Excipients that have been used in presentations of warfarin include:
Tablets, warfarin sodium: allura red AC (E129); powdered acacia; brilliant blue FCF (133); D&C Red No.30; erythrosine (E127); indigo carmine (E132); lactose; magnesium stearate; maize starch; microcrystalline cellulose; polacrilin potassium; quinoline yellow (E104); sunset yellow FCF (E110); talc; tartrazine (E102).
Injections, warfarin sodium: sodium chloride; sodium hydroxide; thiomersal.

REFERENCES

1. Lin S-Y, Yang J-C. Pharm Weekbl (Sci) 1986;8:223–8.
2. Goding LA, West BD. J Org Chem 1968;33:437–8.
3. Hiskey CF, Bullock E, Whitman G. J Pharm Sci 1962;51:43.
4. Benya TJ, Wagner JG [letter]. Can J Pharm Sci 1976;11:70–1.
5. Hiskey CF, Melnitchenko V. J Pharm Sci 1965;54:1298–302.
6. Patel JA, Phillips GL. Am J Hosp Pharm 1966;23:409–11.
7. Moorhatch P, Chiou WL. Am J Hosp Pharm 1974;31:72–8.
8. Illum L, Bundgaard H. Int J Pharmaceutics 1982;10:339–51.

Zinc Oxide   *Astringent*

Flowers of zinc; 'zinc white' is a commercial form of zinc oxide manufactured for use as a pigment.
ZnO = 81.4
CAS—1314-13-2

Pharmacopoeial status

BP, USP

Preparations

Compendial

For extemporaneous preparation of compendial preparations see Formulation, below.
Zinc Cream BP. Contains 32% w/w of zinc oxide in a suitable w/o emulsified basis.
Zinc Ointment BP. Contains 15% w/w of zinc oxide in a suitable water-emulsifying basis.
Zinc and Castor Oil Ointment BP (Zinc and Castor Oil Cream).
Coal Tar and Zinc Ointment BP. Contains 30% w/w of zinc oxide and 10% w/w of strong coal tar solution in a suitable hydrophobic basis.
Zinc and Salicylic Acid Paste BP (Lassar's Paste).
Zinc and Coal Tar Paste BP (White's Tar Paste). Contains 6% w/w each of zinc oxide and coal tar with 38% w/w of starch in a suitable hydrophobic basis.
Compound Zinc Paste BP. Contains 25% w/w each of zinc oxide and starch in a suitable hydrophobic basis.
Zinc and Ichthammol Cream BP. Contains 5% w/w of ichthammol dispersed in a suitable basis of which about 82% w/w is zinc cream.
Elastic Adhesive Bandage BP (Zinc Oxide Elastic Adhesive Bandage).
Extension Strapping BP (Extension Plaster).
Ventilated Elastic Adhesive Bandage BP (Ventilated Zinc Oxide Elastic Adhesive Bandage).
Zinc Paste Bandage BP.
Zinc Paste and Coal Tar Bandage BP.
Zinc Paste and Ichthammol Bandage BP.
Zinc Paste, Calamine and Clioquinol Bandage BP.
Zinc Oxide Ointment USP.
Zinc Oxide Paste USP.

Containers and storage

Solid state

Zinc Oxide USP should be preserved in well-closed containers.

Dosage forms

Zinc Oxide Ointment USP and Zinc Oxide Paste USP should be preserved in well-closed containers, and exposure to temperatures exceeding 30° should be avoided.

PHYSICAL PROPERTIES

Zinc oxide is a soft, white, or faintly yellowish-white amorphous powder; free from grittiness; odourless.

Solubility

Zinc oxide is practically insoluble in water and in ethanol; it is soluble in dilute mineral acids.

STABILITY

When exposed to air, zinc oxide gradually absorbs moisture and carbon dioxide.
Zinc oxide forms cement-like products when mixed with a strong solution of zinc chloride or with phosphoric acid, as a result of the formation of oxy-salts.

INCOMPATIBILITY/COMPATIBILITY

Zinc oxide is incompatible with benzylpenicillin.
Zinc oxide reacts slowly with fatty acids in oils and fats to produce the corresponding fatty acid esters.

Das Gupta[1] noted that when a zinc oxide 'shake lotion' (consisting of zinc oxide 10% and talc 10% in a mixture of glycerol and water) was compounded in Type III clear glass containers, the solids adhered to the containers; complexometric analysis shortly after preparation revealed that the initial concentration of zinc oxide in the lotion had decreased by about 20%. No adherence was apparent in Pyrex glass or plastic (polyethylene resin) containers.

FORMULATION

ZINC CREAM BP

Zinc oxide, finely sifted	320 g
Calcium hydroxide	0.45 g
Oleic acid	5 mL
Arachis oil	320 mL
Wool fat	80 g
Purified water, freshly boiled and cooled sufficient to produce	1000 g

Mix the zinc oxide and the calcium hydroxide, triturate to a smooth paste with a mixture of the oleic acid and arachis oil, incorporate the wool fat and add gradually (with continuous stirring) sufficient purified water to produce 1000 g.

ZINC OINTMENT BP

Zinc oxide, finely sifted	150 g
Simple ointment	850 g

Triturate the zinc oxide with a portion of the simple ointment until smooth, gradually add the remainder of the simple ointment and mix thoroughly.

ZINC AND CASTOR OIL OINTMENT BP

Zinc oxide, finely sifted	75 g
Castor oil	500 g
Cetostearyl alcohol	20 g
White beeswax	100 g
Arachis oil	305 g

Triturate the zinc oxide with a portion of the castor oil until smooth and add the mixture to the remainder of the ingredients previously melted together. Stir while cooling until the temperature is about 40°.

COAL TAR AND ZINC OINTMENT BP

Strong coal tar solution	100 g
Zinc oxide, finely sifted	300 g
Yellow soft paraffin	600 g

Mix the zinc oxide with the strong coal tar solution, triturate with a portion of the yellow soft paraffin until smooth, gradually incorporate the remainder of the yellow soft paraffin and mix.

ZINC AND SALICYLIC ACID PASTE BP

Zinc oxide, finely sifted	240 g
Salicylic acid, finely sifted	20 g
Starch, finely sifted	240 g
White soft paraffin	500 g

Melt the white soft paraffin, incorporate the zinc oxide, the salicylic acid and the starch and stir until cold.

ZINC AND COAL TAR PASTE BP

Emulsifying wax	50 g
Coal tar	60 g
Zinc oxide, finely sifted	60 g
Starch	380 g
Yellow soft paraffin	450 g

Melt the emulsifying wax at 70°, add the coal tar and 225 g of the yellow soft paraffin, stir at 70° until completely melted, add the remainder of the yellow soft paraffin, cool to 30°, add the zinc oxide and the starch, stirring constantly, and stir until cold.

COMPOUND ZINC PASTE BP

Zinc oxide, finely sifted	250 g
Starch, finely sifted	250 g
White soft paraffin	500 g

Melt the white soft paraffin, incorporate the zinc oxide and the starch and stir until cold.

ZINC AND ICHTHAMMOL CREAM BP

Ichthammol	50 g
Cetostearyl alcohol	30 g
Wool fat	100 g
Zinc cream sufficient to produce	1000 g

Melt together the wool fat and the cetostearyl alcohol with the aid of gentle heat, triturate the mixture with 800 g of zinc cream until smooth, incorporate the ichthammol, add sufficient zinc cream to produce 1000 g and mix.

ZINC, STARCH, AND TALC DUSTING POWDER

The following formula was given in the *British Pharmaceutical Codex 1973*:

Zinc oxide	250 g
Starch, in powder	250 g
Purified talc, sterilised	500 g

Suspensions

The physical stability of a suspension of zinc oxide and talc was enhanced by the inclusion of an increasing concentration of Aerosil (colloidal silica; 0.2% to 2.5%) but not by inclusion of an increasing concentration of Tween 80 (0.05% to 1.5%).[2] A combination of Aerosil and Tween 80 was favoured.

Stable suspensions of zinc oxide were prepared with acid tartrates and Veegum; settling was retarded by sodium, potassium, or ammonium acid tartrate.[3]

FURTHER INFORMATION. Effect of deflocculating agents on suspensions of calamine and zinc oxide—Wood AG, Bower MI, Butler CG, Kaye RC. Pharm J 1962;188:557–8.

REFERENCES

1. Das Gupta V. Am J Hosp Pharm 1972;29:724.
2. Muzik M, Turan J, Stachova J. Czeck Farm 1990;39:1–3.
3. Koh YS, Hopponen RE. Drug Standards 1959;27:21.

INDEX